Critical Care Nursing of Infants and Children

Critical Care Nursing of Infants and Children

MARTHA A. Q. CURLEY, M.S.N., R.N., CCRN
Critical Care Clinical Nurse Specialist
Multidisciplinary ICU
Children's Hospital, Boston
Boston, Massachusetts

JANIS BLOEDEL SMITH, M.S.N., R.N., CCRN
Manager
Patient Care Services
Inpatient Cardiology
Vanderbilt University Medical Center
Nashville, Tennessee

PATRICIA A. MOLONEY-HARMON, M.S., R.N., CCRN
Clinical Nurse Specialist, Children's Services
Sinai Hospital of Baltimore
Baltimore, Maryland

W.B. SAUNDERS COMPANY
A Division of Harcourt Brace & Company
Philadelphia London Toronto Montreal Sydney Tokyo

W.B. SAUNDERS COMPANY
A Division of Harcourt Brace & Company

The Curtis Center
Independence Square West
Philadelphia, Pennsylvania 19106

Library of Congress Cataloging-in-Publication Data

Curley, Martha A. Q.

Critical care nursing of infants and children / Martha A. Q. Curley, Janis Bloedel Smith, Patricia A. Moloney-Harmon.

    p.   cm.

ISBN 0–7216–3120–7

1. Pediatric intensive care.   2. Pediatric nursing.   3. Intensive care nursing.   I. Smith, Janis Bloedel.   II. Moloney-Harmon, Patricia A.   III. Title.

[DNLM: 1. Critical Care—in infancy & childhood.   2. Pediatric Nursing—methods.   3. Intensive Care Units, Pediatric—standards.   4. Critical Illness—nursing.   WY 159 C975c 1996]

RJ370.C87 1996   610.73′62—dc20

DNLM/DLC   95-45034

CRITICAL CARE NURSING OF INFANTS AND CHILDREN   ISBN 0–7216–3120–7

Printed in the United States of America.

Last digit is the print number: 9 8 7 6 5 4 3 2 1

To the men in our lives

Jack, Joey, Paul John

Jerry, Scott

Tom

In memory of our colleague

Karen Zamberlan, Ph.D., R.N.

To my nursing colleagues:

It's NOT Invisible

Today, I saw you . . .

> *Make room for more than 20 family members at the bedside all at once, so that everyone could be together with Billy one last time.*
>
> *Ask Billy's grandfather to plug the extension cord in; you knew he needed to do something—anything.*
>
> *Give options to Billy's parents about "being there" during resuscitation attempts and help them choose words to talk with him, considering he was only 8-years-old.*
>
> *Speak very softly to Stephen while removing the tape from his eyelids only to find his pupils blown and unequal . . . you didn't even change your facial expression—you didn't want to upset mom . . . not any more . . . not just then.*
>
> *Ask Stephen's mom what she was thinking as she stood near his bed looking out the window just before support was withdrawn. . . . "He was always very quiet, but I knew something was wrong; I should have taken him to the hospital—but, he didn't want to go". . . . wipe your tears as you listened and convincingly say that she did the best that she could.*
>
> *Take a deep breath before you spoke up at team conference . . . "We ought to be more vigilant about the conversations we hold at the bedside—we don't know what Stephen's level of consciousness is under the sedation and chemical paralyzing agents". . . . whisper in Stephen's ear that the new ventilator might be scary because of the noise it made, then dry his tears.*
>
> *Take the time to sit with Rachel's mom while others resuscitated her daughter, your patient, because you knew she was alone . . . . her husband was on his way in.*
>
> *Resuscitate Rachel because you knew that Rachel's mom needed your colleague right then.*
>
> *Care enough to take the time to "orchestrate" death . . . to make the worst-thing-in-the-world anyone could ever experience . . . a little more tolerable.*

It may be very hard for others to hear what we do . . . it can just be so sad. We eventually stop telling them. Eventually, we might think that our caring becomes invisible. But, it is not invisible—not to Billy, not to Stephen, not to Rachel, or their parents, or to one another.

MARTHA A. Q. CURLEY, RN, MSN, CCRN

CONTRIBUTORS

Mary Allen, M.S.N., R.N.
Clinical Nurse Specialist, Adult and Pediatric
Patient Services, National Institutes of Health,
Warren Grant Magnuson Clinical Center, Bethesda,
Maryland
Host Defenses

Craig Alter, M.D.
Assistant Professor of Pediatrics, University of
Massachusetts Medical School; Pediatric
Endocrinologist, University of Massachusetts
Medical Center, Worcester, Massachusetts
Endocrine Critical Care Problems

June Levine Ariff, M.S.N., R.N., C.N.A.
Vice President Operations/Nursing, Huntington
East Valley Hospital, Glendora, California
In the Best Interest of the Child: Ethical Issues

Annette L. Baker, M.S.N., R.N.
Clinical Research Nurse Coordinator, Department of
Cardiology, Children's Hospital, Boston, Boston,
Massachusetts
Cardiovascular Critical Care Problems

M. Claire Beers, M.S.N., R.N.
Nurse Manager, The Pediatric Intensive Care Unit,
The Johns Hopkins Hospital, Baltimore, Maryland
Oxygenation / Ventilation

Anne Milligan Browne, M.S.N., R.N., CCRN
Clinical Nurse Specialist, Pediatric Surgery, Cooper
Hospital/University Medical Center, Camden, New
Jersey
*Critical Illness and Intensive Care During Infancy
and Childhood*

Cheryl Cahill-Alsip, M.S.N., R.N.
Staff Nurse, Level II, Neurology Department,
Children's Hospital, Boston, Boston, Massachusetts
Hematologic Critical Care Problems

Elaine Caron, R.N.
Staff Nurse, Level III, Multidisciplinary ICU,
Children's Hospital, Boston, Boston, Massachusetts
Oxygenation / Ventilation

Sylvia Chin-Caplan, J.D., B.S.N., R.N.
Former Assistant General Counsel, Children's
Hospital, Boston, Boston, Massachusetts
Legal Implications of Pediatric Nursing Practice

Martha A. Q. Curley, M.S.N., R.N., CCRN
Critical Care Clinical Nurse Specialist,
Multidisciplinary ICU, Children's Hospital, Boston,
Boston, Massachusetts
*The Essence of Pediatric Critical Care Nursing; The
Impact of the Critical Care Experience on the
Family; Tissue Perfusion; Oxygenation / Ventilation;
Intracranial Dynamics; Shock; Resuscitation of
Infants and Children*

Christine M. Dickenson, M.S.N., R.N., CCRN
Clinical Nurse Specialist, Pediatric Intensive Care
Unit, The Children's Hospital of Philadelphia
Philadelphia, Pennsylvania
Toxic Ingestions ·

Patricia Dillman, M.S.N., R.N.
Pediatric Critical Care Clinical Nurse Specialist,
United—The Children's Hospital of New Jersey,
Newark, New Jersey
HIV in the Critically Ill Child

Kathryn M. Dodds, M.S.N., R.N., C.P.N.P., CCRN
Advanced Practice Nurse Practitioner, Division of Pulmonology, A.I. duPont Institute, Wilmington, Delaware
Tissue Perfusion

Neil Ead, M.S.N., R.N., CCRN, C.E.N.
Assistant Professor, Yale University School of Nursing; Clinical Nurse Specialist, Pediatric Critical Care, Children's Hospital at Yale–New Haven, New Haven, Connecticut
Resuscitation of Infants and Children

E. Marsha Elixon, M.S., R.N.,C., CCRN
Pediatric Cardiovascular Clinical Nurse Specialist, Case Manager, Massachusetts General Hospital, Boston, Massachusetts
Tissue Perfusion

Arthur J. Engler, D.N.Sc.(c.), R.N.,C., N.N.P.
Clinical Instructor, University of Maryland at Baltimore School of Nursing, Baltimore, Maryland
Thermal Regulation

Mary J. Fagan, M.S.N., R.N., CCRN
Director, Critical Care Programs, Children's Hospital San Diego, San Diego, California
Leadership in Pediatric Critical Care

Barbara J. Few, M.S.N., R.N.
Quality Improvement Coordinator, Yale–New Haven Hospital, New Haven, Connecticut
Pulmonary Critical Care Problems

Barbara Gill, M.N., R.N.
Abilene Intercollegiate School of Nursing—Adjunct Faculty; Clinical Nurse Specialist, Hendrick Medical Center, Abilene, Texas
Organ Transplantation

Peggy C. Gordin, M.S., R.N.,C., F.A.A.N.
Director, Neonatal Nursing, The Children's Hospital of Philadelphia, Philadelphia, Pennsylvania
Pain and Aversive Stimuli

Donna H. Groh, M.S.N., R.N.
Adjunct Clinical Faculty, University of California, Los Angeles, Los Angeles, California; Vice President/Chief Operating Officer, Irvine Medical Center, Irvine, California
In the Best Interest of the Child: Ethical Issues

Nancy Hagelgans, M.S.N., R.N., E.T.N.
Urology Clinical Nurse Specialist, Rocky Mountain Pediatric Urology, Denver, Colorado
Skin Integrity

Twila W. Harmon, M.S.N., R.N.
Former Adjunct Faculty–Clinical Preceptor, University of Pennsylvania School of Nursing; Former Clinical Nurse Specialist, Pediatric Surgery and Urology, The Children's Hospital of Philadelphia, Philadelphia, Pennsylvania
Gastrointestinal Critical Care Problems

Carol J. Howe, M.S.N., R.N.
Nursing Projects Coordinator, The Children's Hospital of Philadelphia, Philadelphia, Pennsylvania
Pain and Aversive Stimuli

Diane S. Jakobowski, M.S.N., R.N., C.R.N.P.
Adjunct Clinical Faculty, The University of Pennsylvania; Clinical Nurse Specialist, Pediatric Surgery, The Children's Hospital of Philadelphia, Philadelphia, Pennsylvania
Gastrointestinal Critical Care Problems

Kimmith M. Jones, M.S., R.N., CCRN
Faculty Associate, University of Maryland School of Nursing; Clinical Nurse Specialist—Critical Care/ED, Sinai Hospital of Baltimore, Maryland
HIV in the Critically Ill Child

Patricia Lawrence Kane, M.S.N., R.N.
Clinical Nurse Specialist, Pediatric Cardiology and Cardiac Surgery, The Johns Hopkins Hospital, Baltimore, Maryland
Cardiovascular Critical Care Problems

Lori J. Kozlowski, M.S., R.N.
Clinical Nurse Specialist/Case Manager, Pediatric Oncology, The Johns Hopkins Hospital, Baltimore, Maryland
Oncologic Critical Care Problems

Mary Berry LeBoeuf, M.S.N., R.N., CCRN
Advanced Nurse Practitioner/Clinical Nurse Specialist, Pediatric Cardiothoracic Surgery, Children's Hospital of New Jersey, Newark, New Jersey
HIV in the Critically Ill Child

S. Jill Ley, M.S., R.N., CCRN
Assistant Clinical Professor, Department of Physiological Nursing, University of California, San Francisco; Outcomes Coordinator, Cardiac Surgery, California Pacific Medical Center, San Francisco, California
Tissue Perfusion

Patricia Lincoln, M.S., R.N.
Staff Nurse, Level III, Cardiac Intensive Care Unit, Children's Hospital, Boston, Boston, Massachusetts
Cardiovascular Critical Care Problems

Cathleen B. Longo, M.S.N., R.N., CCRN, C.E.N.
Pediatric Clinical Instructor, University of Pennsylvania School of Nursing; Staff Nurse, Emergency Room, The Children's Hospital of Philadelphia, Philadelphia, Pennsylvania
Toxic Ingestions

Wendy Ludwig, M.S., R.N.
Staff Development Specialist, Children's Hospital, Boston, Boston, Massachusetts
Professional Development

Patricia M. Lybarger, M.S.N., R.N.,C.
Lecturer, Paramedic Program, Northeastern University, Burlington, Massachusetts; Staff Development Coordinator, Shriner's Hospital for Crippled Children, Burns Institute–Boston Unit, Boston, Massachusetts
Thermal Injury

Susan Morgan Madder, M.S.N., R.N.
Staff Nurse, Pediatric Intensive Care Unit, The Children's Hospital of Philadelphia, Philadelphia, Pennsylvania
Renal Critical Care Problems

Sarah Martin, M.S., R.N.
Staff Nurse, Wyler Intensive Care Unit, The University of Chicago Hospitals, Wyler Children's Hospital, Chicago, Illinois
Organ Transplantation

Kimberly Mason, O.N.C., R.N.
Clinical Nurse Specialist—Orthopaedics, The Children's Hospital of Philadelphia, Philadelphia, Pennsylvania
Pain and Aversive Stimuli

Beth McDermott, B.S.N., R.N., CCRN
Staff Nurse, Level III, Multidisciplinary Intensive Care Unit, Children's Hospital, Boston, Boston, Massachusetts
Hematologic Critical Care Problems

Elaine C. Meyer, Ph.D., R.N.
Instructor of Psychology, Harvard Medical Schools, Boston, Massachusetts; Clinical Assistant Professor of Pediatrics, Brown University School of Medicine, Providence, Rhode Island; Staff Psychologist, Multidisciplinary Intensive Care Unit, Children's Hospital, Boston, Boston, Massachusetts; Research

Psychologist, Department of Pediatrics, Women and Infants' Hospital, Providence, Rhode Island
The Impact of the Critical Care Experience on the Family

Pamela M. Milberger, M.S.N., R.N., CCRN
Clinical Nurse Specialist, Pediatric Critical Care, Children's Healthcare–Minneapolis, Minneapolis, Minnesota
Renal Critical Care Problems

Joyce Molengraft, B.S.N., R.N.
Staff Nurse, Level II, Multidisciplinary Intensive Care Unit, Children's Hospital, Boston, Boston, Massachusetts
Oxygenation/Ventilation

Patricia A. Moloney-Harmon, M.S., R.N., CCRN
Clinical Nurse Specialist, Children's Services, Sinai Hospital of Baltimore, Baltimore, Maryland
Trauma

Paula J. Moynihan, B.S.N., R.N., CCRN
Staff Nurse, Level III, Clinical Coordinator and Quality Improvement Coordinator, Cardiac Intensive Care Unit, Children's Hospital, Boston, Boston, Massachusetts
Cardiovascular Critical Care Problems

Regina Muir, M.S., R.N.
Unit Manager, Pediatric Trauma Intensive Care Unit, Parkland Memorial Hospital, Dallas, Texas
Trauma

Kathryn M. Murphy, Ph.D., R.N.
Lecturer, University of Pennsylvania; Co-Director, Diabetes Center for Children, The Children's Hospital of Philadelphia, Philadelphia, Pennsylvania
Endocrine Critical Care Problems

Patricia O'Brien, M.S.N., R.N., P.N.P.
Cardiovascular Clinical Nurse Specialist, Cardiovascular Program, Children's Hospital, Boston, Boston, Massachusetts
Organ Transplantation

Kathleen M. Ouzts, Ph.D., R.N.
Former Assistant Professor, School of Health Sciences, Clayton State College, Morrow, Georgia
Fluid and Electrolyte Regulation

Susan N. Peck, M.S.N., R.N., C.R.N.P.
Adjunct Clinical Faculty, University of Pennsylvania School of Nursing; Clinical Nurse

Specialist in Gastroenterology, The Children's
Hospital of Philadelphia, Philadelphia,
Pennsylvania
Gastrointestinal Critical Care Problems

Ann Powers, M.S., R.N., C.S., P.N.P.
Clinical Faculty (Adjunct), Saint Joseph College,
West Hartford, Connecticut; University of
Connecticut, Storrs, Connecticut; Yale University,
New Haven, Connecticut; Pediatric Care Manager,
Connecticut Children's Medical Center, Hartford
Connecticut
Acid-Base Balance

Wendy Roberts, M.S.N., R.N.
Clinical Nurse Specialist, Shriners Hospital for
Crippled Children, Burns Institute–Boston Unit,
Boston, Massachusetts
Thermal Injury

**Cathy Rosenthal-Dichter, Ph.D.(c), R.N.,
CCRN, F.C.C.M.**
Doctoral Candidate and Teaching Assistant,
University of Pennsylvania, School of Nursing,
Philadelphia, Pennsylvania; Formerly Clinical
Nurse Specialist, Pediatric Critical Care, National
Institutes of Health; Warren Grant Magnuson
Clinical Center, Critical Care Nursing Department,
Bethesda, Maryland
Host Defenses

Cindy Hylton Rushton, D.N.Sc., R.N., F.A.A.N.
Assistant Professor of Nursing, The Johns Hopkins
University, Baltimore, Maryland; Nurse Ethicist,
Children's National Medical Center, Washington,
DC
Thermal Regulation

Linda F. Samson, Ph.D., R.N.,C., C.N.A.A.
Dean, School of Health Sciences, Clayton State
College, Morrow, Georgia
Fluid and Electrolyte Regulation

Janis Bloedel Smith, M.S.N., R.N., CCRN
Manager, Patient Care Services, Inpatient
Cardiology, Vanderbilt University Medical Center,
Nashville, Tennessee
*Critical Illness and Intensive Care During Infancy
and Childhood; Tissue Perfusion; Cardiovascular
Critical Care Problems*

Mary Fallon Smith, M.S.N., R.N.
Clinical Nurse Specialist, Emergency Department,
Children's Department, Children's Hospital, Boston,
Boston, Massachusetts
Professional Development

Claire E. Sommargren, M.S., R.N., CCRN
Instructor, Education Department, Dominican
Santa Cruz Hospital, Santa Cruz, California
Environmental Hazards

Patricia Srnec, M.S., R.N., C.N.A.
Director, Emergency/Ambulatory Nursing, St. Louis
Children's Hospital, St. Louis, Missouri
Trauma

Judith J. Stellar, M.S., C.S., C.R.N.P.
Clinical Preceptor, School of Nursing, Graduate
Division, University of Pennsylvania; General
Surgery Clinical Nurse Specialist, The Children's
Hospital of Philadelphia, Philadelphia,
Pennsylvania
Gastrointestinal Critical Care Problems

John E. Thompson, R.R.T.
Associate in Anesthesiology, Harvard Medical
School; Director of Clinical Technology, Children's
Hospital, Boston, Boston, Massachusetts
Oxygenation/Ventilation

Michele Topor, R.N.
Formerly Clinical Coordinator, Renal Transplant
Program, Children's Hospital, Boston, Boston,
Massachusetts
Organ Transplantation

Judy Verger, M.S.N., R.N., C.R.N.P., CCRN
Clinical Lecturer, Pediatric Critical Care Nurse
Practitioner Program, School of Nursing, University
of Pennsylvania; Pediatric Nurse Practitioner,
Emergency Department, The Children's Hospital of
Philadelphia, Philadelphia, Pennsylvania
Nutrition

Paula Vernon-Levett, M.S., R.N., CCRN
Family Care Nurse, Pediatric Intensive Care Unit,
The Children's Memorial Medical Center, Chicago,
Illinois
*Intracranial Dynamics; Neurologic Critical Care
Problems*

Darlene Whitney, B.S.N., R.N., CCRN
Staff Nurse, Level II, Multidisciplinary Intensive
Care Unit, Children's Hospital, Boston, Boston,
Massachusetts
Skin Integrity

Karen Zamberlan, Ph.D., R.N.
Late Clinical Nurse Specialist, Pediatric Liver
Transplant Services, Children's Hospital of
Pittsburgh, Pittsburgh, Pennsylvania
Organ Transplantation

FOREWORD

The publication of *Critical Care Nursing of Infants and Children* is an important milestone in the rapidly evolving development of pediatric critical care nursing. It often surprises students and colleagues when I discuss my experiences in the days "before pediatric intensive care units." They cannot conceive of a time when these specialized units, along with their highly technological treatments, were not available to facilitate the care of critically ill children. During this "before" period, seriously ill children were cared for on regular hospital units with minimal technology. Staff nurses were often assigned to "special" the child, unless the family provided a private duty nurse. Sometimes a special room was set aside for care of several seriously ill children so that one nurse could care for several children. The level of expertise of these staff and private duty nurses, however, was not adequate for the intensive care needs of critically ill children. Obviously, children with serious health problems or children recovering from major surgery were at high risk of dying because adequate treatments and monitoring measures were not available.

The development of pediatric critical care units alongside the development of more sophisticated treatments and related technology was highly effective in reducing the mortality of acutely ill children. As these units developed, it soon became obvious that the nurses working in these units needed advanced training to adequately monitor and care for these seriously ill children. It was essential that nurses have access to the developing knowledge about critical care and develop the skills to apply that knowledge. Staff education, advanced critical care modules, and graduate education were some of the approaches used to prepare nurses for roles in pediatric critical care. In addition, nurses themselves began to become involved in the development of knowledge about critical care nursing through the conduct of nursing research and the synthesis and application of knowl-

edge through the publication of clinical articles and textbooks.

The publication of *Critical Care Nursing of Infants and Children* is another important step in the evolution of nursing knowledge related to pediatric critical care. This state-of-the-art textbook is unique in being developed from a strong nursing perspective, and the organization of the textbook is highly innovative. The first two sections provide a comprehensive background for the book including a focus on historical, developmental, and family issues as well as issues related to the practice environment. The next section on phenomena of concern thoroughly covers the major phenomena that pediatric critical care nurses must deal with on a daily basis. This content is then pulled together differently by focusing in depth on problems involving the major body systems as well as multisystem problems. Finally, standards and practice guidelines are introduced. The end result is a reference and teaching textbook that provides comprehensive and holistic content related to pediatric critical care nursing. Furthermore, the book has very high standards for scholarship. Content is well validated through reference to research and the latest clinical and theoretical knowledge in the field. Putting this material together in an organized, cohesive, reader friendly manner was truly a challenging and exciting endeavor.

Having watched and participated in the evolution of pediatric critical care nursing over the past 35 years, I am astounded at the knowledge explosion in the field and at the comprehensive and complex scope of this specialty area of nursing. To be a pediatric critical care nurse indeed takes knowledge and skills in both the art and the science of nursing. All nurses who take the step toward becoming pediatric critical care nurses should have a copy of this book to guide their development as professionals in this exciting and ever-challenging field. Nurses who are already experienced pediatric critical care nurses would gain new ways of conceptualizing their practice and would find the book extremely valuable as a resource in caring for challenging patients on their units. The text will also be invaluable for students enrolled in advanced practice pediatric graduate programs. One would also hope that every pediatric intensive care unit in the country would have copies available for staff reference.

Critical Care Nursing of Infants and Children is a milestone in nursing textbooks by its excellence and creativity. It may well serve as a model for future approaches in knowledge synthesis for practice. It certainly can serve to strengthen the specialty of pediatric critical care nursing by providing a strong framework and background for practice.

MARGARET S. MILES, Ph.D., R.N., F.A.A.N.
Professor, Health of Women and Children
School of Nursing
The University of North Carolina at Chapel Hill

PREFACE

Critical Care Nursing of Infants and Children is a state-of-the-art textbook, written to provide a comprehensive reference for experienced nurses caring for critically ill pediatric patients and their families. It is based on the broad clinical experiences of its contributors in the care of seriously ill or injured children and in nursing research aimed at improving and perfecting care. The strong nursing focus of this book is apparent in its structural approach using *phenomena of concern* and *final common pathways*. Phenomena of concern address nursing care issues common to all critically ill pediatric patients regardless of their primary problem. Final common pathways cluster patient problems in such a way that allows them to be reframed from a perspective that guides nursing care. Also featured are pediatric critical care standards of care and practice guidelines that can be used to decrease unnecessary variation in care and stimulate clinical research.

Pediatric critical care nursing has experienced extraordinary development since the advent of intensive care units designed specifically for the care of critically ill children. Nurses who care for critically ill infants and children are continuously challenged by diversity in patient age and diagnosis. Skilled clinical practice requires knowledge about a wide variety of illnesses and injuries integrated with an awareness of the continuums of growth and development. Pediatric critical care nurses also require comprehensive information about normal anatomy and physiology, physical and psychosocial development, pathophysiology and disease, critical instrumentation and patient management, and the most current pediatric critical care research findings.

The foundation for the text is provided in the chapters that detail children's and families' responses to the experiences of critical illness and intensive care, as this aspect of pediatric critical care nursing is inherent to practice. Practical information supporting the evolving role of nurse as tender of the care milieu is unique. Chapters on nutrition, host defenses, skin integrity, and pain and adversive stimuli management provide hard-to-find, clinically relevant information specific for the critically ill pediatric patient. A comprehensive review of physiology, with emphasis on the impact of maturation on system structure and function, is provided for each body system. The pathophysiologic mechanisms, clinical manifestations, and diagnosis of disease in infants and children are also presented in detail. Multisystem problems, including organ transplantation, HIV, shock, trauma, burns, toxic ingestions, and resuscitation, are presented separately. Instrumentation appropriate to caring for critically ill children and critical care management of infants and children is discussed from a collaborative framework. Appendices are provided as a clinically useful reference. A complete reference list is found at the end of each chapter, and tables and figures provide support to the entire text.

Critical Care Nursing of Infants and Children is divided into six sections, which encompass all aspects of pediatric critical care nursing.

Section 1: Holistic Pediatric Critical Care Nursing presents essential concepts that provide a foundation for the practice of pediatric critical care nursing. The evolution of pediatric critical care nursing as a specialty is presented. Discussion of the impact of critical illness on children and families provides nurses with an appreciation of the magnitude of this experience and guides interventions aimed at mitigating stress and promoting individual and family growth.

Section 2: The Practice Environment focuses on the milieu affecting nursing care delivery. The broadening professional responsibilities of nurse as leader, teacher, and mentor are acknowledged and supported. Ethical and legal issues are illuminated from a pediatric critical care nursing perspective. Nurses also face occupational hazards in the practice environment, which are also addressed in this section.

Section 3: Phenomena of Concern focuses on the unique care needs of all pediatric patients regardless of their primary problem. Nurses play a major role in optimizing the patient's potential outcome through a deliberative proactive process that integrates skilled clinical knowledge about tissue perfusion, oxygenation and ventilation, acid-base balance, intracranial dynamics, fluid and electrolyte regulation, nutrition, thermal regulation, host defenses, skin integrity, and pain and aversive stimulation. Within each phenomenon of concern, essential embryology, maturational anatomy and physiology, and instrumentation are discussed.

Section 4: Final Common Pathways presents state-of-the-art nursing care for patient problems within each body system. A focus on the final common pathways of many disease states is presented so that system dysfunction is viewed broadly and addressed within a nursing framework. For example, the numerous pathophysiologic states that result in increased intracranial pressure become fairly academic to the bedside nurse who is responsible for managing moment-to-moment changes in cerebral compliance in an effort to prevent secondary brain injury. The etiology, incidence, and pathogenesis of specific disorders that lead to development of a final common pathway are also presented when appropriate. Critical care management, including both independent and collaborative nursing care measures, is focused on the final common pathways of system dysfunction and specifically on patient care unique to a particular disorder.

Section 5: Multisystem Problems addresses the needs of patients experiencing multiple system dysfunction and their complicated demands and unique needs. Because these patients' illnesses involve more than a single body system, they present a distinctive challenge to the care team.

Section 6: Nursing Practice Guidelines for Pediatric Critical Care presents guides for optimal care of critically ill infants, children, and their families. Clinical practice guidelines are presented by nursing diagnosis identified as important by the American Association of Critical-Care Nurses (AACN). These can be reproduced or computerized, then individualized to serve as the patient's management plan. This section also provides guidelines and levels of care for pediatric intensive care units established by the Society for Critical Care Medicine (SCCM).

Critical care nursing of infants and children is a dynamic specialty, necessitating that nurses assure their practice be evidenced based. Our purpose in writing this text will be realized if readers are provided the knowledge they need to assure excellent care to critically ill children and their families. The goal of excellence in the critical care nursing of infants and children is based on commitment to children as our most precious resource and to families as the agents of developing human potential. Also necessary is genuine respect for the unique contributions of each member of the multidisciplinary team and for our nursing colleagues as sources of immeasurable humanity and healing.

MARTHA A. Q. CURLEY

JANIS BLOEDEL SMITH

PATRICIA A. MOLONEY-HARMON

ACKNOWLEDGMENTS

Because all three editors/authors of this text are practicing clinicians in the care of critically ill infants and children, it has been some time reaching reality. Having stretched the patience of family, friends, and colleagues with talk of "the book," work on "the book," editing "the book," etc., we are indebted to you for your endurance and support. We express our gratitude to the clinical experts who are our contributors. The excellence of your work is evident in the pages that follow, in which you share the wealth of your knowledge and expertise. We are grateful to our reviewers, who took the time and made the effort to comment constructively and thoughtfully on the manuscript. We are also grateful to the diligence of the research librarians and graphic artists who either found or created the impossible. To Ilze Rader, our editor at WB Saunders, and Marie Thomas, editorial assistant, specific thanks for your guidance throughout the process. Thanks also to Frank Polizzano, Production Manager, and Tom Stringer, Copy Editing Supervisor. Finally, inspiration has always come from the children, families, and professionals with whom we have worked while this project was ongoing. Some of you may work with us still, perhaps others have a memory of some time or some experience we shared, others may be unaware that we carry your echoes with us. Thank you all.

MARTHA A. Q. CURLEY
JANIS BLOEDEL SMITH
PATRICIA A. MOLONEY-HARMON

CONTENTS

Holistic Pediatric Critical Care Nursing

This section presents essential concepts that provide a foundation for the practice of pediatric critical care nursing. The evolution of pediatric critical care nursing as a specialty is presented. Discussion of the impact of critical illness on children and families provides nurses with an appreciation of the magnitude of this experience and guides interventions aimed at mitigating stress and promoting individual growth.

CHAPTER *1*

The Essence of Pediatric Critical Care Nursing

MARTHA A. Q. CURLEY

EVOLUTION OF THE DISCIPLINE
First Units
Patient Population
Levels of PICU Care
Literature
Professional Organizations
THE CHANGING HEALTHCARE ENVIRONMENT
Our Vision: Driven by the Needs of Patients
Impact Upon the Nursing Profession
Redefining Critical Care Nursing: Patient Needs
   Drive Nurse Characteristics

OUR UNIQUE CONTRIBUTIONS: THE ESSENCE OF PRACTICE
Competent Pediatric Critical Care Nursing Practice
Caring Practices
Family-Centered Care
Evidence-Based Appropriate Practice
Leadership
Advocacy
OUR FUTURE: INNOVATION AND CHANGE

Nurses are privy, like almost no one else, to the body's secret bruises and disfigurements, the mind's unuttered worries, the heart's sweetest emotions, and the spirit's last glimmer.

ANGELA MCBRIDE (1994)

Pediatric critical care nurses create an environment in which critically unstable, highly vulnerable infants and children benefit from the vigilant care and the coordinated efforts of a team of highly skilled pediatric healthcare professionals. Indeed, the art and science of pediatric critical care have grown tremendously in recent years. Still vivid are memories of small rooms, minimum technology, changing boundaries of professional practice, and little clinical expertise. As noted by Diers (1985), nursing is what is intense about ICU care; the constant within the pediatric critical care environment is pediatric critical care nurses. This chapter introduces the reader to both the genesis and essence of the practice of pediatric critical care nursing.

EVOLUTION OF THE DISCIPLINE

Nursing's historical practice of watchful vigilance and triage provided the model for the care of critically ill patients in intensive care units (Fairman, 1992). In the late nineteenth century, Louisa May Alcott (1863) wrote:

My ward was divided into three rooms. . . . I had managed to sort out the patients in such a way that I had what I called "my duty room, my pleasure room, and my pathetic room," and worked for each in a different way. One, I visited, armed with a dressing tray, full of rollers, plasters, and pins; another, with books, flowers, games, and gossip; a third, with teapots, lullabies, consolation, and, sometimes, a shroud. . . . wherever the sickest or most helpless man chanced to be, there I held my watch.

First Units

North Carolina Memorial Hospital opened the first "special care unit" for acutely ill patients in 1953

3

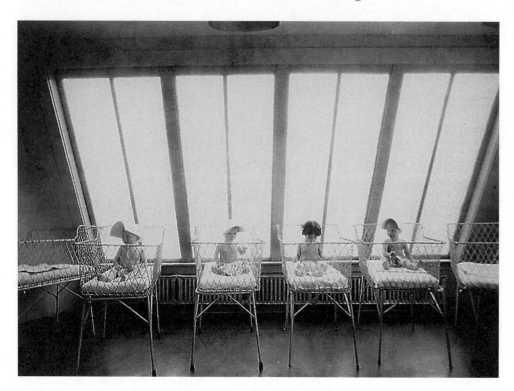

Figure 1-1 ● ● ● ● ● ●
Sun room where babies in sun bonnets received the benefit of natural lighting through large windows, 1930. (Courtesy of Children's Hospital, Boston.)

(Cadmus, 1954). This unit was created to meet the challenge of improving patient care while simultaneously saving time for nursing personnel. Before creating the special care unit, patients were assigned beds by virtue of their financial status. Nurses would care for patients with varying levels of acuity on the same unit; the almost constant attention required of acutely ill patients prevented nurses from adequately caring for less acute patients (Cadmus, 1954). Of interest to pediatrics, the idea of putting all critically ill patients in one room with everything available in case of an emergency was generated by an assistant director of nursing, chief of anesthesia, medical director of the hospital, and otolaryngologist after a near-miss life-threatening respiratory event involving a 4-year-old patient (Cadmus, 1980). This young patient

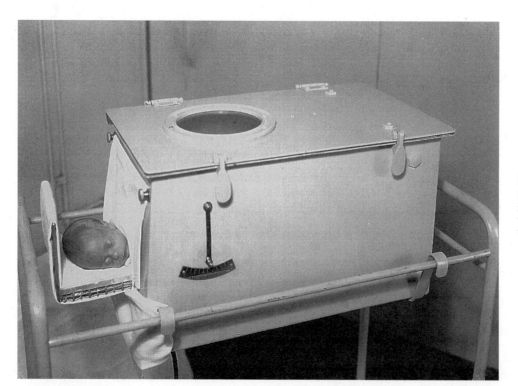

Figure 1-2 ● ● ● ● ● ●
Infant in respirator, 1934, Infant's Hospital, Boston. (Courtesy of Children's Hospital, Boston.)

survived only by chance; a nurse passed her door (a private room at the end of a hallway), noted her distress, and gave her emergency treatment.

The first pediatric-specific ICUs opened after improved patient outcomes were realized when specialized care was provided critically ill neonates and adults. From the 1920s to early 1950s, epidemics of acute poliomyelitis necessitated the use of assisted ventilation for polio victims (Fig. 1–2). First described was negative-pressure ventilation by Drinker and Shaw (1929) in Boston, followed by tracheal intubation and positive-pressure ventilation by Lassen (1953) in Copenhagen. James Wilson, a pediatrician at the Children's Hospital of Boston, designed the four-bed negative-pressure ventilator in 1932 (Smith, 1983a) (Fig. 1–3). As noted by Downes (1992), this was "probably the first unit in the world to cohort and support pediatric patients with vital organ failure." Later in Scandinavia, it was recognized that children had higher mortality rates than adults in these special poliomyelitis respiratory units. Responding to this, separate pediatric respiratory units were developed to specifically care for children in Uppsala and Stockholm (DeNicola & Todres, 1992).

In January 1967, John J. Downes and his colleagues from Children's Hospital of Philadelphia opened the first multidisciplinary PICU in the United States (Downes, 1990) (Table 1–1). This unit consisted of six fully monitored beds with an adjacent procedure room and intensive care chemistry labora-

Table 1–1. EARLY PEDIATRIC ICU PROGRAMS

Abroad

1955 Children's Hospital of Goteburg, Sweden
1961 Stockholm, Sweden
1963 Hospital St. Vincent de Paul, Paris
1963 Royal Children's Hospital, Melbourne
1964 Alder Hey Children's Hospital, Liverpool

United States

1967 Children's Hospital of Philadelphia
1969 Children's Hospital of Pittsburgh
1969 Yale–New Haven Medical Center
1971 Massachusetts General Hospital, Boston

From Downes, J. J. (1992). The historical evolution, current status, and prospective development of pediatric critical care. *Critical Care Clinics of North America*, 8 (1), 1–22.

tory (Fig. 1–4). As recalled by J. Downes, Erna Goulding, then Director of Nursing, became convinced that opening the intensive care unit would be the right decision. Willing to err on the side of what was best for patients, Ms. Goulding recruited a number of high-caliber nursing staff for the unit. The unit's first Nurse Manager was Janet Johnson, followed by Joan Alessio. According to Downes, Johnson's tenure was short. Alessio contributed creativity, drive, and spark to build a self-directed cohesive team that adapted well to the new PICU environment (personal communication, June 17, 1994).

By the end of the 1970s, medical training programs for pediatric intensivists developed. By the mid-1980s, advanced practice nursing programs to prepare clinical nurse specialists in acute care pediatrics were established at Yale University, the University of Pennsylvania, and the University of California at San Francisco. Currently, pediatric intensive care units are found in every major center that provides care to seriously ill pediatric patients. In 1992, 328 pediatric intensive care units were listed by the American Hospital Association (1993).

Patient Population

Although many PICUs care for critically ill surgical neonates and/or maturing young adults with a congenital or childhood disease, the pediatric critical care population traditionally consists of patients who range in age from full-term neonates to adolescents and their families. Unlike system-specific adult critical care units, a wide spectrum of illnesses are found in most PICUs. Both extremes, age and illness, require pediatric critical care nurses to function as generalists within a subspeciality area.

Levels of PICU Care

While patients with a wide variety of illness can be found in most PICUs, the intensity of services may, and perhaps should, be specifically delineated.

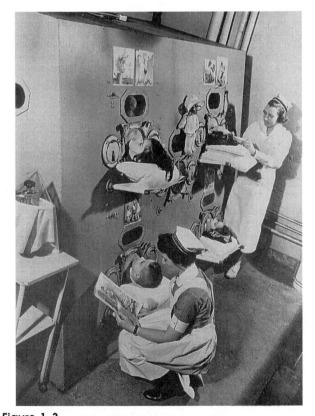

Figure 1–3 ● ● ● ● ● ●
Nurses reading to children in a four-unit respirator, c. 1955. (Courtesy of Children's Hospital, Boston.)

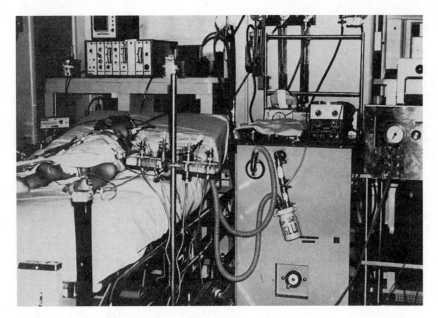

Figure 1–4 ● ● ● ● ● ●
A patient in the first pediatric intensive care unit in the United States (Children's Hospital of Philadelphia, 1970.) Note the Emerson PV-1 ventilator, Gorman-Rupp water mattress, Stratham monitoring system, and strain gauge transducers. (From: Downes, J. J. (1992). The historical evolution, current status, and prospective development of pediatric critical care. *Critical Care Clinics of North America,* 8 (1), 1–22.)

With participation from the Society of Pediatric Nurses, Guidelines and Levels of Care for Pediatric Intensive Care Units (1993) have been proposed by the Pediatric Section of the Society of Critical Care Medicine, the American Academy of Pediatrics Section on Critical Care Medicine, and the Committee on Hospital Care (see Section Six, Standards and Practice Guidelines). The guidelines recommend that level I PICUs provide definitive care for a wide range of complex, progressive, rapidly changing illnesses, often requiring a multidisciplinary approach in pediatric patients of all ages, excluding neonates. The guidelines also recommend that level II PICUs provide stabilization of critically ill children before transfer to a level I unit and care to infants or children with less complex, low-acuity, highly predictable disorders to avoid long-distance transfer. Level II units should be located in geographically isolated regions with a small population base. Formal and informal regionalization of PICU services creates an organized system of care that distributes scarce and expensive resources in an efficient manner to benefit the greatest number of patients (Yeh, 1992).

Literature

The rapid evolution of pediatric critical care required nurses to be self-motivated learners accountable for their own education. Before the early 1980s, educational materials specific to pediatric critical care nursing were nonexistent. Pediatric critical care nurses would occasionally find an additional chapter on pediatrics or an appendix on normal pediatric vital signs placed at the end of a critical care nursing text. In 1981, the first pediatric critical care nursing texts were published: *Pediatric Critical Care Nursing,* edited by Katherine W. Vestal; and the American Association of Critical-Care Nurses (AACN) spon-

sored *Critical Care Nursing of Children and Adolescents,* edited by Annalee R. Oakes. This was followed by Janis Bloedel Smith's (1983b) *Pediatric Critical Care;* then Mary Fran Hazinski's AACN-endorsed, first edition (1984) of *Nursing Care of the Critically-Ill Child.* Journal articles about pediatric critical care nursing are sporadically found in both pediatric and critical care journals.

Professional Organizations

The American Association of Critical-Care Nurses (AACN), first organized in 1969 as the American Association of Cardiovascular Nurses (Lynaugh, 1990), has a long history of supporting critical care nursing across the lifespan. In 1982, the AACN introduced Special Interest Groups (SIGs) to respond to members' expressed needs for specialized information, networking, and education (Disch, 1982). The pediatric SIG, later known as the Neonatal and Pediatric Special Interest Group (NAP SIG), provided the first opportunities for pediatric critical care nurses to collectively gather and share their expertise. The first members of this group included MaryFran Hazinski (Coordinator), Nan Smith-Blair, Margaret Slota, Karen Killian, Holly Weeks-Webster, Janet Wintle, Linda Miers (AACN Board liaison), and James Niebuhr (AACN Staff liaison).

Priorities for the NAP SIG included the provision of high-level programming to meet the specific educational needs of its members. Before this initiative, pediatric critical care nurses attended adult or neonatal programs and extrapolated perceived relevant information when caring for the pediatric patient population. Other priorities of the NAP SIG included developing a resource file of consultants, audiovisual programs, policies and procedures, care plans, and teaching programs (Christopherson, 1982) and support of separate critical care certification exams for neonatal and pediatric critical care nurses (Griffin, Hitchens, & Smith-Blair, 1984).

CCRN Certification

In 1975, AACN Certification Corporation was established to formally recognize the professional competence of critical care nurses. The mission of the AACN Certification Corporation is to certify and promote critical care nursing practice that optimally contributes to desired patient outcomes. The program establishes the body of knowledge necessary for CCRN certification, tests the common body of knowledge needed to function effectively within the critical care setting, recognizes professional competence by granting CCRN status to successful certification candidates, and assists and promotes the continual professional development of critical care nurses.

Certification is attractive to both the critical care nurse and the consumer of critical care nursing services. Whereas state licensure signifies that an individual has the basic knowledge needed for the general practice of nursing, certification provides a means of recognizing professionals who have specialized knowledge and experience, and assures the public that they are receiving care from practitioners who meet a defined level of competence (Niebuhr, 1993).

Because critical care nursing practice is constantly changing, a Role Delineation Study (RDS) is conducted every 3 to 5 years to define the dimensions of current critical care nursing practice and identify the actual tasks required of a competent critical care nurse. The tasks serve as a framework for the CCRN examination blueprint. Exam questions are linked to the study data and evaluate the knowledge and skills required of a nurse to perform the tasks at a competent level of critical care nursing practice.

Before 1992, content and construct validity of the CCRN examination was established for critical care nurses who primarily care for adult patients. Pediatric critical care nurses who sat for the CCRN exam were tested on content that did not reflect their practice. For example, the cardiovascular system, which reflected 19% of the CCRN exam, contained questions on myocardial infarctions and angina/atherosclerosis, a rare phenomenon in pediatric critical care. For years, pediatric critical care nurses recognized both the similarities *and* differences between their practice and that of neonatal and adult critical care but found them difficult to articulate.

In 1989, AACN Certification Corporation began a new Role Delineation Study (RDS). The purpose of the 1989–1990 study was to refine the existing adult CCRN examination and define the tasks, knowledge, and skills fundamental to neonatal and pediatric critical care nursing. Major differences among neonatal, pediatric, and adult critical care nursing practice were identified in the types of patient care problems for which direct bedside care is provided and in the amount of time spent caring for the patients with specific problems (Table 1–2). The results, *for the first time ever,* described the practice of pediatric critical care nursing and justified the need for separate pediatric, neonatal, and adult CCRN examinations. The 1989–1990 RDS described the diverse practice of pediatric critical care nursing and communicated it in terms that could be equated with neonatal and adult critical care nursing practice. The first CCRN exam, specific for pediatric critical care nursing, was administered in July 1992. Almost 75% of the first 848 pediatric critical care nurses who sat for the exam passed it (Ramseyer & Jones, 1992).

In 1989, AACN also restructured all SIGs into a national network of Special Interest Consultants (SICs). Acknowledging the unique and separate needs of neonatal and pediatric nurses, distinct Neonatal and Pediatric SIC positions were established. Pediatric SICs now specifically focus upon issues related to pediatric critical care nursing and are readily available to AACN as regional experts on issues related to pediatric critical care nursing practice.

Other organizations of interest to pediatric critical care nurses include the Society of Pediatric Nurses (SPN), the Association of Care of Children's Health (ACCH), and the Society of Critical Care Medicine (SCCM). Established in 1990, the purpose of the SPN is to improve the nursing care of children and their families and to further the development of pediatric nursing as a subspeciality within the profession of nursing. Established in 1965, ACCH is a multidisciplinary educational and advocacy organization promoting family-centered care policies and practices that are responsive to the unique developmental and psychosocial needs of children, youth, and their families. Established in 1970, the purpose of the SCCM is to improve the care of the critically ill patient with life-threatening illness and promote the development of optimal facilities for care and to bring together leaders from various medical disciplines, nursing, basic sciences, medical technology, bioengineering, and allied health professions.

THE CHANGING HEALTHCARE ENVIRONMENT

America's healthcare system is neither healthy, caring, nor a system (Weisberg, 1990). For years,

Table 1–2. PERCENTAGE OF TIME CARING FOR PATIENTS WITH ALTERATIONS IN BODY SYSTEMS

System Dysfunction	Pediatric Practice	Neonatal Practice	Adult Practice
Pulmonary	28%	39%	22%
Cardiovascular	24%	15%	39%
Neurologic	15%	6%	8%
Multisystem	12%	22%	10%
Hematology/immunology	7%	5%	4%
Renal	5%	3%	5%
Gastrointestinal	5%	7%	8%
Endocrine	4%	3%	4%

Data from Certification Corporation, American Association of Critical-Care Nurses (1990). *Role delineation study.* Laguna Niguel, CA.

critical care nurses have been challenged to maintain the delicate balance between working the system and making the system work for patients. Healthcare reform provides an unparalleled opportunity for critical analysis of the entire healthcare system so that the system can be redesigned to do what it is supposed to do—work for patients and their families.

Our Vision: Driven by the Needs of Patients

AACN articulated a vision of creating a healthcare system driven by the needs of patients in which critical care nurses can make their optimal contribution. Because of nursing's strong history of patient advocacy, patients and families have come to trust that nurses will do the right thing for them. As a profession, nursing has remained focused on patients and supporting a system driven by the needs of patients. Without question, what is right for patients intuitively feels right for nurses.

Impact Upon the Nursing Profession

Healthcare reform will result in rapid growth for the nursing profession. Nursing's traditional focus on patients, wellness, disease prevention, and holism is consistent with the goals of healthcare reform. Our historical framework provides the profession its point of leverage for future growth. The Pew Health Professions Commission (1993) predicts a growing demand for nurses throughout the early years of the next century. The demand for nurses will exceed supply by at least 100,000 per year until 2005; after that, the gap between supply and demand will widen.

The Pew Health Professions Commission (1993) also predicts that as care in hospitals becomes more complex (in terms of technology, information management, and patient care demands), new opportunities for differentiated practice will emerge. No longer will a nurse–be a nurse–be a nurse. The multiple educational pathways that have caused over 30 years of debate will finally be appreciated as we come to rely upon the unique knowledge and skills of associates degree-, diploma-, and bachelor-prepared nurses. In order for this to be accomplished, the profession will have to differentiate, more definitively, the practice and education patterns of various levels of nurses (AACN, 1992). Advanced practice nurses, from clinical nurse specialists to acute care nurse practitioners, will continue to grow in number and take on the responsibility of highly specialized care. The "right" advanced practice role will be determined by the needs of patients within specific units.

By today's standards, patients have to be physiologically unstable to be admitted to and stay in hospitals—as well they should be. Patients are and will continue to move out of the ICU earlier than ever before. Care, traditionally provided in inpatient settings, is being transferred to the outpatient setting. Much of the technology used in the ICU has been adapted for use in the home.

Redefining Critical Care Nursing: Patient Needs Drive Nurse Characteristics

Considering that inpatient acuity will be extremely high, equated to giant ICUs, describing critical care nursing practice by location or by the technology seems passé. In a patient-driven system, nursing practice is described from a patient needs perspective. Critically ill patients are characterized by the presence of, or being at high risk for developing, life-threatening problems (AACN, 1990). Benner notes that critically ill patients need astute clinical judgment applied to problems that have very little margin of error (Gordon, 1994). These extremely vulnerable patients require a high level of nursing vigilance. From a patient's perspective, vigilance is a highly valued caring practice unique to critical care. Our vigilance preserves, protects, and enhances human dignity. Our alert and constant watchfulness, attentiveness, and reassuring presence are necessary to limit potential problems and/or complications. Redefining critical care nursing from a concept of vigilance allows us to maintain our focus on the patient's needs and not on geography and technology.

Critical illness is just one point on the health-illness continuum. It is in the patient's best interest to reengineer our fragmented care processes into a seamless system. Desperately needed is a balanced healthcare system that equally values prevention; health maintenance and education; and primary, chronic, and acute care. Pediatric critical care practitioners have long supported the value of primary prevention (e.g., pool and bicycle safety and helmet legislation). Having cared for chronically ill infants and children during acute episodes of their illness, pediatric critical care practitioners have come to appreciate the continuum of care. Caring for patients in isolation from where they came or where they are going will only continue to interrupt the fluidity of care.

OUR UNIQUE CONTRIBUTIONS: THE ESSENCE OF PRACTICE

Angela McBride (1994) wrote:

As a profession nursing is big enough to express all aspects of one's personality and committed enough to assume the challenges of a changing healthcare system peopled by individuals who don't want to lose sight of old fashioned caring values.

Pediatric critical care nurses do create the environment in which critically unstable, highly vulnerable infants and children benefit from vigilance and the coordinated efforts of a multidisciplinary team of highly skilled pediatric healthcare professionals.

Competent Pediatric Critical Care Nursing Practice

Compassion is no substitute for competence (Beckham, 1993). Competent pediatric critical care nursing practice is based upon a unique body of knowledge that integrates the individual effects of system maturation on physiology, pathophysiology, sociology, psychology, and human development. Clinical expertise—that is, skilled clinical knowledge, use of discretionary judgment, the ability to integrate complex multisystem effects and understand the expected trajectory of illness and human response to critical illness—embellishes competent practice. In critical care, Funk notes that the clinician first masters then transcends the technology and uses it as a means to an end in providing holistic care (Gordon, 1994). With experience, personal mastery develops, enabling the competent nurse to balance the art and science of care. The expert nurse anticipates the needs of patients, predicts the patient's trajectory of illness, and envisions the patient's level of recovery. For the expert, "agency"—an expression of responsibility for a patient's outcome—includes reading the situation based on expected changing relevance, including action based on the significance inherent in the situation, and a practical grasp of other clinicians' perception of the situation (Benner, Tanner, & Chesla, 1992).

Caring Practices

Caring practices optimize and make clinical competence/expertise more visible. As a basic value, caring embodies a spiritual and metaphysical dimension concerned with preserving, protecting, and enhancing human dignity (Caine, 1991). Caring practices include not only *what* nurses do but also *how* they do it. From the patient's perspective, caring practices are expressive activities that help the patients *feel cared for* (Brown, 1986). Essential to the process of caring is nurse recognition and appreciation of the patient's/parent's worth and competency to know and attend to self and congruence of the nursing action with the patient's/parent's perception of need (Brown, 1986).

Demonstration of professional knowledge and skill, surveillance, and reassuring presence have been identified as important caring practices when there is perceived threat to an individual's physical wellbeing (Brown, 1986). In critical care, caring is vigilant behavior that embodies nurturance and highly skilled and technical practices (Burfitt, Greiner, Miers, Kinney, Branyon, 1993).

The unique significance of what nurses do is in making a difference for patients; understanding the impact of critical illness on the infant's or child's person, development, and entire family; and helping so that the experience can be tolerated by patients and their families. This aspect of practice, our *presence* with patients, is unique to nursing.

Nurses coordinate the patient's and family's experiences by continuously focusing upon the person beneath all the high technology. Our concept of vigilance includes the "illness perspective," or the patient's experience of being ill. It takes courage to acknowledge the person of someone critically ill—those patients, surrounded by technology, therapists, physicians, and nurses, chemically paralyzed, narcotized, and apparently lifeless except for the rhythm of monitors, ventilators, and occasional alarms. We acknowledge their person by surrounding them with their possessions—for example, family pictures, cards from friends, their music. We make them human by talking with them, orientating them, and telling them what's going on. Occasionally the communication is not only one-way. The person responds by increasing heart rate, blood pressure or dropping intracranial pressure; sometimes by just shedding a tear. Not only are nurses sensitive to this level of communication, but also they take it one step further by teaching this level of communication to family members so that they too can interact with their critically ill loved one.

Through our vigilance, we coordinate the individual experience of illness and create the environment, making it bearable. Not only do we make it bearable, but also in some cases we make it growth provoking. Numerous nursing research studies now exist to help guide nursing practice in the neonatal ICU to support the development of preterm infants. Nursing research has changed the environment from one that was provider suited to one that is patient driven. The bright, noisy, and sterile neonatal ICUs of long ago now facilitate "kangaroo care"—the practice of giving preterm infants skin-to-skin contact with their parents, enabling them to share warmth and natural closeness. In addition to easing the pain associated with parent-infant separation, kangaroo care helps premature infants grow; leave their Isolettes sooner; and achieve a deeper, more peaceful sleep (Ludington, 1990). Lights are dimmed, isolettes are covered with blankets to decrease both light and noise, and blankets provide appropriate boundaries. Patient survival mandates that neonatal critical care nurses be responsive to the behavioral clues of newborns and assist parents in interpreting and responding to their baby's behavior. Care is focused at supporting the entire family unit, not just a piece of it that can be biologically, but never emotionally, separated from the rest.

Family-Centered Care

Critical care nurses have always prided themselves on having empathetic practices that value the family and provide close, attentive care to the patient (Alspach, 1994). More than any other subspeciality, pediatric critical care nurses have made significant progress in role modeling family-centered care in critical care. There is an abundance of nursing research that describes family stress associated with critical illness. Regardless of the population, the themes are similar: the need for hope, information, proximity; to believe that their loved one is receiving the best care possible; to be helpful; to be recognized as important; and to talk with others with similar issues.

Pediatric critical care nurses have moved beyond just describing what is upsetting to families to describing interventions that the recipients of our care, themselves, find helpful (Curley, 1987, 1988; Curley & Wallace, 1992). We have improved our dialogue with families so that we provide families what they need to make responsible care decisions—to be educated consumers of critical care. Parents note that the most significant contribution pediatric critical care nurses make in their care is to serve as "interpreter" of their critically ill child's responses and of the PICU environment (Curley, 1987).

When nurses develop mutually respectful trusting relationships with parents, families become empowered to choose and to take responsibility for their choices. Creating a humanistic, empowered environment that recognizes parents as unique autonomous individuals who, when supported, are capable of providing vital elements of care to their children forms the foundation for family-centered care. Different for each individual, humane care incorporates the hopes, dreams, values, cultural preferences, and concerns of patients and their families into the daily practice of critical care (Harvey et al., 1993). The only time parents should ever have to be placed in a situation in which they must ask permission to see their children is when the privacy of other patients must be protected. But, ICUs should be designed to provide all patients with privacy. Parents are not visitors to their children (Curley & Wallace, 1992). Family-centered care implies more than just that open visiting hours exist (Curley, 1988).

Part of the problem in dealing with families is that nurses may fail to see the significance of what nursing does. Our work may appear to be similar day after day, but the individuals we care for change—what we do with these individuals will be remembered for their lifetime. Our clinical research on families mandates major changes in our tradition-based practice.

Evidence-Based Appropriate Practice

Nationally, AACN has helped us move toward evidence-based practice in supporting multicenter research studies on endotracheal suctioning, the use of heparinized flush solutions on arterial lines, and weaning patients from mechanical ventilation. As we continue to push the science within our own discipline, we must look for opportunities to integrate our

work across disciplines to ensure that our accomplishments make sense to patients.

When instituting new therapies, the nursing focus is on the illness aspect of care—the human response to disease and therapy. For example, while our medical colleagues may design a randomized study to investigate the effects of high-frequency oscillatory ventilation in pediatric patients with diffuse alveolar disease and air-leak syndrome, nursing may focus upon what bed to nurse the patient on—the chest shakes differently on an air and on a conventional mattress; the noise level, which is still quite high with this mode of ventilation; how to maintain skin integrity, which is challenging with the rigid arm of the ventilator; and how to suction the patient without compromising lung volume.

In isolation, many disciplines function near excellence, but collectively things may approach mediocrity. Necessary for survival in a reformed system is the evidence, the data, necessary to identify and support our contributions to patient outcomes. Inefficient systems and processes—not people—are the prime force driving escalating healthcare costs. Quality improvement methods must continue to progress from single-department joint commission mandates to multidisciplinary teams working together to integrate systems in the best interests of patient care. Parallel processes working with outdated management tools (e.g., nursing care plans) will, it is hoped, give way to collaborative practice groups working with clinical practice guidelines.

Clinical practice guidelines (CPGs), patient-centered multidisciplinary multidimensional plans of care, will help the team move toward evidence-based practice and improve the process of how care is delivered. CPGs encourage practitioner accountability, encourage highly coordinated care, decrease unnecessary variation in practice patterns, increase high-quality cost-effective services, and provide a mechanism to systematically evaluate the quality and effectiveness of practice in moving patients toward desired outcomes.

To be effective, CPGs must be driven by the patient needs (not wants and not what nursing says those needs are) and the evidence that the intervention truly does makes a difference in patient outcomes. CPGs guide the appropriate use of resources in that, if any intervention does not directly benefit the patient, it's probably not worth doing.

The days of whatever it takes and whatever it costs are over. The goal is high-quality care at moderate cost. Prestigious center or not, payors are not interested in spending more for similar clinical outcomes. Outcomes tracking will help determine where to draw the line between cost and quality. Strong data serve as the safety net to protect against too little care. Our goal is balance between societal cost and individual healing (Health Care Advisory Board, 1993).

To survive economically, hospitals must tighten resources and maintain quality that is collaboratively defined by both users and providers of the system.

Labor is the single biggest expense for all service organizations. Cutting nursing positions can be one answer in cutting costs, but improving the processes of care and tightening nonlabor resources is another. By reducing mortality rates, length of stay, costs, and complications, and by increasing family satisfaction and readiness and ability to function upon discharge, nurses make significant contributions to both the quality of hospital services and the containment of hospital costs (Prescott, 1993).

Leadership

Nurses are leaders in creating and managing systems. Back in the 1960s, only nurses who gave direct patient care were considered "real" nurses. Today, as Angela McBride (1994) notes, real nurses also design, implement, and evaluate whole programs of caregiving; manage units in which care is provided; monitor whether the healthcare system as a whole is sensitive to patient needs; and play a role in ethical decision-making around caregiving.

Current expectations for professional nursing practice are high. Whereas professional skill and technologic capability are vital, these essential traits need to exist in a patient-centered culture that emphasizes strong leadership, coordination of activities, continuous multidisciplinary communication, open collaborative problem solving, and conflict management (Zimmerman et al., 1993). Managing multidisciplinary high-performance teams focused on outcomes requires systems savvy. Whereas nurses have learned to manipulate the system to work for the patients, systems thinking—the ability to understand the interrelationships and patterns involved in complex problem solving—is a new but required skill in assuming overall responsibility for the environment in which care is provided.

Working smarter within a reformed system mandates a major transformation in the way nurses work. Future redesigned care delivery models will build upon what was learned from providing team nursing in the 1970s and primary nursing in the 1980s. Integrated multidisciplinary teams mandate individuals to function comfortably as team leaders, team members, and colleagues while providing supervision of unlicensed employees. Delegation is a new concept to those educated within a primary nursing model.

The evolving role of case/care manager "ups the ante" on professional practice (Zander, 1988) by ensuring a level of professional accountability not always apparent within the actual, not intended, primary nursing model. The case management model outlines and activates strategic management of quality patient outcomes and costs. Transforming primary nurses into case managers moves the focus of practice from the nursing process to multidisciplinary outcomes. Benner notes that cost-effective care will exist only in situations in which the patient is known and where there is continuity of care provided

by *expert* caregivers (Gordon, 1994). Excellence results when nurses provide intuitive, scientific care to patients and families.

While it is critically important for the novice nurse to learn, come to know, then articulate nursing's independent contributions, only through the work of the entire team will patient outcomes be optimized. Optimal collaboration requires multidisciplinary socialization. Interpersonal team skills include conflict resolution and consensus building. Senge (1990) notes that team learning begins with dialogue, in which members suspend assumptions and think together to solve problems or chart the future.

Knaus and others (1986) found an inverse relationship between actual and predicted patient mortality and the degree of interaction and coordination of multidisciplinary intensive care teams. Hospitals with good collaboration and communication and a lower mortality had a comprehensive nursing educational support program that included a clinical nurse specialist and specific educational programming to support the use of clinical protocols in which staff nurses were independently responsible. AACN's demonstration project also documented a low mortality ratio, low complication rate, and high patient satisfaction in a unit that had a high perceived level of nurse-physician collaboration, highly rated objective nursing performance, positive organizational climate, and job satisfaction and morale (Mitchell, Armstrong, Simpson, & Lentz, 1989). Pollack and others (1988) demonstrated that a pediatric intensivist improved patient mortality and the efficiency of PICU bed utilization. Similar studies, investigating similar nursing roles within the PICU environment, do not exist.

Advocacy

Each discipline offers a *unique* and *necessary* perspective in advocating for patients. Visintainer (1986) applied an analogy of maps to contrast each discipline's unique approach to clinical problem solving. Various maps exist to describe a geographic location, for example, road maps, air traffic maps, weather maps, and mineral distribution maps. Although all of these maps represent the same geographic area, they differ in what they represent as relevant. A traveler would find a mineral distribution map completely irrelevant, as would an air traffic controller when using a road map. Similar to geographic maps, maps of a discipline provide a framework for selecting and organizing information. In determining what is relevant and what is not relevant for that specific discipline, the nursing map reflects an illness perspective—to care. The medical map reflects a disease perspective—to cure.

In the PICU, it is especially challenging to balance technology with values that emphasize the quality of life, consumer choice, risk-benefit decisions, access, and integrity of human life (Pew Health Professions Commission, 1991). Nursing's moral sensitivity reflects a holistic view of the patient. Nursing practice values and empowers the patient's and families' right to make informed choices consistent with autonomy, personal values, lifestyles, plans, or self-determination.

When cure becomes futile, nurses assume a leadership role in focusing care to ensure death with dignity and comfort. When parents must make difficult decisions about their child's life, what they require from nursing is a real presence that will support them, empower them, and give them the courage to decide (Marsden, 1990). Through experience, we know what activities might be helpful to families, and we provide options when death is imminent. Nurses "orchestrate" death, caring enough to make the worst thing in the world anyone could ever experience, the death of a loved one, a little more tolerable.

It is extremely difficult to "orchestrate death," then continue on with the day as if nothing happened. Often nurses are not able to share their day (like the rest of the world) with non-nurse friends because it is very difficult to talk about and to listen to. As one continues to experience the death of patients, one personally recovers much more quickly—death may become too routine, although it shouldn't be. It's emotionally exhausting to orchestrate death. Traditionally, we have learned how to orchestrate death by watching our colleagues. This almost never talked about intimate aspect of our care, which is learned through role modeling—colleague to colleague—is nursing's most profound contribution to mankind.

OUR FUTURE: INNOVATION AND CHANGE

To restructure what we do requires innovation, an imagination to see what is possible, and a willingness to try something new. When creating new realities, everyone is accountable for innovation and change. Start by *challenging the givens,* which are fundamentally unsupportive to a patient-driven system and unsupported by clinical research. The "givens" are similar to what Senge (1990) describes as mental models—notions or assumptions that have the power to move us forward or hold us back. Stellar changes have occurred when the status quo and/or basic "givens" were challenged—e.g., fathers in the delivery room, admission the day of surgery, patient- or parent-controlled analgesia.

Innovation requires both risk-taking and collegial support. Nursing and risk-taking appear to be dichotomous terms (Gillam, 1991). The American Nurses Association Code for Nurses (ANA, 1985) states that the nurse acts to "safeguard the client," which may be perceived as limiting opportunities in taking risks. However, the code also challenges us to participate in the development of new knowledge and in improving our standards of care. This aspect of practice definitely involves risk-taking in identifying innova-

tions or changes in the care we deliver to groups of patients.

Change—any change—can be risky. Advocating for change, especially when it may appear to buck the system or be unpopular with colleagues, is risky. However, in taking risks, having the courage to move out of your "comfort zone" to value diversity in thought is the essential element for both personal growth and innovations in care. Defeo (1990) notes that personal and professional growth requires courage to move ahead despite doubts or opposition. Three types of courage have been described (Nyberg, 1989): (1) social courage, to invest in open relationships; (2) creative courage, the willingness to instigate change and allow innovation; and (3) moral courage, the courage to care enough to become involved, the courage to take a risk for a matter of principle.

Many nurses have never learned how or when to take risks. Critically important is timing—being strategic in taking risks for what is really important to the profession. Again, what is right for patients and their families is right for the profession. Ask, then really listen to the consumers of care—they know their needs. Be a leader. True nursing leaders support a learning environment, because, as Burns (1989) points out, successful leaders are comfortable enough with their own fallibility in that they allow themselves to be vulnerable and are willing to take risks. Giving oneself permission to make mistakes empowers one to take risks.

In its Agenda for Action, The Pew Health Professions Commissions (1991) recommended that the nation have practitioners with expanded abilities and new attitudes to meet society's evolving healthcare needs (Table 1–3). When the healthcare system is truly a system, all competencies will be relevant to pediatric critical care nursing. AACN (1992) has described critical care nurse competencies for the fu-

Table 1–3. COMPETENCIES FOR PRACTITIONERS FOR THE YEAR 2005

Care for the communities' health
Expand access to effective care
Provide contemporary clinical care
Emphasize primary care
Participate in coordinated care
Ensure cost-effective and appropriate care
Practice prevention
Involve patients and families in the decision-making process
Promote healthy lifestyles
Assess and use technology appropriately
Improve the healthcare system
Manage information
Understand the role of the physical environment
Provide counseling on ethical issues
Accommodate expanded accountability
Participate in racially and culturally diverse society
Continue to learn

From Pew Health Professions Commission. (October, 1991). Healthy America: Practitioners for 2005. (Available from UCSF Center for the Health Professions, 1388 Sutter St, Suite 805, San Francisco, CA 94109.)

Table 1–4. THE NURSE OF THE FUTURE

Practitioners in a system driven by patient needs:
Able to articulate the unique role of nursing.
Integrated thinker.
Autonomous decision-maker.
Systems thinker, with a broad perspective on care provision.
Brain is sought after (and paid for) as major commodity.
Self-motivated learner, accountable for own education.
Focused on outcome-driven practice.
On the cutting edge of new clinical knowledge.
Knowledgeable about the patient care benefits that can be achieved through advanced technology.
Manages, facilitates, and coordinates patient experiences.
Expert in planning patient care.
Understands and integrates economic implications of care into goals and outcomes of practice.
Provides valid practices through research, innovation, and continuous questioning.
Role models well-developed caring practices.
Leader and manager.
Possesses well-developed interpersonal skills.
Not limited by unit or shift: committed to 24-hour accountability.
Expert delegator.
Seeks out resources.

Advanced practitioner in critical care (graduate degree in nursing):
Approaches care from a global perspective; sees beyond the individual.
Integrates education, research, management, leadership, and consultation into the primary clinical role.
Identifies the clinical impact of the system on the patient. Works for solutions in an interdependent way.
Displays expert judgment in immediately recognizing, understanding, and responding to phenomena of nursing concern.
May have overlapping functions with other disciplines but integrates information in the nursing domain.
Innovates by seeing new ways to care for patients; continuously improves quality and prevents quality waste.
Develops new clinical knowledge.
Contributes to the profession at large.

From: American Association of Critical-Care Nurses (1993). *The nurse of the future* (AACN position statement). Aliso Viejo, CA.

ture (Table 1–4). Again, this raises the expectations for professional nursing practice in the years to come.

In conclusion, as Donna Diers pointed out in 1984:

Believe in nursing, in the wildest possible expanse of role and function, and believe so strongly that your beliefs can sustain you through the battles with the unknowing, unthinking, deluded, and barefoot pragmatists who wish to restrain the ideas and talents of nurses.

References

AACN (1990). *Outcome standards for nursing care of the critically ill.* American Association of Critical-Care Nurses, P.O. Box 30008, Laguna Niguel, CA 92607.
AACN (1992). *Critical care in the nursing curriculum: Selecting and integrating essential content.* American Association of Critical Care Nurses, P.O. Box 30008, Laguna Niguel, CA 92607.
Alcott, L. M. (1863). *Hospital sketches* (p. 47). Boston: James Redpath Pub.
Alspach, G. (1994). Giving voice to the vision—achieving the patient-driven system. *Critical Care Nurse,* Supplement, June, 2.

American Hospital Association (1993). *Hospital statistics* 1993–1994 edition (p. 231, Table 13A). Chicago.
(ANA) American Nurses Association (1985), *Code for nurses with interpretive statements,* Washington, DC.
Beckham, D. J. (1993). Andrew's not so excellent adventure. *Health Forum,* 36 (3), 90–96.
Benner, P., Tanner, C., & Chesla, C. (1992). From beginner to expert: Gaining a differentiated clinical world in critical care nursing. *Advances in Nursing Science,* 14 (3), 13–28.
Brown, L. (1986). The experience of care: Patient perspectives. *Topics in Clinical Nursing,* 8 (2), 56–62.
Burfitt, S. N., Greiner, D. S., Miers, L. J., Kinney, M. R., & Branyon, M. E. (1993). Professional nurse caring as perceived by critically ill patients: A phenomenologic study. *American Journal of Critical Care,* 2 (6), 489–499.
Burns, S. P. (1989). Determining the qualities of a leader. *Aspen's Advisor for Nurse Executives,* 4 (12), 4–5, 8.
Cadmus, R. R. (1954). Special care for the critical case. *Hospitals.* JAHA 28 (9), 65–66.
Cadmus, R. R. (1980). Intensive care reaches silver anniversary. *Hospitals,* 54 (2), 98–102.
Caine, R. M. (1991). Incorporating CARE into caring for families in crisis. *AACN Clinical Issues in Critical Care Nursing,* 2 (2), 236–241.
Christopherson, D. (1982). Priorities established for special interest groups. *Focus on AACN,* August, 35.
Committee on Hospital Care and Pediatric Section of the Society of Critical Care Medicine (1993). Guidelines and level of care for pediatric intensive care units. *Pediatrics,* 92 (1), 166–175.
Curley, M. A. Q. (1987). *Effects of the nursing mutual participation model of care and parental stress in the pediatric intensive care unit.* Unpublished master's thesis: Yale University School of Nursing, New Haven, CT.
Curley, M. A. Q. (1988). Effects of the nursing mutual participation model of care and parental stress in the pediatric intensive care unit. *Heart & Lung,* 17 (6, 1), 682–688.
Curley, M. A. Q., & Wallace, J. (1992). Effects of the nursing mutual participation model of care on parental stress in the pediatric intensive care unit—a replication. *Journal of Pediatric Nursing,* 7 (6), 377–385.
Defeo, D. J. (1990). Change: A central concern for nursing. *Nursing Science Quarterly,* 3 (2), 88–94.
DeNicola, L. K., & Todres, I. D. (1992). History of pediatric intensive care in the United States. In B. P. Fuhrman & J. J. Zimmerman (Eds.). *Pediatric critical care* (pp. 45–47). St. Louis: Mosby–Year Book.
Diers, D. (1984). Commencement address. *Yale Nurse,* Fall, 3.
Diers, D. (1985, September 20). *Nursing: Implementing the agenda for social change.* Paper presented at the Fiftieth Anniversary Symposium: Nursing as a Force in Social change. University of Pennsylvania School of Nursing, Philadelphia, PA.
Disch, J. (1982). Special Interest Groups—providing opportunities for AACN members. *Focus on AACN,* April, 41–43.
Downes, J. J. (1992). The historical evolution, current status, and prospective development of pediatric critical care. *Critical Care Clinics of North America,* 8 (1), 1–22.
Drinker, P., & Shaw, L. A. (1929). An apparatus for the prolonged administration of artificial respiration. *Journal of Clinical Investigation,* 7, 229.
Fairman, J. (1992). Watchful vigilance: Nursing care, technology, and the development of intensive care units. *Nursing Research,* 4 (1), 56–60.
Gillam, T. (1991). Legal notes: Risk-taking: A nurse's duty. *Nursing Standard,* 5 (39), 52–53.
Gordon, S. (1994). Inside the patient-driven system. *Critical Care Nurse,* Supplement/June, 3–28.
Griffin, J., Hitchens, M., & Smith-Blair, N. (1984). Certification for pediatric intensive care nurses. *AACN: Neonatal and Pediatric SIG Newsletter,* December, 1,6.
Harvey, M. A., Ninos, N. P., Adler, D. C., Goodnough-Hanneman, S. K., Kaye, W. E., & Nikas, D. L. (1993). Results of the consensus conference on fostering more humane critical care: Creating a healing environment. *AACN Clinical Issues in Critical Care Nursing.* 4 (3), 484–507.
Hazinski, M. F. (1984). *Nursing care of the critically ill child.* St. Louis: C. V. Mosby Co.

Health Care Advisory Board (1993). *Line of fire: The coming public scrutiny of hospital and health system quality.* Advisory Board Company, The Watergate, 600 New Hampshire Ave, N. W., Washington, DC 20037.

Knaus, W. A., Draper, E. A., Wagner, D. P., & Zimmermann, J. E. (1986). An evaluation of the outcome from intensive care in major medical centers. *Annals of Internal Medicine,* 104 (3), 410–418.

Lassen, H. C. A. (1953). A preliminary report on the 1952 epidemic of poliomyelitis in Copenhagen with special reference to the treatment of acute respiratory insufficiency. *The Lancet,* January 3, 37–41.

Ludington, S. M. (1990). Energy conservation during skin-to-skin contact between premature infants and their mothers. *Heart & Lung,* 19 (5, pt. 1), 445–451.

Lynaugh, J. (1990). Four hundred postcards. *Nursing Research,* 39 (4), 254–255.

Marsden, C. (1990). Real presence. *Heart & Lung,* 19 (5), 540–541.

McBride, A. B. (1994). How nursing looks today. *Indiana University Alumni Magazine,* January–February, 64.

Mitchell, P. H., Armstrong, S., Simpson, T. F., & Lentz, M. (1989). American Association of Critical-Care Nurses Demonstration Project: Profile of excellence in critical care nursing. *Heart & Lung,* 18 (3), 219–237.

Niebuhr, B. S. (1993). Credentialing of critical care nurses. *AACN Clinical Issues in Critical Care Nursing,* 4 (4), 611–616.

Nyberg, J. (1989). Roles and rewards in nursing administration. *Nursing Administration Quarterly,* 13 (3), 36–69.

Oakes, A. R. (1981). *Critical Care Nursing of Children and Adolescents.* Philadelphia: W. B. Saunders Co.

Pew Health Professions Commission (October, 1991). Healthy America: Practitioners for 2005. (Available from Pew Charitable Trusts, 1388 Sutter St, Suite 805, San Francisco, CA 94109.)

Pew Health Professions Commission (February, 1993). The nursing profession. In *Health professions education for the future: Schools in service to the nation.* (Available from Pew Charitable Trusts, 1388 Sutter St, Suite 805, San Francisco, CA 94109.)

Pollack, M. M., Katz, R. W., Ruttimann, U. E., Getson, P. R. (1988). Improving the outcome and efficiency of intensive care: the impact of an intensivist. *Critical Care Medicine,* 16 (1), 11–17.

Prescott, P. A. (1993). Nursing: An important component of hospital survival under a reformed health care system. *Nursing Economics,* 11 (4), 192–199.

Ramseyer, K., & Jones, P. (1992). Passing point determined for neonatal and pediatric exam. *CCRN News,* Fall, 6.

Senge, P. M. (1990). *The fifth discipline: The art and practice of the learning organization.* New York: Doubleday.

Smith, C. A. (1983a). *The Children's Hospital of Boston: "Built better than they knew."* Boston: Little, Brown.

Smith, J. B. (1983b). *Pediatric critical care.* New York: Wiley Medical.

Vestal, K. W. (1981). *Pediatric critical care nursing.* New York: Wiley Medical.

Visintainer, M. A. (1986). The nature of knowledge and theory in nursing. *IMAGE: The Journal of Nursing Scholarship,* 18 (2), 32–38.

Weisberg, R. (Author, Producer, Director). (1990). *Borderline medicine* [Documentary—aired by Public Broadcasting Service December 17]. Public Policy Productions, 356 West 58th St., NY, NY 10019.

Yeh, T. S. (1992). Regionalization of pediatric critical care. *Critical Care Clinics of North America,* 8 (1), 23–35.

Zander, K. (1988). Nursing case management: Strategic management of cost and quality outcomes. *Journal of Nursing Administration,* 18 (5), 23–30.

Zimmerman, J. E., Shortell, S. M., Rousseau, D. M., Duffy, J., Gillies, R. R., Knaus, W. A., Devers, K., Wagner, D. P., & Draper, E. A. (1993). Improving intensive care: Observations based on organizational case studies in nine intensive care units: A prospective, multicenter study. *Critical Care Medicine,* 21 (10), 1443–1451.

CHAPTER 2

Critical Illness and Intensive Care During Infancy and Childhood

JANIS BLOEDEL SMITH
ANNE MILLIGAN BROWNE

IMPORTANT CONCEPTS IN CRITICAL CARE NURSING OF CHILDREN
Stress
Coping
Adaptation and Mastery
THE CRITICALLY ILL INFANT
Developmental Characteristics of the First Year of Life
Dealing With Stress
THE CRITICALLY ILL TODDLER
Developmental Characteristics of Toddlers
Dealing With Stress
CRITICAL ILLNESS DURING THE PRESCHOOL YEARS
Developmental Characteristics of the Preschool Period
Dealing With Stress

CRITICAL ILLNESS DURING THE SCHOOL-AGE YEARS
Developmental Characteristics of School-Age Children
Dealing With Stress
THE CRITICALLY ILL ADOLESCENT
Developmental Characteristics of Adolescents
Dealing With Stress
SPECIAL PROBLEMS IN CRITICAL CARE NURSING OF CHILDREN
The Chronically Critically Ill Child
Death in the Pediatric Intensive Care Unit

Hospitalization during childhood is recognized as a situational crisis for children and their families. The emotional development of children is threatened by illness, disability, disfiguring treatment, disrupted family relationships, and unsupportive environments. Behavioral disturbances after brief, scheduled hospital admissions are not uncommon and include altered sleep and rest cycles, feeding difficulties, regression in achievement of developmental milestones, and temper tantrums (Fagin, 1966; Petrillo & Sanger, 1980). Comparatively less information is available regarding the impact of critical illness and

intensive care on growing and developing children. Little data are available that compare the experiences of children in the pediatric intensive care unit (PICU) with those of their less ill agemates or with critically ill adults.

Despite the lack of scientific data, nurses have been actively involved in identifying the aspects of hospitalization that are particularly difficult for children and their families and in implementing interventions aimed at mitigating stress during the experience. In fact, managing the emotional aspects of critical illness and intensive care is uniquely the role of nurses. A foundation for effective intervention to meet the emotional needs of children in the PICU is an appreciation of the impact of development on the individual child's experience. This chapter discusses the concepts of stress, coping, and mastery as they are related to critical care hospitalization. Presented also are the stressors of an intensive care hospitalization and their significance for children from infancy through adolescence, and interventions aimed at assisting children in the PICU and their families to manage stress, cope successfully with the illness, and achieve mastery.

IMPORTANT CONCEPTS IN CRITICAL CARE NURSING OF CHILDREN

Stress

Stress is the result of a problem or an especially demanding situation that cannot be easily solved, that taxes or exceeds an individual's resources, and endangers personal well-being (Lazarus & Folkman, 1984). Selye (1952, 1956, 1971, 1974, & 1976a) and Lazarus (1966) have provided the foundation for understanding the human response to stress from both physiologic and psychological perspectives.

Physiologic Stress Response

Stress results in a complex physiologic response. Selye (1952) initially described the physiologic response as first being mediated by the action of the stressor on the anterior pituitary, which stimulates production of somatotropin and adrenocortical stimulating hormone (ACTH). Somatotropin augments the inflammatory response and combats the pathogen; ACTH stimulates the adrenal cortex to produce both mineralocorticoids and glucocorticoids. Catecholamine production by the adrenal medulla is also increased. Epinephrine and norepinephrine production increases in stressful experiences, increasing metabolic rate and influencing a wide range of physiologic functions. The autonomic nervous system also influences production of the catecholamines by the adrenal medulla in the stress response (Selye, 1971).

The physiologic stress response can be measured by pituitary-adrenal functioning, but many factors determine the overall biologic stress response. Variation in the physiologic stress response occurs with exposure to different stressors and between individuals. Designed to regulate physiologic defense mechanisms, the stress response is a multifactoral hormonal and nervous system protective reaction (Selye, 1971).

Psychological stressors activate the same pituitary-adrenal response (Hill et al., 1956). Early research demonstrated increased ACTH production in response to failing ego defenses (Monat & Lazarus, 1971), punishment, sleep deprivation, noxious stimulation (Mason, 1959a), and general anxiety (Mason, 1959b). The protective influence of defense mecha-

nisms has been demonstrated to decrease stress hormone production in parents of children with leukemia. Lower levels of stress hormones were present in those parents who effectively defended against the threatened loss of their child (Tecce et al., 1966).

Psychological Stress Response

Although physiologic responses to stress are complex and variable, they are somewhat predictable. However, psychological sources of stress and the individual's psychological responses are less uniform. As a consequence, it is impossible to define stress in completely objective terms. Reference must always be made to the characteristics of the individual experiencing stress (Lazarus & Folkman, 1984). The unique relationship between the individual and the stressful experience is mediated by the cognitive process by which the event is evaluated. Lazarus (1966) defined this process as *cognitive appraisal*. The individual's interpretation and evaluation of an event determines whether it is stressful.

Stress Appraisal

Cognitive appraisal is an evaluative process that ultimately determines the meaning of an event for an individual and that, consequently, shapes the emotional and behavioral response to it. Through cognitive appraisal individuals evaluate the significance of what is happening in terms of their own well-being.

Lazarus and Folkman (1984) identify three kinds of cognitive appraisal: primary, secondary, and reappraisal. Primary appraisal consists of making the judgment that a situation is either irrelevant (having no implication for the individual's well-being), benign-positive (preserving or enhancing well-being), or stressful. Stressful appraisals include circumstances in which the person has already sustained harm or loss, anticipates threatened harm or loss, or is challenged by the possibility of mastery and gain.

Secondary appraisal is a judgment about what might and can be done in a stressful situation. Included in secondary appraisal is evaluation of available coping options, the individual's chances of applying a strategy successfully, and the consequences of one particular strategy versus another. Reappraisal refers to a change in the original appraisal of a situation based on either new information or the results of coping. Cognitive appraisals are not always conscious, obvious mental operations. Individuals may be unaware that a threat has been appraised as a result of the operation of defense mechanisms or routine problem-solving processes.

Stress appraisal is influenced by a number of factors related to the individual experiencing the stressful event and by characteristics of the event itself. The most important personal factors that influence cognitive appraisal are commitments and beliefs. Commitments are expressions of that which an individual holds important; they underlie the choices the individual makes. The more meaningful and important an individual's commitment, the greater the threat and challenge in a stressful situation that menaces that commitment. Greater threat also can motivate the person to action and help sustain hope.

Beliefs, particularly those about personal control and existential convictions, influence stress appraisal. Appraisals of control over the stressful event and of one's self affect emotion and coping. Existential beliefs enable individuals to find meaning and maintain hope in difficult situations.

Interdependently influencing the cognitive appraisal processes are characteristics of the stressful situation. Situations that are uncertain are often appraised as threatening. When situations are uncertain or ambiguous, individual characteristics are key in shaping how the person defines the situation. Individual tolerance of ambiguity or uncertainty varies widely between persons. Ambiguity can intensify threat because it limits the individual's sense of control over the situation and increases feelings of helplessness. On the other hand, ambiguity can reduce threat because it permits individuals to consider alternative interpretations of a situation and maintain hope.

The timing of a stressful event influences its appraisal. Imminent events are generally appraised as more urgent. Delay before a stressful event can heighten anxiety, but delay also provides opportunity for people to marshall coping efforts and reduce stress. The duration of an event, if lengthy, may lead to exhaustion but also permits emotional habituation through coping.

The timing of events over the life cycle can affect cognitive appraisal. Neugarten (1968) pointed out that normal life events may be stressful crises if they occur "off time." When events occur off time or out of sequence, they are often unexpected and individuals do not have the opportunity to prepare. In addition, they may not have the support of compatible peers.

The timing of a stressful event in relation to other events may magnify the cumulative stress experienced. The Holmes-Rahe schedule of recent experiences (1967) is a well-known tool for evaluation of the accumulated stress of life events within a specified time period. Coddington (1972) developed life event scales for children based on Holmes and Rahe's work. Stressful events may accumulate in terms of general distress and the added weight of additional stressful events, or because of links between events (Brown & Harris, 1978). Thus, the meaning of a single stressful situation must be related to what else is going on in the individual's life.

An individual's perception of a stressor is also influenced by past experience in coping, both with a particular stressor and by general coping ability. Kobasa (1979) found that stress-resistant people have a certain "hardiness"—a set of attitudes that leaves them open to change, feeling involved, and in control of events. These characteristics, even under very stressful circumstances, are linked to positive coping ability.

The perceived magnitude of the stressor also influences coping ability. Perception of a stressor as small and requiring only a simple response is likely to result in effective coping behaviors. When the stressor is perceived as complex and large, the coping response must be similarly complex. The individual's coping abilities may be overwhelmed, unless the stressor can be divided into more manageable pieces.

In children, the ability to appraise a stressful situation is tied to their level of cognitive development. In addition, each developmental phase is characterized by concerns unique to that stage. Consequently, the appraisal of a situation is determined by both cognitive maturity and developmental age and stage. Each child's view of a stressful situation or event is most meaningful from the vantage point of the child's development.

Stressors Common During Hospitalization

Despite the individual nature of stress, some generalizations with regard to events characteristic of critical illness and intensive care are possible. Predictable stressors include the PICU environment itself and the experiences of separation from family and significant others, pain and intrusive procedures, and loss of self-control.

THE PICU ENVIRONMENT

Little in the intensive care environment bears resemblance to the everyday world of infants and children. The environment is one of high activity around the clock and is crowded with equipment and people. The noise level is often excessive, especially in large, open units; as equipment alarms sound, telephones ring. The voices of caregivers—sometimes raised in anxiety—contribute to a technologic symphony. The noise level recorded in a busy PICU was measured at 45 to 85 decibels (Baker, 1984), significantly in excess of the 35 decibels considered necessary for adequate rest (Slota, 1988). In addition to excessive noise, PICU sounds are unfamiliar and, as a result, may be threatening. Unlike the critical care nurse, who knows the significance of each beep and buzz, children in a PICU can make no sense of these sounds. The sounds are a source of sensory overload.

Along with the noise of the PICU environment are unfamiliar sights and people. Children in the PICU are aware of other patients and are concerned for their welfare (Barnes, 1975). When patients are in close proximity to one another, they may witness distress or fear of procedures in others. Unable to understand the meaning of that which they observe, children may become anxious for another child and concerned that they too may undergo a painful or distressing procedure.

Visual stimulation is also excessive because of continuous overhead lighting. Lights can create sensory confusion, cause patients to lose day-night orientation, and interrupt sleep. Sleep-wake cycles are disturbed, not only by lighting and other sources of environmental stimulation, but also by caregiving interventions. Sleep deprivation is a common problem for children in the PICU (Richards & Bairnsfather, 1988; Slota, 1988; Fontaine, 1989).

Exposed to excessive and threatening environmental overstimulation, children in the PICU also experience sensory and emotional deprivation. Emotional deprivation occurs in a highly technical environment dominated by machines, when patients lose precedence to the technology (Roberts, 1976). It is also related to the loss of meaningful stimulation, to immobilization, confinement, and interpersonal isolation. Deprivation may involve the senses of sight, hearing, and touch. Sensory and emotional deprivation may result in confused, disoriented, and withdrawn behavior.

The PICU syndrome has been described in adult patients. Contributing factors include sensory overload or monotony, sleep deprivation, and use of medications (McKegney, 1966; Helton et al., 1980; Fisher & Moxham, 1984; Kleck, 1984). Manifestations include fear, anxiety, depression, hallucinations, and delirium. In the PICU environment, children have been subjectively described as withdrawn, passive, anxious, egocentric, negative, and demanding (May, 1972; Carty, 1980; Thompson, 1985). Objectively measurable behavioral expression of anxiety, depression, agitation, and withdrawal occurs in children in the PICU (Jones et al., 1992). PICU patients in the study exhibited apprehension about routine nonpainful procedures, anxiety and worry, detachment with staff, sadness and weeping, and tremulousness and shakiness. Positively correlated with the presence of these behaviors were the duration of the intensive care hospitalization, the number of previous hospitalizations, increasing severity of illness, and preexisting psychiatric disorders.

Critically ill children are at high risk for the development of stress-related behavioral disturbances. Loud noises, bright lights, the constant presence of strangers, sudden physical touch, and unanticipated procedures cause distress that is indicative of the high level of uneasiness characteristic of patients in a critical care environment.

SEPARATION

Despite the fact that pediatric nurses have been instrumental in assuring liberal visiting policies for parents of children who are hospitalized, children in the PICU often experience periods of separation from those who are their most important source of emotional support. Parents may be asked to leave the unit when procedures are performed on their child or others and are often excluded during resuscitation. In addition, parents may have responsibilities to other family members and to their jobs, which require that they leave their hospitalized child. Parents also must eat, rest, and care for themselves.

Separation is a painful experience at any age. The normal passages of life include leaving familiar and comforting people and surroundings as individuals move through school, career, intimate relationships, and the eventual death of parents and other older relatives and friends. It is difficult to give up the comfort and security of familiar people, places, and circumstances. Despite the many experiences most adults have with separation, it is significant to note that in a 1984 study of patients followed after having acute myocardial infarction, social isolation played a causal role, independent of other variables, in cardiac death (Ruberman et al., 1984). All human beings are dependent on meaningful relationships with others.

The significance of parents for children has been demonstrated in both animal and human studies. Harlow and Zimmerman (1965) showed that newborn monkeys provided adequate nutrition from a cloth and wire-mesh "mother" became antisocially aggressive and unable to interact within a clan. Spitz (1945) observed children separated from their mothers for both short and long periods in penal nurseries and orphanages. After 6 months of separation the children had fixed changes: they were silent, their measured intelligence fell, previously acquired motor skills were lost, and their faces were rigid and expressionless. Although these children were fed and kept clean, by age 4 years only one of 21 children still in the institutions could talk in sentences, six could not talk at all, five could not walk, and 16 walked only by holding onto furniture.

Robertson (1958), in his study of hospitalized children, provided the labels for the stages of separation that Spitz had observed. Young children in the hospital demonstrated three stages of "separation anxiety," characterized by protest, despair, and resignation (Table 2–1). Bowlby (1966) studied children who had been separated from their London families during World War II and placed in physically safe English countryside homes when nightly bombing raids threatened. These children, although physically safe, suffered deprivation and were characterized as emotionally flat and expressionless. Children deprived of parental contact demonstrate persistent long-term manifestations of their deprivation: impaired trust, diminished intellectual and motor functioning, and disturbed behavior.

Table 2–1. PHASES OF SEPARATION ANXIETY IN INFANTS AND YOUNG CHILDREN

Phase of Anxiety	Behavioral Responses
Protest	Loud, vigorous protest at the absence of parents Restlessness, expectant watching for the parents' return Refuses care or attention from others
Despair	Loud crying ceases Less activity, withdrawn, disinterested in play or food Apathetic and isolated appearance Hopeless and grieving
Resignation/detachment	Resigned to loss and appears to have adjusted Shows some interest in surroundings, begins new relationships but is detached

Although it is unlikely that hospitalization of children at the end of the 20th century will include extremes of separation of children from their parents, historical studies illustrate the importance of a continuing, close relationship between children and parents. Children are dependent on the close and reliable presence of their parents under normal circumstances; their need for parental closeness when they are ill is still greater.

Fagin (1966) noted that the quality of the parent-child relationship influenced children's responses to separation. Assured of the fact that parents return after they have "disappeared," through the development of object permanence (the knowledge that persons and objects continue to exist even when out of sight), older infants and young children learn to tolerate periods of separation from reliable parents who always return after a period of absence. When parents have an inconsistent relationship with their child and are unable to provide consistent substitute caregivers, the child may have difficulty learning to tolerate periods of separation. As a consequence, separation may affect the child who has an insecure relationship with parents to an even greater extent than those children with a secure and confident relationship with their parents.

PAIN AND INTRUSIVE PROCEDURES

Pain and painful or invasive procedures are potentially destabilizing and demoralizing experiences for critically ill patients.

Pain has been identified as a source of stress in the newborn infant and remains so throughout life. Newborns demonstrate wakefulness, irritability, arousal, and decreased ability to quiet themselves following painful procedures. By 6 months of age infants display fearful behavior in response to impending pain. Established in early life experiences, fear of pain persists across the lifespan.

Pain is an unpleasant symptom common to most ailments. Pain induces fear, not only because it evokes unpleasant physical sensations, but also because of the emotional responses common to the experience of pain. Adults describe pain with terms that connote the emotional aspects of the experience, including "agonizing," "demoralizing," "unbearable," and "terrifying." Children in pain are afraid not only of physical sensations but also of threats to self-integrity and self-esteem, which are a clear part of the pain experience.

Children in the PICU may be unable to accurately report and describe pain because of developmental immaturity and limited verbal ability and because of the severity of their illness. Assessment of nonverbal responses to pain is crucial to assuring that it is adequately treated. In addition, the physiologic reactions of the stress response are evoked by acute pain and can be identified.

Pain that is persistent or repetitive may exhaust the neurohormonal responses of the stress reaction. As a consequence, the physiologic signs characteristic of activation of the sympathetic nervous system decline. Adaptation to chronic pain involves the development of physical and psychological responses that are protective in nature. For example, the child may protect a painful area from touch and may develop regressed, demanding, irritable, and uncooperative behavior. Neither physical nor psychological responses afford pain relief. The toll on children who deal with daily pain cannot be ignored or underestimated.

Fear of body intrusion and mutilation is a stressor related to pain and is common to the experience of critical illness and intensive care. Like pain, intrusive procedures threaten self-esteem and self-integrity. As a consequence, children respond similarly to both. They fear that body injury and mutilation may result from invasive procedures and equipment. Mutilation anxiety is high in children at the end of the preschool and start of the school years and during adolescence. However, all sick children require reassurance regarding the intactness of their bodies when they undergo intrusive procedures.

LOSS OF SELF-CONTROL

Self-control is an essential part of ego integrity. The ability to control one's emotions and actions develops across the early years of childhood and is a marker of self-confidence and self-esteem; that is, children who feel confident and proud of themselves and their abilities are more likely to be self-controlled. New situations challenge an individual's ability to maintain self-control, particularly when the situation is threatening. Children, by virtue of their age and its limitations on life experiences, are more vulnerable to the stressors inherent in new, challenging situations. They are more likely to have difficulty maintaining self-control in the face of altered routines, the unknown, physical restriction, enforced dependency, and loss of productive roles.

All individuals establish routines that provide a sense of order in their daily lives. Young children are dependent on routines and rituals to view the world as safe, predictable, and subject to their control. However, the need to maintain an orderly and predictable environment safe from threat is ageless. So universal is the need for a stable environment that Maslow (1954) ranked safety just above the need for food, water, shelter, and other physiologic needs. Routines for daily life and the environment itself are tremendously altered by serious illness and intensive care. The ability of children to maintain self-control despite the loss of trusted people, objects, and routines relied upon for stability is tenuous.

Fears of the unknown are related to stress for children who are hospitalized. Children actively engage their world by learning about it and mastering its sometimes complex, challenging parts. When understanding is achieved, control follows. Young children in the hospital often have vague, generalized fears related to their stage of development, whereas older children tend to have more specific fears related to events or procedures for which they are unprepared. An event or procedure does not need to be potentially or actually painful to induce stress; unfamiliar settings, equipment, and machines are potentially viewed as threatening and challenge children's ability to maintain self-control.

Coping during childhood is aided by the discharge of anxious energy in physical activity. Illness necessitates some restriction of activity to conserve energy for recuperation, whereas a variety of procedures required by a critically ill child may necessitate actual physical restraint and immobility. Physical restrictions limit sensory stimulation and threaten self-control. Physical restraints to prevent the child from dislodging needed critical care paraphernalia and immobilization techniques used by healthcare providers during a procedure have the potential to produce high anxiety and near panic.

Infants and young children are accustomed to depending on others for care. Consequently, the enforced dependency of hospitalization, particularly if familiar caregivers play a substantial role in providing aspects of care, may not threaten the self-esteem and self-control of these youngsters. On the other hand, even toddlers assert their independence when they are well, as their sense of autonomy develops. Older children and adolescents, accustomed to independence in self-care activities, have increased stress by the necessary dependence of the sick role. Maslow (1964) defined the healthy person in terms of "ability to master the environment, to be capable, adequate, competent in relation to it, to do a good job." By the school-age years, these characteristics are often an internal source of self-control and may lead to feelings of inadequacy, powerlessness, and anxiety when illness requires dependency on others. Illness must not only require that sick children be dependent. The environment must permit and recovery provide opportunities to regain independence (Vessey et al., 1991).

Children also experience feelings of loss of self-control and powerlessness because they are unable to enact the social roles that provided them status in their families, their school settings, and peer groups. Sick children fear that their status and position within the family may be preempted by a sibling if they are not present to perform certain tasks, just as the career executive worries about job security when hospitalized. Loss of status with schoolmates and peers is feared by children absent from these social groups.

Clearly, critical illness and intensive care are stressful for infants and children. Mitigating the effects of the stress imposed by the PICU environment, separation from family and significant others, pain and intrusive procedures, and loss of self-control falls to the critical care nurse. Pain and illness are not simply physiologic phenomena, leaving the mind and the spirit unaffected. The total patient—physiologic, psychological, sociocultural, and developmental—is the concern of nursing. Instrumental in the efforts made by nurses to mitigate the stress of serious illness is an understanding of the concept of coping.

Coping

Coping involves constantly changing cognitive and behavioral efforts to minimize, reduce, tolerate, or manage external or internal demands that tax or exceed the individual's resources (Lazarus & Folkman, 1984). Coping is process-oriented rather than tied to specific personality traits or styles. Although individual characteristics influence the coping process, specific demands and conflicts may require complex and variable responses.

Coping involves effort. Murphy (1974) makes a distinction between the coping process and ready-made adaptational devices such as reflexes. Automatic behaviors or thoughts that do not require effort are useful in situations that do not tax or exceed an individual's resources.

Coping is not equated with adaptational success. Coping is viewed as the efforts to manage stressful demands regardless of the outcome. Consequently, no strategy can be considered inherently better or worse than another. Some situations cannot be mastered and require that the individual minimize, avoid, deny, tolerate, and accept the stressful conditions (Lazarus & Folkman, 1984).

Coping during childhood is influenced by a variety of factors. Most significant is the individual child's developmental stage, which largely determines the range of responses available to the child. As young children come to understand the world, they learn complex ways of coping. However, despite changes in the details of coping that are related to maturation and development, there is evidence that patterns in coping responses are apparent early in life and remain constant across life (Murphy, 1974; Murphy & Moriarty, 1976). Likewise, sources of stress change with age, but it is doubtful that coping changes in basic ways across the lifespan.

Coping Resources

The way in which individuals cope is determined in part by their resources. Resources include health and energy, problem-solving skills, social skills, social support and commitments, beliefs, and material resources. Coping is also determined by constraints that impede the use of resources. Personal constraints are internalized cultural values that define ways of behaving. Environmental constraints include institutions that thwart coping efforts. In addition, when a high level of threat is present, individuals are prevented from using coping resources effectively. The intensive care environment is one that may well interfere with coping without modification of the stressors described earlier. This is of particular concern because the critically ill patient obviously lacks fundamental coping resources: health and energy.

Figure 2–1 illustrates factors found to protect children from undue distress. The sections that follow detail important coping resources for critically ill children. Included is a discussion of defense mechanisms and their role in coping.

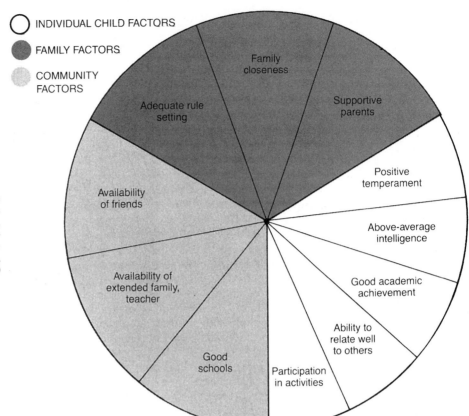

Figure 2-1 ● ● ● ● ● ●

Factors found to contribute to positive coping in children. (From Byrne, C., & Hunsberger, M. (1994). Stress, crises, and coping. In C. L. Betz, M. Hunsberger, & S. Wright (Eds.). *Family-centered nursing care of children* (2nd ed., p. 635). Philadelphia: W. B. Saunders.)

Parental Coping

The level of parental coping during the stress of a child's illness and hospitalization affects how children cope. Because of the close relationship generally shared by parents and their children and the dependence on parents normally experienced by children, children tend to accept what their parents accept. Parental anxiety, despite attempts to conceal it, is often transmitted to children. Termed "emotional contagion," the transmission of parental anxiety to children has been identified and effectively treated by providing parents information about that which will occur and how they can assist their child in learning coping skills (Skipper & Leonard, 1968). These interventions are not only effective in reducing the child's distress but also in increasing the parents' feelings of comfort and competence (Patterson & Ware, 1988; Skipper & Leonard, 1968).

Because parents are the most important individuals in a child's support system, characteristics of the parent-child relationship are correlated with the child's coping abilities. When the relationship is characterized by a high degree of compatibility, parents are able to provide their children with a great deal of emotional support. They are likely to respect and foster their children's abilities. Conversely, parent-child relationships that are unreliable and tenuous may result in children receiving limited support from their parents (Fagin, 1966). There is no likely substitute for parental love, encouragement, and support.

Previous Coping Experiences

Cognitive maturation permits children to recall previous experiences with stressful or challenging situations. A child who has coped successfully with a demanding situation in the past is able to recall the experience with pride and self-confidence. Similar coping strategies are likely to be useful in a new stressful situation. However, the child who has had little opportunity or has been unsuccessful in attempts to master new experiences may lack the confidence necessary to succeed when challenged. Doubtful about their personal abilities, these children are likely to react negatively to new or challenging situations.

Temperament

Innate qualities that determine individual temperament can be identified during infancy (Thomas et al., 1970). Level and extent of motor activity, regularity of daily schedule, response to new objects and people, adaptability to change, sensitivity to stimuli and intensity of response, general mood, degree of distractibility, and attention span or persistence in a given activity are individual characteristics remarkably stable across a lifespan. Regularity of body functions and daily schedule, confident responses to new stimuli, pleasant mood, and persistence in challenging activities characterize the child who copes well with new situations. A child with the opposite temperament is likely to respond negatively to new situations and to need more support in coping.

Murphy (1974) identified four resources that, if part of a child's individual temperament, are likely to be associated with positive coping. The first is a varied range of sources of gratification. The environment must provide and the child must be able to accept alternative sources of gratification and alternative solutions to problems when frustrated. Second, the child who has a positive, outgoing attitude toward life is likely to have a broader range of positive coping resources and the pride, courage, and resilience to mobilize resources despite disappointment and frustration. The third characteristic of positive coping ability is flexibility of coping mechanisms, which allows the child to select from a variety of available defense mechanisms. Finally, the child must be tolerant of retreat and regression. This requires that the child feel secure about self and certain of acceptance by those in the environment, despite regressed behavior.

Defense Mechanisms

Defense mechanisms are intrapsychic ways of thinking or behaving unconsciously employed in coping with stressful situations. Because the range of defense mechanisms increases with cognitive development (Table 2–2), young children have a limited repertoire of mechanisms available for coping. Some are often considered undesirable or even pathologic in older children, adolescents, and adults. However, the stress inherent in critical illness justifies, at least for limited periods of time, the use of any mechanism that assists with coping.

For example, *regression* is a defense mechanism frequently identified in children that may be difficult for others to accept. Regression is a temporary retreat or reversion to an earlier stage of behavior to retain or regain mastery of a stressful, anxiety-producing, or frustrating situation, thus achieving self-gratification and protection (Audette, 1974). Regression allows the child to conserve energy and strength for recuperation and accept caring provided by others. The child who regresses during a period of stress usually gives up the most recently acquired skill. Toilet training may be forgotten, for example, or the child may revert to thumb-sucking or a bottle. The regressed child may also cry a great deal, especially when parents are present. Rather than constituting a negative behavior, crying with parents permits the child to release tension and demonstrates a feeling of safety in relating strong emotions. Lost skills are generally rapidly relearned as recuperation and recovery restore available energy. Regression is an unhealthy response to a stressful situation only if the child is unable to remaster previously learned skills and is fixed at a previously abandoned developmental stage.

Denial is a second example of a defense mechanism often regarded as pathologic. However, when stress is acute, denial is necessary for at least short periods.

Table 2–2. DEFENSE MECHANISMS AVAILABLE BY DEVELOPMENTAL AGE

Stage	Defense Mechanism
Infants	Discrete defense mechanisms not identifiable
Toddlers and preschoolers	Regression: Return to an earlier stage of development in thought, feeling, or behavior Denial: Mental refusal to acknowledge a stressful reality Repression: Unpleasant experiences or thoughts are barred from conscious awareness Displacement: Transfer of emotionally charged thoughts or feelings to a more acceptable substitute object
School-age children	Above plus: Projection: Attribution of unacceptable thoughts or impulses to another person or out into the environment Reaction formation: Expression of an unacceptable impulse or feeling by transforming it into the polar opposite Sublimation: Transformation of unpleasant, blocked, or unacceptable thoughts or wishes into socially acceptable pursuits
Adolescents	Above plus: Rationalization: Application of logical, socially acceptable reasons for behavior or events that do not reflect the real reasons behind the action Intellectualization: Excessive reasoning is applied to allay disturbing feelings or thoughts and to permit isolation

It allows the child to ward off aspects of the environment that are excessively threatening to maintain hope. Denial is evident, for example, in the child who closes or covers the eyes during a stressful procedure such as suctioning the endotracheal tube, or one who indicates dismissal, turning the head away when a parent must leave. Like regression, denial is an unhealthy defense only if it persists unreasonably and interferes with a child accepting a permanent aspect of reality.

Adaptation and Mastery

Adaptation implies that an individual experiencing stress undergoes change that facilitates interaction with the environment. Assimilating aspects of the environment that are new, different, or challenging into previously learned behaviors and accommodating or modifying behavior in response to new or different demands are essential aspects of adaptation. In fact, Piaget (1952) viewed the ability to adapt as key to the survival and subsequent development of the human infant. Adaptation is based on *accommodation* (modification to conform to environmental demands) and *assimilation* (incorporation of previously learned activities in current behavior). The two processes together comprise the key techniques that children, as well as adults, use to interact successfully with the world.

Nursing theorists, notably Levine (1969) and Roy (1971), view ability to respond to environmental changes as dependent on adaptive capacity. They see adaptation as the key process in maintaining health. Other theorists have developed models that incorporate the concepts of development, stress, and adaptation in a view emphasizing change as the constant feature of life and health as complete biologic, social, and emotional well-being, not simply the absence of illness (Chrisman & Riehl, 1974).

Mastery is a more elusive concept. It does not refer to global health and wellness, but rather to possession or development of the skills needed to overcome and defeat a specific challenge. For critically ill children, the challenge is the experience of a critical illness or injury and the subsequent intensive care hospitalization, with all its inherent stressors. Adaptation may well be required in this circumstance; but when mastery is the desired outcome for the child, the focus of nursing interventions is to identify and supply the tools necessary for each individual child to experience a level of success that equates with mastery. That is, the child has the feelings of pride, self-esteem, and self-reliance associated with sure success in a challenging encounter.

Tables 2–3 and 2–4 summarize Piaget's view of cognitive development and Erikson's description of social and emotional development. Effective interventions with critically ill infants and children are guided by knowledge of the tools likely to provide the necessary support for patients in the PICU.

THE CRITICALLY ILL INFANT

During infancy (the period from birth to 1 year of age) the characteristic rapid development and the magnitude of change occurring across the first year of life warrant considering this stage in several phases. These are the neonatal period (the first month of life) and two stages of infancy: preattachment (birth to 6 months of age) and postattachment (the second 6 months of the first year). The section that follows outlines the most significant aspects of development from the perspective of critical illness and intensive care during each phase.

Developmental Characteristics of the First Year of Life

Parent-Infant Attachment

During the neonatal period, the foundations for parent-infant attachment that were established dur-

Table 2-3. PIAGET'S STAGES OF COGNITIVE DEVELOPMENT

Stage	Approximate Age	Characteristics
Sensorimotor	*0–2 years*	
Stage 1	Birth–1 month	No thought, language
		Continual practice of reflexes leads to a sense of order
Stage 2	1–4 months	Primary circular reactions stimulate effort to repeat a behavior
Stage 3	4–8 months	Secondary circular reactions to re-create an interesting effect in the environment. The basis for play
Stage 4	8–12 months	Coordination of secondary circular reactions to intentionally form new, more complex behaviors
Stage 5	12–18 months	Tertiary circular reactions to attain a goal
		Rudimentary trial-and-error behavior with active experimentation
		Object permanence achieved
Stage 6	18–24 months	Can remember, plan, imitate, and imagine
		Uses mental symbols
		See themselves as separate from others
Preoperational	*2–7 years*	
Stage 1	2–4 years	Preconceptual stage, reason dominated by perception
		Play is symbolic and imitative
		Egocentrism influences perception of objects and events
Stage 2	4–7 years	Intuitive stage, reason is not governed by logic
		Reasoning is transductive, from one particular to the next
		Able to focus on one aspect of an object or event only
Concrete Operations	*7–11 years*	Reasons with inductive logic, comprehends conservation and reversibility
		Able to classify and order, comprehends multiple aspects of object, event, or situation
		Problem-solving requires that the problems involve identifiable (concrete) objects
		The future and the abstract are still beyond comprehension
Formal Operations	*11 years on*	Logical reasoning based on deductive logic
		Able to consider the hypothetical and abstract
		Problem analysis is systematic
		Can think about past, present, future
		Develops strong idealism

Table 2–4. ERIKSON'S STAGES OF PSYCHOSOCIAL DEVELOPMENT

Stage/Age	Tasks and Subtasks	Negative Counterpart
Infancy (0–1 year)	Sense of trust is gained in consistent, quality care Hope is realized as small doses of frustration are tolerated	Mistrust
Toddler (1–3 years)	A sense of autonomy and realization of will develop given opportunities to attain some self-control Acceptance of reality begins	Shame and doubt
Preschool (3–6 years)	A sense of initiative and the realization of purpose develop given opportunities to do for self A period of questioning, exploring the environment and own body Sexual differences noted	Guilt
School age (6–12 years)	The sense of industry is gained given opportunities to achieve success and recognition Competence, responsibility, social and work skills, cooperation and fair play are learned Relates closely with same-sex peers	Inferiority
Adolescence (12–? years)	Sense of identity is established through experiences that build self-esteem and foster independence Fidelity is realized Moves toward heterosexuality, selects vocation, begins separation from family	Identity diffusion
Late adolescence/young adult	Intimacy and solidarity are established in close, shared relationships Love is realized with individuals of the same and the opposite sex Creativity and productivity are achieved	Isolation

ing the prenatal period are solidified and strengthened. Parent-infant attachment is a reciprocal process in which the parents and their infant become acquainted with, attached to, and bonded with one another. Attachment is a process, not a spontaneous occurrence. It does not occur instinctively, but is the result of the unique relationship that develops between parents and their children.

From the perspective of the infant, the process of attachment permits a view of the world as reliable and trustworthy. When parents reliably respond to their infant's needs, the baby learns that expressions of discomfort and hunger or the need for human contact bring consistent relief. The social and emotional developmental consequence is the establishment of a sense of trust. Mistrust is the negative counterpart of the task of infancy (Erikson, 1964).

The innate, awakening senses of infants equip them for interaction with their parents and their environment. Tactile sensation is obvious at birth, as demonstrated by the rooting reflex and sensitivity to pain and temperature extremes. Affectionate and comforting touch from parents confirms feelings of reassurance and builds trust. Touch is positive. Through touch and reaching out to touch, infants find comfort and establish trusting associations with their surroundings and the individuals in them.

Within 4 months infants are able to fixate, conjugate, differentiate size and shape, and see clearly at a distance. However, even at birth, infants demonstrate a preference for staring into a human face rather than at an inanimate object. In addition, the senses of taste, smell, and hearing are present within hours of birth. The infant sucks when a pleasant taste is introduced. Babies can differentiate between the smell of their mothers and others and prefer the familiar maternal scent. Hearing is present even before birth. The healthy infant is equipped from the moment of birth to engage in the processes that promote attachment and the development of trust.

The Neonatal Period. In the first month, infants spend as much as 80 percent of their time sleeping. Their waking hours are spent exercising the activities with which they are born: sucking, looking, grasping, and crying. These activities have obvious survival functions but are also important for cognitive development. Through repeating and perfecting these activities, the infant gains control over small aspects of the environment and becomes expert at a limited repertoire of activities by the end of the first month. Still, the coordination between activities is undeveloped. The infant can look at a visually appealing object, but is, as yet, unable to reach out for it.

The Preattachment Period. During the preattachment period, from birth through several months of age, infants are engaged in establishing the differences between themselves and the rest of their world. By the middle of the first year, infants recognize themselves as separate from their parents. Simultaneously, parents become the strongly preferred caregivers. Early in the first year of life infants may not demonstrate distinct reactions to separation from their parents. By 4 to 6 months of age, the attachment of infants for their parents has grown beyond the assurance that needs for food and comfort will be met. Infants begin to prefer their parents for the sake of their company alone, apart from the satisfaction of physical needs. The responsive smile that greets familiar caregivers signals infants' preference for these individuals.

Their developing physical abilities permit infants to have greater interaction with the world that surrounds them. Infants learn new behaviors as the result of accidental responses. For example, the baby accidentally gets a hand or finger or thumb into the mouth, triggering the sucking response and the sensation of the thumb in the mouth. The response and the sensation lead to repetition of the behavior until it is intentional, rather than accidental. Similarly, infants learn that kicking makes a mobile sway and move. Piaget (1952) identified that the baby has learned behaviors designed to make interesting sights and sounds persist.

The Postattachment Phase. Tremendous learning takes place in the second half of the first year of life. Infants learn to use signs to anticipate events. For example, putting on an infant's jacket signals that the family is going out. Rituals at bedtime—a bath, putting on pajamas, stories in the rocking chair—become increasingly important as the infant learns to view the world as reliable and predictable.

Infants in the second 6 months of life are able to coordinate their activities to bring about a desired end. They can now look at an object, reach for it, grasp it, and bring it to the mouth. An important consequence is the development of the realization that objects exist separately and apart from the actions of the baby. Piaget (1952) termed this development the "acquisition of the object" concept.

The beginnings of the cognitive knowledge of object permanence follow. "Object permanence" refers to the ability of infants to separate objects from their perception of them and realize that an object continues to exist even when unperceived. The delight that infants in the first year demonstrate at peek-a-boo games provides evidence of their progress at mastering this concept. However, children only gradually construct an objective world that is coherent and stable and in which comings and goings, and appearances and disappearances, are subject to their own physical laws (Fraiberg, 1959). Infants have not sufficiently mastered the concept of object permanence to face separation from their parents with relaxed ease.

"Stranger anxiety" is very often evident in infants between 6 and 9 months of age. The anxiety displayed by infants toward strangers is actually related to anxiety regarding separation from parents who are not established as having a permanent existence when out of sight. Under usual circumstances, infants in the last part of the first year of life awaken at night and cry for the comfort and reassurance of their parents. Most are comforted by the sound of the voice of a parent when otherwise safe and secure in familiar settings.

Dealing With Stress

Little in the experience of critical illness and intensive care is likely to support the developmental needs of infants in the first year who are striving to establish a sense that their world is trustworthy and reliable. The sections that follow review the stressors inherent in this experience and outline critical care nursing interventions aimed at mitigating the stress of infants in a PICU experience.

The PICU Environment

Research with neonates has demonstrated the impact of the stressful, hectic PICU environment on newborns (Als et al., 1986; Gorski, 1983; Gunderson & Kenner, 1987). Stress during intensive care hospitalization affects physiologic and neurobehavioral outcomes. Bright lighting, noise, and caregiving activities have been linked to stress in the newly born intensive care patient. Strategies to mitigate stressful aspects of the PICU environment by structuring caregiving and modifying the environment have been associated with improved outcomes for neonates (Als et al., 1986). Although they have not been evaluated with full-term newborns or older infants, the experimental strategies implemented with premature and low birth weight infants make sense intuitively for the care of bigger and/or older infants.

Broadly termed *individualized developmental care* or *individualized supportive care,* the principles that guide interventions include, first, identification of signs of stress in the infant and, second, stress reduction through modification of the PICU environment and caregiving activities.

Signs of distress in the infant resulting from environmental overstimulation are nonspecific, requiring that the critical care nurse be alert to their presence. Distressed newborns may be jittery, frequently agitated, and unable to quiet themselves. Vital signs are simultaneously altered; heart rate, blood pressure, and respiratory rate are elevated. Breathing may be irregular and oxygenation and skin color altered. Digestion is altered and feeding intolerance may develop. Level of consciousness may change, with some infants demonstrating "shut down"—that is, becoming unreactive to the environment (Lawhon & Melzar, 1988).

These nonspecific signs of stress are no different from those exhibited in response to physiologic instability, such as those seen in very early sepsis. The critical care nurse systematically rules out potential sources of physiologic distress, including pain, and then assesses the care environment for potential disturbances. Consistency in the assignment of caregivers to critically ill infants assists each to know individual patients on a more sophisticated level and enables the accurate identification of subtle behavioral and physical signs of distress.

As the infant proceeds from the newborn period across the first year of life, recognition of signs the baby is distressed becomes steadily clearer. Often parents can recognize easily distinguishable differences in how the baby cries when hungry, tired, fearful, in pain, or when needing comfort and support for some other reason. Critical care nurses can receive valuable input from parents to assist them in recognizing signs that an infant is distressed. In addition, infants experience tremendous refinement of fine and gross motor skills across the first year, enabling them to express distress, dismay, and displeasure far more articulately than earlier in their development.

Turning away from an unpleasant stimulus is a simple coping tool. Older infants even attempt to remove a noxious stimulus. Autonomic nervous system stability develops steadily across the first months of life. Characteristic changes in vital signs persist in the face of overstimulation and distress, but changes in oxygenation and skin color are not anticipated beyond the newborn period, unless the infant is premature or gravely ill.

Modifying the PICU environment is a necessity. Overhead lighting is dimmed and is augmented with individually controlled bedside lighting. When procedures necessitate bright lighting, a light blanket shielding the infant's eyes mitigates distress. Staff awareness of the auditory impact of loud conversation, phones, stereo equipment, overhead intercom announcements, and mechanical equipment and alarms on each infant is crucial. Monitor and equipment alarms are kept at a safe minimum volume, which ensures that they are heard, but does not startle infants when they sound. Reduction of the overall noise level effectively calms and minimizes stress for infants (Als et al., 1986). An environmental assessment by each nurse at the start of each shift assures that the environment is appropriately modified for infants in the PICU.

The isolette or infant bed requires modification to avoid overstimulation. Isolettes shield infants from the environment, especially if partially covered with a heavy blanket to decrease both light and noise stimulation. Parents can assist the critical care staff to create a bedspace that is personalized and soothing for their infant. The goal is to enhance the infant's ability to rest and sleep between caregiving episodes. A calm, relaxing environment is the ideal. Toys, music, and pictures are selected to comfort, not overstimulate.

Positioning the infant diminishes stress. The prone position, possible even with acutely ill infants who require mechanical ventilation, facilitates lung expansion and improves oxygenation (Martin, 1979). The side-lying position, with support provided by blanket rolls, is preferable to the supine position. If physiologic instability necessitates that the infant be positioned supine, flexion of the extremities can be provided with blanket rolls and other supports. Supports not only maintain the infant in a flexed position, but also provide boundaries for containing the baby.

Light swaddling of the infant with hands free to reach the face enables hand-to-mouth maneuvers. Successfully bringing the hands to the mouth assists in the development of motor organization and the ability to self-comfort. Light swaddling or clothing the infant with a diaper and a tee shirt does not interfere with adequate assessment of most and normalizes what the infant feels during hospitalization.

Direct caregiving activities are best begun slowly and gently, particularly if the baby has been asleep. Maintaining containment and flexion and allowing the infant to grasp or suck are calming interventions during care. Stressful procedures, such as blood sampling or endotracheal tube retaping, usually require that the infant be provided a period of rest and recovery before another intervention is carried out. Swaddling during stressful procedures helps to maintain physiologic stability (Lawhon & Melzar, 1988).

Involving parents in the care of their infant assists them to learn parenting skills and increases their sense of confidence in their caregiving abilities, as well as enhancing the parent-infant relationship. Initially, parents may need guidance to recognize when and how their infant demonstrates signs of distress so that they learn to tailor their interactions with the baby.

Intervening to alleviate environmental stress in the older infant is predicated on involving parents in their baby's care. Infants require the close and reliable presence of their primary caregivers to relax, rest, and recuperate. Assuring that the environment is warm, quiet, and dimly lit also minimizes environmental stress for infants beyond the newborn period. Comforting and familiar objects from home may support an infant's coping abilities during distressing procedures, as does distraction with a rattle or small toy and use of a pacifier or the fingers or thumb for sucking, rocking, and swaddling. Parents should always have the option to remain with their infant during procedures, because they are best positioned to provide support and reassurance.

Separation

Regardless of the age of the infant who requires critical care hospitalization, separation from parents imposes severe stress. Very young infants, as well as those who are very ill, cannot demonstrate distinct behavioral responses to separation from their parents. Nonspecific changes in behavior, such as increased gross motor activity, frequent crying, poor feeding, insomnia, emotional withdrawal, and self-stimulating behaviors may indicate distress. Older infants, if well enough, are likely to demonstrate the phases of separation anxiety described by Robertson (1958) (see Table 2–1).

Parents of infants in a critical care setting warrant assessment of their reactions to their baby's illness and hospitalization. The information they have received about the illness and hospitalization and their understanding of it requires evaluation. Their plans to remain with their infant or visit frequently and regularly are elicited. Parents need resources if they are to remain with their hospitalized infant. Personal, family, and community sources of help and support are assessed.

Parents can also provide data regarding how their infant has responded in the past to strangers and new situations. With that information in mind, the critical care nurse develops an approach to the individual baby and assesses the response to separation from parents and to substitute caregivers. Subtle cues indicating distress are evaluated, as the baby may well be too young or too ill to protest at separation.

Nursing intervention to prevent or minimize the effects of separation is an important aspect of the critical care of infants and their families. Critical care nurses demonstrate to parents that they clearly recognize that parental presence is crucial to the well-being of the ill infant. Welcoming parents in the PICU and including them in both the planning and implementation of the care required by their infant facilitates their being assured of their importance to their baby.

Infants are assisted to cope with temporary separation from their parents when consistent substitute caregivers are assigned. In addition, a quiet, gentle approach to the sick infant helps to establish trust, as does the prompt and consistent response of caregivers to signs that the infant is distressed. Trust develops with a combination of consistency, continuity, and sameness (Washington, 1990). Transitional or security objects can ease periods of separation for the infant, as can familiar musical or story tape recordings.

Pain and Intrusive Procedures

Behavioral responses to pain vary with age. The newborn responds with generalized body movement and loud crying, when well. Serious illness often blunts the infant's response. The ability to localize pain is refined across the first year of life; but even in the first several months pain related to a specific site is well localized. For example, the baby withdraws an extremity quickly when the heel is lanced for capillary blood sampling. Memory of previous painful events and anticipatory fear develop in the second half of the first year. Older infants react to the threat of pain and the painful event itself with intense physical resistance when they are well. Intrusive procedures do not elicit distress in young infants unless they produce discomfort. Older infants may demonstrate fearfulness in anticipation of an intrusive procedure and resist intensely, even if the procedure is not painful.

Astute assessment skills are required to evaluate the infant's responses to pain, because direct communication is not possible and critical illness and its treatment may limit the physiologic and behavioral signs typically demonstrated by infants in pain. It is generally safe to assume the presence of pain for an infant whose care or treatment would produce pain for an older person.

Pain management strategies are founded on the assurance that analgesia is administered when needed to maintain comfort. In addition, nonpharmacologic strategies are useful in the care of the critically ill infant. Distraction, eliciting the sucking reflex, and gentle stroking and vocalizing to the infant all support the infant during periods of distress.

Light swaddling and well-supported positioning to decrease tension on painful incisions enhance comfort. Gentle sensory stimulation, such as rocking, may be soothing. Human contact, particularly with parents or a trusted caregiver, is comforting. Parents are permitted to remain with the infant during procedures if they wish to. Some parents may find this distressing and prefer to return immediately after the procedure is completed to comfort and reassure their infant. Transitional or security objects can aid coping during a distressing procedure for the older infant.

Loss of Self-control

Infants are the least susceptible of all children to stress related to loss of self-control because they are, by nature, dependent on others for their care and well-being. However, illness and hospitalization result in both physical restriction and altered daily routines, disrupting the infant's usual existence. Regularity and reliability in the environment and freedom to explore the environment are important features in the development of trust in themselves and others that engages infants across the first year. Predictable daily routines provide infants the stability necessary for them to view their environment as safe and reliable.

The primary mode of activity during infancy is sensorimotor. Motor control is developed through nearly constant muscle activity during an infant's waking hours. Motor activity is also the primary mechanism by which the infant learns to distinguish between self, others, and the environment. Immobilization and restraint limit motor activity and alter the amount and the variety of environmental stimuli the infant receives.

Asking parents about the routines and schedule with which their infant is familiar is an important aspect of the nursing admission history. The response of infants to alterations in the predictability of their daily routines is often subtle and may not be detectable in the very ill. For example, the infant may not be able to establish a regular sleeping and waking pattern or may not eat well. Often these problems are identified as the infant recovers from a serious illness.

Very ill or very young infants respond to immobilization and restraint with little physical resistance. However, infants recovering from critical illness and those who are older may protest vigorously when restrained. Nurses assess the amount of physical restriction required by an individual infant to maintain safety and perform procedures effectively.

Not only is motor activity limited by physical restraint, but the infant is unable to move away from sources of environmental sensory overload or appreciate fully a range of sensory experiences. Assessing the PICU environment for factors that contribute to sensory overstimulation or deprivation is a first step in the process of evaluating the infant for distress related to physical restriction.

Providing consistent caregivers and incorporating all possible aspects of the infant's usual routine in their nursing plan of care is standard. Parents are invaluable in affording familiarity in routines and limiting the stress experienced by the hospitalized infant. Familiar items from home provide comfort and security.

Assuring appropriate infant stimulation is an important corollary to the physical care of the baby in the PICU. While the infant is ill, stimulation must be gently planned to protect the baby from environmental overstimulation. As the infant recovers, social stimulation is of particular importance because it encourages relationship formation and trust in others. All stimulation is designed to mitigate sensory deprivation with sights, sounds, or activities that appeal to infants. Stimulation is evaluated in terms of the individual baby's response to avoid overstimulation.

When restraints are necessary for safety, they are regularly removed to permit the infant to move freely while supervised. Restraints are applied in a manner that permits the infant to self-comfort (for example, to get thumb to mouth) whenever feasible. Infants who are ill require frequent position changes within their bed.

THE CRITICALLY ILL TODDLER

Developmental Characteristics of Toddlers

Toddlers are among the most challenging children cared for in the critical care setting. The period from 12 through 36 months of age represents only about 3 percent of the average human lifespan, but encompasses more physical, intellectual, and emotional change than any other period.

Physical growth includes an average weight gain of 11 pounds, an average increase in height of 8 inches, and the eruption of 12 new teeth. Mobility progresses from crawling, or the characteristic unsteady gait of the 1-year-old, to the confident running of a 3-year-old.

Intellectual growth is reflected in the toddler's vocabulary, increasing from several words to approximately 900 by age 3 years. The beginning of toddlerhood is marked by the development of object permanence, an elementary concept of cause and effect, and actions that demonstrate deliberate intention.

Toddlers experience the environment in a steadily more mature manner. Through assimilation, tactile stimulation, manipulation, and interaction with the environment, toddlers are intent on figuring out how things work. In the 2 years of the toddler period, learning progresses from predominantly cause-and-effect to the beginning of thinking about solutions and consequences from retained mental images and anticipation of what will happen as a result of certain actions (Piaget, 1952). Toddlers are driven by nearly

insatiable curiosity. Nonetheless, verbal ability is limited, and toddlers tend to act out much of what they feel. Their thinking is egocentric and their world view absolute and animistic.

The social and emotional task of individuating and separating from parents, with the ultimate goal of independence, evolves over the 2 years of the toddler period. The struggles for independence characteristic of toddlers are evidenced in battles over holding their own spoon and squirming against a restraining parent's hand. The inevitable passage through a "no" stage also marks the quest for independence. The successful establishment of toddlers' independence of their parents permits the gain of a sense of autonomy, as opposed to feelings of shame and doubt (Erikson, 1964).

Individuating, separating, and becoming independent of parents requires tremendous emotional growth and change, which often produces ambivalence and aggression in toddlers. Change is managed by dependence on aspects of daily life that are stable and consistent. The sense of security derived from the sameness of certain routine aspects of living is so important to toddlers that routines become rituals. Repetition and mimicking are commonplace in both language and action.

Dealing With Stress

Hospitalization is likely to be particularly threatening in the evolution of autonomous toddlers. Their limited intellectual ability renders preparatory explanations of upcoming events ineffective. Logical explanations likewise prove ineffective, because toddlers are not logical. However, toddlers understand cause and effect to a small extent and learn through mimicry. Because newly acquired independence is founded on the security of a trusting relationship with their parents, this relationship is key to managing the stress inherent in a critical care hospitalization.

The PICU Environment

In the PICU, the consistency and comfort of home are displaced by unfamiliar sights and sounds. A cold chrome crib replaces the familiar warmth of a wooden crib filled with comforting quilts and toys. The surrounding environment is intimidating with bright lighting, strange noises—often loud and offensive—and unknown equipment and people around the bed. Toddlers, who adventure out into the unknown on short excursions from the safely known, are thrust into a completely foreign environment.

If physically able, toddlers may cry fearfully. Some may react to the unfamiliarity of the environment with increased vigilance, rarely closing their eyes even when exhausted. Sicker toddlers are likely to withdraw from the environment. Their withdrawal, a form of denial, is essential to coping because it allows them to take in the environment a little at a time, as they are able.

Toddlers require the close and consistent presence of their parents to manage distress related to the PICU environment. The security of their relationship with trusted parents permits them to rest and recuperate.

When the critical care environment must intrude on the toddler, in the form of a strange person, a new piece of equipment, or a necessary procedure, the approach to the child is less intimidating if caregivers move slowly and talk quietly and calmly about what will occur just prior to the event.

Separation

Separation from parents is a major source of stress for toddlers who are hospitalized. Children at this stage require the close, reliable presence of their parents to successfully individuate and separate from them. When separation is unexpected and enforced, toddlers fear abandonment—a primary fear during this period of development. In addition, egocentric thinking may lead toddlers to conclude that some misdeed of theirs is the cause of their parents' absence.

If they are physically able, toddlers react to impending separation from their parents with vigorous verbal protest and clinging, particularly if the environment is intimidating. The seriously ill toddler lacks the ability to protest, but may cry inconsolably when left alone. When a behavioral response is impossible for the toddler, separation is no less frightening. Toddlers who are denied the dependable and consistent presence of their parents for an extended period may demonstrate the behaviors associated with separation anxiety: protest, despair, and resignation. Even when parents are reliably present, toddlers are not relieved of all distress. Parents may be subjected to avoidance behaviors, aggression, and ambivalence.

Toddlers have a limited repertoire of defense mechanisms to aid their attempts at coping with separation. Denial and regression are the primary mechanisms available to these youngsters. Denial is evidenced in avoidance of the parents when they are present. Behaviors including gaze aversion and refusal to seek physical comfort or initiate contact with their parents may be observed, particularly as critically ill toddlers recover. Regression, marked by a temporary cessation of newly acquired skills, is necessitated by the stress of critical illness and high anxiety.

Hospitalized toddlers are best cared for when parental presence is encouraged. The sustained continuity of the relationship between toddlers and their parents supports the development of individual autonomy and is, more immediately, crucial to avoiding distress that impedes rest and recuperation. Assignment of consistent caregivers assists both toddlers and their parents.

When parents cannot be with their toddler, comfort is often derived from transitional or security objects, although protest is still likely if the child is well enough to muster the response. Familiar toys and family photos can also be helpful.

Parents may need assistance and support in dealing with negativity or aggression directed toward them by their toddler. With the understanding that they are safe individuals to whom the toddler can express strong negative emotion, they are supported in assisting their child's coping with fearfulness and distress. Regression can also be troubling to parents, who need assurance that newly gained developmental skills have been only temporarily lost and will be remastered quickly.

Pain and Intrusive Procedures

Toddlers generally react to acutely painful experiences with vigorous physical resistance and intense emotional upset. However, when critically ill, these responses are often blunted.

Because toddlers have limited concepts of their body image and boundaries, intrusive procedures are as frightening for them as are painful events. Restraint is frequently required during intrusive procedures, heightening the toddler's anxiety and increasing the perception of pain.

Toddlers in the PICU are unlikely to have the physical reserve for the intense reactions that characterize their response to pain when they are well. More often, discomfort evokes responses including whimpering or crying, restlessness or tense body posture, poor appetite, resistance to being left alone, and inability to be comforted. Toddlers' responses to pain are also influenced by the extent of physical restraint applied, separation from their parents, the emotional reactions of those around them (particularly their parents), and their individual temperament.

Toddlers can generally localize pain well, but their ability to describe it is limited by their communication skills. Complaints of pain are taken seriously because children in this age group rarely imagine discomfort.

Preparation for painful or intrusive events can assist the toddler in coping, but is best provided just before the event. The procedure is then carried out without delay. Parents are prepared fully and further in advance of the event so that they are able to consider how best to support and comfort their child. Reassurance includes clarifying that the toddler is not and has not been bad, because the older toddler may perceive pain as punishment.

Loss of Self-control

The ability of the hospitalized toddler to maintain self-control is threatened by altered routines and physical restriction. The development of an autonomous toddler who is able to separate from parents is dependent on the toddler's ability to move away from them physically. Toddlers' insatiable curiosity encourages exploration and manipulation of the environment beyond their parents. As the growing toddler's world widens, self-control is maintained chiefly through routine and ritual, which permit these youngsters to view their expanding world as reliable and subject to control.

Illness and hospitalization restrict the toddler's ability to exercise newly developed physical skills. Exploration of the environment is not only intimidating, but also unsafe. The usual routines toddlers rely on to maintain self-control separate from their parents are likely to be totally disrupted. The world is no longer reliable. Fear of the unknown and enforced dependency may affect the older toddler in particular.

Little in the critical care environment is familiar to the toddler. Nurses learn of the individual child's routines and habits, particularly those related to eating, sleeping, bathing, and toileting, from the toddler's parents. Disruption in all of these areas is likely during a PICU admission. Bedtime is an especially vulnerable time for the toddler, with difficulty settling for sleep and sleep disturbances common among these young children. Regression is a common response to altered routines. Negativism may also be evidenced as toddlers protest disruption.

Toddlers lack the cognitive development necessary for specific fears of the unknown aspects of hospitalization. However, the unfamiliarity of the entire environment is likely to intimidate even the bravest toddler. Toddlers can recall past experiences that were painful or frightening, and fearful anticipation often precedes a procedure or event. Regression is common. In fact, fearfulness may prevent the toddler's maintaining much, if any, self-control.

Illness slows the typical active pace of the toddler's life, but immobilization and restraint result in protest if physical energy is available. Sensory deprivation and immobilization are likely to result in regression and aggression in toddlers. Aggression may be evidenced by general restlessness, physical resistance, or struggling. Aggression, which permits the release of tension and energy, may be impossible until the toddler is less ill.

Some toddlers assert their independence and ability to master their environment by insisting on self-feeding or dressing. When these attempts are thwarted, toddlers usually respond negatively. Enforced dependency may account for outbursts of negativism, but regression generally permits toddlers to accept care from others and conserve energy for recuperation.

Incorporating as many of the toddler's routines and habits into the hospital schedule as is possible provides the foundation for individualized care. Parents play a key role in maintaining routine and are the greatest source of stability for their child. When parents cannot be present, transitional objects and tape recordings, particularly of bedtime stories or songs, assist toddlers to relax and maintain self-control.

Transitional or security objects also provide a measure of reassurance in the unfamiliar PICU environment or when new and unknown procedures or events occur. Preparation of toddlers for events is best provided only shortly before the experience, and because of the egocentric nature of toddlers' thought processes, is depersonalized. Parents are thoroughly prepared for the events their child will experience to facilitate their support and comfort of the child.

Limiting immobilization and restraint whenever possible diminishes their impact on the recuperating toddler in the PICU. Parents can provide watchful eyes and ensure that their child is safe. Recuperation can also provide outlets for aggression if the toddler is permitted activities such as throwing soft balls, exploring, manipulating toys, and the like.

Enforced dependency can be mitigated by providing toddlers with choices when there is an option they can safely choose. Choices are not offered when none exist. Recuperation also permits the toddler to accomplish some aspects of care independently, such as self-feeding. Liberal praise is in order when toddlers complete tasks.

CRITICAL ILLNESS DURING THE PRESCHOOL YEARS

Developmental Characteristics of the Preschool Period

Preschool children, through the development of initiative, become active members of their world. Successful transition through the toddler years produces a self-confident and separate person who has overcome fears of abandonment and separates from family with less distress. Across the next 3 years, from age 3 through age 5 years, children gain an average of 10 pounds and grow 6 inches. Rapid progress in motor abilities, cognitive function, and language development leads to the acquisition of a distinctive, individual personality. Each preschooler develops a "self."

Cognitive development is reflected in increasing awareness of themselves and others. The preschooler's vocabulary increases from 900 words at age 3 years to 2100 words used in meaningful sentences at 5 years. Preschoolers learn to count, identify colors and geometric shapes, and memorize nursery rhymes. They are aware of their own sex and that of others and, at 5 years, understand kinship and become aware of cultural differences. However, preschool logic is precausal and preconceptual. Animism, magical thinking, and fantasy characterize the preschooler's view of the world. They are unable to separate fantasy from reality and may fear ghosts, monsters, supernatural forces, robbers, and kidnappers. Consequently, preschoolers are most often not as mature as might be thought from their verbal ability.

Emotional and social development is characterized by egocentrism and is related to the preschooler's developing sense of self. Preschoolers are unable to see the viewpoint of others and unable to understand another's inability to see their own point of view. Their sense of self provides security and competence, which motivates them to accomplish the tasks and activities that lead to the development of initiative. Initiative is the boldness or courage to take on great projects. If initiative does not develop and the preschooler lacks the self-confidence to tackle new opportunities, guilty feelings are the negative counterpart of preschool developmental tasks (Erikson, 1964).

Conscience begins developing during the preschool years, and is tied to identification of what behaviors are acceptable to parents. Behavior is refined in taking turns, sharing, and following the rules to games. Rules are absolute during the preschool years, determined by parents who are always right. Preschoolers strive to be similar to their parents, particularly the parent of the same sex.

Sexual curiosity is characteristic of the preschool years. The development of longing for the opposite-sex parent and its resolution in identification with the same-sex parent occurs. Children do experience castration anxiety and penis envy, but the Freudian explanation of the Oedipus and Electra complexes are not considered valid explanations of preschoolers' motivations or behaviors (Anderson, 1989).

Dealing With Stress

Hospitalization interrupts the preschooler's efforts to master control of the environment and develop independence through mastery of physical and social skills. The restrictive hospital environment causes considerable distress for preschoolers who experience guilt when their accomplishments are obstructed. Guilty feelings may also be related to egocentric thinking, which leads to the conclusion that "wrong" or "bad" thoughts or actions have caused their illness. Treatment and hospitalization are seen as punishment. Preconceptual and magical thinking create exaggerated fears. Self-care skills and control of body functions, often recently acquired, may be threatened.

The PICU Environment

The critical care environment remains a source of distress for hospitalized preschoolers. Egocentricity, magical thinking, and preconceptual logic may lead to exaggerated fears of equipment, procedures, and personnel. Older preschoolers are more aware of others and may, as a consequence, have fears from information they overhear and do not understand or for other patients around them. Sleep disturbances persist among these young children who are exquisitely sensitive to sensory input (sights, sounds, odors) and still reasonably dependent on bedtime routines.

Fearful behaviors may not be detected in those preschoolers who are very ill. During recuperation, some exhibit fearfulness related to the PICU environment, procedures, or personnel by tense behaviors

such as nail-biting or whining. Others exhibit distress in regressed behavior, such as clinging to their parents or a security object, dependency, and withdrawal. Concrete evidence of the fears some preschool children experience is sometimes obtained from their drawings or by requesting that they tell a "story" about hospital procedures or experiences. Nightmares occurring after recovery and hospital discharge are sometimes related to lingering fears and are reported by many parents after young children are hospitalized. Sleep or night terrors in preschoolers following hospitalization occur when usual sleep patterns have been disorganized (Ferber, 1985; Slota, 1988).

Preschoolers can be protected from at least some of the fears associated with the critical care unit. All procedures are explained in concrete, understandable terms, with emphasis on events to be expected. This practice is assured even when a child's condition is critical, neurologic status unclear, and responses prohibited by chemical sedation or paralysis. When preschoolers are less ill, they benefit from therapeutic play and education.

Shielding preschoolers from disturbing sights and sounds also offers protection from the PICU environment. They may need to be shielded from other patients around them if the environment is an open-unit design. Conversation between staff members or with parents, within the earshot of the preschooler, is not about the child unless the child is included in the conversation. Not only may overheard conversations be frightening to preschoolers who are unable to completely understand the content, but they may inadvertently induce guilty feelings. For example, consider comments such as "She failed that wean," in reference to a patient's inability to tolerate a decrease in mechanical ventilation, or "He's certainly not doing any better," to describe a patient's condition. The preschooler may feel guilty and responsible. It is crucial to remember that the preschooler understands concretely and literally.

Separation

Preschoolers are far more secure than either infants or toddlers in interpersonal relationships and have generally had some experience with separating from parents. When ill, however, they are much less able to cope with separation. Children in this age group fear being left alone, despite resolution of fears of abandonment.

Separation anxiety is expressed more subtly by preschoolers than by younger children. Protest when parents must leave is less aggressive. Distress may be evidenced in sleep disturbances, feeding difficulties, quiet crying, and withdrawal from others. Without parental presence, preschoolers may be unable to cooperate with healthcare personnel during procedures. They may not cooperate with their parents, either, if the parent leaves for a period of time. Aggression is usually not experienced with this age group, although younger preschoolers may still have temper tantrums.

Regression is the most common coping response for preschoolers dealing with separation. Often, mastery of control of body functions is lost, particularly in the face of serious illness. Thumb-sucking may be resumed or baby talk may replace the typical language of the preschooler.

Preschoolers require the close and consistent presence of their parents when ill. Because they have learned to extend trust to other adults, providing consistent caregivers is especially advantageous for this age group, particularly when parents must leave. Transitional or security objects are valuable to ease distress when separation from parents occurs. Familiar toys and family photos are tangible signs that the preschooler is loved. Parental participation in caretaking is comforting for these young children. Parents can also assist their preschooler to maintain contact with siblings and peers through audio or video tape recordings. These can be valuable in combatting loneliness. Even the sickest child can benefit from the comforting voices or images of family members and friends.

Pain and Intrusive Procedures

Preschoolers' reactions to acute pain are only somewhat less vigorous than those of toddlers. Reactions are, however, less generalized and more goal-directed. Preschoolers may attempt to grab equipment or push away the person about to perform a painful procedure. Verbal aggression or pleading with personnel required to perform a procedure is common. Because of their close identification with their parents, the responses of these key individuals influence how preschoolers respond.

The concept of body integrity remains poorly developed among preschoolers. An increased awareness of body image and the psychosexual development of this age group increases the vulnerability and distress experienced with intrusive procedures. Increasing awareness of sexual identity causes concern for the intactness and safety of the genitals.

Preschoolers in the PICU are unable to respond vigorously or directly to painful experiences. Persistent discomfort results in tense body posture; refusal to move; and strained facial expression and whimpering, crying, or moaning, if the child can verbally respond. Preschoolers can describe the nature of their discomfort or point to the area that hurts and rate the intensity of their pain. Pain intensity assessment scales are highly useful with this age group. Loneliness or fear of being left alone intensifies pain among preschoolers.

Cognitive development characteristic of the preschool years results in misconceptions about the cause of pain among this age group. Pain as punishment is a persistent theme that is assessed in preschool children.

Vulnerability and distress with intrusive procedures may be evidenced in resistance. Preschoolers are threatened by removal of their underwear; intrusive procedures in the genital area, such as catheter insertion, are extremely distressing.

Regression is common in the face of either severe or enduring pain and with repeated intrusive procedures. Dependency and withdrawal are frequently observed in the seriously ill preschooler, as are loss of previously mastered self-care skills and control of body functions.

Preschoolers require consistent reassurance that their bodies are intact and no one is to blame for their illness or hospitalization. They need to be assured that only necessary treatments will be done and they will always be told before treatments are performed. Thoughtful explanation of and preparation for painful or intrusive procedures before they occur assists preschoolers to maintain self-control during the procedure. Successes in self-control are consistently praised. Parental preparation aids their ability to assist their child and limits their own anxiety, as well.

Assuring privacy and maximizing comfort during procedures is crucial. In addition, successful pain management is necessary for all children with acute or persistent discomfort.

Loss of Self-control

Because of the tremendous cognitive development that occurs during the preschool years, children of this age group who are successfully gaining initiative feel extremely powerful. These feelings are instrumental in the preschooler's ability to maintain self-control despite serious illness and hospitalization in an unfamiliar and threatening environment. Loss of self-control may result when preschoolers' omnipotent feelings are confronted by fears of the unknown and enforced dependency. Physical restriction and altered routines continue to contribute to distress for preschoolers in the PICU.

Preschoolers have increasing experiences with a variety of environments and social settings, allowing them to be less dependent on routines and rituals for maintenance of self-control. However, dependency on routines diminishes across the preschool years, and bedtime remains a vulnerable time even for 5- and 6-year-olds. All preschoolers relate their sense of time to routine daily activities, and thus they may feel disruption of their sense of time and may need routine and ritual more than when well. Regression also increases dependence on rituals.

Fears of the unknown are closely tied to preschoolers' inability to maintain self-control when distressed. Little in the cognitive development of these preoperational children is likely to prepare them for serious illness and intensive care. Consequently, their fears are vague and generalized and may be exaggerated by the thought processes characteristic of the age group (magical thinking, animism, etc.).

Physical restrictions related to illness and its treatment limit mobility needed for mastery at each developmental level. Restraint may be perceived as punishment. Both limited mobility and restraint in the critical care environment result in altered sensory stimulation.

Preschoolers are actively pursuing mastery of initiative through the independent performance of self-care skills and control of body functions, as well as a variety of other physical and social tasks. Preschoolers are proud of their accomplishments, and relinquishing them when they are ill and under enforced dependence threatens their self-esteem and ability to maintain self-control.

It is essential to obtain information from preschoolers' parents about daily routines and particular rituals that are relied on in the family, for example, those used to settle and quiet the household at bedtime. Data about self-care and elimination routines is also helpful, although the information may not be useful until the preschooler is recuperating. At that point, caregivers can plan interventions that promote the remastery of developmentally appropriate skills.

Although most preschool children have generalized and vague fears about hospitalization, some will have had personal previous experience with illness and hospitals. The child and family health history provides nurses the opportunity to determine whether the child has had prior experience with hospitalization. The preschooler who, for example, has had a grandparent die in the hospital is likely to have very specific fears that require attention.

The impact of physical restriction and restraint may not be significant if only briefly necessary. Longer periods of immobilization may result in quiet, passive submission or active protest and aggressive behavior. Withdrawal from contact with others or regression may be detected.

Enforced dependency also often results in extremes of behavior if illness and critical care are lengthy. Preschoolers may become overly dependent as a consequence of regression, or may actively protest and aggressively act out their frustration with lost independence.

Even in the face of critical illness, promoting rest among preschoolers aids recuperation. Parental participation in the routines the family follows at home assists in settling young children. Parents may also wish to assist with aspects of care for their child, which helps to normalize hospital routines.

Preschoolers require explanation of the equipment around them and of all procedures prior to their being carried out. Information about what they are experiencing and who the people are around them orients them to reality and helps to avoid or correct fantasy and misperception. Preschoolers who are well enough to interact verbally are encouraged to ask questions. They can be questioned to elicit fears or misconceptions about illness and its treatment. Parental preparation also assists them in helping their youngsters accurately interpret what is happening to them so parents can provide reassurance.

Limiting physical restriction and restraint, while maintaining a safe environment, encourages coopera-

tion and self-control. When restraint is necessary, its need is defined simply and the child reassured that immobilization is not a punishment. Restraint during procedures may be limited if the preschooler can be adequately prepared. Preschoolers can cooperate if they are calm, have had adequate explanation, and are permitted to participate.

Child participation in self-care of hygiene and participation in treatments encourages maintenance of self-control and mastery of the environment while it limits dependency. With the exception of the most seriously ill children, it is likely that all children can participate in some aspect of their care. When serious illness or lengthy hospitalization results in regression, caregivers are tolerant of the child's retreat while encouraging remastery of temporarily lost skills.

CRITICAL ILLNESS DURING THE SCHOOL-AGE YEARS

Developmental Characteristics of School-Age Children

Although physical growth and neuromuscular development are fairly slow and steady from ages 6 through 12 years, cognitive and social skills expand tremendously. Height increases 2 inches per year on average, often in spurts of growth. Weight gain averages 5 to 7 pounds per year. Many girls experience a spurt in growth and begin to develop secondary sex characteristics at around age 10, nearly 2 years before their male agemates. The primary teeth are lost and most permanent teeth erupt during these years.

The school-age period is a time of mastering an ever-expanding world as the foundation for adult roles is established. Cognitive development is characterized by dramatic shifts. The young school-age child uses intuitive thought, according to Piaget (1976). Intuitive thinking is based on immediate, unanalyzed relationships between particular elements of the environment and the child. Reasoning is not logical. Thought processes become concrete at 7 or 8 years of age, and by the end of the school-age years, cognitive operations have moved toward formal operations.

Concrete operations strongly influence knowledge acquisition. School-age children work hard to discover how the world around them functions. They can consider the various parts of a whole while retaining the concept of the whole. Conservation of matter, weight, and volume are achieved. Classification, seriation, and numerical concepts are mastered.

Language development progresses rapidly during the school-age period. Beginning with a vocabulary of 2500 words, school-age children learn to read, learn correct grammar, and use language as a tool in riddles, jokes (sometimes disparaging or cruel), chants, and word games. Their vocabulary expands steadily, and words are used in complex sentences.

During the stage of concrete operations, children emerge from their egocentric view of the world and realize that their way of thinking is not the only way. Not only can they mentally retrace the steps they took to reach a conclusion, but also they realize that there may be more than one way of reaching the same end-point. They also recognize the role of chance in the occurrence of events as egocentricity diminishes. They are no longer the cause of every action and reaction around them. The world becomes a kinder and gentler place.

Concrete operations also profoundly influence emotional and social development. The major challenge of Erikson's fourth stage of development is the establishment of a sense of industry, that is, a sense of being useful and able to make and do things well, even perfectly. The negative counterpart of this stage is a sense of inadequacy or inferiority, rather than competence, which may develop if children see their physical and intellectual skills as deficient. Clearly, all children are "inferior" in some area of activity. School-age children learn to recognize their limitations and accept them, as they also recognize and capitalize on their abilities to develop a sense of competence and self-esteem.

The peer group, especially same-sex peers, increases in importance across the school-age years. Interest in the opposite sex begins at the end of the school-age period, but a best friend is more important at this stage and almost always is a same-sex companion. Clubs, teams, camp, and group projects are enjoyed. Team loyalty is intense at the end of the school years. The competent and industrious school-age child becomes productive within a social group of peers in preparation for being a productive member of society as an adult. Cooperation and collaboration based on mutual respect are evidenced in the pride school-age children feel for each other's accomplishments, as well as those of the group. Group activities teach children that individual strengths and weaknesses are balanced in a group.

The absolute rules that guide action for the preschooler become tempered by the realization that the same act can be viewed differently by different individuals. Intentions prompting an act are taken into consideration. Through cooperative and competitive interaction with peers, school-age children develop rules by consensus and mutual consent. Rules are no longer unbendable but can be changed in a democratic process or by extenuating circumstances. Moral judgment becomes increasingly independent of adults as peer groups grow in solidarity. Morality is based on cooperation, developed in discussion with peers.

Increasing independence from adults peaks at age 11 or 12, with the child wanting unreasonable independence and demanding privacy. Relationships with parents and family are ambivalent; children are often self-conscious about their parents. Unruliness, sloppiness, and secretive behavior may impede reasonable increases in the independence permitted

children in the transitional period that concludes the school-age years.

Dealing With Stress

School-age children are better equipped, from a developmental perspective, to cope with the stresses associated with hospitalization. Short-term hospital admissions are associated with less distress for children older than 5 years of age. Less specific data are available regarding the responses of seriously ill school-agers. Although intellectually more mature and capable of sophisticated language and communication, school-age children are reality-based and unlikely to have had specific experiences that will mitigate all the stress of hospitalization. Their abilities to problem-solve and learn are likely to be thwarted when they are seriously ill. Illness restricts opportunities for individual achievement, as well as group accomplishments.

School-age children have low rates of mortality and serious morbidity when compared with other age groups. Chronic illness, which may be a factor in a school-age child's admission to the PICU, places concomitant demands on the child and family and may influence the coping responses of both when critical care is necessitated.

The PICU Environment

The unfamiliar PICU environment is less intimidating, generally, for school-age children than it is for those who are younger. During the school years unreasonable fears and fantasies lessen, and these children actively master that which is unknown or unfamiliar through concrete cognition. However, school-age children do fear bodily injury, loss of self-control, and death, and may be intimidated by the critical care environment. In addition, school-age children in the PICU have been demonstrated to worry for other patients there (Barnes, 1975). Anxiety, depression, agitation, and withdrawal have been reported among school-age children requiring intensive care. These occur with greater frequency in the PICU environment than in other hospital settings (Jones et al., 1992).

Little overt fearfulness is demonstrated by children past the earliest school-age years (6 or 7 years of age). Maintenance of self-control is of vital importance, but anxiety may lead to nail-biting or hair-twirling in children who are well enough. Behavioral expression of anxiety may be exhibited in apprehension with routine nonpainful procedures, worried detachment with staff, sadness, and weeping. Some patients demonstrate tremulousness, shakiness, and motor agitation. Length of hospital stay correlates positively with these findings. Increasing severity of illness is correlated positively with the presence of confusion and disorientation, apprehension with staff and apprehension about routine procedures (Jones et al., 1992). Serious illness may necessitate regression, with behaviors and fears similar to those of pre-schoolers. Crying, excessive fearfulness, or difficulty separating are examples of regressive behaviors.

School-age children rely on their ability to master their environment and are assisted in this process by accurate explanations of that which is happening to and around them. Thinking remains concrete, and thus teaching is aimed at clear and factual explanations. An explanation and a rationale for procedures assist school-age children to maintain self-control and are important even when verbal or physical interaction is prevented by illness or its treatment.

School-age children are accustomed to external appraisal of their accomplishments and are supported in coping with the PICU environment when they receive praise. Regression is tolerated without negative comment or criticism, and the child is reassured that crying or fearfulness is not unusual when someone is very ill.

Severe anxiety or marked agitation may necessitate pharmacologic therapy, as well as consultation with the psychiatric service.

Separation

School-age children are able to tolerate parental separation despite stress during hospitalization, as they tolerate separation and academic stress in their school settings. A concrete concept of time develops across these years, permitting more accurate appraisal of time spent alone. Despite this developmental progress toward independence, school-age children continue to need close, reliable contact with parents. Behavioral reactions to intensive care are more severe and persistent when children are separated from their parents (Fiser et al., 1984).

Separation from siblings, friends, and schoolmates, which includes the concomitant loss of their productive roles in the family, neighborhood, and classroom affects hospitalized school-age children. They are likely to be fearful of losing their friends or their status within their social groups during an absence necessitated by illness.

Familiar articles from home remain important to school-age children, particularly during the early school years. About one-half of school-agers continue to have a special object to which an attachment was formed during early childhood.

Young school-age children may have lingering fears of being left alone and demonstrate fearfulness when their parents leave them, clinging to a transitional object, if available, or crying. If able, they may beg their parents not to leave them. By the middle school years, such fearfulness is less common, but when alone, older school-age children may feel threatened, rejected, isolated, depressed, lonely, and bored. Their tolerance of the PICU environment and necessary procedures diminishes without the supportive presence of their parents. Anxiety or hostility may be evidenced in irritability or verbal aggression. Some children withdraw from contact with others, longing

to ask their parents to stay but afraid of appearing to be "a baby."

The provision of consistent caregivers helps school-age children to maintain self-control when their parents are absent, because trust is extended in other settings beyond the immediate family. However, close bonds to parents are key to managing distress during hospitalization, and school-age children continue to need reliable parental support. The family may also serve as a conduit for information about friends and classmates, easing school-agers' sense of absence from important social groups. Letters and cards from classmates or video tapes of family and school activities assure school-age children they have not been forgotten if hospitalization is lengthy.

Pain and Intrusive Procedures

School-age children generally maintain a great deal of composure when confronted with painful procedures while they are well. Prolonged discomfort associated with illness or injury, however, is demoralizing and results in regression with loss of self-control. School-age children, except for the youngest, have the cognitive ability to recognize that pain is a feature of illness or injury and do not view pain as punishment. They also recognize both physical and psychological sources of pain (Hurley & Whelan, 1988).

Intrusive procedures of a routine nature are not upsetting to school-age children who are accustomed to physical examinations. However, disrobing or being unclothed is anxiety-producing, as are procedures around the genital area.

When well, school-age children maintain self-control during painful procedures by clenching their teeth or jaws, tensing their bodies, self-distraction, or deep breathing. Humor may also be used and verbal protest remains common. They are adept at describing their pain, sometimes in dramatic terms. The seriously ill school-ager may manifest tension only during procedures, but some are extremely apprehensive and behavioral self-control may disintegrate.

Most school-age children still prefer a parent's presence during painful procedures. They may seek contact only with their eyes if too ill to verbally request it or if they believe they should be brave. Intrusive procedures are judged differently, particularly at the end of the school years. If disrobing is necessary or the procedure involves the genitals, the same-sex parent may be supportive, whereas the other's presence is a source of embarrassment and distress. Thoughtful assessment and discussion with the child and parents is necessary to determine the most supportive intervention for each individual. When the child is too ill to participate in the discussion, parents can anticipate interventions that would most likely be helpful based on their relationship with their child.

Pain may result in unstable moods and temperament, leading to angry outbursts of temper. Demanding behavior is also common among some school-age children, whereas others become passive and withdrawn, avoiding eye contact. An anxious facial expression is a potential symptom of pain. Regression may occur if pain is chronic, unremitting, or intense.

School-age children may maintain composure and cooperate during painful procedures when offered a hand to squeeze, diversion in counting or conversation, or other tactics. Outbursts or crying are quietly accepted and the child assured that such behavior is not unusual when children are ill. If they are well enough to participate in procedures, active participation permits them to feel a measure of personal control. The presence of a supportive adult offers comfort, as long as privacy is assured. Adequate analgesia is consistently provided, particularly for children too ill to express pain either verbally or behaviorally. School-age children may benefit from patient-controlled analgesia.

Information is consistently provided to school-age children about that which will be done to them, how long it will take, and how it is likely to feel. Reducing anxiety by providing information can alter the perception of pain and enhance coping. Information is important even if the school-age patient is too ill to indicate hearing or understanding.

Loss of Self-control

School-age children are actively and powerfully engaged in their world. Self-control is normal for them. Serious illness and hospitalization result in altered routines, fear of the unknown, physical restriction, enforced dependency, and loss of productive roles, threatening the maintenance of self-control.

School-age children, who are accustomed to a variety of social settings and routines, are less dependent than younger children on regularity in routines. New experiences carry with them a high sense of adventure for school-agers when they are well. However, independence is limited by hospitalization. Hospitalized school-agers are also denied their productive roles within their families and schools. These factors are influential in the sense of powerlessness and resultant loss of self-control experienced by school-age children who are ill.

School-age children usually have very specific fears related to the unfamiliar aspects of hospitalization and are anxious about matters they do not know or understand. Enhancing their sense of personal control through cognitive mastery of the unknown is an essential component of caring for them.

Immobility or physical restraint limits the discharge of energy and anxiety in physical activity. The sensory burden of the PICU may be overwhelming to immobilized children who are unable to turn away from it.

Industrious school-age children thrive on their steadily increasing ability to be independent. Feelings of loss are experienced when they are placed in the dependent role of a hospitalized patient for a period of time beyond a day or two. Self-control is diminished by limited opportunities for independence in self-care and the pursuit of industry and its associated feelings of worthiness and importance.

School-age children value the roles they play within their families, peer groups, and schools. Actual or perceived changes in the roles they play threaten self-esteem and self-control. Fear of being displaced from their usual position within their families and among friends provokes stress and anxiety. Fear of falling behind or failing at school is the consequence of the student role being disrupted during hospitalization.

The nursing history provides data regarding routines to which a school-age child is accustomed. Their incorporation into the hospital routine assists the youngest school-age children maintain self-control and normalizes the PICU environment to an extent.

School-age children are information seekers. The ability of children to understand their illness, treatment, and procedures increases steadily across the school years. The youngest children may still relate illness to bad behavior, a misunderstanding that requires assessment. The information that school-age children have received in preparation for hospitalization is also assessed to develop an effective teaching plan. The child's perception of events to come is elicited, if possible, and verbalization of fears and questions is encouraged.

Immobilization or physical restraint may result in depression, frustration, or hostility among school-age children. If physical restraint is viewed as a significant threat, anger, hostility, and aggression are common responses. Regression is likely if physical restriction is prolonged or permanent. Likewise, enforced dependence often results in frustration and aggression in school-age children. When dependency is prolonged, regression and over-dependency are common responses. Serious illness may limit displays of hostility and aggression, but not the angry, hostile feelings. Their release in agitated behavior or their sublimation in regressed behavior may be detected.

Being displaced from productive roles at home and school results in feelings of sadness and fearfulness about school failure. Withdrawal and depression are common responses.

Positive feedback is a primary intervention with school-age children in the PICU; it builds self-esteem and encourages self-control. Praise is offered for efforts at cooperation, self-care, and participation in procedures or treatments. Providing opportunities for success several times daily gives the child a sense of accomplishment.

Maintenance of routines related to home, body functions, and self-care is desirable, but may not be possible in the face of serious illness. Bedtime routines may be important for young school-age children and warrant special effort. Recuperation provides increased opportunity to incorporate the child in developing comfortable daily patterns like those followed at home.

Fears of unknown aspects of illness and critical

care are addressed by providing concrete but scientific descriptions of illness and its treatment. Because school-age children may be disturbed by unfamiliar body responses, these too are explained in scientific terms. Patients in the PICU are likely to hear and appreciate explanation of what they are experiencing, even if unable to participate in discussion. As recovery occurs, children are encouraged to verbalize concerns and ask questions. Misinformation or misunderstanding is corrected with complete, truthful information provided in a caring and supportive manner. Truthfulness is an essential feature of the trust required in professional relationships with patients and indicates respect for the child's personal rights and individual autonomy.

Physical restrictions are limited to those imposed by illness, as well as those necessary for safety, because it is usually reasonable to assume that school-age children will cooperate. Thorough preparation for procedures and treatments may limit the amount of restraint necessary. When actively held down for a procedure, the school-age child may abandon all attempts at self-control and cooperation. During recovery, quiet activities are enjoyed, but creative outlets for frustration normally discharged in physical activity are also needed.

School-agers can direct procedures, participate in self-care, and make decisions regarding their care to mitigate the negative aspects of enforced dependence as soon as they are physically able. A model for children's participation in treatment decisions has been developed that can guide their involvement (Erlen, 1987). Children aged 7 years or older, in the stage of concrete operations, are able to assent (agree or concur with a decision made by others). Maturation through the school years increases knowledge, understanding, and competence, preparing children by about age 10 to dissent. With dissent there is a lack of agreement and withholding of assent. Dissent should be taken seriously when there is evidence that the child has sufficient knowledge and understanding of illness and its treatment (Leiken, 1983). At least additional discussion is necessary when school-age children indicate disagreement with their treatment plan.

Involving children in healthcare decisions is not without practical problems, including determining competence and cognitive development, legal ramifications, and potential conflict with parental rights. While these issues remain unsettled, healthcare professionals can promote independence among school-age children by protecting their right to participate in treatment decisions whenever possible.

Anxiety related to loss of productive roles within the family and with friends is mitigated by encouraging continued contact with the school-ager's siblings and friends as recuperation occurs. If hospitalization is lengthy, peer relationships within the hospital setting are fostered. Although usually not feasible in the critical care unit, provision for continuing schoolwork is also important during lengthy hospitalization.

THE CRITICALLY ILL ADOLESCENT

Developmental Characteristics of Adolescents

Adolescence begins at approximately 12 years of age and ends when the child is independent of the family. Physical growth, which once marked the end of adolescence, is complete at about 19 years of age. Cognitive, emotional, and social development are considered to extend the period of adolescent life until the emancipation of an independent young adult.

Physical growth increases significantly during adolescence. Around puberty, both males and females attain the final 20 percent of their mature height. Boys average an increase in height of 8 inches, peaking with a 4-inch increase in 1 year around age 14 years. Girls increase in height by an average of 6 to 9 inches and may grow more than 3 inches per year during the growth spurt, which occurs around age 12 years. At 18 years, nearly all growth is complete. Few adolescents grow more than an inch taller afterward.

Growth is typically uneven, with the legs lengthening first, followed by broadening of the thighs and then the shoulders, and trunk growth occurring last. Coordination is often affected by the uneven growth characteristic of adolescence. Periods of clumsiness are common.

Sexual maturation, the development of both primary and secondary sexual characteristics, is generally not completed until 20 or 21 years. The hormones produced by the ovary and testes are the consequence of hypothalamic and pituitary secretion and are responsible for the development of the secondary sexual characteristics. Tanner (1962) described and labeled these stages as guidelines to the progression of normal development.

Piaget (1976) describes the cognitive development of the adolescent years as a progression and reconstruction of concrete operations to a new level termed "formal operations." With formal operations, adolescents can imagine possibilities, form and test a hypothesis, and interpret the results. Unexpected results are not as confusing as they are to school-age children, because the adolescent has considered several possibilities (Ginsberg & Opper, 1979). Adolescents are able to mentally reverse a sequence of events to understand why something has happened. Piaget (1976) notes that in addition to the ability to form hypotheses and the capacity for deductive reasoning, adolescents' thought processes become more flexible and new problems stimulate the use of previous learning.

Adolescents are able to understand symbolism and abstract concepts. As they contemplate the future, they construct ideals, sometimes leading to a critical view of the adults around them. Their ability to think about thinking leads to introspection, accompanied by a resurgence of egocentricity and preoccupation with self. Adolescents believe that everyone is observing their appearance and behavior, noting their flaws and taking measure of their assets. Hours are spent perfecting every aspect of appearance and holding silent conversations in the mirror.

Teenage egocentricity also leads adolescents to consider their experience as completely unique. They accuse adults of lack of understanding, believing that no one has ever been through what they are experiencing. Egocentricity diminishes by late adolescence as young adults discover that, although they are individuals, their experiences and emotions are not unique. The audience teens once believed was watching fades, enabling them to act and react genuinely.

The formal thought processes of adolescents enable their emotional and social development. Erikson (1964) described the central task of adolescence as the development of identity, with role confusion the possible negative outcome of unsuccessful negotiation of teen social and emotional development. Formal operations permit the internalization of self-image, self-concept, or identity. Potential sources of confusion are the rapid body changes with which the adolescent must come to terms and the reality of the future and adulthood, with the accompanying loss of the comfortable familiarity of childhood (Erikson, 1964).

Peer alliances formed in early adolescence ease the way toward comfort with their own bodies for young teens. Joking and teasing about voice changes or discussing menstrual cramps assure most adolescents that their experiences are normal. However, the invariable comparisons with those around them may produce anxiety in those who develop slightly earlier or later than the majority of the peer group.

Peer relationships help the adolescent avoid role confusion. Peer alliances are firmly established in middle adolescence, but early in the adolescent years changes in groups of friends, as well as the accepted style of dress and manner of speech, are common. Once established, the peer group provides a sort of safety net for teens trying out social roles and behaviors. By late adolescence, the peer group diminishes in importance, and roles and behavior are individually determined.

Independence from parents and family assists adolescents to develop their individuality and identity. Early adolescents have incorporated the values and standards of their parents, usually viewing them as role models and accepting their authority. However, adolescence is a progressive test of parental limit-setting, as more and more independence is demanded. Some adolescents engage in rebellious behavior.

Middle adolescents also frequently confide in an adult other than one of their parents, limiting the influence parents exert as their adolescent progresses. Older adolescents may return to parents for consultation, once they are secure outside the home when parents are no longer seen as a threat to independence or autonomy. Parents and their children ideally develop an adult relationship across the years of adolescence.

Dealing With Stress

Critical illness during adolescence is a potentially serious threat to the successful transition from childhood to adulthood. There is variation in the degree of threat experienced across the adolescent years. Young adolescents are less troubled by enforced dependency and better able to permit their parents and others to care for them. Middle adolescents (14–18 years of age) tolerate illness the least well, because their drive for independence is at its peak. Older adolescents have often achieved sufficient maturity to tolerate some temporary dependence and are individually secure enough to use their families for support (Hunsberger, 1989).

Young and middle adolescents experience anxiety related to physical appearance, function, and mobility when ill. Older adolescents fear that illness will disrupt their career and other future goals. All are distressed by disruption of their usual lifestyle. Fear of death is pervasive across the adolescent years.

The PICU Environment

Although adolescence marks the development of adult-like responses to distress, such reactions take years in development. However, even at the beginning of the adolescent years, anxiety related to the critical care environment is most often related to realistic, rather than fantasized, worries. Adolescent patients can recognize and control anxiety and are almost universally able to maintain self-control despite concerns for disfigurement, disability, and death. In fact, the potential for loss of self-control is a predominant fear.

Staff communication about personal topics within earshot of the adolescent is particularly distressing because it depersonalizes the individual patient. Individual identity is threatened, particularly if the adolescent needs to communicate with staff. Adolescents may be embarrassed by overhearing details of the personal lives of staff who are caring for them.

Like adult patients, any adolescent ill enough to require admission to a PICU will manifest an emotional response. Anxiety and fear are usual emotional responses to critical illness and intensive care. Adolescents realize there is a danger of death. Anxiety may be evidenced by agitation, excessive verbosity, or complete withdrawal (Kleck, 1984). High anxiety is not tolerable, usually resulting in some degree of denial, which is indicated by withdrawal or regression.

When illness and intensive care are prolonged, anxiety is often followed by despondency and depression. When anxiety is relieved by adaptation, an underlying despondency or depression is manifested. Again, behaviors at both ends of the spectrum may be noted. Some adolescent patients deal with stress and depression by constant talk, whereas others withdraw. Serious illness requiring lengthy critical care is also associated with disorientation.

Withdrawing from contact with others may also

indicate feelings of depersonalization. Adolescents in the PICU are isolated from their important peer associations and activities and are at high risk for such feelings.

Like adult patients, adolescents require orientation to their environment, as well as to date and time. Some relief of anxiety and distress is provided by verbal explanation of what is happening, how it is anticipated to feel, what it will accomplish, and how long it will last. Even when patients cannot communicate, explanation is reliably provided. When adolescent patients are able to communicate, they are encouraged to verbalize questions and concerns. Some may need their caregivers to broach the topics of anxiety, fear, or feelings of sadness to begin to express their own concerns. Positive reassurance can be therapeutic.

Feelings of depersonalization are avoided when staff attend to the emotional needs of patients with the same energy and commitment demonstrated in the intense care of physical needs. Willingness to talk and listen to patients and know them as individuals is essential.

Pharmacologic management of anxiety and psychiatric consultation may be indicated for adolescents who have marked emotional reactions in the PICU.

Separation

Separation from home and family is usually tolerated without distress by adolescents who require hospitalization. Separation from the peer group, however, causes significant anxiety. Illness and hospitalization are clear deviations from the accepted group norm. Adolescents feel deprived when separated from their peers and are threatened by potential loss of status within their social groups, particularly if they have achieved leadership status and must relinquish that position. The absence of peer acceptance and approval may threaten emerging individual identity.

Chronic illness ties adolescents to their families—physically, emotionally, and financially. Some respond with active rebellion, whereas others are passive and overdependent. The chronically ill adolescent in the PICU may react to separation from the family more intensely than others. The stress of critical illness may delay progress at learning to manage a chronic illness independently, a vital transition for the chronically ill teenager.

When very ill, adolescents are unlikely to manifest distress at separation from their peers or family. During recovery, evidence of distress may become apparent. Once fears of death are allayed, adolescents' thoughts turn toward the important people in their lives, and feelings of deprivation and despondency are detected. Separation anxiety may be evidenced by withdrawal, uncooperativeness, and ambivalence about visitors, especially family members. Defense mechanisms may mask the verbal acknowledgment of the importance of peers or family, because the adolescent is adept at intellectualization and rationalization. Regressed behavior is not uncommon

among chronically ill adolescents who may, for example, want their parents to stay with them until they fall asleep.

Mitigating the stress associated with separation from peers and family members can be accomplished in several ways. Assuring contact with parents is important, but liberal visitation guidelines are recommended, particularly if an adolescent has a prolonged PICU stay. Peer visitation is a significant event for these patients.

Critical illness may exacerbate overdependency for chronically ill adolescents. When survival itself is at question, independence is a low priority. Although regression is tolerated during serious illness, recuperation provides an opportunity to encourage adolescents and parents to pursue physical and emotional independence.

Pain and Intrusive Procedures

Adolescents are likely to react to pain with stoic self-control when they are well. Pain is an acknowledged part of illness or surgery and is a concern identified by adolescents anticipating surgery (Stevens, 1986). Although approaching adult-like responses to stress, many adolescents lack the maturity for consistently mature responses. Vacillation between maintenance of self-control and a wide range of behavioral responses to pain is common when adolescents are ill.

Adolescents are particularly sensitive about intrusive procedures. Vulnerability increases when illness is severe, hospitalization lengthy, and the number of invasive procedures required is high.

Pain and intrusive procedures threaten adolescents' ability to maintain self-control. As a consequence, teenagers are uniquely intolerant of delays in pain management and may become verbally aggressive and angry if they do not think that their reports of pain are taken seriously. Regression is a fairly common response to severe or long-term pain, leaving the adolescent unable to maintain typical self-control or very dependent on others for comforting. Some adolescents, however, remain stoic throughout illness and an intensive care hospitalization. Physiologic responses to pain are carefully assessed.

Anxiety related to intrusive procedures may be evidenced by verbosity or the use of humor if adolescents in the PICU can verbalize. It is unusual for them to specifically relate their anxiety to procedures, however, because most attempt to appear stoic and undisturbed. Tense facial expression or clenching the fists is common as adolescents struggle to maintain self-control during procedures. Adolescents may attempt to delay either painful or intrusive procedures to maintain or regain self-control. Excessive delay may actually increase anxiety.

If physically able, adolescents benefit from the ability to manage their own pain with the use of patient controlled analgesia (PCA). PCA reduces adolescents' sense of powerlessness and enhances control, because they are in charge of their pain management. Adolescents benefit from education about the medications they are receiving and the effects they can anticipate from their administration.

Painful or intrusive procedures are better tolerated when adolescents are prepared for their occurrence. Adolescents are informed fully regarding diagnostic and therapeutic procedures and tests, including why they are performed, how long they will take, and what will be felt during the procedure. Assuring privacy during procedures is important.

Loss of Self-control

Maintenance of self-control among hospitalized adolescents is threatened by alterations in typical daily routines, fear of the unknown aspects of hospitalization, physical restrictions, enforced dependency, and loss of productive roles. All of these factors, as well as illness itself, are obstacles to attaining independence and individual identity. Dependence and depersonalization may result in the adolescent being unable to maintain self-control.

Adolescents generally adapt to brief interruption of their typical routines without difficulty, but are threatened by the possibility that their lifestyle may be permanently altered. Anxiety is produced by the fact that seriously ill adolescents can do little to exert control over the events happening around and to them. Routines for every aspect of life are altered and controlled. Loss of control of daily routines forces dependency on an age group struggling for independence.

Fear of unknown events and procedures in the critical care environment is stressful. For some, the uncertainty of treatment efficacy and eventual recovery is even more significant, heightening anxiety. Serious illness forces adolescents to reexamine their present and future lifestyle, as well as their potential for adult fulfillment.

Adolescents are unlikely to be unduly anxious about brief periods of immobility or limited physical restrictions. Most procedures do not require restraint if the adolescent is aware of events that will occur and is sufficiently cognizant to cooperate. Immobility that persists beyond a brief period or repetitive procedures may cause distress for even the most resilient adolescent.

Although serious illness necessitates a great deal of dependence, it is unlikely to be distressing during the acute period of physiologic dysfunction. As recovery occurs, depersonalization and continued dependency evoke stronger responses from adolescents, who are deterred from emancipation from their families and the establishment of independence and identity.

The roles that adolescents play in their peer group, as well as in their families, are instrumental in the development of individual identity. Productivity prepares adolescents for adult roles within society. Serious illness results in the loss of both the status achieved in group roles and the productivity such roles provide.

Critical illness or injury permits adolescents to temporarily release self-control to others. However, if recovery does not provide opportunity for reexerting control, most adolescents will demonstrate distress. For example, overly rigid hospital routines or regulations are likely to result in resentment, anger, and hostility as adolescent patients protest the alterations in their usual lifestyle. The unknown or uncertain aspects of illness and treatment heighten anxiety. Anxiety may result in withdrawal from contact with others; camouflage of true feelings in humor, intellectualization, or rationalization; or uncooperativeness, acting out, and other regressive behaviors.

Adolescents facing lengthy immobilization often are angry and aggressive during the early stages of dealing with their illness or injury. Withdrawal and depression often follow, particularly when dependence on others is necessary. Enforced dependence, and the concomitant depersonalization experienced by adolescents, may result in episodes of resentment, anger, and acting out from an otherwise withdrawn teenager. Loss of productive roles contributes to feelings of depersonalization and may exacerbate depression or anxiety.

Adolescents are assisted to maintain self-control when hospital routines are sufficiently flexible and patients are allowed to exercise as much control as possible over daily activities. Setting flexible limits and encouraging participation in self-care as adolescents recover restore a measure of control over daily routines. Adolescents are also provided with opportunities to participate in setting goals, planning their care, and choosing options to promote self-control and independence.

Preparation for events and procedures in the hospital is specific, detailed, accurate, and scientific when adolescents are the audience. As progress across adolescence is made, teenagers develop the cognitive skills necessary for informed consent for treatment and procedures (Erlen, 1987). The stage of formal operations encourages a sense of internal control and recognition that decision-making authority about events in an individual's life should lie with the individual. Formal operations permit teenagers to project into the future, consider cause-and-effect relationships, and identify consequences of proposed actions and choices. Informed consent requires that adolescents receive sufficient information, comprehend it, and voluntarily consent. Adolescents are assured opportunities to exert control over decisions regarding their treatment regimen.

Adolescents need to express frustration via physical activity. Innovation is necessary to develop ways for adolescents to move out of bed and around the unit as they recover from serious illness. Physical and occupational therapy are encouraged to build independence, strength, and mobility during recuperation. When immobilization is the permanent consequence of illness or injury, significant adaptation is required. Long-term rehabilitation deals with the emotional aspects of this life change, as well as its physical consequences.

Assignment of consistent caregivers for adolescent patients in the PICU can mitigate some of the depersonalization and dependence experienced by patients there. Trust is established and a personal, but respectful, relationship develops, providing an atmosphere for optimal recognition of individual identity. Most adolescents strive to regain self-control and independence after serious illness has enforced dependency. Their efforts are complimented and supported.

When serious or chronic illness prolongs enforced dependency, some adolescents regress, because the need to be cared for outweighs the need to be independent. Regression is a necessary and acceptable response to severe threats to the establishment of individual identity and independence. Extensive intervention is required to promote developmental progress.

During recuperation, peer contact and support, in addition to family support, is important for adolescent patients. Opportunities for friends to call or visit are assured. Flexible limits on visitation are necessary to assure adolescents necessary support during a period of feeling they do not belong. Self-esteem and independence are fostered in the peer group.

SPECIAL PROBLEMS IN CRITICAL CARE NURSING OF CHILDREN

The Chronically Critically Ill Child

Advances in technology continue to result in decreased mortality among the most seriously ill infants and children. However, no small number of lives are saved without extended critical care hospitalization and, for some, continued dependence on technology. The Presidential Task Force on Technology Dependent Children (1988) gauged that some 2300 to 17,000 children in the United States were dependent on ventilator assistance, parenteral nutrition, intravenous medications, or other respiratory or nutritional support. Feldman and coworkers (1993) examined the incidence and etiology of hospitalization longer than 30 days for children younger than age 3 years outside the neonatal intensive care unit at a children's hospital. They reported that 2 percent of the inpatient population were infants and children who required lengthy hospitalization and that nearly one third required technologic assistance at the time of discharge. The hospital stays for the children identified represented 23 percent of the patient days for children from newborn to 3 years and 11 percent of the total patient days for children of all ages. Chronically ill children are frequently patients in the PICU.

Children who require lengthy intensive care are often the sickest and smallest patients. Chronically ill children who require intensive care present special

issues in the PICU. Their social and emotional needs are challenging, as are the needs of their families. The life experiences of children who require extended hospitalization are distorted and put them at risk for developmental and emotional sequelae (Rae-Grant, 1985). This section briefly examines the impact of chronic illness on developing children from the perspective of their care in the PICU.

Impact of Chronic Illness on the Child

Chronic illness influences the physical, cognitive, social, and emotional development of children. The nature of the symptoms, treatment, and prognosis determines, in large part, its impact on the child. When specialized care or frequent hospitalizations are required, children face separation from their parents, home, and other social environments. Experiences in the hospital, particularly in the critical care unit, are unlikely to be of a nature that furnishes experiences necessary for developmental progress. Although the critically ill patient obviously appropriately adopts a "sick role" and illness behaviors, children with chronic illness are unable to fully recover and discard the sick role.

Chronic illness shapes a child's foundation and limits developmental opportunities at every age and stage. During infancy, repeated hospitalizations may interfere with parent-infant attachment and the acquisition of trust. Chronically ill toddlers and preschoolers may experience stifling limitations in social, cognitive, and physical development. Acquiring autonomy and initiative is difficult, at best, because illness erects barriers to beginning independence. Preschoolers who are chronically ill become aware that they are different from their peers. By school age, chronically ill children are described by their parents as lacking skills for social interaction and self-care, noncompliant, aggressive, and self-destructive (Beavers et al., 1986). School is often a source of distress for children with chronic illnesses, rather than an environment in which they thrive. Academic and social progress may be interrupted frequently to manage the illness. Peers are most often unsupportive, if not unkind. Adolescents with a chronic illness may be blocked from establishing independence and forced to consider limitations on educational, vocational, and social plans.

Impact of Chronic Illness on the Family

Chronic illness affects many aspects of family life: financial, social, emotional, behavioral, and cognitive. Chronic illness brings increased expenses, tasks, and commitments to the family. Social isolation may occur; chronically ill children may cause anxiety and confusion in social settings when others are uncertain how to interact with the child or family.

Parents often have feelings of guilt, blame, and personal grief at their child's physical vulnerability.

The grieving process is continual and often reactivated by either new issues in the child's condition or new developmental stages, such as school entry. Hospitalization, when required, often brings renewed or additional sadness. Mastering guilt and grief is necessary for each parent's emotional well-being and influences the self-esteem and emotional development of the chronically ill child and siblings.

Families need to be knowledgeable about the chronically ill child's illness, treatment, and expected course. Patterns of daily living and family activities require modification to accommodate treatment regimens.

Impact of Critical Care

When acute illness necessitates intensive care for a child and family already stressed by chronic illness, the potential for distress is high. Special attention to the child's and family's care in the PICU can mitigate distress. Chronically ill children in the PICU require an environment that will support and protect the child and family's growth and development. Lengthy critical care hospitalization, especially for those children who are technology-dependent, necessitates care by a multidisciplinary team. Managing and directing the multidisciplinary team is the shared responsibility of the primary physician and nurse. Nurses identify specific patient and family outcomes and plan comprehensive strategies with many disciplines to make steady progress toward outcome achievement.

Care for the Child

Environmental factors in the PICU affect care of long-term or chronically ill patients. When the child's care does not necessitate continuous surveillance and frequent intervention, the patient's location in the PICU can be reconsidered. Locating the child's bed in a corner, near a window and out of the busiest area of the unit, offers some protection from the environment.

Developmentally supportive care is enhanced by the involvement of other disciplines. Infants and children who require lengthy hospitalization may meet the criteria for early intervention services based on federal law (PL 99-457) and state regulations. Ideally these services begin in the hospital (Feldman et al., 1993). Nurses are knowledgeable about services that will benefit chronically ill children and are in a position to consult with psychologists and social workers to ensure appropriate consultation and referral.

Common responses to the demands of a chronic illness are regression to an earlier and safer period of development or inability to progress in development. Critical illness necessitates some degree of regression, but motivation for developmental progress may be nearly nonexistent even during recovery. Exclusion from activities, learned inferiority, and nonacceptance take a toll on the emotional well-being of children who are chronically ill (Siemon, 1987). Table

2–5 lists patterns of responses commonly identified among chronically ill children and outlines needs that, if met on a consistent basis, encourage adaptive responses. At a minimum, the critical care staff encourages adaptation.

Table 2–5. RESPONSES TO CHRONIC ILLNESS FROM CHILDREN

Child's Behavior	Child's Needs
Fear	
Frightened of everything	Self-confidence
Exaggerated normal fears	Independence
Few friends	
Gives up easily	
Fantasy	
Creates imaginary world	Reality
Escapes undesired thoughts	Problem-solving skills
Neglects real needs	
Helpless, dependent	
Alone	
Invisibility	
Unobtrusive	Security
Indifferent, passive	Structure
Withdrawn	Encouragement
Humor	
Appears happy	Express anger, sadness
Keeps everyone laughing	Closeness
Insecure, immature	Independence
Fears others do not like him/her	
Keeps a distance from others	
Overinvolvement in Medical Care	
Aloof, rigidly independent	Express anger, depression
Adept at medical jargon	Normal peer relationships
Verbally assertive	
Pleases others	
Friendships with healthcare personnel	
Explosive Anger	
Temper tantrums and rages	Understand anger
Clings to others	Reasonable expectations
Blames others, jealous of others	
Believes life is unfair	
Irresponsible	
Giving Up	
Unmotivated, helpless	See personal potential
Ostracized by peers	Realistic goals
Blames others	Gain attention in achievement
Expects to be waited on	
Overdependence	
Extreme awareness of limitations	Encouragement, praise
Afraid to try	Independence
Fear of failing	

Data from Siemon, M. (1987). Patterns of impairment: Cognitive/emotional. In M.H. Rose & R.B. Thomas (Eds.). *Children with chronic conditions: Nursing in a family and community context.* Orlando, FL: Grune & Stratton; Stevens, M. (1986). Adolescents' perceptions of stressful events during hospitalization. *Journal of Pediatric Nursing*, 1, 303–313.

Table 2–6. THE FAMILY POWER RESOURCES MODEL

Power Resource/Definition	Interventions
Positive Self-Concepts	
Family emphasis on the normality of the sick child	Recognize coping skills Support maintenance of "normalcy"
Physical Strength and Reserve	
Family physical functioning, strength of the marriage, strength of sibling support, health of the family system	Promote family involvement in child's care Promote parent/child control
Psychological Stamina	
Psychological strength and resiliency of individual family members and the family system	Encourage family sharing of the child's illness Divide and share family tasks
Support Networks	
Significant others in the community, parent groups, social services	Identify sources of strength Maximize support systems
Energy	
Capacity to do work	Assure adequate nutrition, rest, equitable distribution of labor
Knowledge	
Information, realistic view of the child's situation	Provide detailed, up-to-date information Provide question and answer sessions
Motivation	
Spiritual or philosophical orientation that overcomes inevitable losses, maximizes potential and develops positive self-esteem	Provide support Recognize achievements Focus on the present Support family decisions

Adapted from Ferraro, A.R., & Longo, D.C. (1985). Nursing care of the family with a chronically ill, hospitalized child: An alternative approach. *Image: Journal of Nursing Scholarship, 17,* 77–81.

Care for the Family

Families are not only an asset to the chronically ill child in the PICU but also are a crucial source of support. However, when their child requires hospitalization, parents often experience conflict with staff. When parents care for a chronically ill child at home, they must become knowledgeable and skillful in areas of the child's care that are within the scope of practice of professional healthcare providers. In fact, an estimated 70 to 90 percent of illness episodes in families with a chronically ill child are handled at home, outside the formal healthcare system (Anderson, 1981). Clearly, parents are well equipped to make management decisions for their child.

Parents' expectations for complete and accurate information are sometimes seen as excessively demanding by staff in a busy PICU. Their insistence on care being performed in a manner they designate is viewed as inappropriate or even uncooperative. Their emphasis on normal routines for their child is seen as unrealistic. Nurses who must balance the demands of more physiologically unstable patients and the expectations of parents of chronically ill patients may need assistance.

Ferraro and Longo (1985) have described a model of family power resources, including the knowledge, skills, and adaptive capacities of families coping with a chronic, disabling illness in a child. Components

of the model are summarized in Table 2–6, with suggestions for nursing interventions to strengthen the family's power resources when their chronically ill child is hospitalized. Critical care nurses may find them useful in therapeutic interventions with families of chronically ill or technology-dependent patients in the PICU.

Death in the Pediatric Intensive Care Unit

The death of a child is an intense experience and not uncommon in pediatric critical care. Knowledge of the experiences of terminally ill children (Bluebond-Langner, 1978), adult responses to terminal illness (Kübler-Ross, 1969), and theories about grief and mourning (Lindemann, 1944; Engel, 1964) guide practices in the PICU. However, it is important to note that we have little concrete information about the experiences of children who die in the intensive care setting from critical illness or injury.

Development of Concepts About Death

Children learn about death through the course of regular life events. Their understanding of death changes with age and stage of development. Children younger than 2 years of age have little awareness of death. Between the ages of 3 and 5 years, death is usually thought of as temporary and reversible, like sleep (Lonetto, 1980; Betz & Poster, 1984). Although death is seen as departure, those who have died are thought of as existing in some other place, most often in heaven, and are attributed with life processes and thoughts. Most often death is associated with old age.

School-age children gradually move toward the concept of death as permanent and irreversible when they gain experiences and exposure to death. Death is most often identified with the dead object; the process of death remains elusive for these children. Death is linked to external forces and violence or associated with illness and old age. Because death is recognized as a source of sadness, it is also characterized as dangerous, scary, or mean.

Near the end of the school years, children who are 10 to 12 years old recognize that death is universal and final. Death happens to all living things. The process of dying is identified and associated with pain. Death is fearful for children, bringing feelings of sadness and loneliness.

Adolescent cognitive development permits teens to understand death as adults do, as a final and universal experience that is intensely personal. Their capacity to think about the future allows them to consider impending death. The periods of rapid physical and emotional change that occur during adolescence are often periods of vulnerability to fears about loss. Adolescents are especially fearful about death (McCown, 1988).

Talking to Children About Death

Terminally ill children come to know that they are dying, although no one may tell them. Often they conceal this information from their families and from healthcare personnel (Waechter, 1971; Bluebond-Langner, 1978). Because children do not often tell what they know or ask questions about what will happen to them, some adults believe that children do not know they are gravely ill or, if they do, that they do not want to talk about it or that they are silent because they sense the reluctance of the adults around them to discuss the situation. However, children interpret the behavior of others to obtain a view of themselves. Even very young children are adept at identifying inconsistencies between verbal and nonverbal messages. Tearful, anxious parents and staff speaking in hushed voices come to have meaning across time and with experiences in healthcare settings.

Evidence that children are knowledgeable about death does not ease the task of talking with them about their own impending death. Few guidelines are available. Children who are dying need to share their knowledge and they need to have their parents with them. Terminally ill children conceal their knowledge of their prognosis from their parents; therefore, a logical conclusion is that their need for parental closeness is greater than their need to talk about dying. However, their preoccupation with death is evidenced in their play and art, in avoidance of talk about the future and concern that things be done immediately, in anxiety, and in the establishment of distance from others by acting out or withdrawing (Bluebond-Langner, 1978).

Children do share their knowledge if given the opportunity. They talk with those adults who listen to them carefully, taking cues from the child and answering only what is asked on the child's terms. Parents and healthcare professionals are guided by that information in a task that is monumental.

Application in the PICU

Some patients in the PICU may be physically and neurologically able to talk with parents and caregivers. Discussion with them is particularly important if, for example, an aggressive treatment plan is considered. However, many children in the critical care unit are too ill to participate in discussion. Death most often occurs only after aggressive, life-saving interventions have been attempted and ultimately are deemed futile. Death is unavoidable and imminent, expected within moments to days, and aggressive intervention no longer appropriate.

Families and caregivers may not know what to say to these children. There is no way of knowing with certainty whether they can hear or understand. Some parents continue to talk with their unconscious children, often acknowledging that the child is dying and that they are saying good-bye. Caregivers can follow the parents' lead in talking with children who are dying in the PICU. In addition, caregivers can use their personal and caring resources to provide humane care to dying children.

When aggressive intensive care is discontinued, care is directed toward maintaining the child's comfort and dignity. Dying children, if they are able, maintain some sense of control by choosing care or therapies that enable them to participate in making each day as comfortable as possible. Pain control is a priority, because fear of pain with death is common among children and is a worry for parents of dying children. Parents are logically the individuals who also benefit from participating with their child or for their child in care that assures comfort. Caring tasks may best be performed by parents, who may wish for this sort of physical closeness to their child.

Helping After a Child's Death

Parents may need practical assistance with making funeral arrangements and contacting their extended families. They face the sizeable task of talking with their other children. Siblings are best told about the death as soon as possible in truthful and clear terms. A parent or another trusted adult shares information, as well as their feelings of sadness, in a controlled manner. Some parents may find books that describe talking to children about death helpful or may be assisted by books written for them. Others may find community support groups, such as the Candlelighters or Compassionate Friends, beneficial in the mourning process. A bereavement program established by PICU caregivers for families who lost a child in death was beneficial for families and caregivers alike (Stidham, 1993).

References

Als, H., Lawhon, G., & Brown, E., et al. (1986). Individualized behavioral and environmental care for the very low birth weight preterm infant at high risk for bronchopulmonary dysplasia: Neonatal intensive care and developmental outcome. *Pediatrics,* 78, 1123–1132.

Anderson, J.M. (1981). The social construction of illness behavior: Families with a chronically ill child. *Journal of Advances in Nursing,* 6, 427–434.

Anderson, J.J. (1989). Families with preschoolers. In R.L.R. Foster, M.M. Hunsberger, & J.J.T. Anderson (Eds.). *Family-centered nursing care of children.* Philadelphia: W.B. Saunders.

Audette, M.S. (1974). The significance of regressive behavior for the hospitalized child. *Maternal-Child Nursing Journal,* 3, 31–40.

Baker, C.F. (1984). Sensory overload and noise in the ICU: Sources of environmental stress. *Critical Care Quarterly,* 7, 66–79.

Barnes, C. (1975). School-age children's recall of the intensive care unit. *ANA Clinical Sessions.* Norwalk, CT: Appleton-Century-Crofts, 73–79.

Beavers, J., Hampson, R.B., Hulgus, Y.F., & Beavers, W.R. (1986). Coping in families with a retarded child. *Family Process,* 25, 365–378.

Betz, C.L., & Poster, E.C. (1984). Children's concepts of death. *Nursing Clinics of North America,* 19, 341–349.

Bluebond-Langner, M. (1978). *The private worlds of dying children.* Princeton, NJ: Princeton University Press.

Bowlby, J. (1966). *Maternal care and mental health.* New York: Schocken Books.

Brown, G.W., & Harris, T. (1978). *Social origins of depression: A study of psychiatric disorder in women.* New York: The Free Press.

Carty, R.M. (1980). Observed behaviors of preschoolers to intensive care. *Pediatric Nursing,* 6, 21–25.

Chrisman, M., & Riehl, J. (1974). The systems-developmental stress model. In J. Riehl & C. Roy (Eds.). *Conceptual models for nursing practice.* New York: Appleton-Century-Crofts.

Coddington, R.D. (1972). The significance of life events as etiologic factors in the diseases of children, I and II. *Journal of Psychosocial Research,* 16, 7–18, 205–213.

Engel, G. (1964). Grief and grieving. *American Journal of Nursing,* 64, 93.

Erikson, E.H. (1964). *Childhood and society.* New York: W.W. Norton.

Erlen, J.A. (1987). The child's choice: An essential component in treatment decisions. *Child Health Care,* 15, 156–160.

Fagin, C. (1966). Pediatric rooming-in: Its meaning for the nurse. *Nursing Clinics of North America,* 1, 83–93.

Feldman, H.M., Ploof, D.L., Hofkosh, D., & Goehring, E.L. (1993). Developmental needs of infants and toddlers who require lengthy hospitalization. *American Journal of Diseases of Children,* 147, 211–215.

Ferber, R. (1985). *Solve your child's sleep problems.* New York: Simon & Schuster.

Ferraro, A.R., & Longo, D.C. (1985). Nursing care of the family with a chronically ill, hospitalized child: An alternative approach. *Image,* 17, 77–81.

Fiser, D.H., Stanford, G., & Dorman, D.J. (1984). Services for parental stress reduction in a pediatric ICU. *Critical Care Medicine,* 12, 504–507.

Fisher, M.E., & Moxham, P.A. (1984). ICU syndrome. *Critical Care Nurse,* 4, 39–45.

Fontaine, D.K. (1989). Measurement of nocturnal sleep patterns in trauma patients. *Heart & Lung,* 18, 402–409.

Fraiberg, S.H. (1959). *The magic years.* New York: Charles Scribner's Sons.

Ginsberg, H., & Opper, S. (1979). *Piaget's theory of intellectual development,* 2nd edition. Englewood Cliffs, NJ: Prentice-Hall.

Gorski, P.A. (1983). Premature infant behavioural and physiological responses to caregiving intervention in the intensive care nursery. In J.D. Call, E. Galenson, & R.L. Tyson (Eds.). *Frontiers in infant psychiatry.* New York: Basic Books.

Gunderson, L., & Kenner, C. (1987). Neonatal stress: Physiologic adaptation and nursing implications. *Neonatal Network,* 5, 37–42.

Harlow, H.F., & Zimmerman, R. (1965). Affectional responses of the infant monkey. In P. Mussen, J. Conger, & J. Kagan (Eds.). *Readings in child development and personality.* New York: Harper & Row.

Helton, M.C., Gordon, S.H., & Nunnery, S.L. (1980). The correlation between sleep deprivation and the intensive care unit. *Heart & Lung,* 9, 464–468.

Hill, S.R., Goetz, F.C., Fox, H.M., et al. (1956). Studies on adrenocortical and psychological responses to stress in man. *Archives of Internal Medicine,* 97, 269–298.

Holmes, T.H., & Rahe, R.H. (1967). The social readjustment rating scale. *Journal of Psychosocial Research,* 11, 213–218.

Hunsberger, M.M. (1989). Nursing care during hospitalization. In R.L.R. Foster, M.M. Hunsberger, & J.J.T. Anderson (Eds.). *Family-centered nursing care of children.* Philadelphia: W.B. Saunders.

Hurley, A., & Whelan, E.G. (1988). Cognitive development and children's perception of pain. *Pediatric Nursing,* 14, 21–24.

Jones, S.H., Fiser, D.H., & Livingston, R.L. (1992). Behavioral changes in pediatric intensive care units. *American Journal of Diseases of Children,* 146, 375–379.

Kleck, H.G. (1984). ICU syndrome: Onset, manifestations, treatment, stressors, and prevention. *Critical Care Quarterly,* 1 (1) 21–28.

Kobasa, S.C. (1979). Stressful life events, personality, and health: An inquiry into hardiness. *Journal of Perspectives on Social Psychology,* 37, 1–11.

Kübler-Ross, E. (1969). *On death and dying.* New York: Macmillan.

Lawhon, G., & Melzar, A. (1988). Developmental care of the very low birth weight infant. *Journal of Perinatal and Neonatal Nursing,* 2, 56–65.

Lazarus, R.S. (1966). *Psychological stress and the coping process.* New York: McGraw-Hill.

Lazarus, R.S., & Folkman, S. (1984). *Stress, appraisal, and coping.* New York: Springer Publishing.

Leiken, S.L. (1983). Minor's assent or dissent to medical treatment. *Journal of Pediatrics,* 102, 169–176.

Levine, M.E. (1969). The pursuit of wholeness. *American Journal of Nursing,* 69(1), 96–101.

Lindemann, E. (1944). Symptomatology and the management of acute grief. *American Journal of Psychiatry,* 101, 141–148.

Lonetto, R. (1980). *Children's conceptions of death.* New York: Springer Publishing.

Martin, R.J. (1979). Effect of supine and prone position on arterial oxygen tension in the preterm infant. *Pediatrics,* 63, 528–531.

Maslow, A.H. (1954). *Motivation and personality.* New York: Harper & Row.

Maslow, A.H. (1964). Synergy in the society and the individual. *Journal of Individual Psychology,* 20, 153–164.

Mason, J.W. (1959a). Psychological influences on the pituitary-adrenal-cortical system. *Recent Progress in Hormonal Research,* 15, 345–378.

Mason, J.W. (1959b). Visceral functions of the nervous system. *Annual Review of Physiology,* 21, 353–380.

May, J.G. (1972). A psychiatric study of a pediatric intensive therapy unit. *Clinical Pediatrics,* 11, 76–82.

McCown, D. (1988). Helping children face death in the family. *Journal of Pediatric Health Care,* 2, 14–19.

McKegney, F.P. (1966). The intensive care syndrome. *Connecticut Medicine,* 30, 633–636.

Monat, A., & Lazarus, R.S. (Eds.) (1971). *Stress and coping—an anthology.* New York: Columbia University Press.

Murphy, L.B. (1974). Coping, vulnerability, and resilience in childhood. In G.V. Coelho, D.A. Hamburg, & J.E. Adams (Eds.). *Coping and adaptation.* New York: Basic Books.

Murphy, L.B., & Moriarty, A.E. (1976). *Coping and growth*. New Haven, CT: Yale University Press.

Neugarten, B.L. (1968). *Middle age and aging: A reader in social psychology*. Chicago: University of Chicago Press.

Petrillo, M., & Sanger, S. (1980). *Emotional care of hospitalized children*. Philadelphia: J.B. Lippincott.

Piaget, J. (1952). *The origins of intelligence in children*. New York: International Universities Press.

Piaget, J. (1976). *The psychology of intelligence*. Totowa, NJ: Littlefield, Adams & Co.

Rae-Grant, Q. (1985). Psychological problems in the medically ill child. *Pediatric Clinics of North America, 8*, 653–663.

Report of the Task Force on Technology Dependent Children. (1988). US Government Printing Office, 1988–210–048/80264.

Richards, K.C., & Bairnsfather, L. (1988). A description of night sleep patterns in the critical care unit. *Heart & Lung, 17*, 35–42.

Roberts, S.L. (1976). *Behavioral concepts and the critically ill patient*. Englewood Cliffs, NJ: Prentice-Hall.

Robertson, J. (1958). *Young children in hospitals*. London: Tavistock.

Roy, Sr. C. (1971). Adaptation: a basis for nursing practice. *Nursing Outlook, 19*, 254–260.

Ruberman, W, Weinblatt, E, Goldberg, JD, et al. (1984). Psychosocial influence on mortality after myocardial infarction. *New England Journal of Medicine, 311*, 552–557.

Selye, H. (1952). *The story of the adaptation syndrome*. Montreal: Acta.

Selye, H. (1956). *The stress of life*. New York: McGraw-Hill.

Selye, H. (1971). *Hormones and resistance* I. New York: Springer Publishing.

Selye, H. (1974). *Stress without distress*. Philadelphia: J.B. Lippincott.

Selye, H. (1976a). *The stress of life* (rev. ed.). New York: McGraw-Hill.

Selye, H. (1976b). *Stress in health and disease*. Boston: Butterworth.

Siemon, M. (1987). Patterns of impairment: Cognitive/emotional. In M.H. Rose, & R.B. Thomas (Eds.). *Children with chronic conditions: Nursing in a family and community context*. Orlando, FL: Grune & Stratton.

Skipper, J.K. & Leonard, R.C. (1968). Children, stress and hospitalization. *Journal of Health and Social Behavior, 9*, 275–287.

Slota, M.C. (1988). Implications of sleep deprivation in the pediatric critical care unit. *Focus on Critical Care, 15*, 35–43.

Spitz, R.A. (1945). Hospitalism: an inquiry into the genesis of psychiatric conditions in early childhood. *Psychoanalytic Study of the Child, 1*, 53–66.

Stevens, M. (1986). Adolescents' perceptions of stressful events during hospitalization. *Journal of Pediatric Nursing, 1*, 303–313.

Stidham, G. (1993). A bereavement follow up program for families who lose a child: A new tool to foster humanism among caregivers. *AACN Clinical Issues in Critical Care Nursing, 4*, 536.

Tanner, J.M. (1962). Growth at adolescence. Oxford: Blackwell Scientific Publications.

Tecce, J.J., Friedman, S.B., & Mason, J.W. (1966). Anxiety, defensiveness, and 17-hydroxycorticosteroid excretion. *Journal of Nervous and Mental Disease, 141*, 549–554.

Thomas, A., Chess, S., & Birch, H. (1970). The origin of personality. *Scientific American, 223*, 102–109.

Thompson, R.H. (1985). *Psychological research on pediatric hospitalization and health care* (pp. 108–119). Springfield, IL: Charles C Thomas.

Vessey, J.A., Farley, J.A., & Risom, L.R. (1991). Iatrogenic developmental effects of pediatric intensive care. *Pediatric Nursing, 17*, 229–232.

Waechter, E. (1971). Children's awareness of fatal illness. *American Journal of Nursing, 71*, 1168–1171.

Washington, G.T. (1990). Trust: A critical element in critical care nursing. *Focus, 17*, 418–421.

CHAPTER **3**

The Impact of the Critical Care Experience on the Family

MARTHA A. Q. CURLEY
ELAINE C. MEYER

FAMILY-CENTERED CARE

CHANGING AMERICAN FAMILY DEMOGRAPHICS

BASIS FOR INTERVENTION

SOURCES OF PARENTAL STRESS
Crisis Theory
Stress Unique to the PICU
Trajectory of Parental Stress
Identified Parental Needs and Coping
  Strategies

INTERVENTION STRATEGIES

NURSING MUTUAL PARTICIPATION MODEL OF CARE
Admission: Critical Time for Intervention
Daily Bedside Contact

FAMILY CONTEXT OF CHILDHOOD CRITICAL ILLNESS
Professional Relationships
Collaborative Relationships With Psychosocial
  Support Staff
Preparing for Patient Transfer
Coping With Bereavement Issues

SUMMARY

"It is a good professional rule to let a mother work at her own level, supporting her in her skills and understanding and bolstering her confidence in herself, quietly supplementing her effort instead of giving detailed directions and cautions which may undermine her confidence."

JAMES ROBERTSON (1958)

Inherent in the practice of pediatric critical care nursing is helping families to endure the stressful and unspeakable experience of their infant's or child's critical illness. This humanistic aspect of practice is essential so that families can continue to function in vitally important roles that are therapeutic to them and their critically ill children. This chapter reviews the principles of family-centered care and

the rationale for psychosocial intervention in the intensive care setting. We then review the research on PICU-related parental issues, the trajectory of parental stress, and parental needs during the critical illness and hospitalization of their children. The unique role of nursing in helping families to alleviate stress and to cope is emphasized. The Nursing Mutual Participation Model of Care is presented, which provides a framework for supportive psychosocial interventions for parents of critically ill children. This is followed by a brief review of issues of particular concern to nursing staff including the support of other family members, transition from the PICU to the general unit, bereavement in the context of the intensive care setting, and referral and collaboration with ancillary psychosocial support personnel.

FAMILY-CENTERED CARE

The parental role in the care of hospitalized infants and children has been an evolving process. Not too long ago, parents were neither welcomed nor allowed in pediatric inpatient units primarily because of concerns about infection control. Bowlby (1952, 1973) and Robertson's (1958) classic work describing the separation trauma experienced by young children in hospitals—protest, despair, then detachment—supported the hypothesis that parent-child separation is detrimental to the child and to the parent-child relationship. We now acknowledge that parents are crucial to a child's healthy psychosocial and physical well-being and that parental support during a stressful event, especially critical care hospitalization, is essential for the child's continued socioemotional growth and development.

Family-centered care is currently considered best practiced in pediatric healthcare settings. The central tenet of family-centered care is that the family is the constant in the child's life and, ultimately, holds the responsibility for managing the child's physical, social, and emotional needs (Shelton & Stepanek, 1994). Thus, parents are now encouraged to stay and continue parenting during the entire period of their infant or child's hospitalization.

The Association for the Care of Children's Health (ACCH) has delineated several principles of family-centered care to guide clinical practice (Table 3–1). Family-centered care is a philosophy of care that recognizes, respects, and supports the essential role of the family in the lives of children. It is a philosophy that acknowledges and supports diversity among families—diversity that encompasses varied family structures and sociocultural backgrounds; family goals and priorities; strategies and actions; as well as diversity in family support, service, and informational needs (Ahmann, 1994). Family-centered care strives to support families in their natural caregiving roles by building upon their unique strengths as individuals and families. It is a philosophy that views parents and professionals as equals in a partnership committed to excellence at all levels of healthcare (Shelton & Stepanek, 1994).

Although pediatric nurses have long recognized the fundamental importance of caring for infants and children within a family context, the operationalization or "how to" of family-centered care in the clinical setting is less clear, and is often based on intuition and untested assumptions with few empirical guidelines (Meyer & Bailey, 1993; Rushton, 1990). At times, particularly in intensive care settings, parents may be only marginally involved in the decision-making process and care of their children. Parents may be considered as "visitors," thus forcing a temporary or perhaps permanent disruption in the parent-child relationship. Rushton (1990) has identified several barriers to family-centered care in pediatric critical care settings. Barriers include the highly technologic environment, ethical dilemmas, the range in patient population from hyperacute to

Table 3–1. THE KEY ELEMENTS OF FAMILY-CENTERED CARE

Incorporating into policy and practice the recognition that the *family is the constant* in a child's life, while the service systems and support personnel within those systems fluctuate

Facilitating *family/professional collaboration* at all levels of hospital, home, and community care
  Care of an individual child
  Program development, implementation, evaluation, and evolution
  Policy formation

Exchanging complete and unbiased information between families and professionals in a supportive manner at all times

Incorporating into policy and practice the recognition and *honoring of cultural diversity*, strengths, and individuality within and across all families, including *ethnic, racial, spiritual, social, economic, educational, and geographic diversity*

Recognizing and respecting *different methods of coping* and implementing comprehensive policies and programs that provide *developmental, educational, emotional, environmental, and financial supports* to meet the diverse needs of families

Encouraging and facilitating *family-to-family support* and networking

Ensuring that *hospital, home, and community service and support systems* for children needing specialized health and developmental care and their families are *flexible, accessible, and comprehensive* in responding to diverse family-identified needs

Appreciating families as families and children as children, recognizing that they possess a wide range of strengths, concerns, emotions, and aspirations beyond their need for specialized health and developmental services and support.

From Shelton, T.L., & Stepanek, J.S. (1994). *Family-centered care for children needing specialized health and developmental services,* Association for the Care of Children's Health, 7910 Woodmont Avenue, Suite 300, Bethesda, MD 20814, 301/654-6549.

chronically critically ill, staff shortages, professional attitudes, the intensive care organizational culture, and economic trends.

Paternalistic attitudes and behaviors can be prevalent within the PICU setting, with the underlying assumption that parents are incapable of complex decision-making under the circumstances. There may be the tendency to "protect" parents and to present a "consistent picture," which, although well-intended, limits parents from fully participating as equal-status partners in the decision-making process and care of their child (Meyer & Bailey, 1993; Zaner & Bliton, 1991). Information that is incomplete, biased, or otherwise nonunderstandable diminishes the parents' status relative to professionals, and cripples full participation in healthcare decision-making. Bogdan and coworkers (1982) address the complexities of parent-professional communication within the intensive care setting and advise that professionals be "honest but not cruel." Parental needs, their role with their critically ill child, and the basis for establishing therapeutic nurse-parent relationships are aspects of family-centered care that continue to present challenges to pediatric critical care nurses.

CHANGING AMERICAN FAMILY DEMOGRAPHICS

Any discussion of family-centered care would be incomplete without recognition of the great variability among families with respect to family structure, function, and role responsibilities. The "traditional" two-parent family is no longer the norm in which mother served as child caregiver, nurturer, and homemaker, and father served as economic breadwinner, protector, and disciplinarian. Indeed, many of our assumptions about family membership and organization are no longer applicable and must be adjusted to effectively serve and support children and their families. It is recommended that in psychosocial assessments nurses inquire directly about family member composition, parental role assignments, employment, and childcare arrangements rather than inaccurately assuming traditional family structure and function.

Consider the following facts as evidence of changing American family demographic characteristics (Shelton et al., 1987). It is estimated that only 22% of American families are structured in which the father is employed outside of the home and the mother stays at home full-time. One in five families currently has a female head of household. Twenty-five percent of all infants are born to unwed mothers. Approximately 500,000 infants each year are born to teenage mothers. Twenty-one percent of our nation's children are being reared amid poverty conditions. Chronic, persistent poverty is overrepresented among minority children and families in the United States (United States Current Population Reports, 1991). From conception, minority children are directly or indirectly exposed to a host of problems associated with socioeconomic disadvantage, including differential access to healthcare, residential segregation, unsafe neighborhoods and violence, substandard housing, and parental unemployment or underemployment (Garcia Coll et al., 1995). As further evidence of the changing parental role responsibilities within families, approximately 73% of all mothers with children between the ages of 6 and 13 years are employed outside of the home.

The projections of population growth for the next millennium emphasize the need for healthcare providers to understand the parenting processes and family characteristics among ethnic and minority families. Demographers project that the proportion of minority children and families will continue to increase over the next 20 years, partially the result of immigration and partially because of higher fertility rates in those groups (United States Bureau of Census, 1989, 1990). African-Americans currently comprise approximately 12% of the population, and constitute the largest ethnic minority group in the country. Hispanic Americans now constitute approximately 8% of the population but are projected to become the largest minority group by the turn of the century.

The values, attitudes, and parenting behaviors of ethnic and minority parents vary widely and influence their experience and coping with childhood critical illness and intensive care hospitalization. Factors that are important to consider include the family's cultural heritage and ancestral world views, language preference, degree of acculturation, access to societal institutions, socioeconomic status, exposure to poverty, and other life stressors in the context of racism, prejudice, and discrimination (Garcia Coll et al., 1995). It is beyond the scope of this chapter to fully discuss issues relevant to changing demographic characteristics of American families and ethnic and minority families, but several recent reviews are available (Lynch & Hanson, 1992; Harrison et al., 1990; McLoyd, 1990).

BASIS FOR INTERVENTION

It is simply impossible to care for infants and children without caring for them in the context of their families. From a family systems perspective, family members are interconnected and, consequently, events that befall a single member affect all family members (Berger, 1978; von Bertalanffy, 1968; Bowen, 1978; Minuchin, 1974; Watzlawick et al., 1967). Although infants and children can be physically separated from their parents, emotionally and legally, under ordinary circumstances, they cannot. Mahler and colleagues (1975) proposed that mothers and infants are psychologically inseparable until completion of the separation-individuation process, which occurs at about 3 years of age. She notes that "the biological birth of the human infant and the psychological birth of the individual are not coincident in time. The former is a dramatic, observable, and well-circumscribed event; the latter a slowly unfolding intrapsychic process." Mahler notes that developmental readiness for independent functioning is the driving force behind this normal process.

Historically, parents have served as the primary decision-makers for their infants and children (Zaner & Bliton, 1991). From a legal perspective, parents who have custody must provide consent for their child's procedures. For parents to provide informed consent, they must understand their child's condition and the proposed treatment plan and procedures, and must have the opportunity to ask questions.

In general, critical illness is extremely stress-provoking for infants, children, and their families. Parents are forced, perhaps for the first time, to be separated from their child and to confront the possibility or actual mortality of their offspring. Intensive care hospitalization violates the parents' usual role in caring for and protecting their child, which may be experienced by parents as displacement, enforced passivity, and profound helplessness. Circumstances surrounding the child's admission (e.g., accident, planned surgery, new diagnosis) and the family's previous experience with illness and hospitalization influence the parental experience of stress and coping responses (Rothstein, 1980). The most prominent sources of parental stress include the fear of death, brain damage, and physical handicap (Miles, 1979; Youngblut & Jay, 1991). Specific fears depend upon the child's illness characteristics including acuity, condition, and prognosis. Uncertainty, that is, ambiguity, lack of clarity, conflicting information, and unpredictability over various aspects of the illness or outcome can also be extremely stress-provoking for parents (Comoroff & Maguire, 1981; Mishel, 1983; Turner et al., 1990).

Parental anxiety and stress may be transferred to the infant or child through what Skipper and Leonard (1968) first described as the "emotional contagion" hypothesis. Infants and children can be exquisitely sensitive to the emotions and moods of their parents. Children's moods often reflect their own internal states, as well as the feelings of their parents. Nursing care that facilitates adaptive functioning in the parents will, theoretically, decrease both parents' and child's emotional disequilibrium and stress.

The crisis inherent in hospitalization can severely impair parental sense of confidence and control, thereby compromising parental coping and performance. Hebb (1972) described the relationship between stress and behavioral functioning as an inverted U-shaped curve. That is, moderate degrees of stress are related to optimal behavioral functioning and performance, and very low and very high degrees of stress are related to poor functioning and performance. Thus, helping parents to reduce their own levels of stress into the moderate range enables parents to better fulfill their natural parenting roles, which can be therapeutically useful at the bedside (Wolfer & Visintainer, 1975).

Effective parental functioning can be both supportive and stabilizing to critically ill children. We now have some preliminary evidence that supports the therapeutic value of parental involvement in the PICU environment. For example, Mitchell and colleagues (1985) noted that parental stroking reduced children's intracranial pressure (ICP). Compared with investigator touch, the researchers noted an occasional, rather profound decrease in the ICP with apparent stabilization following parental touch. Similarly, increased parental caregiving and visitation with preterm infants in the neonatal intensive care unit has been found to improve weight gain and reduce the length of hospitalization (Zeskind & Iacino, 1984). Nursing research studies have also supported "kangaroo" care, in which mothers have early and regular skin-to-skin contact with their preterm infants, and its positive effects on neonatal growth and development (Anderson, 1991).

SOURCES OF PARENTAL STRESS

The critical illness of an infant or child is clearly recognized as stressful to parents. Understanding the basis and progression of that stress is necessary

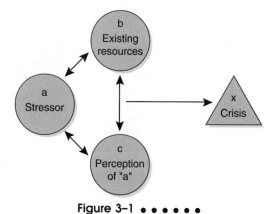

Figure 3–1 ● ● ● ● ● ●
ABCX model of crisis.

so that care can be focused to help parents modulate PICU-related stress. The nature of the nurse-family relationship can be instrumental in reducing the stress experienced by parents of critically ill children, enabling parents to function effectively in their supportive and therapeutic roles with their children.

Crisis Theory

Hill's (1949) ABCX model of crisis provides a basis for understanding the individual responses and needs of parents of critically ill infants and children (Fig. 3–1). Hill described family crises as those situations that create a sense of sharpened insecurity or that block the usual patterns of action and/or call for new ones. Three interacting variables determine whether and to what degree an event becomes a crisis (X) for a family. The variables are the hardship of the situation or the event itself (A); the family's crisis-meeting resources such as role structure, flexibility, and previous history with crises (B); and the meaning the family ascribes to the event according to their goals, sociocultural background, and religious affiliation (C).

Thus, the ABCX model of crisis can help to explain individual differences among family members and why family members have different perceptions, needs, and coping styles when confronting similar illnesses in their children. It is important to note that parental responses to the PICU admission of their child are not well predicted by objective measures of the child's severity of illness (Youngblut & Shiao, 1992). Rather, parental perceptions of the child's illness and hospitalization appear to have greater utility in understanding and predicting parental responses and coping. Hospitalization often precipitates changes in a family's social support network and views of themselves as protector and nurturer, and disrupts the balance between available resources and presenting demands (Broome, 1985).

Expanding upon Hill's work, the double ABCX model proposed by McCubbin and Patterson (1983) incorporates post-crises events that may affect family stress and coping over time (Fig. 3–2). The double ABCX model provides a useful conceptual model for families of chronically critically ill children who require ongoing treatment and periodic hospitalization. This model includes the cumulative nature or pile-up of demands for change within a family as the crisis extends over time (aA); family system resources that may include family members, the family unit, and the community (bB); and the family's perception of the illness-related experience, which includes the family's definition of the major stressor event, the meaning of the resulting hardships, and the family's effort to redefine the event (cC). The resultant crisis (X) may be perceived differently by family members as an opportunity, challenge, or an overwhelming burden. Coping strategies, which are defined as the cognitive, behavioral, and/or emotional processes that individuals use to adapt to the demands of stressful and associated events, result from an interaction between aA, bB, and cC.

Through cognitive appraisal of the perceived meaning of the event, a crisis sets forth basic adaptive tasks to which varied coping skills can be applied (Moos, 1986). Five major adaptive tasks to be confronted in managing crises have been identified (Table 3–2). Coping skills focus upon the meaning of the crisis, the reality of the crisis, or the emotions associated with the crisis. Parents of critically ill children typically use both problem-focused and emotion-focused forms of coping almost equally (Lazarus & Folkman, 1984; Miles & Carter, 1985; LaMontagne & Pawlak, 1990). Problem-focused coping behaviors include attempting to modify or eliminate the source of stress, to deal with the tangible changes, to actively change oneself, and to develop

Table 3–2. ADAPTIVE TASKS IN MANAGING CRISES

1. Establish the meaning of and understand the personal significance of the crises
2. Confront reality and respond to the requirements of the crises
3. Sustain relationships with family and friends and others who may be helpful in resolving the crises
4. Maintain a reasonable emotional balance by managing upsetting feelings
5. Preserve a positive self-image and maintain a sense of competence and mastery

Data from Moos, R. H. (1986). *Coping with life crises: An integrated approach* (pp. 3–28). New York: Plenum Medical Books.

a more satisfying situation. Emotion-focused coping behaviors include managing the emotions aroused by the stressors. The constellation of coping strategies used by parents varies according to parental age, perception of the illness, locus of control, anxiety level, and parental involvement in caregiving activities (LaMontagne et al., 1992). Philichi (1989) noted that an important role for nurses is the identification and facilitation of the various coping strategies used by families.

Stress Unique to the PICU

Rothstein (1980) noted that the family's stress is increased when the illness is severe, when little or no preparation for hospitalization has occurred, when the etiology is unclear, and when the outcome is uncertain. Miles and Carter (1982) were the first to empirically describe parental stress in the PICU setting. They identified three major sources of stress

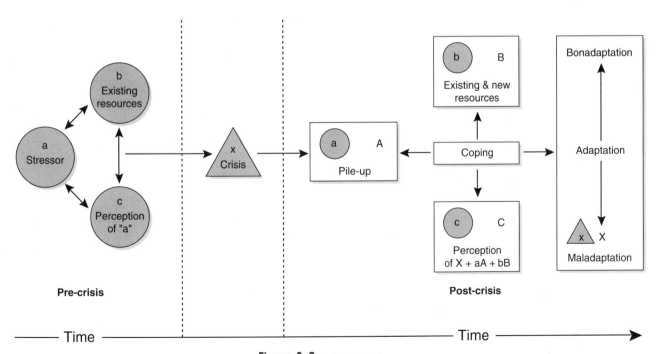

Figure 3–2 ● ● ● ● ● ●
Double ABCX model of crisis.

specifically experienced by parents of children in the PICU. These include situational variables, personal characteristics, and the PICU environment. The first two sources of stress identified by Miles and Carter are congruent with Hill's ABCX model of crises. Situational variables correspond to Hill's "A" component of the model, for example, the child's critical illness and hospitalization. Personal characteristics correspond with Hill's "B" and "C" components of the model, for example, the family's existing resources and individual perceptions of what is occurring. The third factor, environmental sources of stress, is unique to the PICU setting and potentially within nursing's role to manipulate.

Miles and Carter (1982) delineated seven dimensions of the PICU environment that parents find stressful (Table 3–3). These dimensions, derived from observational data, parent and staff nurse interviews, and the literature, form the basis of the Parental Stressor Scale: Pediatric Intensive Care Unit (PSS:PICU). These dimensions may be conceptually divided into two major categories of stress including (1) the physical aspects of the intensive care environment, and (2) the psychosocial aspects, which include parent-staff relationships and the parent-child relationship. Alterations in parental role, and the subsequent disruption in the parent-child relationship, have consistently been identified as the most stressful aspect of the PICU environment (Carter et al., 1985; Eberly et al., 1985; Curley, 1987, 1988; Curley & Wallace, 1992; Miles et al., 1984). Changes in the child's behavioral and emotional reactions, which challenge the parents' ability to know and care for their child, are ranked second in degree of stressfulness following parental role alteration. Rennick (1986) noted that when the parental role is threatened, the parent as a whole person is at risk.

Table 3–3. ENVIRONMENTAL SOURCES OF PICU-RELATED STRESS

Dimension	Items
Sights and sounds	Monitors, alarms, other sick children
Child's appearance	Puffiness, color changes, appearing cold
Child's behaviors and emotional responses	Confusion, uncooperative, crying, demanding, pain, restless, inability to talk, frightened, angry, sad
Child's procedures	Injections, tubes, suctioning, IV, pulmonary care, ventilator, incisions
Staff communication	Explaining too fast, using words that are not understood, inconsistent information, not saying what is wrong, not talking enough
Staff behavior	Not introducing themselves, laughing, joking, too many people
Parental role revision	Not seeing, not holding, not taking care of the child themselves, not visiting, not with crying child, not knowing how to help child

Data from Carter, M. C., & Miles, M. S. (1983). *Parental stressor scale: Pediatric intensive care unit.* Kansas City, KS: School of Nursing, University of Kansas.

Under usual circumstances, parents provide a safe and constructive environment for their children, which fosters their growth and development. Parents nurture, protect, educate, and advocate for their children. Parents are usually considered to be the "expert" on their child, in that they know their child better than anyone else. Although parents take for granted their usual control over their children's lives, critical illness and hospitalization often threaten that sense of control, competence, and stability (Harrison, 1983). Parents find themselves displaced from their familiar roles and, in many cases, dependent upon healthcare providers for the very survival of their child. It is not uncommon for parents to lose confidence in their ability to know or to comfort their child in a meaningful way.

Typically, the critically ill child does not look or act the same to the parent when, for example, paralyzing agents distort the child's facial features. Parent-child interactions are often compromised as a result of barriers created by life support equipment, sedating medications, precaution policies designed to reduce the risk of infection (e.g., surgical masks), prolonged hospitalization, and visitation restrictions (e.g., during change of shift) (Minde, 1984; Resnick et al., 1987). If, for example, the child responds to the parent with an increased heart rate, monitoring alarms may sound, which are not only unnerving but also serve to squelch attempts to communicate. It can be very frustrating to parents that the usual methods of comforting their child are not feasible or effective. Parents may become unsure of themselves during caregiving activities and tasks that they had previously completed hundreds of times. Not only must parents face the uncertainty of their child's critical illness, but also they may feel helpless and ineffectual because they believe that they cannot do anything to improve the situation.

Susan Jay (1977) first identified role-revision, the process of giving up the familiar role of "parent-to-a-well-child" and taking on a new role as "parent-to-an-acutely-ill-child," as a stressor to parents of critically ill infants. Jay noted that during the crisis of a sudden acute illness parents first grieve for their previous role and "need time to resolve the fact that others have their child's life in their hands, that they are no longer in control, and that they may no longer know what is best for their own child." Transition to their new role occurs by first mimicking the caretaking responses of others available to them. They watch parents of other children in the PICU and also watch nurses caring for their own infant or child. Parents slowly assume their revised identity as parent-to-an-acutely-ill-child. Variability in parental role attainment will normally occur. The spectrum is wide and ranges from abandonment, keeping a distance, passive involvement, active involvement, to hypervigilance. Although parents experience an initial grieving process, Rennick (1986) questioned whether role revision would occur in parents who spent only brief periods of time in the PICU before transfer of the infant or child to another unit.

Mothers generally report higher levels of stress than fathers; stress is associated with alterations in parental role and is the result of changes in the child's behavior and emotional reactions (Miles et al., 1984). Parents who experience an unexpected PICU admission of their child are usually more stressed than parents who are prepared for their child's admission (Eberly et al., 1985; Curley, 1987, 1988). Similarly, parents who are unprepared for the admission are more stressed than parents who had formal preparation before the experience (Carter et al., 1985).

Advanced preparation for parents whose children will be hospitalized typically includes providing parents with information about (1) a child's anticipated response to the illness/procedure based upon their developmental stage; (2) a preadmission tour, informal interview, or information session; (3) preadmission parent-child interaction guidelines; and (4) printed resources for the child and parent (Pass & Pass, 1987). Miles and Mathes (1991) noted that parents of critically ill children were seldom prepared for the perceived alterations in the parent-child relationship, which is the most stressful aspect of the PICU hospitalization.

Trajectory of Parental Stress

Research to date has delineated phases and characteristics of the trajectory of parental stress in the PICU. Awareness of the normal trajectory of PICU-related parental stress enables nurses to focus intervention strategies and to identify extreme parental behavior. Parents who experience stress responses that are outside the expected range or extreme may benefit from early consultation and/or referral for more intensive intervention with psychosocial support staff.

Rothstein (1980) studied parents of children admitted to the PICU after catastrophic illnesses and describes a pattern of parental reactions. Within the first 12 hours of admission, parents frequently exhibit overwhelming shock associated with feelings of helplessness. Within 24 hours, this period is followed by a phase in which parents grapple for explanations. This behavior supports the parent's search for explanations to ascribe meaning to the illness (Comoroff & Maguire, 1981; Turner et al., 1990). Rothstein (1980) noted that parents are "responsible" for their children and, thus, may experience real or imagined guilt or blame themselves for their child's critical illness.

Rothstein (1980) next described an anticipatory waiting phase, lasting hours to days, which coincides with the child's medical stabilization. During this phase, parents frequently express concerns about the long-term effects of the illness, focus upon insignificant changes hoping to see improvement, and become more demanding of and perhaps angry at the staff. Specific uncertainties during this time include the child's likelihood of survival, future appearance, an-

ticipated level of functioning, and duration of illness and hospitalization. Parental helplessness continues during this period of waiting. Anticipatory waiting is then followed by either the elation of discharge, or the bereavement process if the outcome is death.

Lewandowski (1980) was the first to describe the initial responses and coping strategies of parents of children undergoing open-heart surgery. Lewandowski reported that despite preoperative teaching and a preadmission tour of the PICU, parents frequently express shock and feel unprepared for their first postoperative visit at the bedside. Parents may experience helplessness and powerlessness because they are unable to function in their familiar role of protector. Lewandowski described several parental coping strategies, which are presented in Table 3–4. Restructuring, sometimes referred to as a time to focus on little things, allows the parent to focus upon one thing at a time, which prevents parents from becoming overwhelmed by the overall condition of the child.

Curley (1987, 1988) found that changes in a child's appearance and PICU-related procedures were more stressful to parents during the first few days of hospitalizations than later in the course of hospitalization. As the hospitalization progresses, issues related to staff communication and behavior become greater contributors to the parental experience of stress. Supporting Rothstein's (1980) notion of the anticipatory waiting phase, Curley (1987, 1988) documented an overall increase in parental stress after the first few days of PICU hospitalization. Most importantly, parental stress related to role alterations was significant throughout the entire PICU hospitalization. Parents, accustomed to their protector role, report helplessness in protecting their child from pain and in knowing how best to help their child. Curley and Wallace (1992) noted that the trajectory of child illness, and concomitantly the trajectory of parental stress, vary across different patient populations. The "typical" trajectory of parental stress differs significantly between parents of surgical patients and medical patients. The trajectory for surgical patients often begins with a hyperacute phase that predictably improves over time, whereas the trajectory for medical patients is often just the opposite.

Table 3–4. INITIAL COPING STRATEGIES

Immobilization	Delay in parental approach to the bedside
Visual survey	Visually scanning the environment and orienting self before attending to verbal explanations
Withdrawal	Nonresponsive passive behaviors or actual physical withdrawal from the bedspace
Restructuring	Focusing on one physical detail or on the care provided
Intellectualization	Dealing with the child's illness on an intellectual level

Data from Lewandowski, L. A. (1980). Stressors and coping styles of parents of children undergoing open heart surgery. *Critical Care Quarterly*, 3, 75–84.

As the child's condition stabilizes or the parents gradually adjust to the role of parent-to-a-critically-ill-child, parents frequently express the need to become personally involved in their child's care. Although parents may initially have been relieved that they were not solely responsible for the care of the child, they wish to play a more active role as their child improves (Miles, 1979) or as they gain self-confidence within the PICU setting (Curley, 1987, 1988). Curley (1987, 1988) has postulated that increases in perceived parental stress relate specifically to nursing communication and nursing behavior, and in general, may reflect parents' unmet needs to participate in caregiving and to fulfill a meaningful role. Parents may experience displacement by staff and usurpment of their traditional parental caregiving role. Similarly, Rothstein (1980) noted that the helplessness experienced by parents is heightened when parents are excluded from taking an active role in the care of their child. Despite the high levels of technology in the PICU environment and the seriousness of the child's illness, parents wish to be informed, to have input into the plan of care, to help with their child's physical care, and to be recognized as important in their child's recovery (Kirschbaum, 1983, 1990).

Identified Parental Needs and Coping Strategies

Numerous researchers have described the perceived needs of parents during the course of PICU hospitalization. Perceived needs support parents' individual coping efforts and, ultimately, the ways in which they are able to manage the threat of their infant's or child's illness. Psychosocial intervention that addresses the parents' identified needs serves to support their individual coping. Frequently cited parental needs are summarized in Table 3–5.

Even when parents are stressed within the PICU setting, Kirschbaum (1983, 1990) found that they are still readily able to identify their own needs when asked. Needs that are most important to parents included believing that there is hope, knowing that the child is receiving the best care possible, and believing that they are getting as much information as possible. One half of the 10 most important needs identified by parents are informational in nature.

Table 3–5. IDENTIFIED PARENTAL NEEDS

Getting as much information as possible
Assurance that their child is receiving the best possible care
Feeling that there is hope
Vigilance
Being near their child as much as possible
Help with physical care
Being recognized as important to child's recovery
Talking with other parents
Prayer
Instrumental resources (e.g., transportation, meals)

Thus, excellence in clinical care and provision of information are major factors that support families. Accurate information is necessary for parents to cognitively appraise the situation, to construct meaning of the illness, to make informed decisions, and to help their children understand events. Rothstein (1980) noted that parental trust develops when information is honest, consistent, and anticipatory in nature.

Parents of acutely ill children report a greater need to be recognized as vital to their ill child's recovery, to visit anytime, and to help with the patient's physical care than relatives of adult acutely ill patients (Kirschbaum, 1983, 1990; Farrel & Frost, 1993). These findings make intuitive sense because parents normally "take care of" their children. Parents need to feel important to their children regardless of how sick they are. For example, parents generally tend to put their child's needs above their own needs. Parents consistently rate their own personal needs (e.g., "having someone concerned about my health") as less important than any child or parent-child need (Kirschbaum, 1990). Some parents, however, do acknowledge a physiologic and psychological need to curtail the amount of time they spend with their child in the PICU (Kasper & Nyamathi, 1988).

Miles and Carter (1985) identified five coping strategies perceived as most helpful to parents of critically ill children. Coping strategies included (1) seeking help or comfort from others; (2) believing that the child is getting the best possible care; (3) seeking as much information as possible; (4) having hope; and (5) being near the child as much as possible. The use of prayer, asking questions of the staff, and talking with other parents were also cited as important. Similarly, Kasper & Nyamathi (1988) identified the most common parental needs as proximity to the child; frequent, accurate, and truthful information about the child's condition; participation in the child's caregiving; sleeping accommodations near the PICU; and reassurance that the child is receiving needed care and treatment.

In addition, parents need to know that their child is being treated as a person (Jay & Youngblut, 1991). Parents assessed this parameter by noting whether staff called their child by name and/or talked to their child on an appropriate developmental level, even if their child was comatose or heavily medicated. Verbally preparing even the unresponsive child for all procedures conveyed the message to parents that the nurse cared about, not just for, their child. Parents perceived staff efforts to treat their children with such dignity as the "best possible care."

Although parents have consistently identified proximity to their infants and children as a very important need, most PICUs limit parental access to children several times during the day. Notwithstanding 24-hours-a-day visitation policies, nurses and other staff excuse parents from the bedspace during activities such as nursing report, medical rounds, and procedures (Tughan, 1992). This is inconsistent with family-centered, humane care in the PICU. Furthermore, mothers who have the benefit of individualized visitation have significantly lower anxiety scores and perceive their child's illness as less severe than mothers who experience structured visitation (Proctor, 1987). The most salient component of family visiting guidelines is flexibility. An individual approach that enables the family's informal social support system to be involved during the hospitalization is also recommended (Wincek, 1991). This includes not only parents, but also siblings, grandparents, and childcare workers, among others, whom the family identifies as important.

Vigilance serves to reduce parental sense of helplessness and to maintain the protective parental role (Miles, 1987). The vigilant parent of a critically ill infant or child is one who stays with the child as much as possible, but who is also able to leave to meet the needs of self and family. The vigilant parent asks questions to keep informed, checks to ensure that the child is receiving proper care, and may request to remain with the child during procedures for the purpose of supporting the child. Vigilant parental behavior increases when the child and parents are exposed to many different caregivers (Curley, 1987).

In some cases, parents may manifest hypervigilance in which the positive aspects of vigilance are outweighed, or even the well-being of the child is jeopardized (Miles, 1987). Several factors have been associated with hypervigilance (Table 3–6). The hypervigilant parent overuses or exaggerates the use of vigilance. Parents never or rarely leave the bedside. They may demand detailed information before agreeing to even minor changes in the child's treatment plan, sometimes delaying or denying medications or treatments. Hypervigilant parents may continually

Table 3–6. FACTORS THAT INFLUENCE PARENTAL VIGILANCE

Parent-family issues	Parent's personality Family relationships Cultural/parental role
Parent-child issues	Child's meaning to parent
Illness-related issues	Parent's perception of the infant's or child's vulnerability Parent's usual level of responsibility for the child's care at home Parent's understanding about the illness Acuity of the illness Illness trajectory Pain; painful/invasive procedures
Environmental issues	Parent-staff communications Level of trust Quality of communication Quality of care History of misdiagnosis, improper care or treatment Continuity of nurses/physicians Response of the staff to vigilant behaviors

Data from Miles, M. S. (1987). Vigilance as a parental coping strategy when a child is seriously ill. Abstract for poster presentation. Biennial meeting of the Society for Research in Child Development, Baltimore, MD.

monitor staff, attempt to control how care is provided, or assume total care of the child. These parents may trust only a few staff and wish to control which nurses take care of their child. They might examine the medical record to identify problems or discrepancies and then record them in a logbook.

Our society generally values and rewards the vigilant parent, but not necessarily in the PICU setting. Hypervigilant parents can be unnerving or even threatening to nursing staff. Nursing interventions should be focused to decrease the parent's sense of helplessness and provide the parent with some degree of control. Positive nursing interventions include welcoming parents and their assistance at the bedside, reinforcing parental questioning, providing information on a consistent basis, reinforcing the parental role, and being receptive to their telephone calls. Nurses need to support each other when providing care for hypervigilant parents and to remember that, although it may be difficult, the parents are doing the best that they can under the circumstances. Negative interventions include behaving defensively, withholding information, maintaining power and control, failing to include parents in the decision-making process, avoiding the parents, and resenting their questions.

Parents have also identified the importance of parent-to-parent support. Parents can offer perspectives and support to each other that professionals are not able to provide (Shelton et al., 1987). Although parents spontaneously interact in waiting rooms, Halm (1990) studied the effect of formal support groups on the anxiety levels of family members during critical illness. Family members perceived many benefits of the group milieu such as sharing with other people in similar situations, instilling hope, reducing anxiety, and learning new coping strategies. Nursing staff can be instrumental in facilitating parent-to-parent support (Rushton, 1990).

Parent-professional trust is the necessary foundation from which all supportive care can build. Trust develops in the context of the parents' perception that their child is receiving excellent care, from the nurses' reassuring presence, and through recognition of parents as unique autonomous individuals. Continuity of nursing and medical care allows strong alliances to form with parents, which further contribute to the development of trust (Rennick, 1986).

Although competence is the most highly valued quality of nursing care, parents also prefer nurses who are sensitive and caring (Beckham, 1993). For example, nurses are considered caring when they talk with parents, provide information without asking, do not make parents feel intrusive, help parents feel that they are part of the team, enable parents to feel comfortable in leaving, and reassure them that everything will be taken care of and communicated (Curley, 1987). In general, parents can more willingly relinquish their child's care to someone they trust.

INTERVENTION STRATEGIES

Most of the nursing research generated on parental stress has been descriptive in nature. Many consistent recommendations for interventions intended to minimize parental stress in the PICU setting have been offered. Interventions may be divided into three major categories: (1) those that nurture a trusting environment, in parents themselves, their children, and PICU staff; (2) those that establish effective communication patterns and provide information and anticipatory guidance; and (3) those that limit parental powerlessness by reestablishing a parental relationship through visitation and participation in caregiving activities. Such interventions are consonant with the Parents' Bill of Rights delineated by the Association for the Care of Children's Health (1991) (Table 3–7).

Nurses tend to intervene in a similar manner with all families whose needs are perceived to be essentially the same (Jacono et al., 1990). This is problematic because there is significant variability in parental perceptions and experiences, stress levels, and needs among individuals that requires individualized nursing interventions. That which may be helpful to one parent may not be helpful, or even useful, to another parent, even within the same family.

Nursing perceptions and interventions may be well-intended but may not be accurate. Researchers have noted that there are differences between that which nurses perceive parental needs to be and that which parents perceive as their own needs within the PICU setting (Johnson et al., 1988). Indeed, additional parental stress may result from mismatches between nurses' understanding of parental needs and parents' own understanding (Hayes & Knox, 1984). Generalized or generic family supportive intervention strategies intended to meet nonexistent needs or needs already met by others frequently lead to much wasted time and energy (Molter, 1979).

NURSING MUTUAL PARTICIPATION MODEL OF CARE

Models that emphasize an individual approach to nursing interventions are preferred, given the individualized nature of PICU-related parental stress and findings that generic family support models are not adequate and may even exacerbate parental stress. The Nursing Mutual Participation Model of Care (NMPMC) represents such an example (Table

Table 3–7. A PEDIATRIC BILL OF RIGHTS

> In this hospital you and your child have the right to:
> Respect and personal dignity
> Care that supports you as a family
> Information you can understand
> Quality health care
> Emotional support
> Care that respects your child's growth and development
> Make decisions about your child's care

Data from Association for the Care of Children's Health. (1991). Bill of rights for parents. *A Pediatric Bill of Rights.* Bethesda, MD: Association for the Care of Children's Health.

Table 3–8. NURSING MUTUAL PARTICIPATION MODEL OF CARE

Admission

Extend our care to include parents
Acknowledge their importance

Daily Bedside Contact

Enabling strategies that provide parents with system savvy
1. Information—teach & clarify
2. Anticipatory guidance—illness trajectory
3. Provide instrumental resources

Facilitate transition to "parent-to-a-critically-ill-child"
1. Enhance parent-child unique connectedness
2. Role model interactions
3. Invite participation in nurturant activity
4. Provide options during procedures

Communication pattern
1. Establish a caring relationship with the parent
   How are you doing today?
2. Assess parental perception of the child's illness
   How does s/he look to you today?
3. Determine parental goals, objectives, and expectations
   What troubles you most?
4. Seek informed suggestions and preferences, and invite
     participation in care
   How can I help you today?

Data from Curley, M. A. Q. (1988). Effects of the nursing mutual participation model of care and parental stress in the pediatric intensive care unit. *Heart & Lung,* 17(6,1), 682–688; Curley, M. A. Q., & Wallace, J. (1992). Effects of the nursing mutual participation model of care on parental stress in the pediatric intensive care unit—A replication. *Journal of Pediatric Nursing,* 7(6), 377–385.

3–8). Szasz and Hollender (1956) first described a "mutual participation" model for use with chronically ill adults. The model, fundamentally different from others practiced at the time, was based on the premise that the healthcare provider could not profess to know what is best for an individual. The search for that which may be considered individually helpful was the essence of the therapeutic interaction. The individual was assisted to help himself as his own experiences and beliefs provided reliable and important clues to therapy.

In 1980, Brody further described the model as a four-step process for use with adults in outpatient settings. The foundation of the intervention process was conceptualized as agenda-seeking; the patient was enlisted and invited into the healthcare decision-making process by asking, "How can I help you today?"

Curley (1987, 1988) adapted the model for nursing care of critically ill children and their parents because it provided the philosophical foundation to incorporate many of the therapeutic interventions recommended from descriptive research. The model supports the view that the nature of PICU-related stress requires individualized nursing interventions. The model is based on the premise that nurses have something of value to offer parents, and acknowledges that parents also have something of value to contribute to the caregiving process and to their children. Nurses, through their expertise, know what might be helpful to parents as a population who are experiencing the critical illness of a child, but nurses do not specifically know what might be best for an individual parent. Parents, on the other hand, know what may be helpful to them and their infant or child, but they do not know what is unique about the PICU.

The NMPMC provides a framework for individualized nursing interactions. It clarifies the parental role, supports active parental involvement with their critically ill child, and fosters parental confidence in performing their role in a foreign setting. The process is individually determined and evolves to meet the expressed needs of each parent. Nurse-parent relationships are characterized by a high degree of empathy and partnership, and expert knowledge is imparted to limit perceived helplessness and passivity. Critical features of the model include equal status of parent and professional in the relationship, mutual interdependency, and mutual satisfaction between nurses and parents.

The effects of the NMPMC on helping parents to alleviate their stress have been supported in two separate nursing research studies. In the first study (Curley, 1987, 1988), the principal investigator, functioning in the role of a clinical nurse specialist, implemented the model. Parents reported significantly less overall stress in the areas of child's behavior and emotions, parental role revision, child's procedures, and nursing communication and behavior. In the second study (Curley & Wallace, 1992), primary nurses implemented the model. Parents who had the benefit of NMPMC intervention reported significantly less stress associated with the hospitalization, particularly in the area of parental role alteration.

The NMPMC is consistent with Greeneich and Long's (1993) nursing taxonomy of family satisfaction (NTFS). Within the NTFS model, family satisfaction results from an interaction between the family, nurse, and healthcare system. Nurses can influence family satisfaction by (1) optimizing critical juncture incidents; (2) accommodating parental personality styles; (3) determining family expectations; and (4) adapting the environment to the family's needs. Critical juncture incidents are episodes in which a nurse's behavior and intervention significantly affects the patient at a time when the family perceives the patient to be most vulnerable. Nurse personality attributes include social courtesy, acceptance, kindness, helpfulness, empathy, and advocacy. The ability of the nurse to develop a trusting relationship with the family is also considered to be an element of personality fit. Trust is inherently linked to effective communication (matched to the family's style) and nursing proficiency. Nurses create a milieu to adapt to the family's expectations and needs. Family satisfaction results when the parent's expectations of care match with the reality of care.

Admission: Critical Time for Intervention

Admission is a very stressful period for parents during which they experience a significant loss of

control (Skipper & Leonard, 1968; Wolfer & Visintainer, 1975). Acknowledging the parent's valuable and irreplaceable role in actions and words during this critical period helps to set the tone for the entire PICU hospitalization. The nurse should state the obvious, for example, "Here at Children's Hospital we believe parents to be very important to their children, especially when they're sick. We would like to work with you to help you find ways that you can continue to be important to your child while s/he is in the ICU." These words broaden the perspective of care to include parents. Right from the start, parents are invited as partners into the caregiving process, thus establishing an atmosphere in which parents feel that their contributions are essential. Parents feel less anxious when they sense that their role is valued, that their child still belongs to them, and that someone will help them to get through the experience with their child as a welcomed participant.

As soon as information is available, it should be provided by the nurse and the physician. This demonstrates multidisciplinary collaboration and communication for the family. After any period of separation or change in their infant's or child's appearance and/or behavior, parents require preparation for that which they will see or hear before reuniting them. Information may need to be repeated because high levels of parental stress can interfere with the parent's ability to hear, understand, and remember.

If parent-child separation is necessary, parents are provided with privacy and a telephone so that they may contact extended family members. During this period of separation, it is imperative that nursing staff maintain contact with the parents. Right from the beginning, staff should seek the parent's preference about the level of information and frequency of contact. Parents usually request information about stabilizing methods, and they wish to be reunited with their infant/child as soon as possible. If prolonged periods of separation are unavoidable, opportunities are sought to provide parents with brief updates or visits between procedures.

Daily Bedside Contact

After acknowledging the importance of the parental role, the model provides a framework for daily interventions that are supportive to and guided by the perceived unique needs of each parent. The model (1) incorporates enabling and empowering strategies to equip the parent with healthcare system savvy, (2) facilitates the parent's transition to parent-to-a-critically-ill-child, and (3) delineates a consistent nurse-parent communication pattern. An accurate family assessment helps to guide effective intervention strategies (Table 3–9). Family characteristics such as the degree of adaptability (rigid, structured, flexible, chaotic) and cohesion (disengaged, separated, connected, enmeshed) are important considerations in psychosocial intervention planning (Philichi, 1989).

Table 3–9. PARAMETERS OF A FAMILY ASSESSMENT

1. Past history of child's illness: when and how diagnoses were made; previous hospitalizations and treatments
2. Parental perception and understanding of illness
3. Feelings engendered by the child's illness: fear, guilt, remorse, helplessness, hopelessness, anger
4. Family history and significant events: past experiences with illness, divorce, death
5. Current family functioning: family membership, structure, and roles, current marital relationship, communication patterns within family, patterns of expressing feelings, siblings and their relationship within the family, religious background, cultural values, financial problems
6. Parental roles and relationships with child: identification of the child as "special" due to having been either the only child, only daughter, only son, youngest, eldest, most vulnerable
7. Unmet parental needs: lack of sleep, lack of privacy, poor nutrition, untreated health problems, poor hygiene, lack of opportunity for sexual expression

Data from Miles, M. S. (1979). Impact of the intensive care unit on parents. *Issues in Comprehensive Pediatric Nursing*, 3, 72–90.

Enabling Strategies That Provide Parents With System Savvy

It has been said that parents do not need to be empowered within the clinical setting; they need their inherent power to be recognized. Socializing parents to the PICU and hospital system, especially providing information that they need to know to get by, serves to empower them.

Provide Information That Instructs and Clarifies. In addition to information about the infant's or child's illness and the standard PICU milieu (monitors, catheters, endotracheal tubes, etc.), specific information is vital about the changes in the child's appearance, behavior, and emotional reactions, and in the parental role. When discussing the technologic devices surrounding the patient it is important to include a discussion about alarm systems. Although nurses know that there is a hierarchy of alarm systems, parents do not necessarily understand these distinctions. Unfamiliar alarms are feared equally by parents, from those that signal hypotension to those that signal the end of an antibiotic infusion or artifact on a cardiac monitor.

After addressing these immediate needs, parents need to understand the PICU and hospital environment. Written materials, such as orientation booklets, are effective in assisting families to remember discrete pieces of information (Henneman et al., 1992). The process of how parents gain access to their infants and children is critically important. It should be stressed that the only reason parents are asked to request permission to see their child in the PICU is for the protection and privacy of other patients.

Information including the routines of the unit, who is in charge of their child's medical and nursing care, and when and where parents get information enables them to effectively function within the system's hierarchy. Parents of children who require multiple services and parents of chronically critically ill children

are at high risk for communication problems related to insufficient or incorrect information about their child's care and management. It is essential that the nurse coordinate the informational needs of parents by delineating, together with the attending physician and parents, a daily communication plan. Routinely scheduled weekly multidisciplinary team meetings are very helpful to the entire team and to parents of chronically critically ill children.

Only after (1) sharing information about their infant or child, (2) providing information about the hospital environment, and (3) answering questions the parents have should dialogue progress to the perceived alterations in parental role and responsibility.

Provide Anticipatory Guidance About the Illness Trajectory. Information about that which parents will see or experience should be shared before it happens, if at all possible. If feasible, nurses should meet with parents and patients prior to a planned admission to the PICU. Describing the illness trajectory, as far as it can be reasonably predicted, is extremely helpful because it allows parents to understand and distinguish that which is "normal and expected" and that which is "life-threatening." Although videotapes may be helpful, tours (except to empty bedspaces) should be avoided because they violate the privacy of existing patients and may frighten the future patient.

Provide Instrumental Resources. Provision of adequate instrumental resources is also necessary so that parents are able to maintain both physical and emotional accessibility to their critically ill child 24 hours a day. Necessary resources include sleep facilities, showers, telephones, nutritious food, transportation, and parking (Fisher et al., 1984). Physical barriers to the welcoming process, including activities that make parents feel like visitors to their own infants and children, should be eliminated.

Facilitate Transition to Parent-to-a-Critically-Ill-Child

Alterations in parental role, and the subsequent disruption in the parent-child relationship, are the most stressful aspects of the PICU environment. Assisting parents to formulate a role with which they are personally comfortable and supporting them in their decision-making capacity helps parents in a successful transition to parent-to-a-critically-ill-child.

Enhance Parent-Child Unique Connectedness. Because of changes in their child's appearance and behavior, parents may need help reconnecting to a child who appears to be so much different. Strategies include finding some characteristic of the child that has not changed (that is, some enduring feature) and emphasizing it to the parents. Examples may include hair or eye color or evidence of the child's increased heart rate in response to the parent's voice. Creativity is sometimes needed to help reestablish the unique parent-child connection when significant disfigurement is present. Parents may need "permission" and demonstrations of how to touch and interact with their critically ill infant or child. Rubin's (1967) maternal touch progression, for example, can be demonstrated in the PICU regardless of the age of the infant or child.

Parents can also be encouraged to bring in the child's favorite blanket, toy, doll, or family pictures to comfort the child and to individualize the bedspaces. All of these reminders of life at home provide nonverbal cues of the valued nature of the family, and they are as important as direct verbal communication.

Role Model Interactions. Parents have reported that their initial fears are lessened by observing and imitating nursing care activities. Parents notice and sort nursing activities into two categories: those that are familiar activity and those that are different activity (Jay, 1977). Acknowledging that one's nursing care activity is being observed (not to ensure correctness, because there is usually no basis for that distinction) provides an opportunity to demonstrate care through nonverbal communication. For example, using touch progression shows where and how to physically touch the critically ill child for the parents, and can help parents feel more comfortable during caregiving activities and interaction with their child.

Invite Participation in Nurturant Activity. Following the initial period of shock and disbelief, parents are usually able to identify those activities in which they wish to participate. When offered caregiving options and opportunity, parents do so consistently to renew their self-esteem and to feel instrumental in their child's recovery. Suggesting ways parents can assist their child in coping helps to reduce parental anxiety (Vulcan & Nikulich-Barrett, 1988). Ideally, special aspects of parental care and comforting can be distinguished from things that others can do for the child (e.g., provide breastmilk, voice, touch). Nursing staff should help parents identify their options by suggesting appropriate diversional, nurturing, comforting, caregiving, and monitoring activities.

The social and emotional needs of infants, in particular, are met in close association with their bodily needs. With a new caregiver, the infant loses much of what is familiar. Physical care constitutes an essential element of the very intimate relationship between parents and infants. Usurping this role from parents is generally not welcomed by the infant, nor is it helpful, especially when the infant is stressed. Nursing practice that directly involves the primary caregiver is more therapeutic than care that replaces the primary caregiver. Efforts should be extended to welcome parents; they should never be made to feel out of place or in competition for their infant or child.

Parents generally enjoy helping with activities that they find personally rewarding and participating in new activities with nursing guidance. A developmental approach is a starting point, for example, considering what parents normally do for their baby, toddler, child, or adolescent (Curley & Wallace, 1992). Reading, massages, bathing, and hairbrushing are familiar and comforting activities for both parents and child. Sociocultural influences will likely affect the parent's selection of activities. Communication, teaching, anticipatory guidance, and mutual trust and support are essential during this process. Parents frequently feel uncomfortable performing tasks with which they were once proficient as a parent of a well child. Clearly, bathing an infant at home is different than bathing an infant who is attached to numerous pieces of equipment. Once the child's condition is stabilized, it is important to incorporate parent-child "private time" in the management plan to sustain the parent-child relationship.

Provide Options During Procedures. Traditionally, parents have been asked to step out of the PICU during their or another child's procedures or treatments. Enforced separations, sometimes lasting hours, and related conflicts in values about the approaches used to obtain the child's cooperation are significant sources of stress for parents (LaMontagne & Pawlak, 1990). Currently, there is great variability among institutions regarding parental presence during special procedures. Inconsistency among staff and unclear policies about visitation and parental presence during procedures can be further anxiety-provoking for parents, as well as staff (Rushton, 1990).

Parents may be dismissed from treatments because of staff fear and apprehension that they may interfere with the procedure or make their child more upset. Sevedra (1981) studied 60 children, ages 2 weeks to 6 years, who had blood drawn in the presence of their parents. The study suggested that even when the procedure was difficult and stressful parents were not disruptive, but instead were supportive of their child as directed by personnel. A variety of verbal and nonverbal strategies were used by parents to help the child to better cope. Similarly, Shaw and Routh (1982) compared 18-month-old and 5-year-old children's reactions to immunizations in the presence and absence of mothers. They found more upset behavior when mothers were present but the researchers hypothesized that the children's increase in negative responses reflected a disinhibitor response. That is, the mother's presence allowed the child greater expression of his or her feelings in an unfamiliar and threatening environment. Upset behavior including crying, terror, uncooperation, or violent protest can be expected when the infant or toddler is stressed by the parent's absence, let alone by a painful procedure. Lack of expected distress responses may reflect a deterioration in the child's level of functioning, detachment, or severe emotional withdrawal. Expecting cooperative behavior or a diminished negative response when parents are present is probably unrealistic.

Parental presence can potentially support the child's coping efforts and provide the child with a familiar source of comfort. It is recommended that parents be offered a choice regarding their presence or participation, and support for their decision. Flexible policies based upon individual patients and parents are ideal.

Developmentally appropriate, honest preparation precedes all procedures. It is important to remember that young children's receptive language generally exceeds their expressive language abilities. Simple explanations that can be easily understood are always offered. For parents to be supportive during a procedure, they need to know the importance of the procedure, what to expect during the procedure, normal age-related reactions that may occur, and how they can best help. Parents should not be placed in a position of restraining their child during any procedure.

Parent support is also important when parents choose to excuse themselves during a procedure. It is probable that parents can anticipate the ways that they and their child can best be helped through a given procedure. Parents may need help to articulate the fears that may block their ability to believe that they are the best possible parent under the circumstances. Parents may find it especially difficult to be present during painful procedures because this seems in conflict with their protective role. Parents may benefit from information that their infant's or toddler's cognitive immaturity prevents a mature level of reasoning and that parents' supportive non-ambivalent presence can potentially emotionally support their child through a procedure.

Parents can also serve as educators for their children. Using parents as the primary source of information for their children may enhance communication and may also limit misconceptions and misinterpretation. Gutstein and Tarnow (1983) found that children's active involvement in preparatory play was significantly related to lower levels of distress after elective surgery. They also found that the child's active involvement in preparatory play with stress-related objects was significantly related to parent helping behaviors.

When parents wait during procedures, they often make assumptions that the longer the wait the more difficult the procedure, or that something is wrong. Parents of sick children spend much time waiting together. This can be a source of either comfort or additional stress. Comfort can be had when another parent is one step ahead and can share in the experience "with someone who really understands." Stress can be exacerbated when another family's child is not doing well. Grieving parents require privacy for themselves and for other parents.

Communication Pattern

The NMPMC delineates a four-step communication process that is helpful and demonstrates caring toward the parent, assesses parental perceptions, determines the parental agenda, and invites participation in care. This communication process is congruent with the ABCX model of crisis in that nursing interventions should be dependent upon the family's perception of the stressful event. This communication strategy is helpful in the PICU because interventions can be specifically focused when time is limited.

When help is rationally directed and purposefully focused at the right time, it is perceived as more effective than more help given at a period of less emotional accessibility.

Establish a Caring Relationship With the Parent. This first aspect adds a humanistic touch by extending the focus of our care to include parents. Asking the parents, for example, "How are you doing? Were you able to sleep?" helps to convey the message that parents, too, are important. It is interesting to note that parents often answer queries based upon their child's state, for example, "I feel better today. Paul was able to get off his blood pressure medication."

Unless assessed and validated, parental affect or behaviors may be misinterpreted in the intensive care setting. For example, a father's body language may be misinterpreted as anger but when queried he may remark how scared and upset he feels. Interventions for angry parents versus scared parents are quite different.

Assess Parental Perception of the Child's Illness. To assess the parental perception of illness severity, ask, "How does your child look to you today? How serious do you think his illness is? How are other family members dealing with everything?" Here, the nurse builds trust by clarifying misconceptions and providing accurate, concise, and complete information. In addition, nurses often make assessments and judgments about a child's pain, activity, and behavior based upon PICU experience, but without familiarity with an individual child. Parents are often well aware of their child's subtle behavioral and communicative cues that can be helpful in individualizing care. Nurses and parents working together can better understand and address an individual child's needs.

Determine Parental Goals, Objectives, and Expectations. The third step helps parents to rank their concerns. It also sanctions the expression of feelings that parents may otherwise consider inappropriate to express. Here, the nurse may ask, "What troubles you most? Do you have any questions? Is this what you expected? Do you have any suggestions or preferences concerning the care your child is receiving? Is there anything that you personally want to do for your child?"

Seek Suggestions and Preferences and Invite Participation in Care. The last step invites parental participation in determining how nursing interventions can be provided. Here, the nurse may ask, "How can I help you? How can we do this together?" Interventions are then focused on parent-specific issues rather than nurse-speculated problems. It should be noted that failure to address a parent's agenda, especially after it has been elicited, may often lead to an increase in stress and parental dissatisfaction.

Providing a humanistic PICU environment that recognizes parents as unique autonomous individuals who, when supported, are capable of providing vital elements of care to their critically ill child helps to alleviate parental stress. The NMPMC is effective in helping to decrease parental stress by assisting parents to formulate a role that is individually comfortable and supportive of them in their decision-making capacity. Not all parents have the desire or capability to actively participate in the care of their child; however, the NMPMC provides a means to assess and individualize psychosocial interventions.

FAMILY CONTEXT OF CHILDHOOD CRITICAL ILLNESS

Traditionally, hospitals have had an approach that emphasizes the treatment of individuals in isolation from their broader family and sociocultural context (Gilkerson, 1990). By contrast, family-centered care embraces a systems approach in which the child's illness is viewed in context. Family-centered care advocates for the child and family as the appropriate focus of healthcare intervention, thus necessarily broadening the care perspective and traditional interventions.

Entire families are affected when an infant or child is critically ill. Parents find themselves thrust into unfamiliar roles including negotiating an often overwhelming healthcare setting, integrating information about the child's illness, and participating in emotionally laden decision-making (Harrison, 1983; Miles & Carter, 1982). Family routines are suddenly disrupted and traditional roles are altered. In addition, parents must balance multiple demands including traveling to the hospital or temporarily residing at the hospital, maintaining a home, caring for other children, meeting financial obligations, and negotiating employment circumstances, among others. Parents may feel torn between the needs of children at home and their critically ill child's immediate needs. As described earlier, parents often experience diminished competence and helplessness relative to their critically ill child, and their inability to adequately meet the needs of their healthy children may compound these self-deprecating feelings. This sense of conflict may be longstanding and particularly difficult for parents when their child is chronically critically ill.

To a great extent, families adjust their priorities and family life when a child requires hospitalization. Hospital staff members tend to view parents primarily as parents of a hospitalized child, however, with less than adequate recognition of the parents' broader family, employment, and community responsibilities (see Table 3-9) (Gilkerson, 1990; Meyer & Bailey, 1993). Problems arise, for example, when staff members assume that parents can be available at any time for meetings and care conferences. Similarly, convenient visiting times for parents may conflict with unit rounds or nursing report. Thus, there must be flexibility and mutual respect on the part of both staff and family members to facilitate the collaborative parent-professional partnership.

For most parents, the most important potentially supportive relationship during this time is with their spouse (Featherstone, 1980; Harrison, 1983). The crisis of critical illness and hospitalization is emotionally charged and represents fertile ground for conflict that may strain even strong spousal relationships. For example, parents may need to come to consensus on issues such as how far to pursue treatment or whether the child's organs may be donated. Aspects of successful adaptation include how parents develop and negotiate their new roles amid the challenges of the PICU, and how they manage to support each other. Parents need to communicate with many healthcare providers and with each other, to grapple with potentially difficult ethical decisions, to negotiate being parents with little privacy, and to keep family and friends informed of the child's condition (Meyer et al., 1993). The unanticipated and fearsome financial burdens inherent in PICU hospitalization may represent an additional, although often unspoken, stressor for parents. Preexisting vulnerabilities in the couple's relationship may be seriously challenged by the child's illness. Spousal conflicts that were present but compensated for before the child's critical illness may now resurface and threaten to disrupt the couple's equilibrium.

Siblings of hospitalized infants and children often have concerns and questions regarding the well-being of their brother or sister, and their parents (Doll-Speck et al., 1993; Maloney et al., 1983). Multiple factors influence the sibling's responses and adjustment to critical illness including the sibling's developmental stage, nature of illness, the sibling's perception of the illness, number and type of other operative stressors, and available situational supports (Lewandowski, 1992). Children may experience disruption in usual family routines, separation from parents, and changes in caregiving arrangements, all of which may contribute to their degree of stress. Siblings may experience feelings of helplessness, fear, guilt, and anger that they may or may not be able to communicate to parents (Newman & McSweeney, 1990).

It is not uncommon for parents to request help for siblings who are perceived to be having difficulty coping with the illness. Parents may also wish guidance about how and how much to explain to their children about the illness, visitation in the PICU, ways to meaningfully involve their other children in the hospitalization, and, in some cases, preparation for the child's death. It may be that enlisting supportive services for their other children is more acceptable to parents than the alternative of direct psychological service for themselves. At the same time, it may also serve to bolster parents in their familiar roles of protector and provider for their children.

In a study investigating the impact of critical care hospitalization on the perceptions of adult patients, spouses, children, and nurses, Titler and colleagues (1988) noted that parents frequently shielded their children from anxiety-provoking information. Parents perceived that their children, ranging in age from 5 to 18 years of age, did not comprehend much about the parental illness or hospitalization. However, children provided accurate descriptions of the hospitalized parent and of both parents' feelings. These findings suggest that children are keenly aware of illness-related experiences and, to the extent possible, construct their own meanings despite limited access to information and healthcare providers.

Formal sibling programs can be facilitated through collaborative efforts between nurses, child life specialists, and volunteers. Educational, supportive visitation programs may include preparation of siblings for visitation, follow-up contact, individual or group activities in the waiting area, and a sibling library (Doll-Speck et al., 1993; Rushton & Booth, 1986; Wincek, 1991). Before visitation, children need to be carefully screened for signs of illness and exposure to communicable diseases. Sibling visitation enables children to experience the reality of the situation first-hand and to participate in family problem-solving and support of their ill brother or sister (Craft, 1986; Newman & McSweeney, 1990; Wincek, 1991). Overall, sibling visitation can contribute to greater family cohesion, adaptation, and satisfaction.

Professional Relationships

Intervening with families while maintaining appropriate professional boundaries has been described by Barnsteiner and Gillis-Donovan (1990). The authors identify the goal of a professional relationship as having caring, well-defined boundaries between a nurse and the patient and family, boundaries that are positive and therapeutic and that promote the family's control over the child's healthcare. They also note that professional nursing is emotionally complicated, requiring the ability to stay meaningfully concerned about a patient and family but, at the same time, separate enough to distinguish one's own feelings and needs. Extremes in inappropriate professional relationships include overinvolvement or underinvolvement with individual patients and their families.

Relatively inexperienced nurses, and those who are new to the intensive care unit, necessarily tend to concentrate on technical skill attainment and mastery rather than psychosocial aspects of care. Within the highly technical and demanding PICU setting, nurses may have little time to devote to psychosocial aspects of care. Moreover, nurses may feel ill-prepared to address the often highly charged emotional aspects of PICU hospitalization. In general, as professionals gain clinical experience, they become increasingly willing and comfortable to formulate collaborative relationships with parents that are consistent with the model of family-centered care (Gill, 1993).

In a study investigating critical care nurses' perceptions of their role with families, in which 20% were pediatric critical care nurses, Hickey & Lewandowski (1988) found that most critical care nurses believed it was emotionally exhausting to repeatedly

become involved with families in need of support. Despite this, nurses report becoming involved with families regardless of their ambivalence and the possible emotional costs to themselves. More than one third of the nurses believed that they did not have the requisite knowledge to meet the emotional and psychosocial needs of families. This underscores the need for ongoing nursing education and collaboration with psychosocial support staff including advanced practice nurses, social work, pediatric psychology, psychiatry, and child life specialists. Among the factors that most influenced nurses' involvement with families were situations relating to the child's death and subjective feelings and responses toward the patient and family.

Collaborative Relationships With Psychosocial Support Staff

Nursing staff who care directly for the child and family generally have the greatest degree of familiarity and regular contact with families. The role of staff nurses in acknowledging and systematically integrating psychosocial aspects of care, as in the Nursing Mutual Participation Model of Care, usefully broadens the focus of intervention from the child alone to the child-in-family. Thus, nurses play a pivotal role in expanding the traditional medical-technologic orientation and language of the intensive care unit to include psychosocial aspects of care (Als, 1992). Through inquiry and attention to parental perceptions and experiences, the nurse emphasizes that these are legitimate aspects of clinical concern and conveys the message that family members, too, are important.

In addition to the nurse's role in psychosocial assessment and intervention, there are several psychosocial support staff members available within the intensive care setting who may play a role in psychosocial service delivery to the family (Table 3–10). Social workers are assigned to each family in the intensive care unit and fulfill a varied role including psychosocial assessment, family support and advocacy, instrumental support, and legal and protective services, if required. Although there is considerable variability among PICUs, other professionals who are available to meet the family's psychosocial needs may include pediatric psychologists, psychiatrists, child life specialists, discharge planners, ethicists, chaplains, child abuse specialists, and parent volunteers. In many cases, the nursing staff and unit-based social worker can adequately address the family's psychosocial needs. However, when the child's or family's needs demand additional services or consultation, support staff should be readily incorporated in the psychosocial planning and intervention efforts.

The nurse plays a pivotal role in contacting and mobilizing these additional services or consultations when needed on behalf of families. It is important that the nurse have a good working knowledge about

Table 3–10. PSYCHOSOCIAL RESOURCES

Advanced practice nurse—clinical nurse specialist
1. Assesses family coping capacities
2. Provides short-term family support
3. Consults with staff regarding expected trajectory of parental stress and coping, interventions with families in crisis related to the critical illness of their child

Social worker
1. Performs psychosocial family assessments
2. Provides family support and advocacy
3. Promotes client access to financial and community services
4. Liaison with child protection team

Child life specialist
1. Provides developmental and therapeutic play activities
2. Supports patient and sibling coping
3. Consults with parents regarding normal child development and adjustment
4. Initiates tutoring referrals

Patient care coordinator
1. Facilitates comprehensive discharge plan
2. Liaison for family with third-party payors
3. Utilization review
4. Accesses community support services for family

Psychologist, psychiatrist
1. Performs diagnostic assessments of children and families
2. Disposition planning of suicidal patients
3. Provides short-term family counseling
4. Provides crisis intervention
5. Facilitates psychopharmacology referrals

Parent volunteer
1. Welcomes family to the PICU
2. Orients parents to the family area
3. Assures family comfort in the waiting area
4. Provides information about hospital resources (meals, telephone, sleep facilities, etc.)

Chaplain
1. Provides spiritual support
2. Performs sacraments as requested by family (e.g., baptism)

Ethics committee
1. Consults with families and staff on ethical issues
2. Educates staff about ethical and legal issues

the various roles of these disciplines, including what they have to offer families and how they may be consulted (Harvey et al., 1993). To facilitate psychosocial service delivery and referral, it is useful for the unit to establish regular psychosocial rounds in which representatives from these disciplines are present. It should be noted that ancillary personnel may provide direct service to children and families, or may merely consult with nursing and social work staff in the context of psychosocial rounds. An organizational chart that delineates the various roles and collaborative relationships of psychosocial support staff and details regarding contact and referral information can be helpful.

Preparing for Patient Transfer

Transition from the intensive care setting to a general hospital unit, or to home, can be fraught with a great deal of apprehension. On one hand, parents may derive comfort from the fact that their child has achieved another step toward recovery (Curley, 1987, 1988; Curley & Wallace, 1992). On the other hand, the transfer requires adjustment to new staff members who do not yet know their child, and to a new environment. Parents may be concerned about their child's readiness for transfer and/or the lower staff-to-patient ratio on the prospective unit. Parents who have come to trust the PICU staff members may be reluctant to reinitiate the process with yet another set of healthcare providers. Anticipatory guidance to assist parents in the transition from the PICU to the general inpatient unit may help to alleviate parental stress related to PICU discharge. Parents need to know that the staff of the receiving unit will be fully informed about the child's history and progress, preferably by the primary nurse or another staff member who knows the child well. This not only ensures optimal clinical care, but also addresses parental anxiety about the transfer.

Formal care conferences that involve the PICU primary nurse, family members, and a nurse from the receiving unit have been demonstrated to significantly reduce the transfer-related anxiety of families (Bokinskie, 1992). In this particular study, the care conference lasted 15 to 30 minutes and consisted of three phases. First, there were introductions and a discussion about the purpose of the meeting. Second, the group discussed the physical environment of the new unit and the child's degree of recovery and progress, and addressed mutual goals and expectations. The third phase provided an opportunity for the group to establish child-centered goals. Conferences such as these serve to mark the transfer from the PICU as a significant event, and have the advantage of focused communication, mutual goal-setting, and parent participation.

Coping With Bereavement Issues

The death of a child is one of the most stressful and traumatic events that a family may ever experience and endure (Schiff, 1977; Miles & Perry, 1985; Rando, 1986). The death of a child is generally perceived in our society as unnatural, untimely, and particularly tragic. Compared to other deaths, the grief of parents can be particularly severe, complicated, and long-lasting, in part resulting from the nature of the parent-child relationship, the circumstances of the death, and societal expectations (Rando, 1986; Sanders, 1978–1980). Parents typically remember the events surrounding the child's death, including the responses of healthcare providers, with great clarity, detail, and emotion (Fischoff & O'Brien, 1976; Jost & Haase, 1989; Schiff, 1977; Strom-Paikin, 1984). The immediate responses and subsequent adjustment of bereaved parents are significantly influenced by the attitudes, psychosocial interventions, and bereavement support offered by healthcare professionals (Cauthorne, 1975; Miles & Perry, 1985; Wortman & Silver, 1989). Thus, positive experiences in the intensive care setting have the potential to facilitate parental bereavement and adjustment, whereas negative experiences may compromise or even derail the parental bereavement and coping process.

Stage models of grief and bereavement have been proposed (Kübler-Ross, 1969; Parkes, 1965), including an adaptation specifically for parents who have suffered the loss of a child (Miles, 1980, 1984, 1985; Miles & Perry, 1985). Expanding upon Parkes' original model, Miles (1980, 1984) has usefully described three broad phases of parental grief including numbness and shock, intense grief, and reorganization. Although stage models offer a "blueprint" with which to understand the bereavement process, it is important to recognize the inherent limitations of linear models to fully explain such complex processes (Featherstone, 1980).

In the intensive care setting, parents may experience emotional turmoil and anticipatory grief before the child's death, and a combination of disbelief, shock, and intense grief responses upon the death of the child. In retrospective semistructured interviews conducted 1 to 3 years following their children's deaths, parents frequently reported "numbness," accompanied by difficulty integrating information, listening to healthcare providers, and making decisions during the time at the hospital (Jost & Haase, 1989). Initial emotional and behavioral responses vary greatly among parents, depending upon personality style, sociocultural background, social support, and circumstances of the death (Miles, 1980, 1984; Rando, 1986). Emotionally, parents may experience sadness, despair, anger, rage, regret, frustration, guilt, resentment, or relief, among others. Behavioral responses may include crying, withdrawal, hysteria, or physical acting out, such as clinging to the child's dead body or aggression towards objects or people (Miles, 1985). During the subsequent phase of intense grief, parents may experience intense loneliness and yearning for the child, helplessness, guilt, anger, fearfulness for the safety and well-being of other children, depressive symptoms including sleep and appetite changes, and disorganization (Miles & Perry, 1985). During the reorganization phase, bereaved parents gradually begin to remember the child with less emotional pain, commemorate the child and focus on happier memories, reinvest in new relationships, and return to their usual life activities and responsibilities. Some bereaved parents report that they never truly recover from the death of their child, but rather that they learn to go on and that, as a result of the loss, they are never truly the same persons again (Schiff, 1977).

When the decision has been made to discontinue intensive treatment efforts, and the child's death has been declared imminent, the burden of comfort care rests with the nursing staff (Davies & Eng, 1993). During this time, the priorities for nursing intervention include comfort and dignity for the dying infant or child and his or her family (Henneman, 1993). The most important aspects of care for families during this time is to demonstrate a caring and genuine attitude, to extend kindness and understanding, and to be present with the family (Jost & Haase, 1989; Mendyka, 1993; Miles & Perry, 1985; Rando, 1986). Although nurses sometimes worry about what to say, and specifically how to say it to families, a caring and genuine approach is most important, and more likely to be remembered by families, than any particular thing that might be said. Johnson and Mattson (1992) have addressed the issue of communication with families before and after the child's death, including suggestions for open-ended questions and responses that may be helpful to families and anxiety-containing for nurses. Key elements include validation of feelings, empathy, and support.

Nurses do indeed help to "orchestrate" the death and early bereavement process for families in the context of the hospital setting. When cure becomes futile, care shifts to ensure death with dignity and comfort. Suggestions for intervention include providing accurate and ongoing information to parents, preparing parents for what to expect relative to the child's bodily functions and the dying process, and listening to and honoring parental stories about the child and parental expressions of grief (Jost & Haase, 1989; Miles & Perry, 1985). Parents often need and seek reassurance from nursing staff that everything possible has been done for the child, and that the child will not experience pain. Parents remember and acknowledge the importance of caring for the child with respect, addressing the child by name, attending to the "little kindnesses" (e.g., combing the child's hair), welcoming family members and friends, and individualizing aspects of care according to the family's wishes (e.g., child wearing own pajamas, favorite sleeping positions). Nurses may facilitate referrals for hospital chaplains; however, parents emphasize that it is important to be given a choice about this beforehand (Jost & Haase, 1989).

Choices relative to holding and viewing the body during discontinuation of life support equipment, and following death, are highly individual decisions for parents that are remembered long after the death. Parents should be offered an explanation of the procedure, including what they may expect and who, if anyone, may be in attendance, according to their wishes. Parents report that viewing the child's dead body serves as a means of closure (Jost & Haase, 1989). Parents may also like the infant's footprints, lock of hair, or hospital identification band as keepsakes. The parents' final good-bye to staff and exit from the unit, with its symbolic finality, may be eased with the escort of a familiar nurse.

Many units have developed standardized care plans for terminally ill patients that may be modified according to the child's circumstances and family wishes (Mendyka, 1993). Care plans such as these serve to assist nursing staff in delivering comprehensive care, facilitate the psychosocial aspects of care, coordinate communication and referrals, and ensure individualized aspects of care. Guidelines such as these help staff to orchestrate the many aspects of providing care to a dying child, and also ease the burden on individual nurses. In addition, in an effort to provide the best practice and to support families during the early bereavement process, many hospitals have implemented bereavement support and follow-up programs (Johnson et al., 1993; McClelland, 1993; Murphy, 1990). In general, families and staff alike note the benefits of bereavement support programs as a means to cope with childhood death. Educational and support programs, designed specifically to address the needs of staff nurses, have also been developed with the goals of better preparing nurses for caring for dying children and their families, and preventing "bereavement overload" (Pazola, 1988; Richmond & Craig, 1985; Vachon, 1987).

SUMMARY

Continued nursing research is needed to describe the possible differences in perceived parental stress in relation to the age of the parent and in relation to a constant primary nurse provider, and the trajectory of parental involvement in relation to the child's clinical status. Studies investigating the relationship between nursing staff attitudes toward parental involvement on parental stress and participation in care are also needed. Studies that illuminate how specific parental involvement can be therapeutic in the PICU setting can guide clinical practice. The long-term effects of PICU hospitalization on parents and children have yet to be investigated.

Pediatric critical care nurses must continue to challenge traditional practice. Nurses traditionally serve as the gatekeepers, the people who directly control parental access and involvement with their children. Parents are the ultimate consumers of pediatric healthcare. It is imperative that parental- and consumer-driven satisfaction be accomplished to economically survive in a highly competitive healthcare delivery system. Care must be inherently supportive to parents. Parental involvement must be encouraged and welcomed because family-centered care implies a partnership, not merely that 24-hour visitation is allowed (Curley, 1987, 1988). Nurses must continue to accept the challenge of developing strategies that assess parental needs, establish therapeutic nurse-parent relationships, provide care that is flexible and individualized, and support the parents' role in the care of their critically ill child. Nurses can make a significant positive difference for parents of critically ill children. By providing care that is inherently supportive to parents we help to make the experience of parent-to-a-critically-ill-child tolerable.

References

Ahmann, E. (1994). Family-centered care: The time has come. *Pediatric Nursing,* 20(1), 52–53.

Als, H. (1992). Individualized, family focused developmental care for the very low birthweight preterm infant in the NICU. In S.L. Friedman & M. Sigman (Eds.). *Advances in applied developmental psychology. The psychological development of low birthweight children* (pp. 341–388). Norwood, NJ: Ablex.

Anderson, G.C. (1991). Current knowledge about skin-to-skin (kangaroo) care for preterm infants. *Journal of Perinatology,* 11(3), 216–226.

Association for the Care of Children's Health. (1991). Bill of rights for parents. *A Pediatric Bill of Rights.* Bethesda, MD: Association for the Care of Children's Health.

Barnsteiner, J., & Gillis-Donovan, J. (1990). Being related and separate: A standard for therapeutic relationships. *Maternal Child Nursing,* 15(4), 223–228.

Beckham, J.D. (1993). Andrew's not-so-excellent adventure. *Healthcare Forum Journal,* May/June, 90–98.

Berger, M.M. (Ed.). (1978). *Beyond the double bind: Communication and family systems, theories, and techniques with schizophrenics.* New York: Brunner/Mazel.

Bertalanffy, L. von (1968). *General systems theory.* New York: George Braziller.

Bokinskie, J.C. (1992). Family conferences: A method to diminish transfer anxiety. *Journal of Neuroscience Nursing,* 24(3), 129–133.

Bogdan, R., Brown, M.A., & Foster, S.B. (1982). Be honest but not cruel: Staff/parent communication on a neonatal unit. *Human Organization,* 41, 6–16.

Bowen, M. (1978). *Family therapy in clinical practice.* New York: Jason Aronson.

Bowlby, J. (1973). *Attachment and loss* (Vol. 2: Separation). New York: Basic Books.

Bowlby, J. (1952). *Maternal care and mental health.* Geneva: World Health Organization.

Brody, D.S. (1980). The patient's role in clinical decision making. *Annals of Internal Medicine,* 93(5), 718–722.

Broome, M.E. (1985). Working with the family of a critically ill child. *Heart & Lung,* 14(4), 368–372.

Carter, M.C., & Miles, M.S. (1983). *Parental stressor scale: Pediatric intensive care unit.* Kansas City, KS: School of Nursing, University of Kansas.

Carter, M.C., Miles, M.S., Buford, T.H., & Hassanein, R.S. (1985). Parental environmental stress in pediatric intensive care units. *Dimensions of Critical Care Nursing,* 4, 180–188.

Cauthorne, C.V. (1975). Coping with death in the emergency department. *Journal of Emergency Nursing,* 1(16), 24–26.

Comoroff, J., & Maguire, P. (1981). Ambiguity and the search for meaning: Childhood leukaemia in the modern clinical context. *Social Science Medicine,* 15B, 115–123.

Craft, M.T. (1986). Effect of visitation upon siblings of hospitalized children. *Maternal-Child Nursing Journal,* 15(1), 47–59.

Curley, M.A.Q. (1987). *Effects of the nursing mutual participation model of care and parental stress in the pediatric intensive care unit.* Unpublished master's thesis: Yale University School of Nursing, New Haven, CT.

Curley, M.A.Q. (1988). Effects of the nursing mutual participation model of care and parental stress in the pediatric intensive care unit. *Heart & Lung,* 17(6,1), 682–688.

Curley, M.A.Q., & Wallace, J. (1992). Effects of the nursing mutual participation model of care on parental stress in the pediatric intensive care unit—A replication. *Journal of Pediatric Nursing,* 7(6), 377–385.

Current Population Reports (1991). Washington, DC: Department of Commerce, Economics and Statistics.

Davies, B., & Eng, B. (1993). Factors influencing nursing care of children who are terminally ill: A selective review. *Pediatric Nursing,* 19(1), 9–14.

Doll-Speck, L., Miller, B., & Rohrs, K. (1993). Sibling education: Implementing a program in the NICU. *Neonatal Network,* 12(4), 49–52.

Eberly, T.W., Miles, M.S., Carter, M.C., Hennessey, J., & Riddle, I. (1985). Parental stress after the unexpected admission of a child to the intensive care unit. *Critical Care Quarterly,* 8(1), 57–65.

Farrel, M.J., & Frost, C. (1993). The most important needs of parents of critically ill children: Parents' perceptions. *Intensive and Critical Care Nursing,* 8, 1–10.

Featherstone, H. (1980). *A difference in the family: Living with a disabled child.* New York: Basic Books.

Fischoff, J., & O'Brien, N. (1976). After the child dies. *Journal of Pediatrics,* 88(1), 140–146.

Fisher, D.H., Stanford, G., & Dorman, D.J. (1984). Services for parental stress reduction in a pediatric ICU. *Critical Care Medicine,* 12(6), 504–507.

Garcia Coll, C.T., Meyer, E.C., & Brillon, L. (1995). Ethnic and minority parenting. In M.H. Bornstein (Ed.). *Handbook of parenting* (Vol. II, pp. 189–209). Mahwah, NJ: Lawrence Erlbaum Associates.

Gilkerson, L. (1990). Understanding institutional functioning style: A resource for hospital and early intervention collaboration. *Infants and Young Children,* 2(3), 22–30.

Gill, K.M. (1993). Health professionals' attitudes toward parent participation in hospitalized children's care. *Children's Health Care,* 22(4), 257–271.

Greeneich, D.S., & Long, C.O. (1993). Using a model to assess family satisfaction. *Dimensions of Critical Care Nursing,* 12(5), 272–278.

Gutstein, S.E., & Tarnow, J.D. (1983). Parental facilitation of children's preparatory play behavior in a stressful situation. *Journal of Abnormal Psychology,* 11(2), 181–191.

Halm, M. (1990). Effects of support groups on anxiety of family members during critical illness. *Heart & Lung,* 19(1), 62–71.

Harrison, H. (1983). *The premature baby book: A parent's guide to coping and caring in the first years.* New York: St. Martin's Press.

Harrison, H. (1993). The principles for family-centered neonatal care. *Pediatrics,* 92(5), 643–650.

Harrison, A.O., Wilson, M.N., Pine, C.J., Chan, S.Q., & Buriel, R. (1990). Family ecologies of ethnic minority children. *Child Development,* 61, 347–362.

Harvey, M.A., Ninos, N.P., Adler, D., Goodenough-Hanneman, S.K., Kaye, W., & Nikas, D.L. (1993). Results of the consensus conference on fostering more humane critical care: Creating a healing environment. *AACN Clinical Issues in Critical Care Nursing,* 4(3), 484–507.

Hayes, V.E., & Knox, J.E. (1984). The experience of stress in parents of children hospitalized with long-term disabilities. *Journal of Advanced Nursing,* 9, 333–341.

Hebb, D.O. (1972). *Textbook of psychology,* 3rd edition. Philadelphia, W.B. Saunders.

Henneman, E. (1993). Multidisciplinary care plan for the dying patient: A strategy to promote humane caring in ICU. *AACN Clinical Issues in Critical Care Nursing,* 4(3), 527.

Henneman, E.A., McKenzie, J.B., & Dewa, C.S. (1992). An evaluation of interventions for meeting the informational needs of families of chronically ill patients. *American Journal of Critical Care,* 1(3), 85–93.

Heuer L. (1993). Parental stressors in a pediatric intensive care unit. *Pediatric Nursing,* 19(2), 128–131.

Hickey, M., & Lewandowski, L. (1988). Critical care nurses' role with families: A descriptive study. *Heart & Lung,* 17(6, part 1), 670–676.

Hill, R. (1949). *Families under stress.* New York: Harper & Row.

Jacono, J., Hicks, G., Antonioni, C., O'Brien, K., & Rasi, M. (1990). Comparison of perceived needs of family members between registered nurses and family members of critically ill patients in intensive care and neonatal intensive care unit. *Heart & Lung,* 19(1), 72–78.

Jay, S.S. (1977). Pediatric intensive care involving parents in the care of their child. *Maternal Child Nursing Journal,* 6(Fall), 195–204.

Jay, S.S., & Youngblut, J.M. (1991). Parent stress associated with pediatric critical care nursing: linking research with practice. *AACN Clinical Issues in Critical Care Nursing,* 2(2), 276–284.

Johnson, L., & Mattson, S. (1992). Communication: The key to crisis intervention in pediatric death. *Critical Care Nurse,* December, 23–27.

Johnson, L.C., Rincon, B., Gober, C., & Rexin, D. (1993). The development of a comprehensive bereavement program to assist families experiencing pediatric loss. *Journal of Pediatric Nursing,* 8(3), 142–146.

Johnson, P.A., Nelson, G.L., & Brunnquell, D.J. (1988). Parent and nurse perceptions of parental stress in the pediatric intensive care unit. *Child's Health Care,* 17(2), 98–105.

Jost, K.E., & Haase, J.E. (1989). At the time of death: Help for the child's parents. *Children's Health Care,* 18(3), 146–152.

Kasper, J., & Nyamathi, A. (1988). Parents of children in the pediatric intensive care unit: What are their needs? *Heart & Lung,* 17, 574–581.

Kirschbaum, M.S. (1990). Needs of parents of critically ill children. *Dimensions of Critical Care Nursing,* 9(6), 344–352.

Kirschbaum, M.S. (1983). *Needs of parents of critically ill children.* Unpublished master's thesis, University of Illinois.

Kübler-Ross, E. (1969). *On death and dying.* New York: Macmillan.

LaMontagne, L.L., Hepworth, J.T., Pawlak, R., & Chiafery, M. (1992). Parental coping and activities during pediatric critical care. *American Journal of Critical Care,* 1(2), 76–80.

LaMontagne, L.L., & Pawlak, R. (1990). Stress and coping of parents of children in a pediatric intensive care unit. *Heart & Lung,* 19(4), 416–421.

Lazarus, R.S., & Folkman, S. (1984). *Stress, appraisal, and coping.* New York: Springer.

Lewandowski, L.A. (1992). Needs of children during the critical illness of a parent or sibling. *Critical Care Clinics of North America,* 4(4), 573–585.

Lewandowski, L.A. (1980). Stressors and coping styles of parents of children undergoing open heart surgery. *Critical Care Quarterly,* 3, 75–84.

Lynch, E.W., & Hanson, M.J. (Eds.). (1992). *Developing cross-cultural competence: A guide for working with young children and their families.* Baltimore, MD: Paul H. Brookes Publishing Company.

Mahler, M.S., Pine, F., & Bergman, A. (1975). *The psychological birth of the human infant.* New York: Basic Books.

Maloney, M.J., Ballard, J.L., Hollister, L., & Shank, M. (1983). A prospective, controlled study of scheduled sibling visits to a newborn intensive care unit. *Journal of the American Academy of Child Psychiatry,* 22(6), 565–570.

McCubbin, H.I., & Patterson, J.M. (1983). Family transitions: Adaptation to stress. In H.I. McCubbin, & C.R. Figley (Eds.). *Stress and the family: Coping with normative transitions* (Vol. 1, pp. 5–25). New York: Brunner/Mazel.

McClelland, M.L. (1993). Our unit has a bereavement program. *American Journal of Nursing,* January, 62–68.

McLoyd, V.C. (1990). The impact of economic hardship on black families and children: Psychological distress, parenting, and socioemotional development. *Child Development,* 61, 311–346.

Mendyka, B.E. (1993). The dying patient in the intensive care unit: Assisting the family in crisis. *AACN Clinical Issues in Critical Care Nursing,* 4(3), 550–557.

Meyer, E.C., & Bailey, D.B. (1993). Family-centered care in early intervention: Community and hospital settings. In J.L. & R.J. Simeonsson (Eds.). *Children with special needs: Family, culture, and society.* New York: Harcourt Brace Jovanovich College Publishers.

Meyer, E.C., Zeanah, C.H., Boukydis, C.F.Z., & Lester, B.M. (1993). A clinical interview for parents of high-risk infants: Concept and applications. *Infant Mental Health Journal,* 14(3), 192–207.

Miles, M.S. (1979). Impact of the intensive care unit on parents. *Issues in Comprehensive Pediatric Nursing,* 3, 72–90.

Miles, M.S. (1980). *The grief of parents when a child dies.* Oak Brook, IL: Compassionate Friends.

Miles, M.S., & Carter, M.C. (1982). Sources of parental stress in pediatric intensive care units. *Children's Health Care,* 11(2), 65–69.

Miles, M.S. (1984). Helping adults mourn the death of a child. In H. Wass & C. Corr (Eds.). *Children and death.* New York: Hemisphere.

Miles, M.S. (1985). Emotional symptoms and physical health in bereaved parents. *Nursing Research,* 34(2), 76–81.

Miles, M.S. (1987). Vigilance as a parental coping strategy when a child is seriously ill. Abstract for poster presentation. Biennial meeting of the Society for Research in Child Development, Baltimore, MD.

Miles, M.S., & Carter, M.C. (1985). Coping strategies used by parents during their child's hospitalization in an intensive care unit. *Child Health Care,* 14(1), 14–21.

Miles, M.S., Carter, M.C., Spicher, C., & Hassanein, R.S. (1984). Maternal and paternal stress reactions when a child is hospitalized in a pediatric intensive care unit. *Issues in Comprehensive Pediatric Nursing,* 7, 333–342.

Miles, M.S., & Mathes, M. (1991). Preparation of parents for the

ICU experience: What are we missing. *Children's Health Care,* 20(3), 132–137.

Miles, M.S., & Perry, K. (1985). Parental responses to sudden accidental death of a child. *Critical Care Quarterly,* 8(1), 73–82.

Minde, K.K. (1984). The impact of prematurity on the later behavior of children and their families. *Clinics in Perinatology,* 11(11), 227–244.

Minuchin, S. (1974). *Families and family therapy.* Cambridge, MA: Harvard University Press.

Mishel, M.H. (1983). Parent's perception of uncertainty concerning their hospitalized child. *Nursing Research,* 32(6), 324–330.

Mitchell, P.H., Johnson, F.B., & Habermann Little, B. (1985). Promoting physiologic stability: Touch and ICP. *Communicating Nursing Research,* 18, 93.

Molter, N.C. (1979). Needs of relatives of critically ill patients: A descriptive study. *Heart & Lung,* 8(2), 332–339.

Moos, R.H. (1986). *Coping with life crises: An integrated approach* (pp. 3–28). New York: Plenum Medical Books.

Murphy, S.A. (1990). Preventive intervention following the accidental death of a child. *Image: Journal of Nursing Scholarship,* 22(3), 174–179.

Newman, C.B., & McSweeney, M. (1990). A descriptive study of sibling visitation in the NICU. *Neonatal Network,* 9(4), 27–31.

Parkes, C.M. (1965). Bereavement and mental illness: A classification for bereavement reactions. *British Journal of Medical Psychology,* 38, 13–26.

Pass, M.D., & Pass C.M. (1987). Anticipatory guidance for parents of hospitalized children. *Journal of Pediatric Nursing,* 2(4), 250–258.

Pazola, K. (1988 Winter). Remembrance: A strategy to prevent bereavement overload. *Caring,* 4.

Philichi, L.M. (1989). Family adaptation during a pediatric intensive care hospitalization. *Journal of Pediatric Nursing,* 4(4), 268–276.

Proctor, D.L. (1987). Relationship between visitation policy in a pediatric intensive unit and parental anxiety. *Children's Health Care,* 16(1), 13–17.

Rando, T.A. (1986). *Parental loss of a child.* Champaign, IL: Research Press Company.

Rennick, J. (1986). Reestablishing the parental role in a pediatric intensive care unit. *Journal of Pediatric Nursing,* 1(1), 40–44.

Resnick, M.B., Eyler, F.D., Nelson, R.M., Eitzman, D.V., & Bucciarelli, R.L. (1987). Developmental outcome for low birthweight infants: Improved early developmental outcome. *Pediatrics,* 80(1), 68–74.

Richmond, T., & Craig, M. (1985). Timeout: Facing death in the ICU. *Dimensions in Critical Care Nursing,* 4(1), 41–45.

Robertson, J. (1958). *Young children in hospitals.* Great Britain: Tavistock Publications.

Rothstein, P. (1980). Psychological stress in families of children in the pediatric intensive care unit. *Pediatric Clinics of North America,* 27(3), 613–620.

Rubin, R. (1967). Attainment of the maternal role. *Nursing Research,* 16(3), 83–91; 16(4), 324–346.

Rushton, C.H. (1990). Family-centered care in the critical care setting: Myth or reality? *Children's Health Care,* 19(2), 68–78.

Rushton, C.H., & Booth, P. (1986). The role of siblings during pediatric hospitalization. Presented at the 21st Annual Association for the Care of Children's Health Conference, San Francisco, CA.

Sanders, C.M. (1978–1980). A comparison of adult bereavement in the death of a spouse, child, and parent. *Omega,* 10(4), 303–322.

Schiff, H.S. (1977). *The bereaved parent.* New York: Crown.

Sevedra, M. (1981). Parental responses to a painful procedure performed on their child. In P. Azarnoff & C. Hardgrove (Eds.). *The family in child health care.* New York: John Wiley & Sons.

Shaw, E.G., & Routh, D.K. (1982). Effect of mother's presence on children's reactions to aversive procedures. *Journal of Pediatric Psychology,* 7(1), 33–42.

Shelton, T.L., Jeppson, E.S., & Johnson, B.H. (1987). *Family centered care for children with special health care needs.* (2nd ed.) Washington, DC: Association for the Care of Children's Health.

Shelton, T.L., & Stepanek, J.S. (1994). *Family-centered care for children needing specialized health and developmental services.* (3rd ed.). Bethesda, MD: Association for the Care of Children's Health.

Skipper, J.K., & Leonard, R.C. (1968). Children, stress, and hospitalization. *Journal of Health and Social Behavior,* 9, 275–287.

Strom-Paikin, J. (1984). Our son is dead. *Nursing Life,* 4, 18–20.

Szasz, T.S., & Hollender, M.H. (1956). A contribution to the philosophy of medicine. *Archives of Internal Medicine,* 97, 585–592.

Titler, M., Craft, M., & Cohen, M. (1988). Impact of a critical care hospitalization: Perceptions of patients, spouses, children, and nurses. *Heart & Lung,* 17(3), 314–315.

Tughan, L. (1992). Visiting in the PICU: A study of the perceptions of patients, parents, and staff members. *Critical Care Nursing Quarterly,* 15(1), 57–68.

Turner, M.A., Tomlinson, P.S., & Harbaugh, B.L. (1990). Parental uncertainty in critical care hospitalization of children. *Maternal-Child Nursing Journal,* 19(1), 45–62.

United States Bureau of Census (1989). U.S. children and their families: Current conditions and recent trends. Projections: 1988–2080. Washington, DC: Government Printing Office.

United States Bureau of Census (1990). U.S. population estimates by age, sex, race and Hispanic origin, 1980–1988. *Current Population Reports,* Series P-25, No. 1045. Washington, DC: U.S. Government Printing Office.

Vachon, M.L.S. (1987). *Occupational stress in the care of the critically ill, the dying, and the bereaved.* New York: Hemisphere Publishing.

Vulcan, B.M., & Nikulich-Barrett, M. (1988). The effect of selected information on mothers' anxiety levels during their children's hospitalization. *Journal of Pediatric Nursing,* 3(3), 97–102.

Watzlawick, P., Beavin, J.H., & Jackson, D.D. (1967). *Pragmatics of human communication.* New York: W.W. Norton & Company.

Wincek, J.M. (1991). Promoting family-centered visitation makes a difference. *AACN Clinical Issues in Critical Care Nursing,* 2(2), 293–298.

Wolfer, J.A., & Visintainer, M.A. (1975). Pediatric surgical patients' and parents' stress responses and adjustment. *Nursing Research,* 24(4), 244–255.

Wortman, C.B., & Silver, R.C. (1989). The myths of coping with loss. *Journal of Consulting and Clinical Psychology,* 57(3), 349–357.

Youngblut, J.M., & Jay, S.S. (1991). Emergent admission to the pediatric intensive care unit: Parental concerns. *AACN Clinical Issues in Critical Care Nursing,* 2(2), 329–337.

Youngblut, J.M., & Shiao, S.Y.P. (1992). Characteristics of a child's critical illness and parents' reactions: Preliminary report of a pilot study. *American Journal of Critical Care,* 1(3), 80–84.

Zaner, R.M., & Bliton, M.J. (1991). Decisions in the NICU: The moral authority of parents. *Children's Health Care,* 20(1), 19–25.

Zeskind, P.S., & Iacino, R. (1984). Effects of maternal visitation to preterm infants in the neonatal intensive care unit. *Child Development,* 55, 1887–1893.

The Practice Environment

This section focuses on the milieu affecting nursing care delivery. The broadening professional responsibilities of nurse as leader, teacher, and mentor are acknowledged and supported. Ethical and legal issues are illuminated from a pediatric critical care nursing perspective. Occupational hazards, a reality in the practice environment, are also addressed.

CHAPTER 4

Leadership in Pediatric Critical Care

MARY J. FAGAN

EMPOWERING PROFESSIONALS
Classic Management Theory
Humanistic Management Theory
Theory Z
Empowerment in Nursing
Shared Governance
Collaborative Governance
Other Empowerment Strategies
LEADERSHIP DEVELOPMENT
Listening Skills
Assertive Communication
Dealing with People in Difficult Situations and
  Resolving Conflict

Developing Effective Work Groups
Motivating People and Evaluating Performance
Problem-solving and Decision-making
Stress Management
Time Management and Delegation
**THE DELIVERY OF COST-EFFECTIVE,
  QUALITY CARE**
Quality Improvement
Cost-effectiveness
ON LEADERSHIP

Healthcare is in the midst of a revolution. Autocratic and authoritarian management styles are being abandoned in favor of empowerment through visionary leadership. Quality assurance has been replaced by the introduction of total quality management and continuous quality improvement; and cost-effectiveness has moved from being a lofty ideal to become the minimum expectation of an educated consumer. All healthcare leaders are being asked to rethink old ideas and pioneer the unexplored and new.

This shift in the way that things have been done has bought about immense challenges. As Machiavelli (1469–1527) has written in *The Prince,* "It ought to be remembered that there is nothing more difficult to take in hand, more perilous to conduct, or more uncertain in its success than the introduction of a new order of things. Because the innovator has for opposition all who have done well under the old conditions, and lukewarm defenders among those who may do well under the new."

The goal of this chapter is to provide an overview

of the major components of pediatric critical care management. Management's purpose is to provide effective leadership to empower a group of specialized healthcare professionals to deliver cost-effective, quality care to critically ill children and their families. The chapter's main sections are empowerment; leadership skill development; and the delivery of cost-effective, quality care.

EMPOWERING PROFESSIONALS

The evolution of hospital management practices has paralleled the development of management theory in general. Albeit slowly, hospitals have been moving away from classic management beliefs and are becoming committed to empowering employees through shared values and consensual decision-making.

Classic Management Theory

Classic theorists such as Taylor (1911) and Fayol (1949) emphasized the importance of centralized authoritarian management. It was their belief that there was only one way to accomplish a task and that management must determine which way things should be done. Then, management must communicate directions down to the front line and ensure that employees comply with the directions. Classic theorists also believe that employees are inherently lazy people who are motivated by money or fear of losing their jobs, and that they are naturally resistant to change.

Classic beliefs have been incorporated widely in hospital and nursing management. One need not be a student of nursing history to be aware that for centuries classic approaches espousing strict authoritarianism have been the norm in hospital management. The efficacy of this approach has been questioned, especially as it applies to managing and organizing professionals (Shamansky, 1989).

Humanistic Management Theory

McGregor (1960) disagreed with the negative assumptions classic theorists espoused about employees and argued that employees are complex individuals who are motivated by different reward systems. He believed that organizations would be more successful if they understood the human needs of employees, supported them, and used their potential. McGregor referred to the classic management theories as Theory X and his humanistic management theory as Theory Y. Theory Y opposes the belief that people are naturally lazy. It states that people have potential, and that they like to be active, productive, and involved.

Supportive management has been proven effective in the management of nursing professionals. Studies have demonstrated that supportive supervision has many positive effects, including decreasing job stress and burnout, and increasing job satisfaction (Duxbury et al., 1984; Cronin-Stubbs & Rooks, 1985; Blegen & Mueller, 1987; Norbeck, 1985).

Theory Z

Theory Z, the Japanese management theory, involves mutual trust, a participative process, and consensual decision-making based on shared values (Ouchi, 1981). In this framework all employees in an organization contribute to and evaluate proposals, creating a sense of collective responsibility for decisions. Shared organizational productivity and quality goals and a commitment to lifetime employment are hallmarks of this theory. Although the process of decision-making takes longer, changes are received with greater support.

This type of power structure recognizes the exper-

tise and commitment of the employee. It has been implemented in some hospitals through the development of shared governance programs that focus on empowering the professional. Hospitals are learning that there is much to be gained in an organization from this approach to management.

Empowerment in Nursing

In the 1980s and 1990s there has been an empowerment explosion in nursing. Studies have demonstrated that systems that empower bedside nurses increase job satisfaction and have low turnover and vacancy rates (Task Force on Nursing Practice in Hospitals, 1983; Kramer & Schmallenberg, 1988a,b; Kramer, 1990). In addition, it has been shown that systems promoting nurses' autonomy have improved patient outcomes (Knaus et al., 1986).

Magnet Hospital Study

A prime example of the results of nursing empowerment is the magnet hospital study originally conducted in 1982 (Task Force on Nursing Practice in Hospitals, 1983). This study identified 41 hospitals across the United States that were known for their excellent nursing care, for being places where nurses wanted to work, and for having low turnover and vacancy rates.

In 1986, Kramer and Schmallenberg conducted a follow-up study on a representative sample of 16 hospitals from this group. The results indicated that these hospitals were not experiencing problems from the nursing shortage that was occurring at that time and that they had remained institutions of excellence in the delivery of healthcare (Kramer & Schmallenberg, 1988a,b). A common thread was identified among the institutions—the hospitals, and their nursing staffs, were value-driven. The values are highlighted in Table 4–1.

In 1989, Kramer revisited the magnet hospitals and learned that they were still centers of nursing excellence (Kramer, 1990). She found that these institutions had remained value-driven, and identified seven other common threads among these institutions.

Staff Mix: Still Moving Toward More RNs. These hospitals were increasing the percentage of

Table 4–1. MAGNET HOSPITAL VALUES

Quality care
Nurse autonomy
Informal, nonrigid communication
Innovation
Bringing out the best in each individual
Valuing education
Respect and caring for the individual
Striving for excellence

Data from Kramer, M., & Schmallenberg, C. (1988). Magnet hospitals: Institutions of excellence. *Journal of Nursing Administration*, 18(1), 13–24.

RNs by decreasing the use of licensed vocational nurses (LVNs). They were also increasing the use of nursing assistants under various titles. The important component of the nursing assistant's role was that they were not assigned to patients; instead, they were assigned to a registered nurse. Their duties involved non-nursing patient care and environmental activities.

Organizational Structure: Middle Managers Had Been Removed From Clinical Decision-making. At these hospitals, the staff RNs were respected for their education, clinical competence, autonomy, and decision-making abilities. With a competent, autonomous RN staff less supervision was needed, and the nurse manager role was redesigned. The role of the nurse manager was changed from that of controller to leader. The span of leadership responsibility was increased, so that one person often had more than one unit to manage.

Salaried Status: Treating Nurses as Professionals. The trend toward having nurses become salaried employees was increasing. In 1986, nurses in five of the 16 magnet hospitals studied were on salaried status. In 1989, nurses in nine were either salaried or moving toward salaried status.

Self-governance: Minding Their Own Stores, but Participating in Department-Wide Issues. The trend toward self-governance in 1986 was continuing. The change noted was that at this time many of the chief nurse executives were distinguishing between the concepts of shared and self-governance. Most of the magnet hospitals had a system of autonomous self-governed operation at the unit level and participative, representative involvement in department-wide issues.

Nursing Care Delivery Systems: More Flexibility According to Patient Needs. Probably the biggest difference seen in the years from 1982 until 1989 was in the delivery systems used. In 1982 almost all of the magnet hospitals were using the primary nursing model, but in 1986 the shift moved toward total patient care. As the patients' length of stay was decreasing and flexible scheduling (with 10- and 12-hour shifts) found nurses working fewer days, there was a push to individualize the delivery system to meet the needs of the patient population and the unit. Case management was gaining popularity as a delivery system, and primary nursing, for the most part, was on its way out. One chief nurse executive was quoted as saying, "Primary nursing has taken a real beating" (Kramer, 1990; p. 70). The hospitals were committed to the philosophy of primary nursing and wanted to continue to achieve the positive results that primary nursing brought about, but changes in the care delivery structure were needed.

Maximizing the Practice of Available Nurses. In the magnet hospitals, more than 50% of the RNs were BSN prepared. This mix provided the opportunity for nurses to work with other nurses who were clinically competent, experienced, and educated.

In addition, 12 of the 16 hospitals had a "no floating policy," which represents an increase from 10 of 16 in 1986. The hospitals were trying to stop or limit the use of agency nurses. There was a slight increase in the use of agency nurses in the magnet hospitals from 1986, but 11 used either none or fewer than four full-time equivalents (FTEs) per month.

The hospitals used RNs predominantly; they were committed to holding to selective hiring values and practices in the face of the nursing shortage. New graduate employment was also being limited. In nine hospitals, only 25% or less of the new hires were new graduates. Units were being self-managed. Nine of the 16 hospitals report self-managed units.

Innovative New Programs. The hospitals were seeking to redesign or further develop new nursing care delivery systems. They were differentiating nurses' roles and setting up programs and activities to enable or empower staff. These institutions were focusing on strengthening nurse-physician practice relationships, flattening the organizational structure, and expanding computerization programs, particularly for documentation.

APACHE Study

The renowned APACHE study demonstrated significant correlation between nurse-physician collaboration and patient outcomes (Knaus et al, 1986). The study reported on the mortality rates in 13 selected intensive care units when patients were stratified for severity of illness and probability of outcome. Actual patient outcomes were compared with predicted outcomes based on the severity of the patient's degree of illness. The most significant finding of this study was that the involvement and interaction of critical care nurses and physicians had a significant correlation with patient outcomes. The intensive care units in which there was a high degree of nurse-physician collaboration and where the bedside nurses were highly involved in patient care decisions had better patient outcomes.

AACN Demonstration Project

The American Association of Critical Care Nurses (AACN) demonstration project participants studied one intensive care unit instead of a group of units (Mitchell et al., 1989). They wanted to see if a unit within an organization that had the aforementioned values of decentralized nursing services, participatory management, staff nurse clinical expertise (as demonstrated by an all-RN staff with 50% registered nurses certified in critical care [CCRNs]), and a high degree of nurse-physician collaboration would deliver high quality nursing care (as the APACHE study had demonstrated). In addition, they wanted to know if this type of nursing care could be delivered in a cost-effective manner. The outcomes of the project indicated that higher quality care was delivered in a cost-effective manner.

Table 4–2. SECRETARY'S COMMISSION ON NURSING'S RECOMMENDATIONS

Recommendation #7
Policy-making, regulatory, and accreditation bodies that have an impact on health care at the national, state, or local levels should foster greater repesentation and active participation of the nursing profession in their decision-making activities.

Recommendation #8
Employers of nurses should ensure active nurse participation in the governance, administration, and management of their organizations.

Recommendation #9
Employers of nurses, as well as the medical profession, should recognize the appropriate clinical decision-making authority of nurses in relationship to other healthcare professionals, foster communication and collaboration among the healthcare team, and ensure that the appropriate provider provides the necessary care. Close cooperation and mutual respect between nursing and medicine is essential.

Data from Department of Health and Human Services (1988). Secretary's Commission on Nursing: *Final Report* (Vol. 1).

Secretary's Commission on Nursing Final Report

Three recommendations from the Secretary's Commission on Nursing final report published in 1988 are germane to empowering nurses (Department of Health & Human Services, 1988). Fifteen recommendations pertaining to education, healthcare financing, utilization of resources, and compensation were offered. Those that specifically related to empowering nurses by way of participation in decision-making are listed in Table 4–2.

Final reports on the magnet and APACHE studies, AACN demonstration project, and the Secretary's Commission on Nursing all indicate that systems that empower staff are effective in recruiting and retaining nurses and in delivering excellent cost-effective care. Still, the change to a philosophy of empowerment in healthcare has been slow. This may be explained partially with a look back at the history of nursing and hospitals, which have their roots in the military and religious orders of medieval times. Changing practices that have been taking place for centuries does not happen overnight.

Military and religious orders are perhaps the most authoritarian organizational structures ever known. Both espouse strict adherence to rules and the preservation of hierarchies that insist on the total subservience and compliance of subordinates.

The problem becomes clear: On one hand there is a group of individuals, with education and expertise, who want to be treated in a professional manner. On the other hand, there exist hospital organizational systems with deep historic foundations adhering to a traditional bureaucratic philosophy and value system. Conflict is inevitable. The conflicts between bureaucratic and professional models are summarized in Table 4–3.

The key to resolving the conflicts inherent in the professional and bureaucratic systems is identifying goals and values that both groups hold. When common goals and values are identified between the professional staff and the organization, the conflicts become insignificant.

Authors of best-selling business books have been espousing this philosophy for years. Peters, who has written *In Search of Excellence, A Passion for Excellence,* and *Thriving on Chaos,* three excellent books on business trends, wrote in 1982 that the best run companies in America were using the following eight basic principles (Peters & Waterman, 1982).

1. A bias for action. A preference for doing something, anything, rather than sending a question through cycles and cycles of analysis and committee reports.
2. Staying close to the consumer. Learning their preferences and catering to them.
3. Autonomy and entrepreneurship. Breaking the corporation into small companies and encouraging them to think independently and competitively. In hospitals, this is called *decentralization.*
4. Productivity through people. Creating in all employees the awareness that their best efforts are essential and that they will share in the rewards of the company's success.
5. Hands-on, value-driven. Insisting that executives keep in touch with the firm's essential business.
6. Stick to the knitting. Remaining in the business that the company knows best.
7. Simple form, lean staff. Few administrative layers, few people at the upper levels.
8. Simultaneous loose-tight properties. Fostering a climate in which there is dedication to the central values of the company combined with a tolerance for all employees who accept those values.

In 1986, Marlene Kramer's second magnet hospital article focused on whether the excellent hospitals identified in the magnet study had the same charac-

Table 4–3. CONFLICTS BETWEEN BUREAUCRATIC AND PROFESSIONAL MODELS

	Bureaucratic	Professional
Loyalty to	The organization	The profession
Decisions made on the basis of	The goals of the organization	The goals of the organization and professional standards
Authority is based on	Position	The profession
Careers are sought in	The organization	The profession
Responsibility is felt to	The organization	The organization and professional ethics
Status is based on	Position	Professional competency

Table 4–4. TOM PETERS' PRESCRIPTION FOR A ''WORLD TURNED UPSIDE DOWN''

1. Creating total customer responsiveness
2. Pursuing fast-paced innovation
3. Achieving flexibility by empowering people
   a. Involve everyone in everything
   b. Use self-managing teams
   c. Listen/Celebrate/Recognize
   d. Spend time lavishly on recruiting
   e. Train and retrain
   f. Provide incentive pay for everyone
   g. Provide an employment guarantee
   h. Simplify/Reduce structure
   i. Reconceive the middle manager's role
   j. Eliminate bureaucratic rules and humiliating conditions
4. Learning to love change: A new view of leadership at all levels
5. Building systems for a world turned upside down

From THRIVING ON CHAOS by Tom Peters. Copyright © 1987 by Excel, a California Limited Partnership. Reprinted by permission of Alfred A Knopf Inc.

teristics as Peter's "excellent" companies (Kramer & Schmallenberg, 1988). The answer was yes.

In *Thriving on Chaos* (Peters, 1988), the author identifies five more prescriptions for success in what he refers to as a "world turned upside down" (Table 4–4).

From the business sector, John Naisbitt and Patricia Aburdene offer a traditionally female profession some very good news in *Megatrends 2000* (Naisbitt & Aburdene, 1990). Chapter seven of *Megatrends 2000* is titled "The 1990's: Decade of Women in Leadership." In this chapter, Naisbitt and Aburdene suggest that the corporations that we have known to date were created for men by men and that the new, successful corporations, with characteristics such as those identified by Peters, give women the distinct advantage in leadership. They write, "It is no longer an advantage to have been socialized a male, women may even hold an advantage because they do not

have to unlearn old authoritarian behavior to run their departments and companies" (Naisbitt & Aburdene, 1990; p. 217). "The primary challenge of leadership in the 1990's is to encourage the new, better-educated worker to be more entrepreneurial, self-managing, and oriented toward lifelong learning" (Naisbitt & Aburdene, 1990; p. 228).

Organizational structures based on the philosophy that empowerment of employees is a powerful management tool have been successful. In nursing, one of the mostly widely acclaimed management concepts is shared governance.

Shared Governance

The first published reports of shared governance in hospital nursing departments came from Rose Medical Center in Denver and St. Joseph's Hospital in Atlanta in the early 1980s. Porter-O'Grady and Finnigan co-authored *Shared Governance for Nursing: A Creative Approach to Professional Accountability* (1984), describing their experience with the model at St. Joseph's. Porter-O'Grady and Finnigan employed a councilor structure wherein responsibility and accountability rest with the same individuals or groups. Decision-making occurs at the councilor level (Fig. 4–1). There is a council on practice, a council on management, a council on quality improvement, and a council on education. A coordinating council integrates and coordinates the governance structure.

The major role of the council on nursing practice is the establishment of professional nursing practice standards. O'Grady and Finnigan warn that to be successful, the composition of this council must be carefully planned. It should incorporate clinical specialists, educators, and managers, but staff nurse members should represent the majority.

The council on quality assurance should also have

Figure 4–1 ● ● ● ● ● ●

Nursing operational framework—organizational structure. (From Porter-O'Grady, T., & Finnegan, S. (1984). *Shared governance for nursing.* ©1984, Aspen Publishers, Inc.)

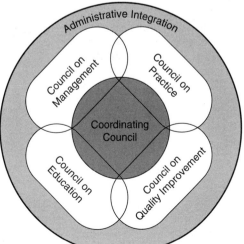

NURSING OPERATIONAL FRAMEWORK
Organizational Structure

Functional Accountability
Practice
Governance
Quality Improvement
Nursing Professional
  Development
Peer Behavior

a staff nurse majority and include other nursing practitioners. The function of this council is to review all nursing practices in the institution to ensure that the standards identified by the council on nursing practice are carried out and ensure their appropriateness.

The council on education is responsible for ensuring that the educational needs of the staff are met and that the mechanisms to maintain high levels of competence are in place. This council has accountability at both the unit and the corporate level, and membership is broad, including all unit-level services.

Membership on the council on management consists of the traditional management representatives, but the scope of responsibility changes dramatically from traditional management role. This council is responsible for giving support to the nursing staff and allowing them to make decisions. Often, the role of the management council is to institute measures to ensure that the decisions of the councils are carried out.

The coordinating council consists of chairpersons of each of the governance councils and the nursing administrator. This council focuses on all nursing activities, assuring their congruence with the nursing department's philosophy, goals, and objectives.

In addition to the councils, Porter-O'Grady and Finnigan describe a unit-based component to their model, the unit-level practice committees. These committees are subsets of the council on nursing practice and work under the leadership of the council. They are responsible for developing quality working relationships between physicians and nurses. These committees focus on the collaborative development of practice parameters, care plans, and intervention strategies.

Porter-O'Grady's shared governance system has its basis in ensuring accountability through the use of credentialing and privileging, and writing nursing bylaws (Porter-O'Grady, 1985). Similar to the manner in which most medical staffs are organized, credentialing and privileging is the process by which new members of the nursing staff are accepted and approved. The credentials review process involves ensuring each applicant has the appropriate licenses, diplomas, degrees, and certifications for the position sought, and that the applicant has successfully interviewed for the desired nursing staff position. After a successful 90-day probationary period, full nursing staff privileges are granted. Nursing bylaws are written statements that describe the relationships between members of the nursing staff and the responsibilities of each nursing staff member in relation to governance activities (Porter-O'Grady, 1985).

Collaborative Governance

Roseville Hospital in Roseville, CA, developed a management strategy called *collaborative governance* (Jacoby & Terpstra, 1990). This is a unit-based par-

ticipative governance structure that has its roots in the 12 shared beliefs of the nursing department (Table 4–5).

These values provide the basis for consensual decision-making in the Roseville structure and make bylaws unnecessary. The unit is the heart of collaborative governance, and there is a central structure to assure that unit activities are coordinated with departmental and hospital activities and goals.

Other institutions have described ways to implement the concepts of participative decision-making into governing nursing departments (Pinkerton & Schroeder, 1988; Ortiz et al., 1987; Jones & Ortiz, 1989; Shindler et al., 1989; Peterson & Allen, 1986a,b), and nursing units (Fagan, 1991, Zelauskas & Howes, 1992; Davis, 1992; Skubak et al., 1994).

Other Empowerment Strategies

In addition to new organizational structures, a number of other strategies have been employed in an attempt to empower bedside nurses.

Salaried Status

Based on the philosophy that true professionalism means control over one's hours as well as one's work, many hospitals (such as 9 of the 16 magnet hospitals) have converted from hourly pay practices to salaried status. Most of the programs have been successful, with nurses reporting increases in professionalism, self-concept, and self-esteem (Salaried status, 1988; Sills, 1993; Sierk, 1994).

It is important when changing from an hourly to a salaried status that nurses be paid a fair salary, typically one that would equal what the nurse would make with incremental overtime. In addition, nurses

Table 4–5. TWELVE SHARED BELIEFS OF COLLABORATIVE GOVERNANCE

1. Knowledge is power.
2. Given adequate information, people will make appropriate decisions.
3. Individuals are unique in their contributions.
4. A sense of purpose results when organization and personal values are congruent.
5. Maximum productivity results when organizational and personal goals are congruent.
6. Risk-taking, with or without success, is growth.
7. People are honest and trustworthy and will work hard to achieve their full potential.
8. Individuals are accountable and responsible for their practice.
9. All problems identified are mutually owned, and responsibility for resolution begins with problem identification.
10. Weaknesses and strengths are the same characteristics used differently (Weaknesses are strengths in excess).
11. Our decisions will acknowledge federal and state regulations and reasonable economic restraints.
12. Full cooperation with other divisions must be maintained to fulfill the hospital's mission.

need to have control over their hours by having input into scheduling policies and practices.

The pediatric critical care unit at University Children's Hospital in Hermann, TX, devised a salaried status program that met the needs of the nursing staff and the hospital (Murphy et al., 1989). The plan, professional reimbursement for nurses (PRN), allowed each nursing staff member to be available for six 12-hour shifts with two on-call shifts in a 2-week time period. The nurse's compensation was based on 84 hours of work and includes usual shift differentials and overtime observed for the hours over 80. The nurse's salary, as a result, was based on 86 hours of work every 2 weeks. This schedule allowed the nurse to work a minimum of 72 hours per pay period or as many as 96 while receiving a salary based on 86.

Evaluation of the PRN program by staff and management was favorable. Ninety-one percent of the staff wanted to continue the plan. The staff cited reasons such as relief from floating, provision of reliable unit coverage with trained staff, more time off (actual hours worked often less than number paid), improved unit teamwork and professionalism, more suggestions from staff with regard to scheduling, and consistent quality care.

Management evaluation revealed many advantages: (1) unit coverage was more consistent for a variable census; (2) cost per patient day remained within the targeted goal (the salaried plan did not increase labor costs, a major concern of hospital administration); (3) individual nurses became more accountable for unit coverage, independently solving scheduling problems; and (4) staff participated more broadly in unit activities.

Turnover rate in the unit dropped 14 percent after initiation of the program, and as a result, orientation hours decreased. Overtime utilization decreased significantly, and sick leave utilization was reduced by 19 sick hours per employee per year. Overall, the plan was budget-neutral, and patient care quality and unit morale were reported to be significantly improved.

In another institution, Zelauskas and Howes (1992) report the results of implementing a professional practice model on an adult and adolescent chemical dependency unit. The model included participative governance, peer review, and the introduction of a salaried structure. The exempt status salary of nurses increased between $4200 and $8000 annually, depending on shift. Actual amounts were determined by incorporating shift differential, holiday pay, projected overtime pay, and other pay incentives specific to their organization.

Three years later, an analysis of salary and nonsalary costs, sick time use, and turnover data demonstrated cost savings trends in the professional practice model unit as compared with those in a control unit. In addition, the authors describe the benefits of the employees adopting a philosophy of working until their job was completed, rather than just the hours mandated. They found the nurses worked more flex-

ible schedules to accommodate the times the unit was busy and the times when the unit was slow.

Two other units evaluating the shift from hourly to salaried status are reported by Blouin (1992). She describes pilot programs in a nine-bed cardiac intensive care unit and a large urban perinatal unit. The cardiac ICU had these results:

Despite increased patient census, total payroll costs were $30,000 less than budgeted
External agency costs were eliminated
Sick (nonproductive) hours were reduced by about 20%
Staff nurse vacancies dropped from 16.9% to 7.2%
Staff nurse turnover decreased from 10.5% to 4.7%
Quality assurance evaluation demonstrated increased quality of patient care documentation
Nurse managers spent 50% less time on biweekly payroll

In the perinatal unit, these results were reported 6 months after salaried status was implemented:

Pretest and post-test staff satisfaction was measured using the Minnesota satisfaction questionnaire and demonstrated significant positive change
Staff nurse turnover decreased from 17% to 0%
Overtime expense for the same time period fell from $7077 and $5551 paid the 2 previous years to $647 during the pilot

In addition, Blouin noted that in both experiences, staff perceived the salary program to be equitable and beneficial and it had resulted in staff nurses' perceptions of increased autonomy, personal control, and professionalism.

Despite these reports, salaried status is only a successful empowerment tool if it is set up to give nurses more control over their environment (Salaried status, 1988). If a hospital changes to salaried status solely as a means to save on overtime, or if there is only lip service about professionalism accompanying salaried status, the system will fail. In becoming salaried employees, nurses must have the benefits and responsibilities attendant with being exempt employees. These include discussions on decision-making processes and scheduling practices.

Incentive Plans

Incentive programs also serve as successful empowerment tools. Like other businesses, many hospitals are incorporating incentives and rewards for top performance. Clinical ladders and merit systems tied to performance provide these rewards. This trend has continued to reward employees at the top of their range with a lump sum merit pay or a bonus for top performance. In some institutions, the cap on the salary range has been removed, and merit increase of up to 10 percent is possible for excellent performance. Intangible rewards, such as recognition among peers for a job well done, also provide performance incentives.

In addition, employee incentive plans, long used by industry to boost productivity, have been implemented successfully in hospitals. Administrators of these incentive programs report that giving workers a cash interest in cutting costs can raise staff performance all around. In addition to containing expenditures, the incentive plans are said to strengthen morale, improve management-employee communications, reduce staff turnover, and provide a useful mechanism for measuring output (Hospitals find, 1979).

Mission Bay Hospital in San Diego, CA, developed an autonomous incentive program known as PRO/ Nurse. The program was based on the belief that quality nursing care and the highest standards promote growth of the hospital in the marketplace more than any other strategy. It provides nurses the opportunity to have a voice in the management of their hospital while receiving an incentive for managing the unit cost-effectively (Basante, 1991).

In this institution, nurses were seen as "owners" of their units, each having a personal interest in the success of the program. A board of directors that consisted of staff nurses and an ex-officio administrator provided direction and motivation for the operation of the nursing units and the earning incentive program. The incentive portion of this program was based on making nurses aware of their nursing costs and challenging them to provide quality care with a cost-effective attitude. When the department was able to care for more patients in a cost-effective manner, a percent of the cost savings went to the nurses giving the care (Basante, 1991).

Zelauskas & Howes (1992) included an incentive component in their professional practice model in which all nonsalary budget dollars saved by more efficient nursing practices were shared with the unit. As the nonsalary dollars per patient day declined, the unit was able to reallocate 50% of the savings to go back into the unit budget for future expenses. Unit committees then voted on how to spend the saved dollars.

The disadvantage of incentive programs has been that the Internal Revenue Service was hesitant to support "nonprofit" institutions participating in "profit-sharing" schemes. But in reality, the schemes are not profit-sharing but cost-saving programs and should result in a benefit to the patient and the payor, as well as the hospital and the motivated staff member. In addition, quality measurement must be instituted to ensure that cost-savings plans will not have a negative impact on patient care.

In designing a successful incentive program, several key points have been identified (Employee incentive plans, 1979): (1) keep the plan simple; (2) provide rewards in short-term intervals; (3) launch a well-planned promotional campaign before the program begins and continue promotion along the way to maintain interest; (4) institute a quality improvement plan along with the incentive program to en-

sure that cost-containment activities do not have an adverse effect on patient care; and (5) gain grassroots support by including key medical, nursing, and other staff in the planning and promotion of the program.

Many hospitals, such as the one described by Blouin (1992), have struggled with the ability to clearly identify measurable quality indicators for their incentive plans. Cost savings are easily identified and measured, whereas objective quality improvement indicators are not. Although they are more elusive, objective quality indicators are essential and must be incorporated into hospital incentive programs.

Unit-Level Strategies

Strategies such as changing to a salaried status or developing a hospital-wide incentive program may not be appropriate to undertake at the individual nursing unit level, but many empowerment activities can occur on nursing units. Simply adopting the philosophy that nurses should have the power to make decisions that affect them or their practice is a start. At the unit level, nurses can have the opportunity to participate in almost every decision that is made. Incentive programs as simple as offering recognition to those who are performing at a high level serve to empower individuals (Keyes, 1994), and shared governance programs have been instituted by staff nurses on individual nursing units (Fagan, 1991); Davis, 1992; Skubak et al., 1994).

In any unit-based empowerment program, it is absolutely essential to ensure that the basic values espoused at the unit level coincide with the values of the nursing department and the institution. This can be determined by reviewing the philosophy of the institution or department and the mission and goals of these groups. If the basic goals and values do not coincide, failure is certain.

LEADERSHIP DEVELOPMENT

Perhaps the most powerful technique in empowering nurses is to provide assistance and training in leadership skill development. Leadership is a learned behavior, and contrary to popular opinion, great leaders are "made," not "born." Essential to being effective, nurse managers must develop high level leadership skills, and they should use these skills to empower staff nurses to become strong leaders. This aspect is especially important in governance systems that seek to empower the bedside nurse.

In *Megatrends 2000* (1990), Naisbitt and Aburdene espouse the notion that "the dominant principle of organization has shifted, from management in order to control an enterprise to leadership in order to bring out the best in people and to respond quickly to change." They conclude that there are many managers, but few leaders. Effective leadership, according to Naisbitt and Aburdene, is recognizing that it is people who make or break an organization and that their power needs to be acknowledged. Leaders differ from managers in values, assumptions, behaviors, and, ultimately, results. The leaders with positive results are those who inspire commitment in employees and empower them by sharing authority.

In participative governance structures, consensual decision-making implies that all members of a group have the opportunity to participate in group leadership. For those who are unaccustomed to leadership roles, this can be threatening. Again, it is important to remember that leadership is learned, and developing nursing leaders requires learning the appropriate skills. Leadership skills can be divided into the areas listed on Table 4–6.

Listening Skills

Peters (1988) believes that listening is the best tool for empowering others, and has referred to the widely held notion that listening may be the chief distinguisher between leaders who succeed and those who fail. Active, engaged listening is the goal. This kind of listening demonstrates respect for an individual, exhibits genuine concern, and encourages people to express their views in return. Developing active listening skills requires that one internalize what a speaker has said. This means that the time the person is speaking is not spent formulating a response. An excellent method to use in improving listening skills is to practice hearing what others mean to be saying. Repeating or validating a message is a useful tool. For those who are experiencing difficulty with listening skills, a helpful exercise is to have the listener repeat exactly what the speaker has said before responding. This is a time-consuming operation, but it serves to ensure active listening and can lead to the development of this important skill.

Assertive Communication

Assertiveness is another learned skill that must be practiced. To be assertive is to be positive or confident in a persistent way. It is based on self-esteem and respect for self and others. Assertive behavior is standing up for one's rights to express one's feelings, reactions, or expectations without alienating the other person. Assertive communication is honest, direct, and appropriate. It is behavior-focused rather than personal criticism.

Assertion needs to be discussed in relation to its contrast to both passivity and aggression. Passive communicators do not stand up for themselves. They allow others to speak up for them, to push them around, and because of this, they may harbor resentment and anger. Aggressive people stand up for their individual rights, but in a manner that infringes on the rights of others. Aggression gets a person what they desire, but often alienates others in the process.

Baillie and coworkers offer the following suggestions to assist in cultivating assertiveness skills:

Practice Positive Self-communication. Expressions of positive regard such as "I am confident," "I am an effective nurse and leader," and "I am fun to be with" help us better deal with conflict and stressful situations that affect our self-worth.

Learn to Deal with Criticism. People who have difficulty dealing with criticism are those who feel that it is essential to be liked and approved of by everyone or that they must never make a mistake. Many see criticism as a rejection of self instead of a rejection of an action. It is essential to separate the problem from one's integrity, and then to respond to the criticism. There are negative ways of responding to criticism: (1) apologizing more than is necessary, (2) becoming defensive, (3) attacking the critic, (4) internalizing the stress and saying nothing. By contrast, one may deal with criticism in a productive and assertive manner. Options include (1) accept it, (2) disagree with it, (3) set limits for the critic, (4) fog, and (5) delay.

Accepting justified criticism from a respected individual is assertive as long as it is accepted without being considered an insult. Disagreeing with the critic is appropriate when the criticism is unjustified. It is important to back up a disagreement with a statement of self-affirmation. Setting limits with the critic is appropriate when the critic is behaving in an inappropriate manner such as using foul language or yelling. In this situation it is fitting to tell the individual to stop, to wait until a more suitable time for the interaction, or to leave the area. Fogging is a technique in which the individual acknowledges the critic, but then immediately changes the subject. Delaying is simply responding to criticism with a statement that the person needs more time to gather information before responding.

Setting Limits and Saying "No." In being assertive, it is important to set limits and say "no" when it is meant. Expectations must be made clear. Saying "no" and setting limits requires allowing negative feelings to be expressed. With practice, one can learn to set limits and say "no" because it fits with one's values, and in this way people teach others how to treat them.

Making Requests and Expressing Initiative. Knowing what is wanted and asking for it are hallmarks of this strategy. It requires risk-taking, a knowledge of self, and the ability to take no for an

Table 4–6. LEADERSHIP SKILLS COMPONENTS

1. Listening skills
2. Assertive communication
3. Dealing with people in difficult situations and resolving conflict
4. Developing healthy work groups
5. Motivating people and evaluating performance
6. Problem-solving and decision-making
7. Stress management
8. Time management and delegation

Data from Baille, V.K., Trygstad, L., & Cordoni, T.I. (1989). *Effective nursing leadership: A practical approach.* Rockville, MD: Aspen.

answer. Taking initiative and asking for what is wanted improves self-esteem and self-actualization, but it does not mean always getting what is asked for.

Expressing Anger. Expressing anger in an assertive manner requires being in touch with the feelings associated with anger and expressing them in a manner that allows further communication to occur. Using "I" instead of "you" statements allows the expression of anger without closing communication pathways.

Dealing with People in Difficult Situations and Resolving Conflict

A common problem for nurses developing their leadership skills is dealing with difficult people and resolving conflict (Freedman, 1993). Perhaps because of a desire to make things run smoothly or keep everyone happy, many nurses avoid dealing with these issues. A common notion is that certain people have always been difficult and will continue to be difficult, and it is a waste of time to try to solve the problem. There are several types of difficult people: the hostile aggressive, the complainer, the silent and unresponsive, the super agreeable, the negativist, the know-it-all expert, and the indecisive. To effectively deal with these types of people, Bramson (1981) offers the following suggestions: (1) do not simply wish that the person were different, (2) consider reasons for the difficult person's behavior, (3) achieve distance from the difficult person, (4) develop a plan to cope with the individual, (5) implement the plan using support from others and principles from behavior modification, and (6) evaluate and update the plan as necessary. These suggestions are also valuable for management teams or groups of nursing staff. If a particular person is seen as difficult by an entire group, developing a plan to cope with the person that is implemented consistently with group support can be very powerful. Especially if the plan incorporates principles of behavior modification and is evaluated and updated regularly, positive results can be achieved.

Conflict is inevitable in organizations and in life. Certainly, in the emotionally charged atmosphere of the pediatric intensive care unit, conflict is a daily occurrence. Conflict can be seen as a negative occurrence, or it can be seen as an exciting opportunity for learning and growth. When conflict is resolved successfully, positive change has occurred. There are five possible responses to conflict: competition, accommodation, avoidance, compromise, and collaboration. Competition is an aggressive and uncooperative approach to conflict. It creates a win-lose situation where the loser is left feeling angry and antagonistic. Accommodation is cooperative but unassertive, and it creates a lose-win situation leaving the accommodator feeling resentful and angry. Avoidance is unassertive and uncooperative. It creates a lose-lose situation. Pretending a conflict does not exist when it has

surfaced serves no one well. Compromise has some aspects of cooperation and some of assertion. Each side makes concessions in a win-lose situation in which both sides win a little and lose a little. Compromise is preferable to competition, accommodation, and avoidance but it is a weak conflict resolution technique. Compromise results in decisions that both sides can live with, but not necessarily the best solution that could have come from the interaction. Collaboration is both assertive and cooperative, creating a win-win situation. In this method both sides work together to find the best solution to a problem (Todd, 1989).

According to Douglass (1988), collaborative conflict resolution requires (1) clear definitions of values and goals, (2) open and honest communication, (3) a sense of responsibility of all who participate, and (4) an environment of trust and a commitment to achieving the best solution.

The following is an example of the use of collaboration in conflict resolution: A physician is troubled with the presence of parents in a busy, open PICU when a child is being admitted, rounds are in progress, or a procedure is being performed on another child. The nurses are concerned that parents would never be able to be with their children if they are asked to leave for all of the reasons cited. Because of his concerns, the physician is asking parents to leave the unit on his own. The nurses are upset with these actions. In collaborating with this physician, Douglass' (1988) steps were followed: (1) Present clear definitions of goals and values; it was agreed that the goals of the PICU with respect to this issue were to provide parents the opportunity to be with their child as often as possible and to afford privacy for the other patients and families in the unit. (2) Engage in open and honest communication; the parties verbalized concerns that space limitations and the open unit design did not provide the optimal environment in which to accomplish both of the stated goals, and that everyone needed to be aware of the goals. (3) Presenting a sense of responsibility of all who participate. Everyone agreed to work together to accomplish both goals to the best of their abilities; physicians would inform the nurses when procedures were about to be performed so that bedside nurses could ask parents if they wanted to stay with the curtains pulled for the duration of the procedure or take an opportunity to leave, and a movable screen would be available to provide privacy at the bedspace where procedures were being performed. Physicians would not independently ask visitors to leave; they would instead discuss the issue with the bedside nurse. Douglass also espouses the need for (4) an environment of trust and commitment to achieving the best solution. In this situation there was trust and commitment from all involved to attempt to accomplish both unit goals, and through this collaborative approach a positive outcome resulted.

Developing Effective Work Groups

High-functioning work groups or teams are essential to survive in today's environment. Common characteristics define these groups and set them apart from others. Buckholz and Roth (1987) describe eight attributes that identify high-performance teams. They demonstrate: a participative leadership style that empowers members; a shared responsibility for group activities and their outcomes; an alignment of purpose with clearly delineated group goals; high levels of communication characterized by mutual trust and respect; a future focus; a task focus; encouragement and support of creative talents; and a penchant for rapid responses, or as Peters (1982) describes it in his book, *In Search of Excellence,* a "bias for action."

Perhaps the biggest barrier to healthy work groups and teamwork is the absence of trust. Work groups in which there is little trust between members may go through the motions of teamwork, but will not be effective. In *The 7 Habits of Highly Effective People* (1990), Covey describes the natural process of growth and development that groups must go through to establish trust and become high-functioning. The process involves developing such principles as fairness, integrity, honesty, human dignity, service, excellence, potential, growth, patience, nurturance, and encouragement. Attempting to short-cut the process will result in disappointment and frustration. As a group leader Covey states "If you want to be trusted, be trustworthy." This process takes time and patience. Heider (1985) has similar beliefs about the role of group leaders (Table 4–7).

A tool known as the DISC profile has been used in numerous organizations to learn more about how individuals contribute to group dynamics. The tool measures four behavior dimensions that have an effect on team functioning: Dominance, Influence, Steadiness, and Compliance (Table 4–8).

High-D (Dominance) people are those who are results-oriented. They take authority, define what is to be done, and solve problems. Their focus is on the task at hand, and this can lead to losing sight of

Table 4–7. DOING LESS AND BEING MORE

Run an honest, open group.
Your job is to facilitate and illuminate what is happening. Interfere as little as possible. Interference, however brilliant, creates dependency on the leader.
The fewer the rules, the better. Rules reduce freedom and responsibility. Enforcement of rules is coercive and manipulative, which diminishes spontaneity and absorbs group energy.
The more coercive you are, the more resistant the group will become. Your manipulations will only breed evasions. Every law creates an outlaw. This is no way to run a group.
The wise leader establishes a wholesome climate in the group room. In the light of awareness, the group naturally acts in a wholesome manner.
When the leader practices silence, the group remains focused. When the leader does not impose rules, the group discovers its own goodness. When the leader acts unselfishly, the group simply does what is to be done.
Good leadership consists of doing less and being more.

From Heider, J. (1985). *The Tao of leadership.* Atlanta; Humanics Publishing Group.

Table 4–8. DISC PROFILE CHARACTERISTICS

D Dominance/Directness
Emphasis on shaping the environment by overcoming opposition to achieve desired results
I Influencing/Interactive
Emphasis on shaping the environment by bringing others into alliance to accomplish results
S Steadiness/Stability
Emphasis on cooperating with others to carry out the task
C Compliance/Competence
Emphasis on working with existing circumstances to promote quality in products or service

people, detail, and the pros and cons of a project. Those who rank high on the I-scale (Influence) demonstrate a people orientation. They are enthusiastic, motivate others, and relate well to the group. High-I people focus on people, and because of this they can lose sight of the task, detail, timing, and organization. People who demonstrate a propensity toward the steadiness (S) dimension have a procedural orientation. They focus on systematic, organized activity. They are good listeners and provide a stabilizing force, but can lose sight of the need for change or variety. The last dimension is (C) Compliance. These team members are detail oriented, analytical thinkers who control quality and check for accuracy. They are diplomatic and courteous, but can lose sight of the need to delegate, the need to make decisions, and the need to assume authority. Everyone has some degree of each dimension, and no dimension is better or worse than another. An important part of team building is to try to achieve a blend of the various dimensions in work groups. It is also helpful for group members to be aware of their dominant personality dimensions and those of their peers so that differences will be appreciated and individual strengths supported.

In addition, leaders can use this information in decision-making. For example, the policy and procedure council would be best chaired by a high-C person who will enjoy the detail of the work and have high standards for quality. If this person also demonstrates a high-S dimension, the committee will move steadily along in a systematic manner (Hargis, 1990).

Motivating People and Evaluating Performance

Attempting to better understand this important principle, many scholars have offered theories of motivation. Among them are Herzberg (1966), Maslow (1962), McClelland (1961), Skinner (1953), and Gordon (1982). Herzberg believes that people are driven by rewards that are both intrinsic and extrinsic. The extrinsic rewards, referred to as hygienes, include supervision, money, work conditions, relationships with peers, safety, and security. Intrinsic rewards, or motivators, are the challenge of the job itself, achievement, recognition, responsibility, advancement, and growth. Maslow's five levels of needs are represented as a pyramid of importance with basic survival needs at the most fundamental levels. According to McClelland's theory, people have three basic human needs: achievement, power, and affiliation. Achievement is the need to accomplish more than is expected; power is the need to persuade people to act in a way that they would not have under other circumstances; and affiliation is the need to have positive relationships. McClelland believes that everyone is motivated by one of these needs, each to a different degree. The key to motivation, according to McClelland, is to decipher and use the motivators that comprise the driving force behind a particular individual or group. Skinner believes that people are motivated by reinforcement of behaviors in a positive or negative manner. He would argue that it is the feedback that an individual receives from others, especially supervisors, that determines whether or not a behavior will be repeated. Gordon would disagree that direct supervisors can have much of an effect on motivating employees but rather asserts that each person has a set of internal motivators that only the person can comprehend. She suggests that the goal of management should be to create a motivating environment, or one that would afford the employees an opportunity to express and satisfy their own aspirations and contribute to the achievement of organizational goals.

More recent authors assert that to motivate people it is essential to develop "shared vision" (Senge, 1990), or as Covey contends, "to begin with the end in mind." These authors believe that one of the most powerful leadership tools available is the capacity to hold a shared picture of the future. Shared visions, according to Senge, emanate from personal visions. He encourages leaders to give up the traditional notion that visions must come from the top of an organization, or that it is appropriate for the leaders to go off and write a "vision statement" that will then be shared with and adopted by others. Although shared visions may come from the top of an organization, Senge suggests that visions that are truly shared take time to emerge, and are most often the result of ongoing conversations wherein people feel free to discuss their dreams and are inspired to truly listen to the dreams of others. People need not give up their personal visions, but instead, over time, multiple visions begin to coexist, and shared visions are the result.

Senge sees the development of a shared vision as one piece of a set of "governing ideas" that are necessary for organizations. These include the organization's vision, purpose or mission, and core values. A vision that is not consistent with the values people live from day to day will not be successful. The governing ideas are simply the answers to three basic questions: "What?" "Why?" and "How?" The vision is the What, the purpose or mission is the Why, and the core values are the How.

An organization's values describe how it wants life to be on a daily basis, how people will treat each other, and how the work will get done. Including everyone in the development of core values is essential. An example of a questionnaire that was used in the PICU at Children's Hospital, San Diego, to determine individual and group core values is a tool called "Systematic Multiple Level Observation of Groups" (SYMLOG). The SYMLOG tool measures current values held by a group or organization—those the group would like to see held in the future, values the group feel they are rewarded for displaying, and those they expect their customers would rate the group as showing toward them (Jensen, 1993). An important learning opportunity for the PICU was the analysis of present and future values, which presented a clear picture of where the group wanted to go—their motivators. In this PICU the unit was viewed as the "organization" for the survey and results were interpreted from the unit as a whole as well as from four identified groups—nurses, physicians, respiratory therapists, and others (unit secretaries, floor aides, pharmacists, social workers).

For the group as a whole, it was identified that an environment that was more friendly and slightly more task-oriented were values held for the unit in the future. With respect to the individual groups, the most striking differences were between the nurses and the physicians. The physicians desired a future orientation that was just *slightly* more friendly and *significantly* more task-oriented. The nurses favored an environment that was *much* more friendly and just *slightly* more task-oriented. This knowledge has helped each group understand some of the inherent differences in the motivation of nurses and physicians of this unit and has provided a basis for the development of unit goals.

The most successful method for evaluating performance is to have people evaluate themselves. If they participate in establishing the criteria by which they are evaluated, this method of evaluation can eliminate awkward and emotionally exhausting traditional methods. Covey (1989) conveys experiences in self-evaluation with college students that he describes as his best: He starts with a shared understanding of the goal up front: "This is what we are trying to accomplish. Here are the requirements for an A, B, or C grade. My goal is to help every one of you get an A. Now you take what we've talked about and analyze it and come up with your own understanding of what you want to accomplish that is unique to you. Then let's get together and agree on the grade you want and what you plan to do to get it." This type of evaluation is possible in nursing units. Specific criteria-based evaluation tools can be created in collaboration with those being evaluated and can still be tailored to meet the needs of each person. In addition, if leaders are committed to help each person achieve their agreed-upon individual objectives, the evaluation process can be a very positive experience.

Feedback from others provides a powerful learning opportunity that may be incorporated into the evaluation process. Many institutions use peer review as a component of each team member's performance appraisal. Feedback of any type is most helpful if it is provided continuously, however, rather than only at the time of one's annual appraisal. And although most commonly referred to as either positive feedback or negative feedback, it is also most effective when it is not simply one-way but circular, and is incorporated into a "feedback loop" in which change and growth take place.

Problem-solving and Decision-making

Covey (1989) describes three types of problems: direct control (problems involving a person's own behavior); indirect control (problems involving other people's behavior); or no control (problems that nothing can be done about, such as the past or situational realities). He offers an approach to solve all three types of problems.

For *direct control* problems, the solution lies in working on personal habits. If a problem is a result of a person's behavior, the solution is to develop new habits that will resolve the problem.

Indirect control problems are solved by changing the methods used to influence others. Everyone has methods of influence in their repertoire, but most people use only a few. People usually start with reasoning, and if this does not work they move straight to fight or flight. Covey has described over 30 methods of human influence that can be incorporated to achieve positive results. Among them are empathy, persuasion, example, and confrontation, and each may be used effectively in appropriate situations. The key is being flexible to change an approach when necessary.

Solving *no control* problems involves accepting them genuinely and peacefully, and learning to live with them. Even though no control problems are disliked, if they are accepted they are not empowered to control the individual.

According to Rubin (1985), the majority of the population are abdicators, giving up their freedom to make decisions. Most are not aware of how they abdicate; they doubt or criticize decisions they were once committed to, make so-called decisions out of panic, or let others decide for them. Dwyer and co-workers (1992) report that nurses may differ considerably in their preferences for autonomy in decision-making. They indicate that nurses who need a high level of autonomy will be more productive and satisfied in an environment that fosters participation in decision-making and primary nursing, and those with lower autonomy needs may desire more concrete direction. It is the responsibility of the nurse manager to attempt to motivate and energize this group, and not to settle into the routine of directing because the group does not want to make a decision. By motivating each other we are working toward empowering the profession.

Most people who abdicate their decision-making power probably do so for fear of having to be responsible for the possible negative repercussions of their decisions. They think of decisions as dichotomies: strong or weak, good or bad, win or lose. Covey (1989) believes that this thinking is fundamentally flawed, and that in decision-making, the result does not have to be "your way or my way," but instead can be a different way or a better way, in which all parties feel good about the decision and the action plan. This is called the Win/Win philosophy of human interaction. Win/Win is contrasted with the other possible paradigms of interaction: Win/Lose—"I get my way, you don't get yours"; Lose/Win—"Go ahead, have it your way"; Lose/Lose—"If I can't win, I'll be sure no one does"; Win—"I've secured my own future, the others can secure theirs"; and Win/Win or No Deal—"If we can't come to a decision that benefits both of us, we agree to disagree." In reality, there may be some times when the options other than Win/Win are appropriate. Such a case is when the issue is not that important and the relationship with the other person is highly valued; in this case it may be appropriate to do it the other person's way. But the best choice is always to try to come to Win/Win (Covey, 1989).

Getting to Win/Win is not an easy process. It grows out of high-trust relationships, and comes from a character of integrity, maturity, and the *abundance mentality*—the belief that there is enough out there for everyone. Once these are in place, Covey recommends a four-step process to achieve Win/Win:

1. See the problem from the other's point of view. Really try to visualize and understand the other person's point of view as well or better than the other person does.
2. Identify the important issues and concerns involved. This is not to be a list of the separate positions that people hold, but the real issues that are being discussed.
3. Determine the results that would mean a fully acceptable solution.
4. Identify some possible new options that would result in that fully acceptable solution.

Through the use of the Win/Win approach to decision-making, a synergistic process occurs. Decisions then change from being something many people choose to abdicate, to instead become an opportunity to create great solutions—solutions neither party would have been able to come to independently.

Stress Management

A conceptual model that addresses the stressors that occur in the intensive care unit has been described by Steinmetz and coworkers (1984). It includes three components: external stressors, internal stressors, and conflict avoidance. External stressors are those occurring as a result of crowded work places or confusing organizational policies. Internal stressors are created by role ambiguity, professional bureaucratic conflict, and situations such as dealing with angry people or believing that perfection is necessary. Conflict avoidance is a stressor brought on by failing to deal directly with conflicts or problem situations.

In a study focusing on PICU nurses, Gilmer (1981) identified the death of a child as the most stress-producing event. Other situations that were highly stressful to PICU nurses included dealing with families who were attempting to cope, problems involving interpersonal relationships, inefficient unit design, and the absence of necessary equipment.

Oehler and Davidson (1992) measured the predictors and incidence of job stress and burnout in PICU and nonacute unit nurses and found that although burnout was more of a problem in critical care nurses, 22% of all pediatric nurses reported symptoms associated with burnout. Particularly troublesome was the high incidence of burnout associated with personal accomplishment. Thirty-nine percent of nonacute unit nurses and 59% of acute care nurses reported a low sense of personal accomplishment.

In relation to the contributors to burnout, results indicated that job stress makes the most significant contribution to feelings of burnout. The death of a child was the highest source of job stress, followed by workload. Conflict with physicians and uncertainty regarding treatment were the third and fourth factors. Oehler and Davidson also found that state anxiety (the level of anxiety a person is experiencing at the present time), and trait anxiety (the amount of anxiety they usually experience) are powerful indicators of burnout. Coworker support was also a predictor of burnout, with groups perceiving low coworker support demonstrating higher levels of burnout. In this study the amount of experience the nurse had was the weakest predictor of burnout, with less experience being associated with higher rates of burnout.

To reduce stress and burnout, Oehler and Davidson (1992) recommend programs to help all personnel cope with death, creative solutions to managing patient assignments and monitoring of individual work load, and work on strategies for improving nurse-physician communication (particularly on the issues of patient management). With respect to anxiety levels, they suggest referrals to personal assistance programs if available. In the area of coworker support, work to develop a supportive work environment with group cohesiveness is recommended. They also suggest that less experienced nurses, because of their increased incidence of burnout, be targeted for special attention.

Fein (1987) has recommended strategies categorized as stress reducing, altering the perception of stress, managing physical well-being, and enhancing coping skills. Strategies to reduce stress include learning to say "no," distinguishing work from home activities, spending time efficiently, and developing friendship networks outside of work. In altering the perception of stress, Fein recommends increasing self-awareness through introspection, reevaluating personal and professional goals, determining what is important, and accepting that which cannot be changed. Managing physical well-being includes taking time out, treating oneself with love and respect, learning to relax without drugs or alcohol, exercising regularly, and eating for health. And in enhancing coping skills one may develop time-management skills; incorporate creative problem-solving; and develop communication, assertiveness, and listening skills. In addition, organizational strategies aimed at managing stress and preventing burnout are described in Table 4–9.

Time Management and Delegation

Time management is really self-management. The challenge is not to manage time, but to manage oneself. Covey (1989) has identified four ways that time is spent involving the concepts of urgent and important. He has described a matrix with four quadrants in which urgent and not urgent are on the horizontal axis and important and not important are on the vertical axis. "Urgent" means that something requires immediate attention, and "Importance" has to do with results—something that will contribute to accomplishing high priority goals. Urgent matters are something to which people react, and important matters are those in which is it necessary to consciously act, to make things happen.

Activities that are both urgent and important are commonly referred to as "crises" or "problems." Everyone has some critical activities in their lives, but others seem to spend all of their time thrown from one crisis to another. They are often referred to as "crisis managers." As a relief from the stress of constantly solving crises, they sometimes seek relief in activities that are neither urgent nor important.

Table 4–9. ORGANIZATIONAL STRATEGIES TO MANAGE STRESS AND PREVENT BURNOUT

Provide adequate staffing.
Institute staff psychosocial rounds.
Allow participatory decision-making.
Periodically review all policies, procedures, and guidelines.
Experiment with flexible scheduling.
Support and encourage creativity.
Increase personal accountability.
Recognize performance.
Establish professional support groups.
Encourage staff to express feelings.
Establish a nurses' journal club.
Promote personal growth by encouraging reading, writing, teaching, and research.
Adequately orient new staff.
Teach stress management as part of orientation.
Encourage continuing education at all levels.

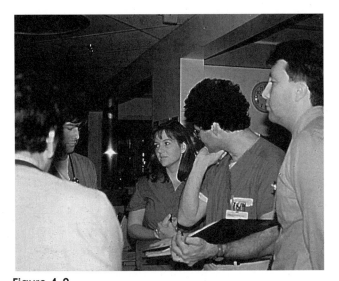

Figure 4–2 ● ● ● ● ●
The leadership role of the nurse is significant during multidisciplinary rounds.

They can thus run the risk of neglecting important yet not urgent activities as well as those that are urgent but not important.

Covey also describes people who spend much of their time dealing with urgent unimportant tasks. While they may think they are dealing with the highest priority items, they are in fact reacting to the priorities of others, not their own.

People who deal mostly with unimportant issues—whether "urgent" or not—never address the highest priorities and basically lead irresponsible lives. Effective people avoid dealing with unimportant issues and spend most of their time on the important priorities.

Effective people spend most of their time dealing with issues that are important but not urgent. This is how they can reduce the amount of time spent with important-urgent issues ("crises")—by dealing with important issues before they become matters of critical urgency. Important, nonurgent concerns include such things as vision, building relationships, long-range planning, exercising—things people know they need but often cannot seem to find the time to do.

To spend more time on the important nonurgent issues, it is necessary to spend less time on all the unimportant ones. This will involve learning to say "no" to some activities, some of which may appear urgent. This means deciding what one's priorities are, and sticking to them. It may then be necessary to kindly and courteously say "no" to some other things.

In organizing to spend as much time as possible dealing with important nonurgent issues, Covey has found that four key activities are involved: identifying roles, selecting goals, scheduling, and daily adapting. As a method to understand his principles, he recommends that people try this experience by organizing 1 week.

Identifying roles is simply the practice of listing key roles. These will include the role of being an individual, and may include being a parent or a spouse, son or daughter, professional, manager, committee member, volunteer, neighbor, or church member, among others. After the roles have been identified, the next step is to think of two or three important results that should be accomplished during the next 7 days in each of the roles. These will be listed as goals and should contain some quadrant II activities. For scheduling, the recommended process is to look ahead at the week and schedule time to achieve each of the listed goals. Previous commitments that are in line with established goals should then be added to the schedule, and those that are not in line should be rescheduled or cancelled. Daily adapting is then the process of prioritizing activities and responding to unanticipated events in a meaningful way.

Covey believes that this type of organizing allows people the freedom and flexibility to handle unanticipated events, to shift appointments if necessary, and to enjoy relationships and interactions with others while still knowing that their week has been organized to accomplish key goals in every area of their life.

Delegation is used to get work done efficiently and with optimal use of human resources (Fig. 4–2). Effective delegation requires knowledge and skill. It is often said that it is easier to do a task oneself than to delegate, which may be true for those who have not acquired the knowledge and skill necessary to delegate effectively. Initially, the work to be done must be identified and defined. The individual to whom the work is being delegated must be aware of the definition and description of the work and the timeframe in which it is to be accomplished. It is helpful to establish controls and checkpoints so that the work can be evaluated, and to have open lines of communication and mutually agreed upon goals (McAlvanah, 1989).

Stewardship delegation, as described by Covey (1989), is focused on results instead of methods. This type of delegation involves clear, direct mutual understanding and commitment regarding expectations in five areas. It takes more time in the beginning, but the time is well spent.

The five areas Covey is referring to are desired results, guidelines, resources, accountability, and consequences. With desired results, it is important that there be a clear, mutual understanding of what needs to be accomplished. This is not telling the person how to do the project, but rather stating that which needs to be accomplished and the timeframe that is involved. Guidelines refer to parameters within which the individual should operate. These should not be overly restrictive, but should provide assistance so that the person does not violate long-standing values or practices or have to re-create the wheel. Be honest—let the individual learn from previous mistakes and experiences. Do not tell people how to accomplish their objective, just give them a start. In the area of resources, Covey is referring to the human, financial, technical, or organizational resources people can use to accomplish their goals. Accountability means that specific standards of performance and timeframes for evaluation should be determined in advance. Consequences are the specific things that will happen, good and bad, as a result of the evaluation. This could mean financial rewards, psychic rewards, promotions, or other consequences.

With a stewardship type of delegation, even when it takes more time initially, both parties benefit and ultimately more work is done in less time. Stewards becomes their own boss, governed by agreed-upon results, and they have the potential to use their own creative energies to achieve the desired results. In the words of Covey "effective delegation is perhaps the best indicator of effective management because it is so basic to both personal and organizational growth" (p. 179).

THE DELIVERY OF COST-EFFECTIVE, QUALITY CARE

Quality has been a buzz word. It seems that everyone is interested in quality. Top corporations such as Ford Motor Company for whom "quality is job one" have recognized that continuous quality improvement, not simply quality assurance, is necessary to survive in a competitive marketplace. Healthcare organizations have been learning this as well.

In *Thriving on Chaos* (1988) Peters quotes Beckman in *Healthcare Forum* discussing quality in healthcare. Beckman conveys his amazement at the manner in which the healthcare industry has been confronting quality, as if all hospitals were "roughly equivalent." This, according to Beckman, "is a ridiculous contention." In 1986 the healthcare industry learned graphically that the quality of care on adult critical care units was not "roughly equivalent" from institution to institution. The APACHE study (Knaus, et al., 1986) rated 13 intensive care units based on predicted and actual mortality rates. The differences were impressive (see page 73).

Hospitals are now in the midst of a quality revolution. A transformation is occurring from the age-old practice of attempting to assure quality to actually measuring and improving the quality of care.

The Joint Commission on the Accreditation of Healthcare Organizations (JCAHO) introduced new nursing service standards in 1991 and wrote that quality is "a journey, not a destination" (JCAHO, 1990).

The transformation is necessary because now, more than ever in the healthcare industry, financial pressures and competition have forced the industry to make changes to ensure their survival. Continuous quality improvement is one of the changes.

Quality Improvement

Continuous quality improvement was introduced to business and industry by an American statistician W. Edwards Deming, who, as a consultant to Japan during its rebuilding stage after World War II, led the quality campaign that has resulted in the huge success of Japanese industrial efforts. Deming helped the Japanese develop an industrial culture that was concerned first and foremost with quality and continuous improvement. He identified 14 points to consider in achieving this goal. Gillem (1988) has applied these principles to the healthcare environment:

1. Create constancy of purpose for service improvement. This most important point describes the leader's role in the improvement of healthcare. Leaders must be future-oriented, define their goals, and communicate them to all employees.
2. Adopt the new philosophy. The new philosophy is "do things right the first time," and nothing less than this should be expected.
3. Cease dependence on inspection to achieve quality.
4. End the practice of awarding business on price alone; make partners out of vendors.
5. Constantly improve every process for planning, production, and service.
6. Institute training and retraining on the job.
7. Institute leadership for system improvement.
8. Drive out fear.
9. Break down barriers between staff areas.
10. Eliminate slogans, exhortations, and targets for the workforce.
11. Eliminate numeric quotas for the workforce and numeric goals for the management.
12. Remove barriers from pride in workmanship.
13. Institute a vigorous program of education and self-improvement for everyone.
14. Put everyone to work on the transformation.

By incorporating these principles into the healthcare arena, hospitals can strive to meet the emerging demands of patients and payors that quality healthcare be provided at the best value. Meeting customer needs must be the primary concern of this process (Gillem, 1988).

As part of their endeavor to foster quality improvement, the JCAHO mission is "to enhance the quality of health care provided to the public." They have related a fundamental principle of quality—that it can not be inspected into a product or service, but it must be built in as the product or service is designated and produced (JCAHO, 1990). The Joint Commission describes quality as including five major components: (1) good professional performance by physicians and other practitioners, (2) efficient use of resources, (3) minimal risk to the patient of injury or illness associated with care, (4) patient satisfaction, and (5) compassionate care.

Most quality assurance activities of the past focused on auditing to ensure that everyone was in compliance with an established standard and then counseling those who were not in compliance. The focus was on finding the "bad egg," and getting that person out, or instituting training to ensure that everyone knew the standard. The shortfall of this approach was that the vast majority of problems facing hospitals today are not problems with compliance of personnel or inadequate training, but instead are problems related to entire systems. In fact, the JCAHO estimates that as many as 85 percent of the problems in hospitals are systems issues instead of personnel problems.

In addition to the fact that they are the majority of problems in hospitals today, other reasons to focus on systems issues include the reality that looking at individuals and counseling people creates an environment of fear, defensiveness, and isolation. Staff who believe they will be punished for errors seldom report them; thus, data become distorted and opportunities for improvement concealed. The strategy of finding problems and fixing them also usually does not improve overall quality. Even if one person changes an old practice, the problems generally continue. The goal of quality improvement is to raise the norm of performance by focusing on processes.

The three main components of quality improvement are (1) studying and understanding processes that contribute to care; (2) measuring performance of processes and their outcomes using valid statistical methods, and (3) taking action to improve the way processes are designed and carried out. For example, a children's hospital had been closed to trauma admissions with increasing frequency because of no ICU nursing, no ICU beds, and no hospital beds. This resulted in patients having to be treated at a hospital that was not the designated pediatric trauma center and also resulted in a loss of revenue to the children's hospital. The statistics related to the closures were presented at various hospital committee meetings and, with the observation that the hospital was expanding its bed capacity, recommendations were made to increase the number of nursing staff.

Using a quality improvement approach to this problem, the first step was to *study and understand the processes that contribute to care*. Contributions were gathered from nursing staff, managers, staffing coordinators, physicians, and the trauma program manager, and a new data collection tool aimed at gathering information about why the hospital was refusing trauma admissions was devised and implemented. Next, performance was measured using *valid statistical tools*. Concurrent data from the new tool were collected and presented using numerators and denominators. Last, the group took *action to improve the way processes were carried out*. Based on the new data, it was evident that nursing staff members and bed availability were not the only reasons the hospital was referring trauma patients elsewhere. Other reasons included evaluating the appropriateness of the patients that were in the PICU, establishing systems to speed up the discharge process on the floors to open beds, and the inadequacy of the present per diem float pool. By improving the way these processes were carried out, more global improvement was possible.

Tools can be used in quality improvement to help understand the processes that are being studied and to clearly present the data that have been collected. Reliable data are essential to all quality improvement activities. Useful tools in understanding processes include brainstorming, the "fishbone" technique, and flow charts. Brainstorming is a technique for generating ideas about an issue from a group. It involves defining the subject of the brainstorming session, allowing time for everyone to think about the issues, and setting a time limit. One way to implement brainstorming is for each group member to call out ideas with someone noting each idea. During this time no one may comment or react to an idea. After all ideas have been shared, the group clarifies the ideas that were presented.

The "fishbone" technique is also known as a cause-and-effect diagram. This is a diagram showing a large number of possible causes for a problem, which, when constructed, looks something like a fishbone (Fig. 4–3). To construct a cause-and-effect diagram, a problem statement is placed to the right of a horizontal line with an arrow pointing to the problem. Major categories that contribute to the problem are then written on diagonal lines that point at the original horizontal line. If applicable, subcategories (or causes) may be listed that affect the main categories. The intent is to begin to understand the root causes of problems, and, once listed, the diagram can be used to determine obvious areas for improvement.

Flow charts are graphic representations of the sequence of steps that are performed in a specific work process. They can be used to identify an actual path that a service follows to see if there are any redundancies, inefficiencies, or misunderstandings; to identify an ideal path for a product or service; or to create a common understanding of how a work process should be done. To implement a flow chart it is necessary to decide on a starting and ending point for the process. Next, activities and decision points are arranged in the order of occurrence, and analysis of the flow chart serves to determine areas for improvement or explain the steps of a newly created process.

Tools that can be used to present data in an easily understandable fashion include histograms and run charts. Histograms are graphic representations of the frequency with which something occurs. They

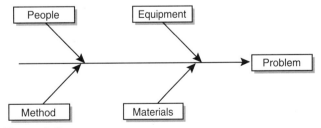

Figure 4–3 ● ● ● ● ● ●

Fishbone Diagram. (Used with permission from *The Memory Jogger: A Pocket Guide of Tools for Continuous Improvement.* ©1988 GOAL/QPC, 13 Branch Street, Methuen, MA 01844-1953. Tel: 508-685-3900)

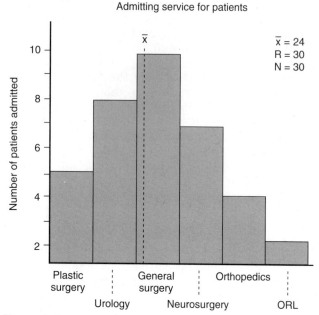

Admitting service for patients

$\bar{x} = 24$
R = 30
N = 30

Figure 4–4 ● ● ● ● ● ●

Example of a histogram. (Used with permission from *The Memory Jogger: A Pocket Guide of Tools for Continuous Improvement.* ©1988 GOAL/QPC, 13 Branch Street, Methuen, MA 01844-1953. Tel: 508-685-3900)

involve listing possible scores on one axis of a graph and the actual count for each category on the other axis (Fig. 4–4).

A run chart is a collection of points plotted on a graph in the order in which they became available over time. A graph is established with the horizontal axis representing time or sequence of the data and the vertical axis indicating increments of measure. Points are then plotted on the graph and connected with a line. The chart can be evaluated to identify meaningful trends or shifts in the average (Fig. 4–5).

These statistical tools are all incorporated to accomplish the goal of presenting accurate, understandable data. Without the use of statistical quality control measures, unsystematic data collection and

subjective evaluation of care can render quality improvement activities futile.

It is essential that all departments and groups participate in quality improvement activities. For example, if a problem is identified that involves patient medications, it is essential that the pharmacy and nursing cooperate with other departments involved to study the processes that lead to medication administration and discover ways to improve current processes. A single department cannot conduct meaningful quality improvement activities in a vacuum.

Quality improvement must be undertaken in a spirit of respect and support. This requires the belief that all people in the organization are committed to doing their best. A quote from the *JCAHO Manual on Quality Improvement in Special Care Units* (1992) emphasizes this point. "A clear message must be communicated to the organization. Management and quality improvement are here to help—not to slap wrists. The leaders will commit resources to reduce double work, eliminate wasted effort, and improve communication so that the organization's competent, caring, hard-working staff can perform with the fewest obstructions."

Cost-Effectiveness

With the adoption of the 1965 Medicare and Medicaid acts, healthcare costs in the United States have increased in relation to the gross national product from 5.2% to 11%. In addition, hospital costs have been increasing annually at about twice the rate of inflation (Kerr et al., 1991). Consumers and payors of healthcare are no longer willing or able to pay these escalating rates and are demanding that costs be contained. This trend has created a fervent search on the part of the healthcare industry for the most cost-effective method of delivering quality care.

In PICUs, large disparities in the efficiency of care have been reported (Pollack et al., 1987). In this report, 1668 patients representing 6962 patient days were studied in eight PICUs. The contributors to inefficiency of two patient groups—low risk moni-

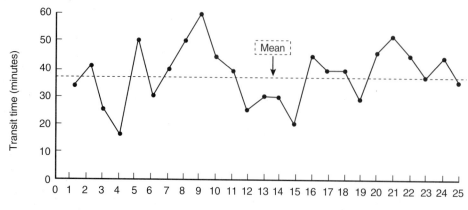

Figure 4–5 ● ● ● ● ● ●

Patient Transfer Process Run Chart. (Used with permission from *The Memory Jogger: A Pocket Guide of Tools for Continuous Improvement.* ©1988 GOAL/QPC, 13 Branch Street, Methuen, MA 01844-1953. Tel: 508-685-3900)

tored patients (who never received a unique PICU therapy) and potential early-discharge patients (whose last days of their PICU stay were judged to be unnecessary)—were quantified using measures of daily mortality risk and therapeutic assessments. Efficiency ratings varied significantly between the PICUs, with low-risk patients constituting 16 to 58 percent of the PICU patient population and potential early-discharge varying from 12 to 29 percent of the population. These findings suggest that there is a great deal of variability in the types of patients seen in PICUs and in the resources these patients use. Controlling this variability may be the key to controlling costs.

Case management is a care delivery method that has been reported to improve the quality of care patients receive and to reduce and control variability in resource utilization (Cohen, 1991; Weilitz & Potter, 1993). With the introduction of case management and clinical practice guidelines into practice settings, many institutions have been able to report a controlled connection between the quality and cost of care. This has been achieved by standardizing the appropriate use of resources for patients within an appropriate length of stay, aimed at specific patient care outcomes. Case management has also been reported to promote collaborative team practice among disciplines; facilitate coordinated continuity of care over the course of an illness; and promote job satisfaction and job enrichment for caregivers, patient and physician satisfaction with care delivery, and the minimization of costs (Olivas et al., 1989).

Whether in a case management environment or not, Rhea (1986) has suggested that the following steps be instituted to begin to achieve the results of decreasing variability in resource use: (1) accurate data must be compiled regarding resource use by case type; (2) a resource utilization standard should then be developed for each case; (3) the resource use of actual patients can be compared with the standards; and (4) variations are analyzed to determine their cause. Then, (5) cases are ranked in terms of the potential for reduction in resource utilization, and (6) research and experimentation with the process must continue.

In addition, Civetta and Hudson-Civetta (1985) have outlined 10 ways in which they reduced the costs of care in an adult intensive care without having a negative effect on quality. They are:

1. Principles of management. "Thinking, not widespread screening, discovers abnormalities." Changes were made in any existing arbitrary practice if it had no scientific basis.
2. Elimination of standing orders. All standing orders for laboratory tests were eliminated because they often resulted in unnecessary breadth and frequency of testing.
3. Classification of patients. Three categories of ICU patients were defined: (a) monitoring/observation, (b) intensive nursing care, and (c) intensive medical care. Although only 10% to 20% of

the patients fell into the last category and may have benefited from extensive testing, the same orders were often written for all patients in the unit.
4. Written guidelines. With the elimination of standing orders designed to minimize oversights, written guidelines were developed so that a unique set of laboratory tests could be ordered for each patient.
5. Mandatory communication. All teams caring for the patient were required to communicate about which tests have been ordered.
6. No repetitive orders. Holding the belief that ordering tests at repeated intervals usually resulted in testing that continued far beyond the clinical utility of the information, the practice was eliminated.
7. Single written orders. Verbal orders were only accepted in true emergencies.
8. Only catheters necessary for monitoring purposes were allowed. Those that simply provided easy access for specimen retrieval were removed.
9. Constant administrative attention. With the forces of insecurity, inexperience, habit, training patterns, traditions, and fatigue resulting in the proliferation of testing, it was essential for the responsible physicians and nurses to maintain constant attention to care practices as a demonstration of their commitment and concern.
10. Feedback. Because they differ significantly from existing practices, these changes were difficult to implement and maintain. Positive individual feedback and group meetings were necessary to guide the process.

By instituting these changes, Civetta and Hudson-Civetta (1985) were able to decrease ICU laboratory charges by a calculated 53% per patient. In 1983, this savings, extrapolated to a year's population in their 12-bed surgical ICU, achieved an anticipated savings of $2 million annually.

Nursing care delivery and RN mix also have a profound effect on the costs of hospitalization. Using a national multihospital data set, Glandon and coworkers (1989) learned that the care delivery model, percentage of RN staff, and the unit size all influenced the cost of patient care. Small primary care units with a high mix of RNs were found to be the most costly, even after controlling for differences in acuity. Costs varied most significantly (14.5%) based on the percentage of RNs, next (11.7%) based on the nursing care delivery model (team, modular, total patient care, and primary care were evaluated), and least by unit size (7.0%). This study did not attempt to measure differences in the quality of care, however.

A consensus on the best approach to providing cost-effective quality care for PICU patients has yet to emerge. Still, most PICUs are investigating various approaches to cost containment, including case management, changes in staffing mix with RN practice partners, or changing practice guidelines. It is essential that everyone who practices in the PICU take a proactive stance in controlling costs and eliminating waste.

ON LEADERSHIP

Leadership and management in the PICU is tremendously challenging. It is important to know, however, that with these challenges and changes come many rewards. The innovations brought forth by gutsy nursing leaders in the past 10 years have helped move the profession of nursing forward at a tremendous pace. Those who persevered in the face of adversity have contributed immensely to the growth of nursing as a profession.

If one area is singled out as that which will make or break leaders in a changing environment, it has to be the establishment of trust. Trust is defined as the "firm belief or confidence in the honesty, integrity, reliability, and justice of another person." (Webster, 1983). Most of the struggles people encounter in providing effective leadership have to do with a lack of trust. This concept can be especially difficult for new nurse managers or those who have been recently promoted, because the need to move forward at a rapid pace and make necessary changes is countered by the necessity to move slowly in establishing trust. A delicate balance must be achieved between spending time developing trusting relationships and spending time planning and acting on future goals. Most importantly, as Covey has stated, "If you want to be trusted, be trustworthy."

In conclusion, this chapter has focused on empowering nursing professionals, developing nursing leadership skills in all team members, and providing quality care at a reasonable cost. It has addressed some of the changes in management beliefs and healthcare financing that have had a dramatic impact on the PICU. In this constantly changing environment, the challenge for the PICU nurse manager is to maintain a sense of stability by adhering to established core values and establishing a sense of trust while incorporating innovative practices into unit operations. By focusing on the exciting challenges that lie ahead and concentrating on empowerment, leadership skill development, quality improvement, and cost containment, PICU goals will be achieved. For even amidst the uncertainty surrounding healthcare management in the 1990s, the overriding value of pediatric intensive care will remain constant—to provide the best possible care for pediatric patients and their families.

References

Baillie, V.K., Trygstad, L., & Cordoni, T.I. (1989). *Effective nursing leadership: A practical guide.* Rockville, MD: Aspen.

Basante, J.T. (1991). PRO/Nurse: An autonomous incentive-based concept. *Nursing Administration Quarterly,* 15(2), 59–63.

Blegen, M.A., & Mueller, C.W. (1987). Nurses' job satisfaction: A longitudinal analysis. *Research in Nursing and Health,* 10, 227–237.

Blouin, A.S. (1992). Exempt salary administration: Redesigning staff nurse compensation. *Journal of Nursing Administration,* 22(6), 24–28.

Bramson, R. (1981). *Coping with difficult people.* New York: Ballantine Books.

Buckholz, S., & Roth, T. (1987). *Creating the high performance team.* New York: John Wiley & Sons.

Civetta, J.M., & Hudson-Civetta, J.A. (1985). Maintaining quality of care while reducing charges in ICU. *Annals of Surgery,* (October), 524–530.

Cohen, E.L. (1991). Nursing case management. Does it pay? *Journal of Nursing Administration,* 21(4), 20–25.

Covey, S.R. (1989). *The 7 habits of highly effective people: Powerful lessons in personal change.* New York: Simon & Schuster.

Cronin-Stubbs, D., & Rooks, C.A. (1985). The stress, social support and burnout of critical care nurses: The results of research. *Heart & Lung,* 14(1), 31–39.

Davis, P.A. (1992). Unit-based shared governance: Nurturing the vision. *Journal of Nursing Administration* 12, 46–50.

Department of Health & Human Services. (1988). Secretary's commission on nursing: *Final report,* Volume I.

Douglass, L.M. (1984). *The effective nurse: Leader and manager* (2nd ed.). St. Louis: C.V. Mosby.

Duxbury, M.L., Armstrong, G.D., Drew, D.J., & Henly, S.J. (1984). Head nurse leadership style with staff nurse burnout and job satisfaction in neonatal intensive care units. *Nursing Research,* 33(2), 97–101.

Dwyer, D.J., Schwartz, R.H., Fox, M.L. (1992). Decision-making autonomy in nursing. Journal of Nursing Administration 22(2), 17–23.

Employee incentive plans. The newest idea: Give employee a share of what they save. (1979). *Cost Containment,* 1(6), 3–6.

Fagan, M.J. (1991). Unit based shared governance: Can it thrive on its own? *Nursing Management,* 22(7), 104L–104P.

Fayol, H. (1949). *General and industrial management.* London: Sir Isaac Pitman & Sons.

Fein, S.L. (1987). Burnout in nursing: Prevention and management. In I.A. Fein & M.A. Strosberg (Eds.). *Managing the critical care unit* (pp. 96–110). Rockville, MD: Aspen Publishers.

Freedman, M. (1993). Dealing effectively with difficult people: learn how to prevent differences from becoming difficulties. *Nursing 93,* Sept, 97–103.

Gillem, T.R. (1988). Deming's 14 points and hospital quality: Responding to the consumer's demand for the best value health care. *Journal of Nursing Quality Assurance,* 2(3), 70–78.

Gilmer, M. (1981). Nurses' perceptions of stresses in the pediatric intensive care unit. In S. Kramptitz & N. Pavlovitch (Eds.). *Readings in nursing research* (pp. 235–245). St. Louis: C.V. Mosby.

Glandon, G.L., Colbert, K.W., & Thomasma, M. (1989). Nursing delivery models & RN mix: Cost implications. *Nursing Management,* 20(5), 30–33.

Gordon, G.K. (1982). Motivating staff: A look at assumptions. *Journal of Nursing Administration,* 12(11), 27–28.

Hargis, C.L. (1990). Recruiting and retaining team players. In A. M. Brooks (Ed.). *Team building* (pp. 63–87). Baltimore: Williams & Wilkins.

Heider, J. (1985). *The Tao of leadership.* Atlanta: Humanics Publishing Group.

Herzberg, F. (1966). *Work and the nature of man.* New York: J.B. Lippincott.

Hospitals find suggestion programs thrive when employees receive a share of the savings. (1979). *Cost Containment,* 1(21), 1–2.

Jacoby, J., & Terpstra, M. (1990). Collaborative governance: Model for professional accountability. *Nursing Management,* 21(2), 42–44.

Jensen, D.B. (1993). Interpretation of group behavior. *Nursing Management,* 24(3), 49–54.

Joint Commission on Accreditation of Healthcare Organizations. (1990). Quality improvement in special care units. Oakbrook Terrace, IL: Joint Commission on Accreditation of Healthcare Organizations.

Jones, L.S., & Ortiz, M.E. (1989). Increasing nursing autonomy and recognition through shared governance. *Nursing Administration Quarterly,* 13(4), 11–16.

Kerr, M.E., Rudy, E.B., & Daly, B.J. (1991). Human response patterns to outcomes in the critically ill patient. *Journal of Nursing Quality Assurance,* 5(2), 32–40.

Keyes, M.A. (1994). Recognition and reward: A unit-based program. *Nursing Management,* 25(2), 52–54.

Knaus, W.A., Draper, E.A., Wagner, D.P., & Zimmerman, J.E. (1986). An evaluation of outcome from intensive care in major medical centers. *Annals of Internal Medicine,* 104, 410–418.

Kramer, M. (1990). Trends to watch at the magnet hospitals. *Nursing90,* June, 67–74.

Kramer, M., & Schmallenberg, C. (1988a). Magnet hospitals: Institutions of excellence, Part I. *Journal of Nursing Administration,* 18(1), 13–24.

Kramer, M., & Schmallenberg, C. (1988b). Magnet hospitals: Institutions of excellence. Part II. *Journal of Nursing Administration,* 18(2), 11–19.

McAlvanah, M.F. (1989). A guide to delegation. *Pediatric Nursing,* 15(4), 379.

McClelland, D. (1961). *The achieving story.* New York; Van Nostrand.

McGregor, D. (1960). *The human side of enterprise.* New York: McGraw-Hill.

Machiavelli, The Prince.

Maslow, A.H. (1962). Toward a psychology of being. New York: Van Nostrand.

Mitchell, P.H., Armstrong, S., Simpson, T.F., & Lentz, M. (1989). American association of critical care nurses demonstration project: Profile of excellence in critical care nursing. Heart & Lung, 18, 219–237.

Murphy, C.A., Walts, L., & Cavouras, C.A. (1989). The PRN plan: Professional Reimbursement for nurses. *Nursing Management,* 20(10), 64Q–64X.

Naisbitt, J., & Aburdene, P. (1990). *Megatrends 2000: Ten new directions for the 1990's.* New York: William Morrow.

Norbeck, J.S. (1985). Types and sources of social support for managing job stress in critical care nursing. *Nursing Research,* 34(4), 225–230.

Oehler, J.M., & Davidson, M.G. (1992). Job stress and burnout in acute and nonacute pediatric nurses. *American Journal of Critical Care,* 1(2), 81–89.

Olivas, G.S., Del Togno-Armanasco, V., Erickson, J.R., & Harter, S. (1989). Case Management: A bottom-line care delivery model Part 1: The concept. *Journal of Nursing Administration,* 19(11), 16–20.

Ortiz, M.E., Gehring, P., & Sovie, M.D. (1987). Moving to shared governance. *American Journal of Nursing,* July, 923–926.

Ouchi, W.G. (1981). *Theory Z.* Reading, MA: Addison-Wesley.

Peters, T. (1988). *Thriving on chaos.* New York: Knopf.

Peters, T., & Austin, N. (1985). *A passion for excellence: The leadership difference.* New York: Warner Books.

Peters, T.J., & Waterman, R.H. (1982). *In search of excellence: Lessons from America's best-run companies.* New York: Warner Books.

Peterson, M.E., & Allen, D.G. (1986a). Shared governance: A strategy for transforming organizations (Part I). *Journal of Nursing Administration,* 16(1), 9–12.

Peterson, M.E., & Allen, D.G. (1986b). Shared governance: A strategy for transforming organizations (Part II). *Journal of Nursing Administration,* 16(2), 11–16.

Pinkerton, S., & Schroeder, P. (Eds.). (1988). *Commitment to excellence: Developing a professional nursing staff.* Rockville, MD: Aspen.

Pollack, M.M., Getson, P.R., Ruttimann, U.E., Steinhart, C.M., Kanter, R.K., Katz, R.W., Zucker, A.R., Glass, N.L., Spohn, W.A., Fuhrman, B.P., & Wilkinson, J.D. (1987). Efficiency of intensive care: A comparative analysis of eight pediatric intensive care units. *Journal of American Medical Association,* 258(11), 1481–1486.

Pollack, M.M., Ruttimann, U.E., Getson, P.R., and members of the multiinstitutional study group. (1987). Accurate prediction of the outcome of pediatric intensive care: A new quantitative method. *New England Journal of Medicine,* 316(3), 134–139.

Porter-O'Grady, T. (1985). Credentialing, privileging, and nursing bylaws: Assuring accountability. Journal of Nursing Administration, 15(12), 23–27.

Porter-O'Grady, T., & Finnigan, S. (1984). *Shared governance for nursing.* Rockville MD: Aspen.

Rhea, J.T. (1986). Long-term improvement in cost and quality within hospitals. *Hospital & Health Services Administration,* 31(4), 64–73.

Rubin, T.I. (1985) *Overcoming indecisiveness: The eight stages of effective decision-making.* New York: Avon Books.

Salaried status: a boost to professionalism? (1988) *OR Manager,* 4(12) 6–7.

Senge, P.M. (1990). *The fifth discipline: The art and practice of the learning organization.* New York: Doubleday.

Shamansky, S.L. (1989). Who governs? *Public Health Nursing,* 6(1), 1–2.

Shidler, H., Pencak, M., & McFolling, S.D. (1989). Professional nursing staff: A model of self-governance for nursing. *Nursing Administration Quarterly,* 13(4), 1–9.

Sierk, T.A. (1994). Implementation of a salary model for staff nurses. *Nursing Management,* 25(1), 36–37.

Sills, L.R. (1993). Implementation of a salaried compensation program for registered nurses. *Journal of Nursing Administration,* 23(1), 55–59.

Skinner, B.F. (1953). *Science and human behavior.* New York: Macmillan.

Skubak, K.J., Earls, N.H., & Botos, M.J. (1994). Shared governance: Getting it started. *Nursing Management,* 25(5), 80I-J, 80N, 80P.

Steinmetz, J., Proctor, S., Hall, D., Blankenship, J., Greene, L., & Miller, G. (1984). *Rx for stress: A nurse's guide.* Palo Alto, CA: Bull Publishing.

Task Force on Nursing Practice in Hospitals. (1983). *Magnet hospitals: Attraction and retention of professional nurses.* Kansas City, MO: American Academy of Nursing.

Taylor, F.W. (1911). *The principles of scientific management.* New York: Harper and Brothers.

Todd, S.S. (1989). *Coping with conflict.* Nursing, 19(10), 100–106.

Webster (1983) Webster's New Twentieth Century Dictionary, 2nd ed.

Weilitz, P.B., & Potter, P.A. (1993). *A managed care system. Financial and clinical evaluation.* Journal of Nursing Administration 23(11), 51–57.

Zelauskas, B., & Howes, D.G. (1992). The effects of implementing a professional practice model. *Journal of Nursing Administration,* 22(7/8), 18–23.

CHAPTER 5

Professional Development

WENDY LUDWIG
MARY FALLON SMITH

The activity and process of staff development is the joint responsibility of the staff nurse, nurse manager, clinical nurse specialist, unit educator, and staff development department. Even though professional growth and development is facilitated by those in leadership positions, the ultimate responsibility is assumed by the individual staff nurse. Opportunities for professional growth and development are best used when the staff development plan for a unit is designed to support and enhance a well-defined clinical advancement program.

A successful critical care unit–based professional advancement program recognizes varying levels of staff nurse knowledge and expertise and fosters advancement through a wide range of clinical learning and professional development activities. Essential components of this program include an orientation

program, a continuing education plan, an in-service education schedule, and an array of other opportunities for clinical and professional development. Unit-based advancement programs are most effective when they coordinate with the nursing department's professional advancement program. In departments without central professional advancement programs, the philosophy and goals of a unit-based program should be congruent with the nursing department's stated philosophy and goals.

This chapter describes how professional development in critical care nursing is facilitated through a staff development plan that reflects a professional advancement model. Based on the understanding that novices in practice focus, interpret, and apply information differently than experts, a unit-based plan that recognizes developmental "levels" of practice best facilitates the professional advancement of *all* staff members.

A professional advancement program for the facilitation, recognition, and reward of expertise contains elements of both clinical and professional development strategies. For the purposes of this discussion, clinical development includes all the knowledge and skills used in the direct care of patients; professional development refers to the skills and knowledge used outside direct patient care, but connected to practice activities (e.g., peer review, certification, research, publishing, public speaking, poster presentation, political action for healthcare legislation, etc.). Critical care professional development strategies should therefore include multiple opportunities for the promotion of both clinical and professional growth. Although many of these opportunities are ultimately interrelated for the advanced practitioner, planning a comprehensive unit-based program that fosters advancement necessitates separate consideration of these two areas.

To best accomplish this objective, levels of practice as defined by the professional advancement program at Children's Hospital in Boston are used to illustrate aspects of clinical development. Implications for planning and implementing a program of professional advancement based on these levels are then discussed and broad performance characteristics are described for each level. In addition, specific examples are given to illustrate critical care behaviors typical of each performance level.

RECOGNIZING CLINICAL DEVELOPMENT

Benner's work, using the Dreyfuss model of skill acquisition, serves as a useful framework for understanding how nurses integrate knowledge and skill over time and, with repeated experience, progress from a novice to an expert practitioner. Benner (1984) describes five levels of practice: novice, beginner, advanced beginner, competent practitioner, and expert practitioner.

For each level of practice, Benner identifies performance characteristics and teaching and learning needs. Benner's work is particularly important in the design and implementation of a unit-based advancement program, as well as unit-based continuing education, because she notes which specific aspects of a clinical experience each level of nurses focuses on. Thus, clinical knowledge development can be enhanced and facilitated by assisting the nurse at any particular level of development to focus on the kinds of knowledge and experience characteristically associated with that level of practice. Unit-based indicators for meeting advancement criteria can be developed to help staff identify specific unit- and patient population–based examples of expected behaviors. It is important that staff understand these examples as *one* way, rather than the *only* way, to meet advancement criteria.

The description of "levels" of clinical nursing practice can be used as the foundation for a professional advancement program. As illustrated in Table 5–1, three levels of practice are described using broad criteria statements within four practice domains. These domains include clinical practice, clinical leadership, professional growth and continuing education, and research/quality assurance.

Level I Practice

Level I practice is based on Benner's description of the novice and advanced beginner, those with little or no experience in the clinical area (see Table 5–1). The rule-governed behavior that is typical of this level practitioner is strict and limited. Level I staff nurses tend to apply rules equally to all situations with very little or no ability to consider the context in which the rules are applied (Benner, 1984). At this level, staff focus on one aspect of a situation (or of care) and tend to weigh all assessment data equally because of lack of prior experience.

New graduates, relatively new graduates, those who have never practiced in critical care, and new orientees can be considered level I practitioners. As new orientees who have experience in critical care nursing become oriented to the patient population, the environment, and the unit policies and procedures, basic competence can be validated and characteristics of more advanced practice emerge. Orientation expectations remain consistent for all staff new to the unit; the rate at which orientation competencies are demonstrated varies between individuals, depending on past experience.

As level I staff complete orientation, learning experiences from actual patient care situations that illustrate one aspect of care can be examined. This level of practitioner can begin to see how the rules are influenced by the situation but continues to need help to integrate the parts into the whole. A level I staff nurse benefits from repeated experiences with similar aspects of patient care and from an educator who can point out similarities and salient aspects of a patient's response to care. This beginner, although competent to provide safe care, benefits from assistance in weighing assessments and in setting priorities.

For example, if a patient requires emergency intubation, the level I staff nurse can focus only on the airway during the crisis. This nurse performs bag mask ventilation with 100 percent oxygen as taught, has suction available, and has the appropriate endotracheal tube and laryngoscope blade ready. Typically, the level I nurse responds to the situation according to rules, focuses on one aspect of the situation only, and needs help in setting priorities if the patient's response is not the one anticipated.

Expectations for level I staff in the area of clinical practice development include assuming responsibility for meeting their own learning needs and staying abreast of professional literature that pertains to their practice. A well-designed staff development

Table 5–1. CLINICAL ADVANCEMENT CRITERIA

Staff Nurse Level I Criteria	Staff Nurse Level II Criteria	Staff Nurse Level III Criteria
	Clinical Practice	
I. DELIVERS COMPETENT, SCIENTIFICALLY BASED NURSING CARE TO PATIENT AND FAMILIES WHOSE NEEDS RANGE FROM UNCOMPLICATED TO COMPLEX 1. Systematically assesses patient needs from a holistic viewpoint 2. Engages the patient and family in the formation of an individualized plan of care based upon scientific principles, in which needs are identified and goals are set 3. Implements nursing care plan in an organized manner; establishes and re-orders priorities as necessary 4. Reevaluates plan of care as needed to achieve identified goals 5. Documents in accordance with established standards 6. Daily practice conveys a personal concept of the nursing role	I. DELIVERS PROFICIENT, SCIENTIFICALLY BASED NURSING CARE TO PATIENT AND FAMILIES WHOSE NEEDS RANGE FROM UNCOMPLICATED TO COMPLEX 1. Systematically assesses patient needs from a holistic viewpoint 2. Engages the patient and family in the formation of an individualized plan of care based on scientific principles and experiential background; needs are identified and goals are set 3. Interventions and documentation reflect a continuous reassessment of the patient's changing condition and desired outcomes 4. Acknowledges and uses expertise of others, through formal and informal consultation in planning and evaluating patient care 5. Conveys, through nursing practice, a clear sense of professional role and identity	I. DELIVERS EXPERT, SCIENTIFICALLY BASED NURSING CARE TO PATIENT AND FAMILIES WHOSE NEEDS RANGE FROM UNCOMPLICATED TO COMPLEX 1. Assessment includes recognition and interpretation of subtle clues 2. Integrates current status with theoretical and own experiential background to formulate specific and detailed goals and interventions 3. Reassessment includes recognizing subtle changes or trends in patient status; responds to unforeseen situations with efficient use of personal and institutional resources 4. Contributes to systematic knowledge development and research by integrating scientific inquiry into all areas of practice and decision-making 5. Models, through nursing practice, a clear sense of professional role and identity
II. ESTABLISHES A HELPING RELATIONSHIP WITH THE PATIENT AND FAMILY USING A HOLISTIC APPROACH 1. Interacts with patients and families in a compassionate and humanistic way 2. Develops an awareness of the boundaries of the therapeutic relationship 3. Identifies learning needs of the patient and family, and develops a teaching plan to meet these needs	II. ESTABLISHES A HELPING RELATIONSHIP WITH THE PATIENT AND FAMILY USING A HOLISTIC APPROACH 1. Has a committed and involved stance with the patient and family that validates them as "whole persons" 2. Develops relationships with the patient and family that facilitates mutual involvement in the planning of care	II. ESTABLISHES A HELPING RELATIONSHIP WITH THE PATIENT AND FAMILY USING A HOLISTIC APPROACH 1. Has an intuitive and comprehensive grasp of a clinical situation that allows identification of the essential problem(s) so that the real issues emerge and artifact is reduced 2. Has the ability to use oneself and the patient relationship to elicit patient involvement and strengths 3. Develops and uses innovative approaches to problem-solving and meets the individual needs of the patients and families
III. SUPPORTS THE CLIMATE FOR FORMULATING AND ACHIEVING GOALS BENEFICIAL TO PATIENT CARE AND PROFESSIONAL PRACTICE 1. Demonstrates evidence of understanding and participation in programmatic goals of the unit 2. Demonstrates a willingness to be a team member and to work collaboratively and interdependently 3. Practice reflects awareness of the short-term needs of the unit, the ability to prioritize, and the appropriate and timely use of resources	III. STRENGTHENS THE CLIMATE FOR FORMULATING AND ACHIEVING GOALS BENEFICIAL TO PATIENT CARE AND PROFESSIONAL PRACTICE 1. Participates in defining and implementing programmatic goals of the unit that are consistent with the philosophy and goals of the Department of Nursing 2. Fosters an environment that facilitates professional collaboration among inter- and intra-disciplinary colleagues 3. Possesses an awareness of the comprehensive needs of the unit. Assumes leadership in establishing priorities, managing resources and modifying environment to meet changing needs	III. COLLABORATES IN THE FORMULATION AND ACHIEVEMENT OF GOALS BENEFICIAL TO PATIENT CARE AND PROFESSIONAL PRACTICE 1. Assumes a leadership role in defining goals and developing programmatic solution 2. Integrates and supports group processes for making decisions among inter- and intra-disciplinary colleagues 3. Guides staff in making clinical/management decisions that consider available resources as well as desired outcomes of practice
IV. SUPPORTS AN ENVIRONMENT THAT FACILITATES GROWTH AND DEVELOPMENT 1. Shares own knowledge with colleagues. Participates in unit-based staff education sessions and staff meetings 2. Identifies own leadership qualities and learning needs; seeks opportunities to enhance personal growth 3. Identifies appropriate leadership role models and seeks their support and counsel	IV. FACILITATES GROWTH AND DEVELOPMENT OF COLLEAGUES 1. Manner invites utilization by staff for problem-solving. Assumes formally designated resource role for colleagues in the clinical management of patients 2. Provides formal and informal staff education in areas of own expertise 3. Demonstrates an awareness of learning needs of others in clinical and/or management areas. Assists throughout the process of meeting defined needs	IV. CREATES AN ENVIRONMENT THAT FACILITATES GROWTH AND DEVELOPMENT OF COLLEAGUES 1. Recognizes own sphere of influence; uses self and the relationship with colleagues to elicit their expertise and strengths 2. Uses an individualized approach to assist staff in the process of prioritizing goals and identifying resources to meet educational needs 3. Pursues diverse avenues in which to share nursing expertise with colleagues

Table continued on opposite page

Table 5–1. CLINICAL ADVANCEMENT CRITERIA *Continued*

Staff Nurse Level I Criteria	Staff Nurse Level II Criteria	Staff Nurse Level III Criteria
Professional Growth/Continuing Education		
V. DEMONSTRATES COMMITMENT TO THE PROFESSION AND COMMUNITY AT LARGE 1. Establishes and maintains membership in professional organizations 2. Daily practice reflects a personal concept of the nursing role 3. Demonstrates awareness of current healthcare policies that may influence practice	V. DEMONSTRATES COMMITMENT TO THE PROFESSION AND COMMUNITY AT LARGE 1. Establishes and maintains active membership in professional organizations 2. Articulates a personal concept of the nursing role; promotes peer and public awareness of the scope of contemporary nursing practice 3. Collaborates in preparing professional reports, articles and presentations within Children's Hospital and community 4. Demonstrates an awareness of the effect of public policy on healthcare delivery	V. DEMONSTRATES COMMITMENT TO THE PROFESSION AND COMMUNITY AT LARGE 1. Maintains membership and contributes to the goals of professional organizations 2. Exemplifies contemporary role of nursing; interprets aspects of nursing role to peers, colleagues, and those outside the profession 3. Prepares reports, articles, and presentations for professional/public policy on healthcare delivery 4. Interprets for peers and public the impact of public policy on healthcare delivery
VI. ASSUMES RESPONSIBILITY FOR OWN LEARNING 1. Assumes responsibility for self-evaluation 2. Formulates yearly goals and objectives and methods for accomplishing these with the nurse manager 3. Participates in the peer review process; identifies areas of merit and need for growth for self and others 4. Attends conferences, workshops, and seminars; shares information gained with collegues 5. Reads professional literature that pertains to current practice 6. Seeks out formal and informal contacts with professional colleagues	VI. ASSUMES RESPONSIBILITY FOR OWN LEARNING; CONTRIBUTES TO THE PROFESSIONAL GROWTH OF COLLEAGUES 1. Formulates both short- and long-term professional goals and objectives and methods for accomplishing these with the nurse manager 2. Acts as a role model in the peer review process; identifies areas of merit and need for growth for self and others 3. Attends conferences and formally critiques information gained with colleagues 4. Reads and analyzes articles from professional journals to assess whether information is transferable to patient care 5. Seeks out formal and informal contacts with professional colleagues within the institution and community	VI. ASSUMES RESPONSIBILITY FOR OWN LEARNING AND FACILITATES THE DEVELOPMENT AND ACHIEVEMENT OF PROGRAM GOALS 1. Professional goals demonstrate commitment to the advancement of unit goals 2. Facilitates professional growth by acting as a mentor for staff in the peer review process 3. Applies experiential background to knowledge gained from publications and professional meetings to advance nursing practice 4. Seeks new opportunities to promote professional growth; is a recognized resource by professional colleagues
Research/Quality Improvement		
VII. DEMONSTRATES COMPETENCY IN THE UTILIZATION OF CLINICAL STUDIES 1. Identifies reported clinical studies that have implications for practice 2. Identifies clinical nursing problems that may be appropriate for scientific testing 3. Participates in on-going research and quality improvement studies 4. Attends research conferences	VII. DEMONSTRATES PROFICIENCY IN THE UTILIZATION OF CLINICAL STUDIES 1. Critically analyzes clinical studies to justify the inclusion/exclusion of findings in practice 2. Evaluates existing practice to identify areas of potential study 3. Collaborates in the clinical studies of colleagues 4. Communicates with colleagues in conferences, poster sessions, and discussion	VII. DEMONSTRATES EXPERTISE IN THE UTILIZATION OF CLINICAL STUDIES 1. Generates enthusiasm for scientific inquiry in clinical studies 2. Collaborates in the design and implementation of clinical studies 3. Presents clinical studies to colleagues at professional meetings 4. Publishes clinical studies

With permission from Children's Hospital, Boston, Department of Nursing, Clinical Advancement Committee; Anne Jenks Micheli, RN, MSN, Chair.

plan provides regular opportunities for level I staff to identify learning needs through discussion of actual patient care experiences and then identify education or practice resources to meet those needs. Moreover, care-focused discussions allow more experienced staff to act as role models of professional development in activities such as presentations, group facilitation, discussion of current literature, and self-directed learning. In this way, level I staff begin to internalize values related to continuous clinical learning.

Level II Practice

Level II nurses, Benner's competent and proficient levels, are characterized by their organizational abil-ities and skills in coping with the competing demands and shifting priorities of clinical practice. Level II nurses gain efficiency and the ability to understand and react to a situation as a whole rather than in parts, basing current decisions and judgments on relevant past experience. In addition, level II nurses have developed the ability to recognize an unexpected turn of events and identify which aspects of a situation are more important than others.

In the situation of the child who requires emergency intubation mentioned earlier, the level II nurse responds in a more organized and proactive manner than the level I nurse. The level II staff nurse assists in airway management and has the appropriate equipment and drugs ready. The patient's response to therapy is anticipated; the family is informed and supported. This nurse demonstrates some mastery and ability to cope with the potential events that may be encountered during emergency intubation. The level II nurse understands the situation as a whole and responds based on past experience and recent events.

Level II nurses learn best from case presentations and interactive situations and from simulations that allow them to practice prioritizing, delegating, decision-making, negotiating for resources, and problem-solving in complex and sometimes ambiguous patient care situations. These nurses learn inductively from case studies and by reflecting on their own experiences over time. "When situations [case studies] are introduced that exhaust the performers' [Level II] way of understanding and approaching the situation, then a fruitful area of necessary learning has been uncovered" (Benner, 1984). Establishing this "need to know" for level II staff paves the way for continued clinical and professional development.

Level III Practice

Level III staff or expert performers have a vast background of experience and do not rely solely on rules, guidelines, or the like to make decisions related to patient care. This "expert is able to zero in on the accurate region of the problem without wasteful consideration of a large range of unfruitful alternative diagnoses and solutions" (Benner, 1984). The expert takes the entire situation and past experience into account in responding to patient care situations. This response is often characterized as "intuitive" and is an example of mastery: the ability to perceive and recognize a wide range of subtle cues and meanings, and to intervene decisively based on those cues and meanings.

In the example of the child who requires intubation, the level III nurse may first recognize the need to electively intubate very early and enlist a physician-colleague's assistance before the child's condition further deteriorates. The nurse is able to recognize a cluster of subtle cues as predictive and meaningful. Even if unsuccessful in convincing the physician to act, the level III staff nurse is able to anticipate the patient's needs and responses. Through this expert, often anticipatory intervention, the level III nurse is able to make the patient's illness trajectory smoother by pre-empting precipitous events. Expertise at this level results from repeated similar experiences that prompt the nurse to begin to make predictions based on the patient's responses.

The clinical nurse specialist (CNS) serves as a resource for nurses at all levels, but provides important advanced practice learning opportunities for level III staff. In collaboration with the CNS, the educator uses case studies to discuss the many factors, subtle cues, and contextual meanings that the nurse takes into account to make clinical decisions. In this way, they assist the level III staff in the recognition and documentation of their clinical learning. As an important resource person, the CNS further pinpoints the subtle early warning cues that expert nurses identify and respond to. Discussion of these cues is instructive for staff at many levels and may provide rich material for nursing research. Level III nurses can participate in research on clinical problems with the CNS and offer unique contributions to this process.

Clinical Advancement Process

A structured, well-defined clinical advancement process facilitates growth. Advancement of staff from one level to another is based on a variety of factors including nurse manager support, peer review and support, and self-evaluation. As illustrated in Table 5–1, nurses who meet the criteria in all four domains on a consistent basis may seek advancement.

The clinical advancement process can be completely centralized or completely unit-based or a combination of the two. For example, the process may be unit-based for advancement to level I and level II, but centralized for level III for purposes of consistency and consensus related to the identification of expert practice throughout the nursing department.

Examples of suggested minimum requirements for advancement in the pediatric critical care setting and recommendations for documents required from the nurse requesting advancement are listed in Table 5–2. The process for promotion from one level to the next should be clear and consistently applied to all applicants. A written guide to promotion at each level facilitates advancement and enhances understanding of the program as a whole.

Facilitating Clinical Learning

Educators who recognize levels of practice and apply knowledge of instructional strategies appropriate to each level facilitate clinical learning. Benner suggests that the way in which nurses approach problems is similar within each level of skill acquisition. She suggests that learning situations that pair a learner of one level with a preceptor closest to the learner's own skill level are most successful (Benner, 1984). Adult learning theory (Knowles, 1970) supports this hypothesis because it takes into account the teacher's awareness of the learner's readiness to learn and need to know the information or skill being taught or demonstrated.

Facilitation of professional advancement in a pediatric critical care setting can be realized through a well-designed unit-based staff development program. This program is a key element in the advancement process and promotes the knowledge and skills necessary for continued professional development.

A staff development program that reflects professional advancement criteria offers nurses the means to achieve professional advancement objectives. Fur-

Table 5–2. MINIMUM REQUIREMENTS AND DOCUMENTATION REQUIRED FOR ADVANCEMENT

Level I	Level II	Level III
Requirements		
• Successful completion of orientation • 1 year nursing practice • 6 months pediatric nursing practice • 6 months pediatric critical care nursing practice	• 2 years nursing practice • 1 year pediatric practice • 2 years pediatric critical care experience	• 5 years nursing practice • 2 years pediatric practice • 1 year pediatric critical care practice
• Meets staff nurse I criteria in all domains	• Meets staff nurse II criteria in all domains	• Meets staff nurse III criteria in all domains
Documentation		
• Nurse manager approval • Portfolio from the nurse requesting promotion: Statement of intent Goals and objectives Documentation of performance, using two exemplars that demonstrate level I performance Letter of peer support from one level II staff	• Nurse manager approval • Portfolio from the nurse requesting promotion: Statement of intent Goals and objectives Documentation of performance using two exemplars that demonstrate level II performance Peer review and peer letters of support (two letters, one from a level II or level III staff)	• Nurse manager approval and written evaluation • Portfolio from the nurse requesting promotion: Statement of intent Curriculum vitae Statement of practice Documentation of performance, using two exemplars that demonstrate level III performance Peer review and peer letters of support (three letters of support, one from a level II or level III, two from colleagues outside the unit)

With permission from Children's Hospital, Boston, Department of Nursing, Cardiac Intensive Care Unit; Patricia Hickey, RN, MSN, Nurse Director.

thermore, when these two important programs complement each other, nursing practice as a whole is strengthened.

DESIGNING STAFF DEVELOPMENT PROGRAMS FOR PROFESSIONAL ADVANCEMENT

The fundamental aim of staff development programs for critical care nurses is safe, competent practice. Sound programs for staff development provide the essential resources to support and promote this goal. Similarly, healthcare laws, regulations, and accreditation requirements focus on the basic importance of safe, competent patient care in an effort to protect the healthcare consumer. Professional nursing standards of practice likewise serve as guides for ensuring safe practice and consumer protection. To ensure that the institution meets all current standards, those responsible for designing critical care education programs must be familiar with all of these prerequisites. The establishment of a sound staff development program is key to the success of a professional advancement program.

The first step in establishing a staff development program is the acquisition of firm support from both nursing and hospital administration. This requires a commitment to provide the human, financial, material, and environmental resources necessary to implement the program. Once this commitment is secured, the nurse educator may begin to structure the program.

Hospital-based critical care staff development programs may be centralized or decentralized. Centralized programs offer the advantage of maximizing resources within the entire nursing department and standardizing programs across units; whereas unit-based, or decentralized, programs maintain separate budgets to specifically respond to the needs of a particular unit.

Regardless of which option is chosen, the reporting relationship between the critical care nurse educator and nursing administration must be clear. Once the administrative structure is in place, the program philosophy, goals, policies, and organizing framework may be developed.

Developing a Program Philosophy

A philosophy statement consists of a set of beliefs related to a specific issue. A comprehensive critical care staff development philosophy reflects the beliefs and values of the critical care area, the department of nursing, and the hospital. This consistency reinforces the program's integration within overall hospital and nursing programs and verifies a commitment to common goals. In addition, an essential component of the critical care staff development philosophy is a clearly stated philosophy of adult education that defines learning and the factors that distinguish both the role of the educator and the role of the learner. For instance, a well-accepted learning theory states that learning only takes place when there is a change in learner behavior, and that the responsibility for learning lies with the learner; the educator's role is to provide the learner with opportunities to learn

(Jiricka, 1987). It is important that these underlying beliefs be clearly communicated in the program philosophy statement.

Overview of Adult Learning Theory

To develop a philosophy statement that reflects adult education principles requires a working knowledge of adult learning theory and the specific characteristics of adult learners. Pike (1988) describes adults as, "babies in big bodies," which connotes that they expect much and like to play while they learn. Nurses, as adult learners, seek out learning experiences that meet personal needs or are interesting to them relative to their practice; they typically prefer to learn by doing rather than by observation.

Knowles (1970) and other theorists of adult learning describe common characteristics of adult learners. They are self-directed, problem-oriented learners who are guided by their own values and come from a heterogeneous experience. Unlike children, adult learners hold an independent self-concept and value their personal time (Jiricka, et al., 1987). Principles of adult learning are derived from these characteristics.

The four principles of adult learning that are most applicable to critical care nurses are those concerning reinforcement, readiness to learn, goals, and the learning environment (Morrow, 1984). Reinforcement in the learning process may be positive or negative. If a newly learned behavior stimulates a positive response, the chances of the behavior recurring is increased. Likewise, if a behavior leads to the elimination of an undesirable response, that behavior will most likely be repeated. For example, a level I nurse who correctly manages a patient's slow cardiac rhythm by implementing a newly learned treatment protocol is likely to follow that protocol again.

Adults are more apt to learn if they perceive societal or professional pressure, a reflection of their developmental tasks. Today, most nurses fall into the middle adult age range, a time in which adults typically strive to maintain an income and achieve recognition. (Tobin, et al., 1979). Hence, they will seek learning experiences that enable them to attain higher nursing credentials and ensure job stability and security.

Adults learn better if they perceive that an educational program meets their personal goals. If program content relates to their current concerns, they are more motivated to learn. For example, nurses interested in working with patients with a congenital diaphragmatic hernia will be more motivated to learn about extracorporeal membrane oxygenation (ECMO) than nurses with other interests.

The learning environment has a definite impact on the adult learning process. The learner must feel comfortable both physically and emotionally if learning is to take place. Some of the most common negative comments found on formal education program evaluations include that the room is too hot or too cold or the seats are uncomfortable. These adverse environmental factors distract the learner.

Environmental factors also affect the clinical learning environment. An environment that causes sensory overload from an unusually high census or an emergency situation is not conducive to learning. The learner focuses on the noise and activities rather than on what is being taught.

Organizing Framework for Staff Development

Critical care staff development programs are designed to educate staff nurses within the domains of clinical practice, clinical leadership, research, and continuing education. Each of these domains comprises a tract in the overall staff development program design and serves as the link that connects the staff development program to the professional advancement program. The program is designed to build upon the nurse's prior education and professional nursing experience to facilitate attainment and maintenance of competence. Concepts inherent to the educational process and to critical care nursing are defined and used as a framework around which educational programs and professional development opportunities are organized. Once defined, the organizing framework serves as the structure within which all critical care nursing staff development programs are designed.

Three essential concepts in critical care education are knowledge, competence, and role (College of Nursing Faculty, 1991). Each of these concepts can be threaded throughout the staff development program's organizing framework (Table 5–3). *Knowledge* serves as the foundation for practice and encompasses the comprehensive scientific understanding as it relates to the critically ill patient, the critical care nurse, and the critical care environment. Critical care nurses acquire this knowledge through core educational programs specific to critical care nursing. *Competence* relates to the qualities and abilities to practice according to current standards and encompasses cognitive, affective, and psychomotor skills. Critical care nurses develop competence through their practice. *Role* relates to expected professional behaviors within the realm of critical care nursing practice. Role development is fostered by the professional socialization process, role modeling, and formal staff development programs.

Steps in Program Development

The steps in the process of program development for all types of nursing education programs are assessment, planning, implementation, and evaluation. Following these steps in an organized manner with specific time lines for each ensures quality programming.

Table 5–3. ORGANIZING FRAMEWORK

Domain	Clinical Practice	Clinical Leadership	Research/Quality Assurance	Professional Growth/ Continuing Education
Knowledge	Pathophysiology Critical care concepts Policies and procedures Nursing theory	Management theory Change theory Role theory	Research process/methods Statistics Quality improvement	Adult learning theory Educational concepts Career development
Competence	Technical skills Knowledge application Time management Communication skills Assessment skills	Organizing Budget management Counseling Staffing Collaboration Directing Performance evaluation	Measurement tool development Data collection Data analysis Evaluation	Program development Teaching skills Audio-visual aids design Writing for publication Professional presentations
Role	Staff nurse Patient care coordinator Clinical nurse specialist	Clinical coordinator Nurse manager	Principal investigator Co-investigator Staff nurse	Preceptor Patient/family teacher Unit teacher Nurse educator

Assessment

The first step in developing an educational program is conducting a needs assessment to identify staff nurses' educational needs, as well as those of the institution or unit as a whole. The methodology used may be simple or sophisticated, depending on the resources available. Five methodologies commonly used are: (1) interviews with the leadership group; (2) nursing care audits, (3) quality assurance results; (4) Joint Commission for Accreditation of Health Care Organizations recommendations; and (5) staff surveys (Bell, 1986). Drawing the information from more than one source allows for a broader perspective of needs and strengthens the validity of the data obtained. Key elements to consider when developing a needs assessment include patient population and nursing population characteristics. Knowledge and skills necessary to provide care to the patient population must be identified in the tool. This ensures that the specific needs of the units are addressed. The nurse educator then analyzes the data and ranks identified needs. Once the priorities are established, the resources necessary to meet these needs are determined.

The needs assessment process should be continuous to meet the changing needs of staff and the institution. This may be accomplished in part by incorporating needs assessment questions into individual program evaluation tools.

Planning

Once the data from the needs assessment is analyzed, program planning may begin. Overall goals for each program are established first and behavioral objectives flow from these. "Behavioral objectives describe observable changes in learner behavior that reflect progress toward or achievement of the goals of the offering" (O'Connor, 1986). They serve as a framework for program design and guide the educator in selecting appropriate instructional methods. Behavioral objectives also provide a means for evaluating whether outcomes were achieved and learning took place.

Writing behavioral objectives involves the technique of clearly and concisely stating expected behaviors that are observable and measurable. It is important to avoid subjective terms such as "understand" or "know" in writing behavioral objectives because it is unclear how to observe and measure those behaviors. There are several lists of action verbs available in the literature for use as guidelines in writing behavioral objectives. Bloom (1956) describes a taxonomy of education objectives that fall into three domains: cognitive, affective, and psychomotor. Table 5–4 lists verbs according to the behavioral categories within each domain.

Behavioral objectives provide the nurse educator with the basis for program format and design. The program content and timeframe are related directly to the objectives.

Implementation

Program implementation varies according to the teaching methods selected to meet program objectives. The learners should be allowed to select the type of teaching methods that best match their learning style. A critical aspect of the educator's role is to ensure an environment that is conducive to learning both physically and psychologically.

Evaluation

Nursing education programs are evaluated in relation to the program goals, objectives, and other predetermined criteria. All those involved in the program should participate in the program evaluation. Nurse educators and managers evaluate the relevance of each offering to overall program goals, specific objectives, and the current scope of practice.

Table 5–4. BEHAVIORAL VERBS

COGNITIVE DOMAIN

Knowledge	Comprehension	Application	Analysis	Synthesis	Evaluation
					contrast
					criticize
					defend
				restate	support
				summarize	attack
				relate	avoid
			analyze	generalize	seek out
		plan	separate	conclude	reorder
		record	break down	derive	weigh
	explain	employ	discriminate	organize	modify
	associate	revise	distinguish	design	verify
	give examples	formulate	detect	deduce	decide
select	draw	apply	categorize	classify	evaluate
describe	illustrate	show	compare	formulate	judge
recall	interpret	demonstrate	contrast	propose	
define	translate	investigate	diagram	compose	
state	extrapolate	perform		modify	
identify	interpolate	relate		combine	
recognize	predict	develop		plan	
name	transform	transfer			
list	rearrange	construct			
	reorder	infer			

AFFECTIVE DOMAIN

Receiving	Responding	Valuing	Organization of Values	Characterization by Value
				acts consistently
				is accountable
				stands for
			defends	
		respects	argues	
		accepts	debates	
	selects	acclaims	declares	
	acts willingly	agrees	takes a stand	
	discusses willingly	assists	formulates a position	
shows awareness	practices	assumes responsibility	is consistent	
acknowledges	responds	cooperates with		
shares	is willing to support	supports		
	listens	helps		
	expresses satisfaction with	participates in		
	seeks opportunities			
	shows interest			

PSYCHOMOTOR DOMAIN

follows example	carries out according to procedure	carries out	practices
follows lead of	follows procedure	is skillful in using	uses

Adapted from Dains, J. (1987). Education. In ENA Emergency Nurses Association Core Curriculum (4th ed.) (p. 838). Philadelphia, W. B. Saunders.

Learners evaluate the program content and teaching strategies relative to both the stated objectives and individual learner objectives. The most common tool used for this purpose is a questionnaire with a three- to five-point scale using qualitative descriptors such as agree/disagree or excellent/poor. This method of evaluation is subjective in that it focuses on learner satisfaction rather than learning outcomes. However, it provides valuable feedback for nurse educators.

Tools that evaluate whether learning took place are more quantitative than qualitative. Paper and pencil tools measure cognitive achievement, and performance checklists measure achievement of psychomotor skills. Although these tools provide a more objective evaluation of learner achievement, they can be anxiety-provoking for the learner and require more resources to develop and implement.

Learning evaluation tools must be reliable and valid. One way of determining the reliability of an evaluation tool is to test it for inter-rater reliability. This examines whether two or more observers of the same situation record the same behaviors (Barnard, 1982). Another way to assess reliability is through a test-retest method in which testing the tool in one population is correlated with testing it in another. Validity is determined by several means. Criterion-related validity looks at how well the evaluation tool measures the stated criteria as compared with another previously established tool. Content validity refers to the ability of the evaluator to recognize elements in the tool simply by reviewing it.

Developing valid evaluation tools is a difficult and time-consuming process. The type of tool used depends on the purpose and level of the evaluation, and thus an existing tool with established validity is often more desirable. Once the validity of the tool is established, the results may be considered with confidence.

COMPONENTS OF STAFF DEVELOPMENT

Staff development programs can be divided into three major categories: orientation, inservice, and continuing education programs. Each of these programs has its own scope, purpose, goals, and objectives. It is important that those responsible for nursing education programs distinguish and understand the difference between each category.

Orientation

The American Nurses Association (1978) describes orientation as, "The means by which new staff members are introduced to the philosophy, goals, policies, procedures, role expectations, physical facilities, and special services in a specific work setting." This implies that all nurses who begin employment in a critical care setting need to participate in some aspects of orientation regardless of their level of experience. For example, a nurse who transfers into a critical care area from another area in the same hospital needs to be oriented to the critical care nursing role expectations, special procedures, and services of the critical care unit. A nurse hired from outside the institution who has previous experience in critical care needs to be oriented to the new working environment. The challenge for the critical care educator is to design an orientation program that meets both the individual needs of nurses from a variety of backgrounds as well as unit-specific needs.

One way to accomplish this is to design a competency-based orientation program. "Competency-based education can be perceived as a very broad concept that is used as the conceptual framework for a total curriculum, or it can be interpreted in a very narrow way, as a framework for an individual unit of instruction such as a self-learning module" (DelBueno, 1978).

A competency-based orientation model has six characteristics: (1) an emphasis on outcomes, (2) use of self-directed learning activities, (3) flexibility and time allowed for achievement of outcomes, (4) use of the teacher as facilitator, (5) assessment of previous learning, and (6) assessment of learning styles (Del-Bueno, et al., 1981). A competency-based approach to orientation facilitates a more positive experience for the orientee through recognition of previously

acquired knowledge and skills. For example, an experienced critical care nurse would find it very frustrating to have to sit through electrocardiogram recognition classes if the nurse had mastered that competency. A competency-based approach allows orientees to select those learning activities that meet their individual learning needs and demonstrate mastery of certain required competencies.

As some of these needs are satisfied or reprioritized as a lesser need, others needs will arise in a Maslowian sequence (Buickus, 1984). A new nurse orientee first seeks safety in the environment and then progresses through stages to attain membership in the work group. At the end of a well-designed orientation, orientees should feel comfortable in the environment and integrated into the staff.

Designing a Competency-based Orientation Program

The steps to follow in designing a competency-based orientation are the same as those discussed earlier for program development, with emphasis on details specific to orientation.

Assessment. During the needs assessment phase, the competencies expected of an orientee in critical care are identified. "The competencies identified should represent realistic expectations of *general* categories of performance for a *beginning level* staff nurse on that unit" (Alspach, 1984). The orientee should not be expected to function at the same level as senior staff by the end of the orientation period.

The process of identifying required competencies necessitates a comprehensive exploration of the specific field of practice. Resources to assist in identifying entry level competencies include: (1) staff nurse position descriptions, (2) JCAHO requirements, (3) professional standards of practice (for example American Nurses Association [ANA], American Association of Critical Care Nurses [AACN]), (4) review of the literature, (5) needs of the patient population on the specific unit, and (6) consensus of expert practitioners. Analysis of the information compiled from these resources provides the nurse educator with a foundation for formulating orientation competency statements. The greatest challenge in this process is to gain consensus from preceptors, staff, and managers regarding levels of competence to expect from orientees. Once this is achieved, the nurse educator ensures that these competencies are clearly stated and attainable by all orientees.

A competency statement is not the same as a behavioral or instructional objective. It is a much broader sample of behavior that integrates knowledge, psychomotor skills, and attitudes. These broad competency statements are then broken down into specific terminal performance criteria that are observable and measurable examples of expected behaviors for demonstration of competency.

Competency statements and performance criteria are developed collaboratively with all those involved in orienting and evaluating new staff. This strength-

Table 5–5. SAMPLE COMPETENCY STATEMENT WITH RELATED PERFORMANCE CRITERIA

Competency:
Provides safe nursing care for the patient who requires temporary cardiac pacing

Performance criteria:
1. Identifies clinical indications for temporary pacing
2. Labels wires A & V
3. Dresses insertion sites with occlusive dressing
4. Secures wires with 2-inch piece of tourniquet
5. Changes battery
6. Documents pacemaker function, settings, and patient response
7. Supports patient and family throughout the period of temporary cardiac pacing

---

ens the validity of the competencies identified. Table 5–5 illustrates an example of a competency statement with its related performance criteria.

Planning. The next step in the orientation process is to consider which methods of evaluation to use for determining attainment of performance criteria. The educator may choose between a written test, a skills laboratory inventory, a performance checklist, or a case study depending on the nature of the criteria; sometimes a combination of two or more methods is used.

Prerequisites may exist for certain competencies before they can be achieved (e.g., knowledge of institutional policies or basic knowledge in critical care nursing). These prerequisites, along with the identified competencies, dictate the core content for critical care orientation.

The content outline for orientation should be structured in an orderly manner that reflects the organizing framework of the staff development program. Performance criteria may be arranged according to knowledge, competence, and role, and integrated into the core content outline. The instructional methods for teaching this core content are then delineated.

Whenever possible, more than one instructional design should be provided to allow orientees to select their own learning methods. Table 5–6 lists appropriate instructional techniques according to the type of behavioral outcome expected. The timeframe for achievement of orientation competencies is also negotiated. Depending on the orientee's level of competence, and the complexity of the unit, this may range from 6 weeks to 6 months. All these negotiated conditions may be written into a learning contract to serve as a guide for implementation and ongoing evaluation.

Implementation. A competency-based orientation program may be implemented using a variety of formats. The role of the nurse educator is to facilitate the acquisition of required competencies. This may involve some formal classes or skills laboratories depending on the orientee's needs and learning styles. A novice critical care nurse requires close supervision and continuous instruction (Benner, 1984). An expert critical care nurse may demonstrate knowledge on written tests and validate current competence in performance of identified skills but may need instruction on role expectations specific to the institution. In each case, goals may be set for every day or week of orientation, which serve as guidelines for ongoing feedback for the orientee.

It is critical that during the implementation phase of orientation the expected level of competence be clear to the orientee and educator. For example, competence in hemodynamic monitoring involves setting up equipment, assisting with insertion, identifying wave forms, troubleshooting, interpreting data, and analyzing the data concurrently with the clinical assessment of a specific patient. This can be overwhelming to an orientee. A well-designed orientation program will allay some of a new orientee's anxiety by making specific expectations clear. Specific behaviors expected of an orientee relative to all competencies must be stated explicitly.

Evaluation. Program elements to be evaluated at the end of the orientation period are the program itself, the educator, and the orientee. The orientee may be evaluated using the methods outlined in the planning phase of the program. An evaluation of overall job performance may also be included.

Table 5–6. BEHAVIORAL OUTCOMES

Type of Behavioral Outcome	Most Appropriate Technique
Knowledge	
Generalizations about experience; internalization of information	Lecture, videotape, debate, dialogue, interview, symposium, panel, group discussion, book-based discussion, reading
Understanding	
Application of information and generalization	Audience participation, demonstration, dramatization, problem-solving, discussion, case study, games
Skills	
Incorporation of new ways of performing through practice	Role playing, games, participative cases, skill labs
Attitudes	
Adoption of new feelings through experiencing greater success with them than with old	Experience-sharing discussion, group-centered discussion, role playing, critical incident process, case method, games
Values	
The adoption and priority arrangement of beliefs	Videotape, lecture, debate, dialogue, symposium, dramatization, guided discussion, experience-sharing discussion, role playing, critical incident process, games
Interests	
Satisfying exposure to new activities	Videotape, demonstration, dramatization, experience-sharing discussion, exhibits

Orientees also evaluate the orientation program in terms of whether it met their individual needs. The quality and appropriateness of instruction are part of that evaluation.

All those involved in the orientation process evaluate the program as a whole in terms of outcomes. This process should occur formally each year. The relationship of the orientation program outcomes to expected outcomes for the unit or the nursing department should be evident. Based on the evaluation data, recommendations for revisions may be made.

Preceptor Programs

For several years, preceptorship has been a popular approach to unit-based clinical orientation of critical care nurses. "A preceptor is an experienced nurse providing instruction and guidance for a novice" (Hamilton, 1981). This person oversees the new staff nurse's orientation process in conjunction with the nurse manager and nurse educator for the unit. The preceptor negotiates a learning contract with the orientee based on identified learning needs. During this process, the preceptor introduces the orientee to both written and unwritten policies and practices of the unit.

Preceptors act as role models, socializers, and educators (Alspach, 1988). They introduce the orientee to staff nurse role expectations by demonstrating clinical competence, good communication skills, and strong organizational skills. The preceptor socializes the new staff member into the work group through introductions to other nurses and providing formal and informal opportunities for interactions with several members of the healthcare team during the orientation period.

The chief component of the preceptor role is that of educator. The preceptor must assess, plan, implement, and evaluate an individualized orientation plan with the orientee. At this point, the preceptor may clarify the expectation that the responsibility for meeting orientation requirements rests with the orientee. The preceptor acts as a resource and facilitates the orientee's accomplishment of program requirements. Selection criteria for preceptors should be clearly defined before embarking on such a program. Common criteria include (1) clinical competence, (2) exemplary interpersonal skills, (3) teaching ability, (4) leadership ability, (5) conflict resolution ability, (6) commitment to the program, and (7) a positive attitude (Greipp, 1989; Begle & Willis, 1984).

The role of the nurse educator during the unit-based orientation is to establish ongoing communication and facilitate a trusting preceptor-orientee relationship. This may be achieved through weekly meetings with the preceptor and orientee to review accomplishments, set goals for the following week, and give feedback to the orientee. It also is an opportunity for the nurse educator to assess the preceptor-orientee relationship.

Many institutions require preceptor experience as one criterion for clinical advancement. Others see it as professional recognition and responsibility without related promotional or financial reward. Whatever the institution's philosophy, some mechanism of positive reinforcement of the preceptor role must exist to avoid burnout. Alspach (1987) proposed a preceptor's bill of rights, which includes the right to role preparation (Alspach, 1987). This is best done by providing a preceptor development workshop. Workshop content should include: (1) a description of the preceptor role, (2) an overview of adult learning principles, (3) steps in orientation needs assessment, (4) communication skills, (5) conflict resolution strategies, and (6) evaluation strategies.

The workshop design should be highly interactive and give participants opportunities in role playing and clarifying expectations. It is also essential to review both central and unit-based orientation programs at the workshop. Preceptors need a clear understanding of the orientation program's goals and objectives to maintain program consistency. This preceptor development workshop serves as a prerequisite to each preceptor's role in program evaluation and revision.

Follow-up sessions or "advanced" preceptor workshops are provided to continue to support the development of expert preceptors. These sessions provide experienced preceptors with an opportunity to clarify issues and meet the changing needs of orientees. It also recognizes the preceptors' commitment to the program. Nurse managers and nurse recruiters may be invited to participate at these meetings to offer feedback to the preceptor group. These sessions should be continuous and responsive to the needs of preceptors if they are to support the preceptors in fulfilling role expectations. Moreover, this kind of support from the leadership group enhances retention of these vital staff members and promotes collaboration between educators and managers.

Critical Care Nursing Inservice Education

Inservice education programs, the most frequently occurring type of staff development activity, involves learning experiences provided in the workplace to assist staff to perform assigned functions and maintain competency (American Nurses Association, 1978). These programs are usually informal and narrow in scope. Often, they are unplanned, spontaneous sessions that arise from new situations on the unit in settings such as patient rounds or staff meetings. Examples of planned inservices are demonstrations of new equipment, procedure reviews, and patient care conferences.

These activities are the most unrecognized types of education programs and subsequently often are not documented. The astute nurse educator develops a mechanism for documenting these learning activities as part of the unit-based education program. The documentation substantiates ongoing efforts to ensure competence and of compliance with JCAHO and other regulatory requirements.

It is crucial to point out, however, that inservice education does not meet the criteria for continuing education credit in nursing. The scope of these programs is limited to the specific work setting and not necessarily to overall professional development of individual nurses. This distinction should be clarified with nursing staff who may be expecting continuing education credit from fire safety classes or other institution-specific inservices.

Continuing Education

The category of staff development activity that is in highest demand is continuing education. This need has been fueled by legislation, regulations, professional standards, and expectations of healthcare consumers. Continuing education programs include planned, organized learning experiences designed to build on previously acquired knowledge and skills (American Nurses Association, 1978). The focus is on knowledge and skills that are not specific to one institution. Examples of continuing education programs include formal conferences, seminars, workshops, and courses.

Accreditation of continuing education programs is the process by which an approving body recognizes that a program meets its required standards. The accreditation process in nursing is accomplished primarily through the ANA. The ANA Board on Accreditation has specific criteria that must be met for approval of continuing education credit. ANA also has a mechanism for nursing associations to become accredited as approvers of continuing education so that an organization can approve the programs of its constituents. The AACN is one such accredited approver.

The measure by which continuing education credit is awarded is the 50-minute contact hour. For every 50 minutes of a planned, organized learning activity, 1 contact hour may be awarded. To calculate the number of contact hours in a learning activity, one adds up the total number of minutes and divides by 50. A minimum of 50 minutes is required to obtain credit. However, partial credit may be awarded over that timeframe. For example, 1 hour of learning experience equals 1.2 contact hours. Three categories of continuing education may be approved for continuing

education credit: an offering, program, or independent study. A summary of definitions and examples of each is provided in Table 5–7.

The educational design criteria for all three categories of continuing education are similar. All of the defined criteria must be met to obtain continuing education credit. Each criterion is listed on the application for approval for continuing education credit. These criteria are:

1. Resources. A person must be identified as administratively responsible for the learning activity. Two registered nurses, one who holds at least a baccalaureate degree in nursing, must be involved in program planning.
2. Target audience and needs assessment. The target audience for the learning activity must be identified and the means by which their needs were assessed must be documented. The needs assessment may be formal or informal.
3. Objectives. The objectives for the learning activity must be stated in behavioral terms.
4. Content/timeframe. A brief content outline with appropriate timeframes for each content unit must be submitted. The relationship between the content and the objectives must be clear.
5. Faculty. Evidence that the faculty is knowledgeable about the content must be provided.
6. Teaching methods. The teaching methods must be appropriate for the content and must reflect the application of adult learning principles.
7. Physical facilities. The site for the learning activity must accommodate the teaching methods described.
8. Coprovidership. If the learning activity is provided by more than one institution, a written agreement regarding each party's role and responsibilities must be explained.
9. Evaluation. The method used to evaluate the learning activity must be defined. Six criteria are evaluated: achievement of stated objectives, teaching effectiveness, relevance, teaching methods, physical facilities, and achievement of personal objectives.
10. Verification of attendance. This is better known as the contact hour certificate, which the participant receives to verify attendance at the program.
11. Record-keeping system. Records must be kept

Table 5–7. CATEGORIES OF CONTINUING EDUCATION

CE Category	Definition	Examples
Offering	A single educational activity that may be presented once or repeated	ECG Workshop Nursing grand rounds
Program	A series of offerings that have a common theme and common overall goal	National Teaching Institute CCRN Core Review Program
Independent study offering	A self-paced learning activity developed for use by an individual learner	Professional journal CEU articles Computer-assisted learning modules

for a period of 5 years. This includes all the information from criteria 1–10, plus a summary of evaluations, and the names and addresses of participants who attended (American Nurses Association, 1986).

The institution's provision of ongoing continuing education reflects two commitments to the nursing staff and to the public they serve. The first is to ensure that patients are cared for by nurses who are current in their practice. The second is a commitment to meet the changing learning needs of the nursing staff so that they are able to maintain competence.

The establishment of a comprehensive staff development program sustains varying levels of knowledge and skill in the educational preparation of nursing staff. It provides a climate that supports career development and fosters excellence in clinical practice. Nurses who practice in this type of environment are encouraged to accept new challenges in clinical and professional arenas and are supported through the growth process on the road to advancement.

Fostering Professional Advancement

Fostering professional advancement includes stimulating growth in clinical knowledge and skills as well as promoting development of the nurse as an active participant in the profession of nursing. Supporting this type of growth and professional involvement requires that the educator be in touch with a variety of professional activities, opportunities, and resources appropriate for staff at all levels. These opportunities can and should be identified at the unit and institutional level (e.g., unit or interdepartmental councils, committees, or task forces), at the state level (e.g., state nurses associations, state political movements or organizations related to healthcare policy, healthcare program grants administered at the state level), and nationally (e.g., national nursing organizations, federal grants, and national policy agendas related to healthcare).

Formal and informal opportunities exist for staff to participate in professional development activities at the unit, institutional, local, state, or national level including activities such as clinical role modeling, formal education, development of areas of expertise, certification, leadership role development, peer review, professional presentations, writing for publication, and participation in nursing research related to critical care. Some of these activities are discussed in the following section.

STRATEGIES FOR PROMOTING PROFESSIONAL DEVELOPMENT

Professional development activities for new graduates and newly hired staff can be made accessible, but cannot be made mandatory. This group of staff are focused on learning to give safe and effective care

in a critical care setting. Emphasis should be placed on exposing new staff to ongoing professional development opportunities and on the unit's and institution's values and expectations related to professional development activities. It is best to introduce new employees to the formal advancement program early so that the idea of advancement can be incorporated into their self-expectations from the start.

As nurses progress to proficient and expert level staff (levels II and III), they are comfortable with their ability to perform clinical care and often are eager for involvement in professional advancement activities appropriate for their level of expertise and personal interests (see Table 5–1). For example, level II and III nurses often become interested in a specific clinical nursing phenomenon and begin to raise questions for research. Opportunities to participate in the research process at the appropriate level can be facilitated by a clinical nurse specialist in critical care. This process enhances clinical practice on the unit and allows staff to gain new skills and knowledge. If educators and managers recognize and capitalize on this readiness, they can enhance job satisfaction and increase retention of skilled staff.

Role Modeling

Clinical role modeling is a very basic but powerful professional development strategy. Nurses take part in important professional activities on a daily basis. Examples include role modeling for clinical practicum students; precepting new staff; and demonstrating collaboration between nurse, physician, and family. Level II staff can assist beginning level staff to view themselves as clinical role models by discussing this activity as it is related to the provision of patient care according to established nursing practice standards or use of departmental policies and procedures in the delivery of safe and effective care. Level II and III staff can serve as role models and discuss examples of clear and effective verbal and written communication and effective use of appropriate resources and problem-solving behaviors for new, unexpected, or problematic situations (Alspach, 1988). All staff members serve as role models for each other, patients, families, and other healthteam members.

Professional Presentations

A wide array of opportunities exist for the presentation of projects, clinical information, new ideas, and research findings. The real challenge lies in helping staff to find the right forum for presentation of the idea, project, or research findings. Other considerations to take into account include the staff members' past experience with a particular method of presentation, the type of audience to be addressed, the knowledge and expertise of the staff related to the topic, and resources (both time and money) available to support professional presentations.

Poster Sessions

Poster sessions are frequently included as a part of an educational or scientific meeting and are an efficient way to present information in a manner that allows quick review of the most salient points in a visually appealing layout (Mottet & Jones, 1988).

A poster presentation allows nurses to discuss their findings or ideas informally with small groups or individuals. Thus, this type of situation is often more comfortable for those without extensive public speaking experience because it allows a dialogue between the presenter and the viewer. As a result of a poster presentation, staff may be offered opportunities to participate in other types of professional development opportunities. The poster session can serve as an important experience in assisting the staff nurse to gain confidence in (and even enjoy) public speaking opportunities.

Oral Presentations

Staff at all levels can learn to communicate clearly and professionally about their practice. Educators can facilitate this process by encouraging or organizing frequent informal and formal clinically focused presentations, first with peers and "safe" groups of colleagues, and later with larger, more diverse audiences. There are a variety of traditional and nontraditional teaching formats that can be used to discuss practice and present clinical topics.

Clinical Rounds and Case Presentations. These, with time for discussion on the unit, should be an expectation of all staff on a regular basis. This type of presentation allows participants to closely examine a specific patient care issue or clinical learning opportunity. It often fosters a rich exchange between different level caregivers and promotes collaborative learning in the midst of patient care. Presenters can ask for feedback regarding the style and format of the presentation that assist them in improving future presentations.

"Mini Topics." Mini topics (Sheehy, 1987) are short topic presentations that are scheduled to occur just before or after shift-to-shift report or during a quiet time on the unit. These presentations are designed to be fun and informative; they last no longer than 10 minutes and should contain an interesting tidbit of information that is new or obscure. Topics can include brief presentations on procedures, equipment updates, or a recent development in clinical care. Staff who perform a procedure particularly well or have become familiar with infrequently used equipment can be encouraged to share their expertise in this informal way.

Formal Lectures. These include presentations that are more structured and are scheduled to occur at a certain time and place. The topic is clearly identified and speakers are expected to have some experience or expertise related to the topic. The process of planning a formal lecture includes the same steps in program development discussed previously.

Assessment is focused on identification of the timeframe and objectives for the lecture, which are often predetermined. Other relevant information includes the size and general characteristics of the audience. Planning involves a complete literature review to ensure that the material to be presented is current. A literature review is invaluable in lending some perspective on the ways others have presented and discussed the topic. It offers ideas on how to begin a lecture, what content to include, and how to summarize the material (Sheehy, 1987). Organizing content in a logical progression of concepts enhances the audience's ability to understand and follow the presentation.

Implementation includes choosing and employing teaching methodologies that meet the stated objectives for the lecture. Choosing audiovisual techniques for enhancement of lecture content depends on the speaker's preference, the size of the audience, the size and configuration of the room available, equipment, and the speaker's familiarity with equipment. Audiovisual media can add or detract from a presentation and must be chosen and developed carefully. Advice for the development of frequently used visual aids appears in Table 5–8.

Rehearsing the presentation many times in private and at least once in front of a small audience is important. Educators can advise staff that the goal is to be natural, not perfect. Practice allows repetition of the sequence of the main points of the presentation, not memorization of the content. It allows the speaker some level of comfort and increases the speaker's ability to interact with the audience.

Table 5–8. DEVELOPING VISUAL AIDS

Flip Charts
- Use colored markers—underline, highlight, or box key words/titles
- Lettering should be readable: 1½–2 inches tall with 2 inches between lines
- Use as few words as possible
- Use the upper ⅔ of the chart
- Use pictures or shapes to increase interest
- Write quickly, capturing key ideas
- Perforate or score flip chart pages prior to the meeting/presentation
- Have tape or tack set up prior to presentation

Overheads
- Use ½-inch letters or larger
- Six lines or less per visual
- Six words or less per line (across)
- Use a variety of colors
- Put captions on top, not underneath
- Use upper and lower case lettering

Slides
- Use strong body type, not all capital letters
- Design slides for those in the back row
- Five to six words per line, no more seven lines in height
- Use graphics when possible
- Choose single words
- Start and end with a solid dark slide to avoid blinding lights
- Keep it simple—slides are only a tool

Evaluation provides information concerning how well the content met both the stated objectives and the learner's individual objectives. In addition, it provides important information to the presenter on the effectiveness of teaching style and visual aids.

Certification

Certification is another avenue for promotion of professional development and is an important means of recognizing and validating standards for a registered nurse's qualifications and knowledge for practice in a specific area. The pediatric CCRN certification program validates the knowledge and qualifications for practice as a critical care nurse in a pediatric critical care setting. CCRN certification is awarded to those critical care nurses who pass a CCRN examination in neonatal, pediatric, or adult critical care nursing.

Writing for Publication

Many journals publish guidelines for authors in each issue, and others provide an address for guideline requests. Author's guidelines review the focus of the journal, the type of manuscript accepted, and manuscript length requirements and format. Usually, the guidelines help authors narrow the scope of their article and select a journal appropriate for publication.

Experienced authors encourage staff who are writing for publication to begin with a skeleton outline and add details in each area. An outline serves to organize the content in a logical progression or sequence of events that enhances readability and understanding. A rough draft is developed from the outline and serves as the basis for further drafts.

Multiple revisions of the manuscript may be necessary to correct inconsistencies in style, organization, and grammar. Resources helpful in improving writing clarity, style, and grammar include *The Elements of Style* (Strunk & White, 1995), *On Writing Well* (Zinsser, 1994), and the *Publication Manual of the American Psychological Association* (1994).

Once a manuscript is submitted to a journal, the average review time is approximately 2½ months (Swanson & McCloskey, 1986), although timeframes vary widely. The outcome of the review is communicated as an acceptance, tentative acceptance pending revisions, or rejection.

Staff receiving a tentative acceptance or a rejection need encouragement and support. Tentative acceptance is often mistaken for a rejection, and many manuscripts returned for revision are never resubmitted (Massachusetts Nurses Association, 1991). If a manuscript is rejected because the content had been covered recently or was inconsistent with the focus of the journal, the educator can encourage the author to submit to another more appropriate journal.

SUMMARY

Professional development activities abound in pediatric critical care and can serve to enhance and enrich clinical practice. Advanced practice activities can be made available to all staff by educators, clinical nurse specialists, and nurse managers who facilitate a program of professional advancement. Resources for clinical and professional development activities appropriate for critical care professionals are available through AACN and other professional nursing organizations.

A professional advancement program for pediatric critical care nurses reflects a nursing department's commitment to quality healthcare for consumers and to the protection of critically ill pediatric patients who are cared for by highly skilled and knowledgeable staff. A program that combines opportunities for professional growth and development with a professional advancement program that recognizes and supports nursing staff at all levels of practice can best meet these goals.

References

AACN Certification Corporation (1991). *Neonatal CCRN examination: A blueprint for study.* Aliso Viejo, CA: Certification Corporation.

AACN Certification Corporation (1991). *Pediatric CCRN examination: A blueprint for study.* Aliso Viejo, CA: Certification Corporation.

Alspach, J.G. (1984). Designing a competency based orientation for critical care nurses. *Heart & Lung,* 13(6), 655–662.

Alspach, J.G. (1987). The preceptor's bill of rights. *Critical Care Nurse,* 7(1), 1.

Alspach, J.G. (1988). *Preceptor handbook.* Secaucus, NJ: Hospital Publications.

American Association of Critical Care Nurses (1990). *1990 National teaching institute speaker's handbook.* Irvine, CA: American Association of Critical Care Nurses.

American Nurses Association (1978). *Guidelines for staff development.* Kansas City: American Nurses Association.

American Nurses Association (1975). *Standards for nursing education.* Kansas City: American Nurses Association.

American Nurses Association (1986). *Manual for accreditation as an approver of continuing education in nursing.* Kansas City: American Nurses Association.

Barnard, K. (1982). Measurements: Reliability. *American Journal of Maternal/Child Nursing,* 7(2), 101, 165.

Bell, E. (1986). Needs assessment in continuing education: Designing a system that works. *The Journal of Continuing Education in Nursing.* 17(4), 112–114.

Benner, P. (1984). *From novice to expert: Excellence and power in clinical nursing practice.* Menlo Park, CA: Addison-Wesley.

Bloom, B.S. (1956). *Taxonomy of education objectives: Handbook 1, cognitive domain.* New York: David McKay.

Buickus, B.A. (1984). Orientation: We're with you all the way. *Nursing Management.* 15(4), 40–45.

College of Nursing Faculty (1991). *Self-study report.* Boston: Northeastern University.

DelBueno, D. (1978). Competency based education. *Nurse Educator,* 3(3), 10–14.

DelBueno, D., Barker, F., & Christmyer, C. (1981). Implementing a competency based orientation program. *The Journal of Nursing Administration,* 11(2), 24–29.

Dutton, J.L. (1987). *How to be an outstanding speaker.* Appleton, WI: Life Skills Publishing.

Greipp, M.E. (1989). Nursing preceptors—looking back—looking ahead. *Journal of Nursing Staff Development,* (4), 183–185.

Hamilton, M.S. (1981). Mentorhood: A key to nursing leadership. *Nursing Leadership,* 4, 4–13.

Harris, C.C., et. al. (1986). The Troubleshooter's guide to media. *Nursing Outlook,* 34(1), 28–33.

Hofland, S.L. (1987). Transparency design for effective oral presentations. *The Journal of Continuing Education in Nursing,* 18(3), 83–88.

Jiricka, M.K., et al. (Eds.) (1987). Principles of adult learning. In M.J. Jiricka, et al. (Eds.), *Critical care orientation: A guide to the process* (pp. 2–7). Newport Beach, CA: AACN.

Knowles, M.S. (1970). *The modern practice of adult education.* New York: Association Press.

Massachusetts Nurses Association (1991). *Getting the word out. A guide to sharing research results.* Canton, MA: The Cabinet on Nursing Research.

Mottet, E.A., & Jones, B.L. (1988). The poster session: An overlooked management tool. *Journal of Nursing Administration,* 18(7,8), 29–33.

Morrow, K.L. (1984). Principles of adult education. In K.L. Morrow, *Preceptorships in nursing staff development* (pp. 135–137). Rockville, MD: Aspen.

O'Connor, A.B. (1986). Writing behavioral objectives. In A.B. O'Connor, *Nursing staff development and continuing education* (pp. 105–117). Boston: Little, Brown.

Pike, R. (1989). *Creative training techniques handbook.* Minneapolis, MN: Lakewood Books.

Publication Manual of the American Psychological Association (4th ed.) (1994). Washington, D.C.: American Psychological Association.

Sheehy, S.B. (1987). Nurse educator: Ways to present clinical topics. *Journal of Emergency Nursing,* 13(6), 377–379.

Sheehy, S.B. (1988). Nurse educator: Preparing visual material for your presentation. *Journal of Emergency Nursing,* 14(1), 41–43.

Strunk, W. Jr., & White, E.B. (1995). *The elements of style* (3rd ed.). New York: Macmillan.

Swanson, E., & McCloskey, J. (1982). The manuscript review process of nursing journals. *Image,* 14(3), 72–76.

Swanson, E., & McCloskey, J. (1986). Publishing opportunities for nurses. *Nursing Outlook,* 34(5), 227–237.

Tobin, H., Wise, P., & Hull, P. (1979). *The process of staff development.* St. Louis: C.V. Mosby.

Winslow, E. (1991). Overcome the fear of speaking in public. *American Journal of Nursing,* 91(5), 51–53.

Zinsser, W.K. (1994). *On writing well: An informal guide to writing non-fiction* (4th ed.). New York: Harper & Row.

CHAPTER 6

Legal Implications of Pediatric Nursing Practice*

SYLVIA CHIN-CAPLAN

. . . Justice is an abstract, undefinable, thing, about which men disagree.

PROSSER

Healthcare institutions are under increasing pressure to operate under market conditions and constraints. No longer do third-party payors unquestionably reimburse healthcare providers for wide variances in healthcare practices. Today, insurers pressure healthcare providers to contain costs while maintaining the quality of patient care and the development of innovative techniques.

As part of the federal government's efforts to control costs, hospital stays have shortened. This mandate for shorter hospital stays will translate into shorter ICU stays. The desire to control healthcare costs is promoting the use of ancillary personnel to provide basic nursing care, which in turn increases the nursing supervisory role and potential exposure to liability. With so many simultaneous changes occurring, legal duties, responsibilities, and obligations are also in flux. The need to adapt professional conduct to societal demands is critical. The nurse's ability to adjust will depend upon a sound understanding of the legal framework upon which professional nurses operate so that reasoned decisions can be made to guide future practice.

SOURCES OF LAW

The origin of the majority of the laws in the United States is primarily two sources: laws that are the

---

*Attorney Mary Ann Malloy shared her knowledge and expertise on Advanced Directives and the Adolescent Patient.

creation of duly elected political figures, and those that are derived from judicial authority.

The United States Constitution is the supreme law of the land (*Marbury v. Madison*, 1803). It is the result of the Continental Congresses that convened in the years immediately following the Revolutionary War. The duly designated delegates to the Congresses were charged with the responsibility of developing the framework by which the newly independent nation could govern itself. The tension between "state's rights" advocates and those who favored the creation of a strong federal government "federalism" is reflected in the key legislative piece of law that embodies the nascent nation's opposing viewpoints.

The Constitution reserves the authority to declare war, negotiate treaties, and impose tariffs on imports and exports solely to the federal government. All other powers are expressly reserved for the states. While the "separation of powers" appears clearly defined, there is shared governance in many arenas by both federal and state governments. It is within this area where the powers of the federal and state governments overlap that constitutional challenges are frequently encountered in the courts. The states cannot abrogate or contradict laws enacted by the federal government, nor can the states usurp powers that have been expressly granted to the federal government. Thus, any laws that seek to regulate conduct in an area expressly reserved to the federal government is preempted by the Constitution (*McCulloch v. Maryland*, 1819). Under the 10th Amendment to the Constitution, areas of law that are not deemed federal in scope pass to the states for regulation. The conduct of professionals is one area thus designated.

The nurse practice acts of most states are statutory creations of state legislatures. The legislatures, in turn, delegate authority to a state agency to promulgate rules and regulations to govern specific conduct. In the areas of social welfare and healthcare, the federal government has historically deferred to the discretion of the individual states.

Nurse Practice Acts

The state's right to regulate the licensure of its healthcare personnel emanates from the police powers delegated to it by the Constitution. Police powers are not defined anywhere within the Bill of Rights or the Constitution (*Railroad Company v. Husen*, 1877). However, it is universally acknowledged that police powers are intrinsic to the sovereignty of the states and, as such, permit each state to codify laws for the protection of the health, safety, and welfare of its community as well as to regulate public order and morals (Id). The Constitution places limitations on the states' exercise of their police powers to ensure that state laws do not infringe impermissibly on constitutional rights. These rights, however, are not absolute and often require a "balancing of interests" by the judiciary.

State licensure of nurses attempts to protect the public from unsafe, incompetent practitioners. The nurse practice acts of most states, today, sets forth the minimum requirements for entry into practice, defines the scope of nursing practice, and regulates the conduct of practitioners by its requirements for licensure and relicensure. Most nurse practice acts, codified by the respective legislatures of each individual state, delegate the authority to develop rules and regulations to govern the practice of nursing to an administrative agency such as the board of nursing. It is the responsibility of the board to investigate claims filed against individual nurses and conduct hearings in accordance with agency practice and procedure to establish findings of fact and conclusions of law. When warranted, sanctions are imposed that are commensurate with the substantiated claim.

Common Law

Common law constitutes that body of principles that reflects the evolution of judicial decisions to challenged conduct. Prior to the Revolutionary War, common law was derived from English common law and applied uniformly throughout the colonies. After the Revolution, the continued clash between proponents of the continuance of a uniform application of law and those who desired decentralization led to a compromise. Each state was permitted to adopt, revise, and adapt the existing common law to the needs of its jurisdiction provided the adaptation of that law did not conflict with those laws expressly reserved in the Constitution to the federal government. Thus, common law may differ from state to state.

An important element to the embodiment of common law is the principle of stare decisis, or precedent. Judicial adherence to stare decisis has its roots in centuries of English practice that sets forth that well-settled points of law that have previously been adjudicated should not be reexamined. The principle of stare decisis, however, is not without controversy. In at least one instance, the Supreme Court's reliance on precedence led to the enforcement of inequitable laws for an additional 54 years (*Plessy v. Ferguson*, 1896). The value of precedential principles continues to be debated in the present day. In *Planned Parenthood v. Webster*, 1992, Justice Scalia openly called for the reversal of *Roe v. Wade*, 1972, declaring that its decision rested on unrecognized principles of constitutional protection.

NEGLIGENCE

Standard of Care

Over the years, negligence actions have been premised upon a belief that a yardstick existed by which one's conduct is measured. The *reasonable man*, a standard of behavior that courts have used as a barometer of proper conduct, is a fictitious judicial creation that has never existed in any material form

(Prosser, 1984). Negligence involves conduct, not intent. An actor need not desire to bring about the consequences that ensue, nor does he need to know that they are substantially certain to occur or that they will occur. For legal purposes, it is sufficient that the risk is apparent enough that one must guard against it. The greater the risk, the greater the care required.

Duty

Negligence is the failure to act as a reasonable person would under the same or similar circumstances that cause harm to another (*Union P.R. Co. v. McDonald*, 1894). For a valid claim to lie, a legal duty must exist (*Becker v. Schwartz*, 1978). Duty is generally defined as an affirmative obligation to conform one's conduct to that expected of a reasonable person in light of the risks presented (*Caldwell v. Bechtel, Inc.*, 1986).

[It] refers to an affirmative obligation imposed by law to do a particular thing, to perform a particular act. It is a requirement of specific conduct. The essence of that duty is not to do, or refrain from doing, a particular act, but rather to act in a particular way—to exercise reasonable care—whenever it is foreseeable that one's conduct may cause harm to another.

(*Walker v. Bignell*, 1981). The degree of duty owed a person is directly proportional to the harm that will result from lack of due care (*Harding v. Philadelphia Rapid Transit Co.*, 1907). The Restatement of Torts 2d §297 (1965) notes that

a negligent act maybe one which involves an unreasonable risk of harm to another (a) although it is done with all possible care, competence, preparation, and warning, or (b) only if it is done without reasonable care, competence, preparation or warning, thus distinguishing between acts which are regarded as dangerous in themselves and acts which are dangerous only because of the improper manner in which they are done.

Therefore, the degree of risk associated with the challenged conduct establishes not only the protected class of persons but also delineates the extent to which the injury will be attributed to the negligent act—i.e., the care required in any given situation is directly proportional to the anticipated harm (*Thompson v. Ohio Fuel Gas Co.*, 1967).

For professionals, such as nurses, the duty to act reasonably arises from the nurse-patient relationship and is rarely, if ever, disputed. For others, duty can arise from operation of law such as a statutory enactment or municipal ordinance (Restatement of Torts 2d § 285, Comment b & c, 1965), as a result of contractual obligations (*Randolph's Adm'r v. Snyder*, 1910), from judicial opinions (*Elbert v. Saginaw*, 1961), or simply be a creation of living in a complex

modern society (*The T.J. Hooper*, 1932). Once a professional nurse undertakes to provide care to a patient, a duty is created and the caregiver cannot terminate that care unless the patient no longer requires it or she is replaced by another equally as competent (see *Rose v. Hakim*, 1971 *infra*). Withdrawal for any other reason may constitute abandonment (*Czubinsky v. Doctor's Hospital*, 1981). Upon the recognition that a duty has been created, the need to determine what would comprise the proper standard of care to guide the inquiry into the complained of conduct must be established.

In nursing malpractice actions, the standard of care can be established by various methods. Expert testimony is the most common. To support and augment the live testimony, many seasoned plaintiffs' attorneys have utilized documentary evidence, such as nursing treatises or texts and journal articles, to demonstrate the appropriate standard of care within the profession. Particularly persuasive, if available, are the standards promulgated by national organizations such as the American Association of Critical-Care Nurses.

Under certain circumstances, a violation of the nurse practice act of one's own state leads to a presumption of negligence, which, unless rebutted, is conclusive for negligence. In those states in which a violation of the nurse practice act is *negligence per se*, the plaintiff must prove (1) that the intent of the act was to protect a certain class of people (public); (2) that the plaintiff is a member of the protected class; and (3) that the harm suffered by the plaintiff was that which the enactment of the statute was intended to prevent.

The evidentiary treatment of statutory violations varies from jurisdiction to jurisdiction. In Massachusetts, once evidence is presented that rebuts the presumption of a statutory violation, the matter is then submitted to the jury to draw whatever inferences it would infer from the factual evidence before it (Leach & Liacos, 1984).

For instance, in Massachusetts, the Nurse Practice Act (M.G.L. c. 112 § 80B & 80E) sets forth that the minimum statutory requirements for an advanced practice nurse who seeks prescriptive rights in the Commonwealth include graduation from an accredited program, certification as an advance practice nurse, the development of collaborative guidelines agreed upon by the practitioner and the supervising physician for the treatment of common disorders, and inclusion of the name of the supervising physician on the written prescription.

The Board of Registration in Nursing, a state agency delegated to oversee the promulgation of regulations to implement the enabling legislation, has enacted detailed rules to guide the practitioner in advanced practice. At a minimum, an advanced practitioner with prescriptive rights must have 24 additional hours of pharmacotherapeutics in addition to that provided in a basic graduate program, develop joint guidelines agreed upon by the practitioner and the supervising physician for the treatment of common disorders, and have a quarterly review by the supervising physician of the patients evaluated by the practitioner. Thus, under the evidentiary rules of Massachusetts, a violation of a statutory and regulatory requirement is evidence of improper care, which a practitioner must rebut by establishing either that the plaintiff was not within the protected class or that the harm suffered was not that which the statute was designed to guard against.

For example, if an advanced practice nurse ordered medication for treatment that was not in accordance with the guidelines agreed upon by the practitioner and physician, the jury would review not only the presumption of improper care (the violation of statute and regulations), but also its rebuttal (reasons put forth by the practitioner explaining why she failed to follow the guidelines). This shifting burden of persuasion permits the jury to assign the evidentiary significance, if any, it would in support of each party's burden of proof. Thus, in Massachusetts, violation of a statutory requirement, under the evidentiary rules developed by the Supreme Judicial Court (hereinafter SJC), becomes merely another piece of evidence to consider. The weight a jury accords to evidence of a statutory violation is collectively derived during jury deliberations.

Breach of Care

Once the existence of a duty is recognized and the appropriate standard of care is determined, a plaintiff must prove that the nurse breached the applicable standard of care. Once again, expert testimony is necessary to establish that a nurse's conduct was improper. Adherence to one's institutional policy and procedure manual may be utilized to establish that the conduct complained of was in accordance with acceptable practice. However, if the policy is unsound and not recognized within the profession as constituting proper care, the imposition of liability will not be avoided (*Vanstreenburg v. Lawrence Memorial Hospital*, 1984).

The third element that must be established in a professional negligence action is causation. The most simplistic definition of causation is a reasonably close causal connection between the challenged conduct and the resulting injury. Unfortunately, simplicity has never been an attribute of law.

Proximate Cause

Proximate cause, historically, has denoted proximity in time (Prosser, 1984). It is a distinction that has disappeared as the law has evolved. Currently, it is widely utilized to mean legal cause. Proximate causation turns on the question whether the conduct was so significant that public policy requires a finding of liability, thereby focusing the inquiry on the extent of the original obligation and the consequences associated with its continuance (Id). Simply

stated, was the invasion of the plaintiff's interests by the defendant entitled to legal protection? Courts have developed three methods to determine whether an injury is proximately caused by the challenged conduct.

The "but for" test or "sine qua non" rule (Prosser Torts §41 1984) focuses on whether the injury would have occurred in the absence of the wrongdoer's act. It is a rule of exclusion, for the jury must find that the injury would not have occurred but for the conduct of the defendant. Ordinarily, the "but for" rule is sufficient to establish the legal cause of an injury. However, it fails in situations where the actions of two or more wrongdoers, occurring in concert, cause the plaintiff harm, either of which alone would have yielded the same result. To compensate for the inability of the "but for" rule to resolve the latter situation, Minnesota courts have applied the "substantial factor" rule (*Anderson v. Minneapolis St. Paul & SSMR Co.*, 1920). Briefly stated, the "substantial factor" rule permits a jury to find liability if the defendant's conduct was a material element in bringing about the harm (Second Restatement of Torts § 433, 1965). It need not be the sole cause of the injury but must be a major contributor to the harm suffered by plaintiff.

To remedy the shortcomings engendered by the "substantial factor" rule, courts have attempted to limit liability by determining whether the harm that occurred was foreseeable. The determination of foreseeability balances an assessment of the gravity of the consequences of the challenged conduct with an evaluation of its social utility. The issue of whether an injury is proximately related to the tortious conduct is a jury question.

Damages

The final element that must be proven in a negligence action is damages. If there is a failure of proof in establishing damages, or harm, there can be no recovery. Because the issue of damages is within the common experience and knowledge of the lay person, expert testimony is not necessary. When a jury calculates damages, the computation is intended to compensate an individual for the harm he has suffered. Compensatory damages include the value of past, present, and future lost earnings. The costs associated with the provision of past, present, and future medical care are considered special damages. The award for exemplary/punitive damages differs depending upon the jurisdiction of each action. In Massachusetts, punitive damages can only be awarded in death actions where wanton, willful, reckless disregard for human life is demonstrated (M.G.L. c. 229 § 2). Lastly, a jury can compensate a plaintiff for her conscious pain and suffering (M.G.L. c. 231 § 60B). In actions where the plaintiff is a minor child, the award for lost earnings varies from jurisdiction to jurisdiction. At least one court has held that an award by a jury for the lost earning capacity of a

CHAPTER 6 ■ Legal Implications of Pediatric Nursing Practice 113

minor was proper despite the evidence that the party was not gainfully employed prior to the alleged, disabling tortious conduct (*Nelson v. Patrick*, 1985).

In addition, traditional tort law has allowed the parents of a minor plaintiff to seek damages for the loss of the child's love, affection, society, and companionship, commonly known as consortium. When that child becomes an adult, however, that loss is theoretically no longer compensable. Also, depending upon the jurisdiction, some family members can be compensated for the emotional distress they suffer as a result of witnessing an injury caused to a loved one. To prevail in Massachusetts, a party must also establish the development of the physical manifestation of an illness that can be temporally related to the negligent act. Thus, a mother who suffered a myocardial infarction after witnessing a car accident involving her 14-year-old son could establish a cause of action for negligent infliction of emotional distress (*Dziokonski v. Babineau*, 1976). Other jurisdictions, such as California, however, have abandoned the requirement of proof of a temporally related physical injury (*Accounts Adjustment Bureau v. Cooperman*, 204 Cal Rptr 881 (Cal. App. 1984); Braemer v. Dotson, 1993).

Burden of Proof

Contrary to common perception, because nursing malpractice suits are civil actions and not criminal actions, a plaintiff need only establish by a preponderance of evidence that the harm she suffered was substantially caused by a deviation in the acceptable standard of care by the defendant. In Massachusetts, substantial evidence does not equate with scientific certainty. So long as the scales of justice tip in favor of one party after the jury has reviewed all the competent evidence, a party has established its burden of proof.

For example, despite the age of the decision, the underlying legal analysis engaged in by the court remains valid in *Rose v. Hakim*, 1971. The court made the following findings of fact. Hakim, an otolaryngologist, was retained by the plaintiff's father to perform a tonsillectomy and adenoidectomy (T&A) in a 5-year-old child for recurrent otitis media. The child was admitted preoperatively to Washington Hospital Center on February 21, 1968.

During surgery, the anesthesia was provided by a member of the group that had contracted to provide anesthesia services to the hospital. Approximately 3 minutes prior to the completion of the T&A, the defendant, Hakim, noted that the child's blood had darkened and requested the anesthesiologist to administer more oxygen. This episode recurred, and oxygen was again administered with a resultant return of oxygenation. Prior to performing the myringotomy, Hakim asked the circulating nurse to check the child's pulse. None was found. Resuscitation efforts commenced immediately, and the child's cardiac rhythm returned two and one-half minutes after it was first noted that he was pulseless.

In the recovery room, Hakim ordered, among other things, a cooling blanket to prevent a rise in the child's body temperature above 90°F. Continued hypothermia was recommended to decrease cerebral oxygenation requirements. Later that day, Hakim ordered a transfer to the intensive care unit. Prior to the transfer, the child was found by Anesthesia to be more alert and reactive, breathing on his own, and in satisfactory condition. It was anticipated that the child would make a complete recovery from the cardiac arrest he had sustained in the operating room. As per the custom at that institution, a nurse from the ICU went to the recovery room to obtain report on the child.

Despite the knowledge that the child required a thermometer that could register below 94°F, no such equipment was available in the ICU upon his arrival from the recovery room. In addition, while the hypothermia machine had an attached probe for continuous assessment of body temperature, it was known to the nursing staff that the apparatus was not accurate. Moreover, despite the knowledge that the child had suffered a cardiac arrest in the operating room, he was not placed on a cardiac monitor upon his arrival into the ICU.

In the ICU, he was cared for by Nurse A, a registered nurse. For the night shift, he was assigned Nurse B, who, unbeknownst to the hospital, had not passed her nursing boards. At no time prior to the night of surgery did the hospital inquire whether Nurse B was a registered nurse.

Shortly after the child's arrival to the ICU, seizures were noted along with a concomitant rise in body temperature. The seizures, which were initially minor, occurred every 15 minutes and were duly recorded by Nurse B, who failed to notify anyone about the development of seizure activity in her patient. At 1:45 A.M., the child suffered his first tonic-clonic seizure and had a respiratory arrest.

From the time of the child's arrival in the ICU, his temperature was monitored by the probe attached to the cooling blanket. The following probe temperatures were recorded:

10:45 P.M.: 92°F
11:00 P.M.: 91.5°F
12:00 midnight: 92°F
1:00 A.M.: 93.5°F
1:30 A.M.: 95.4°F

When a glass thermometer was finally obtained from the emergency room at 6:30 A.M., it became known that the probe recording of the temperature was 4.6° less than that obtained using a rectal thermometer. At the time of the respiratory arrest that was precipitated by the seizure, the child's temperature, in actuality, was 100°F.

Unfortunately, when the child experienced the arrest, no ventilator was available in the unit, and mouth-to-tube resuscitation was administered for 10 to 15 minutes until an operating ventilator could be obtained. The child subsequently suffered two additional seizures that night. Shortly before the shift ended, Nurse B noted that the child was hypoxemic. When respiratory therapy arrived, it was discovered that the cause of the inadequate oxygenation was a kink in the ventilator tubing. The defendant Hakim did not learn of the three seizures and the prolonged period of anoxia (10 minutes) until he was notified later that morning by his department that the child had been transferred to the neurosurgical service. Later that day, a note by an intern and a cardiac consult indicated that the child had suffered a cardiac arrest during the night.

The events that transpired in this case raise several nursing liability issues. When the ICU nurse went to get report from the recovery room nurse, she learned that the child required a thermometer capable of registering below 94°F. While the probe attached to the hypothermia blanket could automatically record temperatures, nursing staff had knowledge that it had malfunctioned previously on more than one occasion, and could not be correlated with manual temperatures. A prudent nurse in the exercise of due care should have recognized that the underlying circumstances were fraught with danger for her patient and would have acted accordingly to prevent or minimize the danger. Nurse A failed to appreciate the dangerousness of the situation.

Moreover, a prudent nurse who has knowledge that her patient had previously suffered a cardiac arrest would, as a precaution, place that patient on a cardiac monitor. These acts of nonfeasance by Nurse A, who accepted the patient into the unit, were unacceptable and substantially contributed to the severity of the child's injury.

Liability also existed for the malfeasance committed by Nurse B. The failure to pass her nursing boards was a clear indication that she lacked the minimum standards necessary to practice nursing within her state. While not conclusive of negligence, a jury would be warranted in drawing a strong inference that the lack of proper certification was an indication that Nurse B was not competent to practice nursing, much less ICU nursing (for a discussion of the evidentiary treatment of statutory violations, see supra).

Assuming for the sake of argument that a jury does not infer that Nurse B's lack of proper credentials was a factor in the second arrest of this child, a jury would be hard pressed to excuse Nurse B's subsequent failure to notify the treating physician of the ominous onset of frequent seizure activity so that timely intervention could take place to prevent the child's first tonic-clonic seizure and subsequent respiratory arrest. After this arrest, the child suffered two additional tonic-clonic seizures, which again went unreported and untreated. To compound Nurse B's liability, after the child had experienced the arrest, a nurse in the exercise of due care should have known, and understood, the basic operation of a functioning ventilator sufficiently well to notice an obvious kink in the tubing of the ventilator, which could further compromise the child's precarious respiratory status

by causing hypoxemia. These acts of malfeasance and nonfeasance by Nurse B substantially contributed to the severe damage suffered by the child.

Not surprisingly, the court had little difficulty in finding the actions of the nursing defendants improper. The disputed issue at trial was whether the negligent nursing actions caused the child's brain damage, cortical blindness, and near total quadriplegia. Absent a finding of causation, the most wanton, reckless conduct will be excused.

In reviewing the facts, it had previously been noted that the child had suffered a cardiac arrest in the operating room. Two and one-half minutes after the arrest, a cardiac rhythm was reestablished. As part of the child's postoperative care, neuro vital signs were ordered by Hakim but never recorded by nursing staff until 4 days after the chain of adverse occurrences had occurred in the ICU. At issue was when the onset of decerebrate and decorticate movements were first noted.

If observed initially in the recovery room, the improper nursing care could not have contributed to the child's neurologic dysfunction, and could only be traced back to the mishap that occurred in the operating room. If noted after the critical events in the ICU, the logical conclusion would be that the poor nursing care had caused the severe neurologic deficits suffered by the patient.

During trial, evidence was introduced that the first notation of decorticate movements was made by nursing staff 4 days after the child's misadventure in the ICU. Testimony was elicited that the onset of decerebrate, decorticate movements was a significant event, and a prudent nurse in the exercise of due care would have charted these abnormal neurologic findings when they were observed. Despite the absence of any documentation, two nurses testified that they had observed decerebrate movements in the recovery room on the evening of the child's surgery. In addition, despite the awareness of both nurses about the need to document this critical observation, both failed to do so and also failed to notify any physician of their observations, leading to the inference that the symptoms had not occurred until the time that was actually noted in the record.

Moreover, the court did not find the testimony of one of the nurses credible, for she was the individual, Nurse A, who had obtained report from the recovery room nurse and had failed to ensure that the proper equipment was available that could have averted, or minimized, the critical events that occurred in the ICU. A good trial attorney would not fail to show that Nurse A's testimony was biased, and thus suspect, for her interest in the outcome of the trial was not impartial. The court found the testimony of both nurses to be not credible and concluded that the proximate cause of the child's devastating neurologic dysfunction was improper nursing care. The court further held that if any neurologic injury occurred after the cardiac arrest in the operating room, it was minor and reversible and did not contribute to the profound deficits suffered by the minor plaintiff.

The inadequate documentation found in the care of this child supported a finding of improper nursing care. If the nurses had charted the neuro vital signs that they presumably were assessing, the onset of decerebrate and decorticate movements would have been readily apparent and could have supported a finding that the substandard nursing care was not the proximate cause of this child's neurologic devastation. The absence of any findings led to the inference that the neuro signs were not performed, as required, and added to the general impression of incompetent nurses, and also permitted the jury to infer that the neurologic dysfunction was not apparent until the fourth day after surgery. Interestingly, if this case were tried today, a good plaintiff attorney would obtain an expert to testify that the cardiac arrest sustained in the operating room substantially contributed to the neurologic injuries the child displayed during trial. Despite the court's finding that the child's cardiac rhythm was timely restored two and one-half minutes after asystole was first noted, the opinion is notably absent for failing to address the possibility that the child might have been asystolic for some time before it was observed.

While not addressed in the court's opinion, events such as this, occurring in the present day, would have provoked an inquiry into the role of hospital administration as a causative agent of this child's brain damage. Not only had the hospital failed to provide adequate equipment necessary for a properly functioning ICU, also the equipment that was operational was not functioning optimally. In addition, its failure to ensure that all nursing personnel met the minimum statutory requirements to practice nursing was not proper. Both these acts, alone, or in conjunction, substantially contributed to the harm suffered by the minor plaintiff.

Interestingly, certain facts that the court found probative in its opinion have since been disproven and are no longer considered valid practice. In urban, tertiary care facilities, such as the site of the Hakim action, patients would not be accepted into the ICU until adequate functioning equipment was available. Thus, the acts of nonfeasance of Nurse A would not have been an issue at trial, for the equipment she failed to obtain for her patient is now considered standard operating equipment for a proper ICU. Also, hypothermia is no longer considered an accepted treatment to decrease cerebral oxygenation requirements. While the specific facts are obsolete, the underlying principles remain intact.

A nurse who fails to recognize the needs of her patient, or a nurse who recognizes the needs of her patient but does not intervene in a timely manner, is not acting in accordance with acceptable practice. An ICU nurse is expected to have a minimum degree of knowledge for each piece of equipment that she will encounter in patient care. She is expected to know how to recognize when a piece of equipment is malfunctioning and when she must obtain a replacement. If assigned a patient for whom she does not feel competent to give care, she must make her needs

known so that alternative arrangements can be made to ensure the safety of the patient (see discussion of refusing an assignment, infra). Clearly, when new signs are noted, such as the onset of seizure activity, a physician must be notified in order to obtain treatment. While the seizures here were most likely evidence of hypoxic damage to the brain, rather than hypoxia causing seizure activity, timely intervention could have prevented the prolonged period of anoxic insult and perhaps improve the patient's outlook.

COMMON LEGAL PRINCIPLES

Informed Consent

In 1914, Justice Cardoza of the New York Supreme Court articulated the principle that "[e]very human being of adult years and sound mind has a right to determine what shall be done with his own body . . . ." (*Schloendork v. Society of New York Hospital*, 1914). This thoughtful statement by the preeminent jurist was the nascent underpinning for the doctrine of informed consent.

Informed consent is rooted in the common law tort of battery (*Kohoutek v. Hafner*, 1986). From the earliest days, any unpermitted touching constituted a battery for which an individual could seek compensation (Prosser, 1984). For a battery to take place, one must demonstrate intent or a "desire to bring about the physical consequences, up to and including death" (Prosser, 1984). If a third person is injured rather than the intended target, the intent to commit the act is likewise transferred to the third party. For an action to lie in battery, a patient need not prove that harm ensued from the unpermitted touching, only that the touching was not permitted.

In cases that allege a lack of informed consent, a patient must establish not only that a material risk of harm was not disclosed that a reasonable person under the same or similar circumstances would have disclosed, but also that the failure to disclose this information caused the individual to suffer harm. Thus, while it is easier to establish a cause of action for battery rather than informed consent, courts have rarely applied the simpler burden of proof to medical negligence actions.

In Massachusetts, the first case to articulate the principles underlying the doctrine of informed consent occurred in *Harnish v. Children's Hospital Medical Center*, 1972. In this action, the plaintiff filed suit against a hospital and three maxillofacial surgeons associated with it, for an almost total loss of lingual function as a result of a severed hypoglossal nerve that occurred during surgery for removal of a recurrent neck tumor. At a pre-screening panel, the court found insufficient evidence to raise a question appropriate for judicial inquiry (M.G.L. c. 231, § 60B) and dismissed the action when the plaintiff failed to post the requisite bond, necessary to proceed, within the statutory period (Id). On appeal, the Supreme Judicial Court of Massachusetts affirmed the dismissal against the hospital and one assisting surgeon but reversed as to the remaining two defendants.

In a cogently worded opinion, which relied heavily on the seminal case *Canterbury v. Spence* (1971), the Massachusetts high court stated "[t]he extent to which a [physician] must share . . . information with his patient depends upon what information he should reasonably recognize is material to the plaintiff's decision." Further, in quoting from a 1972 Rhode Island case, *Wilkinson v. Vesey*, the court stated

Materiality may be said to be the significance a reasonable person in what the physician knows or should know is his patient's position, would attach to the disclosed risk or risks in deciding whether to submit or not to submit to surgery or treatment.

The *Harnish* Court adhered to the opinion set forth in *Canterbury v. Spence* that a lay person, in the absence of an expert, could determine whether the proposed treatment or surgery constituted a material risk of harm. To guide future courts in their deliberations, the *Harnish* Court enumerated the following criteria as examples of what lay persons might consider material information warranting disclosure:

1. The nature of the patient's condition
2. The nature and probability of risks involved
3. The benefits to be reasonably expected
4. The inability of the physician to predict results
5. Irreversibility of the situation
6. The likely result of no treatment
7. Available alternatives including their risks and benefits

The *Harnish* decision, however, was premised upon a finding of competency, an individual capable of giving legal consent to the performance of a procedure.

Competency and Incompetency

A competent individual is one over the age of 18 who possesses the ability to understand the basic information necessary to make a decision whether he will agree to the recommended treatment or not (*Saikewicz*, infra 1977). Grounded in common law, individuals have a "strong interest in being free from nonconsensual invasion of [their] bodily integrity" (Id). This right is also set forth in the penumbras of the constitutional amendments which guarantee a right to privacy (*Roe v. Wade*, 1973, *Griswold v. Connecticut*, 1965), as well as a liberty interest under the due process clause to refuse undesired medical treatment (*Jacobson v. Massachusetts*, 1903). "The law protects [a person's] right to make her own decision to accept or reject treatment, whether that decision is wise or unwise" (*Lane v. Candura*, 1978). An incompetent individual, whether because of age or mental incapacity, cannot legally refuse treatment. For children, parents or legal guardians are normally

the proper individuals to assent to or refuse treatment. The presumption is, of course, is that parents/legal guardians have the best interests of their children at heart. Where parents have refused to provide treatment that is life-saving, courts have historically ordered healthcare providers to render treatment over the objections of the parents (see generally, American Jurisprudence, Infants, 1985).

For those individuals deemed incompetent, courts have engaged in different methods of analysis to determine what the incompetent's decision would be if he had been competent to render one. In Massachusetts, the courts have applied the doctrine of substituted judgment. First articulated in *Superintendent of Belchertown State School v. Saikewicz*, 1977, the Supreme Judicial Court, confronted by a case of first impression, held that a mentally incompetent 52-year-old man who had resided his entire life in state institutions would have refused treatment for his leukemia when the hope of a cure was minimal. In explaining its decision, the SJC stated "[i]t does not advance the interest of the State or the ward to treat the ward as a person of lesser status of dignity than others. To protect the incompetent person within its power, the State must recognize the dignity and worth of such a person and afford to that person the same panoply of rights and choices it recognizes in incompetent person[,]" (Id at 746) with the explicit goal of "determin[ing] with as much accuracy as possible the wants and needs of the individual involved" (*Saikewicz, supra* at 750).

To establish how the court is to substitute its decision for that of the now incompetent, the SJC looks to the words and actions of the individual to determine what his subjective decision would have been, if competent. The incongruity of the *Saikewicz* decision lies in the fact that Saikewicz had never expressed any opinion about the circumstances under which he would have refused treatment, for he lacked the mental competency to understand the consequences of that decision. While defined as "substituted judgment," a subjective standard, the *Saikewicz* court, in actuality, applied an objective standard, for it would have been impossible for it to determine what Saikewicz's previously expressed wishes and desires were, absent any statements to support the process.

For those jurisdictions that require "clear and convincing" evidence before treatment can be withdrawn from an incompetent, an incompetent's previously expressed wishes is a factor in the court's deliberation that may, or may not, be determinative. In the landmark case *Cruzan v. Director, Missouri Dept. of Health*, 1990, the parents of a 22-year-old woman, diagnosed as being in a persistent vegetative state, petitioned the Supreme Court of the United States to permit them to authorize the withdrawal of a feeding tube that was maintaining their daughter's life. The High Court reviewed the lower court's decision and refused to grant the parents of Mary Beth Cruzan the authority to withdraw the life sustaining treatment. In explaining the rationale behind its decision, the court held that there was insufficient documentation to determine what decision Mary Beth Cruzan would make if she were capable of speaking. In support of its decision, the court examined various statements made by Mary Beth Cruzan, prior to the accident that led to her persistent vegetative state, and found that they lacked definitive proof of Mary Beth Cruzan's "not-fully expressed desires," and rejected the parents' petition. *Saikewicz* and *Cruzan* involved patients with incomplete or absent documented desires. In circumstances involving minor patients, the court rulings have demonstrated more unanimity and uniformity.

Advanced Directives and the Adolescent Patient

To counter the hardship engendered by the Supreme Court's decision in *Cruzan*, Congress passed the Health Care Determination Act in 1990 in response to dicta authored by Justice Brennan, who asserted that previously expressed wishes of a now incompetent patient were to be accorded the same constitutional protection as a competent patient's wishes, including the right to refuse treatment.

The Act provides that (1) all adult patients must be offered written information as well as summaries of pertinent institutional policies regarding their rights under state and federal law to accept or refuse treatment and to make advanced directives; (2) there must be documentation in the patient's record to indicate whether the patient has an advanced directive; (3) institutions may not discriminate against or condition care provided to a patient on the basis of whether the patient has executed an advanced directive; (4) institutions have an affirmative obligation to comply with the requirements of state and federal law regarding advanced directives; and (5) institutions must provide individually, or with others, education to staff and community regarding issues associated with advanced directives.

As a practical matter, however, to ensure that one's wishes are followed in the event of incompetency, written documents, such as an advanced directive, would serve as evidence of a patient's previously expressed desires. "Advanced directive" is a broad term that encompasses documents such as living wills, durable power of attorney for healthcare, and healthcare proxies. These documents are executed by competent adults in order to appoint a surrogate decision-maker for healthcare decisions in the event the person later becomes incompetent. The type of document that constitutes a healthcare directive varies in each jurisdiction. The existence of documentary proof of the patient's choice, when competent, avoids needless conflicts between healthcare providers and family members. More importantly, it "empower[s] people to take part in the decisions that affect the duration and condition of their lives" (Rouse, Fenella, 1991).

Currently, patients under the age of 18 are pre-cluded from executing an advanced directive. Nurses who care for the chronically and/or critically ill adolescent are aware that these patients desire to have an active role in making treatment decisions. "As patient advocates, critical care nurses are concerned about how to promote the interest of [these] adolescents in decisions about their health care" (Rushton, Cindy Hylton, et al., 1992). At present, only parents and guardians have the right to make healthcare decisions for adolescents.

Though deemed legally incompetent because of chronologic age, it can be argued that many adolescents are sufficiently competent to make healthcare decisions. At least one commentary has alluded that critical care nurses realize that chronically ill adolescents, such as those suffering from cancer, cystic fibrosis, or cardiac or pulmonary diseases, demonstrate a greater degree of emotional maturity than their chronologic ages would indicate because of the psychological demands of coping with their diseases (Uustal, Diann, 1991). Thus, age alone should not be the sole determination of the ability to render a legal decision.

While most adolescents are legally precluded from executing an advanced directive, an adolescent's expectations with respect to treatment decisions should still be solicited. To obtain valid data, it is essential for nurses to have a thorough understanding of adolescent cognitive development and how this contributes to the adolescent's ability to participate in the treatment decision making process. Utilization of a process such as obtaining a "values history" would elicit information about the adolescent's attitudes towards his present health, hopes for the future, thoughts about death, religious beliefs, and the person he trusts to make treatment decisions for him (Rushton, Cindy Hylton et al., 1992). Providing a conducive environment for the adolescent to express deep, personal emotions is essential to obtain this critical information. Preservation of autonomy and providing a forum for open communication are important nursing interventions which must be considered when caring for these patients.

Jehovah's Witness

As a general rule, neither a parent nor a guardian of a minor is free to refuse life-saving treatment for the minor (American Jurisprudence, Infants). In instances where a minor child of Jehovah's Witnesses has required treatment that the parents have refused to authorize, most courts have ordered the life-saving treatment administered over the objection of the parents *(Id)*. Emergency blood transfusions are always warranted when treating the minor child of a Jehovah's Witness. After the emergent situation has resolved, a hearing must be conducted to obtain a court order to administer blood and blood products on an ad hoc basis.

In *In the Matter of Elisha McCauley* 1991, the Supreme Judicial Court (SJC) of Massachusetts upheld the decision of a trial court judge who had, over the objections of both parents, who were devout Jehovah's Witnesses, authorized physicians at Children's Hospital to "provide all reasonable medical care which in their judgment [was] necessary to preserve the patient's life and health, including but not limited to the administration of blood and/or blood products throughout the entire course of her treatment for leukemia and related conditions." In affirming the lower court judgment, the Massachusetts SJC acknowledged that the private realm of family life was constitutionally protected from unwarranted state interference and reasserted its oft-stated support for the free exercise of one's religion. Having thus reaffirmed that the right to practice one's religion was a fundamental right protected by the Constitution, the court then tempered its statement by asserting that "[t]he right to practice religion freely does not include [the] liberty to expose the [child] to ill health or death." Thus, "[w]hen a child's life is at issue, it is not the rights of the parents that are chiefly to be considered. The first and paramount duty is to consult the welfare of the child."

The court analyzed the four competing interests involved when a parent refuses medical treatment for an ill child: (1) the "natural interests" of the parents; (2) the interests of the child; (3) the interests of the state (parens patriae); and (4) the interests of the medical profession and commented further on those competing factors.

In support of its decision to allow the administration of blood and blood products, the court cited "(1) the child's age; (2) the risk to the child's health and life if the requested treatment was not ordered; (3) the real probability that the child's illness would be in remission if she were given the requested treatment; . . . (4) the substantial chance for a cure and a normal life for the child if she underwent the recommended treatment; and (5) the minimal risks to the child's health which would result from the treatment" (Id at 138). The court acknowledged the sincerely held religious beliefs of both parents, and to the extent possible, the religious beliefs of the 8-year-old minor, and proceeded to an analysis of the State's interests. The SJC delineated the parens patriae analysis enunciated in previous cases and commented on the state's interest in protecting the welfare of children residing within its borders (*Prince v. Massachusetts*, 1944), the preservation of life, particularly for curable illnesses (*Superintendent of Belchertown State School v. Saikewicz*, 1977), and "[t]he maintenance of the ethical integrity of the medical profession" (*Custody of a Minor*, 1978), and concluded that the administration of blood and blood products was in the best interests of the child (*McCauley* at 138–139, 1991).

As always, a competent adult may refuse to allow the administration of blood products to herself. When that refusal, however, endangers the life of a fetus, courts have ordered the treatment despite the objections of the competent adult. Until very recently in Massachusetts, a competent adult could not refuse life-saving treatment if that decision would lead to the "abandonment" of the child. In *Norwood Hospital v. Yolanda Munoz & another*, 1991, Yolanda Munoz, a competent 38-year-old woman with a long history of gastric ulcers, was admitted to Norwood Hospital for an upper gastrointestinal bleed that had been precipitated by the ingestion, for 1 week, of two aspirin every 4 hours for arm pain. The UGI bleed was stopped by the administration of drugs, with a resulting hematocrit of 17% after stabilization. In the opinion of her attending physician, Mrs. Munoz had a 50% chance of rebleeding and would face certain death unless blood and blood products were administered. Mrs. Munoz refused.

At that time, Norwood Hospital had a written policy that in nonemergency situations, if a competent adult, who was not pregnant or the parent of minor children, refused to consent to the receipt of blood, that refusal would be honored. However, if the patient was a minor or the parent of minor children, a judicial determination of the rights and obligations of the parties would be sought. Because Yolanda Munoz had a 6-year-old child at home, the hospital sought a court order to administer blood. After a full evidentiary hearing in the Probate Court, the judge granted the hospital's motion to give blood. In its decision, the court acknowledged that competent adults could refuse life-saving treatment. However, allowing Yolanda Munoz to do so could lead to her death and "the emotional abandonment of Ernesto Jr., which would, more probably than not, be detrimental to [her son's] best interests." The judge concluded that the State's interest in protecting the well-being of Ernesto Jr. outweighed Ms. Munoz's right to refuse medical treatment (Id).

In support of its decision, the court made the following factual findings: Yolanda Munoz was the principal caretaker of Ernesto Jr. While her husband assisted in his son's care, he worked 16-hour days in his own business. Ernesto Jr.'s grandfather, while willing to care for his grandson, was elderly, did not speak English, was unemployed, lacked a driver's license, and had not participated significantly in his grandson's care in the past. In addition, the court found that the willingness of Ernesto Jr.'s maternal aunt to care for him should his mother die lacked substance and refused to allow "this most ultimate of voluntary abandonments" to occur (Id). On appeal, the SJC reversed the lower court. In balancing the competing interests involved in allowing Yolanda Munoz to refuse treatment, the court found that "the State's interest in preserving the patient's life, in maintaining the ethical integrity of the medical profession, and in protecting the well-being of the patient's child did not override the patient's right to refuse life-saving medical treatment" (Id at 130). To some healthcare providers, the failure by a parent to obtain care for his child because of religious beliefs constitutes a form of child abuse.

Child Abuse

In the United States, all states have enacted mandatory reporting statutes requiring healthcare professionals to report instances of suspected child abuse. In Massachusetts, the statute requires a report when "reasonable cause [exists] to believe that a child under the age of eighteen years is suffering physical or emotional injury resulting from abuse inflicted upon him which causes harm or substantial risk of harm to the child's health or welfare including sexual abuse, or from neglect, including malnutrition or who is determined to be physically dependent upon an addictive drug at birth" (M.G.L. c. 119 §51A). Under the Massachusetts statute, a report must be orally communicated via a telephone "hotline" and followed within 48 hours by a written report. Further, if photographs are taken, they may be taken without the consent of the family and should be appended to the written report filed with the appropriate social service agency. Failure by a provider of healthcare to comply with the statutory reporting requirements is punishable by a fine of $1000 (M.G.L. c. 119 § 51B).

While the mandate to report is clear, for certain types of healthcare personnel, such as social workers and psychotherapists, the duty to report is complicated by a statutorily imposed duty to maintain the confidentiality of privileged communications. Massachusetts' courts, however, have addressed this conflict conclusively. In *Commonwealth v. Southier*, 1991, the Appeals Court asserted that the apparent dissonance between a statute requiring a psychotherapist to maintain privileged communications confidential and the mandatory child abuse reporting statute was in actuality a conscious legislative mandate in favor of reporting by statutorily conferring civil and criminal immunity for any report of neglect or abuse by mandated reporters.

For critical care nurses, the need to report is seldom present, for by the time a child has arrived in the ICU, a report has either been filed or called into the hotline as required. The issues that arise in the ICU relate to the ability to divulge confidential information after a report has been filed.

In Massachusetts, a healthcare provider can release confidential information only if he is authorized to do so by either the patient or the legal representative (M.G.L. c. 111 §70E). The filing of a 51A confers immunity only as to the contents contained within the report. The Department of Social Services (DSS), the agency designated to investigate allegations of child abuse and neglect in the Commonwealth of Massachusetts, is empowered with the authority to review medical records and speak to healthcare providers to determine whether the claim of abuse/neglect can be substantiated. However, DSS's right to obtain confidential information is not necessarily transferred to the police and/or the district attorney's office. In many instances, the relevant state agency such as DSS has obtained legal custody of the child and has granted the police and the office of the district attorney the right to obtain medical evidence in support of their quest for a return of a "true bill" from the grand jury. Where legal custody is not sought, a healthcare provider cannot disclose information to

the police or district attorney absent the consent of the legal guardian. Should the legal guardian refuse to cooperate with state authorities, and those authorities are insistent upon obtaining the necessary medical information to support their indictment, hospital counsel should be consulted immediately to compel the district attorney to obtain a court order for the release of medical information. While a Massachusetts healthcare provider is mandated to cooperate with the state's child protection agency, the duty to cooperate does not necessarily extend to police and the district attorney. Thus, the critical care nurse may be placed in the awkward position of obstructing justice by denying access to medical information necessary to support an indictment for child abuse or find herself subjected to an action alleging breach of confidentiality for the unauthorized release of medical information.

Patient's Bill of Rights

The Joint Commission on Accreditation of Health Care Organizations (JCAHO) is a private institution that conducts surveys of hospitals to determine whether healthcare institutions have complied with the standards it issues. Contrary to the belief of many persons, the Joint Commission is not a governmental agency charged with ensuring the safety and quality of patient care. Rather, its authority is derived from the fact that the Health Care Financing Administration, an agency within the Department of Health and Human Services, utilizes the results of Commission surveys to determine whether a hospital should receive reimbursement from federal programs for healthcare provided to the elderly and the needy. There are few hospitals, if any, today that could survive financially absent federal reimbursement funds.

Under the many standards set forth by the Joint Commission, a section in the preamble enumerates the rights and responsibilities of patients that the Commission intended to be an expression of the "relationship between hospitals and patients" (JCAHO, 1991, p. XI). JCAHO has enumerated the following statements as illustrative of the rights and responsibilities of patients.*

Patient Rights

1. **Access to care:** Individuals shall be accorded impartial access to treatment of accommodations that are available or medically indicated, regardless of race, creed, sex, national origin, or sources of payment for care.
2. **Respect and dignity:** The patient has the right to considerate, respectful care at all times and under all circumstances, with recognition of his personal dignity.
3. **Privacy and confidentiality:** The patient has

*Taken from the Joint Commission on the Accreditation of Hospitals, Standards, Chicago, 1991.

the right, within the law, to personal and informational privacy, as manifested by the following rights: to refuse to talk with or see anyone not officially connected with the hospital, including visitors, or persons officially connected with the hospital but not directly involved in his care.

4. **Hospital charges:** Regardless of the source of payment for his care, the patient has the right to request and receive an itemized and detailed explanation of his total bill for services rendered in the hospital. The patient has the right to timely notice prior to termination of his eligibility for reimbursement by any third-party payer for the cost of his care.

5. **Hospital rules and regulations:** The patient should be informed of the hospital rules and regulations applicable to his conduct as a patient. Patients are entitled to information about the hospital's mechanism for the initiation, review, and resolution of patient complaints.

Patient Responsibilities

1. **Provision of information:** A patient has the responsibility to provide, to the best of his knowledge, accurate and complete information about present complaints, past illnesses, hospitalizations, medication, and other matters relating to his health. He has the responsibility to report unexpected changes in his condition to the responsible practitioner. A patient is responsible for reporting whether he clearly comprehends a contemplated course of action and what is expected of him.

2. **Compliance with instruction:** A patient is responsible for following the treatment plan recommended by the practitioner primarily responsible for his care. This may include following the instruction of nurses and allied health personnel as they carry out the coordinated plan of care, implement the responsible practitioner's orders, and enforce the applicable hospital rules and regulations. The patient is responsible for keeping appointments and when he is unable to do so for any reason, for notifying the responsible practitioner or the hospital.

3. **Refusal of treatment:** The patient is responsible for his actions if he refuses treatment or does not follow the practitioner's instructions.

4. **Hospital charges:** The patient is responsible for ensuring that the financial obligation of his healthcare is fulfilled as promptly as possible.

5. **Hospital rules and regulations:** The patient is responsible for following hospital rules and regulations affecting patient care and conduct.

6. **Respect and consideration:** The patient is responsible for being considerate of the rights of other patients and hospital personnel and for assisting in the control of noise, smoking, and the number of visitors. The patient is responsible for being respectful of the property of other persons and of the hospital.

Massachusetts has codified its Patient's Bill of Rights at M.G.L. c. 112 § 70E.

Unlabeled Use of Medication

The use of medication outside of the indications noted on the package insert is a widely accepted practice. There are many drugs currently on the market that are used for unlabeled indications. The primary reason is that it takes a minimum of 18 months for the Food and Drug Administration (FDA) to approve changes to package inserts once a supplemental new drug application is filed. Approval by the FDA would be contingent upon the pharmaceutical manufacturer's ability to demonstrate the effectiveness of the drug for new uses. Often times that occurs by the presentation of medical literature that reports findings of efficaciousness under circumstances not recognized by the manufacturer during its clinical trials. Pharmaceutical companies, needless to say, prefer to devote their energies in obtaining FDA approval to distribute new drugs rather than seeking official approval for uses that the medical profession considers accepted practice. However, simply because a drug is not listed within the package insert as an approved use does not mean that a physician cannot prescribe it for uses outside of the package insert. The determination must be made whether prescribing the medication under the set of circumstances described could be construed as reasonable.

If, during the course of drug administration, a physician observes that the medication is efficacious for disorders not noted in the package insert, it may be reasonable to prescribe a course of therapy for the anecdotally recognized efficacy, despite the fact that the proposed use is an unlabeled one. The determination whether the prescription is reasonable requires an examination of the circumstances surrounding its use. The prescription of a drug outside its packaging is particularly appropriate when journal articles support the unlabeled use of the drug. Indeed, the serendipitous observation that a drug is effective for an unlabeled use often leads to validation of the observation in clinical trials, which then provides the manufacturer with the scientific data needed to substantiate a petition to the FDA to add additional indications for use to the labeling.

In many pediatric ICUs, the use of anesthetic agents such as fentanyl for sedation is currently in vogue. If a practitioner were to review the package insert for indicated uses, the manner for which ICUs utilize the medication would not be found. However, in applying the reasoning set forth above, if support in the medical literature can be found for sedating pediatric patients with anesthetic agents, the practice would be entirely defensible. To the FDA, the contents of the package insert are meant to be only informational (FDA Drug Bulletin, April 1982).

Malpractice Insurance

A recurrent issue for professional nurses is the question of whether malpractice insurance should be purchased. Most nurses are employed by institutions. In common law, the liability of a servant (employee) is vicariously imputed to the master (employer).

Under the Restatement of Agency 2d, §228, 1958, [the] conduct of a servant is within the scope of employment if, but only if: "(a) it is of the kind he is employed to perform; (b) it occurs substantially within the authorized time and space limits; (c) it is actuated, at least in part, by a purpose to serve the master; and (d) if force is intentionally used by the servant against another, the use of force is not unexpected by the master." [If] conduct of a servant is not within the scope of employment, if it is different in kind from that authorized, far beyond the authorized time or space limits, or too little actuated by a purpose to serve the master, § 229 of the Restatement asserts that "[t]o be within the scope of the employment, conduct must be of the same general nature as that authorized, or incidental to the conduct authorized. In determining whether or not the conduct, although not authorized, is nevertheless so similar to, or incidental to, the conduct authorized, as to be within the scope of employment, the following . . . of fact are to be considered: (a) whether or not the act is one commonly done by such servant; (b) the time, place and purpose of the act; (c) the previous relations between the master and the servant; (d) the extent to which the business of the master is apportioned between different servants; (e) whether the act is outside the enterprise of the master or, if within the enterprise, has not been entrusted to any servant; (f) whether or not the master has reason to expect that such an act will be done; (g) the similarity in quality of the act done to the act authorized; (h) whether or not the instrumentality by which the harm is done has been furnished by the master to the servant; (i) the extent of departure from the normal method of accomplishing an authorized result; and (j) whether or not the act is seriously criminal." For nurses, there should be no dispute that their professional conduct falls within the ambit of agency and as such would be protected conduct and covered by the institutional malpractice insurance.

There are currently two types of insurance policies available for coverage: claims made and occurrence policies. In a claims made policy, an insured is covered for claims that are made during the covered period. Courts have broadly construed claims and have declared an insurer to have notice of a duty to defend when any action gives rise to a potential claim (*Manacare Corp v. First State Inc., Co.,* 1979). For coverage to be provided under a claims made policy, the claim must be made during the year in which the premium is paid.

Occurrence policies provide coverage for the time period when the alleged negligence occurred. Thus, even though a professional may not be aware that a suit has been filed against her until many years after the alleged injury-producing conduct, under an occurrence policy, the terms of the policy dictate that the insurer will defend the professional regardless of when the claim is made. For pediatric practitioners, the issue of whether coverage exists for the alleged negligent conduct is particularly important, as many states have statutes that extend the statute of limitations for minors beyond that of adults. In Massachusetts, if the child who is injured by nursing negligence is under the age of 2, the statute of limitations does not expire until the child's seventh birthday. For those minors whose injuries occur over the age of 2, the statute of limitations is tolled until the child's ninth birthday (M.G.L. c. 231 § 60B). Other authorities provide that a minor's cause of action does not commence until 2 years after the appointment of a guardian (M.G.L. c. 260 § 10; *Gaudette v. Webb,* 1972). For persons deemed incompetent at the time of their injury, the law tolls the statute of limitations until 3 years after the disability has been lifted. Persons declared mentally ill or mentally retarded may never become competent. Thus, their statute of limitations could conceivably never expire.

Problems arise when coverage is changed from a claims made policy to an occurrence policy or when an insured retires and discontinues coverage. To protect personal assets from potential litigants after discontinuance of coverage under a claims made policy, insurance companies offer a "reporting endorsement" or "tail coverage policy" that protects against future claims by, as yet, unknown plaintiffs.

The issue for most nurses is when to purchase a policy for professional liability. Under most institutional policies, a nurse's action is protected conduct provided the injury causing conduct that constitutes the alleged negligence occurs within the scope of the professional nurse's employment. For nurse practitioners who practice in an outpatient setting, within a private partnership, or in a physician's office, prudence dictates that the practitioner request either having the policy reviewed by an attorney experienced in the interpretation of insurance policies or specifically request that (s)he be added as a named insured (*National Union Fire Insurance Co. of Pittsburgh v. Medical Liability Mutual Insurance Co.,* 1981). Failure to do so may leave the nurse's personal assets exposed in a nursing negligence action, for it is not the intent of the parties that will guide the courts in rendering a decision, but the language contained within the policy. Thus, a named insured must be precisely that—a name inscribed as a covered party under the insured section. For critical care nurses, coverage should never be an issue, unless the conduct that is the basis of the cause of action is not sanctioned by their institutional employer.

In instances such as this, an insurer could legitimately "disclaim" coverage, thereby leaving the nurse unprotected and her personal assets subject to a potential plaintiff's verdict. In *Hakim* (supra), the hospital's insurer could have legally "disclaimed" coverage for Nurse B because she had failed to disclose to administration that she had not passed the nursing boards. For various reasons, specific to the facts unique to that case, a disclaimer of coverage was unlikely. Under the proper circumstances, however, "disclaimers" are legal and denials of coverage have been upheld on appeal.

RISK FACTORS AFFECTING THE DELIVERY OF HEALTHCARE

Unfortunately, as critical care nursing becomes increasingly technologically oriented, external factors, such as healthcare reform, have placed critical care nurses in the uncompromising position of responding to the needs of high-technology patient care with decreasing resources. While most hospital administrators recognize the need for maintaining adequate nurse:patient ratios, they must also respond to market-driven forces that are dictated by the level of reimbursement for patient care. The boom times of the 1980s when primary nursing attained ascendancy now give way to the sobering 1990s where the provision of quality healthcare involves the delegation of tasks and functions to assistive personnel. As cyclical as history is, so too is the concept of team nursing and nursing assistants. The debate over what constitutes professional nursing cannot be dictated or defined by tasks and functions. Many current nursing functions in critical care areas would have been considered the practice of medicine when intensive care areas were first conceptualized in the 1960s (*Commonwealth v. Porn*, 1907). To adapt to the economy of the twenty-first century, the model of critical care nursing will, in all probability, resemble that of critical care medicine in which tasks and functions will be delegated to assistive personnel of varying levels of ability and the supervision and planning of care becomes the primary focus of professional nursing. With the delegation of tasks comes the greater responsibility of assessing the capabilities and competencies of the assistive personnel to perform the acts delegated to them. Not only will nursing remain responsible for the failure to meet the standards of its own profession, but it will also assume the mantle of oversight for the actions of third parties. That oversight will require a constant ongoing assessment of skills and intervention when the skill level threatens the provision of quality patient care.

A recurrent theme in nursing journals during the 1980s involved the ability of a professional nurse to refuse an assignment when she believed she lacked the proper credentials to provide the degree of care necessary for the needs of her patient. To the author's knowledge, absolute refusal by a nurse to care for patients, regardless of the validity of the refusal, has led to disciplinary action by the institution and, in some circumstances, termination. While refusing an assignment is rarely a viable option, it behooves the professional nurse to discuss the scope of the assignment first so that alternative arrangements can be negotiated for others to provide the care for which the assigned nurse is clearly not qualified to do safely.

By negotiating the assignment, a professional nurse puts hospital administration on notice that the skills required to care for the particular patient may not be met by the individual assigned to that patient and records the objections of the professional to the assignment while indicating a willingness to assist hospital administration to develop a viable, safe alternative. In short, the image that is projected is not that of an obstructionist, but of a professional who recognizes her limitations and the need to achieve a satisfactory solution that does not compromise patient care (Florida Nurses Association, 1989).

Just as the nurse:patient ratio is affected by market forces, so too will the makeup of critical care units as they now exist. Rather than the explosive growth that specialty ICUs saw in the 1980s, the dawning of the twenty-first century will oversee the consolidation and dismantling of many of those units, with the formation, once again, of multidisciplinary ICUs as replacement. Pediatric ICUs, unless contained specifically in pediatric institutions, will in all probability merge with adult critical care units. Thus, to meet the challenges of nursing in the next century, critical care nurses will find it necessary to attain and maintain a greater skill mix for professional practice. Cross-training in the care of both adults and pediatrics will, in all likelihood, be inevitable. The attainment of basic competencies necessary to provide quality patient care in all specialty areas must be identified and maintained if nursing expects to provide leadership in the development of healthcare policy and participate in the debate of how healthcare will be provided in a fiscally responsive manner.

As greater autonomy and authority are achieved, the responsibility to keep abreast of trends in the profession will increasingly become the duty of the professional. It will become an expectation that, as a profession, nursing, like law and medicine, will be responsible for participating and engaging in continuing education with minimal or no support from the institution. For the present, every attempt must be made to match the skill levels of the practitioner to the needs of the patient and once the immediacy of the situation has passed, the professional nurse must make provisions for attaining the knowledge and skills necessary to provide the care warranted by patient needs. The law does not examine how minimum competency is obtained; it simply requires it. The failure of an institution to provide the support necessary for clinical practice does not relieve a critical care nurse from her legal duties and responsibilities. Acting proactively, rather than reactively, will be essential if nursing hopes to gain a voice in the direction of how healthcare should be provided in the future. Once an institution undertakes the responsibility to provide continuing education, however, it is under an obligation to do so in a non-negligent manner. In the event that an institution decides that it can no longer support continuing education efforts, it should provide advance notice to individual practitioners to allow them to develop contingency plans to meet their mandatory and professional requirements.

As the scope of critical care nursing increases exponentially, so too does the concept of what constitutes critical care nursing. The presence of critical care nurses as members of transport teams is not questioned. Some institutions have developed transport teams composed solely of nurses. For these teams, a cautionary note must be sounded to alert nurses that they must examine the nurse practice acts of their respective states to ensure that their actions cannot be construed as the practice of medicine. Institutionally sanctioned actions, such as the insertion of central lines by nurses, may, nonetheless, violate state law. For nurses who practice in tertiary care facilities, it is a natural progression for skilled nurses to assume responsibility for more complex technical skills as technologic advances enable medicine to venture beyond the frontiers of what was considered inconceivable. But in those institutions where primary care has ascendancy, tension will inevitably arise between nurses who are technologically proficient and physicians who adhere to more traditional concepts of the divisions between nursing and medicine. Problems will also arise for nurse transport teams when codes occur en route to the tertiary care facility. In Massachusetts, with the exception of some statutorily created exclusions, only physicians can pronounce a patient dead. Thus, should a nurse transport team be unable to revive a patient, that team would be required to continue CPR until a physician is available to pronounce the patient dead (see M.G.L. c. 45 § 9).

For nurse transport teams that travel to adjoining states, a recurrent issue will be the scope of what is permissible practice if the individual nurse is not licensed to practice within that state. Physicians, to some extent, have managed to avoid this quagmire by defining the nonlicensed transport physician as a consultant, a role that is specifically recognized statutorily. (See laws and statutes of the 6 New England states.) Such protection is not extended to the purely nurse transport team. Any institution that contemplates a transport team composed solely of nurses must do so with caution and assess the legality of such a development, for the laws of few states, if any, are supportive of this advance given the historical perspective of the profession. Many states have enacted regulations to guide advanced practice nurses. (In Massachusetts, see 244 CMR § 4.00 et seq.) Under this requirement, the scope of practice is clearly defined along with the need for the development of collaborative guidelines and physician supervision. The needs of transport nurses are much more fluid, however, and the advanced practice regulations do not support the flexibility necessary for nurse transport teams to operate autonomously. Flexibility is essential to cover all possible situations that can develop during the transport of critically ill patients, and any future statutory and regulatory developments must recognize these needs if the intent is to utilize nurses in expanded healthcare roles.

CONCLUSION

As nursing stands at the dawn of a new century, the decisions it makes, and the steps it takes, in the development of the profession will determine the role it plays in the provision of healthcare needs in the future. Anticipating legal consequences before they occur will prevent the interdisciplinary battles. For nursing, the future has never been brighter. For legal unsophisticates, however, the path is fraught with pitfalls.

GLOSSARY OF LEGAL TERMS

Abandonment: Unilateral termination of a nursing:patient relationship, by the nurse, without adequate arrangements for follow-up care.

Agency: Relationship between persons in which one party authorizes the other to act on his behalf.

Allegation: Statement of a party in a pleading setting forth the facts that he expects to prove.

Appeal: The process by which a decision of a lower court is brought for review before a court of higher jurisdiction. The party seeking the appeal is the appellant, and the party opposing the appeal is the appellee.

Assault: An intentional act that places one in apprehension of immediate bodily harm.

Battery: Any intentional and unauthorized touching of a person.

Causation: A nexus between the act or omission of the defendant and the injury suffered by the plaintiff.

Cause of Action: Set of facts that give rise to a legal right at law.

Civil action: A suit that involves a trial either at law or equity that is not criminal in nature.

Common Law: Rules and principles derived from usage and customs that are based on Anglo-Saxon law and developed from court decisions based on such law. It is distinguished from statutes enacted by legislatures and all other types of law.

Consent: Agreement by one person to allow another person to do something. "Express consent" is an agreement that is given, either orally or in writing. "Implied consent" is that consent which is derived from signs, actions, or facts that give rise to a presumption that the consent has been given.

Damages: The amount awarded to a plaintiff to compensate him for his losses in a civil trial. "Compensatory" damages are to compensate the injured party for the injury sustained and nothing more. "Special" damages are the actual out-of-pocket losses incurred by the plaintiff, such as medical expenses, and are part of the compensatory damages. "Nominal" damages are a trifling sum awarded to plaintiffs in a civil action where there is no substantial injury. "Punitive" damages are awarded to punish a defendant who has acted wantonly or in reckless disregard of the plaintiff's rights. Massachusetts does not allow "punitive damages" except in wrongful death actions.

Defendant: The person against whom a civil or criminal action is brought.

Expert Witness: Person qualified to offer an opinion by reason of his special training, skill, or familiarity with the subject, that is beyond the average person's knowledge.

Guardian: Person appointed by a court to manage the affairs and to protect the interests of another who is adjudicated incompetent to do so whether because of age or physical or mental infirmity.

Incompetency: Lack of ability, legal qualifications, or fitness to manage his or her own affairs because of mental or physical infirmities.

Independent Contractor: Person who contracts to work for another for which the person is not expected to be under the direct supervision or control of the hiring party.

Informed Consent: Patient's voluntary agreement to accept treatment based upon the patient's awareness of the nature of his or her disease, the material risks and benefits of the proposed treatment, the alternative treatments and risks, or the choice of no treatment at all.

Injunction: An equitable remedy issued by the court commanding a person or entity to perform or refrain from performing a certain act.

Malfeasance: Committing an act that is wrong or improper. Any wrongful conduct that affects, interrupts, or interferes with the performance of official duties.

Malice: The intentional doing of a wrongful act without just cause or excuse, with an intent to inflict an injury, or under such circumstances that the law will imply an evil intent.

Malpractice: Failure to meet a professional standard of care resulting in harm to another.

Negligence: The failure to act as a reasonable person would under the same or similar circumstances that causes harm to another.

Nonfeasance: The failure to perform a required act.

Pain and Suffering: An element of damages that allows recovery for the mental anguish and/or physical pain endured by the plaintiff as a result of injury caused by the defendant.

Perjury: Lying under oath.

Plaintiff: Party who brings a civil lawsuit that seeks relief or compensation for damages.

Prima Facie Case: A complaint that apparently contains all the necessary legal elements for a recognized cause of action that will suffice unless disproven by some evidence to the contrary.

Prima Facie Evidence: Evidence that is sufficient to establish a fact and, if not rebutted, becomes conclusive of the fact.

Probate Court: Court having juridiction of the estates of deceased persons and persons under guardianship.

Proximate Causation: Essential element in a legal cause of action for negligence. The dominant and responsible cause, the one that necessarily sets other causes in operation that is not interrupted by some intervening cause.

Respondeat Superior: A doctrine in which the employer (master) is responsible for the legal consequences associated with the lack of due care on the part of his employee (servant) toward those to whom the employer owes a duty to use care provided the breach of duty occurs within the scope of employment.

Statute of Limitations: Statutes that limit the time period in which an action can be filed once knowledge of the harm becomes known.

Subpoena: A process that requires a person to appear to give testimony for a party.

Summons: Notice to the defendant that an action has been instituted against him and that he is required to answer it at a time and place named.

Tortfeasor: A wrongdoer. One who commits or is guilty of a tort.

Torts: Civil wrong in which there has been some violation of a duty to the plaintiff.

Vicarious Liability: Secondary liability in which the liability is imputed to an individual or entity who has control over the actual tortfeasor.

Witness: One who testifies about what he has seen, heard, or otherwise observed.

Adapted from Black's Law Dictionary, 6th ed., St. Paul, Minn., West Publishing, 1990.

Legal Citations

Accts. Adj. Bureau v. Cooperman, 204 Cal Rptr 881 (Cal. App. 1984)

American Jurisprudence, Vol. 42, Infants, 2nd ed. Lawyers Cooperative Publishing Co., San Francisco, Calif. (1969)

American Law Institute Restatement of Agency 2d, West Publishing Co., St. Paul, Minn. (1958)

American Law Institute Second Restatement of Torts, West Publishing Co., St. Paul, Minn. (1965)

American Nurses Association, Standards of Clinical Practice, Standard VI, Collaboration, Kansas City, Mo., 1, 16 (1991)

Anderson v. Minneapolis St. Paul & SSMR Co., 146 Minn. 430 (1920)

Becker v. Schwartz, 386 NE2d 807, 46 NY2d 401 (1978)

Braemer v. Dotson, No. 21661 W. Va. Sup. Ct. of App. (Dec. 23, 1993)

Caldwell v. Bechtel Inc., 203 App DC 407, 631 F2d 909 (1986)

Canterbury v. Spence, 464 F2d 772 (D.C. Cir. 1972), cert. den. 409 U.S. 1064 (1972)

Commonwealth v. Southier, 31 Mass. App. Ct. 219 (1991)
Commonwealth v. Porn, 196 Mass 326 (1907)
Cruzan v. Director, Missouri Dept. of Health, 497 U.S. 261 (1990)
Custody of a Minor, 375 Mass. 733 (1978)
Czubinsky v. Doctor's Hospital, 188 Cal Rptr 685 (Cal. App. 1981)
Dziokonski v. Babineau, 375 Mass 555 (1976)
Elbert v. Saginaw, 363 Mich 464, 109 NW2d 879, 1961
FDA Drug Bulletin, April 1982
Gaudette v. Webb, 362 Mass. 60 (1972)
Griswold v. Conn, 381 U.S. 479 (1965)
Harding v. Philadelphia Rapid Transit Co., 66 A. 151 (1907)
Harnish v. Children's Hospital Medical Center et al., 387 Mass. 152 (1982)
In the Matter of Elisha McCauley, 409 Mass. App. Ct. 134 (1991)
Jacobson v. Mass., 197 U.S. 11 (1903)
Kohoutek v. Hafner, 38 SW2d 295 (1986)
Lane v. Candura, 6 Mass. App. Ct. 377, 383 (1978)
Leach & Liacos, Evidence, Little, Brown Publishing Co., Boston, MA (1984)
M.G.L. c. 119 §51A
M.G.L. c. 112 §80B
M.G.L. c. 119 §51B
M.G.L. c. 112 §80E
M.G.L. c. 229 §2
M.G.L. c. 11 §70E
M.G.L. c. 46 § 9
M.G.L. c. 231 §60B
M.G.L. c. 260 § 10
M.G.L. c. 205 § 12
Manacare Corp. v. First State Inc. Corp, 374 SO2d 1100 (1979)
Marbury v. Madison, 1 Cranch 137 (1803)
McColloch v. Maryland, 4 Wheat 316 (1819)
National Union Fire Insurance Co. of Pittsburgh v. Medical Liability Mutual Ins. Co., 446 N.Y.S.2d 480 (1981)
Nelson v. Patrick, 326 SE2d 45 (N.C. App. 1985)
Norwood Hospital v. Yolanda Munoz & another, 409 Mass. 116 (1991)
Planned Parenthood v. Casey, 505 US—, 112SCT 2791, 120LED 2nd 674 (1992)
Plessy v. Ferguson, 163 U.S. 537 (1896)
Prince v. Mass., 321 U.S. 158 (1944)
Prosser, William L., Law of Torts 4th ed., West Publishing Co., St. Paul, Minn. (1971)
Railroad Company v. Husen, 95 U.S. 465 (1977)
Randolph's Adm'r v. Snyder, 129 S.W. 562 (1910)
Roe v. Wade, 410 U.S. 113 (1973)
Rose v. Hakim, 335 F. Supp. 1221 (1971)
Schloendork v. Society of N.Y. Hosp., 105 NE2d 92 (1914)
Superintendent of Belchertown State School v. Saikewicz, 373 Mass. 728 (1977)
The T.J. Hooper, 60 F2d 737 (1932), cert. den. 287 U.S. 662
Thompson v. Ohio Fuel Gas Co., 9 Ohio St. 2d 116, on remand 11 Ohio App2d (1967)
Union PR Co. v. McDonald, 152 U.S. 262 (1894)
Vanstreenburg v. Lawrence Memorial Hospital, 481 A2d 750 (1984)
Walker v. Bignell, 100 Wis 2d, 256, 301 NW2d 447 (1981)
Wilkinson v. Vesey, 110 R.I. 606, 627 (1972)

References

Florida Nurses Association. *Guidelines for the registered nurse in giving, accepting, or rejecting a work assignment.* Orlando: Florida Nurses Association, May 1989.
Joint Commission on the Accreditation of Hospitals, Standards, Chicago, Ill. (1991).
Rouse, F. (1991). Patients, providers, & the PSDA in practicing the PSDA. *21 Hastings Center Report* 5, Supp. 2.
Rushton, C. H., & Lynch, M. E. (1992). Dealing with advanced directives for critically ill adolescents. *Critical Care Nurse,* 12 (5), 31–37.
Uustal, D. (1991). Ethical issues in caring for patients who have suffered water related injuries. *Nursing Clinics of North America,* 3 (2), 361–371.

CHAPTER *7*

In the Best Interest of the Child: Ethical Issues

JUNE LEVINE ARIFF
DONNA H. GROH

BIOETHICAL DILEMMAS
What Is Morally Right to Do
Ethical Principles for Decision-making
Who Decides
Informed Consent
To What Extent Can Minors Decide Treatment?

STRATEGIES TO CREATE AN ETHICAL ENVIRONMENT
For Patients and Families
For Caregivers
A MODEL FOR ETHICAL DECISION-MAKING
Use of the Model
Steps of the Model

Being a very ill child or the parent of a very ill child must test the outermost limits of human tolerance; . . . being involved in the care of very ill children must be one of the most demanding responsibilities in the world, the failures more awful, the triumphs more rewarding than in almost any other kind of job. The stakes are so high: whole lifetimes.

PEGGY ANDERSON (1985)

Nurses working in pediatric critical care may experience frustration and anguish as they watch children struggle against formidable odds and observe parents grapple with some of the most difficult decisions a family can ever confront. Nurses watch children bear the consequences of disease, injury, and technology. A perceived inability, by the nurse, to minimize or eliminate tragic outcomes brings on feelings of powerlessness and helplessness. The demands of the critical care unit are hectic and at times unrelenting. Tasks are accomplished under high personal and professional tension. Ethical dilemmas grow as some children's lives end before potential is reached and other children's lives hang on too long.

Andrew Jameton (1984) sorts the moral problems

nurses face in the hospital environment into three different categories:

- Moral uncertainty—when one is unsure of which principles or values apply, or even what the moral problem is.
- Moral dilemmas—when two or more clear moral principles apply, but they support mutually inconsistent courses of action.
- Moral distress—when one knows the right thing to do but is prevented by institutional constraints from pursuing the right course of action.

The problems are similar in that psychological suffering results, but they are different as to the cause of that suffering. Moral uncertainty and moral dilemmas produce discomfort because of the nurse's inability to decide what is right. Moral distress, on the other hand, produces negative feelings because of the nurses' inability to maneuver through the environment, to do what they believe is the right thing toward an outcome.

Most healthcare professionals encounter moral uncertainty and moral dilemmas. The nurse, because of often conflicting loyalties (to the patient, family,

126

physician, institution, profession, and colleagues) may also experience moral distress.

The ethical issues that occur in a pediatric critical care unit raise questions concerning the rights of children to make their own treatment decisions, the status of parental rights, the obligations of nurses and other healthcare professionals to prevent and relieve suffering, and society's beliefs about how people should live and how they should die. It is within this complex environment that nurses experience moral uncertainty, moral dilemmas, and moral distress.

This chapter describes the specific moral issues that arise in the care of sick children. The principles of beneficence, nonmaleficence, autonomy, and veracity will be discussed from both the child's and parent's perspective. Coupling these principles with a model for decision making should provide the nurse with practical assistance to sort through the ethical dilemmas typically present in the pediatric critical care unit.

BIOETHICAL DILEMMAS

Traditionally, hospitals have been seen as places where patients were provided all of the treatment options available to them. The development of the intensive care unit (ICU) provided an environment where advances in science and technology can be implemented. Technologic achievements removed life and death decisions from the privacy of the home and exposed them to public scrutiny. Unanticipated dilemmas resulted as powerful diagnostic techniques, sophisticated surgical procedures, effective drugs, and expedient therapeutic interventions interrupted the usual course of illness and disability. Problems became magnified because life could be sustained for a significant period if the patient accepted dependence on a specific procedure or machine.

Medical technology is usually beneficial in the care of sick or injured persons, sometimes dramatically so. However, since it is often intrusive, occasionally cruel, sometimes of little value, and almost always expensive, its use must be assessed critically, particularly in ICUs.

DUFF (1979, p. 17)

The uncertainties and ambiguities that result from disease, injury, and the use of technology often force healthcare professionals to demand cure, in the absence of otherwise compelling evidence to choose a different course. The inevitable conflicts that arise produce questions such as these: Can treatment be stopped once initiated? Who gives consent for medical treatment? Can patients be forced to go along with a recommended treatment plan? Do all patients have to be resuscitated? Who judges the quality of someone's life? When is a patient considered dead? The indecision that occurs reflects a growing uneasi-

ness with the consequences of scientific advances, especially when death is not imminent but the quality of life is greatly impaired. In pediatric critical care, the problems are complicated further by the child's developmental stage, chronological age, and family situation.

It is helpful, however, to remember that bioethical issues are not new. They have always been a part of clinical practice. Ethical considerations lie on or just below the surface of many clinical activities, yet are rarely noticed. It is only when decisions feel uncomfortable or when alternatives seem equally unsatisfactory that the finer issues of moral decision-making are considered.

Consider these two examples: A mother brings her 5-year-old child into the emergency room of a local hospital. The child remained disoriented and extremely lethargic after falling off of a bicycle. The physician orders a computed axial tomography (CAT) scan and draws blood for a complete blood count (CBC) and electrolytes. The nurse offers comfort to the child and the mother as intravenous (IV) infusions are started and tests are explained. A diagnosis of concussion is made. The physician wants the child observed overnight in the pediatric critical care unit. The mother believes that her child is being helped and willingly accompanies her to the critical care unit. Because there was no disagreement over what was to be done or who was to decide, the moral content remained hidden.

In another case, a 10-year-old boy with diseased kidneys has had dialysis since age 3 years. After two transplants the child is back on dialysis, both prior organs having been rejected. Dialysis is taking its toll; the child's bones are demineralized and beginning to fracture under modest stress. The physician does not believe that the child can have a reasonable length or quality of life on dialysis. The physician does not necessarily believe another transplant is the correct course of action. The child's parents care very much about their child and have been conscientious about medical follow-up and care at home but have not yet grasped the seriousness of their son's present circumstances.

Even though both cases present apparently dissimilar situations, they both raise two consistent questions:

1. What is the morally right thing to do?
2. Who should decide?

The differences in the cases lie in whether both or either question is of concern to the patient and family or the healthcare providers. Moral questions are present in both cases. However, the first case did not raise the issues to the surface, thus no moral dilemma occurred.

In the latter case, treatment decisions are less clear because the probable outcomes for the child are less certain. In addition, there may be disagreement between the parents and the physician over which course of medical treatment or nontreatment should be followed. Thus, who decides what treatments the child will receive may become a question of concern.

What Is Morally Right to Do

Most people have a sense of what is right and what is wrong. These values are developed while growing up within a society that teaches specific social rules, expectations, and prohibitions. "Morality tells us not to harm others, not to kill, to be good persons, to keep promises, and to tell the truth" (Fowler, 1985, p. 24). Morality provides us with general rules of conduct; it tells us whether the consequences of actions are good or bad. Thus, people form opinions about how one ought to act and what one ought to believe in certain situations.

Ethics, however, refers to the systematic study of principles and values. It is a discipline that looks at the way people act and asks whether their actions are good or harmful. The study of ethics goes beyond what is and asks what ought to be. In asking these questions, ethical inquiry helps form and change moral conduct.

Ethical Principles for Decision-making

Ethical inquiry in healthcare situations is guided by a number of principles. These are considered in the following sections.

Beneficence and Nonmaleficence

Nurses have a desire to do good and do no harm to the patients they care for. In fact, as healthcare providers, nurses have a duty to comply with the bioethical principles of beneficence and nonmaleficence. Looking at these two principles together, they state that:

1. One ought to do or promote good
2. One should prevent harm
3. One should remove harmful conditions
4. One should not inflict harm (Beauchamp & Childress, 1989).

The first three statements apply directly to beneficence and the last to nonmaleficence. Beneficence, being a more active principle, requires that the nurse promote good, remove harmful conditions, and prevent harm. On the other hand, nonmaleficence merely requires the nurse to do no harm. The Code for Nurses of the American Nurses Association (ANA) stresses the alleviation of suffering as a nursing duty, over saving life. The ANA Code for Nurses states: "Nursing encompasses the promotion and restoration of health, the prevention of illness and the alleviation of suffering" (American Nurses Association, 1976).

When promoting good such as health, relief from pain and suffering, and the prevention of illness,

nurses may seek answers to these difficult questions: How do you know what is good in a specific situation? Can circumstances alter the perception of what is good? When does doing good become harm? Who decides what is good? Is one doing good when one continues to treat a critically ill child for whom there is no hope? Is one doing good when a child in a persistent vegetative state continues to receive antibiotics, food, and fluids? Is one doing good when a 15-year-old child is forced to continue chemotherapy against her wishes?

Benefits and Burdens

Historically, to do good and not do harm, healthcare professionals did not consider a patient's or family's wishes, beliefs, and values. Wanting to protect patients from their own lack of knowledge and subsequent bad judgment, healthcare professionals did not involve patients or families in healthcare decisions. The norm that functioned promoted the belief that healthcare professionals knew what was best for patients. Patients were not to know too much about their diagnosis or prognosis and were not to interfere with treatment plans. This paternalistic attitude was often justified on the basis of doing no harm. Duff (1979) called this "ethical elitism" and noted that when paternalism thrives, the dictum of do no harm may be violated. Caring for others requires consideration of *their* values and contributions (Mayeroff, 1971). Healthcare professionals who believe that they know best foster family dependency and increase feelings of loss of control. Healthcare professionals must remember that to accept or reject recommended medical treatment is a moral decision and is not the healthcare professional's responsibility.

In caring for critically ill children there are always potential harms, even when the outcome promotes good. Pain and discomfort are the usual burdens one associates with illness. However, for children in particular, other burdens such as fear, immobilization, isolation from family and friends, and various individual physiologic and emotional side effects must be considered. Nurses are obligated to prevent or minimize such burdens. Ensuring that adequate pain medication is administered, giving antiemetics on a timely basis, explaining what is going to happen next, facilitating broad visiting guidelines, and assuring that a favorite toy is present all promote good and prevent harm. Benefits such as cure, correction, or relief from pain and suffering must be weighed against burdens, such as prolongation of pain, quality of life, and ability to participate in society, which are identified by the individual child and the family.

When decisions must be made for adults who lack decision-making capacity, a surrogate decision-maker, usually a family member, tries to make decisions from the perspective of what the adult would want if still able to make a decision. In other words, the surrogate decision-maker attempts to determine the preferences the person would state, if able, about having or not having certain treatments. A number of methods can be used to determine preferences. Adults may have told their surrogates exactly how they wish to be treated if certain health problems occur. The adult patient may have signed a durable power of attorney for healthcare or completed a living will (depending on state legislation) that indicates preferences in writing. Finally, the surrogate may know that adult well by knowing how the adult lived life, what that person valued and how that person reacted to similar situations.

In the case of minors, the benefits and burdens are not so easily weighed. "Decision-making for children is more complex since children generally lack the capacity to make independent decisions, and they have not expressed life goals and values upon which such decisions would be based" (Rushton & Glover, 1990, p. 206). The healthcare professional, the parents, and the child may not all agree on whether the outcomes of treatment or nontreatment are beneficial or burdensome. Clearly, choices among alternative treatment options ought to benefit the child and outweigh the associated burdens.

To help distinguish whether the outcome of a treatment is beneficial or burdensome, questions such as these might be asked:

What is the degree of intrusiveness, risk, and discomfort of treatment?
Will the intervention minimize or relieve pain?
Will the treatment prolong an inevitable death?
Can the patient's prognosis be improved?
What is the individual's capacity to experience and enjoy life?
What are the possibilities of a return to a cognitively and physically functioning life? (Levine-Ariff & Groh, 1990, p. 34).

These questions suggest that pain and suffering are not the only burdens that can befall a person.

Best Interest

A "best interest" standard recognizes the possibility that medically indicated treatment may result in a profoundly burdensome life for the child. The "best interest" standard recognizes that death may not be the "greatest evil to befall a person" (Arras, 1984, p. 27). Thus, it presumes that prolongation of life may not always be in the child's best interest. Focusing on what is best for the child avoids morally dubious justification based on the interests of other involved parties such as the parents, siblings, healthcare professionals, or the institution.

One of the most difficult clinical situations for determining the child's best interests occurs when there is medical uncertainty—when the precise diagnosis and/or prognosis is unclear. As a consequence, it is more difficult to understand the precise benefits or burdens that will result from treatment or nontreatment. Sometimes additional tests or consultations minimize this uncertainty. In other cases, only the passage of time makes clear the likely extent of re-

covery. It is important that parents be helped to understand the uncertainties of disease, injury, and treatment so that they can make a decision truly in the best interest of their child. Determining the benefits and burdens of treatments, as well as deciding which interventions are in the best interest of the patient, aids the nurse in determining the morally right thing to do in a given situation.

Who Decides

In the United States there is presumption of parental moral and legal authority in matters of concern for their minor children. This is based on a belief that parents generally have a sincere concern to protect their child's life. Parents are in the best position to know their child's wants and desires. They have a tendency to place their child's interests ahead of their own. As a result of a long-term specific relationship with their child, parents have a commitment to ongoing care. Thus, parents should have responsibility for their children's healthcare decisions. After all, they bear the financial, emotional, and medical consequences for those decisions. Long after well-meaning healthcare professionals have gone home "the family will be remembering and incorporating this momentous decision into the fabric of their lives" (Rushton & Glover, 1990, p. 208). In practice, the issue of who decides is not usually raised to the surface. Only when disagreement arises over what measures will serve the child best does the question of who decides become a thorny one.

For example, during the past two decades, the question of parents' rights to make medical decisions for their children has gained national attention. It began in 1975 with the case of Karen Ann Quinlan (In re Quinlan, 1976), whose parents had to go to the New Jersey Supreme Court to be allowed to remove their comatose daughter from the ventilator. The Baby Doe cases in 1982 prompted an attempt by the federal government to take decision-making power away from parents who refused any medical intervention for seriously handicapped newborns (Child Abuse Amendments, 1984). Then, in 1989, a father in a Chicago pediatric intensive care unit held hospital staff at bay with a shotgun while he unplugged the respirator from his son, who was diagnosed to be in a persistently vegetative state (Lantos, et al., 1989).

Limits to Parental Authority

The social policy of the United States gives a great deal of discretion to parents and permits supplanting their authority only when the child's interests are clearly and severely threatened by parental action. Children exist and develop within the context of their family. As long as parents do not neglect those people under their care, society should not intervene. However, society has a responsibility to intervene when parents refuse to give care to children that would clearly benefit them or when parents subject children to clear harm. For example, parental rights do not include the right to abandon or endanger a child. However, when parents insist on undertreatment or overtreatment in situations in which the healthcare team is in disagreement, the responsibility for decision-making is less certain.

There is no easily applied standard for determining when family decisions are appropriate. Such decisions should be based on the benefits and burdens the child may encounter. However, as Arras (1984) has noted, that standard begs the question of who shall determine what is in a child's best interest. Thus, it becomes more important to view the parents' decision in light of the child's diagnosis, expected outcome with and without treatment, degree of uncertainty about the outcome, quality of the child's life, probability of benefits from treatment and presumed burdens if treatment occurs or does not occur. Unless a child is in imminent danger of dying, the healthcare team has a duty to both the child and family to take the time and effort necessary to reach consensus on treatment decisions.

Physicians should use their knowledge of the child's healthcare status to attempt to resolve disagreement with the family rather than supplant the family's decision-making authority. The physician must be certain that to withhold a specific treatment or a specific procedure would result in serious harm that would threaten the child's life. The process of informing parents often causes pain and anguish for them. Yet, to avoid giving parents all the information available about their child's diagnosis and prognosis does not show respect for their right to make informed healthcare decisions and provide their child with needed support. Informed consent demands being given the information and then being allowed to make a choice.

The Courts

Although there is wide latitude given to families to practice various religions and lifestyles, courts have intervened to protect children and have not permitted refusal of standard medical treatment in life-threatening situations, for example, by Jehovah's Witness and Christian Scientist parents. The courts justify this interference by invoking the "parens patriae" doctrine; that is, the state's legitimate interest in the welfare of children and its right and duty to protect vulnerable people from harm. The "parens patriae" doctrine is often used in legislation and authorizes the state to intervene when parents fail to provide necessary medical care (Larsen, 1954).

Ultimately, a court must decide when parents will be disqualified as decision-makers and another person designated to act in their stead. It is incumbent upon the healthcare team to show the court convincing evidence of why the parents should be removed as the child's decision-maker. It has been argued that when parents appear unable to make decisions in the best interest of their child, a healthcare professional,

usually the physician, ought to make the healthcare decisions. However, healthcare professionals are not necessarily unbiased participants. Personal feelings of defeat and helplessness become interwoven with their own individual beliefs about life and death. Conflicts among the various agendas of research, education, and treatment may slant their perspective.

A court may appoint a surrogate decision-maker, who can be another family member or a person who is not a member of the healthcare team. The surrogate decision-maker should have knowledge of the facts of the child's case and should be free of serious conflicts of interest. It is important that the healthcare team understand the circumstances under which the surrogate was appointed, which decisions the surrogate can make, and what other judicial action may be occurring.

If the state removed itself completely from such situations, the consequences could be devastating for many children. Yet, because of a primary belief that parents want to and do act in their child's best interest, the healthcare team should guard against reaching premature conclusions about parental intentions.

Informed Consent

The legal and ethical standard for informed consent comes from the ethical principle of autonomy. Autonomy refers to individual self-determination and freedom of choice. "It requires that we respect the rights of others to make autonomous decisions. To violate a person's autonomy is to treat that person merely as a means to an end that is in accordance with one's own beliefs and values" (Levine-Ariff & Groh, 1990, p. 29).

Informed consent is also the legal standard by which permission is sought for medical treatment of an individual. The only acceptable legal exception to this law is that in which the need for medical treatment constitutes an emergency; that is, when the patient would suffer irreversible harm if not treated. Thus, when consent cannot be obtained because the patient is not competent and a surrogate decision-maker is not immediately available, the treatment can proceed. However, in all other instances, the patient or the patient's surrogate must consent to or may refuse treatment.

Consent by Minors

In caring for children, special ethical issues arise because children are not consenting adults. Competent adults have the right to refuse life-sustaining treatment for themselves, and their decisions must be respected. Adults are generally permitted to make autonomous decisions (i.e., to consent to or refuse treatment based on their own wishes and interests). The Patient Self Determination Act (PSDA) (Table 7–1) currently only supports the right of adults to accept or refuse medical treatment (Omnibus Reconciliation Act, 1990). This limitation is based on the

Table 7–1. KEY POINTS OF THE PATIENT SELF DETERMINATION ACT (PSDA) OF 1990

As part of the Omnibus Reconciliation Act of 1990, Congress enacted the Patient Self Determination Act, which became effective December 1, 1991. The major thrust of the Act supports the right of adults to make their own decisions regarding medical care including the right to accept or refuse all medical interventions. The legislation charges all health care institutions that receive Medicare and Medicaid funding with the following requirements:

1. Patients are to be provided at the time of admission to a health care facility written information concerning their rights under state law to make decisions regarding medical interventions, including the right to withhold or withdraw treatment.
2. Patients are to be provided with written information specifying the health care institutions' policies regarding the implementation of these rights.
3. It must be documented in the patient's medical record whether or not they have executed an advance directive.*
4. Health care providers are not to discriminate against an individual based on whether he or she has executed an advance directive. Care is to be given to patients whether or not they have executed an advance directive.
5. Education is to be provided to staff and the community about issues concerning advance directives.
6. Health care providers are to ensure compliance with state law with respect to advance directives.

*Advance Directive: A written document in which an adult specifies their wishes for medical treatment should they become unable to make their own decisions. State law should be consulted as to the type of advance directive(s) recognized and the conditions under which it can be executed.

Congressional Record. Title IV, Section 4206, October 26, 1990.

premise that only adults have the capacity to determine what should be done to their bodies. Minors, of all ages, generally do not have the legal autonomy afforded adults and, as a consequence, the law assumes they do not have the capacity to give consent. Decisions are made for them based on others' perceptions of what is right and good. Young children do not have the cognitive ability to provide informed consent or refusal. Thus, parents or legal guardians are usually responsible for treatment decisions for their children. As a child nears adolescence, parents' rights to make healthcare decisions may be limited by both the increase in the minor's cognitive ability and precepts of law.

The concept of the "mature minor" has received increasing judicial approval. A mature minor statute recognizes that a young person (14 or 15 years of age or older) can understand the nature and consequences of certain proposed treatments. The treatment must not involve very serious risks and the physician must believe that the minor could give the same degree of informed consent as an adult (Holder, 1985). Treatment for venereal disease, drug and alcohol abuse, pregnancy, and communicable diseases may fall into this area. In fact, California state law recommends that it may be appropriate to seek legal advice if a minor aged 14 or older objects when parental consent is given for a procedure that involves a significant risk of severe adverse consequences (California Hospital Association, 1990).

Specific state statutory provisions "emancipate" minors for the purpose of making their own healthcare decisions. Generally, an emancipated minor is someone younger than 18 years of age who is not living at home and/or is self-supporting, married, in the military, or an unmarried mother. An emancipated minor statute reflects the judgment of a particular state that, when certain conditions are met, these minors are capable of consenting to their own healthcare. In particular, provisions that grant adult status to minor parents consenting to treatment for

their own child have significant implications in the care and treatment of children.

State laws may need to be clarified in situations such as when a minor is in the custody of juvenile court or foster parents and when minors are suspected victims of child abuse. Legally, some minors have been given the authority to give consent for medical treatment in specific situations. Although the PSDA involves only adults making decisions for themselves, the spirit of the law reinforces the involvement of minors, especially adolescents, in their own treatment decisions and encourages the creation of an atmosphere in which children, with their parents, can make informed decisions (Rushton & Lynch, 1992).

Assuring Informedness

Although full informed consent has been said to be a theoretical ideal, reality must come as close as is possible to that ideal for parents to make decisions in the best interests of their child. Informed decisions are made with full knowledge of that which needs to be done and why. An atmosphere of open discussion must exist, free from fear of reprisal. Informing patients and their families is a dialogue, not a lecture, wherein the provision of information helps to clarify understanding.

To make a decision about medical treatment requires that the same information to be provided to either an adult or a child. The physician must provide all the information necessary for the patient or their surrogate to make a reasoned, free choice about treatment. The risks of doing or not doing a procedure must be explained, as well as any alternative choices that are available. The information given should focus on the child and what life will be like with and without treatment. Parents should be asked questions about their goals and desires for the child; their values regarding disease, disability, and death; and their desire to be involved in healthcare decision-making. It is within this fuller context of communication that informedness can be assured.

Information must be conveyed in a quiet atmosphere in which optimal communication can occur. The critical care unit can be a frightening place for parents and children alike. Constant artificial light, ceaseless activity, frequent emergencies, and the ever-present threat of death unnerves the sturdiest of families. Information should be provided in the language of the decision-maker, minimizing the use of medical terminology. For example, "unconsciousness," "mental retardation," and "life-support" are words that must be explained. Parents must be helped to understand that what they see as movement, for example, is actually involuntary motion indicating the child's level of neurologic damage. Whether a child has an 80 percent chance of survival or a 20 percent chance of dying has little meaning for many parents. Healthcare professionals must explain these serious discussion points in clear language and avoid using them to sway the parents' decision. Written materials should be offered to further clarify the circumstances whenever possible.

Obviously, no single information session assures informedness, especially when decisions about life and death are involved. Thus, frequent meetings may be necessary. The nurse plays a vital role in assuring informedness by arranging to have medical specialists, nurses, and social work professionals available for on-going discussion with the patient and family.

Finally, the physician should provide a recommendation for care. The recommendation should be stated in light of the benefits and burdens anticipated for the individual patient. The physician who does not explain the proposed treatment plan fully enough risks having the parents acquiesce to authority and later raise questions of concern or refuse treatment out of a lack of understanding.

Nurses assure informed consent through ongoing discussion of the situation with the child and family and by providing support, clarification, and understanding as decisions are reached. Nurses tend to view informed consent as a series of interactions. Davis (1989) defined the role of nurses in the process as including (1) monitoring informed consent, (2) advocating for patients to the physician, (3) providing patients with explanations and information about alternatives, (4) coordinating consent processes with families and patients, and (5) negotiating between involved parties when there are differences of opinions. Clearly, the involvement of nurses is critical as parents and their children grapple with serious issues.

To What Extent Can Minors Decide Treatment?

It used to be said that children should be seen and not heard. Historically, children were considered property, completely under the control of their parents. However, public and legal opinion have shifted away from viewing children as parental possessions and toward recognizing children as having individual interests and rights. Parents are now encouraged to develop their child's decision-making skills at an early age, beginning with choosing the foods they eat and clothes they wear, and advancing toward more weighty decisions such as providing ideas regarding their own healthcare decisions. Even when the child is not the ultimate decision-maker, being given some choices reinforces the senses of autonomy and self-control and indicates respect for the individual child.

Developing Children's Decision-making Capacity

The capacity to consent to medical treatment requires a person's ability to understand the treatment options and consequences, reason about them, and freely choose from various alternatives. Two factors that influence a child's level of participation in healthcare decisions are cognition and competence. As these develop, a child is able to take on increased responsibility for treatment decisions. Children do not suddenly develop decision-making capacity when they reach 18 years of age. Children's ability to recognize their own best interest and to choose or refuse treatment follows a developmental process like any other normal path of growth and development. This ability develops gradually throughout childhood, at a pace that varies from one child to another.

How then does one weigh the child's ability to choose or refuse treatment? The normal childhood developmental processes have been fully explored by Erikson (1963) and Piaget (1926). They describe milestones or points at which a child masters certain tasks or processes. Although most children pass through these milestones at a steady pace, some children advance, stop, or even fall back as environmental conditions, such as their home life, limits in mental intelligence, and illness, interfere with normal progress. In particular, chronic or terminal illness often influences a child's developmental progress. Capacity for healthcare decision-making is not an all or none concept. Capacity may be situational. For example, an individual child may be able to decide to discontinue chemotherapy but not have the capacity to decide to go home and die. Thus, each child must be viewed individually, taking into account developmental, as well as chronologic, age and the particular characteristics of the situation.

Before the age of 11 or 12, children believe illness is caused by something external to their bodies or something they ingest (Bibace & Walsh, 1980). Very young children who are sick are principally concerned with separation from their parents and the unpleasantness of the procedures that they must undergo. At about age 6 or 7 the child often believes that illness is retribution for bad thoughts or actions. By 12 years of age children develop the capacity to think abstractly. At this stage of development a child is able to consider multiple factors, hypothesize, and predict future consequences. The child is able to understand illness as a process caused by a malfunctioning of an internal organ system. The child is able to understand the long-term risks of chronic disease, instead of just focusing on whether the disease will interfere with their immediate routine. Cause and effect relationships become more understandable. By the time adolescents reach the age of 15, they are less likely to acquiesce to their parents' wishes. Thus, the ability to freely assent to treatment or nontreatment has developed.

The term "assent" recognizes a child's significant contribution to healthcare decision-making, when they are legally unable to give consent. Assenting to treatment means that the minor has agreed to proceed with a specific course of therapy or has decided to withhold certain therapies, with the approval of the parents. The process of obtaining assent confers respect for a child by encouraging involvement in care and increasing control at a time when dependency needs are strong because of illness.

Understanding a child's views of illness and the developing capacity to reason aids the nurse to initiate interventions for comfort, explain procedures appropriately, provide opportunities to participate in care, and ultimately assure an environment in which the child's developmental needs are integrated into daily activities.

Truthtelling: The Ethical Principle of Veracity

Whether to inform children about the seriousness of their illness and encourage their participation in treatment decisions is an issue with which both parents and healthcare professionals wrestle. The idea of having children actively participate in health-related decisions can be intimidating. Yet, when the child is able to reason and understand the consequences of actions, withholding information or lying is an act of paternalism and requires justification.

Parents and healthcare professionals who practice such deception do so because they believe that they are allaying fear and anxiety on the part of the child. "An overwhelming wish to protect the sick child from disturbing information, guilt feelings, or the emotional threat posed by the imminent death of their child may overshadow parental recognition or acceptance of the juveniles' autonomy or even his or her welfare" (Leiken, 1989, p. 18). There is no certainty, however, that being honest, even when the situation is a difficult one, will cause a significant negative reaction. Knowing the full extent of the illness is often less anxiety-provoking to the minor than receiving no or false information (Chester & Barbarin, 1987). Furthermore, withholding from children accurate and appropriate information denies them the opportunity to discuss their feelings and come to terms with what is happening to their body and mind. Family relationships may become strained at a time when both the child and the parents need each other. Talking and explaining helps children to see the reasons for medical treatment and under-

stand the various treatment or nontreatment alternatives. In fact, researchers have demonstrated that children older than 5 years of age with cancer have an understanding of the finality of death and should be openly provided information and be involved in treatment decisions (Nitschke, et al., 1982).

Trust is at the foundation of the ethical principle of veracity. Veracity teaches us that truthfulness is fundamental to establishing trust between individuals. Sick children depend upon the trusting relationship they have with their parents and their healthcare providers, especially at a time when dependency needs are at their highest. Withholding information or lying threatens the trusting relationship and, consequently, children's ability to rely on the adults on whom they depend. As with adults, children may not want to hear certain information and may want their parents to make decisions. Such requests should be respected. However, it is necessary for ongoing dialogue to occur so that the children are certain that any information they request will be provided truthfully.

Obviously, the developmental context in which a child's questions arise aids the nurse in ensuring that the child's best interests are met. Essentially, at all ages, children should have their questions answered in ways most helpful to them. The child's own thoughts, feelings, values, and wishes should be considered at all times. "To respect a child is to acknowledge the importance of his or her world and the relationships that are central to it" (Rushton & Glover, 1990, p. 207). To do otherwise is to minimize the emotional and social influences on any person's well-being.

STRATEGIES TO CREATE AN ETHICAL ENVIRONMENT

For Patients and Families

One of the best things any healthcare professional can do for families is to create an environment wherein parental decision-making is supported and parents are encouraged to be involved in their child's care. Making the family a partner in the healthcare team minimizes distrust and facilitates the child's care. Family partnership in the care of critically ill children is at the foundation of providing an environment that is ethical. Several strategies can be implemented to assure the creation of such an environment.

Minimize Environmental Stressors

Lack of understanding, coupled with unfamiliar sights, sounds, and people, may compromise a parent's ability to think clearly and make rational decisions. Added to the disorientation parents often experience in the PICU environment are fears about their child's welfare. Parents are confronted by strangers speaking in hushed tones, asking for decisions about often unheard-of medical problems. The critical care environment requires the healthcare professional's sensitivity to these factors. Such matters are common, everyday occurrences in the ICU but unique and unsettling for individual families. Orienting parents to the unit and the hospital helps them focus their energies on their child. Parents must be helped to know who people are, what their roles are, and how to get in touch with them when the need arises. Many critical care units and hospitals provide this information in written form. Yet, a written document should only be an adjunct to verbal explanation so questions can be asked and current information or clarification provided.

Enhance Communication

The critical care environment is a strained and unnatural arena in which to discuss personal concerns. The healthcare provider can help to diffuse the natural tensions that are present by ensuring a calm environment and allowing the time necessary for discussion of issues. Discussion may need to occur away from the bedside. Clinicians may need to reschedule a planned meeting if they are unprepared or adequate time cannot be allowed. Similarly, if parents are assessed to be in a state of severe emotional turmoil, information provided should be precise, clear, and brief. Plans should be made to meet with the parents again to discuss the situation further. At other times, however, it may be vital to communicate certain complex information immediately to parents. In these situations, especially, the clinician should periodically pause and ask the parents for feedback about what has been said and then take additional time, as needed, to ensure that the explanations are understood.

Information provided often must be repeated or clarified. For example, parents' refusal to consent to a certain treatment should be considered an opportunity to ask why consent is denied rather than make assumptions regarding their rationale, potentially pitting the healthcare team against the family. Parents should be encouraged to write down questions as they arise and assured that no question is too trivial to ask about their child.

Information must be provided in the parent's own language, using interpreters when necessary. The language of medicine can serve to render vital information inaccessible to parents. Healthcare professionals could have an entire conversation with laypersons in which few words and concepts are understood. Unfortunately, healthcare professionals who feel uncomfortable with discussion about these kinds of issues often use extensive technical explanations. Not only does this discourage questions but it may give the impression that the healthcare professional is in charge and controls the situation. If the goal is communication and not intimidation, the words used must be simple and clarification provided for any technical terms that must be conveyed. For example, mental retardation may have different

meanings for parents and healthcare professionals. Words and phrases like "vegetative state," "brain death," "resuscitation," "coding," and a "30 percent chance of surviving" must be explained. Asking parents if they want everything done for their child must include information on what everything includes. Parents are exposed to sometimes inaccurate usage of medical terms in the movies, on television, and in everyday life. It is important to ask them to explain terms that they use to ensure clear understanding.

Provide Continuity and Coordination of Care

Healthcare professionals can help children and their families anticipate issues about care and treatment and allow time for deliberation. Families often seek out anyone who will listen to them. Appointing a nurse and physician as the primary contacts for information facilitates continuity. Because a single person cannot be present 24 hours a day, the primary caregivers must communicate to the entire healthcare team the information they are sharing with the family. Medical record documentation, up-to-date care plans, and periodic team conferences help to avoid misconceptions and facilitate consistent and accurate communication. Because nurses have continuous contact with children and families in the ICU, sensitivity to the need for consistent caregivers can facilitate communication as continuity and coordination of care are enhanced.

Provide Emotional Support

The range of emotions parents of a critically ill child experience may be confusing to them. They may experience intense anger at themselves, their spouse, at God, the healthcare team, and even at their child. The events leading to the hospitalization may aggravate feelings of guilt or powerlessness. It is important for parents to be helped to sort through their intense emotions so that they can make reasoned decisions for their child. Obviously, for individual parents, the range of emotions experienced, their severity, and the timeframe over which adaptation occurs will vary. Parents can be assured that the peaks and the valleys of emotion they experience are normal. Support can often be obtained by talking with other parents who have a child with a similar diagnosis or is also in the critical care unit. The need for referral to a social worker, clergy, psychologist, or psychiatrist must be identified to support the family in crisis.

Focus on the Child

The constant demands of caring for a critically ill child can allow the child's interests to get buried under sophisticated medical procedures and technically demanding treatments. Uncertainty in diagnosis and/or prognosis may perpetuate burdensome evaluations and treatments. It is necessary to stop and ask whether what is being done will affect the course of the disease or whether a specific treatment or intervention is actually helping the child. The goals of treatment may change and need to be reviewed periodically. Is the goal curative, palliative, to provide comfort, or to ensure a peaceful death? Clarifying the goal of treatment may help the team resolve conflict and focus on the child.

Parental involvement in treatment decisions can be cut to a minimum in several ways. For example, not telling parents about the significance of various signs and symptoms, being overly optimistic in presenting data, and not informing parents of treatment options, including withholding or withdrawing life-sustaining treatment, minimizes their participation. The healthcare team must exercise caution as they communicate with families. Providing certain information in a positive light may give families false hope. For instance, the fact that a child's serum electrolyte values are normal may have little to do with the child's overall prognosis.

Finally, healthcare professionals must remember that whether a particular treatment should or should not be implemented is a function not only of the physiologic needs of the patient, but also of the beliefs, commitments, and values held by the patient and family. No amount of medical expertise permits others to make the decisions which are the family's. Effective decision-making requires that the entire healthcare team develop an understanding of the beliefs held by patients, parents, and team members. In an ethical environment, where patient and parental decision-making is valued and encouraged, healthcare professionals serve as advisors, share specific information, offer recommendations and, finally, act as advocates for children if a decision is made that is truly not in a child's best interest.

For Caregivers

Nurses are not required to participate in patient care they cannot accept for professional or ethical reasons. However, withdrawing from a patient's care is morally permissible only if qualified healthcare professionals can be substituted, and the withdrawal will not be perceived by the patient and family as abandonment during a time when the nurse's support and solace is needed (American Nurses Association, 1985). Pediatric critical care nurses are likely to encounter situations that produce moral uncertainty and distress. Strategies to minimize personal and professional distress and strengthen the ability of nurses to participate meaningfully in the resolution of ethical dilemmas are described in the next sections.

Ethics Education

Healthcare professionals who work in critical care units have been expected to be experts in the moral issues that surround life and death. Unfortunately, most have received little education in ethics. Many

professionals still practice with the belief that one's desire to do good is directly proportional to how much good is actually done. Thus, when called upon to buffer the powerful reality of disease and disability and to make sense out of alternative courses of action, healthcare professionals may not be successful.

Nurses can enhance their decision-making ability by taking advantage of educational opportunities that focus on ethical analysis and the specific moral issues faced by critical care nurses. Ethics education helps practitioners make moral choices based upon reason rather than intuition. Hospitals can provide a variety of educational opportunities for both nurses and physicians that enhance their knowledge of ethics and their collaboration. Grand rounds, unit-based rounds, and journal clubs are excellent additions to formal educational seminars.

Ethics Rounds

Ethics rounds are similar to other formal case discussions. However, in ethics rounds, the clinical aspects of the case become the backdrop for an organized discussion of the ethical dilemma and possible solutions. Ethics rounds can be multidisciplinary or confined to a homogeneous group, such as nurses in the pediatric critical care unit. To be helpful, these rounds must be regularly scheduled and conducted by a skilled leader with knowledge in bioethics. It is helpful if this individual is also a nurse or is a person experienced in working with nurses on resolving ethical issues so that nursing concerns are raised and discussed. Ethics rounds can be a discussion of retrospective or concurrent cases. They offer an opportunity to consider ethical concerns prospectively, rather than operating from a crisis position. The goal of these rounds is not to make clinical decisions, but to discuss moral problems confronting caregivers.

Institutional Ethics Committees

Institutional ethics committees are another tool for promoting individual and institutional sensitivity to the ethical issues faced at the bedside. Ethics committees can provide a forum of impartiality to assist parents and healthcare professionals in the process of ethical decision-making. Complex issues coupled with obvious disagreement about what the treatment should be or who should decide invite ethics committee consultation. Most ethics committees provide (1) education about ethical principles that guide decision-making; (2) a forum for airing feelings and conflicts about dilemmas; (3) a system for emotional support for healthcare professionals and families; and (4) an interdisciplinary group to formulate policies that guide decision-making. Generally, the actions of the committee are purely consultative and are not binding on any professional. However, submitting ethical dilemmas to uninvolved parties for consideration allows for objective discussion of various viewpoints.

The generic makeup of an ethics committee is not

universally agreed upon. However, it should be reflective of the diversity of the services provided by the institution. Generally, physicians and nurses make up the majority of the membership. For example, a full-service community hospital may have a surgeon, an obstetrician, a pediatrician, a neurologist, and an internist. An ethics committee at a children's hospital may have as members a pediatrician, a neonatalogist, an intensivist, a neurologist, a surgeon, and a geneticist. In turn, nursing membership could include representatives from like nursing specialties. These individuals should also represent the broad range of nurses in the institution (i.e., clinical nurse specialists, staff nurses, and nursing managers). A broad perspective enhances contributions on issues that may require knowledge about organizational systems and external resources that may aid decision-making. Other committee members may include social workers, clergy, lawyers, ethicists, and community members. It is most important that all committee members be willing to look beyond their own values and preferences and view issues from the patient's perspective. The members should have a desire to be informed about ethical theory and principles, as well as current issues. The members must be willing to listen to each other; accept ambiguity; and be reflective, critical thinkers.

Access to the ethics committee should be available to any hospital employee, physician, family member, or patient. The committee should develop procedures to ensure timely and effective consultation. Written information that outlines the committee's roles should be provided to staff and families.

A MODEL FOR ETHICAL DECISION-MAKING

In a clinical situation, the issues pertinent to determining the morally right thing to do and identifying who makes the decision are critical to resolving treatment dilemmas. A dilemma may arise when there are conflicting loyalties, duties, values, and/or rights. Choices may not be readily apparent, may require further delineation, or may be equally unsatisfactory. Smith and Davis (1980, p. 1463) describe four basic situations that may give rise to an ethical dilemma:

1. When there is conflict between two equally unsatisfactory alternatives.
2. When there is conflict between two ethical principles.
3. When there is conflict between one's ethical principles and one's role obligations.
4. When there is a demand for action and a need for reflection.

The key to analyzing an ethical dilemma lies in knowing which questions to ask. A systematic approach to asking those questions helps guide the practitioner through the knotty process of sorting

Table 7–2. A MODEL FOR ETHICAL DECISION-MAKING

I. Define the dilemma
II. Identify the medical facts
III. Identify the nonmedical facts
A. Patient and family factors
B. External factors
IV. Separate assumptions from facts
V. Identify items that need clarification
VI. Identify the decision-makers
VII. Review underlying ethical principles
VIII. Define alternatives
IX. Follow-up

From Levine-Ariff, J., & Groh, D. H. (1990). *Creating an ethical environment.* Baltimore: Williams & Wilkins.

through the issues, clarifying critical factors, and delineating possible alternatives. Using a systematic process can serve to minimize individual biases and decrease the risk of incomplete or inaccurate information influencing the final decision. One suggested model is presented here (Table 7–2). Its application in clinical case studies will demonstrate the process.

Use of the Model

Initially, following the model step by step may seem awkward and artificial. There may be a tendency to skip over some steps. As confidence with the model, and with ethical discussion, is gained, some steps may require only brief consideration and need not be followed in a rigid sequence. However, imposing a sense of order when first learning something new encourages precise application and facilitates learning.

Using an ethical decision-making model such as this one can facilitate group problem-solving; however, not all dilemmas need to be, nor should be, subjected to group process. It may be one nurse, two nurses, or a nurse with another colleague who discuss the issues. When immediate decisions are required, it may be impossible to spend the time necessary for group discussion. However, as one works with the model in both concurrent and retrospective case review, it will serve as an aid for quickly processing the known and the unknown pieces of information and arriving at alternatives for action.

It is also recommended that the model be used as an educational tool in workshops and in ethics rounds, using either hypothetical cases or a retrospective review of actual cases. Participants then become familiar with the process and are able to move more quickly through the steps when confronted with a dilemma in practice. By using the model for multidisciplinary ethics rounds, more open dialogue between disciplines is promoted and an environment in which there is enhanced recognition of different perspectives can be created. When using the model for group work, it is useful to have an experienced facilitator for the process.

Steps of the Model

I. Define the Dilemma

The first step of any algorithm is to identify the problem. Because ethical issues are not always easy to state succinctly, it is best to voice the concern in plain language. Sometimes the dilemma is formulated as a question; at other times it is expressed as a statement of concern. For example, "Has Dr. James told Erin's parents that if he resects her entire small intestine she will need total parenteral nutrition for the rest of her life?" or "Kevin's parents have always said they don't want to continue therapy if he has suffered serious neurologic damage, but they don't seem to understand what Dr. Anthony has told them about his intraventricular hemorrhage."

Different individuals may perceive an ethical dilemma in different ways. If a group is analyzing the situation together, it is important to allow everyone an opportunity to verbalize their view of the dilemma in their own words. A particular situation may present different dilemmas to different individuals, whereas a situation that is problematic to some may not be troublesome for others. Hearing one individual's perception of the problem may, in fact, help someone else focus on what is most distressing in the situation.

II. Identify the Medical Facts

As the medical facts are delineated, it may become apparent that individuals differ in their understanding of the facts. Some facts that were thought to be accurate may not be. The likely benefits and associated burdens of current therapies should be delineated. Conflicts in opinion between different medical specialists must be acknowledged and explored. Diagnosis and prognosis should be confirmed and understood by all.

The discussion of medical facts must be relevant to the issue at hand. Too often, when learning ethical decision-making, nurses and physicians get bogged down in the medical model and spend a great deal of time discussing specific test results, the latest ventilator settings, or the pros and cons of repeating a certain study. Discussion can too easily stray into issues that are not pertinent to the issue at hand—that is, the ethical concerns of the dilemma.

III. Identify the Nonmedical Facts

There are two separate groups of nonmedical facts that must be explored, those that apply directly to the patient and family and those that are external to the family but may affect the resolution of the dilemma.

Patient and Family Factors. Family demographics, cultural factors, religious beliefs, and the social and psychological history of the patient and family are all important aspects of an ethical issue and should be identified. What the patient and family "know" about the issue at hand should be openly discussed. Sometimes, what some healthcare providers believe the family knows is not always based on fact.

With the advent of the Patient Self Determination Act, some states are looking for ways to adapt this legislation in the care of children and adolescents. The existence of advance directives such as living wills, durable powers of attorney for healthcare, or verbal statements made by emancipated minors indicating values or preferences in such situations is applicable. Some parents with chronically critically ill children may have already formulated a directive.

As when reviewing the medical facts, relevancy is a key factor here as well. It is very easy to get caught up in the intricacies of the psychosocial data. The statement of the dilemma should be periodically reinforced so that relevancy is maintained and gossip is minimized.

External Factors. Administrative policies, federal and state laws, practice acts, regulations, professional codes of ethics, and nursing and medical standards of care should be considered, as applicable to the situation. Conflicts between the values of the healthcare providers or the healthcare system and the patient and family's value system must be acknowledged. It is imperative that healthcare providers not attempt to answer ethical dilemmas by asking the question, "What would you do if this were your child?" The facts are that this is not their child under discussion and that the question can be answered by 10 different people in 10 different ways. What is reasonably certain is that each parent would want the autonomy to make decisions about his/her own child's care.

When stating facts of policies, procedures, laws, and regulations in the course of an ethical discussion, one must recognize that ethics asks what "ought to be" and weighs current practices in that light. Perhaps the situation under consideration will alter a now-current institutional practice or eventually lead to new laws or regulations. The law can be a tool or a barrier, and what is legal is not always ethical. Simply establishing the legality of an action does not speak to its morality, yet known laws or legal precedents must be acknowledged and discussed. Certainly, if a state or federal law clearly forbids a certain action, legal counsel should be sought and potential risks and consequences identified. The reality is that current healthcare practices are presenting new ethical issues that will often be ahead of changes in the law and institutional policies. This can cloud the issue. Although offering no constraints, there is also no guidance from others who have addressed the issue and made decisions. It is important to remember that while the law requires us to do no harm, ethics goes beyond that by also requiring us to do good.

IV. Separate Facts from Assumptions

As the medical and nonmedical facts are identified, it becomes clear that certain "facts" are really just assumptions. Often patients' and families' statements are misinterpreted. One must listen carefully and assure separation of fact and assumption. For example, a family's statement "We don't want him to suffer" could be misinterpreted to mean they want life support withdrawn or no resuscitation, when their concern was focused on assuring adequate pain relief. At times, by virtue of an individual's stated religion, assumptions may be made regarding that person's expected decisions, when the parents may have entirely different preferences.

V. Identify Items That Need Clarification

Often, assumptions require clarification. In addition, other information needed is usually identified as part of the process in steps II and III, earlier.

VI. Identify the Decision-makers

Identification of the decision-maker is an important step toward fitting the pieces of the puzzle together. In the past, the decision-maker was often automatically assumed to be the physician. Nurses are now recognizing their role as decision-makers in nursing practice dilemmas. However, it must be remembered that while many dilemmas place the physician and nurse in positions of concern and in an advisory capacity to the patient and family, it is the parents and patients' right to make the choices of whether to undergo treatment or not. It is helpful to distinguish between medical decisions and those decisions that are moral in nature. Decisions that require medical diagnosis, prognosis, and proposed treatment are ones in which physicians have specific expertise. Decisions about whether to proceed with recommended treatments are moral ones that must be made by the patient and family based on their values.

When identifying the decision-makers, it is important to review whether the preferences of the child patient have been taken into account. As previously discussed, a child's chronologic as well as developmental age must be considered when treatment decisions must be made. Reviewing state laws provides guidance as to the legal rights a minor patient may have.

VII. Review Underlying Ethical Principles

Principles of bioethics can be employed as guides for making moral decisions and as standards for the evaluation of actions and policies. These principles help clarify what is actually happening. If it is said that a child has had an intracerebral bleed, certain mental images are formed. Questions are formulated and, based on their answers, certain interventions are anticipated. In the same way, when an issue of patient autonomy is identified, certain questions will

surface, and a potential direction to resolve the issue emerges.

Most ethical dilemmas do not have a single principle operating. Discussion may identify one principle as the most important; however, individual practitioners may give greater weight to certain principles than to others. For example, for some practitioners, doing no harm may be more important than doing good. Evaluation of the benefits and burdens for the patient may reveal that different principles are primary. Remembering that it is the patient and family's values that ought to guide decision-making assists in making clear the most important ethical principles in a given situation.

VIII. Define Alternatives

It may be that only one alternative is identified as the natural and obvious course of action in a situation. However, discussion may reveal multiple alternatives. To determine the appropriate actions, the options generated need to be weighed against the principles and values involved.

It is important not to immediately squelch alternatives that seem unacceptable. It may be that they are unacceptable only on the surface or only to some members of a group. In reality, that which initially seems to be an unacceptable alternative may be possible, except for institutional barriers such as arbitrary or outdated policies. It may be that these barriers need to be eliminated or minimized, and the process to do so may be listed as an alternative. Those options that are truly identified as unacceptable must be raised for discussion and then dismissed. Acknowledgment of unacceptable alternatives is just as important as acknowledgment of reasonable ones. This process may help the healthcare team to understand the issue more fully.

IX. Follow-up

As the initial steps of the model are followed, responsibility for various tasks, such as clarifying facts and seeking information, should be defined with a timeframe for completion. If all the information needed is brought forth during the discussion and a clear direction chosen, responsibility for carrying out that alternative must be clearly defined. To whom, and how, the conclusions will be communicated must be defined.

In addition, thought should be given to education needs and to policies or guidelines necessary to assist in addressing similar issues in the future. Ideally, the group should come back together after final resolution of the issue so as to "debrief" and discuss how the problem-solving process evolved and whether there were aspects that could have been improved. Particularly when there has been a tragic outcome, there needs to be recognition by the participants that a good process was used to address the issue. Unfortunately, there are not always happy endings to these dilemmas, but feeling comfortable with the decision-making process can be the difference between internal peace and moral distress for the involved caregivers.

CASE STUDY

• • • • • •

A 1½-year-old male child was brought to the emergency room following an accident in which he had fallen off the child seat of his father's bicycle. He was found to have a large subdural hematoma, requiring a bone flap for treatment. The child was hospitalized in the PICU. Initial therapy included intubation, continuous monitoring of systemic arterial pressure, central venous pressure measurement, intracranial pressure monitoring, and an electroencephalogram, as well as supportive cardiovascular therapy, pentothal, mannitol, and 3 percent saline infusions. Over a 2-month course, the child developed sepsis and adult respiratory distress syndrome (ARDS). Increased supportive therapy included a Swan-Ganz catheter for monitoring, multiple antibiotics, and an epinephrine drip. As the ARDS worsened, ventilation became more difficult and increasingly higher FiO_2 concentrations, inflating pressures, and positive end-expiratory pressures were required. The patient developed pneumothoraces and a pneumomediastinum, requiring insertion of chest tubes. The parents were insistent that everything possible be done. They had a strong belief in God and felt sure that with God's help, their son would recover. The nursing staff experienced feelings of distress, as if they were inflicting harm, and thought that recovery with reasonable quality of life for this child was impossible.

The issue of concern to the healthcare team centered around whether the parents were able to make decisions that were in the best interests of their child or whether the emotional issues related to the father's stated guilty feelings and sense of responsibility for the accident, along with their religious beliefs, prevented them from accepting the possibility of his death.

Case Study Analysis

DEFINE THE DILEMMA. *In this case the dilemma may be stated as "Are we giving treatment that is futile?" or, "Who should decide what is best for this child?" or, for an individual nurse, "I can't keep hurting this child."*

IDENTIFY THE MEDICAL FACTS. *As this case is stated, it is known that the child had a subdural hematoma that required a bone flap. He has ARDS and continues to require high levels of mechanical ventilation and extensive supportive care. He has been treated for sepsis. There are no stated facts about the child's neurologic status, nor is the actual prognosis clearly defined.*

IDENTIFY THE NONMEDICAL FACTS.

PATIENT AND FAMILY. *The child is 1½ years old. The injury occurred while the father was giving him a ride on the back of his bicycle, and the father has expressed guilt feelings over the circumstances of the accident. The parents have strong religious beliefs.*

EXTERNAL FACTORS. *Factors external to the patient and family that would be pertinent here are related to whether healthcare professionals are obligated to provide care they believe is futile. The matter of making decisions based on a judgment of futile treatment is currently a subject of some controversy. The definition of the word "futile" is that which is ineffectual or useless. Futility implies hopelessness in addition to uselessness. A pronouncement of futile treatment, when determined by a physician, reflects a clinical judgment that a specific treatment or procedure will not achieve the desired end. The controversy in healthcare today, of course, arises over the patient and family's right to demand life-supporting care which a physician has deemed futile but from which the patient or family perceives some benefit.*

SEPARATE ASSUMPTIONS FROM FACT. *There seems to be an assumption in this case that the child has suffered extensive permanent neurologic damage. There may be an assumption on the part of some caregivers that the parents do not have the best interests of the child at heart.*

IDENTIFY ITEMS THAT NEED CLARIFICATION. *These are some of the questions that may have arisen as the first four steps of the model were followed.*

MEDICAL FACTS. *What is the child's neurologic status? An assumption that is implied in the case is that the child is in a persistent vegetative state, but not brain dead. What studies have been done to confirm or refute this? What is the prognosis for his recovery from ARDS? Are there other treatment options here or at another facility that may be beneficial?*

NONMEDICAL FACTS: A. *What is the social situation of the family? Are there other family members involved and what is the nature of their relationship? Is this an only child or are there siblings? What has been discussed with the family about the child's severity of illness and prognosis for recovery? Is the family's verbalization about the child's severity of illness and prognosis inconsistent with what has been explained to them? How is the healthcare team perceived by the family—is the team perceived as having the best interests of the child at heart or has the relationship become adversarial? Is there some real basis for the father's guilt feelings—was there carelessness on his part that contributed to the injury? What counseling support has been offered to the family? Have their religious advisors been involved?*

NONMEDICAL FACTS: B. *Are there community standards that would help to define the limits of futile treatment in this case? What are the expressed values and biases of the healthcare team members? Are these in conflict with those expressed by the family?*

IDENTIFY THE DECISION-MAKERS. *Who is the decision-maker in any situation is related directly to the statement of the dilemma. If the dilemma is viewed as that of providing futile treatment, then the physician becomes a decision-maker. Healthcare workers are not expected to deliver care that is indeed futile. While* the Code for Nurses states that nurses "must take all reasonable means to protect and preserve human life when there is hope of recovery or reasonable hope of benefit from life-prolonging treatment" (American Nurses Association, 1985), it clarifies that the nurse need not proceed with treatment that is indeed futile. Unfortunately, it is often difficult to determine when use of the modern arsenal of technology reaches the endpoint of providing benefit, becomes futile, and, in fact, creates a situation of inflicting harm.

If the dilemma is viewed as one of "who should decide," the determining factors need to be those that are in the best interests of the child. Seeking legal intervention for appointment of a surrogate decision-maker to help weigh benefits and burdens of the treatment and determine what is in the child's best interests is one avenue to aid decision-making.

If the dilemma is that of an individual nurse saying "I can't continue hurting this child," there needs to be peer and unit support that permits the nurse to have a break from being a caregiver. Over time there will be situations in which different nurses need to be excused from providing care to specific patients. There need to be mechanisms in place to assure both ongoing care to the patient and support to nurses.

REVIEW ETHICAL PRINCIPLES. *Two of the ethical principles at work here are those of beneficence and nonmaleficence, the conflict of inflicting harm in an effort to do good. Autonomy also is at issue. The situation described places the healthcare givers in a dilemma wherein they must weigh the principle of autonomy against the principles of beneficence and nonmaleficence. The restriction of the parents' right to choose treatment options can be viewed from one perspective as limiting their autonomy. However, does anyone have the right to insist on treatment that is futile? What about the autonomy of the caregivers? Can they be forced to provide treatment that they believe is not only futile but, in fact, harmful? While a full exploration of the issues relating to futile treatment is clearly beyond the scope of this chapter, there are numerous articles available in the current literature. Healthcare providers who find themselves confronting these issues should familiarize themselves with the available resources.*

DEFINE ALTERNATIVES. *Other opinions can be sought about treatment options for the child's ARDS, such as extracorporeal membrane oxygenation or high frequency ventilation. A multidisciplinary patient care conference, including the parents, could be held to discuss the case, focusing on the benefits and burdens of the current treatment. The case could be reviewed by the hospital ethics committee. Legal opinion could be sought about the steps to petition for a surrogate decision-maker.*

FOLLOW-UP. *Depending on the alternative chosen, follow-up varies. In this particular case, it is likely that several or all of the alternatives identified above will be pursued. The case conference could end with a decision to take the case to the ethics committee or, perhaps, the case conference can be combined with the ethics committee review. Before holding these* meetings, information from other centers regarding alternative therapies should be gathered and the hospital's legal counsel consulted regarding the surrogate decision-maker, so that all necessary information is available at the time of the meeting.

● ●

SUMMARY

Ethical principles are relevant in all clinical issues nurses face. Ethical dilemmas occur when there is conflict about what is the morally right thing to do and who decides. Understanding current ethical issues and the process of ethical decision-making allows the nurse to participate appropriately on the healthcare team in a supportive role to patients and families. Creating an ethical environment for professional practice and patient care involves establishing an environment in which communication and coordination of care are optimized, where the focus remains on the best interests of the child, and there are continual efforts to encourage the child's participation in decision-making. Providing ongoing education through ethics rounds and participation on ethics committees will immeasurably enhance the ability of the healthcare team to support patients and families, as well as one another, when addressing the ethical issues that arise in the course of practicing pediatric critical care.

References

American Nurses Association (1985). *Code for nurses with interpretive statements*. Kansas City: American Nurses Association.

Anderson, P. (1985). *Children's Hospital*. New York: Harper & Row.

Arras, J.D. (1984). *On the care of the imperiled newborn*. The Hastings Center Report, 14(2), 27.

Arras, J.D. (1984). *Toward an ethic of ambiguity*. The Hastings Center Report, 15(2), 25–33.

Beauchamp, T.L., & Childress, J.F. (1989). *Principles of biomedical ethics* (3rd ed.). New York: Oxford University Press.

Bibace, R., & Walsh, M. (1980). *Development of children's concept of illness*. Pediatrics, 66, 912–917.

California Hospital Association (1990). *California consent manual* (p. 22). Sacramento, California Hospital Association.

Chester, M., & Barbarin, O. (1987). *Childhood cancer and the family: Meeting the challenges of stress and support*. New York: Brunner/Mazel, 1987.

Child Abuse Amendments (P.L. 98–457). (1984). (42. U.S. Code, 5101). Interpretative Guidelines (45 CFR Part 1 1340.15 et seq.).

Davis, A.J. (1989). *Clinical nurses' ethical decision making in situations of informed consent*. Advances in Nursing Science, 12, 63–69.

Duff, R.S. (1979). *Guidelines on deciding care of critically ill or dying patients*. Pediatrics, July 17, 64(1).

Erickson, E.H. (1963). *Childhood and society* (2nd ed.). New York: W.W. Norton.

Fowler, D.M. (1985). Introduction to ethics and ethical theory: A road map to the discipline. In D.M. Fowler & J. Levine-Ariff (Eds.). *Ethics at the bedside: A source book for the critical care nurse*. Philadelphia: J.B. Lippincott.

Holder, A. (1985). *Legal issues in pediatrics and adolescent medicine* (2nd ed.). New Haven: Yale University Press.

In re Quinlan, 70 N.J. 10,A.2d 647, 1976.

Jameton, A. (1984). *Nursing practice: The ethical issues.* Englewood Cliffs, NJ: Prentice-Hall.

Lantos, J.D., Miles, M., & Cassel, M.E., et al. (1989). The Linares affair. *Law, Medicine, and Health Care,* 17(4), 308–315.

Larsen, G. (1954). Child neglect in the exercise of religious freedom. *Kent Law Review,* 32, 283.

Leikin, S. (1989). A proposal concerning decisions to forego life-sustaining treatment for young people. *Journal of Pediatrics,* 115(1), 18.

Levine-Ariff, J., & Groh, D.H. (1990). *Creating an ethical environment.* Baltimore: Williams & Wilkins.

Mayeroff, M. (1971). *On caring.* New York: Harper & Row.

Nitschke, R., et al. (1982). Therapeutic choices made by patients with end-stage cancer. *Journal of Pediatrics,* 101, 471.

Omnibus Reconciliation Act of 1990. Title IV, Section 4206. Congressional Record. October 26, 1990: h12456–h12457.

Piaget, J. (1926). *The language and thought of the child.* New York: Humanities Press.

Rushton, C.L., & Glover, J.J. (1990). Involving parents in decisions to forego life-sustaining treatments for critically ill infants and children. In J.M. Clochesy, et al. (Eds.). *AACN Clinical Issues in Critical Care Nursing.* Philadelphia: J.B. Lippincott, 1(1):206–208.

Smith, S.J., & Davis, A.J. (1980). Ethical dilemmas: Conflicts among rights, duties, and obligations. *American Journal of Nursing,* 80, 1463–1466.

CHAPTER 8

Environmental Hazards

CLAIRE E. SOMMARGREN

CHEMICAL HAZARDS
Soap, Solvents, and Cleaning Agents
Compressed Gases
Waste Anesthetic Gases
Pharmacologic Agents
PHYSICAL HAZARDS
Ionizing Radiation

BIOLOGIC HAZARDS
Hepatitis Viruses
Human Immunodeficiency Virus
Mycobacterium tuberculosis Infection (Tuberculosis)
Herpes Viruses
Neisseria meningitidis Infection
SUMMARY

Discussion of pediatric critical care includes not only the issues of professional practice, but the working environment as well. The pediatric critical care environment presents actual and potential occupational hazards to nurses employed in this area.

The phrase "occupational hazards" may bring to mind images of workers in a coal mine, pesticide factory, or construction project. These people are at high risk for work-related injury or toxic exposure. Until recently, only infrequently have nurses considered their own professional risks. Indeed, nursing presents many occupational health hazards. Some, such as heavy lifting and exposure to ionizing radiation, have long been acknowledged as potentially dangerous. Other hazards are more subtle, and not as readily identified, but can be just as dangerous.

Hospitals are among the most complex of workplaces. The working environment of nurses, particularly in pediatric critical care units, is subject to rapid change. Almost daily, new diagnostic tests, therapeutic procedures, or pharmacologic agents are introduced. Along with these technologic advancements comes the potential for increased exposure of nurses to health hazards.

Occupational diseases and injuries are potentially preventable. Nurses *can* protect themselves by becoming informed about the occupational risks they face.

Hazards in the workplace can be classified into one of five broad categories: chemical, physical, psychological, ergonomic, and biologic. The hazards discussed in this chapter are components of chemical, physical, and biologic risks. However, Table 8–1 presents an overview of all five classifications.

A simple method of identifying hazards in a critical care unit is the walk-through inspection, which should be carried out on a periodic basis. This is done by physically walking through the unit, following the flow of operations from start to finish, and recording potential hazards that are observed. Areas inspected include work stations, hallways, and utility rooms. It is often useful to observe a nurse working in a typical patient care area, noting the nurse's position, the workspace, lighting, and arrangement of equipment. Critical care nurses, because of their keenly developed observational and assessment skills, can become quite adept at evaluating their units for hazards using this method. Actual or potential hazards discovered during the walk-through inspection should be reported promptly.

Once health or safety hazards have been identified, control methods are instituted to reduce or eliminate the risk of exposure. These control methods include substitution, engineering controls, work practice modifications, personal protective equipment, administrative controls, and medical surveillance programs.

Substitution is considered the best way of dealing

Table 8-1. CLASSIFICATION OF HAZARDS

Hazard	Type	Examples
Chemical hazards	Soaps	
	Solvents	Acetone
		Benzoin
		Alcohol
	Cleaning agents	Glutaraldehyde
		Household bleach
	Compressed gases	
	Waste anesthetic gases	
	Pharmacologic agents	Antineoplastic agents
		Ribavirin
		Pentamidine
Physical hazards	Radiant energy hazards	Visible light inappropriate lighting
		Phototherapy sources
		Ionizing radiation x-rays gamma rays
		Lasers
	Electricity	
	Noise	
Ergonomic hazards	Work station hazards	
	Manual lifting	
Psychological hazards	Stress	
	Shift work	
	Violence	Physical violence
		Verbal abuse
Biologic hazards	Hepatitis viruses	Hepatitis A virus (HAV)
		Hepatitis B virus (HBV)
		Hepatitis C virus (HCV)
		Hepatitis D virus (HDV)
	Human immunodeficiency virus (HIV)	
	Mycobacterium tuberculosis	
	Herpes viruses	Herpes simplex virus
		Varicella zoster virus
		Cytomegalovirus
	Neisseria meningitidis	
	Intestinal pathogens	*Salmonella*
		Shigella
		Campylobacter
	Sarcoptes scabiei	

with workplace hazards. It consists of simply replacing the dangerous substance or piece of equipment with another that is less hazardous. For example, an instrument cleaning solution that can cause respiratory irritation is replaced by a less toxic agent.

Environmental hazards in the clinical setting can also be controlled by *engineering methods*. This involves the modification of equipment or the workspace. For instance, staff complaints of chronic eye strain may be eliminated by installation of a more appropriate lighting system, or noise levels in a unit may be significantly reduced by the installation of acoustic materials.

Some workplace hazards are simply the result of unsafe *work practices* of personnel. An example of this is the nurse who fails to report a damaged electric outlet or improperly discards needles. Such behaviors are promptly discouraged by means of education and reinforcement to prevent unnecessary risk not only to the offending nurse but also to other members of the nursing and support staffs.

Personal protective equipment is the least satisfactory control method, because it places the burden of protection on the nurse. However, its use cannot be avoided in situations when substitution or engineering controls do not completely eliminate an exposure, such as when the nurse is faced with certain biologic or physical hazards. Gowns, gloves, goggles, and lead aprons are examples of personal protective equipment. Adequate supplies of personal protective equipment and education of staff members in its proper use are key factors in encouraging compliance with an occupational health and safety program.

If the previously described control methods are not applicable or appropriate, it may be necessary to remove a worker from a hazardous situation for a period of time. For example, scheduling may be changed because the nurse has experienced physical disturbances caused by rotating shift work. This is an example of an *administrative control*.

Medical surveillance programs in hospitals should take into consideration the risk of workplace exposure to hazards, with appropriate monitoring of actual exposures on an ongoing basis. It is essential that critical care nurses support their hospital's employee health and safety program. This includes communicating openly and working closely with occupational health and infection control professionals with the goal of creating a workplace that is safe and healthful.

CHEMICAL HAZARDS

Critical care nurses use a wide variety of chemicals in their practice. These range from such seemingly benign substances as handwashing soaps to obviously hazardous materials, such as cytotoxic drugs. A toxic agent is defined as an agent that is capable of producing a negative health response that can lead to serious injury or dysfunction, or death (Travers, 1986b).

It is important to know certain facts about all chemical substances used in the critical care environment. The first is the identity of the agent. Proper labeling is crucial. Unlabeled substances should never be used and should be removed from the unit. Other essential information includes the agent's toxicity, its route of entry into the body, associated health hazards, and applicable precautions or control measures that are to be used.

The Federal Hazard Communication Standard and state "right-to-know" legislation have mandated that hospitals inform all employees about the substances with which they work. This is accomplished through training and educational programs, and by accessibility to Material Safety Data Sheets (MSDS), informational documents that give brief overviews of potentially toxic substances present in the workplace. Critical care nurses should read the MSDSs on the unit to become familiar with these substances. Nurses should also know where to obtain more detailed information on chemical agents. Some excellent resources and references for this purpose are listed at the end of this chapter.

Nurses may be exposed to toxic substances by several routes. The most important route to consider is that of inhalation, which can enable a substance to enter the bloodstream rapidly. Chemicals may also be absorbed through the skin. Although broken skin, such as chapped hands, speed this method of entry, even intact skin allows the absorption of some chemicals. The third route of exposure is ingestion. Although this risk may seem unlikely, it can easily occur when a nurse eats, smokes, or applies cosmetics after handling toxic agents.

Exposure to chemical hazards may or may not produce adverse health effects. Some of the variable factors that can affect the outcome of an exposure include the form and concentration of the agent, and the duration and frequency of the exposure. In addition, individual susceptibility and work practices of the exposed person, the working conditions under which the exposure occurs, and any other exposures the worker may have experienced will influence the outcome of the exposure (Travers, 1986a).

Adverse health effects experienced as a result of exposure to toxic agents may be categorized as acute or chronic. Acute effects are those that appear shortly after exposure and are of relatively short duration, such as skin irritation, vertigo, or nausea. Chronic effects, on the other hand, may not be recognized until years after exposure. Liver and lung disease are examples of chronic health effects.

A number of substances used in critical care may be classified into one of several categories. These include *carcinogens,* capable of inducing cancer; *teratogens,* causing abnormal fetal development; or *mutagens,* adversely affecting genetic material.

Soaps, Solvents, and Cleaning Agents

A common chemical exposure of nurses in clinical areas is to soaps and cleaning agents. Frequent handwashing, a necessary part of nursing care, may lead to dried, chapped, and cracked skin, breaking down an important barrier to the entry of chemical and biologic agents. Some nurses may also develop an allergic reaction to soaps, including inflammation, rash, and blistering. It is best to have more than one type of soap available to offer an alternative

for sensitive individuals. Effects of soaps should be countered by frequent use of moisturizing lotions.

A variety of cleaning agents can be found in critical care units. Substances used to clean instruments, such as glutaraldehyde and related compounds, may cause irritation of the eyes, skin, and respiratory tract, as well as headache, nausea, and lightheadedness. Problems such as these can be avoided by adequate ventilation in areas of use. The use of protective clothing and goggles is recommended if skin contact or splashing of the chemical is anticipated (National Institute for Occupational Safety and Health, 1988).

Solvents, carbon compounds that can dissolve other substances, are another class of chemical agents commonly found in critical care units. Isopropyl alcohol, acetone, and benzoin are examples of solvents. The routes of entry into the body for these substances are skin absorption and inhalation. Known toxic effects are limited to short-term symptoms such as localized skin drying and irritation, and central nervous system disturbances including vertigo, fatigue, headache, insomnia, concentration difficulties, feelings of exhilaration, memory problems, and mood changes (Baker & Fine, 1986).

Direct skin contact with solvents can be avoided by using gloves. Containers of solvents should be kept tightly capped when not in use to prevent accidental inhalation of vapors.

Compressed Gases

Cylinders of oxygen, and less frequently helium and carbon dioxide, can be found in critical care units. Compressed gases present potential safety hazards. Care must be taken to store containers away from sources of temperature extremes. If exposed to excess heat, the gas within these cylinders expands and the cylinder eventually explodes if the pressure becomes excessive. It is also important to keep compressed gas cylinders carefully secured in a rack or specially designed holder to prevent them from falling and breaking. Such breakage could allow the sudden escape of the pressurized gas, turning the cylinder into a missile. If it is not possible to secure a cylinder, it should be placed flat on the floor until it can be moved. Special caution should be taken to secure oxygen cylinders during the transport of patients.

Oxygen, whether contained in cylinders or "piped in" from a central source, may also present a fire hazard. Although not flammable itself, oxygen accelerates the combustion of flammable materials. Caution must be taken to eliminate open flame in the vicinity of an oxygen source.

Waste Anesthetic Gases

The health effects of anesthetic gases on operating room and anesthesia personnel have been the subject of many studies in the past few years. Nurses in the critical care unit may also, however, have low levels of exposure to waste anesthetic gases that are exhaled by their post-anesthesia patients. Even low level exposures have been shown to cause toxic effects (Rogers, 1986). Acute effects can include impairment of judgment and coordination, depression, irritability, headache, nausea, and fatigue (National Institute for Occupational Safety and Health, 1977). Long-term effects have not been precisely defined, but past studies have reported such health effects as cancer, spontaneous abortion, congenital anomalies, and liver damage (Foley, 1993).

Most problems related to waste anesthetic gases can be controlled in critical care units by the presence of adequate air exchange in patient care areas. Avoidance of close or prolonged contact with the exhaled air from patients who have recently received general anesthesia also helps to prevent exposure. If symptoms of acute exposure are noted, the nurse should leave the area. It is particularly important to report any symptoms of acute toxicity to encourage the institution of control methods that may prevent long-term effects.

Pharmacologic Agents

Critical care nurses are exposed to a wide variety of pharmaceuticals on a daily basis. In general, there are very few data available on acute and chronic health effects of pharmacologic agents for those who prepare and administer them. Until such information is known, nurses should adhere to work practices that limit exposure to these substances as much as possible. Specifically, nurses should avoid introducing aerosolized medications into the environment during preparation of injectable drugs; avoid skin contact with medications; clean away spilled medications immediately; wash hands thoroughly after preparation of medications; limit as much as possible the inhalation of medications being administered to patients by the aerosol route; refrain from eating or drinking in areas where medications are stored or prepared.

Antineoplastic Agents

Perhaps the most widely studied potentially hazardous pharmacologic agents are antineoplastic drugs. Introduced in the 1940s, these agents interfere with the growth and development of cancerous cells by acting directly on a cell's genetic material or upon its protein synthesis mechanism. Antineoplastic, or cytotoxic, agents can affect normal cells as well as malignant cells.

Exposure to antineoplastic drugs can be by inhalation, skin contact or absorption, ingestion, or accidental needlestick. Acute health effects have been recognized since these drugs were first introduced. Effects include nausea; headache; eye, skin, and mucous membrane irritation; and local tissue necrosis.

Chronic effects suggested by recent studies include carcinogenesis, teratogenesis, and mutagenesis (Rogers, 1987).

Because of the high potential for adverse health effects, the Occupational Safety and Health Administration (OSHA) has issued guidelines that outline proper techniques for the preparation, administration, handling, and disposal of antineoplastics. This document points out two key elements to ensure proper workplace practices: (1) education and training of all staff involved in the handling of any aspect of antineoplastic drugs; and (2) use of vertical flow containment hoods (also called biologic safety cabinets) during preparation of these agents (Yodaiken, 1986). It is important that nurses not handle or administer antineoplastic drugs unless they have received special education and training, and unless specialized equipment, as outlined by OSHA, is available (Mayer, 1992.)

Ribavirin

In recent years, several other kinds of drugs have been implicated as potential health hazards to personnel who administer them. Of particular concern in pediatric critical care is the antiviral drug ribavirin. It was approved by the Food and Drug Administration in 1986 for aerosol use in the treatment of severe respiratory syncytial virus (RSV) infections in children.

Acute symptoms of coughing and throat irritation have been reported after exposure to aerosolized ribavirin. In nurses with pre-existing respiratory conditions, symptoms may be more serious, including lung irritation, wheezing, and shortness of breath. Eye irritation has also been reported by contact lens wearers (California Department of Health Services, 1990). Some studies suggest that ribavirin may be mutagenic, and further research is directed toward determining if it has carcinogenic properties. There are currently no reports of birth defects in humans resulting from exposure, but animal studies have shown that ribavirin is teratogenic and embryolethal, and also causes testicular atrophy (Centers for Disease Control [CDC], 1988).

Because the drug is administered via the aerosol route, much of the drug may not actually be delivered to the patient, but rather is released into the environment. It has also been suggested that ribavirin precipitate, which tends to form in aerosol equipment and accumulate on the patient, bed linens, and nearby supplies, may become airborne during routine nursing care. In addition, respiratory secretions of patients receiving ribavirin may contain the drug and may be another source of exposure (Prows, 1989). Based on the results of animal studies, these environmental exposures may pose a serious reproductive threat to women who are pregnant or attempting to conceive.

Patients receiving ribavirin should be placed in a private room or grouped with others receiving the medication. This room should have static or negative pressure, and the door should remain closed to minimize exposure to nearby patients and personnel. Specially designed delivery systems, as well as scavenging equipment, should be used wherever possible (Fig. 8–1). Warning signs should be used to make others aware of the hazard (California Department of Health Services, 1990).

Data are incomplete regarding the efficacy of personal protective clothing, but it has been recommended that gown, gloves, and hair and shoe covers be worn by all persons entering the room, including housekeeping personnel. Hands must be thoroughly washed after glove removal. Contact lens wearers are advised to wear goggles. It is doubtful that surgical or dust masks prevent exposure.

Although many questions remain unanswered at this time, it is recommended that personnel and visitors who are pregnant or may become pregnant be warned of the potential reproductive risks of exposure to aerosolized ribavirin (CDC, 1988). Personnel with underlying respiratory problems should keep to a minimum their contact with ribavirin. The availability of alternative work assignments has been recommended (California Department of Health Services, 1990).

Based on data from animal studies, ribavirin exposure may place the nurse at risk. In the past, emphasis was placed on the use of protective clothing as a means to limit exposure. However, now the emphasis

is on improved delivery systems that limit environmental exposure.

Pentamidine

Pentamidine, a pharmaceutical agent used as prophylaxis against *Pneumocystis carinii* pneumonia in patients infected with human immunodeficiency virus (HIV), has also been identified as potentially hazardous to those who administer it. Pentamidine can be given intravenously or by aerosol. The risk to caretakers is greatest when it is given in aerosol form.

When used correctly, a filter system on the nebulizer used to administer pentamidine prevents most of the drug from entering exhaled gases. However, if the nebulizer is not used properly, significant amounts of pentamidine can reach the environment and nearby persons. Exposure to aerosolized pentamidine may cause the nurse to experience the same adverse effects as the patient, including coughing and wheezing (CDC, 1989b). It must also be kept in mind that the safety of pentamidine in pregnancy is not known at this time. Early animal studies have reported embryocidal effects (Harstad, et al., 1990).

Pentamidine may also play a role in transmission of *Mycobacterium tuberculosis* to nurses. This is because pentamidine may cause profuse coughing episodes during its administration, enhancing the airborne spread of the bacterium from infected patients to nearby staff. For this reason, CDC recommendations are that active pulmonary disease be ruled out before treatment with pentamidine is initiated (CDC, 1989b).

If pentamidine is administered to a patient with known or suspected pulmonary tuberculosis, special respiratory isolation precautions must be taken. These include administering such treatments in negative pressure rooms or booths with external air exhaust systems and adequate air exchange (CDC, 1990a).

PHYSICAL HAZARDS

A variety of physical hazards face the pediatric critical care nurse, including radiant energy, electrical energy, and noise. Ionizing radiation, a form of radiant energy, deserves special discussion because of the nurse's high risk of exposure.

Ionizing Radiation

Critical care nurses are at risk for exposure to ionizing radiation from such sources as portable x-ray machines, fluoroscopy equipment, and body substances of patients who have received radioactive preparations during diagnostic procedures. The level of exposure to ionizing radiation is rarely high enough to cause acute effects to personnel in the hospital setting. The danger lies chiefly in low doses

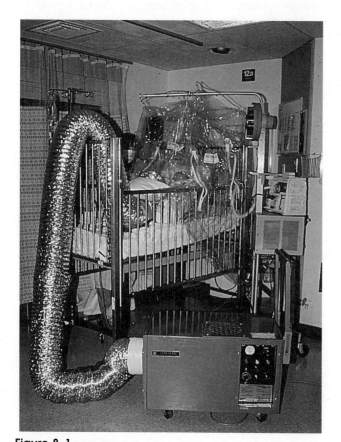

Figure 8–1 ● ● ● ● ● ●
Ribavirin administration equipment.

over a long period of time. The amount of ionizing radiation that is hazardous has not been firmly established, but it is generally believed that *any* exposure involves some risk (National Institute for Occupational Safety and Health, 1988).

The effects of low-level ionizing radiation are primarily on cells that divide rapidly, such as the skin, eye lenses, blood-forming tissues, and gonads. At the cellular level, effects can include genetic mutation and disturbances of cell division and metabolism. It can result in cancer, cataracts, sterility, aplastic anemia, radiation dermatitis, and fibrosis of the lungs and kidneys. The developing fetus is particularly susceptible to damage. Prenatal exposure to ionizing radiation can cause small head size, mental retardation, and fetal death resulting from leukemia or abnormalities in organ development (Beebe, 1981; Myer & Tanascia, 1981).

Recommendations for controlling ionizing radiation hazards have been issued by the National Council on Radiation Protection and Measurements (NCRP). These recommendations are enforced through state and federal laws. The NCRP has established maximum permissible dose (MPD) limits for radiology workers and the general public. The unit used to express dose is the rem. Currently, the MPD for personnel working in radiology departments is 5 rem/year. The MPD for nurses outside radiology departments is 0.5 rem/year, whereas the dose limit for fetuses of occupationally exposed women is 0.5 rem during the entire pregnancy (National Institute for Occupational Safety and Health, 1988). Workers who are actually or potentially exposed to more than 1.25 rem/year must wear a film badge to monitor the dose received (US Nuclear Regulatory Commission, 1984).

It is important for critical care nurses to take measures to protect themselves as much as possible from ionizing radiation exposure. This can be accomplished by using the principles of time, distance, and shielding:

- Time. The ionizing radiation dose received is directly proportional to the length of the time of exposure. Therefore, it is important to keep to an absolute minimum the duration of exposure to a source, even when shielding devices, such as lead aprons, are worn.
- Distance. The nurse can further decrease dosage of ionizing radiation by increasing distance from the source. Ten feet is the minimum recommended distance from an ionizing radiation source, such as the x-ray machine during portable x-ray examination.
- Shielding. Ideally, diagnostic films are performed in the radiology department where engineering controls are in place. Portable x-ray devices should be used only when it is not feasible to transport the patient to the radiology department.

If it is necessary for the nurse to remain closer than 10 feet to the radiation source, for example, to position or restrain an infant during taking of a portable film, shielding is necessary. This shielding includes any part of the body (including the hands) in the direct field or nearby, where scatter radiation levels are high. No part of the body should ever be directly exposed to ionizing radiation.

Shielding is usually accomplished by means of lead garments. Lead aprons should cover both the front and back of the body, and lead gloves should be used to shield hands from exposure. It is also recommended that for long exposures, such as those that occur during angiography and other diagnostic procedures, lead glasses and thyroid shields be worn (National Institute for Occupational Safety and Health, 1988).

Portable x-ray and fluoroscopy devices are obvious sources of ionizing radiation, but patients who have received radioactive materials during diagnostic procedures may also serve as a source of exposure for up to 24 hours after the test. Such patients must be clearly identified to all personnel responsible for their care. Although most of these procedures use only small amounts of radioactive materials with short half-lives, the patient's body substances, such as urine and feces, are considered radioactive. It is necessary for the nurse to avoid contact with body wastes by wearing waterproof gloves when disposing of these substances.

BIOLOGIC HAZARDS

Virtually every environment abounds with microorganisms, but most of these do not pose a danger to persons with normally functioning immune systems. It is important for critical care nurses to recognize, however, that several infectious agents definitely do present the threat of transmission to them, possibly resulting in negative health effects. These are known as biologic hazards, and include viruses, bacteria, and parasites.

Transmission of infectious agents can occur by a variety of routes, including contact transmission, direct or indirect (droplet, percutaneous/blood-borne, skin or mucous membrane, sexual contact, oral/fecal, contact with contaminated object); airborne transmission (droplet nuclei or dust particles, spreading more than 3–4 feet from the source); vehicle-borne transmission (contaminated food or water); or vector-borne transmission (insects).

Contact of a host with an infectious agent may result in varying degrees of invasion. The microorganism can grow and multiply without actually entering body tissues. This is referred to as "colonization." Infection occurs if the agent gains entry and multiplies in body tissues. At this stage the person may or may not have symptoms. If signs and symptoms do occur, the stage is described as "infectious disease." Infectious agents are often transmitted to nurses by persons who appear to be well, but who are either colonized or asymptomatically infected with that agent.

There is a common misconception that pregnancy places a person at greater risk for acquiring infection. Studies have shown repeatedly that this is not the case, and pregnant healthcare workers need not avoid assignment to infectious patients. However, some infections, such as cytomegalovirus, hepatitis B virus (HBV), and rubella can have negative health effects on both the mother and the fetus. For this reason, it is especially important that female nurses of childbearing age be knowledgeable regarding biologic hazards and effective control strategies and adhere strictly to recommended infection control measures at all times (Valenti, 1986; Williams, 1983).

Several strategies can be employed to prevent the transmission of infectious agents to healthcare workers. Perhaps the most important of these is the continuing education of personnel regarding the presence of biologic hazards and appropriate control methods. The currency of this knowledge base helps personnel keep pace with the ever-expanding body of knowledge on infectious disease. The hospital's infection control nurse can be invaluable in assisting critical care nurses to keep their environment and daily practice as safe as possible.

Immunization is an extremely effective control method. Safe, effective vaccines are used to prevent hepatitis B, as well as most common childhood disease (hepatitis B vaccine will be discussed later). The CDC of the United States Public Health Service and others have recommended that all medical personnel who have patient contact be immune, either by documented medical history or by vaccination, to measles and rubella (CDC, 1990d; Greaves, et al., 1982; CDC, 1989c; Davis, et al., 1986). These immunities become particularly important for nurses working with infants and children, who are the most common source of these illnesses.

Another preventive strategy is the removal of infectious agents through the washing of the hands and skin. Hands should be washed before and after contact with the patient or patient-care items, and upon leaving the patient care area. Proper care of the hands should include preservation of an intact skin barrier. The use of moisturizing skin lotions prevents chapping and cracking of the skin that can occur with frequent handwashing. Careful care of the fingernails should focus on preventing breaks in the cuticle, a common site for entry of infectious agents.

Contact with infectious agents can be prevented by employing methods to cover the microorganism's portal of exit or entry with personal protective equipment, such as gloves, goggles, or gowns. Engineering controls, such as negative airflow and outside exhaust of air from isolation rooms, can help control airborne microorganisms.

OSHA, in its standard on Occupational Exposure to Bloodborne Pathogens, has mandated use of "universal precautions" by workers giving direct care. These precautions are based on the potential infectiousness of blood and certain body fluids of *all* patients for HIV, HBV, and other blood-borne pathogens. The OSHA standard contains not only general precautions regarding prevention of injuries from sharp devices, the use of protective barriers, and immediate washing of contaminated hands and other body surfaces, but also regulations concerning HBV vaccination, management of exposures, management of infected healthcare workers, and environmental control strategies. Body fluids covered under universal precautions include amniotic fluid, cerebrospinal fluid, synovial fluid, pleural fluid, pericardial fluid, peritoneal fluid, and other body fluids or secretions that contain visible blood. Universal precautions do not apply to breast milk, because it has not been implicated in the transmission of blood-borne pathogens to healthcare workers (OSHA, 1991). It is essential that all critical care nurses become knowledgeable regarding universal precautions, and integrate these principles into all patient care activities. Universal precautions do not eliminate the need for other types of precautions, such as enteric precautions, isolation for pulmonary tuberculosis, or other disease-specific protective techniques.

Hepatitis Viruses

A number of infectious agents are responsible for the occurrence of viral hepatitis, an inflammatory disease of the liver seen primarily in young adults. Different types of viral hepatitis have clinical similarities, but their etiologies and epidemiologies are quite different. Taken as a whole, almost 60,000 cases of viral hepatitis were reported in the United States in 1988, and the actual number of cases is estimated to be several times the number of reported cases (CDC, 1990b).

Hepatitis A Virus

This virus is responsible for approximately one half of the reported cases of hepatitis in the United States. Transmission of hepatitis A virus (HAV) occurs primarily from person to person through the oral/fecal route. Epidemics have been caused by contaminated food or water.

Symptoms are of abrupt onset and include malaise, fever, abdominal pain, nausea, jaundice, and dark urine. The severity of symptoms is variable and increases with age; however, children infected with HAV are commonly asymptomatic. Among reported cases, the case-fatality rate is approximately 0.6% (CDC, 1990b). Sequelae or asymptomatic carrier states do not appear with HAV as they do with some other types of viral hepatitis. Transmission of HAV from patients to nurses can be prevented by consistent use of gloves and diligent handwashing whenever there is contact with feces.

Hepatitis B Virus

Of all the biologic hazards, HBV presents perhaps the most immediate and important threat to critical care nurses. This is because of two factors: (1) HBV is relatively easily transmissible because it is found in high concentrations in the body fluids of infected persons; and (2) because estimates are that in the United States 750,000 to 1 million people are infectious carriers of HBV, many of whom are asymptomatic and unaware of their carrier status.

The primary mode of transmission of HBV is percutaneous or permucosal contact with infective blood or body fluids. Transmission can occur during the birth process, through sexual contact, during transfusion of blood or plasma products, or by contaminated needles.

HBV causes serious disease, primarily in young adults. It is estimated that each year in the United States 300,000 persons become infected with HBV. Of these, 10,000 are sufficiently ill to require hospitalization, and 250 die of fulminant hepatitis.

Among adults, 6% to 10% of those infected develop chronic HBV infection. This can lead to chronic active hepatitis, cirrhosis, and primary liver cancer. These chronic states lead to the majority of fatalities. It has been estimated by the CDC that 4000 persons suffering from chronic HBV infection die each year from cirrhosis and 800 from liver cancer (CDC, 1990c).

HBV presents a real threat to critical care nurses. An estimated 6000 to 8000 new HBV infections occur annually among healthcare workers (CDC, 1990c). Of these, 250 workers die from either fulminant hepatitis, cirrhosis, or liver cancer. Studies have shown that 10 to 30 percent of healthcare and dental workers may show serologic evidence of past or present HBV infection (CDC, 1989a).

Because HBV infection is often unrecognized in hospitalized patients, nurses must strictly adhere to universal precautions when caring for all patients. In addition, it is strongly recommended that all critical care nurses become immunized against HBV. A safe and effective vaccine has been available since 1982, and OSHA has mandated that employers provide this vaccine at no cost to nurses and other healthcare workers who are at risk of exposure to HBV.

All significant exposures to HBV, such as needlestick injuries or mucosal splashing, must be reported to the hospital employee health professional immediately. Reporting ensures that appropriate post-exposure testing, treatment, and counseling proceed without delay.

Hepatitis C Virus

Serologic tests to detect the presence of hepatitis C virus (HCV) became available in 1990. HCV is transmitted via the parenteral route, but it is currently unclear whether it may also be spread by the sexual or perinatal routes. Studies have implicated this agent as the most common cause of parenterally transmitted non-A, non-B hepatitis (CDC, 1991).

Infection with HCV is clinically similar to that with HAV and HBV. Sequelae include chronic active hepatitis and cirrhosis. Research is continuing to clarify the incidence, transmission, and long-term health implications of HCV.

Currently, there is no HCV vaccine. Adherence to universal precautions can prevent exposure to HCV.

Hepatitis D Virus

This agent (HDV), also called the delta virus, replicates only in the presence of HBV. Infection with HDV occurs as a coinfection in persons with acute HBV infection, or as a superinfection of HBV carriers. The symptoms and routes of exposure of HDV are the same as those for HBV. Because HDV infection occurs only in conjunction with HBV, it can be prevented by immunization with HBV vaccine.

Human Immunodeficiency Virus

Infection with HIV results in the depletion of a subset of T lymphocytes with subsequent disruption of the body's immune system functions. People infected with HIV frequently do not exhibit symptoms for months, or even years, after infection, although occasionally a mild flu-like syndrome is reported early in the course of the disease. Initial symptoms include weight loss and persistent lymphadenopathy, followed by opportunistic infections and neoplasms. Acquired immune deficiency syndrome (AIDS) is a progressive illness, defined by specific criteria (CDC, 1992), that results from HIV infection.

HIV infection is transmitted in the same manner as HBV, that is, by percutaneous or permucosal contact with infected blood or body fluids. HIV is much less readily transmissible than HBV, probably resulting from a lower concentration of HIV in body fluids of infected persons.

Prevention of exposure to HIV is primarily accomplished by implementation of universal precautions at all times. Again, as with all blood-borne pathogens, great care must be taken to avoid accidental injury with contaminated needles or other sharp instruments. There is currently no HIV vaccine available. Significant exposures to blood or body fluids should be reported promptly and followed by hospital employee health professionals according to OSHA regulations.

Mycobacterium tuberculosis Infection (Tuberculosis)

Mycobacterium tuberculosis (MTB) is the bacterium that causes tuberculosis. It is denoted as an acid-fast bacillus (AFB) because of staining properties that allow its identification. Infection with tuberculosis can occur in many organs of the body, but it is pulmonary or laryngeal tuberculosis that presents the greatest risk of transmission to the nurse.

Transmission of MTB occurs when the bacteria are spread by microscopic airborne particles (droplet nuclei) generated when an infected person coughs, sneezes, laughs, or speaks. The droplet nuclei are distributed throughout an area by normal air currents, and can be inhaled into the lungs of persons in the vicinity. Nurses are particularly at risk for exposure to MTB during procedures that stimulate patients to cough, such as endotracheal suctioning or administration of aerosolized medications. Treatment with aerosolized pentamidine, in particular, has been implicated in placing healthcare workers at risk (see p. 146).

Tuberculosis infection can be asymptomatic, or it can produce symptoms including weight loss, fever, cough, and night sweats. Tuberculosis should be suspected in any patient who exhibits these symptoms. People with unrecognized infection who are not taking antituberculosis drugs and have not been placed in AFB isolation present the greatest risk to nurses.

Diagnosis of tuberculosis is generally based on the results of a tuberculin skin test, chest radiograph, and bacteriologic studies of sputum. Drug therapy may include one or more antituberculosis agents, such as isoniazid and rifampin.

Strategies to control the transmission of MTB include the early identification and treatment of those infected with MTB and isolation of those with active disease. The goal of AFB isolation is to prevent the spread of infectious droplet nuclei into the air of the hospital unit. The CDC has presented clear guidelines for the institution of AFB isolation (CDC, 1993). The patient should be instructed to cover all coughs and sneezes with a tissue, if at all possible. If the patient is not capable of doing this, masks must be worn by all those entering the patient's room.

There has recently been increased concern because of the occurrence of outbreaks of tuberculosis caused by strains of MTB that are resistant to more than one of the usual antituberculosis drugs. Because of this multidrug-resistant tuberculosis, one can no longer assume that a patient is noninfectious simply because customary drug therapy has been instituted.

There has also been concern about higher than average rates of occurrence of tuberculosis among patients with HIV infection. These patients are at greater risk for both new infection with MTB and reactivation of latent tuberculosis, although they constitute the minority of tuberculosis patients in most areas of the country. Critical care nurses must be aware that tuberculosis may be difficult to diagnose in persons with HIV infection. The patient frequently presents with another pulmonary infection, such as *Pneumocystis carinii*. Because of impaired immune system function, the tuberculin skin test in the HIV-infected patient may give a false-negative result, and the chest x-ray may not present the typical pattern of lung cavitation. Sputum smears in HIV patients with tuberculosis are less likely to be positive for AFB than those from persons with normal immune systems. Noninfectiousness can only be truly determined by negative findings on sputum smears for three consecutive days for a patient on antituberculosis drug therapy (CDC, 1990a).

Herpes Viruses

Herpes viruses are ubiquitous in the environment, and exposure to them is almost universal before adulthood. Herpes viruses are frequently shed by immunocompromised patients. Infected persons may have lesions, or they may be asymptomatic.

The herpes viruses include herpes simplex viruses, cytomegalovirus, and herpes zoster virus. They all can cause active disease but may also lie dormant in the body for prolonged periods of time and later become reactivated. New infection or reactivation of dormant herpes viruses during pregnancy or the perinatal period can cause serious illness or congenital defects in the newborn.

Herpes Simplex Virus

Herpes simplex virus (HSV) infection can cause a variety of health effects, which include lesions of the oral mucosa, the genital mucosa, or the skin. Transmission from patient to nurse usually occurs from contact with infectious oral, respiratory, or genital secretions. It may also result from contact with skin or mucous membrane lesions.

Herpetic whitlow, also called paronychia, is a painful infection of the cuticle which is not uncommon (Fig. 8–2). It is usually caused by contact with oral or respiratory secretions from an infected patient.

Herpes simplex transmission can be controlled by frequent handwashing and the use of gloves *on both hands* whenever contact with oral, respiratory, or genital secretions is anticipated. The avoidance of direct contact with herpetic lesions also will prevent transmission.

Cytomegalovirus

Most persons are exposed to cytomegalovirus (CMV) during childhood or adolescence, and transmission is believed to occur frequently in daycare

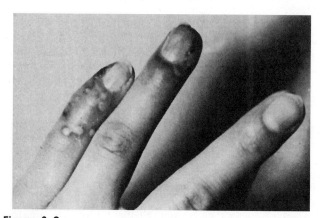

Figure 8–2 ● ● ● ● ● ●

Herpetic whitlow on the finger of a dental technician. (From Crumpacker, C.S. (1987). Herpes simplex. In Fitzpatrick, T., et al. (Eds.). *Dermatology in general medicine: Textbook and atlas* (3rd ed., p. 2308). With permission of The McGraw-Hill Companies.)

centers. CMV is present in the respiratory secretions, urine, saliva, tears, feces, breast milk, semen, and cervical secretions of infected persons. The virus is most commonly spread by respiratory droplets or by direct contact with urine or respiratory secretions. There is evidence that transmission may also occur by ingestion or by sexual contact. CMV is shed by apparently healthy infants and toddlers and by immunocompromised patients.

Infection with CMV may cause a mild flu-like illness but is most often asymptomatic. The greatest concern regarding CMV is its ability to cause negative health effects in the developing fetus. CMV infection occurs in 1% to 2% of live births but causes symptoms in only 10% of those infected. These can range from mild to severe neurologic disorders and defects. Congenital CMV infection may result from either new CMV infection or reactivation of previous infection during pregnancy. Studies of nurses employed in children's hospitals have shown that these nurses do not have a greater incidence of CMV than the general population, and that working in such a setting is not considered to be a major risk factor for acquiring CMV infection (Lipscomb, et al., 1984; Balcarek, et al., 1990).

Prevention of transmission of CMV can be effectively accomplished by adhering to basic good hygiene and routine infection control practices. Perhaps the most important element is thorough handwashing after contact with all patients, especially their body fluids or secretions. Gloves should be used if contact with mucous membranes or body fluids is anticipated. Nurses should refrain from kissing infant and toddler patients.

Varicella Zoster Virus

Both chickenpox (varicella) and shingles (herpes zoster) are caused by varicella zoster virus (VZV). Chickenpox is a common childhood disease. Almost 90% of persons have acquired immunity by adulthood. Chickenpox is usually a mild and self-limiting disease, but occasionally it causes complications such as pneumonia. Symptoms include a vesicular rash, malaise, and slight fever. Chickenpox is easily transmissible, usually by respiratory droplets, but possibly also by direct contact with fluid from lesions. Both chickenpox and shingles are considered communicable until skin lesions are dried and crusted.

Shingles is characterized by a vesicular rash which is localized to one or more dermatomes. Generalized rash occurs occasionally in patients with impaired immune function. Shingles is caused by a reactivation of dormant virus that has resided in the body since a previous infection.

Nurses who do not have a history of chickenpox and who are serologically negative should not care for patients with known VZV infection. However, because VZV shedding occurs for 48 hours before the rash appears, inadvertent exposure of susceptible personnel is not unusual. VZV exposure should be reported immediately to the infection control profes-

sional to avoid an outbreak in the hospital. Nonimmune personnel who have been exposed to VZV are considered potentially infective and must not have direct contact with patients during the incubation period (up to 21 days after exposure).

Neisseria meningitidis Infection

Neisseria meningitidis is a fragile, fastidious, and usually benign bacterium. Rarely, however, it causes serious disease such as meningitis, meningococcal pneumonia, or meningococcemia.

Nosocomial transmission of *N. meningitidis* from patients to healthcare personnel is rare. For such transmission to occur, there must be direct contact with oropharyngeal secretions such as that which might occur during unprotected mouth-to-mouth resuscitation. Droplet spread may be possible in cases of meningococcal pneumonia, particularly if the patient has a productive cough (Williams, 1983).

Symptoms of meningococcal meningitis include fever, headache, irritability, photophobia, stiff neck, and decreased level of consciousness. Meningoccal pneumonia is clinically similar to lower respiratory infections of bacterial origin.

Until *N. meningitidis* has been ruled out as the causative agent, nurses should wear masks whenever they are within 3 feet of the patient with meningitis of unknown etiology. All significant exposures should be reported promptly so that prophylactic antibiotics such as rifampin can be provided within 48 hours of exposure.

SUMMARY

Nurses working in pediatric critical care units face many occupational health and safety hazards. Concern in recent years about exposure to HIV and HBV has precipitated a renewed, strong interest in the entire spectrum of hazards that critical care nurses face every day.

Much research has been done on the topic of occupational hazards, but very little of it is specific to those hazards encountered by nurses in the clinical setting. For example, there is currently no information on the long-term effects on nurses of repeated exposures to low levels of ionizing radiation. Future research on occupational hazards may provide information leading to new and effective preventive strategies.

A general overview of some of the health and safety hazards in the critical care unit has been presented, but to effectively protect themselves and their colleagues, nurses must seek out more detailed information. Critical care nurses must develop a good working knowledge of the hazards they face, so that they can work effectively with hospital administration to assure a safe and healthful workplace for all.

References

Baker, E.L., & Fine, L.J. (1986). Solvent neurotoxicity: the current evidence. *Journal of Occupational Medicine, 28*(2), 126–129.

Balcarek, K., et al. (1990). Cytomegalovirus infection among employees of a children's hospital: No evidence for increased risk associated with patient care. *Journal of the American Medical Association,* 263(6), 840–844.

Beebe, G. (1981). The atomic bomb survivors and the problem of low-dose radiation effects. *American Journal of Epidemiology,* 114(6), 761–783.

California Department of Health Services (1990). *HESIS hazard alert: Ribavirin.* Berkeley, CA: California Department of Health Services.

Centers for Disease Control and Prevention (1988). Assessing exposures of health-care personnel to aerosols of ribavirin—California. *Morbidity and Mortality Weekly Report,* 37(36), 560–563.

Centers for Disease Control and Prevention (1989a). Guidelines for prevention of transmission of human immunodeficiency virus and hepatitis B virus to health-care and public-safety workers. *Morbidity and Mortality Weekly Report,* 38(S-6), 1–37.

Centers for Disease Control and Prevention (1989b). Guidelines for prophylaxis against *Pneumocystis carinii* pneumonia for persons infected with human immunodeficiency virus. *Morbidity and Mortality Weekly Report,* 38(S-5), 1–9.

Centers for Disease Control and Prevention (1989c). Measles prevention: Recommendations of the Immunization Practices Advisory Committee (ACIP). *Morbidity and Mortality Weekly Report,* 38 (no. S-9),

Centers for Disease Control and Prevention (1990a). Guidelines for preventing the transmission of tuberculosis in health-care settings, with special focus on HIV-related issues. *Morbidity and Mortality Weekly Report,* 39 (RR-17), 1–27.

Centers for Disease Control and Prevention (1990b). Protection against viral hepatitis: Recommendations of the Immunization Practices Advisory Committee (ACIP). *Morbidity and Mortality Weekly Report,* 39 (RR-2), 1–23.

Centers for Disease Control and Prevention (1990c). Public health burden of vaccine-preventable diseases among adults: Standards for adult immunization practice. *Morbidity and Mortality Weekly Report,* 39(41), 725–729.

Centers for Disease Control and Prevention (1990d). Rubella prevention: Recommendations of the Immunization Practices Advisory Committee (ACIP). *Morbidity and Mortality Weekly Report,* 39(RR-15), 1–16.

Centers for Disease Control and Prevention (1991). Public Health Service inter-agency guidelines for screening donors of blood, plasma, organs, tissues, and semen for evidence of hepatitis B and hepatitis C. *Morbidity and Mortality Weekly Report,* 40(RR-4), 1–13.

Centers for Disease Control and Prevention (1992). 1993 revised classification system for HIV infection and expanded surveillance case definition for AIDS among adolescents and adults. *Morbidity and Mortality Weekly Report,* 41 (no. RR-17), 1–18.

Centers for Disease Control and Prevention (1993). Draft guidelines for preventing the transmission of tuberculosis in health-care facilities (2nd ed.). *Federal Register,* 58(195):52810–52852.

Davis, R., et al. (1986). Transmission of measles in medical settings 1980 through 1984. *Journal of the American Medical Association,* 255(10), 1295–1298.

Foley, K. (1993). Update for nurse anesthetists—occupational exposure to trace anesthetics: Quantifying the risk. *AANA Journal,* 61(4):405–412.

Greaves, W., et al. (1982). Prevention of rubella transmission in medical facilities. *Journal of the American Medical Association,* 248, 861–864.

Harstad, T.W., Little, B.B., Bawdon, R.E., Knoll, K., Roe, D., & Gilstrap, L.C., III (1990). Embryocidal effects of pentamidine isethionate administration to Sprague-Dawley rats. *American Journal of Obstetrics and Gynecology,* 163(3):912–916.

Lipscomb, J., et al. (1984). Prevalence of cytomegalovirus antibody in nursing personnel. *Infection Control 1984,* 5(11), 513–518.

Mayer, D.K. (1992). Hazards of chemotherapy. Implementing safe handling practices. *Cancer,* 70([Suppl] 4):998.

Myer, M., and Tanascia, J. (1981). Long-term effects of prenatal xray of human females. II. Growth and development. *American Journal of Epidemiology,* 114(3), 317–326.

National Institute for Occupational Safety and Health (1977). *Criteria for a recommended standard: Occupational exposure to waste anesthetic gases and vapors.* Publ. no. 77–140. Washington, D.C.: National Institute for Occupational Safety and Health.

National Institute for Occupational Safety and Health (1988). *Guidelines for protecting the safety and health of the health care worker.* Publ. no. 88–119. Washington, D.C.: National Institute for Occupational Safety and Health.

Occupational Safety and Health Administration (1991). 29 CFR Part 1910.1030, Occupational exposure to bloodborne pathogens; Final rule. *Federal Register,* 56 (235), 64004–64182.

Prows, C. (1989). Ribavirin's risks in reproduction—how great are they? *Maternal Child Nursing,* 14(6), 400–404.

Rogers, B. (1986). Exposure to waste anesthetic gases. *AAOHN Journal,* 34(12), 574–579.

Rogers, B. (1987). Health hazards to personnel handling antineoplastic agents. *Occupational Medicine: State of the Art Reviews,* 2(3), 513–516.

Travers, P.H. (1986a). Application of toxicological concepts to the occupational history. *AAOHN Journal,* 34(11), 524–529, 562–568.

Travers, P.H. (1986b). Toxicology: An overview of fundamental principles. *AAOHN Update Series,* 2(19).

US Nuclear Regulatory Commission (1984). United States Nuclear Regulatory Commission Rules and Regulations (Title 10, Chapter 1, Code of Federal Regulations—Energy. Part 20, Standards for Protection Against Radiation). Washington, D.C.: US Nuclear Regulatory Commission.

Valenti, W. (1986). Infection control and the pregnant health care worker. *American Journal of Infection Control,* 14(1), 20–27.

Williams, W. (1983). Guideline for infection control in hospital personnel. *Infection Control,* 4(4), 326–349.

Yodaiken, R.E. (1986, January 29). Dealing with cytotoxic (antineoplastic) drugs. In *Work practice guidelines for personnel.* Washington, D.C.: Office of Occupational Medicine, Directorate of Technical Support, Occupational Safety and Health Administration (OSHA).

Phenomena of Concern

Critical care nurses are concerned with tissue perfusion, oxygenation and ventilation, acid-base balance, intracranial dynamics, fluid and electrolyte regulation, nutrition, thermal regulation, host defenses, skin integrity, and pain and aversive stimulation in each critically ill infant and child for whom they provide care. These phenomena are the focus of the chapters in this section. Universal care needs, rather than specific primary problems, are examined where nurses play a major role in optimizing patient outcomes through a deliberate proactive process that integrates clinical knowledge and skillfull assessment and intervention. Within each phenomenon of concern for critical care nurses, essential embryology, maturational anatomy and physiology, and instrumentation are discussed.

CHAPTER 9

Tissue Perfusion

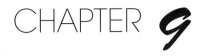

JANIS BLOEDEL SMITH
S. JILL LEY
MARTHA A.Q. CURLEY
E. MARSHA ELIXSON
KATHRYN M. DODDS

The function and survival of cells, organ systems, and the individual are dependent on the maintenance of adequate tissue perfusion. The production of energy for the multitude of functions required for homeostasis is dependent on the delivery of sufficient oxygen and nutrients to cells throughout the body.

Although cells in the human body vary widely in structure and function, mitochondria in all cells are responsible for the production of energy. In the presence of oxygen, the mitochondria synthesize significant quantities of adenosine triphosphate (ATP) from glucose. ATP forms adenosine diphosphate (ADP), releasing cellular energy in the process. Constant energy is available, because ADP can recombine with a phosphate group to form another ATP. Without oxygen (that is, under anaerobic conditions) only a fraction of ATP normally synthesized from glucose is produced. Clearly, if a pathophysiologic process interferes with the delivery of oxygen to cells, all the processes that require energy can be disrupted.

The cardiovascular system is responsible for the delivery of oxygen and nutrients to tissues. Not only does the heart pump continuously to ensure that the billions of cells within the body are adequately perfused, but the cardiovascular system is responsive to demands for more or less blood to tissues.

This chapter provides a foundation for understanding the complex physiology of the cardiovascular system in infants and children. Fetal development of the heart is presented as a basis for understanding the defects in structure seen in congenital heart disease. Essential anatomy of the cardiovascular system is reviewed, and the physiology of cardiovascular performance is developed in greater detail, with attention to the maturational changes that are characteristic of infancy and childhood. Assessment of the cardiovascular system is related to the care of infants and children who are seriously ill and require intensive care. Pharmacologic support of cardiovascular function, pacemaker therapy, and mechanical support of circulation are discussed. Cardiovascular dysfunction is detailed in Chapter 19.

ESSENTIAL EMBRYOLOGY

Cardiac embryologic development begins just prior to the third week of gestation and is normally completed by the seventh week. The cardiovascular system is the first system to function in the embryo; its early development is most likely a response to the high metabolic demands of the rapidly developing fetus.

Development of the Heart

The origin of cardiac tissue is the mesoderm of the embryo. At day 18, during the third gestational week, a crescent, or arch, of mesoderm is formed from a pair of endothelial tubes. The endothelial tubes fuse and grow, establishing a single, straight "heart tube" at about day 20. The primitive heart is characterized by the rhythmic ebb and flow of blood that precedes heart beating.

Continued cellular development around the cardiac

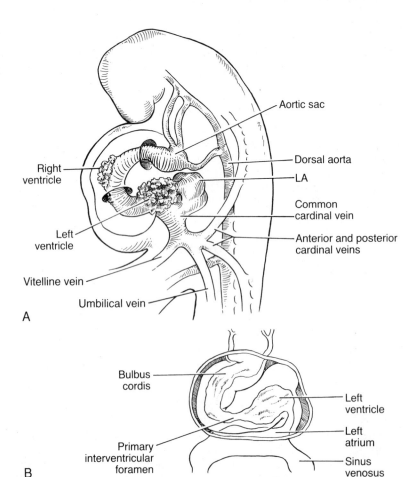

Figure 9–1 ● ● ● ● ● ●

A and *B,* The early embryonic heart. The straight tube has looped; the ventricle is left and posterior; and the bulbus cordis is right and anterior. The definitive right ventricle is noted to bud out of the bulbus cordis. The earliest connection between the primitive (left) ventricle and the evolving right ventricle is the primary interventricular foramen (bulboventricular foramen). (From Holbrook, P.R. (1993). *Textbook of pediatric critical care,* p. 243. Philadelphia: W.B. Saunders.)

tube results in the formation of distinct myocardium and endocardium. By day 22, contractile activity of the heart is evident, and forward blood flow is achieved. Between day 24 and 26, heart beating is evident, as is the regulation of heart rate, vascular tone, and cardiac output through cardiac sympathetic nervous system innervation and action of circulating catecholamines (Ruckman, 1993).

Bulbus Cordis

Because the anterior (arterial) and posterior (venous) ends of the cardiac tube are fixed in place, growth of cardiac tissue occurs in a confined space, causing torsion and flexion of the cardiac tube. At approximately 25 days' gestation, the straight tube has flexed into a loop with the rightward expansion forming the bulboventricular mass—the future right ventricle (Fig. 9–1A). Looping to the right is referred as dextro or D-looping and results in the right ventricle lying to the right of the primitive left ventricle. (Looping to the left is called levo or L-looping, which results in ventricular inversion.)

Differentiation of the ventricles begins as continued hyperplasia of the cardiac tube occurs (see Fig. 9–1B). Growth of the proximal bulbus cordis gives rise to the right ventricle. The midportion of the bulbus cordis, referred to as the conus cordis, gives rise to the outflow portions of both ventricles. The distal portion of the bulbus cordis, the truncus arteriosus, divides into the aortic and pulmonary roots.

Septation of the Heart

The primitive ventricles are connected by the primary interventricular foramen, which is the only route for blood flow into the developing right ventricle because the atrioventricular (AV) canal is associated only with the left ventricle. As the ventricles enlarge, the muscular septum develops from the floor of the ventricles. The endocardial cushions, which initially appear as heaped up masses of endocardium, develop from the walls of the AV canal. The cushions grow toward each other, eventually fusing in a process that results in the origin of two AV valve orifices, each aligned with one ventricle. The tricuspid and mitral valves evolve from the processes, which divide and align the AV canal. A communication between the two ventricles, referred to as the secondary interventricular foramen, persists until the sixth week of gestation (Fig. 9–2). The secondary interventricular foramen closes through contributions from the muscular septum, endocardial cushion tissue, and conus cordis.

The atria are separated by a series of partitions (Fig. 9–3). The first to form is the septum primum, which grows toward the endocardial cushions. Communication between the atria persists through the ostim primum. As septum primum joins the AV septal portion of the AV canal, perforations of the septum primum join to give rise to the septum secundum. Growth of the septum secundum leads to the

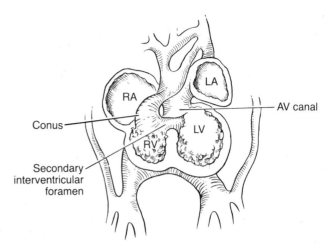

Figure 9–2 ● ● ● ● ●

Septation of the ventricles. The two ventricles are well formed and are connected by the secondary interventricular foramen. The outflow region of the heart is defined by the conus. (From Holbrook, P.R. (1993). *Textbook of pediatric critical care*, p. 243. Philadelphia: W.B. Saunders.)

obliteration of any communication between the atria except for the foramen ovale—the flap-like valve that is covered by a portion of septum primum and permits right-to-left blood flow across the atrial septum throughout gestation.

Conotruncal Development

The truncus arteriosus is the common outlet for blood flow from the heart. It is ultimately separated into an aortic and a pulmonary trunk. Ridges from the bulbus cordis form proximally as truncal ridges form distally. The ridges grow and fuse into the aorticopulmonary septum. Under the influence of streaming blood flow, the common truncus arteriosus spirals and divides into the great arteries, the aorta and pulmonary artery, around day 34 of gestation. Spiraling results in a right-to-left reversal of the aorta from above the right ventricle to the left ventricle. If the aorticopulmonary septum fails to align with the interventricular septum, a ventricular septal defect results. In addition, unequal partitioning or alignment can result in an undersized aorta or pulmonary artery. Persistence of the truncus arteriosus can also result, if aorticopulmonary septation fails, associated with ventricular septal defect, because the bulbar ridges contribute to ventricular septation as well.

The conus cordis, the midportion of the developing bulbus cordis, is important in right ventricular development, particularly in the development of the right ventricular outflow tract. The distal tissues of the conus also participate in septation of the truncus arteriosus. Development of the midportion of the conus results in the establishment of definitive continuity between the left ventricle and the aorta. The right side of the conus establishes the outflow tract or infundibulum of the right ventricle associated with

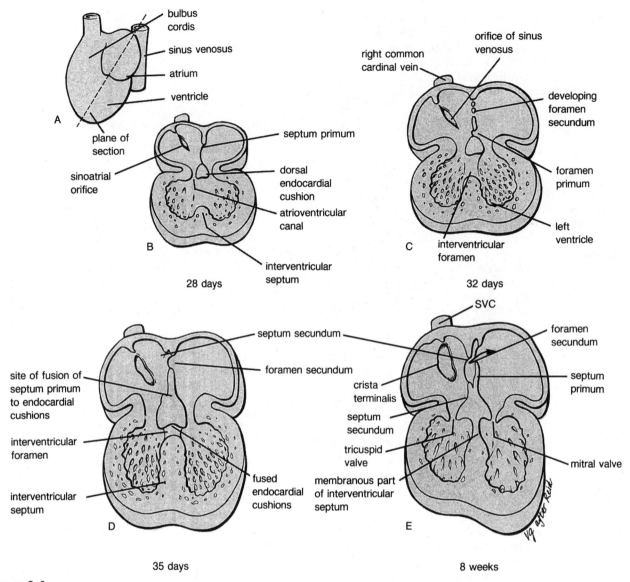

Figure 9–3 ● ● ● ● ● ●

Drawings of the developing heart, showing partitioning of the atrioventricular canal, primitive atrium, and ventricle. *A,* Sketch showing the plane of the coronal sections. *B,* During the fourth week (about 28 days), showing the early appearance of the septum primum, interventricular septum, and dorsal endocardial cushion. *C,* Section of the heart (about 32 days), showing perforations in the dorsal part of the septum. *D,* Section of the heart (about 35 days) showing the foramen secundum. *E,* About 8 weeks, showing the heart after it is partitioned into four chambers. (From Moore, K.L., Persaud, T.V.N., & Shiota, K. (1994). *Color atlas of clinical embryology,* p. 185. Philadelphia: W.B. Saunders.)

the pulmonary trunk. If the conus is inverted, transposition of the great arteries results. Double outlet right ventricle or Taussig-Bing malformation can result when the subaortic conus is not absorbed.

Pulmonary and Systemic Veins

The common pulmonary vein grows from the posterior atrial wall as atrial septation is developing (Fig. 9–4). It forms connections with the splanchnic plexus, which is associated with both the developing lungs and the cardinal venous system, which in turn drains into the umbilical vein. Growth and expansion of the common pulmonary vein establishes four drainage channels from the lungs. As the individual pulmonary veins are defined and enlarged, the left atrium enlarges as well, incorporating the pulmonary veins directly into its posterior wall. Connections of the systemic veins into the splanchnic plexus are separated as the individual pulmonary veins are defined. Consequently, all pulmonary venous drainage from the splanchnic plexus flows to the left atrium via the pulmonary veins. Persistence of connections between the cardinal venous and pulmonary venous systems results in partial or total anomalous pulmonary venous connection or drainage.

The sinus venosus is the proximal end of the cardiac tube, the inlet chamber of the primitive heart.

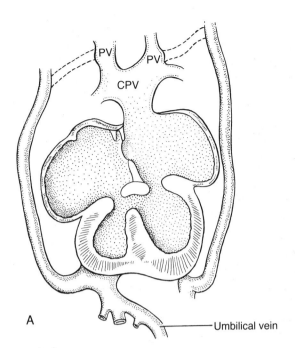
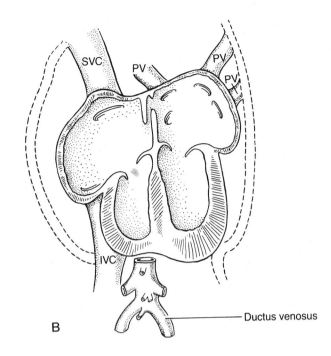

Figure 9–4 ● ● ● ● ● ●

A, Development of the common pulmonary vein. As the individual pulmonary veins are defined, connections to the systemic veins are lost. During this time, ventricular and atrial septation are proceeding. *B,* Connection of the pulmonary veins. The common pulmonary vein becomes incorporated into the back of the left atrium, allowing connection of four individual veins. Septation is complete, and the cardinal system has atrophied. (From Holbrook, P.R. (1993). *Textbook of pediatric critical care,* p. 244. Philadelphia: W.B. Saunders.)

The right sinus horn ultimately forms the superior vena cava (SVC). The coronary sinus is formed from the proximal left sinus horn and the connection of the two sinus horns. By the end of the sixth week of gestation, the establishment of the SVC and separation of pulmonary drainage of the splanchnic plexus result in involution of the left common cardinal vein and the distal portion of the left sinus horn. The left innominate vein develops from the left common cardinal system. The right common cardinal system may persist as the azygous vein.

Atrioventricular Valves

The mitral and tricuspid valves develop primarily from the ventricles, with small contributions to the anterior leaflets of both derived from the tissue that surrounds the developing AV valve orifices. Sheets of tissue are formed along ventricular trabeculations that subsequently create definitive valve leaflets with supporting tendons and muscles. The anterior leaflet of the mitral valve receives an important contribution from the superior endocardial cushion. The tricuspid valve develops almost exclusively from the right ventricle. Mitral valve development is complete before development of the tricuspid valve, which continues into 12 weeks of gestation.

Semilunar Valves

Partitioning of the truncus arteriosus into the aorta and pulmonary trunk has occurred by 33 days of gestation. Paired swellings of truncus cushion tissue form the primitive aortic and pulmonic valves. Blood flow through the valves results in evacuation and migration of the valves through 6 weeks of gestation.

Aortic Arch

Six pairs of aortic arches develop from the truncus arteriosus, giving rise to major arteries and the aortic arch itself. Head and neck arteries develop from the third and fourth pair of arches. The fourth arch also develops into the aortic isthmus or the definitive aortic arch. The right and left sixth arches form the right and left pulmonary arteries. The distal portion of the left sixth arch persists as the ductus arteriosus. Incomplete involution of the aortic arch vessels can result in coarctation of the aorta, interrupted aortic arch, and other defects.

Congenital Cardiac Defects

There is no single classification system that separates cardiac malformations into major etiologic groups. One classification system divides congenital heart defects (CHD) into four groups (Table 9–1): (1) anomalies of the three major cardiac segments; (2) defects of cardiac septation; (3) congenital defects of the arterial wall and intracardiac connective tissue; and (4) congenital abnormalities of the endomyocardium (Neill, 1972).

Table 9–1. ETIOLOGIC CLASSIFICATION OF CONGENITAL HEART DISEASES

Defects of the Major Cardiac Segments
Dextrocardia
Levocardia
Corrected transposition
Tetralogy of Fallot
Transposition of the great arteries
Defects of Cardiac Septation
Atrial septal defect
Ventricular septal defect
Endocardial cushion defect
Aortic stenosis (valvar and subvalvar)
Pulmonic valve stenosis
Defects of the Arterial Wall and Cardiac Connective Tissue
Persistent ductus arteriosus
Coarctation of the aorta
Interrupted aortic arch
Peripheral pulmonary stenosis
Supravalvar aortic stenosis
Aortic, pulmonary or mitral insufficiency
Defects of the Endomyocardium
Endocardial fibroelastosis
Glycogen storage disease
Idiopathic hypertrophic subaortic stenosis
Cardiac conduction disorders

Defects of Cardiac Segmentation

Van Praagh and Pvlad (1967) described the heart as consisting of three major segments: visceroatrial situs, the ventricular loop, and the conotruncus. Defects of the **visceroatrial situs** include dextrocardia and levocardia. Dextrocardia, or a structurally normal but malpositioned heart that is the mirror image of the usual position, is inherited by a recessive gene. Levocardia may also be similarly inherited, but is associated with complex structural malformations of the heart. In both, situs inversus of the abdominal viscera coexists.

The developing ventricle normally loops towards the embryo's right, making a dextro or D loop. **Abnormal ventricular looping** results in CHD such as corrected transposition of the great arteries, which is associated with defects in cardiac septation and abnormalities of the atrioventricular (AV) valves.

All the major cyanotic CHDs are most likely the result of **anomalies of the developing conotruncus.** Abnormal development of this vital area of the fetal heart may result in tetralogy of Fallot or transposition of the great arteries, the two most common cyanotic heart defects. Abnormal development of the conus almost invariably leads to secondary defects, including defects of the ventricular septum.

Defects of Cardiac Septation

Defects of the atrial septum are among the most common CHDs. Most are compatible with multifactoral inheritance. Defects of the ventricular septum are even more common. This is probably the case because the ventricular septum closes over a long period of time (as compared with other developmental occurrences in the fetal heart), leaving it susceptible to adverse environmental conditions over a lengthy time period.

The endocardial cushions play a role in both atrial and ventricular septation, as well as in the formation of the AV valves. Defects in their development result in severe CHD, including ostium primum atrial septal defect and complete AV canal defect. Infants with trisomy 21 have about a 40% incidence of CHD, almost all involving defects of atrial or ventricular septation and maldevelopment of the endocardial cushions. Although the precise reason for this association is not known, the other major autosomal trisomies (15 and 18) also show endocardial cushion anomalies and ventricular septal defects.

Bicuspid aortic valve is a common CHD that is most often evidenced in adulthood. Pulmonic valvular stenosis is a common defect with origins in malformation of the endocardial cushions. Localized, fibrous subaortic stenosis is also related.

Defects of the Arterial Wall and Intracardiac Connective Tissue

Patency of the ductus arteriosus is most likely the result of both prenatal and perinatal influences. Premature infants and those infants with congenital rubella syndrome have a higher incidence of patent ductus arteriosus. Perinatal hypoxia plays a role in persistent patency of the ductus, although its exact role is unclear. There is increased incidence of persistent patent ductus arteriosus among infants born at high altitude, and the ductus remains patent somewhat longer in infants with cyanotic heart disease than in the normal.

Coarctation of the aorta and interrupted aortic arch may be the result of reduced flow across the left ventricular outflow tract. Patients with interrupted aortic arch usually have a large ventricular septal defect and may have other associated complex cardiac anomalies, such as transposition of the great arteries and double outlet right ventricle. These cases reflect complex events during cardiogenesis related to altered migration of neural crest cells, which contribute to the development of the aortic arch and the conotruncal region of the heart. Neural crest cells are also important in the development of the thymus. The association of interrupted aortic arch and DiGeorge syndrome (congenital absence of the thymus) may be related to neural crest abnormalities.

Coarctation of the aorta may occur as an isolated defect, suggesting that the events contributing to its development may occur after development of the heart is complete. Coarctation usually involves a shelf of tissue that extends in the aortic wall around its circumference. The shelf may be related to the orifice of the left subclavian artery or to the insertion of the ductus arteriosus at the site of the narrowing.

Congenital rubella syndrome is associated with generalized hypoplasia of the pulmonary artery branches, which results in peripheral pulmonic stenosis. Supravalvular aortic stenosis is often a familial problem.

Abnormalities of intracardiac connective tissue may lead to aortic, pulmonary, or mitral insufficiency. In patients with Marfan's syndrome, myxomatous degeneration of valve leaflets most often affects the aortic and mitral valves.

Congenital Anomalies of the Myocardium, Endocardium, and Conducting System

Endocardial fibroelastosis (EFE) is a sequel to perinatal viral infection. Glycogen storage disease is a metabolic disorder in which the myocardium is infiltrated with glycogen. It is the result of a recessive gene. Antenatal diagnosis is possible because the enzymatic abnormality has been defined. Idiopathic hypertrophic subaortic stenosis (IHSS) is a progressive cardiomyopathy usually manifested in early adult life and associated with left ventricular failure, cardiomegaly, and rhythm disturbances. The degree of left ventricular outflow obstruction varies between individuals. It is most likely transmitted by a dominant gene, but shows variable and delayed expressivity.

Several disorders of cardiac conduction, including Wolff-Parkinson-White (WPW) syndrome, have been reported in families. However, the mode of inheritance of WPW syndrome is unclear. The Nielsen-DeLange syndrome, in which a long QT interval is associated with recurrent episodes of ventricular fibrillation, is genetically transmitted by a dominant mode of inheritance.

Fetal Circulation

Structure and function of the fetal cardiovascular system not only support fetal life and development, but also permit nearly instantaneous transition to extrauterine life at birth. During fetal life, the placenta is the source of oxygenated blood, which flows from the placenta via the umbilical vein to the fetal liver (Fig. 9–5). Here, flow is divided. Some blood is directed to the developing liver and abdominal viscera, while most is shunted through the ductus venosus to the fetal inferior vena cava (IVC). The most oxygen-rich blood passes up the IVC where it preferentially streams across the foramen ovale to the left atrium and left ventricle, aortic arch, and to the developing heart (via the coronary circulation) and brain.

Blood from the coronary circulation, brain, and upper body of the fetus returns to the fetal heart via the superior vena cava (SVC). Flow from the SVC, which is less oxygen-rich than IVC blood, drains into the right ventricle and is ejected into the pulmonary artery. Flow here is again divided. The majority flows across the ductus arteriosus to the descending aorta. All but 7% to 8% is shunted away from the fetal lungs. SVC blood mixes with a smaller volume of blood descending from the aortic arch and supplies

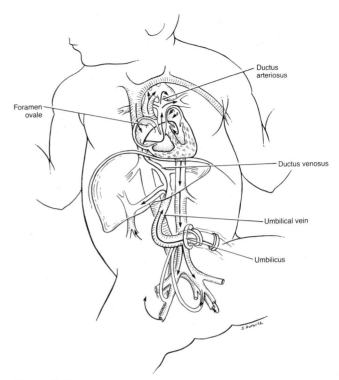

Figure 9–5 ● ● ● ● ● ●
The fetal circulation. Flow from the placenta is directed into the umbilical vein, through the liver via the ductus venosus, and into the right atrium. Streaming, aided by venous valves, carries the oxygenated blood through the foramen ovale to the systemic circulation. Smaller flows proceed through the right heart and ductus arteriosus to the descending aorta. (From Holbrook, P.R. (1993). *Textbook of pediatric critical care*, p. 246. Philadelphia: W.B. Saunders.)

the lower body of the fetus and returns to the placenta via the umbilical arteries.

Fetal oxygenation is unique. Blood from the placenta is 70% to 80% saturated with oxygen (Po_2 32–35 mmHg). Blood ejected from the left ventricle, perfusing the heart, head, and brain, is 65% to 70% oxygenated (Po_2 28–30 mmHg). Oxygen saturation in the descending aorta is 60% to 65% (Po_2 20–22 mmHg). Blood returning to the placenta in the umbilical arteries is less than 60% saturated (Po_2 14–21 mmHg). Polycythemia and fetal hemoglobin, which has an increased affinity for oxygen, permit compensation for the relative hypoxia of the fetal environment.

The largest volume of flow to the fetal heart is through the IVC. Therefore, the hepatic circulation and the ductus venosus are significant regulators of the total venous return. During periods of fetal stress or hypoxia, the ductus venosus dilates to preserve delivery of oxygenated blood to the heart. As a consequence, less blood is directed through the hepatic veins. In addition, a larger percentage of SVC blood flows across the foramen ovale rather than streaming almost exclusively into the right ventricle. Both factors allow more efficient delivery of oxygen and nutrients to vital organs (Ruckman, 1993).

Fetal Cardiac Output

During fetal life, cardiac output is regulated by mechanisms that are similar to those that function in the mature cardiovascular system. However, fetal response to regulatory mechanisms is different. As is true of the infant after birth, the capacity for change of stroke volume is limited. Thus, the heart rate response to demands for increased cardiac output is especially important. Similarly, although the relationship between end-diastolic volume and stroke volume holds, the fetal heart, like that of the infant, functions near the top of the Frank-Starling curve. Because fetal myocardium does not readily distend, changes in filling volume or pressure result in little change in cardiac performance. Finally, as is also true in the infant, afterload is the primary regulator of cardiac output. When afterload is increased, cardiac output falls because of the limited capacity for increased contractility related to limited numbers of myofibrils and less efficient calcium exchange across the myocardial cell membrane.

Fetal Stress Response

Hypoxia is the major stress to the fetal heart. The mature cardiovascular system responds to hypoxia via neurohormonal and local vascular pathways, which result in tachycardia, vasoconstriction, increased cardiac output, and redistribution of blood flow to the brain and myocardium. However, in the fetus, hypoxia leads to bradycardia rather than tachycardia. Bradycardia results from both vagal action and decreased myocardial oxygenation. In addition, because hypoxia stimulates vasoconstriction in the fetus, afterload is increased and both right and left ventricular output falls.

Circulatory Changes at Birth

Rapid adaptation to extrauterine life occurs at birth as the neonate takes a first breath and the umbilical cord is clamped. The establishment of respiration is associated with increased Po_2. In addition, the onset of breathing stimulates synthesis of pulmonary vascular prostacyclin, which is undetectable in fetal life. Both prostacyclin and increased Po_2 have pulmonary vasodilatory effects. As a consequence, pulmonary vascular resistance (PVR) falls acutely within 15 minutes and pulmonary blood flow (PBF) increases. Pulmonary venous return to the left atrium is increased, raising left atrial pressure and forcing closure of the foramen ovale. Only functionally closed, the foramen ovale may open and permit right-to-left blood flow if PVR increases abruptly, as occurs with crying.

The ductus arteriosus, which diverts blood away from the pulmonary circuit during fetal life, may permit a persistent right-to-left shunt for up to 3 days in the normal newborn as a consequence of nearly equal pulmonary artery and aortic pressures.

More commonly, PVR decreases rapidly, such that mean pulmonary artery pressure decreases from 60 to 30 mmHg during the first 10 hours of life. Right-to-left shunting is normally observed for about 6 hours after birth. Thereafter, flow across the ductus arteriosus is reversed because systemic vascular resistance (SVR) and pressure are greater than that in the pulmonary circuit. Left-to-right shunting persists for an additional 9 hours. At about 15 hours, the ductus demonstrates physiologic (functional) closure. Ductal closure is partially a response to increased Po_2, which induces constriction of the duct. In addition, prostacyclin synthesis, responsible for pulmonary vasodilation, decreases significantly by 5 hours of life. Thrombosis and fibrosis of the ductus, which result in anatomic closure into the ligamentum arteriosum, take several more days and may extend into the first few weeks of life. During this time, the ductus may open and close physiologically.

Ductal patency may be reestablished or maintained by an intravenous infusion of the potent vasodilator prostaglandin E_1. Conversely, agents such as indomethacin, which inhibit prostacyclin, stimulate ductal closure.

Cardiac output (CO) increases steadily following birth as the right and left ventricles begin functioning in circular series and as a consequence of increased left ventricular end-diastolic volume. The increase in left ventricular volume is the result of several factors: decreased PVR and right ventricular afterload and increased PBF with subsequently increased pulmonary venous return to the left ventricle. The drop in PVR over time is exponential. By 6 weeks of age, resistance in the pulmonary circuit falls to levels near the normal adult range.

The normal adaptation of the cardiovascular system, which occurs at and following birth, may be delayed or severely impaired in sick newborns. Infants with hypoxemia, hypercarbia and acidosis, hypothermia, sepsis, low gestational age, hematologic abnormalities, and left-to-right cardiac shunting are at risk for delayed adaptation of the cardiovascular system to extrauterine life. Persistence of fetal circulatory pathways (i.e., the right-to-left shunts at the ductus arteriosus and foramen ovale) are related to continuing high PVR.

ESSENTIAL ANATOMY AND PHYSIOLOGY

Structure and function of the cardiovascular system are designed to deliver metabolic nutrients to cells and remove the end-products of metabolism. The system is composed of the heart, which is divided into two coordinated pumps (the right ventricle and the left ventricle), and two circulations. The pulmonary circulation is between the right and left sides of the heart and the systemic circulation between the left and right sides of the heart.

The heart is divided longitudinally by the interatrial and interventricular septa. The right and left atria are thin-walled chambers that function primarily as reservoirs for blood returning to the heart. Atrial contraction at the end of ventricular diastole propels a small percentage of the end-diastolic volume into the ventricles. The atria are separated from the ventricles by the AV valves: the tricuspid valve on the right and the mitral valve on the left. During ventricular diastole, the AV valves are open and blood flows through each into the relaxed muscular ventricles. During ventricular systole the ventricular muscle contracts and blood is propelled through the semilunar valves, the pulmonary valve on the right and the aortic valve on the left, into the pulmonary artery and the aorta.

Because the pulmonary circulation is short and broad, resistance to flow through it is low. In contrast, the systemic circulation is longer and has higher resistance to flow. As a consequence, right heart and pulmonary pressures are low as compared with left heart and systemic pressures. However, it is important to note that these characteristics are present in the mature cardiovascular system. The transition from fetal circulation to neonatal circulation includes changes in the resistance and pressure in the pulmonary circulation and the right heart.

Ventricular contraction produces a pressure pulse that propels blood through the arteries. The arteries branch into arterioles and capillaries, which distribute blood to the microcirculation where oxygen and nutrients are delivered to tissues and metabolic waste products are removed. The venules and veins coalesce as they return blood to the heart. The arterioles are the primary regulators of vascular resistance. As they branch, the total cross-sectional area of the circulatory system is high and flow decreases. The veins are capacitance vessels that serve as reservoirs for blood, and they contain nearly two-thirds of the total blood volume. As they coalesce, the cross-sectional area of circulation decreases and flow increases as blood returns to the heart.

Blood moves from the arterial to the venous side of the circulation along a pressure gradient. Pressure steadily declines along the circulatory pathway. Mean arterial pressure in children is approximately 60 mmHg, central venous pressure about 6 mmHg, and right ventricular end-diastolic pressure 0 to 2 mmHg. The pulmonary system has similar arterial-venous pressure differences, although the magnitude of the difference is less (Fig. 9–6).

The Heart

The heart is located within the thoracic cavity in the mediastinal space, and is covered by the loosely fitting fibrous pericardium. The pericardium provides the heart with physical protection and a barrier to infection. It limits, to a degree, overdistension of the heart chambers. The pericardium consists of an inner serous layer and an outer fibrous layer. Between the layers is the pericardial space, a potential space that normally contains a small volume of serous fluid that

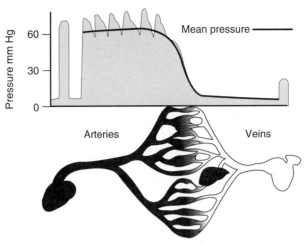

Figure 9–6 ● ● ● ● ● ●
Resistance and resulting loss of pressure within the circulation. Arterial pressure diminishes very rapidly in the small resistance vessels of the circulation. In the venous vessels the pressure gradient is very low. (Redrawn from Kinney, M.R., et al. (1988). *AACN's clinical reference for critical care nursing,* [2nd ed.] St. Louis: Mosby–Year Book.)

acts as a lubricant during cardiac contraction and relaxation.

The heart is suspended by the great vessels and is positioned obliquely, so that the right atrium and ventricle are almost fully anterior to the left. Only a small portion of the lateral left ventricle is on the frontal plane of the heart.

Fibrous Skeleton

The cardiac skeleton consists of four interconnecting valve rings and surrounding connective tissues. It forms a rigid support for attachment of the heart valves and for insertion of cardiac muscle and separates the atria from the ventricles.

Cardiac Musculature

The walls of the heart are composed of two layers in the atria and three in the ventricles. Atrial muscle fibers originate in and insert on the fibrous cardiac skeleton. Deep muscle fibers within each atria propel blood through the AV valves with atrial contraction. Superficial muscle fibers pass through both atria and produce lateral constriction of the chambers and coordinated contraction between them.

The walls of the ventricle consist of three layers. The endocardium lines the ventricular chambers and is continuous with the lining of the blood vessels that leave the heart and with the myocardium. The myocardium is the middle layer and the epicardium the outermost layer. The muscle fibers of the ventricle arise from the fibrous skeleton and the roots of the aorta and pulmonary artery. The muscle fibers in each ventricle are interlocking and change orientation as they pass from the epicardium, through the myocardium to the endocardium. The interlocking arrangement of the fibers produces both circumferential and longitudinal compression of the ventricular chamber during cardiac contraction, which propels blood into the great arteries.

The Heart Valves

Unidirectional flow of blood through the heart and into the great arteries is provided by the heart valves. The opening and closing motion of the valves is most likely the passive result of pressure changes between the heart chambers and between the ventricles and great arteries. During ventricular systole, the valve leaflets, valve annulus, papillary muscles, chordae tendineae, and atrial wall all function to ensure closure and competency of the AV valves. The valve leaflets begin to close when pressure in the ventricle exceeds atrial pressure. The valve annulus narrows as the ventricular chamber becomes smaller with contraction. Contraction of the papillary muscles exerts tension on the chordae tendineae to prevent eversion of the valve leaflets.

The aortic and pulmonic valves have three cusps, permitting them to open widely with ventricular ejection. During ventricular diastole the cusps collect the retrograde flow of blood in the great arteries, ensuring complete closure of the valve.

There are no valves where blood enters the heart from the systemic and pulmonary veins. When outflow from either atria is impeded, the venous system becomes congested.

The Coronary Circulation

The blood supply for the heart is provided by the coronary arteries, which arise in the aortic root just above the aortic valve and traverse the heart's surface in the epicardium. The major epicardial vessels are the right coronary artery and the left main coronary artery, which divides near its origin to form the left anterior descending branch and the circumflex branch. The epicardial coronary arteries give off penetrating branches that perfuse the myocardium. Although the usual origin and course of the coronaries arteries is well described, a number of variations are recognized to occur fairly commonly. Figure 9–7 illustrates the usual route of the coronaries.

The right coronary artery runs laterally and posteriorly from its origin in the atrioventricular sulcus between the right atrium and right ventricle. The acute marginal branches perfuse the right ventricular freewall. The right coronary artery turns downward in the posterior right ventricular epicardium in the posterior interventricular sulcus and becomes the posterior descending coronary artery. The posterior descending artery perfuses the posterior aspect of the interventricular septum and a portion of the posterior left ventricle.

The left main coronary artery is very short and branches into the left anterior descending and the circumflex arteries. The left anterior descending runs in the anterior interventricular sulcus in an inferior

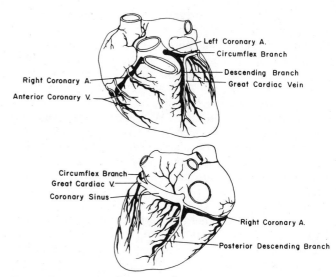

Figure 9–7 ● ● ● ● ● ●

Diagram showing location of major coronary arteries and veins on anterior (*top*) and posterior (*bottom*) surfaces of the heart. (From Little, R., Little, W. (1985). *Physiology of the heart and circulation.* By permission of Mosby–Year Book, Inc.)

direction, branching into septal perforates that perfuse most of both the interventricular septum and the conduction system. The anterior and lateral walls of the left ventricle are perfused by diagonal branches. The circumflex artery runs posteriorly in the atrioventricular sulcus and with its major branches perfuses the posterior wall of the left ventricle.

After passing through the arteries and capillary beds, venous blood from the myocardium drains through the cardiac and coronary veins and the coronary sinus into the right atrium.

Coronary artery blood flow is regulated by the metabolic needs of the heart muscle. When cardiac work is increased, generalized coronary artery vasodilation occurs. The precise mediators of the vasodilation have not yet been fully determined, but carbon dioxide, reduced oxygen tension, lactic acid, hydrogen ions, and other metabolites have been suggested. The sympathetic nervous system (SNS) also plays a role in regulating coronary blood flow. Both alpha and beta receptors are known to exist in the coronary arteries.

Cardiac contraction affects blood flow through the coronary arteries. Unlike flow in other arteries, coronary blood flow occurs during ventricular diastole rather than during systole. During systole, the muscular contraction compresses the coronary arteries and reduces flow.

Metabolic Needs of the Myocardium

Under normal conditions the heart extracts and consumes 60% to 80% of the oxygen delivered by the coronary arteries, compared with the approximately 25% consumed by skeletal muscle. As a consequence, there is little oxygen reserve in coronary venous blood. Demands for increased oxygen are met by increased coronary flow. During strenuous exercise, coronary blood flow increases four to five times to meet the energy requirements of the heart.

The oxygen demands of the heart are a function of the ventricular wall tension generated to pump blood, the stroke volume that is ejected, the contractile state of the myocardium, and the heart rate. When wall tension is greater, as occurs with ventricular dilation, the heart expends more energy to overcome the tension and decrease its size in contraction. Stroke work is the effort the heart expends to pump blood. The stroke work of the heart is determined by the volume of blood ejected with each beat and the pressure the ventricle must develop to eject blood against the resistances to flow. The contractile state of the myocardium refers to the heart's inherent ability to modulate its force of contraction without a change in end-diastolic volume, heart rate, or arterial pressure. Heart rate reflects the frequency with which the heart repeats the energy-consuming process of contraction. A higher heart rate increases oxygen demand.

The Conduction System

A unique rhythmic property of the heart allows it to beat independent of nervous system stimulation. Unlike skeletal muscle, the heart generates and conducts its own electrical impulses (action potentials). The conduction system of the heart is composed of modified myocardial tissue that forms the sinus (sinoatrio [SA]) node, the atrial internodal tracts, the AV node, the His (common) bundle, the right and left bundle branches, and the Purkinje fibers (Fig. 9–8). These specialized tissues both generate and transmit electrical impulses more rapidly than other cardiac tissue, allowing control of heart rate and rhythm.

Normally, cells in the SA node initiate an electrical impulse that spreads to other cells via low-resistance pathways in the specialized conduction tissues throughout the atria to the AV node. Transmission of the impulse is slowed through the junctional fibers of the AV node to approximately 1/25th the speed of conduction in other cardiac tissues. The delay in the transmission of electrical impulses at the AV node permits atrial contraction to occur before ventricular contraction begins. The impulse then spreads to the His bundle, bundle branches, Purkinje fibers, and, finally, from cell to cell in the ventricles. Transmission of the action potential in the ventricle is very rapid, allowing for simultaneous excitation of the right and left ventricle and rapid ejection of blood from the heart.

Mechanisms of Contraction

Cardiac muscle fibers are composed of a number of independent cylindrical elements called myofibrils. Each myofibril consists of smaller units that contain thin actin and thick myosin filaments. Each unit is a

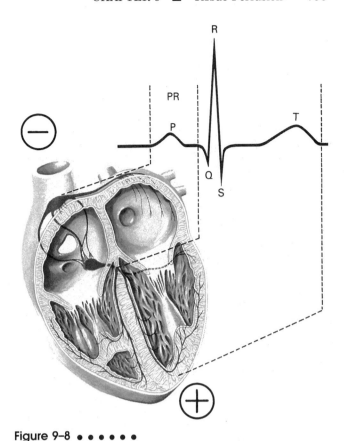

Figure 9–8 ● ● ● ● ● ●

The conduction system and corresponding normal waveforms utilizing lead II. (From Curley, M.A.Q. (1985). *Pediatric cardiac dysrhythmias,* p. 43. Bowie, MD: Brady Communications.)

sarcomere, the functional unit of the contractile system in muscle. The actin and myosin filaments are embedded in the sarcoplasmic reticulum, an intracellular system of longitudinal tubules (T tubules) that conduct action potentials across the myofibrils and lateral sacs, which store calcium for release during muscle contraction.

When cardiac myofibrils are relaxed, the active binding sites for myosin on actin are blocked or inhibited by regulatory proteins. An action potential propagated along the T tubule triggers the release of calcium from the lateral sacs of the sarcoplasmic reticulum and increases calcium diffusion from the interstitial fluid into the cytosol, the area of the actin and myosin filaments. The calcium ions bind with regulatory proteins in the myofibril, exposing the binding sites for myosin on actin. The myosin attaches to the actin, using energy from ATP. The binding, or crossbridging, of actin and myosin pulls the actin fiber past the myosin fiber toward the center of the sarcomere and results in fiber shortening. This process is repeated many times during a single contraction, as long as calcium and ATP are available.

During muscle relaxation, calcium influx ceases and active calcium pumps in the sarcoplasmic reticulum and T tubule remove calcium from the cytosol. The active binding sites on the actin filaments are again inhibited. Calcium is also removed by means of the nonenergy-dependent sodium-calcium exchange, in which two internal calcium ions are exchanged for one external sodium ion.

The strength and rate of contraction and the rate and degree of relaxation are both determined by intracellular calcium concentration, the rate of calcium exchange, and the resting myofibril length. Each of these factors influences the number of actin and myosin crossbridges that form. At rest, maximal crossbridge formation does not occur and there is considerable systolic or contractile reserve. When sympathetic nervous system stimulation occurs, however, the amount of calcium that enters the cell and the rate of calcium exchange through energy-dependent channels are both increased. The strength of contraction, as well as the rate of contraction and relaxation, are greater. Medications that block calcium exchange channels decrease contractility and slow the rate of contraction and relaxation. In addition, in heart failure or intravascular volume overload with excessive myofibril stretch, crossbridge formation is decreased. Chronic heart failure results in depletion of endogenous catecholamine stores, which decreases calcium transport, further impairing contractile performance. Digitalis drugs, which block the sodium channels, increase the amount of calcium available and improve contractility. Myocardial ischemia and hypoxemia impair calcium transport out of the cytosol, diminishing ventricular relaxation and decreasing compliance.

The Heart's Electrical Activity

The electrical activity of myocardial cells depends primarily on changes in cell membrane permeability to the cations sodium, potassium, and calcium. Membrane permeability to these and other ions is dependent on the electrochemical gradient of the ions on each side of the membrane and the function of ionic pumps in the cell membrane. Movement of ions across the cell membrane occurs both passively along the electrochemical gradient and via energy-dependent ion pumps in the cell membrane, which actively transport ions against their electrochemical gradient.

Electrical activity or action potential in cardiac cells is divided into five phases, which are illustrated in Figure 9–9 and are summarized as follows:

Phase 0: depolarization, characterized by the rapid upstroke of the action potential
Phase 1: the brief period of repolarization
Phase 2: the plateau, which causes the action potential of cardiac muscle to persist far longer than in other muscle, resulting in a correspondingly increased period of contraction
Phase 3: the period of repolarization
Phase 4: the resting membrane potential

The cardiac cell membrane in a resting state is permeable to potassium and slightly permeable to sodium and calcium. Potassium slowly diffuses out

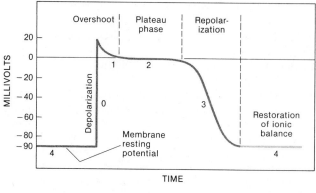

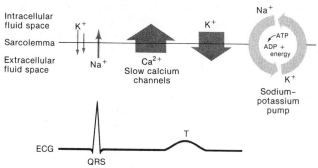

Figure 9–9 ● ● ● ● ● ●

Transmembrane potential in the resting, depolarized, and repolarized states. (Redrawn from Lipman, B.S., Dunn, M., & Massie, E. (1984). *Clinical electrocardiography,* 7th ed., p. 35. By permission of Mosby–Year Book, Inc.)

of the intracellular compartment along its electrochemical concentration gradient, leaving the inside of the cell increasingly negative in charge. The resting membrane potential of the cell is -90 mV, which is established by the passive movement of potassium out of the cell and minimal influx of sodium and calcium ions. With electrical excitation of the membrane during phase 0, the cell membrane permeability to sodium increases rapidly as the voltage-regulated fast sodium channels open. There is rapid influx of sodium into the cell, as well as slowing of the efflux of potassium, so that the membrane potential rises to $+30$ mV. In phase 1, the fast sodium channels close, abruptly decreasing the membrane's permeability to sodium. Slow efflux of potassium continues, bringing the membrane potential to near 0 mV.

Partial depolarization of the cell membrane results in the opening of the slow sodium and calcium channels in phase 2. The influx of calcium and sodium matches the efflux of potassium, and the cell membrane remains depolarized. The influx of calcium stimulates actin and myosin crossbridge formation, and mechanical contraction results. In the phase 3 repolarization period, the influx of sodium and calcium ceases as the slow channels close and membrane permeability to potassium rises sharply. The efflux of potassium from the cell restores the resting membrane potential at phase 4, which corresponds mechanically with ventricular diastole.

Following an action potential there is a period during which the cell membrane is not polarized and cannot accept another electrical stimulus. During phases 0, 1, and 2, the cell is absolutely refractory or completely insensitive to stimulation. As the cell membrane potential is reestablished during phase 3, the cell is relatively refractory. That is, a more intense stimulus is required to initiate an action potential. At the end of phase 3, a supernormal period permits stimulation of an action potential by a weak stimulus. In cardiac muscle, the absolute refractory period is prolonged. Because this period is nearly as long as the heart's contraction, a second contraction cannot be stimulated until the first is over. The length of the absolute refractory period permits the alternating contraction and relaxation of cardiac muscle essential for its pumping action.

Sinus Node Action Potential

Electrical activity in the sinus node differs from that described above (which is characteristic of the cells of the atria, ventricles, interatrial conducting fibers, and Purkinje fibers) in several important ways (Fig. 9–10). In the sinus node, the resting membrane potential is −55 to −60 mV. The fast sodium channels are inactive at this membrane charge. During phase 0 of the sinus action potential, the rise is relatively slow because it is the result of opening of the slow calcium and sodium channels. There is no plateau phase (phase 2). Instead, when the slow calcium and sodium channels are inactivated and potassium efflux occurs, repolarization is permitted.

The third difference between the two cardiac action potentials is the spontaneous rise of phase 4 in the action potential of the sinus node. This rise is the basis of automaticity in the pacemaker cells of the heart, which produces an action potential without an outside stimulus such as is required for skeletal muscle. During phase 4 in these cells there is a slow

decrease in the efflux of potassium from the cell, which limits the negativity of the cell's interior, or an increase in influx of sodium and calcium, which exerts the same effect or both (Guyton, 1991). As a consequence, the cells automatically (or spontaneously) reach the threshold for depolarization and initiate depolarization of the entire heart.

The slope of the rise in phase 4 of the heart's pacemaker cells is influenced by the autonomic nervous system. The neurotransmitters epinephrine and norepinephrine, released when the SNS is stimulated, increase the slope of phase 4 to firing threshold by increasing cell membrane permeability to calcium. Sinus node firing is increased as a consequence. These neurotransmitters act along the entire length of the conduction system, increasing conduction velocity. Contractile cardiac cells are affected as well.

Conversely, the neurotransmitter acetylcholine, which is released with parasympathetic nervous system stimulation, causes the resting membrane potential to be more negative and slows the rate of spontaneous depolarization in the SA node and the rate of conduction in the AV node. The increased negativity of the action potential is the result of slowed sodium influx in the face of persistent potassium efflux. As a consequence, it takes longer for the cell membrane to reach firing threshold and longer for the electrical stimulus to be conducted through the AV node. Extreme vagal stimulation of the parasympathetics can produce complete conduction block at the AV node. Carotid massage may evoke such an extreme stimulus.

The action potentials of cardiac cells outside the SA and AV nodes can be converted to those of the specialized conduction nodes under certain abnormal circumstances. For example, myocardial ischemia and electrolyte imbalances predispose to premature ectopic beats and cardiac rhythm disturbances.

The Cardiac Cycle

The cardiac cycle is the relationship between the electrical events, mechanical events, and blood flow that occurs with each heart beat (Fig. 9–11). The electrical events are recorded and can be evaluated on the electrocardiogram (ECG). Measurement of atrial, ventricular, and aortic pressure and volume requires cardiac catheterization or echocardiography. However, atrial and arterial pressure can be monitored at the bedside and provide data that can be used in clinical evaluation of critically ill patients. The phonocardiogram records the heart sounds.

The cardiac cycle is divided into two parts: ventricular systole, the period during which the ventricles are contracting and blood is ejected from the heart, and ventricular diastole, the period when the ventricles are relaxed and are filled with blood. Atrial systole occurs late in ventricular diastole. During the cardiac cycle, electrical events precede mechanical events. The heart sounds are produced by mechanical events.

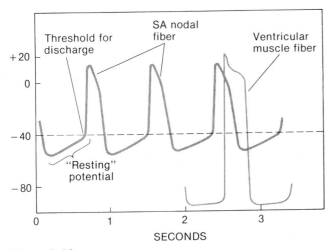

Figure 9–10 ● ● ● ● ● ●

Action potential of SA nodal fiber and ventricular muscle fiber. (Redrawn from Guyton, A.C. (1991). *Textbook of medical physiology*, 8th ed., p. 112. Philadelphia: W.B. Saunders.)

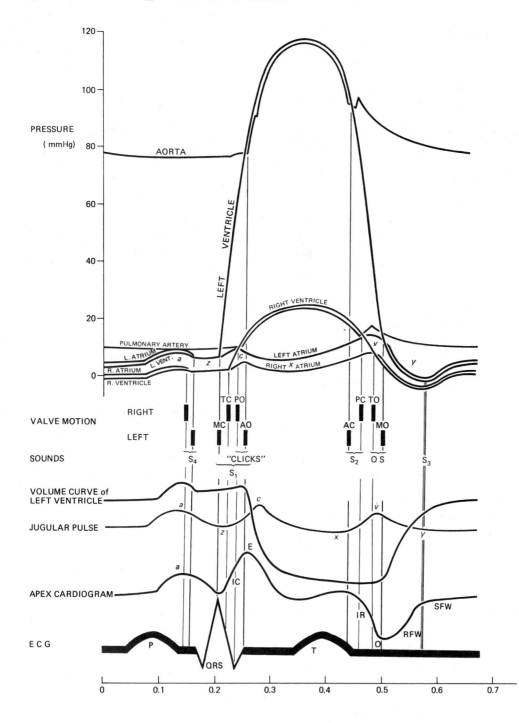

Ventricular Systole

As a wave of depolarization passes through the ventricle, it is recorded on the ECG as the QRS complex. Mechanical contraction is stimulated and begins in the middle of the QRS complex. As the ventricles begin to contract, ventricular pressure exceeds atrial pressure almost immediately and the AV valves close, producing the first heart sound (S_1). The aortic and pulmonic valves remain closed as pressure in the ventricles is less than pressure in the aorta and pulmonary artery. The ventricles continue to contract, increasing the intraventricular pressure.

Because all of the heart valves are closed, there is no change in ventricular volume during this period, a condition termed "isovolumetric contraction." Ninety percent of myocardial oxygen consumption occurs during this phase of systole. The ventricle shortens from base to apex and becomes more spherical in shape. The AV valves bulge into the atria, producing the c wave on the atrial pressure waveform. Continuing increases in ventricular tension pull the floor of each atria downward, increasing their size and decreasing their pressure, which is evidenced on the atrial waveform as the x descent.

When ventricular pressure exceeds pressure in the

aorta and pulmonary artery, the semilunar valves open and blood is rapidly ejected from the heart. Ventricular contraction continues during ejection. The myofibrils shorten circumferentially and longitudinally, ventricular wall thickness increases, and chamber size decreases. Peak ejection produces systolic pressure in the aorta and pulmonary artery. More than 50% of the stroke volume is ejected in the first quarter of systole. The atria continue to fill with blood during ventricular systole. The subsequent increase in atrial pressure produces the v wave on the atrial pressure waveform.

As each ventricle empties, the volume of blood ejected decreases and pressure in the ventricular chambers, aorta, and pulmonary artery falls. At the end of systole there is a sudden fall in intraventricular pressure as the ventricles relax. Retrograde flow in the aorta and pulmonary artery results, catching the cusps of the semilunar valves and closing them. Mechanical closure of the valves produces the second heart sound (S₂) and the dichrotic notch (or incisura) in the arterial pressure waveforms. Arterial pressure continues to decline to the diastolic level as blood runs off toward the periphery.

The ventricle does not empty completely with any contraction. Blood left in the heart at the end of systole is called the residual or end-systolic volume (ESV). Stroke volume, the amount of blood ejected per beat, is the difference between end-diastolic volume (EDV) and ESV. The ejection fraction is the measure of the stroke volume as a percentage of the EDV. Normal ejection fraction is 65% to 70%. In the healthy heart, the ESV provides a reserve that can increase stroke volume and cardiac output with more vigorous contraction. In the failing myocardium, the ESV is typically elevated because of the poor contractile performance of the heart.

Ventricular Diastole

Following closure of the aortic and pulmonic valves, the heart continues to relax with all the valves closed. There is no change in intraventricular volume during this period of isovolumetric relaxation, and ventricular pressure falls below atrial pressure. The AV valves open and blood that has filled the atria during systole pours into the ventricles, resulting in the y descent on the atrial pressure waveform. Ventricular relaxation continues; consequently, ventricular pressure continues to fall despite the rapid filling of the chambers. A third heart sound (S₃) may be auscultated during the period of rapid ventricular filling if the ventricles are noncompliant or distended. In some children an S₃ is not indicative of cardiac pathology, but it is a finding in a normal child. Slow filling of the ventricle continues through the middle third of the diastolic period. The ventricular chambers do not relax further; but, as the AV valves remain open, the ventricles continue to distend with blood that returns to the heart. An increase in ventricular pressure is seen on the ventricular pressure waveform.

The P wave on the ECG indicates atrial depolarization, which is followed by atrial contraction at end-diastole. The final component of the ventricular EDV is delivered to the ventricles, marked by the a wave on the atrial and ventricular pressure waveforms. In the normal, mature individual atrial contraction contributes 10% to 15% of the EDV. The contribution is less in pediatric patients, who are less dependent on "atrial kick." However, in patients of any age with ventricular failure or excessively rapid heart rate, which limits the diastolic filling time, the atrial contribution to EDV is more significant. The propulsion of blood into the ventricle with atrial contraction may produce a fourth heart sound (S₄) if ventricular compliance is poor.

Regulation of Cardiac Performance

The efficiency or performance of the heart is often measured in terms of cardiac output. Cardiac output (CO) is the volume of blood that is ejected from the heart in 1 minute. It is the product of heart rate (HR) and stroke volume (SV), the amount of blood pumped from the heart with each beat:

$$CO = HR \times SV$$

CO varies with body size, so it is indexed to reflect that variation by dividing CO by body surface area (BSA). BSA is determined on a normogram or can be calculated from the equation

$$0.007184 \times \text{weight (kg)} \times \text{height (cm)}$$

Normal cardiac index is

$$3.5 \pm 0.7 \text{ L/min/m}^2$$

Cardiac output varies with the physiologic demands of metabolizing tissues. The determinants of CO, HR, and SV are sensitive to a number of physiologic influences. In addition, both are affected by maturation in growing infants and young children. The sections that follow detail the impact of HR and heart rhythm and the factors that control SV (i.e., preload, ventricular compliance, afterload and ventricular contractility) on CO and describe the maturational factors that influence cardiac performance.

Determinants of Cardiac Output

Heart Rate

The expression "children are heart rate–dependent" is frequently heard in pediatric critical care. In fact, HR is one-half of the CO equation and is crucial to cardiac performance in all individuals. However, infants and young children are less able to vary SV in response to increases in demand for CO because cardiac performance in the young is near maximal under basal conditions. As a consequence, SV is less dynamic and HR influences CO to a greater extent than is the case in mature individuals.

When HR is normal for age, the systolic component of the cardiac cycle occupies about 30% of the time that elapses in the cycle and diastole about 70%. When the HR increases, the systolic component remains fairly constant because ventricular contraction is an efficient process, but the diastolic period of the cycle is progressively shortened. Figure 9–12 illustrates the shortening of the diastolic component of the cardiac cycle with elevation of HR to one and one-half and twice the normal.

The potential pathophysiologic consequences of the shortened diastolic period are twofold. First, the period of time during which the ventricles fill with blood is shorter. Ultimately, excessively rapid HR will diminish CO because preload is inadequate. Secondly, myocardial oxygen supply decreases during tachycardia because the coronary arteries are filled and the myocardium is perfused during diastole. This decrease in supply occurs in the face of increased demand because a higher HR results in increased myocardial oxygen consumption. The outcomes of prolonged tachydysrhythmia are myocardial failure and inadequate tissue perfusion.

Slow HR easily diminishes CO in infants and young children because SV is relatively fixed. In fact, inadequate HR necessitates active resuscitation in the infant. Infants are at risk for bradycardia because sympathetic innervation of the SA node and myocardium is incomplete at birth, whereas parasympathetic innervation is complete well before term. Consequently, vagal stimulation can result in bradycardia mediated by parasympathetic stimulation of the SA node, which is not adequately balanced by sympathetic impulses that would increase the heart rate.

Heart Rhythm

The sequential relationship between the electrical and the mechanical events of the cardiac cycle result

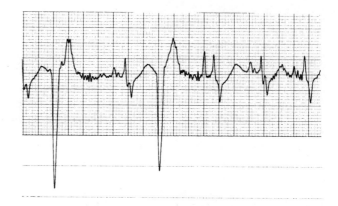

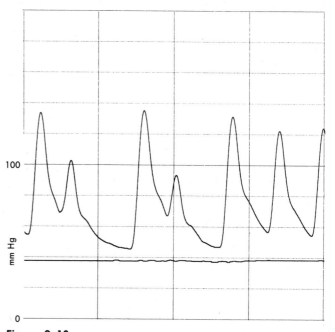

Figure 9–13 ● ● ● ● ● ●

PVCs producing altered stroke volume as reflected in the arterial pressure waveform. (From Daily, E.K., & Schroeder, J.S. (1989). *Techniques in bedside hemodynamic monitoring.* St. Louis: C.V. Mosby.)

from orderly electrical stimulation of the heart, which is followed by mechanical contraction and ejection of blood into the systemic and pulmonary circulations.

Whenever the electrical wave of depolarization that produces the mechanical contraction (excitation-contraction coupling) is disturbed, mechanical performance is influenced. Stroke volume is altered when ventricular ejection occurs early, as with a premature ventricular contraction (PVC), or if it occurs without the preceding atrial contraction, as in a junctional rhythm. Figure 9–13 demonstrates the altered SV as reflected in the arterial pressure waveform as a narrow pulse pressure that is the consequence of abnormal electrical stimulation of ventricular contraction.

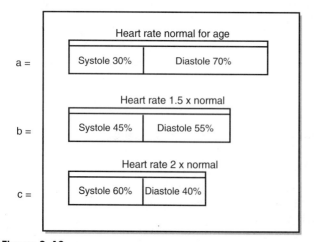

Figure 9–12 ● ● ● ● ● ●

Effect of tachycardia on the diastolic period of the cardiac cycle.

Preload

Preload is the distending force or the stretch on myocardial muscle fibers just prior to electrical stimulation and ventricular contraction. As with skeletal muscle fibers, the force of myocardial muscle contraction is a function of the initial length of the muscle fibers. At the end of the 19th century, the length-tension relationship was demonstrated by Frank and in later work by Starling, and the well-known Frank-Starling law of the heart was defined. The law states that the more the diastolic volume or fiber stretch at end diastole, the greater the force of the next contraction during systole (Fig. 9–14).

Preload determines the force and efficiency of ventricular contraction because it regulates the resting sarcomere's length, determining the number of actin and myosin crossbridges formed during systole. Most alterations in CO in the patient with a normal heart are related to the volume of venous return to the heart. Optimal stretch on the sarcomere facilitates crossbridge formation. The number of crossbridges formed directly relates to the muscular tension generated in the myocardium and, therefore, to the force of ventricular contraction. Modifications of venous return through volume administration, for example, contribute to relatively large changes in CO. Patients with heart failure have higher ventricular end-diastolic volume and pressure for measured ventricular performance (Fig. 9–15). Administration of additional volume in the face of myocardial failure is far less efficacious and may worsen the patient's clinical status.

Venous tone has a significant effect on venous return to the heart and, therefore, on CO. Vascular tone on the venous side of the circulation is dependent on a number of nervous system and hormonal factors. Venoconstriction results from SNS stimulation, muscular exercise, anxiety, and marked hypotension, as well as from medications including the cardiac glycosides and sympathomimetic agents. Venous constriction has a profound effect on improving venous return and CO. However, even marked venous constriction does not adversely increase systemic vascular resistance (SVR) because the venous system is normally highly compliant. Venous dilation can cause pooling of blood in the venous system outside the thorax. Generally, venodilation is the consequence of medications such as nitrates, beta-blockers, or calcium channel blockers.

Ventricular end-diastolic volume is affected by total blood volume and by how blood is distributed in the intravascular compartment. Acute or massive reduction of the total blood volume causes stroke volume to fall. However, gradual reduction or loss of less than 10% to 15% of the total blood volume does not result in perceptible decreases in CO.

Body position affects blood distribution. In the supine position blood pools in the lower extremeties. Trendelenburg position increases the venous return and CO. Military antishock trousers (MAST) and intermittent liver compression improve CO by the same mechanism.

Normal respiration results in negative intrathoracic pressure during inspiration. This negative pressure pulls blood into the intrathoracic cavity, augmenting venous return. In addition, pulmonary artery pressure is lower during inspiration, enhancing pulmonary blood flow. Positive pressure ventilation reverses both these phenomena, especially in combination with positive end-expiratory pressure.

Compliance

Compliance is the ability of the ventricle to relax and distend, that is, to fill, during diastole. Compliance is defined by the relationship between end-diastolic pressure and end-diastolic volume (Fig. 9–16). The normal, mature ventricle is highly compliant, allowing it to accept large increases in EDV without a significant increase in pressure. However, as ventricular EDV increases, additions of more volume result in larger changes in end-diastolic pressure. In addition, if the ventricle is stiffer or less distensible (i.e., compliance is low), the pressure change is greater for any change in intracardiac volume.

At birth, infants have a greater proportion of noncontractile myocardial fibers than contractile elements. As a consequence, the ventricle is relatively less compliant than is the case in the adult. Reduced diastolic compliance limits diastolic reserve. In clinical practice, little improvement in cardiac performance can be achieved in the very young by volume loading, unless the patient is clearly hypovolemic. Instead, additions of volume produce an acute rise in ventricular end-diastolic pressure and may result in myocardial failure. In addition, the degree of filling of one ventricle has a greater inhibitory influence on filling of the other, again limiting the ability to increase CO in the small infant by additions of volume.

A number of clinical problems reduce ventricular compliance. Most common are myocardial hypoxemia and acidosis, which may be the consequence of a variety of pathophysiologic processes. In addition, compliance is diminished in congestive heart failure (CHF), with ventricular hypertrophy and with pericardial tamponade.

Unavoidable decreases in ventricular compliance are evidenced in patients who require the administration of positive inotropic agents or the application of high levels of positive end-expiratory pressure (PEEP). Conversely, compliance can be enhanced by assuring adequate myocardial oxygenation and acid-base balance or by the administration of afterload-reducing agents. In addition, compliance is high in individuals with dilated cardiomyopathy.

Afterload

Afterload is the amount of resistance or impedance to ventricular ejection. The forces opposing ventricu-

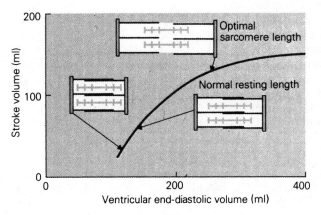

Figure 9–14 ● ● ● ● ● ●

Frank-Starling law of the heart. This graph illustrates the relationship between stroke volume and changes in ventricular end-diastolic volume. The insets showing diagrammatic sarcomeres illustrate the relationship between end-diastolic volume and myofilament overlap. At normal resting ventricular volumes, sarcomere length is less than the optimal length for contraction. (From Rhoades, R., Pflanzer, R. (1992). *Human physiology,* 2nd ed. Copyright ©1992 by Saunders College Publishing.)

Figure 9–15 ● ● ● ● ● ●

Frank-Starling ventricular performance curves. In the normal ventricle when end-diastolic volume is increased, there is a concomitant increase in ventricular performance until a plateau is reached. Patients with myocardial dysfunction and heart failure demonstrate a shift of this curve downward and to the right. In heart failure, an increase in end-diastolic volume produces less of an increase in ventricular performance and a "plateau" is reached at a much lower level of ventricular performance. (From Chernow, B. (1988). *Pharmacologic approach to the critically ill patient,* p. 347. Baltimore: Williams & Wilkins.)

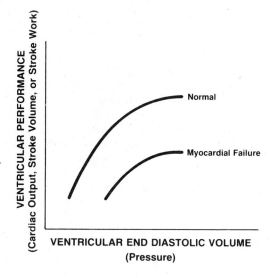

Figure 9–16 ● ● ● ● ● ●

Diastolic pressure-volume relationship of the left ventricle. At low ventricular volumes, substantial changes in volume produce little change in ventricular pressure. At higher ventricular volumes, small changes produce exponentially greater increases in pressure. Increasing ventricular compliance with vasodilator therapy shifts the curve to the right, allowing a greater end-diastolic volume at a lower pressure. (From Chernow, B. (1988). *Pharmacologic approach to the critically ill patient,* p. 347. Baltimore: Williams & Wilkins.)

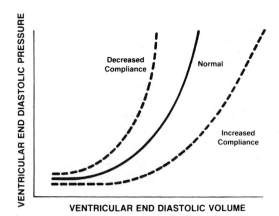

lar fiber shortening include ventricular size and shape (the law of La Place), aortic and pulmonary artery impedance, and systemic and pulmonary vascular resistance. Stroke volume is inversely proportional to afterload, whereas ventricular work and oxygen consumption are directly proportional to afterload.

The forces that oppose ventricular fiber shortening are determined by EDV and the radius of the ventricle. When EDV is high, as it is in CHF or volume overload, a greater intraventricular pressure must be overcome before fiber shortening can begin. The period of isovolumetric contraction is longer and more oxygen is consumed. Thus, preload contributes to the force of ventricular afterload.

Aortic and pulmonary artery impedance, the stiffness of the great arteries, and the inertia of the column of blood in each must be overcome before ejection of blood from the ventricles can occur. The more distensible the great arteries, the less the force that must be generated by the ventricles in order to eject their stroke volumes.

Vascular resistance is the major variable determining afterload and is a measure of the degree of constriction in the arterioles of either the systemic or the pulmonary circulation. Systemic vascular resistance varies with tissue metabolic demands, the degree of autonomic nervous system stimulation, and the level of circulating catecholamines.

In the mature cardiovascular system, SVR is the major determinant of afterload. However, in some pathophysiologic states and with some congenital heart defects it is important to note that the pulmonary vascular resistance (PVR) may be the factor that limits cardiovascular performance.

The pulmonary vascular bed is maintained in a vasoconstricted state in the fetus by a mechanism or mechanisms that remain unknown despite many years of investigation. At birth, both oxygenation and expansion of the lungs are independently effective in decreasing PVR. Recruitment of peripheral arteries, which were closed in fetal life for pulmonary blood flow, dilation of the normally muscular proximal arteries, and growth of peripheral vessels all contribute to decreased PVR from the first moments through several months of life.

PVR will not fall at birth and persistent pulmonary artery hypertension will result as the consequence of several problems (Rabinovitch, 1989). Maladaptation of the pulmonary vascular bed results if pharmacologic maturation has not occurred and the arteries are unresponsive to the mediators that cause the drop in PVR at birth. A perinatal insult such as hypoxia may sustain the vasoconstricted state of the fetus, as does acute or chronic hypoxia in utero. Finally, structural maldevelopment of the pulmonary vascular bed and conditions that result in pulmonary hypoplasia, such as congenital diaphragmatic hernia, may also result in persistent pulmonary hypertension.

Pulmonary hypertension can also be induced by a number of factors (Rabinovitch, 1989). High oxygen concentration used in the treatment of neonatal lung disease is associated with abnormally muscularized pulmonary arteries and hypertrophy of the medial layer of the proximal pulmonary arteries.

Heart defects such as ventricular or atrioventricular septal defects, which cause a left-to-right shunt as PVR begins to fall in the postnatal period, result in high pulmonary blood flow and pressure. Structural changes in the pulmonary vascular bed result, ultimately, in pulmonary vascular disease, which is progressive and associated with pulmonary hypertension and increased reactivity of the pulmonary vascular bed.

Fat embolism syndrome, most often a complication of traumatic injury with long-bone fractures, is manifested primarily by severe respiratory insufficiency (Reed & Keegan, 1993). PVR may be increased sharply and may result in hemodynamic instability, as well, if myocardial failure is the consequence.

If EDV (preload), contractility, and HR are held constant, an acute increase in pulmonary or systemic afterload decreases SV and CO or results in increased myocardial work to maintain SV. With normal cardiac function, the acute increase in afterload decreases SV, which increases ESV and thus the preload for the next cardiac contraction. Contractility is increased for subsequent contractions and CO is maintained, although at the expense of increased work.

Gradual increases in SVR or PVR, as occurs with chronic systemic or pulmonary hypertension, do not decrease SV or CO acutely (Fig. 9–17). CO is maintained by an increase in contractility, which over-

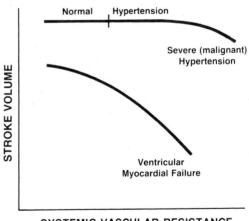

Figure 9–17 ● ● ● ● ●

Relationship of systemic vascular resistance to stroke volume in a normal and dysfunction ventricle. Increases in afterload do not cause a decrease in stroke volume in a normal ventricle (*upper curve*) except at very high levels of afterload when severe hypertension caused ventricular decompensation. In a failing ventricle (*lower curve*), however, an increase in afterload causes a progressive depression of stroke volume and cardiac output. Thus, vasodilator-induced reductions in afterload enhance stroke volume in patients with severe ventricular dysfunction. (From Chernow, B. (1988). *Pharmacologic approach to the critically ill patient,* p. 348. Baltimore: Williams & Wilkins.)

comes the increased vascular resistance. However, malignant hypertension leads to heart failure.

When ventricular function is impaired, afterload is the most influential factor affecting SV and CO as myocardial contractility is diminished. Similarly, infants are exquisitely sensitive to increases in afterload because myocardial immaturity limits the ability of the heart to enhance its contractile performance.

Contractility

The inotropic capacity of the heart refers to its inherent capacity to modulate its contractile performance, the rate and force of fiber shortening, independent of fiber length. Increased contractility results in increased CO independent of preload and afterload although inverse changes in afterload produce very important clinical effects (Fig. 9–18). Contractility is influenced by SNS activity, circulating catecholamines, metabolic imbalances, exogenous pharmacologic agents, loss of contractile mass, and maturity.

Sympathetic stimulation increases cardiac contractility as a result of direct release of norepinephrine in cardiac tissue. Catecholamines are also released by the adrenal medulla and extracardiac sympathetic ganglia and circulate in the blood. Circulating catecholamines also enhance contractility, but do so more slowly than cardiac norepinephrine. However, when cardiac stores of catecholamine are depleted, as is the case with chronic severe CHF, circulating catecholamines become more important. Catecholamines increase the rate of both calcium influx during stimulation and efflux during repolarization, increasing

both the force and the rate of contraction and relaxation.

The metabolic environment of the myocardium influences its contractile performance. Hyponatremia slows depolarization and decreases contractility. Hyperkalemia decreases contractility. In addition, inotropy is impaired by acidosis, hypoxia, and ischemia.

Pharmacologic agents can either augment or depress cardiac contractility. The cardiac glycosides, sympathomimetic agents, caffeine, and theophylline all have positive inotropic effects. Conversely, beta-adrenergic and calcium channel blockers, anesthetic agents, and barbiturates depress cardiac contractility.

Loss of functional cardiac muscle, as occurs with myocardial infarction, results in a loss of contractile mass necessary for ventricular contractile performance. Common in the adult population, myocardial infarction, although clearly unusual in infants and children, does occur. Most often, abnormalities in coronary artery anatomy or familial lipid metabolism are implicated.

Relative immaturity is characteristic of the infant heart. Compared to that of the adult, the infant's heart differs in its mechanical properties, autonomic nervous system innervation, and in the appearance of its ultrastructure. Myocardial cells in the very young are smaller in diameter and contain fewer contractile elements than later in life. As a consequence, the force generated and the degree and velocity of fiber shortening are less. In situations wherein resistance to ventricular emptying (afterload) is increased, the functional capacity (systolic reserve) of the immature heart is limited. In addition, the newborn myocardium lacks complete development of sympathetic (adrenergic) innervation, whereas parasympathetic (cholinergic) innervation is complete at birth. Releasable stores of norepinephrine in ventricular myocardium are fewer, also decreasing the inotropic response that increases contractility in the mature heart. The infant heart may be functioning near capacity, limiting its ability to increase contractility.

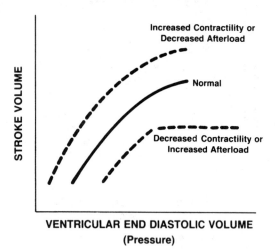

Figure 9–18 ● ● ● ● ● ●

Ventricular function curves demonstrating the effects of changes in contractility or afterload. If afterload is held constant, an increase in contractility of the ventricle will shift the functional curve upward and to the left, demonstrating improved ventricular performance at any given level of end-diastolic volume. If ventricle contractility is left unchanged, a decrease in afterload will produce a similar shift in the ventricular function curve. (From Chernow, B. (1988). *Pharmacologic approach to the critically ill patient*, p. 349. Baltimore: Williams & Wilkins.)

Regulation of Tissue Perfusion

The volume of blood circulated to the various tissues of the body is dependent on the metabolic needs of each tissue. The cardiovascular system responds to differences among tissues and to changes in metabolic demand. Autoregulation, humoral factors, and the autonomic nervous system permit acute control of the circulation.

Autoregulation of Blood Flow

Autoregulation of blood flow is governed by factors that are, as yet, not precisely known. Autoregulation may be governed by local metabolic needs that control blood flow. When metabolic needs in a tissue are increased, vasodilation occurs and blood flow increases. The reverse is the case when metabolic needs are low. Decreased demand results in vasoconstriction and reduced flow.

Increased metabolic activity causes local formation of substances including carbon dioxide, lactic acid, hydrogen ions, adenosine, and bradykinin, which are all vasodilators. Tissue hypoxia is responsible for the release of these substances. Their release stimulates vasodilation and increased blood flow (Guyton, 1991). Tissue oxygen deficiency may directly cause vasodilation. Oxygen is necessary to maintain normal vascular tone; thus, hypoxia allows vascular smooth muscle to dilate (Guyton, 1991).

Active hyperemia is the term that describes the increase in blood flow to an area at a time of increased demand. *Reactive hyperemia* is the surplus blood flow that occurs when flow to an area that was abruptly obstructed is reestablished. Reactive hyperemia may continue for minutes to hours following the release of the obstruction. Hyperemia in both cases illustrates the relationship between metabolic demand and blood flow.

Changes in vascular tone may result from changes in arterial tone, which are caused by increases or decreases in mean arterial pressure. When mean arterial pressure falls, arteriolar tone is decreased and the vessel dilates, allowing increased flow to the area. Autoregulation may well be the result of a combination of all these factors.

Autonomic Nervous System Regulation of Blood Flow

The autonomic nervous system operates both globally and locally to regulate blood flow through sympathetic and parasympathetic functions. Sympathetic innervation of the heart and blood vessels arises from neurons located in the reticular formation of the brainstem. The axons of these neurons descend into the spinal cord. Outflow from the SNS is transmitted to the cardiovascular system by cell bodies in the paravertebral ganglia and their postganglionic axons. Sympathetic control of cardiovascular function is mediated by the catecholamines, which are released from the sympathetic nerve terminus (norepinephrine) and the adrenal medulla (epinephrine). Thus, the catecholamines exert their effects locally at the receptor site and globally as a circulating hormone (Zaritsky & Chernow, 1984).

Fibers of the SNS are widely distributed throughout the myocardium, the SA and AV nodes, and both arterial and venous smooth muscle. Their origin in the vasomotor center of the medulla is composed of three major areas: the vasoconstrictor area, the vasodilator area, and the cardioaccelerator area. The primary role of the vasodilator area is to inhibit vasoconstriction.

Stimulation of the cardioaccelerator and vasoconstrictor areas of the vasomotor system elicits SNS response. The results are increased cardiac inotropy and chronotropy, increased venous return by venous

vasoconstriction, and increased SVR and blood pressure by generalized arteriolar constriction (Guyton, 1991).

The vasomotor centers of the medulla are stimulated by baroreceptors in the aortic arch, atria, large arteries, and veins. Baroreceptors respond to decreased mean pressure or pulse pressure, which decreases their stretch by decreasing their rate of firing. The vasomotor center responds by increasing SNS output and decreasing the output from the parasympathetic nervous system (PNS). CO increases through the Starling mechanism as venous return to the heart is augmented by venoconstriction, increasing EDV. Increased arteriolar tone maintains central blood pressure and diverts flow from the peripheral vascular beds to essential organs. Increased HR and force of contraction maintain CO despite the increase in SVR.

Parasympathetic innervation of the heart originates in the vagal nucleus in the medulla and is transmitted via the cardiac branches of the vagal nerve. Parasympathetic stimulation inhibits the SA node firing, slows conduction through the AV node, and decreases myocardial contractility. Normally, the PNS is tonically active and has a constraining effect on HR. Strong vagal stimulation can stop impulse formation at the SA node or block impulse transmission at the AV node. PNS effects on the vascular system are negligible.

Humoral Regulation of Blood Flow

The catecholamines and other substances described above, which influence local blood flow (carbon dioxide, hydrogen ions, lactic acid, etc.), are humoral factors that regulate blood flow. In addition, other hormones and vasoactive substances regulate blood flow and tissue perfusion. These are listed in Table 9–2. It is important to note that vasodilating substances in the systemic side of the circulation have the reverse effect on the pulmonary vasculature. This circumstance has clear clinical implications in the management of conditions in patients with some forms of complex congenital heart disease.

Table 9–2. HUMORAL REGULATION OF BLOOD FLOW

Vasodilators	Vasoconstrictors
Systemic	*Systemic*
Carbon dioxide	Epinephrine
Lactic acid	Norepinephrine
Hydrogen ions	Angiotensin II
Adenosine	Vasopressin (ADH)
Bradykinin	
Histamine	
Serotonin	
Prostaglandins	
Pulmonary	*Pulmonary*
Nitric oxide	Carbon dioxide
Oxygen	Hypoxia
Prostaglandins	Hydrogen ions

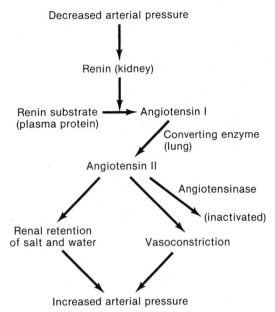

Decreased arterial pressure

Renin (kidney)

Renin substrate ⟶ Angiotensin I
(plasma protein)

Converting enzyme
(lung)

Angiotensin II

Angiotensinase

(inactivated)

Renal retention   Vasoconstriction
of salt and water

Increased arterial pressure

Figure 9–19 ● ● ● ● ● ●

The renin-angiotensin constrictor mechanisms for arterial pressure control. (From Guyton, A.C. (1991). *Textbook of medical physiology,* 8th ed. Philadelphia: W.B. Saunders.)

Angiotensin II is a potent vasoconstricting substance that causes a sharp increase in SVR and blood pressure. Angiotensin II is synthesized when renal blood flow is decreased via the renin-angiotension system (Fig. 9–19). Decreased renal blood flow, an early consequence of inadequate tissue perfusion and the SNS stimulation that results, causes the release of renin from the juxtaglomerular cells of the kidney that produce and store it. Renin acts on angiotensinogen to release angiotensin I, which, in the presence of a converting enzyme, results in the formation of angiotensin II. Angiotensin II has two major effects on blood flow and pressure. The first is a rapid and generalized arteriolar vasoconstriction. Second is a decrease in sodium and water excretion by the kidney. Water and sodium retention increases the blood volume, increasing blood pressure as well. The renal effects of angiotensin II persist far longer than its vasoconstricting effects, although they are less immediate.

Vasopressin, or antidiuretic hormone (ADH) is an even more potent vasoconstrictor than angiotensin II. However, it is released from the posterior pituitary gland in such small quantities that it has little short-term impact on blood flow or blood pressure.

PHYSICAL ASSESSMENT OF THE CARDIOVASCULAR SYSTEM

The child's cardiovascular system responds quickly to the stress of illness, as is evident on even a cursory physical examination. However, adequate cardiovascular response to critical illness or injury cannot be

assumed. Detailed and accurate assessment of the cardiovascular system is a necessity in the care of critically ill infants and children.

General Health and Appearance

A child's general health and appearance often reflect the status of the cardiovascular system. However, it is erroneous to assume a connection in all cases. For example, a child whose growth has been limited and who has poor appetite and little energy may have a serious disorder, but it may not be of cardiovascular origin. On the other hand, anorexia in a child with known heart disease is a signal for concern and additional investigation. Similarly, a child who has frequent "chest colds" does not necessarily have cardiovascular disease, although this finding is related to increased pulmonary blood flow (PBF) in children with congenital heart defects. The presence of cardiovascular disease and an accurate assessment of cardiovascular status cannot be established on the basis of general health and appearance alone; however, careful assessment and thorough questioning of parents may elicit information that leads to further investigation and provides broad evidence of cardiovascular adequacy. Table 9–3 lists areas of assessment that are closely related to cardiovascular function and are assessed or investigated with the family as a foundation for more specific cardiovascular assessment.

Table 9–3. GENERAL HEALTH ASSESSMENT

Physical growth: Height and weight are measured serially and plotted on a standard growth chart. Both inadequate cardiac output and cyanosis can impair growth.

Appetite: Intake of food and fluid is assessed. Sources of dietary or supplemental iron are noted; anemia can increase breathlessness and exercise intolerance in children, with or without concomitant cardiac disease.

Exercise tolerance: An estimate of the functional limitation* imposed is obtained. The occurrence of chest pain with exertion is noted. Chest pain may be related to aortic outflow obstruction.

Frequency of colds or other infections: Frequent respiratory infections may be related to increased PBF. Infection requires aggressive treatment in children with cardiac disease.

Breathing pattern: Tachypnea and dyspnea are signs of pulmonary vascular congestion. Some infants with limited PBF may experience paroxysmal hyperpnea.

*Functional capacity of people with heart disease is classified into four groups based on the severity of the patient's symptoms:
Class I Patients with heart disease who have no symptoms of any kind. Ordinary physical activity does not cause fatigue, palpitation, dyspnea, or anginal pain.
Class II Patients who are comfortable at rest but have symptoms with ordinary physical activity.
Class III Patients who are comfortable at rest but who have symptoms with less than ordinary effort.
Class IV Patients who have symptoms at rest.
Data from New York Heart Association.
PBF, pulmonary blood flow.

Families are questioned about medications the child may be taking. Careful inquiry regarding dosage and administration is made. Asking parents if there is a concern or question that they have about their child may elicit important information that might otherwise go unmentioned.

Vital Signs

Heart Rate

Heart rate in infants and children is particularly variable, increasing rapidly in response to excitement, stress, activity, pain, or fever. With fever, HR increases 15 to 20 beats per minute (bpm) with each centigrade degree of temperature rise above normal. Because of the high variability in HR, tachycardia is especially significant if it persists when the child is relaxed or asleep.

Blood Pressure

Indirect blood pressure measurement is best achieved by auscultation or the use of noninvasive automatic equipment, the two techniques that provide both systolic and diastolic pressures and allow calculation of pulse pressure and mean arterial pressure. Palpation of the radial pulse while an arm blood pressure cuff is deflated approximates only the systolic pressure. The flush method approximates the mean arterial blood pressure at the reading obtained when color returns to a blanched extremity as the blood pressure cuff is deflated. These measurements are inadequate.

Accurate indirect blood pressure measurement requires judicious selection of an appropriately sized blood pressure cuff. The inflatable bladder should be long enough to completely encircle the extremity without overlapping or leaving a gap, although use of a cuff with an inflatable bladder that half encircles the extremity may also be accurate if the bladder is centered over the compressible artery.

The bladder should be wide enough to cover two-thirds of the upper arm, thigh, or calf. Appropriate cuff width is estimated from the diameter or circumference of the extremity. The width of the cuff should be 20% greater than the diameter of the arm, or, for ease of estimation, extend around 40% of the extremity. A blood pressure cuff that is too narrow results in a falsely high reading; a cuff that is too wide underestimates the true systolic reading, although this margin of error is less than that obtained with too narrow a cuff.

Ideally, blood pressure is measured in the right upper extremity. Although use of this site may not always be possible, it is the standard because arterial flow to the right arm is derived from the first vessels that branch from the aortic arch. In certain congenital heart defects, such as interrupted aortic arch and coarctation of the aorta, it may be the only pressure that approximates that in the aorta. Measurement of blood pressure in all four extremities is indicated if hypertension is detected in the right arm measurement and in some children with CHD (i.e., those with an anatomic obstruction to left ventricular outflow). The systolic pressure in the thigh is equal to arm pressure in infants and young children. After the first year of life, the systolic pressure in the leg rises steadily until it is 10 to 20 mmHg higher than that in the arm. Diastolic pressure in the upper and lower extremities is nearly equal. It is important to note that there are no established normal ranges for blood pressure measured peripherally, particularly in the distal lower extremities. The extremity that is used for blood pressure measurement is noted.

Four factors of technique are important in accurate and reproducible auscultation of indirect blood pressure. They are (1) cuff placement, (2) rate of cuff deflation, (3) identification of systolic and diastolic pressure points, and (4) function of the auscultatory equipment.

Cuff Placement. The inflatable bladder within the cuff is to be centered over the artery to be compressed. The measured pressure is erroneously higher when the cuff is misplaced.

Deflation Rate. The cuff is to be deflated at a rate of 2 to 3 mmHg per heart beat or per second. In patients with a slow heart rate, rapid cuff deflation can result in significant measurement error. The systolic pressure may be underestimated simply because the sounds are not heard at their true pressure reading but at a lower pressure because of rapid cuff deflation (e.g., 10 mmHg per second). Accurate assessment of diastolic blood pressure is impossible when the cuff is deflated rapidly.

Systolic and Diastolic Points. Systolic pressure corresponds to audible pulsations that occur with distension of a previously collapsed artery. It is recorded when the first sound appears during blood pressure cuff deflation, as it has been since it was first suggested by Korotkoff. Diastolic pressure measurement is more controversial. Should the diastolic pressure be recorded when the Korotkoff sounds muffle and become dull or when the sounds disappear? Members of The American Academy of Pediatrics Task Force on Blood Pressure Control in Children (1977) recommend that the point of muffling be accepted as the diastolic pressure. If muffling and disappearance of the Korotkoff sounds can be clearly identified, both are recorded (e.g., 120/82/60).

Auscultatory Equipment. Korotkoff sounds are low-frequency sounds just above the normal hearing threshold. Normal hearing and a good quality stethoscope are prerequisites for accurate auscultation of blood pressure.

Respiratory Assessment

The cardiovascular and respiratory systems are closely linked. Cardiovascular pathophysiology may be evidenced in the respiratory system. Consequently, both must be carefully assessed in the critically ill child.

Inspection

Examination of the cardiovascular system proceeds with inspection. While assessing the infant or child, an impression is also established regarding level of consciousness, capacity for activity, and degree of comfort.

Color. Color is best assessed in natural lighting and in an environment at a comfortable temperature. Artificial lighting may create a blue or yellow cast to the skin color, and peripheral vasoconstriction due to cold (or pain and fear) influences the child's peripheral color. Vasoconstriction also occurs when cardiac output is inadequate, but the presence of tachycardia, tachypnea, and other signs of physiologic distress are noted as well in this situation.

Color is best assessed in the most highly vascularized areas of the head and neck, the earlobes, and the mucous membranes. Nowhere, however, does skin actually derive its color from arterial blood. This bedside assessment is an indirect means of judging arterial oxygen saturation, but it may alert caregivers to a change in the patient's condition when based on careful and continuous observation of the critically ill child. Continuous noninvasive pulse oximetry provides early warning of hypoxemia.

Central cyanosis, if detected, is confirmed with arterial blood gas analysis or noninvasive pulse oximetry. When cyanosis is a persistent problem, other abnormalities typically accompany it, including clubbing of the finger- and toenails; dry skin; and dry, brittle hair. Persistent cyanosis also results in polycythemia.

Edema. Detection of visible edema is a second general aspect of inspection of the cardiovascular system. Generalized edema is rare in children, except in nephrotic syndrome. Periorbital edema and, more rarely, ankle, tibial, and sacral edema are detected in infants and children with CHF.

Visible Pulsations. The internal and external jugular veins are inspected for distension and abnormal pulsations. When the child is supine, the jugular veins are normally distended and visible. When the child's head is elevated 35° to 45°, the veins should no longer be visible. Persistent neck vein distension is seen with CHF or volume overload. The typically rapid HR of infants and children often prevents visualization of the double pulsations in the jugular veins that are detected in the adult and correspond to the a and v waves. The short neck of most infants also may interfere with assessment of the jugular veins.

Carotid pulsations are normally visible in children in the supine position. They too are not visually detectable when the head is elevated. Visible, bounding carotid pulsations may occur with hypertension, hypoxia, anemia, or anxiety.

Chest Inspection. When the anterior chest wall is inspected, both sides of the rib cage are compared. Obvious bulging over the precordium is caused by chronic cardiac enlargement. In young or thin children the apical pulse may be visible as a precordial impulse. The visible pulsation normally corresponds to the point of maximal impulse (PMI). This is usually the apex of the heart and is located at the left midclavicular line (or 1–2 cm to the right of it) in the fifth intercostal space (ICS) in children age 8 years or older. In infants and younger children, the heart is normally positioned more horizontally and its apex is higher. The precordial impulse is visible in the third or fourth intercostal space to the left of the left midclavicular line. The visible precordial impulse is generally a normal finding, but, if it becomes apparent in a child in whom it was previously undetectable, left ventricular volume or pressure overload may be present. Finally, the visible precordial impulse is differentiated from a precordial lift or heave, which are abnormal findings involving the actual movement of the chest wall with contraction of the underlying cardiac muscle. Chronic cardiomegaly is usually the cause of each.

Palpation

Precordial palpation is performed to confirm and qualify visible findings and to detect other normal and abnormal pulsations and vibrations. Vibrations are produced by abnormally turbulent blood flow. Referred to as a cardiac thrill, these vibrations are palpable heart murmurs (Table 9–4). Palpation is begun by placing the palms of the hands and the fingers over visible areas of pulsation. The fingers are used to detect the rate, rhythm, and intensity of the pulsations. Figure 9–20 illustrates the cardinal areas for palpation and auscultation of the heart.

The PMI is palpated over the apex of the heart in the position described above. Other positions indicate cardiomegaly, malposition of the heart, or mediastinal shift. The PMI is normally a single pulsation. Double or paradoxical impulses may indicate CHF. A notably prominent impulse may also be indicative of CHF or of increased left ventricular systolic pressure.

Moving to the base of the heart, the aortic area is palpated for pulsations, thrills, or heaves. Palpation of the aortic area is improved when the patient sits up or leans forward. Pulsations in this area are not normal. A thrill in this area may indicate aortic stenosis.

In the pulmonic area, a single, slight, brief pulsation may be palpated simultaneous in timing to the

Table 9–4. PALPABLE CARDIAC THRILLS

Defect	Description of Associated Thrill
Ductus arteriosus	Palpable throughout the cardiac cycle at the LSB; 2nd and 3rd ICS
Ventricular septal defect	Palpable during systole at the LSB; 4th, 5th and 6th ICS; may radiate to axillary line
Aortic stenosis	Palpable during systole at RSB; 2nd ICS; may radiate to right neck
Pulmonic stenosis	Palpable during systole at the LSB; 2nd ICS; may radiate to left neck

ICS, intercostal space, LSB, left sternal border, RSB, right sternal border.

PMI. This is a normal finding in the child with a thin chest wall. It may be evident, as well, in children following exertion or in the presence of fever or anemia. A slow, sustained, forceful pulsation in this area may indicate pulmonary hypertension or mitral stenosis.

Erb's point, located in the third ICS at the left sternal border, is palpated next. Murmurs of either aortic or pulmonic origin are often referred to this location.

Palpation is continued over the parasternal area until the tricuspid or right ventricular area is reached. Pulsation in the tricuspid area may indicate right ventricle (RV) enlargement. A significant lift or heave in this location accompanies RV enlargement or increased pressure in the RV.

A pericardial friction rub may be palpated as a scratchy or grating sensation over the precordium. Unlike a pleural friction rub, it does not vary with respiration. It is always an abnormal finding.

Abdominal Palpation. Palpation of the abdomen is included in the cardiovascular examination because CHF in infants and young children is associated with liver enlargement. The liver cannot usually be palpated in adolescents or adults because it is located well above the right costal margin. However, in the infant the liver edge is normally as much as 3 cm below the costal margin. The size of the liver relative to the child's size decreases with age: at age 1 year, the liver edge is palpable 2 cm below the

Table 9–5. PULSE INTENSITY

Pulse	Normal Intensity
Temporal	+2
Carotid	+2
Brachial	+2
Radial	+1 to +2 (age-dependent)
Femoral	+2
Popliteal	+1 to +2 (age-dependent)
Posterior tibial	+1
Dorsalis pedis	+1

Intensity scale: 0 = absent
                 +1 = weak, easily obliterated
                 +2 = normal, easily palpated, cannot be obliterated
                 +3 = full
                 +4 = full, bounding

costal margin, and by 4 or 5 years of age it is located 1 cm below the costal margin. Palpation of a normal liver reveals a sharp edge, in contrast to the blunted edge of the liver distended in patients with CHF. In addition, the distended liver is usually tender.

The epigastric area is palpated to detect pulsations present in that area. Pulsation of the aorta in children can often easily be detected and is not abnormal. Pulsation of the liver may be detected in the epigastric location, indicating CHF.

Pulses. Central and peripheral pulses are evaluated for their intensity (Table 9–5) and compared with one another in both timing and intensity. Intensity is graded on a scale from 0 to +4. An absent pulse receives a 0; a pulse that is weak and easily obliterated with fingertip pressure receives a +1; an average or normal pulse can be palpated with ease and cannot be obliterated and is graded +2; a full pulse receives +3; and a full and bounding pulse receives +4. The carotid, brachial, radial, and femoral pulses occur simultaneously. The brachial and femoral pulses are approximately equal in intensity. Careful palpation of pulses is important in evaluating systemic vasoconstriction and in determining the presence of obstruction to aortic blood flow.

Percussion

Percussion in examination of the cardiovascular system is limited to estimation of heart and liver size and approximate location. Because the chest radiograph provides definitive information about cardiac size, shape, and position, percussion is often eliminated from cardiovascular assessment.

Auscultation

Normal heart sounds are produced by the flow of blood through the heart and great arteries, which results in the orderly and sequential closure of the cardiac valves. The sounds are associated with mechanical events in the cardiac cycle. Briefly, these events and the associated sounds are as follows:

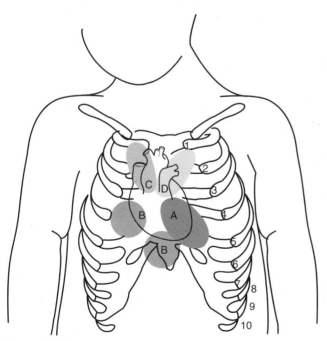

Figure 9–20 ● ● ● ● ● ●

Areas for auscultation and palpation of the heart. A, Mitral or apical area, where the first heart sound is loudest and where the third and fourth heart sounds may be heard. B, Tricuspid area, where a split in the first heart sound may be heard. C, Aortic area where the second heart sound is heard well. D, Pulmonic area, where a split in the third heart sound may be heard.

1. Systemic and pulmonary venous blood returning to the right and left atria flows directly into the relaxed right and left ventricles. At this point in the cardiac cycle, the ventricles are in diastole and the AV valves are open.
2. Following atrial electrical stimulation and the resultant contraction, pressure in both ventricles rises as they are filled with blood. The rapid increase in end-diastolic pressure in the ventricle causes the AV valves to close just before ventricular systole, preventing regurgitation of blood into the atria.
3. Closure of the mitral and tricuspid valves occurs almost simultaneously. The first heart sound (S_1) is heard as a single sound in most individuals.
4. Electrical stimulation of the ventricles follows AV valve closure, resulting in ventricular contraction. The aortic and pulmonic valves (semilunar valves) are forced open and blood fills the aorta and pulmonary artery.
5. When the ventricles have completed ejection, higher pressure in the aorta and pulmonary artery causes the semilunar valves to close, preventing retrograde flow of blood into the ventricles.
6. Closure of the semilunar valves produces the second heart sound (S_2). The aortic and pulmonic components of S_2 differ in intensity and do not always occur simultaneously.

Each heart sound is reflected to a specific area of the chest wall where it is best heard (see Fig. 9–20). The mitral component of S_1 is best heard at the apex of the heart near the position of the PMI, although it is audible over the entire precordium. Tricuspid S_1 is best heard in the fifth ICS just to the right, just below, or just to the left of the sternum. The aortic component of S_2 is heard best in the right second ICS. Pulmonic S_2 is best heard in the second left ICS. Both S_1 and S_2 are high-pitched sounds, although S_1 is slightly lower in pitch than S_2, and is also longer in duration than S_2.

As each component of S_1 and S_2 is heard, other heart sounds remain audible. It requires concentration and practice to develop the skill of listening to only one aspect of each heart sound at a time. It is also helpful to develop a routine method of auscultating heart sounds and to follow it faithfully. A suggested routine is:

1. Listen to the mitral component of S_1 (M_1).
2. Listen to the tricuspid component of S_1 (T_1).
3. Listen to the aortic component of S_2 (A_2).
4. Listen to the pulmonic component of S_2 (P_2).

This routine is based on the sequence of mechanical events during the cardiac cycle and, therefore, seems logical; but others are also practiced. For example, head-to-toe patient assessment directs auscultation of both components of S_2, followed by auscultation of both components of S_1. The key is to listen to heart sounds in the same way each time to develop the skill necessary to distinguish normal from abnormal sounds.

Split Heart Sounds. Both S_1 and S_2 are usually heard as single sounds. However, a split S_2 is not uncommon in children and does not usually indicate pathology. A physiologically split S_2 is audible at the pulmonic or aortic area when the aortic valve (A_2) closes before the pulmonic valve (P_2). It is wider on inspiration than exhalation because venous return to the right heart is enhanced during inspiration. Right ventricular ejection is prolonged, delaying the closure of the pulmonic valve. The asynchronous closure of the two semilunar valves results in splitting of the second heart sound.

If the width of the split of the second heart sound does not vary with respiration (a "fixed" split) or is wider on exhalation than on inspiration (a "paradoxical" split), the finding is considered pathologic and warrants further evaluation. For example, a fixed split of S_2 occurs with atrial septal defect (ASD) and with pulmonic stenosis (PS). Paradoxical splitting may occur when left ventricular contraction is delayed because of a left bundle branch block and the aortic valve closes after the pulmonic valve during exhalation. Right bundle branch block delays right ventricular contraction and pulmonic valve closure, producing a widely split S_2.

Splitting of S_1 (i.e., an audible separation between the mitral and tricuspid components of the first heart sound) is best heard in the tricuspid location. Because of the greater pressure gradients on the left side of the heart, the mitral valve may close just ahead of the tricuspid in some individuals. A split S_1 is not considered pathologic if it is narrow.

Accentuated Heart Sounds. Each component of the second heart sound is also assessed for its intensity. An accentuated pulmonic component of S_2 is a marker of pulmonary hypertension. P_2 may also be accentuated in heart failure and with ASD. A_2 is accentuated with systemic hypertension. The aortic component of S_2 may be diminished when arterial pressure is low, as in hypovolemia or shock.

Extra Heart Sounds. Extra heart sounds include ejection clicks, S_3 and S_4. Ejection clicks are heard in early, middle, or late systole and are associated with abnormalities of the AV or semilunar valves. These crisp sounds are well localized to the valve areas. Pulmonic and aortic ejection clicks are heard most often in early systole. A pulmonary ejection click may diminish in intensity during inspiration. It is associated with pulmonary stenosis or pulmonary hypertension. An aortic ejection click does not vary with respiration and is associated with aortic valve stenosis, coarctation of the aorta, and aortic aneurysm. Mitral valve prolapse produces a midsystolic click. This is not an uncommon finding in the general population, and, although not a critical care problem, it may be detected in adolescents in the PICU.

A third heart sound (S_3) is sometimes produced by the rapid entry of blood into an empty or dilated ventricle and is referred to as a ventricular flow sound. S_3 is a dull, low-pitched sound best heard at

Table 9–6. INTENSITY OF CARDIAC MURMURS

Grade	Description
I	Faintest murmur audible, often undiscovered initially
II	Faint, but heard without difficulty
III	Soft, but louder than II
IV	Loud, but not as loud as V, associated with a palpable thrill
V	Loud, still audible when stethoscope is lifted partially off the chest, associated with a palpable thrill
VI	Loudest murmur, remains audible when stethoscope is lifted away from the chest

the apex early in diastole, just after S_2. Although it can be the consequence of decreased left ventricular compliance and is heard in both children and adults with CHF, S_3 is often normal in children and athletic teens or adults.

A fourth heart sound (S_4) may also occasionally be heard normally in children but is more often associated with cardiovascular abnormality. It is usually an abnormal sound that is produced by the acceleration of blood into the ventricles with atrial contraction and is referred to as a late ventricular filling sound. Like S_3, S_4 is a dull, low-pitched sound that is best heard at the apex. S_4 is distinguished from S_3 by its timing in the cardiac cycle, occurring just before S_1. S_4 is often associated with hypertension, anemia, or CHF.

"Gallop rhythm" is the term used to describe the heart sounds when an S_3, S_4, or both sounds are detected on auscultation. The presence of an S_3 sound produces a protodiastolic gallop. When a presystolic S_4 and a protodiastolic S_3 combine to form a single, loud, evenly spaced extra sound in diastole, the term "summation gallop" is used to describe the abnormality. Gallop rhythms are best heard at the apex with the bell of the stethoscope.

A pericardial friction rub is a transient scratching, grating, or squeaking sound that is high in pitch. Indicative of pericarditis, it is best heard between the apex of the heart and the LSB. The friction rub is associated with cardiac movement as the heart contracts. If the HR is slow, three components of the sound may be detected that correspond to atrial systole, ventricular systole, and ventricular diastole.

Cardiac Murmurs. Murmurs are the result of abnormally turbulent blood flow within the heart, at the heart valves, or within the great arteries. The location at which a murmur is best heard depends, like other characteristics of the murmur (timing, duration, intensity), on the defect that produces the abnormal blood flow. The location at which the murmur is heard best, as well as its radiation to other areas of the chest or neck, is described.

The timing of a murmur is related to the cardiac cycle. Systolic murmurs occur between S_1 and S_2, during ventricular systole. Diastolic murmurs occur after S_2, during ventricular diastole. Continuous murmurs occur throughout the cardiac cycle.

Cardiac murmurs are evaluated for characteristics

that include intensity, pattern, pitch, and quality. Intensity of murmurs is graded on a scale from I to VI (Table 9–6). Grade I murmurs are the faintest murmurs audible, whereas grade VI murmurs are the loudest. A grade VI murmur continues to be audible even when the examiner lifts the stethoscope away from the child's chest wall. Assigning a specific intensity to a murmur is subject to individual interpretation, and there are sometimes discrepancies between different examiners. When a single person assesses a child with a cardiac murmur across time, changes in the intensity of the murmur are of note and are evaluated further.

The intensity of a murmur often has a particular variation or pattern. The most common are:

1. Ejection murmur (usually systolic ejection murmur): Loudest at midsystole or mid-diastole
2. Holosystolic or holodiastolic (usually holosystolic, because holodiastolic murmurs are rare): Heard throughout systole or diastole in equal intensity
3. Crescendo murmur: Marked by increasing intensity during systole or diastole
4. Decrescendo murmur: Marked by decreasing intensity during systole or diastole
5. Crescendo-decrescendo (diamond-shaped) murmur: Marked by increasing, then by decreasing, intensity during systole or diastole

Pitch of heart murmurs is described as high, medium, or low. The quality of the murmur is described with terms including harsh, musical, blowing, or rumbling.

Heart murmurs that are produced by defects in cardiac structure are referred to as organic murmurs. A number of children who do not have heart defects have innocent, or functional, heart murmurs. Functional murmurs are generally quiet (grade I or II/VI), systolic murmurs of short duration that are best heard at the pulmonic area and do not radiate or transmit sound to other areas. These murmurs are heard in children with normal growth and development.

NONINVASIVE EVALUATION AND DIAGNOSIS

A number of noninvasive diagnostic tests are routine in the evaluation of infants and children with a potential for cardiac dysfunction. Included are cardiac rhythm monitoring, radiographic evaluation of the heart, and echocardiography.

Monitoring and Evaluating the Rhythm Strip

Patients at risk for the development of cardiac dysrhythmias require careful monitoring, accurate diagnosis of the dysrhythmia, and assessment of the hemodynamic consequences of the rhythm disturbances. Primary cardiac dysrhythmias, like primary cardiac arrest, are unusual among infants and children. Infants and children at risk for a primary cardiac rhythm disturbance are those with congenital or acquired heart disease (particularly following cardiac surgical procedures), severe electrolyte imbalance, ingestion of a toxic substance, congenital complete heart block, and vagal sensitivity.

The clinical significance of a disturbance in cardiac rhythm for any patient is twofold: (1) what is the potential lethality of the rhythm disturbance and, (2) what is the dysrhythmia's potential for decreasing cardiac output and tissue perfusion.

Compared with adults, there is equal potential lethality among pediatric patients with similar dysrhythmias. Figure 9–21 illustrates the rapid (6-second) deterioration of supraventricular tachycardia (SVT) to ventricular tachycardia (VT) and ventricular fibrillation (VF) in a 9-month-old with viral myocarditis. In addition, pediatric patients may be at greater risk than adults for the potential of decreased CO when cardiac rhythm is disturbed because they are less able to adjust SV when cardiac rate or rhythm changes.

Accurate assessment of cardiac rhythm disturbances requires practice and understanding of four general principles. First, it is important to adopt a systematic approach to cardiac rhythm analysis and apply it consistently so that nothing is overlooked. Second, changes that are observed are followed for trends over time to evaluate their clinical significance. Third, observed changes are compared with age and maturationally related normal values (see Table 9–5). Finally, the rhythm disturbance is considered in terms of the patient's clinical situation (for example, recent acid-base or electrolyte values).

In addition, it is important to consider some fundamental principles of accurate bedside ECG monitoring.

Monitoring Leads

Most PICUs use bedside cardiac monitors with three lead wires designated RA and LA for right arm and left arm and LL for left leg. These bipolar leads monitor the leads I, II, and III via a positive, a negative, and a ground electrode. MCL_1 and MCL_6 leads can also be monitored via three bipolar electrodes. The MCL leads are more valuable than lead

II in evaluating abnormal ventricular conduction. To obtain MCL_1, the positive electrode is placed at the fourth intercostal space to the right of the sternum, the negative electrode is placed in the area of the left shoulder, and the ground lead is placed anywhere else. Figure 9–22A and B compares the position of the positive and negative electrodes in lead II and MCL_1. MCL_6 is obtained by placing the positive electrode at the fifth intercostal space at the midaxillary line, whereas the negative and ground electrodes are placed as in MCL_1.

Most rhythm disturbances among infants and children are disorders of rate, which produce bradycardia or tachycardia. Because bradycardia has a dramatic effect on cardiac output in young patients if not promptly recognized and treated, the most common goal of cardiac rhythm monitoring in critically ill infants and children is immediate recognition of progressive HR changes. In these instances, monitoring of lead I, II, or III is based on which lead provides the cleanest cardiac rhythm trace with clearly visible QRS complexes that are accurately counted by the monitor. Monitoring of the MCL leads is reserved for patients with ventricular conduction abnormalities.

Second-generation bedside cardiac monitors offer five-lead cardiogram monitoring, which makes it possible to monitor V_1 and V_6. Monitoring the cardiac rhythm from the V_1 or V_6 lead permits more reliable detection of right bundle branch block and clearer distinction between VT and SVT with aberrant ventricular conduction.

Electrode Placement

Regardless of the lead that is monitored, accurate positioning of the electrodes in their precise anatomic locations improves the accuracy of the cardiac rhythm tracing. The exception to this principle is the placement of limb electrodes in the 12-lead ECG, which may be placed anywhere on the extremity. Moving a chest electrode a short distance from its designated location can alter the appearance of the cardiac rhythm tracing dramatically. The RA and LA electrodes should be placed at the respective shoulder and the LL electrode on the left lower torso. When electrodes are moved close to the heart, the cardiac rhythm tracing is inaccurate. However, protecting the skin of critically ill infants and children and avoiding surgical incisions or chest tube insertion

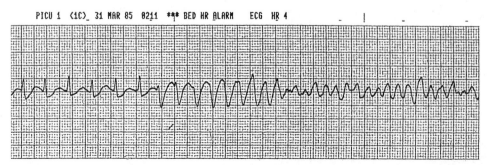

Figure 9–21 ● ● ● ● ● ●

Rapid (6-second) deterioration of supraventricular tachycardia (SVT) to ventricular tachycardia (VT) and ventricular fibrillation (VF) in a 9-month-old with viral myocarditis.

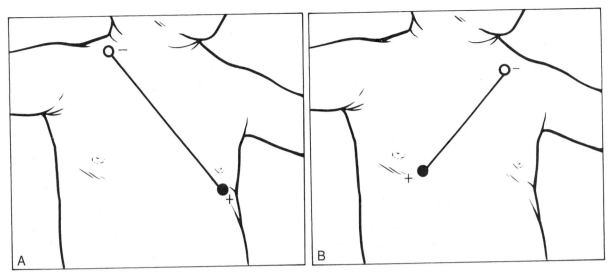

Figure 9–22 ● ● ● ● ● ●
A, Placement of the positive and negative electrodes for lead II monitoring. *B*, Electrode placement for MCL₁. (From Curley, M.A.Q. (1985). *Pediatric cardiac dysrhythmias*, p. 33. Bowie, MD: Copyright ©1985 Brady Communications Company, Inc.)

sites may necessitate moving electrodes from their designated spot.

Cardiac Rhythm Assessment

Ten factors are systematically assessed when evaluating a rhythm strip. Applying this approach permits accurate detection and diagnosis of rhythm disturbances.

The First Parameter to Evaluate Is Heart Rate. Heart rate (HR) is determined by the patient's metabolic demands, age, and clinical status. There is a gradual increase in average HR during the first month of life, followed by an even more gradual decrease across childhood and adolescence. Table 9–7 presents normal ranges for HR across infancy and childhood.

Sinus bradycardia and sinus tachycardia are individually defined as HRs beyond the normal range for age. They are, however, evaluated according to the child's activity level and clinical status. For example, a sinus tachycardia of 220 is not an unexpected or

Table 9–7. NORMAL VALUES IN PEDIATRIC CARDIAC RHYTHM ASSESSMENT

Age Interval	Heart Rate (range) bpm	P Wave Height (mm)/ Duration (seconds)	Maximum PR Interval Heart Rate (bpm)	Maximum PR Interval Interval (seconds)	QRS Duration (seconds)	QTc (seconds)
0–24 hours	119 (94–145)	<3.0/0.06		<0.11	0.04–0.05	<0.49
1–7 days	133 (100–175)	"			"	"
8–30 days	163 (115–190)	"			"	"
1–3 months	154 (124–190)	<2.5/0.08	91–110	<0.14	"	
			111–130	<0.13		
			131–150	<0.12		
			>150	<0.11		
3–6 months	140 (111–179)	"	"	"	"	"
6–9 months	140 (112–177)	"	"	"	"	<0.425
9–12 months	140 (112–177)	"	91–110	<0.15	0.05–0.06	"
			111–150	<0.14		
			>150	<0.10		
1–3 years	126 (98–163)	"	"	"	"	"
3–5 years	98 (65–132)	"		<0.16	0.06–0.08	"
5–8 years	96 (70–115)	"	<90	<0.18	"	"
			>90	<0.16		
8–12 years	79 (55–107)	"	"		0.08–0.10	"
12–16 years	75 (55–102)	"	"		"	"

bpm, beats per minute.
Adapted from Curley M.A.Q: Pediatric cardiac dysrhythmias. In S. J. Kelly (ed.). *Pediatric emergency nursing* (2nd ed., p. 231). Norwalk: Appleton & Lange, 1994.

abnormal finding in a stressed, febrile, anemic infant. Conversely, a sinus bradycardia of 90 can also be observed in a sleeping infant.

Generally speaking, extremes in HR are of no concern in pediatric patients unless the HR is incongruent with the patient's clinical needs. Slow rhythms in infants and young children are typically regarded as "code rhythms," that is, requiring emergency intervention. Most often, bradycardia is the result of hypoxia and acidosis or vagal stimulation.

Faster inherent rates are present in all of the potential pacemaker sites scattered throughout the myocardium. As a consequence, infants and children have faster escape rhythms than those seen in adults. Therefore, it is not possible to accurately diagnose an ectopic rhythm on the basis of HR alone.

When rapid heart rhythms are detected, the first element in accurate interpretation of the rhythm is consideration of the patient's history and current clinical situation. For example, sinus tachycardia (ST) is most often associated with fever, anemia, or extracellular fluid volume losses. Infants with SVT most often present with a several-day history of poor feeding and lethargy and demonstrate signs of CHF such as increased respiratory rate, sweating, liver enlargement, and others. Atrial flutter (AFl) most often occurs in patients with a significant history of congenital heart disease most often involving the atria. VT is most often seen in patients with history of severe metabolic or electrolyte imbalance, toxic ingestion, cardiomyopathy, or cardiac surgery.

ST is a secondary rhythm disturbance that reflects the need for more cardiac output in patients with increased metabolic demands. Primary tachycardias, which include SVT, AFl, and VT, are present in children with signs of cardiac dysfunction. Although poor perfusion is often present, it is the consequence of the rhythm disturbance, not the result of a demand for more cardiac output.

A key factor used to differentiate rapid HRs is the onset of the tachycardia. ST is characterized by a somewhat gradual acceleration of the heart rate. SVT and AFl, on the other hand, are tachydysrhythmias with abrupt acceleration of heart rates to 230 to 320 bpm, which most often is a result of a reentry mechanism.

A reentry circuit (Fig. 9–23) is formed from two functionally discrete conduction pathways that are joined proximally and distally to form a closed circuit, but that possess different refractory periods. When a premature atrial impulse reaches the reentry circuit, it is conducted slowly down the pathway with the shorter refractory period and blocked at the pathway with the longer refractory period. When the impulse arrives at the distal bifurcation of the two pathways, it is conducted down to the ventricles and conducted in a retrograde direction back up the pathway that was initially blocked. As a result of perfect reciprocal timing of both limbs of the reetry circuit, the impulse stimulates repetitive ectopic impulses that are conducted similarly and sustain very rapid heart rates.

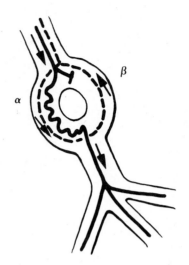

Figure 9–23 ● ● ● ● ● ●

Reentry circuit. (From Holbrook, P.R. (1993). *Textbook of pediatric critical care,* p. 386. Philadelphia: W.B. Saunders.)

The Second Parameter for Evaluation of a Rhythm Strip Is the Regularity of the Rhythm, as Well as the Presence of Grouped Beats. Sinus rhythm is fairly regular, but some variability is normally detected because of changes in vagal tone at the SA node. Sinus rhythm variability is best observed in young, sleeping children who demonstrate so-called "sinus arrhythmia." Figure 9–24 demonstrates the variation typical in sinus dysrhythmia during inspiration and exhalation. SVT and AFl are monotonously regular, because of the reentry circuit that perpetuates these dysrhythmias. Monotonous regularity can be easily identified using the trend recordings of HR over time available on some cardiac monitors; the rapid rates typical of SVT and AFl occur suddenly and are extremely consistent. Grouping of QRS complexes (i.e., clustering of QRS complexes identified by examination of a long rhythm strip) can be observed with sinus arrhythmia and with type I second degree heart block. Patterned irregularity is seen with type II second degree heart block.

The Third Parameter to Assess Is the P Wave. The P wave is evaluated for amplitude (height), duration, and consistency. P wave size and duration correspond to the relative size (mass) of the atria. Normally the P wave is no taller than 2.5 mm in children or 3 mm in newborns. The duration of the P wave is normally slightly shorter in the newborn, approximately 0.06 seconds, whereas 0.08 seconds is normal in children (see Table 9–7). Tall, peaked P waves may indicate right atrial hypertrophy. Wide, notched P waves are characteristic of left atrial hypertrophy. Bilateral atrial hypertrophy is indicated by P waves that are both wide and tall and perhaps notched. However, it is important to note that atrial hypertrophy may not be detected by a lead II rhythm strip.

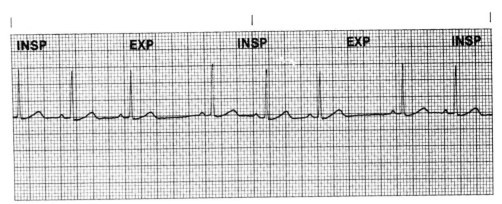

Figure 9–24 ● ● ● ● ● ●
Sinus arrhythmia in a 3-year-old. (From Curley, M.A.Q. (1985). *Pediatric cardiac dysrhythmias,* p. 70. Bowie, MD: Copyright ©1985. Brady Communications Company, Inc.)

Figure 9–25*A* illustrates P waves that are 5 mm tall and 0.12 seconds in duration, well beyond normal range for pediatric patient.

P waves should be upright and consistent in appearance in lead II. If they are not, an ectopic rhythm is suspected. For example, normal P waves are re-

placed by flutter or fibrillation waves in AFl or atrial fibrillation, respectively (Fig. 9–25*B*). In junctional rhythms, the P wave may occur before the QRS complex and look different than the sinus P wave, or the P waves may be buried within or occur after the QRS complex (Fig. 9–25*C*).

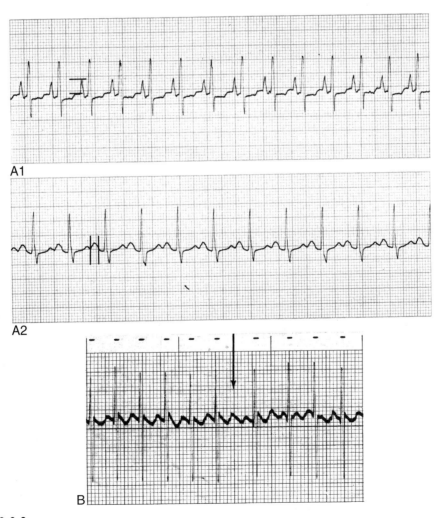

A1

A2

B

Figure 9–25 ● ● ● ● ● ●
A, Abnormal P waves in a pediatric patient. 1, Right atrial hypertrophy, P waves measure 5 mm. 2, Left atrial hypertrophy, P wave duration measures 0.12 second. *B,* Normal P waves replaced by flutter waves in atrial flutter.
Illustration continued on following page

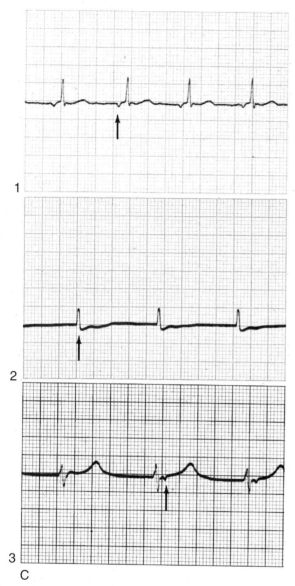

Figure 9–25 *Continued* ● ● ● ● ●

C, Altered P wave morphology and location in junctional heart rhythms. 1, Inverted P waves before the QRS complex atrial depolarization first, then ventricular depolarization. 2, Buried P wave within the QRS complex atrial ventricular depolarization at the same time. 3, Inverted P wave after the QRS complex ventricular depolarization first, then atrial depolarization. (From Curley, M.A.Q. (1985). *Pediatric cardiac dysrhythmias,* pp. 59, 88, 101, 102. Bowie, MD: Copyright ©1985 Brady Communications Company, Inc.)

The Fourth Parameter for Evaluation Is the PR Interval. The length of the PR interval varies both with age and HR; it is shorter in younger patients and with more rapid HRs (see Table 9–7). The PR interval is measured to ascertain whether it is normal, too short, or prolonged. First degree heart block is defined as a PR interval longer than the normal for age and HR. It is seen in approximately 10% of the population in whom it is indicative only of parasympathetic dominance at the SA node, but no pathophysiology. In patients receiving digoxin, first degree heart block is a sign of digoxin effectiveness in slowing conduction. In atrial ectopic rhythms, conduction of the atrial impulse does not follow the normal pathways. The PR interval may be prolonged as a consequence. Occasionally, a long PR interval is detected in patients with myocarditis and in patients with endocardial cushion defects, Ebstein's anomaly of the tricuspid valve, or L-transposition (also called "corrected transposition").

Conversely, the PR interval may be excessively short—less than 0.08 seconds in those younger than 3 years of age, less than 0.10 seconds in children between the ages of 3 and 16 years, and less than 0.12 seconds in those over 16 years. The short PR interval demonstrates accelerated conduction to the ventricles. For example, in junctional rhythms the PR interval is short if the P wave occurs before the QRS complex, because the impulse is initiated closer to the ventricular conduction system than impulses initiated in the SA node. The rhythm strip in patients with WPW syndrome typically demonstrates a short PR interval because conduction from the atria to the ventricles is more rapid than normal because of the presence of accessory fibers that connect the two (Fig. 9–26). As a result, conduction from the atria bypasses the AV node. The early activation of the ventricles also produces a short, sloped PR interval known as a delta wave (Fig. 9–27). Occasionally, a short PR interval is detected in people with glycogen storage disease, related to the low electrical impedance characteristic of the myocardial effects of the disorder, and in patients with tricuspid atresia.

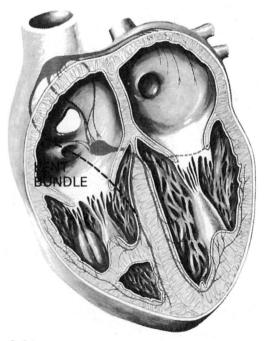

Figure 9–26 ● ● ● ● ● ●

Accessory fibers that connect the atrium and ventricle in Wolff-Parkinson-White (WPW) syndrome. (From Curley, M.A.Q. (1985). *Pediatric cardiac dysrhythmias,* p. 86. Bowie, MD: Copyright ©1985. Brady Communications Company, Inc.)

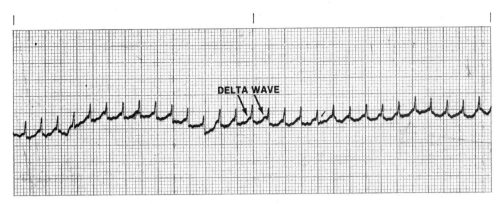

Figure 9-27 ● ● ● ● ● ●
Delta wave in the ECG of a patient with WPW syndrome. (From Curley, M.A.Q. (1985). *Pediatric cardiac dysrhythmias*, p. 87. Bowie, MD: Copyright ©1985. Brady Communications Company, Inc.)

The Fifth Parameter for Assessment Is the P:QRS Relationship. Every P wave that occurs after a T wave should be conducted to the ventricles and produce ventricular depolarization, which is demonstrated by a QRS complex. If a one-to-one P:QRS relationship does not exist, heart block or AV dissociation is suspected.

In patients with second degree heart block, the rhythm strip reveals more than one P wave for each QRS complex. Second degree heart block is classified in two groups. In patients with Mobitz type I heart block (also called Wenckebach phenomenon), there is progressive prolongation of the AV node refractory period and slowing of AV node conduction. Eventually, an atrial impulse arrives at the AV node during its absolute refractory period and cannot be conducted. The rhythm strip reveals progressive lengthening of the PR interval and concomitant shortening of the RR interval until a P wave is not followed by a QRS complex (Fig. 9–28). Characteristic grouping of complexes is evident. Mobitz type I second degree heart block may reflect AV node dysfunction in patients following intracardiac surgical procedures near the AV node or in those with digoxin, beta-blocker, calcium channel blocker, or quinidine toxicity. It is, however, detected in people without pathophysiology, especially during sleep. Mobitz type I second degree heart block does not usually progress to third degree (complete) heart block. No treatment is indicated unless the ventricular rate is excessively slow and CO is compromised as a consequence. In these patients, administration of atropine may be helpful because it accelerates AV node conduction and the rate of SA node impulse formation.

In patients with Mobitz type II second degree heart block, analysis of the rhythm strip reveals an occasional or a patterned block of AV conduction. The P wave is not followed by a QRS complex (Fig. 9–29). This type of heart block is related to bundle of His or bundle branch dysfunction, usually as a result of surgical injury. Progression to third degree heart block is more common. Intravenous isoproterenol or epinephrine accelerates the ventricular rate and may be helpful in stabilizing the rhythm until pacemaker therapy is available.

Third degree or complete heart block (CHB) may be either congenital or acquired. Regardless of the etiology, the SA node paces the atria, whereas either a junctional or ventricular escape rhythm paces the ventricles. CHB in the area of the AV node is characterized by a narrow complex, junctional escape rhythm (Fig. 9–30). In contrast, complete block at the His bundle results in a wide complex, ventricular escape rhythm. Junctional escape rhythms often increase in response to stress or exercise, whereas ventricular escape rhythms are more often fixed at a low rate that does not respond to demand for increased cardiac output. Figure 9–30 represents the rhythm strip of an infant with septic shock who developed CHB.

Acquired CHB may result from severe metabolic derangement such as hypoxia; acidosis; hypothermia; hypoglycemia; electrolyte imbalance (especially of potassium or calcium); drug toxicity; acquired myocardial disease, including myocarditis; or as a consequence of surgical procedures around the ventricular conduction system.

While efforts to identify and correct the underlying cause of acquired CHB are initiated, administration of intravenous isoproterenol or epinephrine (0.05–0.1 mcg/kg/min) to increase the ventricular rate is usually necessary. Temporary pacing may be accomplished with a transcutaneous or transvenous pacemaker or via surgically placed epicardial wires. Permanent pacing is necessitated if acquired CHB persists, because the escape rhythm is generally unresponsive to demand for increased CO. Demand for increased HR often is detected on the rhythm strip as an increase in atrial rate, without an increase in ventricular rate, or by a widened QRS complex.

Congenital CHB is frequently associated with maternal collagen vascular diseases such as systemic

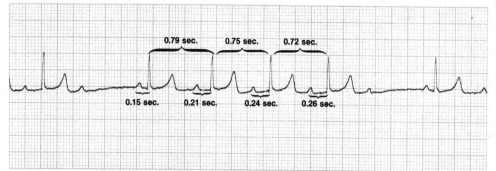

Mobitz type I second degree heart block with progressive lengthening of the PR interval and shortening of the RR interval until no QRS complex follows the P wave. (From Curley, M.A.Q. (1985). *Pediatric cardiac dysrhythmias*, p. 136. Bowie, MD: Copyright ©1985. Brady Communications Company, Inc.)

Mobitz type II second degree heart block with 2:1 atrioventricular conduction. (From Curley, M.A.Q. (1985). *Pediatric cardiac dysrhythmias*, p. 137. Bowie, MD: Copyright ©1985. Brady Communications Company, Inc.)

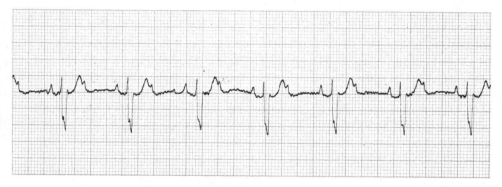

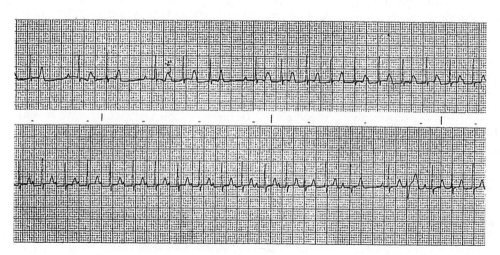

Complete heart block in an infant with sepsis.

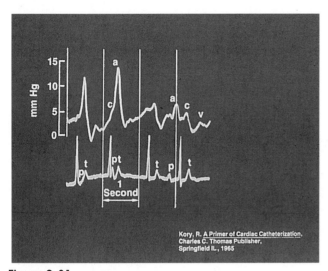

Figure 9–31 ● ● ● ● ● ●

Cannon A waves in AV dissociation as the atria contract against a closed tricuspid valve.

lupus erythematosus. In addition, some 25% of infants with congenital CHB have congenital heart defects; including L-transposition, univentricular heart, AV canal, and tricuspid atresia.

Infants with CHB are most often diagnosed during the prenatal period when an excessively slow HR is detected. Fetal echocardiography reveals that the semilunar valves are opening and closing at a rate far slower than the AV valves. In some, the HR is so slow that severe CHF is present at birth. Mortality is high among this group. Those infants who are asymptomatic at birth, except for the slow HR, generally have an escape rhythm of 60 to 70 bpm.

Initial management of infants with CHB may necessitate administration of atropine or isoproterenol to increase HR. The infant is carefully evaluated for the development of CHF or activity intolerance. If either is present, or if the ventricular rate cannot increase when metabolic demand increases, placement of a permanent pacemaker is indicated. If the HR is able to increase, the infant may be discharged without intervention, but with close follow-up. Both HR and SV may increase over time; CHF, exercise intolerance, and Stokes-Adams attacks are managed by pacemaker insertion.

The P-QRS relationship may also be useful in analysis of tachydysrhythmias, although it is often difficult to detect P waves from the lead II rhythm strip because ectopic rhythms in infants and children occur at very rapid rates. Supraventricular pacemakers are usually conducted to the ventricle in a one-to-one ratio. In junctional ectopic tachycardia (JET) or VT, AV dissociation is present.

A number of diagnostic tools are available to assist in the assessment of the AV relationship during tachycardia. First, AV dissociation can be assessed from the RA hemodynamic waveform. In Afl, flutter waves replace the normal a, v, and c waves in the RA waveform. Cannon A waves are present in AV dissociation, occurring when the atria contract against a closed tricuspid valve (Fig. 9–31).

Second, assessing the P-QRS relationship in more than one lead is often useful. Figure 9–32 is a 12-lead ECG in a 9-year-old with wide complex tachycardia. In lead V-1 the AV dissociation is evident, aiding the diagnosis of VT.

Finally, the rhythm strip can be recorded using a transesophageal electrode or from transthoracic atrial wires, if they were placed during a cardiac

Figure 9–32 ● ● ● ● ● ●

Wide complex tachycardia with AV dissociation evidence in lead VI.

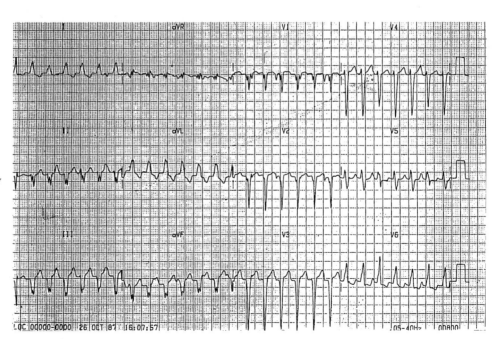

surgical procedure. Atrial depolarization is detected with the transesophageal electrode because the lower esophagus lies posterior to the left atrium (LA). Here, a 4 or 6 French bipolar pacing catheter or a swallowed pill electrode is placed like a nasogastric tube and slowly withdrawn to provide optimal visualization of atrial waves (Fig. 9–33). An epicardial rhythm strip is recorded directly from the wires placed on the RA and LA to clearly demonstrate the AV relationship. In addition, atrial overdrive pacing to interrupt a tachydysrhythmia can be accomplished via either transesophageal or atrial epicardial wires. Less traumatic than traditional cardioversion, atrial overdrive pacing is useful when the patient is resistant or intolerant of drug therapy or until the patient's condition is stabilized on antidysrhythmic medications.

Duration of the QRS Complex Is the Sixth Assessment Parameter Evaluated in Rhythm Strip Analysis. QRS duration correlates with ventricular mass and becomes wider as the infant or child grows (see Table 9–7). Wider-than-expected QRS complexes occur when ventricular impulse conduction is aberrant. For example, premature ventricular contractions (PVCs) and bundle branch blocks (BBB) result in abnormally long conduction pathways. PVCs are often insignificant in infants and children; however, in the face of cardiac dysfunction or other rhythm disturbances, they warrant careful assessment. In all cases, the hemodynamic significance of the premature beats is evaluated. Degree of block (that is, partial or complete BBB) is not differentiated in pediatrics. Conduction blocks occur in either the right or the left bundle branch because of congenital heart defects or myocardial inflammation. Right BBB is common after right ventriculotomy.

The QRS duration is typically described as the index that, in conjunction with HR, is most useful in differentiating VT from SVT. However, VT in pediatric patients may produce a faster rate and shorter QRS duration than is seen in adults patients, making the distinction between VT and SVT with aberrant ventricular conduction difficult. A number of factors are considered in making the distinction between the two:

1. Rate. VT can occur at rates more rapid than SVT; VT between 230 and 425 bpm have been reported (Garson, 1987). In infancy, VT is suspected if the rate is in excess of 300 bpm, whereas SVT occurs at rates between 230 and 300. Out of infancy, rates greater than 230 are thought to be SVT.
2. Rhythm. VT is an irregular rhythm, with beat-to-beat variation. SVT is monotonously regular.
3. P-QRS relationship. In SVT the relationship is one-to-one (1:1), whereas AV dissociation exists in VT.
4. QRS duration. The duration of the QRS complex is the most critical assessment parameter in pediatric patients with an uncertain tachydysrhythmia. In the vast majority of patients with SVT,

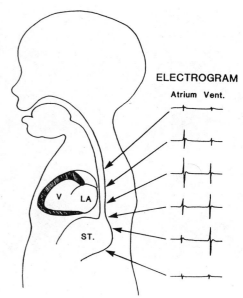

Figure 9–33 ● ● ● ● ● ●

The anatomic relationship between the esophagus and the cardiac chambers in infants. The ideal electrogram at midesophagus has an atrial spike that is equal to, or larger than, the ventricular signal. V, ventricle; LA, left atrium; ST, stomach. (From Walsh, E.P. (1992). Electrocardiography and introduction to electrophysiological techniques. In Fyler, D.C. (ed.). *Nadas' pediatric cardiology*, p. 147. Philadelphia: Hanley & Belfus.)

the QRS complex is normal or only slightly abnormal (a few have RBBB or AV bypass tracts). Aberrant conduction is rarely rate-related in pediatric patients. As a consequence, any wide complex tachycardia in infants or children is considered VT until proved otherwise.
5. Initial deflection. If the first beat of a tachydysrhythmia is observed or recorded, it may hold a valuable diagnostic clue. In VT the initial abnormal beat is deflected in the direction opposite the normal QRS complex. In SVT the direction of the deflection is the same as that of the QRS complex.
6. Fusion complexes. Fusion complexes are aberrently conducted QRS complexes that are created from a fusion of a supraventricular and ventricular initiated beats; thus, they resemble a combination of both. They may be present at the start of a run of VT.

Figure 9–34 shows rhythm strips in which wide complex tachycardia is noted. The most crucial assessment in each case is the impact of the rhythm disturbance on CO and tissue perfusion.

Ingestion of tricyclic antidepressants results in prolongation of the QRS complex. Prolonged QRS duration provides a bedside guide to predict patients at risk for significant complications of tricyclic medication overdosage (i.e., seizures, ventricular dysrhythmias, and death). Figure 9–35 is an illustration of the change in QRS duration across 8 hours' time in a 14-year-old patient who ingested a tricyclic antidepressant.

The QRS duration, finally, is a useful assessment

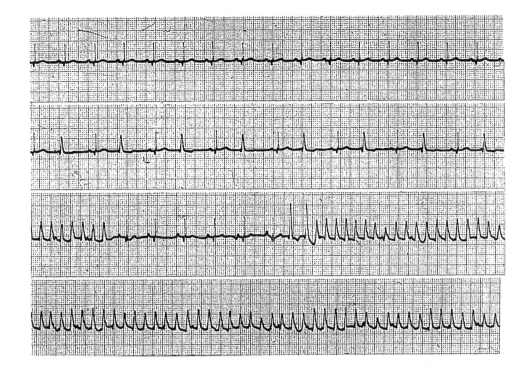

Figure 9–34 ● ● ● ● ● ●
Wide complex tachycardia.

tool in patients with hyperkalemia. The first rhythm strip change noted with hyperkalemia is tenting of the T wave. However, if the serum potassium level continues to rise, cardiac conductivity is decreased. The rhythm strip appears stretched; the QRS duration is lengthened, the PR interval is excessively long, and the P wave is broad. Figure 9–36 represents the rhythm strip of a patient with acute adrenal insufficiency and a serum potassium level of 10 mEq/L.

The Seventh Assessment Parameter Is the ST Segment. The ST segment is evaluated from the J point (the junction of the QRS complex and the ST segment) and compared with the isoelectric line or baseline of the rhythm strip. Normally there is less than a 1-mm deviation from the baseline in a lead II rhythm strip, and the ST segment rises from the J point. Abnormalities include both a horizontal ST segment and a downward slope from the J point.

Depression of the ST segment is associated with

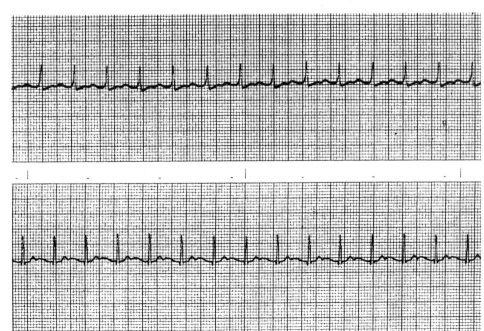

Figure 9–35 ● ● ● ● ● ●
Prolonged QRS duration in tricyclic antidepressant ingestion; changes in a patient's ECG over 8 hours time. (From Kelley, S.J. (1994). *Pediatric emergency nursing,* 2nd ed., p. 234. Norwalk, CT: Appleton & Lange.)

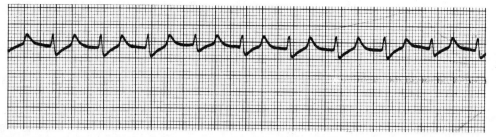

Figure 9–36 • • • • • •

Hyperkalemia prolongs cardiac conduction: the QRS duration and PR interval are prolonged, the P wave broad. (From Curley, M.A.Q. (1985). *Pediatric cardiac dysrhythmias,* p. 153. Bowie, MD: Copyright ©1985. Brady Communications Company, Inc.)

ventricular strain or ischemia and is sometimes seen with tachycardia (Fig. 9–37). Rapid HR shortens the diastolic period of the cardiac cycle and decreases the time for coronary artery filling. Patients with SVT who undergo cardioversion may demonstrate persistent ST segment depression for several days, indicating the stress sustained by the myocardium during the tachycardia. Elevation of the ST segment is seen in patients with pericarditis or other cardiac inflammatory processes.

The ST segment may be deformed by an Osborn wave, also called a J wave or hypothermic hump. This positive deflection near the J point is indicative of late ventricular depolarization. It is detected in patients with severe hypothermia or in those who are brain dead.

The Eighth Parameter for Assessment Is the T wave. The direction of T wave deflection is normally the same as the QRS deflection. The T wave is generally about 1/5 the height of the QRS complex. Abnormalities in the T wave are the result of abnormal depolarization (such as that which occurs with PVC) or when repolarization is abnormal (as in patients with myocarditis).

Whereas serum potassium levels may be misleading, the rhythm strip graphically represents potassium shifts across the excitable cell membrane. The rhythm strip is a useful tool in the assessment of total body potassium. For example, in diabetic ketoacidosis (DKA), shifts in serum potassium are common. Figure 9–38 shows the rhythm strip changes that resulted when serum potassium fell from 7.9 to 2.1 mEq/L in a patient with DKA.

The Ninth Parameter Evaluated Is the QT Interval. The QT interval represents the total time elapsed in ventricular systole. Because duration of the QT interval varies with HR, increasing with slower rates and decreasing with rapid rates, the duration is corrected by the following calculation:

$$\text{QTc} = \text{measured QT interval} \div \text{square root of the RR interval}$$

Generally, the corrected QT interval is calculated only if the T wave ends beyond two-thirds of the distance in the RR interval. Normally, it is less than 0.49 seconds in infants younger than 6 months of age and less than 0.425 seconds in all other children.

Shortening of the QT interval is detected in patients receiving digoxin and in those with hypercalcemia. Prolonged QT interval occurs with hypocalcemia, myocarditis, hypothermia, organophosphorus

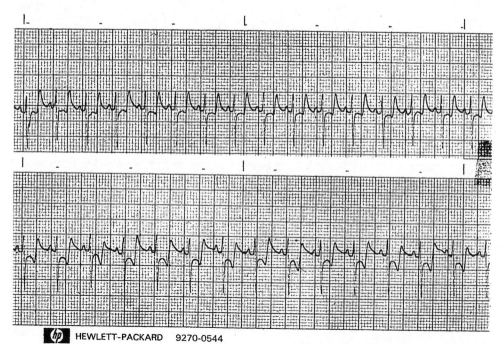

Figure 9–37 • • • • • •

Depression of the ST segment with tachycardia.

HEWLETT-PACKARD   9270-0544

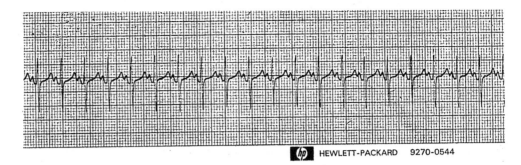

HEWLETT-PACKARD   9270-0544

Figure 9-38 • • • • • •

T wave changes with shifts in serum potassium in a patient with diabetic ketoacidosis.

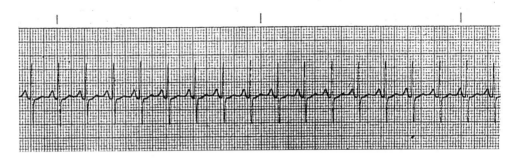

insecticide poisoning, and medication toxicity (i.e., with quinidine, procainamide, ecainide, and amiodarone). In addition, a potentially lethal disorder, prolonged QT interval syndrome, is recognized.

Patients with prolonged QT interval syndrome have a genetic disorder in which a trigger event such as emotional stress, physical activity, or auditory startle increases SNS activity and an imbalance of right and left sympathetic ganglion activity occurs. Left sympathetic ganglion activity, which lengthens the QT interval, is increased. As a consequence, ventricular depolarization is prolonged and the person is at risk for ventricular dysrhythmias and sudden death. Tosades de pointes, a polymorphic form of VT, is seen in these patients.

Treatment is aimed at restoring SNS balance to shorten the ventricular depolarization period. Cardioversion is required immediately for conversion of VT. Medical treatment with antidysrhythmics or implantation of an internal pacemaker are required for long-term management.

The Tenth Parameter Assessed Is the Presence of U Waves. The significance of this late electrical event is uncertain. It may represent delayed depolarization of the terminal Purkinje network. Hypokalemia, which also prolongs ventricular depolarization, is evidenced by a depressed ST segment, a flat T wave, and the presence of U waves. Ventricular ectopy is increased in the presence of hypokalemia.

Radiographic Evaluation

Chest radiographs of the seriously ill pediatric patient provide important information about heart size,

specific chamber enlargement, and the volume of pulmonary blood flow. Most of these data are obtained from a standard posteroanterior (AP) chest film. Oblique and lateral films may be helpful in the detection of specific changes in cardiac shape and size.

Detection of cardiac enlargement is an important goal of chest radiography. This determination is often made by measuring the transverse diameter of the heart and comparing it with the width of the thorax. Cardiomegaly is present when the heart size is greater than one-half the width of the thorax. Also significant is a change in heart size detected when one radiograph is compared with previous films. Although this technique reliably reveals left ventricular enlargement, right ventricular enlargement is not appreciated in the AP view, but rather is best seen in the lateral view.

Assessment of the vascular markings on the chest radiograph detects alterations in pulmonary blood flow. With a large left-to-right shunt, PBF is increased, resulting in increased size and prominence of the pulmonary blood vessels well into the peripheral lung fields. Patients with heart defects that result in decreased PBF have diminished vascular markings in the lung fields.

The skeletal aspects of the chest radiograph are examined because of the association of congenital heart defects with other congenital anomalies, including vertebral and other skeletal abnormalities. The pulmonary parenchyma is inspected because pneumonia is a significant problem in children with increased pulmonary blood flow. Atelectasis may also occur in children who have large left-to-right shunts, especially in the postoperative period following cardiac surgery.

Barium swallow and magnetic resonance imaging (MRI) add substantially to the cardiac evaluation. Barium swallow esophagrams are useful in the detection of atrial enlargement and coarctation of the aorta. However, MRI has largely replaced the barium swallow for these indications. Barium swallow remains useful in detecting vascular rings that result in airway or esophageal obstruction, although MRI provides specific anatomic detail. MRI is also useful in older children suspected to have coarctation of the aorta and in postoperative evaluation of the reconstructed aorta (Fig. 9–39). MRI has added fine anatomic detail to the evaluation of intracardiac and great vessel structure and orientation.

Echocardiography

Echocardiography provides the most complete noninvasive assessment of cardiac structure and function. Echocardiography uses high frequency ultrasonic waves from a transducer. Waves are directed toward cardiac structures and reflected back to the transducer by even very small structures. The sound waves reflected back can be recorded. Although physical examination may not always exclude structural heart defects, echocardiography has been shown to accurately reveal abnormalities and guide the care of patients with CHD.

Two-dimensional (2-D) echocardiograms record sound waves reflected from cardiac structures on a planar image, permitting a spatial orientation or view of the heart. Atrial and ventricular septal defects can be identified by 2-D echocardiography, as can most other abnormalities of cardiac structure.

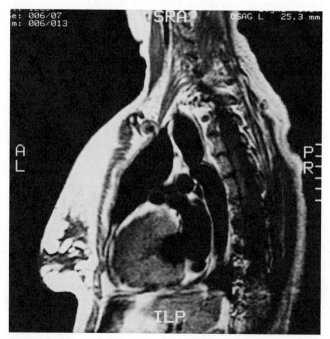

Figure 9–39 ● ● ● ● ● ●
MRI demonstrates coarctation of the aorta in an adolescent patient.

Doppler echocardiography records the velocity of moving objects and can accurately assess blood flow within the heart, at the heart valves, and in the great vessels. Pulsed Doppler echocardiography can accomplish the same things, but also provides a recording of the heart structures (Fig. 9–40A and B). It can determine the presence, timing, and direction of an intracardiac shunt, as well as the pressure differences between cardiac chambers. In patent ductus arteriosus, Doppler echocardiography detects the turbulent flow in the pulmonary artery during both systole and diastole and indicates the direction of shunting through the ductus. The same data can be obtained for surgically created shunts.

In addition to revealing structural cardiac defects, echocardiography is useful in the evaluation of cardiac function. The simplest measures of cardiac performance are the dimensions of the cardiac chambers at end-systole and end-diastole. The end-diastolic diameter of the ventricle provides a measure of the patient's intravascular volume status. Ventricular shortening fraction, a measure similar to ejection fraction, is a predictor of ventricular systolic performance. It is calculated by dividing the difference between ventricular end-diastolic diameter and end-systolic diameter by the end-diastolic diameter

$$VED - SED \div VED, \%$$

The velocity of ventricular shortening and the ventricular systolic time also can be measured and are good indicators of the heart's systolic performance.

Measurement of the heart's diastolic function can also be achieved with echocardiography. The ventricles fill with blood in a predictable pattern during diastole. Abnormalities in filling can be identified, as can alterations in end-diastolic chamber size and wall thickness. A small-chambered, thick-walled ventricle is characteristic of poor ventricular diastolic function and may be seen in severe heart failure, hypertrophic cardiomyopathy, and end-stage heart disease.

Cardiac output measurements made by Doppler echocardiography correlate well with other measures of CO (Alverson et al., 1982). Doppler CO measurement is based on measurement of the left ventricular outflow tract and the velocity of blood flowing through the aortic valve. Errors in measurement are the result, most often, of inaccuracies in measurement of the outflow tract. Despite this limitation, Doppler measures of CO are particularly useful in following trends in a patient. Even if there is error in measurement of the outflow tract, relative changes in cardiac output can be followed (Martin & Holley, 1993).

Occasionally, transthoracic echocardiography does not provide adequate images for accurate diagnosis. Obesity, prior cardiac surgery, ventilator therapy, and chest wall deformity can prohibit adequate transthoracic imaging. A transesophageal echocardiogram can be performed in the intensive care unit. The transesophageal echocardiogram uses a flexible endo-

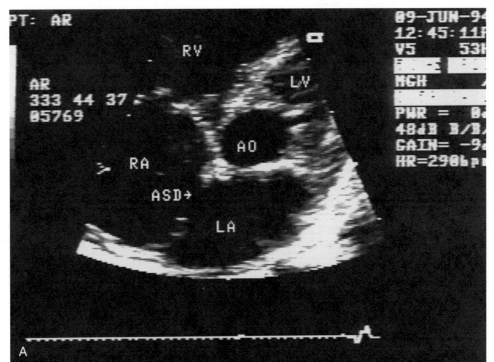

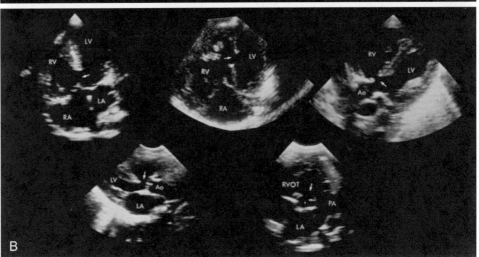

Figure 9–40 ● ● ● ● ● ●

A, Doppler echocardiography demonstrates an atrial septal defect (ASD). *B,* Five different types of ventricular septal defect are demonstrated with Doppler echocardiography.

scope with a high-resolution ultrasonic transducer at the tip. Cardiac structures viewed from the transesophageal position are visualized with substantially improved images. Intracardiac vegetations, small cardiac tumors or clots, and intraoperative or postoperative repair of structural heart defects can be assessed via the transesophageal route.

In the postoperative cardiac surgery patient, pericardial tamponade is a potentially life-threatening development. Patients with thoracic trauma may also develop cardiac tamponade. Patients with myocarditis and those recovering from the Fontan procedure may develop pericardial effusion. In each case the diagnosis can be made by echocardiography and the introduction and position of a pericardiocentesis

needle guided and confirmed by echocardiography prior to aspiration of the fluid.

Fetal Echocardiography

Prenatal ultrasonography has become routine for many. Ultrasound provides a global view of the fetal heart, revealing its presence and rhythmic contraction, and demonstrating the great arteries arising from the heart. Fetal echocardiography using continuous Doppler imaging has become an established technique for detecting abnormal intra- and extracardiac anatomy. Fetal echocardiography yields reliable information at 16 to 18 weeks gestation if the technician is able to obtain an adequate window to view the fetus. Fetal position or movement may make the examination difficult, requiring the mother to ambulate or return for reexamination.

INVASIVE EVALUATION AND DIAGNOSIS

Definitive diagnosis of cardiac structure and function may require invasive diagnostic techniques. In the intensive care unit, hemodynamic monitoring provides valuable information regarding cardiovascular function. Definitive structural and functional information about the heart is obtained, in some instances, only by cardiac catheterization.

Hemodynamic Monitoring

Invasive hemodynamic monitoring of infants and children in the PICU is routine. Although the ability to measure, monitor, and calculate many physiologic parameters related to cardiovascular performance is valuable in the care of critically ill pediatric patients, numeric hemodynamic data alone is inadequate for clinical decision-making. The sections that follow focus on the measurement of hemodynamic parameters and the calculation of derived hemodynamic data. The correlation of hemodynamic data with clinical assessment information and the effects of various modes of therapy are integrated. Accurate clinical decision-making is based on the integration of hemodynamic monitoring data and sound clinical assessment.

Fundamentals of Hemodynamic Monitoring

Invasive hemodynamic monitoring systems use a transducer to convert one energy form to another. The physical energy of blood pressure is converted to an electrical signal that is amplified and displayed. Most often disposable transducers are used, which eliminate the risks of patient infection from reusable equipment. Disposable transducers are cost-effective, rugged, and highly accurate. They do not drift with time or temperature and are calibrated to within ± 2% or 1 mmHg, whichever is greater.

Figure 9–41 illustrates one example of an arterial blood pressure monitoring system. A radial artery catheter is connected through a short piece of pressure tubing to a stopcock. The stopcock near the insertion site is connected to a second stopcock at the transducer with a longer pressure tube. The transducer is connected to a flush device that delivers a controlled volume of solution on a continuous basis (e.g., a syringe pump) and to the monitor that displays the pressure waveform and the numeric measurement of the blood pressure. Basic transducer setups vary among institutions. For example, use of

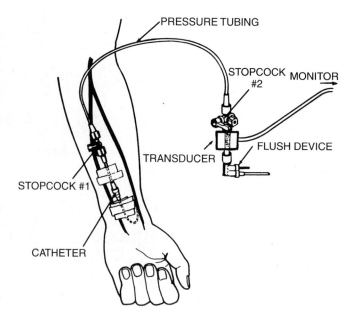

Figure 9–41 ● ● ● ● ● ●

An arterial blood pressure monitoring system. (From Gardner, R.M., Hujcs (1993). Fundamentals of physiologic monitoring. *AACN Clinical Issues in Critical Care Nursing,* 4:19.)

needleless systems that eliminate the stopcocks in the system is increased.

Setting the Zero Point for the Monitoring System. Setting the zero point or "zeroing" the pressure monitoring system is the *single* most important step in setting up the monitoring system. The proper technique for setting the zero point for a pressure monitoring system is illustrated in Figure 9–42. The transducer must be carefully positioned at the fourth intercostal space-midaxillary-line or phlebostatic reference point. Inaccurate transducer position can result in large errors in pressure measurement, especially when pressures are low, as is the case when central venous or pulmonary artery wedge pressures

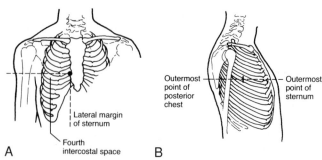

Figure 9–42 ● ● ● ● ● ●

The phlebostatic axis. The crossing of two imaginary lines defines the assumed position of the monitoring catheter tip within the body i.e., right atrial level. *A,* A line that passes from the fourth intercostal space at the lateral margin of the sternum down the side of the body beneath the axilla. *B,* A line that runs horizontally at a point midway between the outermost portion of the anterior and posterior surfaces of the chest. (From Darovic, G.O. (1987). *Hemodynamic monitoring: Invasive and non-invasive clinical applications,* p. 126. Philadelphia: W.B. Saunders.)

are monitored. For example, a transducer positioned 15 cm above the phlebostatic reference point will result in a venous pressure reading 11 mmHg lower than is actually the case; a transducer located 15 cm below the midaxillary line will result in a venous pressure reading 11 mmHg above the actual pressure. These inaccuracies are the consequence of the effects of hydrostatic pressure on the blood pressure reading. When more than one pressure is monitored, all transducers are placed in one holder to ensure accuracy when correlating data.

When the transducer is accurately positioned, either the stopcock at the patient end of the system or the stopcock at the transducer is opened to air and the monitor zeroed. Care must be taken to ensure that excessively long lengths of tubing from the flush device or between the patient and the transducer are avoided and that the tubing does not hang below the transducer.

Unusual pressure readings should always prompt reassessment of the system position and re-zeroing of the monitoring system, especially if treatment changes are anticipated based on the pressure measured. Changes in the transducer or amplifier related to time and temperature and changes in the patient's position relative to the transducer can produce zero changes.

System Calibration. Transducer manufacturers calibrate the system sensitivity to within ± 1%. Thus, only zeroing is required when using standardized, disposable transducers. Checking the calibration with a column of air or mercury is unnecessary and may introduce risk of system contamination or embolism.

Optimizing System Accuracy. Hemodynamic pressure waveforms are dynamic, not static. The accuracy and reliability of the system's transmission of a pressure waveform to the transducer is crucial. To ensure accuracy of invasive pressure monitoring, the following procedures are necessary, in addition to the zeroing procedure described (Gardner & Hujcs, 1993; Quaal, 1993b):

1. All air bubbles in the system are eliminated. Air bubbles result in underestimation of the systolic pressure and overestimation of the diastolic pressure. Air bubbles frequently are located in stopcocks, when all the ports have not been filled with fluid, and at connection points between tubings and between tubings and stopcocks.
2. Blood clots are prevented by the continuous infusion of flush solution. Thrombus formation on the catheter has the same effects described when air bubbles are present in the system.
3. Only noncompliant pressure tubing, in the shortest lengths possible (no longer than 3 to 4 feet), is used. Venous tubing, which is excessively compliant, or long lengths of tubing result in the same errors described above.
4. The number of tubing connections is minimized. All loose-fitting connections are corrected.

Assuring that pressure monitoring equipment is properly set up and maintained provides accurate and valuable data to critical care personnel. Attention to detail assures the acquisition of accurate physiologic data.

Dynamic Response Validation. The ability of the hemodynamic monitoring system to accurately transmit a pressure waveform is a function of both the system's "natural frequency" (analogous to a car tire bouncing on a highway) and its "damping coefficient" (how quickly the car stabilizes after each bounce) (Gardner & Hollingworth, 1986). The fast-flush test stimulates the hemodynamic monitoring system with high pressure so that the natural frequency and damping coefficient can be observed. The fast flush test is performed by opening and quickly closing the fast flush device to temporarily interrupt the physiologic pressure waveform. A "square wave" pressure, followed by oscillations that revert to the pressure waveform being monitored, is observed (Fig. 9–43A and B). Daily and Schroeder (1989) detail the fast flush test procedure.

Performing the fast flush test necessitates brief but rapid infusion of flush solution into the vascular catheter. Small arteries in patients with inadequate tissue perfusion may spasm in response to rapid flushing. In this circumstance, it is impossible to perform the fast flush test. However, natural frequency is maximized in every patient's monitoring system by meticulous attention to the factors listed earlier that enhance system accuracy.

Arterial Blood Pressure Monitoring

Continuous invasive monitoring of arterial blood pressure is frequently necessary in the pediatric intensive care setting to ensure accurate evaluation of changes in patient status and the effects of therapies prescribed. Direct blood pressure measurement is preferred in patients with circulatory dysfunction, because impaired peripheral circulation and vasoconstriction render indirect measurement inaccurate or impossible to obtain. In addition, arterial cannulation for direct blood pressure measurement provides reliable access for blood sampling when frequent laboratory evaluation, such as of arterial blood gases, is required.

Arterial Cannulation Sites. The choice of an arterial pressure monitoring site is based on the identification of an artery that has adequate collateral circulation. The Allen test is performed when the radial artery is selected for cannulation. Both the radial and ulnar arteries are compressed until the hand blanches. The ulnar artery only is released and the hand is assessed for return of color in 5 to 7 seconds. If perfusion is delayed for more than 15 seconds, collateral circulation is considered inadequate and another arterial site is selected for cannulation (Fuhrman et al, 1992; VanRiper & VanRiper, 1987). Similar technique for evaluating other arterial sites is necessary. For example, the posterior tibial

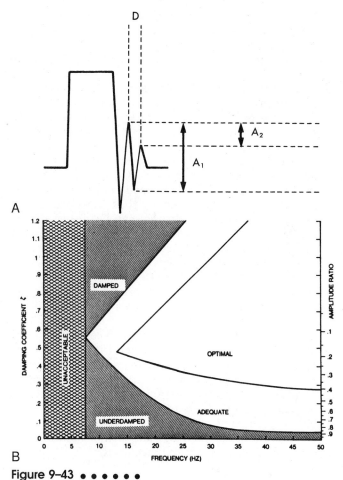

Figure 9–43 ● ● ● ● ● ●

A, Schematic illustration of a fast flush test. The natural frequency is determined by measuring the distance (D) between two consecutive oscillating peaks. This interval (mm) is divided by the paper speed (usually 25 mm/s). Damping coefficient is determined by calculating the ratio between the amplitude of two consecutive peaks (A_1/A_2). This ratio is then plotted on the scale illustrated to obtain the damping coefficient. (From Daily, E.K., Schroeder, J.S. (1989). *Techniques in bedside hemodynamic monitoring.* St. Louis: C.U. Mosby.) *B,* Scale for determining damping coefficient. The amplitude ratio on the right is referenced across to the damping coefficient on the left. Optimal systems have a high natural frequency (20–25 Hz) and a damping coefficient between 0.5 and 0.75. (From Gardner, R.M. (1981). Direct BP measurement: Dynamic response requirements. *Anesthesiology, 54:*227–236.)

and dorsalis pedis artery combination is assessed when either is considered for cannulation.

Other considerations in the selection of an arterial pressure monitoring site include easy access for blood sampling, care of the line and assessment of the insertion site; avoidance of areas likely to be contaminated or where wounds exist; and selection of an artery large enough to permit blood flow around the catheter (Gorny, 1993). Arterial catheters are not placed in extremities with vascular prostheses such as those used for hemodialysis.

Possible sites for arterial cannulation include the radial, dorsalis pedis, posterior tibial, femoral, brachial, axillary, temporal, and umbilical arteries. The umbilical arteries can be cannulated for the first

several days of life before they become obliterated. In the young infant they provide reliable and safe arterial access. Verified by radiographs, optimal position of the distal catheter is either high, above the diaphragm at T4 to T10, or low, at L3 to L4. These positions avoid the renal and mesenteric arteries. In either position, perfusion of the lower extremities is carefully assessed.

The radial artery is the most common site for arterial cannulation because it is easy to access and is associated with few serious complications. The arteries of the foot may be used, but access is often more difficult to obtain in small children. In addition, maintaining the catheter in either the dorsalis pedis or posterior tibial artery in position for proper functioning is more difficult. Often the foot cannot be positioned comfortably.

Femoral arterial lines are presumed to expose the patient to increased risks of contamination. In pediatric patients fecal contamination is a risk, and open, infected abdominal wounds may also be a potential source of contamination. Massive occult bleeding may occur if the femoral arterial line bleeds down into the retroperitoneal space.

The brachial artery is used only for short-term arterial cannulation when other sites are unavailable (Gorny, 1993). Joint immobility adversely affects patient comfort. The femoral and axillary arteries are large superficial vessels that provide a central pathway for cannulation and are often selected in patients with severe vasoconstriction resulting from progressive circulatory dysfunction. The right axillary artery communicates fairly directly with the cerebral circulation; the left artery communication is less direct. Often, the left axillary artery is selected first to avoid central nervous system sequelae of arterial embolization. Documented use of axillary arterial lines in pediatric patients is limited, but their safety and efficacy has been established in small studies (Lawless & Orr, 1989).

The temporal artery has been reported as a useful site for monitoring in small children with no alternative site (Gorny, 1993). However, its use has been associated with cerebral infarction and is, consequently, avoided.

Arterial Pressure Analysis. Invasive blood pressure measurement provides a moment-to-moment picture and a visual display of systolic, diastolic, and mean arterial pressure. Systolic arterial blood pressure (SAP) is the pressure exerted within the arterial vasculature during ventricular contraction. Diastolic arterial pressure (DAP) reflects the pressure of the heart during ventricular relaxation. Pulse pressure (PP) is the arithmetic difference between the systolic and diastolic measurements and is a function of stroke volume (SV) and arterial capacitance. For example, PP is typically decreased or narrowed when intravascular volume is inadequate. Mean arterial blood pressure (MAP) is the average pressure throughout the cardiac cycle. It is calculated by one of two formulas (all measures are in mmHg):

$$MAP = SAP + 2(DAP) \div 3 \text{ or } MAP = DAP + PP \div 3$$

MAP is not the mathematical mean of the systolic and diastolic blood pressures because diastole normally persists for approximately two-thirds of the cardiac cycle. Electronic monitoring equipment performs the calculation of MAP automatically and provides a visual display of SAP, DAP, and the mean pressure. MAP is dependent on blood volume and the elasticity of the arterial walls and is representative of the perfusion pressure throughout the capillaries.

The pressure wave that results from contraction of the ventricle begins in the aorta. Arterial systole begins with the opening of the aortic valve and rapid ejection of blood into the aorta. Runoff of blood from the proximal aorta to the peripheral arteries follows. The arterial pressure waveform shows these events as a sharp rise in pressure that is followed by a decline in pressure. As the ventricles relax and the aortic valve closes, a small rise in arterial pressure occurs, resulting in the dichrotic notch on the downstroke of the arterial pressure waveform. Figure 9–44 shows a normal arterial waveform.

The arterial pressure differs both in contour and in measured value in various arterial locations. Impedance increases as the pressure wave travels toward the periphery, causing an increase in amplitude. The height of the pressure wave and the measured systolic pressure are greater distally than centrally. In addition, the more distal the location of the arterial catheter, the sharper the systolic upstroke and the less defined the dichrotic notch. The normally higher systolic pressure in the lower extremeties that is normal in older children results in higher systolic pressures in the femoral artery than in the arteries of the upper extremities.

The systolic arterial pressure rises immediately after ventricular depolarization, that is, after the QRS complex on the rhythm strip. Delay is related to the catheter location and the length of tubing between the catheter and transducer. The dichrotic notch occurs after the T wave of the rhythm strip.

A decrease in the slope of the arterial pressure upstroke reflects a decrease in the velocity with which blood is ejected from the left ventricle, which is consistent with a decrease in ventricular contractility. Ventricular outflow obstruction, produced by aortic stenosis or pericardial tamponade, also decreases the slope of the arterial pressure upstroke. A rapid, exaggerated upstroke and little area under the pulse contour correspond to decreased SV and increased vascular resistance, even when systolic blood pressure is "normal" for age. Decreased CO and increased SVR also elevate the diastolic blood pressure and narrow the PP. In patients who require mechanical ventilation, excessive positive pressure and/or inadequate intravascular volume are evidenced by arterial pressure that decreases with mechanical inspiration, which restricts venous return to the heart.

Damped waveforms occur when obstacles prevent the pressure wave from being transmitted freely along the system. Damped waveforms have a characteristic smoothed out appearance and are identified by a gradual upstroke, rounded out peak-systole, poor dicrotic notch, and narrow PP. Troubleshooting includes assessment of the entire system from cannula to solution for catheter obstruction, clot formation, air in the system, and arterial spasm. Overzealous flushing is avoided because it has been associated with complications such as cerebral emboli.

Overshoot, resulting from high flow within a narrow artery or high resonance within the catheter system, produces a more than 20 mmHg pressure gradient. In this case, dP/dT (the rate of the pressure rise over the time interval) is high. This may be caused by rapid HRs, excessive length of pressure tubing from the patient to the transducer, use of compliant tubing (including a T piece), and air that amplifies the wave. Overshoot can be avoided by using only noncompliant tubing of the shortest possible length.

Arterial spasms may occur with catheter manipulation, especially if peripheral perfusion is poor. Spasms are usually self-limiting. During cannula insertion lidocaine without epinephrine may be used to flood the area, or 10 mg may be injected.

Cardiac rhythm abnormalities alter the arterial pressure waveform. For example, in atrial fibrillation the arterial pressure varies considerably depending on the RR intervals and the corresponding time in any one cardiac cycle for ventricular filling (Fig. 9–45). When a premature ventricular contraction (PVC) occurs, ventricular contraction is initiated early. The result is diminished SV, reflected in a lowered arterial systolic pressure. Isolated occasional PVCs are usually well tolerated because of the increased SV and arterial pressure with the subsequent ventricular contraction.

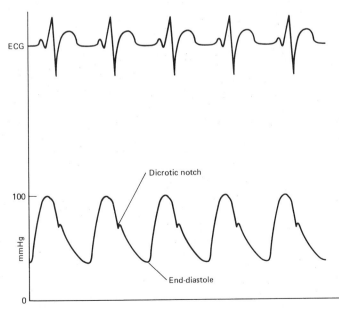

Figure 9–44 ● ● ● ● ● ●

Normal arterial pressure tracing. ECG, electrocardiogram. (Reproduced by permission from Smith, J.B. *Pediatric critical care,* p. 111. Delmar Publishers, Albany, NY, ©1985.)

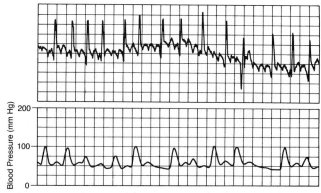

Figure 9–45 ● ● ● ● ● ●

Effect of altered cardiac rhythm on the arterial pressure wave-form. (From Darovic, G.O. (1987). *Hemodynamic monitoring: Invasive and non-invasive clinical applications*, p. 111. Philadelphia: W.B. Saunders.)

Complications. Neurologic and vascular function of the extremity can be compromised in the extremity with an arterial catheter in place. Necrosis of the overlying skin is characterized by skin that blanches during catheter flushing progressing to skin that remains blanched. The distal forearm is perfused by small offshoots of the radial artery that lack collateral circulation. The tip of the cannula or the thrombus that forms around the cannula within 48 hours may occlude these vessels. Repositioning or removal of the cannula may be necessary.

Ischemia and necrosis of digits have occurred. Assessments of pain, blanched or pale areas beyond the cannulation site, pulselessness distal to the catheter, numbness and tingling, or motor impairment are essential to avoid or minimize these complications.

Infection is a potential complication, because bacteremia is associated with invasive hemodynamic monitoring (Simmons, 1983). Increased risk of infection occurs with catheters placed by cutdown technique rather than percutaneous insertion, catheters in place longer than 4 days, and catheters that require manipulation and repositioning to maintain function. Application of povidone iodine at the cannulation site is often practiced; however, routine dressing changes have not influenced the incidence of infection. Dressings that are wet are changed.

Infection is best prevented by maintenance of a sterile, closed system and use of heparized normal saline solution for catheter flushing. The flush solution is changed every 24 hours, the tubing system every 48 to 72 hours (Simmons, 1983). The Centers for Disease Control (1983) also recommend that if the vascular catheter is suspected as a source of infection it be removed and, if necessary, placed at another site. The patient is assessed for unexplained fever and other signs of infection.

Thrombosis of an artery can develop while an invasive arterial pressure monitoring catheter is in place, after the catheter has been removed, or as a consequence of multiple arterial punctures, either to establish invasive monitoring or sample arterial blood.

Multiple arterial punctures increase the risk of thrombosis, as does catheterization beyond 4 days, intermittent (versus continuous) flushing of the catheter, and catheter size larger than 20 gauge. Patients who experience hematoma formation at the arterial catheterization site and those with inadequate tissue perfusion, particularly if the administration of vasoactive medications is required, are at increased risk to develop thrombosis (Clark & Harman, 1990). After an artery has been cannulated for invasive monitoring, recannulation of the vessel can extend from days to several weeks (Gorny, 1993).

Thrombosis of an artery or at the catheter tip interferes with accurate blood pressure measurement and blood sampling. Thrombosis can be minimized by avoiding the problems that are recognized to increase the incidence of thrombosis when possible and by the use of tapered-tipped, Teflon-coated catheters. When thrombosis is suspected, gentle aspiration of the catheter is indicated. Forceful flushing can result in embolization of the thrombus. If the catheter cannot be aspirated, it is discontinued.

Air embolism can develop from air in the flush system or when the system is opened to sample blood. Care in preparation and maintenance of the system can prevent the problem.

Catheter Removal. When the arterial catheter is removed, pressure is applied at the insertion site for as long as necessary to achieve complete hemostasis; this is followed by application of a pressure dressing. Some recommend that a syringe be attached to the catheter and negative pressure applied while removing the catheter to minimize the risks of leaving thrombus on the catheter tip within the blood vessel (Gorny, 1993). Peripheral neurovascular function is assessed. The insertion site is assessed for signs of infection, ecchymosis, and local ischemia and necrosis. The catheter tip may be sent for culture if infection is suspected.

Central Venous Pressure Monitoring

Catheterization of the central venous circulation may by undertaken in critically ill infants and children for a variety of reasons, including obtaining venous access when peripheral veins are inaccessible and administering fluid and medication infusions into the central circulation to maximize effect and avoid peripheral vascular injury. Central venous catheters may to used to administer hypertonic parenteral nutrition solutions and to obtain blood samples. Hemodynamic monitoring of CVP reflects the pressure in the great veins as blood returns to the heart and is a reliable indicator of intravascular blood volume. In addition, CVP monitors right ventricular function directly and accurately reflects left ventricular function in individuals without cardiopulmonary disease. However, there are many situations that invalidate the relationship between CVP and left ventricular end-diastolic pressure (LVEDP). Severe respiratory disease and the use of positive pressure ventilation at high pressures, hypothermia, and massive blood transfusion alter the relationship between CVP and LVEDP. Pathophysiologic factors that increase PVR, such as hypoxemia and acidosis, alter the relationship. Use of pulmonary artery catheters or direct left atrial catheters (for example, in the postoperative cardiac surgery patient) for evaluation of LVEDP and left heart function is necessary in these situations.

Central Venous Cannulation. Central venous access in pediatric patients is obtained either by cutdown or percutaneous technique following the administration of sedation. The most commonly used sites are the internal jugular, femoral, subclavian, and antecubital veins. Ideally, the catheter is advanced to the caval-atrial junction. In this position, there is little motion of the catheter with respect to the heart, improving the accuracy of hemodynamic monitoring; less chance of inducing dysrhythmias than when the catheter is advanced within the right atrium; less chance of cardiac perforation; and less thrombus formation because blood flow is rapid and the vessel caliber is large (Martin & Holley, 1993). Central venous catheters can be placed in the umbilical vein of the newborn infant.

In patients younger than 1 year and weighing less than 6 kg, the internal and external jugular veins are often considered for venous access because they enter the superior vena cava with a straight course. The subclavian veins enter the central venous circulation at acute angles, which become less acute as the child grows (Schwenzer, 1990). The infraclavicular approach to the subclavian vein is sometimes preferred for long-term central venous catheterization in children, although there is risk of pneumothorax, hydrothorax, and hemothorax.

The femoral vein provides a large vessel that is easily identified and cannulated in both infants and children. The basilic vein in the antecubital space is also easily palpable, but the success rate in reaching the central venous circulation is limited in small children. This site provides successful central venous placement more frequently in children weighing more than 20 kg (Schwenzer, 1990).

Monitoring of intravascular volume status and right ventricular function can also be accomplished via a transthoracic right atrial (RA) catheter inserted, most commonly, at cardiac surgery. The RA line is used exclusively for hemodynamic monitoring, rather than for infusion of fluids or medications, unless other venous access is unobtainable or in the case of an emergency.

Venous Pressure Waveform Analysis. The normal central venous waveform is diagrammed in Figure 9–46. The pressure changes within the right atrium are small, consisting of three positive deflections—the *a, c,* and *v* waves—each followed by a descent in pressure. The *a* wave is the pressure rise produced by atrial contraction. The *c* wave may appear as a distinct positive deflection, as a notch on the *a* wave, or may be absent altogether. The *c* wave reflects the slight increase in intra-atrial pressure that occurs with closure of the AV valve leaflets. It may be absent in pediatric patients because the atria are very distensible in youngsters. The *v* wave is produced by increased atrial pressure resulting from contraction of the ventricles, which causes the AV valve leaflets to bulge into the atria with concomitant atrial filling.

The descents that follow the *a* and *c* waves (the *x* and *x'* descents) are produced by the decrease in pressure during atrial relaxation and the downward pulling of the floor of the atrium at the onset of ventricular systole. The descent following the *v* wave (the *y* descent) is produced by the opening of the AV valve leaflets and emptying of the atria into the relaxed ventricles.

The pressure rises during atrial systole (the *a* wave) and atrial diastole (the *v* wave) are nearly the same. As a consequence, atrial pressure is monitored as the average or mean of both pressure rises. However, right atrial pressure waveforms are characterized by a dominant or larger *a* wave, compared with

Figure 9–46 ● ● ● ● ●

Normal central venous pressure waveform. Central venous pressure waveform with simultaneous electrocardiogram. (From Clochesy, J.M., Breu, C., Cardin, S., Rudy, E.B., Whittaker, A.A. (Eds.) (1993). *Critical care nursing,* p. 159. Philadelphia: W.B. Saunders.)

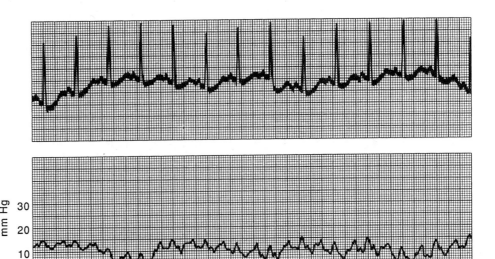

the v wave, whereas the reverse is true of the left atrial waveform. The v wave is dominant on the left atrial pressure tracing and higher mean pressure is found in the left atrium (4–12 mmHg) compared with that of the right (3–7 mmHg).

Correlation of the atrial pressure tracing with the ECG is helpful in differentiating the positive pressure deflections. The a wave immediately follows the P wave on the ECG, generally occurring in the PR interval. The c wave corresponds to the RS-T junction of the ECG. The v wave occurs during the TP interval.

Atrial fibrillation results in the absence of uniform atrial contraction, and no a wave is visible on the atrial pressure tracing as a consequence. Only the v wave produces a distinct positive deflection. If the atria contract while the AV valves are closed (AV dissociation), a large or cannon a wave results.

Increased atrial pressure and elevation of the a wave are also seen with ventricular dysfunction and hypertrophy. Other causes of increased resistance to ventricular filling, such as AV valve stenosis or pulmonary hypertension, also exaggerate and elevate the a wave (Fig. 9–47). Severe AV valve regurgitation, which may occur with severe ventricular failure or structural valve incompetence, produces marked elevation of the atrial v wave (Fig. 9–48). In addition, atrial septal defects, which increase flow into the right atrium during ventricular systole, increase the size of the v wave. Both the a and v waves are elevated in cardiac tamponade.

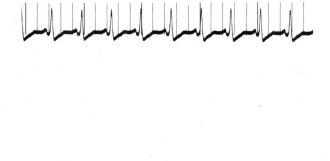

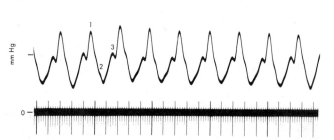

Figure 9–47 ● ● ● ● ● ●

Elevated RA pressure with exaggerated a wave (1) in a patient with RV failure and increased resistance to ventricular filling. (2 = x descent; 3 = v wave.) (From Daily, E.K., & Schroeder, J.S. (1989). *Techniques in bedside hemodynamic monitoring*, p. 102. St. Louis: C.V. Mosby.)

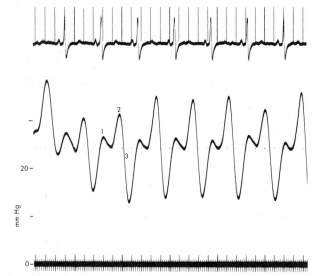

Figure 9–48 ● ● ● ● ● ●

Elevated RA pressure with exaggerated v wave (2) and rapid y descent (3) in a patient with tricuspid regurgitation as a result of acute RV failure. The a wave (1) of approximately 26 mmHg reflects an elevated RVEDP and RV failure. (From Daily, E.K., & Schroeder, J.S. (1989). *Techniques in bedside hemodynamic monitoring*, p. 103. St. Louis: C.V. Mosby.)

Changes in intrathoracic pressure with ventilation are readily transmitted through the relatively thin-walled atria and great veins and are reflected in the CVP and atrial pressure. During spontaneous and negative pressure ventilation, inspiration lowers the CVP (Fig. 9–49). Positive pressure ventilation increases the CVP during inspiration, as does coughing and Valsalva manuever. The application of PEEP to a patient's airway is also transmitted to the central vasculature and increases RAP and CVP. These circumstances can make the interpretation of high venous pressure difficult in isolation. Other clinical findings regarding the adequacy of venous return, intravascular volume, and cardiac function are key to accurate interpretation of numeric data.

Complications. During insertion of a central venous catheter there is potential for local tissue injury of adjacent tissues and blood vessels. Inadvertent arterial puncture is the most common injury, which is usually not significant if the needle is immediately withdrawn and local pressure applied. Localized hematoma formation may develop from inadvertent arterial puncture or some venous punctures. This problem is minimized by use of a small-gauge needle to locate the central vein, by attention to proper technique, and by experience with central venous catheterization procedure.

Pneumothorax or hemothorax may be associated with needle puncture of the pleura during central venous catheter insertion. The subclavian approach is associated with risks of injury to mediastinal structures as well, resulting in pneumomediastinum, hemomediastinum, pneumopericardium, and pericardial tamponade.

Figure 9-49 ● ● ● ● ● ●

Effect of spontaneous breathing on the CVP waveform. (From Clochesy, J.M., Breu, C., Cardin, S., Rudy, E.B., & Whittaker, A.A. (Eds.) (1993). *Critical care nursing,* p. 159. Philadelphia: W.B. Saunders.)

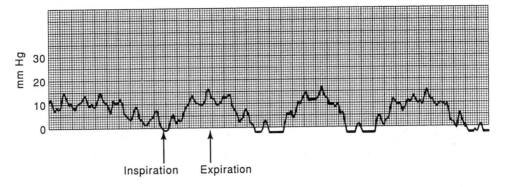

Air embolism is a potentially fatal complication of central venous catheterization, which can occur during insertion of the catheter if the needle is not capped with a syringe. It can also occur when intravenous (IV) tubings are changed or if they are inadvertently disconnected. Proper attention to detail at insertion and meticulous care of central venous catheters and associated IV or hemodynamic monitoring tubings prevent air embolism.

Complications that may occur after insertion of a central venous catheter include infection and thrombosis. Perforation of vascular or cardiac structures is a potential risk but is extremely rare.

Local and systemic infection may develop in patients with central venous catheters, because these invasive lines are important potential sources of nosocomial infections and sepsis. Contamination can occur at the time of insertion if sterile technique is breached and secondary migration of bacteria from the skin develops. Contamination can also occur from hematogenous spread from distant infected foci or from infected IV fluids, tubings, or transducers. Once the central venous catheter is colonized, it may become a source for disseminated infection, particularly in critically ill and immunocompromised patients. The risk of catheter-related bloodstream infections is approximately 4% when central venous catheters are used, compared with a 1% risk for peripheral IV catheters (Maki, 1982).

Most bloodstream infections related to IV catheters originate from either the patient's bacterial flora or from organisms on the hands of caregivers. Scrupulous attention to aseptic technique at the time of catheter insertion and during dressing changes is necessary to prevent the invasion of organisms. Careful maintenance of sterile IV solutions, tubings, and transducers is necessary.

Catheter-associated bacteremia can be identified while the infection is localized. Generally, a positive result upon culture of blood drawn through the catheter with more than 15 colonies denotes infection, even if a peripheral blood culture result is negative. The patient is at clear risk for catheter-related septicemia. Most often the catheter is withdrawn and replaced, if necessary.

Venous thrombosis and thrombophlebitis are associated with the presence of a central venous catheter. Most patients with thrombosis demonstrate edema of the arm, neck, and face, which is localized to the involved side. When central vein thrombosis is present, microembolization and pulmonary embolism can occur. If the patient's clinical situation indicates pulmonary embolism, thrombosis of the central veins is suspected. Venogram may be necessary to confirm thrombosis, although treatment may be initiated without radiographic confirmation. Treatment requires removal of the catheter and consideration of IV heparin therapy.

Catheter Removal. The central venous catheter is removed when the hemodynamic data obtained from it is no longer necessary for clinical decision-making and the patient's condition permits administration of necessary IV fluids via a peripheral catheter. Aseptic technique and universal precautions must be ensured when the catheter is removed. Air entry into the central vein is prevented by having patients perform a Valsalva manuever, if they able to cooperate and the manuever is not contraindicated (for example, by increased intracranial pressure). In all patients, the catheter is most safely removed at the end of inspiration, when intrathoracic pressure is highest. The catheter is clamped and withdrawn with a steady motion. After removal, manual pressure is applied to the insertion site until hemostasis is ensured. The insertion site is assessed for signs of inflammation or infection and the catheter is inspected to ensure that it has been removed in its entirety. The tip of the catheter may be sent for culture if line sepsis is suspected.

Pulmonary Artery Pressure Monitoring

Pulmonary artery catheters were first introduced in 1970 and were used enthusiastically in critically ill adults during the 1970s and early 1980s. Recognition of serious potential complications has resulted in more conservative use; that is, a pulmonary artery catheter is indicated only when the data obtained will improve clinical decision-making. Small, flexible catheters are available for use in pediatric patients.

The pulmonary artery catheter is valuable in the diagnosis and treatment of critically ill patients with cardiopulmonary failure. It measures right atrial pressure (RAP); pulmonary artery systolic, diastolic, and mean pressures (PAS, PAD, and PAM); and the pulmonary artery wedge pressure (PAW). The PA catheter can be used for rapid determination of CO using the thermodilution technique. Other parameters, such as cardiac index, systemic and pulmonary vascular resistance, and ventricular contractility indicators, can be derived from these data. The catheter can be used to sample mixed venous blood for intermittent analysis or, if equipped with a fiberoptic lumen, to continuously monitor mixed venous oxygen saturation.

PA Catheter Description. The multiple lumens of the PA catheter provide the means to assess a variety of physiologic characteristics of the cardiovascular system (Fig. 9–50). The standard quadrilumen PA catheter is available in two sizes: 5 and 7 French. The 5 French size is suitable for children weighing less than 18 kg; the 7 French is used for larger children and adults. The distal tip of the PA catheter is open and associated with a lumen that runs the entire length of the catheter. The inflatable balloon is positioned just proximal to the tip of the catheter. When the balloon is inflated through its lumen, it covers the tip of the catheter, reducing irritation of

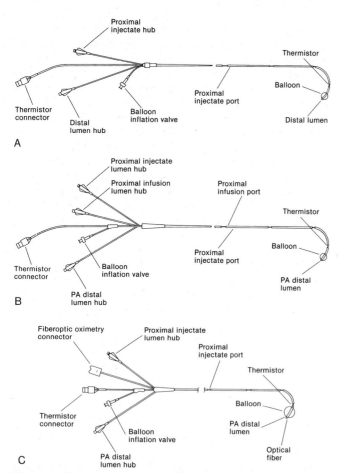

Figure 9–50 ● ● ● ● ● ●

Types of pulmonary artery catheters. *A,* Triple lumen catheter. *B,* Quadruple lumen catheter. *C,* Oximetry catheter. (Redrawn from Baxter Healthcare Corporation, Edwards Critical-Care Division. All rights reserved. In Clochesy, J.M., Breu, C., Cardin, S., Rudy, E.B., Whittaker, A.A. (Eds.) (1993). *Critical care nursing,* p. 164. Philadelphia: W.B. Saunders.)

the endocardium during catheter insertion. The thermistor is positioned 4 cm from the tip of the catheter. Its insulated wires run through a third lumen to the thermistor hub, which connects to the cardiac output computer. The proximal lumen of the PA catheter is located 30 cm from the catheter tip, which is a position designed to locate it in the RA when the distal lumen opening is in the PA. In patients weighing less than 10 kg, the proximal port is frequently outside the RA, and thus a 5 French catheter with a proximal lumen located 15 cm back from the catheter tip is used.

Pulmonary Artery Cannulation. Before inserting the PA catheter, the patient's serum electrolyte (especially potassium, calcium, and magnesium), acid-base, and coagulation study results are evaluated. Hypoxemia, acidosis, hypokalemia, hypocalcemia, and hypomagnesemia place the patient at increased risk for the development of serious dysrhythmias. Abnormal coagulation can result in hemorrhage or extensive hematoma formation (Gardner, 1993). A lidocaine bolus (1 mg/kg) is also prepared; the defibrillator is positioned for easy access.

Catheterization of the PA is most often accomplished from the internal jugular vein, although the subclavian, femoral, or external jugular veins may be selected. The internal jugular is preferred because of a lower incidence of pneumothorax associated with this approach and because the catheter is easily secured in the neck area. Before catheter insertion, each catheter lumen is flushed with heparinized solution, balloon integrity is assessed by inflating and inspecting the balloon, and thermistor integrity is assessed by connecting the therminstor hub to the CO machine and watching for a temperature. Two pressure transducers are prepared, leveled with the patient's phlebostatic axis, connected to the monitor, and zeroed. The distal lumen of the catheter is connected to the transducer to permit waveform assessment during catheter insertion.

Insertion of the catheter is usually performed through an introducer (dilator) sheath that remains in place with the catheter. A sterile sleeve is placed over the catheter and attached to the introducer, permitting positioning and manipulation of the catheter without contamination.

The catheter is advanced from the internal jugular vein to the right atrium. When location within the RA is identified from the pressure waveform, the balloon is inflated to its full volume (0.5–1.5 mL). With continuous waveform monitoring (Fig. 9–51) the catheter is carefully advanced through the right ventricle and into the pulmonary artery. Ultimately the PA catheter wedges, or is in the occlusion pressure position, in a pulmonary artery branch. The balloon is then deflated and the PA systolic and diastolic pressures are continuously monitored. The pressures and waveforms assessed during catheter insertion are documented as baseline data. Documentation of the length of catheter inserted and the external markings at the exit site are helpful in assessing and ensuring maintenance of the desired catheter position.

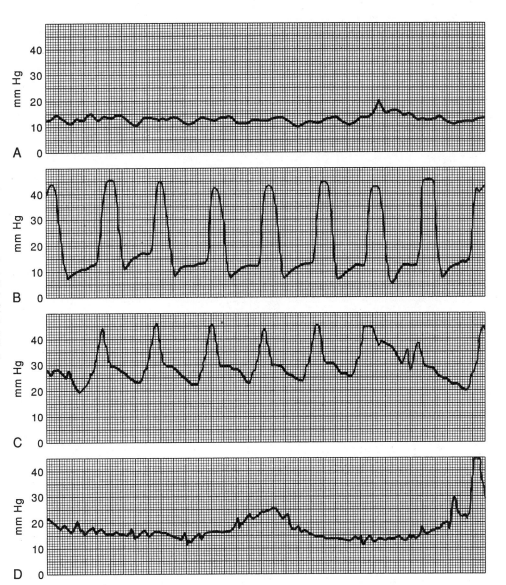

Figure 9–51 ● ● ● ● ● ●

Waveforms observed during insertion of a pulmonary artery catheter. *A*, Right atrial pressure. *B*, Right ventricular pressure. *C*, Pulmonary artery pressure. *D*, Pulmonary artery wedge pressure. (From Clochesy, J.M., Breu, C., Cardin, S., Rudy, E.B., Whittaker, A.A. (Eds.) (1993). *Critical care nursing*, p. 165. Philadelphia: W.B. Saunders.)

Waveform Analysis. Measurement of the RA mean pressure and analysis of the RA waveform during PA catheterization is the same as that described earlier. As the catheter passes through the tricuspid valve, the peak systolic RV pressure and the RV end-diastolic pressure (RVEDP) are measured. The characteristic RV pressure waveform reflects the dynamic pumping action of that chamber. Figure 9–52 depicts the normal RV pressure waveform, with the specific events that occur during ventricular systole and diastole illustrated. The normal peak RV systolic pressure range is 20 to 30 mmHg. RVEDP is measured after atrial systole (the *a* wave on the pressure waveform) and normally ranges from 2 to 8 mmHg. The systolic portion of the RV pressure waveform corresponds to ventricular depolarization and occurs during the QT interval of the ECG. The diastolic portion of the waveform occurs in the TQ period of the EKG.

Although RV pressure is not routinely monitored at the bedside, it is important to note the initial pressure levels as a reference. The RA pressure should be equal to the RVEDP, whereas the PA systolic and RV systolic pressures are also normally equal. As a result, the RV pressure is monitored indirectly via these two pressures. It is important to accurately identify the RV pressure waveform on the oscilloscope if it occurs at a time other than during insertion of the PA catheter. Its detection requires withdrawal of the central venous, RA, or PA catheter into the atrium. In the case of a PA catheter, the balloon is then inflated for reflotation out to the PA.

RV systolic pressure may be increased by a number of clinical problems. Any condition that increases PVR results in increased RV pressure, including pulmonary artery hypertension (PAH), hypoxemia, adult respiratory distress syndrome, pulmonary embolism, obstructive pulmonary disease, or pulmonary venous hypertension, most often the result of left ventricular dysfunction. RV systolic pressure may also be ele-

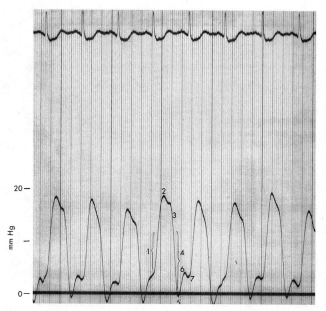

Figure 9–52 ● ● ● ● ● ●

Normal RV pressure waveform (1 = isovolumetric contraction; 2 = rapid ejection; 3 = reduced ejection; 4 = isovolumetric relaxation; 5 = early diastole; 6 = atrial systole; 7 = end-diastole). (From Daily, E.K., & Schroeder, J.S. (1989). *Techniques in bedside hemodynamic monitoring,* p. 108. St. Louis: Mosby–Year Book.)

vated by pulmonic stenosis (because of increased resistance to ventricular ejection) or ventricular septal defect (due to left-to-right shunting of blood under high pressure). RVEDP approximates RA pressure if the tricuspid and pulmonic valves are normal. Increased RV diastolic pressure is the consequence of the same factors that increase the atrial pressure. Most often increased RVEDP is the consequence of the ventricular dysfunction characteristic of heart failure.

PA Pressure. The pressure waveform in the pulmonary artery is divided into three phases: systolic, diastolic, and mean. Systolic pressure is representative of the rapid ejection of blood into the pulmonary artery following RV contraction and opening of the pulmonic valve. This is depicted as a sharp rise in pressure on the waveform, followed by a decline in pressure as the volume of blood ejected declines (Fig. 9–53). Normal PA systolic pressure is the same as RV systolic pressure, 20 to 30 mmHg.

When RV pressure falls below the pressure in the pulmonary artery, the pulmonic valve closes, creating the dichrotic notch on the downslope of the waveform. Diastole follows closure of the pulmonic valve, as runoff of blood into the pulmonary vascular system occurs without any further blood flow from the RV. The PA diastolic pressure is measured immediately before the next systole and corresponds closely to the LVEDP, in the absence of pulmonary and mitral valve disease. The normal PA diastolic pressure is 4 to 12 mmHg. Pulmonary artery mean pressure (PAM) is calculated, as is mean systemic arterial pressure. Normally the PAM pressure is 7 to 18 mmHg.

The systolic pressure in the PA corresponds with ventricular depolarization. However, the length of the PA catheter and monitoring tubing delay the signal somewhat. PA systole occurs in the QT interval of the ECG.

High systolic PA pressures are the consequence of either increased pulmonary blood flow, as in CHD with a left-to-right shunt, or increased resistance to blood flow. Increased PVR is seen in pulmonary diseases, pulmonary artery hypertension, pulmonary embolism, and severe heart failure. The PAD pressure may not accurately reflect the LVEDP in patients with pulmonary disease or pulmonary embolism. Tachycardias, which shorten the diastolic period of the cardiac cycle, falsely elevate the PAD pressure.

PA Wedge Pressure. When a PA catheter is properly positioned, inflation of the balloon results in movement of the catheter to a small branch of the pulmonary artery. The balloon then occludes and obstructs blood flow in that blood vessel. The pressure measurement that is obtained is referred to as the PA wedge (PAW) or PA occluded pressure (PAOP). This pressure, transmitted across the pulmonary veins to the catheter tip, is approximately the same as LA pressure, an indicator of LV filling pressure. The PAW pressure waveform is similar to the RA or LA waveform (*a* and *v* waves; most often the *c* wave cannot be seen) because the pressure is produced by the same physiologic events (Fig. 9–54). Normal, resting PAW pressure is the same as LA pressure (i.e., 4–12 mmHg) and is measured as a mean pressure because the *a* and *v* waves are normally approximately the same.

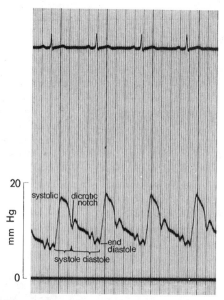

Figure 9–53 ● ● ● ● ● ●

PA pressure waveform showing phases of systole, dicrotic notch (pulmonic valve closure), and end diastole. Normally, PA end diastole closely represents LVEDP. (From Daily, E.K., & Schroeder, J.S. (1989). *Techniques in bedside hemodynamic monitoring,* p. 110. St. Louis: Mosby–Year Book.)

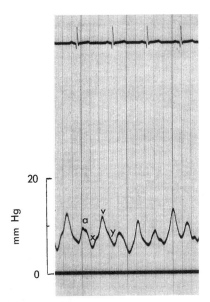

Figure 9–54 ● ● ● ● ●

Normal pulmonary artery wedge pressure waveform showing *a* and *v* waves and *x* and *y* descents. (From Daily, E.K., & Schroeder, J.S. (1989). *Techniques in bedside hemodynamic monitoring*, p. 116. St. Louis: Mosby–Year Book.)

As with atrial pressure monitoring, the *a* wave follows the P wave of the ECG and the *v* wave follows the T wave. However, in PAW pressure monitoring, a longer delay between the electrical and mechanical events is frequently noted because of the distance between the mechanical event and its retrograde measurement in the PA, as well as the length of the catheter and tubing. The effects of rhythm disturbances on the PAW pressure measurement are the same as described with atrial pressure monitoring.

Abnormal PAW pressure occurs with a number of clinical problems. The *a* wave may be elevated with LV failure or mitral stenosis, because these conditions increase the resistance to LV filling. The *v* wave is elevated with mitral insufficiency and regurgitation, which may be the consequence of either structural abnormality or severe LV failure (Fig. 9–55). Elevated PAW pressure may also be the result of intravascular volume overload, cardiac tamponade, or pericardial effusion. Decreased PAW pressure is seen in patients with hypovolemia.

The PA diastolic pressure and the PAW pressure are usually within 1 to 5 mmHg of each other when pulmonary vascular resistance is low, pulmonary function is normal, and the mitral valve is competent. An increase in the PA diastolic pressure to the point that the gradient between it and the PAW pressure is greater than 5 mmHg can result from tachycardia, pulmonary artery hypertension, cor pulmonale, or pulmonary embolus. PAW pressure exceeds the PAD pressure only in patients with mitral regurgitation.

Technical Problems in PA Monitoring. Mechanical problems may interfere with accurate PA pressure monitoring. Dampening of the pressure waveform is the most common problem. The overdamped waveform loses sharp definition and appears rounded, the dichrotic notch is absent or poorly defined, the systolic pressure is measured falsely low, and the diastolic pressure is overestimated. Overdampening may be the result of simply corrected technical problems. Examples are the use of an excessive number of stopcocks between the PA catheter and the transducer (no more than three are recommended [Gardner, 1993]); the presence of air bubbles, blood, loose connections, or kinked tubing in the monitoring system; and the use of excessive lengths of tubing or tubing that is excessively compliant in the monitoring system. A pressure waveform that is overdamped prompts an evaluation of the monitoring system to detect and correct these simple problems.

Overdamped pressure waveforms are also the consequence of problems with the catheter itself. Kinking of the catheter can occur at the insertion site or internally, the catheter can be wedged against the vessel wall, or fibrin can be deposited on the tip of the catheter. Problems with catheter kinking or position may be resolved by repositioning the catheter. However, if fibrin or clot deposition is suspected, urokinase may clear the catheter or it will have to be replaced.

Exaggerated oscillations of the pressure waveform, referred to as catheter "fling" or "whip," can occur

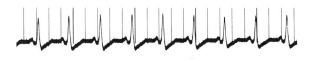

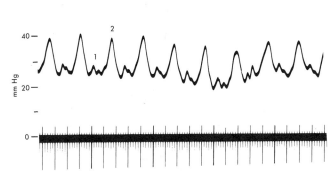

Figure 9–55 ● ● ● ● ●

Elevated pulmonary artery wedge pressure with a dominant and elevated *v* wave (2) as a result of mitral regurgitation. The *a* wave (1) is also elevated indicating LV failure. In this case, the mitral regurgitation is most likely functional secondary to LV failure and dilation. (From Daily, E.K., & Schroeder, J.S. (1989). *Techniques in bedside hemodynamic monitoring*, p. 119. St. Louis: Mosby–Year Book.)

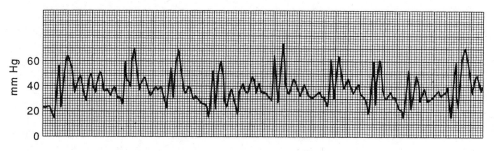

Figure 9–56 ● ● ● ● ● ●

Pulmonary artery pressure waveform with catheter "whip" or "fling." (From Clochesy, J.M., Breu, C., Cardin, S., Rudy, E.B., & Whittaker, A.A. (Eds.) (1993). *Critical care nursing*, p. 171. Philadelphia: W.B. Saunders.)

when blood flow is turbulent (Fig. 9–56). This may occur if the catheter is located near the pulmonic valve or coiled in the RV or in patients with PAH or dilated pulmonary arteries (Daily & Schroeder, 1989). Catheter repositioning will correct the problem if its location was the source of the difficulty. In the latter situations, accurate PA pressure monitoring is difficult, at best, and may be impossible. When catheter fling does not resolve, only the PAM pressure is measured (the PAD continues to be monitored for RV fallback).

Catheter migration can result in several technical problems during PA pressure monitoring. The catheter may spontaneously or accidentally be withdrawn into the RV. The usual signs of this development are the detection of the lower diastolic pressure reading characteristic of the RV and the presence of ventricular dysrhythmias (usually PVCs). The catheter can most often be repositioned by withdrawing the catheter into the RA, reinflating the balloon and manipulating the catheter. Balloon inflation while the catheter is in the RV may impair CO in small pediatric patients, but it is noted to decrease ventricular irritation and ectopy in adult patients as the tip of the catheter is engulfed by the balloon.

Catheter migration into small pulmonary vessels can result in spontaneous wedging of the catheter. In spontaneous wedging there is potential for loss of blood supply to a PA branch vessel and risk of pulmonary infarction. Overwedging of the PA catheter, caused by overinflation or uneven inflation of the balloon of the catheter, may result in PA rupture.

Overwedging is avoided by careful assessment of the PA waveform as the balloon is inflated. The balloon is inflated only until the morphology of the atrial waveform is clearly appreciated (i.e., the *a* and *v* waves). Overinflation results in loss of the waveform characteristics and a linear increase or decrease in the pressure (Fig. 9–57). If the catheter wedges at an unexpectedly low inflation volume or if spontaneous wedging occurs, prompt repositioning of the catheter is necessary.

Accurate pressure measurement is dependent on maintenance of the monitoring system. It is crucial that the phlebostatic axis reference point be accurately determined and that the transducer be accurately leveled at the phlebostatic axis. Changes in hemodynamic data may be the result of a change in the patient's condition; however, before treatment measures are undertaken, it is important to assess the system for potential sources of error. A rapid assessment of the transducer position, and re-zeroing of the system, as well as reassessment of the pressure waveform morphology, ensures that the data is accurate.

Clinical Factors in PA Monitoring. A number of physiologic and clinical factors affect PA pressure measurement. The first is *pulmonary blood flow*. Three physiologic zones of blood flow have been identified in the lungs (West et al., 1964). These zones are not anatomic divisions, but correspond to the interaction between alveolar, pulmonary arterial, and pulmonary venous pressures in each zone and the resulting blood flow in each (Fig. 9–58). Accurate

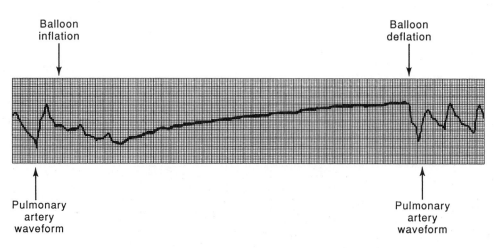

Figure 9–57 ● ● ● ● ● ●

Overwedging of the pulmonary artery catheter during balloon inflation. (From Clochesy, J.M., Breu, C., Cardin, S., Rudy, E.B., & Whittaker, A.A. (Eds.) (1993). *Critical care nursing*, p. 172. Philadelphia: W.B. Saunders.)

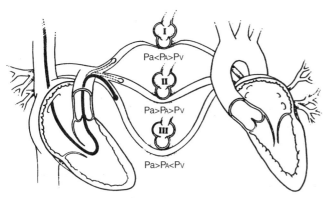

Figure 9–58 ● ● ● ● ● ●

Lung zones. PAW estimates LAP only when the catheter is in lung zone 3 (capillaries below left atrium level), allowing for a continuous column of blood to exist from catheter tip to left atrium. LAP, left atrial pressure; PAW, pulmonary artery wedge pressure; Pa, pulmonary arterial pressure; PA, pulmonary alveolar pressure; PV, pulmonary venous pressure. (Reprinted with permission from O'Quin, R., Marini, J.J. (1983). Pulmonary artery occlusion pressure: Clinical physiology, measurement and interpretation. *American Review of Respiratory Disease,* 128:319–326.)

PA pressure determination necessitates that the catheter be positioned where pulmonary blood flow is continuous, in zone 3 of the lung. Only in this position does the PA reflect LA pressure. In zones 1 or 2, where flow is absent or intermittent, the PA pressure reflects alveolar pressure.

Location of the catheter in zone 3 is confirmed by waveform analysis and chest radiograph. Lateral chest radiograph most accurately reveals that the tip of the PA catheter is below the level of the left atrium. Catheter location in zone 3 is also verified by the appearance of the characteristic atrial waveform when the PA catheter is wedged. If the catheter is located in zone 1 or 2, wedging produces marked respiratory variation and loss of the characteristic atrial pressure waveform (Gardner & Woods, 1989).

PAP varies with both *spontaneous and mechanical ventilation.* During spontaneous breathing, the pressure in the PA follows intrathoracic pressure (i.e., both the PA and PAW pressures fall during inspiration and rise with exhalation). All hemodynamic

pressures are read at one point in the respiratory cycle; traditionally at end-exhalation.

The application of PEEP with mechanical ventilation may be transmitted from the airways to the pulmonary blood vessels and alter all intrathoracic pressure readings. However, discontinuing PEEP is not recommended to obtain pressure readings. First, if pressure readings are obtained without PEEP, the patient's clinical situation is not accurately depicted. Second, discontinuing PEEP can result in alveolar collapse, rapid movement of interstitial fluid into the alveoli, and deterioration in the patient's condition (Lookinland, 1989). Instead, an estimate of the effects of PEEP can be calculated: every 5 cm of PEEP results in a 1.5 mmHg increase in PAW pressure (Fig. 9–59). Alternatively, the effects of PEEP can be disregarded and the patient's PA pressures followed for trends without mathematical correction of the measured pressure reading. If correction is made for the effect of PEEP on the PA pressure, it is important that all caregivers be consistent in the practice so that hemodynamic data is not misinterpreted.

Complications. Because central venous access is achieved for insertion of a PA catheter, the potential complications of adjacent tissue damage are present during PA catheterization. In addition, during flotation of the PA catheter, dysrhythmias, heart valve damage, and knotting of the catheter can occur. Intracardiac knotting of the catheter has been reported, requiring manipulation of the catheter under fluoroscopy, withdrawal of the catheter or, occasionally, surgical intervention (Dach et al., 1981; Thomas, 1982). Tricuspid and pulmonary valve damage has been associated with prolonged PA catheterization (Elliot et al., 1979).

Cardiac rhythm disturbances that occur during insertion of the PA catheter are usually self-limited. PVCs most often cease when the catheter has exited the right ventricle. If PVCs are sustained or if they progress to ventricular tachycardia (VT), the catheter is withdrawn into the right atrium until the dysrhythmia stops. Dysrhythmias can reoccur after catheter insertion, usually associated with either looping of the catheter in the right atrium or ventricle or displacement of the catheter tip from the PA into the ventricle. A continuous infusion of lidocaine

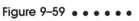

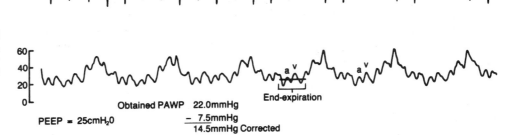

Figure 9–59 ● ● ● ● ● ●

Effects of PEEP on measured PA pressure. (From Gardner, R.M. (1993). Pressure monitoring. *AACN Clinical Issues in Critical Care Nursing,* 4:113.)

Obtained PAWP 22.0mmHg

PEEP = 25cmH₂O

− 7.5mmHg

14.5mmHg Corrected

End-expiration

increases the dysrhythmia threshold and may allow the patient to tolerate the PA catheter. Repositioning or removal of the catheter may be necessary if the rhythm disturbance is resistant to management with lidocaine.

Improper position of the PA catheter places the patient at risk for pulmonary infarction and pulmonary artery rupture. Pulmonary infarction is most often the result of persistent wedging of the catheter in a peripheral pulmonary arteriole or obstruction of a more central artery by an inflated balloon. Prolonged balloon inflation is avoided and the catheter is repositioned if spontaneous wedging occurs because of peripheral migration of the catheter.

Pulmonary artery rupture leads to massive hemorrhage and death. Risk factors for serious pulmonary artery injury include PAH and hypothermia (Schwenzer, 1990). Imminent rupture may be preceded by only a small amount of pulmonary bleeding evidenced by hemoptysis or the presence of bloody secretions with airway suctioning. Fatal hemorrhage may occur without pulmonary artery rupture in patients receiving anticoagulants. Usually PA bleeding and rupture are associated with distal migration of the catheter and subsequent balloon inflation. In patients with PAH, extreme caution is necessary during all measurements of PAW pressure. The balloon is inflated for only two or three respiratory cycles, a time period not to exceed 10 to 15 seconds. If the PAD and PAW pressures correlate well, the PAD pressure is substituted for the PAW and balloon inflation is limited.

Local and systemic infection can develop in patients with PA catheters. Bacteremia is increasingly likely when the catheter is in place for more than 72 hours, in the presence of inflammation at the insertion site, or when the catheter is inserted in a patient with bacteremia (Lange et al., 1983). Diagnosis of a catheter-related infection and care of the patient with an infection is the same as for patients with infection related to a central venous catheter.

Catheter Removal. The PA catheter is removed once the data obtained with it are no longer needed to guide clinical decision-making and patient care. The catheter is removed in the same manner as a central venous catheter. In addition, as the catheter is withdrawn using a steady motion, the patient's ECG is observed for the presence of dysrhythmias. Rhythm disturbances may occur while the catheter is located within the right ventricle, usually abating as soon as it is withdrawn further. If any resistance is encountered as the catheter is withdrawn, the procedure is discontinued until the patient can be assessed with fluoroscopy for knotting or kinking of the catheter, which may ensnare it on intracardiac structures. When the catheter is completely withdrawn, hemostasis is achieved and the insertion site is assessed and dressed with a dry, sterile dressing. The catheter is assessed to ascertain that it was removed in its entirety. The PA catheter is often exchanged for a multilumen central venous catheter placed over a wire in order to maintain central venous access.

Left Atrial Pressure Monitoring

Direct measurement of left atrial pressure (LAP) is reserved for cardiac surgical patients in whom a transthoracic catheter is placed at the time of operation. These catheters are only used for continuous, accurate assessment of left ventricular filling pressure and function during weaning of the patient and discontinuation of cardiopulmonary bypass and throughout the acute postoperative period (Gold et al., 1986). RA and PA pressures may also be directly monitored following cardiac surgery.

LA Waveform Analysis. Analysis of the LA waveform is the same as was described for monitoring venous pressures. Given the proximity of the catheter to the mechanical events produced by the heart's electrical activity, the correlation between the ECG and the pressure waveform is close.

Complications and Catheter Removal. Direct intracardiac monitoring of RAP and LAP in postoperative cardiac surgery patients has been associated with dysrhythmias related to catheter malposition in either ventricle, with difficult removal and intrapericardial accumulation of blood after catheter removal (Gold et al., 1986). Although the incidence of complications is low, their potential risk is high and necessitates special caution at the time of catheter removal.

Malposition of the catheter is evidenced by ventricular rhythm disturbances, usually PVCs, and an abrupt change in the monitored pressure. The catheter must be repositioned or removed. When the LA or RA catheter is removed, the potential for accumulation of blood in the pericardial space is anticipated. Adequate drainage of the area via a mediastinal or chest tube must be ensured, as is the availability of blood for volume resuscitation if hemodynamic compromise occurs.

Cardiac Output Determination

In the intensive care setting, CO is measured by techniques that are based on the Fick principle, an application of the law of conservation of mass. The Fick principle uses the following relationships to determine CO:

$$CO \text{ (mL/minute)} = V_{O_2} \div [CaO_2 - CvO_2] \times 100$$

The Fick principle states that the difference between the arterial and venous oxygen content reflects oxygen uptake or consumption per unit of blood as it flows through the lungs. In the equation above, cardiac output (the amount of blood flowing through the lungs) is equal to oxygen consumption divided by the difference between the oxygen saturations of mixed venous blood (flowing into the lungs) and arterial blood (leaving the lungs).

Calculation of CO with the Fick method requires collection and measurement of exhaled air volume and oxygen content over at least a 3-minute period. It is rarely used for bedside measurement of CO. However, it is often referred to as the standard

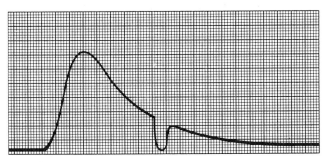

Figure 9–60 ● ● ● ● ● ●
Time-temperature cardiac output curve. (From Clochesy, J.M., Breu, C., Cardin, S., Rudy, E.B., Whittaker, A.A. (Eds.) (1993). *Critical care nursing*, p. 172. Philadelphia: W.B. Saunders.)

against which other methods of CO calculation are measured. Error in CO determination by the Fick method is estimated to be 10% (Visscher & Johnson, 1953). Inaccuracies are related to errors in sampling mixed venous blood or exhaled gases, the length of the time over which the measurements are made, and the presence of cardiac or pulmonary shunts (Lake, 1990).

Indicator-dilution Method. The indicator-dilution method of CO determination is based on the principle that if a known amount of indicator is added to an unknown quantity of flowing blood and the concentration of the indicator is measured downstream, the timing and concentration of the downstream measurement provide a quantitative index of flow.

$$CO = \text{indicator dose} \div \text{average concentration} \times \text{time (seconds)}$$

The usual indicator for CO determination is a nontoxic dye, indocyanine green, which is measured with a photodensitometer. A bolus of the dye is injected into the venous circulation and blood is withdrawn from an artery through the densitometer to measure its concentration. Use of the indicator-dilution method for determining cardiac output has been refined to use a thermal indicator rather than dye. Dye dilution is rarely used in the critical care setting.

Thermodilution Method. The use of a thermal indicator was introduced by Fegler in 1954 (Fegler, 1954). Ganz and colleagues developed the thermodilution technique for CO determination in 1971 (Ganz et al., 1971). The technique's advantages are that it is simple and rapid, results are reproducible, and it employs a safe indicator that mixes rapidly with blood and does not require blood sampling.

Thermodilution is a modification of the indicator-dilution technique in which cool 5% dextrose or normal saline solution is injected into the right atrium or central veins through the proximal lumen of a PA catheter or central venous catheter. A thermistor in the pulmonary artery measures the decrease in the temperature of the blood as the cool solution passes through the heart and a time-temperature curve is

produced (Fig. 9–60). A computer calculates the area under the curve and displays the CO in a measurement of liters per minute. The values obtained using thermodilution correlate well with those obtained by Fick or dye-dilution technique. However, as with other CO measurement techniques, there are a number of potential sources of error in thermodilution CO determination (Table 9–8).

Technical Consideration. Accurate CO measurement by thermodilution requires that the PA catheter be properly positioned to ensure that the thermistor can measure the temperature change occurring when the cold injectate is instilled. The PA waveform is assessed for damping or wedging due to catheter migration or position against the wall of the vessel.

A computation constant and the temperature of the blood in the patient's PA, if not automatically measured and recorded, are entered into the CO computer. These values are incorporated into the computer's calculations to correct for a number of

Table 9–8. POTENTIAL SOURCES OF ERROR IN THERMODILUTION CO MEASUREMENT

Source of Error	Resulting Problem/Error
Faulty computer or cables	Wide discrepancy in CO measurements
Cable connection not secure	No readings
	PA or injectate temperature does not register
PA Catheter	
Clotted proximal lumen	Difficulty injecting solution, may be impossible to inject
Catheter malposition	Thermistor lying against small vessel wall because of catheter migration, CO curve has low amplitude
	Tip of catheter not in zone 3 lung, measured CO affected by ventilation
Catheter kinking at entrance site or within the heart	Difficulty injecting solution
Fibrin growth on catheter	Difficulty injecting solution, variations in core temperature measurements
Technique-related	
Incorrect injectate volume	CO values do not correspond to the patient's clinical condition
Incorrect computation constant entered in computer	
Injectate temperature outside specified range	
Uneven, prolonged injectate delivery	
Patient-related	
Patient movement during measurement	Variation in serial CO measurements
Cardiac dysrhythmias	Oscillations of the baseline
Mechanical ventilation	
Low CO states	Recirculation of thermal indicator, prolonged baseline drift
Hypothermia	Low amplitude CO curve because of small temperature difference between blood and injectate

variables that affect the measurement, such as the inherent warming of the injectate as it travels down the catheter and rate of temperature change in PA blood anticipated for a specific volume and temperature of injectate (Loveys & Woods, 1986). The connections between the injectate probe cable, the thermistor coupling and the catheter-connecting cable, and the computer are secured.

The patient is usually positioned supine with conservative elevations in the head of the bed (0–20 degrees). Flat positioning has not been demonstrated to be necessary, as high correlation between flat supine and modest head elevation CO measurement has been found (Grose et al., 1981; Kleven, 1984).

Rapid, even injection within 4 seconds is essential to ensure a smooth time-temperature curve (Loveys & Woods, 1986). The volume of injectate is an important factor in accuracy because volumes less than 5 mL or greater than 10 mL have been demonstrated to underestimate or overestimate CO in adults (Enghoff & Sjogren, 1973; Pearl et al., 1986). Minimum and maximum injectate volumes for determining CO in infants and children are not known.

Both iced and room temperature injectate are used. Iced injectate produces a thermal signal two to three times larger than room temperature solution (Lake, 1990). However, similar CO measurements are obtained with either temperature injectate in adults (Vennix et al., 1984; Pearl et al., 1986). Even in hypothermic adult patients, room temperature injectate CO correlated well with iced injectate determinations in one group of patients (Shellock et al., 1983). Both 5 and 10 mL injectate volumes at room and iced temperature have been found to have high intercorrelation in adults (Vennix et al., 1984; Pearl et al., 1986). Most clinicians prefer to use iced injectate for injections less than 10 mL to maximize the thermal signal.

Timing of the injection with end-expiration produces less variable results, because the effects of the phase of respiration on PA temperature are eliminated. End-expiration is judged most convenient and is most often used.

The CO computer displays the calculated CO approximately 15 seconds after the injection. A second and a third determination of CO are made, separated by 45 to 90 seconds. The three measurements are averaged, unless a measurement falls outside 10% of the middle value. In a series, a CO value that falls outside the standard error of the estimate (10%) is discarded and the remaining two are averaged or a fourth measurement is made.

Accuracy of the measurement is also assessed by inspection of the thermodilution curve. The configuration should be smooth with a rapid up slope to peak and a gradual down slope to the baseline (Fig. 9–60).

Hemodynamic Calculations. CO, calculated in liters per minute (L/min), is the basis for calculation of a number of additional, derived hemodynamic indices (Table 9–9). The first is cardiac index. Calculations are performed automatically by the CO computer, necessitating that data entry be accurate.

Table 9–9. DERIVED HEMODYNAMIC PARAMETERS

Cardiac Index (CI)
Normal = 2.8 to 4.2 L/minute/m²

$$CI = \frac{Cardiac\ output}{Body\ surface\ area}$$

Stroke Volume (SV)
Normal = 60 to 90 mL/beat

$$SV = \frac{Cardiac\ output \times 1000}{Heart\ rate}$$

Stroke Volume Index (SVI)
Normal = 30 to 60 mL/beat/m²

$$SVI = \frac{Stroke\ volume}{Body\ surface\ area}$$

Stroke Work (SW)
Normal LV = 60 to 80 g. Normal RV = 10 to 15 g.*

$$LVSW = (MAP - PAWP) \times SV \times 0.0136$$
$$RVSW = (PAM - CVP) \times SV \times 0.0136$$

where CVP = central venous pressure
MAP = mean arterial pressure
PAM = mean pulmonary artery pressure
PAWP = pulmonary artery wedge pressure
SV = stroke volume
0.0136 = conversion factor for pressure to work (measured in g)

Systemic Vascular Resistance (SVR)
Normal = 1000 to 1300 dyn-sec/cm⁻⁵

$$SVR = \frac{MAP - CVP}{CO} \times 80$$

where MAP = mean arterial pressure
CVP = central venous pressure
CO = cardiac output

Systemic Vascular Resistance Index (SVRI)
Normal = SVRI: 800–1600 dyn-sec/cm⁵/m²

$$SVRI = \frac{SVR}{Body\ surface\ area}$$

Pulmonary Vascular Resistance (PVR)
Normal = 150 to 250 dyn-sec/cm⁻⁵

$$PVR = \frac{PAM - PAWP}{CO} \times 80$$

where PAM = mean pulmonary artery pressure
PAWP = pulmonary artery wedge pressure
CO = cardiac output

Pulmonary Vascular Resistance Index (PVRI)
Normal = PVI: 80–240 dyn-sec/cm⁵/m²

$$PVRI = \frac{PVR}{Body\ Surface\ Area}$$

*LVSWI: 56 ± 6 g-m/m²
RVSWI: 6.0 ± 0.9 g-m/m²

SV is equal to CO divided by the heart rate during the CO determination. Normal SV depends on the patient's size and activity level. SV index is obtained by dividing SV by the patient's body surface area. As with cardiac index, this normalizes the measurement to the patient's size.

The stroke work of the ventricle is a measure of the ventricle's work during any one cardiac contraction, as well as an indicator of the effectiveness of the heart's pumping function or functional capacity.

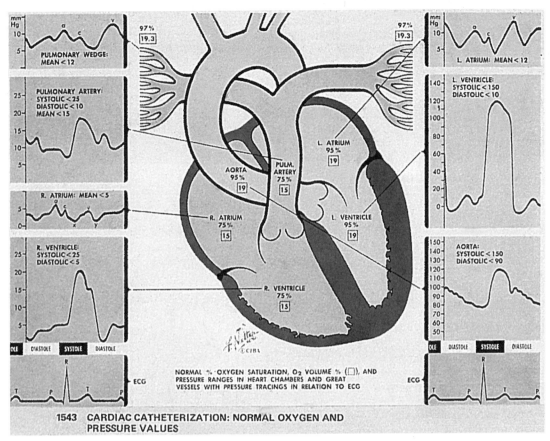

1543 CARDIAC CATHETERIZATION: NORMAL OXYGEN AND PRESSURE VALUES

Figure 9–61 ● ● ● ● ● ●

Hemodynamic indices and oxygen saturation normal values measured at cardiac catheterization. (© Copyright 1996. CIBA-GEIGY Corporation. Reprinted with permission from the Ciba Collection of Medical Illustrations, illustrated by Frank Netter, M.D. All rights reserved.)

Stroke work is the product of the average pressure generated by the ventricle during contraction multiplied by the SV ejected with that beat. Stroke work can also be indexed to the size of the patient. Hypertension or increased vascular resistance, as well as hypervolemia, increases the ventricle's stroke work. Stroke work is decreased with poor myocardial contractility, as is seen in patients with CHF or shock.

Vascular resistance is another index of ventricular work, representative of the force a ventricle must overcome to eject its SV. For SVR, the mean arterial pressure in a large peripheral artery and CVP or RAP are used in the calculations. Pulmonary vascular resistance (PVR) calculations use mean PAP and PAWP or LAP. Both SVR and PVR measurements can be indexed to the patient's size.

Cardiac Catheterization

Cardiac catheterization provides the most complete hemodynamic evaluation of cardiovascular function. In addition, detailed information about the structure of the heart and great vessels is achieved by angiography. Despite the refinement of noninvasive techniques for cardiovascular evaluation, the number of cardiac catheterizations performed in infants and children has not decreased, because of the increase in the number of interventional procedures performed in the cardiac catheterization laboratory (Lock et al., 1987). Cardiac catheterization, although an invasive procedure, can be performed safely and with few complications (Cohn et al., 1985).

At cardiac catheterization, a catheter introduced into a peripheral vein or artery is advanced through the vascular system to the heart. In infants and children the femoral or saphenous veins are most frequently selected for access to the right heart. The left heart is accessed from the right via the atrial septum or retrograde from the femoral or brachial artery.

Both hemodynamic and angiographic measures are obtained during cardiac catheterization. Hemodynamic indices include measurement of the pressures in the heart chambers, great vessels, and across the cardiac valves; pressure differences across obstructions; and calculation of vascular resistances. Oxygen saturation in the heart chambers and great vessels is measured (Fig. 9–61); and calculations of cardiac performance, including cardiac output and index (by Fick method or thermodilution) and shunt detection and quantification are performed (Table 9–10).

Angiography is used to provide anatomic informa-

Table 9–10. NORMAL HEMODYNAMIC VALUES OBTAINED AT CARDIAC CATHETERIZATION

	a Wave	v Wave	Mean	Systolic	End-diastolic	Mean
Pressures (mmHg)						
Right atrium	2–10	2–10	0–8			
Right ventricle				15–30	0–8	
Pulmonary artery				15–30	3–12	9–16
PAW, left atrium	3–15	3–12	1–10			
Left ventricle*				100–140	3–12	
Systemic arteries*				100–140	60–90	70–105

Oxygen consumption index (mL/min/m²) 110–150
Arteriovenous oxygen difference (mL/L) 30–50
Cardiac output index (L/min/m²) 2.6–4.2
Resistances (dyn-sec/cm⁻⁵)
  Pulmonary vascular 20–130
  Systemic vascular 700–1600

*Age-dependent.
PAW, pulmonary artery wedge.

tion about structural heart defects. Chamber size and functioning are shown, as is valvular function. Septal patency and vessel patency and origin are evaluated.

Cardiac catheterization can be used to provide direct evaluation and manipulation of the electrical activity of the heart by special catheters equipped with electrodes that are placed inside the cardiac chambers. Cardiac electrophysiology studies provide information on sinus node function, AV conduction and tachydysrhythmias; guide therapy by assessment of the effectiveness of antidysrhythmic medications; and can map the conduction system, revealing the origin of dangerous and repetitive dysrhythmias. These data can direct surgical or catheter intervention in the management of patients with dangerous dysrhythmias.

In addition to management of critical rhythm disturbances, cardiac catheterization can be used to provide definitive treatment of specific congenital heart defects. Both persistent ductus arteriosus and atrial septal defect have been successfully closed with devices inserted via a cardiac catheter. Balloon atrial septostomy also can improve oxygenation and provide hemodynamic stability in infants with transposition of the great arteries. Coarctation of the aorta has been successfully treated with balloon angioplasty (Lock et al., 1987).

PHARMACOLOGIC SUPPORT OF CARDIOVASCULAR FUNCTION

Management of cardiovascular dysfunction is multifaceted and often requires (1) restoration of adequate intravascular fluid volume; (2) improvement of myocardial contractility; (3) treatment of abnormal vascular capacitance and resistance; (4) correction of abnormal cardiac rate or rhythm (Notterman, 1993).

Intravascular Volume Restoration

Volume expansion to restore preload and ventricular filling is essential in circumstances involving ei-

ther absolute (abnormal fluid losses) or relative (maldistributed fluid volume) hypovolemia. Vascular access is of primary importance, followed by the timing and volume of fluid administered. It is critical to restore tissue perfusion before irreversible tissue ischemia occurs. Aliquots of 10 to 20 mL/kg can be safely administered over 1 to 15 minutes to pediatric patients with two important exceptions: patients in cardiogenic shock and premature infants at risk for intraventricular hemorrhage (McCrory & Downs, 1993).

The patient's response to fluid administration is assessed immediately. Important initial responses are a decrease in HR, broadening of the pulse pressure or increase in blood pressure if hypotension was detected, and improvement in the quality of peripheral pulses. Fluid administration is continued until perfusion of the skin, kidneys, and central nervous system is also improved, as evidenced by brisk capillary refill and warm extremities, adequate urine output, and appropriate level of consciousness. Infusion of 60 to 100 mL/kg of fluid may be required over a brief time period.

Cardiogenic shock requires prompt recognition and unique management when compared with absolute or relative hypovolemia. Importantly, the child's history reveals no abnormal fluid losses. Physical examination detects hepatomegaly, venous engorgement, a gallop rhythm, and rales. Cardiomegaly seen on chest radiographs confirms the likely diagnosis. Treatment is directed at inotropic, vasodilator, or antidysrhythmic therapy.

Inotropic Therapy

Cardiac glycosides and catecholamines have been used for centuries. The catecholamines augment cardiac contractility by action that simulates the sympathetic nervous system (SNS); hence, the term "sympathomimetic." Digitalis glycosides also enhance contractility. A group of inotropes that modify phosphodiesterase activity, the bipyridines, have been developed.

Adrenergic Stimulation

Sympathomimetic agents interact with cell surface adrenergic receptors. Adrenergic receptors are glycoproteins that are structurally and genetically related. They extend between the internal and external surfaces of the cell membrane and are transducers of signals or information across the cell membrane. That is, stimulation of an adrenergic receptor elicits a cellular response. Table 9–11 is a classification of the adrenergic receptors and indicates the physiologic responses to stimulation of each. The medications that are receptor agonists are listed in order of their potency. With the exception of the alpha$_1$-receptor, adrenergic receptors affect cell function by altering the intracellular concentration of cyclic adenosine monophosphate (cAMP). An increase in the intracellular concentration of cAMP ultimately affects intracellular calcium concentration, which, in turn, affects myocardial systolic and diastolic function and HR.

Changes in the sensitivity of adrenergic receptors to stimulation has been documented. Exposure of the receptors to sympathomimetics mediates receptor desensitization. Desensitization has also been related to endotoxin, tumor necrosis factor, and CHF.

Phosphodiesterase Inhibition

Phosphodiesterase (PDE) activity is inhibited by the methylxanthines (theophylline) and the bipyridines (amrinone, milrinone), resulting in increased intracellular cAMP. The rise in the concentration of cAMP in myocytes enhances contractility. The bipyridines selectively inhibit only one type of PDE, whereas the methylxanthines inhibit all three known types of PDE. The consequence may be the more selective inotropic action of amrinone, as compared with the limited inotropic and marked chronotropic actions of theophylline (Lawless et al., 1989).

Adenosine Triphosphate Inhibition

The digitalis glycosides act on the heart through a different mechanism than those described above, but the final outcome, increased intracellular calcium, is similar (Notterman, 1993). Digitalis glycosides inhibit the sodium-potassium pump, secondarily increasing intracellular calcium concentration and enhancing contractility.

Special Issues in Pediatric Pharmacotherapy

Immature animals and humans respond differently to inotropes than do adults (Driscoll et al., 1978). This may be the consequence of developmental differences in the concentration of adrenergic receptors in a variety of target organs (Whitsett et al., 1982; Boreus et al., 1986). Differences including reduced ventricular compliance, greater ventricular interdependence, and reduced myocardial contractile protein in the immature heart also point to structural and ultrastructural differences that are potentially important. Consequently, the young infant's heart does not tolerate or respond well to volume loading, when compared with that of older children and adults.

Care of critically ill infants and children necessitates that caregivers appreciate both the limited response to augmented preload and the reduced sensitivity of the heart and vasculature to adrenergic agents characteristic of some patients in the PICU. However, Notterman (1993) notes that the practical consequences of these differences have not been established. An age-based paradigm for pharmacotherapy is not yet possible.

Table 9–11. ADRENERGIC RECEPTORS, PHYSIOLOGICAL RESPONSES, SYMPATHOMIMETIC AGONISTS

Receptor	Physiologic Responses	Agonist
Alpha$_1$	Increase intracellular Ca, muscle contraction, vasoconstriction, inhibit insulin secretion	Epinephrine Norepinephrine Dopamine
Alpha$_2$	Decrease cAMP, inhibit NE release, vasodilation, negative chronotropy	Epinephrine Norepinephrine
Beta$_1$	Increase cAMP, inotropy, chronotropy, enhance renin secretion	Isoproterenol Epinephrine Dopamine Norepinephrine
Beta$_2$	Increase cAMP, smooth muscle relaxation, vasodilation, bronchodilation, enhance glucagon secretion, hypokalemia	Isoproterenol Epinephrine Dopamine Norepinephrine
D1	Increase cAMP, smooth muscle relaxation	Dopamine
D2	Decrease cAMP, inhibit prolactin and beta-endorphin	Dopamine

D = dopamine, NE = norepinephrine, Ca = calcium.
Modified from Notterman, D. A. (1989). Pharmacologic support of the failing circulation: An approach for infants and children. *Problems in Anesthesia*, 3:288–294.

Digitalis Glycosides

Cardiac glycosides are prescribed in the PICU for control of some supraventricular dysrhythmias and for patients in whom poor myocardial contractility is expected to persist beyond a few days. In patients with chronic CHF, digoxin remains the mainstay of pharmacologic therapy.

Digoxin increases myocardial contractility in normal and diseased hearts. When CHF is present, digoxin increases SV and reduces elevated ventricular filling pressures. When digoxin is administered to infants, contractility increases, as judged by echocardiographic examination (Berman et al., 1983; Park, 1986). Adult patients with acute heart failure who were given a single dose of digoxin experienced a 69% increase in LVSWI, a 25% reduction in PAWP, and a 16% to 28% increase in CI (Rackow et al., 1987). Similar invasive hemodynamic measurements have not been made in infants or children.

The elevated HR associated with CHF is reduced by digoxin. Digoxin is also useful to treat atrial fibrillation or flutter and recurrent paroxsymal atrial tachycardia.

Digoxin is eliminated by the kidney. Renal dysfunction that impairs glomerular filtration interferes with elimination. Hypokalemia increases digoxin binding to cell receptor sites, accounting in part for digoxin-induced cardiac rhythm disturbances during hypokalemia (Lewis, 1990).

Dosage and Administration

Infants and young children eliminate digoxin rapidly and have a large volume of distribution for the drug (Park, 1986). As a consequence, they require higher doses of digoxin than do adults to achieve a therapeutic plasma level of 1 to 2 ng/mL.

Dosage is based on the age of the patient, the indication for therapy, the route of administration, and the presumed sensitivity of the myocardium to potential toxicity (Notterman, 1993). Table 9–12 indicates the recommended intravenous digoxin doses for pediatric patients. It is important to note that the presence of inadequate renal function or electrolyte imbalance or evidence of myocardial irritability (i.e., dysrhythmia) necessitates that the doses be reduced and, during digitalization, the pace of digitalizing be slowed. When digoxin is used to treat supraventricular tachycardia, higher doses may be necessary.

Serum digoxin levels are of limited benefit as a guide to therapeutic response, because there is wide variability in the serum concentration required to achieve the desired response. Serum digoxin levels are of benefit to ensure that the dose given is sufficient to achieve a measurable blood concentration and to confirm the clinical suspicion of toxicity.

Digoxin Toxicity

Toxic levels of digoxin are capable of producing virtually every cardiac rhythm disturbance known.

Table 9–12. RECOMMENDED DIGOXIN DOSES FOR PEDIATRIC PATIENTS

Intravenous Digitalization	Enteral Digitalization
Total digitalizing dose = 30 mcg/kg/24 hours	Total digitalizing dose = 40 mcg/kg/24 hours
Maximum Dose = 800 mcg IV	Maximum dose = 1 mg po/ng
Digoxin 15 mcg/kg IV	Digoxin 20 mcg/kg po/ng
Digoxin 7.5 mcg/kg IV 8 hours after first dose	Digoxin 10 mcg/kg po/ng 8 hours after first dose
Digoxin 7.5 mcg/kg IV 8 hours after second dose	Digoxin 10 mcg/kg po/ng 8 hours after second dose
Begin maintenance digoxin (7.5 mcg/kg/day) 12 hours after third dose	Begin maintenance digoxin (10 mcg/kg/day) 12 hours after third dose

Infants and children are most likely to develop bradycardia and AV conduction delay. Sinus bradycardia is produced by digoxin suppression of sinus node discharge. All degrees of AV block can occur, sometimes associated with ectopic atrial beats or junctional ectopic tachycardia. Ectopy and tachydysrhythmia are more common in adult patients, probably because of myocardial irritability from ischemia. However, the myocardium of infants and children is not less sensitive to digoxin than that of older patients (Park, 1986).

Digoxin toxicity can occur because of accidental or intentional ingestion. One study reported fatal digoxin overdose in one-half the cases of acute ingestion (Ordog & Beneron, 1987). Toxicity can also occur because of dosing error or because of a change in the patient's sensitivity to the drug or in its pharmacokinetics. Assessment of the patient for predisposing factors (hypokalemia, renal dysfunction) is an important initial step in treatment. Hypomagnesemia, hypoxemia, myocarditis, and coadministration of catecholamines or calcium all exacerbate digoxin toxicity. As cardiac disease worsens or metabolic disturbances develop, digoxin toxicity can develop in patients receiving constant digoxin doses with stable serum concentration (Notterman, 1993).

Catecholamines and Other Inotropes

Epinephrine

Epinephrine is an endogenous catecholamine that is produced and released from the adrenal gland in response to stress. Its direct cardiac effects are the result of stimulation of the beta-adrenergic receptors. Epinephrine shortens systole by improving contractility and speeding conduction through the AV node and Purkinje system. It accelerates SA node firing. Epinephrine increases coronary blood flow, but also increases myocardial oxygen demand, so that the potential for a mismatch exists. It also decreases the refractory period of ventricular muscle, predisposing to dysrhythmias.

The clinical effects of epinephrine vary with the rate of infusion. At low dose (0.05–0.2 mcg/kg/min) peripheral vasodilation and increased HR and contractility are the consequence of $beta_1$ and $beta_2$–adrenergic stimulation. The pulse pressure is widened, systemic and pulmonary vascular resistance decrease, and SV and CO increase if the patient's intravascular volume is adequate.

Increasing infusion rates result in stimulation of the alpha-adrenergic receptors. Increased SVR and elevated blood pressure occur. Afterload is increased and may ultimately affect CO if the myocardium is unable to maintain SV.

Epinephrine is a potent renal artery vasoconstrictor, potentially reducing renal blood flow and urine output. However, the improvement in CO achieved with epinephrine may increase renal blood flow.

Dosage and Administration. In pediatric patients, infusion rates of 0.05 to 0.3 mcg/kg/minute are recommended in treatment of shock associated with myocardial dysfunction (Zaritsky & Chernow, 1984). Epinephrine may be most useful when combined with a vasodilator for afterload reduction. When catecholamine stores are depleted, epinephrine may be the inotrope of choice.

Epinephrine is best administered through a central venous line, because infiltration from peripheral venous administration can cause local tissue ulceration. Infusion rate is controlled with a constant infusion pump. Epinephrine is compatible with both dextrose and normal saline solutions; alkaline solutions are avoided because catecholamines are inactivated at higher pH.

Toxicity. Epinephrine may induce central nervous system excitation marked by restlessness, fear, anxiety, or dread and throbbing vascular-type headache. Tachycardia is always produced, with atrial and ventricular ectopy and tachydysrhythmias a risk at increasing infusion rates. Severe hypertension and anginal pain can occur. Severe mismatching of myocardial oxygen delivery with oxygen consumption and subsequent ischemia may be detected on ECG.

Norepinephrine

Norepinephrine is the hormone precursor of epinephrine and is the neurotransmitter of the SNS. Norepinephrine raises blood pressure and improves tissue perfusion in hypotensive patients who have normal or elevated cardiac index. Although norepinephrine possesses both alpha- and beta-adrenergic receptor activity, its alpha-adrenergic effects predominate at all but the lowest infusion rates. SVR rises sharply because of alpha-adrenergic mediated vasoconstriction. The peripheral, renal, splanchnic, and hepatic vascular beds are constricted, as is the pulmonary vasculature. Cardiac contractility is augmented and SV and cardiac index rise, if the increase in afterload can be tolerated. Chronotropy is opposed by reflex vagal activity, which slows the rate of sinus node discharge.

The hemodynamic effects of norepinephrine limit its use in pediatric critical care almost exclusively to treatment of patients with septic shock. It is most often used after volume repletion and administration of other inotropes have been ineffective in raising the blood pressure (Notterman, 1993; Zaritsky & Chernow, 1984).

Dosage and Administration. Initial infusion rates are 0.05 to 0.1 mcg/kg/minute. Successful treatment results in improved perfusion pressure, which maintains vital organ function. The lowest possible dose that achieves improved skin color and temperature, tissue pH and urine output are used. Invasive monitoring that includes a pulmonary artery catheter is useful to evaluate both systemic and pulmonary vascular resistance. The rate of infusion is titrated up to 1 mcg/kg/minute.

Toxicity. Careful monitoring is necessary during norepinephrine administration to prevent excessive increases in ventricular afterload and organ ischemia. If norepinephrine elevates blood pressure, but does not improve clinical evidence of tissue perfusion, continuing its infusion may lead to ischemic injury of the extremities, widespread organ failure, and death (Notterman, 1993). Profound hypertension can result from inadvertent boluses or excessive infusion rates, resulting in myocardial infarction or cerebral hemorrhage (Weiner, 1985).

Isoproterenol

Isoproterenol is a synthetic catecholamine structurally related to epinephrine and norepinephrine. It has beta (beta$_1$ and beta$_2$) specificity and does affect alpha-adrenergic receptors. Its potent effects on the heart include an increase in cardiac contractility, HR, and conduction velocity. Stimulation of peripheral beta$_2$ receptors results in vascular smooth muscle relaxation, decreased SVR, and a fall in diastolic blood pressure. Widened pulse pressure is detected, because the systolic blood pressure increases. Tachycardia may be extreme because the decline in diastolic pressure augments the chronotropic effect of the drug. In the face of hypovolemia, hypotension may develop when isoproterenol therapy is initiated. An increase in cardiac output is assured only if circulating blood volume is adequate. Because heart rate and contractility are increased, isoproterenol increases myocardial oxygen consumption. Simultaneous decreases in both diastolic filling time and diastolic perfusion pressure as a result of the drug may impair oxygen supply and result in myocardial ischemia. Myocardial ischemia, myocardial infarction, and fatal myocardial necrosis have been reported in adolescents receiving continuous isoproterenol infusion (Page et al., 1986).

Isoproterenol also relaxes pulmonary vascular and bronchial airway smooth muscle. Refractory or rapidly worsening status asthmaticus is the primary indication for continuous IV isoproterenol infusion. Once used to treat a variety of shock states, newer drugs and an improved understanding of the pathophysiology of shock have made isoproterenol obsolete for this purpose. It is, however, still employed to treat hemodynamically significant bradycardia. In heart block resistant to atropine, isoproterenol may be used until definitive treatment with pacemaker placement occurs. Low-dose epinephrine infusion may be better tolerated, however, because it maintains diastolic coronary perfusion pressure better than isoproterenol.

Dosage and Administration. Isoproterenol infusion is initiated at a rate of 0.01 mcg/kg/minute and adjusted to a rate of 0.05 to 0.1 mcg/kg/minute until the desired chronotropic or hemodynamic effect is achieved. Heart rate and blood pressure are closely monitored, as is evidence of myocardial ischemia. Often, daily measurement of cardiac enzyme levels is ordered. Isoproterenol can be safely administered via a peripheral vein because extravasation of the drug does not produce tissue necrosis.

Toxicity. Sustained tachycardia and the risk of myocardial ischemia limit isoproterenol's utility. It is effective for respiratory failure due to status asthmaticus, although its use in older children and adolescents is questioned (Notterman, 1993).

Dopamine

Dopamine is a neurotransmitter in the central and sympathetic nervous systems and is found in the adrenal medulla, where it is the immediate precursor of norepinephrine. Dopamine stimulates dopamine receptors (D-1 and D-2) in the vascular beds of the kidney, mesentery, and coronary arteries at low plasma concentrations, producing vasodilation. As the plasma level of dopamine increases, beta- and then alpha-adrenergic receptors are activated. In addition to these direct sympathomimetic effects, dopamine stimulates release of norepinephrine from sympathetic nerve terminals, resulting in indirect sympathetic stimulation.

Renal blood flow and urine output increase with infusion of dopamine at 0.5 to 2 mcg/kg/minute because of the selective action at DA receptors that occurs at these two doses. Dopamine also inhibits tubular reabsorption of sodium and promotes sodium excretion by the increase in renal blood flow. Infusion of dopamine at 2 to 5 mcg/kg/minute increases cardiac contractility and cardiac output, with little change in HR or vascular resistance. At doses of 5 to 6 mcg/kg/minute, both blood pressure and HR increase, although the tachycardia is less than that seen with isoproterenol. Doses up to 10 mcg/kg/minute further increase cardiac output. At doses in excess of 10 mcg/kg/minute, increasing alpha-adrenergic effects are seen with increases in SVR and tachycardia. The salutory effect on the renal vascular bed may be lost when alpha-adrenergic effects predominate at doses greater than 20 mcg/kg/minute.

There are data suggesting that infants have reduced sensitivity to dopamine. However, the evidence for this is not strong (Notterman et al., 1989). Notterman also notes, importantly, that dopamine crosses the blood-brain barrier in preterm neonates and warns against its use for trivial indications in this age group. Although low-dose infusion of dopamine is frequently administered to augment renal function among critically ill patients, there is no evidence of the influence of this practice on the incidence of renal failure resulting from poor perfusion.

Although dopamine is used widely in pediatric critical care practice, there is little systematically collected data regarding its use. Dopamine has both inotropic and vasopressor properties, as well as the potential to enhance renal blood flow. Shock with cardiovascular dysfunction and mild to moderate hypotension is improved with dopamine infusion. At moderate infusion rates it is unlikely to produce excessive tachycardia or dysrhythmias, compared with either epinephrine or isoproterenol. When hypotension is marked and cardiac index is very low, epinephrine is the drug of choice. Dopamine is not the agent of choice in distributive shock when cardiac index is high and vascular resistance low. If blood pressure is normal but cardiac contractility abnormal, a pure inotrope such as dobutamine or amrinone is preferable (Notterman, 1989).

Dosage and Administration. As with other catecholamines, dopamine is not mixed with alkaline IV solutions and is administered into a central vein using a continuous infusion device. Significant skin injury from extravasation is a risk with peripheral administration. Dextrose and normal saline solutions are compatible.

Infusion rates of 0.5 to 2 mcg/kg/minute result in selective DA actions on vascular beds. Infusion rates between 5 and 10 mcg/kg/minute produce dominant beta-adrenergic effects; doses between 10 and 20 mcg/kg/minute have mixed alpha- and beta-adrenergic effects. Infusion doses in excess of 20 mcg/kg/minute have predominantly alpha-adrenergic effects.

Toxicity. Limb ischemia, gangrene, and extensive loss of skin are associated with dopamine infusion in peripheral veins and with extravasation because dopamine both releases norepinephrine from synaptic terminals and is converted to norepinephrine when metabolized. Extravasation requires immediate treatment with phentolamine administered locally with a fine hypodermic needle.

Dopamine, like other inotropes, increases myocardial oxygen demand as increased contractility increases myocardial work. It is likely to produce less oxygen supply and demand mismatch than epinephrine or isoproterenol, because it is associated with less tachycardia; however, it is more likely to do so than dobutamine or amrinone.

Dobutamine

Dobutamine is synthesized to model a catecholamine that has specific, selective inotropic action with limited chronotropic or vasopressor activity. Infusion of dobutamine produces prompt improvement in cardiac performance. With improved contractility a decrease in SVR and left atrial pressure follow. A decrease in PVR is associated with dobutamine (Leier & Unverferth, 1983). Tachycardia is unusual. Improved CO improves renal blood flow and urine output.

Dobutamine is most useful when the primary disturbance impairing tissue perfusion is cardiac. Typical indications include viral myocarditis, cardiomyopathies, or myocardial infarction (Kawasaki disease). Positive inotropic effect and little increase in HR have been demonstrated in children given dobutamine for a variety of shock states. Dobutamine is less effective in septic shock than in cardiogenic shock. In postoperative cardiac surgery patients, results have been uneven; children with some congenital heart defects had a positive inotropic response, whereas others did not (Berner et al., 1983). Others demonstrated improved cardiac output only because HR increased (Bohn et al., 1980). Contractility may not have been significantly impaired, as is the case in most children undergoing surgery for congenital heart defects, in those who did not demonstrate inotropic response (Notterman, 1993).

In adults with CHF, dobutamine increased myocardial oxygen demand. However, in the absence of coronary obstruction, coronary blood flow and oxygen supply also increased, favorably affecting oxygen balance (Marjerus et al., 1989). A similar response can reasonably be expected in children with depressed contractility and patent coronaries. Because heart rate increases only modestly with dobutamine, the metabolic demand anticipated is less than with inotropes associated with greater tachycardia. Dobutamine is also less likely to produce atrial and ventricular dysrhythmias than other inotropes, although these problems can occur.

Dosage and Administration. Dobutamine therapy is initiated with a continuous IV infusion at 2 to 5 mcg/kg/minute. Maximal effects are generally seen at doses of 10 to 15 mcg/kg/minute. The maximal therapeutic dose is not known. Infusion is generally recommended via a central venous line, although dobutamine does not have significant vasoconstricting effects.

Toxicity. Side effects include excessive HR and dysrhythmias, although both are less common than is the case with other inotropes. Headaches, anxiety, tremors, and excessive fluctuations in blood pressure have been reported (Leirer & Unverferth, 1983).

Amrinone

Amrinone possesses positive inotropic actions on the heart and has potent vasodilating effects. It is the first bipyridine to be widely used in the United States for infants, children, and adults with impaired myocardial contractility. In patients with CHF, amrinone increases SV and cardiac index, while simultaneously decreasing systemic vascular resistance, central venous pressure, and LVEDP. Tachycardia is not observed. Both systolic myocardial contractility and diastolic relaxation are improved (Colucci et al., 1986a; Lawless et al., 1988; Lawless et al., 1991; Skoyles & Sherry, 1992).

Amrinone is a selective PDE inhibitor that increases myocardial cAMP content and provides a positive inotropic effect. It also has profound vasodilating action, via increased cAMP. At the heart, intracellular calcium is increased; it is blocked at the level of the vascular smooth muscle (Skoyles & Sherry, 1992). Unlike every other inotrope, PDE inhibitors improve cardiac performance in the failing heart with unchanged or reduced oxygen demand. This is in part because systemic vasodilation reduces ventricular wall stress. In addition, myocardial perfusion is increased because coronary resistance is decreased.

Amrinone is useful in the treatment of both chronic CHF and acute myocardial failure. It has been used preoperatively in patients with pulmonary artery hypertension to improve hemodynamics (Hess, 1989) and in patients with end-stage heart disease awaiting cardiac transplantation (Watson et al., 1990). PDE inhibitors act synergistically with other catecholamines and are particularly useful in those patients whose symptoms are refractory to catecholamine therapy because of excessive sympathetic nervous system activation or adrenergic receptor downregulation from lengthy exposure to catecholamines (Skoyles & Sherry, 1992).

Dosage and Administration. Amrinone is mixed in normal saline (glucose solutions are *not* used) and is administered by continuous IV infusion following a bolus IV dose administered over 10 minutes. Critically ill pediatric patients have a larger volume of distribution for the drug and require a loading dose of at least 3 mg/kg (Lawless et al., 1988; Lawless et al., 1991). (It should be noted that the recommended loading dose for adults is 0.75–1.5 mg/kg.) When followed by a continuous infusion, steady state is obtained within 1 hour of initiating therapy (Lawless et al., 1991). The usual infusion dose is 5 to 10 mcg/kg/minute.

Toxicity. Hypotension is the principal concern, particularly during administration of the loading dose. Hypotension is more likely in patients with low central venous pressure. It is important to note that ventricular filling pressures may be high in patients with heart failure, but when SVR is reduced, intravascular volume is actually low. If hypotension occurs, fluid therapy corrects the problem. Hypotension is avoided by slow administration (over 10 minutes) of the loading dose and by ensuring adequate intravascular volume.

Amrinone, and the other PDE inhibitors, may cause cardiac rhythm disturbances. In adult patients, ventricular ectopy and brief episodes of ventricular tachycardia were seen in approximately 10% of patients and sustained ventricular tachycardia or ventricular fibrillation in 1% (Naccarelli et al., 1984). Dysrhythmias may be related to the patient's underlying pathophysiology.

Thrombocytopenia is a common adverse effect of amrinone when it is administered orally. With IV therapy, the incidence of thrombocytopenia is far lower. When amrinone is discontinued, the platelet count returns to normal within several days.

Milrinone

Milrinone is a slightly newer member of the bipyridine inotropic/vasodilating agents with PDE inhibiting action. Its actions and indications for use are like those of amrinone. When compared to both dobutamine and nitroprusside in adult patients with severe heart failure, milrinone demonstrated potent inotropic effects and a greater effect on both right and left heart filling pressures, consistent with a greater degree of vasodilation (Colucci et al., 1986a).

Dosage and Administration. Milrinone is administered with a loading dose of 50 mcg/kg infused over 10 minutes and followed by a continuous IV infusion of 0.375 to 0.75 mcg/kg/minute. The volume of distribution of milrinone may be different in pediatric patients, as it is for amrinone, but this has not yet been systematically investigated and reported. Milrinone is administered in normal saline or 5% dextrose solutions. Dosing information for patients with impaired renal function is available from the manufacturer.

Toxicity. Hypotension and cardiac rhythm disturbances occur with milrinone administration, as is the case with amrinone. The incidence of thrombocytopenia with milrinone is less than that seen in patients receiving amrinone.

Vasodilating Agents

Myocardial failure results in activation of a number of compensatory mechanisms designed to maintain systemic blood pressure and perfusion of vital organs. Regardless of the cause of myocardial failure, attempts at compensation are the same in all. First, the ventricle dilates to increase end-diastolic volume. Increased end-diastolic volume eventually exceeds the optimal level and is inappropriately elevated, as is end-diastolic pressure. Second is an increase in adrenergic stimulation of the heart, augmenting cardiac contractility and HR. Finally, SVR increases in response to low SV and as a consequence of sympathetic stimulation, increased renin-angiotensin activity, and other factors. In many patients with heart failure, SVR is inappropriately elevated and actually depresses SV.

In patients with reduced SV and systemic vasoconstriction, inotropic support alone may be ineffective in restoring adequate cardiac output. In addition, inotropes (with the exception of the new PDE inhibitors) may exact a significant penalty by increasing myocardial oxygen consumption.

Vasodilating agents in these patients are highly effective (Friedman & George, 1985; Artman & Graham, 1987; Schneeweiss, 1990). Venous vasodilators increase the capacitance of the venous sytem, reducing elevations in ventricular end-diastolic volume and pressure. By reducing arterial vasoconstriction and afterload, arterial vasodilators increase SV and CO. Heart rate does not increase in most patients treated with vasodilators. Blood pressure decreases only slightly or not at all, as a result of increased SV.

Vasodilators exert their positive effects on cardiac performance while also decreasing myocardial oxygen consumption. By decreasing preload and reducing ventricular size, in addition to decreasing ventricular systolic pressure, myocardial oxygen needs are also reduced.

Although the mechanism of action is not clearly known, vasodilators also enhance ventricular compliance. Vasodilators shift the volume-pressure curve to the right where there is a greater increase in end-diastolic volume at a lower end-diastolic pressure.

Vasodilators are classified based on their primary site of action on either the arterial or venous or both (balanced) sides of the systemic vascular bed (Table 9–13). It is important to note that all vasodilators,

Table 9–13. CLASSIFICATION OF VASODILATORS BASED ON PREDOMINANT SITE OF ACTION

Venous	Arterial	Balanced
Nitroglycerin	Diazoxide	Nitroprusside
	Nifedipine	Phentolamine
	Tolazoline	Captopril
	Hydralazine	Enalapril
		Prazosin

regardless of classification, exert some effect on both the venous and arterial circuits.

Table 9–14 summarizes the hemodynamic effects of various vasodilating agents. Not all are discussed in detail here. The focus is on those used most frequently in pediatric critical care practice.

Nitroprusside

Sodium nitroprusside is a balanced vasodilator, with approximately equal actions on the venous and arterial circuits. It is useful to treat acute, severe hypertension, but is used more frequently as adjunctive therapy in severe CHF or cardiogenic shock. Its role in pediatric critical care may be modified as experience with the PDE inhibitors expands.

Infusion of nitroprusside results in rapid, widespread, and marked vasodilation affecting both the arterial and venous systems. If SVR is not elevated, SV and cardiac index decline and blood pressure is reduced. Heart rate increases reflexively. However, when SVR is high and contractility depressed, as is the case in patients with severe ventricular failure, the reduction in afterload and preload that is achieved with nitroprusside results in increased SV and cardiac index. The increase in SV is proportional to the decrease in SVR. Heart rate declines and blood pressure is unchanged. Nitroprusside is useful for treating CHF and cardiogenic shock and as adjunctive therapy for impaired ventricular perfor-

Table 9–14. HEMODYNAMIC EFFECTS OF VASODILATING AGENTS

	CO	HR	PAP	RAP	SVR	PVR	BP
Captopril	0	0	0	0	↓↓	0–↓	↓
Diazoxide	↑	↑	0	0	↓↓	↓	↓
Hydralazine	↑	↑	0	0	↓↓	↓	↓
Nifedipine	0–↑	0–↑	↓↓	↑	↓↓	↓	↓↓
Nitroglycerin	0–↑	0	↓↓	↓	0–↓	↓↓	↓
Nitroprusside	0–↑↑	↑	↓	↓	↓↓	↓↓	0–↓
Phentolamine	↑	↑	0–↓	?	0–↓	0–↓	0–↓
Tolazoline	↑	↑	0–↓	?	0–↓	0–↓	0–↓

Reproduced with permission from Packer, M. (1985). Vasodilator therapy for primary pulmonary artery hypertension: Limitations and hazards. *Annals of Internal Medicine* 103:258.

BP, blood pressure; CO, cardiac output; HR, heart rate; PAP, pulmonary artery pressure; PVR, pulmonary vascular resistance; RAP, right atrial pressure; SVR, systemic vascular resistance.

mance in the immediate postoperative period following open heart surgery.

Dosage and Administration. Nitroprusside has an extremely rapid onset and short duration of action. Peak effects are noted within 2 minutes and effects dissipate within 3 minutes of stopping an infusion (Notterman, 1993). Administered by continuous IV infusion, the beginning dose is 0.5 mcg/kg/minute. SVR is generally reduced with doses between 1.5 and 2 mcg/kg/minute. Occasionally doses as high as 5 to 10 mcg/kg/minute are required if vasoconstriction is profound.

Nitroprusside is administered in 5% dextrose solution with an infusion pump. The solution is light-sensitive, requiring that only fresh solutions be used (i.e., within 24 hours) and that the administration container and tubing are opaque or covered.

Toxicity. Hypotension is the most common problem encountered with nitroprusside administration. It is rapidly corrected by a reduction in the infusion rate, but should always prompt a reevaluation of the patient's intravascular volume status as well.

Nitroprusside undergoes intravascular decomposition into both nitric oxide, the agent responsible for its vasodilating effects, and cyanide. Cyanide is metabolized in the liver to thiocyanate, which is then excreted by the kidney. Accumulation of thiocyanate can develop in patients with inadequate renal function, resulting in central nervous system excitation evidenced by confusion, delirium, and seizures. Blood thiocyanate levels are determined in patients with poor renal function and those who receive nitroprusside for longer than 72 to 96 hours. Thiocyanate is cleared by dialysis.

Cyanide poisoning is the cause of death in animals given massive doses of nitroprusside and has been reported in humans. However, concern for cyanide accumulation has probably been overstated (Notterman, 1993). Because an early sign of cyanide poisoning is lactic acidosis, it is prudent to monitor serum lactate levels in patients receiving high dosage or prolonged infusions of nitroprusside.

Nitroglycerin

Nitroglycerin is a venous vasodilator employed extensively in the critical care of adult patients. Its major indication for use is myocardial ischemia from coronary artery disease. Only in the last 10 to 15 years has nitroglycerin been used to treat patients with CHF and pulmonary edema. Another occasional indication includes pulmonary artery hypertension (PAH).

The primary effect of nitroglycerin in patients with heart failure is to reduce ventricular filling pressures by dilation of systemic and pulmonary veins. Enlarging the venous capacitance results in decreased volume in the left and right ventricles and improved ventricular compliance. Central venous, atrial, and PAW pressures are reduced, without systemic hypotension. In patients with acute CHF and pulmonary edema, nitroglycerin may be the drug of choice, particularly if systemic blood pressure is marginal.

Nitroglycerin does decrease arterial vascular resistance, but to a far lesser extent than does nitroprusside.

Nitroglycerin has been investigated in children with acquired PAH and increased PVR related to congenital heart defects with left-to-right shunts. Children with preoperative PAH experienced a decrease in PVR and an increase in cardiac output in response to nitroglycerin (Ilbawi et al., 1985). The utility of nitroglycerin for treatment of idiopathic or primary PAH is uncertain.

Dosage and Administration. Nitroglycerin migrates into many plastics, resulting in substantial loss of medication potency when conventional polyvinyl chloride (PVC) IV administration sets are used. Dosage recommendations for pediatric patients also are difficult to make, because investigators have not reported whether special non-PVC infusion sets were used. Experience with adult patients leads to a suggested starting dose of 0.1 mcg/kg/minute, increasing the dose by 0.1 to 0.2 mcg/kg/minute until the desired effect is achieved. Administration of nitroglycerin with non-PVC infusion sets is recommended to minimize variation in dosage and the potential for error.

The nitrate pastes used among adult patients with coronary artery disease have not been systematically investigated in pediatric patients.

Toxicity. Nitroglycerin administration increases intracranial pressure; adults report severe headache that persists for several days with continued therapy. Cautious use is necessary in patients in whom increased intracranial pressure is a potential problem. More commonly, as with nitroprusside, hypotension complicates nitroglycerin administration. Temporary cessation of the infusion or reduction in the infusion dosage restores blood pressure, because the duration of action of nitroglycerin is short. Adequate intravascular volume is assured, as well.

Nifedipine

Nifedipine is a vasodilator that blocks the calcium channels in vascular smooth muscle and inhibits contraction. There are limited data about its efficacy in acute heart failure in pediatric patients, but it has been used in adults with cardiogenic pulmonary edema and in those with chronic CHF. In pediatric critical care nifedipine has been used in hypertensive emergencies (Ruley, 1993) and to treat patients with primary PAH (Rich & Brundage, 1987).

Dosage and Administration. Nifedipine administered sublingually has a rapid onset of action. Effects are seen in 10 to 15 minutes, with peak action at 60 to 90 minutes. A dose of 0.25 mg/kg/dose (every 4 to 6 hours) can be withdrawn from the capsule with a 1 mL syringe and squirted under the tongue.

Toxicity. Calcium channel blockers have a direct depressant effect on the myocardium and have had limited use in patients with heart failure. However, nifedipine has more profound vasodilating effects than myocardial depression. Still it has not been investigated in pediatric patients with heart failure.

Patients given nifedipine for systemic or pulmonary hypertension may experience headache and other symptoms and signs of vasodilation: sweating, flushing, feelings of warmth, tachycardia, and palpitations.

Captopril

Moderate to severe heart failure results in activation of the renin-angiotensin-aldosterone system, causing compensatory fluid retention to maintain blood pressure. However, the vasoconstrictor substance angiotensin II contributes to inappropriately elevated afterload in advanced heart failure. Inhibition of the renin-angiotensin system reduces afterload and improves cardiac performance. Captopril inhibits the enzyme that converts angiotensin I to angiotensin II, producing vasodilation. Its exact mechanism of preload reduction is not known. It has been postulated that because captopril also inhibits the enzyme that degrades bradykinin, circulating levels of this potent vasodilator are increased. Other angiotensin-converting enzyme (ACE) inhibitors are also available (enalapril, lisinopril, enalaprilat).

In patients with chronic heart failure, captopril provides reduction in both afterload and preload. The hemodynamics produced are similar to those seen with nitroprusside: cardiac output increases proportionately to the decrease in afterload achieved. Because angiotensin II is inhibited, aldosterone release is not stimulated and potassium is spared from renal excretion. Captopril has been used in treatment of adult patients with heart failure due to myocardial ischemia and cardiomyopathy (Abramowicz, 1993; Pfeffer et al., 1992). Use in pediatric patients with heart failure includes those with Kawasaki disease, cardiomyopathy, myocarditis, and those with end-stage heart disease awaiting transplantation.

Captopril is also particularly useful in renovascular hypertension and in treating patients with hypertension related to immunosuppression following organ transplantation. It lowers blood pressure without causing postural hypotension or a reflex increase in sympathetic nervous system activity. HR is usually not affected.

Dosage and Administration. Captopril is available only in oral tablets of 12.5, 25, 50, and 100 mg. These must be crushed and the powder mixed with glucose or tap water for administration to small children or infants. Blood levels peak in 30 to 90 minutes of oral administration. A dose of 0.1 to 2.0 mg/kg is administered every 8 to 12 hours.

Toxicity. Hypotension may occur in volume-depleted patients. Captopril can cause immunologic side effects; the most common is a pruritic rash, which is sometimes accompanied by fever. Neutropenia occurs in some patients and may be severe, necessitating that therapy be discontinued. Occasionally, because ACE inhibitors impair the breakdown of bradykinin, life-threatening angioedema develops.

Increased levels of bradykinin in the circulation may result in chronic cough. Renal side effects include proteinuria. Potassium supplements and potassium-sparing diuretics are avoided in patients receiving captopril.

Antidysrhythmic Agents

Cardiac dysrhythmias are the result of abnormal impulse formation, abnormal impulse conduction, or a combination. Determining both the site of origin and the electrophysiologic mechanism of a cardiac rhythm disturbance is necessary to select pharmacologic therapy. Antidysrhythmic drugs exert their effects by interaction with the ion channels in myocardial cells. When channels are in the drug-bound state, the ion regulated and conducted by that channel is inhibited.

The classification system for antidysrhythmic drugs is based on their predominant effect on electrophysiology in isolated normal cardiac cells (Vaughn-Williams, 1984). The system allows grouping of agents with similar mechanisms of action and potential clinical use, but (like all classification systems) cannot predict the efficacy of a given drug in an individual patient (Table 9–15).

Class I agents are local anesthetics that block the fast sodium channel, slowing conduction and prolonging refractoriness. They are further subclassified by their primary effect on the duration of the action potential. Class II agents block adrenergic receptors. Class III drugs block the potassium channels and prolong repolarization. Drugs in class IV block the slow calcium channels.

Antidysrhythmic drug levels are measured just before the next dose a patient is to receive; that is, a trough level is obtained. The only exception to this is digoxin, which is measured at steady state 6 to 12 hours after a dose is administered and after digitalization is complete. The most commonly used drugs in each category are reviewed in the sections that follow.

Class IA Antidysrhythmic Agents

Quinidine and procainamide are class IA agents that act at the sodium channel and prolong the action potential and refractory period of atrial, ventricular, and Purkinje cells. AV nodal and His-Purkinje conduction times are prolonged. The drugs also decrease normal automaticity except at high concentrations. ECG monitoring of patients receiving these drugs reveals prolongation of the PR interval, QRS duration, and QTc interval.

Class IA agents are effective in treating AV reentrant tachycardias related to accessory pathways because they slow conduction in the accessory pathway. Because they suppress abnormal automaticity, they may be effective in treating atrial, junctional ectopic, and ventricular tachycardia. When used in patients with atrial fibrillation or flutter, improved AV nodal

Table 9–15. CLASSIFICATION OF ANTIDYSRHYTHMIC DRUGS

Class	Major Action	ECG Effects	Examples
I	Sodium channel blockade	Ia: moderate decrease in conductivity, moderate increase in repolarization	Quinidine Procainamide Disopyramide
		Ib: mild increase in conductivity, shorten effective refractory period	Lidocaine Phenytoin Mexiletine Tocainide
		Ic: Marked decrease in conductivity, little effect on repolarization	Flecainide Encainide Propafenone
II	Beta-adrenergic blockade	Antagonizes endogenous catecholamines	Propranolol Nadolol Atenolol Acebutolol Esmolol
III	Potassium channel blockade	Prolongs action potential and repolarization	Amiodarone Bretylium
IV	Calcium channel blockade	Slows conduction at AV node, decreases SA, AV nodal automaticity	Verapamil
Other	Digitalis glycosides	Slows conduction at AV node, decreases SA node discharge rate	Digoxin
	Purinergic agents	Decreases automaticity, slows conduction in SA, AV nodes	Adenosine

conduction may facilitate transmission of atrial impulses and result in a rapid ventricular rate and hemodynamic instability. Previous administration of digoxin or propranolol is used to block AV nodal conduction and counteract the secondary vagolytic effects of the class IA agents.

Dosage and Administration. Both quinidine and procainamide are available in IV form. However, IV quinidine is not generally used because it produces profound hypotension. Procainamide is administered by continuous IV infusion at 30 to 80 mcg/kg/minute, following a loading dose of 10 to 15 mg/kg.

Both these class IA agents are also available in tablets and capsules, which are tolerated by older pediatric patients. The IV form of procainamide can be administered orally to young children and is less erratically absorbed than when the powder from a capsule is suspended in solution for oral administration (Vetter, 1993). The usual oral dose of procainamide is 50 to 100 mg/kg/day administered every 6 hours. Dosages up to 150 mg/kg may be required by infants, who with young children require high doses to maintain adequate blood levels. Quinidine is administered at 30 to 60 mg/kg/day. Both medications are given in doses to obtain a therapeutic response with as little toxicity as possible.

Side Effects. Quinidine exerts alpha-adrenergic blocking effects that decrease peripheral vascular resistance and may result in hypotension. Because these effects are profound when the drug is given IV, the parenteral route is rarely used and limits the overall prescription of quinidine in the PICU.

Both quinidine and procainamide can prolong the QTc interval excessively, resulting in a Torsades de pointes type of polymorphic ventricular tachycardia. Children are less likely than adults to develop this serious side effect (Vetter, 1993). This type of dys-

rhythmia production is less common with procainamide than with quinidine. An increase in the QTc interval of more than 25% to 30% or to more than 0.5 seconds is considered an indication of high risk for dysrhythmia development, and the medication is discontinued or the dose reduced. In addition, both class IA drugs can cause AV block.

Additional side effects include gastrointestinal complaints (abdominal pain, anorexia, and diarrhea) with quinidine. Central nervous system toxicity includes visual disturbances, hearing loss, confusion, and delirium. Procainamide can produce a lupus-like syndrome with gastrointestinal symptoms, especially diarrhea; confusion; disorientation and depression; blood dyscrasias; decreased myocardial contractility; and hypotension. Signs and symptoms are reversible and the drug is generally discontinued. Myocardial depression can be particularly significant in patients in whom performance is already impaired.

Class IB Antidysrhythmic Agents

Lidocaine is the most commonly used class IB agent prescribed in the pediatric critical care setting. Lidocaine suppresses automaticity in Purkinje fibers, making it the most effective agent used to treat ventricular dysrhythmias. Its effect is greater in patients with acidosis and hyperkalemia and in ischemic states.

Mexiletine and tocainide are similar to lidocaine but can be given orally. They are used for maintenance therapy in patients with ventricular dysrhythmias responsive to lidocaine who require long-term therapy.

Phenytoin has electrophysiologic effects similar to those of lidocaine, which may be effective in the treating digoxin-related ventricular dysrhythmias. It has also been effective in treating the ventricular tachycardia associated with congenital long QT interval syndrome.

Dosage and Administration. Lidocaine is administered as a continuous IV infusion following a loading dose of 1 to 3 mg/kg. The typical infusion rate to control ventricular ectopy or dysrhythmia is 20 to 50 mcg/kg/minute. Both the loading and maintenance infusion rates are decreased by one-third to one-half with myocardial and/or hepatic dysfunction.

Mexiletine is given at 4 to 15 mg/kg/day, administered every 8 hours. Tocainide is given at 20 to 40 mg/kg/day, but is rapidly metabolized and may require administration every 4 hours in children (Vetter, 1993).

Phenytoin is administered with an IV loading dose of 10 to 15 mg/kg. The oral maintenance dose is 4 to 8 mg/kg/day administered every 8 to 12 hours, following decreasing total daily oral doses of 15 mg/kg and 7.5 mg/kg.

Side Effects. Lidocaine, mexiletine, and tocainide are associated primarily with gastrointestinal and central nervous system (CNS) side effects. Nausea and abdominal pain are seen most frequently. CNS effects with continuous lidocaine infusion include drowsiness, agitation, slurred speech, tinnitis, disorientation, seizures, coma, and paresthesias. Serum levels are monitored carefully because they correlate well with the development of side effects. The oral preparations, mexiletine and tocainide, can produce dizziness, headache, visual disturbance, tremor, and convulsions. Blood dyscrasias and hepatic toxicity may occur.

Phenytoin may cause myocardial depression with rapid IV administration, as well as vasodilation and systemic hypotension. Its myocardial depressant effects are more common in patients also receiving lidocaine or inderal. An allergic rash is a fairly common side effect of phenytoin. CNS effects are ataxia, drowsiness, nystagmus, and coma. Long-term administration results in gingival hyperplasia and hirsutism.

Class IC Antidysrhythmic Agents

Flecainide is the most frequently used class IC medication. It is used for maintenance therapy in patients with SVT or ventricular tachycardia, following acute management of the dysrhythmia. In children, its greatest efficacy is in the treatment of SVT related to an accessory pathway (Perry et al., 1989; Chang et al., 1990).

Flecainide is a potent inhibitor of the rapid sodium channel, slowing conduction in the atria, ventricles, and Purkinje fibers. AV node conduction is also slowed. Automaticity in Purkinje fibers is inhibited; SA nodal automaticity is unaffected by flecainide. Long-term therapy with flecainide increases the PR interval and QRS duration.

Dosage and Administration. Flecainide is administered orally every 12 hours at a dose of 3 to 6 mg/kg/day.

Side Effects. Life-threatening cardiac toxicity is possible with flecainide, particularly in patients with abnormal ventricular function. These patients may experience negative inotropic effects and demonstrate new or worsened congestive heart failure. These patients, as well as those with pre-existing rhythm disturbance, are also at risk for the development of prodysrhythmias. Polymorphic ventricular tachycardia resistant to cardioversion has resulted in death in adult patients (Podrid & Morganroth, 1985). Complete AV block has been reported in patients with preexisting AV conduction system disease. Careful ECG monitoring of the PR interval and QRS duration is recommended for several days when therapy with flecainide is initiated.

In patients with stable ventricular function, flecainide produces a range of mild extracardiac side effects. CNS effects include blurred vision, dizziness, and headache. Nausea and abdominal pain are also reported. Most are managed by dosage adjustment.

Class II Antidysrhythmic Agents

The beta-adrenergic blocking agents used most frequently to treat rhythm disturbances in children include propranolol, nadolol, atenolol, and esmolol. Beta-blockers inhibit catecholamine binding at the beta-receptor sites, depressing inward sodium flux and membrane responsiveness in Purkinje fibers. Automaticity in all cardiac fibers is diminished. The sinus rate is slowed, as is AV nodal conduction, prolonging the PR interval on ECG.

Patients with cardiac rhythm disturbances mediated by excessive sympathetic nervous system (SNS) stimulation (for example, long QT interval syndrome and exercise-induced dysrhythmia) may be prescribed a beta-blocker. Because these drugs increase AV nodal refractoriness, they may control the ventricular rate in atrial fibrillation or flutter and prevent supraventricular tachycardia in patients with WPW syndrome.

Dosage and Administration. Atenolol and nadolol are administered only in oral form, both prescribed at a daily dose of 1 to 2 mg/kg. Nadolol is administered in a single daily dose, atenolol every 12 to 24 hours.

Propranolol may be administered IV for loading purposes or in patients with supraventricular or ventricular tachycardia and deteriorating hemodynamics. Cardiac side effects are common with the IV route of administration, necessitating careful assessment during administration. The IV dose of propranolol is 0.01 to 0.15 mg/kg, administered by slow IV push.

Esmolol is an ultra–short-acting beta-blocker administered intravenously for the acute reduction of ventricular rate in atrial fibrillation or flutter. An IV bolus dose of 500 mcg/kg administered over 10 minutes is followed by a maintenance infusion of 50 to 200 mcg/kg/minute.

Side Effects. Beta-blockers are negative inotropes and may impair ventricular function, worsening heart failure in some patients. Acute negative inotropic effects are most common with IV administration of propranolol. AV block, severe bradycardia, hypotension, and asystole can occur. An isoproterenol infusion or a temporary external pacemaker is readied when IV propranolol is required. Bradycardia and hypotension can occur with the oral forms of the beta-blockers as well.

Because adrenergic receptors in other organs are also blocked, side effects in various systems are seen. Bronchospasm may occur in patients with reactive airway disease. CNS effects include lethargy, fatigue, sleep disturbance, depression, and personality change. Although atenolol is more cardioselective (i.e., it is a beta$_1$-blocker) and nervous system effects are less, it still has cardiac and airway side effects.

Gastrointestinal effects include abdominal pain, diarrhea, and anorexia. Hypoglycemia may occur.

Class III Antidysrhythmic Agents

Medications in class III prolong cardiac refractoriness and slow conduction. The agents in this class have variable and mixed actions on cardiac cells, but all prolong the action potential.

Amiodarone. Amiodarone prolongs action potential duration (especially phase 3) by blocking potassium channels and prolonging repolarization. As a result, refractoriness is prolonged and conduction slowed. Amiodarone also has a nonspecific inhibiting effect on sympathetic stimulation, blocking alpha- and beta-adrenergic receptors. Sodium channels are inactivated, decreasing automaticity and slowing the rate of SA node firing.

Amiodarone is effective in children in suppressing refractory rhythm disturbances; especially supraventricular or ventricular tachycardia, atrial flutter, and junctional ectopic tachycardia (Garson et al., 1984). These resistant dysrhythmias may occur in the presence of organic cardiac disease including congenital heart defects, myocardial tumor, cardiomyopathy, or myocarditis.

Dosage and Administration. Amiodarone is generally administered orally, because it is less effective via the IV route. The oral loading dose is 10 mg/kg/day administered every 12 hours for 1 to 3 weeks. Its onset of action is delayed; effects are not apparent for 2 to 3 days in children because of the drug's deposition in adipose tissue. In older pediatric patients or obese children, onset may be delayed as long as 10 days, as is the case with adult patients. With long-term therapy, amiodarone dose is decreased to 5 to 10 mg/kg daily.

Serum levels of amiodarone are not particularly useful as a guide to therapy. Myocardial concentration of the drug may be 50 times the concentration in plasma with long-term use. Elimination is extremely slow when therapy is discontinued; in adult patients a mean of 53 days is reported (Naccarelli et al., 1985). Pediatric patients eliminate the drug more rapidly, usually within 3 weeks, because less is deposited in adipose tissue (Garson et al., 1984).

Side Effects. Cardiac side effects are most likely during initiation of therapy because of amiodarone's profound effects on all areas of the conduction system. Marked sinus bradycardia, AV block, and polymorphic ventricular tachycardia may occur, necessitating close monitoring as treatment is begun. Patients with sinus node dysfunction or AV conduction delay may require temporary external pacing. Hypotension can also complicate treatment initiation, because amiodarone is a potent skeletal muscle vasodilator. The potential severity of cardiovascular side effects is high. Amiodarone is reserved for treatment of refractory and life-threatening cardiac rhythm disturbances. Effects of amiodarone can be assessed in the ECG: the PR interval, QRS duration, and QT interval are all prolonged. Pulmonary fibrosis is a significant side effect occurring in adults that has not been reported in pediatric patients. Liver function disturbance, rash, photosensitivity, bluish-gray skin discoloration, and corneal deposits of the drug are noted fairly commonly. Amiodarone inhibits conversion of T$_4$ to T$_3$. Chronic inhibition may affect growth, although these data are not yet available. Elevated levels of T$_3$ correlate with the development of toxicities and are useful for screening. Pediatric patients receiving chronic amiodarone are monitored with chest radiography, liver function tests, and thyroid function evaluation on a regular basis, usually every 3 to 6 months.

Mild gastrointestinal side effects (nausea, vomiting, constipation) occur in children. Weakness, ataxia, and headache have also been noted.

Bretylium. Bretylium has complex sympathetic nerve terminal interactions. Initially, administration of the drug releases norepinephrine from adrenergic neurons. Subsequently, bretylium accumulates in the nerve ending, depleting norepinephrine stores, inhibiting further norepinephrine release, and blocking reuptake of catecholamines.

Initial administration results in a transient increase in the sinus rate, AV conduction, and ventricular automaticity. These effects, resulting from myocardial norepinephrine release, may aggravate some cardiac rhythm disturbances. Blood pressure also increases. Chronic administration prolongs the action potential duration and increases refractoriness. The ventricular fibrillation threshold is increased, producing an antifibrillatory effect. Bretylium is generally used in pediatric patients with recurrent ventricular fibrillation or tachycardia, after lidocaine, procainamide, and beta-blockers have been judged unsuccessful therapeutic agents.

Dosage and Administration. In patients with ventricular fibrillation or tachycardia, an IV dose of 5 to 10 mg/kg is administered. A continuous IV infusion at 15 to 30 mcg/kg/minute follows for maintenance. These doses are extrapolated from those prescribed for adult patients, because no specific pediatric data exist.

Side Effects. Initial therapy requires monitoring for cardiovascular collapse because transient hypertension, increased automaticity in the sinus node or in ectopic foci, and increased myocardial oxygen demand may all produce deleterious effects. Subsequently, severe hypotension is commonly observed with continued therapy. Acute hypotension may necessitate intravascular volume administration. Nausea and vomiting are also noted with bretylium.

Class IV Antidysrhythmic Agents

Class IV drugs selectively bind with the slow calcium channels in myocardial tissue in the SA and AV nodes. As a consequence, sinus automaticity is suppressed and conduction through the AV node is prolonged.

Verapamil. Verapamil is the prototype of the group of drugs that selectively affect calcium transport (i.e., the calcium channel blockers). It is the calcium channel blocker used most often to treat dysrhythmias. When the slow inward calcium channel is blocked, sinus and AV node refractoriness is prolonged. Early and late extrasystoles are also suppressed.

Verapamil is most effective in treating supraventricular tachycardia (SVT), especially AV nodal or AV reentrant SVT. In patients with atrial flutter or fibrillation and those with WPW syndrome, verapamil is avoided. When the AV nodal refractory period is increased in these patients, a rise in ventricular response over the accessory pathway often develops.

Dosage and Administration. In patients older than 1 year with normal ventricular function monitored in the PICU, verapamil is administered via the IV route in the presence of SVT and signs of inadequate CO and tissue perfusion. A dose of 75 to 150 mcg/kg is administered over 1 minute. The onset of action with verapamil occurs in 3 to 5 minutes; its half-life is correspondingly brief. The IV dose of verapamil may be repeated once in 15 minutes if SVT persists. Occasionally, patients with persistent SVT are given a continuous IV infusion at 5 mcg/kg/minute. Long-term oral doses of verapamil are administered at 5 to 15 mg/kg daily, every 8 hours.

Side Effects. Verapamil depresses myocardial function. Its calcium channel blockade interferes with excitation-contraction coupling. In addition to its negative inotropic effects, IV administration causes severe bradycardia, AV nodal block, and asystole. These effects are especially pronounced in young children and infants, and death has been reported (Epstein et al., 1985). Verapamil is not recommended in children younger than 1 year of age or in patients with impaired ventricular function. In addition, concomitant therapy with beta-blockers or quinidine may intensify the potentially pronounced side effects. Treatment of cardiovascular collapse consists of IV administration of atropine, isoproterenol, and calcium.

Other Antidysrhythmic Agents

Two additional medications are sometimes useful in the management of pediatric patients with SVT. The digitalis glycosides are classified as Class V antidysrhythmic agents. Adenosine is a class VI, purinergic agent.

Digoxin. Digoxin is a positive inotropic agent. Its antidysrhythmic effects are the consequence of both direct action on myocardial cells and indirect action mediated by the parasympathetic nervous system (PNS). The sinus rate is slowed and AV nodal conduction is prolonged, lengthening the effective refractory period.

Digoxin is most effective in treating AV nodal reentrant SVT or reentrant SVT resulting from a concealed accessory pathway. It is avoided in patients with manifest accessory pathways (as those with WPW syndrome), because as AV nodal refractoriness is increased, refractoriness in the accessory pathway may decrease. The result is increased ventricular response to atrial flutter or fibrillation. Patients with WPW who are given digoxin for its inotropic effects in myocardial failure undergo electrophysiologic study to determine the effect of digoxin on the accessory pathway refractory period (Vetter, 1993).

Dosage and Administration. (See Table 9–12.) When digoxin is administered IV, its onset of action is 30 minutes with peak effects in 2 hours. In patients with asymptomatic SVT, vagal manuevers to convert the rhythm are sometimes successful when reattempted after one-half the digitalizing dose has been administered. Coadministration of other antidysrhythmics—quinidine, verapamil, and amiodarone—increase serum digoxin levels. Digoxin doses are generally decreased, the serum levels followed, and the ECG evaluated with care during concomitant use of these drugs.

Adenosine. Adenosine decreases automaticity and slows conduction in the sinus and AV nodes. It terminates reentrant SVT by blocking the impulse at the AV node. This fairly new medication recently proved safe and effective in terminating SVT in infants and children (Overholt et al., 1988).

Dosage and Administration. In patients with symptomatic SVT, adenosine is administered by rapid IV push. Its onset of action is nearly immediate and its half-life less than 10 seconds. These features are a benefit in the pediatric critical care setting because repetitive doses can be administered and side effects, if they occur, are short-lived. An initial dose of 50 to 100 mcg/kg is administered, followed by increasing doses of an additional 50 mcg/kg at 2-minute intervals until an effect is achieved. The maximum dose is 350 mcg/kg or 12 mg.

Side Effects. Adenosine may produce transient shortness of breath and dyspnea due to bronchospasm. Cardiovascular side effects include AV block, marked sinus bradycardia, flushing, and hypotension. Irritability is sometimes noted. Generally these effects are short-lived, but measures to support circulation and ventilation are ensured until a normal sinus rhythm resumes.

MANIPULATION OF DUCTAL PATENCY AND PULMONARY VASCULAR RESISTANCE

The first hours and days after birth are characterized by stabilization of the respiratory and cardiovascular systems. Closure of the ductus arteriosus is one of the important events during this period of time, as is the establishment of "normal" vascular resistances in both the pulmonary and the systemic circuits. However, infants with some complex congenital heart defects (CHD) depend on patency of the ductus arteriosus for survival following birth. In addition, a variety of problems can impede the fall in PVR that normally occurs after birth. Cardiovascular collapse and death can be the result in either situation.

In 1981, the Food and Drug Administration approved prostaglandin E_1 (PGE$_1$) for use in neonates with CHD to maintain patency of the ductus arteriosus in lesions that depend on ductal patency for either systemic or pulmonary blood flow. Administration of PGE$_1$ permits delay of surgical intervention until the infant with a critical CHD can be transferred to a tertiary care center specializing in congenital cardiac surgery. In additionally, inhaled nitric oxide (NO) and inhaled carbon dioxide (CO_2) are new methods of manipulating PVR and pulmonary blood flow (PBF) in these infants and others who have sustained pulmonary hypertension.

Developmental Physiology of the Pulmonary Vasculature

Fetal pulmonary vascular development parallels development of the lungs. From the sixteenth week of gestation, the pulmonary arteries and the preacinar arteries that accompany the terminal bronchioles are present. Throughout the remainder of gestation, respiratory units develop from the terminal bronchioles and are accompanied by developing intraacinar arteries and pulmonary capillaries. The preacinar arteries have a muscular wall, as do the arteries at the level of the terminal bronchioles. The intraacinar arteries are largely nonmuscular (Rabinovitch, 1989, 1992).

The pulmonary vascular bed of the fetus is maintained in a vasoconstricted state throughout gestation. Only about 8% of the CO from both the right and left ventricles perfuses the fetal lungs because of high PVR. Conversely, SVR is low, owing to the low-pressure placenta.

Within minutes of birth, this situation reverses. PVR drops, although the mechanism responsible is unknown. Oxygenation and expansion of the lungs are independently effective at decreasing PVR, and other factors have been identified as instrumental in the drop in pressure, but how these stimuli are mediated is not yet understood. Previously closed peripheral arteries are recruited for circulation; there is dilation of the proximal, muscular arteries; and the peripheral vessels continue to grow and branch. Although dilation of the smallest and most distal vessels occurs across months and muscle extension into the walls of the peripheral arteries takes years (Rabinovich, 1989, 1992), PVR decreases by 80% in the first hour after birth and reaches adult levels during the first months of life. Simultaneously, SVR

increases owing to separation of the newborn from the placenta. The consequences of the resistance changes at birth (and other factors) are increased PBF, improved oxygenation, and eventual closure of the fetal shunts at the foramen ovale and ductus arteriosus.

Normal pulmonary vascular development can be disrupted by a number of problems. Abnormal structure and function may be the consequence of maladaptation (the fetal lung does not mature appropriately), maldevelopment (increased muscularization may be the consequence of intrauterine insult or a CHD that obstructs pulmonary venous drainage), or underdevelopment (pulmonary hypoplasia results from a condition such as diaphragmatic hernia (Rabinovitch, 1989). Either acute or chronic fetal or postnatal hypoxia prevents the anticipated fall in PVR after birth. Hypoxia sustains the vasoconstricted state, and PVR and pulmonary artery pressure remain high. CHD associated with decreased PBF may result in hypoplasia of the pulmonary vascular bed and may increase PVR as a consequence. Those CHDs with increased PBF induce pulmonary vascular changes resulting in increased PVR as the consequence of high flow and high pressure in the pulmonary circuit. High oxygen concentrations used in the treatment of neonatal lung disease may be detrimental to both alveolar and arterial growth and development.

Maintaining Ductal Patency

In newborns with a CHD who are dependent on patency of the ductus for systemic or pulmonary blood flow, administration of PGE$_1$ restores or maintains ductal patency and can improve arterial oxygen saturation, enhance tissue perfusion, correct tissue hypoxia and acidosis, and maintain systemic blood pressure (Freed et al., 1981; Schneeweiss, 1986; Noerr, 1991). Table 9–16 lists CHD types in which PGE$_1$ is indicated.

Infants with pulmonary atresia, tricuspid atresia, and severe pulmonary stenosis may be far better oxygenated after PGE$_1$ is initiated. Improvement in

Table 9–16. CONGENITAL HEART DEFECTS IN WHICH PGE$_1$ IS RECOMMENDED

To Improve Pulmonary Blood Flow or Arteriovenous Mixing	To Maintain Systemic Perfusion
Pulmonary atresia	Interrupted aortic arch
Critical pulmonary stenosis	Critical coarctation of the aorta
Tricuspid atresia	Hypoplastic left heart syndrome
Transposition of the great arteries with intact ventricular septum	Critical aortic stenosis
Tetralogy of Fallot with pulmonary atresia or pulmonary artery hypoplasia	

Adapted from Rickard, D. H. (1993). Reproduced by permission of *Neonatal Network*, 12 (4), 17–22.

these severely cyanotic infants is generally seen within 30 minutes of the PGE_1 infusion's initiation. Lack of dramatic improvement may indicate that the ductus has maximally dilated, but pulmonary vasodilation with PGE_1 often enhances PBF and provides at least a modest increase in arterial oxygen saturation (Freed, 1981). Infants with other cyanotic CHDs, including transposition of the great arteries, truncus arteriosus, and total anomalous pulmonary venous return may benefit by PGE_1 infusion to improve arteriovenous mixing.

Infants with left-sided obstructive lesions may develop cardiovascular collapse because ductal closure prevents systemic perfusion. In those with interrupted aortic arch (IAA), severe coarctation of the aorta, hypoplastic left heart syndrome, and severe aortic stenosis, PGE_1 obtains maximal ductal patency and reverses tissue hypoxia and acidosis. Infants with these obstructive CHDs may not respond as rapidly to PGE_1 as do cyanotic infants. Freed (1981) found that infants with IAA had maximal response in 90 minutes, whereas those with severe coarctation did not respond maximally for 3 hours. In the case of a critically ill newborn in whom either a cyanotic or obstructive heart lesion is suspected, PGE_1 is instituted quickly. The infusion is maintained while definitive echocardiographic diagnosis is obtained.

Dosage and Administration. PGE_1 can be administered via central or peripheral IV or via the umbilical artery. Intravenous therapy is preferred, because cutaneous vasodilation may be more pronounced with intraarterial administration (Lewis et al., 1981). The initial recommended infusion rate is 0.05 to 0.1 mcg/kg/minute. When improvement in arterial oxygenation or systemic perfusion have been achieved, the lowest dose that maintains the response is administered. Typically, 0.05 to 0.2 mcg/kg/minute achieves the desired clinical effect. The infusion is continued until surgical intervention is provided or until further assessment shows no need to maintain ductal patency.

Toxicity. Side effects to PGE_1 infusion are fairly common. Respiratory depression, evidenced by apnea and/or hypoventilation, is thought to be related to CNS effects and is very common. Airway management, including intubation and mechanical ventilation, is provided for all infants receiving PGE_1, when necessary. Cardiovascular side effects including bradycardia, tachycardia, and hypotension are most likely related to vasodilation and are anticipated. Infants weighing less than 2 kg at birth experience the most significant respiratory and cardiovascular side effects (Lewis et al., 1981). Less frequently observed toxic effects include seizures, jitteriness, hypoglycemia, hypocalcemia, diarrhea, renal failure, and clotting abnormalities (Lewis et al., 1981).

Manipulating Pulmonary Vascular Resistance

Pulmonary vascular resistance in the newborn is labile, and the pulmonary vascular bed reacts intensely to a number of stimuli. Stimuli are listed in Table 9–17 and provide a foundation for the conventional management or control of pulmonary vascular reactivity.

Reducing Pulmonary Vascular Resistance

PVR is reduced by assisted ventilation with high inspired concentrations of oxygen, which increase oxygen diffusion across the alveolar membrane and promote pulmonary vasodilation. The pulmonary vasodilation associated with breathing oxygen may be mediated through endothelium-derived relaxing factor (Roberts & Shaul, 1993). Assisted ventilation also facilitates gas delivery even when airway resistance is increased and pulmonary compliance is decreased owing to parenchymal disease. Mechanical ventilation is facilitated by neuromuscular blockade and the administration of IV narcotics.

Hyperventilation to a systemic $PaCO_2$ of 25 to 35 mmHg further reduces pulmonary artery pressure and improves oxygenation (Peckham & Fox, 1978). It is not clear whether the decrease in carbon dioxide or the respiratory alkalosis that results is operational in reducing pulmonary vasoconstriction. Systemic alkalosis can also be induced by IV administration of sodium bicarbonate, reducing the degree of hyperventilation required and limiting the potential for barotrauma. Excessive sodium bicarbonate administration, however, may result in hypernatremia and increased serum osmolarity.

Intravenous vasodilating agents have been used experimentally and clinically to reduce pulmonary vasoconstriction (Kulik & Lock, 1984). However, currently available IV vasodilators are not specific for the pulmonary vasculature and all reduce systemic vascular resistance, resulting in significant systemic hypotension. Hypotension may decrease coronary perfusion pressure and result in cardiac ischemia. In addition, vasodilation in nonventilated segments of the lung results in increased ventilation and perfusion mismatching, which may actually reduce alveolar gas exchange.

Extracorporeal membrane oxygenation (ECMO) has been used to support full-term newborns with persistent PAH who are not successfully treated with maximal ventilatory and medical support. With ECMO, gas exchange occurs independent of pulmo-

Table 9–17. FACTORS INFLUENCING PULMONARY VASCULAR RESISTANCE

Vasoconstriction (↑ PVR)	Vasodilation (↓ PVR)
Hypercarbia	Hypocarbia
Alveolar hypoxia	Alveolar hyperoxia
Acidosis	Alkalosis
Hypothermia	
Agitation	Analgesia, sedation
Alveolar overdistension	
Vasoconstrictive mediators	Vasodilating agents

nary blood flow. Since the first survivor in 1975, thousands of infants have been successfully supported on ECMO (Stork, 1989). However, the risks of potentially serious complications have stimulated the continued search for a pulmonary vasodilator.

Nitric Oxide. Nitric oxide (NO) is produced by vascular endothelium. Endogenous NO diffuses into adjacent vascular smooth muscle, producing vasodilation by stimulating the production of cyclic GMP (cGMP). It is important in mediating the decrease in PVR that normally occurs after birth.

Inhalation of low levels of exogenous NO reverses hypoxic pulmonary vasoconstriction in lambs (Frostell et al, 1991) and adult volunteers (Frostell et al., 1993). PVR is decreased with NO therapy in adults with primary PAH (Pepe-Zaba et al., 1991) and ARDS (Rossaint et al., 1993). Roberts and coworkers (1993a) demonstrated that inhaled NO selectively reduced PVR in full-term infants with persistent pulmonary hypertension of the newborn (PPHN) and improved systemic oxygenation. NO has also been shown to reduce pulmonary vasoconstriction in pediatric patients with congenital heart disease complicated by PAH (Roberts et al., 1993b). Inhaled NO produces selective pulmonary vasodilation without systemic hypotension because NO that diffuses into the pulmonary circulation is inactivated rapidly by combination with hemoglobin.

Investigations of the utility of NO in reducing PVR and pulmonary artery pressure have included its lengthy use in infants with PPHN. In infants who were considered ECMO candidates, NO was administered for as long as 24 days (Roberts et al., 1993a). Prolonged NO inhalation improved the clinical condition of patients considered for ECMO by Kinsella and coworkers (1992).

The short-term use of NO during cardiac catheterization of pediatric patients with PAH from CHD demonstrated that NO can dilate pulmonary vasoconstriction that is not caused by hypoxia (Roberts et al., 1993b). The investigators suggest that inhaling NO during cardiac catheterization is likely to aid the assessment of the vasodilatory capacity of the pulmonary vascular bed in children with PAH.

Case study reports of the potential benefit of NO include its use in the intraoperative management of a patient with low cardiac output associated with high PVR following Fontan-type repair of a complex CHD (Miller et al., 1993). Hemodynamic improvement in this patient included a significant increase in systemic blood pressure, which accompanied the fall in PVR, as would be anticipated with Fontan physiology. Abram and coworkers (1993) reported on the use of inhaled NO in the management of a premature infant with severe respiratory distress and PAH, demonstrating that the immature pulmonary circulation is responsive to exogenous NO.

Dosage and Administration. NO is administered with inhaled gases to maintain the concentration of oxygen in room air (0.21%). The gases are administered via the ventilator circuit to critically ill patients or via a pediatric face mask in situations such as the investigation with children with CHD

(Roberts et al., 1993b). NO gas is administered in parts per million (ppm) and is quantified by chemiluminescence. Inhalation of as little as 20 ppm produced pulmonary vasodilation in infants with PPHN (Kinsella et al., 1992). Roberts and coworkers (1993b) demonstrated that breathing 80 ppm NO at FiO_2 0.9 produced the greatest reduction in mean pulmonary artery pressure and lowered PVR to the lowest levels in patients with PAH undergoing cardiac catheterization.

Patients receiving NO do not experience systemic vasodilation and subsequent hypotension. Prolonged inhalation of NO does not decrease responsiveness to the gas (Roberts et al., 1993a; Kinsella et al., 1992).

Toxicity. NO is oxidized to nitrogen dioxide (NO_2). Inhalation of gas mixtures containing high levels of NO and NO_2 produces severe, acute pulmonary injury with pulmonary edema. However, evidence suggests that inhaling low levels of NO in the absence of NO_2 is safe. Chemiluminescence measures the concentration of both NO and NO_2 in inhaled gases, so that the oxides can be chemically absorbed. In addition, high flow rates reduce the conversion of NO to NO_2 (Frostell et al., 1991).

NO that diffuses into the intravascular space and combines with oxygen produces methemoglobin. At high concentrations of NO (i.e., 5000–20,000 ppm), critical reduction of arterial oxygen content caused by methemoglobin results in death. At low concentrations, methemoglobin levels may increase, but not to a level that interferes with tissue oxygenation. Mice exposed to 10 ppm NO for 6 months displayed signs of increased red blood cell turnover with enlarged spleens and elevated serum billirubin levels. The duration and level of NO exposure that will produce red cell degeneration in humans is unknown (Frostell et al., 1991).

Increasing Pulmonary Vascular Resistance

Infants with left-sided obstructive CHD (see Table 9–16) are dependent on patency of the ductus arteriosus for systemic circulation. Closure of the ductus produces rapid cardiovascular collapse. Reestablishing patency of the ductus with PGE_1 restores systemic perfusion, but control of the ratio of blood flowing to the pulmonary and systemic circuits (Qp:Qs) can be difficult to achieve and maintain. Balanced flow (a Qp:Qs ratio of 1) ensures adequate systemic blood flow and tissue perfusion.

When PBF is increased, systemic hypoperfusion and metabolic acidosis result. Because many infants with left-sided obstructive lesions are not identified prior to cardiovascular collapse, metabolic acidosis is common among these patients. Metabolic acidosis triggers compensatory hyperventilation, which decreases $PaCO_2$ and PVR, increases PBF at the expense of systemic perfusion, and sets in motion a vicious cycle.

Pulmonary overcirculation will result in death in infants with a left-sided obstructive cardiac lesion if not rapidly corrected. This is also the case in other infants with parallel circulations, such as those with truncus arteriosus. It is important to recognize that ventilation with an FiO_2 greater than 0.21 does not improve systemic oxygenation and may decrease PVR. Additional control of PVR is achieved, when necessary, by controlling ventilation. Infants are intubated and given a neuromuscular blocking agent. Administration of a bolus dose of IV sodium bicarbonate raises $PaCO_2$ acutely when compensatory hyperventilation is prevented. Controlled hypoventilation increases PVR and redistributes blood flow across the ductus more evenly between the systemic and pulmonary circulations. The addition of PEEP and hyperinflation also increase PVR.

Carbon Dioxide. Hypoventilation, even when controlled, can result in atelectasis and hypoxemia. The administration of CO_2 gas at concentrations of 1% to 4% has been demonstrated to allow additional control of pulmonary and systemic blood flow (Jobes et al., 1992).

Dosage and Administration. The usual concentration of CO_2 in room air is 0.03%. CO_2 gas is administered to the infant in the PICU via the ventilator circuit or in the oxygen hood to increase the concentration of CO_2 to 1% to 4% (Smith & Vernon-Levett, 1993). Intraoperative administration of CO_2 has been accomplished with administration of the gas through the anesthesia bag (Jobes et al., 1992). The concentration of CO_2 necessary to balance Qp:Qs is determined by arterial blood gas analysis. Generally, maintaining the infant's $PaCO_2$ at 40 to 50 mmHg increases PVR sufficiently to ensure adequate systemic blood flow, evidenced by adequate systemic blood pressure and peripheral pulses and by acid-base balance.

Toxicity. Experience with the administration of CO_2 gas is limited. A report of its clinical use in approximately 200 infants with complex CHD described the advantages of early and more precise control of $PaCO_2$, an important variable in determining PVR, in preoperative and postoperative care. Toxicity was not observed (Jobes et al., 1992).

PACEMAKER THERAPY

Advances in pacemaker technology over the past 25 years have made permanent cardiac pacing in infants and children a safe, practical therapy. Permanent cardiac pacemakers have been miniaturized and can be programmed or reprogrammed noninvasively. Lithium batteries have extended the life of the permanent pulse generator and surgical placement techniques have been improved. Temporary external pacing in acute illness has also been refined.

The majority of pediatric patients requiring either temporary or permanent cardiac pacing have bradydysrhythmia. In a few patients, pacemaker therapy is used to control tachydysrhythmia.

Indications

Bradydysrhythmias

Sinus or AV node dysfunction following intracardiac repair of a CHD is the most common cause of bradydysrhythmia in infants and children (Table 9–18). Transient cardiac conduction disturbances may be the result of surgical manipulation or suturing near the conduction system, but they are also related to hypothermia or electrolyte imbalance in some patients. Depending on the type of cardiac surgical procedure performed, temporary atrial and/or ventricular epicardial pacing wires are placed at operation to promptly manage postoperative dysrhythmias. Bradycardia related to surgical manipulation of the heart usually resolves within 2 or 3 weeks, and an intrinsic HR adequate for cardiac output is restored. When conversion does not occur and temporary external pacing is required for an extended period of time, permanent pacemaker implantation is planned.

Congenital complete heart block (CHB) occurs in infants with structurally normal hearts, as well as in some with abnormal cardiac structure. When associated with a structural CHD, complete AV block has a far higher mortality than is the case in infants with isolated CHB (Machado et al., 1988).

Once diagnosed, close monitoring for signs of fetal distress, including growth retardation and fetal hydrops, is required. After delivery, the infant is monitored and observed for several days in an intensive care setting to assess hemodynamic stability and determine the need for intervention. Neonatal pacemaker implantation is currently recommended for all symptomatic infants and for asymptomatic infants with a resting heart rate less than 55 bpm (Smith, 1990; Frye et al., 1984).

Conduction disturbances and bradycardia may be related to infection. Viral myocarditis is associated with SA node dysfunction, diffuse ST-T wave changes, interventricular conduction delays, and variable AV block. Sinus and AV node dysfunction may be permanent sequelae necessitating pacemaker placement or transient problems with conversion to sinus rhythm occurring with resolution of the infection. Table 9–19 lists the causes of bradydysrhythmia in infants and children.

Table 9–18. POTENTIAL CARDIAC DYSRHYTHMIAS AFTER SURGICAL REPAIR OF CHD

Sinus node and atrial dysrhythmias
Total anomalous pulmonary venous connection
Atrial septal defect
Fontan procedure
Mustard/Senning procedures
Atrioventricular conduction block
Mitral valve repair/replacement
Endocardial cushion defect
Ventricular septal defect
Tetralogy of Fallot

Table 9-19. CAUSES OF BRADYDYSRHYTHMIAS IN INFANTS AND CHILDREN

Intracardiac repair of congenital heart defects
Congenital complete heart block
L-transposition of the great arteries
Viral myocarditis
Lyme disease
Sick sinus syndrome
Long QT interval syndrome
Myotonic dystrophy
Orthotopic heart transplantation

From Lawrence P. A., (1991). Cardiac pacing in children. *AACN Clinical Issues in Critical Care Nursing*, 2:150–155.

Other Rhythm Disturbances

Although less common than bradydysrhythmias in infants and children, other cardiac rhythm disturbances may be treated with temporary or permanent cardiac pacing. Included are both supraventricular dysrhythmias (atrial fibrillation, atrial flutter, atrial tachycardia, and junctional tachycardia) and ventricular dysrhythmias (PVCs, ventricular tachycardia, and Torsades de pointes, associated with a prolonged QT interval) (Sulzbach & Lansdowne, 1991).

Temporary External Cardiac Pacing

Temporary external cardiac pacing is most often needed in the diagnosis and management of rhythm disturbances in infants and children with CHD who require cardiac surgical procedures. In addition, some sustained tachydysrhythmias can be successfully converted with an external pacemaker, and noninvasive pacing has recently become an accepted therapy in advanced life support.

Temporary Pacing Lead Selection

Pacing in postoperative cardiac surgical patients is achieved via epicardial wires placed in the atria or ventricles at the time of the operation. Transvenous pacing is possible in larger pediatric patients and transesophageal pacing in patients of any size. These pacing modes are most often used for overdrive pacing to convert tachydysrhythmias. Transcutaneous pacing is a fairly new technique used to restore cardiac rhythm in emergency situations.

Temporary Epicardial Pacing. Epicardial pacing wires are swedged stainless steel Teflon-coated wires placed at the conclusion of a cardiac surgical procedure. Two pairs may be placed on the free wall of both the right atrial and ventricular epicardia. Placement of ventricular wires only is not uncommon following intracardiac repair of CHD, because young pediatric patients appear less dependent than adults on AV synchrony. However, the presence of AV block precludes the use of atrial wires alone in most patients. The epicardial wires are brought out through the chest wall on either side of the sternum. When both atrial and ventricular wires are placed, the atrial wires are generally secured to the right of the sternum and the ventricular wires to the left.

Epicardial pacing is used to treat bradydysrhythmias that are the consequence of sinus node dysfunction or complete heart block. Less frequently, they are used to suppress irritable dysrhythmias or ectopy, terminate or slow supraventricular tachydysrhythmias, enhance CO by achieving AV synchrony, or to produce overdrive suppression of refractory ventricular dysrhythmias. In addition, epicardial pacing wires can be used for dysrhythmia identification using an atrial or ventricular wire ECG (Sulzbach & Lansdowne, 1991; Bumgarner, 1992).

Temporary Transvenous Pacing. Transvenous pacing wires are placed via the superior vena cava in either the right atrium or ventricle. The pacing impulse is most often conducted via the endocardium to a single location only. Transvenous pacing wires are sometimes placed prophylactically in patients at high risk for cardiac rhythm disturbances before major surgical procedures, provided the patient is of sufficient size and has normal cardiac anatomy. More frequently, transvenous pacing is elected to manage persistent tachydysrhythmia.

Transesophageal Pacing. Bipolar pacing catheters designed for positioning in the esophagus just behind the left atrium permit recording of a transesophageal ECG, as well as overdrive pacing, which is often successful in the conversion of atrial flutter or reentrant SVT.

Temporary Pulse Generator

Temporary external pacemakers are classified based on a three-letter code developed by the Inter-Society Commission for Heart Disease (ISCHD) in 1974. The first letter describes the chamber that is paced; the second, the chamber that is sensed, and the third, the pacer's response to sensing. The code was revised in 1984 and expanded to five positions (Table 9–20).

In both codes, the first letter indicates the chambers paced; the second letter, the chambers sensed; the third letter, the response to sensing; the fourth, the programmability of the unit; and the fifth, the antitachycardia function of the unit. The fourth and fifth modalities are available on internal permanent pulse generators (Bernstein, et al. 1987). The most common pacing modes for pediatric patients are atrial demand (AAI), ventricular demand (VVI), atrioventricular triggered or inhibited (DDD), or atrioventricular triggered or inhibited, rate responsive (DDDR) (Kugler & Danford, 1989).

Children with bradydysrhythmias due to isolated sinus node dysfunction who have normal AV conduction and those with bradycardia-tachycardia syndrome who develop SVT are recommended for AAI pacing. The noncompetitive single-chamber unit recognizes the child's intrinsic atrial rate and triggers

Table 9–20. PACEMAKER MODALITY CODES AND MODES

1974 Three Letter ICHD Code

Chamber Paced	Chamber Sensed	Response	
V	O	O	VOO, Ventricular fixed rate, asynchronous
V	V	I	VVI, Ventricular demand
A	A	I	AAI, Atrial demand
D	V	I	DVI, AV sequential demand
V	D	D	VDD, Atrial triggered
D	D	D	DDD, Automatic, universal

1984 Revised Five Position ICHD Code

I Chamber(s) Paced	II Chamber(s) Sensed	III Modes of Response	IV Programmable Functions	V Antitachycardia
	O = none	I = inhibited	O = none	B = bursts
A = atrium	A = atrium	T = triggered	P = simple (rate/output)	N = normal rate competition
V = ventricle	V = ventricle		M = multiple (complex)	S = scanning
D = dual	D = dual		C = communicating	
			R = rate modulation	

an atrial impulse only when the atrial rate falls below the programmed level.

Ventricular demand pacing (VVI) is the most common pacing modality in pediatric patients, owing to the the incidence of AV block following intracardiac repair of CHD. VVI pacing is accomplished with a simple, single-chamber unit with sensing and pacing occurring in the ventricle. Symptomatic bradycardia resulting from intermittent or complete AV block in children who are hemodynamically stable without an atrial contraction is treated with this pacing mode.

DDD and DDDR pacing mimic physiologic antrioventricular synchrony with dual-chambered cardiac activity. Atrial *and* ventricular pacing leads are required for pacemaker response to a variety of intrinsic cardiac rates and rhythms. Basic operation consists of the following steps:

1. A low heart rate limit is programmed.
2. If the pacemaker does not sense an intrinsic atrial impulse within the low heart rate limit, a pace impulse is triggered and delivered to the atria.
3. A preset delay is programmed, during which ventricular activity is anticipated.
4. If spontaneous ventricular depolarization occurs, the pacemaker is inhibited and no ventricular pacing impulse is generated; if there is no spontaneous ventricular activity, the pacemaker fires a paced ventricular beat.

DDD and DDDR pacing provide optimal cardiac performance necessary in those patients who require atrioventricular synchrony.

Pacing Modes

Asynchronous, or fixed rate, pacemakers function in either the AOO or VOO pacing mode. Pacing impulses are discharged to the atrial or ventricular pacing electrodes at a preset rate, regardless of the patient's intrinsic electrical activity. Patients with CHB may be paced in an asynchronous ventricular mode.

Pacemakers that can sense the patient's inherent cardiac electrical activity and both inhibit or discharge an impulse paced on the intrinsic HR are termed "demand" or "synchronous" pacers. Ventricular demand (VVI), atrial demand (AAI), and demand AV sequential pacing (DVI, VDD, or DDD) can be accomplished with an external pacemaker.

Figure 9–62 illustrates a demand dual-chamber pacemaker. The sensitivity control adjusts the level at which the sensing electrode can detect (or sense) the patient's inherent atrial or ventricular activity. The output control regulates the amount of energy discharged by the pulse generator. Generally, the stimulation threshold (the minimum amount of energy required to consistently elicit cardiac depolarization) is determined and the output, in milliamperes (mA), is set approximately 5 mA higher to ensure consistent pacing. The AV interval control sets the time between atrial sensing/pacing and ventricular sensing/pacing. Like the native PR interval, it is measured in milliseconds. The rate control determines atrial and ventricular rate. The on/off control, which serves the obvious function, is locked in position when turned to "on" to prevent accidental or inadvertent discontinuation of pacing. Alternatively, the temporary pulse generator can only be turned off by simultaneously depressing more than one control.

Nursing Care of Patients With Temporary External Pacemakers

Patients who require temporary external cardiac pacing are closely monitored to ensure the effectiveness of pacemaker therapy. Potential pacemaker problems include those that may suddenly and significantly reduce cardiac output. These problems—

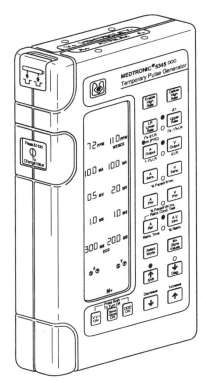

Figure 9–62 ● ● ● ● ● ●

Temporary external demand, dual-chamber pacemaker. (Copyright ©1990 Medtronic, Inc. Reprinted with permission.)

undersensing, oversensing, failure to capture, and loss of pacemaker output—can occur with either temporary or permanent pacing. They are described here because the condition of the patient requiring temporary external pacing may be physiologically unstable and uniquely dependent on adequate pacemaker function. The critical care nurse ensures effective pacemaker function by careful monitoring of the patient's ECG and thorough assessment of tissue perfusion, oxygenation, and acid-base and electrolyte balance.

Troubleshooting Pacemaker Dysfunction

Patients with either temporary or permanent pacemakers may develop interference with electrical signals traveling between the pulse generator and the heart, which affect the pacemaker's performance. Some problems may result in an immediate, significant decline in cardiac output and obvious signs and symptoms of difficulty in the patient. In other patients, the onset of a pacemaker problem is less obvious. For example, an exhausted pacemaker battery or broken lead will result in loss of pacing, but some children are asymptomatic and only the routine HR check performed by a parent alerts them to the problem.

Battery depletion or lead fracture or displacement require surgical intervention. Other pacemaker problems may be addressed at the bedside, either by

adjusting the controls of the temporary external pacer or reprogramming the implanted pacer. The most common problems are failure of the pacemaker to sense the heart's electrical activity (undersensing or competition), failure to pace in the absence of cardiac activity (oversensing), and loss of capture. In addition, patients with temporary external pacemakers require special protection from electrical hazards, particularly in the hospital environment.

Undersensing. If the pacemaker is unable to respond to the electrical signals from the patient's heart, it behaves as if the signals were absent: it delivers pacing impulses. Loss of sensing is recognized on the patient's rhythm strip as late pacemaker artifact (Fig. 9–63) or because the patient experiences the sensation of extrasystoles that are initiated by the pacemaker. Undersensing results in competition between native myocardial activity and the pacemaker's activity. The pacemaker stimulus, if delivered during the relative refractory period, can provoke ventricular tachycardia or fibrillation.

Undersensing may occur during temporary external pacing if the sensitivity of the pulse generated is inappropriately set or inadvertently readjusted. Loose connections between the pacing leads and the pulse generated may prevent accurate sensing, as can magnetic or electrical interference. Undersensing of atrial activity with temporary epicardial wires in postoperative cardiac surgery patients is a common problem (Sulzbach & Lansdowne, 1991), limiting the usefulness of temporary demand atrial pacing. The external pulse generator is not sensitive enough to detect P waves, although permanent atrial demand pacing is possible.

Undersensing may be corrected by adjusting the sensitivity of the pulse generated upward, by ensuring tight connections between the pacing electrodes and the temporary external pacemaker, and by eliminating sources of interference. If these measures fail with the temporary external pacemaker, another generator is substituted.

Oversensing. The pacemaker may be overly sensitive to electrical stimuli, interpreting other electrical signals as the R wave. The pacemaker may sense the T wave, P wave, or chest or abdominal muscle activity as myocardial activity. Electromagnetic in-

Undersensing

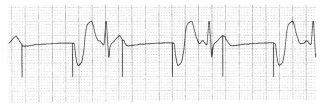

Figure 9–63 ● ● ● ● ● ●

Pacemaker loss of sensing (undersensing). (Copyright ©1990 Medtronic, Inc. Reprinted with permission.)

Oversensing

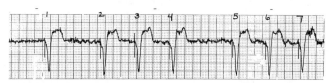

Figure 9–64 ● ● ● ● ● ●

Pacemaker oversensing (failure to pace). Shivering produces fasciculations in the ECG baseline interpreted as myocardial electrical activity. (Copyright ©1990 Medtronic, Inc. Reprinted with permission.)

terference or loose connections may prevent the pacemaker from accurately sensing.

The risk in oversensing is loss of pacemaker activity when it is required, with subsequent reduction in cardiac output. Patients may report dizziness with intermittent oversensing or may actually lose consciousness. Oversensing is confirmed with a rhythm strip (Fig. 9–64).

Rapid intervention may be necessary for patients dependent on a pacemaker for adequate HR and CO. Oversensing is corrected by ensuring secure connections between the pacing electrodes and the temporary pacemaker. Electromagnetic interference is eliminated. If oversensing persists, the sensitivity of the pacemaker is decreased to ensure that it fires when necessary.

Loss of Capture. When the pacemaker delivers an impulse that fails to result in depolarization, capture has been lost. Loss of capture is recognized on the ECG, which demonstrates the generator's pacing spikes without cardiac electrical activity in response (Fig. 9–65). Some patients demonstrate dramatic signs of reduced CO and require emergency intervention.

Patients with permanent pacemakers and sudden complete or intermittent loss of capture most often

have battery depletion, pacing lead fracture or displacement, a loose connection to the pulse generator, or increased pacing threshold. Investigation necessitates chest radiography to evaluate the pacing leads and pulse generator evaluation and attempts at reprogramming. It may be necessary to support the patient's HR and ensure hemodynamic stability with a continuous medication infusion of isoproterenol or epinephrine. Temporary transesophageal or noninvasive temporary pacing may be used until the problem is corrected.

Loss of capture with a temporary external pacemaker may be the result of pacing lead displacement, loose connections with the pulse generator, battery depletion, or change in pacing threshold. Pacing threshold is anticipated to increase with temporary epicardial pacing electrodes because of fibrous tissue deposition at the wire insertion site. Pacing threshold may also change with acid-base imbalance, electrolyte imbalance, or as a consequence of medication administration. While these potential causes of loss of capture are investigated, the pacing stimulation threshold is assessed and the output from the pulse generator is increased to ensure that pacer firing results in myocardial response. A new battery or replacement pacemaker may be required.

Loss of Output. Failure of the pacemaker to fire when necessary is detected by the absence of pacing spikes on the ECG. A permanent pacemaker may have battery exhaustion or lead disconnection, fracture, or displacement, necessitating surgical intervention. With a temporary pacemaker, the on-off switch is checked, as are all connections, to ensure that no inadvertent change has occurred. A new battery is inserted in the pulse generator or the pacemaker is replaced with another. The patient may require emergency intervention to maintain cardiac output.

Electrical Safety. Patients with temporary external pacemakers in place are uniquely sensitive to environmental electrical hazards. The pacemaker unit itself is shielded to prevent contact with sources

Loss of Capture

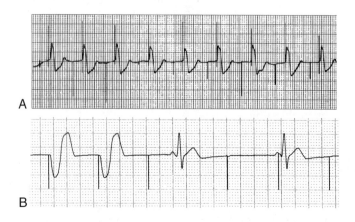

A

B

Figure 9–65 ● ● ● ● ● ●

Loss of pacemaker capture. *A*, Loss of atrial capture. *B*, Loss of ventricular capture. (Copyright ©1990 Medtronic, Inc. Reprinted with permission.)

of 60-cycle current that may cause serious ventricular dysrhythmias. In addition, the unit cannot be exposed to fluids, which pose an immediate electrical hazard. Often, when the pacemaker or pacing electrodes are manipulated, caregivers wear gloves to avoid static electrical discharges being transmitted to the patient. All mechanical equipment in the patient's room or at the bedside is grounded and the use of extension cords is avoided. Staff conscientiously avoid simultaneous contact with any electrical equipment and either the pacemaker or the patient.

Temporary Noninvasive (Transcutaneous) Pacing

Temporary noninvasive cardiac pacing was added to the Advanced Cardiac Life Support (ACLS) algorithms in 1986. Noninvasive pacing is a recommended intervention for adults with symptomatic bradycardia or asystole when atropine and epinephrine administration are unsuccessful. Noninvasive pacing has been used successfully in both infants and children (Beland et al., 1987). In addition to treatment of bradycardia and asystole, noninvasive transcutaneous pacing (NTP) has been used for overdrive suppression of sustained tachycardia (Luck & Davis, 1987).

NTP is achieved via multifunction electrodes that permit ECG evaluation and either pacing or defibrillation via the same electrodes with only the turn of a switch on the pacemaker-defibrillator. In an emergency there is the choice of either pacing or defibrillation with the same electrodes. NTP can be used in the demand mode because the multifunction electrodes permit sensing of the patient's inherent ventricular rate. Other relatively new improvements include refinements in NTP technology that minimize the electrical current needed for capture and advances in electrode construction that diminish the threshold for stimulation. Comfort of NTP in conscious patients has been maximized (Appel-Hardin, 1992).

Indications for NTP

The clearest indications for NTP are medication-resistant bradycardia and asystolic cardiac arrest. In these situations, NTP can be used to maintain a cardiac rhythm until a more permanent pacemaker (transvenous or transthoracic) can be established. NTP has been used for overdrive pacing of SVT or ventricular tachycardia.

Implementation of NTP

The posterior multifunction electrode is applied first in a position on the patient's back to the left of the spine and below the scapula (Fig. 9–66). Positioning the electrode over substantial bone is avoided, because bone conducts the pacing current poorly. The

anterior electrode is placed in the V_2 to V_5 position on the precordium. In the vernacular, a "heart sandwich" is made with the pacing electrodes.

In situations when NTP electrodes have been applied prophylactically, it is advisable to determine the pacing threshold by setting the pacing rate 10 to 20 beats higher than the patient's intrinsic HR and slowly increasing the milliamperes of the pacemaker until capture is obtained (Appel-Hardin, 1992). The pacemaker can then be operated in the demand mode. In cardiac arrest situation, the pacing rate is set at 100 and the milliamperes adjusted upward until ventricular pacing occurs. In adult patients, output of 60 to 100 mA was required for reliable pacing (Heller et al., 1989). Normal values for pediatric patients have not been established. The effectiveness of ventricular capture is assessed clinically by palpating a pulse and evaluating tissue perfusion.

Troubleshooting Common NTP Problems

The most common clinical problems encountered with NTP are painful stimulation, unnecessary pacing (undersensing), and failure to or loss of pacemaker capture.

Painful Stimulation. Contraction of the chest wall muscles during pacing can result in pain, a sensation that is also frightening to the patient. Pain is minimized if the pacing threshold is set at the lowest effective level. Discomfort is also reduced by

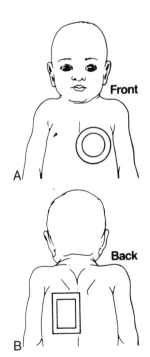

Figure 9–66 ● ● ● ● ● ●

Positions of the multifunction electrodes for noninvasive transcutaneous pacing. *A,* A "heart sandwich" is made with the pacing electrodes. *B,* A posterior electrode is applied to the back left of the spine and below the scapula. (Courtesy of Zoll Medical Corporation, Burlington, MA.)

ensuring that the pacing electrode is in good contact with the skin. Changing the position of the pacing electrode may reduce discomfort if other measures are unsuccessful (Appel-Hardin, 1992).

Undersensing. Unnecessary pacing may occur when the pacemaker does not sense the patient's intrinsic HR. Most often, contact between the electrode and the patient's skin is inadequate. Adherence may lessen across time, especially in the presence of diaphoresis. Adherence of the electrode is checked regularly to ensure that the pacemaker does not interpret loss of the ECG signal as bradycardia or asystole and commence firing at the preset rate. Patient position changes may also affect electrode adherence and sensing capability. When the multifunction electrodes are changed, it is important to remember to turn off all pacemaker controls or turn the function control knob to "monitor only" to avoid accidental electrical shock.

Loss of Capture. Changes in patient position, which may decrease electrode adherence to the back or chest or loosen pacer connections, may be associated with failure to capture. Measures to prevent poor contact between the electrode and the patient's skin are crucial.

Because the pacing output in NTP is set just 5 to 10 mA above the patient's pacing threshold, changes in the patient's physiologic status can influence pacemaker capture. With all types of cardiac pacing, the pacing threshold may change with electrolyte imbalance, acid-base imbalance, myocardial ischemia, hypoxia, and with new drug therapy. Reassessment of the pacing threshold with any of these changes is necessary to avoid loss of capture.

Permanent Cardiac Pacing

In 1984, a joint task force of representatives from the American College of Cardiology and the American Heart Association developed guidelines for permanent pacemaker implantation in children and adults (Table 9–21). Bradydysrhythmia is the most common finding necessitating pacemaker implantation. Evaluation of the bradycardic infant or child for signs and symptoms indicative of inadequate cardiac output or unstable cardiac rhythm may reveal CHF, ventricular ectopy, bradycardia-tachycardia syndrome, syncope, activity intolerance, or poor exercise performance. Pacemaker implantation is indicated in all sympotomatic patients.

Permanent Pacemaker Selection

The first implantable pediatric pacemaker became available in the 1960s. By today's standards it was large and had a short-lived battery. It fired only in an asynchronous mode and was not programmable. Currently, selecting an appropriate permanent pacemaker requires consideration of multiple issues: endocardial vs. epicardial lead system; single vs. dual-chambered pulse generator; anticipated pro-

Table 9–21. GUIDELINES FOR PACEMAKER IMPLANTATION

Class I: Pacemaker indicated (noncontroversial)
(a) Second or third degree AV block with symptomatic bradycardia
(b) Second or third degree AV block with ventricular dysrhythmias
(c) Second or third degree block with marked exercise intolerance
(d) Symptomatic AV block and CHF not responsive to medical management
(e) Sinus node dysfunction with symptomatic bradycardia
(f) Congenital AV block with HR <55 bpm
(g) Congenital AV block with wide QRS complex
(h) Bradycardia-tachycardia syndrome requiring digoxin and other antidysrhythmic drugs

Class II: Pacemaker indicated (controversial)
(a) Transient postsurgical AV block reverting to a bifascicular block
(b) Asymptomatic second or third degree AV block

Class III: Conduction disturbances not requiring a pacemaker
(a) Transient postsurgical AV block reverting to sinus rhythm 2–3 weeks after surgery
(b) Asymptomatic postoperative bifascicular block
(c) First degree AV block

Data from the American College of Cardiology and the American Heart Association, 1984.

grammability needs; the child's anticipated somatic growth and activity level; and the long-term prognosis. Pacemaker reliability and longevity and maximal hemodynamic benefit are the primary goals of the selection process.

Pacing Lead Selection. Epicardial and endocardial lead systems are used for permanent cardiac pacing in pediatric patients. Epicardial leads are secured directly on the outer wall of the heart via either a thoracotomy or a subxyphoid approach. Epicardial lead placement is necessary in small patients (weighing less than 10 kg), in patients with abnormal cardiac structure precluding transvenous placement (e.g., univentricular heart or cavopulmonary connection), and in patients with right-to-left intracardiac shunt (because of the risk of systemic thromboembolism with endocardial leads) (Lawrence, 1991). Pacing via epicardial leads is anticipated to result in buildup of fibrous tissue at the lead attachment site, which is associated with increased impedance to the pacing current, necessitating high pacing thresholds. Eventual inability to pace because of lead dysfunction is a fairly common problem.

Endocardial, or transvenous, leads are threaded into the subclavian vein from a small anterior chest incision, advanced through the right atrium, and wedged into the right ventricular trabeculae. Adequate venous access and suitable cardiac anatomy (with the superior vena cava in communication with the right atrium) are required for effective endocardial lead placement. Generally, patient weight of at least 10 to 15 kg is anticipated as the minimum weight necessary for successful transvenous location of the pacing electrodes.

Advantages of transvenous endocardial lead placement include: (1) implantation in the cardiac catheterization laboratory with sedation and local anesthesia, rather than general anesthesia; (2) brief hospital stay; and (3) potentially lower pacing threshold and longer pulse generator life (Lawrence, 1991). Because long-term pacing is anticipated, the major disadvantage of this pacing system is the technical difficulty associated with repositioning, replacing, or removing the lead once it is anchored in the right ventricle.

Regardless of which pacing lead system is selected, lead replacement may be necessitated because of linear growth, lead fracture, change in pacemaker technology, or development of a superior pacing system. Transvenous lead systems increase the risk of bacterial endocarditis, which may require lead removal.

Current pacemaker implantation techniques anticipate spurts in a child's growth and an active lifestyle. Loops of lead wire are tucked into a subcutaneous tissue pocket to extend with growth and avoid stressing and dislodging the epicardial or endocardial leads and allow a longer interval between operations for lead replacement. Insulated, highly flexible lead wires are tunneled through subcutaneous tissue to the pacemaker generator to help avoid lead fracture. Antibiotic prophylaxis may be provided for patients with transvenous leads during dental or surgical procedures, although this not stipulated in the American Heart Association guidelines.

Pulse Generator Selection. The pulse generator itself is surgically implanted in a pocket of subcutaneous tissue beneath the clavicle, in the subpectoral muscle, or in the upper left quadrant of the abdominal wall. A number of pacing modalities are available. Selection of the most appropriate unit is based on consideration of the underlying cardiac rhythm disturbance and the physiologic and hemodynamic needs of the patient.

Nursing Care After Pacemaker Placement

Children who require pacemaker implantation are often monitored and cared for in the PICU for 12 to 24 hours after surgery. Initial nursing assessment is focused on the patient's hemodynamic stability in response to pacing and on pacemaker function. On admission to the PICU, vital signs are measured and recorded and a chest radiograph is obtained to verify pacing lead placement and to document the absence of hemopneumothorax. Ongoing postprocedure care includes continuous ECG monitoring, ensuring adequate hydration and pain management, maintaining bedrest to avoid accidental lead displacement, and broad spectrum antibiotic administration (Lawrence, 1991). The surgical wound is routinely assessed; only routine wound care is anticipated. Patient and family education, begun before implantation, becomes more focused as discharge is anticipated. Documentation of the type of pacing electrode (endocardial or epicardial, unipolar or bipolar); the pacemaker manufac-

turer, model number and serial number; the pacing mode selected; and programmed pacing parameters are ensured.

MECHANICAL SUPPORT OF CARDIOVASCULAR FUNCTION

Indications and Experience With Pediatric Patients

During the last decade, major strides have been made in the application of mechanical circulatory support technology for adult patients suffering from severe cardiac failure. Gains in available devices, clinical management strategies, and technical refinements have led to widened applications and improved outcomes for these critically ill patients (Shiono, 1993). However, cardiovascular device technology has not been widely applied to pediatric patients. Few mechanical circulatory support devices are available to accommodate small children and infants, and variable results have been achieved in terms of complication and mortality rates. Despite these limitations, the number of patients supported with devices has doubled in the last decade, and significant gains in survival are reported (Pennington & Swartz, 1993). Wider applications of pediatric device technology seem certain in the near future.

The use of mechanical devices for circulatory support is considered a last resort for all patients, exhausting fluid and pharmacologic interventions that restore CO before their initiation. The majority of patients needing device intervention are those requiring temporary cardiovascular support pending myocardial recovery. This group includes patients following cardiac surgery, those with acute myocarditis or reversible cardiogenic shock, or those with severe rejection episodes following cardiac transplantation. A second group includes those with irreversible cardiac failure awaiting transplantation whose clinical condition deteriorates before location of a suitable organ donor (i.e., bridge-to-transplant). In these patients, the goal of treatment is not myocardial recovery but maintenance of tissue and end-organ perfusion despite severe cardiac compromise until cardiac transplantation can occur. Hemodynamic criteria for device placement have been described and are included in Table 9–22, but for each patient an assessment of the potential risks and benefits of this treatment modality is needed before initiation of mechanical support (Veasy, 1993).

Noninvasive External Assist Devices

Venous return to the heart is enhanced by the use of external venous assist devices. Reduction of third-space fluid loss in the lower body is also accomplished (O'Brien & Elixson, 1990). A variety of venous assist devices including pneumatic trousers (MAST suit),

Table 9–22. HEMODYNAMIC CRITERIA FOR MECHANICAL CIRCULATORY SUPPORT IN PEDIATRIC PATIENTS*

Cardiac index ≤ 2 L/min/m^2
Persistent hypotension with inadequate perfusion
Persistent metabolic acidosis
Worsening hypoxemia
Elevated cardiac filling pressures
Mixed venous oxygen <30 mmHg
Urine output <1 mL/kg/hr

*Despite adequate preload and pharmacologic support
Adapted from Veasey, L.G. (1993). Pediatric adaptation in blood pumping. In S.J. Quaal (Ed.). *Comprehensive intraaortic balloon counterpulsation*, (2nd ed). St Louis: C.V. Mosby.

intermittent lower body compression, abdominal compression with a MAST suit, lower extremity boot, and right atrial balloon pump have been described (Heck & Doty, 1981; Milliken et al., 1986; Jacobs & Vlahakes, 1987). All phasic compression devices provide improved ventricular filling pressures by redistributing peripheral venous fluid into the central circulation. When the lower body is compressed, increases in carotid and coronary flow have been measured with coincident decreases in femoral flow in adults treated with the MAST garment (Wangensteen et al., 1968).

Abdominal compression with simultaneous chest compression during standard cardiopulmonary resuscitation in adults provides an increase in aortic pressure (Barranco et al., 1990). Phasic compression of the lower body and abdomen has been described in the postoperative management of pediatric patients who underwent Fontan procedure (Milliken et al., 1986; Jacobs & Vlahakes, 1987; Tobias et al.,

1990). Improvement in patient condition and outcome is attributed to increased venous return leading to increased pulmonary blood flow, ventricular filling pressure, and CO. Increased systemic blood pressure, improved peripheral perfusion, and decreased third spacing or fluid retention are the positive results of phasic compression devices in the immediate perioperative period (O'Brien & Elixson, 1990).

Intraaortic Balloon Counterpulsation

Intraaortic balloon counterpulsation augments CO and improves coronary artery perfusion via intermittent inflation of a small balloon catheter within the descending thoracic aorta. Because the balloon deflates when the heart is in systole and inflates when the heart is in diastole, its pumping action is counter to that of the heart. Thus the term *counterpulsation* (Fig. 9–67A and B).

Cardiac function can be assisted via the intraaortic balloon pump (IABP) during both phases of the circulation. When the balloon inflates during diastole, blood volume is displaced proximally to the aortic arch and coronary arteries, and distally to the renal and lower extremity vessels. This *diastolic augmentation* leads to increased diastolic pressure as well as improved tissue perfusion. Additional benefits are obtained by rapid deflation of the balloon just prior to systole, which results in afterload reduction or *systolic unloading*. Intraaortic volume and pressure decrease with rapid balloon deflation, reducing myocardial impedance to ejection and decreasing myocardial workload (Quaal, 1993a).

Despite widespread use of this device in adult pa-

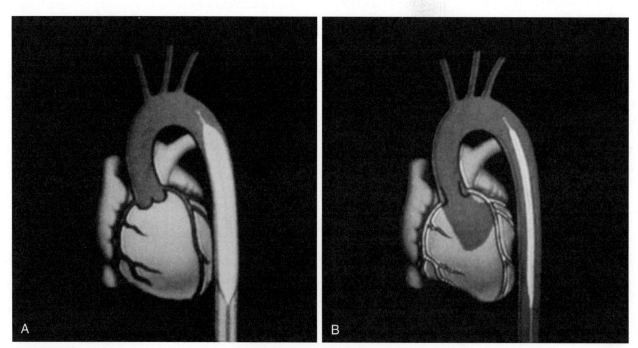

Figure 9–67 ● ● ● ● ● ●
Intraaortic balloon position during inflation *(A)* and deflation *(B)*. (Courtesy of Datascope Corporation.)

tients, pediatric IABP use has been limited for several reasons. First, unlike the percutaneous insertion technique used for adults, infants and small children require surgical intervention to correctly place the device. Second, the range of available balloon sizes for small patients is limited and inappropriate sizing may negate appreciable benefit of the device. Blood displacement may be minimal in the highly compliant pediatric aorta, which also may negate both systolic and diastolic benefits of the device. Use of oversized balloons has been reported as a possible solution to this problem (Dunn, 1989). Finally, CO increases with pediatric IABP support have not been quantified and reported, but presumably do not exceed the 10% gains reported for adult patients (Smith & Cleavinger, 1991). For severely ill patients, more aggressive therapy with a ventricular assist device (VAD) may therefore be warranted.

Contraindications

Use of the IABP is reserved for patients with a competent aortic valve and healthy aorta. Aortic valve insufficiency is an absolute contraindication, because regurgitant blood flow from aorta to left ventricle, as the path of least resistance, is likely to increase during balloon inflation. Aortic coarctation is a concern, because blood displacement against the anatomic narrowing during balloon inflation efforts is limited. Coagulation disorders are a relative contraindication, potentially leading to uncontrolled bleeding at the insertion site. Finally, use of the device is advocated *before* the onset of irreversible cardiac dysfunction, defined as a cardiac index (CI) less than 1.2 L/min/m² (Veasy, 1993).

Equipment and Insertion

The balloon pump consists of two components: the balloon itself and the console that regulates balloon inflation and deflation. Pediatric balloons range from 2.5 to 20-mL inflation volumes, mounted on catheters from 4.5 to 7.5 French (Table 9–23). Ideal balloon size is based on body surface area (BSA), and can be estimated from the following formula, using the patient's heart rate (HR) and an assumed CI of 2.0, if unknown (Veasy, 1993).

$$\frac{CI \times BSA}{HR} \times 0.5 = \text{balloon size}$$

Other guidelines offered by this author include use of a balloon with a volume of at least one-half the patient's SV, as well as selecting the largest balloon size possible to optimize cardiac support benefits.

The IABP console regulates the pumping of helium gas into the balloon chamber. Helium is used because its light weight allows it to be displaced rapidly in and out of the balloon. The console controls allow the operator to regulate triggering and timing of the device. A variety of ECG or arterial pressure signals can be used to regulate the balloon *triggers,* or what the pump should recognize as systole and diastole. The operator can then fine-tune the balloon *timing,* including both inflation and deflation points, to optimize hemodynamic parameters.

The balloon may be inserted in the critical care unit, cardiac catheterization laboratory, emergency department, or operating room. The femoral artery is the most common insertion site, although the internal iliac artery may also be used. A percutaneous approach is rarely possible in the pediatric patient because of small vessel size, warranting a vascular cutdown procedure. A synthetic side-arm graft is sutured directly to the artery, which houses the catheter entry site into the vessel (Anella et al., 1990). The catheter is then sutured in place and covered with a sterile occlusive dressing. Rarely, a surgeon places the balloon directly into the aorta when the chest is open during surgery. This transaortic approach requires a return to the operating room for balloon removal upon discontinuing IABP support.

Regardless of the initial approach, the balloon is positioned in the thoracic aorta approximately 1 to 2 cm distal to the left subclavian artery and above the renal arteries. Once correctly positioned, the catheter is connected to the gas line of the IABP console and pumping is started.

Balloon Timing

Optimal timing of balloon inflation and deflation in concert with native cardiac events requires console adjustments by a specially trained nurse or IABP technician. Achieving optimal hemodynamic benefits with counterpulsation relies on careful timing of bal-

Table 9–23. PEDIATRIC INTRAAORTIC BALLOON PUMP CATHETERS

Volume (mL)	Catheter (French)	Balloon Length (cm)	Balloon Diameter (mm)
2.5	4.5	10.7	6.0
5.0	5.5	12.8	8.0
7.0	5.5	14.2	9.0
12.0	6.5	15.8	10.0
20.0	7.5	17.8	12.0
(4.0 mL available by special order)			

Data from Datascope Corp., Paramus, NJ.

loon events using the ECG and arterial pressure waveform, with the understanding that there is a slight time delay between the electrical and mechanical events of the heart. A variety of triggering modes is available with current IABP technology, but the R wave of the ECG continues to be used in most situations. In this mode the IABP uses ECG signals to determine systole and diastole, automatically deflating with R wave sensing to avoid balloon inflation during systole. Balloon inflation is timed to occur with the midpoint of the T wave, which coincides with the onset of diastole (Quaal, 1993a). To provide this electrical signal, a second set of ECG electrodes must be connected to the IABP console.

Manual IABP timing adjustments allow for fine tuning beyond basic triggering, and are made with the IABP inflating every other beat (1:2 augmentation). This allows for comparison of augmented (balloon-assisted) and nonaugmented beats on the arterial waveform. The rapid heart rates seen in pediatric patients require special timing considerations. Timing of balloon inflation just *before* the dicrotic notch (i.e., before the onset of diastole) has been advocated by Veasy and coworkers (1993) to increase the duration of assisted diastolic perfusion. Echocardiography demonstrated that forward flow from the aorta ends before the dicrotic notch on the arterial blood pressure tracing. Others advocate maintaining 1:2 balloon assistance (rather than full 1:1 support) when the HR exceeds 160 bpm, to optimize helium exchange and pump efficiency at rapid heart rates (Dunn, 1989).

When optimal timing has been achieved, hemodynamic benefits are evident both clinically and on the arterial blood pressure tracing. Diastolic augmentation should reach suprasystolic levels, meaning that the balloon assisted diastolic pressure becomes the highest point on the waveform. Afterload reduction is evidenced by a decreased systolic pressure

following balloon inflation (assisted systole), as well as by lowered aortic end-diastolic pressures (Fig. 9–68). In reality, these "ideal" tracing landmarks are not always evident, despite clinical improvements in CO and tissue perfusion. Young patients are less likely to achieve suprasystolic augmentation, which was reported to occur in less than 50% of patients under the age of 2 years, versus 88% to 100% of older children (Christensen et al., 1991).

Continuous hemodynamic and HR monitoring provides evidence of the need for IABP timing adjustments, which should be made for signs of deteriorating clinical status, a change in cardiac rhythm, or HR changes greater than 10 bpm (Anella et al., 1990). Improper IABP timing can result in less cardiac support than intended, at best, or severely compromised cardiac ejection, at worst.

Nursing Care

Care of the pediatric IABP patient requires high level nursing skills applicable to any critically ill child, as well as an appreciation of the unique problems that can occur with device technology. These patients typically require mechanical ventilation and invasive monitoring, as well as tremendous psychosocial support for themselves and their families. The nurse must also focus on problems related to continued cardiac failure, as well as potential complications of the device itself. These include impaired tissue perfusion, bleeding related to anticoagulation, and infection.

Patients who require IABP support are at risk for impaired CO and tissue perfusion resulting from either continued progression of their underlying cardiac disorder or from balloon-related problems. Frequent assessment of hemodynamic parameters should reveal the anticipated benefits of IABP counterpulsation, including increased CO and mean arte-

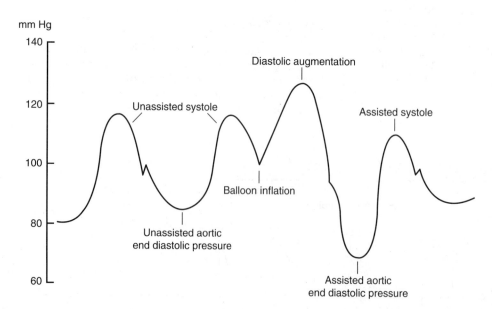

Figure 9–68 ● ● ● ● ● ●
Arterial pressure waveform characteristics during intraaortic balloon counterpulsation therapy.

rial pressure, decreased SVR and filling pressures, and improved end-organ perfusion. Failure to achieve these parameters may be the result of improper IABP timing, dysrhythmias, or damage to the balloon catheter.

IABP timing should be assessed at least every 4 hours and reassessed as indicated earlier. Dysrhythmias may affect the efficiency of IABP triggering, leading to an impaired CO, which may warrant appropriate antidysrhythmic therapy. The balloon catheter itself may be another source of CO impairment, if it becomes dislodged or damaged by excessive movement or thrombus formation. Leg restraints and sedation are often needed to prevent excessive movement, especially hip flexion that could cause catheter crimping. Anticoagulation is usually warranted to prevent thrombus formation on the balloon and is initiated once intraoperative bleeding has subsided. Continuous heparin infusions are adjusted to maintain the partial thromboplastin time (PTT) at 1.5 to 2 times control values, warranting initiation of bleeding precautions (Anella et al., 1990).

Catheter migration may result in decreased perfusion of either the kidneys or left arm. The urine output is assessed hourly as an indicator of adequate renal perfusion. An abrupt cessation of urine flow may indicate downward balloon migration with obstruction of the renal arteries. Upward balloon displacement can result in obstruction of the left subclavian artery, resulting in impaired arm perfusion. Correct IABP position can be evaluated with a daily chest radiograph, because the catheter tip is radiopaque.

The most frequent complication of IABP therapy is ischemia of the cannulated extremity, below the insertion site. Christensen and coworkers (1991) reported a 10% incidence of this complication in children. The quality of peripheral pulses should be assessed before and after balloon placement to note changes from baseline. Asymptomatic loss of distal pulses occurs frequently after IABP insertion and often does not progress to severe limb ischemia. Signs of more severe obstruction to blood flow, including pain, pallor or mottling, and decreased sensation or loss of motor function, warrant physician notification.

The IABP insertion site is a potential source of infection that requires preventive measures and careful observation of site integrity. Measures to decrease infections include meticulous handwashing and daily (or unit-specific) sterile dressing changes to the IABP cannulation site using an occlusive dressing. Surveillance for systemic infection includes monitoring of body temperature every 2 to 4 hours and daily white blood cell counts. Antibiotic prophylaxis may be administered immediately after IABP insertion and continued as needed based on risk of infection.

Few people outside the critical care arena have heard of IABP or its effects on cardiac function, which warrants educational preparation of families and older children. A study examining family percep-

tions of the adult IABP experience revealed that 13 of 27 family members (48%) had the device explained by a nurse (Goran, 1989). In the same study, all families understood the device "helped the heart," but many confused the IABP with an angioplasty balloon. These families requested information about the anticipated duration of IABP use, its complications, if the patient can feel it, how the pump is removed, and if the patient can go home with the pump in place. Additional information about cardiac anatomy and intraaortic balloon placement was deemed very helpful for these families.

Weaning From The IABP

Attempts at weaning from the IABP are initiated when hemodynamics become stable, usually within 24 to 48 hours of insertion. Inotropic requirements should be minimal or absent before device weaning, offering the ability to resume pharmacologic support if mild cardiac dysfunction recurs after device removal. Weaning is achieved by decreasing the frequency of augmentation from every beat (1:1) to every 2nd, 4th, or 8th beat (1:2, 1:4, 1:8). During the weaning process the nurse should assess for signs of intolerance to decreased support, including decreased CO, increased filling pressures, ventricular ectopy, or other signs of impaired perfusion. If weaning is tolerated, the physician will remove the device surgically by trimming the side-arm graft and closing the incision (Anella, 1990). Careful assessment of perfusion to the distal extremity is important after IABP removal, because thrombus formation or distal embolization can occur.

Ventricular Assist Devices

For patients with profound cardiac failure, a 10% augmentation in CO may be insufficient to meet organ perfusion needs. Although more invasive than an IABP, ventricular assist devices (VADs) can provide up to 100% of cardiac pumping function for these critically ill patients (Smith & Cleavinger, 1991). More than a dozen types of VAD systems have been used for adult patients; however, one device, the centrifugal pump, has shown promising results in providing circulatory support to infants and children.

Principles of Support

The Medtronic Bio-medicus centrifugal pump has been used for cardiopulmonary bypass (CPB) during open heart surgery as well as more extended cardiac support out of the operating room environment. Although current Food and Drug Administration (FDA) clearance is for CPB durations of 6 hours or less, both ECMO and LVAD support of 190 hours have been reported (Galantowicz & Stolar, 1991; Karl et al, 1991). This device uses centrifugal force, such as that created by a tornado, to propel blood through the circulation. Blood is drawn from the patient, via cannulae connections, into an acrylic pumphead containing two or three cylindrical cones (Fig. 9–69). When magnetically coupled to the device console, the pumphead spins at a rapid rate, propelling blood out of the pumphead and into the patient in a nonpulsatile manner (Quaal, 1991).

Cardiac support is initiated intraoperatively following a median sternotomy, using large-bore CPB cannulae to divert blood around the heart. A typical venoarterial CPB circuit (from right atrium, to a pump and oxygenator, with return to the aorta) may be continued postoperatively to provide ECMO support for severe cardiac failure. In contrast, VAD support provides a unilateral (either systemic or pulmonary) circuit, without an oxygenator in place. Left-sided (LVAD) cannulation diverts blood from the left atrium to the pumphead and console, where rotating blades then propel it back to the systemic circulation via the aorta (Fig. 9–69). Right-sided (RVAD) or biventricular (BVAD) support can be provided by cannulating the right atrium and pulmonary artery in a similar fashion. Two pump sizes are available for support, including the standard sized pumphead and tubings containing a 200 to 250 mL blood circuit volume, which may be used for larger children. The Medtronic Bio-medicus Model BP50 Bio-Pump is designed for the smallest patients, containing a 50 mL

pumphead with 1/4-inch tubings. Keeping the circuit length to a minimum has been advocated to prevent excessive extracorporeal blood volumes and limit heat loss in the neonate or small child. Pump tubings may also be covered with foil or warm heating pads to maintain normothermia, but heating lamps are not recommended.

Once the blood flow circuit is complete, console controls are adjusted to initiate support. Pump flow rates (L/min) are adjusted via manipulation of the magnet rotation speed, in revolutions per minute (rpm), based on patient size and CO requirements. Although flow rates up to 6 L/minute are possible with the larger pumphead, initial flows of 2.5 L/minute/m^2 have been reported for patients with weights ranging from 3.4 to 45 kg (Karl, et al; 1991). Once pumping has commenced, closure of the sternotomy incision around the cannulae is attempted, although it is not always possible even in adult patients, because of size constraints. A rubber dam or other occlusive material may then be used to cover the mediastinum, providing a barrier to infection. Incomplete heparin reversal is advocated, followed by continuous heparin infusion to an activated clotting time (ACT) of 150 seconds (Karl, et al., 1991) to 200 to 250 seconds (Moat, et al., 1990) to prevent clotting of the extracorporeal circuit.

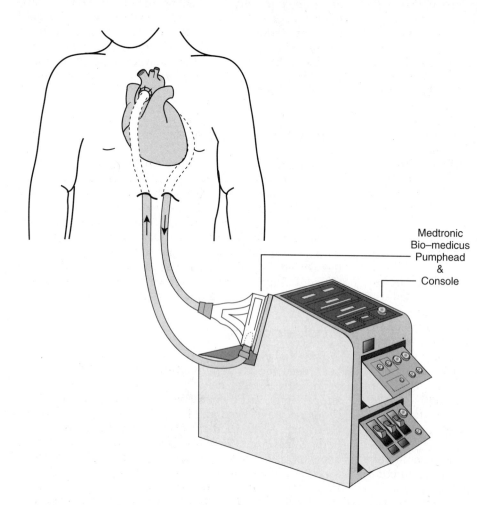

Medtronic
Bio–medicus
Pumphead
&
Console

Figure 9–69 ● ● ● ● ● ●
Left ventricular assist device support with Medtronic Bio-medicus centrifugal device. (Copyright ©1990 Medtronic, Inc. Reprinted with permission.)

Nursing Care

Care of the patient requiring centrifugal VAD support requires a highly skilled, multidisciplinary approach to provide a safe environment, minimize complications, and promote optimal recovery. Unlike the IABP, which requires frequent and precise timing adjustments, the centrifugal pump typically requires minimal rpm changes to provide needed flows. Physiologic principles do apply, however, in that the pump cannot deliver an adequate stroke volume if it is not adequately filled or if it must eject against high resistance. Monitoring device operations includes documenting VAD flow rates and the rpms required to *generate* that flow. Acceptable values are patient-specific, but the need for increasing rpms to generate constant device flow rates warrants investigation. The most frequent cause of inadequate flow is hypovolemia. Appropriate volume therapy often restores pump flow rates and corrects tubing "chatter," or excessive tubing vibration (Quaal, 1991).

Monitoring of the pediatric patient with VAD includes assessment of typical indicators of tissue perfusion such as CO, filling pressures, skin color and temperature, and organ perfusion indices. Several monitoring techniques will be altered with use of the device. Pulse oximeters rely on pulsatile signals to calculate arterial oxygen saturation, which may be inadequate when using the nonpulsatile centrifugal VAD. Nonpulsatile flow will also lead to narrowed arterial and venous waveform tracings, making the mean arterial pressure the most accurate indicator of systemic blood pressure. The use of thermal dilution CO measurements will be unaffected by LVAD, but will invalidate CO determinations in patients with RVAD because of an altered path for injectate volumes. Estimations of native heart function can be made by subtracting VAD flow rates from the thermal dilution CO value. Ventricular recovery will be indicated by rising native heart CO values, tolerance of gradually decreasing VAD flow rates, as well as improved tissue perfusion. While *brief* periods of minimal or absent flow to assess native heart recovery are acceptable, clamping of VAD tubings is not recommended because it may lead to thrombus formation within the circuit (Pennington et al., 1988).

Specific guidelines for nursing care vary significantly depending on whether the sternum has been surgically closed after device placement. Turning is not advised for patients with an open chest or those with only skin closure around device cannulae (Quaal, 1991). These patients may require high doses of sedatives or paralyzing agents to maintain integrity of the VAD circuit, as well as meticulous skin care and pressure control mattresses to avoid decubitus formation. Measures to ensure that VAD tubings are secure and emergency electrical power is maintained are also warranted to ensure patient safety. Emergency resuscitation with external cardiac compressions poses a high risk of cannulae disruption and is not advised. Although the risk of accidental circuit disruptions is extremely unlikely with careful attention to patient and tubing positioning, clamps are kept at the bedside *exclusively* for prevention of hemorrhage with a disconnection.

Recognition and Management of Potential Complications

Karl and coworkers (1991) report that bleeding (42%), infection (42%), and renal dysfunction (33%) were the most common complications seen in their series of 12 pediatric patients requiring postcardiotomy VAD support. Data from the combined ECMO-VAD pediatric registry failed to show a relationship between the occurrence of a specific complication and survival rates (Pennington & Swartz, 1991).

Bleeding is the most prevalent complication of mechanical circulatory support in both adult and pediatric patients, often necessitating reoperation to control hemorrhage (Pae, 1993). Factors that contribute to postoperative bleeding include preoperative hepatic congestion, prolonged CPB times, multiple cannulation sites, and platelet interaction with biomaterial surfaces. Decreases in both platelet number and effectiveness can be anticipated in any patient following CPB, with more pronounced platelet dysfunction often occurring after prolonged support (Copeland et al., 1989). Hemodilution of coagulation factors also contributes to hemostatic abnormalities. Strategies to minimize postoperative bleeding include prompt and aggressive correction of coagulopathies, use of topical agents to facilitate hemostasis, as well as a policy of keeping patients in the operating room until bleeding is well controlled (Ley & Hill, 1993). The site of ECMO cannulation, neck versus chest, has not been shown to affect the incidence of bleeding episodes, which are reported to be 35% and 33%, respectively (Galantowicz & Stolar, 1991).

Assessment for bleeding complications includes strict monitoring of chest tube output, hematocrit (Hct), and coagulation tests, as well as noting signs of excessive bleeding from line sites and incisions. Packed red cells and fresh frozen plasma are administered to maintain a desired Hct, PT, and PTT. If bleeding is excessive, platelets may be administered despite a relatively normal laboratory count to counteract platelet dysfunction. Cryoprecipitate and vitamin K are generally avoided because of the potential for catastrophic thrombotic occlusion of the device circuit (Reedy et al., 1990).

Thrombus formation within the extracorporeal circuit or native heart may be precipitated by blood contact with biomaterial surfaces and/or low flow states. The presence of artificial heart valves may be an additional risk factor for thrombosis. Karl and coworkers (1991) reported a 33% incidence of incomplete prosthetic valve thrombosis during VAD support, which was treated successfully with thrombolytic therapy in one patient. To prevent this potentially catastrophic event, anticoagulation is initiated once initial bleeding has been controlled. Heparin is administered as a continuous infusion to maintain the desired ACT and coagulation parameters. The low flow rates used in pediatric patients makes monitoring of anticoagulation an *extremely* important aspect of care, requiring frequent assessment and adjustment to prevent clot formation or excessive bleeding.

Hemolysis may also be a concern during prolonged support, especially at high flow rates (Quaal, 1991). Traumatic destruction of red cells may occur from turbulent flow related to the device. Daily monitoring of the plasma free hemoglobin level is indicated, with elevations greater than 40 mg/dL (normal 2–7 mg/dL) confirming red cell lysis (Reedy, 1990). Lowering VAD flow rate (if tolerated) may correct the hemolysis, and red cells are transfused as needed.

Infectious complications were reported in 13% to 22% of pediatric ECMO-VAD registry patients (Pennington & Swartz, 1993). Potential predisposing factors to infection include preoperative sources (i.e., endocarditis, sepsis), use of invasive monitoring lines and catheters, open sternotomy wounds, and prolonged ventilatory support. A decrease in circulating T-cell levels has been noted following CPB, leaving patients with VAD with impaired host defense mechanisms during the immediate postoperative period (McBride et al., 1987). Avoidance of infection is a primary goal for all patients but achieves special significance in bridge-to-transplant patients, because even a minor infection can delay or preclude lifesaving transplant procedures in this population.

Measures to decrease infection include frequent handwashing, strict aseptic technique during contact with invasive lines, prompt removal of nonessential lines and catheters, aggressive pulmonary hygiene measures, and use of sterile technique during VAD dressing changes. Protective isolation does not appear to be warranted, having been shown to have no impact on the incidence,morbidity, or mortality from infection in adult and pediatric heart transplant recipients (Gamberg et al., 1987). Broad-spectrum antibiotics are initiated intraoperatively for several days, followed by organism-specific antibiotics as needed, based on positive culture results. Surveillance for infection includes a daily leukocyte count and temperature assessment every 2 to 4 hours.

Profound shock before initiation of VAD support can lead to persistent renal insufficiency requiring peritoneal dialysis, which occurs in 30% to 100% of patients (Pennington & Swartz, 1993; Moat et al., 1990). Once device flows have restored tissue perfusion, improvements in renal function may be seen if irreversible organ damage has not yet occurred. Unfortunately, current methods for evaluating renal function are not sensitive enough to identify when this line has been crossed. Complete renal recovery in dialysis-dependent patients has been reported to be 50% to 66% (Karl et al, 1991; Moat et al., 1990). Despite these encouraging findings, measures to optimize renal perfusion both before and after device support are warranted to avoid this potential complication. Strategies to maintain CO, limit the duration of low flow states, and use of dopamine to augment renal perfusion have been advocated (Pierce et al., 1993).

Results and Future Directions

Although the application of IABP technology in the pediatric population has been limited, several centers are reporting excellent results with this therapy. The Toronto Hospital for Sick Children reported a 37% survival rate for 38 patients over a 10-year experience with their IABP program (Del Nido et al., 1988). In a more recent report, Christensen and coworkers (1991) reported a 41% survival rate in 29 children at Primary Children's Hospital of Salt Lake City. Survival rates were highest in children over the age of 5 years (88%), compared with younger patients (11%–33%). The inability to achieve near-systolic diastolic augmentation in more than 50% of their smallest patients indicates inadequate cardiac assistance and a need for greater circulatory support.

The use of ECMO for *cardiac support* in a collective series of 453 patients reported to the pediatric ECMO registry resulted in a cumulative survival rate of 43%. Some centers report improved survival rates recently, exceeding 50% in the last 3 years (Pennington & Swartz, 1993).

Reported results following VAD support include some encouraging survival rates, ranging from 50% at Royal Children's Hospital in Melbourne, Australia (Karl et al., 1991) to 55% at Children's Hospital in Boston. A combined registry experience of 32 postcardiotomy pediatric patients with VAD reports a 28% survival, with the most frequently cited complications in nonsurvivors being biventricular failure (43%) and bleeding (39%) (Pennington & Swartz, 1993). Severe RV failure following univentricular left heart support is a common problem in adults as well, occurring in 36% of patients (Pierce et al., 1989). The use of minimal LVAD flow rates to avoid RV overload may decrease this complication in some patients.

Despite the invasiveness and potential complications related to IABP and VAD, their use is on the rise with broader applications anticipated in the future (Pennington & Swartz, 1993). The reality is that few other options currently exist for infants and children with severe cardiac failure. The adult VAD experience has revealed that optimal benefits can be gained with devices designed for longer use, allowing time to reverse organ dysfunction, improve nutritional status, and strengthen muscles prior to device weaning or transplantation. Preliminary work with a pediatric total artificial heart capable of longer support is ongoing, although it is not yet available for clinical use, and may show promise for these children in the future (Pennington & Swartz, 1993).

In the meantime, optimal patient selection criteria are still evolving, creating a compelling argument to offer these therapies to desperately ill children with no other options for survival. Nurses caring for these patients will be challenged to provide state-of-the-art technical care, while maintaining the human touch that only they can provide. Few publications exist to guide nursing care delivery for this relatively new and complex patient population. As our experience continues, nursing must continually refine and document proven strategies for providing safe, effective, and holistic care to these critically ill children.

SUMMARY

This chapter has provided a review of fetal development of the heart and fetal circulation and the circulatory changes that occur at birth. Normal fetal cardiovascular development provided a mechanism to introduce congenital heart disease. The physical properties of the cardiovascular system were reviewed next; including an overview of essential anatomy, the function of the heart's electrical system, the cardiac cycle, and regulation of cardiac output. Attention was directed at the effects of maturation on cardiovascular function.

The second major focus of the chapter was assessment of the cardiovascular system. Both physical assessment and noninvasive evaluation were reviewed. Discussion of intensive care unit monitoring of cardiovascular function and cardiac catheterization followed.

The chapter was concluded by sections that detailed cardiovascular support to maintain adequate tissue perfusion. Pharmacologic support, pacemaker therapy, and mechanical support were discussed. Because cardiovascular failure and inadequate tissue perfusion are the final common pathophysiologic pathways in a variety of critical illnesses and injuries in infants and children, critical care nurses are motivated to master complex therapies and technologies aimed at restoring health to these youngsters.

References

Abram, S.H., Kinsella, J.P., Schaffer, M.S., et al. (1993). Inhaled nitric oxide in the management of a premature newborn with severe respiratory distress and pulmonary hypertension. *Pediatrics,* 76:606–609.

Abramowicz, M. (1993). Drugs for chronic heart failure. Medical Letter, 8:40–42.

Alverson, D.C., Eldridge, M., Dillon T., et al. (1982). Noninvasive pulsed doppler determination of cardiac output in neonates and children. *Journal of Pediatrics* 101:46–51.

Anella, J., McCloskey, A., & Vieweg C. (1990). Nursing dynamics of pediatric intraaortic balloon pumping. *Critical Care Nurse* 10(4):24–36.

Appel-Hardin, S. (1992). The role of the critical care nurse in noninvasive temporary pacing. *Critical Care Nurse,* 12:10–19.

Artman, M., & Graham, T.P. (1987). Guidelines for vasodilator therapy of congestive heart failure in infants and children. *American Heart Journal,* 113:994–1005.

Barranco, F., Lesmes, A., Irles, J.A., et al. (1990). Cardiopulmonary resuscitation with simultaneous chest and abdominal compression: Comparative study in humans. *Resuscitation,* 20:67–76.

Beland, M., Hesslein, P., Finlay, C., et al. (1987). Noninvasive transcutaneous cardiac pacing in children. *PACE,* 10:1262–1270.

Berman, W., Yabek, S.M., Dillon, T., et al. (1983). Effects of digoxin in infants with a congested circulatory state due to a ventricular septal defect. *New England Journal of Medicine,* 308:363–366.

Berner, M., Rouge, J.C., & Friedli, B. (1983). The hemodynamic effect of phentolamine and dobutamine after open heart operations in children: Influence of the underlying heart defect. *Annals of Thoracic Surgery,* 35:643–646.

Bernstein, A.D., Camm, A.J., Fletcher, R.D., et al. (1987). The generic code for antibradyarrhythmia and adaptive rate pacing and antitachy-arrhythmia devices. *PACE,* 10:794–799.

Bohn, D.J., Poirier, C.S., & Edmunds, J.F. (1980). Hemodynamic effects of dobutamine after cardiopulmonary bypass in children. *Critical Care Medicine,* 8:367–371.

Boreus, L.O., Hjemdahl, P., & Lagercrantz, H. (1986). B-adrenoceptor function in white blood cells from human infants: No relation to plasma catecholamine levels. *Pediatric Research,* 20:1152–1158.

Bumgarner, L.I. (1992). Diagnostic uses of epicardial electrodes after cardiac surgery. *Progress in Cardiovascular Nursing,* 7:21–24.

Chang, A.C., Zappalla, F.R., Kurer, C.C., et al. (1990). Clinical outcome in children with the permanent form of junctional reciprocating tachycardia. *Journal of the American College of Cardiology* 15:176a.

Christensen, D.W., Veasy, L.G., McGough, E.C., et al. (1991). Intraaortic balloon counterpulsation in children: A review of 29 patients. *Critical Care Medicine,* 19(4):S75.

Cohn, H.E., Freed, M.D., Hellenbrand, W.F., et al. (1985). Complications and mortality associated with cardiac catheterization in infants under one year: A prospective study. *Pediatric Cardiology,* 6:123–128.

Colucci, W.S., Wright, R.F., & Braunwald, E. (1986a). New inotropic agents in the treatment of congestive heart failure. *New England Journal of Medicine,* 314:290–299.

Colucci, W.S., Wright, R.F., Jaski, B.E., et al. (1986b). Milrinone and dobutamine in severe heart failure: Differing hemodynamic effects and individual patient responsiveness. *Circulation,* [Suppl III]: 175–183.

Copeland, J.G., Harker, L.A., Joist, J.H., et al. (1989). Panel 3: Bleeding and anticoagulation, Circulatory Support Symposium: Society of Thoracic Surgeons. *Annals of Thoracic Surgery,* 47:88–82.

Dach, J.L., Galbut, D.L., & Lepage, J.R. (1981). The knotted Swan-Ganz catheter: New solution to a vexing problem. *American Journal of Roentgenology,* 137:1274–1275.

Daily, E.K., & Schroeder, J.S. (1989). Techniques in bedside hemodynamic monitoring. St. Louis: C.V. Mosby.

Del Nido, P.J., Swan, P.R., Benson, L.N., et al. (1988). Successful use of intra-aortic balloon pumping in a 2-kilogram infant. *Annals of Thoracic Surgery,* 46:574–576.

Driscoll, D.J., Gillette, P.C., Ezrailson, E.G., et al. (1978). Inotropic response of the neonatal canine myocardium to dopamine. *Pediatric Research,* 12:42–47.

Dunn, J.M. (1989). The use of intra-aortic balloon pumping in pediatric patients. *Cardiac Assists,* 5(1):2–4.

Elliot, C.G., Zimmerman, G.A., Clemmer, T.P. (1979). Complications of pulmonary artery catheterization in the care of critically ill patients. Chest, 76:647–652.

Enghoff, E., & Sjogren, J. (1973). Thermal dilution for measurement of cardiac output in the pulmonary artery in man in relation to choice of indicator volume and injectate time. *Upstate Journal of Medical Science* 78:33–37.

Epstein, M.C., Kiel, E.A., & Victoria, B.E. (1985). Cardiac decompensation following verapamil therapy in infants with supraventricular tachycardia. *Pediatrics,* 75:737–742.

Fegler, G. (1954). Measurement of cardiac output in anesthetized animals by thermodilution method. *Quarterly Journal of Experimental Physiology,* 39:153–164.

Freed, M.D., Heymann, M.A., Lewis, A.B. et al. (1981). Prostaglandin E-1 in infants with ductus arteriosus-dependent congenital heart disease. *Circulation,* 64:899–905.

Friedman, W.F., & George, B.L. (1985). Treatment of congestive heart failure by altering loading conditions of the heart. *Journal of Pediatrics,* 106:697–706.

Frostell, C., Blomquist, H., Hedenstierna, H., et al. (1993). Inhaled nitric oxide selectively reverses human hypoxic pulmonary vasoconstriction without causing systemic vasodilation. *Anesthesiology.*

Frostell, C., Fratacci, M.D., Wain, J.C., et al. (1991). Inhaled nitric oxide: A selective pulmonary vasodilator reversing hypoxic pulmonary vasoconstriction. *Circulation,* 83:2038–2047.

Frye, R.L.,Collins, J.J., DeSanctis, R.W., et al. (1984). Guidelines for permanent cardiac pacemaker implantation. *Circulation*, 70:331–339a.

Fuhrman, T.M., Pippin, W.D., Talmage, L.A., & Reilly, D.O. (1992). Evaluation of collateral circulation of the hand. *Journal of Clinical Monitoring*, 8:28–32.

Galantowicz, M.E., & Stolar, C.J.H. (1991). Extracorporeal membrane oxygenation for perioperative support in pediatric heart transplantation. *Journal of Thoracic and Cardiovascular Surgery*, 102(1):148–152.

Gamberg, P., Miller, J.L., & Lough, M.E. (1987). Impact of protection isolation on the incidence of infection after heart transplantation. *Journal of Heart Transplantation*, 6(1):147–149.

Ganz, W., Donoso, R., Marcus, H.S., et al. (1971). A new technique for measurement of cardiac output by thermodilution in man. *American Journal of Cardiology*, 27:392–396.

Gardner, P.E. (1993). Pulmonary artery pressure monitoring. *AACN Clinical Issues in Critical Care Nursing*, 4, 98–119.

Gardner, R.M., & Hollingsworth, K.W. (1986). Optimizing the electrocardiogram and pressure monitoring. *Critical Care Medicine*, 14:651–658.

Gardner, R.M., & Hujcs, M. (1993). Fundamentals of physiologic monitoring. *AACN Clinical Issues in Critical Care Nursing*, 4:11–24.

Gardner, P.E., & Woods, S.L. (1989). Hemodynamic monitoring. In S.L. Underhill, S.L. Woods, E.S. Froehlicher, et al. (Eds.). *Cardiac nursing* 2nd ed., pp 451–481. Philadelphia: J.B. Lippincott.

Garson, A., Jr. (1987). Medicolegal problems in the management of cardiac arrhythmias in children. *Pediatrics*, 79:84–88.

Garson, A., Jr, Gillette, P.C., McVoy, P. et al. (1984). Amiodarone treatment of critical arrhythmias in children and young adults. *Journal of the American College of Cardiology*, 4:479–485.

Gold, J.P., Jonas, R.A., Lang, P., et al. (1986). Transthoracic intracardiac monitoring lines in pediatric cardiac surgical patients: A ten year experience. *Annals of Thoracic Surgery*, 42:185–191.

Goran, S.F. (1989). Family perceptions of the intra-aortic balloon pumping experience. *Critical Care Nursing Clinics of North America* 1:475–477.

Gorny, D.A. (1993). Arterial blood pressure measurement technique. *AACN Clinical Issues in Critical Care Nursing*, 4:66–80.

Grose, B.L., Woods, S.L., & Laurent, D.J. (1981). Effect of backrest position on cardiac output measurement by the thermodilution method in acutely ill patients. *Heart & Lung*, 10:661–665.

Guyton, AC. (1991). *Textbook of medical physiology* (8th ed). Philadelphia: W.B. Saunders.

Heck, H.A. Jr, & Doty, D.B. (1981). Assisted circulation by phasic external lower body compression. *Circulation*, 64 [Suppl II]: 118.

Heller, M., Peterson, J., Ikanpamipour, K. et al. (1989). A comparison of five transcutaneous pacing devices in unanesthetized human volunteers. *Prehospital Disaster Medicine*, 4(1):15–18.

Hess, W. (1989). The effects of amrinone on the right side of the heart. *Journal of Cardiothoracic Anaesthesia*, 3[Suppl 2]:38–44.

Ilbawi, M.N., Idriss, F.S., DeLeon, S.Y., et al. (1985). Hemodynamic effects of intravenous nitroglycerin in pediatric patients after heart surgery. *Circulation* 72[Suppl II]:101.

Jacobs, M.L., & Vlahakes, G.J. (1987). Augmentation of pulmonary blood flow by a right atrial balloon pump after the Fontan operation. *Circulation*, 76[Suppl III]:72.

Jobes, D.R., Nicholson, S.C., Steven, J.M., et al. (1992). Carbon dioxide prevents pulmonary overcirculation in hypoplastic left heart syndrome. *Annals of Thoracic Surgery*, 54:150–151.

Karl, T.R., Sano, S., Horton, S., et al. (1991). Centrifugal pump left heart assist in pediatric cardiac operations. *Journal of Thoracic and Cardiovascular Surgery*. 102, 624–630.

Kinsella, J.P., Neish, S.R., Shaffer, E. et al. (1992). Low-dose inhalational nitric oxide in persistent pulmonary hypertension of the newborn. *Lancet*, 340:819–820.

Klem, S.A. (1993). Cardiovascular support—mechanical. In P.R. Holbrook (Ed.). *Textbook of pediatric critical care*. Philadelphia: W.B. Saunders.

Kleven, M. Effects of backrest position on thermodilution cardiac output in critically ill patients receiving mechanical ventilation with PEEP. *Heart & Lung*, 13:303–304.

Kugler, J.D., & Danford, D.A. (1989). Pacemakers in children: An update. *American Heart Journal*, 117:665–678.

Kulik, T.J., & Lock, J.E. (1984). Pulmonary vasodilator therapy in persistent pulmonary hypertension of the newborn. *Clinical Perinatology*, 11:693–701.

Lake, C.L. (1990). Monitoring ventricular function. In C.L. Lake (Ed.) (pp. 237–279). *Clinical monitoring*. Philadelphia: W.B. Saunders.

Lange, H.W., Galliani, C.A., & Edwards, J.E. (1983). Local complications associated with indwelling Swan-Ganz catheters. *American Journal of Cardiology*, 52:1108–1111.

Lawless, S.T., Burckart, G., Diven, W., et al. (1988). Pharmacokinetics of amrinone in neonates and infants. *Journal of Clinical Pharmacology*, 28:283–284.

Lawless, S.T., Orr R. (1989). Axillary arterial pressure monitoring in pediatric patients. *Pediatrics*, 84, 273–275.

Lawless, S.T., Zaritsky, A., & Miles, M. (1991). The acute pharmacokinetics and pharmacodynamics of amrinone in pediatric patients. *Journal of Clinical Pharmacology*, 31:800–803.

Lawrence, P.A. (1991). Cardiac pacing in children. *AACN Clinical Issues in Critical Care Nursing*, 2:150–155.

Leier, C.V., & Unverferth, D.V. (1983). Dobutamine. *Annals of Internal Medicine*, 99: 4–12.

Lewis, R.P. (1990). Digitalis: A drug that refuses to die. *Critical Care Medicine*, 18:85–89.

Lewis, A.B., Freed, M.D., Heymann, M.A., et al. (1981). Side effects of therapy with prostaglandin E-1 in infants with critical congenital heart disease. *Circulation*, 64:893–897.

Ley, S.J., & Hill, J.D. (1993). The Thoratec VAD. In S.J. Quaal (Ed.). *Cardiac mechanical assistance beyond balloon pumping*. St Louis: C.V. Mosby.

Lock, J.E., Keane, J.F., & Fellows, K.E. (1987). *Diagnostic and interventional catheterization in Congenital Heart Disease*. Boston: Martinus Nijhoff.

Lookinland, S. (1989). Comparison of pulmonary vascular pressures based on blood volume and ventilator status. *Nursing Research*, 38:68–72.

Loveys, B.J., & Woods, S.L. (1986). Current recommendations for thermodilution cardiac output measurement. *Progress in Cardiovascular Nursing*, 1:24–32.

Luck, J., & Davis, D. (1987). Termination of sustained tachycardia by external pacing. *PACE*, 10:1125–1129.

McCrory, J.H., & Downs, C.E. (1993). Resuscitation of the child. In P.R. Holbrook, (Ed.). *Textbook of pediatric critical care*. Philadelphia: W.B. Saunders.

Machado, M.V., Tynan, M.J., Curry, P.L., et al. (1988). Fetal complete heart block. *British Heart Journal*, 60:512–515.

Maki, D.G. (1982). Infections associated with intravascular lines. In M. Schwatrz, & J. Remintion (Eds.). *Current topics in clinical infectious disease*. New York: McGraw-Hill.

Marjerus, T.C., Dasta, J.F., Bauman, J.L., et al. (1989). Dobutamine: Ten years later. *Pharmacotherapy*, 9:245–250.

Martin, G.R., & Holley, D.G. (1993). Cardiovascular monitoring and evaluation. In P.R. Holbrook (Ed.). *Textbook of pediatric critical care*. Philadelphia: W.B. Saunders.

Miller, O.I., James, J., Elliot, M.J. (1993). Intraoperative use of inhaled low-dose nitric oxide. *Journal of Thoracic and Cardiovascular Surgery*, 105:550–551.

Milliken, J.C., and Laks, H., & George, B. (1986). Use of a venous assist device after repair of complex lesions of the right heart. *Journal of the American College of Cardiology*, 8:922–929.

Moat, N.E., Pawade, A., Lewis, B.C., et al. (1990). Circulatory support in infants with post-cardiopulmonary bypass left ventricular dysfunction using a left ventricular assist device. *European Journal of Cardio-thoracic Surgery*, 4(12):649–652.

Naccarelli, G.V., Gray, E.L., & Dougherty, A.H. (1984). Amrinone: Acute electrophysiologic and hemodynamic effects in patients with congestive heart failure. *American Heart Journal*, 54:600–604.

Neill, C.A. (1972). Etiology of congenital heart disease. *Cardiovascular Clinics*, 4(3):137–148.

Nelson, L.D., Houtchens, B.A. (1982). Automatic versus manual injections for thermodilution cardiac output determination. *Critical Care Medicine*, 10:190–192.

Noerr, B. (1991). Prostaglandin E-1. *Neonatal Network*, 9:66–67.

Notterman, D.A. (1989). Pharmacologic support of the failing circulation: An approach for infants and children. *Problems in Anesthesia*, 3:288–294.

Notterman, D.A. (1993). Cardiovascular support—pharmacologic.

In P.R. Holbrook (Ed.). *Textbook of pediatric critical care.* Philadelphia: W.B. Saunders.

Notterman, D.A., DeBruin, W., & Metakis, L. (1989). Plasma catecholamine levels in critically ill children—evidence of early B-adrenergic receptor desensitization. *Pediatric Research,* 25:42–44A.

O'Brien, P., & Elixson, E.M. (1990). The child following the Fontan procedure: Nursing Strategies. *AACN Clinical Issues in Critical Care Nursing,* 1:46–58.

Ordog, G.I., & Beneron, S. (1987). Serum digoxin levels and mortality in 5,100 patients. *Annals of Emergency Medicine,* 16:32–36.

Overholt, E.D., Rheuban, K.S., Gutgesell H.P., et al. (1988). Usefulness of adenosine for arrhythmias in infants and children. *American Journal of Cardiology,* 6:336–340.

Pae, W.E. (1993). Ventricular assist devices and total artificial hearts: A combined registry experience. *Annals of Thoracic Surgery,* 55(1):295–298.

Page, R., Gay, W., & Friday, G. 1986. Isoproterenol associated myocardial dysfunction during status asthmaticus. *Annals of Allergy,* 57:402,429.

Park, M.K. (1986). Use of digoxin in infants and children. *Journal of Pediatrics,* 108:871–876.

Pearl, R.G., Rosenthal, M.H., Nielson, L., et al. (1986). Effect of injectate volume and temperature on thermodilution cardiac output determination. *Anesthesiology,* 64:798–801.

Peckham, G.J., & Fow, W.W. (1978). Physiologic factors affecting pulmonary artery pressure in infants with persistent pulmonary hypertension. *Journal of Pediatrics* 93:1005–1010.

Pennington, D.G., Kanter, K.R., McBride, L.R., et al. (1988). Seven years' experience with the Pierce-Donachy ventricular assist device. *Journal of Thoracic and Cardiovascular Surgery,* 96(6):901–911.

Pennington, D.G., & Swartz, M.T. (1993). Circulatory support in infants and children. *Annals of Thoracic Surgery,* 55(1):233–237.

Pepe-Zaba, J., Higenbottam, T.W., Dinh-Xuan, A., et al. (1991). Inhaled nitric oxide as a cause of selective pulmonary vasodilation in pulmonary hypertension. *Lancet,* 338:1173–1174.

Perry, J.C., McQuinn, R., Smith, R.T., et al. (1989). Flecainide acetate for resistant arrhythmias in the young: Efficacy and pharmacokinetics. *Journal of the American College of Cardiology,* 14:185–191.

Pfeffer, M.A., Braunwald, E., Moye, L.A., et al. (1992). Effect of captopril on mortality and morbidity in patients with left ventricular dysfunction after myocardial infarction. *New England Journal of Medicine,* 327:669–677.

Pierce, W.S., Gray, L.A., McBride, L.R., et al. (1989). Panel 4: Other postoperative complications; Circulatory support symposium, Society of Thoracic Surgeons. *Annals of Thoracic Surgery,* 47:96–101.

Pierce, W.S., Hershon, J.J., Kormos, R.L., et al. (1993). Management of secondary organ dysfunction. *Annals of Thoracic Surgery,* 55(1):222–226.

Podrid, P.J., & Morganroth, J. (1985). Aggravation of arrhythmia during drug therapy: Experience with flecainide acetate. *Practical Cardiology,* 11:55–70.

Pollack, M.M., Getson, P.R., Ruttiman, U.E., et al. (1987). Efficiency of intensive care a comparative analysis of eight pediatric intensive care units. *Journal of the American Medical Association,* 258:1481–1486.

Quaal, S.J. (1991). Centrifugal ventricular assist devices. *AACN Clinical Issues in Critical Care Nursing,* 2(3):515–526.

Quaal, S.J. (1993a). Basic principles of IABC. In S.J. Quaal (Ed.). *Cardiac mechanical assistance beyond balloon pumping.* St Louis: C.V. Mosby.

Quaal, S.J. (1993b). Quality assurance in hemodynamic monitoring. *AACN Clinical Issues in Critical Care Nursing,* 4:197–206.

Rabinovitch, M. (1989). Structure and function of the pulmonary vascular bed: An update. *Cardiology Clinics,* 7:227–238.

Rabinovitch, M. (1992). Developmental biology of the pulmonary vascular bed. In R. Freddom, L. Benson, J. Smallhorn J (Eds.). *Neonatal heart disease.* London: Springer-Verlag.

Rackow, E.C., Packman, M.I., & Weil, M.H. (1987). Hemodynamic effects of digoxin during acute cardiac failure. *Critical Care Medicine,* 12:1001–1007.

Reed LJ, Keegan MJ. (1993). Fat embolism syndrome: A complication of trauma. Critical Care Nurse, 13:33–38.

Reedy, J.E., Ruzevich, S.A., Noedel, N.R., et al. (1990). Nursing care of the ambulatory patient with a mechanical assist device. *Journal of Heart Transplantation* 9(2):97–105.

Rich, S., & Brundage, B.H. (1987). High dose calcium channel blocking therapy for primary pulmonary hypertension: Evidence for long term reduction in pulmonary arterial pressure and regression of right ventricular hypertrophy. *Circulation,* 76:135–143.

Rikard, D.H. (1993). Nursing care of the neonate receiving prostaglandin E-1 therapy. *Neonatal Network,* 12:17–22.

Roberts, J.P., & Shaul, P.W. (1993a). Advances in the treatment of persistent pulmonary hypertension of the newborn. *Pediatric Clinics of North America,* 40:983–1004.

Roberts, J.P., Lang, P., Bigatello, L., et al. (1993b). Inhaled nitric oxide in congenital heart disease. *Circulation,* 87:447–453.

Rossaint, F., Falke, K.J., Lopez, F., et al. (1993). Inhaled nitric oxide in adult respiratory distress syndrome. *New England Journal of Medicine,* 328:399–405.

Ruckman, R.N. (1993). Development and maturation of the cardiovascular system. In P.R. Holbrook (Ed.). *Textbook of pediatric critical care.* Philadelphia: W.B. Saunders.

Ruley, E.J. (1993). Hypertension. In P.J. Holbrook (Ed.). *Textbook of pediatric critical care.* Philadelphia: W.B. Saunders.

Schneeweiss, A. (1986). Prostaglandin E. In *Drug therapy in infants and children with cardiovascular diseases.* Philadelphia: Lea & Febiger.

Schneeweiss, A. (1990). Cardiovascular drugs in children II: ACE inhibitors in children. *Pediatric Cardiology,* 11:199–207.

Schultz, C.K., & Woodall C.E. (1989). Using epicardial pacing electrodes. *Journal of Cardiovascular Nursing,* 3:25–33.

Schwenzer, K.J. (1990). Venous and pulmonary pressures. In C.L. Lake (Ed.). (pp. 147–196). *Clinical monitoring.* Philadelphia: W.B. Saunders Co.

Shellock, F.G., Riedinger, M.S., Bateman, T.M., & Gray, R.J. (1983). Thermodilution cardiac output determination in hypothermic postcardiac surgery patients. *Critical Care Medicine,* 11:668–670.

Shiono, M., Noon, G.P., Coleman, C.L., & Nose, Y. (1993). Overview of ventricular assist devices. In S.J. Quaal (Ed.). *Cardiac mechanical assistance beyond balloon pumping.* St Louis: C.V. Mosby.

Simmons, B.P. (1983). CDC guidelines for the prevention of nosocomial infections. Guidelines for prevention of intravascular infections. *American Journal of Infection Control,* 11:183–193.

Skoyles, J.R., & Sherry, K.M. (1992). Pharmacology, mechanisms of action and uses of selective phosphodiesterase inhibitors. *British Journal of Anaesthiology,* 68:293–302.

Smith, J.B., & Vernon-Levett, P. (1993). Care of infants with hypoplastic left heart syndrome. *AACN Clinical Issues in Critical Care Nursing,* 4:329–339.

Smith, R.G., & Cleavinger, M. (1991). Current perspectives on the use of circulatory assist devices. *AACN Clinical Issues in Critical Care Nursing,* 2(3):488–499.

Smith, R.T. (1990). Pacemakers for bradycardia. In A. Garson, Jr, & J.T. Bricker (Eds.) (pp. 2135–2155). *The science and practice of pediatric cardiology.* Philadelphia: Lea & Febiger.

Stork, E. (1989). Extracorporeal membrane oxygenation in the newborn and beyond. *Clinical Perinatology,* 15:815–829.

Sulzbach, L.M., & Lansdowne, L.M. (1991). Temporary atrial pacing after cardiac surgery. *Focus on Critical Care,* 18:65–74.

Thomas, H.A. (1982). The knotted Swan-Ganz catheter: A safer solution. (Letter). *American Journal of Roetgenology,* 183:986–987.

Tobias, J.D., Schleien, C.L., & Reitz, B.A. (1990). Use of the MAST suit in the postoperative care of patients after the Fontan procedure. *Critical Care Medicine,* 18:781–785.

Van Praagh, R. & Pvlad. (1967). Dextrocardia, mesocardia and levocardia. In J.D. Keith, R.D. Rowe, & P. Vlad (Eds.). *Heart disease in infancy and childhood.* New York: Macmillan.

VanRiper, S., VanRiper, J. (1987). Arterial pressure monitoring. In G.O. Darovic (Ed.). *Hemodynamic monitoring: Invasive and noninvasive clinical methods.* Philadelphia: W.B. Saunders.

Vaughn-Williams, E.M. (1984). A classification of antiarryhthmic actions reassessed after a decade of new drugs. *Journal of Clinical Pharmacology,* 24:129–147.

Veasy, L.G. (1993). Pediatric adaptation in balloon pumping. In S.J. Quaal (Ed.). Comprehensive intraaortic balloon counterpulsation (2nd ed.). St Louis: C.V. Mosby.

Vennix, C.V., Nelson, D.H., & Pierpoint, G.L. (1984). Thermodilution cardiac output in critically ill patients: Comparison of room-temperature and iced injectate. *Heart & Lung,* 13:574–578.

Vetter, V.L. (1993). Arrhythmias. In P.R. Holbrook (Ed.). *Textbook of Pediatric critical care.* Philadelphia: W.B. Saunders.

Visscher, M.D., & Johnson, J.A. (1953). The Fick principle: Analysis of potential errors in its conventional application. *Journal of Applied Physiology,* 5:635–638.

Wangensteen, S.L., Ludewig, R.M., & Eddy, D.M. (1968). The effect of external counterpressure on the intact circulation. *Surgery, Gynecology and Obstetrics,* 125:253–258.

Watson, D.M., Sherry, K.M., & Weston, G.A. (1990). Milrinone: a bridge to heart transplantation. *Anaesthesia,* 46:285–288.

Weiner, N. (1985). Norepinephrine, epinephrine and the sympathetic amines. In A.C. Gilman, L.S. Goodman, T.W. Rall, F. Murad (Eds.). The pharmacologic basis of therapeutics. New York: Macmillan.

West, J.B., Dollery, C.T., & Naimark, A. (1964). Distribution of blood flow in isolated lung; Relation to vascular and alveolar pressures. *Journal of Applied Physiology,* 19:713–724.

Whitsett, J.A., Noguchi, A., & Moore, J.J. (1982). Developmental aspects of alpha and beta-adrenergic receptors. *Seminars in Perinatology,* 6:125–131.

Zaritsky, A., & Chernow, B. (1984). Use of catecholamines in pediatrics. *Journal of Pediatrics,* 105:341–350.

CHAPTER *10*

Oxygenation/ Ventilation

MARTHA A.Q. CURLEY
JOHN E. THOMPSON
JOYCE MOLENGRAFT
ELAINE CARON
M. CLAIRE BEERS

Support of oxygenation and/or ventilation is integral to the practice of pediatric critical care nursing because the majority of critically ill infants and children require interventions to stabilize the pulmonary system (AACN, 1991). Although general principles of care are similar within all age groups, striking differences do exist among them.

Pulmonary system functioning continues to mature throughout childhood. Developmental immaturity of the pulmonary system places the infant and young child at risk for organ system dysfunction. Respiratory failure is the number one factor contributing to cardiopulmonary arrest in the pediatric population (Chameides, 1990).

This chapter discusses principles of oxygenation and ventilation as they pertain to critically ill or injured children. Essential embryology, anatomy, and physiology are reviewed. Pulmonary assessment is presented, followed by a discussion of pulmonary intensive care monitoring, diagnostic testing, and mechanical support of ventilation. The chapter concludes with a discussion of nursing care issues related to infants and children who require alternative modes of pulmonary support.

ESSENTIAL EMBRYOLOGY

The human lung is designed for the single purpose of gas exchange across an intact alveolar-pulmonary capillary membrane. The lungs enrich blood with oxygen and eliminate carbon dioxide. Pulmonary function is immediately essential to extrauterine life. Embryonic development is detailed below (Fig. 10–1).

Pulmonary development is divided into five stages, named to reflect histologic maturation of the lung (O'Brodovich & Haddad, 1990). The duration of each stage can only be approximated, as fetal growth is somewhat individualized. The lung first appears as a ventral outpouching of the primitive foregut in the *embryonic period,* day 26 to 52 of gestation. The foregut is eventually divided into a dorsal portion, the esophagus, and a ventral portion, the trachea and the lung buds. The primary bronchial buds split into two buds on the left and three buds on the right, thus giving shape to the developing bronchial tree (Charnock & Doershuck, 1973). The left lung bud develops into two main bronchi and two lobes. The right bud forms three main bronchi and three lobes.

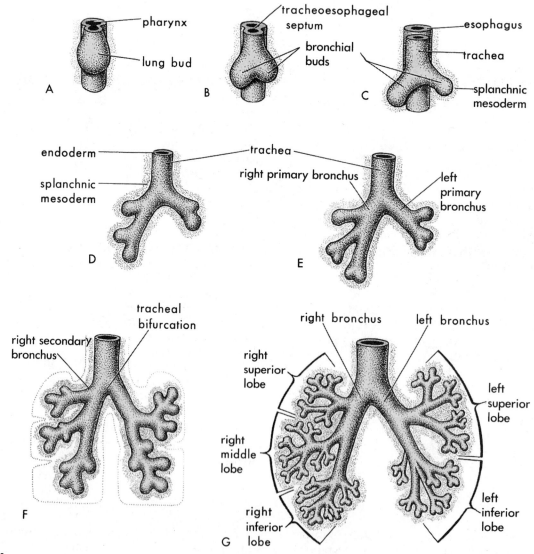

Figure 10–1 ● ● ● ● ●

Successive stages in the development of the bronchi and lungs. *A to C,* Four weeks. *D and E,* Five weeks. *F,* Six weeks. *G,* Eight weeks. (From Moore, K.L., & Persaud, T.V.N. (1993). *The developing human* (5th ed., p. 230). Philadelphia: W.B. Saunders.)

Table 10–1. CHANGES IN RESPIRATORY SYSTEM DIMENSIONS WITH GROWTH

	Newborn to 1 Month	Infant	1–5 Yr	6–8 Yr	12–14 Yr	Adult
Chest, diameter, cm						
Transverse	10	14	15.5	19	25	28
Anteroposterior	7.5	9	10	11.5	14.5	16.5–18
Trachea, length, mm	40/57	42/67	45/81	57	64	90–150
Diameter, mm	4	5	8	10	11	15–16
CSA, mm²	26	34	50	79	112	200–250
Mainstem bronchi diameter, mm	4	4	6	8	—	12
CSA, right/left	—	20/13	38/20	65/44	81/56	138/116
Bronchioles, diameter, mm	0.3	0.4	0.5	—	—	0.7
CSA	0.07	0.12	0.2	—	—	0.4
Terminal bronchioles, diameter, mm	0.2	0.3	0.3	—	—	0.5–0.6
Internal diameter, mm	0.1	0.12	0.14	0.15	0.17	0.2
CSA	0.03	0.07	0.07	—	—	0.2
Alveoli, diameter, mm	0.05	0.06–0.07	0.08–0.10	0.10–0.20	0.15–0.25	0.3
Surface area, M²	2.8	6.5	12	32	—	64–75
Body length, cm	50	—	—	123	—	175
Weight, kg	3.4	—	—	24	—	70
Surface area, M²	0.21	0.3	0.46	0.56	—	1.8

CSA, cross-sectional area.
From Polgar, G., & Weng, T. R. (1979). The functional development of the respiratory system. *American Review of Respiratory Disease,* 120, 677.

This early developing bronchial tree is nourished by the main pulmonary artery.

The *pseudoglandular period* follows the embryonic period from day 52 to week 16 of gestation. During this period, all major conducting airways including terminal bronchioles are formed. Arterial supply throughout the bronchial tree becomes more evident. The diaphragm, derived from the fusion of the pleuroperitoneal folds, is formed during the eighth to tenth week of gestation (Sadler, 1990).

Development of respiratory bronchioles characterizes the *canalicular period,* week 17 to 24 of gestation. Each bronchiole ends in two or three thin-walled dilations referred to as terminal sacs or primitive alveoli (Moore and Persaud, 1993). The rich pulmonary vascular bed continues to develop as capillaries proliferate around the terminal bronchioles.

The *saccular period,* characterized by intense vascularization of the lung and loss of its glandular appearance, occurs during the 28th to 36th week of gestation. Elastic fibers, important in true alveolar development, begin to develop. For the first time, close contact between the air spaces and the pulmonary capillaries is established. There is concurrent active development of the lymphatic capillaries. The first true alveoli are present at 34 weeks; gas exchange is possible but not optimal.

The final period of development is the *alveolar period,* week 36 to term. Here, further refinement of the terminal sacs and formation of the walls of the true alveoli occur (Fig. 10–2). Columnar cells within the alveolar wall differentiate into type I and type II cells. Type I cells provide the alveolar surface area necessary for gas exchange. Type II cells secrete surfactant, a complex lipid substance that forms a monomolecular film over the walls of alveoli and is responsible for lowering alveolar surface tension. Surfactant is necessary for sustained inflation of the lung. Surfactant production increases during the later stages of pregnancy, especially during the last 2 weeks of gestation. Infants born prematurely are at risk for surfactant deficiency, which results in respiratory distress syndrome (RDS).

It is important to note that the pulmonary system continues to mature after birth. Postnatal maturation continues until at least the eighth year of life and perhaps into early adolescence. Although alveoli increase in size after birth, pulmonary maturation is primarily due to an increase in the number of respiratory bronchioles and primitive alveoli—alveoli that have the potential for forming additional alveoli (Table 10–1). During the postnatal period, tracheal diameter triples, alveolar dimensions increase fourfold, and alveoli numbers increase 10-fold, resulting in 24 million alveoli present at birth and 200 to 600×10^6 alveoli present in the adult (Polgar & Weng, 1979).

Congenital anomalies or malformations of the lower respiratory tract are relatively rare. Congenital diaphragmatic hernia occurs in approximately 1:2000 births, whereas tracheoesophageal fistula occurs in 1:2500 births (Moore & Persaud, 1993). A congenital diaphragmatic hernia occurs when the diaphragm fails to completely separate the pleuroperitoneal cavity into the abdominal and thoracic cavities. As the herniated abdominal viscera continue to grow and develop within the chest throughout gestation, pulmonary development is compromised. A tracheoesophageal fistula or communication between the trachea and esophagus results from incomplete division of the foregut into the respiratory and digestive systems. Pulmonary agenesis or absence of one lung results from the failure of a lung bud to develop. Congenital cysts of the lung form by dilatation of the terminal or larger bronchi (Salzberg, 1977). If multiple cysts are present, the lung may have a honeycomb appearance on x-ray.

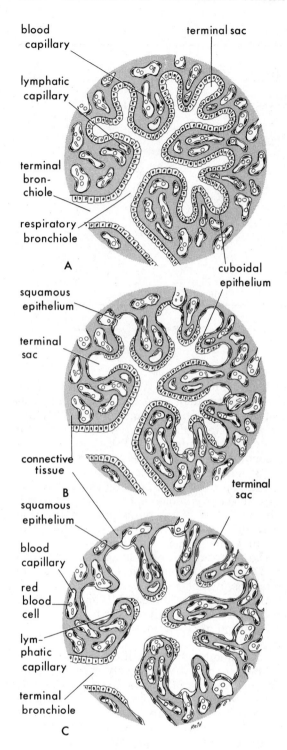

Figure 10–2 ● ● ● ● ● ●

Diagrammatic sketches of histologic sections, illustrating progressive stages of lung development. *A,* Late canalicular period (about 24 weeks). *B,* Early terminal sac period (about 26 weeks). *C,* Newborn infant (early alveolar period). Note that the alveolar-pulmonary capillary membrane is thin and that some of the capillaries have begun to bulge into the terminal sacs (future alveoli). (From Moore, K.L., & Persaud, T.V.N. (1993). *The developing human* (5th ed., p. 231). Philadelphia: W.B. Saunders.)

ESSENTIAL ANATOMY AND PHYSIOLOGY

Airways

The airway can be divided into three major areas: the supraglottic airway, the glottis, and the intrathoracic airway. The supraglottic airway includes the nose, the naso-oropharynx, and the epiglottis. The glottis includes the vocal cords, subglottic area, and cervical trachea. The intrathoracic airway includes the thoracic trachea, the mainstem bronchi, and the lungs. Each of these areas has unique features in the infant and young child.

Supraglottic Airway

The nose, lined with ciliated mucous epithelium, serves as the passageway for air. The nasal structures are protective in that they heat, humidify, and filter inspired air. The nasal passages are narrow, and any factor that further decreases the diameter, e.g., secretions, edema, or bleeding, will increase airway resistance and compromise ventilation. The newborn is considered an obligate nose breather for at least the first few months of life. Some infants do not mouth breathe until 5 to 6 months of life. Therefore, any obstruction to the infant's nares will cause respiratory distress, for example, choanal atresia. The area from the nasal cavity to the nasopharynx is abundantly lined with lymphoid tissue, the adenoids or pharyngeal tonsils, which can also obstruct the upper airway.

The mouth of the young child is small and the tongue is large in relation to the mandible. The palatine tonsils are located at the junction of the mouth and oropharynx. Although the tonsils are thought to prevent upper airway infection, large tonsils can potentially obstruct the airway. In addition to the small mouth and large tongue, the infant has a large head, soft neck, and weak shoulder girdle. In total, these factors predispose infants to airway obstruction by position alone. To maintain an open airway in an infant with an altered level of consciousness, the head is placed in a neutral position and a small roll is placed under the shoulders.

Glottis

The infant's epiglottis is omega shaped and floppy. The epiglottis enters the anterior pharyngeal wall at a 45-degree angle and projects more posteriorly than is the older child. These factors make visualization of the glottis difficult in the infant and young child (Backofen & Rogers, 1992). The epiglottis is also very susceptible to trauma and infection, which may cause edema and airway obstruction.

The larynx of the infant is more cephalad than in the older child. The glottis, the area between the vocal cords, is located between the second and third vertebrae in infants and descends to the fourth and fifth cervical vertebrae in adults. The infant vocal cords are approximately 50% cartilage and thus are less distensible than the older child. The cricoid ring, the only complete ring of cartilage in the pediatric airway, is the narrowest portion of the upper airway in infants and children, while the glottis is the narrowest portion of the adult upper airway (Fig. 10–3). In the newborn, the cricoid ring is approximately 6 mm in diameter, which places infants at particular risk for airway obstruction in this area.

Thoracic Airway

From the larynx, air passes through the trachea, which is short in the infant, approximately 4 to 5 cm long from the cricoid to the carina. The trachea is approximately 7 cm in the young adolescent. The bifurcation of the trachea at the carina forms the right and left mainstem bronchi. Because the right mainstem angles down more vertically and is somewhat larger that the left, objects aspirated into the airway more frequently lodge in the right mainstem bronchus.

The lower airways are smaller and less developed than in the adult. Airway obstruction results in in-

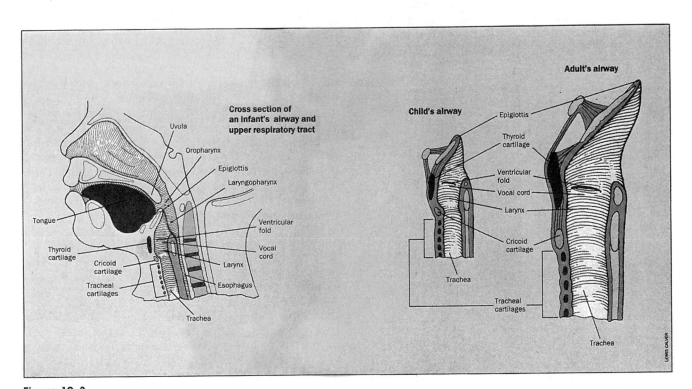

Figure 10–3 ● ● ● ● ● ●
Comparative anatomy of the adult and infant airways. (From Thomas, D.O. (1986). The ABCs of pediatric emergencies. *RN*, March 1986. Reprinted by permission of Medical Economics/RN magazine/Lewis E. Calver.)

creased airways resistance. Factors that impact airways resistance include the length and radius of the airway. Critically important in infants and children is airway radius. According to Poiseuille's law, resistance to airflow is inversely proportional to the fourth power of the radius for laminar flow ($1/r^4$) and to the fifth power for turbulent flow ($1/r^5$). Thus, a reduction in diameter by half reduces laminar flow to 1/16th of its former level. To maintain the same flow requires a 16-fold increase in pressure, which significantly increases the work of breathing (Thompson, Farrell, & McManus, 1992). As noted in Figure 10–4, minor reductions in the already small diameter pediatric airway result in a large reduction in the cross-sectional area.

The walls of the tracheobronchial tree are composed of smooth muscle. The airways of the newborn contain little smooth muscle; however, by 4 to 5 months of life, enough smooth muscle is present to cause airway narrowing in response to an irritating stimulus. Smooth muscle development by 1 year of age is comparable with that of an adult.

Developmental changes also take place in the alveoli and the terminal bronchioles. The terminal bronchioles continue branching during the first year of life. The number and size of alveoli continue to increase until at least 8 years of age. These changes are responsible for the increased respiratory surface area available for gas exchange in the older child and adult. At birth, the interstitium of the lung contains little collagen and elastin. This may explain the frequency of alveolar rupture in the premature infant. Collagen and elastin production increases in the postnatal period (Wohl & Mead, 1990).

Little collateral ventilation exists in infants and young children. Pores of Kohn, which allow interalveolar communication, first appear between the first

and second years of life (Macklem, 1971). Canals of Lambert, which allow bronchiole-alveolar communication, start to form after age 6 (Boyden, 1977). With age, both structures allow ventilation of alveoli distal to an obstructed airway. Absence of collateral pathways contributes to patchy atelectasis when airway disease is present in infants and young children (Wohl & Mead, 1991).

Thoracic Cavity

The ribs, vertebrae, and sternum provide the bony framework of the thoracic cavity. Within the thoracic cavity lie three lobes of lung on the right, two lobes of lung on the left, and the mediastinum, which is off center to the left containing the heart, great vessels, esophagus, and trachea. The entire thoracic cavity is lined with parietal pleura, whereas the lungs are encased by visceral pleura. In health, the potential space between the pleura is filled with just enough fluid to allow the two pleura to glide over each other during ventilation. In illness states, the pleural space may fill with air (pneumothorax), fluid (pleural effusion), blood (hemothorax), lymph (chylothorax), or pus (empyema).

The contour of the thoracic cavity changes shape over time. The infant's thorax is round at birth with the anteroposterior diameter equal to the transverse diameter (1:1). This gradually changes, so that by 6 years of age the thorax reaches the adult diameter (1:2). In infancy, the chest wall is thin, with little musculature, and is highly compliant. The muscles of respiration include the diaphragm, intercostal, accessory, and abdominal muscles. The diaphragm is the most important muscle of respiration, as it is responsible for most of the inspiratory effort. The phrenic nerve, formed by components of the third, fourth, and fifth cervical spinal nerves, supplies the diaphragm with both motor and sensory innervation. The intercostal and accessory muscles are poorly developed in infants, so they contribute little toward respiratory effort. The infant uses abdominal muscles to assist with ventilation. This combination of muscle use gives the appearance of seesaw breathing—that is, a paradoxic movement of the chest and abdomen. Seesaw breathing becomes exaggerated when intrapulmonary compliance decreases.

The infant's chest wall is very compliant, which allows for (1) passage through the birth canal and (2) removal of intrapulmonary fluid before the first breath. In the presence of respiratory disease, the diaphragm contracts and the chest wall moves inward on inspiration. In the older child or adolescent, the chest wall is rigid. When the diaphragm contracts, the rib cage is elevated and the chest wall moves outward (Fig. 10–5). The soft, flexible rib cage of the infant makes retractions a prominent feature in respiratory distress and prevents the generation of high intrathoracic pressures needed to reexpand collapsed alveoli.

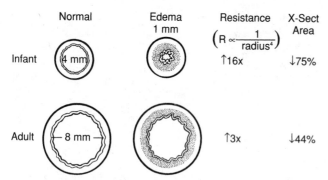

Figure 10–4 ● ● ● ● ●

The effects of edema on airway resistance in the infant versus the adult. Normal airways are represented on the left; edematous airways (1 mm circumferential edema) on the right. Resistance to flow is inversely proportional to the radius of the lumen to the fourth power for laminar flow, and the fifth power for turbulent flow. The net result is a 75% decrease in cross-sectional area and a 16-fold increase in resistance in the infant versus 44% and 3-fold, respectively, in the adult. (From Coté C., Todres, I.D. (1986). The pediatric airway. In Ryan, J.F., Todres, I.D., Coté, C., & Goudsouzian, N. (eds). *A practice of anesthesia for infants and children* (p. 39). New York: Grune & Stratton.)

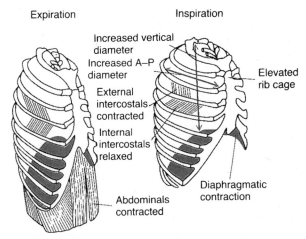

Expiration Inspiration

Increased vertical diameter
Increased A–P diameter
External intercostals contracted
Internal intercostals relaxed
Abdominals contracted
Elevated rib cage
Diaphragmatic contraction

Figure 10–5 ● ● ● ● ● ●
Expansion and contraction of the thoracic cage during expiration and inspiration, illustrating especially diaphragmatic contraction, elevation of the rib cage, and function of the intercostals. (From Guyton, A.C. (1991). *Textbook of medical physiology* (8th ed.). Philadelphia: W.B. Saunders.)

Pulmonary Circulation

The lungs receive blood from both ventricles. Unoxygenated blood flow from the right ventricle reaches the lungs by way of the pulmonary arteries. The pulmonary arteries divide into two systems: the conventional and the supernumerary. Conventional arteries travel with the airways, dividing as the airways divide. Supernumerary arteries, which exceed the conventional arteries in number, provide blood supply directly to the gas-exchanging units. Pulmonary vessels, similar to airways, develop with growth. (Please refer to Chapter 9 for an indepth discussion of pulmonary vascular development and resistance.)

The left ventricle provides oxygenated blood to the lungs by way of three bronchial arteries. The bronchial arteries perfuse the bronchi, bronchioles, lymph nodes, and visceral pleura. Pulmonary venous drainage returns to the right and left atria. The right atrium receives blood via the bronchial veins, and the left atrium receives blood via the pulmonary veins. Bronchial arteries do hypertrophy in the presence of pulmonary infection. Hemoptysis may begin in these bronchial vessels in disorders such as cystic fibrosis (O'Brodovich & Haddad, 1990).

Lymphatic System

The major function of the lymphatic system is to return interstitial fluid to the systemic circulation. As blood flows through the pulmonary capillaries, plasma is filtered into the interstitium where it collects in lymphatic channels and is returned to the circulation by the lymphatic system. Lymphatic drainage can significantly increase in certain disease states, for example, in patients with pulmonary

edema. Whereas most fluid is returned to the systemic circulation by the lymphatic system scattered throughout the lung parenchyma, another set of lymphatic vessels returns lymphatic drainage over the surface of the lung within the pleura. In conditions in which the major lymphatic drainage through the thoracic duct is blocked, lymph may back up to form a chylous effusion.

Pulmonary Metabolism

The lungs have the only capillary bed in which the entire blood volume passes. Considering this, the pulmonary capillary circulation is uniquely suited for exercising a controlling influence on a number of circulating vasoactive agents. These include activation of angiotensin I to angiotensin II; inactivation of bradykinin, serotonin, PGE, and PGF_2; and partial inactivation of norepinephrine and perhaps histamine. In addition to modulating bronchial and pulmonary vascular diameter, the systemic effects of these agents include increased capillary permeability, platelet aggregation, and peripheral vasodilation.

Control of Respiration

The neural and chemical control of respiration involves an intricate balance of numerous factors that serve to maintain PaO_2, $PaCO_2$, and pH at levels that promote optimal cellular functioning. Nervous system control of breathing includes the cerebral cortex through the corticospinal tracts to the respiratory muscles and autonomic control through the medulla and pons of the brainstem.

Expansion of the thoracic cavity on inspiration occurs by stimulation of the phrenic nerve, which innervates the diaphragm, and stimulation of the spinal nerves, which innervate the external intercostal muscles. If expiration must be facilitated, stimulation through the spinal nerves causes contraction of the internal intercostal and abdominal muscles.

Rhythmic discharge of neurons in the medulla oblongata produces spontaneous respiration. Although specific pacemaker cells that drive respiration have not been identified, two groups of respiratory neurons in the medulla influence respiration: the dorsal respiratory group (DRG) and the ventral respiratory group (VRG). The DRG is the source of rhythmic drive to the contralateral phrenic motor neurons, and the VRG innervates ipsilateral accessory muscles and provides inspiratory and expiratory input to the intercostal muscles. Rhythmic discharge of the medullary neurons is modified by centers in the pons and by afferent information from the vagus nerve stretch receptors in the chest.

The pneumotaxic center is located in the rostral section of the pons. Stimulation of the expiratory neurons inhibits the inspiratory center in the medulla; thus, the pneumotaxic center works with the medulla to generate regular cyclical respirations. The apneustic center is located in the middle and caudal pons. Stimulation of this center along with a vagotomy produces apneustic respiration, a respiratory pattern characterized by extremely prolonged inspiratory periods.

Scattered throughout the upper airway, trachea, and lungs are mechanoreceptors that provide information to the respiratory center via the vagus nerve. These receptors include slowly adapting stretch receptors, rapidly adapting stretch receptors, and C fibers. Slowly adapting receptors (SAR) are activated by increases in lung volume; when stimulated, the SAR are responsible for prolonging expiratory time. Rapidly adapting receptors (RAD) are activated by lung inflation and a variety of chemical substances (histamine and prostaglandin) and cause an increase in respiratory rate. C fibers are also activated by chemical substances (histamine, prostaglandin, bradykinin, and serotonin) and cause apnea followed by rapid, shallow breathing.

Central chemoreceptors, responsible for the dramatic increase in minute ventilation (V_E) when $PaCO_2$ levels are elevated, are located in the medulla. Medullary chemoreceptors monitor H^+ ion concentration of cerebrospinal fluid and brainstem interstitial fluid. Although H^+ and HCO_3^- ions are unable to cross the blood-brain barrier easily, CO_2 readily penetrates and immediately hydrates to form carbonic acid (H_2CO_3), which dissipates into H^+ and HCO_3^-. The H^+ ion concentration in the brain interstitial fluid parallels $PaCO_2$ and acts as a stimulus to increase respiration.

The peripheral chemoreceptors include the carotid body located near the bifurcation of the internal and external carotid arteries and the aortic bodies located near the arch of the aorta. The carotid bodies are sensitive to PaO_2 and potentiated by H^+ ion and $PaCO_2$ concentration; aortic bodies are sensitive to circulatory changes. Afferent nerve fibers from the carotid and aortic bodies ascend to the medulla to increase ventilation as necessary. Chronic sustained hypoxia decreases the carotic bodies' response to low PaO_2.

Oxygen Transport

"Adequate" oxygenation can only be defined when tissue oxygen supply matches tissue oxygen demand. Essential factors to be considered include (1) alveolar-pulmonary capillary oxygen transport, (2) oxygen transport in the blood, and (3) cellular respiration. Table 10–2 provides a summary of oxygenation profile parameters.

Alveolar-Pulmonary Capillary Oxygen Transport

Between the extremely thin alveoli walls is an almost solid network of interconnecting capillaries. Gas exchange occurs throughout the alveolar-pulmonary capillary membrane of all the terminal portions of the lungs. Oxygen and CO_2 move across the seven-layer alveolar-pulmonary capillary membrane by passive diffusion from an area of high partial pressure to an area of low partial pressure (Fig. 10–6). Diffusion is directly proportional to the gradient of partial pressure across the alveolar-pulmonary capillary membrane, the alveolar-pulmonary capillary surface area, and the gas solubility. Diffusion is inversely proportional to the thickness of the alveolar-pulmonary capillary membrane and the molecular weight of the gas.

According to Dalton's law of partial pressures, the total pressure of a mixture of gases is equal to the sum of the pressures of the individual gases. The total pressure of gas in the atmosphere, the atmospheric pressure, is 760 mmHg at sea level. Thus, partial pressures of a component gas depend on the fraction of the total mixture occupied by that gas. Room air contains 21% oxygen; thus, oxygen exerts a partial pressure of 21% of 760 mmHg, which is 160 mmHg. At high altitudes, the percent concentration of oxygen doesn't change but the absolute number of molecules in a given volume does. For example, at 5000 feet, atmospheric pressure is 632 mmHg; 21% of 632 mmHg is 133 mmHg.

As gases are inhaled into the upper airway, they are warmed and humidified. The pressure of water vapor depends upon the temperature of atmospheric gas. At high temperatures, atmospheric gas has more water in vapor form, whereas the opposite is true with low temperatures. Water vapor exerts a pressure of 47 mmHg at 30°C. Water vapor reduces the partial pressure of inspired oxygen; $760 - 47 = 713$; 21% of 713 is 149.7 mmHg.

Alveolar ventilation refers to the portion of ventilation that undergoes gas exchange. Inspired gas is mixed in the alveoli with gas that contains water vapor and CO_2. Alveolar partial pressure of oxygen

Table 10–2. NORMAL OXYGENATION PROFILE VALUES

Parameter	Calculation	Norms
CaO_2	$CaO_2 = (Hgb \times 1.34 \times SaO_2) + (PaO_2 \times 0.003)$	20 mL/dL
CvO_2	$CvO_2 = (Hgb \times 1.34 \times SvO_2) + (PvO_2 \times 0.003)$	15 mL/dL
a-vDO_2	$CaO_2 - CvO_2$	3.5–5 mL/dL
DO_2	$DO_2 = CaO_2 \times CI \times 10$	620 ± 50 mL/min/M^2
VO_2	$VO_2 = (CaO_2 - CvO_2) \times CI \times 10$	120–200 mL/min/M^2
O_2ER	$(CaO_2 - CvO_2)/CaO_2 \times 100$	25 ± 2%
SvO_2		75% (60–80%)

CaO_2, arterial oxygen content; Hgb, hemoglobin; SaO_2, arterial oxygen saturation; CI, cardiac index; DO_2, oxygen delivery; PaO_2, arterial partial pressure of oxygen; CvO_2, venous oxygen content; SvO_2, venous oxygen saturation; PvO_2; venous partial pressure of oxygen; a-vDO_2, arteriovenous oxygen difference; VO_2, oxygen consumption; O_2ER, oxygen extraction ratio.

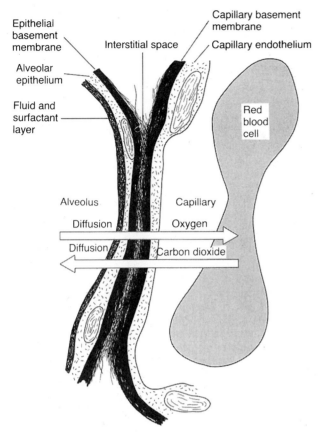

Epithelial basement membrane

Interstitial space

Capillary basement membrane

Capillary endothelium

Alveolar epithelium

Fluid and surfactant layer

Red blood cell

Alveolus

Capillary

Diffusion Oxygen

Diffusion Carbon dioxide

Figure 10–6 ● ● ● ● ● ●

Cross-section of the pulmonary capillary membrane. (From Guyton A.C. (1991). *Textbook of medical physiology* (8th ed.). Philadelphia: W.B. Saunders.)

(PaO$_2$) is calculated using the *alveolar gas equation:* PAO$_2$ = PiO$_2$ − PaCO$_2$/RQ. The inspired partial pressure of oxygen (PiO$_2$) is corrected for water vapor (47 mmHg) and is PiO$_2$ = (P$_B$ − 47) × FiO$_2$. The value of CO$_2$ is corrected by the respiratory quotient (RQ), which takes into consideration that more O$_2$ is consumed than CO$_2$ is produced. In room air, at normal barometric pressure and normal PaCO$_2$, with a respiratory quotient (RQ) of 0.8, the PAO$_2$ is equal to 99.7 mmHg; PAO$_2$ = (760 − 47) × 0.21 = 149.7 mmHg − 40/0.8.

The partial pressures of alveolar gases equal atmospheric pressure; any increases in one alveolar gas is associated with a decrease in another. Decreases in pulmonary uptake of oxygen are related to either diffusion or ventilation-perfusion deficits. For example, diffusion defects occur secondary to problems affecting the diffusion of gases over the alveolar-pulmonary capillary membrane (interstitial edema), whereas ventilation-perfusion deficits occur secondary to problems affecting alveolar ventilation (atelectasis) or alveolar perfusion (cardiovascular collapse).

Considering that the PAO$_2$ is close to 100 mmHg and the normal venous partial pressure of oxygen (PvO$_2$) is 40 mmHg, the alveolar-capillary diffusion gradient for oxygen is about 60 mmHg. The capillary-alveolar diffusion gradient for CO$_2$ is significantly

less (46 mmHg − 40 mmHg = 6 mmHg), but CO$_2$ is 24 times more soluble than oxygen and its molecular weight is greater than oxygen. Differences in solubility and size make CO$_2$ 20 times more diffusible than oxygen. Whereas PaO$_2$ better reflects ventilation to perfusion matching, PaCO$_2$ better reflects the adequacy of alveolar ventilation.

Oxygen Transport in the Blood

Oxygen is carried in the blood in two forms: in combination with hemoglobin and dissolved in plasma. Oxygen binds rapidly and reversibly with hemoglobin to form oxyhemoglobin (HbO$_2$). Almost all oxygen is carried as oxyhemoglobin.

The *arterial oxygen content* (CaO$_2$) describes the total amount of oxygen carried by arterial blood. CaO$_2$ (mL/dL) = (Hgb × 1.34 × SaO$_2$) + (PaO$_2$ × 0.003). For example: with a hemoglobin (Hgb) concentration of 15 g/100 mL of blood, arterial saturation (SaO$_2$) of 98%, and a PaO$_2$ of 100 mmHg, CaO$_2$ (mL/dL) = (15 × 1.34 × 98%) + (100 × 0.003); CaO$_2$ = 19.7 + 0.3; CaO$_2$ = 20 mL/dL. When fully saturated, 1 g of hemoglobin carries 1.34 mL of oxygen; plasma carries only 0.003 mL of oxygen per mmHg O$_2$ per dL. Whereas the PaO$_2$ gives excellent information regarding lung function, PaO$_2$ assumes an insignificant role in oxygen transport. The CaO$_2$ clearly demonstrates the highly significant role of hemoglobin in oxygen transport. Alternative shortened formulas for CaO$_2$ calculation eliminate the PaO$_2$ portion of the equation. Note that once hemoglobin is fully saturated at 100%, the only way to dramatically improve CaO$_2$ is through erythrocyte administration, increasing hemoglobin concentration.

Oxygen-Hemoglobin Affinity: Oxyhemoglobin Dissociation Curve (ODC). The oxygen-carrying capacity of blood is directly related to hemoglobin concentration and the affinity of oxygen for hemoglobin. Although PaO$_2$ contributes little to CaO$_2$, PaO$_2$ plays a major role in determining the affinity of oxygen for hemoglobin as described by the sigmoid-shaped ODC (Fig. 10–7A).

The S-shaped curve facilitates alveolar capillary uptake of oxygen (the association process) and tissue release of oxygen (the dissociation process). Over the upper flat portion of the curve (>70 mmHg → ∝), hemoglobin bond to oxygen is favored. A large change in oxygen tension results in a small change in oxygen saturation/content. Hemoglobin remains fully saturated, providing a consistent oxygen content/saturation over a wide range of oxygen tensions commonly found in the alveolar capillary bed. Over the steep portion of the curve (PO$_2$ of 10–40 mmHg), hemoglobin release of oxygen is favored. A small drop in oxygen tension results in a large drop in oxygen saturation/content. This ensures delivery of large quantities of oxygen to the tissue capillary beds.

The affinity of oxygen for hemoglobin may change and shift the position of the ODC to the right or left. The PO$_2$ at which hemoglobin is 50% saturated, the P$_{50}$, is used as a marker for the relative position of

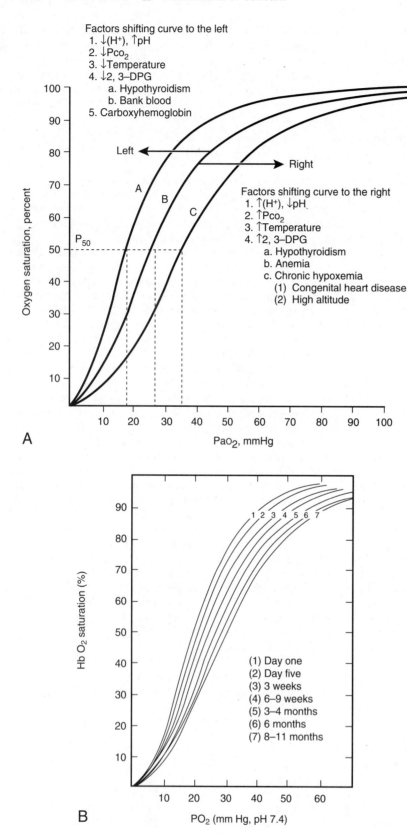

Factors shifting curve to the left
1. ↓(H⁺), ↑pH
2. ↓Pco₂
3. ↓Temperature
4. ↓2, 3–DPG
   a. Hypothyroidism
   b. Bank blood
5. Carboxyhemoglobin

Factors shifting curve to the right
1. ↑(H⁺), ↓pH
2. ↑Pco₂
3. ↑Temperature
4. ↑2, 3–DPG
   a. Hypothyroidism
   b. Anemia
   c. Chronic hypoxemia
      (1) Congenital heart disease
      (2) High altitude

A

Figure 10–7 ● ● ● ● ● ●

A, The S-shaped oxyhemoglobin dissociation curve facilitates alveolar capillary uptake of oxygen (the association process) and tissue release of oxygen (the dissociation process). (Redrawn from Kinney (1993). *AACN's clinical reference for critical care.* St. Louis: Mosby–Year Book.) *B,* Age-dependent ODCs. (From Oski, F.A. (1973). Reproduced by permission of Pediatrics 51:494. © Copyright 1973.)

(1) Day one
(2) Day five
(3) 3 weeks
(4) 6–9 weeks
(5) 3–4 months
(6) 6 months
(7) 8–11 months

B

the ODC. At a pH of 7.4 and temperature of 37°C, P_{50} for hemoglobin A is 27 mmHg. A *shift to the left* (decreased P_{50}) means that oxygen is more tightly bound to hemoglobin; a *shift to the right* (increased P_{50}) means that oxygen is readily released from hemoglobin (Fig. 10–7A). A shift to the right has little effect on the association process, but the dissociation process is enhanced. For example, at the upper flat portion of the curve, slightly less than 100% saturation occurs; but at the steep portion of the curve, significantly more oxygen is unloaded to the tissues. The opposite is true of a shift to the left; the association process is enhanced, whereas the dissociation process is diminished.

Principal modulators of oxygen-hemoglobin affinity include temperature, P_{CO_2}/pH, and the concentration of red blood cell 2,3-diphosphoglycerate (DPG) (an enzyme that accumulates in response to sustained periods of impaired oxygen delivery).

Hyperthermia results in a decreased oxygen affinity (right shift), whereas hypothermia results in a increased oxygen affinity (left shift). Clinically, oxygen becomes more available to the tissues when there is an increased metabolic need marked by hyperthermia.

Known as the Bohr effect, increased H^+ ion concentration shifts the ODC to the right. Associated with the hydration of CO_2 to carbonic acid (HCO_3), acidosis results in decreased oxygen affinity. Clinically, a shift to the right favors the release of oxygen for aerobic metabolism in the more acidotic CO_2-rich environment of tissue capillary beds.

The organic phosphate 2,3-DPG decreases oxygen affinity for hemoglobin, resulting in an increased oxygen release to the tissues. Increased levels of 2,3-DPG are associated with chronic anemic and/or hypoxic states, for example, in patients with cyanotic heart disease and chronic lung disease; decreased levels are found with inorganic phosphate deficiency and in sepsis. Also, 2,3-DPG concentrations decrease with advanced red blood cell age, for example, in banked blood.

In infants and children, a cluster of ODCs exist (see Fig. 10–7B). As mentioned, at a pH of 7.4 and temperature of 37°C, the P_{50} for hemoglobin A is 27 mmHg. Hemoglobin A, adult type hemoglobin, consists of two α-chains and two β-chains with each containing a heme group with iron. Fetal hemoglobin, hemoglobin F, consists of two α-chain and two γ-chain units. The transition from fetal to adult hemoglobin starts to occur just before birth in full-term infants and is complete by 6 months of age. Term newborns have approximately 70% hemoglobin A and 30% hemoglobin F. Compared with hemoglobin A, hemoglobin F has an increased oxygen affinity. Under similar conditions, P_{50} at birth for hemoglobin F is 19.4 mmHg. P_{50} then shifts to approximately 30 mmHg by 11 months of age. The left shift of fetal hemoglobin allows higher oxygen saturation at lower oxygen tensions. This is crucial for adequate oxygenation of the fetus, as placental blood normally provides a P_{O_2} of 35 to 40 mmHg.

Oxygen delivery (DO_2), the amount of oxygen delivered to the tissues, is equal to CaO_2 × cardiac index (CI) × a conversion factor of 10, which changes the CaO_2 measurement from deciliters to liters; $DO_2 = CaO_2 \times CI \times 10$. Normal DO_2 is 620 ± 50 mL/min/M^2. Barcoft (1920) identified three separate causes of inadequate DO_2: hypoxia, anemia, or stagnant flow. Hypoxia occurs secondary to a low arterial oxygen saturation, for example, hypoxia associated with ventilation-perfusion mismatch. Anemia occurs secondary to low hemoglobin concentration, for example, anemia after hemorrhage. Stagnant flow occurs secondary to low cardiac output, for example, shock states. The clinical significance of alterations in the determinates of DO_2 are reviewed in Table 10–3. Deficits occur in isolation or in combination. Also, parameters compensate for the other; for example, tachycardia increases after hemorrhage. Clinical management strategies are directed toward correction of the primary problem and supporting compensatory mechanisms.

Cellular Respiration

Tissue oxygenation is dependent upon microcirculation regulated by arteriolar and precapillary sphincter tone and DO_2. Capillary oxygen moves from erythrocytes, through plasma, and into tissue by diffusion.

Adjustments in microcirculation can enhance oxygen extraction and preserve organ metabolism. Precapillary sphincters, located at the arterial end of each capillary, maintain capillaries open or closed depending upon the metabolic requirements of the specific tissue bed. Local increases in H^+ ion concentration shifts the ODC to the right to augment hemoglobin release of oxygen.

All cells are dependent upon a continuous supply of oxygen to support aerobic metabolism necessary for the synthesis of high-energy compounds (ATP) essential for cell life and function. Most cellular oxygen is consumed by the mitochondria to drive oxidative phosphorylation (Fig. 10–8). In the absence of oxygen, there is a decrease in electron transport activity and cells start to produce ATP anaerobically from the conversion of pyruvate to lactate. Not only

Table 10–3. CLINICAL SIGNIFICANCE OF ALTERATIONS IN THE DETERMINATES OF DO_2

		$DO_2 = CaO_2 \times CI \times 10$, where CaO_2 (mL/dL) = (Hgb × 1.34 × SaO_2) + (PaO_2 × 0.003)				
State	Hgb (g/100 ml)	SaO_2 (%)	PaO_2 (mmHg)	CaO_2 (mL/dL)	CI (L/min/M^2)	DO_2 (mL/min/M^2)
Normal	12–15	95–100	80–100	20	3.5–5.5	620 ± 50
Hypoxia	15	**85**	**50**	17	4.0	680
Anemia	**8**	100	100	11	4.0	440
Stagnant flow	15	100	100	20	**2.0**	400

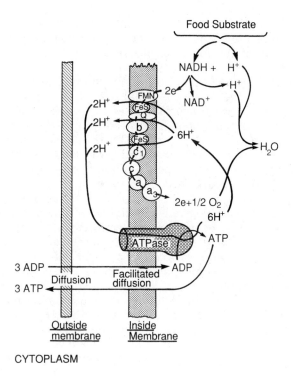

Food Substrate

Figure 10–8 ● ● ● ● ● ●
Oxidative phosphorylation produces massive quantities of ATP. (From Guyton, A.C. (1991). *Textbook of medical physiology* (8th ed.). Philadelphia: W.B. Saunders.)

is this process less efficient (20 times less ATP is produced), but also lactic acid lowers tissue pH and depletes cellular NAD^+ necessary for aerobic glycolysis.

Oxygen delivery does not provide information about the adequacy of tissue oxygenation. For example, in septic shock DO_2 is high but blood is shunted across tissue-capillary beds without unloading oxygen. Indirect methods of assessing the adequacy of tissue oxygenation include monitoring mixed venous oxygenation, oxygen consumption, and oxygen extraction ratio.

Blood returning from various regions of the body becomes well mixed in the right ventricle. To avoid regional contamination, true mixed venous oxygenation is monitored from the pulmonary artery. Pulmonary artery catheters, designed specifically for continuous SvO_2 monitoring, are available in sizes designed specifically for the pediatric population. The interrelationship between SvO_2 values and VO_2 is noted in Table 10–4.

Reflecting metabolic requirements, *oxygen consumption* (VO_2) is the amount of oxygen used by tissues. VO_2 is assessed as the net oxygen difference between the amount of oxygen entering tissue and the amount of oxygen leaving tissue. VO_2 can be approximated by using a modified version of the Fick equation: $VO_2 = (CaO_2 - CvO_2) \times$ cardiac index $\times$ 10. Where $CvO_2 = (Hgb \times 1.36 \times SvO_2) + (pvO_2 \times 0.003)$; CvO_2 norm is 15 mL/dL or vol%. The conversion factor of 10 is necessary to change deciliters to

liters. Resting VO_2 in infants and young children is almost twice that of an adult. The significantly higher VO_2 reflects the metabolic requirements of continued growth—that is, growth adds a metabolic burden. Factors that affect VO_2 are noted in Table 10–5.

Oxygen extraction ratio, O_2ER, is a ratio of VO_2 to DO_2 (oxygen consumption to oxygen delivery or availability). The O_2ER represents the proportion of DO_2 that is actually utilized by the tissues. O_2ER is calculated by: $O_2ER = (CaO_2 - CvO_2)/CaO_2 \times 100$. The O_2ER is normally 25%. This means that only

Table 10–4. INTERRELATIONSHIP BETWEEN SvO_2 AND VO_2

Normal SvO_2 and increased VO_2
Compensation effective—increased supply (DO_2) to preserve venous reserve
Decreased SvO_2 and increased VO_2
Compensation ineffective or impossible—patient using venous reserve
Increased SvO_2 and decreased VO_2
Decreased need
Increased supply
Decreased utilization (sepsis, L shift to ODC, cyanide toxicity)
L → R shunting (CHD, AV malformations, AV fistulas, loss of autoregulation of blood flow, vasodilated states)

Table 10–5. FACTORS THAT AFFECT TISSUE OXYGEN CONSUMPTION

%	Activity–Clinical State
Increase VO_2	
138%	Head injury, nonsedated
100%	Burns
50–100%	Sepsis
50–100%	Shivering
89%	Head injury, sedated
20–80%	Multiple system organ dysfunction
60%	Chest trauma
40%	Work of breathing
25–40%	Nasal ETT intubation
36%	Patient weight
35%	Bronchial hygiene
31%	Position change
10–30%	Orthopedic injuries
27%	ETT suctioning
25%	Chest x-ray
23%	Bath
20%	Physical examination
18%	Agitation
16%	EKG
10%	Fever (increase for each °C)
10%	Dressing change
7%	Routine postoperative procedures
Decrease VO_2	
50%	Anesthesia in burned patients
25%	Anesthesia
25–50%	Sleep, relaxation, pain relief, paralysis, hypothermia

Data from White, K. M., Winslow, E. H., Clark, A. P., & Tyler, D. O. (1990). The physiologic basis for continuous mixed venous oxygen saturation monitoring. *Heart & Lung*, 19 (5, part 2), 548–551.

25% of the oxygen delivered to the tissues is actually utilized. This apparently low O_2ER is protective in that significantly more O_2 can be extracted if necessary to maintain adequate tissue delivery when V_{O_2} increases or D_{O_2} decreases. The O_2ER increases when the demand for O_2 increases (fever, pain) or the supply of O_2 falls (decreased hemoglobin, Sa_{O_2}, or cardiac index); the O_2ER decreases when demand for O_2 decreases (hypothermia, adequate sedation, chemical paralysis) or when supply, relative to demand, increases. The O_2ER is not a valid measure when the Cv_{O_2} is contaminated with R→L blood shunted across anatomic cardiac defects.

Physiologic oxygen supply dependency describes the *normal* biphasic relationship between D_{O_2} and V_{O_2} (Fig. 10–9). Initially when D_{O_2} falls, oxygen extraction increases to maintain V_{O_2} until a critical level of D_{O_2} is reached. At this critical level of D_{O_2}, referred to as critical oxygen transport, V_{O_2} progressively decreases and becomes linearly dependent on D_{O_2}. Metabolic demands are thought to be met on the flat portion of the curve as long as the O_2ER can increase to meet tissue demands for oxygen.

In contrast, *pathologic oxygen supply dependency* describes an *abnormal* relationship between D_{O_2} and V_{O_2}; O_2ER remains low, and V_{O_2} is linearly dependent on D_{O_2} over a wide range of values (Fig. 10–9). This abnormal V_{O_2}-D_{O_2} relationship is thought to occur in several disease states, for example, adult respiratory distress syndrome (ARDS) and sepsis (Lister, 1991).

Under normal circumstances, organ blood flow (oxygen supply) is distributed to match organ metabolic need (oxygen demand). Control of oxygen flow to match metabolism is regulated by the resistance of capillary vessels. This along with alterations in hemoglobin affinity enhance peripheral oxygen extraction to sustain tissue metabolism. When D_{O_2} decreases or if V_{O_2} increases *and* systemic blood flow is distributed to match metabolic need, the O_2ER (an average of each individual organ oxygen extraction) should increase. If systemic blood flow is not distributed to match metabolic need, hypoxia and a low O_2ER results.

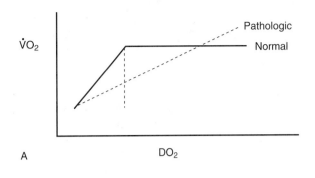

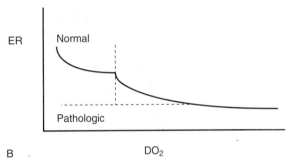

Figure 10–9 ● ● ● ● ●

A, The normal and pathologic relationships of oxygen consumption (V_{O_2}) and oxygen delivery (D_{O_2}). The normal critical D_{O_2} is shown as the vertical line separating the independent and the dependent portions of the normal V_{O_2} and D_{O_2} relationship. The pathologic relationship is characterized by a greater critical D_{O_2} compared with the normal relationship. In animal models, the pathologic relationship has a plateau of V_{O_2}, and increased critical D_{O_2} is clearly identified. However, clinical studies have not shown a plateau of V_{O_2} in individual patients who have pathologic dependence of V_{O_2} on D_{O_2}. *B,* The normal and pathologic relationships of oxygen extraction ratio (ER) and D_{O_2}. The critical oxygen ER is the extraction ratio at the critical D_{O_2} shown as the vertical line corresponding to the critical D_{O_2} determined by the D_{O_2}/V_{O_2} relationship above. In the normal relationship, the oxygen ER continues to increase below the critical oxygen ER, but not enough to maintain V_{O_2} constant. In the pathologic relationship, the oxygen ER remains relatively constant and, therefore, V_{O_2} is dependent on D_{O_2}. In animal models, pathologic dependence of V_{O_2} on D_{O_2} is characterized by a lower critical oxygen ER than normal. (Adapted from Russell JA, Phang PT (1994). The oxygen delivery/consumption controversy: Approaches to management of the critically ill. *American Journal of Respiratory and Critical Care Medicine,* 149, 533–537.)

Pulmonary Ventilation

Ventilation, the process of inspiration followed by expiration, is accomplished when the diaphragm functions to move air in and out of the lungs. When the thoracic cavity changes in size, pressure gradients are created between the intrapleural space, intra-alveolar space, and the atmosphere. The external pressure exerted on the thorax is atmospheric at 760 mmHg. Intra-alveolar pressure, which is in direct communication with the atmosphere, is also 760 mmHg. Intrapleural pressure, the pressure between the visceral and parietal pleura, is subatmospheric at 757.5 mmHg or a −2.5 mmHg.

Inspiration is an active process in that energy is required for the contraction of inspiratory muscles that expand the thoracic cavity. As the thoracic cavity expands, intrapleural pressure becomes increasingly subatmospheric at −6 mmHg. Intra-alveolar pressure also becomes subatmospheric and air moves in bulk flow from the atmosphere to alveoli where diffusion can occur.

Expiration is a passive process in that the muscles of respiration relax and the size of the intrathoracic cavity decreases. When the muscles relax, the elastic properties of the lung followed by the elastic properties of the chest wall pull the thoracic cavity back to a resting position. As the size of the intrathoracic cavity decreases, intra-alveolar pressure becomes supra-atmospheric and air moves in bulk flow from the alveoli to the atmosphere. Because of normal increased airways resistance during expiration, passive expiration requires more time than inspiration.

Compliance

Compliance refers to the stretchability, distensibility, or elasticity of the lungs and thoracic structures. The elastic properties of the lungs and chest wall allow the thoracic cavity to return to a resting state after inspiration. Compliance describes the relationship between volume (V) and pressure (P) ($\Delta V/\Delta P$) and is an indicator of elastic recoil and surface tension of the lung. Total compliance is the product of lung compliance and chest wall compliance. Clinically, total compliance is approximated by dividing the plateau pressure minus the positive end-expiratory pressure (PEEP) into measured tidal volume (V_T): $\Delta V/\Delta P = V_T \div P_{plat} - PEEP$. (The plateau pressure is a pause pressure obtained at end-inspiration.) For example, if the V_T/plateau pressure − PEEP were 60 mL ÷ 15 cm H_2O, the total lung compliance is approximately 4 mL/cm H_2O.

Lung compliance is measured in either a dynamic or static state. *Dynamic compliance* is equal to V_T divided by the transpulmonary pressure. The transpulmonary pressure (PL) is the difference between the alveolar pressure and the intrapleural pressure. Because dynamic compliance is measured during breathing, it is influenced by airway resistance and respiratory rate. *Static compliance* (Cst) is equal to V_T divided by PL at the cessation of airflow. Because Cst is measured under zero-flow conditions, it reflects the elastic properties of the lungs (Behnke & Koff, 1993). Clinically, PL can be approximated by subtracting intraesophageal pressure (as measured by an esophageal catheter/balloon placed in the lower third of the esophagus) from proximal airway pressures (using an adapter placed on the ETT) at the same point in a single breath. Similar results can also be achieved by measuring volume and flow by respiratory inductance plethysmography. A curve relating ΔV to ΔPL is constructed; the slope of the curve describes lung compliance (Fig. 10–10).

The pressure/volume characteristics of the lungs are not linear; at very high and very low lung volumes, changes in pressure produce little change in volume (the flatter the curve, the stiffer the lungs). Volume/pressure relationships also differ during inspiration and exhalation; more pressure is required to increase volume during inspiration than the reciprocal during exhalation.

Lung compliance changes with age, normally decreasing with increasing age and changes with disease, e.g., surfactant-deficient ARDS. Thoracic compliance can be significantly reduced in many clinical states, for example, in patients with scoliosis, muscular dystrophy, obesity, and in the postoperative patient with surgical splinting.

Airways Resistance

Total pulmonary resistance is affected by (1) radius, length, and number of divisions of bronchi; (2)

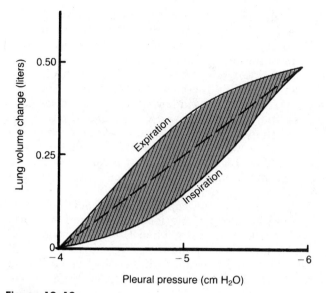

Figure 10–10 ● ● ● ● ● ●

A curve relating ΔV to ΔPL is constructed; the slope of the curve describes lung compliance. (From Guyton, A.C. (1992). *Textbook of medical physiology* (8th ed.). Philadelphia: W.B. Saunders.)

diameter and length of the endotracheal tube; (3) gas flow; and (4) character of gas flow. Airways resistance, or the rigidity of the bronchioles and thoracic structures, refers to the ease of air movement through conducting airways. Airways resistance is the pressure required to move a volume of gas at a given flow rate. Airways resistance is the product of the peak inspiratory pressure (PIP) minus the plateau pressure divided by the gas flow ($R_{aw} = PIP - P_{plat} \div V$).

The volume of gas that is pulled into the lungs and forced out of the lungs is inversely related to airways resistance. Until 5 or 6 years of age, small peripheral airways contribute up to 50% of total airways resistance compared with only 20% in adults (Hogg, Williams, Richardson, 1970). Diseases that affect the small airways, for example, asthma and bronchiolitis, can cause a significant increase in airways resistance and work of breathing in the younger, more vulnerable age group.

During normal spontaneous ventilation, the airways widen during inspiration and become narrow on exhalation. Autonomic nervous system regulation of bronchiolar smooth muscle can decrease (sympathetic) or increase (parasympathetic) airways resistance. Bronchiolar smooth muscle is also very sensitive to chemicals, such as histamine and low CO_2 levels, causing bronchoconstriction, whereas high CO_2 levels cause bronchodilation.

Time Constants

The tidal flow of gas into and out of the lung depends upon the compliance of the alveoli and the resistance of the airways. The relationship between compliance and resistance determines the actual rate of alveolar filling and emptying. The relationship between these two properties can be expressed mathematically as the time constant (Fig. 10–11; time constant = resistance × compliance). The time constant is expressed in seconds as the product of compliance and resistance. One time constant is the measure of the time necessary for the alveolar pressure to reach 63% of the total change in airway pressure. About 99% of pressure equilibration occurs within three to five time constants. The longer the time constant, the longer alveolar filling and emptying will take (Fig. 10–12).

Increased airways resistance prolongs the time necessary to fill an alveoli with air; likewise, a region of low compliance takes more time to fill with air than an area of high compliance. Pulmonary disease affecting either airways resistance or lung compliance exhibits nonhomogeneous time constants—that

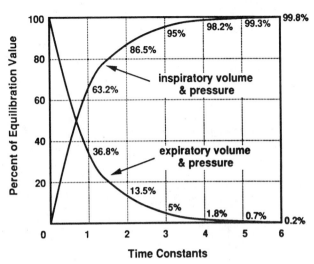

Figure 10-12 ● ● ● ● ● ●

The exponential rise and fall of lung pressure and volumes during inspiration and expiration in terms of time constants. (From Chatburn, R.L. (1991). Principles and practice of neonatal and pediatric mechanical ventilation. *Respiratory Care, 36*, 6, 578.)

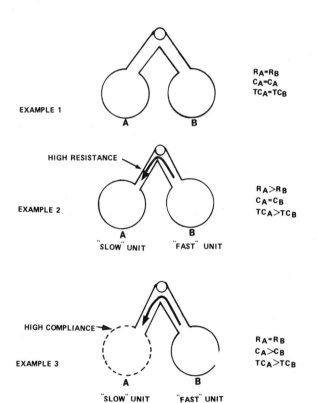

Figure 10-11 ● ● ● ● ● ●

Effect of changes in resistance and compliance on the distribution of gas between lung units. In example 1, the resistances (R) and compliances (C) and thus time constants (TC) between lung units A and B are equal and no redistribution of gas occurs if inspiration ends before the lung units are filled to maximal capacity. In example 2, the TC of A is lengthened by increasing its resistance. Both will eventually attain the same volume because the compliances are the same but unit A will take longer to fill. If inspiration ends prematurely, gas will be redistributed from B to A. In example 3, the TC of A is lengthened by increasing its compliance relative to B while the resistances of both remain equal. The less compliant unit B will never inflate to as great a volume as A. If inspiration ends prematurely, gas will be redistributed from B to A. (From Helfaer, M.A., Nichols, D.G., & Rogers, M.C. (1992). Developmental physiology of the respiratory system. In Rogers, M.C. (Ed.). *Textbook of pediatric intensive care* (2nd ed., p. 112). Baltimore: Williams & Wilkins.)

is, areas with both prolonged and normal time constants. Alveoli with normal time constants fill with air first followed by alveoli with prolonged time constants. As respiratory rates increase, alveoli with normal time constants may overfill and compress alveoli with prolonged time constants. Overdistended alveoli become less compliant because they have reached their elastic limit.

An appreciation of time constants is especially important when managing the infant or child who requires mechanical ventilation because a wide range of ventilator settings can be employed to manage clinical conditions with different combinations of resistance and compliance states (Table 10–6).

Pulmonary Volumes

Pulmonary volumes and capacities are defined and illustrated in Figure 10–13. Changes in body position

Table 10-6. THE EFFECT OF VARYING COMPLIANCE AND RESISTANCE STATES ON THE TIME CONSTANT AND ASSOCIATED CONDITIONS

Compliance	Resistance	Time Constant	Clinical Conditions
Decrease	Normal	Short	Pneumonia Pneumothorax Atelectasis
Increase	Normal	Long	Neuromuscular disease
Normal	Decrease	Short	Post-bronchodilator
Normal	Increase	Long	Airway obstructions Intubated patient
Increase	Increase	Long	BPD, COPD
Decrease	Increase	Long/short	Bronchiolitis

BPD, bronchopulmonary dysplasia; COPD, chronic obstructive pulmonary disease.

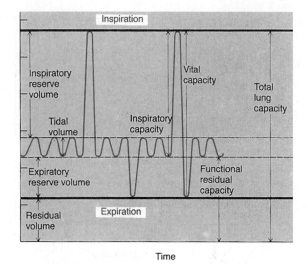

Figure 10–13 ● ● ● ● ● ●

Pulmonary volumes and capacities. *Tidal volume (VT):* The volume of air entering and leaving the lungs during a single breath in a resting state; 6–8 mL/kg. *Inspiratory reserve volume (IRV):* The amount of air that can be inspired over and above resting tidal volume. *Expiratory reserve volume (ERV):* The air remaining in the lungs at the end of a normal expiration that can be exhaled by active contraction of expiratory muscles. *Residual volume (RV):* The amount of air remaining in the lungs after maximal expiration. *Vital capacity (VC):* The sum of normal tidal volume, inspiratory reserve volume, and expiratory reserve volume; infants, 33–40 mL/kg; adults, 52 mL/kg. *Inspiratory capacity (IC):* The sum of inspiratory reserve volume and tidal volume. *Functional residual capacity (FRC):* The sum of the expiratory reserve volume and the residual volume; infants, 30 mL/kg; adults, 34 mL/kg. *Total lung capacity (TLC):* The amount of air in the lungs after a maximal inspiration; infants, 63 mL/kg; adults, 86 mL/kg. (From Guyton, A.C. (1991). *Textbook of medical physiology* (8th ed., p. 285). Philadelphia: W.B. Saunders.)

can affect pulmonary volumes and capacities. In a prone position, values decrease because the abdominal contents exert pressure on the diaphragm and, to a lesser extent, increased pulmonary blood volumes decrease available space for pulmonary air.

Dead space is the volume of inhaled air that does not participate in gas exchange. *Anatomic dead space* includes the volume of conducting air that fills the nose, mouth, pharynx, larynx, trachea, bronchi, and the distal bronchial branching that does not participate in gas exchange (Fig. 10–14). Normal anatomic dead space is approximately 2 mL/kg. *Alveolar dead space* refers to the volume of gas that fills alveoli whose perfusion is abnormally reduced or absent. Factors that contribute to alveolar dead space include hypotension, compression of the alveolar capillary bed, and pulmonary embolus. Physiologic dead space is the sum of both anatomic and alveolar dead space. *Dead space ventilation* (V_D) refers to the amount of gas ventilating physiologic dead space per minute. Physiologic dead space is usually expressed as a fraction of tidal volume (V_D/V_T). The normal V_D/V_T ratio is 0.3, that is, 30% of the volume of each breath does not participate in gas exchange.

Minute ventilation (V_E) is the volume of air that moves in or out of the lungs per minute. Minute ventilation is the product of tidal volume and respiratory rate. *Alveolar ventilation* (V_A) is the volume per minute that ventilates all perfused alveoli and is the difference between minute ventilation and dead space ventilation ($V_A = V_E - V_D$). Whereas CO_2 production is dependent upon metabolic rate, CO_2 elimination from the lungs is determined by the effectiveness of V_A (TV, RR, V_D). Adequate alveolar ventilation is present when the $PaCO_2$ is maintained less than 40 mmHg with a normal V_E. With hyperventilation, V_E is high, driving down the $PaCO_2$; whereas with hypoventilation, V_E is low driving up the $PaCO_2$.

Forced vital capacity (FVC) is the volume of air forcibly exhaled after inhaling to total lung capacity. The volume of gas exhaled over time is usually plotted out to include the volume exhaled in 1 second (FEV_1) and the volume exhaled in 3 seconds (FEV_3). Patients with airway obstruction show a reduced rate of airflow on exhalation. The smaller the ratio of FEV_1 to FVC, the more difficult it is to exhale. Pre- and post-expiratory FVC measurements are used to assess the effectiveness of bronchodilating drugs in patients with obstructive airways disease.

Functional residual capacity (FRC) is the amount of air remaining in the lungs at the end of normal expiration. With atelectasis, FRC falls as the number of alveoli that participate in gas exchange decreases. Airway closure occurs in dependent areas of the lung at low volumes. The lung volume at which airway closure occurs is referred to as *closing capacity*. In adults, closing capacity is usually at residual volume (amount of air remaining in the lungs after maximal expiration). In infants, closing capacity is at FRC due to reduced elastic tissue, so closing capacity may be present during normal tidal breathing (Fig. 10–15). Pulmonary diseases that affect the relationship between tidal volume, FRC, and closing capacity contribute significantly to ventilation-perfusion mis-

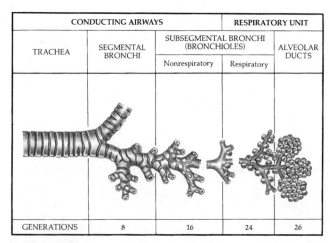

Figure 10–14 ● ● ● ● ● ●

Dead space ventilation continues down to the respiratory unit. (Modified from Weibel, E.R. (1963). *Morphemetry of the human lung.* Berlin: Springer-Verlag; in Thompson, J.M., McFarland, G.K., Hirsh, J.E., & Tucker, S.M. (1993). *Mosby's clinical nursing* (3rd ed., p. 123). St. Louis: Mosby–Year Book.)

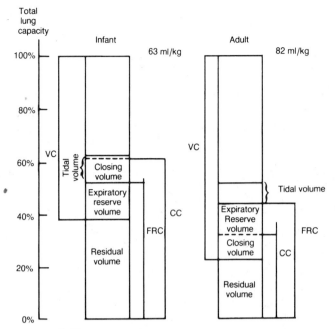

Figure 10–15 ● ● ● ● ●

Lung volumes in infants and adults. Note that tidal breathing in the infant takes place in the range of the closing capacity (CC) of the lung. VC, vital capacity; FRC, functional residual capacity. (From Smith, C.A., & Nelson, N.M. (1976). *The physiology of the newborn infant* (4th ed., p. 207). Springfield, IL: Charles C Thomas.)

match and hypoxemia. Positive end-expiratory pressure (PEEP), which increases FRC above closing capacity, helps to limit alveolar collapse.

Work of Breathing

Work of breathing, defined as the pressure generated by the respiratory muscles to move a volume of gas, can be divided into three components: (1) compliance work—required to expand the elastic forces of the lung; (2) resistance work—required to overcome the viscosity of the lung and thoracic cage; and (3) airways resistance—work required to overcome resistance to gas flow (Fig. 10–16). Under normal situations, most of the work of breathing is expended during inspiration to overcome the elastic properties of the lung.

Pulmonary disease can increase the work of breathing of any or all of the three components. Rapid respirations and increased airways resistance can cause expiratory work to surpass inspiratory work. Small changes in the work of breathing can significantly increase the metabolic rate and oxygen demand, resulting in respiratory muscle fatigue.

Ventilation-Perfusion Ratio

Gas exchange becomes optimal when both ventilation and pulmonary blood flow are equally matched. Under normal conditions, the *ventilation-to-perfusion ratio* (V/Q) is not equal to 1.0. This discrepancy is

due to gravitational forces that create regional differences in intrapleural pressures and pulmonary vascular pressures.

During spontaneous breathing, a greater proportion of air and perfusion is directed toward dependent areas of the lung. In the upright patient at rest between breaths, intrapleural pressures at the top of the lung are more negative than at the base of the lung, creating larger alveoli at the apex and smaller, more compliant alveoli at the base. During spontaneous inspiration, ventilation is preferentially distributed to the more compliant alveoli at the base rather than the apex. Similarly, gravitational forces distribute perfusion of the lung greatest in the base, and lowest in the apex. However, in total, ventilation is greater than perfusion at the apex and perfusion is greater than ventilation at the base. This results in an overall V/Q of 0.8.

West and others (1964) described regional differences in lung perfusion in upright adults (Fig. 10–17). West's zone I conditions occur when the mean pulmonary artery pressure is less than or equal to alveolar pressure (PA > Pa > Pv). Zone I conditions are present in the apices of an upright adult and are characterized by a lack of pulmonary blood flow and gas exchange. West's zone II conditions are characterized by pulmonary artery pressures greater than alveoli pressure (Pa > PA > Pv). Zone II conditions are present in the midportion of the lung and blood flow is determined by a balance of arterial and alveolar pressures, not influenced by venous pressures. West's zone III conditions are characterized by pulmonary artery and venous pressures that exceed alveolar pressures (Pa > Pv > PA). Zone III conditions are located at the base of the lung, and blood flow is a function of the two vascular pressures. Although

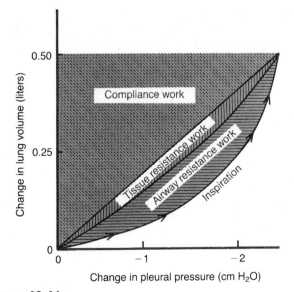

Figure 10–16 ● ● ● ● ● ●

Graphic representation of the three different types of work accomplished during inspiration. (From Guyton, A.C. (1991). *Textbook of medical physiology* (8th ed.). Philadelphia: W.B. Saunders.)

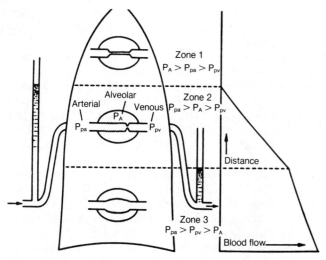

Figure 10–17 ● ● ● ● ● ●

Zones of perfusion in the lung. (From West, J.B., Dollery, C.T., & Naimark, A. (1964). Distribution of blood flow in isolated lung: Relation to vascular and alveolar pressures. *Journal of Applied Physiology, 19,* 713.)

similar research in the pediatric population does not exist, it is reasonable to assume that zone II and III conditions are similar in younger age groups. Because the height of the lung is reduced when lying flat, zone I conditions probably do not exist in the supine position, especially in the infant population (Helfaer, Nichols, & Rogers, 1992).

Ventilation-Perfusion Abnormalities

Intrapulmonary shunting is the major cause of clinical hypoxemia. Characterized by a low V/Q ratio, a *shunt* refers to venous blood that travels from the right to left side of the circulation without ever coming in contact with ventilated lung. Two categories of shunts exist: an anatomic shunt and a capillary shunt. An *anatomic shunt* refers to normal or abnormal R→L connections, for example, bronchial, pleural, and thebesian veins (the pulmonary circulation) or R→L congenital heart defects. A *capillary shunt* occurs when alveolar-capillary blood flow comes in contact with nonventilating alveoli, for example, atelectasis, pneumonia, and pneumothorax. As expected, mixing oxygenated and unoxygenated blood significantly impacts oxygenation and hypoxemia results (see Fig. 10–18).

Normally, an almost immediate diffusion of gases occurs over the alveolar-capillary membrane, so that arterial and alveolar gas concentrations are similar. Venous blood passing nonfunctional alveoli creates an admixture of venous and arterial blood, decreasing PaO_2. *Venous admixture* represents the ratio of shunted blood (Qs) to total pulmonary blood flow (Qt). The Qs/Qt ratio is calculated using the shunt equation: $Qs/Qt = (CpcO_2 - CaO_2)/(CpcO_2 - CvO_2)$, where $CpcO_2$, CaO_2, and CvO_2 are the pulmonary capillary, arterial, and mixed venous oxygen contents,

respectively. The $CpcO_2$ is computed using the alveolar gas equation ($PAO_2 = PiO_2 - PaCO_2/RQ$; where $PiO_2 = [760 - 47] \times FiO_2$ and the $RQ = 0.8$). The Qs/Qt normally ranges from 3% to 7%; changes greater than 5% are considered significant. Work of breathing significantly increases when the Qs/Qt is greater than 15%.

When a pulmonary artery catheter is not available to provide the mixed venous blood specimen necessary for calculating an intrapulmonary shunt, an alveolar-arterial PO_2 difference (A-aDO_2) or PaO_2/FiO_2 ratio can be used to estimate the percent shunt. The alveolar partial pressure of oxygen (PAO_2) is again calculated using the alveolar gas equation: $PAO_2 = PiO_2 - PaCO_2/RQ$ and the PaO_2 is obtained from a standard ABG report. To obtain an A-aDO_2, the PaO_2 is subtracted from the calculated PAO_2. Normally, the A-aDO_2 should be less than 20 mmHg. The PaO_2/FiO_2 ratio calculation is straightforward; the norm is greater than 286.

The magnitude of the shunt helps to determine what effect increasing the FiO_2 might have on the PaO_2. If the shunt is insignificant, changes in the PaO_2 will occur in direct proportion to changes in FiO_2. If the shunt is significant, increases in FiO_2 will not impact PaO_2. PEEP is used to increase FRC, which potentially decreases Qs/Qt and the risk of oxygen toxicity associated with the use of high FiO_2. Continuous assessment of the entire oxygenation profile is required to balance excessive PEEP, which may contribute to cardiac depression, and inadequate PEEP, which may contribute to progressive pulmonary hypoxemia.

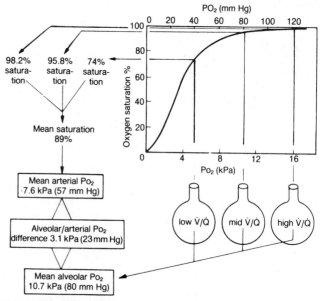

Figure 10–18 ● ● ● ● ● ●

The effect of V/Q scatter on PaO_2 and SaO_2. Three lung units with low, mid, and high V/Q ratios and PAO_2 of 40, 80, and 120 mmHg. Because of the shape of the ODC, the mean PaO_2 is only 57 mmHg and the mean saturation is only 89%. (From Nunn, J.F. (1977). *Applied respiratory physiology* (2nd ed., p. 284). London: Butterworths.)

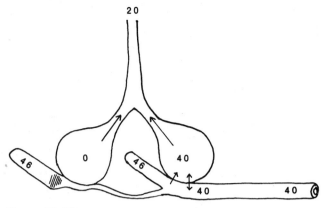

Figure 10-19 ● ● ● ● ●

Dead space unit. (From Swedlow, D.B. (1986). Capnometry and capnography: The anesthesia disaster early warning system. *Seminars in Anesthesia,* V (3), 194–205.)

In addition to the actual amount of shunted blood, the $C\bar{v}O_2$ of shunted blood also impacts CaO_2. The CaO_2 will fall if the shunted blood ($C\bar{v}O_2$) is more hypoxic secondary to increases in $\dot{V}O_2$ or decreases in $\dot{D}O_2$.

Characterized by a high V/Q ratio, *dead space* refers to alveoli that are ventilated but not perfused (Fig. 10–19). As discussed, $PaCO_2$ is determined by alveolar ventilation in relation to CO_2 production. Alveolar ventilation is compromised by increased dead space ventilation.

Physiologic dead space is calculated by the physiologic dead space/tidal volume ratio: $V_D/V_T = (PaCO_2 - PECO_2) \div PaCO_2$. This is measured by drawing an arterial sample to obtain a $PaCO_2$ and by collecting the patient's expired air in a Douglas bag or similar device for several minutes to obtain a P_ECO_2 (partial pressure of carbon dioxide in the mixed expired air).

Dead space ventilation can also be approximated by calculating an end-tidal CO_2-$PaCO_2$ gradient, the A-aDCO_2. In dead space units, mixed venous CO_2 is approximately 46 mmHg; alveolar CO_2 is 40 mmHg in the perfused unit, as is the pulmonary vein draining that unit. The alveolar CO_2 in the unperfused lung is zero because no blood has supplied it with CO_2. Downline, the arterial CO_2 is an average of only the units perfused (40/1 = 40 mmHg), and $ETCO_2$ is an average of all units ventilated (40/2 = 20 mmHg). Thus, with 50% dead space ventilation, the A-aDCO_2 will be 20 mmHg.

To compensate for increasing V_D/V_T, V_E must increase. Increases in V_E increase the work of breathing in direct proportion to increasing V_D/V_T. Thus, assessment of V_E (respiratory rate and tidal volume) and $PaCO_2$ levels are helpful tools in assessing dead space. If V_E increases, $PaCO_2$ levels should decrease if V_D/V_T is normal; if V_E increases and $PaCO_2$ remains the same, V_D/V_T is probably increased or pulmonary blood flow is decreased. The $PaCO_2$ is maintained at normal levels as long as the V_A can be maintained.

Various pulmonary diseases accentuate ventilation-perfusion abnormalities resulting in significant alterations in oxygenation and CO_2 removal. In fact, positive-pressure ventilation alone immediately contributes to V/Q mismatching; preferential ventilation is switched to nondependent areas, while preferential perfusion continues to dependent areas. Various physiologic mechanisms attempt to match ventilation to perfusion. For example, ventilation is altered by high CO_2 levels, which result in bronchodilation, whereas low CO_2 levels result in bronchoconstriction. Pulmonary arteriolar smooth muscle is very sensitive to the partial pressure of oxygen; increased alveolar oxygen results in vasodilation, and decreased alveolar oxygen results in vasoconstriction. This mechanism, known as *hypoxic pulmonary vasoconstriction* (HPV), attempts to enhance perfusion of well-ventilated alveoli and limit perfusion to unventilated alveoli. Many drugs used in the ICU can attenuate HPV. Propranolol and dopamine enhance HPV, whereas calcium channel blockers, vasodilators, beta-agonists, and anesthetic agents diminish HPV. Pulmonary arteriolar smooth muscle is also very sensitive to H^+ ion concentration, which is directly related to CO_2 concentration. An increase in H^+ ion concentration results in vasoconstriction and shunting of blood away from poorly ventilated alveoli with high alveolar CO_2 levels to better ventilated alveoli.

ASSESSMENT OF PULMONARY FUNCTIONING

History

Patient assessment begins with data collection to describe the scope of the patient's problem, to identify the progression of illness, and to help delineate the initial management plan. Often, especially in patients with chronic respiratory illnesses, parents provide excellent data particularly regarding the success of past management strategies.

When obtaining a medical history, interview depth and content are individualized to the age of the patient, the relevancy of information as it relates to the present illness, and the urgency of the current problem. For example, prenatal, natal, and postnatal history is relevant for infants admitted with a respiratory illness within the first year of life. If a perinatal history were significant, knowledge of whether the infant ever required assisted ventilation is important. Extensive questions about medication and environmental allergies are critical in patients with reactive airways disease. Questions related to fever are important if infection is suspected. Questions related to dietary intake, exercise tolerance, and school work may give clues related to the chronicity of the illness. As a general rule, infants and young children should not experience more than five uncomplicated upper respiratory infections per year. In patients with chronic respiratory illness, activity tolerance, oxygen dependency, home ventilator settings, and successful coping strategies provide meaningful baseline information.

Questions related to the onset of the present illness are also important. Acute-onset illnesses include asthma, pneumonia, and upper airway obstruction. Aspiration of a foreign body is suspected when the onset of distress is acute, especially in the inquisitive toddler. Chronic or recurrent illnesses suggest infection or an unresolved foreign body, but also allergic or immunologic problems, late-presentation congenital anomalies, or extrapulmonary problems such as heart disease or cancer.

Physical Assessment

Inspection

When first approaching an infant or young child, note the child's position of comfort. Infants and children normally assume a wide variety of positions to enable ventilation and limit the work of breathing. Classic positions include that of a drooling 3-year-old with epiglottitis whose survival depends on maintaining an upright position, usually tripod, with neck extended. Also classic is the older child with cystic fibrosis who while exhaling through pursed lips prefers to sit forward with arms supported on an overbed table. As a general rule, support the patient's attempts to find and maintain his or her own position of comfort.

Note the patient's facial expression; even young infants will appear tense, tired, and anxious when gas exchange is inadequate. Integrate the patient's level of consciousness into the examination; hypoxia will be reflected as anxious, restless, and irritable behavior, whereas hypercapnia produces drowsy and obtunded behavior. Note the presence of pallor or cyanosis. Skin color should be consistent with the individual's race. Cyanosis, a late sign of respiratory distress, will be evident when more than 5 g of reduced hemoglobin is present per deciliter of blood. Patients who are chronically cyanotic will exhibit clubbing of their distal phalanges.

Assess the rate, rhythm, and effort of breathing. Breathing is usually quiet and effortless; inspiration should be the only active phase of respiration. Respiratory rates in infants and children are highly variable, depending on age, medical history of lung disease, activity, anxiety level, and temperature. Respiratory rates are determined while the patient is at rest. Norms range from 30 to 60 in newborns, 20 to 40 in early childhood, and 15 to 25 during late childhood, reaching adult levels by age 15. Tachypnea is often the first sign of respiratory distress. With time, infants especially will fatigue and decrease their respiratory rates. The pattern of tachypnea followed by bradypnea with intermittent periods of apnea is a ominous sign.

Abnormal respiratory patterns are described in terms of rate, depth, and pattern (Table 10–7). Respiratory patterns vary considerably during the first year of life, that is, one minute the infant breathes slowly, then the next minute more rapidly. Apnea

Table 10–7. ABNORMAL RESPIRATORY PATTERNS

Type	Description	Etiology
Apnea	Absent	
Bradypnea	Slow for age	Hypothermia
		Drug-induced respiratory depression
		Increased ICP
		Metabolic alkalosis (intestinal obstruction)
Dyspnea	Difficult or labored breathing	Acute distress (pneumothorax)
		Chronic distress (cystic fibrosis)
		Intermittent distress (asthma)
Hyperpnea	Deep and rapid for age	
Kussmaul	Deep (fast or slow)	Diabetic ketoacidosis
Orthopnea	Intolerant of supine position	Asthma
		Pulmonary edema
Tachypnea (with respiratory distress)	Rapid for age	Pulmonary disease
Tachypnea (without respiratory distress)	Rapid for age	Nonpulmonary disease
		Metabolic acidosis
		Increased metabolic need
		Anxiety
		Severe diarrhea
		Salicylate toxicity
		Chronic renal insufficiency
		Inborn errors in metabolism
Apneustic	Extremely prolonged inspiratory periods	Stimulation of the apneustic center (located in the middle and lower pons) along with a vagotomy
Ataxic	Unpredictable, irregular	Cerebral dysfunction at the level of the medulla
Central neurogenic hyperventilation	Rapid, deep	Cerebral dysfunction at the midbrain level
Cheyne-Stokes	Cyclic hyperpnea-apnea pattern	Bilateral diencephalon dysfunction
Cluster	Irregular cluster	Cerebral dysfunction at the level of the pons

lasting greater than 15 seconds accompanied by duskiness, cyanosis, or respiratory rates greater than 60 breaths per minute is considered significant in the newborn (Endo & Nishioka, 1993).

Normal inspiratory:expiratory (I:E) ratio is 1:2. Prolonged inspiration occurs with upper airway obstruction, whereas prolonged expiration occurs with lower airway obstruction. Inspiratory stridor may also be present with upper airway disease, while expiratory wheezing is present with lower airways disease. Grunting, forced expiration against a partially closed glottis, accomplishes the same effect as pursed lip breathing in older children. Both occur in an attempt to maintain FRC, thus oxygenation. When present, consider oxygen administration if not already in place.

Note the shape of the chest. Chest deformities can limit vital capacity. Scoliosis is a lateral curvature of the spine at extreme resulting in an S-shaped configuration. Kyphosis is an exaggeration of the normal posterior convexity of the thoracic spine. In pectus carinatum, the sternum is displaced in an anterior position; in pectus excavatum, the sternum is displaced posteriorly.

Note how the chest moves. Early in infancy, diaphragmatic breathing is predominant and thoracic excursion is minimal; this reverses by 7 years of age. Diaphragmatic breathing produces a paradoxic breathing pattern: on inspiration, the lower ribs are pulled in while the abdomen is pushed out; the opposite is true on expiration. Paradoxic breathing becomes exaggerated—that is, it takes on a see-saw appearance—when pulmonary compliance is decreased. If paradoxic breathing is replaced by thoracic breathing in an infant, diaphragmatic dysfunction is suspected; if thoracic breathing is replaced by abdominal breathing in a child, parenchymal disease is suspected.

During a deep breath, confirm symmetric chest excursion. Unequal chest excursion is associated with atelectasis, pneumonia, thoracic trauma, or pneumothorax.

When respirations are labored, accessory muscles are recruited to support ventilation. The sternomastoid, scaleni, pectorals, internal and external intercostals, and abdominal muscles may contract visibly. Head bobbing, or extension of the neck on inspiration, indicates the use of neck accessory muscles. Nasal flaring on inspiration is frequently observed with labored respirations. Suprasternal, substernal, supraclavicular, and intercostal retractions may occur (Fig. 10–20). Retractions of the upper chest are associated with upper airway disease, whereas retractions of the lower chest usually suggest lower airways disease. As the work of breathing increases, so do oxygen requirements. Metabolic acidosis follows respiratory acidosis when the work of breathing exceeds the ability to provide adequate tissue oxygenation (Chameides, 1990).

Assess for the presence of a characteristic cough: for example, gradual/sudden onset, productive/nonproductive, dry/congested, associated with decreased/increased activity, able/unable to sleep, febrile/afebrile. A barking or croupy cough is present with laryngotracheobronchitis or epiglottitis. A progressive cough—that is, from dry to wet—is characteristic of congestive heart failure. Coughs due to bronchitis or pneumonia are congested. If a cough is productive, the sputum is described in terms of color, consistency, and odor. The significance of sputum color is as follows: white or clear with bronchitis or viral infections; yellow or green with bacterial infections; pink/frothy with pulmonary edema; and rust color with tuberculosis.

Palpation and Percussion

The entire chest wall is palpated for tactile fremitus, that is, palpable vibrations transmitted from the lung to the chest wall when the patient speaks or cries. Fremitus should be symmetric. Increased transmission is noted over areas of consolidation, for example, pneumonia or atelectasis. Decreased or absent transmission is noted over areas of decreased airflow, for example, in asthma, pneumothorax, or pleural effusion.

Percussion helps to determine whether the underlying tissue is air filled, fluid filled, or solid. The infant's round chest normally produces a hyperresonant pitch. A resonant pitch, indicating healthy lung, is present by age 6. After age 6, hyperresonance may indicate the pathologic presence of air, for example, with a pneumothorax. A resonant pitch before 6 years of age or a dull pitch thereafter indicates consolidation, for example, atelectasis, pneumonia, or pleural effusion.

Crepitus, or subcutaneous emphysema, occurs when free air enters subcutaneous tissue. When palpated, crepitus feels crunchy, creating a crackling sensation over the skin surface. Subcutaneous air may follow tracheotomy or any disruption in the larynx or trachea. Crepitus may also occur after a thoracentesis around the wound site or dissect large sur-

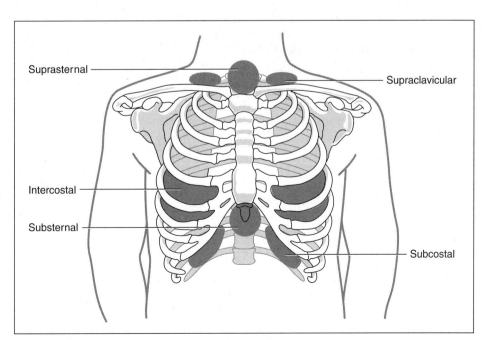

Figure 10–20 ● ● ● ● ●
Locations of retractions. (From Whaley, L.F., & Wong, D.L. (1991). *Nursing care of infants and children* (3rd ed., p. 1386). St. Louis: Mosby–Year Book.)

face areas as in patients with severe air-leak syndrome. Crepitus is usually self-limiting and does not require treatment; resolution occurs by reabsorption after resolution of the primary problem. On rare occasions, tracheal compression may require surgical intervention.

Auscultation

Three types of breath sounds can be auscultated in infants and children: bronchial, bronchovesicular, and vesicular (Table 10–8). Symmetry, comparing right and left sides, allows patients to serve as their own control. Progressing systematically from top to bottom, assess the pitch, intensity, and duration of each breath sound. Assess for (1) the presence and location of normal breath sounds; (2) the presence of normal breath sounds heard over abnormal locations; and (3) the presence of adventitious breath sounds.

Breath sounds are usually louder in infants and young children because the thinner chest wall brings the stethoscope closer to the origin of the sounds. Bronchovesicular sounds are usually auscultated throughout the lung periphery. Although seldom heard in infants, displaced bronchial breath sounds may indicate consolidation. Because breath sounds are easily transmitted throughout the small thoracic cavity, referred breath sounds are prevalent in infants and young children. Even when a significant pneumothorax is present, breath sounds can be auscultated over collapsed areas. Decreased breath sounds do occur in older children with obstructed bronchi, hyperinflated lungs, pneumothorax, or pleural effusion.

Three types of adventitious breath sounds can be identified: crackles, wheezes, and pleural rubs (Forgacs, 1978). Crackles are discrete noncontinuous sounds that can be simulated by rolling a lock of hair between your fingers near an ear. End-inspiratory crackles (previously termed crepitant rales) result from the reopening of previously collapsed alveoli, for example, during pneumonia and congestive heart failure. Early-inspiratory crackles (previously termed rhonchi) may be heard in the airway of patients with obstructive airways disease. Loud inspiratory and expiratory crackles may be heard with bronchiectasis.

Wheezes are musical sounds produced by the rapid passage of air through narrowed airways. Wheezing occurs more frequently in infants because of the size of their airways. Although wheezes are typically ex-

piratory, they may be heard on both inspiration and expiration. During normal spontaneous ventilation, intrathoracic airways widen during inspiration and narrow on exhalation, whereas the opposite is true of extrathoracic airways. Because maximum resistance to airflow occurs during expiration in intrathoracic airways and during inspiration in extrathoracic airways, expiratory wheezes usually indicate lower airway problems and inspiratory wheezes usually indicate upper airway problems. The disappearance of wheezing in a severe asthmatic may be disconcerting, as it may indicate that the patient is no longer moving air through narrowed airways.

Pleural rubs result from the friction generated by the movement of inflamed pleural surfaces over one another. Pleural rubs are usually painful, loud yet low pitched, synchronous with respiration, and confined to a small surface area.

When assessing adventitious sounds, the location and timing—that is, when in the respiratory cycle they are auscultated—are noted.

Assessment of the Intubated Infant/Child

When caring for an infant or child with an endotracheal tube (ETT), assessment priorities include patient safety and comfort. Assess the security of the ETT. Ensure that the tape securing the ETT is adherent to the skin *and* ETT. Compare the ETT exit markings at the lip/nare line with those noted immediately post intubation or after the ETT was last repositioned. Assess for the potential of ETT-induced pressure necrosis to the nare or corner of the mouth. If present, reposition and retape the ETT as soon as possible.

Once ETT security has been addressed, determine whether the ETT itself is causing respiratory distress. Inadequate ETT size will precipitate signs and symptoms of upper airway obstruction. Determine whether there is excessive ETT length that may contribute dead space. If the patient is hypercapnic, consider shortening the ETT to a reasonable length after confirming correct ETT placement on chest x-ray with the patient's head in neutral position.

Assess the comfort level of the infant or child. Provide a level of sedation necessary to ensure airway maintenance. This is highly individual, as patient tolerance may be high or extremely low. Freedom sleeves or limb restraints are essential to prevent unintentional extubation. Ensure that the ETT and tubing are supported to allow head movement but prevent accidental extubation, especially in the active infant and child. Drain oxygen delivery tubing of condensation on a regular basis to prevent inadvertent water entry into the patient's airway and unnecessary weight on the patient's ETT. All equipment necessary to reintubate the individual infant or child as well as an emergency tracheostomy tray should be readily available in the unit.

Patients with oral and nasal ETTs are assessed in

Table 10–8. NORMAL BREATH SOUNDS

Breath Sound	I:E Ratio	Pitch	Intensity	Location
Bronchial	I≤E	High	Loud	Large airways
Bronchovesicular	I=E	Moderate	Moderate	Mid airway and peripheral lung fields
Vesicular	I>E	Low	Soft	Peripheral lung fields

a similar manner. Awake children with oral ETTs may require a bite block to prevent biting down on the ETT. Children with an altered level of consciousness and oral ETT may require an oral airway. Additionally, nasal ETTs can obstruct eustachian tubes, which empty into the nasopharynx. There should be a high index of suspicion for middle ear infections whenever caring for patients with nasal ETTs.

When caring for an infant or child with a new tracheostomy tube (TT), priorities again include patient safety and comfort. Tracheostomy holders are assessed for security. The entire neck is assessed for skin breakdown under the tracheostomy holder. The character of the tracheostomy site is assessed for infection. Dressings or sponges are examined for drainage. If the patient is connected to a ventilator, potential pressure points created by the TT adapter should be cushioned. Finally, an extra same-size tracheostomy tube should be positioned in clear view at the bedside in case of an emergency.

Assessment of the Ventilated Infant/Child

Assessment of the infant or child supported on mechanical ventilation includes (1) assessing patient-ventilator synchrony, (2) validating the ventilator settings and alarm systems, and (3) assessing for the presence of airleaks around uncuffed endotracheal or tracheostomy tubes.

Start by assessing the patient's level of comfort. Does the infant or child appear anxious? Is chest expansion adequate during a delivered breath? Is the I:E ratio normal? Is the inspiratory time (IT) too short? Does the patient have enough time to exhale before receiving another breath? Is the patient able to generate a sufficient number of adequate spontaneous breaths? Is the patient tachypneic?

Next check the ventilator settings to ensure that the patient is on the intended settings. Ensure that alarm settings are activated and are within a tight range to call immediate attention to problems.

Assess for the presence of an airleak on end-inspiration. Airleaks are not uncommon in infants or children with uncuffed ETTs, especially when pulmonary compliance is low. Airleaks should be quantified. When measured tidal volumes are significantly compromised, airleaks can be addressed by ventilator or patient manipulations. Ventilator manipulations include those that result in increasing the delivered tidal volume to compensate for the airleak. Patient manipulations range from simply changing head position to reintubating the patient with a larger ETT or TT.

If a cuffed ETT or TT is in place and delivered tidal volumes are compromised, consider inflating the cuff with just enough volume to eliminate the airleak. This *minimal occlusion volume* (MOV) technique is accomplished by placing a stethoscope over the larynx and slowly inflating the cuff until sounds cease over the larynx. Once the airleak is eliminated, cuff pressures are obtained to ensure that the cuff

pressure is less than 20 mmHg. Most tubes will seal at pressures between 14 and 20 mmHg. The amount of pressure and volume to obtain a seal and prevent mucosal pressure depends on tube size and design, cuff configuration, mode of ventilation, and the individual's airway and arterial pressure. Mucosal ischemia occurs when lateral wall pressure exceeds capillary perfusion pressure resulting in decreasing mucosal blood flow (Boggs, 1993). Iatrogenic complications from cuff inflation include tracheal stenosis, necrosis, tracheoesophageal fistula, and tracheomalacia.

If cuff total occlusion is unnecessary, consider the *minimal leak volume* (MLV) technique. Here a stethoscope is again placed over the larynx. The cuff is inflated then slowly deflated until a small airleak is heard at end-inspiration. Check to ensure that the airleak is occurring at less than 20 mmHg inflating pressure or directly measure the cuff pressure.

When patients are chemically paralyzed, assessments include the adequacy of the paralysis. Initial movements hallmarking the need for additional chemical paralyzing agent include abdominal fasciculations as the patient attempts to inhale. Train-of-four monitoring is becoming increasingly prevalent in the management of the chemically paralyzed patient (see Chapter 20). Table 10–9 provides a summary of the primary and secondary assessment parameters for the ventilated infant/child.

NONINVASIVE PULMONARY INTENSIVE CARE MONITORING

Recognizing the technical difficulties and associated risks of invasive pediatric monitoring, there has

Table 10–9. ASSESSMENT OF THE VENTILATED PATIENT

Primary Survey	
General appearance	**Breath sounds**
Skin color	Equality
Airway—ETT size, cuffed/uncuffed, amount of dead space	Normal and adventitious
Spontaneous respiratory effort	Quality of spontaneous and ventilator breaths
Respiratory excursion—ventilator and spontaneous breaths	
Abdominal distension	
Level of responsiveness/comfort	
Muscle tone	
Respiratory rate	**Airleak**
Ventilator + spontaneous = total	Endotracheal tube
	Chest tubes
Presence of subcutaneous air	**Noninvasive gas monitoring**
	SpO_2; $ETco_2$; tidal volume

Secondary Survey	
Ventilator settings and safety check	**Chest x-rays**
Blood studies	**Hemodynamic and oxygenation profiles**
Arterial blood gases	
Hemoglobin	

been a literal explosion in noninvasive monitoring techniques. It is essential that as alternative monitoring techniques become available for use in the pediatric population, they be valid and reliable. Pediatric monitors must not only accommodate the wide range of sizes but also be sensitive enough to detect both the rapid and small quantitative physiologic changes that frequently hallmark pediatric crisis states. Low arterial pressures, cardiac outputs, and oxygen reserves matched with high oxygen requirements offer little buffer and require rapid detection.

Effective clinical use of any technology requires an understanding of what is actually measured, how it is measured, and the patient care requirements for applying that technology. This section focuses upon these issues as they relate to noninvasive monitoring of pulmonary function.

Pulse Oximetry

Continuous monitoring of oxygen saturation has made a significant impact on patient assessment in the past decade. Unlike measuring arterial blood gases (ABGs), pulse oximetry provides *continuous* arterial hemoglobin saturation (SpO_2) data and almost immediate detection of hypoxemic events.

Since oxygen is primarily transported in blood chemically attached to hemoglobin, SpO_2 monitoring provides a more complete picture of the patient's oxygenation status. Saturation monitoring also provides a more reliable indicator of hypoxemia during extreme shifts of the ODC: inadequate oxygenation in spite of a PaO_2 greater than 50 mmHg during a shift of the ODC to the right or adequate oxygenation in spite of a PaO_2 less than 50 mmHg during a shift of the ODC to the left. In the upper part of the ODC, small changes in SaO_2 correspond to very large and potentially toxic levels of PaO_2. Bucher and others (1989) reported that when SpO_2 was maintained at less than 96%, the PaO_2 was never higher than 100 mmHg. The researchers proposed that maintaining the patient's SpO_2 around 96% would prevent hyperoxia. Manufacturers claim an error factor of less than 3% at an SpO_2 greater than 70%.

Mechanism of Measurement

Pulse oximeters measure the absorption of two wavelengths of light passed through pulsating tissue (Fig. 10–21). Oxyhemoglobin and reduced hemoglobin absorb varying degrees of light. For a given site, the light absorption of bone, tissue, venous blood, and arterial blood remains constant except for the absorption from the added blood volume associated with arterial pulsation. The varying absorption is translated into two waveforms, and the ratio between the amplitude of these waveforms is used to calculate the SpO_2.

Pulse oximeters update SpO_2 with each heart beat. They provide accurate data to heart rates of 250 beats per minute. A high correlation between heart

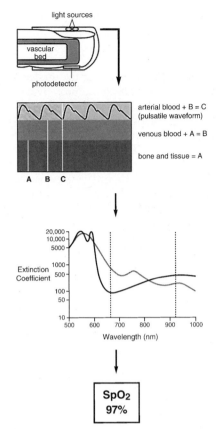

Figure 10–21 ● ● ● ● ● ●

Pulse oximeters measure the absorption of two wavelengths of light passed through pulsating tissue. Oxyhemoglobin and reduced hemoglobin absorb varying degrees of light. For a given site, the light absorption of bone, tissue, venous blood, and arterial blood remains constant except for the absorption from the added blood volume associated with arterial pulsation. The varying absorption is translated into two waveforms, and the ratio between the amplitude of these waveforms is used to calculate the SpO_2. (Reprinted by permission of Nellcor Puritan Bennett, Pleasanton, CA.)

rates obtained from a cardiac monitor and SpO_2 monitor helps to establish the reliability of SpO_2 data. Qualitative analysis of perfusion is also available by assessment of the perfusion bar, which pulsates with each heart beat. An audible tone varies in pitch according to saturation. This feature is very important during procedures that may affect SaO_2; attention can be paid to the procedure while listening for changes in the tone of the pulse oximeter indicating changes in saturation.

Sensors contain three optical components: two light sources (red and infrared) and one light receiver. To function properly, the sensor must be positioned so that the light source and photodetector oppose one another (see Fig. 10–21). Sensors are available in various shapes and sizes to facilitate monitoring at different locations and size patients (Fig. 10–22). If the patient is sensitive to adhesive, it can be removed with adhesive remover. The sensor is then attached using a gauze dressing. All sensor sites are assessed frequently for skin abrasion and circulatory impairment. Pressure necrosis may occur when a sensor is placed too tightly. During magnetic resonance imaging, Bashein & Syrory (1991) reported that the pulse oximeter patient cable can act as an antenna, causing second and third degree burns to the skin. Care should be taken to position cables away from the magnet and patient skin.

To enhance performance, the sensor is placed at the level of the heart on an extremity without a vascular line or blood pressure cuff. In infants with R→L shunting, the right hand is used for preductal SpO_2 and the left hand or either foot is used for postductal SpO_2.

Troubleshooting. Interference with SpO_2 readings typically result from problems related to the signal to noise ratio. Too little signal may result from poor perfusion or improper probe placement; too much noise may result from excessive motion, ambient light, electrocautery, or a venous pressure wave.

Sensors incorporate ambient light protection, but strong light sources—for example, fluorescent, procedural, and bilirubin lights—may interfere with SpO_2 measurement. Problems with ambient light are easily resolved by covering the sensors with a blanket. Patient motion may also affect system performance. Occasionally, a large dicrotic notch may be sensed as a separate arterial pulse resulting in twice the actual heart rate. Models that synchronize SpO_2 readings with the QRS complex are available to limit this problem.

Any event that significantly reduces arterial pulsation will affect SpO_2 readings. Although accurate to extremely low mean arterial pressures, pulsations may be lost with severe hypotension, low cardiac output states, or in patients on VA ECMO. Oximetry may also fail in patients with severe anemia or hemodilution, for example, when the hemoglobin is less than 5 g/dL. High bilirubin levels do not affect SpO_2 readings.

Alkhudhairi and others (1990) evaluated pulse oximetry readings during profound hypothermia associated with cardiac surgery. Ten pediatric patients were cooled to 25°C. Arterial saturation was overestimated by the pulse oximeter between 30° and 36°C, whereas arterial saturation was underestimated by the pulse oximeter when the temperature was less than 30°C. The authors noted that when the starting saturation is low, vasoconstriction may essentially stop flow to the finger but the pulse may be maintained.

Significant venous pulsations can also lead to inaccurate low SpO_2 readings. This occurs when a sensor is wrapped too tightly; when the sensor is placed on a dependent limb; or during decreased venous return states, such as increased intrathoracic pressure, congestive heart failure, or during a Valsalva maneuver. Falsely low readings can also occur if the finger probe is malpositioned beyond the fingertip (Kellehen & Ruff, 1989).

Because of the different ways saturation is measured, pulse oximetry data cannot be exactly validated by other saturation measures. Pulse oximeters are calibrated to read functional hemoglobin or the percentage of hemoglobin available to bind with oxygen. Saturation readings obtained with ABG reports are calculated from PaO_2 values and thus may be invalid due to shifts in the ODC. Specific requests for a measured SaO_2 with a co-oximeter in the labora-

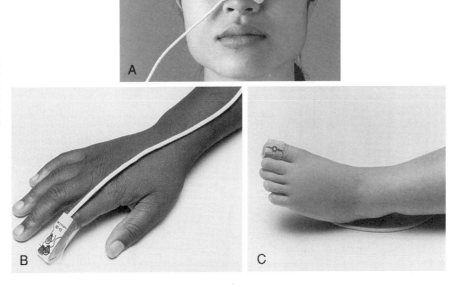

Figure 10–22 ● ● ● ● ● ●

A to *C*, Sensors contain three optical components—two light sources and one light receiver—and are available in various shapes and sizes to facilitate monitoring at different locations and size patients. (Reprinted by permission of Nellcor Puritan Bennett, Pleasanton, CA.)

tory will provide fractional SaO_2 readings, e.g., carboxyhemoglobin and methemoglobin. All carboxyhemoglobin will be counted as oxyhemoglobin by the pulse oximeter. When methemoglobin levels are less than 20%, the pulse oximeter will add one half the actual percent to the SpO_2 reading. When methemoglobin levels are greater than 20%, the pulse oximeter will always read 85%. The impact of methemoglobin levels on pulse oximeter values is important when medications that increase these levels are prescribed (Dapsone and nitric oxide). Lastly, when high concentrations of fetal hemoglobin are present, because of absorption differences, the laboratory co-oximeter reports erroneously high carboxyhemoglobin and low oxyhemoglobin fractions.

Clinical Applications

Saturation monitoring is considered a standard in most pediatric ICUs. SpO_2 readings are particularly helpful as a continuous monitor of intrapulmonary shunt (Qs/Qt) and during pulmonary care and titration of oxygen therapy. Continuous monitoring of SpO_2 levels while weaning FiO_2 eliminates the need for repeated blood gases.

End-Tidal CO_2 Monitoring

Until recently, the only method to quantify the adequacy of ventilation was through assessment of arterial blood gases (ABGs). End-tidal CO_2 monitoring provides a noninvasive continuous real-time measurement of end-exhaled CO_2 gases. Normally, if ventilation and perfusion are well matched, the $ETCO_2$ closely approximates the $PaCO_2$ (Fig. 10–23A). As illustrated, mixed venous CO_2 (blood returning from the systemic circulation) is approximately 46 mmHg. Carbon dioxide rapidly diffuses into the alveolar space until the alveolar pulmonary-capillary CO_2 and the alveolar CO_2 become equal at 40 mmHg. Thus, downline at the sampling points, arterial and $ETCO_2$ should be approximately equal at 40 mmHg. In those with normal lungs, the A-aDCO_2 gradient (difference between alveolar and arterial CO_2) is usually less that 2 to 3 mmHg with $ETCO_2$ lower than arterial PCO_2. Changes in the noninvasive $ETCO_2$ will continuously reflect changes in the invasive $PaCO_2$ or the A-aDCO_2 gradient.

Mechanism of Measurement

The most common device used to measure CO_2 concentration in exhaled gases is the infrared analyzer or capnometer. The analyzer makes use of the fact that gaseous CO_2 absorbs infrared light within a specific wavelength range, specifically waves about 4.3 μm in length. As this narrow band of light is projected through a gas sample, an attenuation of the light beam results and the intensity of attenuated light is measured. The greater the concentration of CO_2, the greater the absorption and less infrared detection by the sample detector cell.

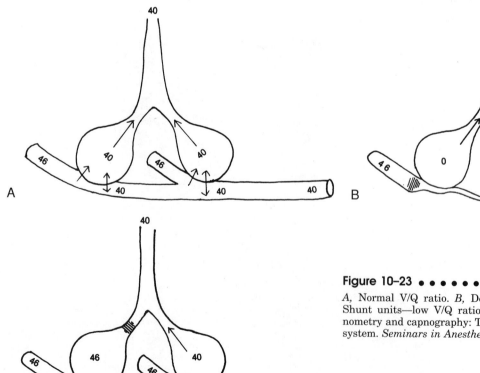

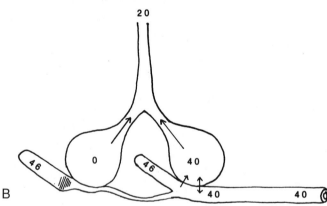

Figure 10–23 ● ● ● ● ● ●

A, Normal V/Q ratio. *B,* Dead space units—high V/Q ratio. *C,* Shunt units—low V/Q ratio. (From Swedlow, D.B. (1986). Capnometry and capnography: The anesthesia disaster early warning system. *Seminars in Anesthesia,* V (3), 194–205.)

There are two basic types of sampling techniques: sidestream or mainstream. With the sidestream capnometer, the gas sample is continuously aspirated from the respiratory circuit through a small-bore tube leading to a sensing chamber within a monitor. With the mainstream capnometer, the sensor is incorporated between the ventilator circuit and an artificial airway.

An advantage to the sidestream monitor is that it can be used in the intubated or non-intubated patient. In the non-intubated patient, the aspirating tube is placed at or a few centimeters into the nare. This technique may not be tolerated by the patient or the results may not be acceptable if mouth breathing is present. Also, if the monitor entrains room air, the readings will be falsely low, providing a false sense of security when alveolar hypoventilation is present. Further disadvantages to the sidestream capnometer include a total delay time (Pascucci, Schena, & Thompson, 1989), a falsely low $ETCO_2$ created by high aspirating flow rates, and potential for analyzer contamination if water and mucus is drawn back into the monitor. An airway adapter with water trap has been designed to address the last problem.

Mainstream capnometers require intubation and have two main advantages. First, delay time is less and water or moisture is less apt to affect sensor function. It has also been reported that mainstream capnometers more accurately reflect $ETCO_2$ data in pediatrics (Pascucci, Schena, & Thompson, 1989). A disadvantage, especially in pediatrics, is that some sensors are heavy and require support to avoid tension on the endotracheal tube and the size may add excessive dead space.

Capnometers differ but may require a two-point calibration: to a zero CO_2 point (100% oxygen) and to a second CO_2 point within the range of CO_2 to be measured (5% CO_2). Capnometers used in the pediatric population must be able to rapidly respond to changes in CO_2, respond to the small exhaled volumes, and be sensitive to track small changes in CO_2.

Clinical Applications

Capnography is the recording and analysis of waveforms produced by changes in the level of exhaled CO_2. Capnograms can be recorded at a slow (12.5 mm/sec) or fast (25 mm/sec) speed (Fig. 10–24). The vertical axis represents CO_2 concentration, whereas the horizontal axis represents time. Slow recordings are suitable for trending baseline and $ETCO_2$ levels. Fast recordings allow individual waveform analysis. Any factor that alters CO_2 production, CO_2 transport to the lungs, alveolar ventilation, V/Q ratio, and CO_2 transport to the sampling site will affect the $ETCO_2$.

Capnogram Analysis: Slow Speed

CO_2 Production. Changes in CO_2 production are usually matched by changes in minute ventilation, so $ETCO_2$ levels should remain constant. In those unable to alter their tidal volumes or respiratory

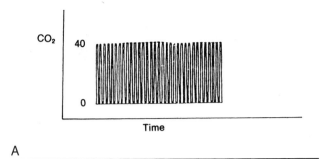

A

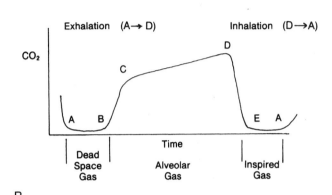

B

Figure 10–24 ● ● ● ● ● ●

A, Slow-speed capnogram recorded at 12.5 mm/second. *B,* Fast-speed capnogram recorded at 25 mm/second. (Reprinted from *Pediatric Nursing,* 1990, Volume 16, Number 4, p. 397. Reprinted with permission of the publisher, Jannetti Publications, Inc., East Holly Avenue Box 56, Pitman, NJ 08071-0056; Phone (609) 256-2300; FAX (609) 589-7463.)

rates sufficiently, increased production will be manifested by increased $ETCO_2$ whereas decreased production will be manifested by decreased $ETCO_2$. Fever, pain, stress, increased muscle activity (seizures and shivering), sodium bicarbonate infusion, increased carbohydrate intake, malignant hyperthermia, and hyperthyroidism all increase CO_2 production. Hypothermia and increased fat intake decrease CO_2 production.

Dead Space. As discussed, alveoli can only eliminate CO_2 that is presented by the pulmonary capillary membrane, so changes in lung perfusion will be reflected in the capnogram (see Fig. 10–23B). The $ETCO_2$ will fall in shock states, when excessive positive end-expiratory pressure (PEEP) is used, or in those with a pulmonary embolus. These states are characterized by a high ventilation/perfusion (V/Q) ratio or dead space units (see previous discussion). The A-aDCO_2 gradient can be followed to detect insidious shock and evaluate response to treatment.

During a cardiac arrest, the $ETCO_2$ acutely disappears, reappearing only when circulation is restored by effective cardiac resuscitation. The extent to which advanced life support measures maintain cardiac output can be rapidly assessed by $ETCO_2$ monitoring (Fig. 10–25A).

Hypo/Hyperventilation. With alveolar hypoventilation, the arterial and $ETCO_2$ both increase. Hypo-

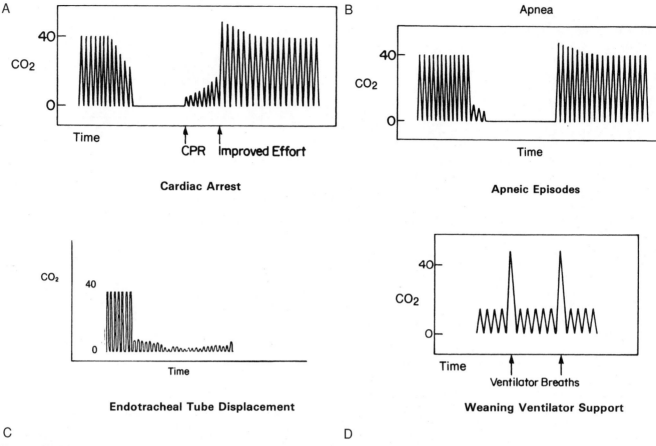

A

Cardiac Arrest

B

Apnea

Apneic Episodes

Endotracheal Tube Displacement

C

Weaning Ventilator Support

D

Figure 10–25 ● ● ● ● ●

Slow-speed capnograms. *A,* Cardiac arrest. Decreased perfusion to the pulmonary vascular bed will gradually decrease the ET_{CO_2}. *B,* Apneic episodes. ET_{CO_2} disappears during apneic episodes, then overshoots previous readings. *C,* Endotracheal tube displacement. ET_{CO_2} will fall to zero when the ETT is displaced. *D,* Weaning ventilator support. Note that the ET_{CO_2} is lower during spontaneous breaths than during ventilator breaths. (Reprinted from *Pediatric Nursing,* 1990, Volume 16, Number 4, p. 397. Reprinted with permission of the publisher, Jannetti Publications, Inc., East Holly Avenue Box 56, Pitman, NJ 08071-0056; Phone (609) 256-2300; FAX (609) 589-7463.)

ventilation may occur in those with central nervous system depression, neuromuscular disease, and in the chemically paralyzed patient with inadequate ventilator parameters.

When hypoventilation is severe (where air only in the conducting airways is moved), the ET_{CO_2} will decrease. With apnea, the ET_{CO_2} disappears completely because CO_2 is no longer transported from the lungs to the gas-sampling point (see Fig. 10–25*B*). Capnography is thus a good apnea alarm because periods of apnea can be confirmed, timed, and documented. The ET_{CO_2} reappears after ventilation is restored and usually overshoots previous readings.

Alveolar hyperventilation decreases ET_{CO_2} and arterial CO_2. An important application of ET_{CO_2} monitoring is in the cerebral hypertensive patient in whom CO_2 retention produces pronounced cerebral vasodilation and further compromises intracranial pressure.

Shunt Unit. The pathophysiologic effects of shunting, characterized by a low ventilation/perfusion (V/Q) ratio, are seen in many pulmonary disease states (see Fig. 10–23*C*). In shunt units, those that are perfused but not ventilated, mixed venous CO_2 is

approximately 46 mmHg. The alveolar CO_2 is 40 mmHg in the ventilated unit, as is the pulmonary vein draining that unit. The alveolar CO_2 in the unventilated unit is 46 mmHg because it is in equilibrium with its pulmonary capillary membrane. Downline, the arterial CO_2 is an average of all the lung units perfused (46 + 40/2 = 43 mmHg) and ET_{CO_2} is an average of all units ventilated (40/1 = 40 mmHg). Thus, with a 50% shunt, the A-aD_{CO_2} will be only 3 mmHg. Shunt units are characterized by an undramatic A-aD_{CO_2} gradient but a dramatic decrease in arterial saturation.

Endotracheal Tube Placement. ET_{CO_2} monitoring of unstable intubated chemically paralyzed patients helps to reduce iatrogenic injury (Eichhorn, Cooper, Cullen et al., 1986). ET_{CO_2} monitoring helps to determine correct endotracheal tube placement, as little or no CO_2 reading can be gained from the esophagus. ET_{CO_2} monitoring also allows for rapid detection of ETT displacement (see Fig. 10–25*C*).

Weaning from the Ventilator. ET_{CO_2} monitoring can be an effective, noninvasive way to monitor alveolar ventilation in patients who are being weaned from mechanical ventilation. Ventilator rates can be gradually decreased to the lowest point at which the patient can comfortably maintain effective alveolar ventilation. If the $ETCO_2$ rises or if the patient appears to be working too hard as evidenced by rapid spontaneous respiratory rates, ventilator rates can be returned to previously acceptable settings.

In patients with chronic pulmonary disease, the $ETCO_2$ of spontaneous breaths may be much lower than the $ETCO_2$ of larger ventilator-initiated breaths (see Fig. 10–25D). Generally, stability of the $ETCO_2$ during spontaneous and ventilator breaths indicates the patient's readiness for weaning ventilator breaths. Use of this assessment parameter is especially helpful in weaning patients where there is uncertainty as to whether they can physiologically resume the work of breathing. Noninvasive gas monitoring is less traumatic for the patient in relation to the pain and anxiety of ABGs.

Capnogram Analysis: Fast Speed

The normal capnogram, recorded at a fast speed, is illustrated in Figure 10–24B. At the beginning of exhalation, the CO_2 concentration is zero as primarily dead space of the conducing airways empties of its CO_2-free gas (A-B). As exhalation continues, there is a steep rise in CO_2 tension when dead space gas mixes with CO_2-rich alveolar gas (B-C). Levels quickly reach a near-constant horizontal plateau representing CO_2-rich alveolar gas that has been in equilibrium with the pulmonary capillary membrane (C-D). The end-point of this segment, the highest value of CO_2 concentration at the end of normal exhalation in the upper right corner of the waveform, is the $ETCO_2$ (D). Immediately following $ETCO_2$, the CO_2 concentration falls, indicating dilution of CO_2-rich gas with CO_2-free inspired gas (D-E). Finally, only inspired gas is present at the gas-sampling port, producing the inspiratory baseline. Capnographic characteristics vary and can be diagnostic of certain disease states.

First assess the baseline CO_2 level. Baseline CO_2 should be zero because it primarily represents previously inspired dead space CO_2-free gas. Any increase in baseline indicates that rebreathing is occurring (Fig. 10–26A).

Next assess the slope where dead space gas mixes with CO_2-rich alveolar gas. The slope should be nearly vertical to the plateau phase. Occasionally, the slope is significant to the point at which the plateau disappears (Fig. 10–26B). This is caused by lung units emptying at different rates, prolonged exhalation secondary to small airway obstruction (asthma), or a partially kinked ETT. A good alveolar plateau ensures that the $ETCO_2$ is a reliable estimate of mixed alveolar gas.

Capnograms can be useful in assessing the effectiveness of bronchodilator treatments in the asthmatic patient and/or racemic epinephrine treatments in the patient with laryngotracheobronchitis. A decrease in the slope, less peaking of the $ETCO_2$, and an increase in plateauing all correlate with a positive

response to treatment in the patient with severe obstruction (Fig. 10–26C).

With atelectasis, a CO_2 blip followed by a sharp terminal rise in $ETCO_2$ appears as trapped air at end-exhalation is released (see Fig. 10–26D). These blips and peaks can be smoothed out when adequate PEEP is applied. Capnography provides rapid feedback on the effects of changing ventilator settings that control minute ventilation, tidal volume, and respiratory rates. The necessity for frequent ABGs can be avoided.

Partial neuromuscular blockade or return of voluntary function will be first seen in capnograms as a cleft in the alveolar plateau (see Fig. 10–26E). This is caused by the rush of CO_2-free gas as the diaphragm contracts. Capnograms can provide early information that more chemical paralyzing agent is needed.

Descending limb analysis also provides information. A staircase effect on the descending limb is seen when a pneumothorax is present (see. Fig. 10–26F). When chest tubes are in place, a staircase effect may indicate chest tube obstruction.

$ETCO_2$ monitoring provides a continuous real-time monitor, thus closer surveillance of the adequacy of ventilation. $ETCO_2$ does not completely replace ABGs because the $ETCO_2$ measure is not the same as the $PaCO_2$ in many clinical situations. $ETCO_2$ monitoring also provides information that is not derivable from ABGs alone. The A-aDCO_2 gradient can render a $ETCO_2$ useful rather than being a limitation. Presence of an appreciable gradient indicates a serious V/Q disturbance, whereas closure of the gradient indicates effective treatment or improvement of lung disease. Capnography provides a useful adjunct to the more frequently used methods of respiratory system assessment and provides early detection of potentially dangerous trends that can be reversed before crises result.

INVASIVE PULMONARY INTENSIVE CARE MONITORING

Critically ill patients require rapid titration of therapy based upon astute and accurate assessments of hemodynamic and oxygenation data. The instruments that provide data have evolved significantly in recent years. What has also developed is how we use hemodynamic and oxygenation profile data to optimize care. For example, the cardiovascular and respiratory systems are interrelated. Alterations in one system often elicit a change in the other. Achieving and maintaining optimal functioning of both systems are fundamental objectives in critical care. This section reviews invasive monitoring of cardiopulmonary function in critically ill pediatric patients, including the clinical significance of direct and derived data and the importance of trending the determinates of DO_2 and O_2 utilization.

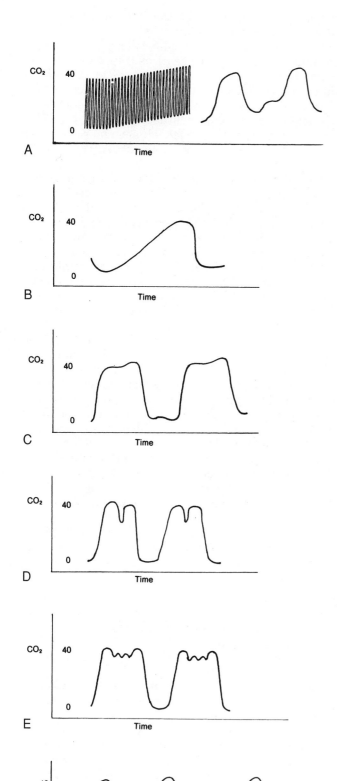

Figure 10–26 ● ● ● ● ●

Fast-speed capnograms. *A,* Rebreathing. Rebreathing will produce a gradual increase in the baseline; recorded at slow and fast speeds. *B,* Plateau disappearance. Asthma: increased slope, peaking of the ET_{CO_2}, and loss of plateau. *C,* Plateau reappearance. Decreased slope, less peaking of the ET_{CO_2}, and better plateau after bronchodilator treatment; *D,* CO_2 blip. Occurs as trapped CO_2 gas is released at end-exhalation. *E,* Cleft in the alveolar plateau. Indicates the return of spontaneous breathing. *F,* Staircase effect. Pneumothorax. (Reprinted from *Pediatric Nursing,* 1990, Volume 16, Number 4, p. 397. Reprinted with permission of the publisher, Jannetti Publications, Inc., East Holly Avenue Box 56, Pitman, NJ 08071-0056; Phone (609) 256-2300; FAX (609) 589-7463.)

Blood Gas Analysis

Blood gases are analyzed for two major reasons: (1) to directly assess the patient's oxygenation and ventilation status, and (2) to provide information regarding the patient's acid/base status. Blood gas analysis can be performed using arterial, venous, or capillary blood. *Arterial blood gas* (ABG) analysis provides primary information about the adequacy of the lungs to oxygenate blood. *Venous blood gas* (VBG) analysis provides indirect information regarding tissue perfusion and Vo_2. *Capillary blood gas* (CBG) analysis provides limited information that can be trended over time when arterial and venous blood gases are unavailable.

Limitations associated with blood gas analysis include the procedure. Unless vascular access is available, a painful and perhaps time-consuming procedure is performed. Blood gases are expensive, require the removal of oxygen-carrying cells from the patient, and provide only intermittent data. Blood gases are also not infallible. They can be altered by the amount of heparin in the syringe, by the amount of time the specimen sits before analysis, and by hyperventilation or breath holding if the patient cries during the procedure.

Arterial Blood Gases

ABGs are obtained through an existing arterial line or by arterial puncture. The sites most commonly used for arterial puncture include the radial, dorsalis pedis, posterior tibial, and femoral arteries. The femoral artery is the last choice, as hemorrhage and hematomas are difficult to control in this area and because of the high potential for limb ischemia if artery damage occurs.

To perform an arterial puncture, a setup typically consisting of a 23 or 25 gauge butterfly needle attached to a 1 to 3 mL heparinized syringe is prepared. Preheparinized syringes are now available and should be used to save pharmacy, nursing, and laboratory expense: pharmacy, to avoid the waste of discarding partially used vials of heparin (1:1000 U/mL concentration); nursing, in the time it takes to prepare a heparinized syringe; and laboratory, in the expense of having to repeat an ABG with an erroneously low pH linked to having too much heparin in the syringe.

Before attempting arterial puncture, the adequacy of collateral circulation is assessed. Allen's test is used to assess the adequacy of ulnar collateral flow when the radial artery is considered for arterial puncture. Here the hand is elevated above the heart, and, while compressing both ulnar and radial arteries, the hand is passively opened and closed. When the hand appears pale, ulnar compression is released while radial compression is maintained. If the hand flushes or if the pulse oximeter Spo_2 on any of the fingers of the hand returns to normal, ulnar competency is considered adequate. A similar evaluation of the foot is accomplished prior to dorsalis pedis puncture. The dorsalis pedis is compressed, and the big toe is blanched by compressing the toenail. Collateral flow is considered adequate if the toenail flushes when pressure is released (Chameides, 1990).

Under controlled circumstances, Emla cream should be used to ease the patient's discomfort. The pain and anxiety associated with arterial puncture will alter the infant's or child's breathing pattern and obscure results. ABGs are obtained using universal precautions. After removing all air from the syringe and capping it with an occlusive barrier, ABGs are sent to the laboratory on ice. Excessive air will distort the gas results, and ice will slow metabolism in the blood sample. Apply firm pressure to the puncture site for 5 minutes or until bleeding stops. Once bleeding stops, apply a pressure dressing. Because of patient discomfort and the potential for vasospasm, hematoma formation, and neurovascular compromise, arterial cannulation should be performed if frequent sampling is required to manage the patient.

Venous Blood Gases

To obtain a representation of systemic perfusion and Vo_2, a true mixed venous blood sample is obtained from the distal port of a pulmonary artery catheter. Venous blood gases obtained from more peripheral sites will vary considerably, depending upon the Vo_2 of nearby organ systems. This is especially true during shock or septic states. When obtaining a mixed venous sample, the mixed flush/blood discard and blood specimen are drawn slowly over 2 minutes from the distal port of a pulmonary artery catheter. This time frame is necessary to prevent "arterialization" of the specimen (that is, pulling blood over the alveolar pulmonary-capillary membrane) that would produce erroneously high mixed venous oxygenation data. The $Pvco_2$ should always be higher than a simultaneous drawn $Paco_2$; if not, the mixed venous specimen is probably arterialized. After drawing the mixed venous sample, care is taken to adequately flush the lumen to prevent clot formation, especially in the smaller PA catheters.

Capillary Blood Gases

If peripheral perfusion is adequate, CBG data will correlate with arterial pH, $Paco_2$, and HCO_3. Because adequate peripheral perfusion is necessary for arterial correlation, capillary blood gases are usually not an option in critical care. To maximize CBG-ABG correlation, an "arterialized" CBG is obtained. This is accomplished by collecting a free-flowing blood specimen from a site that had been wrapped in a warm (45°C) wet cloth for 5 to 7 minutes. Skin-puncturing devices designed for blood glucose monitoring can be used for CBGs. CBGs are usually drawn from the medial or lateral surface of the heel in infants or from one of the digits in older infants and children.

Interpretation

Blood gas analyses typically report the pH, Po_2, Pco_2, So_2, HCO_3, and base excess (BE)/base deficit

(BD). Normal ranges are noted in Table 10–10. According to Dalton's law of partial pressures, the total pressure of a group of gases is equal to the sum of the partial pressures of the individual gases in a mixture. When oxygen and carbon dioxide dissolve in blood, they exert a pressure. The Po_2 and Pco_2 reflect the partial pressures of dissolved oxygen and carbon dioxide in blood. The So_2 is the percent hemoglobin saturation with oxygen; when 100% saturated, each gram of hemoglobin carries a full load of 1.34 mL of oxygen. The Pao_2 and Sao_2 reflect the adequacy of oxygenation, whereas the $Paco_2$ reflects the adequacy of ventilation.

The $Paco_2$ level can only be influenced by pulmonary function. Two abnormal conditions are associated with changes in $Paco_2$: respiratory acidosis and respiratory alkalosis. Respiratory acidosis is evidenced by a decreased pH and increased $Paco_2$. Respiratory acidosis is caused by decreased CO_2 elimination—that is, hypoventilation. Respiratory alkalosis is evidenced by an increased pH and decreased $Paco_2$. Respiratory alkalosis is caused by an increase in CO_2 elimination—that is, hyperventilation.

The pH is inversely proportional to H^+ concentration. As H^+ concentration increases in the blood, the pH falls; when H^+ ion concentration decreases in the blood, the pH rises. Bicarbonate (HCO_3^-) is a base that buffers H^+ concentration. The base excess/deficit mainly reflects an excess/deficit concentration of bicarbonate that can only be influenced by nonpulmonary function.

Donlen (1983) described a three-step method that is helpful in interpreting blood gases. First, the pH is evaluated for acidosis or alkalosis. Next, the origin of the disorder is identified by analyzing HCO_3, BE/BD, and Pco_2 levels. This is followed by an assessment of compensation. Please refer to Chapter 11 for interpretation of acid-base imbalances.

Oxygenation Profile Monitoring

Invasive oxygenation profile monitoring is extremely helpful in patients with acute respiratory failure to help manage Fio_2 and PEEP. Patient management is directed toward resolution of the primary problem while titrating therapy to achieve an optimal physiologic, oxygenation, and hemodynamic state while limiting the potential for iatrogenic injury. Normal parameters may not be optimal in these patients. The most challenging aspect of care is to identify and support optimal parameters (which change almost constantly) for an individual patient. What is also important is to trend the parameters over time and assess whether they make clinical sense in that they correlate with changes in the physical examination.

Monitoring Oxygen Supply and Demand

The goal in managing critically ill patients is to ensure adequate O_2 supply with respect to demand. Each phase of oxygenation is monitored: (1) gas exchange over the pulmonary capillary membrane, (2) oxygen transport in the blood, and (3) oxygen consumption. All three parameters are interrelated in that changes affecting one phase affect the others.

Gas exchange over the pulmonary capillary membrane is assessed by calculating the alveolar-arterial Po_2 difference (A-aDo_2). To obtain an A-aDo_2, the Pao_2 (obtained from an ABG report) is subtracted from the PAo_2 (calculated using the alveolar air equation: $PAo_2 = Pio_2 - Paco/RQ$). Normally, the A-aDo_2 should be less than 20 mmHg.

When mixed venous gases are available, the Qs/Qt ratio, the ratio of shunted blood (Qs) to total pulmonary blood flow (Qt), is calculated using the shunt equation: Qs/Qt = (Cpco_2 − Cao_2)/(Cpco_2 − Cvo_2), where Cpco_2, Cao_2, and Cvo_2 are the pulmonary capillary, arterial, and mixed venous oxygen contents, respectively. The alveolar air equation is used to provide data for the Cpco_2. The Qs/Qt normally ranges from 3% to 7%. Shunt fractions greater than 50% are not uncommon in patients with severe ARDS.

Oxygen transport in the blood refers to the amount of arterial O_2 available for tissue utilization. Do_2 is the amount of O_2 leaving the heart to be delivered to tissues. Oxygen delivery is calculated by: $Do_2 = Cao_2 \times$ cardiac index (CI) $\times$ 10. Normal Do_2 is 620 ± 50 mL/min/M^2.

Oxygen reserve is the amount of oxygen returned to the venous side of the circulation not utilized by the tissues. Oxygen reserve is calculated in a similar manner to Do_2 but includes the Cvo_2. The oxygen reserve = $Cvo_2 \times$ CI $\times$ 10. The high oxygen reserve, more than 400 mL/min/M^2, serves as a protective mechanism to prevent tissue hypoxia during periods of hypermetabolic need.

Oxygen consumption (Vo_2), the total amount of oxygen consumed by the body per minute, is calculated as the difference between the Do_2 and oxygen reserve; that is, ($Cao_2 - Cvo_2$) $\times$ CI $\times$ 10. Normal resting Vo_2 in infants and young children is twice that of adults; varying with age, the Vo_2 ranges from 120 to 200 mL/min/M_2. The higher Vo_2 in the younger age group (approximately 175 mL/min/M^2)

Table 10–10. NORMAL BLOOD GAS VALUES

Parameter	Arterial	Mixed Venous	Capillary
pH	7.35–7.45	7.31–7.41	7.35–7.45
O_2 saturation	95–97%	60–80%	Less than arterial
Po_2	80–100 mmHg	36–42 mmHg	Less than arterial
Pco_2	35–45 mmHg	40–50 mmHg	Same as arterial
HCO_3	22–26 mEq/L	Same as arterial	Same as arterial
Total CO_2 content	23–27 mEq/L	Same as arterial	Same as arterial
Base excess/ deficit	+2 to −2	Same as arterial	Same as arterial

Capillary Po_2 is approximately 10 mmHg less than arterial except when decreased tissue perfusion is present, that is, cardiovascular collapse or hypothermia. In these states, samples will not accurately reflect Pao_2. Total CO_2 content equals HCO_3 plus Pco_2 (0.03 to convert mmHg to mEq/L).

is due to the additional metabolic burden of growth. "Adequate" D_{O_2} is considered to be four times V_{O_2}.

The arterial-venous oxygen difference (a-vD_{O_2} = Ca_{O_2} − Cv_{O_2}) reflects tissue O_2 uptake. Normally, only a 3 to 5.5 mL/dL difference exists between the Ca_{O_2} and the Cv_{O_2}, again reflecting 25% oxygen utilization.

The O_2ER represents the percent of oxygen delivered to tissues that is actually utilized. The O_2ER indicates the adequacy of D_{O_2} with respect to V_{O_2}. The rate of oxygen consumption/availability is calculated by: a-vD_{O_2}/Ca_{O_2} × 10. Normal O_2ER is 25 ± 2%.

Sv_{O_2} Monitoring

Pediatric-size oximetry pulmonary artery catheters allow continuous monitoring of mixed venous oxygen saturation (Sv_{O_2}). The technology is very similar to pulse oximetry except that the sensor sits at the end of a pulmonary artery catheter and continuously monitors Sv_{O_2}. Mixed venous oxygen saturation continuously reflects the interaction among all variables impacting D_{O_2} and V_{O_2}.

As V_{O_2} increases, the body compensates by increasing oxygen supply in an effort to preserve venous reserve. Sympathetic stimulation increases both cardiac output and minute ventilation, so Sv_{O_2} remains unchanged.

If compensation starts to deteriorate or is ineffective or impossible (for example, the cardiac output, Sa_{O_2}, or hemoglobin is or cannot be further maximized), threefold increases in tissue extraction can occur to prevent hypoxemia. A decreased Sv_{O_2} indicates that the patient is using venous reserve; alterations more than 5% lasting for more than 5 minutes are considered significant.

Decreased Sv_{O_2} can result from increased V_{O_2} or decreased D_{O_2}. Factors that impact V_{O_2} are noted in Table 10-5. Factors that decrease D_{O_2} include a myriad of problems affecting cardiac output, hemoglobin concentration, and saturation. Primary interventions are always focused to correct the primary problem followed by interventions focused to support compensatory mechanisms.

Whereas Sv_{O_2} trends are critically important in patient care management, one of the greatest benefits of continuous Sv_{O_2} monitoring is assessment of patient tolerance to care procedures. Patients with little oxygen reserve have negligible tolerance to basic care activities, such as repositioning and physical care. Additionally, these extremely vulnerable patients may desaturate with suctioning, no matter how cautious the procedure is performed. Trending the patient's ability to recover from necessary procedures is helpful in determining how best to administer care, e.g., separating or clustering care.

Increased Sv_{O_2} can result from decreased V_{O_2} or improved D_{O_2}. Factors that decrease V_{O_2} include sleep, adequate sedation and pain relief, normothermia, chemical paralysis, and anesthesia. Pathologic issues that decrease V_{O_2} include R→L shunting associated with sepsis and cyanide toxicity associated with nitroprusside administration. Factors that improve D_{O_2} include interventions that optimize cardiac output, hemoglobin concentration, and saturation.

Convergent oximetry—that is, decreasing Sa_{O_2} and increasing Sv_{O_2}—equates with cell death, whereas divergent oximetry—that is, increasing Sa_{O_2} and decreasing Sv_{O_2}—equates with cell life.

PULMONARY DIAGNOSTIC STUDIES

Radiologic Procedures

Serial chest x-rays are used to monitor the progression of disease and response to therapy, and to confirm various tube placements preventing iatrogenic injury. Although the quality of portable films varies, they are frequently performed in ICU settings. Fundamental skills in x-ray interpretation are necessary, as critical care nurses are often the first individuals to assess the chest x-ray and are responsible for manipulating various tubes into position. Access to films is even more prevalent, given the increased use of computerized systems that directly image films in the ICU.

Just prior to obtaining a chest x-ray, it is important to ensure the best quality film possible by removing anything from the patient's chest that would obscure the image. The head and neck are placed in alignment, and the head is positioned in a neutral position. Neck flexion or extension would displace the ETT. Radiation precautions for patients include gonad shielding.

When evaluating a film, one interprets the characteristics of and relationships between structures of varying density ranging from air, fat, water, to bone. If the structure is not dense (air-filled alveoli, pneumothorax, air in the stomach), the x-ray beam passes through the tissue, resulting in a dark gray or black image on the film. A very dense structure (bone) will block most of the x-ray beam, preventing it from reaching the film and resulting in a light gray or white image. Usually, lung is translucent, while the heart, blood vessels, liver, spleen, and muscle appear opaque on x-ray.

As illustrated in Figure 10–27, the trachea has a tube-like appearance and is visible in the midline of the anterior mediastinal cavity. The trachea bifurcates into the right and left mainstem bronchi at approximately the level of the fourth rib. The bronchi are usually not clearly visible but have a tube-like appearance if surrounded by consolidated lung. The heart is visible in the anterior left mediastinal cavity and should occupy less than one half of the thoracic cavity. The clavicle and ribs are evaluated for continuity. The lung parenchyma is usually not visible throughout the lung fields except for white lines radiating from the hilum, which represent the pulmonary vascular tree. Pulmonary vascular markings are usually visible in the proximal two thirds of the lung. If

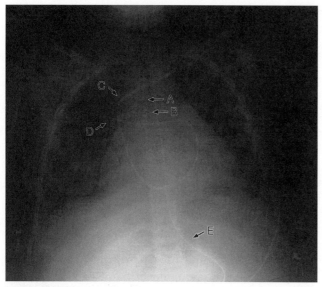

Figure 10–27 ● ● ● ● ● ●

Chest x-ray with landmarks. *A,* Endotracheal tube 1 cm above the carina. *B,* The carina. *C,* Left subclavian introducer tip. *D,* Pulmonary artery catheter tip in the RUL. *E,* Nasogastric tube tip off film in region of the duodenum. (Courtesy of Robert Cleveland, MD. Radiology Department, Children's Hospital, Boston, MA.)

the density of the lung changes, for example, with atelectasis, pneumonia, pulmonary edema, or hemorrhage, the lung will appear more opaque. When structures of similar density, for example, the heart and atelectatic lung, are positioned side-by-side, they cannot be differentiated from each other, so the heart border disappears. The heights of the right and left diaphragm are compared for symmetry. The costophrenic angles should be well defined and taper into points. The dark gastric bubble is seen under the left diaphragm.

Major problems such as a pneumothorax, or a displaced airway, central line, or feeding tube, should be identified so that immediate interventions can occur (Kelly-Heidenthal & O'Connor, 1994). The patient's endotracheal tube should be visualized within the trachea midway between the carina and clavicles. The radiopaque markings on the ETT should end 2 to 3 cm above the carina—the point at which the right and left mainstem bronchi bifurcate. When assessing ETT position, head position is first assessed to ensure a neutral position. If the neck were flexed, the ETT would be displaced downward; if the neck were extended, the ETT would be displaced upward. When the ETT is "too high," the tip is positioned at the level of the clavicles. When the ETT is "too low," the tip is positioned near the carina or down either mainstem bronchi—most often the right because it is more vertical than the left. When the ETT intubates either bronchus, hyperinflation of the affected lung occurs along with hypoinflation and atelectasis of the unintubated lung.

Lung tissue normally fills the chest, so pulmonary markings should be equal and visible out to the rib margins. If the pulmonary markings are replaced

with a dark edge, consider a pneumothorax. When significant, the trachea may deviate away from the collapsed lung. If the mediastinum is encircled by a dark line, consider a pneumomediastinum.

The patient's central line should sit within the right atrium. The patient's pulmonary artery catheter should sit within the main pulmonary artery or proximal within the right or left pulmonary artery. The patient's nasogastric tube should sit within the stomach. Landmarks include the right atrium (RA), which is located to the right of the sternum and extends down to the diaphragm. Above the RA is the superior vena cava (SVC). The left ventricle (LV) is to the left of the sternum and rests on the diaphragm. Above the LV is the left atrium (LA), and above that are the pulmonary arteries (PA). The stomach sits under the left diaphragm.

Other radiologic procedures of the pulmonary system include fluoroscopy, angiography, and V/Q scanning. Fluoroscopy images the dynamic process of ventilation, and thus is very useful during pulmonary artery catheter insertion in a small infant and in assessing diaphragmatic function. Pulmonary angiography is a radiologic study of the pulmonary vessels used to delineate pulmonary arteriovenous malformations and pulmonary embolus. V/Q scanning includes two complementary tests involving the inhalation and intravenous injection of necular material for the purpose of determining the match of ventilation to perfusion. VQ scanning provides valuable information in the lung transplant patient. Before sequential single-lung transplant, a VQ scan is used to help determine the better lung to maintain ventilation while the other lung is being transplanted.

Bronchoscopy

Technologic advances have provided the opportunity for even the smallest of neonates to benefit from bronchoscopy. Two types of bronchoscopic examinations are available: rigid and flexible. Whereas rigid bronchoscopy is often performed in the operating room under general anesthesia, flexible bronchoscopy is often performed within the ICU environment. Bronchoscopes have all or some of the following features: fiberoptics for visualization and ports for ventilation, suction, retrieval of objects, or collection of specimens.

Table 10–11 provides a summary of the potential indications for bronchoscopy. Rigid bronchoscopy offers a large channel, so it is used predominantly for the retrieval of a foreign body and control of bleeding in the presence of massive hemoptysis. The three most common techniques employed through flexible bronchoscopy include bronchoalveolar lavage, transbronchial biopsy, and bronchial brushing.

Nursing care during a bedside bronchoscopic examination is generally supportive; the priority is ensuring a safe environment. Anesthesia, if indicated, is provided by an anesthesiologist. Conscious sedation and coaching the patient through the procedure are

Table 10-11. POTENTIAL INDICATIONS FOR
BRONCHOSCOPY

Rigid Scope

Foreign body removal
Tissue mass removal
Massive hemoptysis
Establishment of an airway in the patients with
 epiglottitis

Flexible Scope

Evaluation of stridor
Persistent or recurrent atelectasis
Identification of infectious organisms
Hemoptysis
Difficult intubation
Abnormal cry or hoarseness
Vocal cord paralysis
Evaluation of a mass lesion

From Behnke, M., & Koff, P.B. (1993). Patient assessment (p. 45). In P.B. Koff, D. Eitzman, & J. Neu (Eds.). *Neonatal and pediatric respiratory care* (2nd ed.). St. Louis: C.V. Mosby.

nursing responsibilities. Prepare emergency medications prior to the procedure and maintain access to a vascular line during the procedure. Potential complications include laryngospasm, hypoxia, cardiac dysrhythmias secondary to hypoxia or vagal stimulation, bronchial tears, pneumothoraces, pulmonary hemorrhage, epistaxis, subglottic edema, contamination of the lower airway with upper airway flora, and oversedation.

RESPIRATORY SUPPORT

Oxygen Therapy

The goal of oxygen therapy is to relieve hypoxemia, decrease the work of breathing, and reduce myocardial stress (Wilson & Desautels, 1993). Oxygen, considered a medication, is administered in the lowest possible concentration to support life while avoiding toxicity. Pulmonary toxic effects of oxygen are progressive and include diminished mucociliary clearance, capillary endothelial damage, interstitial edema, and destruction of type I pneumocytes. Subsequent progression includes hyperplasia of the type II pneumocytes, interstitial fibrosis, then death (Martin, Rafferty, & Gioia, 1992).

Environmental gases are warmed and humidified to 100% relative humidity. Proper humidification of inspired gas prevents drying of the tracheobronchial tree, which may cause impaired ciliary activity, inflammatory changes, and retention of thick secretions (Wilson & Desautels, 1993). Providing warmed humidified gas is particularly important in infants who are sensitive to heat loss as well as in patients with a bypassed upper airway, as in those who are intubated.

When the airway is secure and the patient is spontaneously breathing, oxygen can be delivered as needed by several modalities. These include simple mask, partial or non-rebreathing mask, face tent, nasal cannula, oxygen hood, hut tent, and mist tent. Any of these delivery devices can be regulated to achieve desired oxygen concentrations. Table 10–12 summarizes the advantages and disadvantages of several commonly used oxygen delivery devices.

Oxygen Delivery Devices

Simple Face Mask. The most common type of oxygen delivery device is the simple face mask. Available in a wide variety of sizes, these masks are designed to deliver oxygen through a cone-shaped face piece with open exhalation ports. The FiO_2 is influenced by the size of the mask, the patient's ventilatory pattern and tidal volume, and oxygen flow. As tidal volume increases, FiO_2 is decreased as more

Table 10-12. OXYGEN DELIVERY DEVICES

Device	FiO_2	Flow Rate (L/min)	Advantages	Disadvantages
Simple face mask	.35–.55	3–5 child 5–10 adolescent	Easy to use	Patient may overbreathe flow rate and entrain room air CO_2 retention at low flow rates Patient intolerance
Rebreathing mask	To .60	Variable—adjust to keep reservoir partially filled	Delivers higher FiO_2	Same as for simple face masks
Non-rebreathing mask	To 1.0	Variable—adjust to keep reservoir partially filled	Delivers higher FiO_2 Can be used to administer other gases (HeO_2)	Same as for simple face masks
Nasal cannula	Variable	25 mL/min to 6 L/min	Ease of use Patient tolerance	FiO_2 varies Gastric inflation at high flow rates May occlude with nasal secretions
Oxygen hood Hut tent	To 1.0	10–15	Patient tolerance Patient access	Noise level Limted to infants <1 year
Mist tent	To .5	10–15	Provides cool mist	Limited and variable FiO_2 Cumbersome

Data from Wilson, B.G., & Desautels, D.A. (1993). Oxygen therapy. In P.B. Koff, D. Eitzman, J. Neu (Eds.). *Neonatal and pediatric respiratory care.* (2nd ed.). St. Louis: C.V. Mosby.

environmental air is pulled in (entrained) through the exhalation ports. Too small of a mask will decrease inspired FiO_2; too large will add excessive dead space. An FiO_2 of .35 to .55 can be achieved when oxygen flow rates of 3 to 5 L/min in a child and 5 to 10 L/minute in the adolescent are used (McPherson, 1990).

Face masks are not usually tolerated by infants and small children. This age group will not understand the benefit of a tight-fitting mask blowing moist air on their face. If the patient struggles, hypoxemia will worsen as VO_2 increases while DO_2 remains unchanged. There is also an increased risk of aspiration if the infant or child vomits into the mask.

Partial Rebreathing Mask. A partial rebreathing mask is similar to a simple face mask with an added reservoir bag. The purpose of the reservoir bag is to collect the first third of the patient's exhaled gas, dead space gas that is high in oxygen and low in carbon dioxide. Allowing rebreathing of this gas mixed with a fresh oxygen source will allow an FiO_2 as high as .60 (McPherson, 1990). Entrainment of room air is reduced and rebreathing of carbon dioxide from the mask is prevented by maintaining an oxygen flow rate into the bag that is greater than the patient's minute ventilation. This is determined by adjusting the flow rate high enough to keep the bag from completely deflating during inspiration; generally gas flows at 10 to 12 L/min are required (Chameides, 1990).

Non-rebreathing Mask. A non-rebreathing mask is similar to the partial-rebreathing mask except that one-way exhalation valves are incorporated into the sides of the mask to prevent entrainment of room air and a valve is placed at the reservoir bag to prevent gas flow back into the bag during exhalation. The patient can only draw gas from the oxygen-rich reservoir bag and displace gas through the exhalation valves. In order to achieve maximum oxygen concentration, the mask must fit snugly. When the mask fits properly and the reservoir is inflated, this device can provide an FiO_2 close to 1.0. (McPherson, 1990).

Most disposable non-rebreathing masks are manufactured with one exhalation valve removed. This safety mechanism allows the patient to breathe room air if gas flow into the mask is interrupted. This type of non-rebreathing mask (manufactured with only one exhalation valve) is only slightly more effective in delivering high FiO_2 than a partial rebreathing mask.

Face Tent. Sometimes referred to as a shovel or scoop, a face tent is a soft plastic mask that fits close to the chin but is completely open around the patient's face. This device is better tolerated by infants and children because the face is accessible, allowing the patient to use a pacifier, eat, or talk (Chameides, 1990). The downside of this device is that even at high flow rates, an FiO_2 in excess of .40 is difficult to achieve.

Nasal Cannula. A nasal cannula provides a light weight, less restrictive system for oxygen delivery. The device consists of either soft plastic prongs that are inserted into the nare or slits within soft plastic tubing that direct oxygen toward the posterior naso/oropharynx. It is difficult to predict and control the FiO_2 using these devices. The FiO_2 depends upon the flow rate of oxygen, the patient's spontaneous minute ventilation, peak inspiratory flow, the volume of environmental air inhaled by the patient, cannula position, the proportion of nose to mouth breathing, and the size of the upper airway, which provides an anatomic oxygen reservoir (Wilson & Desautels, 1993). Changes in any of these parameters will result in changes in the FiO_2.

In infants, low-flow flow meters are used to allow more precise titration of gas flow. Titration in flow rates are made based upon the desired SpO_2 and blood gas. Oxygen flow (L/min) should not exceed the patient's predicted minute ventilation ($V_T \times RR$). Excessive flow rates may cause gastric distension and vomiting (Lough & Doershuk, 1985).

Nasal cannulas are useful in clinical situations where the infant or child requires less precise and low FiO_2 concentrations for extended periods of time. Nasal cannulas allow the patient to use a pacifier, eat, or talk while receiving a continuous flow of oxygen. To maintain skin integrity, cannulas can be taped to small pieces of Duoderm placed directly on the maxilla. Potential problems include otitis media, sinusitis, and a local reaction to the plastic prongs.

Oxyhood and Hut Tents. An oxyhood is a clear plastic enclosure that fits over the infant's entire head and neck. A hut tent is a small tent frame with canopy that fits over the infant's upper body. Capable of delivering an FiO_2 of 1.0, both require a flow rate of 10 to 15 L/min to flush out exhaled CO_2. Oxygen may layer within the hood/hut, producing a higher oxygen concentration at the bottom of the device. Oxygen concentrations are continuously monitored close to the infant's head with high and low alarm limits set on the oxygen analyzer (Wilson & Desautels, 1993).

Oxyhoods are well tolerated by infants, as free head movement is allowed in addition to the use of pacifiers and other comfort measures. Hut tents allow the infant hand-mouth self-stimulation. One potential problem is the noise level produced by incoming gas. Also, the delivery of cold gas can result in considerable stress to small infants; therefore, heating and humidification must be provided.

Mist Tent. Mist tents are clear plastic enclosures that fit over the patient's entire body providing cool aerosol and low to moderate concentrations of oxygen. The FiO_2 varies, depending upon total gas flow, tent volume, and the tightness of seal around the bottom of the tent. Again, higher levels of oxygen are found lower in the tent. An FiO_2 of up to .5 can be achieved at flow rates of 10 to 15 L/min if patients are left undisturbed. However, leaving a critically ill patient undisturbed is usually not an option within the ICU environment. In addition to limited patient access, the mist may also compromise caregiver observation of the patient. For comfort, frequent linen changes are necessary. For fire safety, patients are instructed not to play with any electrical or friction toys within the tent.

Resuscitation Bag-Valve-Masks

Bag-valve-mask ventilation provides a method of ventilating a patient with ineffective or absent respirations. Resuscitation bags and face masks are available in a wide variety of sizes to accommodate the wide range in pediatric size. Correct size masks provide an air-tight seal around the patient's face from the bridge of the nose to the cleft of the chin. Whereas round masks function well in small infants, anatomically correct masks reduce the potential for ocular pressure that precipitates vagal stimulation and tend to provide a better seal in older children. Masks should have a small undermask volume to decrease dead space and prevent rebreathing. Clear masks are preferred, as continuous assessment of the patient's color and early identification of regurgitation are possible (Chameides, 1990).

Bag size is selected to accommodate patient lung volume. Two types of resuscitation bags are available: self-inflating and anesthesia.

Self-inflating Bags. Self-inflating bags consist of a standard 15/22 mm connector for mask or endotracheal tube connection, a non-rebreathing valve assembly that also regulates inspiratory and expiratory pressures, a pressure release valve, and a self-inflating bag with distal ports for oxygen and a reservoir to entrain room air. The oxygen gas inlet has a one-way valve that fills the bag with oxygen. At 10 L/min of oxygen flow, the self-inflating bag will deliver an FiO_2 of .3 to .8; higher concentrations can be achieved if a oxygen reservoir is attached to the room air port. The bag automatically fills independent of gas flow.

During bag inflation, the gas valve opens, entraining room air or oxygen from the reservoir. During bag compression, the gas intake valve closes and the patient valve is opened. During patient exhalation, the non-rebreathing valve closes and exhaled volumes are displaced into the environment.

To avoid barotrauma, most self-inflating bags are equipped with a preset (or adjustable) pop-off valve that allows a maximum peak inspiratory pressure of 30 to 35 cm H_2O. While appropriate in the intubated patient, preset valved bag-valve-masks have limited utility in extubated patients with poor lung compliance who require high inflating pressures for adequate tidal volume. Also, because of the bag-valve assembly, self-inflating bags cannot be used to provide supplemental oxygen to a spontaneously breathing patient. Even if the pediatric patient could generate sufficient negative pressure to open the valve, the added work of breathing is not optimal. Also, some self-inflating bags are designed to deliver volume only when the bag is actually compressed.

Anesthesia Bags. Sometimes referred to as flow-inflating or "Mapleson" bags, anesthesia bags inflate when a gas is delivered into the bag. These bags consist of a standard 15/22 mm connector for mask or endotracheal tube connection, a gas inlet port, pressure gauge port with manometer, a corrugated reservoir tube, a non–self-inflating reservoir bag, and a distal adjustable gas escape port or pop-off valve. Careful adjustment of flow is required to maintain volume in the reservoir tube and bag while also flushing out exhaled gases. When the reservoir bag is compressed, the patient receives tidal volume from the oxygen source and corrugated reservoir tube. Flow rates two to three times the patient's V_E are usually adequate to keep the bag half inflated between breaths.

Careful adjustment to gas escape is required to provide adequate tidal volume, peak inflating time and pressure, and end-expiratory pressure. High inflation pressures, continuous positive airway pressure (CPAP), and ventilatory rates are matched by high flow rates to adequately inflate the bag. Improper use may result in pulmonary barotrauma (high-flow, low-escape), insufficient washout of exhaled gases (low-flow, low-escape), or insufficient tidal volumes (high- or low-flow, high-escape). To prevent barotrauma, an in-line manometer should be used to monitor and deliver appropriate levels of peak inspiratory and end-expiratory pressures. Because of the continuous flow, anesthesia bags can be used to provide oxygen and CPAP in the spontaneously breathing patient.

Airway Adjuncts

The goals of airway management include recognition and treatment of obstruction, prevention of aspiration of gastric contents, and promotion of adequate gas exchange (Yaster, 1991). Upper airway obstruction may be relieved by repositioning the patient using a chinlift or jaw thrust. Although endotracheal intubation may be required, nasopharyngeal or oropharyngeal airways are simpler devices when assisted ventilation is unnecessary.

Nasopharyngeal Airways

A nasopharyngeal airway is a soft rubber tube that extends below the base of the tongue. Nasopharyngeal airways rarely induce vomiting, so they can be used in both the conscious and obtunded patient. Available in sizes 12 to 36F, the size chosen should fit snugly within the nare without causing sustained blanching (Chameides, 1990). The 12F size usually accommodates an infant. Appropriate length is determined by measuring the distance from the tip of the nose to the tragus of the ear (see Fig. 10–28A).

Care measures include maintaining skin integrity and tube patency. Potential complications from nasopharyngeal airways include epistaxis and ulceration of the tip of the nose. Laryngospasm may occur if the airway is too long and impinges upon the epiglottis. Nasopharyngeal airways should not be placed in those at high risk for uncontrolled bleeding, e.g., anticoagulated patients and in those with head and/

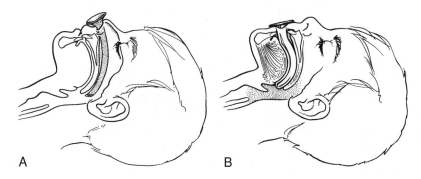

A   B

Figure 10–28 ● ● ● ● ● ●

A, Placement of a nasopharyngeal airway. *B,* The oropharyngeal airway. (Reproduced with permission. © *Textbook of Pediatric Advanced Life Support,* 1994. Copyright American Heart Association.)

or facial trauma at high risk for cribriform plate fracture.

Oropharyngeal Airways

An oropharyngeal airway is a rigid plastic device that curves over the base of the tongue, pulling it forward away from the pharyngeal wall. Because of the potential for induced vomiting and laryngospasm, oropharyngeal airways are placed only in unconscious patients. Oropharyngeal airways are used to (1) relieve airway obstruction caused by the tongue, (2) facilitate oropharyngeal suctioning, and (3) facilitate endotracheal suctioning and ventilation when the patient is biting down on an oral endotracheal tube. The correct size for an oropharyngeal airway is determined by placing the airway next to the patient's face with the phalange next to the teeth. The tip of the airway should reach the angle of the jaw (Fig. 10–28*B*). The airway is inserted by depressing the tongue with a blade and inserting the airway to follow the natural curve of the tongue. Inserting the airway upside down then rotating it 180 degrees may cause damage to fragile oral mucosa.

Care measures include maintaining skin integrity of the lips, tongue, and mouth. A misplaced oropharyngeal airway will result in airway obstruction by pushing the tongue back in the oropharynx. Complications of oropharyngeal airways include trauma to the lips, teeth, tongue, and surrounding soft tissue (Yaster, 1991).

Endotracheal Tubes

Endotracheal tubes (ETTs) are constructed of soft plastic (polyvinyl chloride). The proximal end is fitted with a standard 15-mm male adapter. The tip is beveled to allow smooth passage through the nares, and a side hole ("Murphy eye") provides ventilation in the event of distal obstruction. ETT labeling includes the size of the ETT, a radiopaque line down the entire length of the ETT, and distance hatch markings (in centimeters) that provide reference points to facilitate tube placement. A distal vocal cord marker is placed at the level of the glottic opening to ensure that the tip of the ETT is in a midtracheal position (Chameides, 1990).

Uncuffed ETTs are used in children less than 8

years of age because the cricoid cartilage serves as a physiologic cuff. When airleaks around ETTs become unmanageable, cuffed ETTs may be used. Soft cuffs, low-pressure high-volume cuffs, exert low and equal lateral tracheal wall pressure to minimize the potential for tracheal injury. The inflating tube is constructed with a distal one-way valve and a "pilot" balloon that indicates the presence of air within the cuff.

Approximate ETT size can be calculated using the formula: ID = 16 + age in years ÷ 4 (where ID is the internal diameter in mm). Usually, a 3.0 to 3.5 mm ETT will accommodate term newborns, whereas a 4.0 ETT can be used in infants less than 1 year of age. A quick check can be made by comparing the outside diameter of an ETT with the patient's little finger. Table 10–13 lists recommended sizes per age of the patient.

Endotracheal Intubation. Indications for endotracheal intubation include establishment of a secure airway in patients with a diminished gag or cough reflex and the need for controlled ventilation. Prior to endotracheal intubation, the patient is positioned in a sniffing position and equipment is prepared (Table 10–14). An adequate cardiac and pulse oximetry tracing is ensured. A suction source and Yankauer are made available to clear the oropharynx of thick secretions, vomitus, or blood. An appropriate-sized resuscitation bag and mask are needed to pre/reoxygenate the patient with an FiO_2 of 1.0. To visualize the vocal cords, the large floppy epiglottis in infants and children is raised using a straight Miller laryngoscope blade.

The sedatives, narcotics, anesthetics, and neuro-

Table 10-13. ETT AND SUCTION CATHETER SIZES

Age	ETT Size	Suction Catheter Size
Newborn	3.0–3.5	6–8F
6 months	3.5–4.0	8F
1 year	4.0–4.5	8–10F
2 years	4.5	8–10F
4 years	5.0	10F
6 years	5.5	10–12F
8 years	6.0 cuffed or uncuffed	12F
12 years	6.5 cuffed or uncuffed	12–14F
Adolescent	7.0 cuffed	14F
Adult	7.5–8.0 cuffed	14–16F

Table 10-14. INTUBATION EQUIPMENT CHECKLIST

Patient

Monitoring equipment
  Good cardiac tracing
  Strong SpO₂ pulse indicator
  Good A-line tracing or operational blood pressure cuff/monitor
Medications
  Sedation
  Muscle relaxant

Equipment

Oxygen
  Adequate-sized mask
  Resuscitation bag to provide an FiO₂ of 1.0.
Suction
  Large-bore Yankauer or tonsil-tip suction
  Sterile suction catheters that will fit the selected ETT
Laryngoscope
  Handle, correct size and shape blade, strong light source
Endotracheal tubes
  Calculated size—one size larger and smaller than calculated
  Stylet to fit the selected ETT
  Water-soluble lubricant for nasotracheal intubation
  Magill forceps for nasotracheal intubation
Adhesive tape and skin protector
Appropriate size nasogastric tube with attached catheter tip syringe
Gloves and goggles—universal precautions

muscular blocking agents commonly used to facilitate intubation are noted in Table 10–15. Neuromuscular blocking agents are divided into two groups: depolarizing and nondepolarizing agents. Depolarizing agents mimic the action of acetylcholine but produce prolonged depolarization of the neuromuscular junction. Nondepolarization agents bind to acetylcholine receptor sites, preventing depolarization of the neuromuscular junction. Use of neuromuscular blocking agents are contraindicated when the ability to establish an artificial airway is in question or difficulty in maintaining adequate ventilation is anticipated (Arnold & Castro, 1990). Whereas only time will reverse the effects of a depolarizing agent, pharmacologic reversal of nondepolarizing agents can be obtained by increasing the concentration of acetylcholine at the neuromuscular junction. Administration of an anticholinesterase inhibitor plus muscarinic antagonist will accomplish this (see Table 10–15).

Unless contraindicated, the depolarizing agent succinylcholine is recommended for intubation because of its rapid onset (45–60 seconds) and short duration (5–10 minutes). For intubation, succinylcholine is usually administered with an anticholinergic agent (atropine) to prevent excessive vagal effects related to the initial release of acetylcholine. If succinylcholine is contraindicated, a rapid-acting nondepolarizing agent, for example, either atracurium or vecuronium, can be used. To produce a more rapid effect, a priming dose (1/10th the intubating dose) is administered 5 minutes before the intubating dose.

The technique of endotracheal intubation depends upon the indication for intubation and the condition of the patient. There are many accepted techniques for ETT placement. ETTs may be placed nasally or orally, patients may be fully awake or receive some combination of sedation and analgesia, and patients may be pharmacologically paralyzed or breathing spontaneously. Common approaches in the intensive care setting include nasal, rapid sequence, awake oral, unconscious oral, and fiberoptic bronchoscopy. Whatever approach is used, the patient's vital signs and oxygen saturation are continuously assessed. The intubation procedure is immediately interrupted and the patient is hand ventilated with a bag-valve-mask at the first sign of desaturation.

Nasotracheal intubation is preferred if intubation is anticipated for a long period of time. Nasotracheal ETTs are more comfortable for the patient, allow continued oral stimulation, are easier to secure, and are less apt to be displaced. Complications associated with nasotracheal intubation include epistaxis, trauma to adenoids, pressure necrosis to the nare, and obstruction of the eustachian tube and sinusitis.

If nasotracheal intubation is performed, the endotracheal tube is lubricated, inserted nasally, and gently advanced until the tip is visualized in the pharynx. The laryngoscope is then used to visualize the cords, and the Magill forceps are used to direct the tip of the tube through the vocal cords. Contraindications of nasotracheal intubation include fracture of the cribriform plate with a cerebrospinal leak, bleeding disorders, and nasal deformities.

Orotracheal intubation can be performed rapidly and is associated with minimal complications. A curved Macintosh laryngoscope blade is inserted into the vallecula above the epiglottis, whereas a straight Miller blade is passed over the epiglottis to rest above the glottic opening. Once the vocal cords are visualized, the ETT is advanced. Stylets are used to stiffen and shape ETTs to facilitate insertion. When used, stylets are positioned proximal to the side hole and should not protrude through the end of the ETT, as this may cause vocal cord damage.

Rapid sequence intubation is used to decrease the risk of aspiration of gastric contents. Patients at high risk for aspiration include those with a full stomach due to prior oral intake or decreased gastric emptying, resulting from pain, shock, or increased abdominal pressure. The procedure is accomplished by an intravenous infusion of a rapid-acting anesthetic/sedative, for example, some combination of thiopental sodium (Pentothal), methohexital sodium (Brevital), ketamine, or midazolam with a muscle relaxant, usually succinylcholine. Cricoid pressure is applied to prevent passive regurgitation, and the ETT is inserted orally. If the patient gag and cough reflex is intact, gastric decompression occurs prior to intubation. This technique should not be attempted if anatomic abnormalities that potentially may prevent rapid intubation are present.

Fiberoptic bronchoscopy is used if endotracheal intubation is expected to be difficult. Here, an ETT is threaded over a fiberoptic bronchoscope. Once the

Table 10-15. INTUBATION MEDICATIONS

Drug	Dose (duration)	Comment
Sedatives and Narcotics		
Diazepam	0.1–0.3 mg/kg IV or PR (2–4 hr)	Painful on injection; mild respiratory depression; decreased cerebral blood flow and metabolism
Midazolam (Versed)	0.05–0.1 mg/kg IV (1–2 hr)	May cause respiratory depression
Lorazepam (Ativan)	0.05–0.1 mg/kg/dose (8–12 hr)	
Fentanyl	1–5 μg/kg IV (0.5–1.5 hr)	Respiratory depression; large doses are given rapidly; may cause bradycardia and chest wall rigidity
Morphine	0.1–0.2 mg/kg IV (2–4 hr)	Respiratory depression; histamine release producing bronchospasm and hypotension
Anesthetic Agents		
Ketamine	0.5–2 mg/kg IV (10–15 min) Intubation: administer with glycopyrrolate	Useful in hypotensive patients because of catecholamine release (increases HR and BP); potent bronchodilator; increases ICP; spontaneous respirations maintained but may cause laryngospasm; copious secretions
Thiopental (Pentothal)	2–4 mg/kg IV (5–10 min)	Potent myocardial depressant, decreases peripheral vascular resistance and may precipitate CV collapse in the patient with MC dysfunction and hypovolemia; will produce apnea in doses greater than 4 mg/kg
Methohexital (Brevital)	1–2 mg/kg	
Neuromuscular Blocking Agents		
Depolarizing		
Succinylcholine (Anectine)	2 mg/kg: infants 1–2 mg/kg IV: children 1–1.5 mg/kg: adolescents (5–10 min) Administer with atropine	Decrease HR; may increase intracranial, intraocular, and intragastric pressure; arrhythmias common with second dose; may cause massive elevation in serum potassium in patients with severe burns, crush injuries, spinal cord injury, and neuromuscular disease; known trigger for malignant hyperthermia; myoglobinuria in healthy children
Nondepolarizing		
Atracurium besylate (Tracrium)	0.5 mg/kg IV (15–20 min) 0.3–0.6 mg/kg/hr infusion	Mild histamine release; hypotension; neither renal nor hepatic function necessary for excretion; active metabolites
Vecuronium bromide (Norcuron)	0.1–0.15 mg/kg/dose IV (35 min children and 70 min in infants) 0.06–0.1 mg/kg/hr infusion	Minimal CV effect Elimination: liver
Pancuronium bromide (Pavulon)	0.1–0.15 mg/kg IV (60–90 min)	Hypotension; vagolytic effect increases HR Elimination: liver and kidney
d-Tubocurarine chloride	0.1–0.2 mg/kg IV (25–90 min)	Dose-related fall in blood pressure
Metocurine (Metubine)	0.3 mg/kg IV (60–75 min)	Histamine release Shellfish derivative Elimination: kidney
Reversal Agents		
Anticholinesterase inhibitors		
Neostigmine	0.06 mg/kg (max 2.5 mg)	Reverses the effects of nondepolarizing neuromuscular blockade; always precede with atropine
Pyridostigmine	0.1–0.25 mg/kg (max 10 mg)	
Muscarinic anticholinergics		
Atropine	0.02–0.03 mg/kg (min 0.1 mg/ max 2 mg)	Used to prevent bradycardia, salivation, bronchospasm, and gastrointestinal hypermotility
Glycopyrrolate	0.01 mg/kg	
Miscellaneous		
Lidocaine	1–2 mg/kg IV (max q 1 hr)	Given 2 min before suctioning may prevent elevations in ICP

HR, heart rate; BP, blood pressure; ICP, intracranial pressure; CV, cardiovascular; MC, myocardial.

scope passes through the vocal cords, the previously threaded ETT is advanced forward into position. The flexible fiberoptic scope is also useful in evaluating vocal cord movement prior to extubation (Backofen & Rogers, 1992).

Intubating a patient with *increased intracranial pressure* (ICP) is specifically challenging. The goal is airway access while averting cerebral hypertension associated with increased mean arterial pressure and

hypercapnia. Intubation is accomplished by anesthetizing the patient in an effort to bunt expected cardiovascular responses. After preparing the equipment, an anesthetic dose of thiopental sodium (4 mg/kg) is administered followed by vecuronium (0.1–0.2 mg/kg). Thiopental decreases cerebral oxygen consumption and thereby lowers cerebral blood flow and ICP. Vecuronium is a nondepolarizing neuromuscular blocking agent chosen to avoid histamine release and sympathetic stimulation. Lidocaine (1.5 mg/kg IV) is also administered to diminish cardiovascular reflexes activated with intubation. The patient is then hyperventilated to decrease $PaCO_2$ to the mid-20 range, then intubated.

Also challenging is intubating the patient with a compromised airway secondary to a *large mediastinal mass*. These patients are able to stent their airways open through chest movement. If respiratory muscle function becomes impaired (through sedation, anesthesia, or neuromuscular blockade), a large mediastinal mass can collapse the airway leading to sudden and complete airway obstruction despite positive-pressure ventilation. The goal is to keep the patient breathing spontaneously until the size of the mass can be reduced by radiation or chemotherapy.

Correct Placement. Once the ETT is placed, the patient is cautiously hand ventilated using a resuscitation bag while ETT position is evaluated. Correct ETT positioning is marked by observation of condensation within the ETT, bilateral chest excursion, symmetric breath sounds, and adequate oxygenation. Auscultation of breath bounds is best accomplished at the apex of each axilla; auscultation over the stomach rules out esophageal intubation. Unilateral chest excursion marks mainstem bronchus intubation, whereas breath sounds will not be heard with esophageal intubation. End-tidal CO_2 monitoring helps confirm correct ETT placement; a capnogram is possible only with endotracheal intubation.

After securing the ETT, a chest radiograph (with the head in a neutral position) is obtained to confirm proper tube position in the trachea midway between the carina and clavicles. Care is taken whenever moving an intubated infant or child. Neck flexion shortens the mouth-to-carina distance, thus displacing the uncuffed ETT tip downward and increasing the danger of endobronchial intubation (see Fig. 20–4). Neck extension increases this distance, promoting accidental extubation. Inadvertent extubation is hallmarked by increased respiratory distress, and grunting, crying, or vocalization indicating air movement through the glottis.

Securing the ETT. Once ETT position appears satisfactory, the ETT is secured. The procedure of taping or retaping an ETT is performed by two people to prevent inadvertent extubation. One person is responsible for immobilizing the head and holding the tube with the specific ETT markings at the nare or lip line, while the other person is responsible for the actual taping procedure. Breath sounds are auscultated before and after taping. ETT position is changed from one side of the mouth to the other during a tape change to prevent pressure necrosis.

Numerous methods to secure ETTs in the pediatric population have been described. Benjamin, Thompson, and O'Rourke (1990) reported a relatively low 3% incidence of accidental extubation with the use of white cloth adhesive tape slit down the middle resulting in a Y configuration. For an *oral ETT*, the skin of the upper lip and ETT is prepped with tincture of benzoin then allowed to dry. The ETT is positioned so that it will be attached to the least mobile area of the mouth—that is, the upper lip away from the corner of the mouth. One arm of the Y is attached to the upper lip, and the other arm of the Y is wrapped around the ETT. A second piece, mirroring the first but started from the opposite side of the mouth, can be placed for added security. For a *nasal ETT*, the nose, upper lip, and ETT is prepped with tincture of benzoin then allowed to dry. The untorn piece of tape is applied to the nose; one arm of the Y is applied to the upper lip, while the other arm is wrapped around the ETT. A second Y can be applied, positioning the untorn arm on the cheek; one arm of the Y layers is placed over the first piece on the upper lip, and the other is wrapped over the first piece on the ETT. While taping a nasal ETT, care is taken to avoid excessive pressure to the skin at the nasal septum and outer upper ridge of the nare. Care is also taken to avoid gaps in the tape when wrapping the ETT. Gaps fill with secretions, which will eventually loosen the tape. Tape-sensitive skin may be protected by first applying DuoDerm to the face then attaching the tape to the DuoDerm.

Complications from endotracheal intubation can occur during laryngoscopy, any time during the intubation period, or after extubation. Complications occurring during the intubation procedure include dental and soft tissue trauma, aspiration of gastric contents, esophageal intubation, right mainstem intubation, and cardiac dysrhythmia from hypoxia. Obstruction of the ETT from secretions, kinking, or biting; accidental extubation; and increased resistance to breathing are the common complications during the intubation period (Yaster, 1991). Later complications include laryngeal and tracheal edema or damage, acquired subglottic stenosis, and the inability to extubate.

Extubation. Once the indications for intubation have been resolved, extubation may be considered. The patient is made NPO for 4 to 6 hours before extubation is attempted. Sedation is avoided prior to extubation so that the patient's cough and gag reflexes are intact and active. The ETT is suctioned as well as the oropharynx. Care is taken to remove secretions above the ETT cuff; the cuff is then deflated on exhalation. The ETT is removed on exhalation. Following the removal of the ETT, humidified oxygen is delivered by mask or hood.

Symptoms of hoarseness and croupy cough may occur after extubation. Those at high risk include patients under 4 years of age and those with a cuffed ETT. Also prevalent are patients who have experienced traumatic or repeated intubations, excessive movement of the ETT, or those with airway abnormalities or infection. Post-extubation croup usually resolves with cool mist or humidity as well as the use of racemic epinephrine. The action of racemic epinephrine is unclear; however, benefit may be related to its topical mucosal vasoconstriction effect. Until a wellness trajectory can be predicted, withhold feedings and deep suctioning and provide familiar sources of comfort to avoid vigorous crying. If reintubation is necessary, management of second or subsequent extubation attempts include dexamethasone (Decadron) 0.5 mg/kg up to a maximum of 4 mg, 6 hours before extubation, at the time of extubation and 6 to 12 hours after extubation (Manning & Brown, 1990).

Cricothyrotomy

In an emergency, when other methods of gaining airway access have failed, a cricothyrotomy can be performed. The cricothyroid membrane is a relatively avascular membrane that extends from the cricoid to thyroid cartilage. It is palpated as an anterior and midline transverse indentation between the two cartilages. The membrane can be punctured and the underlying trachea entered percutaneously using a large-bore cannula. The 14-gauge cannula is directed in the midline caudally and posteriorly at a 45-degree angle. A cricothyrotomy can also be accomplished surgically with a short horizontal incision. After incision, a 3.0 ETT can then be threaded into the tracheal opening.

Tracheostomy Tube

Similar to ETTs, tracheostomy tubes (TTs) are available in a wide variety of sizes and styles. Variations in TT specifications are found among manufacturers (Table 10–16). For example, a standard 3.5-mm ETT is comparable with a Shiley pediatric 0 and a Portex pediatric 1 TT. Companies also provide custom TT lengths upon request. As with ETTs, low-pressure high-volume cuffed TTs are used when airleaks become unmanageable. Larger sizes may have an inner cannula that can be removed for cleaning.

Indications for tracheostomy include an acute upper airway obstruction, prolonged need for mechanical ventilation, and prevention of aspiration. TTs are inserted into an incision made below the cricoid cartilage through the second to fourth tracheal rings. Elective tracheostomy is performed in the operating room. When performed within the ICU environment, nursing care and responsibility are similar to those

for any sterile invasive procedure. Priorities include continued patient monitoring and safety.

Postoperative tracheostomy holders are left intact for the first 3 days after surgery and are not changed. For added security, the outer phalange of the TT is often sutured to the skin to avoid inadvertent decannulation. Until the stoma is secure, reinsertion of a TT could be quite difficult. Routine care includes (1) assessing the TT holders for security, (2) assessing the character of the skin under the TT and holders, and (3) stoma care.

Tracheostomy holders should be secure enough to hold the TT in place but not too tight as to cause pressure necrosis of the neck. When assessing skin integrity, the entire circumference of the neck is assessed with particular attention to the infant's skin folds. Available in a wide variety of sizes, soft foam Velcro tracheostomy holders are used because they are less traumatic to the skin (see Chapter 17).

Traditional stoma care includes cleansing the skin with one-half strength H_2O_2 and applying antibacterial water-soluble gel and a dry sterile split gauze tracheostomy dressing. Care is taken to avoid displacing the TT with multilayered tracheostomy dressings. Once the stoma is healed, sterile dressings are replaced with sponges to collect secretions as necessary.

Skin surrounding the stoma and chin is assessed for pressure necrosis secondary to the TT phalange or TT connector. The phalange of the TT may need to be shaved down to eliminate pressure points. Skin around the tracheostomy site and chin can be protected using DuoDerm or moleskin.

Tracheostomy masks provide humidified gases to the airway. General principles are similar to those of face masks, except that tracheostomy masks are secured gently to avoid decannulation in the active patient. Various style trach-to-ventilator or resuscitation bag connections are available. The ideal connector provides little dead space and the greatest range of motion to the head and neck.

Changing a TT may be necessary after inadvertent decannulation, when the inside diameter is compromised by secretions, or routinely per institutional norm. The first TT change is accomplished by the

Table 10–16. TRACHEOSTOMY TUBE SPECIFICATIONS

Size	Shiley Inner Diameter (mm)	Portex Inner Diameter (mm)	Shiley Outer Diameter (mm)	Portex Outer Diameter (mm)	Shiley Length (mm)	Portex Length (mm)
Neonatal 00	3.1	2.5	4.5	same	30	same
0	3.4	3.0	5.0	5.2	32	same
1	3.7	3.5	5.5	5.8	34	same
Pediatric 00	3.1	2.5	4.5	same	39	30
0	3.4	3.0	5.0	5.2	40	36
1	3.7	3.5	5.5	5.8	41	40
2	4.1	4.0	6.0	6.5	42	44
2.5	–	4.5	–	7.1	–	48
3	4.8	5.0	7.0	7.7	44	50
4	5.5	same	8.0	8.3	46	52

Adapted from Scott, A.A., & Koff, P.B. (1993). Airway care and chest physiotherapy (pp. 285–302). In P.B. Koff, D. Eitzman, & J. Neu (Eds.). *Neonatal and pediatric respiratory care* (2nd ed.). St. Louis: C.V. Mosby.

surgeon who originally placed the TT. Any individual variance is noted for future reference. Subsequent TT changes are accomplished by the nurse. If the infant or child is going home with the TT, parents are invited to participate in the procedure. If not for education, the parents' presence can provide a source of comfort for their infant or child. The patient is held NPO for 4 to 6 hours. Sedation is considered per individual infant or child. All equipment, including a correct size face mask and one size smaller TT, is prepared. The new same-size TT is examined, the obturator is removed and replaced, the balloon is tested (if appropriate), and the TT is lubricated with a water-soluble gel. The patient's TT is suctioned, followed by vigilant removal of upper airway secretions. The patient is positioned prone with a small roll behind the shoulders. The patient is preoxygenated with an FiO_2 of 1.0. On exhalation, the existing TT is removed following the natural curve of the tube, then the new TT is immediately inserted in a similar manner. Slight tension should be expected. If the TT cannot be reinserted, the patient is reoxygenated using a face mask and resuscitation bag while gently occluding the stoma with a gloved finger(s). When the patient is adequately reoxygenated, reinsertion of the same size or one size smaller TT is reattempted.

Decannulation of the tracheostomy patient usually occurs as a planned admission to the ICU. In preparation for decannulation, the child's TT may be replaced with a progressively smaller TT. Because of the size of the pediatric airway, this maneuver may not be an option in infants and small children. Removal occurs as per TT change (see above), but the patient is usually held in an upright position on the parent's lap. Sterile gauze is placed over the stoma after TT removal. Supplemental humidified oxygen may be administered. The patient is assessed for increased work of breathing, stridor, and desaturation. Length of ICU observation post-decannulation depends upon the patient, family, and system. The stoma will close in 48 to 72 hours post-decannulation.

Suction Catheters

Numerous types of suction catheters are available in various distal tip configurations. Common features include measured distance markings in centimeters, a blunt tip (beveled or straight), and side holes (one to four). In pediatrics, it is especially important to compare the actual size of the distal opening when comparing manufacturers. Whereas outside diameters of suction catheters are similar, the size of distal openings may vary. Because smaller catheters are used in the pediatric population, smaller distal openings further compromise the ability to suction thick secretions. The amount of suction applied is regulated to prevent hypoxia and mucosal damage. Appropriate negative pressure includes 60 to 80 mmHg in infants under 1 year of age, 80 to 120 mmHg in

children 1 to 8 years of age, and 120 to 150 mmHg in children over 8 years of age.

Nasopharyngeal and oropharyngeal suctioning is indicated in patients who cannot clear secretions in their upper airway or to elicit deep breathing and a cough. The nasopharynx is suctioned first, as it is considered cleaner than the oropharynx. Catheter size should fit comfortably into the nare using a water-soluble lubricant. Appropriate insertion length is determined by measuring the distance from the tip of the nose to the tragus of the ear. To minimize mucosal injury, the catheter is inserted next to the nasal septum and advanced caudally. After inserting to appropriate length, suction is applied and the catheter is slowly withdrawn in a rotating manner.

When suctioning an artificial airway, although ideal, using a catheter size of no more than one half the inside diameter of the tube is impractical in the pediatric population. In reality, the largest suction catheter that can comfortably fit down the ETT or TT is used (see Table 10–13).

Helium

The work of breathing through a narrowed upper airway can be decreased by breathing a low-density gas mixture. Oxygen in helium (HeO_2) is less dense than air or pure oxygen, thus it permits higher inspiratory flow at lower resistance (Thompson, 1992). Different concentrations of HeO_2 are available, usually providing an FiO_2 of 0.4. HeO_2 can be administered through a non-rebreathing mask for upper airway obstruction or through an ETT for intrathoracic airway obstruction.

Bronchial Hygiene

An important intervention for both acute and chronic respiratory disorders is a series of maneuvers referred to as bronchial hygiene. The procedures include postural drainage, chest percussion and vibration, and deep breathing/coughing exercises. The goal of bronchial hygiene is removal of airway secretions, improved matching of ventilation to perfusion, and avoidance of alveolar collapse (Scott & Koff, 1993).

Postural drainage uses gravity to move lung secretions from smaller peripheral lung segments into larger, more central airways where coughing or suctioning clears the secretions. A variety of positions are employed to drain different lung segments (Fig. 10–29). The chest x-ray guides the intervention; the patient is positioned to drain areas identified as needing improvement. The patient is kept in a position for 15 minutes, 5 minutes if combined with percussion and vibration. Patient tolerance often controls the variety of positions used during postural drainage. Also, several positions are contraindicated in some patients, for example, Trendelenburg in the cerebral hypertensive patient or in the patient with gastric reflux.

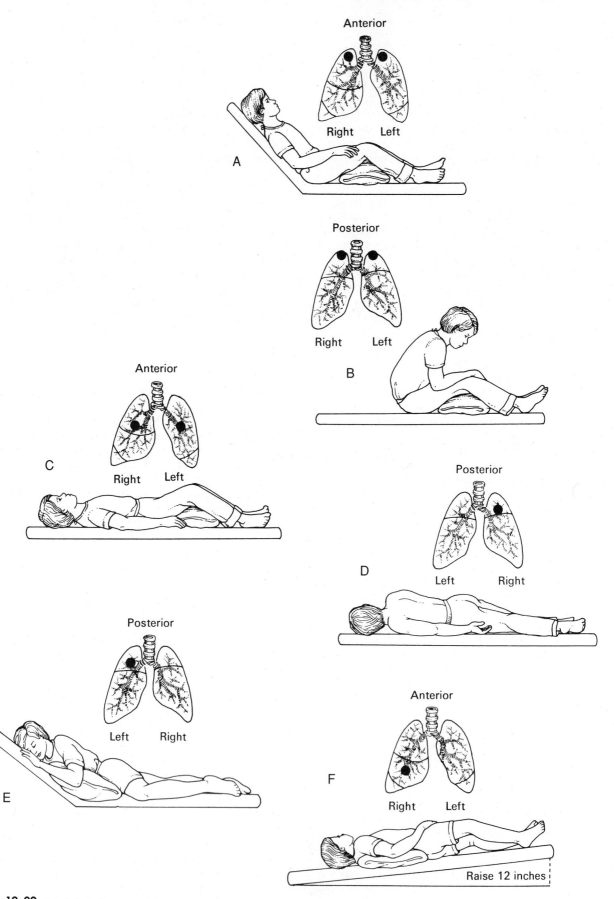

Figure 10–29 ● ● ● ● ● ●

Postural drainage positions. *A,* Anterior apical segment; sitting. *B,* Posterior apical segment; sitting. *C,* Anterior segment; lying flat on back. *D,* Right posterior segment; lying on left side. *E,* Left posterior segment; lying on right side. *F,* Right middle lobe; lying on left side.

Illustration continued on opposite page

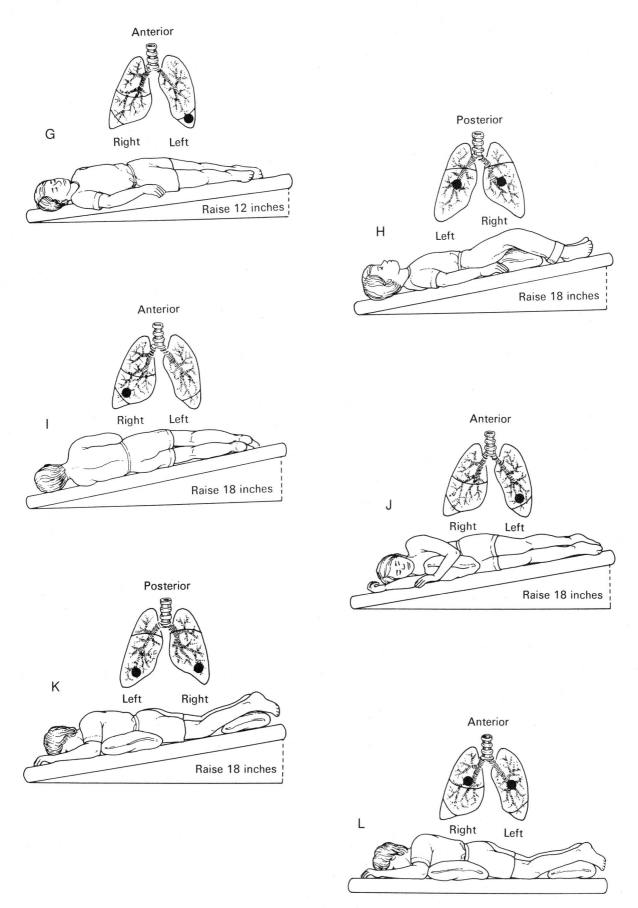

Figure 10–29 ● ● ● ● ● ● *Continued*

G, Left lingula; lying on right side. *H,* Anterior segments; lying on back. *I,* Right lateral segment; lying on left side. *J,* Left lateral segment; lying on right side. *K,* Posterior segments; lying on stomach. *L,* Superior segments; lying on stomach. (From Hirsch, J., & Hannock, L. (1981). *Mosby's manual of clinical nursing procedures.* St. Louis: Mosby–Year Book.)

In conjunction with postural drainage, *chest percussion and vibration* help mobilize secretions from nondependent lung segments to central airways for removal. Chest percussion and vibration may improve the effectiveness of postural drainage. Percussion is performed using a cupped hand or percussion cup and rhythmically "clapping" the chest wall. Chest percussion is performed only over the rib cage and not over a bony prominence, e.g., the clavicle, scapula, vertebrae, and sternum. Vibration is accomplished by shaking the chest on exhalation using the hands in tremor-like movements. Mechanical vibrators can be used in small infants. Gentle chest vibration is used apart from chest percussion in patients with thrombocytopenia or in those at risk for bone injuries or fractures, for example, patients with osteogenesis imperfecta. Both maneuvers are useful in conditions where large amounts of sputum are produced, e.g., cystic fibrosis, bronchiectasis, retained secretions, and lobar atelectasis.

Deep breathing and coughing are useful only in the alert cooperative patient. Games, such as bubble blowing and incentive spirometers, also increase the depth of inspiration in patients who may not take deep breaths on their own. Deep inspiration prevents atelectasis, promotes lung expansion, improves oxygenation, and provides an opportunity for patients to actively participate in their own care (Wigal & Will, 1993). Forced exhalation helps to clear secretions. If patients are unable to cough spontaneously, naso/oropharyngeal or tracheal suctioning may be necessary to stimulate a cough to help remove mobilized pulmonary secretions.

Bronchial hygiene is not a benign procedure. The benefits of selected maneuvers—specifically, percussion and postural drainage—have been challenged (Anderson and Falk, 1991). Transient, yet significant, decreases in PaO_2 may follow chest physiotherapy. Also, the presence of a focal abscess theoretically presents a risk to the contralateral lung for contamination during postural drainage (Martin, Rafferty, & Gioia, 1992). Individualized care is warranted.

Chest Tubes

The primary purpose of a chest tube is to, as rapidly and simply as possible, reestablish full expansion of the lung and evacuate air, fluid, or blood from the pleural space. Chest tubes vary in size from 10 to 36F, 10 to 18 inches long, and consist of vinyl, silicone, or latex nonthrombogenic material. The distal end that sits within the pleura has a number of drainage holes to prevent occlusion; the proximal end is connected to the chest drainage system.

Chest tubes are inserted at the bedside under local anesthesia and sterile conditions. Insertion site depends upon the problem. A chest tube inserted for a pneumothorax will be placed at the second intercostal space midclavicular line because air will rise to the apex. Alternative sites, especially in females, include a more lateral position in the third to fifth intercostal space with the chest tube threaded up into the apex. A chest tube inserted for any type of fluid collection will be placed at the fifth to seventh intercostal space midaxillary line because gravity will pull fluid to the base of the lung. Once in place, the chest tube is sutured to the skin to prevent displacement and taped to prevent lateral movement. An occlusive dressing consisting of petrolatum gauge and a dry sterile split gauze is applied. Placement is confirmed on chest x-ray.

The chest drainage system removes air and/or fluid from the pleural space and prevents the backflow of air and fluid into the pleural space. All connection points are banded to ensure that the system remains airtight. Chest tube milking or stripping is not advised, as transient high negative pressures cause patient discomfort, inflict tissue trauma, and may cause bleeding. Clamping chest tubes is also not advised. Once clamped, trapped air and fluid accumulate in the pleural space and a tension pneumothorax may result. If clamping is necessary to precisely identify the location of an airleak, clamps are left on only for several breaths per test site location.

Closed chest tube drainage systems use gravity and/or suction to restore intrapleural negative pressure. Chest tubes are connected to a underwater seal drainage system so that air can only escape from and not enter the pleural space. A Heimlich flutter valve or bottle of saline can be used as a temporary measure until a chest tube drainage system is available. The early bottle systems have been replaced by disposable triple-chamber chest drainage systems. Basic principles are exactly the same whatever system is used.

The triple-chamber systems consist of (1) a drainage collection chamber connected to (2) a water-seal chamber connected to (3) a vacuum-control chamber. All three are positioned side by side in a molded plastic disposable unit. Step-by-step instructions for setting up these disposable systems vary and are included in the package inset or printed on the unit itself. The units can be hung below the level of the chest on the crib using the attached hanger hooks or are positioned on the floor using the built-in stand.

The first chamber is graduated so that chest drainage can be accurately measured. The second chamber (directly connected to the first) provides the water-seal chamber that prevents air from reentering the chest. When the system is placed on gravity drainage, respiratory fluctuations in the water-seal chamber reflect normal fluctuations in intrapleural pressure and thus indicate an intact system. Bubbling in this chamber indicates a airleak within the system. When all connection points are occlusive, the airleak can come only from the patient. To verify the source of an airleak, the chest tube and connecting tubes are systemically clamped at various levels. Once a clamp is located between the airleak and the water seal, the bubbling will stop. The third chamber controls the amount of suction applied to the chest tube when wall suction is connected to the system. Suction is necessary for rapid pulmonary reexpansion. The amount of suction applied to the chest tube is determined by the fluid level within the unit; usually a negative 15 to 20 cm H_2O is adequate. Wall suction is adjusted to produce continuous bubbling within the suction chamber. Turning up the wall suction will only cause more bubbling within the suction chamber as more air is pulled into the system. Vigorous bubbling creates more noise that can be distracting to the patient and hastens fluid evaporation. Safety features vary but usually include both high-negativity and positive-pressure release valves. See Table 10–17 for trouble-shooting triple-chamber chest drainage systems.

Removal of a chest tube is performed when the lung has reexpanded, the air leak has resolved, and drainage has ceased. After providing adequate analgesia, stay sutures are removed and the chest tube is pulled on exhalation. An occlusive dressing consisting of petrolatum gauge and a dry sterile gauze is then applied.

Inhaled Medications

Inhalation is frequently the most optimal method of delivery of medications into the respiratory tract. Aerosolization of medication is frequently better tolerated, safer, and more effective than systemic administration. Aerosols consist of particulate water suspended in gas. Theoretically, the smaller the size of the aerosol particle, the more distal the particles are deposited into the bronchial tree. Airway resistance and breathing pattern will also influence the amount of medication reaching the airways (Lough, 1990). In the adult population, approximately 10% of nebulized medication reaches the lung periphery in non-intubated patients (MacIntyre et al., 1985), while 1.2% to 4.8% of the nebulized medication reaches the lung periphery in intubated patients (Fuller et al., 1990).

A small-volume nebulizer (SVN) is commonly used to aerosolize medications. Particles are generated by passage of a high-velocity gas stream (usually oxygen) across a tube creating a Bernoulli effect; the medication is pulled from the reservoir and becomes nebulized. A baffle in front of the gas stream removes larger particles, returning them for renebulization, while smaller particles (1 to 5 μm in diameter) are delivered to the patient airway. Flow rates of 6 to 8 L/min are necessary to achieve an adequate particle size to reach the conducting airways. If possible, the patient is instructed to take slow, deep breaths through the mouth and hold at end-inspiration (Koff & Durmowicz, 1993).

Ultrasonic nebulizers generate ultrasonic sound waves directed at the air-liquid surface producing a cloud of fine particles whose diameters vary depending upon the frequency of the sound used. The

Table 10–17. TROUBLE-SHOOTING TRIPLE-CHAMBER CHEST TUBE DRAINAGE SYSTEMS

Drainage tubing: Tight connections; no kinks, compressions, or dependent loops

Fluid-filled dependent loop or kink impedes drainage
  Straighten tubing and anchor to the bed linen

Collection chamber: Positioned below the patient's chest; assess volume and character of drainage

No change in drainage
  None if drainage is stopped
  Check for patency of tubing
  Consider milking chest tube if obvious clots are present
Large volume of drainage accumulated in a short time
  Assess for signs and symptoms of hypovolemia—report drainage
Collection chamber is full
  Change the unit—once prepared, switch units without clamping chest tube

Water-seal chamber: Filled to appropriate level; bubbling present; fluctuations if to gravity

Water seal is underfilled (so no effective seal is present)
  Fill the water seal to the 2-cm level with sterile water or saline
Water seal is overfilled (creating more resistance for air escape from the pleural space)
  Using the self-sealing diaphragm, remove enough fluid to return the water seal to 2 cm
Continuous bubbling in the water-seal chamber (airleak between the patient and system)
  Locate the source by systemically and momentarily clamping the system from the chest wall to unit
  Bubbling will stop when a clamp is placed between the airleak and unit

If the bubbling never stops, the unit may be cracked, so change the unit
  Tighten/reband loose connections
  Report if new bubbling occurs
Intermittent bubbling in water-seal chamber
  Expect bubbling when suction first applied
  Patient may have a small airleak
No fluctuations or bubbling in the water-seal chamber of a patient with gravity drainage and the solution has crept up to a fixed position
  Lung has reexpanded—expect equal breath sounds and easy respirations
  Tubing is obstructed—check for dependent loops or kinks
Large fluctuations in the water-seal chamber of a patient with gravity drainage
  High intrapleural negative pressure on inspiration indicative of increased work of breathing

Suction control chamber: Filled to appropriate level; gentle continuous bubbling; if suction is off, tubing detracted from suction source and open to air

Suction control chamber is underfilled to prescribed level
  Fill to prescribed level with sterile water or saline, then turn on the suction until gentle bubbling occurs
Suction control chamber is overfilled from prescribed level
  Using the self-sealing diaphragm, remove enough fluid to obtain the prescribed level, then turn on the suction until gentle bubbling occurs
Bubbling in the suction control chamber is too vigorous
  Wall suction is set higher than needed—turn down
No bubbling in the suction control chamber
  Reconnect wall suction
  Turn up wall suction until gentle bubbling occurs

Data from Erickson, R.S. (1989). Mastering the ins and outs of chest drainage, part 1. *Nursing 89*, May, 37–43; Part 2, June, 46–49.

small-particle aerosol generator (SPAG) unit is a pneumatically operated nebulizer used for ribavirin therapy. Aerosol therapy for the intubated patient is accomplished by either hand bagging the medication or by placing the nebulizer in the ventilator circuit (Salyer & Chatburn, 1990).

Table 10–18 lists some of the more common agents used for nebulization. Clinical responses to aerosol therapy are closely assessed because of the varying amount of medication reaching the distal airways. Because of variable delivery, optimal dosages are determined by the clinical responsiveness of the individual patient. It is important to note that aerosol therapy also delivers free water to the patient and a mode of bacterial transmission to the lower respiratory tract.

Bronchodilators, affecting sympathetic and parasympathetic airway receptors, are by far the most common. Inhaled sympathetic agents stimulate beta$_2$ receptors producing bronchodilation. Additionally, sympathomimetics inhibit mast cell degranulation,

reduce mucous gland secretion, augment mucociliary clearance, and improve respiratory muscle contractility. Sympathomimetics vary in their peak onset and duration of action. Newer agents are beta$_2$ selective, limiting beta$_1$ cardiovascular side effects. Continuous nebulized bronchodilator therapy is becoming increasingly popular in the ICU setting (Portnoy, Nadel, Amado, Willsie-Ediger, 1992). Continuous nebulization of albuterol (Papo, Frank, Thompson, 1993) and terbutaline (Kelly, McWilliams, Katz, Murphy, 1990) is safe, provides more rapid clinical improvement, and is cost effective.

MECHANICAL SUPPORT OF VENTILATION

The primary objective of mechanical ventilation is to improve the balance of ventilation to perfusion, the most common cause of impairment of oxygenation and CO_2 removal (Chatburn, 1991a). In the

Table 10–18. DRUGS USED FOR AEROSOL THERAPY

Drug	Dose	Peak Onset Duration	Comments
Beta-sympathomimetic			
(Side effects common to class include muscle tremor, tachycardia, hypokalemia, dysrhythmia, hypertension, anxiety, headache, dizziness)			
Albuterol (Proventil 5%, Ventolin)	0.25–0.5 mL in 2.5 mL	0.5–1 hr 6–8 hr	Bronchodilation Beta$_2$-selective
	Continuous nebulization: 0.3 mg/kg/hr to a maximum of 15 mg/hr		
Isoetharine (Bronkosol 1%)	0.2–0.5 mL in 2.5 mL	15–60 min 1–2 hr	Bronchodilation Less cardiac effect than isoproterenol
Metaproterenol (Alupent 5%)	0.1–0.3 mL in 2.5 mL	0.5–1 hr 4–6 hr	Bronchodilation Less cardiac effect than isoproterenol
Terbutaline (Brethine 1 mg/1 mL)	0.25 mg in 2 mL	5–20 min 6–8 hr	Bronchodilation Beta$_2$-selective
	Continuous nebulization: 0.3 mg/kg/hr to a maximum of 15 mg/hr		
Alpha-sympathomimetic			
Racemic epinephrine (Micronefrin, Vaponefrin)	0.25–0.5 mL in 2.5 mL	2–4 min 1–2 hr	Reduces mucosal swelling by vasoconstriction
Parasympathomimetic			
Atropine	0.05 mg/kg (max 2.5 mg)	1 hr 3–4 hr	Synergistic with beta$_2$-agents; more effective in large airway bronchospasm; may cause mucous plugging, tachycardia, hypertension
Ipratropium (Atrovent)	0.25–1 mg	1.5 hr 6 hr	
Mucolytic			
Acetylcysteine (Mucomyst 20%)	1–2 mL in 2.5 mL q 6 hr		Enhanced mobilization of secretions Foul smelling—may cause nausea May cause bronchospasm—administer with a bronchodilator
Antimicrobial			
Gentamicin	20–125 mg in 4 mL; twice daily		Gram-negative bacteria
Tobramycin	80–240 mg in 4 mL; twice daily		Cystic fibrosis; use preservative-free solution
Ribavirin	Nonintubated: 2 g in 33 mL over 2 hours, 3 times/day for 3–5 days Intubated: 6 g in 100 mL over 16 hours for 3–5 days		Respiratory syncytial virus Caregiver precautions are essential
Pentamidine	300 mg in 6 mL (daily for treatment; monthly for prophylaxis)		Prophylaxis against *Pneumocystis carinii* Caregiver precautions are essential

Normal saline is used as the diluent.
Data from Lough, M. (1990). Medicated aerosol therapy. In J.L. Blummer (Ed.). *A practical guide to pediatric intensive care* (pp. 978–980). St. Louis: C.V. Mosby.

presence of disease, ventilation often exceeds the level of perfusion (high V/Q) or perfusion may exceed the level of ventilation (low V/Q). Overventilation results in dead space ventilation (wasted ventilation) and an increased $PaCO_2$. On the other hand, underventilation results in a physiologic shunt and a decreased PaO_2. When mechanical ventilation is instituted, perfusion to well-ventilated regions may decrease from the effects of positive pressure, which may necessitate delivery of larger than physiologic minute volumes to maintain an acceptable $PaCO_2$. Any ventilator maneuver that has the potential to increase intrathoracic pressure may impair cardiac output and tissue perfusion and ultimately impair cellular gas exchange.

Managing the pediatric patient supported on mechanical ventilation presents a particular challenge, as this group of patients will require a wide variety of interventions technology can now offer. It is difficult to uniquely separate pediatric mechanical ventilation from that of neonates and adults, as the practical applications are similar. What is essential to safe and effective ventilation of this population is a knowledge of time constants, V/Q relationships, and ventilator options and strategies. Having previously discussed time constants and V/Q relationships, this section discusses ventilator options and strategies in terms relevant to the pediatric patient.

Indications for Initiating Assisted Ventilation

The indications for mechanical ventilation in the pediatric population are mainly subjective. The younger the patient, the more subjective the indications become. Standard spirometry is seldom used in pediatrics as an indication for mechanical ventilation. Vital capacity requires an alert and cooperative patient not affected by pain, characteristics rarely found in patients under 5 years of age. Vital capacity is affected by muscle function, chest wall disorders, and parenchymal disease. Acute muscle weakness will only slightly affect vital capacity (Maxham, 1990).

Physiologic measurements define respiratory and/or ventilatory failure. Respiratory failure is described as a PaO_2 less than 70 mmHg or a PaO_2 divided by the FiO_2 of less than 150. Ventilatory failure is described as an acutely elevated or rising $PaCO_2$ greater than 60 mmHg with respiratory acidosis. Other physiologic parameters include increased work of breathing. This is described as a respiratory rate twice baseline with the use of accessory muscles.

Types of Ventilators

Technologic advances continue to provide us with numerous options to support the patient in acute respiratory failure. Ventilators are described according to which ventilation variable is controlled in the inspiratory phase of each cycle (Chatburn, 1991b).

Pressure Controlled. Most infant ventilators are pressure controlled, so that peak pressure remains constant, but tidal volumes change as compliance and resistance varies. A continuous gas flow provides the patient a source of fresh gas for spontaneous breathing. Infants less than 10 kg are often ventilated using pressure-limited time-cycled ventilators.

Volume Controlled. Most adult ventilators are designed to deliver a preset tidal volume. Flow is the variable controlled by the ventilator to deliver a consistent volume. Since flow and volume are functions of each other, these machines are referred to as volume controllers. Airway pressure will vary with resistance and compliance during a volume-controlled breath.

Pressure-Controlled and Volume-Controlled. The newest generation of ventilators offer several modes in which pressure or volume can be the control variable. It is the actual operational mode that is most relevant to clinical management, as it best describes the interaction between patient and machine.

Modes of Ventilation

Pressure, volume, flow, and time are used as phase variables that determine the parameters for each ventilatory cycle (Chatburn, 1991b). The trigger variable describes the variable used to initiate inspiration. The limit variable describes the variable in which a preset value cannot be exceeded during inspiration. The cycle variable describes the variable used to end-inspiration. Baseline variables describe the variables that are controlled during expiration. Combinations of these four phase variables describe the various modes of ventilation. The major indications and special considerations for commonly used ventilator modes are summarized in Table 10–19.

Controlled Ventilation (CV). CV generally refers to a volume-controlled mode where all breaths are determined by the preset machine parameters and are completely independent of the patient's respiratory efforts or breathing pattern. This mode is poorly tolerated in spontaneously breathing patients and offers no benefit over other modes that allow the patient to initiate a ventilator breath on demand or to breathe in between mechanical breaths. This mode of ventilation is used in chemically paralyzed patients when spontaneous breathing can be potentially detrimental, for example, in the patient with a flail chest.

Intermittent Mandatory Ventilation (IMV). IMV allows a patient to breathe spontaneously from a continuous flow or demand valve in between preset mandatory breaths that are either pressure controlled or volume controlled. The patient is thereby able to breathe at his or her own rate and comfort level. V/Q matching is mixed because the spontaneous breaths result in increased ventilation to dependent lung regions whereas the mechanical breaths

Table 10–19. INDICATIONS AND SPECIAL CONSIDERATIONS FOR COMMONLY USED VENTILATOR MODES

Mode	Indications	Special Considerations
Controlled ventilation (CV)	Chest wall instability CNS dysfunction Respiratory muscle paralysis	Dynamic patient needs not accounted for Respiratory muscle inactivity leads to muscle atrophy
(S)IMV pressure controlled	Infants approximately < 10 kg where pressure is desired control variable	V_T will vary with patient compliance and resistance V_T delivery may be limited in larger patients Continuous flow available for spontaneous breaths
(S)IMV volume controlled	Older infants or where volume is the desired control variable	The smaller the patient, the more relative V_T lost to the compressible volume of the ventilator tubing V_T may vary in presence of ETT leaks, and changes in compliance and resistance Demand valve spontaneous flow systems may have poor response to high respiratory rates. Addition of continuous flow (2–5 L/min) may help
Pressure control ventilation (PCV)	Patients with low compliance and/or high resistance states (ARDS) Unilateral lung disease Large ETT leaks	V_T should be closely monitored PIP should be lower than in volume-limited modes Mean airway pressure may be higher than in volume-limited modes
Pressure support ventilation (PSV)	Failure to wean Muscle reconditioning Asynchrony	Backup (S)IMV rate may be provided Patients with ETT < 4.0 mm may prematurely cycle breath Patients with large ETT leaks may not cycle off breath appropriately Patient must be able to trigger PS breath with ease
Flow synchronization PSV	Weaning Muscle conditioning Asynchrony	Patient triggered Premature termination prevented with ETT < 4.0 mm Patients with large leaks may not cycle off breath
CPAP	Conditions with decreased FRC	Should provide continuous flow Patient must be spontaneously breathing

result in increased ventilation to nondependent lung regions. This mode is thought to be beneficial for weaning, as the patient is able to maintain the use of his or her respiratory muscles and provide increasing spontaneous support as the IMV or mandatory rate is gradually decreased. The clinician should be aware that the work of breathing may increase as the patient assumes responsibility for more of the ventilatory load.

Synchronized IMV (SIMV). This mode, as with IMV, offers preset mandatory breaths but synchronizes these breaths with a patient effort that is generally detected by a circuit change in pressure or flow. The theoretical advantages are that the patient will not have a mechanical breath superimposed upon a spontaneous one and that patient work will be more synchronous. While virtually all ventilators now offer SIMV, its benefits over IMV are unproved.

Pressure Control Ventilation (PCV). PCV is a mode of ventilation that is comparable with pressure-controlled (S)IMV, in that a preset pressure is reached with every breath. In PCV, however, there is a very high initial flow rate that allows an almost immediate rise to the preset peak inspiratory pressure (PIP). This PIP is then sustained throughout the preset inspiratory time. One theoretical advantage of this mode is that gas distribution is enhanced during the sustained PIP plateau.

Pressure Support Ventilation (PSV). The PSV mode of mechanical ventilation augments only the patient's spontaneous efforts with a preset level of airway pressure. In PSV, the inspiratory pressure plateau is reached early in inspiration and is maintained until inspiratory flow decreases to approximately 25% of initial peak flow. At this point inspiration ends, thus affording the patient control of inspiration and expiration. PSV can be used alone or in conjunction with a mandatory mode such as SIMV and PCV. Pressures of 5 to 30 cm H_2O are typically set; pressures of 5 to 15 cm H_2O are considered ideal. Tidal volumes can be variable as the patient's pulmonary mechanics change.

The pediatric patient unable to tolerate weaning will demonstrate decreased spontaneous tidal volumes leading to atelectasis, increased work of breathing, and an increased respiratory rate. In such patients, PSV may reverse this spiral and decrease patient work. While the benefits of PSV are untested in pediatrics, the authors have found this mode to be useful in achieving patient comfort during a protracted weaning process. Generally, the authors judge PSV to be beneficial if the patient's respiratory rate drops and work of breathing decreases.

There are a few unique problems when PSV is used in infants and small children. First, the increased airway resistance posed by smaller ETTs (less than 4.0) may precipitate premature termination of PS. That is, inspiration ends because of the high resistance created by the airway and not because of the patient's respiratory effort. This will reduce the effectiveness of PSV in augmenting tidal volume (TV). Second, if a significant ETT/TT air leak is present, the ventilator may be unable to sense the decrease in flow that normally occurs at end-inspiration. When this happens, the patient loses control over end-inspiration because the ventilator will automatically use a built-in time limit to end inspiration.

Flow-Synchronized Pressure Support Ventilation. Microprocessors and the evolution of sensor technology have made possible patient-synchronized ventilation in infants and small children. A number of systems are available that allow the patient's spontaneous breathing effort to trigger positive-pressure breaths.

Ventilator breaths can be triggered by a drop in patient airway pressure, the detection of a set inspiratory volume, and even the chest or abdominal movement preceding a spontaneous breath. However, the measurement of inspiratory flow at the patient's airway is one of the most sensitive methods of patient triggering. Flow triggering requires the use of a flow sensor at the patient's airway to detect a spontaneous breathing effort. This sensor generates a flow signal that the ventilator uses to detect a spontaneous breath. A machine-assisted breath is initiated when the ventilator senses an inspiratory flow rate equal to the set trigger sensitivity.

The availability to patient-trigger ventilator breaths provides the option of two patient-triggered modes of mechanical ventilation—SIMV and assist/control (A/C). SIMV delivers a fixed number of mandatory breaths that are synchronized with the patient's spontaneous breathing efforts and allows unassisted spontaneous breathing between mandatory breaths. With A/C, every patient effort that meets the trigger sensitivity criteria initiates a machine-assisted breath.

While the term flow synchronization has generally been applied to the use of flow to trigger ventilator breaths, the inspiratory flow signal can also be used to cycle (terminate) the inspiratory phase of ventilator breaths. The VIP Bird with flow synchronization uses the inspiratory flow signal to both trigger and cycle ventilator breaths. With flow cycling, the inspiratory phase is terminated when the inspiratory flow rate falls to a preset percentage of the peak inspiratory flow rate for that breath. Thus, ventilator rate and inspiratory time are primarily a function of the patient's ventilatory drive and respiratory mechanics. However, inspiratory time can also be influenced by manipulating the flow cycling threshold, which is adjustable from 5% to 25% of peak flow rate. The ability to flow trigger and flow cycle provides a high level of patient regulation of ventilation.

The potential benefits of flow-synchronized ventilation (and patient-synchronized ventilation in general) include enhanced gas exchange (particularly oxygenation), decreased incidence of barotrauma, decreased incidence of intraventricular hemorrhage, decreased need for heavy sedation and paralysis, and a decrease in the duration of mechanical ventilation.

Continuous Positive Airway Pressure (CPAP). CPAP is a spontaneous mode that provides a constant preset distending pressure. This constant pressure increases functional residual capacity (FRC) and prevents atelectasis. Increased lung volume increases pulmonary compliance and thus decreases the work of breathing. Low levels of CPAP are considered "physiologic" whenever the upper airway is bypassed with an ETT or TT. When these low levels—e.g., a CPAP of 3 to 5 cm H_2O—are reached, extubation is usually considered. On CPAP, the resistance imposed by smaller ETTs used in children may result in a higher work of breathing than the patient might experience extubated. Therefore, it is common to extubate from low rates of 4 or 6 breaths per minute.

Pressure-Controlled Inverse Ratio Ventilation (PCIRV). This mode of ventilation describes the delivery of volume at a preset peak inspiratory pressure (PIP) where the time spent in inspiration exceeds that of expiration. In PCIRV, PIPs are reached early in inspiration, creating a decelerating flow wave pattern and square pressure wave pattern. V_T depends upon IT, PIP, and the patient's pulmonary mechanics. The square pressure plateau wave facilitates alveolar recruitment and allows a more even distribution of gases within the lung in patients with nonhomogeneous lung disease (Betit, Thompson, & Benjamin, 1993). Prolonged ITs allow higher MAPs while limiting PIPs and PEEPs and maintaining PaO_2. Shorter ETs deter alveoli from falling below their closing capacity.

Patients supported on PCIRV require nursing assessment of alterations in cardiac output and pulmonary barotrauma occurring secondary to an inadequate expiratory phase, hyperinflation, and the development of autopeep (Juarez, 1992). The altered breathing pattern may also give patients a feeling of fullness that can be uncomfortable, making them anxious and restless, increasing their work of breathing and increasing VO_2 (Briones, 1991). Analgesia, sedation, and chemical paralysis are required for patient comfort and compliance.

Airway Pressure Release Ventilation (APRV). In this mode of ventilation, the patient breathes spontaneously at a positive baseline (CPAP). Periodically, this baseline is released to a lower pressure level for 1 to 2 seconds, allowing CO_2 to be exhaled. APRV is an alternative mode to improve oxygenation with lower mean airway pressures.

Mandatory Minute Ventilation (MMV). Infrequently used, this mode of computer-generated ventilation ensures the delivery of a predetermined minute ventilation distributed between spontaneous and ventilator breaths. If the patient's V_E is calculated to be low, additional breaths are delivered to the patient. One disadvantage of this mode of ventilation is that the quality of the patient's spontaneous breaths is not considered. A rapid, shallow pattern will not be distinguished from a slow, deep pattern because the V_E is the same. Altered respiratory patterns can lead to acid-base disturbances and atelectasis (Boegner, 1990).

Ventilation Parameters

Tidal Volume (V_T). In a volume-limited mode, V_T is set directly in cubic centimeters (cc). In a pressure-limited mode, V_T is determined by the difference between peak inspiratory pressure and PEEP—this is referred to as delta P ($\Delta P = PIP - PEEP$).

Frequency (F). The ventilator rate. Adjustable in breaths/minute.

Inspiratory Time (Ti). Ti together with F determines the inspiratory:expiratory (I:E) ratio. Pro-

longing Ti generally improves oxygenation by increasing the time the alveoli remain distended participating in gas exchange. Faster Ti and longer expiratory times are used to prevent hyperinflation in patients with airways disease. Some ventilators offer an inspiratory hold or pause that prolongs Ti.

Positive End-Expiratory Pressure (PEEP). The pressure that is sustained at the end of expiration. PEEP improves oxygenation by increasing FRC, preventing alveolar collapse, and enhancing the ratio of ventilation to perfusion. Excessive levels of PEEP

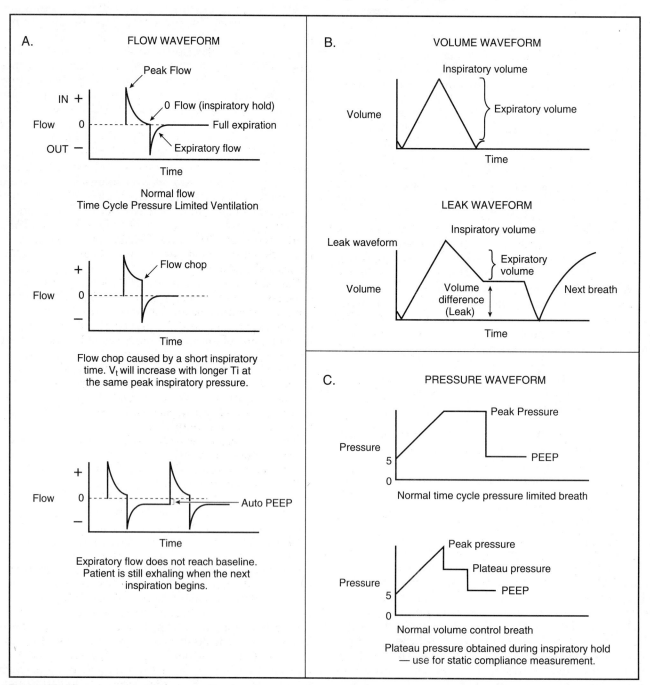

Figure 10–30 ● ● ● ● ● ●

Examples of *A,* flow waveform; *B,* volume waveform; *C,* pressure waveform.

Table 10-20. SUGGESTED INITIAL VENTILATOR SETTINGS FOR VARIOUS TIME CONSTANTS

Ventilator Setting	Long Time Constant	Normal Time Constant	Short Time Constant
V_t	10–12 mL/kg	8–12 mL/kg	8–10 mL/kg
F/min	8–15	10–20	15–30
I:E ratio	>1:4	1:2	1:1
PEEP	0–5	3–5	>5

will cause hyperinflation and CO_2 retention by adding unnecessary dead space. Excessive PEEP will also impede venous return to the chest, which will eventually decrease the patient's cardiac output and oxygen delivery.

Peak Inspiratory Pressure (PIP). The pressure that is reached and sustained during inspiration. PIP is directly adjusted in the pressure-limited modes but varies with compliance and resistance in the volume-limited modes.

Mean Airway Pressure (MAP). Measured in cm H_2O, MAP is the average airway pressure over a respiratory cycle (AARC, 1992). PIP, Ti, PEEP, and F all directly affect MAP. MAPs over 12 cm H_2O are considered significant. This parameter is a monitored value on most ventilators.

Fraction of Inspired Oxygen (Fio2). The inspired oxygen concentration. FiO_2 levels less than 0.6 are generally considered safe (Betit, Thompson, & Benjamin, 1993).

Flow Rate. The continuous flow of ventilator gas adjusted in L/min. Pressure-controlled ventilators require adequate flow rates for the delivery of PIP, for optimal V_T, and for a continuous source of gas for spontaneous breaths. Flow rates determine the time it takes to reach PIP during inspiration. When flow rates are low, PIP is reached at the end of inspiration, decreasing the plateau phase; if flow rates are high, PIP is reached early in inspiration, increasing the plateau phase (Betit, Thompson, & Benjamin, 1993). The inspiratory plateau affects gas distribution; the longer the plateau, the better the distribution of gas throughout the lung (see Fig. 10–30).

Alarm Systems. For patient safety, ventilator alarms remain activated within a tight range at all times. Most ventilators are equipped with an inspiratory line pressure alarm to detect a sudden loss in pressure (disconnect) and a sudden increase in pressure (obstruction). Other alarms include gas supply, FiO_2, gas humidity and temperature, and electricity failure. Ventilator alarms that allow a 10- to 15-second automatic reset are safer for the patient, as the human factor is eliminated.

Initiation of Mechanical Ventilation

Prior to initiating mechanical ventilation, the clinician evaluates the patient's pulmonary mechanics by "feel" during manual hand ventilation using an anesthesia bag and attached manometer. Initial ventilator settings are then matched to those identified as optimal during hand ventilation.

An alternative strategy is to start the patient on the suggested ventilator settings listed in Table 10–20, which take into consideration anticipated time constants. Faster rates without stacking of breaths can be used in patients with lung disease states characterized by short time constants (lungs quickly fill and empty). Slower rates and longer expiratory times are used in patients with lung disease characterized by long time constants (lungs take a long time to fill and empty). Once the patient is on mechanical support, ventilator settings are fine tuned within established ABG parameters and measured pulmonary mechanics.

Ventilator Strategies

Mechanical ventilation has two goals: to maintain mean lung volume and alveolar ventilation. As mentioned, reduction in V/Q imbalance must also be a consideration and although ventilator manipulations may optimize ventilation, the V/Q relationship is best viewed as a dynamic phenomenon. The clinician's challenge is to achieve an acceptable minute ventilation with respect to perfusion in the presence of an adequate mean lung volume. Factors to assess upon initiation of mechanical ventilation are included in Table 10–21.

Making the Right Maneuver

Paco2. $PaCO_2$ is inversely related to minute ventilation (V_E) ($V_E = V_T \times F$). A portion of V_T is com-

Table 10-21. FACTORS TO ASSESS UPON INITIATION OF MECHANICAL VENTILATION

1. Baseline breath sounds (quality, adequate expiratory time)
2. Decreased work of breathing (decreased respiratory rate, severity of retractions, nasal flaring, grunting, etc.)
3. Chest excursion and symmetry
4. Chest x-ray (ETT position, improved lung volume, pathology)
5. Pulmonary mechanics (decreased airway resistance, increased compliance, and FRC [time constants, autopeep])
6. Arterial blood gases (improved oxygenation, decreased $PaCO_2$, improved pH)
7. Need for noninvasive monitoring
8. Need for muscle relaxants, sedation (chemical restraint)
9. Need for pulmonary hygiene
10. Need for aerosolized or systemic bronchodilators

posed of dead space volume (V_D) and therefore will not participate in gas exchange. V_D is related to body surface area and normally accounts for 30% of V_T. In mechanically ventilated patients, V_D may be as high as 50% to 60% from the effects of positive pressure on the airways. Accordingly, changes in ventilator parameters can alter V_D. Any tubing or adapters distal to the patient ventilator will add mechanical dead space, as this volume acts as an extension of the patient's airway. Mechanical V_D should be kept to a minimum.

Pao₂. The most basic control of PaO_2 is FiO_2. The relationship between FiO_2 and PaO_2 is not as straightforward as that between $PaCO_2$ and V_E. This is due to the effects of water vapor pressure in the lung and oxygen diffusibility relative to the (diseased) alveolar-pulmonary capillary membrane. PaO_2 is also affected by the degree and pattern of ventilation and V/Q ratio. The MAP is a very useful index of the overall effect of changes in ventilation variables and is directly related to PaO_2. Any maneuver that alters MAP has the potential to change PaO_2. The five factors that affect the MAP include (1) PIP, (2) PEEP, (3) inspiratory time, (4) inspiratory flow, and (5) increased respiratory rate with same inspiratory time. Optimal MAP is where gas exchange is efficient and beyond which alveolar overdistension occurs (Oakes, 1990).

Chest X-ray. In general, there should be radiologic evidence of improved lung volume. Adequate lung volume is evidenced by the ninth anterior rib above the dome of the diaphragm, although aeration is relative to surrounding structures. Assuming the film is taken during inspiration, the diaphragm should be neither elevated nor flattened. Hypoaeration is managed by increasing PEEP or Ti.

Autopeep. In situations where the F is high or the patient has long time constants, the clinician should check for the presence of autopeep or intrinsic peep. Autopeep refers to the spontaneous development of PEEP at the alveolar level due to insufficient expiratory time (Benson, 1988). Autopeep can be detected in a noncontinuous flow ventilator system and is checked by occluding the expiratory limb of the ventilator at end-expiration. If autopeep is present, the baseline pressure (PEEP) will rise as expiratory flow continues from the patient. The level of autopeep is clinically important, as its presence may contribute to enhanced oxygenation and/or CO_2 retention. While the presence of 1 to 3 cm H_2O of autopeep may not be clinically deleterious, this number should be monitored in appropriate patients, as it is a dynamic number (unlike set PEEP) and can change rapidly.

Blood Gas Monitoring. Whenever possible, ABGs should be obtained in the newly ventilated patient to assess for improved gas exchange. If arterial access is not immediately possible, a venous blood gas may be helpful in assessing acid-base status. Pulse oximeters may be used to continuously and noninvasively assess oxygenation. $ETCO_2$ monitoring is useful; however, the presence of large ETT leaks can result in inaccurate low readings and some monitors will not read accurately at high (>30) respiratory rates.

Bronchial Hygiene. Adequate suctioning is essential in the pediatric patient. Smaller ETT diameters predispose these patients to airway obstruction. The relative small size of the conducting airways places the child at increased risk for significant compromise from the effects of infection, edema, and secretions. Partial or complete obstruction of the bronchioles and bronchi can result in air trapping and atelectasis. What may seem like an insignificant amount of secretions may have a significant impact on airway resistance. In patients with thick secretions, liberal instillation with normal saline is recommended.

Sedation. Ensuring an adequate level of comfort for the mechanically ventilated patient is fundamental to humane care. Artificial airways and imposed breaths are poorly tolerated by the alert child. Because of developmental immaturity, one cannot depend on patient cooperation. In fact, if a toddler, for example, cooperates with a stranger when the parents are not present, one would question the child's level of consciousness. In addition to parents, analgesics and sedatives are frequently used to help the patient tolerate both the ICU environment and the treatments involved. Chemical restraints should be used in combination with physical restraints. In assessing agitation, it is important to determine what comes first—hypoxia or agitation. A distressed infant may be trying to indicate inadequate ventilator settings, an obstructed ETT, a pneumothorax, pain, or the need for a quieter environment. The use of neuromuscular blocking agents may be indicated in the sedated patient if ventilator support is escalating resulting in the use of higher PIP, PEEP, or F, or if the child is asynchronous or fighting the ventilator. These agents are not used indiscriminately because they remove critically important assessment signs, such as activity and comfort levels.

Special Considerations

Endotracheal (ETT) Tube Leaks. Due to the use of uncuffed ETTs in young children, leaks are often present and can compromise ventilation if they are excessive. An ETT leak detected above an inspiratory pressure of 20 cm H_2O is generally desirable, as this may help reduce the occurrence of airway trauma and post-extubation swelling, yet this may in turn limit the ability to deliver an adequate tidal volume in the patient where higher peak inspiratory pressures are needed. Very large ETT leaks may cause autotriggering of mechanical breaths on some ventilators where loss of PEEP may be sensed as the patient's inspiratory effort. It is therefore important to assess ETT leaks periodically by hand ventilating the patient with a manometer inline to note at what pressure the leak begins. Leaks can be further quantified by a volume-monitoring device. Many of the newest ventilators have the capability to measure

CHAPTER 10 ■ Oxygenation/Ventilation **303**

volume at the patient airway, which can accurately quantify an ETT leak. Leaks are notoriously variable and can vary with ETT position, head position, and fluid balance. If it is felt that a leak is compromising ventilation, it may be necessary to re-intubate with a larger tube.

ETT Resistance. Reducing the diameter of a tube by one half results in a 16-fold decrease in flow through that tube. The small ETT diameters used in children cause a substantial increase in flow resistance and therefore a significant increase in the work of breathing. For this reason, children are usually not extubated from ventilator rates less than 4 to 6 breaths per minute. The work imposed by the pediatric ETT is often compared to "breathing through a straw." Attentiveness to this phenomenon is especially important in the child with a history of significant respiratory failure.

Compressible Volume. The compressible volume of a ventilator circuit refers to the amount of the tidal volume that is lost with each breath to displacement and compression of the volume of the ventilator tubing. This portion of the breath never enters the patient's lungs. Ventilator tubing has a measurable compliance or distensibility that can be used to distinguish the actual delivered tidal volume from the lost compressible volume. This is the compressible volume factor. The loss of compressible volume is particularly important in volume-limited ventilation when small tidal volumes are used. For example, in a situation where tubing has a compressible volume factor of 3 mL/cm H_2O and peak inspiratory pressure is 40, the set tidal volume would be reduced by 120 mL (3×40). The loss of volume is quite relevant in pediatric mechanical ventilation because of the small volumes used. For instance, if a tidal volume of 200 mL were set in the above situation, the delivered volume would be only approximately 80 mL.

Ventilator Limitations. Infants and small children may have difficulty using the assist-control mode of ventilation, as they need to inhale a greater proportion of their TV before creating enough negative pressure to trigger the ventilator's sensing mechanism. Once triggered, the response time may be too slow to support the faster pediatric respiratory rate. An inadequate response time can lead to an increased work of breathing. A similar problem occurs during spontaneous ventilation; usually gas flow is delivered to the circuit when a demand valve is activated by negative airway pressure. This demand valve may be too difficult for the pediatric patient, so a continuous-flow reservoir is typically added to the circuit in patients less than 15 kg. Providing a low level of added continuous flow may alleviate the problem, as it will allow the child to spontaneously breathe without triggering the demand valve system.

Volume Monitoring. Monitoring of tidal volume should be considered in the patient where one of the above variables may be compromising the delivery of a consistent tidal volume. This may involve intermittent checks to note changes after setting changes or continuous monitoring in patients with large or

variable ETT leaks. Tidal volume (V_T) monitoring is now easily accomplished with equipment specifically designed for the pediatric population. These include Bournes Neonatal Volume Monitor–NVM (Bear Medical System, Riverside, CA), Bicore (Bear Medical System, Riverside, CA), Ventrak (Novametric Medical Systems, Wallingford, CT), and Partner IIi (Bird Medical Corp, Palm Springs, CA). Ventilator settings can be adjusted to deliver a specific V_T (mL/kg). A constant V_T will stabilize the FRC and allow immediate corrective action for acute changes. Computers, used in conjunction with volume monitors, allow calculation of respiratory mechanics, e.g., compliance, resistance, time constants, T_I/T_{TOT}, work of breathing, flow/volume loops, and pressure/volume curve. Scalar tracings of flow, pressure, and volume of each breath allow for bedside graphic interpretation (see Fig. 10–30).

Complications of Mechanical Ventilation

Rapid deterioration in the pediatric patient is often attributable to one of the factors listed in Table 10–22. The incidence of pneumothorax in pediatrics has been reported to be between 4.5% and 8% and in some studies has been correlated with mortality (Benjamin, Thompson, & O'Rourke, 1990). Certainly, this complication must be recognized promptly and treated. In patients with reactive airways disease, sudden development of bronchospasm may occur in the absence of a precipitating event and result in significant compromise. As previously mentioned, autopeep is a dynamic phenomenon that can have adverse effects and should be periodically checked if the clinical picture is suggestive of its presence. Acute ETT obstruction is common in pediatrics, and if it is suspected, the patient should be reintubated if an attempt to clear the tube is unsuccessful. The instrumented pediatric airway is difficult to maintain because of patient size and lack of cooperation. Slight changes in ETT position can result in right mainstem intubation or accidental extubation. Finally, an increasing ETT leak can occur from resolving airway edema or diuresis resulting in decreased minute ventilation or failure to hold PEEP.

General complications of mechanical ventilation are listed in Table 10–23. The major side effects of CPAP/PEEP include hemodynamic complications and pulmonary barotrauma. Increased intrathoracic

Table 10-22. COMMON RESPIRATORY CAUSES OF RAPID CLINICAL DETERIORATION

1. ETT position change
2. Large or positional ETT leak
3. Secretions
4. Bronchospasm
5. Development of autopeep
6. Pneumothorax

Table 10-23. COMPLICATIONS OF MECHANICAL VENTILATION

Air leak	Pneumothorax
	Pneumomediastinum
	Pneumopericardium
	Pneumoperitoneum
	Subcutaneous emphysema
Infection	Pneumonia
	Septicemia
Airway	Dislodgment
	Occlusion
	Accidental extubation
	Erosion
	Stenosis
Hyperinflation	Air trapping (autopeep)
Cardiovascular	Decrease venous return
	Decrease cardiac output
	Increase pulmonary vascular resistance
Extrathoracic organs	Decrease urine output
	Increase antidiuretic hormone
	Decrease hepatic blood flow
	Increase intracranial pressure
Mechanical	Ventilator malfunction
	Disconnection

pressure leads to decreased systemic venous return resulting in decreased cardiac output. These hemodynamic effects can be easily monitored with a pulmonary artery catheter. Optimal levels of CPAP/PEEP can also be approximated by esophageal pressure monitoring. Esophageal pressure should increase slightly with each increase of CPAP/PEEP until optimal levels are reached. After that, esophageal pressures will increase exponentially with only slight increases in CPAP/PEEP. In addition to producing pulmonary barotrauma, overdistension increases V_D and results in a rising $PaCO_2$. When faced with progressively worsening ABGs, one strategy is to cautiously decrease inflating pressures when the possibility of overinflation is present.

Guidelines for the Weaning Process

Weaning patients involves assessing their readiness to wean, optimizing factors that can facilitate weaning, selecting the appropriate weaning method, and continually assessing the patient progress (Weilitz, 1993). In the adolescent, adult criteria are used as guidelines: a vital capacity of 15 to 20 mL/kg, negative inspiratory force (NIF) of -20 cm H_2O, tidal volume of 6 to 10 mL/kg, and a maximum voluntary ventilation (MVV) of greater than twice the minute ventilation (Henneman, 1991). For all pediatric patients, the best indication of weaning is respiratory rate.

Pediatric patients respond to respiratory compromise by decreasing tidal volume and increasing respiratory rate. During weaning, regardless of the strategy, the respiratory rate should be below two times the baseline. Clinical states that impact patient readiness to wean are listed in Table 10–24.

The modes most commonly used to wean patients include CPAP, SIMV, and pressure support ventilation. Mechanical support is gradually decreased one parameter at a time until a minimal amount of support is reached. Usually, the longer a patient has been ventilated, the longer the weaning process. Because of respiratory muscle atrophy, a period of muscle reconditioning is required before extubation. This is accomplished by progressively exercising the respiratory muscles to rebuild endurance. Chronically ventilated patients are not weaned at night, as adequate rest is critically important to success.

Starting with the most potentially toxic parameter, settings can be gradually weaned or the patient can be switched to pressure support ventilation. Generally, Ti is returned to normal; the FiO_2 is decreased by 2% to 10% to maintain a PaO_2 greater than 60 mmHg; PIPs are decreased by 2 to 5 cm H_2O to the low 20s to maintain TVs in the 7 to 10 mL/kg range; PEEP is decreased to 3 to 5 cm H_2O provided that oxygenation is adequate on low FiO_2; and rate is decreased by 1 to 2 breaths slowly over hours to days (depending upon tolerance) to maintain a $PaCO_2$ within normal limits for the patient and allow spontaneous breaths without excessive work of breathing.

When ventilatory rates are weaned to a low of 6 breaths/min in an infant or 4 in a child, or successful trial of 3 to 5 cm H_2O of CPAP has been accomplished, extubation is considered if criteria are reached—that is, good gases on an FiO_2 less than .5, adequate cough and gag, and thin or moderate consistency in the character of secretions. Note that infants are extubated from higher rates because of the increased airway resistance created by the smaller ETT.

The major benefit of PSV is that it re-establishes the patient's control over breathing, improves patient-ventilator synchrony, decreases diaphragmatic muscle fatigue, and reduces the work of breathing. PSV eliminates the shallow ineffective TVs associated with progressive tachypnea and atelectasis that may occur during more traditional weaning methods.

After extubation, the patient may benefit from a 20% increase in FiO_2 or nasal/facial CPAP if lung volume is a problem. Nasal/facial CPAP may help prevent alveolar collapse and is weaned as tolerated—usually, if the patient struggles more when it

Table 10-24. CLINICAL STATES THAT IMPACT PATIENT READINESS TO WEAN FROM MECHANICAL VENTILATION

1. Cardiovascular stability
2. Adequate oxygen-carrying capacity
3. Fluid balance
4. Electrolyte balance
5. Acid-base balance
6. Optimized nutritional state
   (infants: consistent weight gain > 10–20 g/day)
7. Infection-free
8. Adequate level of comfort and rest
9. Level of consciousness
10. Ability to tolerate environment

is on, it's time to take it off. The patient is observed for long-term endurance failure.

Nasal/Facial Continuous Positive Airway Pressure (CPAP)

Relatively low levels of CPAP can be administered to spontaneously breathing extubated patients using specialty nasal prongs or masks. The success of this strategy is variable but may be used as either a continuous or intermittent bridge to extubation in the chronically ventilated patient. The success of nasal CPAP in infants depends on the degree of mouth breathing and crying present. The success of facial CPAP in the child is dependent upon patient tolerance and a mask that adequately fits the patient. Side effects include gastric distension; a nasogastric tube can be used to continuously vent the stomach.

Specialty Ventilators

Home Care. Home care ventilators are designed for portability for the tracheotomized patient. The ventilator is volume controlled with battery power capability. Modes are kept simplistic for ease of use.

BiPAP (Biphasic Positive Airway Pressure). BiPAP is generally used for assisted ventilation of the non-tracheotomized patient. A nasal mask or pillows are used. The BiPAP system may be totally patient triggered, or a rate may be set. The mode is pressure controlled with continuous flow compensating for leak around the mask.

Negative-Pressure Ventilators (NPVs). Iron lungs, cuirass, and raincoats create negative abdominal pressure, allowing the diaphragm to distend and draw air into the lungs (Fig. 10–31). NPV is pressure controlled; tidal volumes are dependent upon the patient's transthoracic pressure and thoracic compliance. Increased transthoracic pressures augment FRC, limit intrapulmonary shunting, and improve systemic oxygenation. Tidal volumes can be measured at the patient airway using a spirometer.

NPVs are generally used for non-tracheotomized patients who cannot tolerate BiPAP. NPV may be used continuously, intermittently, or at night to permit the patient to rest. Patients with hypercapnic respiratory failure secondary to alveolar hypoventilation syndromes and/or neuromuscular or chest wall mechanical problems may benefit from NPV. NPV may also benefit the postoperative cardiovascular surgery patient who requires assisted ventilation but would benefit from lower pulmonary artery pressures and enhanced pulmonary and central venous return.

Blaufuss and Wallace (1987) delineated the nursing care issues involved in caring for patients supported on NPV. These patients are at risk for airway obstruction and pulmonary aspiration. Nasojejunum tubes are recommended for enteral feedings. Hypothermia secondary to convective cooling as air is pulled through the collar may become an issue. Maintaining skin integrity and vascular access requires

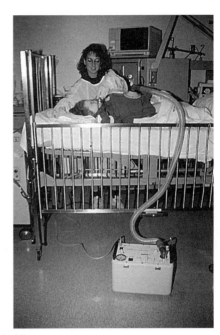

Figure 10–31 ● ● ● ● ● ●
Raincoat negative-pressure ventilator.

proactive interventions. Patients commonly experience claustrophobia, helplessness, and sleep deprivation, so diversional therapy is also very important.

ALTERNATIVE THERAPIES

High-Frequency Ventilation

High-frequency ventilation (HFV) has become increasingly popular in supporting infants and children with acute respiratory failure (ARF) who cannot be ventilated by traditional means. Conventional mechanical ventilation (CMV) is not without risk; the delivery of normal tidal volumes (V_T) to a patient with sick, noncompliant lungs necessitates high inflating pressures. However, decreased compliance is not a global phenomenon and regions of high compliance become overdistended (Chatburn, 1990). These extreme swings in airway pressure, from PIP to PEEP, contribute to the incidence of pulmonary barotrauma and associated airleak syndrome, e.g., pneumothorax, pneumomediastinum, pneumopericardium, pneumoperitoneum, and pulmonary interstitial edema (PIE).

With HFV, small V_Ts (equal to or less than V_D) delivered at high frequencies maintain constant lung volumes at airway pressures just above alveolar closing pressure. The lungs stay inflated while both volume and pressure peaks and valleys associated with continuous forced opening and passive closing of alveoli are avoided. One potential, but unsupported, benefit of HFV is the reduction of iatrogenic ventilator injury while maintaining adequate gas exchange using similar mean airway pressures (MAPs) but lower PIPs associated with CMV.

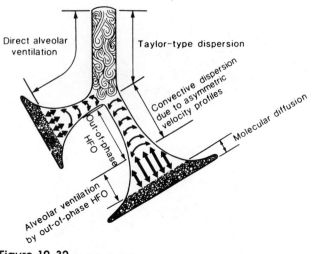

Figure 10–32 ● ● ● ● ● ●

Modes of gas transport during high-frequency ventilation. (From Villar J., et al. (1990). Non-conventional techniques of ventilatory support. *Critical Care Clinics*, 6, 579.)

Definition

HFV is a broad term used to describe numerous techniques of ventilation that deliver tidal volumes less than the patient's dead space at supraphysiologic rates. In adults, HFV is operationally defined as 60 or more breaths per minute (bpm) or 1 hertz (Hz). This definition has obvious limitations in sick infants and children, who normally have respiratory rates within this range. A better definition for the pediatric population is the use of ventilatory rates greater than 150 bpm at V_T that approaches anatomic V_D.

Mechanism of Gas Transport in HFV

CMV attempts to simulate spontaneous ventilation by delivering gas in bulk volume that approximates V_T at physiologic respiratory rates. Gas transport in the larger airways occurs primarily by bulk convec-

tion of three times V_D, whereas diffusion is important in the terminal airways and alveoli.

Traditional physiology, based upon bulk flow, cannot explain the mechanism of gas exchange in HFV. In 1915, Henderson and others noted that when smoke was blown down a tube, it formed a thin spike; the quicker the puff, the thinner and sharper the spike. Correlating their observation to panting dogs, they believed that gas exchange, sufficient to support life, was possible when V_T was less than V_D. Chang and Harf (1984) identified five mechanisms of gas transport thought to be important in HFV: (1) convection, (2) pendelluft flow, (3) Taylor dispersion, (4) asymmetric velocity, and (5) molecular diffusion (Fig. 10–32).

Convection refers to the bulk flow of inspired gas to the level of the alveoli. Unlike CMV, HFV delivers V_Ts equal to at least one half to three quarters anatomic V_D. Direct alveolar ventilation becomes less pronounced as V_T approaches V_D (Coghill, Haywood, Chatburn, & Carlo, 1991). *Pendelluft flow* refers to interregional gas mixing or the movement of gas between neighboring lung units dependent upon time constants. Pendelluft flow is enhanced during HFV and facilitates interregional gas mixing of adjacent lung units. *Taylor dispersion* describes the distribution of gas moving in a column; axial dispersion and radial diffusion. Gas flowing through a straight tube forms a parabolic (bullet-tipped) velocity profile with the highest velocity occurring at the center. This effect disperses gas across the front of the moving column of gas (axial dispersion) and facilitates molecular diffusion around its periphery (radial diffusion). *Asymmetric velocity* is the mixing of inspiratory and expiratory gases in the airway. Inspiratory gas (O_2) moves toward the alveoli in the center of the airway, and expiratory gas (CO_2) moves away from the alveolus along the periphery. *Molecular diffusion,* the process of gas transport across the alveolar pulmonary-capillary membrane, is the primary mechanism of gas transfer between the alveolus and blood. The

Table 10-25. OVERVIEW OF HIGH-FREQUENCY VENTILATION TECHNIQUES

	HFPPV	HFJV	HFFI	HFOV
Flow generator	High-pressure gas source	High-pressure gas source	High-pressure gas source	Piston pump
Fresh gas delivery system	Continuous or valved fresh gas flow	Jet catheter with continuous fresh gas bias flow	Valved flow interrupter	Continuous fresh gas flow
TV	> V_D	> < V_D	> < V_D	< V_D
Expiration	Passive	Passive	Passive	Active
Airway pressure waveform	Variable	Triangular	Triangular	Sine wave
Entrainment	None	Yes	None	None
Frequency	60–120 (1–2 Hz)	60–600 (1–10 Hz)	300–1200 (5–20 Hz)	60–3600 (1–60 Hz)
Ventilator	Siemens	Bunnell Universal	Emerson Infant Star	Hummingbird Sensormedics

Data from Coghill, C.H., Haywood, J.L., Chatburn, R.L., & Carlo, W.A. (1991). Neonatal and pediatric high-frequency ventilation: Principles and practice. *Respiratory Care, 36*(6), 596–609; Martin, L.D., Rafferty, J.F., Walker, L.K., & Gioia, F.R. (1992). Principles of respiratory support and mechanical ventilation (pp. 134–203). In M.C. Rogers. (Ed.). *Textbook of pediatric intensive care*. Baltimore: Williams & Wilkins.

literal shaking of the chest during HFV probably enhances molecular diffusion.

Although gas transport during HFV is thought to be a function of all five mechanisms, observations made in the laboratory setting using rigid uniform cylinders cannot be applied to humans with a complex tracheobronchial tree. The exact mechanisms of gas exchange in HFV are controversial but probably vary in different areas of the lung, in different disease states, and with different techniques employed.

Classification

The early days of HFV were characterized by device confusion, a technology in search of a disease (Arnold, Troug, Thompson, & Fackler, 1993). Since that time, a variety of HFV techniques have been used in clinical trials. Four techniques are in clinical use today: high-frequency positive-pressure ventilation (HFPPV), high-frequency jet ventilation (HFJV), high-frequency flow interruption (HFFI), and high-frequency oscillation ventilation (HFOV). Table 10–25 provides an overview of these techniques. When analyzing research related to HFV, the method of HFV as well as the ventilation strategy is important.

HFPPV, considered by many to be an extension of CMV, employs a standard ventilator modified with low-compliance tubing so that adequate V_T can be delivered using short Ti (Coghill, Haywood, Chatburn, & Carlo, 1991). Flow is intermittently delivered to the patient through a pneumatic valve located at the airway. Effective ventilation can occur within an open or closed system. When closed, the system allows an accurate determination of V_T because environmental air entrainment does not occur. Tidal volume is delivered via a standard ETT with the inspiratory phase the only active phase of the respiratory cycle. Expiration is achieved by passive lung recoil. Ventilation frequency, V_T, FiO_2, and Ti can be controlled. Starting frequencies are usually in the range of 60 to 120 bpm (1–2 Hz), V_T 3 to 4 mL/kg, and inspiratory times (Ti) 20% to 33% (Wetzel & Gioia, 1987). Heijman and others (1972) cautioned that high frequencies may limit V_T and compromise actual alveolar ventilation despite an increase in minute ventilation.

HFJV delivers small bursts of gas from a high-pressure source into the patient's trachea through an injector port of an ETT designed specifically for jet ventilation (Fig. 10–33A). The burst of gas, representing inspiration, is the only active phase of the ventilatory cycle; expiration depends on passive lung recoil. Tidal volumes are generated by the jet volume plus varying volumes entrained by a Venturi effect from a parallel continuous low-pressure flow circuit. Entrainment occurs when the jet burst entering the airway under high pressure creates an area of low pressure behind the entry point. Gas from the upper airway is pulled into the low pressure area, giving additional V_T to each jet pulse. The volume delivered depends on ventilator settings and pulmonary me-

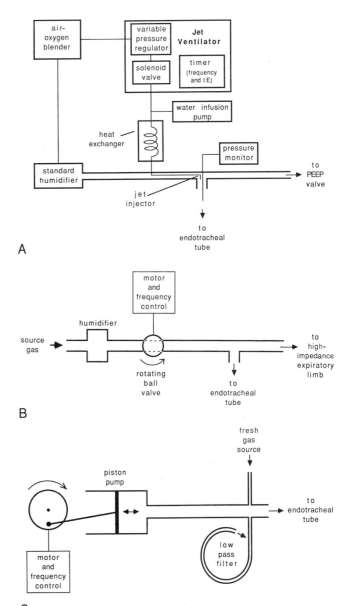

Figure 10–33 ● ● ● ● ● ●

A, Schema of a high-frequency jet ventilation system. *B,* Schema of a high-frequency flow interruption system. *C,* Schema of a high-frequency oscillatory ventilation system. (From Chatburn, R.L. (1990). High-frequency ventilation. In J.L. Blummer (Ed.). *A practical guide to pediatric intensive care* (3rd ed., pp. 957–958). St. Louis: Mosby–Year Book.)

chanics, such as airway resistance. The presence of a large back pressure may impede gas entrainment and jet flow. Frequencies range from 4 to 10 Hz. Concerns with this mode of HFV include providing adequate humidification and the need to reintubate a critically ill patient with the special ETT.

HFFI, considered to be a hybrid of HFJV, provides small bursts of gas at high frequencies into the ventilator circuit rather than the patient's trachea. Ventilation occurs through the interruption of high-pressure gas flow by either a shutter system or rotating ball device (Fig. 10–33B). Compared with HFJV, humidification is better, a special ETT is unnecessary, and gas entrainment does not occur (Tsuzaki, 1990). Frequencies can to adjusted to 20 Hz.

HFOV uses a piston acting across a low-bias flow circuit to deliver small volumes of gas through a standard ETT (Fig. 10–33C). Gas is pushed in, and, as the direction of the piston reverses, similar volumes are extracted from the lung. The primary difference between HFOV and other modes of HVF is that exhalation is active, not entirely dependent on passive lung recoil. Active exhalation not only enhances CO_2 removal but also reduces the incidence of stacking of breaths causing inadvertent increases in lung volume (Weber & Asselin, 1990). Because of the active exhalation phase, very fast rates from 300 to 3000/min or 5 to 50 Hz can be used.

Equal power is applied to both inspiratory and expiratory phases. As long as the inspiratory and expiratory time constants of the lungs are equivalent, equal volumes of gas are delivered and extracted. Time constants are rarely equal, and at 50% Ti at high frequency, air trapping can occur resulting in an increase in lung volume. As long as Ti is less than 40% of the respiratory cycle, mean alveolar pressure will not exceed mean proximal airway pressure (Venegas, 1989).

Oscillatory ventilation holds lung volume constant. This not only eliminates potential mechanical damage from the opening and closing of the delicate small airways and alveoli, but also eliminates the need for high peak pressure breaths needed to reopen closed alveoli. Lung volume is held relatively constant to enhance alveolar recruitment.

Clinical Issues

Coghill and others (1991) noted that, regardless of the technique used, the most consistent observation in HFV is that CO_2 elimination is usually easily accomplished. CO_2 elimination is related to both V_T and frequency; but, unlike CMV, V_T appears to be more important in HFV.

Delivered V_T increases with ETT size and decreases with frequency (Tsuzaki, 1990). In HFPPV and HFJV, $PaCO_2$ increases when the frequency passes a threshold level due to decreased delivered V_T. Insufficient expiratory time (<66%) will cause an increased lung volume and impedance to lung inflation at higher frequencies. During HFOV, increasing the frequency will decrease the $PaCO_2$ until a plateau is reached. HFOV eliminates CO_2 faster than expiratory-passive forms of HFV. In HFJV, the position of the jet cannula tip in the airway is also an important factor; the closer the tip is to the carina, the better the CO_2 elimination.

As in CMV, oxygenation is largely determined by mean airway pressure and its correlate—lung volume. Compared with CMV, some proponents of HFV believe that oxygenation can be accomplished using lower MAPs. However, MAPs measured at the proximal airway are probably different than alveoli pressure (Froese & Bryan, 1987). Comparisons of oxygenation between CMV and HFV at similar proximal airway pressures have not necessarily ensured equivalence of mean alveolar pressure and lung volumes (Wetzel & Gioia, 1987). PIPs are lower with HFV because of smaller delivered V_T.

During CMV, there is a gradual increase in alveolar pressure during inspiration. At end-inspiration, alveolar pressure may become supra-atmospheric and restrain pulmonary capillary blood flow. Increased intrathoracic pressure associated with positive-pressure ventilation also decreases venous return, stroke volume, and cardiac output. Attempts to limit these adverse circulatory effects prompted enthusiasm for HFV. However, studies comparing cardiac output and other hemodynamic variables during HFV and CMV at equal mean alveolar pressures in animals have failed to reveal significant differences (Wetzel & Gioia, 1987).

The effects of HFV on the pulmonary circulation and V/Q matching have not been adequately defined. Humorally mediated attenuation of the hypoxemic pulmonary vasomotor response during HFV may contribute to pulmonary venous admixture and arterial desaturation (Wetzel & Gioia, 1987).

In the setting of intracranial hypertension, the negative impact of high intrathoracic pressure on cerebral circulation is well documented. Decreased respiratory variation in intrathoracic and central vascular pressures during HFV should diminish phasic swings in ICP. Total and regional blood flow does not appear to be different during HFV and CMV.

The early use of HFJV was complicated by necrotizing tracheobronchitis (NTB) characterized by epithelial erosion, loss of ciliated cells, squamous cell metaplasia, and infiltration of the mucosa by neutrophils (Chatburn, 1990). Symptoms of NTB include acute airway obstruction and aspiration of necrotic debris from the airway. Possible pathogenesis of NTB includes inadequate humidification of delivered gas and extremely high velocity jet flows (Tsuzaki, 1990). Even though significant progress has been made in both atomizing and heating inspired gas, HFJV is still associated with significant iatrogenic injury to the airway when compared with both CMV and HFOV. Although there are conflicting data regarding the effect of HFV on mucociliary transport, without adequate humidification mucous clearance becomes a problem.

Studies investigating the effects of HFV on lung water and edema formation have produced contradictory findings. Pulmonary compliance and surfactant activity have been studied and suggest that mechanical pressure-volume relationships and surfactant activity of the lung are not negatively influenced during HFV (Wetzel & Gioia, 1987).

Eucapneic apnea has been observed with HFV. This apneic state associated with HFV is mediated by chest wall receptors and vagal afferent fibers and appears to be independent of chemical respiratory drive and lung volume changes.

Clinical Applications

Compared with the neonatal population, the use of HFV in infants and young children has received less attention. While the benefits of HFV in pediatrics are unproved, pediatric applications include major pulmonary airleaks, interstitial pneumonia, ARDS, and congenital diaphragmatic hernia (Arnold, Troug, Thompson, & Fackler, 1993). While there are sound theoretical reasons to support the use of HFV in numerous clinical situations, clinical trials are lacking. Research is needed to determine when, if, and what type of HFV can improve patient outcome.

The most persuasive indication for HFV is pulmonary airleak. Bronchopleural fistula, major airway disruptions, and pneumothoraces respond favorably to HFV (Gonzalez, Harris, Black, & Richardson, 1987). Healing of disrupted airways occurs more rapidly in the presence of lower tidal swings in airway pressure associated with HFV (Wetzel & Gioia, 1987).

HFPPV and HFJV have been used in short-term support of ventilation during airway procedures such as bronchoscopy and laryngoscopy. Airway visualization is enhanced and ventilatory motion is decreased with these techniques of HFV.

Nursing Care of a Patient on HFOV

Nursing care of the patient on HFOV centers on vigilance in assessment and preventing complications (Curley & Molengraft, 1994). While continuous monitoring is critical, constant vibration of the child's body and noise from the ventilator limit traditional assessment methods. Auscultation of heart, breath, and bowel sounds is difficult if not impossible. The only time auscultation is possible is during a suctioning procedure when the patient is being hand ventilated. Most patients on HFOV are chemically paralyzed and sedated. Because it is difficult to detect fine movements that hallmark the need for additional chemical paralyzing agent, continuous infusions guided by peripheral nerve stimulation provides a more reasonable approach to the use of chemical paralysis in this population. EEGs cannot be used to assess for the presence of seizure activity. Possible autonomic symptoms of seizure activity include increased heart rate, increased blood pressure, dilated pupils, and possibly worsening blood gases.

Subtle changes in patient color, worsening blood gases, decreasing SaO_2, and even slight increases in heart rate and decreases in blood pressure require immediate attention. Continuous assessment of chest wall vibration (wiggle factor) requires attention. Changes in the acoustic characteristics (pitch and rhythm) of the ventilator may indicate ventilator malfunction (Millette, 1988).

Impaired Gas Exchange: Hypoxemia and Hypercapnia. The goal of HFOV is to reduce or eliminate hypoxemia and hypercapnia using similar MAPs but lower PIPs than used with CMV while minimizing the risk of barotrauma and oxygen toxicity. Frequent arterial blood gases are necessary with the initiation of therapy. Changes in ventilator settings may take up to an hour to be reflected in the patient's ABGs. Baseline ABGs are individualized; lower PaO_2 (<50 mmHg) and higher $PaCO_2$ (>80 mmHg) may be tolerated as long as the pH remains greater than 7.25. Acidosis is managed with Tham, a non-CO_2 generating buffer. SaO_2 monitoring provides an ongoing trend of oxygenation. Oxygenation profiles (obtained with a pulmonary artery catheter) provide data regarding the adequacy of DO_2 compared with VO_2.

Improved Oxygenation: Optimize Lung Volume. To ensure adequate alveolar recruitment, the MAP is initially set 2 to 3 cm H_2O higher than what was required on CMV. The MAPs are increased in 1- to 2-cm H_2O increments until the SaO_2 is greater than 90% with a baseline FiO_2 of 0.55 to 0.6 or there is evidence of overinflation on chest x-ray. Whereas appropriate MAPs will increase alveolar recruitment and lung volume and thus oxygenation, excessive MAPs will cause overdistension, air trapping, and V/Q mismatch and impair oxygenation.

Ventilation strategy for the manipulation of MAP varies among disease categories (Arnold, Troug, Thompson, & Fackler, 1993). The goal in a patient with diffuse alveolar disease (DAD) characterized by a noncompliant, surfactant-deficient lung is *high volume*. Alveolar recruitment to maintain optimal lung volume is a priority; thus, high MAPs are used while the FiO_2 is maintained less than 0.6. The goal in airleak syndrome (ALS) is *low volume*, to promote lung healing and recovery. Attempts are made to decrease or maintain MAPs until airleak is resolved tolerating higher FiO_2.

Other factors to be considered include improving DO_2; limiting VO_2; and altering pulmonary mechanics, e.g., sedation, muscle relaxants, repositioning, suctioning, and managing bronchospasm. If chest wall vibration suddenly decreases, decreasing lung compliance, pneumothorax, additional atelectasis, ETT obstruction/malposition, and hyperinflation with V/Q mismatch are considered. Unorthodox positions (i.e., the prone position) may be required to optimize V/Q matching (Fig. 10–34). "Best" positioning is reevaluated daily as patient tolerance permits.

Improve CO_2 Elimination: Frequency and Tidal Volume. As discussed, alterations in V_T will have a much greater effect on CO_2 elimination than changes in frequency. CO_2 elimination is controlled by adjusting the oscillatory amplitude, which is the power control. Power is responsible for the volume of air exchanges with each oscillatory cycle. The power is adjusted until adequate chest wiggle, i.e., ΔP, V_T, is achieved. Given the attenuation of airway pressure from the proximal airway to the distal airways, it is very difficult to predict exactly how much pressure is transmitted to the lungs. Presumably, the larger the ETT the greater the pressure transmission. Oscillatory amplitude has no effect on oxygenation.

Starting frequencies employed with HFOV (which approximates the resonant frequency of lung) are 15

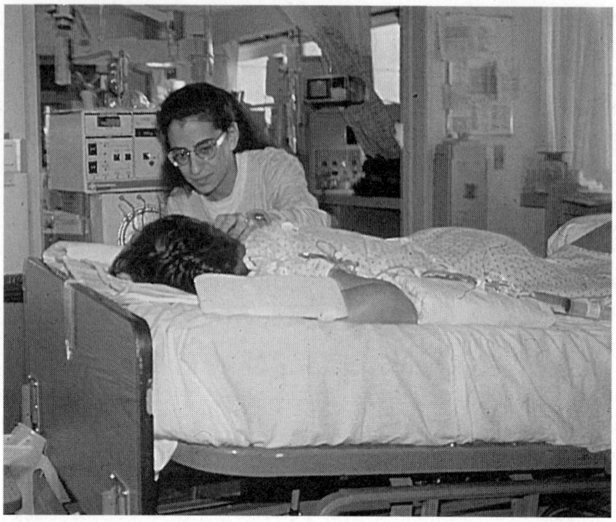

Figure 10–34 ● ● ● ● ● ●
Patient supported on HFOV in prone position.

Hz in neonates and 5 to 10 Hz in older children. If maximum ΔP is unable to improve ventilation in children, a secondary strategy includes decreasing frequency and increasing power to increase V_T and expiratory time. Unlike in neonates, an improvement in ventilation cannot be accomplished by increasing frequency. If an elevated $PaCO_2$ persists, a 10% increase in V_T can be obtained by increasing the Ti toward 50% of the cycle. This maneuver is used with caution because higher frequencies and Ti close to 50% may result in increased lung volume and stacking of breaths. Follow up chest x-rays are used to assess for overinflation.

Weaning. The patient's lung compliance often improves rapidly and requires aggressive weaning of the airway pressure to avoid overdistension and development of pneumothoraces. Signs of improvement are often subtle, i.e., increase in the percent piston displacement using the same power, improved tolerance to hand ventilation and procedures, improving SaO_2 with an FiO_2 less than 0.6, and resolving airleaks. Frequency is not weaned even in the event of an improved patient condition. Airway pressure is decreased by 1- to 2-cm increments followed by close observation. In the event of decreasing SaO_2 and lower PaO_2, a chest x-ray is justified to assess for atelectasis from the decrease in MAP. Increasing the MAPs back to the original settings or perhaps 1 to 2 cm higher will help reexpand collapsed alveoli.

There are no guidelines that help determine the best time to return to CMV. When the MAPs are lower, airleaks are resolved, and the patient is able to tolerate suctioning without prolonged periods of desaturation, CMV may be reinitiated. Some patients have been extubated directly from HFOV without returning to CMV.

Altered Fluid Volume. Patients do become edematous as a result of continued chemical paralysis, production of antidiuretic hormone (ADH), and possible hemodynamic changes (Mikhail, Banner, Gallagher, 1985; Mirro, Massanori, Tashio, 1985). Fluid restriction is usually necessary to optimize lung compliance and prevent fluid overload. Maximizing physiologic function through the scheduling and titration of drug therapies, e.g., diuretics, inotropes, and vasodilators, will help minimize vascular, interstitial, and/or intracellular fluid retention or overload.

Potential for Injury. *Pulmonary toilet* for the patient on HFOV is challenging for several reasons: in addition to the lack of indicators (breath sounds cannot be auscultated, and high peak pressure ventilatory alarms do not exist), patient tolerance is extremely low as demonstrated by prolonged periods of recovery after suctioning. While the patient on HFV does not seem to require more frequent suctioning than the patient on CMV, the effectiveness of HFV is extremely sensitive to a buildup of secretions in the ETT (Weber & Asselin, 1990).

Frequency of suctioning depends on the disease, fluid balance, recent chest x-ray findings, ABGs, and SaO_2. Patients with alveolar disease may require suctioning as often as every 6 hours, whereas patients with airleak syndrome (ALS) may need suctioning as little as every 24 to 36 hours.

Because most patients are intolerant of suctioning, the procedure may include premedicating with lidocaine and preoxygenating on the ventilator by increasing the FiO_2 to 1.0 and MAPs 2 to 4 cm H_2O 15 to 20 minutes before suctioning. Because it is impossible to mimic the ventilatory pattern/rate of HFOV, the oscillator is turned off and the MAP is maintained during the suctioning procedure. A minimal number of suction passes are made using an inline suctioning device. Normal saline is instilled in sufficient amounts to clear the endotracheal tube while avoiding surfactant washout. Vibrations are used if the platelet counts are greater than 50,000 and the patient is hemodynamically stable.

Because oxygenation is critically dependent upon lung volume, re-recruitment procedures may be necessary following the suctioning procedure. After the patient reaches presuctioning SpO_2, the FiO_2 and MAPs are returned to baseline as tolerated.

Patients supported on HVOF are at high risk for *alterations in skin integrity* secondary to immobility. Whereas eggcrates are used, air mattresses are avoided because they may affect the resonant frequency of the chest. The ventilator is moved from one side of the bed to the other every 12 hours so that the patient's head can be turned. This is necessary because any change in the configuration of the tubing will alter the propulsion of air to the airway and change the process of ventilation. Lastly, these patients also experience an increased number of radiologic procedures and require strict maintenance of shielding techniques.

Optimal Sensory Perception. The loud cadence of HFOV along with other ICU monitoring devices often results in an altered sleep/rest pattern. Earshields, earplugs, and music are used in a therapeutic manner to hallmark "safe times."

Altered Comfort: Pain or Agitation. Sedation is used as a comfort measure when the patient must tolerate prolonged periods of intubation with higher pressure support. Adequate sedation reduces the incidence of working against the ventilator with increased airway pressure.

Altered Coping: Child and Family. Stress precautions are taken to help control the environment for these liable infants and children. In addition to the stress related to having their child require an extraordinary level of care, parents require support in understanding the apparently unnatural breathing pattern. Data regarding the memories of children supported by this ventilatory strategy are nonexistent.

Extracorporeal Membrane Oxygenation (ECMO)

Despite significant advances in ventilator therapy, some patients with ARF will fail to respond and die unless alternative therapy is available (Redmond, Loe, Bartlett, & Arensman, 1988). Extracorporeal membrane oxygenation (ECMO) is prolonged cardiopulmonary bypass performed at the bedside. It is an alternative intervention for patients in profound respiratory or cardiopulmonary failure who are refractory to maximal conventional therapies. ECMO supports the cardiopulmonary system so that toxic high positive airway pressures and levels of oxygen can be avoided while permitting resolution of *reversible* pathology.

ECMO is considered "standard rescue therapy" in supporting critically ill neonates in ARF. Based upon its success in the neonatal population, some centers have extended the use of ECMO to a carefully selected group of pediatric patients (Fuhrman & Dalton, 1992). However, some very important differences exist between these two patient populations—pulmonary reactivity significantly decreases after 2 weeks of age; diseases that cause pediatric ARF are not as homogeneous as those that cause neonatal ARF; and most causes of pediatric ARF involve pulmonary parenchymal dysfunction. In the pediatric population, ECMO is not considered "rescue" therapy but a supportive intervention that may prevent iatrogenic injury related to oxygen and ventilator support.

Current Application

There are no precise indications for ECMO in the pediatric population. ECMO may be helpful in a pediatric patient with reversible disease that can be resolved within the feasible time limit for maintaining ECMO. A typical pediatric ECMO course for pulmonary support is usually much longer than a pediatric ECMO course for cardiac support—2 to 4 weeks compared with 4 to 5 days. ECMO may be considered when the disease trajectory is directed toward the patient's demise, the patient is refractory to maximal conventional therapy, and there is still potential for

good neurologic outcome. Maximal conventional therapy, ill defined and controversial among centers, includes optimal ventilator, pharmacologic, or surgical therapy. In describing maximal conventional ventilation, the "process of care" becomes important. Some centers derive excellent results from alternative ventilator management techniques, some with high-frequency ventilation, while others with ECMO. The success of any one therapy at a particular institution may not be able to be replicated in another.

In the pediatric population, ECMO has been used successfully to support the patient after cardiovascular surgery for congenital heart disease. ECMO provides gas exchange and biventricular support, which is important in pediatrics because of the numerous congenital heart defects that primarily result in right ventricular (RV) dysfunction (Kanter, Pennington, Weber, Zambie, Braun, & Martychenko, 1987). ECMO has also been used to support patients before and after cardiac transplantation (Dalton, Siewers, Fuhrman, Del Nido, Thompson, Shaver, & Dowhy, 1993). ECMO criteria for the pediatric cardiac patient are listed in Table 10–26. Poor outcomes have been reported in patients who were placed on ECMO because they were unable to come off intraoperative cardiopulmonary bypass and in cardiac patients who required ECMO support for more than 7 days (Kanter, Pennington, Weber, Zambie, Braun, & Martychenko, 1987).

Pediatric ECMO has been used successfully to support patients with *reversible single-organ failure,* that is, ARF before iatrogenic lung injury or multisystem organ failure (MSOF) develops. Criteria for patients with pulmonary dysfunction are difficult to establish because the specificity of various measures are not exact; most criteria are unit-dependent (Table 10–27). One common theme is that the patient will die of reversible ARF unless ECMO is offered.

Compared with indications, contraindications of ECMO support are easier to identify. Factors include those that preclude a quality outcome or a successful ECMO run (Table 10–28). Identifying reversible pulmonary disease is difficult. In children, diseases that cause respiratory failure leading to interstitial inflammation may result in pulmonary fibrosis and necrosis. Lung biopsy and/or documentation of fixed pulmonary vascular resistance may be necessary to rule out irreversible lung damage. The extent of pulmonary fibrosis is related to the severity and duration of the interstitial inflammation as well as to

Table 10-26. GUIDELINES FOR ECMO IN THE CARDIAC PATIENT

Low CO after and despite optimal pharmacologic and ventilator management
  CI less than 2 L/M²/min × 3 hr
  Metabolic acidosis: base deficit greater than −5 × 3 hr
  Low MAP with oliguria
    Less than 50 mmHg infant or 60 mmHg child
    Urinary output less than 0.5 mL/kg/hr × 3 hr
Unable to come off bypass

Table 10-27. GUIDELINES FOR ECMO IN THE PULMONARY PATIENT

Evidence of a significant intrapulmonary R → L shunting
  >30% during maximal conventional therapy
Static compliance <0.5 mL/cm/H_2O/kg
PaO_2 < 50 mmHg; $PaCO_2$ > 50 mmHg with MAPs > 18 cm H_2O,
  barotrauma, hypotension/arrest
Alveolar-arterial O_2 gradients ($AaDO_2$)
  >580 with PIPs >40 cm H_2O will predict 81% mortality in
    children
Oxygenation index (OI)
  >0.4 predicts 77% mortality in children
  present twice more than 30 minutes apart despite maximal
    conventional therapy

the duration of high positive airway pressures from mechanical ventilation. Typically, a patient's primary problem will shift from respiratory failure to ventilatory failure when fibrosis becomes significant.

ECMO Circuit

There are two options when providing ECMO support: venoarterial (VA) and venovenous (VV). In VA ECMO, blood is drained from the venous circulation via a cannula placed in the right atrium and oxygenated blood is returned to the arterial circulation through a cannula placed in the aortic arch. In VV ECMO, blood is drained in a similar manner but oxygenated blood is returned to the venous circulation through a cannula commonly placed in one of the common femoral veins. A double-lumen cannula (DLC) (1991; Kendall Healthcare Products, Mansfield, MA) placed in the right internal jugular vein has been used successfully to provide VV support (Anderson, Otsu, Chapman, & Bartlett, 1989). Use of the DLC is currently limited by the 14F cannula size, which can only accommodate neonates to 4 kg. Larger sizes are under development.

Although VA ECMO is currently more widely used, VV ECMO is gaining popularity. Table 10–29 contrasts the major differences between VA and VV ECMO support. Contraindications to VV ECMO include the patient in cardiac failure and the patient with inadequate venous access. An advantage of VV ECMO is that it may limit the physiologic conse-

Table 10-28. CONTRAINDICATIONS OF ECMO SUPPORT

Multisystem organ failure
Severe neurologic damage
Irreversible lung damage
  Greater than 7–10 days on high ventilator pressures and FiO_2
  Prolonged period of time since injury occurred
  Slow escalation of therapy
  Bronchoalveolar lavage and biopsy: increased macrophages
Prolonged shock (base deficit −5; oliguria; decreased MAP for
  >12 hours)
Current or prior cardiac arrest with unknown neurologic status
Condition incompatible with normal healthy childhood
  (institutional care, incurable disease, metastatic cancer)

Table 10-29. COMPARISONS OF VA AND VV ECMO

VA ECMO
  Provides cardiac and pulmonary support
  Decompresses the pulmonary vascular bed
  Carotid artery is used
  Potential lethality of emboli
  Coronary artery blood flow is derived from the LV (<PaO_2)

VV ECMO
  Provides only pulmonary support—does not support cardiac
    function
  Normal pulmonary circulation is maintained
    Can still assess PA pressures—cannot use thermodilution
      cardiac output
  Provides higher SvO_2 saturations to the PV bed, so it may
    help decrease PVR and heal the lung
  May require a 20% increase in flow to compensate for "pump
    recirculation"
  Requires standard ventilator management
  Selective perfusion is not a problem—myocardial circulation
    maintained
  Normal pulsatile pulse contour is maintained
  Carotid artery is spared
  May develop problems with the femoral vein related to
    chronic venous insufficiency/edema
  Longer cannulation time—two sites
  Less concern over emboli—returning blood to the venous
    system

quences of microemboli. Most children on long-term VA ECMO support die of MSOF, probably related to microemboli from the ECMO circuit.

Regardless of whether VA or VV ECMO is used, the ECMO circuit remains the same (Fig. 10–35). Blood is drained by gravity from the venous cannula in the right atrium down to a 30- to 50-mL polyethylene bladder that servoregulates the hemopump. This venous reservoir is in direct contact with a microswitch that can sense a decrease in bladder size, indicating a diminished venous blood supply. Insufficient drainage into the bladder causes the bladder to collapse, which automatically shuts off the pump. Known as "bladder chatter," this may be a result of

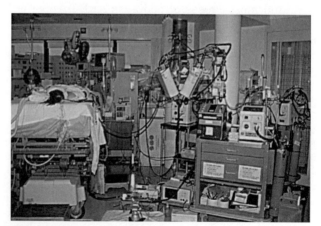

Figure 10–35 ● ● ● ● ● ●

The ECMO circuit: from the right atrium, blood drains by gravity to a blood reservoir, is pumped to the membrane oxygenator, heated, then returned to the patient.

hypovolemia; excessive flow; or a kinked, malpositioned, or inadequately sized cannula. Failure of the pump to shut off in response to a loss of venous blood supply could result in air emboli or right atrial suction.

From the bladder, blood is drawn into a hemopump, where either a centrifuge or roller pump propels the blood forward. Pump flow regulates the volume of blood sent through the oxygenator; as a result, the pump flow also regulates the patient's PaO_2. The flow is usually maintained at 70 to 120 mL/kg/min. The blood is pumped into the membrane oxygenator for oxygenation and CO_2 removal. The membrane oxygenator is a flat silicone envelope tightly wound into a coil that divides the membrane into two compartments; ventilating gas flows down on one side, and blood is pumped up on the other. Oxygen, measured in liters per minute (LPM), is administered via a sweep gas. Because the membrane is six to seven times more permeable to carbon dioxide than oxygen, carbogen (5% carbon dioxide and 95% oxygen) is usually added to prevent or correct hypocapnia. Pre- and postmembrane pressures are monitored for the early detection of circuit malfunction. Premembrane pressures are kept below 300 mmHg to avoid red cell and platelet destruction; postmembrane pressures should be between 200 and 300 mmHg. A rise in postmembrane pressures indicates occlusion or kinking of the return cannula.

Arterialized, the blood leaves the oxygenator and flows into the heat exchanger, which in the pediatric patient may be housed within the oxygenator. Blood flows through seven stainless steel rods that are surrounded by a water bath warmed to 39°C. This temperature allows for ambient cooling as the blood returns to the patient through the return cannula placed in the right common carotid artery (aorta) in VA ECMO or through the selected vein (inferior vena cava) in VV ECMO.

The "bridge" links the drainage and return lines. This connection allows the patient to be excluded from the ECMO circuit without fear of blood stasis and associated clot formation. Clamped during ECMO support, the bridge is opened during ECMO cycling.

Cannulation

ECMO cannulation is a surgical procedure performed in the pediatric ICU. The patient is chemically paralyzed to avoid respiratory movement, which may precipitate an air embolus during venous cannulation. Fentanyl (20 μg/kg) is used for anesthesia, keeping the heart rate and blood pressure within a tight 10- to 20-point range (McDermott & Curley, 1990). The surgical team, including scrub nurse, controls the sterile environment, which includes the surgical space, instrument tables, suction, and electrocautery; caps and masks are worn by all personnel within 6 feet of the operative field. The bed is raised to facilitate venous drainage, and the patient is positioned with a roll under the shoulders and the head

turned to the left. Routine prepping and draping are performed.

The critical care nurse maintains access to the patient, including the airway and preferably a large-gauge central intravenous (IV) line to administer emergency medications, platelets, and heparin. Access to the arterial line is desirable but is not always possible. One unit of concentrated platelets is administered as the sternocleidomastoid incision is opened. The carotid sheath is exposed, and the vessels are isolated. The largest possible venous cannula (16 to 28F) is selected and inserted into the right internal jugular vein. The large cannula size and multiple side ports will usually allow venous drainage equivalent to the normal resting cardiac output of most patients. The arterial cannula (12 to 22F) has one large distal opening and is inserted into the right common carotid artery. Heparin, 30 units/kg, is administered IV as the cannulas are inserted. In VV ECMO, the femoral vein is cannulated by a separate surgical team. An alternate cannulation site in the cardiac surgical patient includes a transthoracic approach. Another unit of concentrated platelets is administered as the incision(s) is(are) closed.

When cannulation is complete, the patient is connected to the ECMO circuit, the clamps are released, and the ECMO flow is started at 100 mL/min. ECMO flow is gradually increased over 5 to 10 minutes to a rate of 80 to 120 mL/kg/min while the adequacy of venous return and SaO_2 are assessed.

As VA ECMO flow increases, inotropic support can be gradually weaned. By increasing the nonpulsatile flow in VA ECMO, it is possible to assume approximately 80% of the patient's cardiac output. This is evidenced by a narrowing of the arterial pulse pressure (Fig. 10–36). Hypertension and bradycardia may result from a too rapid increase in VA ECMO flow or too slow an inotropic wean. Time may resolve these effects, but antihypertensive medications, for exam-

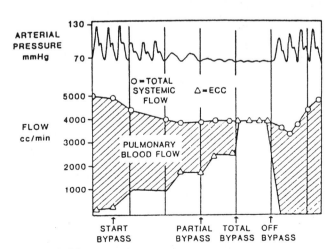

Figure 10–36 ● ● ● ● ● ●

Pulse pressure changes on VA ECMO. (From Bartlett, R.H., et al. (1984). *Extracorporeal membrane oxygenation technical specialist manual* (7th ed., p. 28). Ann Arbor: The University of Michigan Department of Surgery.)

ple, hydralazine 0.1 to 0.4 mg/kg IV, may be necessary.

In VV ECMO, there should be no change in the patient's pulse pressure. Inotropic agents usually cannot be immediately weaned, and continuous mixed venous saturation monitoring (SvO_2) of the drainage line is used to assess for pump recirculation. The goal is less than a 80% SvO_2 in the drainage line. Pump recirculation is suspected when the SvO_2 of the drainage line is equal to or greater than SaO_2.

After the incisions are dressed, the patient is repositioned. The patient's head is placed in a midline position.

Nursing Care of a Patient on ECMO

Care of the patient requires the ability to rapidly assess a complex critically ill patient and intervene appropriately using management protocols and standards of care. Throughout the ECMO course, the nurse works in collaboration with other members of the team and side by side with the ECMO specialist.

The bedside nurse is responsible for the overall care of the patient. The ECMO specialist performs all circuit manipulations, adjusts the level of anticoagulation, and regulates pump flow within the parameters set by the physician (Chapman & Bartlett, 1990). Although medications are administered through the circuit by the ECMO specialist, the nurse is responsible for preparing the correct drug dose, properly diluted and correctly labeled, before giving it to the ECMO specialist for administration.

Impaired Gas Exchange. The patient remains intubated and ventilated while on VA ECMO, but minimal ventilator settings are used to avoid further barotrauma. These settings are individualized but usually include PIPs of less than 35 cm H_2O, PEEP of 8 to 12 cm H_2O, and an FiO_2 of 0.21 to 0.40. The rate may be set at 5 to 10 breaths per minute with a tidal volume of 10 to 12 mL/kg. Patients are not routinely chemically paralyzed, so normocapnia will continue to stimulate respiratory efforts and help to maintain respiratory muscle tone and coordination.

The underlying disease, the patient's immediate condition, and progress dictate individualized pulmonary toilet and airway care. Hand bagging, instillation of normal saline, and suctioning may be needed as often as every 1 to 2 hours or may be therapeutically delayed to once every 12 hours. Manual deep inflation breaths help to maintain alveolar volume. Lung compliance and aeration are assessed with every pulmonary intervention. Aggressive bronchial hygiene is often limited because of systemic heparinization, but with adequate platelet counts may be safely accomplished. Bronchoscopy and bronchioalveolar lavage can be helpful if persistent areas of atelectasis and consolidation are present. Bronchodilators—for example, albuterol and terbutaline—may be helpful in the bronchospastic patient.

Arterial and mixed venous blood gases are closely monitored. With an ECMO flow rate of 100 mL/kg/min, arterial blood saturation should be greater than

95%. The mixed venous blood gases should have a normal pH, a PvO_2 greater than 37, and SvO_2 of 70%. In VA ECMO, adequate PaO_2 levels are accomplished through manipulating the ECMO flow rate. The higher the rate, the more blood that interfaces with the membrane oxygenator, resulting in a higher PaO_2. Adjustments for $PaCO_2$ levels are made through the addition and manipulations of carbogen. With the inclusion or increase of carbogen, there is also an infusion of additional oxygen, so that the oxygen sweep gas may need to be decreased. In summary, to increase the PaO_2, the blood flow is increased; to decrease the $PaCO_2$, the gas flow is increased.

Care of the patient on VV ECMO is similar to the care of the patient on VA ECMO. With normal pulmonary blood flow, the lungs contribute significantly to gas exchange. Ventilator settings are maintained at settings that avoid iatrogenic injury. Pulmonary toilet is aggressive; arterial and venous blood gases dictate changes in ventilator management. There are fewer manipulations of the ECMO flows and sweep gases than on VA ECMO.

Daily chest x-rays reflect the disease process and document patient progress. Complete opacification, or "white out," is common for the ECMO patient. This phenomenon is thought to be related to the sudden withdrawal of distending airway pressure upon conversion to ECMO and to the blood-circuit surface interaction that initially causes the release of vasoactive substances (Keszler, Subramanian, Smith, Dhanireddy, Mehta, Molina, Cox, & Moront, 1989). Both changes are associated with generalized capillary leak and interstitial pulmonary fluid shifts. This may further compromise the pulmonary status during the first 24 to 48 hours of ECMO support.

Iatrogenic complications of maximal mechanical ventilation prior to ECMO—that is, pneumothoraces—are not uncommon. If a pneumothorax were to develop while the patient was on VA ECMO, signs and symptoms would include an increase in PaO_2 and a decrease in peripheral perfusion followed by a decrease in venous drainage and progressive hemodynamic deterioration. The presence or absence of airleaks is documented. Persistent pulmonary airleaks may be managed by decreasing the mean airway pressure to just under the pressure associated with an airleak. Chest tube patency is maintained with water-seal drainage usually at 20 cm H_2O with or without suction. Stripping of chest tubes is controversial, especially in the heparinized patient. All chest tube drainage is documented and may require colloid replacement.

Alterations in Cardiac Output. The ECMO circuit contains approximately twice the blood volume of the patient. VA ECMO flow overrides the patient's inherent cardiac output, which significantly narrows the pulse pressure. Once the pulse pressure is lost, the mean arterial pressure (MAP) guides nursing interventions, inotropic support, and fluid administration. Normal MAP is age-dependent, but greater than 60 mmHg is considered baseline. Even though resuscitative events prior to ECMO frequently leave the patient in a positive fluid balance, equilibration between the patient's own circulation and the ECMO circuit often requires additional colloid.

Hypotension may result from hypovolemia, an insufficient flow rate, sepsis-related vasodilation, or oversedation. Associated clinical signs include pallor; prolonged capillary refill; cool, mottled extremities; and decreased urinary output.

Persistent hypovolemia, evidenced by a decreased MAP, frequent "bladder chatter," and SvO_2 less than 70%, requires volume administration. Packed red cells (PRC), fresh-frozen plasma (FFP), or 5% albumin 10 to 20 mL/kg may be given to maintain the MAP and hematologic parameters. After volume expansion, the use of vasopressors, such as dopamine, may be considered.

Hypervolemia, inadequate sedation, or excessive environmental stimuli may be primary or secondary causes of hypertension. Diuretics, antihypertensives, and/or sedatives are used; stress precautions are enforced; and the underlying cause for hypertension is investigated and managed.

Hypervolemia may result from pre-ECMO resuscitative efforts, fluid retention due to prerenal oliguric states, and/or third spacing from capillary leakage due to sepsis. A diuretic regimen, sometimes accompanied by the use of 25% albumin, may be employed.

Idiopathic hypertension is common in the pediatric ECMO patient. The nonpulsatile flow, characteristic of VA ECMO, downloads baroreceptors. The kidneys may also interpret the nonpulsatile flow as a low-flow or hypotensive state, stimulating renin release and activation of the renin-angiotensin and aldosterone system. The net result is vasoconstriction and sodium and water retention. With normal pulmonary vascular resistance, overriding the patient's inherent cardiac output with VA ECMO may be impossible. Hypertension may result from the two cardiac outputs existing within a single circulatory system. Since oxygenation is determined by the ECMO flow rate, lowering the flow to treat hypertension will compromise oxygenation.

Hypertension exacerbates bleeding, so is aggressively managed in the ECMO patient. Antihypertensive drugs, such as hydralazine or captopril, may be used for blood pressure control. In addition, nitroprusside, nitroglycerin, phentolamine, and diazoxide have been used in refractory situations. Short-acting beta-blockers, which depress the patient's native cardiac output, are used cautiously because if an unexpected interruption of ECMO support occurs, cardiac output would be significantly reduced.

VV ECMO provides no cardiac override; the native cardiac output remains fully pulsatile, thus a normal arterial pulse pressure is maintained. Cardiac output is augmented as with any critically ill patient.

Environmental stimuli, anxiety, and pain contribute to patient stress. Controlling the environment and clustering nursing care to allow for periods of uninterrupted sleep become a nursing priority. Effective nursing intervention requires coordinating respiratory therapists, physicians, and other staff in pro-viding their care in a sequence that maximizes a calm, quiet atmosphere. In addition, minimizing the numbers of bedside personnel and providing adequate sedation aid in reducing anxiety.

Alteration in Fluid and Electrolyte Balance. The goal of fluid management is to promote diuresis while maintaining adequate tissue perfusion, nutrition, and hematologic values (McDermott & Curley, 1990). This requires astute assessment of hypotension, tachycardia, decreased urine output, poor capillary refill, and "bladder chatter." Administration of fluids and drugs is easily accomplished via the ECMO circuit. A multiple-port manifold is used to deliver maintenance IV fluid, parenteral nutrition and 10% intralipids, and numerous medications through a bladder port. The heparin drip is infused through a separate port that allows for minuscule changes in dosage to be recognized immediately independent of the rates of the other solutions.

The patient's total hourly IV rate is usually restricted to three-quarters maintenance to avoid fluid overload, which can compromise ventilation and weaning from ECMO. As with normal ventilation, there is an insensible water loss over the ECMO membrane. The daily volume of this loss is dependent upon the size of the membrane and gas flow.

Prerenal oliguric states may be related to hypotensive insults prior to ECMO support, the dehydrating regimen while on ECMO, or the primarily nonpulsatile VA ECMO blood flow. Blood urea nitrogen (BUN) values frequently increase during ECMO support. Aggressive diuretic therapy with furosemide is employed to return patients to their dry weight. Low-dose dopamine (2.5 μg/kg/min) is often used to augment renal perfusion.

For patients who are resistant to diuretics, ultrafiltration can be incorporated within the ECMO circuit and used for fluid removal. Heparinization and access are nonissues in ECMO. Priming the hemofilter requires approximately 50 mL of blood; therefore, additional colloid is kept available to compensate for this diversion. Blood is diverted from the oxygenator, ultrafiltrated, then returned to the bladder. The volume of ultrafiltrate removed is determined by the patient's condition, dry weight, and estimated volume of fluid excess. The use of the hemofilter has little impact on serum electrolytes. However, rapid removal of excess fluid may result in dehydration with attendant elevations in BUN. The clinical signs of dehydration—that is, sunken eyes, dry mucous membranes, dry skin with poor turgor, and a depressed anterior fontanelle in the infant—are monitored. Accurate documentation of fluid balance is maintained, and the use of an ongoing cumulative balance sheet over the entire ECMO course is helpful in evaluating the total fluid status of the patient. Acute renal failure, as evidenced by anuria, progressive hyperkalemia, and increased BUN and creatinine, is managed with hemodialysis placed similarly within the ECMO circuit.

Alteration in Hemostasis. Activated clotting times (ACTs) are closely monitored to guide the degree of heparinization necessary to avoid clot formation within the circuit and prevent untoward systemic bleeding. When the initial postcannulation ACT is 300 seconds, a heparin drip is started at 10 units/kg/hour. ACTs are performed hourly at the bedside, and the heparin drip is titrated to maintain the ACT between 180 and 220 seconds. Several factors, such as low flow rates, bleeding, renal function, or platelet administration, may alter this range. A low flow rate because of bladder chatter may require higher ACTs; the slower the flow, the greater the chance of clot formation within the circuit. Diuresis and platelet administration will both require an increase in heparin dosage. Heparin is excreted by the kidneys, so a lower ACT can be expected after a large diuresis; the opposite is true in renal failure. Platelets contain heparinase, an enzyme that metabolizes heparin; therefore, the heparin dose is increased when platelets are administered. Prior to platelet administration, a baseline ACT is performed, and if less than 200 seconds, a heparin bolus equal to one half the hourly infusion dose is administered. When half of the platelets have been infused, a repeat ACT is performed and treated. In addition to a bolus dose, the heparin drip rate may need to be increased by 10 to 20 units/hour at this time. Another ACT is checked at the end of the platelet transfusion and is treated if necessary.

Since the membrane and the pump both contribute to platelet destruction, daily platelet transfusions may be necessary to maintain a platelet count greater than 100,000. If fluid volume is an issue, the platelets may be concentrated or "spun," which in itself destroys some platelets. Thus, a greater increase is seen in the post-transfusion platelet count if the platelets are administered in their unconcentrated form. Platelets can be given directly to the patient via a peripheral or central IV or infused through the circuit postmembrane. Infusion into the circuit premembrane results in platelet aggregation within the membrane, which diminishes platelet effectiveness and increases the possibility of clot formation in the membrane.

Prothrombin time is kept below 17 seconds. An elevation of 3 seconds over control will require FFP 10 to 20 mL/kg. Partial thromboplastin times (PTTs) are not followed because they will always be greater than 100 due to heparinization. Large volumes of chest tube drainage may require replacement of FFP at the rate of 0.5 mL per mL of drainage.

Fibrinogen levels are maintained at 200%. One to three units of cryoprecipitate are given to correct low fibrinogen levels, but cannot be infused through the circuit because the factors are destroyed by the heat exchanger.

As with any systemically heparinized patient, precautions are needed to avoid bleeding. Insertion of all vascular lines, nasogastric tube, bladder catheter, or other indwelling tubes should be accomplished prior to the initiation of ECMO. No intramuscular medications should be given, nor should finger or heel sticks be performed. Should manipulation or replacement of an indwelling catheter be necessary while on ECMO, a platelet transfusion prior to the event helps avoid or minimize bleeding. All large catheters should remain in place for the duration of ECMO support to avoid hemorrhage upon removal. Cannula site oozing may be controlled by the topical administration of a microfibrillar collagen hemostat (Avitene) and absorbable gelatin (Gelfoam) with a pressure dressing. Uncontrollable bleeding may require surgical exploration of the wound. All site bleeding should be measured and counted as output.

Unlike the neonatal population, spontaneous intracranial bleeds are rare in the pediatric population. In the United States, there is a 20% incidence of extracranial bleeding in neonates; the incidence more than doubles to 50% in the pediatric population. Assessment of fluids, vasopressors, antihypertensives, diuretics, and blood product replacement requires constant vigilance. Persistent hypovolemia, especially increasing RBC requirements, is a warning sign that there is occult bleeding. Subtle clinical signs include increased pallor, agitation, increased respiratory rate, and decreased capillary refill. All bodily secretions are checked for the presence of blood. Pulmonary hemorrhage is obvious by bright red blood endotracheal secretions or massive chest tube drainage. Mucous membrane bleeding, most often involving the oro-nasopharynx, may require packing. Gastric bleeding becomes evident through nasogastric tube drainage and/or melena. Abdominal girths are monitored; abdominal x-ray and ultrasound may confirm any abdominal bleeding.

Most bleeding can be minimized by maintaining an adequate platelet count and a lower ACT. Unfortunately, the progression of almost any bleeding process while still on ECMO is almost inevitable.

A continuous infusion of aminocaproic acid (Amicar; Lederle Parenterals, Carolina, PR) has been helpful in controlling bleeding in high-risk patients (Wilson, Bower, Fackler, Beals, Bergus, Kevy, 1993). Amicar stabilizes clot formation through inhibition of thrombolysis. Amicar inhibits both plasminogen activator substances and, to a lesser degree, antiplasmin activity. It slows the production of plasmin, which lyses fibrin and fibrinogen.

After cannulation, Amicar, 100 mg/kg, is administered diluted in equal volumes of 5% dextrose in water or normal saline through a peripheral IV over 5 to 10 minutes. A constant infusion of 30 mg/kg/hr is then infused via the ECMO circuit. Therapeutic dosage is achieved when a daily plasminogen activator time is greater than 120 seconds. ACTs remain in the 180 to 200-second range. Amicar is discontinued if bleeding is not a problem after 72 hours.

Potential Alterations in Nutrition. Parenteral nutrition and 10% intralipids provide the child with the necessary 80 to 100 kcal/kg for healing to occur. Ultrafiltration permits earlier initiation of full parenteral nutrition. The ECMO circuit is limited to 10% intralipids at 1 g/kg/day because the fat may interfere with membrane function. Any additional or more concentrated intralipid solution is delivered through a peripheral or central IV. Enteral feedings of the volume necessary for caloric and protein support are impractical due to the potential for pulmonary aspiration and paralytic ileus. The patient is usually started on ranitidine (Zantac) to inhibit gastric acid secretion. Gastric pH is monitored routinely, and antacids are administered to maintain the gastric pH greater than 5. The nutritional status may be evaluated by following serum albumin and total protein levels, by stringently monitoring fluid balances, and by clinical observation.

Alteration in Comfort. With rare exceptions, the pediatric ECMO patient is a previously healthy child who perceives and reacts to pain and is subject to fear and anxiety. The pediatric patient supported on ECMO for ARF lives prone for at least 3 weeks in an overstimulating environment with little opportunity for long periods of undisturbed rest. Constant infusions and bolus doses of narcotics, such as fentanyl or morphine sulfate, are used to alleviate discomfort (Caron & Maguire, 1990). Acute tolerance as well as membrane binding helps to explain why increasing fentanyl doses are necessary. The ECMO circuit continuously binds close to 1000 μg of fentanyl, and tolerance, achieved at different times, increases approximately 10% per day (Arnold et al., 1991).

The ECMO patient is at risk for cannula displacement with excessive head and/or shoulder movement. The head is supported in an optimal position, but sedation *must* be sufficient for patient safety. Benzodiazepines such as lorazepam (Ativan) or midazolam (Versed) are used for sedation and amnesia. The goal is to provide the patient with a comfortable ECMO course while still allowing for neurologic evaluation and periodic social interaction. Depending upon the level of sedation achieved, the patient may require premedication with a narcotic and/or sedative for suctioning, dressing changes, or other noxious procedures.

Maintaining skin integrity can be a particularly challenging when caring for the pediatric ECMO patient. Hypervigilance is essential. A low air-loss bed and gel pillow placed under the occiput are frequently used. It is not impossible to slightly turn the patient on a routine basis in order to minimize pressure points, visualize the back, and provide skin care. Other nursing comfort measures include, but are not limited to, passive range of motion and repositioning of the extremities, hand rolls, and skin and mouth care.

With organization of nursing and medical procedures, there should be periods of time for the patient to simply rest undisturbed. During these times, listening to favorite music or television programs may be relaxing. Radios and tape decks may be used; headphones may be carefully placed on the older child. The presence of the child's family often provides the most comfort.

Preventing Iatrogenic Injury

Sepsis. While the potential for sepsis increases with ECMO support, it is very difficult to detect. The usual first sign of sepsis is fever, but temperature instability is blunted by the heat exchanger. A consistently low platelet count, often an indicator of sepsis, is unreliable due to the degree of platelet consumption by the circuit. A persistent elevation in WBC, with or without a significant shift in the differential, or positive cultures may be the only dependable sign. Blood, urine, and tracheal aspiration cultures are obtained every other day. Prophylactic antibiotics (ampicillin, gentamicin, and oxacillin) are administered throughout the ECMO course. Gentamicin levels are closely monitored. Because of slow gentamicin excretion, higher trough levels result, necessitating the extension of dose intervals to every 18 hours.

Accidental Decannulation. In a properly sedated, carefully monitored ECMO patient, accidental decannulation is rare. The patient becomes most vulnerable during any examination or exploration of the insertion site, being moved for procedures or linen change, or during patient transport. Accidental decannulation can result in death by exsanguination. Emergency action includes applying very firm pressure to the cannulation site and clamping the remaining cannula. There may be no chance for recannulation without entering the thoracic cavity.

Cardiac Arrest. In the event of a cardiac arrest, cardiac compressions are unnecessary in patients supported on VA ECMO because pump flow can be increased to provide optimal cardiac output for organ perfusion. Compressions with ventilations are still necessary in the patient supported on VV ECMO.

Mechanical Failure. Occasionally a portion of the ECMO circuit will malfunction, requiring the patient to be immediately isolated from the system. There is a specific sequence of clamping the ECMO circuit when coming off ECMO: (1) clamp the venous cannula; (2) unclamp the bridge; then (3) clamp the arterial cannula. Clamping in this sequence allows the venous drainage to stop before the arterial return is clamped, increases the patient's blood volume, and helps prevent hypotension. The patient's ventilator settings are increased, and colloid and drugs, including chemical paralyzing agents, are administered as needed. The gas source is removed from the membrane to prevent air emboli; system repairs are performed by the ECMO specialist and therapy resumed as soon as possible.

Normally, the rapid, high volume blood flow through the circuit inhibits clot formation. However, treating hemorrhage in the pediatric ECMO patient requires lower heparin doses, which may result in an increase in clot formation. The bridge is one portion of the system that has the potential for blood stagnation. Periodic opening of the bridge provides a flush of blood that remixes pooled blood and reduces the potential for clot formation. Small clots that form on the membrane may decrease its overall efficiency but may not be life-threatening. Occasionally, a clot will form and enlarge in a portion of the circuit that will require replacement of that section of the circuit, or in some cases, changing the entire ECMO circuit.

The multiple access ports and connectors increase the potential for air emboli. Air on the venous side is allowed to drift down to the bladder, where it may be aspirated from a bladder port. Air on the arterial side is a life-threatening emergency. Here, air can be forced across the bridge into the venous side of the circuit, then aspirated out.

The maximum efficiency of the membrane is often limited to approximately 2 weeks, but may be further restricted in the presence of low flow rates and/or ACT ranges. The premembrane pressure should be less than 300 mmHg to avoid red blood cell and platelet destruction. A rise in this pressure, especially when accompanied with a change in ABGs, indicates a failing membrane. Because CO_2 transfer is dependent upon gas flow and the surface area of the membrane, a rising $PaCO_2$ can be a sensitive indicator of loss of functioning membrane. If the sum of both pre- and postmembrane pressures is greater than 700 mmHg, there is a very real danger of membrane rupture.

The area where the ECMO tubing is compressed by the pump's rollers is called the "raceway." The "raceway" is advanced several times during the ECMO course to avoid constant pressure on the same portion of tubing. Areas of wear could eventually rupture, causing rapid blood loss. It is imperative that all caretakers use eye protection, as delineated by universal precautions, at ECMO bedspaces.

In the event of a pump failure, a hand crank may be used to propel blood manually. In the pediatric patient, the pump volume and rate may be impossible to achieve. A fully charged back-up generator should be at the bedside at all times.

A failure or improper setting of the thermostat of the heater can result in the exchanger's water bath either cooling to room temperature or overheating to unacceptable limits. A cooled water bath will result in a hypothermic, mottled, bradycardiac and hypotensive child. The patient will become feverish, tachycardiac, and hypertensive if the heater temperature becomes excessive.

Alteration in Parental Role. In rapid succession, parents are faced with a PICU admission, information of a grave illness and possible death, and requests for permission to use life-supporting technologies that have no guarantees for outcome and a long list of potential complications. Often, the child must be transported to an ECMO center, separating the parents from home, family, and support systems.

Meeting the parents either precannulation or soon after to explain what they will see and hear in the ECMO bedspace is necessary. The high technology environment is taken to the extreme with ECMO. Seeing your child connected to so many machines with his blood circulating outside his body is frightening. Any parent-oriented ECMO literature is helpful for reinforcing explanations.

Routine time is allotted for the primary medical and nursing team to talk with the parents and answer their questions. Honest, pertinent information is the base upon which the parents will make future decisions regarding changes in life support. Given the potential complications of pediatric ECMO, pre-

dictors are unreliable. Hope is always supported by acknowledging the positive or neutral aspects of the child's condition; accepting the parents' future plans that include the child and by displaying guarded optimism. Only when the decision is made to terminate all support is hope tempered with reality.

While nursing plays an enormous role in parental support, talking with another parent whose child was supported on ECMO may be invaluable. There are several regional ECMO parent support groups with parents of ECMO survivors providing telephone contact with new ECMO parents. The parent support groups provide a supportive forum for the intimate exchange of feelings and ideas.

Coming Off ECMO

It may take as little as 5 days or as long as 4 weeks for indicators of improved pulmonary function to occur. These include a clearing chest x-ray, increasing lung compliance, and normalizing blood gases. On VA ECMO, the child's PaO_2 represents a mixture of pump blood and the blood that traverses his native cardiopulmonary circuit. With flows held constant, any increase in PaO_2 represents an increase in patient contribution. Early in the course of ECMO the patient contributes little, so pump flows are maintained at high levels. As the patient's pulmonary status improves, ECMO support can be titrated in one of two ways.

Weaning. In concert with improved lung function, pump flows are gradually decreased and ventilator settings are increased. Vital signs, pulse oximetry, and arterial blood gases are monitored. The pump flow is weaned down to 20% to 30% of the original rate, and, if tolerated, the patient is clamped off ECMO. With this method, the patient is continuously challenged over many hours or days.

Cycling. Cycling is a time-limited method of trailing off ECMO. The patient is chemically paralyzed and sedated, all ventilator settings are increased, and the flows are gradually turned down until total flow is decreased to 30 mL/kg/min. If this is tolerated, the patient is clamped off ECMO. Following vital signs, pulse oximetery, and arterial blood gases, the ventilator support is gradually decreased. If the patient can realize a PaO_2 greater than 60 mmHg and a $PaCO_2$ less than 45 mmHg on reasonable ventilator settings, the decision is usually made to decannulate. If these parameters cannot be met, the patient is cycled again at a later time, with modified ventilator settings to promote alveolar recruitment, after aggressive pulmonary care to mobilize secretions, or with inotropic support. The goal is to minimize O_2 toxicity and barotrauma but to wean ECMO support as soon as possible. With this method, the patient is challenged only once or twice a day for a short time, and the low flow rates that are associated with thromboemboli can be avoided. After cycling, flows are gradually increased and the patient is observed for rebound hypertension.

In either case, once the patient is excluded from

the ECMO circuit, the bridge between the arterial and venous tubing is opened and ECMO circulation continues. When weaning or cycling is completed, the patient is placed back on ECMO while the decision to continue or stop ECMO support is made. This is unnecessary when weaning or cycling from VV ECMO. In VV ECMO, the ventilator settings are increased as in VA ECMO but the oxygen source to the membrane is capped. The ECMO blood flow continues to circulate through the patient as well as the system.

Nursing responsibilities during cycling include reassuring the patient and parents that all the additional activity is controlled, and assessing the patient's tolerance to weaning. It is also necessary to accurately document vital signs, pulse oximetry, ventilator settings, and laboratory results. If it is likely that the patient will be isolated from the ECMO circuit, all infusions are transferred to a peripheral or central IV. The heparin infusion remains in the circuit, but the dose is reduced by 50% until the patient is back on ECMO and an ACT is rechecked.

Decannulation

Decannulation is a surgical procedure performed in the PICU. The patient is anesthetized and paralyzed, all infusions are transferred to a peripheral or central IV, and the heparin drip discontinued. The patient is prepped and draped, with the nurse maintaining access to a patent IV for any necessary drug administration. Two units of platelets is given postdecannulation. If cannulation and the ECMO course have done minimal damage to the vessels, the surgeon may attempt reconstruction. Otherwise, both are ligated. Advances in cannulas and technique allow vessel repair (Adolph, Bonis, Falteman, & Arensman, 1990). If the carotid artery is ligated, collateral flow to the right cerebral hemisphere is maintained by the external carotid and vertebral arteries. There are no proven complications related specifically to ligation or repair of the carotid artery, but long-term problems are unknown.

Post-decannulation, patient movement is limited until all clotting factors have returned to baseline. Narcotics are slowly weaned; the patient is assessed for iatrogenic physical withdrawal. Fentanyl is immediately weaned by 25% to 50% after ECMO support is discontinued, followed by a 10% wean every 4 to 12 hours as tolerated. A smooth transition can be accomplished by switching the patient over to longer-acting narcotics, for example, methadone in equal analgesic doses.

SUMMARY

Caring for an infant or child who requires support of oxygenation and/or ventilation is inherent to the practice of pediatric critical care nursing. Even so, there isn't a significant amount of nursing research

to help guide it. This chapter presents selected principles of oxygenation and ventilation as they pertain to critically ill or injured infants and children. As discussed, pulmonary system functioning is essential for life and because of developmental immaturity, the pediatric patient is at high risk for system dysfunction.

The next decade brings hope for primary prevention to avoid pediatric critical illness involving the pulmonary system. The next decade also brings new therapies, for example, intratracheal pulmonary ventilation and liquid perfluorocarbon ventilation (Fuhrman, Paczan, & Defrancisis, 1991; Greenspan, 1993). As new therapies become available, what constitutes conventional and unconventional support of the pulmonary system will be redefined.

References

AACN Certification Corporation (1991). Pediatric CCRN examination blueprint. *CCRN News,* Spring, 6.

AARC—American Association for Respiratory Care (1992). Consensus statement on the essentials of mechanical ventilators—1992. *Respiratory Care,* 37 (9), 1000–1008.

Adolph, V., Bonis, S., Falteman, K., & Arensman, R. (1990). Carotid artery repair after pediatric extracorporeal membrane oxygenation. *Journal of Pediatric Surgery,* 25 (8), 867–869.

Alkhudhairi, D., Prabho, R., el Sharkawy, M., & Burtles, R. (1990). Evaluation of a pulse oximeter during profound hypothermia. An assessment of the Biox 3700 during induction of hypothermia before cardiac surgery in paediatric patients. Int Journal Clinical Monitoring Computing, 7, 217–222.

Anderson, J.B., & Falk, M. (1991). Chest physiotherapy in the pediatric age group. *Respiratory Care,* 36 (6), 546–552.

Anderson, H.L., Otsu, T., Chapman, R.A., & Bartlett, R.H. (1989). Venovenous extracorporeal life support in neonates using a double lumen catheter. *ASAIO Transactions,* 35 (3), 650–653.

Arnold, J., & Castro, C. (1990). Endotracheal intubation. In J.L. Blummer (Ed.). *A practical guide to pediatric intensive care* (3rd ed.). St. Louis: Mosby–Year Book.

Arnold, J.H., Truog, R.D., Scavone, J.M., & Fenton, T. (1991). Changes in the pharmacodynamic response to fentanyl in neonates during continuous infusion. *Journal of Pediatrics,* 119 (4), 639–643.

Arnold, J.H., Truog, R.D., Thompson, J.E., & Fackler J.C. (1993). High frequency oscillatory ventilation in pediatric respiratory failure. *Critical Care Medicine,* 21, 272–278.

Backofen, J.E., & Rogers, M.C. (1992). Emergency management of the airway. In M.C. Rogers (Ed.). *Textbook of pediatric intensive care* (Vol. 1, pp. 52–74). Baltimore: Williams & Wilkins.

Barcoft, J. (1920). On anoxaemia. *Lancet,* 2, 485.

Bashein, G., & Syrory, G. (1991). Burns associated with pulse oximetry during magnetic resonance imaging. *Anesthesiology,* 75, 382–385.

Behnke, M., & Koff, P.B. (1993). Chapter 3: Patient assessment. In P.B. Koff, D. Eitzman, & J. Neu (Eds.). *Neonatal and pediatric respiratory care* (2nd ed.). St. Louis: C.V. Mosby.

Benjamin, P.K., Thompson, J.E., & O'Rourke, P.P. (1990). Complications of mechanical ventilation in a children's hospital multidisciplinary intensive care unit. *Respiratory Care,* 35 (9), 873–878.

Benson, M.S. (1988). Autopeep during mechanical ventilation of adults. *Respiratory Care,* pp. 33–37.

Betit, P., Thompson, J.E., & Benjamin, P.K. (1993). Chapter 19: Mechanical ventilation. In P.B. Koff, D. Eitzman, & J. Neu (Eds.). *Neonatal and pediatric respiratory care* (2nd ed.). St. Louis: C.V. Mosby.

Blaufuss, J.A., & Wallace, C.J. (1987). Two negative pressure ventilators: Current clinical application and nursing care. *Critical Care Nursing Quarterly,* 9 (4), 14–30.

Boegner, E. (1990). Pediatric ventilatory support and weaning parameters. *AACN's Clinical Issues in Critical Care Nursing,* 1 (2), 378–386.

Boggs, R.L. (1993). Airway management. In R.L. Boggs & M. Wooldridge-King (Eds.). *AACN procedure manual for critical care* (3rd ed.). Philadelphia: W.B. Saunders.

Boyden, E.A. (1977). Development and growth of the airways: In: W.A. Hodson (Ed.). *Development of the lung* (p. 3). New York: Marcel Dekker.

Briones, T.L. (1991). Pressure controlled inverse ration ventilation in respiratory failure. *Dimensions of Critical Care Nursing,* 10 (5), 254–261.

Bucher, H., Fanconi, S., Baeckert, P., & Duc, G. (1989). Hyperoxemia in newborn infants. *Pediatrics,* 84 (2), 226–230.

Caron, E., & Maguire, D.P. (1990). Narcotic dependency of the infant on ECMO. *Journal of Perinatal and Neonatal Nursing,* 4 (1), 63–74.

Chameides, L. (Ed.). (1990). *Textbook of pediatric advanced life support.* Dallas: American Heart Association.

Chapman, R.A., & Bartlett, R.H. (1990). *Extracorporeal life support for adult and pediatric patients.* Ann Arbor, MI: ELSO & University of Michigan ECMO Team.

Chang, H.K., & Harf, A. (1984). High frequency ventilation: A review. *Respiratory Physiology,* 157, 135–152.

Charnock, E.L., & Doershuk, C.F. (1973). Developmental aspects of the human lung. *Pediatric Clinics of North America,* 20 (2), 275–292.

Chatburn, R.L. (1990). High-frequency ventilation. In J.L. Blummer (Ed.). *A practical guide to pediatric intensive care* (3rd ed., pp. 956–961.). Philadelphia: Mosby–Year Book.

Chatburn, R.L. (1991a). A new system for understanding mechanical ventilators. *Respiratory Care,* 36, 10, 1123–1155.

Chatburn, R.L. (1991b). Principles and practice of neonatal and pediatric mechanical ventilation. *Respiratory Care,* 36, 6, 569–595.

Coghill, C.H., Haywood, J.L., Chatburn, R.L., & Carlo, W.A. (1991). Neonatal and pediatric high-frequency ventilation: Principles and practice. *Respiratory Care,* 36 (6), 596–609.

Curley, M.A.Q., & Molengraft, J.A. (1994). Care of the child supported on high frequency oscillatory ventilation. *AACN: Clinical Issues in Critical Care Nursing,* 5 (1), 49–58.

Curley, M.A.Q., & Thompson, J.E. (1990). End-tidal CO_2 monitoring in critically ill infants and children. *Pediatric Nursing,* 16 (4), 397–403.

Dalton, H.J., Siewers, R.D., Fuhrman, B.P., Del Nido, P., Thompson, A.E., Shaver, M.G., & Dowhy, M. (1993). Extracorporeal membrane oxygenation for cardiac rescue in children with severe myocardial dysfunction. *Critical Care Medicine,* 21 (7), 1020–1028.

Donlen, J. (1983). Interpreting acid-base problems through arterial blood gases. *Critical Care Nurse,* 3 (5), 34–38.

Donn, S.M., & Kuhns, L.R. (1980). Mechanism of endotracheal tube movement with change of head position. *Pediatric Radiology,* 9, 37–40.

Eichhorn, J.H., Cooper, J.B., Cullen, D.J., Maier, W.R., Philip, J.H., & Seeman, R.G. (1986). Standards for patient monitoring during anesthesia at Harvard Medical School. *JAMA,* 256 (8), 1017–1020.

Endo, A.S., & Nishioka, E. (1993). Chapter 17: Neonatal assessment. In C. Kenner, A. Brueggemeyer, & L.P. Gunderson (Eds.). *Comprehensive neonatal nursing.* Philadelphia: W.B. Saunders.

Forgacs, P. (1978). The functional basis of pulmonary sounds. *Chest,* 73, 399.

Froese, A., & Bryan, C. (1987). State of the art: High frequency ventilation. *American Review of Respiratory Disease,* 135, 1363–1374.

Fuhrman, B.P., & Dalton, H.J. (1992). Progress in pediatric extracorporeal membrane oxygenation. *Critical Care Clinics,* 8 (1), 191–202.

Fuhrman, B.T., Paczan, P.R., & Defrancisis, M. (1991). Perfluorocarbon-associated gas exchange. *Critical Care Medicine,* 19 (5), 712–722.

Fuller, H.D., et al. (1990). Pressurized aerosol versus jet aerosol delivery to mechanically ventilated patients: Comparison of dose to the lungs. *American Review of Respiratory Disease,* 141 (5), 440–444.

Gonzalez, F., Harris, T., Black, P., & Richardson, P. (1987). Decreased gas flow through pneumothoraces in neonates receiving high-frequency jet ventilation versus conventional ventilation. *Journal of Pediatrics,* 110, 464–466.

Greenspan, J.S. (1993). Liquid ventilation: A developing technology. *Neonatal Network,* 12 (4), 23–32.

Heijman, K., Heijman, L., Jonzon, A., Sedin, G., Sjöstrand, U., & Widman, B. (1972). High frequency positive pressure ventilation during anaesthesia and routine surgery in man. *Acta Anaesthesiol Scand,* 16, 172.

Helfaer, M.A., Nichols, D.G., & Rogers, M.C. (1992). Developmental physiology of the respiratory system. In M.C. Rogers (Ed.). *Textbook of pediatric intensive care* (2nd ed.). Baltimore: Williams & Wilkins.

Henneman, E.A. (1991). The art and science of weaning from mechanical ventilation. *Focus on Critical Care,* 18 (6), 490–500.

Hogg, J.C., Williams, J., Richardson, J.B., et al. (1970). Age as a factors in the distribution of lower airway conductance and in the pathologic anatomy of obstructive lung disease. *New England Journal of Medicine,* 282, 1283.

Juarez, P. (1992). Mechanical ventilation for the patient with severe ARDS: PC-IRV. *Critical Care Nurse,* 12 (4), 34–39.

Kanter, K.R., Pennington, D.G., Weber, T.R., Zambie, M.A., Braun, P., & Martychenko, V. (1987). Extracorporeal membrane oxygenation for postoperative cardiac support in children. *Journal of Thoracic and Cardiovascular Surgery,* 93, 27–35.

Kellehen, J.F., & Ruff, R.H. (1989). The penumbra effect: Vasomotion-dependent pulse oximeter artifact due to probe malposition. *Anesthesiology,* 71, 787–791.

Kelly, H.W., McWilliams, B.C., Katz, R., & Murphy, S. (1990). Safety of frequent high dose nebulized terbutaline in children with acute severe asthma. *Annals of Allergy,* 64 (2, part 2), 229–233.

Kelly-Heidenthal, P., & O'Connor, M. (1994). Nursing assessment of portable AP chest X-rays. *Dimensions of Critical Care Nursing,* 13 (3), 127–132.

Keszler, M., Subramanian, S., Smith, Y.A., Dhanireddy, R., Mehta, N., Molina, B., Cox, C.B., & Moront, M.G., (1989). Pulmonary management during extracorporeal membrane oxygenation. *Critical Care Medicine,* 17 (6), 495–500.

Koff, P.B., & Durmowicz, A.G. (1993). Chapter 15: Pharmacology (pp. 246–264). In P.B. Koff, D. Eitzman, and J. Neu (Eds.). *Neonatal and pediatric respiratory care* (2nd ed.). St. Louis: C.V. Mosby.

Lister, G. (1991). Oxygen supply/demand in the critically ill. In R. Taylor (Ed.). *Critical care: State of the art* (Vol. 12, pp. 311–350). Fullerton, CA: Society of Critical Care Medicine.

Lough M. (1990). Medicated aerosol therapy. In J.L. Blummer (Ed.). *A practical guide to pediatric intensive care* (pp. 978–980). St. Louis: C.V. Mosby.

Lough, M.D., Doershuk, C.F., & Stern, R.C. (1985). *Pediatric respiratory therapy.* Chicago: Year Book Medical Publishers.

MacIntyre, N.R. et al. (1985). Aerosol delivery in intubated mechanically ventilated patients. *Critical Care Medicine,* 13 (1), 81–84.

Macklem, P.T. (1971). Airway obstruction and collateral ventilation. *Physiol Rev,* 51, 368.

Manning, S.C., & Brown, O.E. (1990). Chapter 36: Sequelae of intubation (pp. 298–302). In D.L. Levin and F.C. Morris (Eds.). *Essentials of pediatric intensive care.* St Louis: Quality Medical Publishing.

Martin, L.D., Rafferty, F.F., & Gioia, F.R. (1992). Principles of respiratory support and mechanical ventilation. In M.C. Rogers (Ed.). *Textbook of pediatric intensive care* (Vol. 1, pp. 132–203). Baltimore: Williams & Wilkins.

Martin, L.D., Rafferty, J.F., Walker, L.K., & Gioia, F.R. (1992). Principles of respiratory support and mechanical ventilation (pp. 134–203). In M.C. Rogers. (Ed.). *Textbook of pediatric intensive care.* Baltimore: Williams & Wilkins.

McDermott, B.K., & Curley, M.A.Q. (1990). ECMO: Current use and future directions. *AACN Clinical Issues in Critical Care Nursing,* 1 (2), 348–364.

McPherson, S.P. (1990). *Respiratory therapy equipment.* St. Louis: C.V. Mosby.

Mikhail, M., Banner, M., & Gallagher, J. (1985). Hemodynamic effects of positive end-expiratory pressure during high frequency ventilation. *Critical Care Medicine,* 13, 732.

Millette, S.W. (1988), High frequency oscillatory ventilation: Neonatal application. *Dimensions of Critical Care Nursing,* 7 (4), 220–225.

Mirro, R., Massanori, T., & Tashio, K. (1985). Systemic cardiac output and distribution during high frequency oscillation. *Critical Care Medicine,* 13, 732.

Moore, K.L., & Persaud, T.V.N. (1993). The respiratory system. *The developing human.* Philadelphia: W.B. Saunders.

Oakes, D. (1990). *Neonatal/pediatric respiratory care.* Old Towne, ME: Health Educator Publications, pp. 15–19.

O'Brodovich, H.M., & Haddad, G.G. (1990). The functional basis of respiratory pathology. In V. Chernick (Ed.). *Kendig's disorders of the respiratory tract in children* (pp. 3–47). Philadelphia: W.B. Saunders.

Papo, M.C., Frank, J., & Thompson, A.E. (1993). A prospective, randomized study of continuous versus intermittent nebulized albuterol for severe status asthmaticus in children. *Critical Care Medicine,* 21 (10), 1479–1486.

Pascucci, R.C., Schena, J.A., & Thompson, J.E. (1989). Comparison of a sidestream and mainstream capnometer in infants. *Critical Care Medicine,* 17 (6), 560–562.

Polgar, G., & Weng, T.R. (1979). The functional development of the respiratory system. *American Review of Respiratory Disease,* 120, 625–695.

Portnoy, J., Nadel, G., Amado, M., & Willsie-Ediger, S. (1992). Continuous nebulization for status asthmaticus. *Annals of Allergy,* 69 (1), 71–79.

Redmond, C.R., Loe, W.A., Bartlett, R.H., & Arensman, R.M. (1988). Extracorporeal membrane oxygenation (pp. 200–212). In J.P. Goldsmith & E.H. Karotkin: *Assisted ventilation of the neonate.* Philadelphia: W.B. Saunders.

Rivera, R.A., Butt, W., & Shann, F. (1990). Predictors of mortality in children with respiratory failure. *Anaesthesia and Intensive Care,* 18 (3), 385–389.

Sadler, T.W. (1990). *Langman's medical embryology.* Baltimore: Williams & Wilkens.

Salyer, J.W., & Chatburn, R.L. (1990). Patterns of practice in neonatal and pediatric respiratory care. *Respiratory Care,* 35 (9), 879–888.

Salzberg, A.M. (1977). Congenital malformations of the lower respiratory tract. In E.L. Kendig, Jr., & V. Chernick (Eds.). *Disorders of the respiratory tract in children* (Vol. 1, pp. 213–252). Philadelphia: W.B. Saunders.

Scott, A.A., & Koff, P.B. (1993). Chapter 17: Airway care and chest physiotherapy (pp. 285–302). In P.B. Koff, D. Eitzman, & J. Neu (Eds.). *Neonatal and pediatric respiratory care* (2nd ed.). St. Louis: C.V. Mosby.

Scott, P.H., Eigen, H., Moye, L.A., Georgitis, J., & Laughlin, J.J. (1985). Predictability and consequences of spontaneous extubation in a pediatric ICU. *Critical Care Medicine,* 13 (4), 228–232.

Thompson, A.E. (1992). Chapter 14: Pediatric airway management (pp. 111–128). In B.P. Fuhrman & J.J. Zimmerman (Eds.). *Pediatric critical care.* St. Louis: Mosby–Year Book.

Thompson, J.E., Farrell, E., & McManus, M. (1992). Neonatal and pediatric airway emergencies. *Respiratory Care,* 37 (6), 582–599.

Tsuzaki, K. (1990). High-frequency ventilation in neonates. *Journal of Clinical Anesthesia,* 2, 387–392.

Venegas, D. (1989). Abstract: Effects of HFV on distribution of ventilation. *6th conference of HFV in infants,* Snowbird, UT.

Weber, K.R., & Asselin, J.M. (1990). High frequency oscillatory ventilation. *Neonatal Intensive Care,* May/June, 20–23.

Weilitz, P.B. (1993). Weaning a patient from mechanical ventilation. *Critical Care Nurse,* 13 (4), 33–41.

West, J.B., Dollery, C.T., & Naimark, A. (1964). Distribution of blood flow in isolated lung: Relation to vascular and alveolar pressures. *Journal of Applied Physiology,* 19, 713.

Wetzel, R.C., & Gioia, F.R. (1987). High frequency ventilation. *Pediatric Clinics of North America,* 34 (1), 15–37.

Wigal, D.T., & Will, M.W. (1993). Incentive spirometry treatments (pp. 79–82). In R.L. Boggs & M. Wooldridge-King (Eds.). *AACN procedure manual for critical care* (3rd ed.). Philadelphia: W.B. Saunders.

Wilson, B.G., & Desautels, D.A. (1993). Oxygen therapy. In P.B. Koff, D. Eitzman, & J. Neu (Eds.). *Neonatal and pediatric respiratory care* (2nd ed.). St. Louis: C.V. Mosby.

Wilson, J.M., Bower, L.K., Fackler, J.C., Beals, D.A., Bergus, B.O., & Kevy, S.V. (1993). Aminocaproic acid decreases the incidence of intracranial hemorrhage and other bleeding complications of ECMO. *Journal of Pediatric Surgery,* 28 (4), 536–540.

Wohl, M.E., & Mead, J. (1990). Age as a factor in respiratory distress. In V. Chernick (Ed.). *Kendig's disorders of the respiratory tract in children* (pp. 175–182). Philadelphia: W.B. Saunders.

Yaster, M. (1991). Airway management. In D.G. Nicholes, et al. (Eds.). *Golden hour: The handbook of advanced pediatric life support* (pp. 9–46). St. Louis: Mosby–Year Book.

CHAPTER 11

Acid-Base Balance

ANN POWERS

All patients who are admitted to the pediatric critical care unit are at risk for acid-base disturbances that may complicate their underlying disorder and further compromise their overall status. Acid-base balance is maintained through a variety of physiologic processes, which may be disrupted with serious illness or injury. Knowledge of acid-base balance is essential to the practice of pediatric critical care nursing so that appropriate assessment, monitoring, and intervention can be provided in a timely manner to optimize the child's outcome.

DEFINITION OF ACID-BASE BALANCE

Normal metabolism results in the production of acids. An acid is a proton or hydrogen ion (H^+) donor, and a base is a proton or hydrogen ion acceptor. There are a large number of potential hydrogen ions in the body, most of which are buffered and therefore not in free form. The normal concentration of free H^+ in the extracellular fluid (ECF) is extremely small, approximately 40 nmEq/L, which is equivalent to one millionth of a mEq/L concentration of sodium. The term pH expresses the negative logarithm of free H^+ concentration. The relationship is inversely proportional in that as free H^+ concentration increases, pH decreases, and vice versa. A normal arterial pH of 7.40 correlates with a free H^+ concentration of 40 nmEq/L. For each .01-unit change in pH from 7.40, H^+ concentration changes 1 nmEq/L in the opposite direction, provided that the pH range is between 7.20 and 7.50 (Brewer, 1990).

Normal metabolism produces hydrogen in the form of volatile and fixed acids. To maintain pH within its normal narrow range of 7.35 to 7.45, acids must be buffered or excreted. A buffer is defined as a substance that reduces the change in a solution's free H^+ concentration when an acid or base is added to it. In other words, the presence of a buffer in a solution increases the amount of acid or base that must be added to change the pH.

The largest amount of acid load in the body is in the form of carbonic acid (H_2CO_3), which is a volatile acid. Carbonic acid is formed, or dissociated, into either hydrogen and bicarbonate or carbon dioxide and water. This is illustrated by the following equation:

$$\begin{array}{ccccc} & & \text{Carbonic acid} & & \\ & & \rightleftharpoons H_2CO_3 \rightleftharpoons & & \\ H^+ & + & HCO_3^- & CO_2 & + & H_2O \\ \text{Hydrogen} & & \text{Bicarbonate} & \text{Carbon} & & \text{Water} \\ & & & \text{dioxide} & & \end{array}$$

Table 11–1. PHYSIOLOGIC EFFECTS OF ALTERATIONS IN pH

	Increase pH
Increase	Insulin-induced glycolysis
	Responsiveness to catecholamines
Decrease	Krebs cycle oxidations in muscles and renal cortex
	Gluconeogenesis in the renal cortex
	2,3-Diphosphoglycerate concentration with a corresponding left shift in the oxyhemoglobin dissociation curve
	Vascular tone and resistance

	Decrease pH
Increase	Krebs cycle oxidations in muscles and renal cortex
	Gluconeogenesis in the renal cortex
	2,3-Diphosphoglycerate concentration with a corresponding right shift in the oxyhemoglobin dissociation curve
	Pulmonary vascular resistance
Decrease	Glycolysis
	Lipolysis
	Quantities of liver glycogen
	Lactate production
	Insulin secretion and binding to receptors
	Pancreatic amylase secretion
	Threshold for ventricular fibrillation
	Responsiveness to catecholamines
	Peripheral vascular resistance
	Mesenteric blood flow
	Pulmonary macrophage function
	Granulocyte function
	Immune response

Data from Baer, C. L. (1988). Regulation and assessment of acid-base balance. In M. R. Kinney, et al. (Eds.). *AACN's clinical reference for critical care nursing* (2nd ed.). New York: McGraw-Hill.

The specific reaction (dissociation or formation of carbonic acid) is determined by the underlying acid-base environment.

Hydrogen that is generated in the form of a fixed acid includes lactic acid, ketoacid, phosphoric acid, and sulfuric acid. These are buffered by extracellular bicarbonate and eventually excreted by the kidneys. Dietary intake of acids and alkali are also metabolized and buffered to prevent changes in pH balance.

Biochemical processes are extremely sensitive to minute changes (0.1–0.2 units) in body fluid pH. Cardiac, central nervous system, and metabolic function may be significantly altered by changes in pH. Table 11–1 summarizes the physiologic effects of alterations in pH. An interval of 1.0 pH unit (6.8–7.8) is the widest range compatible with human life.

REGULATION OF ACID-BASE BALANCE

Three systems function interdependently to regulate and maintain acid-base balance. They are the buffer, respiratory, and renal systems.

Buffer System

The buffer system can be activated within seconds, thus is considered the first line of defense against changes in pH (Table 11–2). The most important of these buffers is the bicarbonate-carbonic acid (HCO_3^--H_2CO_3) pair, which is responsible for buffering ECF. This buffer pair consists of a weak acid (H_2CO_3), which is activated when the pH is threatened by a strong base; and a weak base (HCO_3^-), which is activated when the pH is threatened by a strong acid. Whenever a buffering reaction occurs, the concentration of one member of the pair increases while the other decreases. The bicarbonate-carbonic acid system is assessed clinically by arterial blood gas pH, P_{CO_2}, and HCO_3^-. In clinical settings where arterial plasma HCO_3^- measurement is unavailable, it can be estimated as being approximately 1 mEq/L less than the venous serum total CO_2 content as measured with electrolytes (Narins, 1994). Therefore, an elevated total CO_2 would suggest buffering of a strong base. Arterial blood gas analysis also reveals whether other systems (respiratory or renal) are involved in maintaining or attempting to restore acid-base balance.

The relationship of pH, bicarbonate, and carbonic acid is summarized by the Henderson-Hasselbalch equation:

$$pH = pK + \frac{(HCO_3^-)}{(H_2CO_3)}$$

This equation illustrates that the H^+ concentration (pH) of a solution is determined by the pK (carbonic acid dissociation constant, which is 6.1), and the concentration ratio of the buffer pair. Although useful, the Henderson-Hasselbalch equation is difficult to use clinically. The normal ratio of bicarbonate to carbonic acid is 20:1. This equation illustrates that a solution's pH depends upon the ratio of the concen-

Table 11–2. BUFFER SYSTEM PAIRS

Weak Acid	Weak Base	% Total Buffer Action
Carbonic acid (H_2CO_3)	Sodium bicarbonate ($NaHCO_3$)	53
Hemoglobin (Hb)	Potassium hemoglobinate (KHb)	35
Oxyhemoglobin (HbO_2)	Potassium oxyhemoglobinate ($KHbO_2$)	35
Plasma protein (HPr)	Proteinate (NaPr)	7
Acid organic phosphate ($NaRHPO_4$)	Alkaline organic phosphate (Na_2RPO_4)	3
Acid inorganic phosphate (NaH_2PO_4)	Alkaline inorganic phosphate ($NaHPO_4$)	2

From Baer, C. L. (1993). Regulation and assessment of acid base balance. In M. R. Kinney, et al. (Eds.). *AACN's clinical reference for critical care nursing* (3rd ed.). New York: McGraw-Hill.

tration of bicarbonate to carbonic acid, and not on their absolute value. A simpler and more clinically relevant way of relating pH to alterations in the acid-base ratio is:

$$pH = \frac{base}{acid} = \frac{HCO_3^-}{H_2CO_3} = \frac{20}{1}$$

The second most abundant buffer pair is hemoglobin and oxyhemoglobin, an important buffer of carbonic acid. As blood passes from the arterial to the venous end of a capillary, cellular CO_2 enters erythrocytes and combines with water to form carbonic acid. At the same time, oxyhemoglobin gives up its oxygen to the cells, some of which becomes reduced hemoglobin carrying a negative charge. The hemoglobin ion then attracts the H^+ from carbonic acid, resulting in a weaker acid than carbonic acid. When this system is active, the exchange demonstrates why erythrocytes tend to give up oxygen more rapidly when Pco_2 is elevated (as in respiratory acidosis), resulting in a shift to the right of the oxyhemoglobin dissociation curve. Erythrocytes hold onto oxygen when Pco_2 is decreased (as in respiratory alkalosis), resulting in a shift to the left in the oxyhemoglobin dissociation curve (Fig. 11–1). This is termed the Bohr effect (Antonini & Brunori, 1970).

The protein buffer pair is the most abundant intra-cellular and ECF buffer. Proteins are composed of amino acids, which contain at least one carboxyl and one amine group. The carboxyl group tends to function like an acid, while the amine group tends to act like a base. Thus, proteins can act as both acid and base buffers.

The phosphate buffer pair, which works in the same manner as the bicarbonate–carbonic acid pair, is an important regulator of both erythrocyte and renal tubular pH. This buffer pair consists of acid-alkaline organic and inorganic sodium phosphate.

Respiratory System

Ventilation also plays a major role in maintaining pH balance. The respiratory system can activate changes in pH within 1 to 3 minutes and can eliminate and/or conserve CO_2 (which directly impacts acid-base status) more quickly and efficiently than all the buffer systems combined.

As discussed, when a strong acid is present in the body, the bicarbonate–carbonic acid buffer pair is activated to buffer the acid. This results in a net increase of carbonic acid, which dissociates into CO_2 and H_2O. Carbon dioxide is then eliminated by the lungs (Fig. 11–2). An increase in H^+ concentration in the blood stimulates the breathing center in the medulla to increase respiratory rate, which facilitates CO_2 elimination. If, on the other hand, pH is elevated secondary to an increase in HCO_3^-, the respiratory center is inhibited and the respiratory rate decreases. This results in CO_2 retention, which then becomes available to form carbonic acid, which buffers the excess bicarbonate. The respiratory system is thus able to compensate for changes in pH related to metabolic disorders (e.g., diabetic ketoacidosis) by regulating Pco_2, which alters the bicarbonate-carbonic acid ratio. The respiratory system cannot, however, produce any loss or gain of hydrogen ions. Respiratory compensation is activated within minutes and is usually fully functional within 1 to 2 days.

Renal System

Compared with the respiratory system, which operates by passive CO_2 diffusion, the kidneys control acid-base balance through several highly developed active transport processes. Renal compensation is a slower process, requiring 1 to 2 days for complete activation with disorders resulting in respiratory alkalosis, and 3 to 5 days to be fully functional with disorders resulting in respiratory acidosis. The length of time a primary acid-base disturbance has been present is an important factor in determining the expected degree of renal compensation.

The kidneys react to changes in pH by regulating the excretion or conservation of H^+ and HCO_3^- (Fig. 11–3). A low pH stimulates excretion of H^+ into the urine. As H^+ enters the urine, it displaces another positive ion, usually Na^+. At the same time, HCO_3^- is reabsorbed in exchange for the H^+. The Na^+ is then reabsorbed into the tubule cell, where it combines with HCO_3^- to form $NaHCO_3$, which is then available to buffer other H^+ in the blood. The rate of H^+ excretion, and therefore the rate of HCO_3^- reabsorption, is proportionate to arterial Pco_2. This reaction is reversed for increases in pH.

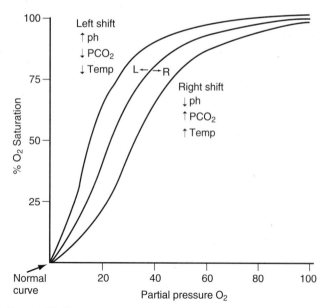

Figure 11–1 ● ● ● ● ● ●

pH effect on the oxyhemoglobin dissociation curve. (Modified from Shapiro, B. (1989). *Clinical application of blood gases* (4th ed.). Chicago: Year Book Medical Publishers.)

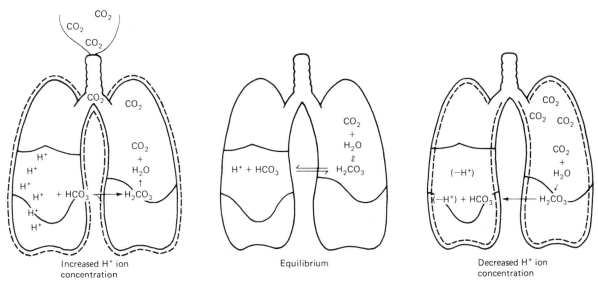

Figure 11-2 • • • • • •
Regulation of hydrogen ion concentration by the respiratory system. (From Baer, C. L. (1993). Acid-base balance. In M. R. Kinney, et al. (Eds.). *AACN's clinical reference for critical care nursing* (3rd ed., p. 211). St. Louis: Mosby–Year Book.)

The transport of H^+ in the renal tubules is facilitated by the buffers phosphate (as previously discussed) and ammonia, which is classified as a base. Most ammonia is converted to urea by the liver and is eliminated from the body in urine. The remaining ammonia combines with H^+ to form the ammonium ion (NH_4^+) in the renal tubules (Fig. 11–4). NH_4^+ also displaces Na^+ and is eliminated in the urine. The Na^+ is then reabsorbed into the tubule cells, where it combines with HCO_3^- to form $NaHCO_3$, which is absorbed into the blood to buffer excess H^+.

The amount of H^+ excreted in the urine can be measured by determining the amount of alkali required to neutralize the urine, and is called titratable acidity. As a result of H^+ and NH_4^+ excretion, urine usually has an acidic pH of 6. In the clinical setting, checking urine pH can be a useful indicator of the degree of renal compensation when assessing acid-base status. For example, a low or acidic blood pH will be accompanied a few days later by a low or acidic urine pH when renal compensatory mechanisms are active. The reverse is true in alkalotic states.

ELECTROLYTES AND ACID-BASE BALANCE

It is extremely important in the clinical setting to recognize how H^+ interacts with other ions so that

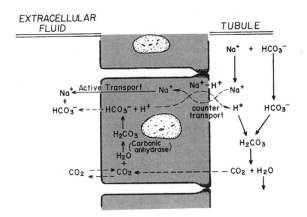

Figure 11-3 • • • • • •
Chemical reactions for (1) secondary active secretion of hydrogen ions into the tubule, (2) sodium ion reabsorption in exchange for the hydrogen ions secreted, and (3) combination of hydrogen ions with bicarbonate ions in the tubules to form carbon dioxide and water. (From Guyton, A. C. (1994). *Human physiology and mechanisms of disease* (5th ed., p. 236). Philadelphia: W. B. Saunders.)

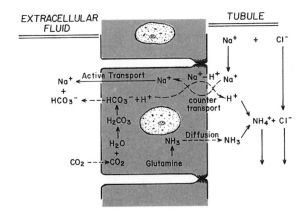

Figure 11-4 • • • • • •
Primary active transport of hydrogen ions through the luminal membrane of the tubular epithelial cell. Note that one bicarbonate ion is absorbed for each hydrogen ion secreted, and a chloride ion is secreted passively along with the hydrogen ion. (From Guyton, A. C. (1994). *Human physiology and mechanisms of disease* (5th ed., p. 237). Philadelphia: W.B. Saunders.)

metabolic and electrolyte imbalances can be anticipated and managed in a timely and appropriate manner. Figure 11–5 illustrates the location of the major concentrations of electrolytes that are affected by acid-base balance. As discussed, an increase in plasma CO_2 results in an increased renal excretion of H^+ and reabsorption of HCO_3^-, which then buffers excess H^+ in the body. This is a very important compensatory mechanism that can stabilize pH.

Potassium (K^+) also interacts in very important ways with H^+; the two share a reciprocal relationship. When H^+ concentration is elevated in the ECF, as occurs in metabolic acidosis, H^+ moves into the cell and K^+ moves out. This exchange allows H^+ access to the intracellular protein buffers, which can minimize changes in pH. However, during this process, the shift in K^+ from the intracellular fluid (ICF) to the ECF results in hyperkalemia. A shift in a very small amount of the ICF K^+ will produce a significant increase in ECF K^+ concentration and may lead

to the potentially lethal cardiac dysrhythmias associated with hyperkalemia (see Chap. 13). When H^+ concentration is decreased (as in metabolic alkalosis), H^+ moves out of the cell, and K^+ moves in, which can result in a hypokalemic state. Cardiac dysrhythmias are also possible with hypokalemia but are usually not life-threatening.

Sodium is affected by H^+ balance, as previously discussed. When H^+ concentration is elevated, Na^+ is displaced in the renal tubules so that excess H^+ can be eliminated in the urine. The displaced Na^+ is reabsorbed, which tends to increase HCO_3^- reabsorption. Normally, this process alone does not affect pH. However, if tubular Na^+ reabsorption is significantly elevated (as in prolonged sodium deprivation), a metabolic alkalosis with hyponatremia may result.

The chloride ion (Cl^-) can also contribute to acid-base imbalance, since it usually follows Na^+ passively. An increase in Cl^- results in a decreased reabsorption of HCO_3^- with Na^+ in the renal tubules,

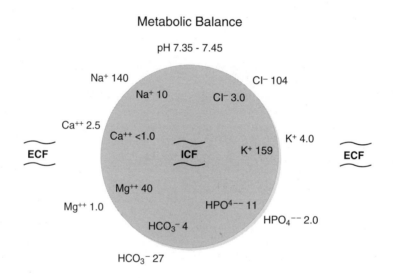

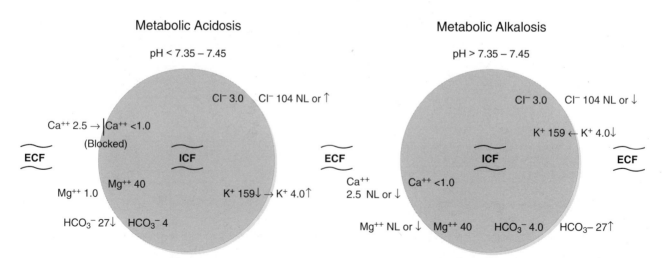

Figure 11–5 ● ● ● ● ● ●

Location of major concentrations of electrolytes that impact on acid-base balance (in mEq/L). (Redrawn from Mathewson-Kuhn, M. (1994). *Pharmacotherapeutics: A nursing process approach*, 3rd ed. Philadelphia: F.A. Davis.)

which can result in a metabolic acidosis associated with hyperchloremia. The reverse of this (increase in HCO_3^- resulting in a decreased reabsorption of Cl^- with Na^+) can result in a hypochloremic metabolic alkalosis.

Calcium (Ca^+) is another ion that is affected by acid-base balance. Maintaining Ca^+ levels within their normally narrow range is critical to normal neuromuscular and cardiac function. When pH is normal, 40% of the total plasma Ca^+ is bound to protein (mostly albumin) and 60% is present as ionized calcium in the plasma. Changes in pH alter the amount of Ca^+ bound by proteins, which, in turn, alters ionized Ca^+ levels. A change in pH of 0.1 unit will effect a corresponding change in protein-bound calcium of 0.12 mg/dL (Bordeau & Attie, 1994). When metabolic alkalosis is present in a child with a low serum Ca^+, the ionized Ca^+ is likely to be very low and can lead to neuromuscular and cardiac dysfunction. In a child with a metabolic acidosis and a low Ca^+ level, the ionized Ca^+ may be within normal limits. Chronic metabolic acidosis increases renal clearance of Ca^+. $NaHCO_3$ administration reestablishes normal calcium reabsorption.

MATURATIONAL FACTORS

The systems that regulate and maintain acid-base balance become fully operational at different developmental time periods. The buffer systems are functional in utero. Respiratory system control of acid-base balance is mature in newborns provided that pulmonary function is adequate. Any respiratory, neuromuscular, or neurologic disorder that alters CO_2 elimination can result in an acid-base disturbance.

Renal system control of acid-base balance is not fully functional at birth. Newborns have a limited ability to excrete hydrogen and ammonium ions. Since H^+ excretion matures rapidly, the ability of the kidney to excrete a maximal acid load is achieved by 2 months of age in both term and preterm infants. Ammonium production may not fully mature until age 2. Newborns also have a low serum bicarbonate level, which is secondary to a lower renal threshold for bicarbonate. The mechanism for this is unknown, but it may be related to an expanded ECF volume and immaturity in the transport capacity for bicarbonate reabsorption. Because of these immature renal functions, infants have a diminished renal capacity for dealing with acid-base disturbances.

ANALYZING ACID-BASE BALANCE

Before discussing specific acid-base disturbances, a review of terminology and guidelines for analyzing acid-base balance will be presented. The terms *base excess* and *base deficit* are frequently used in the clinical setting in relation to acid-base balance. Base excess describes the presence of an excessive amount of base (HCO_3^-), or a deficit in the amount of fixed acid (not including H_2CO_3).

Base excess or deficit can be determined clinically by application of three *Rules* (Chameides & Hazinski, 1994). These rules assist in determining if a disorder is respiratory, metabolic, or mixed. *Rule I* states that an acute change in PCO_2 of 10 torr is associated with an increase or decrease in pH of .08 units. Normally, if pH is 7.40, the PCO_2 would be 40 torr in the absence of metabolic acidosis. Application of Rule I would reveal the following:

$$PCO_2\ 50\ (40 + 10) = pH\ 7.32\ (7.40 - .08)$$

$$PCO_2\ 30\ (40 - 10) = pH\ 7.48\ (7.40 + .08)$$

Rule II states that for every .01-unit change in pH not due to a change in PCO_2, there is a 2/3 mEq/L change in the base. For example, if the pH is 7.26 and the PCO_2 is 50 torr, the increase in PCO_2 would indicate a respiratory acidosis. The calculated pH would be 7.32 (according to Rule I). Since the measured pH is 7.26, there is a pH difference of .06 units. By applying Rule II (6 × 2/3), the calculated base deficit would be 4 mEq/L. Thus, a metabolic and respiratory acidosis are both present.

Rule III is the least helpful in the clinical setting. It states:

Total base deficit = base deficit × weight (kg) × 0.3

HCO_3^- is located primarily in ECF, which is equal to 30% of body weight; thus total base deficit can be determined by multiplying base deficit by body weight by 0.3. In a 10-kg child with a PCO_2 of 50 and a pH of 7.24, the PCO_2 is 10 torr above normal, which would suggest that the pH be 7.32 if the child had a respiratory acidosis. The unexplained pH difference of .08 units must therefore be attributed to a metabolic acidosis with a base deficit of 6 mEq/L (according to Rule II). Application of the above equation would reveal:

Total base deficit = base deficit × wt (kg) × 0.3

$$18 = 6 × 10 × 0.3$$

To avoid overcorrection and a rebound metabolic alkalosis, total bicarbonate correction is not recommended. Half the calculated dose is most often used. In this particular case, 9 mEq of sodium bicarbonate ($NaHCO_3$) would be given. Note that the usual recommended dose of $NaHCO_3$ for correction of moderate metabolic acidosis, 1 mEq/kg (which would be 10 mEq in this case), is very close to the more complicated calculation using Rule III. Therefore, a standard dose of 1 mEq/kg is acceptable for quick determination of bicarbonate replacement (Chameides & Hazinski, 1994).

SODIUM BICARBONATE ADMINISTRATION

$NaHCO_3$ administration increases blood pH by providing additional HCO_3^- to combine with H^+. Again:

$HCO_3^- + H^+ \Rightarrow H_2CO_3 \Rightarrow CO_2 + H_2O$. Note that CO_2 is formed as H^+ is buffered. In order to maintain the buffering capacity of $NaHCO_3$, effective ventilation *must* be present.

$NaHCO_3$ administration will transiently increase PCO_2. Since CO_2 crosses cell membranes more rapidly than HCO_3^-, $NaHCO_3$ administration may temporarily worsen intracellular acidosis. This can seriously impair or further compromise cellular function, for example, myocardial contractility and cerebral acidosis. It is imperative to maintain adequate ventilation or hyperventilation, and to optimize perfusion when administering $NaHCO_3$ to facilitate the CO_2 removal as rapidly as possible. If successful, one can expect the end-tidal CO_2 to increase for a short period of time after $NaHCO_3$ administration (Curley, 1990).

Sodium bicarbonate has been used traditionally in patients with cardiac arrest and ventricular fibrillation. Yet, numerous studies have failed to demonstrate $NaHCO_3$ effectiveness in helping to restore circulation or in improving the success of defibrillation as previously believed (Redding & Pearson, 1968; Telivuo et al., 1968). Other adverse effects associated with $NaHCO_3$ administration include hyperosmolarity, hypernatremia, and iatrogenic metabolic alkalosis. The alkalosis may decrease ionized calcium and potassium levels, shift the oxyhemoglobin dissociation curve to the left (inhibiting O_2 release to the tissues), and predispose the patient to life-threatening dysrhythmias. The potential risks and benefits must be carefully considered in individual clinical situations when deciding if $NaHCO_3$ is indicated. Several clinicians advocate its use only when the pH is less than 7.20 and the patient is at risk for complications associated with acidosis (Brewer, 1990; Kaehny, 1992).

ACID-BASE DISTURBANCES

The buffer, respiratory, and renal compensatory mechanisms function interdependently at specific time intervals to restore acid-base balance. Signs and symptoms and the clinical significance of acid-base disturbances are directly related to the rate at which the pH changes. Disorders that develop slowly, such as chronic renal or respiratory failure, allow time for maximum compensation to occur and thus will be accompanied by minimal changes in pH. Rapidly progressing or sudden insults, such as a cardiac arrest, allow little or no time for compensation to occur, resulting in profound alterations in pH that may be fatal if immediate and effective intervention is not initiated. The arterial blood gas (ABG) is the most useful diagnostic tool in determining acid-base imbalances in the clinical setting. Normal blood gas values are listed in Table 11–3. The steps used to analyze arterial blood gases to determine the acid-base imbalance are illustrated in Figure 11–6.

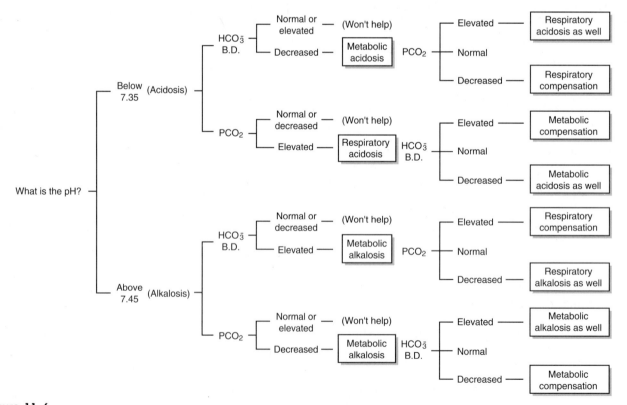

Figure 11–6 ● ● ● ● ● ●

Arterial blood gas analysis to determine the acid-base imbalance. B.D., base deficits. (From Donlen J. Interpreting acid-base problems through arterial blood gases. Reprinted with permission of CRITICAL CARE NURSE®, 3 (5), 38, 1983.)

Table 11-3. NORMAL BLOOD GAS VALUES

Parameter	Arterial	Mixed Venous	Capillary
pH	7.35–7.45	7.31–7.41	7.35–7.45
PO_2	80–100 mmHg	35–40 mmHg	Less than arterial*
O_2 saturation	95–97%	70–75%	Less than arterial
PCO_2	35–45 mmHg	40–50 mmHg	35–45 mmHg
HCO_3	22–26 mEq/L	22–26 mEq/L	22–26 mEq/L
Total CO_2 content	20–27 mEq/L	20–27 mEq/L	20–27 mEq/L
Base excess	+2 to −2	+2 to −2	+2 to −2

*Capillary PO_2 is approximately 10 mmHg less than arterial except when decreased tissue perfusion is present, that is, cardiovascular collapse or hypothermia. In these states, capillary samples will not accurately reflect arterial PO_2.

Respiratory Acidosis

Respiratory acidosis is an excess of ECF carbonic acid that is caused by conditions resulting in hypoventilation and CO_2 retention. These conditions are summarized in Table 11-4. Buffer response to hypercapnia occurs immediately and is complete within 10 to 15 minutes. Renal compensatory mechanisms are activated within 2 to 5 hours but take 3 to 5 days to function at maximum capacity.

Signs and symptoms depend on the severity of the respiratory acidosis (Table 11-5). Changes in respiratory function such as decreased respiratory rate and shallow breathing occur secondary to the underlying problem that has triggered the alveolar hypoventilation. Dyspnea is caused by stimulation of the respiratory center in the medulla and peripheral chemoreceptors that are triggered by a decrease in blood pH. Cardiovascular effects such as tachycardia, increased cardiac output, and increased blood pressure occur secondary to sympathetic stimulation and epinephrine release from the adrenal medulla. This mechanism is stimulated by hypercapnia and a low pH. Although receptor response to catecholamines is blunted in acidosis, this is initially offset by a surge in catecholamine release. Acute hypercapnia has opposing effects on peripheral vasculature. Vasodilation occurs by its direct effect on vascular smooth muscles. Vasoconstriction is simultaneously produced by catecholamine release. This usually results in either a mild vasoconstriction or vasodilation.

Important exceptions to this occur in the pulmonary and cerebral vessels. Whereas cerebral vascular resistance decreases and cerebral blood flow increases proportionately with an increase in PCO_2, the opposite occurs in the pulmonary vascular bed. Increased cerebral blood flow precipitates the headache associated with hypercapnia and respiratory acidosis. An acute increase in PCO_2 may precipitate pulmonary vasospasm, resulting in an abrupt increase in pulmonary vascular resistance and decreased pulmonary blood flow. Any increase in pulmonary vascular resistance may worsen the underlying disorder responsible for the respiratory acidosis.

The pathophysiology of the central nervous system (CNS) effects are unclear. Cerebrospinal fluid (CSF) pH changes in relation to blood pH. CO_2 permeates the blood-brain barrier, so increases in arterial PCO_2 are seen immediately in the CSF. However, the CSF contains fewer buffers than the blood so CSF pH falls more dramatically, which may contribute to the CNS symptomatology that occurs with respiratory acidosis. CNS symptomatology can vary greatly in different individuals. For example, similar increases in PCO_2 cause some children to become somnolent and others to become apprehensive and agitated.

In respiratory acidosis, the arterial pH is less than 7.35, PCO_2 is greater than 45 torr, and the HCO_3^- is normal or elevated (depending on the degree of renal compensation). It is important to note that hypoxemia may be a very late sign of respiratory acidosis; therefore, cyanosis may not be present until the child progresses to respiratory failure. Serum po-

Table 11-4. DISORDERS ASSOCIATED WITH RESPIRATORY ACIDOSIS

Acute Obstructive Airway Disorders
Croup	Asthma
Epiglottitis	Bronchiolitis
Foreign body	

Chronic Obstructive Airway Disorders
Bronchopulmonary dysplasia
Cystic fibrosis

Pulmonary Restrictive Disorders
Pneumonia	Pleural effusion
Aspiration	Pneumothorax
ARDS	Flail chest
Pulmonary edema	Kyphoscoliosis
Interstitial lung disease	Pierre Robin syndrome

Neuromuscular Disorders
Muscular dystrophy	Spinal cord injury or tumor
Multiple sclerosis	Myasthenia gravis
Spinal muscular atrophy	Diaphragmatic paralysis
Guillain-Barré syndrome	Pickwickian syndrome
Brainstem injury or tumor	Poliomyelitis
Botulism	

Central Nervous System Depressants
Narcotics	Cerebral trauma or infection
General anesthesia	Brain tumor
Sedatives	

Circulatory Crises
Cardiac arrest
Severe pulmonary edema
Massive pulmonary embolism

Iatrogenic Causes
Inadequate mechanical ventilation
Hyperalimentation with high carbohydrate content
Sorbent regenerative hemodialysis

Table 11–5. SIGNS AND SYMPTOMS ASSOCIATED WITH ACID-BASE IMBALANCE

Respiratory Acidosis	Respiratory Alkalosis	Metabolic Acidosis	Metabolic Alkalosis
Decreased respiratory rate	Hyperventilation	Tachypnea → Kussmaul respirations	Hypoventilation
Shallow breathing	Breathlessness	Tachycardia → bradycardia	Cardiac dysrhythmias
Dyspnea	Cardiac dysrhythmias	Cardiac dysrhythmias	Decreased perfusion
Tachycardia	Hypotension	Hypotension	Hypotension
Headache	Extremity and perioral paresthesias	Poor perfusion with a grayish pallor	Confusion
Decreased responsiveness	Vertigo	Decreased peripheral pulses	Lethargy
Disorientation	Syncope	Increased capillary refill time	Unresponsiveness
Restlessness	Anxiety	Decreased urine output	Hyperreflexia
Apprehension	Nervousness	Decreased level of consciousness	Muscle cramps
Agitation	Confusion	Congestive heart failure	Twitching
Fatigue	Decreased level of consciousness	Fatigue	Tetany
Weakness	Decreased psychomotor performance	Drowsiness	Seizures
Diminished reflexes	Hyperreflexia	Confusion	Nausea, vomiting, and diarrhea
Seizures	Muscle cramps	Apathy	
Nausea and vomiting	Twitching	Unresponsiveness	
	Tetany	Seizures	
	Seizures	Nausea and vomiting	
		Abdominal distension and pain	

tassium increases 0.1 mEq/L for each 0.1-u decrease in blood pH and therefore would be normal to slightly elevated with respiratory acidosis. Blood lactate levels fall slightly and phosphorus becomes mildly elevated (Gennari, 1994). Urine pH may be decreased, again depending on the degree of renal compensation.

Clinical management of respiratory acidosis is directed toward re-establishing effective ventilation and treating the underlying problem. The child may require intubation, mechanical ventilation, or a change in the ventilation plan while the primary problem is being treated. Oxygen and $NaHCO_3$ may be given based on the ABG. While hypoxemia does not usually affect acid-base balance, a PO_2 of less than 35 torr may induce a lactic (metabolic) acidosis. $NaHCO_3$ is administered only to correct severe metabolic acidosis. Effective ventilation must be established prior to the administration of $NaHCO_3$; otherwise, the acidosis will worsen (see previous discussion on sodium bicarbonate administration).

The *clinical significance* of respiratory acidosis depends upon the child's general health and the physiologic effects of the acidosis and hypoxemia. Nursing assessment parameters include vital signs, noting rate, rhythm, character, and pattern of all parameters; perfusion status, noting skin color and temperature, peripheral and central pulses, capillary refill time, level of consciousness, and urine output; muscle strength and movement; oxygenation status, noting color of nailbeds and mucous membranes, and SaO_2; gastrointestinal function; degree of comfort; and laboratory data.

Nursing interventions include positioning the child to optimize ventilation, administering oxygen, and suctioning to clear the airways and enhance CO_2 elimination. Care is directed to minimize O_2 consumption by providing an environment with minimal stimulation and uninterrupted periods of rest. Inherently important is to provide the child and family

with appropriate explanations, support, and reassurance.

Respiratory Alkalosis

Respiratory alkalosis is an ECF deficit of carbonic acid caused by conditions resulting in alveolar hyperventilation and CO_2 deficit. Rare as a primary problem, disorders associated with respiratory alkalosis in children are summarized in Table 11–6. Buffer response to hypocapnia begins immediately and is

Table 11–6. DISORDERS ASSOCIATED WITH RESPIRATORY ALKALOSIS

Intoxications	
Alcohol	Paraldehyde
Salicylate	Xanthine

Increased Intracranial Pressure	
Meningitis	Vascular accidents
Encephalitis	Brain lesions
Head trauma	

Pulmonary Disorders	
Pneumonia	
Pulmonary edema	
Pulmonary emboli	

Increased Metabolic Rate	
Fever	Anemia
Hyperthyroidism	Gram-negative sepsis
Exercise	Interstitial lung disease

Miscellaneous	
High altitude	Hepatic failure
Voluntary hyperventilation	CHF with hypoxemia
Anxiety	Mechanical ventilation
Hysteria	

complete within 10 to 15 minutes. Renal compensatory mechanisms are activated within 2 to 5 hours in respiratory alkalosis and take 1 to 2 days to be fully functional.

Signs and symptoms associated with respiratory alkalosis are summarized in Table 11–5. Hyperventilation results from stimulation of the respiratory center in the medulla, and stimulation of peripheral chemoreceptors and nociceptive receptors in the lungs. Hyperventilation may also occur when signals from the cerebral cortex override the chemoreceptors, as in voluntary hyperventilation.

Heart rate increases secondary to sympathetic stimulation and the resultant catecholamine release from the adrenal medulla. This can cause atrial and ventricular tachydysrhythmias. There is usually no major change in cardiac output and blood pressure in awake children. Cardiovascular response to hypocapnia differs in anesthetized children. While tachycardia may not develop, cardiac output and perfusion may decrease. This occurs secondary to increased intrathoracic pressures associated with passive hyperventilation, resulting in decreased venous return. Whereas pulmonary vasodilation occurs with hypocapnia, peripheral vasoconstriction also occurs. This results in decreased blood flow to the skin and contributes to paresthesias. Cerebral blood flow (CBF) is also drastically reduced secondary to cerebral vasoconstriction. This vasoconstriction decreases intracranial and intraocular hydrostatic pressure (Gennari, 1994). Cerebral oxygen consumption does not decrease when blood flow is reduced, so cerebral hypoxemia and hypoxia may develop leading to lightheadedness, syncope, anxiety, altered levels of consciousness, and seizures.

Calcium binding, resulting in hypocalcemia, occurs with alkalemia. This also contributes to the development of seizures, as well as neuromuscular irritability, hyperreflexia, muscle cramps, twitching, and tetany.

In respiratory alkalosis, the arterial pH is greater than 7.45, P_{CO_2} is less than 35 torr, and the HCO_3^- is normal or decreased (less than 25 mEq/L). Potassium concentration decreases 0.1 mEq/L for each 0.1-u increase in pH, and therefore should be normal or slightly decreased (Gennari, 1994). Urine pH is normal to increased, depending on the degree of renal compensation.

The *clinical management* of respiratory alkalosis is directed toward restoring effective ventilation and treating the underlying cause. Sedation, breathing exercises, and relaxation with controlled breathing can correct the imbalance (if the child is developmentally capable of participating in such activities). Administration of 3% to 5% CO_2 and neuromuscular paralysis with intubation and mechanical ventilation may also be necessary if respiratory alkalosis is severe and other measures are ineffective (Baer, 1988).

The *clinical significance* of respiratory alkalosis depends on the presence and extent of neuromuscular effects. Seizures from respiratory alkalosis can be life-threatening. Nursing assessment parameters

Table 11–7. DISORDERS ASSOCIATED WITH METABOLIC ACIDOSIS

Increased Anion Gap (Normochloremic)

CARDIOVASCULAR COLLAPSE
Diabetic ketoacidosis
Lactic acidosis (tissue hypoxia)
Starvation
Drugs/toxins (methanol, ethanol, salicylate, fructose, sorbitol, cyanide, carbon monoxide, paraldehyde)
Organic acid metabolism (pyruvate)
Hepatic failure
Renal failure
Congenital enzymatic defects
    Glucose-6-phosphate deficiency
    Fructose 1,6-diphosphatase deficiency
    Pyruvate carboxylase deficiency
    Methylmalonic aciduria

Normal Anion gap (Hyperchloremic)

Diarrhea
Intake of chloride-containing compounds (HCl, NH_4Cl, $CaCl_2$, $MgCl_2$, arginine HCl, cholestyramine)
Hyperalimentation
Pancreatic, small bowel, or biliary tubes or fistulas
Ureterosigmoidostomy, ileal conduit
Carbonic anhydrase inhibitors (acetazolamide)
ECF volume expansion
Mineralocorticoid deficiency (adrenal disorders)
Renal tubular acidosis
Early uremic acidosis

include vital signs, noting rate, rhythm, character, and pattern of all parameters; perfusion status, noting skin color and temperature, peripheral and central pulses, capillary refill time, level of consciousness, and urine output; muscle movement and strength; sensation in the extremities and around the perioral area; and seizure activity.

Nursing interventions with respiratory alkalosis include maintaining seizure precautions. If age and clinical condition indicate, interventions may include assisting with relaxation and slow breathing techniques and/or having the child breathe through a paper bag. Care is directed toward providing a safe environment with age- and condition-appropriate activities, minimal stimulation, and uninterrupted periods of rest.

Metabolic Acidosis

Metabolic acidosis is an ECF deficit of bicarbonate caused by conditions that result in a loss of bicarbonate or an increase in fixed acids. These conditions are summarized in Table 11–7. Note that the most common cause of metabolic acidosis in the pediatric population is insufficient tissue perfusion. Situations that produce an increase in fixed acids result in a normochloremic acidosis with an increased anion gap. Situations that cause a bicarbonate loss result in a hyperchloremic acidosis with a normal anion gap. The normal range for the anion gap is 8 to 16 mEq/L and is calculated using the formula:

$$\text{Anion gap} = Na^+ - (Cl^- + HCO_3^-)$$

Buffer and respiratory compensatory mechanisms are activated within minutes with metabolic acidosis. Respiratory compensation results in an increased respiratory rate to eliminate excess CO_2; however, it is not usually effective in correcting the imbalance.

Signs and symptoms depend on the severity of the metabolic acidosis (see Table 11–5). Tachycardia results from sympathetic stimulation and the subsequent release of epinephrine from the adrenal medulla, which is stimulated by acidosis. As pH falls below 7.10, heart rate progressively slows. This is most likely related to the inhibitory effect acidosis has on the action of catecholamines, or accumulation of acetylcholine caused by the inhibition of acetylcholinesterase. Ventricular dysrhythmias are usually related to the electrolyte imbalances seen with acidosis, particularly hyperkalemia. Acidosis also decreases the fibrillation threshold, so the child is at greater risk for ventricular fibrillation. As pH falls from 7.40 to 7.20, the negative inotropic effect of acidosis and the positive inotropic effect of catecholamine release offset each other so that effective myocardial contraction is maintained. However, as pH falls below 7.20, the negative inotropic effect dominates, which results in poor perfusion and hypotension. Calcium entry into the cell is also inhibited at this point, which further decreases effective myocardial contraction. Although epinephrine facilitates calcium entry into the cells in early acidosis, this becomes inhibited as H^+ concentration increases. Infants and children who are receiving beta-adrenergic antagonists or calcium channel blocking agents as well as those who are chronically stressed and have limited endogenous catecholamine stores are more susceptible to the negative inotropic effects of acidosis. A pH of less than 7.20 also effects arterial and venous tone. The arterial system dilates while the venous system constricts, which forces blood to flow centrally. This increases the workload of the heart and can result in congestive heart failure.

Tachypnea results from stimulation of the respiratory center in the medulla. Kussmaul respirations develop with acute severe metabolic acidosis as the child increases tidal volume as well as respiratory rate to improve oxygenation and eliminate CO_2. Oxygen delivery to the tissues is enhanced by metabolic acidosis as the oxyhemoglobin dissociation curve shifts to the right (see Fig. 11–1). However, if acidosis progresses, glycolysis slows and red blood cell 2,3-diphosphoglycerate (DPG) is depleted, which eliminates the beneficial Bohr effect as previously described. Hypoxemia and tissue hypoxia then progress. Neurologic changes are related to decreased perfusion to the brain, hypoxemia, hypoxia, and metabolic and electrolyte imbalances.

The gastrointestinal symptoms associated with metabolic acidosis are likely related to either ketogenesis, or electrolyte and biochemical changes that accompany acidosis. Normal tone and contraction of the gastrointestinal tract are altered, resulting in abdominal pain, distension, nausea, and vomiting.

In metabolic acidosis, the arterial pH is less than 7.35, the P_{CO_2} is decreased (a normal or elevated P_{CO_2} would indicate failing respiratory compensation and the development of respiratory acidosis), and HCO_3^- is less than 25 mEq/L. Serum potassium is elevated 0.1 mEq/L for each .01-u decrease in pH; chloride is normal or elevated (depending on etiology); and urine pH is normal or decreased, again depending on the etiology of the acidosis.

Clinical management of metabolic acidosis is directed toward identifying and treating the underlying problem. Treatment will, therefore, vary depending on the cause. Bicarbonate losses should be replaced in severe acidosis. $NaHCO_3$ should be administered to achieve a slight undercorrection and thus prevent a rebound metabolic alkalosis from occurring. Adequate ventilation must be established prior to administering $NaHCO_3$ (see previous discussion on $NaHCO_3$ administration).

The *clinical significance* of metabolic acidosis depends on the severity of the disorder. The body does not tolerate changes in H^+ concentration well. Without appropriate intervention, metabolic acidosis will progress to life-threatening alterations in cardiac, neurologic, and metabolic function. Nursing assessment parameters include vital signs, noting rate, rhythm, character, and pattern of all parameters; perfusion status, noting skin color and temperature, peripheral and central pulses, capillary refill time, level of consciousness, and urine output; seizure activity; gastrointestinal function; intake and output; muscle strength; signs of hyperkalemia; the child's level of comfort; and appropriate laboratory data.

Nursing interventions include administering medications and fluids, positioning the child to optimize ventilation, maintaining seizure precautions, and providing comfort measures for gastrointestinal upset. Care is directed to provide a safe environment with age- and condition-appropriate activities, minimal stimulation, and uninterrupted periods of rest.

Metabolic Alkalosis

Metabolic alkalosis is an ECF excess of HCO_3^- caused by conditions resulting in excess base because of loss of H^+, reabsorption of HCO_3^-, or loss of other ions (i.e., chloride, sodium). These conditions are summarized in Table 11–8. Buffer and respiratory compensatory mechanisms are activated immediately with metabolic alkalosis. Respiratory compensation results in a decreased respiratory rate to conserve CO_2; however, this is ineffective and does not correct the imbalance.

Signs and symptoms associated with metabolic alkalosis are summarized in Table 11–5. Hypoventilation results from stimulation of the respiratory center in the medulla, which attempts to conserve P_{CO_2} by decreasing alveolar ventilation. This may result in hypoxemia, which can further compromise the child's status. Cardiac dysrhythmias with a subsequent decrease in cardiac output and blood pressure usually occur secondary to hypoxemia or hypokalemia.

Table 11-8. DISORDERS ASSOCIATED WITH METABOLIC ALKALOSIS

Vomiting	Renal failure
Gastrointestinal suctioning	ECF volume depletion
Cl⁻-wasting diarrhea	Cystic fibrosis
Cl⁻-deficient formula	Excess mineralocorticoid
Diuretics	Hyperaldosteronism,
Hypokalemia	Cushing's syndrome,
Hypocalcemia	adrenogenital
Hypochloremia	syndrome
Exogenous alkali intake: HCO₃⁻,	Laxative, licorice abuse
citrate, lactate, acetate	Excessive tobacco chewing
Excessive steroid use	Bartter's syndrome

Changes in level of consciousness occur secondary to decreased cerebral blood flow, which results from the cerebral vasoconstriction that is associated with alkalosis. Seizures can develop secondary to hypoxemia, hypocalcemia, or hypomagnesemia. Calcium binding increases with alkalemia, resulting in hypocalcemia. Magnesium levels decrease in relation to calcium. Hypocalcemia also contributes to the development of neuromuscular irritability, muscle cramps, and tetany. Gastrointestinal effects are usually associated with the underlying problem, which results in nausea, vomiting, and diarrhea.

In metabolic alkalosis, the arterial pH is greater than 7.45, HCO_3^- is greater than 30 mEq/L, base excess is greater than +2, and the P_{CO_2} is normal or elevated. Serum electrolytes usually reveal a hypokalemia, with a 0.1 mEq/L decrease in potassium for each .01-u increase in blood pH. Hypocalcemia and hypochloremia may also be present. Urine chloride is usually decreased and urine pH is normal or increased; the degree depends on the etiology.

The *clinical management* of metabolic alkalosis is directed toward identifying and treating the underlying cause of the imbalance. This usually involves expanding ECF volume with saline; administering chloride (arginine or ammonium chloride if the NaCl is insufficient to replace the lost ion); correcting hypokalemia with potassium chloride; and facilitating excretion of HCO_3^- with carbonic anhydrase–inhibiting diuretics (i.e., acetazolamide), or dialysis if renal impairment is present.

The *clinical significance* of metabolic alkalosis depends on the severity of the disorder and the accompanying neuromuscular and respiratory effects. Nursing assessment parameters include vital signs, noting rate, rhythm, character, and pattern of all parameters; perfusion status, noting skin color and temperature, peripheral and central pulses, capillary refill time, level of consciousness, and urine output; neuromuscular function; muscle movement and strength; Chvostek's and Trousseau's signs for hypocalcemia; strict intake and output; stooling pattern and characteristics; and laboratory data.

Nursing interventions with metabolic alkalosis include administering medications and fluids, maintaining seizure precautions, and providing comfort measures for gastrointestinal upset. Care is directed to providing a safe environment with age- and condition-appropriate activities, minimal stimulation, and uninterrupted periods of rest.

MIXED ACID-BASE DISORDERS

Mixed acid-base disturbances frequently occur in a variety of infants and children with multisystem problems. Mixed disturbances can result in excessive or diminished compensation. The clinical significance of the imbalances depends upon the net change in pH.

In general, mixed disorders that drive the pH in opposite directions (respiratory acidosis with metabolic alkalosis) are better tolerated because each compensates for the other to keep the pH near, or within, normal limits. Mixed disorders that drive the pH in the same direction (respiratory and metabolic acidosis) have profound effects on pH because compensation is impossible. Since the body is unable to tolerate significant changes in pH, mixed disorders can significantly alter cardiac, neurologic, and metabolic function and be life-threatening without appropriate intervention. It is important to treat each component of the mixed disorder simultaneously in order to avoid exacerbating one while correcting the other. Accurate interpretation of ABGs and monitoring of the child's clinical response to therapy are critical nursing interventions since the patient's response to therapy may be asynchronous.

Respiratory Acidosis With Metabolic Alkalosis

Respiratory acidosis and metabolic alkalosis can occur in children with obstructive pulmonary disease (for example, bronchopulmonary dysplasia or cystic fibrosis) who are receiving diuretics as part of their management plan. Such children usually live in a state of compensated respiratory acidosis secondary to CO_2 retention related to their pulmonary disease. Chronic diuretic therapy with potassium-wasting drugs (such as furosemide) can lead to hypokalemia and metabolic alkalosis. A similar scenario also occurs in children with congestive heart failure and chronic respiratory acidosis who are on long-term diuretic therapy. The pH with this mixed imbalance is usually near or within normal limits because of compensation. If, however, the pH rises with the metabolic alkalosis, respiratory drive may be depressed in the medulla, resulting in a decrease in P_{O_2} and an increase in P_{CO_2}, which can progress to respiratory failure.

Clinical management of this mixed imbalance is directed toward correcting the metabolic alkalosis. This is accomplished by administering sodium and potassium chloride to facilitate renal excretion of HCO_3^-. This must be done cautiously to avoid inducing or exacerbating congestive heart failure. Although pH may fall to acidemic levels, this will stimulate respiration and subsequently increase Po_2 and decrease Pco_2 levels. Oxygen must be administered carefully, since increasing the Po_2 above the patient's normal threshold may depress the respiratory drive in the medulla. It is extremely helpful to know what the baseline ABG status is for the patient with chronic lung disease so that appropriate treatment goals can be established.

Nursing assessment and interventions would be the same as those listed under each disorder. Consideration must be given to these children's underlying disease process, and to what degree they are compromised when planning, implementing, and evaluating clinical management.

Respiratory and Metabolic Acidosis

Respiratory and metabolic acidosis may develop in infants and children with chronic obstructive pulmonary disease who are in shock, who have any type of metabolic acidosis and develop respiratory failure, and in those who suffer cardiopulmonary arrest. Compensation is not possible with this mixed disorder, and the pH will fall dramatically, even when changes in Pco_2 and HCO_3^- are moderate. The clinical significance is related to the fall in pH and can result in cardiac, neurologic, and metabolic dysfunction.

Clinical management of this imbalance is directed toward careful correction of both the respiratory and metabolic component to normalize pH. It is helpful to know the baseline status of the patient with chronic lung disease, as previously discussed. Special consideration must be given to the care of these children, since the goal will be to return them to their baseline compromised status, which will include normalizing pH, but not necessarily other ABG parameters. Mechanical ventilation may be necessary to eliminate excess CO_2 and return these children to their baseline status. $NaHCO_3$ is usually administered after adequate ventilation is established. Nursing assessment and intervention are as discussed under each disorder.

Respiratory Alkalosis With Metabolic Acidosis

The mixed imbalance of respiratory alkalosis with metabolic acidosis may be seen in children with hepatic failure. The respiratory alkalosis is due to hyperventilation (secondary to restrictive lung capacity with liver enlargement), and the metabolic acidosis is due to hepatic failure with lactic acidosis, renal failure, or renal tubular acidosis. This imbalance can also occur in children with chronic renal failure and acute sepsis. The respiratory alkalosis develops secondary to the hyperventilation that accompanies sepsis, and the metabolic acidosis is associated with the

renal failure. Salicylate intoxication also results in a respiratory alkalosis, which is related to stimulation of the breathing center in the medulla; and metabolic acidosis, which occurs secondary to disruption of the Krebs cycle with accumulation of lactic and other organic acids.

Clinical management of the child with this mixed imbalance is directed toward correction of the underlying problem. The pH is usually close to or within normal limits because of effective or excessive compensation and may not require specific treatment. Nursing assessment and interventions are as discussed under each disorder.

Respiratory and Metabolic Alkalosis

The combination of respiratory and metabolic alkalosis is seen in children with chronic hepatic failure who are on diuretics and/or who develop vomiting. The respiratory alkalosis is due to hyperventilation from restrictive lung disease related to hepatic enlargement, and the metabolic alkalosis is due to potassium or fixed acid loss related to diuretic therapy or vomiting (respectively). It is also seen in children with chronic respiratory acidosis (from chronic lung disease) with appropriately elevated HCO_3^- levels, who are placed on mechanical ventilation and are overventilated resulting in a drastic fall in Pco_2 resulting in respiratory alkalosis. Neither disorder is able to compensate for the other, and pH rises dramatically.

Clinical management of this imbalance is directed toward treating the underlying problem and normalizing the pH. The respiratory component is managed by treating the cause of hyperventilation or adjusting the ventilator. The metabolic component is corrected with sodium and potassium chloride. Fluids must be administered cautiously to avoid inducing congestive heart failure or pulmonary edema. Nursing assessments and interventions are as listed under each disorder.

Triple Acid-Base Disorders

Triple acid-base disorders may occur in children with disorders affecting more than one body system, such as those with chronic liver failure. Hyperventilation and respiratory alkalosis result from restrictive lung capacity related to the enlarged abdomen. Metabolic alkalosis occurs if the child is on diuretics, develops vomiting, or requires nasogastric suctioning. Finally, metabolic acidosis may develop secondary to renal tubular acidosis, diarrhea, uremic acidosis, and lactic acidosis. Clinical management of such a complicated disorder involves careful assessment and correction of each component simultaneously to normalize pH. Nursing assessment and intervention would include those listed under each disorder.

SUMMARY

Acid-base disturbances are associated with many disorders and diseases seen in the pediatric critical care unit. It is crucial for the nurse to be able to accurately assess the child's acid-base status, to recognize imbalances, and to anticipate the potentially life-threatening complications that may result from them. Appropriate interventions can then be implemented to prevent or minimize these complications, and thus improve the patient's outcome.

References

Antonini, E., & Brunori, M. (1970). Hemoglobin. *Annual Review of Biochemistry*, 39, 977–1042.

Baer, C. L. (1988). Regulation and assessment of acid base balance. In M. R. Kinney, et al. (Eds.). *AACN's clinical reference for critical care nursing* (pp. 193–248). New York: McGraw-Hill.

Bourdeau, J. E., & Attie, M. F. (1994). Calcium metabolism. In R. G. Narins (Ed.). *Maxwell and Kleeman's clinical disorders of fluid and electrolyte metabolism* (5th ed., pp. 243–306). New York: McGraw-Hill.

Brewer, E. D. (1990). Disorders of acid base balance. *Pediatric Clinics of North America*, 37 (2), 429–447.

Chameides, L., & Hazinski, M. F. (1994). Fluid and medication therapy. In *Pediatric advanced life support* (2nd ed., pp. 6.1–6.18). Dallas: Scientific Publishing, American Heart Association.

Curley, M. A. Q., & Thompson, J. E. (1990). End-tidal CO_2 monitoring in critically ill infants and children. *Pediatric Nursing*, 16 (4), 397–403.

Donlen, J. (1983). Interpreting acid-base problems through arterial blood gases. *Critical Care Nurse*, 3 (5), 34–38.

Gennari, F. J. (1994). Respiratory acidosis and alkalosis. In R. G. Narins (Ed.). *Maxwell and Kleeman's clinical disorders of fluid and electrolyte metabolism* (5th ed., pp. 957–989). New York: McGraw-Hill.

Graf, H., et al. (1985). Metabolic effects of sodium bicarbonate in hypoxic lactic acidosis in dogs. *American Journal of Physiology*, 18 (5), F630–F635.

Kaehny, W. D. (1992). Pathogenesis and management of respiratory and mixed acid base disorders. In R. W. Schrier (Ed.). *Renal and electrolyte disorders* (4th ed., pp. 211–230). Boston: Little, Brown.

Kuhn, M. (1991). IV therapy. In *Pharmacotherapeutics: A nursing approach*. Philadelphia: F. A. Davis.

Narins, R. (1994). Acid base balance: Definitions and introductory comments. In *Maxwell and Kleeman's clinical disorders of fluid and electrolyte metabolism* (5th ed., pp. 755–767). New York: McGraw-Hill.

Redding, J. S., & Pearson, J. W. (1968). Resuscitation from ventricular fibrillation: Drug therapy. *JAMA*, 203 (4), 255–260.

Shapiro, B. (1989). *Clinical Application of Blood Gases* (4th ed.). Chicago: Year Book Medical Publishers.

Telivuo, L., et al. (1968). Comparison of alkalizing agents in resuscitation of the heart after ventricular fibrillation. *Annales Churgiae et Gynaecologiae Fenniae*, 57, 221–224.

CHAPTER 12

Intracranial Dynamics

MARTHA A.Q. CURLEY
PAULA VERNON-LEVETT

Unlike in other organ systems, functional immaturity of the neurologic system is extremely obvious when approaching the infant and young child in the pediatric ICU. Neurologic developmental immaturity impacts every aspect of care; how nurses approach patients, assessment strategies and management priorities.

Neurologic dysfunction may be primary or may occur as a secondary result of dysfunction to other major organ systems, for example, cardiovascular collapse or acute respiratory failure. Compared with other organ systems, the neurologic system is unforgiving. Cells within the central nervous system cannot regenerate; short periods of inadequate perfusion may result in long-term devastating outcomes. Although infants appear to compensate for significant neurologic deficits, older children and adolescents require extensive rehabilitation.

More than in adult or neonatal critical care, approximately 15% of pediatric critical care practice involves caring for patients with neurologic problems

(AACN, 1991). Because of this, requisite knowledge of the neurologic system is essential. This chapter reviews essential neurologic embryology, anatomy, and associated physiology. Neurologic assessment is presented, followed by a discussion of neurologic intensive care monitoring and diagnostic testing.

ESSENTIAL EMBRYOLOGY

The third week of human development is a period of rapid embryonic development with differentiation of the three primitive germ layers: ectoderm, mesoderm, and endoderm. The ectoderm layer gives rise to the central nervous system (CNS), consisting of the brain and spinal cord, and other structures, e.g., the skin.

The notochord, a cellular rod, develops during the third week of gestation, defining the primitive axis of the embryo and giving it some rigidity. The embryonic ectoderm over the notochord (neuroectoderm)

thickens to form the neural plate. On approximately the eighteenth day of embryonic development, the neural plate invaginates to form the longitudinal neural groove with two adjacent neural folds. At the end of the third week, the neural folds move together and begin to fuse to form the neural tube. Fusion of the two neural folds begins centrally and expands toward the future brain (rostrally) and the sacral area (caudally). The rostral end closes first, followed 2 days later by closure of the caudal end. The cranial two thirds of the neural tube develops further to form the future brain, while the caudal one third becomes the spinal cord. The neural tube canal becomes the ventricular system of the brain and the central canal of the spinal cord. The process of embryonic development from neural plate formation to neural tube development is referred to as neurulation and is complete by the fourth week.

As the neural folds fuse, the neural tube separates from the surface ectoderm. During this fusion, groups of neuroectoderm cells lying on the crest of each neural fold separate from the neural tube. These neuroectoderm cells, collectively referred to as the neural crest, form a mass between the surface ectoderm and neuroectoderm. The neural crest cells differentiate into a number of cells in the peripheral nervous system, autonomic nervous system, cranial and skeletal nerves, and some skeletal nerves and muscular components of the head.

During the fourth week and before closure of the caudal and rostral neuropores, three primary brain vesicles begin to appear that later develop into the brain (Fig. 12–1). The most rostral vesicle is the forebrain or prosencephalon, the middle vesicle is the midbrain or mesencephalon, and the most caudal vesicle is the hindbrain or rhombencephalon. During the fifth week, with further development, two of the primary vesicles subdivide to form secondary vesicles. The prosencephalon develops into the telencephalon and the diencephalon, and the rhombencephalon develops into the metencephalon and the myelencephalon. The mesencephalon remains unchanged.

A longitudinal groove, called the sulcus limitans, forms along the lateral surface of the neural tube canal during the fourth week. This groove subdivides the dorsal part (alar plate) of the spinal cord from the ventral part (basal plate). These plates form longitudinal bulges that extend most of the length of the spinal cord. This regional separation is important in terms of spinal cord function. The alar plate is later associated with afferent function, and the basal plate is associated with efferent function.

Most abnormal development of the CNS results from failure of the neural tube to close properly during the fourth week of development. Defective closure of the caudal opening of the neural tube (caudal neuropore) produces malformations of the spinal cord and the overlying tissue. These malformations, collectively referred to as spina bifida, range in severity from minor, clinically insignificant defects (spina bifida occulta) to severe defects with neurologic deficits (myelomeningocele). Defective closure of the rostral opening of the neural tube (rostral neuropore) results in severe malformations of the brain, for example, anencephaly or exencephaly. Other CNS malformations may result from faulty histogenesis of the cerebral cortex, interference with cerebrospinal fluid (CSF) circulation and absorption, and defective formation of the cranium. Table 12–1 summarizes congenital malformations of the CNS.

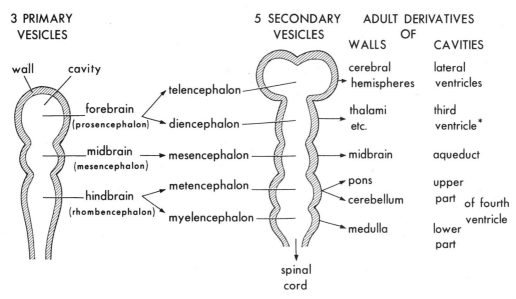

Figure 12–1 ● ● ● ● ● ●

Diagrammatic sketches of the brain vesicles indicating the adult derivatives of their walls and cavities. *The rostral (anterior) part of the third ventricle forms from the cavity of the telencephalon; most of the third ventricle is derived from the cavity of the diencephalon. (From Moore, K.L., & Persaud, T.V.N. (1993). *The developing human: Clinically oriented embryology* (5th ed., p. 401). Philadelphia: W.B. Saunders.)

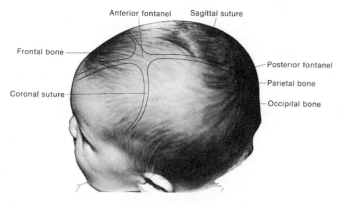

Figure 12–2 ● ● ● ● ●

Location of the anterior and posterior fontanelles. (From Betz, C.L., Hunsberger, M., & Wright, S. (1994). *Family-centered nursing care of children* (2nd ed., p. 124). Philadelphia: W.B. Saunders.)

ESSENTIAL ANATOMY AND PHYSIOLOGY

The nervous system is divided into the peripheral nervous system (PNS) and the central nervous system (CNS). The PNS is composed of the cranial and spinal nerves, and the CNS is composed of the brain and spinal cord. The basic unit of the nervous system is the neuron. The following section briefly discusses each of the above microscopic and macroscopic structures of the nervous system, as well as the CNS coverings, the ventricular system, and cerebral circulation.

Microscopic Structures

The two basic cellular elements of the nervous system are neurons and glial cells. The neuron is the primary cell of the CNS and is responsible for detecting environmental changes and initiating body responses. Neuroglial cells of the CNS and PNS provide nutrition and structural support to the neurons.

Neurons come in a variety of sizes and shapes with a number of different functions. Most neurons have three components: a cell body, dendrites, and an axon. The cell body contains a nucleus but lacks the ability to reproduce itself. The dendrites carry nerve impulses to the cell body, and the axon(s) conducts impulses away from the body. Numerous descriptive terminology exists to classify neurons, based on their location, morphology, and function.

Glial cells (neuroglia) compose approximately 50% of CNS tissue volume and outnumber neurons by a factor of 10. There are different types of glial cells with different functions. Oligodendroglia in the CNS and Schwann cells in the PNS form myelin sheaths around axons to increase the speed of conduction of an impulse. Other types of glial cells assist with metabolic functions, remove cellular debris, and form special contacts between neuronal surfaces and the circulation.

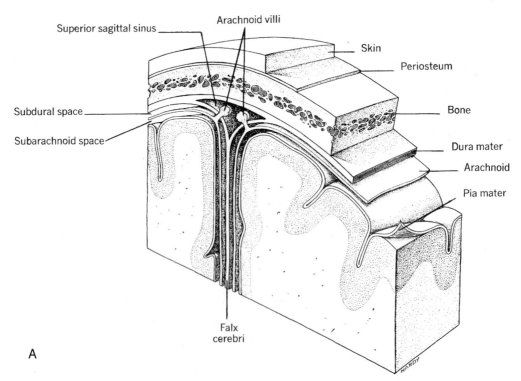

A

Figure 12–3 ● ● ● ● ●

A, The cranial meninges. Arachnoid villi shown within superior sagittal sinus are one site of passage of cerebrospinal fluid into the blood. (From Chaffee, E.E., & Lytle, I.M. (1980). *Basic physiology and anatomy.* Philadelphia: J.B. Lippincott.)

Illustration continued on opposite page

Extracranial Structures

The skull (cranial vault) consists of two components: neurocranium and viscerocranium. The neurocranium is a protective covering of the brain, and the viscerocranium is the skeleton of the jaw. At birth, the newborn's skull is cartilaginous and consists of eight bones: one frontal, one ethmoid, one sphenoid, two temporal, two parietal, and one occipital. The flat bones are separated by dense white fibrous connective tissue membranes called sutures. These sutures accommodate the rapid growth of brain tissue, which is greatest during the first 2 years of life. There are six areas where several sutures join together to form fontanelles (Fig. 12–2). The posterolateral fontanelles and the anterior fontanelle close during the first and second years of life, respectively, from growth of surrounding bone.

Meninges is the term given to describe the three membranous connective tissue layers that cover and protect the brain and spinal cord (Fig. 12–3A). The outermost layer is the dura mater (dura) and consists of two thick, membranous layers. The outer (periosteum) layer adheres to the inner surface of the skull

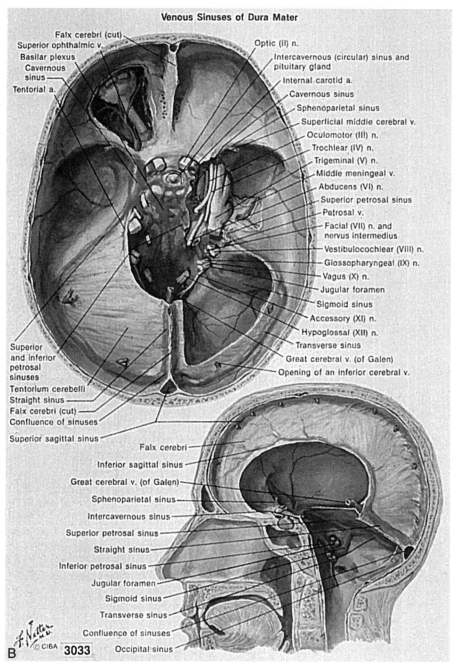

Figure 12–3 ● ● ● ● ● ●

Continued B, Dural folds and venous sinuses. (© Copyright 1996. CIBA-GEIGY Corporation. Reprinted with permission from the Ciba Collection of Medical Illustrations, illustrated by Frank Netter, M.D. All rights reserved.)

Table 12–1. CONGENITAL MALFORMATIONS OF THE CENTRAL NERVOUS SYSTEM

Name	Description
Neural Tube Defects	
Anencephaly	Absence of most of the cerebral hemispheres and calvaria
Exencephaly	Herniation or protrusion of brain and meninges through a defect in the skull
Meningocele	Protrusion of a sac-like cyst containing meninges and spinal fluid through a defect in the vertebral arch
Myelomeningocele	Protrusion of a sac-like cyst containing meninges, spinal fluid, and a portion of the spinal cord with its nerves through a defect in the vertebral arch
Arnold-Chiari malformation*	Downward displacement of the brainstem and cerebellum through the foramen magnum and into the spinal canal. Hydrocephalus from CSF obstruction occurs in the majority of cases
Cranial Deformities	
Acrania	Almost complete absence of the cranial vault. Frequently associated with a vertebral column defect
Craniosynostosis	Premature closure of one or more of the cranial sutures
Microcephaly	Small calvaria and brain with normal-sized face
Miscellaneous	
Agenesis of the corpus callosum	Complete or partial absence of the corpus callosum

*Does not result from defective closure of the neural tube but is frequently associated with a myelomeningocele.

and the vertebral column. The inner layer of the dura divides the two cerebral hemispheres along the median longitudinal fissure (falx cerebri), the cerebral hemispheres from the cerebellum and brainstem (tentorium cerebelli), and the two cerebellar hemispheres (falx cerebelli) (Fig. 12–3B).

The middle covering is named after the Greek word *arachne,* which means spider web. This arachnoid layer is a transparent avascular covering with many thin strands of collagen called trabeculars. It is believed that the trabeculae help suspend the brain within the meninges (Nolte, 1988).

The pia mater (pia) is the innermost meningeal layer. It is a very delicate, clear membrane that directly adheres to the surface of the brain following all of the contours of the brain and spinal cord. The arachnoid and pia layers are collectively referred to as the leptomeninges and are sometimes referred to as the same entity.

The outer layer of the dura normally adheres closely to the inner table of the skull, especially in the infant. A potential space (epidural or extradural) may develop from bleeding that causes separation of

the dura from the skull. The space between the dura and arachnoid layers is the subdural space. It is narrow and contains a small amount of serous fluid that prevents adhesions from forming between the two layers. The subarachnoid space is between the arachnoid and pia layers. This space is relatively large and contains circulating CSF.

Brain

The brain is divided into three gross anatomic units: the cerebrum, the brainstem, and the cerebellum. The cerebrum is further subdivided into the telencephalon and the diencephalon, and the brainstem is subdivided into the mesencephalon (midbrain), the metencephalon (pons), and the myelencephalon (medulla). Each of these macroscopic units are considered in this discussion.

Telencephalon

The telencephalon is composed of the right and left cerebral hemispheres and the basal ganglia. The cerebral hemispheres are mirror images divided from each other by the median longitudinal fissure. The surface of the cerebral hemispheres have convolutions, and each of these ridges is known as a gyrus. Each gyrus is separated by a shallow groove (sulcus) or a deep groove (fissure). The outer layer of the cerebral hemispheres or cortex is gray in color and consists primarily of cell bodies. The inner layer is white in color and consists of myelinated axons. Axons that pass from one lobe to another in the same hemisphere are known as associative fibers. Axons that pass between hemispheres, such as the corpus callosum, are known as commissural fibers. Axons that pass from a cerebral hemisphere to other areas of the CNS are known as projection fibers.

The basal ganglia, including the caudate nucleus, putamen, globus pallidus, claustrum, and amygdala, is a collection of gray matter nuclei located deep in the white matter of the cerebral hemispheres on either side of the midline. General function of the basal ganglia includes unconscious control of lower motor centers. Damage or dysfunction of the basal ganglia may produce disturbances of muscle tone and various abnormal involuntary movements.

Anatomic fissures divide each of the cerebral hemispheres into four lobes: the temporal, parietal, frontal, and occipital (Fig. 12–4). These lobes have some distinct functions; however, they are not precise and there is considerable functional overlap among lobes. Some neuroanatomy texts consider a fifth lobe, called the insula, which is buried deep in the lateral sulcus and has no known function in humans. Although oversimplified, functional descriptions of the four lobes are given for purposes of general orientation. The reader is referred to neuroanatomy references at the end of this chapter for a more detailed discussion of cortical function.

The frontal lobe is the largest lobe of the cerebral

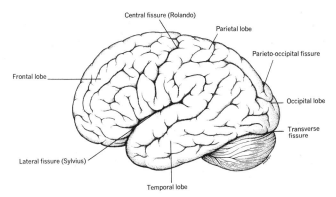

Figure 12–4 ● ● ● ● ● ●

Lateral aspect of the left cerebral and cerebellar hemispheres. (From Hickey, J.V. (1986). *The clinical practice of neurological and neurosurgical nursing* (2nd ed., p. 32). Philadelphia: J.B. Lippincott.)

hemispheres. The central sulcus (fissure of Rolando) divides the frontal lobe from the parietal lobe, and the lateral cerebral fissure (fissure of Sylvius) divides the frontal lobe from the temporal lobe. The frontal lobe has four general functional areas: the primary motor cortex and premotor areas are involved in the initiation of voluntary movements, Broca's area is involved with written and spoken language, and the prefrontal cortex is the origin of "personality." Injury or impairment of the frontal lobe may cause personality changes, altered intellectual functioning, memory deficits, language deficits, or impaired body movements.

The temporal lobe is separated superiorly from the frontal lobe by the lateral cerebral fissure. Posteriorly, it is divided from the occipital lobe by an imaginary line from the parieto-occipital fissure. General functions of the temporal lobe include reception and interpretation of auditory information, expression of emotional and visceral responses, and retention of recent memory. Injury or impairment of the temporal lobe may cause an inability to interpret sensory experiences.

The parietal lobe is separated from the frontal lobe by the central sulcus and from the temporal and occipital lobe by the parieto-occipital fissure. The parietal lobe is associated with three general functions: initial processing of tactile and proprioceptive information, comprehension of language (together with the temporal lobe), and orientation of spatial relationships and time. Injury or impairment of the parietal lobe may result in language dysfunction, aphasia, and motor and sensory loss in the lower extremities.

The occipital lobe is relatively small and sits on the tentorium cerebelli. The rostral border is the parieto-occipital sulcus. The lateral surface is poorly delineated from the parietal lobe and is composed of a number of irregularly shaped lateral occipital gyri. The major function of the occipital lobe is reception and interpretation of visual stimuli. Injury or impairment of the occipital lobe may impair vision.

Diencephalon

The diencephalon is a paired structure on each side of the third ventricle between the cerebral hemispheres (Fig. 12–5). It protrudes over the most rostral end of the brainstem, and some consider it a part of the brainstem. It is divided into the thalamus, the hypothalamus, and the epithalamus.

The thalamus is the largest subdivision of the diencephalon. It is an egg-shaped nuclear mass, part of which surrounds the third ventricle. The enlarged lateral and caudal portions of the thalamus overlie the midbrain structures. A very simplistic description of its function is that of a relay station. However, it also performs complex, interrelated functions; it transfers sensory input to the cerebral cortex, controls electrocortical activity, and assists to modulate motor functions. Damage or dysfunction of the thalamus may result in impaired consciousness.

The hypothalamus, as its name indicates, lies below and anterior to the thalamus forming the floor and walls of the third ventricle (Fig. 12–5B). Although small, it has many vital functions. It plays an important role in physiologic homeostasis by regulating visceral, endocrine, and metabolic activity. It also regulates with such functions as temperature control, sleep, hunger, and emotion. Damage or dysfunction of the hypothalamus may cause alterations in vegetative, endocrine, and metabolic functions, for example, coma and/or diabetes insipidus (see Chapter 25, Endocrine Critical Care Problems).

The epithalamus is made up of the pineal gland and some small neural structures. The pineal gland or epiphysis is a small, cone-shaped body attached to a stalk. It is attached midline to the roof of the third ventricle (Fig. 12–5C). The exact function of this gland is not well understood. However, it appears that it may function as a biologic clock regulating both physiologic and behavioral processes.

Mesencephalon (Midbrain)

The mesencephalon is one of three structures that compose the wedge-shaped brainstem. The mesencephalon is the smallest of all of the five divisions of the brain and is located rostrally on the brainstem between the diencephalon and the metencephalon (Fig. 12–6). The mesencephalon is further divided into three areas: the tectum, the tegmentum, and the paired cerebral peduncles. The tectum is made up of two upper rounded projections (superior colliculi) and two lower rounded projections (inferior colliculi). These four projections are associated with visual and auditory functions. The body of the mesencephalon where fiber tracts pass is referred to as the tegmentum. Also situated in the tegmentum are the nuclei from the oculomotor nerve and the trochlear nerve. At the base of the mesencephalon are a pair of fiber bundles (cerebral peduncles) that are continuations of descending fibers. Damage or dysfunction of the mesencephalon may cause impaired consciousness, decerebrate posturing, and neurologic hyperventilation.

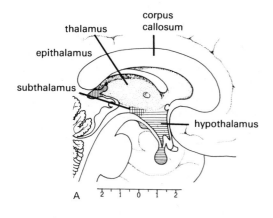

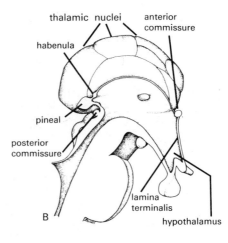

Figure 12–5 ● ● ● ● ● ●

Different views of the diencephalon. *A,* Left midsagittal surface. *B,* Midsagittal surface dissected exposes dorsal surface of thalamus. *C,* Dorsal view of thalamus. *D,* Lateral view of brainstem and diencephalon. (From Romero-Sierra, C. (1986). *Neuroanatomy: A conceptual approach.* New York: Churchill Livingstone.)

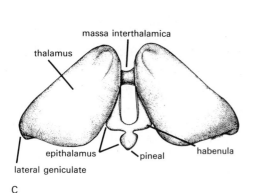

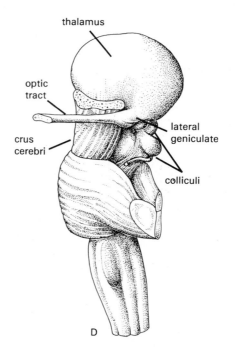

Metencephalon (Pons)

The metencephalon is located between the midbrain and the medulla. It is ventral (anterior) to the cerebellum, separated from it by the fourth ventricle (Fig. 12–6). The ventral portion of the metencephalon is called the basis pontis. It contains longitudinal descending fiber bundles, pontine nuclei, and transverse fibers that connect with the cerebellum. Dorsal to the basis pontis is the tegmental portion of the metencephalon. The tegmentum contains collections of cells and fibers that form the reticular formation that is continuous with the medulla and midbrain. Also within the tegmentum are cranial nerve (CN) nuclei V, VI, VII, and VIII and ascending and descending fiber tracts. Damage or dysfunction of the metencephalon may cause impaired consciousness; deep, rapid, periodic breathing; and impaired muscle function innervated by CN V through VIII.

Myelencephalon (Medulla)

The myelencephalon is also referred to as the medulla or medulla oblongata. It is located below the pons ventral to the cerebellum (see Fig. 12–6). The fourth ventricle is located in the dorsal midline of the myelencephalon. Like the pons and midbrain, the myelencephalon contains ascending and descending fiber tracts. It also contains CN nuclei IX through XII. The reticular formation originates from the medulla containing cardiac, respiratory, and arousability centers. Damage or dysfunction to the myelencephalon may cause impaired vital functions, alteration in consciousness, ataxic breathing, and loss of gag and corneal reflexes.

Cerebellum

The cerebellum is a wedge-shaped structure that lies in the posterior fossa dorsal to most of the brainstem and inferior to the tentorium. It is divided into two lobes or hemispheres by a midline structure, the vermis, and is anchored to the brainstem via three pairs of fiber bundles called the cerebellar peduncles. The dorsal surface is arranged in multiple, small folds, giving it a banded external appearance and increasing its surface area. The cerebellum is primarily concerned with coordination of voluntary movements, control of muscle tone, and maintenance of equilibrium. Damage or dysfunction of the cerebellum may cause a variety of problems with coordination, gait, and general motor function.

Cerebrospinal Fluid and the Ventricular System

Deep within the brain is the ventricular system, which consists of four interconnecting chambers that produce and circulate CSF (Fig. 12–7). The two paired lateral ventricles are the largest of the four chambers and are contained within the cerebral hemispheres. Each lateral ventricle is divided into five parts: an anterior horn, a body, an atrium, a posterior horn, and an inferior horn.

The lateral ventricles communicate with each other and the third ventricle through the interventricular foramen (foramen of Monro). The third ventricle is a small, narrow slit that connects with the fourth ventricle through the aqueduct of Sylvius. Unlike the lateral and third ventricles, which communicate only with other parts of the ventricular system, the fourth ventricle also communicates with the subarachnoid space. Circulation of CSF occurs between

the ventricular system and the subarachnoid space around the brain and spinal cord via three openings: the paired foramina of Luschka (lateral) and the midline foramen of Magendie.

CSF is produced primarily by the choroid plexus, present in all four ventricles, and to a lesser degree by the brain parenchyma. Its primary functions are protection, nutrition, and fluid and electrolyte balance of the CNS tissue. The microscopic structure of the choroid plexus is a three-layer membrane: choroid capillary endothelium, pial cells, and choroid epithelium. CSF is formed by active transport. CSF is a colorless liquid that has an ionic composition similar to that of plasma, but it is low in proteins and cells (Table 12–2). The rate of production of CSF is relatively constant at 0.35 mL/kg/min and is unaffected by systemic blood pressure or intraventricular pressure.

After CSF circulates in the subarachnoid space over the cerebral hemispheres and around the spinal cord, it travels back to the superior sagittal sinus, where it is reabsorbed by the arachnoid villi (see Fig. 12–7). These villi are small arachnoid projections that function as one-way valves between the subarachnoid space and the sagittal sinus. They allow CSF to enter the dural venous blood but prevent blood from entering the subarachnoid space.

Disturbances may occur in CSF production and circulation that may result in dilation of the ventricular system with an excessive increase in head size in the infant (hydrocephalus). The three conditions that produce hydrocephalus are obstruction of CSF circulatory pathways, diminished reabsorption of CSF, and overproduction of CSF. The most common

Figure 12–6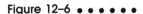

The ventral surface of the human brainstem and diencephalon. (From Gilman, S., & Winans, S.S. (1982). *Manter & Gatz's essentials of clinical neuroanatomy and neurophysiology* (6th ed.). Philadelphia: F.A. Davis.)

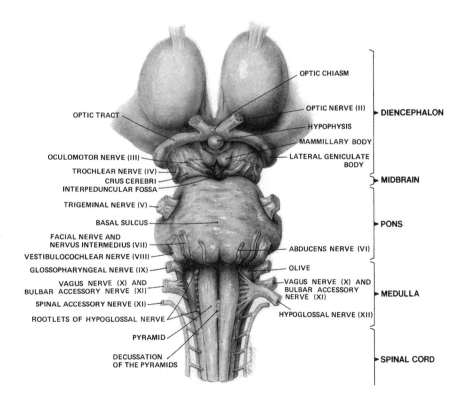

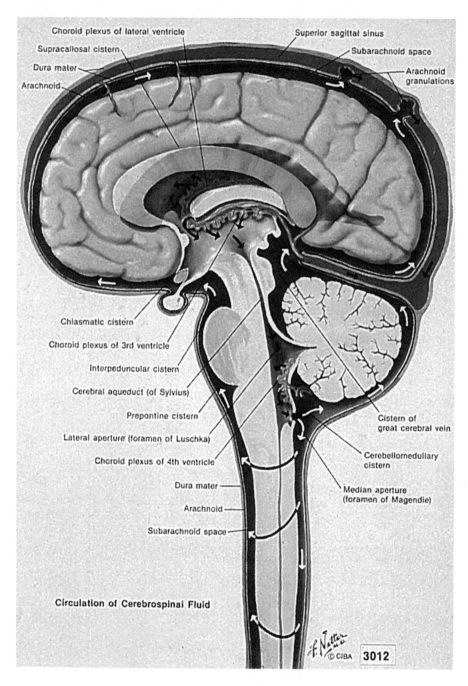

Choroid plexus of lateral ventricle
Supracallosal cistern
Dura mater
Arachnoid
Superior sagittal sinus
Subarachnoid space
Arachnoid granulations

Chiasmatic cistern
Choroid plexus of 3rd ventricle
Interpeduncular cistern
Cerebral aqueduct (of Sylvius)
Prepontine cistern
Lateral aperture (foramen of Luschka)
Choroid plexus of 4th ventricle
Dura mater
Arachnoid
Subarachnoid space

Cistern of great cerebral vein
Cerebellomedullary cistern
Median aperture (foramen of Magendie)

Circulation of Cerebrospinal Fluid

Figure 12–7 ● ● ● ● ● ●

Ventricular system. (© Copyright 1996. CIBA-GEIGY Corporation. Reprinted with permission from the Ciba Collection of Medical Illustrations, illustrated by Frank Netter, M.D. All rights reserved.)

of these etiologies is obstruction of the CSF pathways from either congenital or acquired conditions. Malabsorption of CSF is rare, occasionally seen with a subarachnoid hemorrhage when the arachnoid villi are obstructed from debris. Overproduction of CSF may be caused by a choroid plexus papilloma.

Spinal Cord

The spinal cord is a long, cylindrical structure, encased within the vertebral column. Rostrally, it begins at the foramen magnum and extends caudally to the level of the second lumbar vertebra (L2), where it becomes cone shaped (conus medullaris). The spinal cord is covered with the same three meningeal layers as on the brain.

A cross-sectional view of the cord reveals a centrally located H-shaped area of gray matter that consists of neuronal cell bodies and their processes (Fig. 12–8). The gray matter has two anterior (ventral) horns and two posterior (dorsal) horns. The anterior horns contain motor neurons (lower motor neurons) that supply skeletal muscles, while the posterior horns contain neurons that are associated with sensory input to the spinal cord. The size of the gray matter varies depending on the number of structures innervated at a particular spinal cord level. For ex-

Table 12–2. NORMAL CSF (>1 MONTH OF AGE)

Appearance	Clear
	Colorless
Glucose	2/3 of blood sugar
	>60 mg/dL
Protein	15–45 mg/dL
Cell count	<5/mm³
Leukocytes	≤5/mm³
Pressure	60–160 mm H₂O

Table 12–3. COMMON ASCENDING AND DESCENDING SPINAL TRACTS

Ascending (Sensory)	
Tract Name	**Function**
Dorsal (posterior) spinocerebellar	Proprioception
Ventral (anterior) spinocerebellar	Proprioception
Lateral spinothalamic	Pain, temperature
Ventral (anterior) spinothalamic	Touch, pressure

Descending (Motor)	
Corticospinal (pyramidal tracts)	
Ventral (anterior) corticospinal	Skilled voluntary movements
Lateral corticospinal	Skilled voluntary movements
Rubrospinal	Fine movements, muscle tone
Vestibulospinal	Aid equilibrium, extensor muscle tone
Reticulospinal	Posture, muscle tone
Tectospinal	Mediates optic and auditory reflex movement

ample, the gray matter is larger in the cervical and lumbosacral areas because innervation of the extremities occurs from these areas of the cord.

Surrounding the gray matter is white matter composed of myelinated nerve fibers. The nerve fibers consist of one of three types: long ascending fibers from the spinal cord to the brainstem, cerebellum, or brainstem nuclei; long descending fibers from the cerebral cortex or brainstem nuclei to the spinal cord gray matter; and short fibers that interconnect various segments of the spinal cord. Descending and ascending fibers that have similar functions tend to travel together and are called spinal tracts. Numerous tracts are arranged together to form a funiculus. Table 12–3 summarizes the most common ascending and descending tracts.

Peripheral Nervous System

Spinal Nerves

Within the peripheral nervous system (PNS) are 31 pairs of spinal nerves with related branches and ganglia. They form from the convergence of the ventral (motor) efferent and dorsal (sensory) afferent rootlets that exit the spinal cord through the intervertebral foramen. The paired spinal nerves are di-

vided into 5 segments: (eight) cervical, (twelve) thoracic, (five) lumbar, (five) sacral, and (one) coccygeal. Spinal nerves are numbered after the vertebral level from which they exit. Because there are eight cervical spinal nerves, they take their number from the vertebra level below their exit. The remaining spinal nerves are numbered to correspond to the vertebral level above their exit.

Cranial Nerves

There are 12 pairs of cranial nerves, with their nuclei originating from the CNS. Because they connect the CNS with peripheral structures, they are generally classified as belonging to the PNS. Most of the cranial nerves have both sensory and motor

Figure 12–8 ● ● ● ● ● ●
Cross-section of the spinal cord.

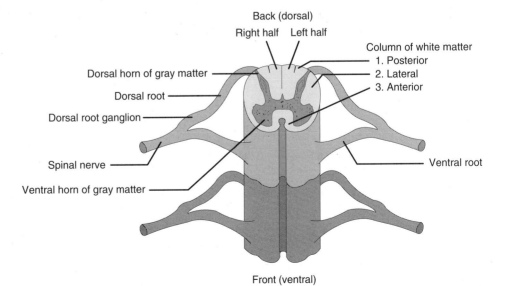

Back (dorsal)
Right half   Left half
Dorsal horn of gray matter
Dorsal root
Dorsal root ganglion
Spinal nerve
Ventral horn of gray matter
Column of white matter
1. Posterior
2. Lateral
3. Anterior
Ventral root
Front (ventral)

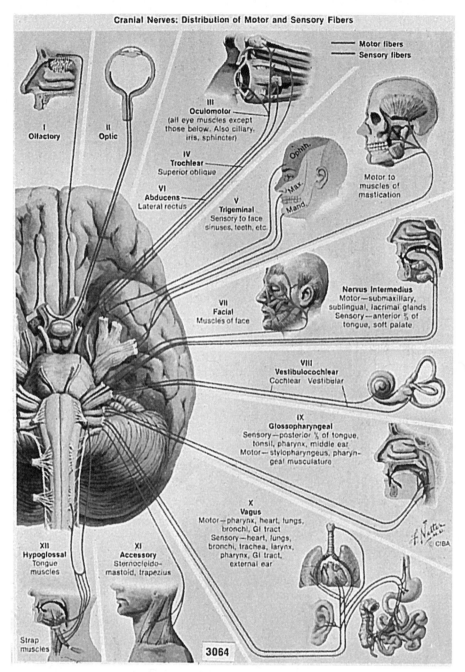

Cranial Nerves: Distribution of Motor and Sensory Fibers

— Motor fibers
— Sensory fibers

I
Olfactory

II
Optic

III
Oculomotor
(all eye muscles except
those below. Also ciliary,
iris, sphincter)

IV
Trochlear
Superior oblique

VI
Abducens
Lateral rectus

V
Trigeminal
Sensory to face
sinuses, teeth, etc.

Ophth.
Max.
Mand.

Motor to
muscles of
mastication

VII
Facial
Muscles of face

Nervus Intermedius
Motor—submaxillary,
sublingual, lacrimal glands
Sensory—anterior ⅔ of
tongue, soft palate

VIII
Vestibulocochlear
Cochlear Vestibular

IX
Glossopharyngeal
Sensory—posterior ⅓ of tongue,
tonsil, pharynx, middle ear
Motor—stylopharyngeus, pharyn-
geal musculature

X
Vagus
Motor—pharynx, heart, lungs,
bronchi, GI tract
Sensory—heart, lungs,
bronchi, trachea, larynx,
pharynx, GI tract,
external ear

XII
Hypoglossal
Tongue
muscles

XI
Accessory
Sternocleido-
mastoid, trapezius

Strap
muscles

3064

Figure 12–9 ● ● ● ● ● ●

The cranial nerves. (© Copyright 1996. CIBA-GEIGY Corporation. Reprinted with permission from the Ciba Collection of Medical Illustrations, illustrated by Frank Netter, M.D. All rights reserved.)

functions, although there are some with purely sensory or motor functions. Damage directly to cranial nerves or to surrounding structures can often be determined by assessing cranial nerve function. Figure 12–9 illustrates the cephalocaudal location of CN nuclei I through XII. Table 12–4 outlines CN function, how each is tested according to age, and the clinical significance of abnormal findings.

Autonomic Nervous System

The autonomic nervous system (ANS) has structures that are located in both the CNS and the PNS; however, most consider it part of the efferent division of the PNS. The ANS unconsciously regulates three types of body tissue: cardiac muscle, smooth muscle, and most glands. The ANS is divided structurally and functionally into two parts: the sympathetic and parasympathetic nervous system. Both systems are based on a two-neuron pathway. The first neuron is referred to as a preganglionic neuron and the second a postganglionic neuron. With few exceptions, these two systems have neurons that stimulate and control the same organs (Fig. 12–10). Because the parasympathetic and sympathetic systems have antagonistic functions, they are usually maintained in balance. An imbalance can occur between the two systems in one of two ways: by increasing the stimulus from one system or by decreasing the stimulus from the other system.

Parasympathetic System

The parasympathetic system is the division of the ANS that usually dominates when a person is resting. The neurotransmitter acetylcholine is released in the synapse between the parasympathetic post-ganglionic neurons and the effector organ. Activation of the parasympathetic system produces responses such as increased peristalsis, decreased heart rate, and secretion of intestinal enzymes. Administration of exogenous sources of acetylcholine or stimulation of a nerve that contains many parasympathetic nerve fibers (for example, the vagus nerve) produces a characteristic parasympathetic response.

Figure 12–10 ● ● ● ● ● ●

Diagram of the autonomic nervous system, including parasympathetic or craniosacral fibers and sympathetic or thoracolumbar fibers. Note that most organs have a double nerve supply. (From Chaffee, E.E., & Lytle, I.M. (1980). *Basic physiology and anatomy*. Philadelphia: J.B. Lippincott.)

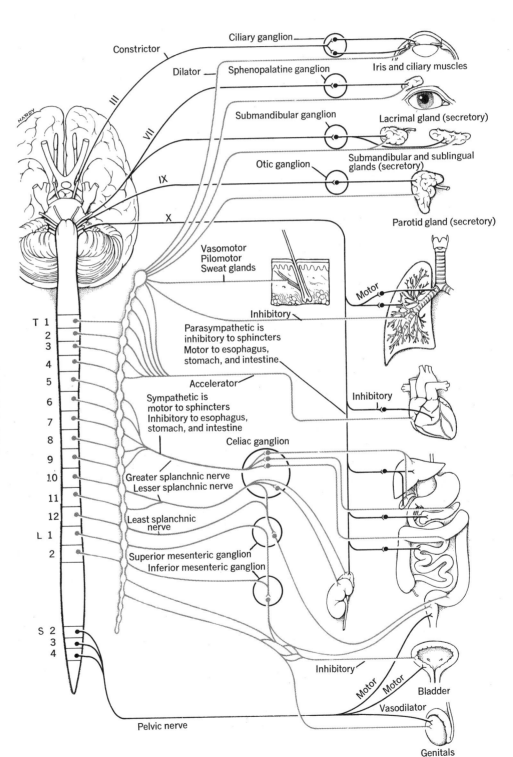

Table 12-4. ASSESSMENT OF CRANIAL NERVE FUNCTION

Cranial Nerve	Function	Testing		Altered Level of Consciousness	Clinical Significance
		Infant	Child		
I Olfactory	Smell	Usually not assessed, young infant responds to strong odors with generalized movement, but testing is unreliable	Assess each nostril separately using common odors (e.g., soap, mints, orange, etc.). Testing is unreliable in very young children	Not tested	Must have patient cooperation. Damage to the nerve or olfactory bulbs can alter or result in loss of smell
II Optic	Vision	Introduce a bright light and observe for a blink response in the newborn. Observe older infants' ability to pick up small objects	Visual acuity tested in young child through recognition of familiar objects at various distances. The older child can be tested with Snellen chart or measuring tape with numbers. Ophthalmoscopic exam performed at end of session in young child. The child is instructed to fixate on a distant object	Assess pupillary response to light	Any abnormality requires further investigation. Lesions in the optic chiasm generally produce bilateral but nonhomonymous defects. Lesions behind chiasm produce homonymous field defects in both fields of vision. Lesion of the eye and optic tract produce visual defects in the visual field of one eye only. Papilledema may indicate elevated intracranial pressure. The optic disc is pale, gray, and poorly developed in the infant. The child's retina is lighter than the adult's. Failure of pupil constriction to light may indicate optic nerve damage or oculomotor nerve paralysis
III Oculomotor	Pupillary constriction, extraocular movements, elevation of upper eyelid	Assess pupillary response; shine a bright light in each eye starting from the outer periphery of the visual field. Assess consensual response by shining a bright light in one eye and observing for constriction in the other eye. Assess accommodation by noting convergence and constriction as a bright light is brought toward the nose. Assess eyelids for ptosis (drooping). Extraocular movements are tested with cranial nerves III, IV, VI (see below)	Same as infant	Assess pupillary response to light	Elevated intracranial pressure may produce unequal pupils; unreactive or sluggish pupillary response to light; or dilated pupil(s). Roving eye movements may be present in the comatose patient with intact nerve

348

Cranial Nerve	Function	Assessment	Assessment	Comatose Patient	Comments
III Oculomotor IV Trochlear VI Abducens	IV—Downward and inward movement of the eye VI—Lateral movement of the eye III—All other extraocular movements	Assess the six fields of gaze; note conjugate movement of the eyes as a bright object is moved from the midline into each of the six fields of gaze (see Fig. 12–18)	Assess the six fields of gaze with the infant	Tested with efferent portion of oculocephalic and oculovestibular responses	Binocular fixation usually present by 3 months of age. Nystagmus normal in premature infants and neonates. Damage to cranial nerve IV can cause diplopia and altered downward movement. Dysconjugate gaze after 6 months of age may indicate a lesion or dysfunction of various parts of the brain. Be prepared to protect airway if oculocephalic or oculovestibular responses absent (negative)
V Trigeminal	Motor division: muscles of mastication Sensory Division: Innervation of the face with three branches (ophthalmic, maxillary, mandibular)	Test strength of muscles by assessing the infant sucking on a finger or nipple. Test rooting reflex. Test corneal reflex by lightly touching the cornea with a cotton wisp. Observe for blinking and tearing	Palpate the temporal and masseter muscles while the child is clenching; assess for strength and symmetry. Observe jaw movement for symmetry while talking, laughing, crying. Test the three regions of the face (eyes closed) for sensation. Test the corneal reflex as in the infant	Assess corneal reflex	Damage to the motor division can result in impaired mastication. Damage to the sensory division may impair facial sensation or cause pain. Tears are usually not present in infants less than 2–3 months of age. Use of contact lenses may diminish or abolish corneal reflex
VII Facial	Motor division: motor innervation of facial muscles and mouth Sensory division: Taste in anterior 2/3 of tongue	Facial tone can best be observed during crying and smiling. Movement should be symmetrical. Testing for discrimination of taste not possible	Motor innervation of the face can be tested by asking the child to make a "mad" face and observe facial tone while smiling or crying. Ask the child to "puff out" his cheeks. Sensation tested by applying various substances to the anterior tongue	Not tested	Damage to the nerve can produce facial paralysis or weakness and loss of taste sensation to the anterior tongue
VIII Acoustic	Cochlear division: hearing Vestibular division: balance	Hearing can be assessed in newborns by testing the acoustic blink reflex: a loud noise by the infant will produce a blink response. Older infants will stop moving when listening to sound or move head in direction of sound. Vestibular function is not routinely tested. Oculovestibular response may be tested in patient with altered mental status	Hearing is tested using a variety of high and low pitched sounds. Vestibular function not routinely tested. Oculovestibular response (caloric testing) may be tested for complaints of tinnitus or vertigo. May also be tested in patient with altered mental status	Tested with afferent portion of oculocephalic and oculovestibular responses	Damage to the nerve can result in impairment of hearing, deafness, vertigo, tinnitus, and nystagmus. A normal response to caloric testing in the awake patient is jerk nystagmus, nausea, and/or vomiting. Caloric testing in the comatose patient with brain stem damage produces no response (i.e., eyes are fixed)

Table continued on following page

Table 12-4. ASSESSMENT OF CRANIAL NERVE FUNCTION *Continued*

Cranial Nerve	Function	Testing			Clinical Significance
		Infant	*Child*	*Altered Level of Consciousness*	
IX Glossopharyngeal	Sensory innervation to the pharynx and posterior 1/3 of the tongue	Assess together with cranial nerve X. Stimulate a gag reflex by touching posterior portion of the tongue. Note hoarse or stridorous crying	Assess together with cranial nerve X. Instruct the child to say "ah" and note movement of the soft palate. Movement should be upward. Stimulate a gag reflex. Observe child's ability to swallow without pain or choking. Note excess drooling or coughing	Assess gag reflex	Damage to the nerve can result in dysphagia, dysarthria, impaired sensation, excessive drooling, stridor, and autonomic nervous system changes related to the vagus nerve
IV Vagus	Sensory division: innervation to the larynx and pharynx Motor division: innervation to the palate and pharynx and parasympathetic functions				
XI Spinal accessory	Motor innervation of the sternocleidomastoid muscle and the upper portion of the trapezius muscle	Observe for normal side-to-side head movement	Ask the child to shrug his/her shoulders against the pressure of your hands. Ask the child to turn his head side to side against the pressure of your hand. Observe for strength and symmetry	Not tested	Fasciculation is occasionally seen in denervating diseases. Damage to this nerve can result in asymmetric shoulder posture, impaired strength, and difficulty moving the head from side to side
XII Hypoglossal	Motor innervation to the tongue	Observe the tongue for fasciculations, asymmetric movement or atrophy	Same as the infant	Not tested	In pyramidal disorders, the tongue may be spastic. Unilateral damage to the nerve or its nucleus can cause deviation of the tongue toward the side of the lesion. Damage to this nerve can cause paresis, paralysis, fasciculations, or atrophy

Reprinted with permission of Slota, M.C. (1983). Neurological assessment of the infant and toddler. CRITICAL CARE NURSE® 3 (5), 87; Slota, M.C. (1983). Pediatric neurological assessment. CRITICAL CARE NURSE,® 3 (6), 106.

Sympathetic System

The sympathetic nervous system is responsible for increasing the overall energy level of the body when necessary to overcome a stressful situation, whether it is physical or psychological. Unlike the parasympathetic system, whose postganglionic neurons secrete acetylcholine, sympathetic postganglionic neurons secrete norepinephrine. Activation of the sympathetic system with release of norepinephrine produces a characteristic response: bronchiolar dilation, increased heart rate and contractility, vasodilation of blood vessels to vital organs, and pupillary dilation. Similarly, if a person is administered an exogenous source of epinephrine or if the parasympathetic system is blocked, the body mimics responses that directly result from sympathetic activation.

Central Nervous System Circulation

In comparison with other organs of the body, the brain's metabolic demands for glucose and oxygen are very high. The amount of glucose and oxygen required by the brain per minute is referred to as the cerebral metabolic rate glucose (CMR glucose) and the cerebral metabolic rate oxygen ($CMRo_2$). The CMR glucose is approximately 4.5 to 5.5 mg/100 g per minute, and the $CMRo_2$ is approximately 3.0 to 3.5 mL/100 g per minute. To meet these metabolic demands, approximately 20% of the body's cardiac output must be continuously delivered to the brain (Sundt, 1979).

Arterial System

The predominant arterial flow to the brain is from two systems: the paired carotid arteries anteriorly and the paired vertebral arteries posteriorly (Fig. 12–11). The majority of cerebral blood flow (CBF) is supplied by the internal carotid arteries, which originate from the (common) carotid arteries. The internal carotid arteries further subdivide into the anterior and middle cerebral arteries. The anterior cerebral artery supplies blood to the basal ganglia of the corpus callosum, the medial surface of the cerebral hemispheres, and the superior surface of the frontal and parietal lobes. The middle cerebral artery supplies blood to the frontal lobe, the parietal lobe, and the cortical surfaces of the temporal lobe. Occlusion of the anterior cerebral artery may lead to weakness or hemiplegia on the contralateral side of the body. Occlusion of the middle cerebral artery may cause aphasia and contralateral hemiplegia.

The paired vertebral arteries originate at the subclavian arteries. They join to form the basilar artery on the ventral surface of the brainstem at the junction of the pons and medulla. The basilar artery proceeds rostrally, and at the level of the midbrain, it divides to form the paired posterior cerebral arteries. The vertebral-basilar arteries supply blood to the posterior sections of the cerebral hemispheres, the cerebellum, and the brainstem. Occlusion of the vertebral-basilar arteries may cause a variety disorders such as sensory loss, visual loss, and contralateral hemiplegia.

At the base of the brain, the posterior cerebral arteries, the posterior communicating arteries, the internal carotid arteries, the anterior cerebral arteries, and the anterior communicating artery fuse to form the circle of Willis. As these large conducting arteries leave the circle of Willis, their diameter becomes smaller to form arterioles and pial arteries. These smaller arterioles branch off at 90-degree angles into the brain parenchyma and are called penetrating or nutrient arteries.

Venous System

The two systems of venous drainage in the brain consist of superficial and deep veins, all of which are valveless (see Fig. 12–3B). In general, the superficial veins drain venous blood from the cerebral hemispheres and empty into the dural venous sinuses. The deep veins drain internal structures and empty centrally into the great cerebral vein (of Galen), which eventually empties into the straight sinus. All venous drainage ultimately exits at the base of the skull via the internal jugular veins. Obstruction of venous outflow may cause headaches, cerebral edema, or cerebral hypertension.

Blood-Brain Barrier

Blood-brain barrier is the term used to describe the anatomic structures and physiologic processes that separate the brain and CSF compartments from the blood compartment. Anatomic barriers include the arachnoid layer, the blood-CSF barrier, and the cerebral capillary barrier. All barrier sites are characterized by cells with tight junctions between them. These tightly connected cells function as a single layer of cells, allowing precise regulation of chemicals between the brain, CSF, and plasma.

The blood-brain barrier protects the CNS by preventing passage of potentially harmful molecules from the blood to the brain. However, this barrier is equally effective in preventing the passage of many antibiotic and chemotherapeutic medications. Consequently, there are a reduced number of therapeutic agents available to treat CNS disorders. The blood-brain barrier may be altered from a number of CNS insults, for example, chemical, physical, biologic, and/or infective insults.

Spinal Cord

The arterial supply of the spinal cord originates from the vertebral arteries and radicular arteries. At the base of the skull, the vertebral arteries give rise to the posterior spinal arteries and the anterior spinal artery, which descend alongside the spinal cord. Radicular arteries originate from the thoracic and abdominal aorta and enter the spinal canal through

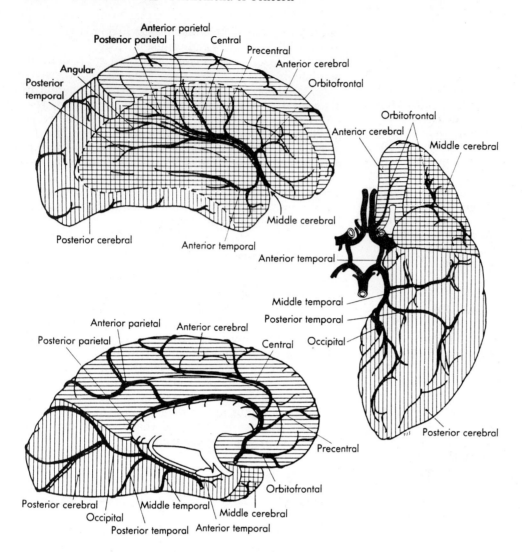

Figure 12–11 ● ● ● ● ● ●
Arterial supply of the brain. (From Mettler, F.A. (1948). *Neuroanatomy* (2nd ed.). St. Louis: C.V. Mosby.)

the intervertebral foramen. The radicular arteries and the spinal arteries eventually connect. Venous drainage of the spinal cord is via a series of plexiform channels, which in turn drain into the radicular veins. There are no valves in the spinal venous network.

INTRACRANIAL PRESSURE DYNAMICS

Modified Monro-Kellie Doctrine

The Monro-Kellie doctrine, which has been modified over the years, provides the basis for understanding the determinants of intracranial pressure (ICP). This doctrine states that the skull and relatively inelastic dural sheath provide a rigid container filled to capacity with nearly noncompressible contents. The three volume components of the intracranial space are brain tissue, CSF, and blood. The most important concept of this doctrine is that if there is a change in any one of the volume compartments, there must be a reciprocal change in one or more of the other volume compartments to maintain equilib-

rium. With reciprocal changes in volume, abnormal increases in ICP can be diverted.

Brain tissue represents the largest volume component of the intracranial space, composing approximately 80% to 90% of the total. This volume may be increased by the presence of neuropathologies such as cerebral edema or a brain tumor. The cerebral blood and CSF compartments each represent 5% to 10% of intracranial volume. The total cerebral blood volume may be altered in the same way that cerebral blood flow is controlled, for example, by arterial carbon dioxide tension ($Paco_2$) and arterial oxygen tension (Pao_2), and/or by local pH. CSF volume may also be increased by mechanisms described earlier (see Cerebrospinal Fluid and the Ventricular System).

Because the skull is not rigid until closure of the fontanelles and fusion of the cranial sutures (which occurs around 5 years of age), it is often thought that the Monro-Kellie hypothesis does not apply in the infant and young child. While it is true that in the first 3 years of life *slow* increases in intracranial volume are accommodated by increasing head circumference, rapid or unabated increases in intracranial volume overburden this adaptive mechanism.

Table 12–5. NORMAL ICP IN INFANTS AND CHILDREN

Age Group	Normal ICP (mmHg)
Newborn	0.7–1.5
Infants	1.5–6.0
Children	3.0–7.5
Adults	<10

Data from: Welch, K. (1980). The intracranial pressure in infants. *Journal of Neurosurgery, 52,* 693–699.

Studies also suggest that expansion of the skull evidenced by increased head circumference occurs only after critical ICPs have been reached (Vidyasagar & Raju, 1977). At best, the non-rigid container in the young child tends to make the signs and symptoms of cerebral hypertension less striking. Astute nursing assessment to detect subtle changes in neurologic status is therefore necessary to avoid secondary neurologic injury.

Volume/Pressure Relationships

Normal ICP varies in different age groups (Table 12–5). Derived from the age-dependent normals, increased ICP is also age-dependent. Clinically, pressures greater than 15 mmHg are considered elevated and pressures between 20 and 40 mmHg moderately elevated, whereas cerebral hypertension is defined as ICPs greater than 40 mmHg.

ICP is dynamic and fluctuates with each heartbeat and respiration. ICP increases momentarily with certain activities and physiologic responses including coughing or sneezing and during Valsalva maneuvers and REM sleep. Temporary increases in intracranial volume and subsequent ICP are normally well tolerated. CSF volume manipulation is a major adaptive mechanism when the subarachnoid space and ventricular outflow tracts are patent. Along with decreased production and increased reabsorption, CSF is translocated from the brain to the distensible spinal subarachnoid space. When compensation is maximized, slit ventricles and absence of sulci are viewed on CT scan. To a lesser degree, reducing total cerebral blood volume or brain mass may also offset an increase in ICP.

The patient's adaptive capacity is dependent upon the volume of the mass lesion, its rate of expansion, the total volume of the intracranial cavity, and the relative volume of blood and CSF that is available for displacement. When adaptive mechanisms are obliterated, ICP will increase rapidly, often with minor changes in cerebral blood volume.

The intracranial volume/pressure relationship curve describes how much intracranial volume produces how great a change in ICP (Fig. 12–12). Elastance is the term used to describe the change in pressure that occurs with a change in volume into the intracranial space; elastance = $\Delta P/\Delta V$. Compliance is the inverse of elastance and is used to describe the same volume/pressure relationship when pressure changes are induced; compliance = $\Delta V/\Delta P$.

The relationship between intracranial volume and ICP is not linear. The intracranial volume/pressure (V/P) curve has three distinct phases: flat, exponential, and increased intracranial pressure. Phase 1, the flat portion of the curve, illustrates normal ICP with good compliance. At this point, compensation is effective in that the volume added is equal to the volume removed from the intracranial compartment. Phase 2, the exponential portion of the curve, illustrates normal ICP with poor compliance. Here, the intracranial compartment is described as "tight," adaptive capacity is reached, and any further small increase in volume produces disproportionately large increases in intracranial pressure that may not return to baseline. Phase 3 illustrates increased ICP with poor compliance. Compensatory mechanisms

Figure 12–12 ● ● ● ● ●

Intracranial volume/pressure curve. (Adapted from Becker, D.P., Mickell, J., & Keenan, R. (1981). In W.C. Shoemaker & W.L. Thomson (Eds.). *Critical care: State of the art* (p. 1). Fullerton, CA: Society of Critical Care Medicine.)

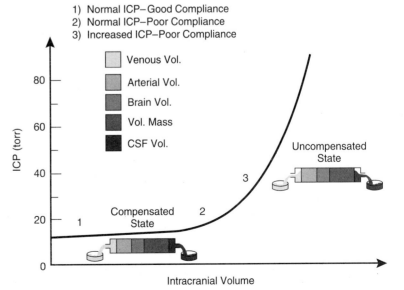

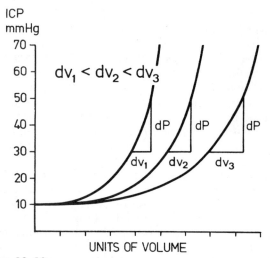

Figure 12–13 ● ● ● ● ● ●

Variation in the volume/pressure curve. Diagram to illustrate how changes in the gradient of the pressure/volume curve mean that different volumetric changes are needed to produce a given pressure change, less where the curve is steep and more where the curve is flatter. Alternatively, the same volume change will produce greater and lesser changes in pressure. (From Miller, J.D. (1984). *Increased intracranial pressure: Theoretical considerations*. In J.M. Pellock & E.C. Myer (Eds.). *Neurological emergencies in infants and children* (p. 65). Philadelphia: Harper & Row.)

have been exhausted. The exponential relationship of the volume/pressure curve explains the variability in ICP response among individuals and also in the same individual at different times.

The critical point when compensation is lost varies and depends on such factors as the rate of volumetric change, systemic arterial pressure, and osmotic therapy. Age has also been found to be a variable, with the younger child having less buffering capacity (Shapiro, Marmarou, & Shulman, 1980a and 1980b). Thus, when speaking of intracranial compliance, a series of compliance curves exist rather than a single curve (Fig. 12–13). For example, the first volume/pressure curve (dv_1) may represent the acute increase in ICP that occurs within 24 to 48 hours after head trauma. The second volume/pressure curve (dv_2) may represent the 48- to 72-hour delay in increased ICP after a hypoxic-ischemic episode. The last volume/pressure curve (dv_3) may represent the slow increase in ICP that results from a patient with a brain tumor. The collaborative management goal is to shift the patient's ICP *down to the right of one curve* or, better yet, to improve intracranial compliance and shift the patient's ICP *to a new volume/pressure curve on the left of the curve.*

Cerebral Blood Flow

A severe and prolonged increase in ICP can cause a lethal reduction in cerebral blood flow (CBF). A progressive increase in intracranial volume causes obstruction of the CSF pathways, eliminating the primary means of buffering increased ICP. In addi-

tion, increased ICP causes venous outflow obstruction and compensatory arterial hypertension. As a consequence, capillary pressure increases, predisposing the brain to cerebral edema. The end result is a further increase in intracranial volume that ultimately may cause herniation of brain structures and a reduction in CBF.

As mentioned earlier, the brain requires constant and consistent delivery of blood flow to meet its high metabolic demands. The determinants of cerebral blood flow are arteriolar radius, blood viscosity, perfusion pressure, and length of the vascular bed. Practically speaking, the length of the vascular bed and blood viscosity remain constant. Therefore, the important variables of CBF are cerebral perfusion pressure and arteriolar radius.

Cerebral Perfusion Pressure

Cerebral perfusion pressure (CPP) represents the pressure drop between the inflow (arterial) pressure and outflow (venous) pressure. Traystman (1983) identified three separate conditions that require consideration (Fig. 12–14). In condition I, the intracranial pressure is greater than the mean arterial pressure (MAP) and both are greater than the central venous pressure (CVP). When these conditions are

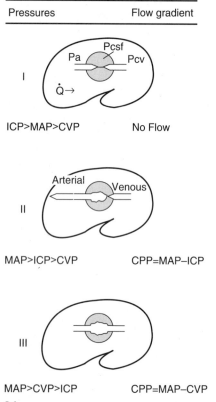

Figure 12–14 ● ● ● ● ● ●

Three separate conditions that require evaluation when calculating cerebral perfusion pressure. (Adapted from Mortillaro, N.A. (1983). *The physiology and pharmacology of the microcirculation* (pp. 237–238). New York: Academic Press.)

present, cerebral blood flow is impossible. In condition II, the mean arterial pressure is greater than the intracranial pressure and both are greater than the central venous pressure. Here, the cerebral perfusion pressure is calculated as mean arterial pressure minus the intracranial pressure (MAP − ICP). In condition III, the mean arterial pressure is greater than the central venous pressure and both are greater than the intracranial pressure. Here, the cerebral perfusion pressure is calculated as mean arterial pressure minus the CVP (MAP − CVP). Clinically, the CPP = MAP − ICP unless the CVP is significantly elevated, then the CPP = MAP − CVP. Because it is possible to have a normal ICP but no blood flow (thus no oxygen extraction) through damaged areas of the brain, some research centers trend cross-brain oxygen consumption and metabolic rates with ICP and CPP.

Normal cerebral perfusion pressure is unknown in the pediatric population, but is thought that a CPP greater than 50 mmHg is necessary for adequate cerebral perfusion. Cerebral perfusion pressures less than 40 mmHg, because of cerebral hypertension or systemic hypotension, are thought to be the cutoff point between good quality survival and poor outcomes. This critical point is much less in the neonate. In this age group, normal CPP is thought to depend upon weight and be about 30 mmHg (Raju, Vidyasagar, & Papazafiratou, 1981).

Cerebral Autoregulation

Normally, cerebral blood flow (CBF) matches the cerebral metabolic rate (CMR). For example, when the CMR increases, there is a concomitant increase in CBF; when CMR decreases, there is a concomitant decrease in CBF. This compensatory process, known as autoregulation, matches CBF with CMR and is accomplished by either cerebral vasoconstriction or vasodilation. This mechanism is believed to occur from a myogenic mechanism located in the muscular arterioles (Folkow, 1964). Changes in arteriolar transmural pressure produce changes in arteriolar radius by vasoconstriction or vasodilation.

Under normal circumstances, autoregulation is maintained when the CPP ranges from approximately 60 to 160 mmHg (Rogers, Nugent, & Traystman, 1980). If these limits are exceeded, CBF is passively dependent on CPP. The upper limit of CPP may be higher in individuals with chronic hypertension. Furthermore, autoregulation may be altered locally or globally with CNS insult. If CBF is greater than the CMR, hyperemia occurs, a common finding after pediatric head trauma. When CBF is less than the CMR, cerebral hypoxia ensues, a common finding during pediatric resuscitation.

Chemical Regulation

In addition to pressure autoregulation, CBF is also affected by chemical autoregulation. Both $Paco_2$ and Pao_2 affect CBF and cerebral blood volume by altering cerebral arteriolar radius. High levels of $Paco_2$ cause vasodilation of the cerebral vasculature with an increase in CBF and therefore an increase in cerebral blood volume. Conversely, a decrease in $Paco_2$ produces a decrease in CBF. Thus, lowering $Paco_2$ with hyperventilation is a clinically useful tool for emergent management of intracranial hypertension.

In contrast to $Paco_2$, the cerebral vasculature seems to be somewhat less sensitive to Pao_2. Hypoxia, Pao_2 less than 50 mmHg, increases CBF by producing a vasodilatory response. Conversely, hyperoxia produces a mild vasoconstrictive response with only a modest decrease in CBF. The critical lower limit of Pao_2 that causes a increase in CBF may be lower in the neonate (Traystman, 1983). Newborns are relatively hypoxic (normal Pao_2 range 65–70 mmHg) compared with infants and young children, and the actual delivery of oxygen to the tissues is affected by the percentage of fetal hemoglobin (Duc, 1971).

NEUROLOGIC ASSESSMENT

Central nervous system development is incomplete at birth, maturing over the first several years of life. Maturation reflects myelinization, dendritic arborization, increases in synaptic connections, increases in glial cell population, and changes in neurochemical properties. As a result, the infant has underdeveloped cortical integrative function and has immature neuromuscular control. Therefore, neurologic assessment of the infant and young child requires a developmental approach that reflects the age and temperament of the child. The following section describes the components of neurologic assessment in the infant and young child.

History

The neurologic history provides the framework for guiding the neurologic examination. The data obtained from the history assist the nurse in formulating preliminary nursing diagnoses that are either supported or rejected by the physical examination. The length of the interview, the specific questions, and the timing depend on whether the child has a static, a progressive, or an acute condition. Taking of history may need to be delayed if the parents are not present and the child is pre-verbal or if the child's physical status is life-threatening.

The first component of the neurologic history is the *chief complaint*. Whenever possible, the school-age child should be asked questions directly. Preschool children are less reliable and, like the pre-verbal child, often require their parents to describe the problem.

Once the chief problem has been stated, questions are asked to obtain information leading up to the *present illness*. Questions should be formulated so that the nurse can determine whether the patient's condition is progressive or static, focal or generalized, and acute or insidious.

Specific questions that need to be addressed regarding the patient's history depend in part on the patient's age and present illness. For the infant and young child, a summary of the antenatal, perinatal, and postnatal courses should be obtained. This includes, but does not exhaust, questions regarding maternal infections, drug intake during pregnancy, gestational age, and Apgar scores. A history of meconium staining, neonatal seizure activity, or oxygen use needs further investigation. Medical history should also include a chronologic list of the child's developmental milestones, which is then compared against established norms (Table 12–6).

For the older child who was previously healthy, questions should be asked to differentiate between metabolic and structural causes of neurologic dysfunction. For example, has the child had a recent fall, been exposed to chemical toxins, or have an endocrine disorder such as diabetes?

The *family history* should include questions regarding neurologic illnesses in family members, as well as specific signs and symptoms that may have a neurologic basis. Most neurodegenerative disorders are transmitted as a recessive gene, and some epilepsies are transmitted as a dominant trait (Menkes et al., 1990).

Table 12–6. DEVELOPMENTAL MILESTONES

Age	Developmental Skills
Newborn (full-term)	Blinks at light and loud sound; turns head from side to side; regards face
4 weeks	Chin held up momentarily; vocalizes, not crying
8 weeks	Smiles responsively; head held up 45 degrees; fixes and follows object 180 degrees
12 weeks	Turns head to sound; laughs and squeals
4 months	Brings hand to midline; rolls over; smiles spontaneously
6 months	Bears weight on legs; sits alone; transfers objects
9 months	Creeps; stands holding on; imitates sounds
15 months	Walks alone; creeps upstairs; stacks 2–3 cubes; knows a few body parts
24 months	Runs; kicks ball; walks up steps
30 months	Jumps; throws ball overhand; follows simple instructions; knows name; identifies objects
36 months	Walks up and down stairs by alternating feet; imitates vertical line; draws circles; independent dressing, except buttons
48 months	Hops on one foot; buttons clothing; recognizes common colors
60 months	Skips; balances on one foot; copies a diamond; counts

Physical Examination

For the awake, stable child, vital signs and height and weight should be measured. The general appearance of the child should be observed—in particular, dysmorphic features, asymmetries, cutaneous lesions (e.g., café au lait spots, angiomas), condition of scalp and hair, palmar creases, and unusual odors.

Skull Examination

For infants, the neurologic assessment includes a skull examination. Head circumference should be measured on admission and repeated at regular intervals determined by the patient's condition. The largest circumference (occipitofrontal) should be consistently measured and plotted on a head growth chart. Since head growth reflects brain growth, a significantly small head circumference may indicate impaired brain growth. In contrast, an unusually large head may be a manifestation of hydrocephalus or some other abnormal fluid accumulation or tissue growth. The normal rate of head growth in the first 12 months of life is 2 cm per month for the first 3 months, 1 cm per month for the fourth through sixth month, and 0.5 cm per month for the remaining 6 months (Jacobson, 1989).

The cranial sutures and associated fontanelles should be palpated gently. The posterior fontanelle usually closes within the first few months of life, and the anterior fontanelle remains open until approximately 12 to 18 months of life. In a United States study (Popich & Smith, 1972), the average diameter of the anterior fontanelle at birth was found to be 2.1 cm. However, an unusually small or large fontanelle may not, by itself, reflect an abnormality in the infant. Its presence should be correlated with other clinical findings. Ideally, the fontanelle should be palpated while the infant is sitting upright and in a quiet state. Normally, the fontanelle feels soft and flat or slightly depressed compared with the surrounding skull.

The cranial sutures should be palpated to determine if they are overriding or widely separated. Overriding sutures from head molding in the birth canal may be a normal finding in the newborn. However, it may also represent premature closure of the sutures (craniosynostosis) or inadequate brain growth. Widely separated sutures may suggest hydrocephalus.

Transillumination is a simple, noninvasive technique used to detect abnormal fluid collection within the scalp and beneath the calvarium. Its use is restricted to the first 9 to 12 months of age because of the thickness of the skull beyond this age. Many commercial instruments are available, but a battery flashlight with a rubber adaptor (fits close to the skull) is very reliable. The light source is placed on the infant's skull, usually starting at the anterior fontanelle. In the normal full-term newborn, there is a larger rim of transillumination in the frontal area (as much as 3 cm) compared with the occipital area

(Haller, 1981). An area of increased or asymmetric transillumination should be noted.

If time and the patient's condition permit, the calvarium should be auscultated for bruits. Although the presence of a bruit in young infants may be normal, a particularly loud or asymmetric bruit may be heard with an intracranial vascular malformation. An extreme downward rotation of the eyes at rest and paralysis of upward gaze are known as the "setting-sun" sign. It may be intermittent and is seen in some children with increased ICP. It is a common clinical characteristic of hydrocephalus. A similar appearance may be seen with abnormal retraction of the upper eyelids (Collier's sign) from lesions affecting the costal midbrain and third ventricle. When the cranial sutures are separated because of increased ICP, Macewen's sign or a "cracked pot" sound maybe heard during percussion of the skull.

Level of Consciousness

Consciousness is a state of awareness of self and environment. There are two physiologic components of consciousness: content and arousal. Content is controlled by cerebral function, and arousal is controlled by physiologic mechanisms that originate in the reticular formation. Dysfunction of the cerebral hemispheres and/or the reticular activating system (RAS) of the upper brainstem, hypothalamus, and thalamus will produce an alteration in consciousness (Plum & Posner, 1982). Altered states of consciousness are on a continuum ranging from the extremes of complete consciousness to coma. For the patient with minimal alteration in consciousness, mental status is assessed. For more severely altered states, coma scales may be required to assess level of consciousness.

Mental Status. Cortical growth occurs both quantitatively and qualitatively within the first 2 years of life. Consequently, the mental status (cerebral function) portion of the neurologic examination is individualized according to the infant and young child's age. Specific areas to assess in the infant and young child include alertness and level of activity, quality of cry, feeding patterns, language development, and presence or absence of primitive reflexes.

Ideally, the young infant's state of alertness is assessed during a period of time when stress is at a minimum. Usual patterns of sleep and wakefulness are assessed and evaluated based on the infant's age, nutritional state, and quality of sleep within the previous 24 hours. In general, extreme states of agitation or lethargy are noted.

Normally, the infant's cry is loud and energetic. Abnormal cries include ones that are difficult to elicit, associated with cyanosis, high-pitched, weak, monotonous, or moaning (Amiel-Tison, 1976).

Normal feeding behavior includes a strong suck and good suck-swallowing coordination. Note if the young child cannot finish a bottle without tiring or becomes cyanotic. Also, note if the child has excessive gagging and choking.

Normal speech and language skills develop over

Table 12–7. SPEECH AND LANGUAGE DEVELOPMENT

Age	Vocalization Skill
Newborn (full-term)	Responds to bell; reflexive cry
2 months	Differentiation of cries; babbles, single vowel sounds
4 months	Laughs aloud and squeals, modulating voice and vocalization of vowels
6 months	Babbles vowels and consonants
8 months	Repetitive utterances (e.g., "dada," "mama")
10 months	Imitates speech sounds
12 months	Use of 2–3 words with meaning
18 months	Combines two different words; three words in addition to "mama" and "dada"
24 months	100–300 word vocabulary; 50% of speech understandable
36 months	Three-word sentences; 80% of speech understandable
60 months	Adult level speech in syntax; 100% of speech understandable

several years (Table 12–7). These skills depend on normal development of motor control of the oral musculature. Therefore, if the child deviates significantly from established norms, the gag reflex and tongue movements are tested for coordination and strength.

In the older awake child, a comprehensive evaluation of mental status includes attention, alertness, orientation, cognition, memory, affect, and perception. Most of the assessment can take place during normal conversation with the child. Care should be taken when determining which questions to ask the child. Questions are individualized according to the child's age and temperament.

Motor Function

Assessment of motor function is adapted to the age of the child. A variety of primitive reflexes are normally present in the infant, and determining their presence or absence is an important component of the neurologic examination. The disappearance of primitive reflexes reflects increasing maturation of the cortex. As myelinization progresses, higher cortical centers become functional and gradually suppress these reflexes. Table 12–8 lists the most common primitive reflexes and the time of their appearance and disappearance. Abnormal findings include the persistence of a primitive reflex significantly beyond the normal time of disappearance or the reappearance of a primitive reflex.

Normal motor development proceeds cephalocaudally and proximodistally. Early in life, movements are more generalized and reflexive. Fine motor control follows development of gross motor control. The infant's extremities are assessed for muscle symmetry, mass, and tone. When examining the young in-

Table 12-8. PRIMITIVE REFLEXES

Reflex	Description	Age of Appearance	Age of Disappearance
Moro	Elicited by a sudden movement of the body that causes a change in equilibrium. There is extension and abduction of the upper extremities (fingers fan), followed by flexion and adduction	28–32 weeks' gestation	3–5 months
Asymmetric tonic neck response	Elicited by rotating the head to the side while the chest is maintained in a flat position. The arm and leg extend on the side the face is rotated and the opposite arm and leg flex	Birth–2 months	4–6 months
Placing	Elicited with infant supported in vertical position with dorsum of one foot pressed against hard surface. The foot will flex and extend, simulating walking	35–37 weeks' gestation	1–2 months
Rooting	Elicited by stroking the perioral skin at the corner of the mouth, moving laterally toward the cheek, upper lip and the lower lip. Infant will turn head toward the stimulated side with sucking movements	28 weeks' gestation	3–4 months
Parachute	Elicited by holding infant in ventral position. A sudden plunge downward produces extension and abduction of arms and fingers	4–9 months	Persists throughout life, but covered up with voluntary movement
Palmar grasp	Elicited by placing index finger of examiner into the ulnar side of infant's hand and pressing against palmar surface. Infant's fingers immediately flex around examiner's finger	28 weeks' gestation	4–6 months

fant, the head is maintained in a midline position to prevent an asymmetric tonic neck reflex. In infants less than 3 months of age, increased flexor tone is normal (Slota, 1983). The newborn's hands are usually closed; however, they may open and close spontaneously while sleeping or when very quiet. Hands that are always closed after 2 months of age represent an abnormal finding, which is correlated with other neurologic findings to determine its significance (Amiel-Tison, 1976). Definite hand dominance is usually not present until the second or third year of life. Hand preference in infants less than 24 months may indicate weakness or spasticity of the other hand (Swaiman, 1989).

Reflexes

Deep Tendon. Testing deep tendon reflexes helps to evaluate both the lower motor neurons and the motor and sensory fibers within a particular spinal level. In the older child, deep tendon reflexes are readily tested and graded narratively or by using a stick figure. The most common reflexes examined are the biceps, triceps, brachioradialis, patellar, and Achilles reflex. Hyperreflexia may indicate corticospinal dysfunction or may be a response from an abnormal "spread" of responses, that is, abnormal contraction of muscle groups that usually do not contract when a reflex is being tested (Swaiman, 1989). Hypo-

reflexia may be seen with lower motor unit dysfunction.

In infants, some deep tendon responses are not present at birth and when present are less reliable due to the immaturity of its corticospinal tracts. In general, responses in the infant that require further investigation include reflexes that are very brisk, asymmetric, or deviate from previous assessments (Slota, 1983; Swainman, 1989). Ankle clonus is often present in the newborn period, but it is rarely sustained and usually disappears by 2 months of age.

Superficial Reflexes. A positive Babinski response, that is, dorsiflexion of the foot and fanning of the toes after stroking the sole laterally from heel to toe, is normally present in the infant. This response disappears in the second year of life at approximately 18 to 24 months of age. Persistence or reoccurrence of this response is pathologic, indicative of dysfunction of the corticospinal tracts or the motor area of the cerebrum. Abdominal and cremasteric responses are present at birth. The abdominal response is elicited by stroking the abdomen from a lateral position moving to the umbilicus in all four quadrants. A normal response is slight muscle contraction and movement of the umbilicus toward the stimulus. The cremasteric response is elicited in males by stroking downward on the inner aspects of the upper thigh. The scrotum should contract and elevate. Unilateral absence of the abdominal response and absence or asymmetry of the cremasteric response may indicate corticospinal dysfunction.

Sensory Function

Responses to sensory testing in the infant are more variable and less reliable than in the older child. However, the infant should respond to light stroking of the extremities. With normal sensory function, the infant will usually withdraw the limb being tested. Vibration sense may be tested by placing a tuning fork over bony areas. In response, the infant will usually stop all movement and display a look of surprise. Proprioception cannot be tested at this age. Pain sensation is tested at the end of the examination by nailbed pressure.

In the older child, sensory function can be tested in the usual fashion. For initial screening, light touch and superficial pain are tested in all four extremities. If abnormalities are suspected or detected, more thorough segmental sensory testing is indicated, including temperature, vibration, pressure, and position sensations. Figure 12–15 is a drawing of segmental sensory innervation of the body.

Cerebellar Function

Cerebellar function of the older child and adolescent can be evaluated in much the same way as in

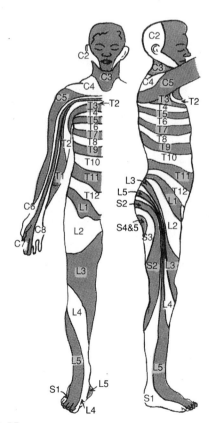

Figure 12–15 ● ● ● ● ● ●

The dermatomes. (Modified from Grinker and Sahs (1966). *Neurology* (6th ed.). Courtesy of Charles C Thomas, Publisher, Springfield, Illinois; in Guyton, A.C. (1991). *Textbook of medical physiology* (8th ed., p. 518). Philadelphia: W.B. Saunders.)

the adult. Rapid alternating movements, as well as finger-to-nose, finger-to-finger, and heel-shin testing, is possible. Maneuvers to evaluate the young child and infant are less precise. Much information can be obtained by observing the young child in play, noting tremors, dysmetria, and truncal swaying. Once again, familiarity with age-dependent motor skills when determining the adequacy in which a child performs a maneuver is important.

Cranial Nerve Function

With the exception of the olfactory nerve, all of the cranial nerves originate in the brainstem. An evaluation of their function provides valuable diagnostic evaluative information about the child's neurologic status. The specific cranial nerves that should be tested and the order in which they are tested will depend on the age and condition of the child. A complete cranial nerve assessment is usually not needed for routine screening. Table 12–4 lists the 12 cranial nerves, how they are tested according to age, and the clinical significance of abnormal findings.

Funduscopic Examination

Normally, the funduscopic examination reveals a red reflex that is orange-red and fairly uniform in color, a creamy pink optic disc with an indented center (physiologic depression) and smooth margins, and veins (slightly wider than arteries) that have no light reflex and manifest slight pulsations. Papilledema, represented as blurring of the nasal and upper edges of the optic disc, is commonly seen with increased ICP in the older child. Papilledema is an unusual finding during infancy because the cranial sutures usually spread and the head enlarges in response to chronic increases in ICP. Retinal hemorrhages may be present with significant head injury and subarachnoid hemorrhage (commonly associated with "shakened baby syndrome" in child abuse). Decreased peripheral retinal vascularity is seen in infants with retrolental fibroplasia.

Assessment of the Neurologically Impaired Child

The child with an altered level of arousal requires frequent clinical assessment of neurologic function. Patterns of pathophysiologic responses and their evolution provide valuable information about the location, extent, and progression of neurologic dysfunction. Five assessment parameters are critical to the neurologic evaluation: level of consciousness, motor function, respiratory patterns, cranial nerve response, and vital signs. The neurologic assessment of the child begins with assessment of level of consciousness. Cerebral hemispheric function is determined by assessing motor function. As neurologic dysfunction progresses caudally, characteristic respiratory patterns may occur. In late stages with lower brainstem dysfunction, abnormal cranial nerve responses occur followed by abnormal vital signs.

Level of Consciousness

Level of consciousness is the most important initial assessment for the neurologically impaired child. Accurate and consistent assessment of level of consciousness can indicate if the patient's condition is improving, worsening, or remaining static. There is a range of altered states of consciousness and a number of ways to label and define these states. Table 12–9 defines commonly used terms to describe various states of consciousness. More important than labels are the patient's actual behaviors and responses.

Numerous coma scales have been developed, most notably the Glasgow Coma Scale (GCS; see Table 12–10). Originally developed as a prognostic tool for patients with head injury, the GCS also helps to identify the depth of coma by standardizing assessments (Jennett & Bond, 1975). Despite its widespread use, the GCS has limited use with pre-verbal infants and intubated patients. As a result, a number of institutions have modified the GCS. Tables 12–11 and 12–12 are examples of coma scales adapted for infants and neonates.

The modified GCS assesses arousibility in relation to three responses: eye opening, verbal response, and motor response. When using a stimulus to assess level of consciousness, the least noxious stimuli is used first. For example, start with a voice stimulus, then progress to touch, and if the patient is still unresponsive, apply a painful stimulus. Care is taken to avoid harming the patient, especially when coagulation factors are abnormal. Nailbed pressure is a reliable stimulus because it can be consistently reproduced by numerous individuals. The exact stimulus that provides a minimal response is documented so that progression of neurologic defects can be easily identified. Careful assessment is necessary to differentiate between appropriate withdrawal to stimuli,

Table 12–9. ALTERED STATES OF CONSCIOUSNESS

Clouding of consciousness	Reduced wakefulness: reduced attention, confused, drowsiness alternating with hyperexcitability
Delirium	Disorientation, fear, irritability, visual hallucinations, agitation. Patients may be loud, offensive and suspicious
Obtundation	Mild to moderate reduction in alertness, reduced interest in environment, increased periods of sleep
Stupor	Unresponsive except to vigorous and repeated stimuli
Coma	No motor or verbal response to environment

Data from Plum, F., & Posner, J.B. *The diagnosis of stupor and coma* (3rd ed.). Philadelphia; F.A. Davis.

Table 12–10. GLASGOW COMA SCORE

Write number in box to indicate status at time of this exam

(A) Eye opening
Spontaneous	=4
To speech	=3
To pain	=2
None	=1

(B) Best motor response (extremities of best side)
Obeys	=6
Localizes	=5
Withdraws	=4
Abnormal flexion	=3
Extends	=2
None	=1

(C) Best verbal response (If patient intubated, give best estimate)
Oriented	=5
Confused conversation	=4
Inappropriate words	=3
Incomprehensible sounds	=2
None	=1

Total GCS
(Best GCS = 15)
(Worst GCS = 3)

From Jennett, B., & Bond, M. (1975). Assessment of outcome after severe brain damage: A practical scale. *Lancet* 1, 480–485. © by The Lancet, Ltd., 1975.

which involves cortical activity, and a spinal cord stretch reflex, which does not.

Motor Function

In addition to assessing motor response with the GCS, motor function is also evaluated in terms of symmetry of response and the presence of pathologic signs. Normally, posture is controlled by the interaction between higher inhibiting brain centers and lower exciting brain centers. In the comatose patient, some degree of cortical control over motor function

Table 12–11. MODIFIED COMA SCORE FOR INFANTS

Activity	Best Response	Score
Eye opening	Spontaneous	4
	To speech	3
	To pain	2
	None	1
Verbal	Coos and babbles	5
	Irritable cries	4
	Cries to pain	3
	Moans to pain	2
	None	1
Motor	Normal spontaneous movements	6
	Withdraws to touch	5
	Withdraws to pain	4
	Abnormal flexion	3
	Abnormal extension	2
	None	1
	Total Score	3–15

From Rogers, M.C. (1992). *Textbook of pediatric intensive care.* © 1992, the Williams & Wilkins Co., Baltimore.

Table 12-12. NEONATAL AROUSAL SCALE

	Scale
Best Response to Bell	
Facial and extremity movements	5
Grimaces/blinks	4
Increase in RR/HR	3
Seizures/extensor posturing	2
No response	1
Best Response to Light	
Blink and facial/extremity movements	4
Blink	3
Seizures/extensor posturing	2
No response	1
Best Motor Response	
Spontaneous	
Periods of activity alternating with sleep	6
Occasional spontaneous movements	5
Sternal rub	
Extremity movements	4
Grimace/facial movements	3
Seizures/extensor posturing	2
No response	1
Total	3-15

RR, respiratory rate; HR, heart rate.
From Duncan, C.C., & Ment, L.R. (1980). A scale for the assessment of neonatal neurologic status. *Child's Brain,* 8, 299–306. S. Karger AG, Basel.

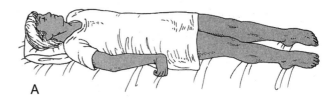

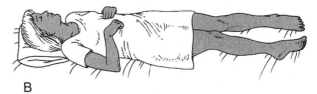

Figure 12-16 ● ● ● ● ● ●
Pathologic posturing occurring in severe brain injury. *A,* Extension posturing (decerebrate rigidity). *B,* Abnormal flexion (decorticate rigidity). (From Betz, C.L., Hunsberger, M., & Wright, S. (1994). *Family-centered nursing care of children* (2nd ed., p. 1726). Philadelphia: W.B. Saunders.)

may be lost, allowing primitive postural reflexes to emerge. Spontaneous motor movement may occur in the unconscious patient. Localization represents movement of an extremity across the midline of the body toward the opposite extremity receiving a painful stimulus. In the comatose patient, both localization and spontaneous movement are favorable prognostic signs.

When there is severe dysfunction of the cortex and subcortical white matter and preservation of the brainstem, decorticate posturing emerges. Typically, decorticate posturing includes flexion of the upper extremities and extension of the lower extremities. Decerebrate posturing represents dysfunction of the cortex and brainstem at the level of the pons. It is manifested by extension of the upper and lower extremities with rigidity. No motor response to noxious stimuli (bilateral flaccidity) in all four extremities is an ominous sign and is one criterion for brain death determination. Care must be taken to rule out

other causes of flaccidity, such as stroke or spinal cord injury. Figure 12–16 schematically illustrates decorticate and decerebrate posturing.

Respiratory Patterns

Alterations in respiratory pattern is an early and reliable sign of neurologic dysfunction. Breathing is primarily regulated by metabolism in the so-called respiratory centers of the brainstem and by behavior in the forebrain. The presence of two major breathing centers at different levels of the brain sometimes produces characteristic breathing patterns that reflect the location of the neuropathology. Table 12–13 describes the most common pathologic respiratory patterns and their neuropathologic location (Plum & Posner, 1982). Even though the presence of characteristic breathing patterns is well described, overlap in patterns may occur or patterns may change very rapidly. The most ominous breathing pattern is one that is irregular and slow progressing to apnea (ataxic).

Table 12-13. PATHOLOGIC RESPIRATORY PATTERNS AND THEIR NEUROPATHOLOGIC LOCATION

Name	Location	Description
Cheyne-Stokes	Bilateral Hemispheric or Diencephalon	Periodic breathing; phases of hyperpnea alternating with apnea
Central neurogenic hyperventilation	Rostral Brainstem Tegmentum	Sustained, rapid, and deep hyperpnea
Apneustic	Mid- or caudal-pontine level	Prolonged inspiration with a pause at full inspiration
Ataxic	Medulla	Irregular pattern; deep and shallow breaths occur randomly

Cranial Nerve Response

Pupil Size and Reactivity. Pupillary size and reactivity are regulated by the autonomic nervous system, an intact afferent connection of CN II, and CN III nucleus. Pupillary size changes almost continuously due to the interaction of parasympathetic and sympathetic fibers. Stimulation of parasympathetic fibers causes the pupil to constrict (miosis), and stimulation of sympathetic fibers causes the pupil to dilate (mydriasis). Because the brainstem contains adjacent areas that control both pupillary reactivity and arousal, testing pupillary response provides valuable information regarding the presence and location of brainstem dysfunction producing coma. Figure 12–17 illustrates autonomic and cranial nerve control of pupillary response.

Both pupils should first be observed and the exact size noted. The usual range in size varies between 2 and 6 mm. The size of the pupil changes with age, being the smallest during infancy and the largest during adolescence (March, 1983; Norman, 1982). Most children have equal-sized pupils, but a 1-mm discrepancy between pupils (anisocoria) may be normal (i.e., for patients with a known discrepancy). Extremely small pupils may indicate opiate affects, pontine hemorrhage, metabolic encephalopathy, or lower brainstem compression. Pupils that are widely dilated and unresponsive result from CN III compression commonly seen with transtentorial hernia-

tion or from the midbrain lesion in the area of the Edinger-Westphal nucleus (March, 1983). The acute appearance of this pupillary finding is an ominous and late sign requiring immediate attention. Other common causes of dilated and unreactive pupils include severe hypothermia, anoxia, ischemia, and ingestion of atropine-like substances.

After observing the pupils for size and equality, reactivity to light is tested. To test the pupils' reaction to direct light, use a light with a narrow, bright beam. Test each eye independently by covering or closing one eye while testing the other. Approach the eye from the periphery to avoid constriction of the pupil by accommodation. Once the eye is exposed to the direct light, the pupil should constrict briskly. Document the pupils' response and grade how briskly the pupil constricts using consistent labels or a numerical scale. For example, both pupils are 3 mm in size and react to light briskly.

Consensual or indirect light response refers to the pupillary constriction that occurs in the eye opposite the eye being stimulated with light. The normal consensual pupillary response represents transmission of light to the brainstem where the Edinger-Westphal nucleus activates the parasympathetic efferent fibers of both pupils (March, 1983). Abnormalities in the direct light response and/or the consensual response can help determine whether there is damage to the optic nerve (CN II) or to the oculomotor nerve (CN III).

Ocular Movements. Eye movements are controlled by both voluntary cerebral hemispheric centers and involuntary control centers in the brainstem. These areas interact with three paired cranial nerves (III, IV, and VI) that innervate the extraocular muscles that control ocular movement (Fig. 12–18). Normally, the eyes move together synchronously, i.e., conjugate eye movements.

Abnormal eye movements include nystagmus, dysconjugate eye movements, and extraocular palsies. Nystagmus refers to a repetitive, involuntary oscillation of one or both eyes. The usual planes of nystagmus are horizontal, vertical, and rotary. Horizontal nystagmus is seen normally with extreme lateral gaze, with the use of certain drugs (e.g., anticonvulsants, barbiturates, alcohol), and sometimes with cerebellar dysfunction (Bishop, 1991; Mein & Harcouty, 1986).

Conjugate eye movement is controlled by several different areas of the brain: frontal gaze center, occipital gaze center, and medial longitudinal fasciculus (MLF). Thus, damage to several parts of the brain can cause dysconjugate eye movements.

Extraocular palsies of cranial nerves III, IV, and VI can also cause abnormal eye movements. However, their presence is less precise in identifying a specific area of brainstem dysfunction because they may also result from increased ICP.

Oculocephalic Response. In the comatose patient, the integrity of the brainstem can also be assessed by testing the oculocephalic response (doll's eye maneuver). This maneuver determines the integ-

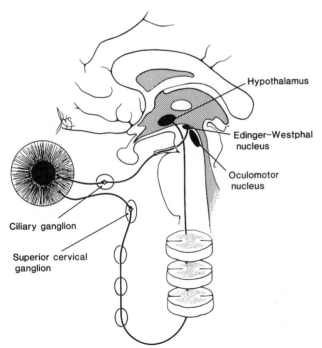

Figure 12–17 ● ● ● ● ● ●

Pupillary responses to light stimulation in differentiating ocular or optic nerve disease from oculomotor nerve dysfunction. (From Vannucci, R.C., & Young, R.S.K. (1984). Diagnosis and management of coma in children. In J.M. Pellock & E.C. Myer (Eds.). *Neurological emergencies in infants and children.* Philadelphia: Harper & Row.)

Hypothalamus

Edinger–Westphal nucleus

Oculomotor nucleus

Ciliary ganglion

Superior cervical ganglion

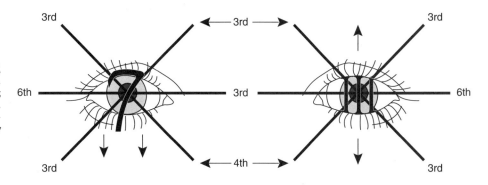

Figure 12–18 ● ● ● ● ●

Three paired cranial nerves—III, IV, and VI—control ocular movement. Cranial nerve VII closes the eyelid; cranial nerve III elevates the eyelid. (Modified from Goldberg (1995). *Clinical neuroanatomy made ridiculously simple.* Miami: MedMaster, Inc.)

rity of cranial nerves III, VI, and VIII. It can only be performed in the unconscious patient or in an infant less than 2 months of age (Moore, 1988). After clearing the cervical spine for injury, the test is performed by briskly turning the head from side to side. With an intact brainstem, the eyes will deviate to the opposite side the head is turned and then slowly turn in the direction the head is rotated (Bishop, 1991; March, 1983; Zegeer, 1989). With severe brainstem injury, the patient's eyes will remain midpositioned or fixed while turning the head.

Oculovestibular Response. Like the oculocephalic response, the oculovestibular response (cold calorics) can be used to assess the integrity of the brainstem. This test is performed by first elevating the head of the bed 30 degrees, confirming an intact tympanic membrane and dura, and removing cerumen from the external canal. The reflex is elicited by injecting water (usually 30°C) into the external canal. With an intact brainstem in the unconscious patient, there is slow conjugate movement of the eyes toward the stimulus followed by fast return to the midline. A patient with a low brainstem lesion would have eyes that remain at midposition and fixed. Figure 12–19 illustrates the oculocephalic and oculovestibular responses.

Vital Signs

Changes in vital signs, indicative of brainstem dysfunction, occur before cardiopulmonary arrest. Cushing's triad includes the classic signs of increased systolic pressure, widened pulse pressure, and bradycardia.

Neurologic Assessment of the Chemically Paralyzed Child

Neuromuscular blocking agents are commonly used as adjunctive therapy in critically ill infants and children. These agents cause skeletal muscle relaxation by altering the response of acetylcholine at the neuromuscular junction (Davidson, 1991; O'Brien, 1989). After an appropriate dose of a neuromuscular agent is injected, the onset of effects is rapid. Motor weakness progresses to flaccid paralysis in the following sequence: eyes and fingers; limbs,

neck, and trunk; intercostal muscles; and finally the diaphragm. Recovery of muscles occurs in the reverse order. The most common indications for use in children are to (1) improve controlled ventilation, (2) stabilize or maintain intracranial pressure, and (3) decrease oxygen consumption.

Despite the advantages of neuromuscular blocking agents, their use precludes most of the neurologic assessment. Because peripheral skeletal muscle paralysis is present, the patient will be unable to respond to commands and is unresponsive to standard tests of motor function, reflexes, and sensation. However, because these agents are unable to cross the blood-brain barrier, consciousness and normal sleep-wake cycles are preserved. These patients are able to hear and feel pain. Consequently, sedatives and analgesics are always administered concurrently. Pupillary reflexes can be tested, and abnormal responses indicate the same clinical significance as in the nonparalyzed patient. Normal oculovestibular and oculocephalic responses are blocked with neuromuscular blocking agents.

Autonomic function is preserved; thus changes in vital signs can be used to assess the patient's responsiveness. An increase in the baseline heart rate may indicate the patient is responding to parents, experiencing pain, anxiety, or a seizure. Pain or anxiety is usually accompanied by a sympathetic response with diaphoresis (sweaty brow). The only clue of a seizure may be an abrupt increase in heart rate and blood pressure. An electroencephalogram (EEG) is used to determine cerebral electrical activity.

If the patient's condition permits, intermittent withdrawal or reversal of the agent allows for determination of the neurologic status. Recovery from neuromuscular blockade may be prolonged due to certain physiologic states and/or concurrent administration with other medications. More precise monitoring of neuromuscular activity, as well as confirmation of patient flaccidity, may be determined by a peripheral nerve stimulator (see Chapter 20, Pulmonary Critical Care Problems) (Davidson, 1991; Fiamengo, 1991; Mylrea et al, 1984).

NEUROLOGIC INTENSIVE CARE MONITORING

Caring for the pediatric patient at risk for neurologic deterioration is uniquely challenging. The col-

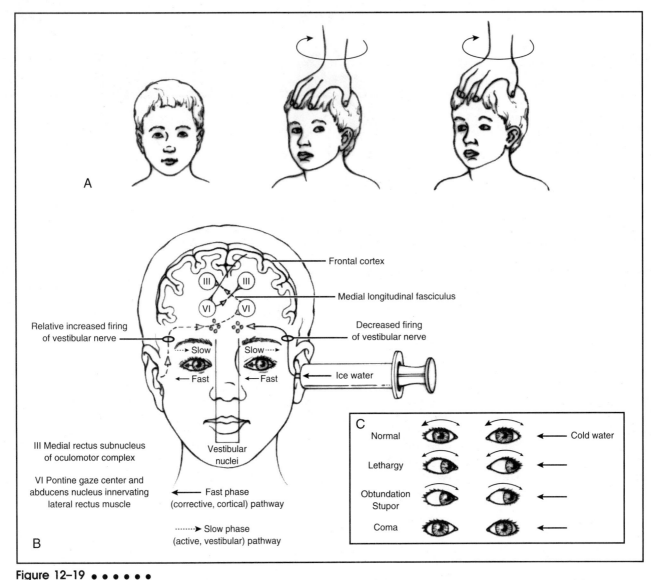

Figure 12-19 ● ● ● ● ● ●

A, Oculocephalic response. *B and C,* Oculovestibular response.

laborative goal is to preserve cerebral functioning. Bedside neurologic monitoring provides continuous insight into the central nervous system environment and actual neuronal functioning. The following section focuses on major monitoring modalities, presenting general principles, current devices, and essential elements of nursing care.

INTRACRANIAL PRESSURE MONITORING

Only when the ICP is known can therapy intended to manage cerebral hypertension be rationally directed. ICP monitoring is considered in acute neurologic disorders with a known potential for the development of intracranial hypertension in which aggressive therapy will improve neurologic outcome. ICP monitoring assists in the (1) detection of increas-

ing ICP and compromised cerebral perfusion pressure (CPP) prior to changes in the neurologic examination, especially when the neurologic examination is diminished by therapy, such as administration of anesthetics and/or chemical paralysis; (2) clinical evaluation of intracranial compliance, for example, volume/pressure response testing; (3) evaluation of the effectiveness of therapeutic interventions; and (4) prognostication of the patient's clinical status.

Knowledge of ICP and CPP allows precise titration of therapy intended to prevent secondary neurologic injury from cerebral ischemia and/or herniation. Successful control of ICP and CPP following hypoxic-encephlopathic injury will not ensure intact neurologic survival. Sustained late increases in ICP are indicative of a profound primary neurologic insult. ICP monitoring in this patient population is used more for prognostication than to avert further neurologic injury (Dean & McComb, 1981; Nussbaum & Galant, 1983).

While an ICP greater than 15 indicates reduced adaptive capacity, a normal ICP does not reliably reflect normal intracranial compliance or adequate adaptive capacity. To determine intracranial compliance or identify where the patient is on the V/P curve, direct or indirect volume/pressure response testing is helpful.

With direct compliance testing, an intensivist injects 0.1 to 1 mL of sterile normal saline without preservative into an intraventricular catheter (IVC) and notes the resultant change in ICP. Although unreliable with enlarged ventricles, the value derived is the ratio of change in ICP to the amount of volume introduced. Miller (1976) noted that reduced cerebral adaptive capacity was present when an injection of approximately 7% of the intracranial volume into an IVC caused a increase in the mean ICP of greater than 4 mmHg/mL. Similar information can be obtained by removing CSF. Currently, indirect methods of testing intracranial compliance are more common because of the potential risks of adding volume into a tight intracranial compartment and infection related to opening the system.

Indirect compliance testing involves trending the patient's response to procedures known to increase ICP. All nursing interventions to some extent affect intracranial pressure in the patient with reduced adaptive capacity. A significant response is defined as a 10-mmHg increase in intracranial pressure lasting more than 3 minutes. The intensivist may also elect to apply unilateral or bilateral internal jugular compression or abdominal pressure to provide a rapidly reversible unquantified volume challenge to the intracranial space.

ICP Monitoring Systems

ICP can be monitored from a variety of locations: intraventricular, intraparenchymal, subarachnoid space, epidural space, and the anterior fontanelle. ICP monitoring systems include either fluid-coupled or fiberoptic systems. Fluid-coupled systems have been used successfully for many years to monitor both intraventricular and subarachnoid pressures. Fiberoptic systems now provide extremely accurate monitoring of ICP from numerous locations, including intraventricular, intraparenchymal, subarachnoid, epidural, and anterior fontanelle pressures.

Fluid-coupled systems are similar to traditional hemodynamic monitoring systems but do not contain a slow continuous infusion device. When used, they should be as uncomplicated as possible and consist of noncompliant Luer-locked tubing of the shortest possible length between the patient and transducer (Fig. 12–20). To prevent cortical necrosis, the system is primed with normal saline without heparin or preservatives.

When calculating CPP, controversy exists on where to reference fluid-coupled transducers. As with hemodynamic monitoring, transducers 1 inch out of position will produce a 2-mmHg deviation in measure-

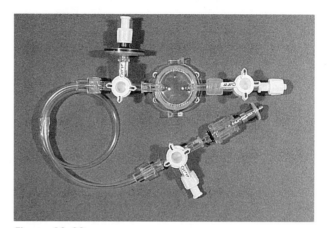

Figure 12–20 ● ● ● ● ● ●
Fluid-coupled bolt system.

ment, higher readings when the transducer is too low and lower readings when the transducer is too high. In the research laboratory setting, most patients are flat with the ICP and MAP transducer leveled at the right atrium. In the clinical setting, most ICP transducers are positioned at an area that approximates the lateral ventricle, either at the external auditory meatus or at the top of a triangle formed by the external auditory meatus, outer canthus of the eye, and behind the hairline. In the clinical setting, care is typically provided with the head of the bed elevated. When the head of the bed is elevated, two different reference points are created: the ICP transducer at the head and the MAP transducer at the right atrium. In this position, ICP may be underestimated and the CPP overestimated. While transducer placement continues to depend upon personal preference, whatever reference point is used, it is extremely important that it be consistent and that the monitored data be used to trend changes in ICP and not as independent decision points. Consistency in readings can be enhanced if the ICP transducer is attached to the head dressing or secured to a fixed position, for example, an armboard that rests upon the patient's shoulder.

With fluid-coupled systems, damped waveforms may result from problems in the fluid path between the patient and transducer. System problems include loose connections, fractures in the plastic components of the line, air bubbles, kinks, and incorrect scale. Occasionally, the system may require tensing with 0.10 to 0.25 normal saline without preservative due to the dissipation of fluid within the system. Fluid-filled systems require recalibration every shift or whenever the position of the transducer is changed.

Fiberoptic systems use catheters that are light-sending and -receiving systems that respond to the movement of a mirror-diaphragm located at the tip. Light is analyzed by a microcomputer and converted to an analog signal that displays the mean ICP. The Ladd sensor and the Camino catheter are two fiberoptic systems that are currently available.

The Ladd fiberoptic sensor (Princeton Medical Cor-

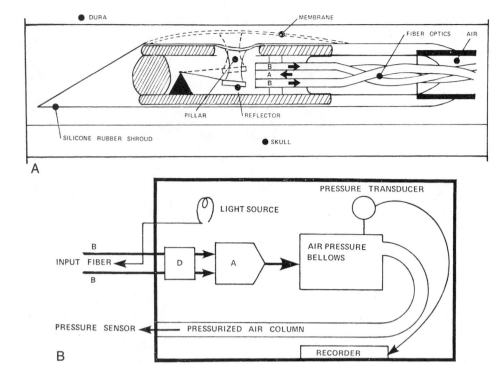

A

B

Figure 12-21 ● ● ● ● ● ●

Ladd fiberoptic sensor. *A,* Cross-section of the pressure sensor. A, input fiber; B, output fiber; *arrows* indicate direction of light. *B,* Monitor control unit. B, output fiber; D, photocell light detectors; A, amplifier. (From Ivan, L.O., Choo, S.H., Ventureyra, E.C.G. (1980). Intracranial pressure monitoring with the fiberoptic transducer in children. *Child's Brain,* 7, 303–313. S. Karger AG, Basel.)

poration, Hudson, NH) consists of a pressure-sensitive membrane with a miniature mirror mounted on its surface (Fig. 12–21). Three fiberoptic columns, contained within a pneumatic tube, connect the sensor to the monitor. Light is transmitted to the mirror, and the monitor compares the amount of light reflected back. The Ladd fiberoptic sensor is used to monitor ICP from the epidural space and/or anterior fontanelle.

The Camino fiberoptic system (Camino Laboratories, San Diego, CA) is a disposable 4F catheter with a miniaturized fiberoptic transducer at the tip (Fig. 12–22). The portable Camino monitor interfaces with a conventional monitoring system for waveform display. Unlike the Ladd, the Camino catheter can be placed at any number of locations: intraventricular, intraparenchymal, subarachnoid, epidural, or the fontanelle. Unlike any fluid-coupled system, the Camino catheter uniquely allows direct intraparenchymal monitoring, providing extremely clear recordings of ICP waveforms (Ostrup, Luerssen, Marshall, Zornow, 1987).

Similar to fluid-coupled systems, advantages and disadvantages vary according to fiberoptic placement. Fiberoptic systems eliminate the need for a fluid path, which typically requires frequent intervention that may place the patient at a higher risk of infection. Because the transducer is located in the tip of the catheter, there is no concern about where to level the transducer. Another advantage is that the fiberoptic catheter slips through the IVC, so that CSF can be drained while also obtaining ICP measurements. One disadvantage is that the fiberoptic catheter requires gentle handling, especially during

insertion and manipulation. The rigid catheter stands straight up from the point of insertion, so it must be protected (Hollingsworth-Fridlund, Vos, Daily, 1988).

Each Camino catheter is calibrated by the manufacturer and is not adjustable. Prior to insertion, the catheter's zero is matched to the Camino monitor by turning a screw at the hub of the catheter. Anytime afterwards, the Camino monitor zero and calibration are matched to the bedside monitor by depressing the "CAL" button on the Camino monitor and simultaneously adjusting the bedside monitor. Once inserted, the catheter cannot be rezeroed; zero drift

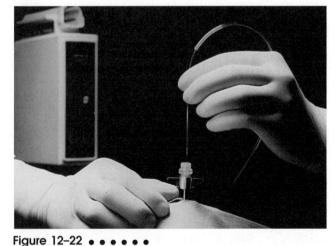

Figure 12-22 ● ● ● ● ● ●

Camino fiberoptic system. (Courtesy of Camino Laboratories, San Diego, CA.)

is much less than the reported 3 mmHg/24 hours (Hollingsworth-Fridlund, Vos, & Daily, 1988).

Another disadvantage is the cost of purchasing an additional monitor. However, the cost may be justified by the other advantages of the system and because the monitor is portable, allowing continuous ICP monitoring during high-risk patient transport.

Intraventricular Catheter

An intraventricular catheter (IVC) is a radiopaque catheter placed within a lateral ventricle for the purpose of ICP monitoring. The IVC provides high-quality waveforms and is considered the "gold standard" of ICP monitoring unless error is introduced through the measurement system.

Under local anesthesia, a radiopaque IVC is inserted through a burr hole on the non-dominant side at the intersection of the level of the pupil and external auditory meatus in the area of the coronal suture. The right side is usually chosen until hand dominance can be identified after 3 years of age. During insertion, the head is steadied; the patient will feel pressure and hear the sound of the turning drill. The IVC is inserted into the frontal horn of the lateral ventricle using a stylet. This area is chosen because it has little or no choroid plexus, which may obstruct the IVC, and also avoids penetration of vital brain areas. Location is verified when CSF is returned. If a fluid-coupled system is used, the stylet is removed and the IVC is tunneled 2 to 3 cm under the scalp and brought out through a separate incision. The separate incision allows the natural defenses of the skin to prevent organisms from gaining access to the CNS. This level of protection is not possible with a Camino IVC. The Camino fiberoptic system is secured directly into the bolt attachment, which is screwed into the skull.

Unlike other ICP monitoring devices, an IVC allows access for CSF sampling, drainage, intrathecal medication, and direct compliance testing. Disadvantages of the IVC include a 1% incidence of catheter-related brain trauma, that is, creation of an epileptic focus or intracranial bleed. Risk of infection—ventriculitis, encephalitis, and meningitis—has been reported to range between 0% and 27% (Mayhill, Archer, Lamb, Spadora, Baggett, Ward, & Narayan, 1984).

Mayhill and others (1984) conducted a prospective study of ventriculostomy-related infections. Identified risk factors for ventriculostomy-related infections included intracerebral hemorrhage with intraventricular hemorrhage, irrigation of the system, ICP greater than 20 mmHg, IVC in for more than 5 days, and neurosurgical operations. Previous ventriculostomy does not increase the risk of infection. There were no significant differences in the incidence of infection when the catheter was inserted in the ICU or operating room. The researchers suggested that ventriculostomy-related infections could be decreased by maintenance of a closed system and early removal of the IVC. If ICP monitoring is required for more

than 5 days, Mayhill and others (1984) recommended that the system should be removed and reinserted at a different site.

In contrast, Kanter and others (1985) reported that after 6 days there was a significant decrease in the infection rate of ICP monitoring devices. These researchers felt that infection was introduced at the time of insertion of the ICP monitoring device. To decrease the incidence of infection, these researchers suggest using a single ICP monitoring device as long as necessary unless malfunction occurred or daily surveillance cultures demonstrated infection.

When the ventricles are compressed or shifted, it may be difficult to place the IVC. Collapsed ventricles are not considered a contraindication to catheter placement, as pressures may be adequately monitored as long as waveforms remain distinct. Occlusion difficulties may occur when the IVC itself becomes occluded with debris from the ependymal lining of the ventricles or when the CSF is bloody or high in protein.

Controlled CSF Venting. Reduction of CSF volume is accomplished through controlled continuous or intermittent CSF drainage. To avoid ventricular collapse, drainage is accomplished against a positive-pressure gradient of at least 15 mmHg. To accomplish this, the intraventricular drainage system drip chamber is placed approximately 27 cm above the reference point of the external auditory meatus. In this position, CSF will automatically drain when the ICP is greater than 20 mmHg. (As mercury is 13.6 times heavier than H_2O, 1 mmHg is equal to 1.36 cm H_2O.) Care is taken to avoid the risk of uncontrolled CSF loss with incorrect stopcock position or drainage position.

Intermittent CSF venting follows preset guidelines that include (1) the level of ICP at which to initiate drainage, usually greater than 15 mmHg after nursing measures to decrease ICP are unsuccessful (see Chapter 21, Neurologic Critical Care Problems); (2) the frequency of drainage, usually every hour; (3) the time interval for drainage, usually 5 minutes; and (4) the maximal amount of CSF, which depends upon CSF production and degree of obstruction. Some institutions prescribe CSF drainage at a rate that matches the rate of CSF production. This is approximately 0.35 mL/minute or 21 mL/hour in an adolescent and 0.30 mL/minute or 18 mL/hour in a young child. A regimen such as this may avoid ventricular collapse with ICP spikes. Drainage also provides a check for IVC patency. Because the amount of drainage reflects the degree of ventricular obstruction, the amount and character of CSF drainage are trended over time. Care is taken to clamp the drainage system prior to changes in the patient's head position in relation to the drainage device (Tilem & Greenberg, 1988).

Subarachnoid Bolt

There are many different types of subarachnoid bolts: for example, the Richmond screw, Philly bolt,

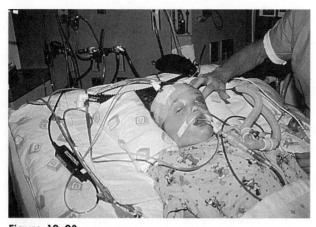

Figure 12–23 • • • • • •
Patient monitoring with a Camino fiberoptic system.

and Leeds screw. In consideration of the thinner skull of infants and children, pediatric bolts are usually shorter (3.5–5 mm) compared with the adult length (5–8 mm) and lighter in weight, consisting of either metal or plastic. Silastic rings are sometimes used to support the longer bolt within the thin pediatric cranial table.

The subarachnoid bolt is inserted under local anesthesia using a twist drill hole in the non-dominant prefrontal cranium behind the hair line 2 cm anterior to the coronal suture. This area is chosen because it is accessible and does not interfere with head rotation. Because the skull and dura lack innervation, only local anesthesia for incisional pain is necessary.

After the bolt is threaded though the skull, the lumen is flushed with normal saline to clear bone fragments and blood. The dura is then widely opened with a spinal needle to allow communication with the subarachnoid space.

Advantages of the subarachnoid bolt include ease of insertion and avoidance of brain tissue penetration (Nussbaum & Maggi, 1985). Disadvantages include bolt-related brain trauma. Although the bolt is less invasive than an IVC, the bolt carries a rare risk of subdural hematoma. Risk of infection is low before 5

days but exponentially increases after 2 weeks or if a subdural hematoma is present (Aucoin, Kotilainen, Gantz, Davidson, Kellogg, Stone, 1986).

Fixation can be difficult in the pediatric patient. The thread on the bolt must match the cranial table. The bolt requires an intact skull, which limits its use when significant skull fractures are present. Also, the accuracy of the subarachnoid bolt in the presence of open fontanelles is unknown. When ICP is high, occlusion difficulties may result from herniation of brain tissue into the bolt. In this circumstance, the bolt may under-read ICP when it is elevated (Mendelow, Rowan, Murray, & Keer, 1983). Finally, the bolt does not permit direct compliance testing or provide an access for CSF drainage.

Intraparenchymal Monitoring

The Camino catheter has redefined the standard in ICP monitoring; high-fidelity ICP waveforms can be recorded from brain tissue. Intraparenchymal monitoring using the Camino catheter has replaced fluid-coupled subarachnoid bolts in many centers (Fig. 12–23).

The Camino catheter allows direct monitoring of intraparenchymal pressures. Catheter insertion is similar to that of a subarachnoid bolt. Once the bolt is placed, the fiberoptic catheter is inserted through the bolt into the brain parenchyma approximately 0.5 to 1 cm beyond the surface of the dura. To prevent kinking or dislocation, the catheter is looped and attached to the head dressing.

Epidural Monitoring

The Ladd fiberoptic sensor is used to monitor ICP from the epidural space. Inserted through a frontal burr hole, the 10 mm × 1 mm sensor is slipped under the skull so that the sensor membrane rests on intact dura. Ivan, Choo, and Ventureyra (1980) recommend that 3 cm around the edge of the burr hole be stripped from the skull's inner table to prevent a wedge effect (Fig. 12–24). The skin is closed and cable secured to scalp.

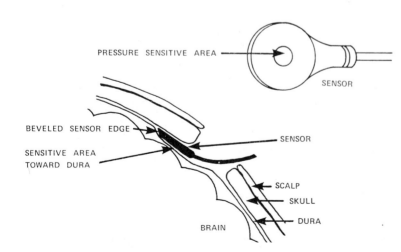

Figure 12–24 • • • • • •
Ladd sensor inserted through a frontal burr hole. (From Ivan, L.O., Choo, S.H., Ventureyra, E.C.G. (1980). Intracranial pressure monitoring with the fiberoptic transducer in children. *Child's Brain* 7, 303–313. S. Karger AG, Basel.)

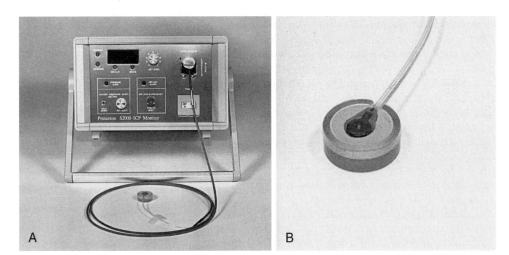

Figure 12–25 ● ● ● ● ● ●

A, Princeton fiberoptic ICP monitor. *B,* Peabody disc holder. (Courtesy of Princeton Medical Corporation, Hudson, NH.)

Advantages of epidural ICP monitoring include ease of insertion and, because the dura is left intact, decreased risk of infection and hemorrhage. The major disadvantage of the system is questionable accuracy. Epidural ICP readings tend to exceed other methods of measurement, especially at higher ICP. This may be minimized by adequate stripping of dura from the skull's inner table or by using epidural ICP data to establish trend information only. Newer sensors provide greater stability and accuracy of readings and are relatively drift-free. Also, disconnection will not affect calibration. Other disadvantages include lack of access for CSF drainage and direct compliance testing and the additional cost of a separate monitor.

Anterior Fontanelle Monitoring

The Ladd fiberoptic transducer can be easily applied to the anterior fontanelle to provide indirect ICP measurements (Vidyasagar & Raju, 1977). The hair is shaved over the anterior fontanelle, and the sensor is applied gently to the skin and held in place by a 4 × 4 cm soft compliant self-adhesive foam material (Hill & Volpe, 1981).

The advantage of using the anterior fontanelle to monitor ICP is that it is noninvasive, simple, and provides useful data trends. Disadvantages of the system are related to its questionable accuracy. ICP measurements are influenced by the amount of external pressure applied to the sensor. Hill and Volpe (1981) then Colditz and others (1988) devised application methods that correlate extremely well (r = .99) with simultaneous IVC measurements. More recently, the Peabody Disc Holder for the fiberoptic sensor head (Princeton Medical Corporation, Hudson, NH) has been developed to correct variation in the amount of external pressure applied to the transducer (Fig. 12–25).

In addition, sudden increases in ICP may not be recorded accurately due to pressure damping because of the inherent limitation in response time of the monitor and unknown compliance characteristics of the fontanelle. The data tend to under-read high ICP. This method also does not allow direct compliance testing or CSF access, and there is an additional cost of the monitor.

ICP Waveform Analysis

ICP waveforms mimic in shape, but are of lower amplitude than the arterial waveform (Fig. 12–26). Respiratory fluctuations alter the baseline through transference of pressure through the venous system. Waveform clarity depends upon the location of the device and the monitoring system used. Because of narrow intracranial pulse pressures, ICP is monitored in the mean mode. The scale that permits adequate waveform definition, usually 20 to 40 mmHg, is used.

The ICP waveform has three or more descending sawtooth peaks. The first three components are always present. Additional peaks vary and are thought to be caused by retrograde venous pulsations. Their clinical significance has not been established. P1, the percussion wave, is a sharp, fairly consistent peak generated primarily by the arterial pulsations of the choroid plexus that are modified by the viscoelastic properties of the brain. P2, the rebound or tidal wave, is variable in shape, ending on the dicrotic notch. P3, the dicrotic wave, immediately follows the notch,

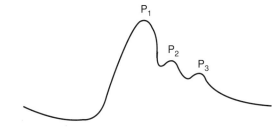

Figure 12–26 ● ● ● ● ● ●

ICP waveforms. (From McQuillian, K.A. (1991). *AACN's Clinical Issues in Critical Care Nursing,* 2 (4), 623–636.)

tapering down to the diastolic portion unless retrograde pulsations add a few more peaks.

Waveform changes have been associated with decreased adaptive capacity (Price, 1981). With cerebral vasodilation, the pulse wave becomes less restrained by the arterioles and is allowed to pass to the compliant capillaries and veins. Signs of decreased adaptive capacity include a P2 equal to or higher than P1, followed by an increase in the waveform pulse pressure (Fig. 12–27). If compliance continues to decrease, the diastolic component will elevate and the waveform will become rounder; then, at higher ICPs, it will assume a triangular shape (Cardoso, Rowan, Galbraith, 1983). Given the predictable, evolving waveform pattern that indicates decreased intracranial compliance (Germon, 1988), rapid therapeutic interventions and environmental adjustment should be possible. Additional nursing research is necessary to confirm this.

ICP Trend Recordings

In addition to continuous ICP waveform assessment, trend recordings (25 mm/min) enable detection of baseline elevations over time, correlation of ICP with therapeutic interventions, and identification of Lundberg A, B, and C waves (Fig. 12–28).

A waves or plateau waves are spontaneous, rapid, irregular increases in ICP 50 to 100 mmHg over baseline lasting 5 to 20 minutes per wave followed by a rapid decrease in ICP. *A* waves progress through four phases generated by a complex interaction between systemic arterial pressure, intracranial compliance, and cerebrovascular autoregulation (Bergman, 1992). The *A* wave begins with the *drift phase,* which is characterized by a progressive decrease in mean arterial pressure. The *plateau phase* follows as hypotension decreases the CPP, stimulating autoregulatory cerebral vasodilation and resulting in an increase in cerebral blood volume and ICP. The *ischemic phase* ensues when progressive cerebral hypertension produces brainstem ischemia and activates the Cushing's response to increase both MAP then CPP. The *resolution phase* terminates the *A* wave when cerebral perfusion improves, decreasing cerebral vasodilation, cerebral blood volume, and ICP.

A waves are clinically significant, reliably signaling reduced intracranial compliance. The more square the shape of the wave, the greater the reduction in intracranial compliance. *A* waves are associated with impaired cerebral blood flow. Patients with cerebral hypertension die of diminished cerebral perfusion during plateau waves. *A* waves may be accompanied by transient neurologic deficits, for example, pupil dilation, headache, and vegetative responses, which include sweating, flushing, and/or bradycardia.

B waves are sharp rhythmic increases in ICP to 50 mmHg lasting 30 seconds to 2 minutes. *B* waves may precede *A* waves, indicating a progressive loss of cerebral compliance. *B* waves may occur prior to a seizure; during headache, posturing, or isometric movement; or accompany respiratory compromise and decreased level of consciousness.

C waves are normal rhythmic ICP fluctuations associated with respirations. They are considered be-

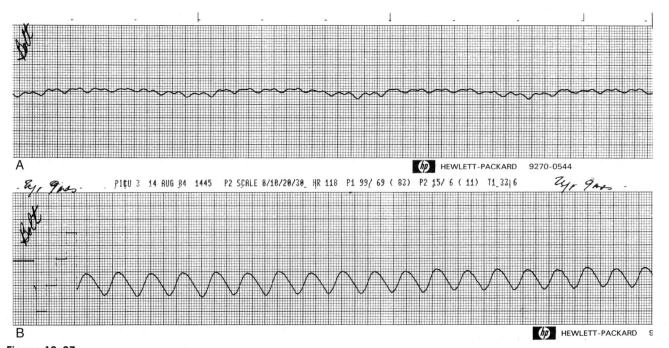

Figure 12–27 ● ● ● ● ●

Signs of decreased adaptive capacity include a P2 equal to or higher than P1 followed by an increase in the waveform pulse pressure. Two-year, 9-month toddler with decreased cerebral compliance. Note waveform change from *A* to *B*.

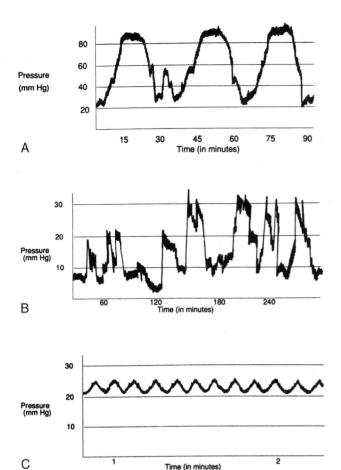

Figure 12–28 ● ● ● ● ●

A to C, Lundberg A, B, and C waves. (From McQuillian, K.A. (1991). *AACN's Clinical Issues in Critical Care Nursing,* 2 (4), 623–636.)

nign but may indicate an increase in venous pressure and/or a decrease in venous outflow.

Monitoring ICP trends allows a proactive management of cerebral hypertension. Anticipating care by using an individualized protocol to decrease ICP may prevent secondary neuronal injury. Pressure waves greater than 20 mmHg, lasting for more than a few minutes, especially if associated with a change in neurologic status or the inability to maintain CPP greater than 50 mmHg or ICP less than 15 mmHg, require *immediate* intervention. Occult seizure activity should be considered as a potential problem when increased ICP is unresponsive to standard management.

Nursing Implications

Priorities for the nursing care of patients who require ICP monitoring implications include (1) keeping the ICP monitoring system intact and operational; (2) ensuring the accuracy of the data; and (3) limiting iatrogenic injury. Both ICP and CPP are constantly assessed throughout any intervention in

order to evaluate the patient's response to therapy. Trends in patient tolerance of care are noted over time.

The accuracy of data obtained from ICP monitoring is assessed from waveform analysis. Good-quality tracings correspond with good measurements, unless the transducer is leveled inaccurately when using fluid-coupled systems. ICP measurements should always correlate with the neurologic examination and appropriately reflect clinical interventions.

Because the cranium is compartmentalized, Weaver and others (1982) found significant differences in ICP measurements (using a fluid-coupled subarachnoid bolt) between the ipsilateral and contralateral side of a focal supratentorial lesion. They recommend that supratentorial subarachnoid pressure be measured ipsilateral to the site of the focal lesion. Pressure increases in nonpathogenic compartments occur only after herniation. Note that with the fiberoptic system, intraparenchymal pressures more accurately reflect ipsilateral and contralateral pressures (Crutchfield, Narayan, Robertson, & Michael, 1990).

IVC and bolts measure supratentorial pressure. Patients with a posterior fossa mass or infratentorial lesion must be observed carefully for the development of respiratory and cardiovascular distress even when normal/low supratentorial ICP is present.

Contraindications to ICP monitoring are few and include a history of bleeding, current anticoagulant therapy, and/or scalp infection. When these conditions are present, the potential risks of ICP monitoring may outweigh the potential benefits.

Currently, there is lack of nursing research to guide clinical practice in the care of patients with these devices. Protocols usually reflect central line protocols. It seems reasonable that ICP devices function under different principles because they exist within a system protected by the blood-brain barrier. The blood-brain barrier limits high antibiotic and immunoglobulin concentration, so there may be added risk of infection.

Until nursing research is available, some recommendations can be made. Site care includes use of an occlusive dry sterile dressing. Dressings are changed every 48 to 72 hours to inspect the insertion site for signs and symptoms of infection and CSF leakage.

Currently, there are no data to suggest that ICP monitor tubing should be changed with the same frequency as arterial and venous pressure lines (Hickman, Mayer, & Muwaswes, 1990). Strict aseptic technique is used whenever the system is opened. Prior to insertion, the monitoring system is prepared in a non-traveled area wearing masks and gloves. All systems should be maintained as closed systems and left intact unless contaminated.

The diagnosis of ventriculitis or meningitis is made on the basis of positive CSF cultures. Mayhill and others (1984) found that CSF pleocytosis was more significantly related to the diagnosis of ventriculitis or meningitis than were fever and leukocytosis. Because of the low predictive value of fever and leukocytosis, CSF cell counts and cultures are obtained daily. Currently, research does not support the potential benefits of using prophylactic antibiotics either systemically, in line, or at the incisional area (Mayhill, Archer, Lamb, Spadora, Baggett, Ward, & Narayan, 1984; Aucoin, Kotilainen, Gantz, Davidson, Kellogg, & Stone, 1986).

MONITORING CEREBRAL FUNCTION

While ICP monitoring provides information about the neurologic environment, EEG and evoked potential monitoring provides information about actual neurologic functioning. The ability to assess neuronal function is critical, especially when the clinical examination is clouded by therapy; for example, when chemical paralysis is used to control ventilation.

Continuous EEG Monitoring

Continuous bedside EEG monitoring provides information about the spontaneous electrical activity produced by the outer 20% or 6-mm surface of cerebral cortex located near the electrodes. The EEG does not provide information on white matter or brainstem function.

EEG monitoring is most frequently used in the PICU for identification of seizure activity (Fig. 12–29A). Undetected and untreated seizure activity can result in neuronal death (Delgado-Escueta, Wasterlain, Treiman, & Porter, 1982). Continuous EEG monitoring is also essential when managing therapeutic barbiturate coma (Sloan, 1988). Barbiturate coma is used to suppress cerebral metabolic rate and requirements. The goal of barbiturate coma is burst suppression—electrical activity progressing to an isoelectric line, then resumption of electrical activity (Fig. 12–29B). Length of burst suppression depends upon drug levels; the higher the level, the longer the isoelectric line. When barbiturate coma is used to manage intractable seizures, cerebral dysactivity is suppressed completely in order to permit the return of normal activity (Orlowski, Erenberg, Lueders, & Cruse, 1989). If inadequate barbiturate doses are used, the therapeutic benefit may not be realized; whereas if excessive doses are used, cardiovascular instability may result.

EEG monitoring also permits direct visualization of the effects of compromised cerebral blood flow associated with significant episodes of cerebral hypertension. When cerebral blood flow is compromised, normal EEG rhythms are reduced in both amplitude and frequency (Sloan, 1988). An isoelectric EEG results when cerebral blood flow is less than 12 to 15 mL/100 g/minute (Fig. 12–29C) (Wiznitzer, 1990).

EEGs also provide a prognostic tool to predict return of cognitive function after an hypoxic-ischemic injury. Poor neurologic outcomes have been correlated with slower frequencies, amplitude suppression, and a static EEG frequency spectrum over time

(Filloux, Dean, Kirsch, 1992). In the absence of barbiturates, burst suppression is a ominous finding after a major hypoxic-ischemic injury to the brain (Johnston, 1992). Although not absolute in drug overdose or hypothermia, cerebral silence (as evidenced by an isoelectric EEG) has been used as a criterion for brain death. EEG activity may persist in some patients with cortical necrosis; survival is possible because EEGs do not assess brainstem activity.

Waveform Analysis

EEG waveforms are described in terms of frequency, amplitude, velocity, distribution, regularity, and specific pattern (Table 12–14, p. 377). The EEG traditionally records voltage over time from 16 channels. Waveform frequency is described in hertz (Hz) or cycles per second. Waveform amplitude, measured from peak to peak, is described in microvolts (μV). Waveform velocity describes the rate of climb and descent of waves; for example, a spike has a duration less than 80 milliseconds, whereas a sharp wave has a longer duration.

As noted in Table 12–14, waveforms correlate with level of consciousness and range from high frequency–low amplitude to low frequency–high amplitude. Background alpha activity is regulated by brainstem neurons know as "pacemaker" cells. Right and left hemispheric symmetry is analyzed by assessing lead pairs clustered down the EEG page.

EEG interpretation is complex, especially in the pediatric population, where individual maturational factors complicate EEG interpretation. For example, in the newborn, cortical activity is irregular in frequency and incidence. Asymmetry and asynchrony may be normal throughout infancy. Alpha rhythms are slow to develop and may not reach adult range until 10 to 12 years of age (Wiznitzer, 1990).

Seizure activity begins with a change in background activity, followed by generalized low-voltage fast activity, which increases in amplitude and slows in frequency. This pattern progresses to generalized polyspikes and wave patterns from 1 to 4 Hz (Orlowski & Rothner, 1992). Different seizure classes generate specific spike and wave patterns. As expected, focal seizures are asymmetric. Focal seizures with secondary generalization can be identified and tracked on the EEG. Postictal activity can be identified as diffuse depression of background activity.

EEG analysis depends upon pattern recognition placed in the context of the patient's changing clinical picture. Accurate interpretation requires years of experience and analysis of enormous amounts of data. This tends to make 16-channel EEG analysis impractical in the PICU.

Two-lead bipolar (pairs) systems can screen for seizure activity (Fig. 12–30). These single-channel systems use five electrodes: two placed over each mastoid process, two placed over each temporal area, and one ground electrode placed over the middle of the forehead. Esposito and Westgate (1987) describe using the Siemens EEG cassette in a PICU setting.

Text continued on page 377

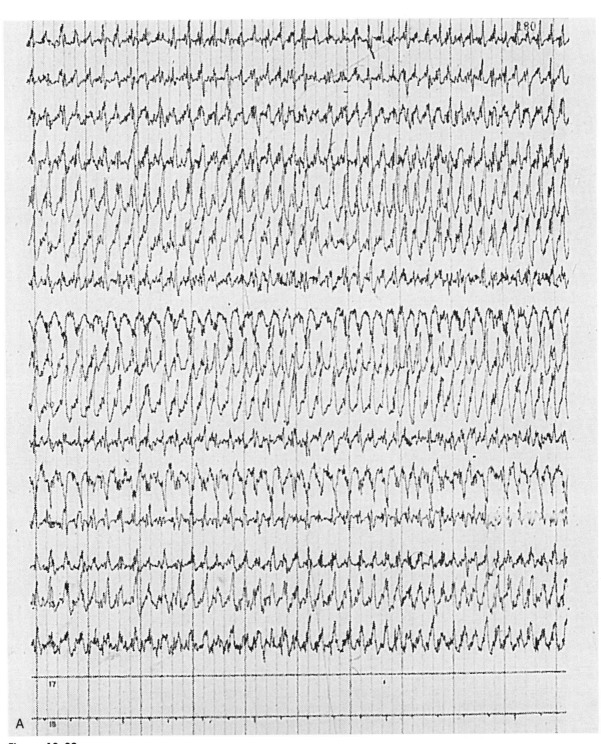

Figure 12–29 ● ● ● ● ● ●

A, Seizure activity.

Illustration continued on following page

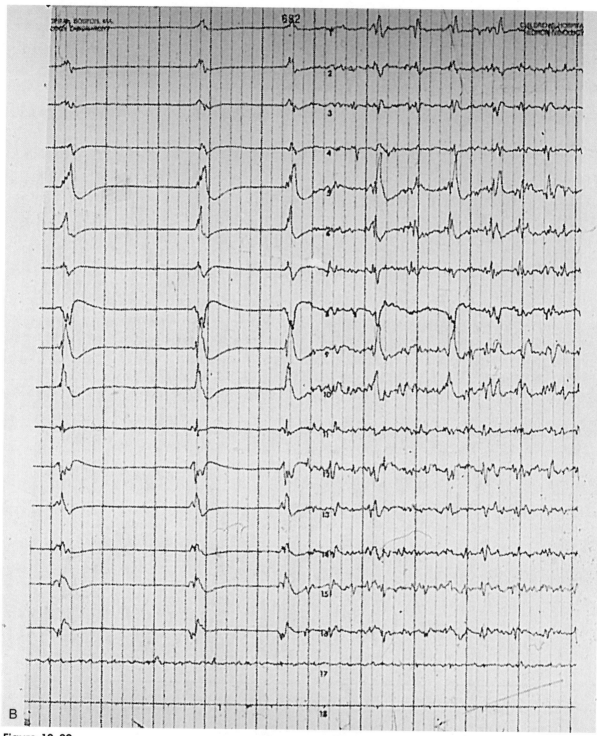

Figure 12–29 ● ● ● ● ● ●

Continued B, Burst suppression—electrical activity progressing to an isoelectric line, then resumption of electrical activity.

Illustration continued on opposite page

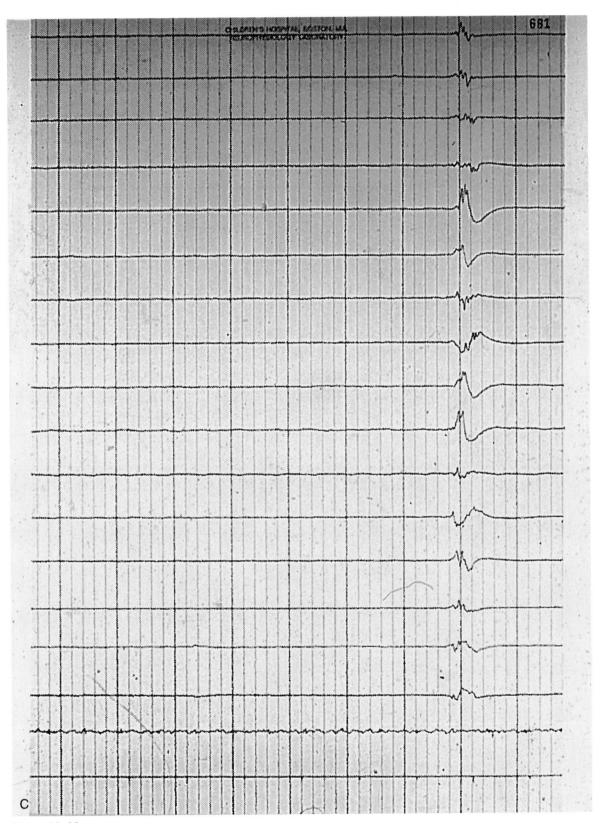

Figure 12–29 ● ● ● ● ● ●

Continued C, Isoelectric EEG.

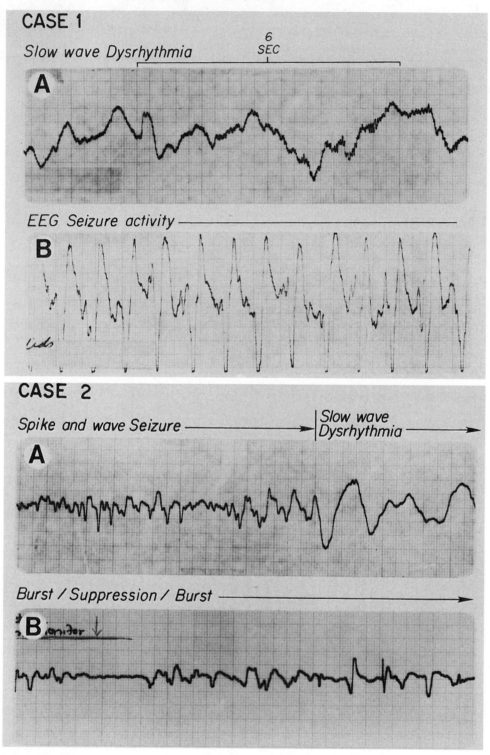

Figure 12–30 ● ● ● ● ● ●

Two-lead bipolar (pairs) systems. (From Esposito, N., & Westgate, P. (1987). *Journal of Pediatric Nursing, 2* (4), 272–277.)

Table 12-14. EEG WAVEFORMS

Rhythm	Frequency (Cycle/sec)	Amplitude (Peak–Peak)	Area	State	Waveform
Beta	13–30Hz	10–20 uV Intermittent	Frontal and Central	Awake Eyes Open	
Alpha	8–13Hz	Infant: 20uV Child: 75 uV Adult: 50 uV	Dominant rhythm of Occipital and Parietal	Awake Eyes Closed	
Theta	4–7Hz	Child: 50 uV Adult: 10 uV	Temporal or Central area in children to age 3	Drowsiness Encephalopathies	
Delta	1–4Hz	100 uV	Frontal	4th stage sleep—coma Structural lesions Normal in young children	

This system will reflect EEG activity only within close proximity of the electrode pairs, one set at a time.

Processed EEG Recordings

Processed EEG recordings are useful for continuous monitoring in the critical care setting because they allow rapid assessment and trending of basic, yet important, parameters. Used only as a trending device, processed EEG recordings do not replace the need for periodic 16-channel EEG assessment.

First-generation processed EEG monitors include the *Cerebral Function Monitor* (CFM; Criticon Inc., Tampa, FL). This system is a single-channel, single-lead bipolar trend recording of EEG amplitude and variability. Three electrodes are used—one placed over each parietal area, and one ground electrode placed over the frontal area. The lower printout records amplitude: 0 to 10 µV, then 10 to 100 µV. The upper printout records frequency: top = 0Hz; bottom = 16 Hz. The paper speed condenses about 2 minutes of EEG activity into a 1-cm tracing. Two characteristics are assessed: the overall amplitude, reflecting the average of cortical activity; and the width, reflecting the degree of variability in cortical activity. High, wide tracings indicate high EEG voltages with considerable variability in peak-peak amplitude. Conversely, a low, narrow tracing results from low voltage with little variability in amplitude. The limitation of this system is that it cannot assess regional activity because only two leads are used.

The CFM is helpful in the PICU to assess EEG trends and identify classic EEG patterns (Stidham, Nugent, & Rogers, 1980). For example, episodic high-voltage activity suggests the presence of seizure activity. Progressive increase in EEG amplitude correlates with improved neurologic outcome following a hypoxic-ischemic event; the opposite is associated with a poor neurologic outcome. Presence of EEG activity during periods of increased ICP suggests that adequate cerebral perfusion pressure is maintained (Sloan, 1988). Finally, a "comb" pattern indicates burst suppression (Talwar & Torres, 1988).

Another first-generation processed EEG recorder is *compressed spectral array* (CSA). Here, raw EEG data are rearranged from voltages versus time to amplitude versus frequency during a sampling period (Fig. 12–31). Frequency is on the horizontal axis with delta waves on the left and beta waves on the right. The power spectrum is then plotted and stacked vertically into a three-dimensional representation for trend analysis.

Because CSA compresses a significant amount of data, critical events may be smoothed together, including, for example, burst suppression and seizure activity. Like the CFM, CSA is helpful in the assessment of EEG trends and identification of classic patterns. CSA is particularly helpful in the prediction of outcome from coma. A fluctuating frequency spectrum carries a more favorable prognosis than an invariable type (Cant & Shaw, 1984).

Aperiodic analysis, *Lifescan* (Neurometrics, Inc., San Diego, CA), is considered a second-generation processed EEG recorder. Aperiodic analysis assesses each wave vector and displays it in a three-dimensional glass box. Two sets of leads are used; the negative electrode is placed behind the ears, the positive electrode in the frontal area, and ground electrode in the center of the forehead. Frequency bands are positioned from left to right: 0.5 Hz to the left, and 30 Hz to the right. To enhance visualization, waves are color coded; beta waves are yellow, alpha waves are green, subalpha are magenta, theta are light blue, and delta waves are dark blue. Waveform amplitude is approximated by vector height. Time is

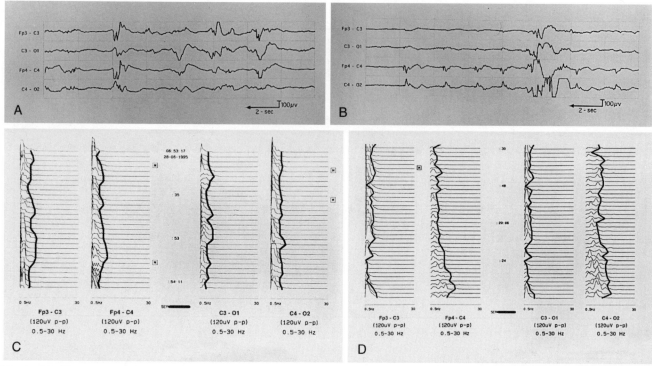

Figure 12–31 ● ● ● ● ● ●

A to D, Cerebral function monitor. *C,* Compressed spectral array (CSA) of raw EEG display shown in *A.* The CSA represents a 2-second update rate with a frequency band of .5 to 30 Hz. *D* presents a CSA of raw EEG display shown in *B.* At the onset of an electrographic seizure, the CSA increases in frequency as the spike and wave activity occurs.

expressed on the diagonal. The activity edge, a white line on the top of the each box, trends changes in both frequency and amplitude over time (Fig. 12–32).

The acronym SAFE can be used to systematically assess the Lifescan recording. "**S**" represents symmetry between the left and right cerebral hemispheres. "**A**" represents vector amplitude. "**F**" represents vector frequency. "**E**" represents activity edge. Vector height should vary over time and from one frequency to another. Vector distribution should also vary over time. The activity edge should reflect symmetry between the left and right hemisphere and vary symmetrically over time.

Narcotics will produce a gradual shift of the activity edge to the left, reflecting an increase in delta activity. Cerebral ischemia will also produce a left shift of the activity edge with a reduction in amplitude at all frequencies. Unilateral ischemia will produce an asymmetric shift to the left, whereas bilateral ischemia produces a symmetric shift to the left. Burst suppression will decrease alpha/beta activity and increase delta/theta activity. The activity edge will shift far to the left then back to the right. Alterations in temperature will produce high or low activity at all levels; the edge will shift bilaterally to the right or left.

Evoked Potential Monitoring

Evoked potential (EP) monitoring provides a computerized summation of the electrical potentials pro-

duced by specific neural pathways in response to an external stimulus. EP monitoring is useful because the nerve pathways tested are less sensitive to drug effects. In addition, the waveforms correlate to the anatomy of the sensory tracts. EP monitoring offers the possibility of assessing structures not seen with EEG (Fig. 12–33).

Each EP is a series of waves plotted as voltage versus time. The amplitude (voltage) and latencies (time) reflect conduction and processing of sensory information through the CNS. The EP is assessed for changes in the presence and absence of waves, individual latencies, interwave latencies, and relative amplitudes. Again, maturational factors are important because development affects interwave latencies in children less than 2 years of age (Mizrahi & Dorfman, 1980).

Loss of transmission or slowed conduction (increased latency) indicates functional injury related to cerebral hypoxia, compression, and/or other factors that affect cerebral metabolism. Decreased amplitudes are related to decreased cerebral blood flow. Loss of transmission after a particular wave identifies the specific level of dysfunction (Table 12–15).

There are three EP modes: visual, somatosensory, and auditory. Multimodal EPs (MEPs) assess several different tracts to provide specific information regarding various components of the CNS.

Generated by a flashing light, *visual evoked potentials* (VEP) assess the integrity of the retinal-occipital pathway. York and others (1981) found that in-

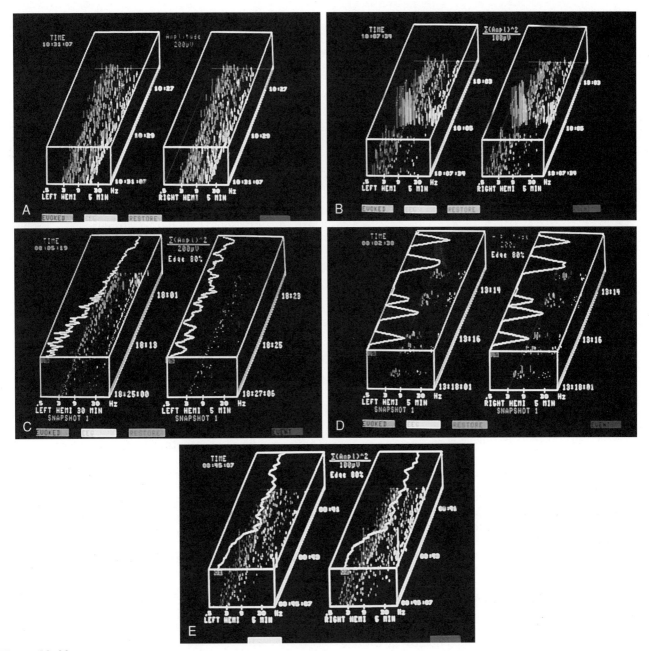

Figure 12–32 ● ● ● ● ● ●

Lifescan Brain Activity Monitor. *A*, Normal display. *B*, Seizure activity. *C*, Barbiturate coma. *D*, Burst suppression. *E*, Bilateral ischemic event. (Courtesy of Diatek Neurometrics, San Diego, CA.)

creases in ICP secondary to either cerebral edema or hydrocephalus produced characteristic alteration in VEPs (increased latency of wave N_2) through compression of intercerebral visual pathways. The relationship establishes a reliable noninvasive method of estimating ICP (York, Legan, Benner, & Watts, 1984).

Somatosensory evoked potentials (SEP) assess the integrity of the sensory pathways from the peripheral nerve to the sensory cortex from either the median nerve in the wrist or the posterior tibial nerve in the ankle to the cerebral hemispheres. SEP is useful in identifying the level of spinal cord injury. An absent

waveform below the region of spinal injury indicates a complete injury, whereas the presence of the wave indicates an incomplete lesion. Presence or return of SEPs often precede clinical improvement and offer a favorable prognosis.

Brainstem auditory evoked responses (BAER) are frequently used in the critically ill patient. BAERs measure the change in EP in the auditory pathways to the brainstem in response to a noise (click). Electrodes are placed on top of the head and in the external auditory meatus. After ensuring patency of the auditory canal and an intact tympanic membrane, repeated clicks are delivered through an ear-

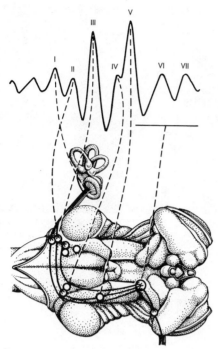

Figure 12–33 ● ● ● ● ● ●

Brainstem auditory evoked potentials (BAEP). Neural generations of the BAEP. It is most likely that each wave has components arising from different generators that include brainstem nuclei and white matter tracts. I to VII, waveforms. (From Wiznitzer, M. (1990). In J.L. Blumer (Ed.). *A practical guide to pediatric intensive care*. St. Louis: Mosby–Year Book.)

piece at about 10 Hz while "white noise" masks stimulation to the other ear. Click intensity is increased about 60 decibels above minimal hearing threshold. The signal is amplified 50,000 times, and averaging is performed over a 10-msec sweep after each click. Usually, over 2000 clicks are averaged.

The time measured from peak to peak, known as the interpeak latency, is unaffected by changes in the intensity of the stimulus and peripheral hearing apparatus. Normal BAERs suggest the absence of lesions when toxic or metabolic comas or a diffuse cortical process is present. BAERs are unaffected by barbiturates, so they are useful to monitor brainstem integrity during therapeutic coma. If BAERs are normal in the comatose patient, nursing care can be planned to provide appropriate auditory stimulation. Decreasing amplitude or increased latency of wave 5

indicates brainstem compression secondary to increased ICP. Loss of wave 5 indicates severe brainstem dysfunction and suggests central herniation. In brain death, BAERs are not conducted past wave 1. Brain death may also include wave 1, but the integrity of the peripheral auditory apparatus cannot be validated.

MEPs combine the use of several EPs for localization of defects and prognostic evaluation (Greenberg & Ducker, 1982). With brainstem dysfunction, SEPs and BAERs are abnormal, while VEPs are normal. With hemispheric dysfunction, VEPs and BAER and SEP *cortical* EPs are abnormal, but BAER and SEP *subcortical* EPs are normal (Fig. 12–34). If all EPs are dysfunctional, global dysfunction is probably present.

As a prognostic indicator in coma, 80% of patients with mild abnormalities in MEP awaken within 30 days and 90% of patients with mild EP abnormalities at 14 days make a good neurologic recovery (Sloan, 1988). Goodwin and others (1991) studied BAERs and SEPs in 41 children ranging in age from 6 weeks to 18 years. When assessing survivor outcome, determined both at discharge and by follow-up examination conducted 1 to 3 years later, no false pessimistic predictions had been made and only two were falsely optimistic.

EP limitations are present when ocular, auditory, or peripheral nerve disease is present. Also, EPs test only specific nerve tracts. The frontal lobes, cerebellum, and cognitive function are not tested.

Computerized processing of multilead EEG and EP allows total *brain mapping*. Moment-to-moment variations in the brain's spontaneous or evoked electrical activity is displayed on a computer monitor in the form of multi-colored maps. Different colors and color shades are used to indicate the magnitude of positive and negative EEG voltages simultaneously measured from various scalp locations. Mapping techniques can be useful in identifying functional abnormalities not distinguished by anatomic or metabolic studies.

Table 12–15 BRAINSTEM AUDITORY EVOKED POTENTIALS

Wave	Location	Level of Pathway
I	Acoustic nerve (CN VIII)	Peripheral receptor
II	Cochlear nuclei	Medulla
III	Superior olivary complex	Pons
IV	Lateral lemniscus	Mid to upper pons
V	Inferior colliculus	Midbrain
VI	Medial geniculate	Thalamus
VII	Auditory radiations	Thalamocortical

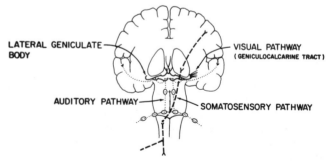

Figure 12–34 ● ● ● ● ● ●

Schematic view of sensory pathways involved in the generation of multimodality evoked potentials. The sensory input generating somatosensory and auditory evoked potentials traverses more caudal regions of the brainstem than does the sensory input for visual evoked potentials. (From *Journal of Neurosurgery*, Vol. 56, January 1982.)

NEURODIAGNOSTIC STUDIES

Under non-emergent circumstances, patient and family preparation precedes *all* procedures. Nursing responsibility includes augmenting the primary information provided by the attending physician. Specific concerns that are often addressed by nurses include how the procedure is performed, what the expectations of the patient will be during the procedure, what the patient will experience during the procedure, the anticipated response of the patient to the procedure, and how the parents might help the patient through the procedure.

A *lumbar puncture* involves the insertion of a spinal needle into the subarachnoid space for the purposes of measuring spinal fluid pressure and obtaining CSF for laboratory analysis (see Table 12–2 for normal CSF characteristics). During the procedure, the nurse continuously monitors the patient while helping the patient maintain a side-lying position with hips and neck flexed. Under local anesthesia, the spinal needle is inserted into the L3–L4 or L4–L5 vertebral interspace. A manometer is used to measure opening and closing spinal pressures. CSF samples are collected in tubes to allow visualization and laboratory analysis. Usually, CSF cell count and Gram's stain are obtained first, followed by CSF chemistries and then CSF culture.

A lumbar puncture should not be performed in patients at high risk for bleeding or in those with increased ICP. In patients with increased ICP, withdrawing CSF from the spinal compartment may create a significant pressure differential between the cerebral and spinal compartments. This disequilibrium will result in further compression and herniation of thalamus and midbrain through the tentorial notch and may eventually cause infraction of these structures (Johnston, 1992).

Cerebral blood flow measurements are very important when monitoring the balance between cerebral oxygen supply and demand, especially when autoregulation is lost. Modifications of the Fick principle (the uptake of a substance by an organ is equal to the amount of the substance that enters it minus the amount that leaves it) can be used to approximate the cerebral metabolic rate (CMR). Cross-brain concentration gradients of glucose (CMR/glu), lactate (CMRL), and oxygen ($CMRo_2$) have been used. For example, the cerebral metabolic rate of oxygen ($CMRo_2$) is equal to the cerebral blood flow (CBF) multiplied by the difference between the cerebral arterial and venous oxygen difference ($avDo_2$).

Normally, CBF matches the $CMRo_2$. When autoregulation is intact, changes in the $CMRo_2$ will be matched by reciprocal changes in CBF and cerebral $avDo_2$ will remain constant. The $CMRo_2$ and CBF are frequently modulated by alterations in temperature, seizure activity, and certain medications—for example, narcotics, sedatives, and analgesics. When autoregulation is lost, for example, after trauma or encephalopathy, changes in $CMRo_2$ do not produce reciprocal alterations in CBF and the $avDo_2$ can

serve as an indicator of an adequacy of CBF (Robertson, Narayan, Gokaslan, Pahwa, Grossman, Caram, & Allen, 1989).

Although cerebral arterial blood can be sampled from any artery, cerebral venous blood should not be contaminated by extracerebral blood. In order to accomplish this, Goetting and Preston (1990) described a method of percutaneous cannulation of the jugular venous bulb by retrograde advancement of a catheter placed into the jugular vein (Fig. 12–35).

Oximetric catheters placed in the jugular venous bulb have been used to continuously monitor cerebral venous saturation. The ratio of $CMRo_2$ to CBF can be expressed as the cerebral extraction of oxygen (CEo_2), which is the difference between arterial saturation (Sao_2) and jugular bulb saturation (Sjo_2) (Cruz, Miner, Allen, Alves, & Gennarelli, 1990). The CEo_2 can serve as a continuous trend monitor of cerebral oxygen supply and demand. Increased CEo_2 indicates either decreased extraction or increased delivery. Decreased CEo_2 indicates either increased extraction or decreased delivery.

Similar to pulse oximetry, cerebral oxygen saturation can be noninvasively evaluated with *near infrared spectroscopy* (NIRS) examination of cytochrome c oxidase and hemoglobin (INVOS 3100; Somanetics, Troy, NY) (McCormick, Stewart, Goetting, Dujovny, Lewis, & Ausman, 1991). Infrared light (650–1100 nm) can penetrate extracerebral tissue and return with valuable information about the attenuation of that light. Intracerebral cells capable of attenuating light include oxyhemoglobin, deoxyhemogloblin, and oxidized cytochrome c oxidase, all of which are important in oxygen delivery.

Inhalation or injection of [133]xenon, a radioisotope, is also used to assess cerebral blood flow. [133]Xenon study is based upon the principle that the rate of uptake of an inert diffusible gas is dependent upon

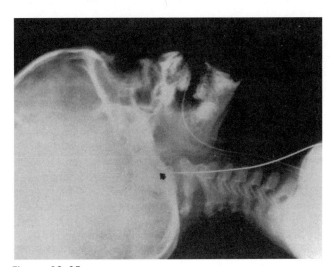

Figure 12–35 ● ● ● ● ● ●

Jugular venous bulb SVo_2 monitoring. Skull x-ray demonstrating proper catheter tip position. *Arrow* indicates jugular bulb. (From Goetting, M.G., & Preston, G. (1990). *Critical care medicine, 18* (11), 1220–1223. © by Williams & Wilkins, 1990.)

blood flow (Johnston, 1992). This study can be accomplished rapidly and provides useful information when cerebral hypoperfusion associated with stroke, massive cerebral hypertension, or brain death is suspected.

Cranial ultrasound uses sound waves to identify cranial structures of different densities. In infants with open fontanelles, serial cranial ultrasound can assist in accurate identification of the ventricular system and is helpful in the rapid identification and management of intraventricular hemorrhage. Ultrasound technology has also been used to monitor CBF by *Doppler ultrasonography* (Hassler, Steinmetz, & Gawlowski, 1988). The velocity of CBF is measured by sound waves reflecting back from moving red blood cells through the anterior cerebral artery. Direction of flow can also be identified with color imaging.

Skull and spine x-rays are the most common radiologic tests performed on the neurologic system. A variety of skull and spine views are selected to identify fractures, abnormal calcification, and tissue densities. Suture lines may appear widened in the patient with cerebral hypertension. In the multiple-trauma patient, spinal cord immobilization is essential until spinal x-rays are read as negative by a radiologist.

Computed tomography (CT) and magnetic resonance imaging (MRI) have revolutionized neurodiagnostic imaging. These noninvasive studies provide clear visualization of neuroanatomy. CT differentiates tissues by x-ray density. Areas of low density (air) appear dark, while areas of high density (bone) appear white. CT with contrast is used to enhance visualization of blood vessels, well-vascularized lesions, and localized alteration in the blood-brain barrier. The use of contrast media is contraindicated in patients with acute renal failure and in those with a positive history of allergy to contrast media. CT scan uses about the same amount of radiation as a standard skull series.

The MRI image is formed by the tissue-specific realignment of protons when short radiofrequencies are applied from a strong external magnetic field to move them out of uniform alignment. When moved, the atoms resonate and emit signals based on nuclear density and realignment time. The signals are tracked on an image revealed on a high-resolution screen image.

CT scans are selected when global neuroanatomic information is needed: for example, ventricular size, shift and distortion of brain tissue in the patient with cerebral hypertension. MRI delineates between tissue structure (for example, white and gray matter differentiation). Thus, MRI can be helpful in evaluating brain tumors, especially when located in the posterior fossa, where x-ray artifact from adjacent bone obstructs the CT view. Because personnel and metal objects cannot be in immediate proximity to the patient during MRI, its use in critical care is extremely limited.

Transporting the critically ill patient to radiology for either CT or MRI places the patient in an extremely vulnerable position. Transport requires forethought and teamwork. Planning for potential emergencies is key. Patients and personnel with implanted magnetic devices should not be near an MRI, as the magnetic field may dislodge or interfere with the function of the device. Expecting infants and young children to cooperate by holding still during the examination, especially during the loud knocking MRI sounds, is unrealistic. Sedation in this age group is often used to accomplish both CT scan and MRI.

During *cerebral angiography,* radiopaque contrast medium is injected into the carotid artery and sequential skull x-rays are taken to track medium flow throughout the cerebral vasculature. Cerebral angiography is used to delineate arteriovenous malformations or to assess the circulation to a brain tumor. Common to any angiographic procedure, there is a potential for arterial spasm, embolism, and thrombosis. Allergic reaction to the contrast medium may occur. Hematoma formation at the injection site is another potential risk. Patients may report a burning or warm sensation for about 20 to 30 seconds when the medium is injected.

Positron emission tomography (PET) scans provide information regarding cerebral metabolic function. Positron-emitting isotopes, which readily cross the blood-brain barrier, are either inhaled or injected. When the positrons (positive electron charge) come in contact with electrons (negative electron charge), gamma rays are released. The intensity of the gamma rays is then measured by a computerized detector that creates an image that indicates the pattern of metabolic activity. The half-life of the nuclides is extremely short, so that there is no radiation exposure risk to either patients or caregivers. Although use in critical care is limited, PET scanning has been found to be valuable in locating epileptic foci in infants and young children prior to excision.

CONCLUSION

In summary, caring of the patient at risk for neurologic compromise is inherent to the practice of critical care nursing. The astute neurologic examination, repeated at frequent intervals by an expert clinician, is the most reliable monitor of neurologic functioning. ICU neurologic monitoring provides additional information that cannot be assessed by conventional methods.

References

AACN Certification Corporation (1991). Pediatric CCRN examination blueprint. *CCRN News,* Spring, 6.

Amiel-Tison (1976). A method for neurologic evaluation within the first year of life. *Current Problems in Pediatrics,* 7 (1), 9–31.

Aucoin, P.J., Kotilainen, H.R., Gantz, N.M., Davidson, R., Kellogg, P., & Stone, B. (1986). Intracranial pressure monitors, epidemiologic study of risk factors and infections. *The American Journal of Medicine,* 80, 369–376.

Bergman, I. (1992). Pediatric neurological assessment and monitoring. In B.P. Fuhrman & J.J. Zimmerman (Eds.). *Pediatric critical care* (pp. 569–576). St. Louis: Mosby–Year Book.

Bishop, B.S. (1991). Pathologic pupillary signs: Self-learning module, part 2. *Critical Care Nurse,* 11 (7): 58–67.

Cant, B.R., & Shaw, N.A. (1984). Monitoring by compressed spectral array in prolonged coma. *Neurology,* 34, 35–39.

Cardoso, E.R., Rowan, J.O., & Galbraith, S. (1983). Analysis of the cerebrospinal fluid pulse wave in intracranial pressure. *Journal of Neurosurgery,* 59, 817–821.

Colditz, P.B., Williams, G.L., Berry, A.B., & Symonds, P.J. (1988). Fontanelle pressure and cerebral perfusion pressure: Continuous measurement in neonates. *Critical Care Medicine,* 16 (9), 876–879.

Crutchfield, J.S., Narayan, R.K., Robertson, C.S., & Michael, L.H. (1990) Evaluation of a fiberoptic intracranial pressure monitor. *Journal of Neurosurgery,* 72, 482–487.

Cruz, J., Miner, M.E., Allen, S.J., Alves, W.M., & Gennarelli, T.A. (1990). Continuous monitoring of cerebral oxygenation in acute brain injury: Injection of mannitol during hyperventilation. *Journal of Neurosurgery,* 73, 725–730.

Davidson, J.E. (1991). Neuromuscular blockade. *Focus on Critical Care,* 18, 512–520.

Dean, J.M., & McComb, J.G. (1981). Intracranial pressure monitoring in severe pediatric near-drowning. *Neurosurgery,* 9, 627–630.

Delgado-Escueta, A.V., Wasterlain, C., Treiman, D.M., & Porter, R.J. (1982). Current concepts in neurology: Management of status epilepticus. *New England Journal of Medicine,* 306 (22), 1337–1339.

Duc, G. (1971). Assessment of hypoxia in the newborn: Suggestions for a practical approach. *Pediatrics,* 48, 469–481.

Esposito, N., & Westgate, P. (1987). Continuous EEG monitoring in the PICU. *Journal of Pediatric Nursing,* 2 (4), 272–277.

Fiamengo, S.A. (1991). Editorial: Use of muscle relaxants in intensive care units. *Critical Care Medicine,* 19, 1457–1459.

Filloux, F., Dean, J.M., & Kirsch, J.R. (1992). Monitoring the central nervous system. In M.C. Rogers (Ed.). *Textbook of pediatric intensive care* (2nd ed., pp. 667–697). Baltimore: Williams & Wilkins.

Folkow, B. (1964). Description of the myogenic hypothesis. *Circulation Research,* 14 & 15 (Suppl. 1), I279–I287.

Germon, K. (1988). Interpretation of ICP pulse waves to determine intracerebral compliance. *Journal of Neuroscience Nursing,* 20 (6), 344–349.

Goetting, M.G., & Preston, G. (1990). Jugular bulb catheterization: Experience with 123 patients. *Critical Care Medicine,* 18 (11), 1220–1223.

Goodwin, S.R., Friedman, W.A., & Bellefleur, M. (1991). Is it time to use evoked potentials to predict outcome in comatose children and adults. *Critical Care Medicine,* 19 (4), 518–524.

Greenberg, R.P., & Ducker, T.B. (1982). Evoked potentials in the clinical neurosciences. *Journal of Neurosurgery,* 56, 1–18.

Haller, J.S. (1981). Skull transillumination. In M. Coleman (Ed.). *Neonatal neurology* (pp. 41–49). Baltimore: University Park Press.

Hassler, W., Steinmetz, H., & Gawlowski, J. (1988). Transcranial Doppler ultrasonography in raised intracranial pressure and in intracranial circulatory arrest. *Journal of Neurosurgery,* 68, 745–751.

Hickman, K.M., Mayer, B.L., & Muwaswes, M. (1990). Intracranial pressure monitoring: Review of risk factors associated with infection. *Heart & Lung,* 19 (1), 84–92.

Hill, A., & Volpe, J.J. (1981). Measurement of intracranial pressure using the Ladd intracranial monitor. *The Journal of Pediatrics,* 98 (6), 974–976.

Hollingsworth-Fridlund, P., Vos, H., & Daily, E.K. (1988). Use of fiber-optic pressure transducer for intracranial pressure measurements: A preliminary report. *Heart & Lung,* 17 (2), 111–120.

Ivan, L.P., Choo, S.H., & Ventureyra, E.C.G. (1980). Intracranial pressure monitoring with the fiberoptic transducer in children. *Child's Brain,* 7, 303–313.

Jacobson, R.I. (1989). Congenital structural defects. In K.F. Swaiman (Ed.). *Pediatric neurology: Principles and practice* (Vol. 1, pp. 317–362). St. Louis: C.V. Mosby.

Jennett, B., & Bond, M. (1975). Assessment of outcome after severe brain damage: A practical scale. *Lancet,* 1, 480–485.

Johnston, M.V. (1992). Development, structure, and function of the brain and neuromuscular systems. In B.P. Fuhrman & J.J. Zimmerman (Eds.). *Pediatric critical care* (pp. 559–587). St. Louis: Mosby–Year Book.

Kanter, R.K., Weiner, L.B., Patti, A.M., & Robson, L.K. (1985). Infectious complications and duration of intracranial pressure monitoring. *Critical Care Medicine,* 13 (10), 837–839.

March, K. (1983). Look into my eyes. *Journal of Neurosurgical Nursing,* 15, 213–221.

Mayhill, C.G., Archer, N.H., Lamb, V.A. Spadora, A.C., Baggett, J.W., Ward, J.D., & Narayan, R.K. (1984). Ventriculostomy related infections: A prospective epidemiologic study. *New England Journal of Medicine,* 310 (9), 533–559.

McCormick, P.W., Stewart, M., Goetting, M.G., Dujovny, M., Lewis, G., & Ausman, J.I. (1991). Noninvasive cerebral optical spectroscopy for monitoring cerebral oxygen delivery and hemodynamics. *Critical Care Medicine,* 19 (1), 89–97.

Mein, J., & Harcouty, B. (1986). *Diagnosis and management of ocular motility disorders.* Boston: Blackwell Scientific Publications.

Mendelow, A.D., Rowan, J.O., Murray, L., & Keer, A.E. (1983). A clinical comparison of subdural screw pressure measurements with ventricular pressure. *Journal of Neurosurgery,* 58, 45–50.

Menkes, J.H., Till, K., & Gabriel, R.S. (1990). Malformations of the central nervous system. In J.H. Menkes (Ed.), *Textbook of child neurology* (pp. 209–283). Philadelphia: Lea & Febiger.

Miller, J.D. (1976). Intracranial pressure-volume relationships in pathological conditions. *Journal of Neurosurgical Science,* 20, 203.

Mizrahi, E.M., & Dorfman, L.J. (1980). Sensory evoked potentials: Clinical applications in pediatrics. *The Journal of Pediatrics,* 97 (1), 1–10.

Moore, P.C. (1988). When you have to think small for a neurological exam. *RN,* 51 (6), 38–44.

Mylrea, K.C., Hameroff, S.R., Calkins, J.M., Blitt, C.D., & Humphry, L.L. (1984). Evaluation of periheral nerve stimulation and relationships to possible errors in assessing neuromuscular blockade. *Anesthesiology,* 60, 464–466.

Nolte, J. (1988). *The human brain: An introduction to its functional anatomy* (2nd ed.). St. Louis: C.V. Mosby.

Norman, S. (1982). The pupil check. *American Journal of Nursing,* April, 588–591.

Nussbaum, E., & Galant, S.P. (1983). Intracranial pressure monitoring as a guide to prognosis in the nearly drowned, severely comatose child. *Journal of Pediatrics,* 102 (2), 215–218.

Nussbaum, E., & Maggi, J.C. (1985). Intracranial pressure monitoring by subarachnoid bolt in comatose children. *Clinical Pediatrics,* 24 (6), 329–330.

O'Brien, D.D. (1989). Review and update of neuromuscular blocking agents. *Critical Care Nurse,* 9 (10), 76–80.

Orlowski, M.P., & Rothner, A.D. (1992). Diagnosis and treatment of status epilepticus. In B.P. Fuhrman & J.J. Zimmerman (Eds.). *Pediatric critical care* (pp. 595–604). St. Louis: Mosby–Year Book.

Orlowski, J.P., Erenberg, G., Lueders, H., & Cruse, R.P. (1989). Hypothermia and barbiturate coma for refractory status epilepticus. *Critical Care Medicine,* 12 (4), 367–372.

Ostrup, R.C., Luerssen, T.G., Marshall, L.F., & Zornow, M.H. (1987). Continuous monitoring of intracranial pressure with a miniaturized fiberoptic device. *Journal of Neurosurgery,* 67, 206–209.

Plum, R., & Posner, J.B. (1982). *The diagnosis of stupor and coma* (3rd ed.). Philadelphia: F.A. Davis.

Popich, G.A., & Smith, D.W. (1972). Fontanels: Range of normal size. *Journal of Pediatrics,* 80, 749–752.

Price, M.P. (1981). Significance of intracranial pressure waveform. *Journal of Neurosurgical Nursing,* 13 (4), 202–206.

Raju, T.N.K., Vidyasagar, D., & Papazafiratou, C. (1981). Cerebral perfusion pressure and abnormal intracranial pressure wave forms: Their relation to outcome in birth asphyxia. *Critical Care Medicine,* 9 (6), 449–453.

Robertson, C.S., Narayan, R.M., Gokaslan, Z.K., Pahwa, R., Grossman, R.G., Caram, P., & Allen, E. (1989). Cerebral arteriovenous oxygen difference as an estimate of cerebral blood flow in comatose patients. *Journal of Neurosurgery,* 70, 222–230.

Rogers, M.C., Nugent, S.K., & Traystman, R.J. (1980). Control of cerebral circulation in the neonate and infant. *Critical Care Medicine,* 8, 570–574.

Shapiro, K., Marmarou, A., & Shulman, K. (1980a). Characterization of clinical CSF dynamics and neural axis compliance using the pressure-volume index: I. The normal pressure-volume index. *Annals of Neurology,* 7, 508–514.

Shapiro, K., Marmarou, A., & Shulman, K. (1980b). A method for predicting PVI in normal patients. In K. Shulman, A. Marmarou, J.D. Miller, et al. (Eds), *Intracranial pressure IV* (pp. 85–87). New York, Springer-Verlag.

Sloan, T.B. (1988). Neurologic monitoring. *Critical Care Clinics,* 4 (3), 543–557.

Slota, M.C. (1983). Pediatric neurological assessment. *Critical Care Nurse,* 8 (9), 106–112.

Stidham, G.L., Nugent, S.K., & Rogers, M.C. (1980). Monitoring cerebral electrical function in the ICU. *Critical Care Medicine,* 8 (9), 519–522.

Sundt, T.M. (1979). Blood flow regulation in normal and ischemic brain. *Current concepts,* The Upjohn Company.

Swaiman, K.F. (1989). Neurologic examination after the newborn period until 2 years of age. In K.F. Swaiman (Ed.), *Pediatric neurology: Principles and practice* (pp. 35–44). St. Louis: C.V. Mosby.

Talwar, D., & Torres, F. (1988). Continuous electrophysiologic monitoring of cerebral function in the pediatric intensive care unit. *Pediatric Neurology,* 4, 137–147.

Tilem, D., & Greenberg, C.S. (1988). Nursing care of the child with a ventriculostomy. *Journal of Pediatric Nursing,* 3 (3), 188–193.

Traystman, R.J. (1983). Microcirculation of the brain. In N.A. Mortillaro (Ed.). *The physiology and pharmacology of the microcirculation* (pp. 237–298). New York: Academic Press.

Vidyasagar, D., & Raju, T.N.K. (1977). A simple noninvasive technique of measuring intracranial pressure in the newborn. *Pediatrics,* 59, 957–961.

Weaver, D.D., Winn, H.R., & Jane, J.A. (1982). Differential intracranial pressure in patients with unilateral mass lesions. *Journal of Neurosurgery,* 56, 660–665.

Welch, K. (1980). The intracranial pressure in infants. *Journal of Neurosurgery,* 52, 693–699.

Wiznitzer, M. (1990) Neuroelectrophysiologic monitoring. In J.L. Blumer (Ed.). *A practical guide to pediatric intensive care* (3rd ed., pp. 891–904). St. Louis: Mosby–Year Book.

York, D., Legan, M., Benner, S., & Watts, C. (1984). Further studies with a noninvasive method of intracranial pressure estimation. *Neurosurgery,* 14 (4), 456–461.

York, D.H., Pulliam, M.W., Rosenfeld, J.G., & Watts, C. (1981). Relationship between visual evoked potentials and intracranial pressure. *Journal of Neurosurgery,* 55, 909–916.

Zegeer, L.J. (1989). Oculocephalic and vestibulo-ocular responses: Significance for nursing care. *Journal of Neuroscience Nursing,* 21 (1), 46–55.

CHAPTER 13

Fluid and Electrolyte Regulation

LINDA F. SAMSON
KATHLEEN M. OUZTS

Fluid and electrolyte imbalances are common in the critically ill child. One of the goals of critical care is to prevent major fluctuation in electrolyte concentrations and to stabilize fluid in the correct compartment.

EMBRYOLOGIC DEVELOPMENT OF THE RENAL SYSTEM

Development of the renal system can be traced through three successive bilateral excretory systems in the embryo: the pronephros, the mesonephros, and the metanephros (permanent kidney) (Fig. 13–1). All of the systems are formed from the nephrogenic cord, which is derived from the mesoderm (Tisher & Madsen, 1991).

The formation of the pronephros begins around the end of the third week after conception (Moore, 1983). The pronephros appears to be nonfunctional in mam-

mals. Approximately seven pronephric tubules are formed. These tubules degenerate as the mesonephric and metanephric tubules are formed. One tubule is retained as a part of the mesonephros (Moore, 1983).

The mesonephros begins developing in the middle of the fourth week after conception in a position caudal to the pronephros (Moore, 1983). The mesonephric tubules are more complex in structure than the pronephric tubules. Each mesonephric tubule possesses a glomerular structure and proximal and distal tubules. Although still evolutionary and primitive, the mesonephros is capable of urine formation.

The mesonephric tubules begin to regress in females during the third month of gestation. In males, the mesonephric tubules remain and further develop to form parts of the male reproductive system, including the vas deferens, epididymis, and ejaculatory duct (Tisher & Madsen, 1991).

The metanephros is the final developmental phase

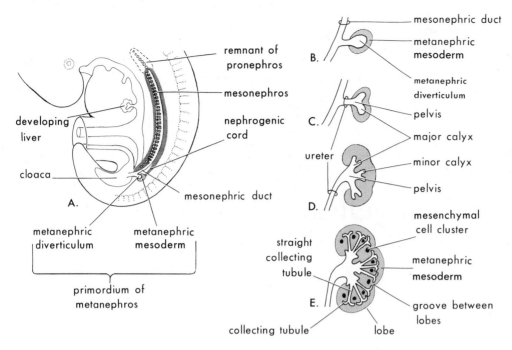

Figure 13-1 ● ● ● ● ● ●

A, Sketch of a lateral view of a 5-week embryo showing the primordium of the metanephros, or permanent kidney. *B* to *E*, Sketches showing successive stages of development of the metanephric diverticulum (fifth to eighth weeks) into the ureter, pelvis, calyces, and collecting tubules. The renal lobes illustrated in *E* are visible in the kidneys of newborn infants. The external evidence of the lobes normally disappears by the end of the first year. (From Moore, K.L. (1985). *Before we are born: Basic embryology and birth defects* (2nd ed., p. 171). Philadelphia: W. B. Saunders.)

of the human kidney. It begins to appear about 2 weeks after the formation of the mesonephros. Although the metanephritic kidney is located in the pelvis, ascent to the abdomen begins by the seventh to ninth week after conception (Andrews & Mooney, 1990).

The metanephros is formed from two different embryonic tissues. The excretory portion, including the collecting ducts, calyces, pelvis, and ureter, develops from the ureteric bud. The metanephric blastema gives rise to Bowman's capsule, most of the glomerulus, and the tubules of the nephrons. The collecting ducts and the tubules then make connections, giving rise to an anatomically complete microstructure by 12 to 16 weeks after conception (Moore, 1983).

Nephron formation begins during the eighth week of gestation. By the time of birth, each human kidney contains approximately one million nephrons in different stages of development. The most mature nephrons are found in the renal medulla. The immature nephrons are located in the outer cortex. Although maturation of the renal system continues after birth, no additional nephrons are formed.

STRUCTURE AND FUNCTION OF THE RENAL SYSTEM

Although the permanent kidney has a complete microstructure by the fourth month of gestation, renal development continues until adolescence. At birth, the kidneys occupy a large portion of the posterior abdominal wall. This is the result of the ascent and rotation of the kidneys during gestation. The ureters are proportionately shorter in infancy than in adults. As renal development continues, the ureters grow to adult proportions. The kidney reaches

adult size by adolescence. The kidney's weight is 10 times greater at maturity than at birth (Andrews & Mooney, 1990).

At birth, the bladder is located in the lower abdomen, close to the abdominal wall. The bladder descends into the pelvis with growth after birth. During the maturational process, it also changes from the cylindrical shape seen in infancy to the pyramidal shape found after maturation is complete.

Macroscopic Anatomy

The kidneys are located in the retroperitoneal space in front and on both sides of the vertebral column. Each kidney is covered by a thin fibrous capsule composed of connective tissue, lymphatics, and blood vessels. The blood vessels, lymphatics, nerves, and ureter enter or exit the kidney in the area known as the hilum.

A cross-section of the mature kidney demonstrates an outer area of renal cortex that is approximately 1 cm wide and an inner area of renal medulla that is approximately 5 cm wide (Fig. 13–2). About 85% of the nephrons in each kidney are located within the renal cortex. The remaining 15% are called "juxtamedullary nephrons" and are located at the junction of the cortex and medulla.

The mature kidney receives 20% to 25% of the cardiac output (Guyton, 1991). Total blood supply circulates through the kidneys approximately 12 times per hour, with 90% of renal blood flow circulating through the cortex and the remaining 10% flowing through the medulla. Because the kidney develops from the center toward the periphery, renal distribution of blood flow in the newborn period is primarily to the medulla. This, along with the immature and shorter loops, leads to a more dilute urine in infants (Andrews & Mooney, 1990).

Microscopic Anatomy

At birth, each kidney contains approximately one million nephrons. Although these nephrons are at varying maturational stages, each has both a tubular and a vascular component. The arcuate artery branches within the kidney to form the afferent arterioles. Afferent arterioles then divide into capillary tufts called glomeruli, which protrude into Bowman's capsule. Filtration occurs across the capillary membrane in Bowman's capsule. The tubular component of the nephron is composed of Bowman's capsule, the proximal and distal convoluted tubules, the loop of Henle, and the collecting ducts.

Structural Abnormalities

It is estimated that variations from normal anatomic structure of the urinary tract occur in 10% to 15% of the population (Andrews & Mooney, 1990). Variations may range from minor ones that do not interfere with normal function, to those that are ei-

ther incompatible with life or life-threatening. Structural abnormalities may or may not be apparent at birth. Failure of the kidneys to ascend may result in ectopic kidneys, an essentially benign abnormality. On the other hand, bilateral renal agenesis (Potter syndrome) is incompatible with life. Structural abnormalities account for 45% of reported renal failure in children (Andrews & Mooney, 1990).

Function

Urine formation begins at a point between 12 and 16 weeks gestation and contributes to the overall volume and composition of the amniotic fluid. The volume of urine produced increases from 2 to 4 mL/hour in the second trimester to nearly 40 mL/hour at term (Moore, 1983). However, urine production may decrease during the first several days of life. Seven percent of normal infants may fail to urinate for up to 24 hours after birth (Engle, 1986; Sherry & Kramer, 1955).

Normal urine output averages between 0.5 mL/kg/hour in a well-hydrated adolescent to 1 mL/kg/hour in the child and 2 mL/kg/hour in the infant. Although normal urine specific gravity is between 1.005 and 1.020, infants and children younger than 2 years

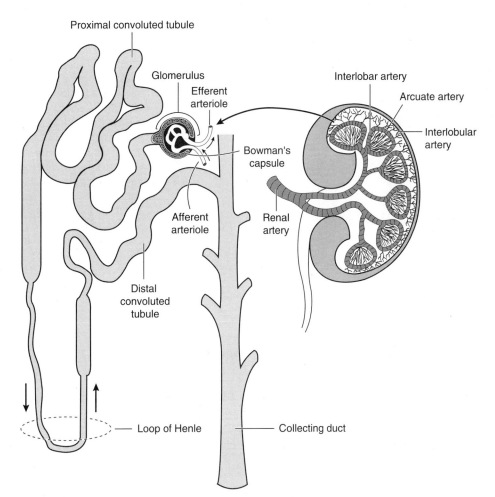

Figure 13–2 ● ● ● ● ● ●
Gross structure of a bisected kidney.

may not present with high specific gravity because of renal maturational factors. Renal blood flow and glomerular filtration rate (GFR) increase linearly with gestational age (Costarino & Baumgart, 1986). Before birth, the increases are related to the growth of new nephrons. After birth, a dramatic increase in GFR occurs as the result of decreased vascular resistance and a rise in systemic blood pressure. Initial GFR values average 20 to 30 mL/1.73 m²/minute. An estimation of glomerular filtration rates in children can be derived using a formula based on body length and plasma creatinine levels (Schwartz et al., 1976; 1984). Calculation of GFR in children ages 1 to 16 is 0.55 × length (in cm)/plasma creatinine (mg %). This yields GFR in mL/min based on body surface area corrected to 1.73 m².

The GFR increases over the first and second years of life, stabilizing in a range between 30% and 50% of adult levels by the end of the first year and reaching adult levels by 2 years (Andrews & Mooney, 1990).

The glomeruli serve to protect the body from filtration of red blood cells (RBCs), white blood cells (WBCs), and protein. Immaturity of the nephrons at birth may prevent complete filtration, causing loss of RBCs, WBCs, and protein, even in the absence of disease states. The proximal convoluted tubules serve to reabsorb a large percentage of the fluid and electrolytes. The distal convoluted tubules serve to reabsorb the remaining electrolytes. Functions in the distal tubules are dependent upon the actions of aldosterone and antidiuretic hormone (ADH). In the infant, the distal tubule is relatively insensitive to aldosterone. Hence, the infant has limited ability to respond to sodium excess or depletion and may experience impaired secretion of potassium and hydrogen ions. These developmental factors continue to play a role in fluid and electrolyte balance during the first 2 years of life and help to explain the sensitivity of infants and young children to fluid and electrolyte alteration.

COMPOSITION OF BODY FLUIDS

Fluid and electrolyte homeostasis occurs when fluid and electrolyte balance is maintained within narrow limits despite a wide variation in dietary intake, metabolic rate, and kidney function.

An electrolyte is a substance that develops an electrical charge (ion) when dissolved in water. Those substances that develop a positive electrical charge are called cations (i.e., potassium, K^+; sodium, Na^+; calcium, Ca^{++}; and magnesium, Mg^{++}). Electrolytes that develop a negative charge are called anions (i.e., chloride, Cl^-, and bicarbonate, HCO_3^-). Electrolytes are regulated by intake, output, acid-base balance, hormonal influence, and cellular integrity. Nonelectrolytes are small solute particles that do not carry an electrical charge when dissolved in water. Examples are simple sugars (i.e., glucose), proteins, oxygen, carbon dioxide, and organic acids.

TOTAL BODY WATER

Water constitutes approximately 65% to 80% of the body weight. Total body water (TBW) varies from person to person and is dependent on several factors: age, gender, skeletal muscle mass, and fat content. The water content of adipose tissue is less than that of other tissues; thus, the amount of fat in the body determines, to a major degree, the amount of water.

TBW, as a percentage of body weight, changes during the first year of life. As the infant becomes older, the total body fluid percentage decreases, with the most rapid change occurring in the first 6 months of life (Metheny, 1987). TBW accounts for 70% of body weight at 6 months and 65% at 1 year of age (40%–45% intracellular and 25% extracellular) (Boineau & Lewy, 1990). In children, the percentage of total weight as body water decreases steadily until the adult percentage (55%–60%) is reached at about 8 years of age (Innerarity & Stark, 1990) (Table 13–1). On the average, obese children and females have lower percentages of TBW as water. TBW is distributed in two separate compartments: the extracellular fluid compartment (ECF) and the intracellular fluid compartment (ICF) (Fig. 13–3).

Extracellular Compartment

The extracellular compartment is divided into three separate compartments: interstitial fluid (ISF), intravascular fluid (plasma), and transcellular water (TSW). The ISF bathes all of the body cells. ISF volume accounts for approximately 15% of the body weight. Plasma is the liquid component of whole blood. Accounting for 5% of the body weight, it is contained within the vascular system. TSW, representing a minute proportion of TBW, is found in a number of spaces and cavities that contain or could contain fluid. Examples of these spaces include the pleural cavity, peritoneal cavity, pericardial cavity, joint spaces, and ventricles of the brain. The function of TSW is to either lubricate (joint) or cushion.

The serum or plasma portion of the extracellular compartment contains the electrolytes found in the ECF and a large amount of protein. The plasma

Table 13–1. CHANGES IN TOTAL BODY WATER (TBW) AND BODY COMPARTMENTS DURING DEVELOPMENT

Age	TBW (% Body Weight)	Extracellular Fluid (% Body Weight)	Intracellular Fluid (% Body Weight)
Premature	75–80		
Newborn	70–75	50	35
1 year	65	25	40–45
Adolescence			
Males	60	20	40–45
Females	55	18	40

From Feld, L., et al. (1988). The approach to fluid and electrolyte therapy in pediatrics. *Advances in Pediatrics* 35:497–536.

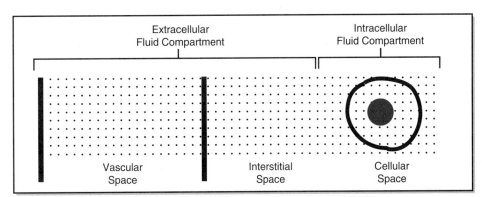

Figure 13–3 ● ● ● ● ●
Fluid distribution—body compartments.

proteins determine colloid osmotic (oncotic) pressure, with the most abundant plasma protein being albumin. Albumin, because of its size, remains in the vascular space and exerts a differential osmotic force or oncotic pressure between the capillary lumen and the interstitial space. The consequence is maintenance of volume in the intravascular space. Oncotic pressure is also important in the kidney, influencing filtration and reabsorption of water and solutes.

The ECF contains large quantities of sodium and chloride ions, reasonably large quantities of bicarbonate ion, and small quantities of potassium, calcium, magnesium, phosphate, sulfate, and organic acid ions. The ECF comprises just 20% of body weight in the adult but 50% in full-term infants (Masiak, 1985). The infant's entire ECF volume is replaced every 3 days. By age 1 year ECF decreases by one half and declines very slowly thereafter (see Table 13–1).

Intracellular Compartment

Intracellular fluid consists of all liquid within the cell membranes of the body and is the largest fluid compartment, accounting for 40% of the body weight of the child by one year of age (see Table 13–1). Much of the ICF is found within muscle cells. ICF contains only small quantities of sodium and chloride ions, and almost no calcium ions. Large quantities of potassium and phosphate and moderate quantities of magnesium and sulfate ions are also found in the intracellular compartment. The cells contain four times as much protein as the plasma.

A dynamic relationship exists between the ECF and ICF compartments, which maintains cellular homeostasis through exchange of fluids and electrolytes. The compartments are kept separate by the structural and functional integrity of cell membranes. The movement of water and solutes across the cell membrane is regulated by both passive and active processes. The selective permeability of the cell membrane and the specific active transport activity of the cell determine the characteristics of ICF and ECF. A profound alteration in any one of the fluid compartments can disrupt cellular health and may result in a fatal systemic response.

Homeostatic maintenance of fluid balance assures that TBW remains constant. The aim is to have intake equal output plus insensible water loss. Intake is composed of water from enteral or intravenous solutions, and fluid metabolically produced through oxidative metabolism (300 mL/24 hours). Intake is regulated mainly through the mechanism of thirst. This mechanism cannot be relied upon to obtain adequate intake in critically ill children because they may not be able to demonstrate or respond to thirst.

Output of fluids and electrolytes is regulated by the integumentary, respiratory, digestive, and renal systems. All work together to protect adequate elimination and retention of body water. Several factors, such as humidity and ambient temperatures, affect the amount of water lost. Factors affecting insensible water loss are presented in Table 13–2.

REGULATION OF WATER AND ELECTROLYTE BALANCE

The kidneys, in conjunction with the endocrine system, are responsible for the regulation of the body's fluid and electrolyte balance. The regulation of fluid and electrolytes in designated compartments (intracellular and extracellular) is dependent on the osmotic pressure, colloid osmotic pressure (COP), hydrostatic pressure (pressure exerted by a liquid) in

Table 13–2. FACTORS KNOWN TO INFLUENCE INSENSIBLE (EVAPORATIVE) FLUID LOSSES

Increased Insensible Loss	Decreased Insensible Loss
Hyperthermia*	Humidified air
Increased activity	Hypothermia
Hyperventilation	Sedation
Radiant warmers+	Decreased activity
Phototherapy=	

*Increases sensible losses by 12% per Celsius degree above 38°C.

+Increases insensible losses by 40% to 50% in infants less than 1500 g; percentage may be higher in larger infants.

=Increases insensible losses by approximately 40% in infants less than 1500 g; percentage may be higher in larger infants.

From Besunder, J.B. (1990). Abnormalities in fluids, minerals, and glucose. In J.L. Blumer (Ed.). *A practical guide to pediatric intensive care* (3rd ed., p. 546). St. Louis: Mosby–Year Book.

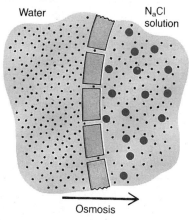

Figure 13–4 ● ● ● ● ●

Osmosis at a cell membrane when a sodium chloride solution is placed on one side of the membrane and water on the other side. (From Guyton, A.C. (1991). *Textbook of medical physiology* (8th ed., p. 45). Philadelphia: W. B. Saunders.)

the spaces, and capillary permeability. Hydrostatic pressure is produced through the action of the cardiovascular and lymphatic systems. Capillary hydrostatic pressure is generated by the force of cardiac contractions.

The term "colloid osmotic pressure" is used to distinguish the osmotic effects of the colloid from those of dissolved crystalloids such as sodium. Colloid osmotic pressure is a pulling force generated by plasma proteins that opposes fluid filtration from the capillaries. The plasma proteins are large colloid molecules that disperse in the blood and sometimes escape into the tissue spaces. Both the intravascular and interstitial compartments contain plasma proteins, including albumin, the globulins, and fibrinogen. Albumin, the smallest and most abundant of the plasma proteins, accounts for about 70% of the total osmotic pressure. Albumin provides for the return of fluid to the vascular compartment from the tissue spaces. When plasma protein concentration falls acutely, plasma oncotic pressure falls and fluid may leave the vascular space, resulting in third spacing of fluid.

MOVEMENT OF FLUIDS AND ELECTROLYTES

For water and electrolytes to function effectively in the body, a regulatory process that controls fluid movement is required. The regulatory process is dependent on the concentration of the specific fluid or electrolyte (osmolality) and on the functioning capacity of the renal system. Fluids move constantly from one body compartment to another and then remain in specific compartments until an inequality in concentration of electrolytes develops and movement once again occurs. Movement is through one of four transport mechanisms: osmosis, diffusion, filtration, and active transport.

Osmosis is the movement of water through a semipermeable membrane from an area of lower solute content to an area of higher solute activity (with lower activity of water molecules) (Fig. 13–4). Osmosis occurs only when the membrane is more permeable to water than solutes. The force of the movement, or shift, of water is dependent on serum osmolality, which controls distribution and movement of water between compartments.

Osmolality refers to the concentration of particles (proteins and electrolytes) per liter of water. The osmolality of a solution does not depend on the size, molecular weight, or electrical charge of the molecules. Osmotic pressure of a solution is described by the terms "osmole" and "milliosmole." The osmolar concentration of a solution is called the osmolality when the concentration is expressed as osmoles per kilogram of water. The terms "tonicity" and "osmolality" are used interchangeably.

Serum osmolality can be estimated by the following formula:

serum osmolality
$$= 2(\text{serum Na}) + \text{glucose}/18 + \text{BUN}/2.8$$

Normally, the amount of water that diffuses in and out of the cell is balanced and ECF and ICF volume remain constant. Because water moves freely between the blood, interstitial fluid, and tissues, changes in the osmolality of one body compartment

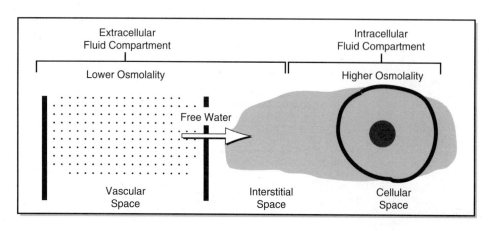

Figure 13–5 ● ● ● ● ●

Fluid movement with changes in osmolality.

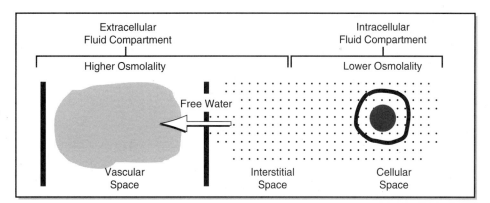

Figure 13–6 ● ● ● ● ● ●

Fluid movement with changes in osmolality.

produce a shift in all body fluids. Consequently, in most cases, the osmolality of the plasma is equal to the osmolality of other compartments (Fig. 13–5).

Water moves from the ECF to the ICF if the ICF osmolality increases (Fig. 13–5). Conversely, if the ECF osmolality increases, water will shift from the ICF into the ECF (see Figs. 13–5, 13–6). When the movement of water causes a concentration difference, the cells either shrink or swell, depending on the direction of the net movement. An isotonic solution (0.9% saline) is one that does not cause cells to either shrink or swell. A hypertonic solution (one with greater than 0.9% saline) is one that causes a cell to shrink by moving water from within the cell to the ECF, which has less sodium than the cell. A hypotonic solution (such as 5% dextrose and 0.2% NS) causes a cell to swell. Table 13–3 describes the most frequently used intravenous solutions in critically ill children.

Diffusion is movement of a substance (electrolytes and nonelectrolytes) from an area of higher concentration to one of lower concentration through a solution or gas (Fig. 13–7). Diffusion ceases when equilibrium occurs. Electrical potential differences and pressure differences across the pores of a semipermeable membrane also influence diffusion, although the most important factor determining the rate of diffusion is the concentration difference. The greater the concentration difference, the greater the rate of diffusion.

Molecules moving via simple diffusion must possess one or two capabilities: lipid solubility and a negative charge. The lipid-soluble molecules, such as oxygen, carbon dioxide, and alcohol, are able to diffuse readily through the lipid component of the cell membrane. Chloride is an example of a negatively charged particle able to pass with ease through the membrane pores.

Filtration is the transfer of water and dissolved substances through a semipermeable membrane from a region of high pressure to a region of low pressure. The force causing filtration is hydrostatic pressure. An example of filtration is the passage of water and electrolytes from the arterial capillary bed to the interstitial fluid in response to blood pressure. The pumping action of the heart causes the hydrostatic pressure (Metheny, 1987).

Movement against a concentration or electrochemical gradient is known as **active transport,** and energy, in the form of adenosine triphosphatase (ATPase), is required for the activity (Fig. 13–8). The transport occurs somewhat like a "pump" in the membrane of the cell, driven by the energy generated by cellular respiration. Regulation and distribution of sodium and potassium within the interstitial and the ICF compartments are via the sodium-potassium pump. Active transport is necessary to move sodium from the cells to the ECF. The active process of pumping sodium out of the cells forces potassium into the cell.

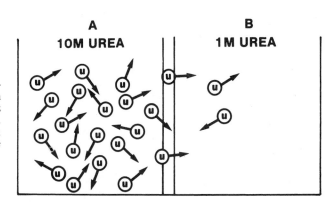

Figure 13–7 ● ● ● ● ● ●

Simple diffusion. A membrane permeable to urea separates two solutions. Side A contains a tenfold greater concentration of urea than side B. Random motion of individual solute molecules results in net movement of urea from A to B. (From Wright, E., & Schulman, G. (1985). Dynamics of body water: Principles of epithelial transport. In M.H. Maxwell, C.R. Kleeman, & R.G. Narins (Eds.). *Clinical disorders of fluid and electrolyte metabolism* (p. 17). New York: McGraw-Hill.)

Table 13–3. COMPOSITION OF COMMON PARENTERAL FLUID SOLUTIONS

Solution	Solute	Concentration (g/100 mL)	pH	Na$^+$	K$^+$	Ca^{2+}	Cl$^-$	Lactate	Calc Osm (mOsm/L)
					Ionic Concentrations (mEq/L)				
Dextrose in water									
5.0%	Glucose	5	4.7	—	—	—	—	—	250
10.0%	Glucose	10	4.6	—	—	—	—	—	505
Saline									
0.45% (hypotonic)	NaCl	0.45	5.3	77	—	—	77	—	155
0.90% (isotonic)	NaCl	0.9	5.3	154	—	—	154	—	310
Dextrose in saline									
2.5% in 0.45%	Glucose	2.5							
	NaCl	0.45	4.9	77	—	—	77	—	280
5.0% in 0.20%	Glucose	5.0							
	NaCl	0.20	4.6	34	—	—	34	—	320
5.0% in 0.45%	Glucose	5.0							
	NaCl	0.45	4.6	77	—	—	77	—	405
5.0% in 0.90%	Glucose	5.0							
	NaCl	0.90	4.6	154	—	—	154	—	560
Polyionic									
Lactated Ringer's (RL)	Lactate	0.31							
	NaCl	0.60	6.3	130	4	3	109	28	275
	KCl	0.03							
	CaCl$_2$	0.02							
Dextrose in polyionic									
2.5% in 1/2 RL	Glucose	2.5							
	Lactate	0.155							
	NaCl	0.30	5.1	65	2	1.5	54	14	265
	KCl	0.015							
	CaCl$_2$	0.01							
4.0% in modified RL	Glucose	4.0							
	Lactate	0.062							
	NaCl	0.12	5.0	26	0.8	0.5	22	5.5	280
	KCl	0.006							
	CaCl$_2$	0.004							
5.0% in RL	Glucose	5.0							
	Lactate	0.31							
	NaCl	0.60	4.7	130	4	3	109	28	515
	KCl	0.03							
	CaCl$_2$	0.02							
5% albumin (Plasmanate)	Albumin	5.0	6.9	154	1		154	—	310
	NaCl	0.9							

From Perkin, R.M., & Levin, D.L. (1980). Common fluid and electrolyte problems in the pediatric intensive care unit. *Pediatric Clinics of North America,* 27:567–586.

An example of the effects of the sodium-potassium pump is seen in children with severe burns. The injury causes more sodium than water to be drawn into the interstitial spaces. This decreases the efficiency of the sodium pump, which allows more water and sodium to enter the intracellular space. The increased osmotic pressure gradient drives potassium out of the cell. The loss of water and sodium from the intravascular space results in the increased secretion of aldosterone and ADH as compensatory mechanisms. This contributes to the retention of sodium and water.

Not only is energy required to move substances against a concentration gradient, but a carrier substance is required for the transport of sodium, potassium, chloride, sugars, and amino acids. Carrier substances are either a protein or a lipoprotein. The protein carriers function by providing an attachment site for the specific substance to be transported. The lipoprotein facilitates the solubility of the substance in the lipid portion of the cell membrane.

FLUID VOLUME REGULATION

Water is the most abundant component of the body. Although serving a vital role in the regulation of body heat through insulation or evaporation, water further serves as the diluent for cell solids and as a message carrier among the cells, tissues, and organs of the body. Water also provides the body with form and structure.

Vasopressin, or ADH, is manufactured in the hypothalamus of the brain and is released by the posterior pituitary gland. ADH acts on the cells of the renal collecting ducts to increase their permeability to water, promoting a simultaneous increase in ECF volume and decrease in urinary output.

There are three major stimuli for the regulation of ADH secretion: (1) plasma osmolality, (2) changes in the ECF volume, and (3) changes in arterial blood pressure. When sufficient water is not being taken in or excessive loss occurs, serum osmolality rises. A small increase in serum osmolality of 1% to 2% is sufficient to cause ADH release, which acts at the nephrons, signaling them to conserve water and produce a more concentrated urine. ADH is released when the osmotic pressure of the ECF is greater than that of the cells (e.g., during hyperglycemic and/or hypernatremic states). When osmotic pressure of the ECF is less than that of the cells, ADH is inhibited, causing renal excretion of water (Metheny, 1987). When the blood pressure falls or there is a decrease in blood volume, ADH is also released.

ADH has a direct vasoconstrictor effect on the blood vessels, resulting in elevation of the blood pressure. Other stimuli affecting ADH secretion are angiotensin II; drugs (opiates, nicotine, barbiturates, alcohol); stress; and severe pain. Release of angiotensin II, stress reaction, and severe pain cause release of ADH and thus increase blood pressure. Opiates, barbiturates, and alcohol reduce ADH secretion and are associated with decreases in blood pressure.

The adrenal cortex secretes aldosterone, which is a mineralocorticoid and a primary influence in fluid homeostasis. Sodium depletion, increases in potassium concentration, angiotensin II, and adrenocorticotrophic hormone (ACTH) stimulate aldosterone release. The distal renal tubules, sweat glands, salivary glands, and intestines are the receptors of aldosterone activity.

Aldosterone influences renal retention and excretion of both sodium and potassium. When the serum level of sodium falls, aldosterone is secreted. This leads to sodium and water retention in the renal tubules. Potassium is then given up by the renal tubules in a further effort to increase sodium levels. When aldosterone secretion is inhibited, potassium is retained and sodium and water are excreted. Aldosterone helps regulate blood volume by regulating sodium retention.

ALTERATION IN FLUID VOLUME

Fluid Deficit

Fluid volume deficit is defined as negative body fluid or water balance. When extracellular volume depletion is present, hypovolemia is said to exist and circulatory collapse can result. In infants and children, "fluid volume deficit" and "dehydration" are terms often used interchangeably. Fluid volume deficit is a common problem in critically ill infants and children. Negative water balance occurs from (1) excess loss of fluids and electrolytes, such as that which occurs as the result of diarrhea or vomiting; (2) shifts of fluids and electrolytes into nonaccessible third spaces, such as in the severely burned child or often following abdominal surgery; and (3) decreased intake of fluid and electrolytes, such as in the child who has nothing by mouth (is NPO) (Baer, 1988; Feld et al., 1988).

Excessive fluid volume loss and loss of electrolytes are major contributing factors to dehydration in infants and children. Increased insensible water loss may occur with burns, hyperventilation, fever, renal or gastrointestinal disease, increased ambient temperature, sweating, and cystic fibrosis (Feld et al., 1988). In children losing fluid because of sweating, as much as 400 to 2000 mL/m² of water may be lost each day (Goldberger, 1986). In cystic fibrosis, not

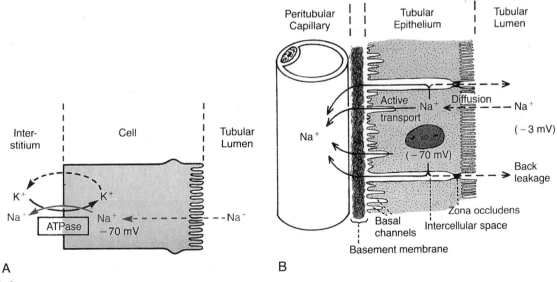

Figure 13–8 ● ● ● ● ● ●

A, Basic mechanism for active transport of sodium through the tubular epithelial cell. This figure shows active transport by the sodium potassium pump, which pumps sodium out of the basolateral membrane of the cell and simultaneously creates a very low intracellular sodium concentration as well as a negative intracellular potential. The low intracellular sodium concentration and the negative potential then cause sodium ions to diffuse from the tubular lumen into the cell through the brush border. *B,* The net mechanism for active transport of sodium from the tubular lumen all the way into the peritubular capillary. (From Guyton, A.C. (1991). *Textbook of medical physiology* (8th ed., p. 299). Philadelphia: W. B. Saunders.)

only is excessive fluid lost, but sodium losses in sweat may vary between 50 and 130 mEq/L (Wood et al., 1975). Increased renal water loss occurs as a result of osmotic diuresis, central diabetes insipidus, impaired tubular response to ADH, renal tubular dysfunction, and in sodium wasting conditions (Feld et al., 1988). Gastrointestinal water loss from diarrheal disease is ordinarily the most common cause of excess fluid volume loss in infants and children.

In the critically ill child, fluid volume loss through "third spacing" is a common cause of fluid volume loss. Third spacing occurs when ECF volume is shifted into cavities where it accumulates and is physiologically inaccessible for use by the body (Baer, 1988). Third spacing develops in ascites, pancreatitis, burns, peritonitis, sepsis, and intestinal obstruction.

Fluid deficit produced by inadequate intake is primarily caused by unreplaced normal insensible water loss. Examples of underlying clinical problems that contribute to decreased intake are coma, dysphagia, debilitation, impaired thirst, or anorexia (Feld et al., 1988). In addition, intake may not be adequate if ongoing losses are undetected or excessive.

Dehydration is usually classified on the basis of the serum sodium level, because the level in dehydrated patients may be low, normal, or high, depending on electrolyte losses. Dehydration is classified as hyponatremic when serum sodium levels are less than 130 mEq/L, isonatremic when serum sodium levels are 130 to 150 mEq/L, and hypernatremic when serum sodium levels are above 150 mEq/L (Barbero, 1992). These forms of dehydration are also hypotonic, isotonic, and hypertonic, respectively, because plasma osmolality reflects sodium concentration. However, the two sets of terms cannot be used interchangeably because changes in tonicity do not always indicate sodium concentration.

Hyponatremic dehydration occurs when there is a proportionately greater loss of sodium compared with fluid loss. This often is the result when a child who is experiencing diarrhea or vomiting at home is given a hypotonic fluid such as water. An osmolar gradient results and produces a fluid shift from the hyponatremic extracellular space into the intracellular space, increasing the ECF loss.

Isonatremic dehydration occurs when equal amounts of fluid and electrolytes are lost. When there is no osmolar gradient and isotonicity exists, the resultant fluid volume depletion is primarily extracellular (Feld et al., 1988).

Hypernatremic dehydration is characterized by an increased osmolality of the ECF, which results in a shift of fluid from within the cells to maintain osmolar equilibrium (Feld et al., 1988). ICF volume is depleted, and ECF loss is less than expected (Barbero, 1992).

The severity of fluid volume depletion can be estimated by change in body weight. Dehydration is considered mild when there is a weight loss of 3% to 5%, moderate when there is a weight loss of 5% to 10% in infants and young children, or 3% to 6% in older children, and severe when weight loss is 10% to 15% in infants and young children, or 6% to 9% in older children (Robson, 1992).

Clinical Assessment

An infant or child with fluid volume deficit may exhibit any of the clinical signs and symptoms presented in Table 13–4. The severity of the physical

Table 13–4. CLINICAL ASSESSMENT OF SEVERITY OF DEHYDRATION

Signs and Symptoms	Mild Dehydration	Moderate Dehydration	Severe Dehydration
General appearance and condition			
Infants and young children	Thirsty, alert, restless	Thirsty, restless or lethargic but irritable to touch or drowsy	Drowsy, limp, cold, sweaty, cyanotic extremities, may be comatose
Older children and adults	Thirsty, alert, restless	Thirsty, alert, postural hypotension	Usually conscious, apprehensive, cold, sweaty, cyanotic extremities, wrinkled skin of fingers and toes, muscle cramps
Radial pulse	Normal rate and strength	Rapid and weak	Rapid, feeble, sometimes impalpable
Respiration	Normal	Deep, may be rapid	Deep and rapid
Anterior fontanelle	Normal	Sunken	Very sunken
Systolic blood pressure	Normal	Normal or low	Less than 90 mmHg, may be unrecordable
Skin elasticity	Pinch retracts immediately	Pinch retracts slowly	Pinch retracts very slowly (>2 sec)
Eyes	Normal	Sunken (detectable)	Grossly sunken
Tears	Present	Absent	Absent
Mucous membranes	Moist	Dry	Very dry
Urine flow	Normal	Reduced amount and dark	None passed for several hours, empty bladder
Body weight loss (%)	4–5	6–9	10 or more
Estimated fluid deficit (mL/kg)	40–50	60–90	100–110

Data from McCarthy, P.L. (1992). General considerations in the care of sick children. In R.E. Behrman (Ed.). *Nelson textbook of pediatrics* (14th ed., pp. 171–211). Philadelphia: W. B. Saunders.

Table 13-5. EFFECTS OF TYPE OF DEHYDRATION ON PHYSICAL SIGNS

Parameter	Isonatremic Dehydration (Proportionate Loss of Water and Sodium)	Hyponatremic Dehydration (Loss of Sodium in Excess of Water)	Hypernatremic Dehydration (Loss of Water in Excess of Sodium)
ECF volume*	Markedly decreased	Severely decreased	Decreased
ICF volume*	Maintained	Increased	Decreased
Physical signs			
Skin			
Color†	Gray	Gray	Gray
Temperature	Cold	Cold	Cold or hot
Turgor‡	Poor	Very poor	Fair
Feel	Dry	Clammy	Thickened, doughy
Mucous membranes	Dry	Slightly moist	Parched§
Eyeball	Sunken and soft	Sunken and soft	Sunken
Fontanelle	Sunken	Sunken	Sunken
Psyche	Lethargic	Coma	Hyperirritable
Pulse†	Rapid	Rapid	Moderately rapid
Blood pressure†	Low	Very low	Moderately low

*ECF, extracellular fluid; ICF, intracellular fluid.
†Signs of shock rather than of dehydration itself.
‡Reflects magnitude of fluid loss from ECF.
§Tongue often has shriveled appearance because of loss of cellular fluid.
Data from McCarthy, P.L. (1992). General considerations in the care of sick children. In R.E. Behrman (Ed.). *Nelson textbook of pediatrics* (14th ed., pp. 171–211). Philadelphia: W. B. Saunders.

changes and abnormalities of vital signs are dependent upon the degree of dehydration. The set of symptoms is altered by the type of dehydration as described in Table 13–5.

A second set of signs is associated with partial compensation by correction with hypotonic fluids, which produce decreased tonicity of body fluids (Naylor, 1985). These symptoms are the result of cellular swelling and are first manifested in the central nervous system. They include confusion, lethargy, disorientation, and seizures (Naylor, 1985).

An estimate of the degree of dehydration should be based on the child's weight loss associated with the illness and graphed on a growth chart. Another estimate of fluid loss can be made by considering that 1 g of weight loss is caused by 1 mL of fluid loss. Additional assessments should include tear production with crying, presence of salivary bubbles under the tongue, and the appearance of the anterior fontanelle, if it remains open.

Systemic perfusion is assessed in fluid volume alterations. With increasing severity of dehydration, the following symptoms may be manifested: tachycardia; cool and mottled skin; cyanotic mucous membranes; weak, thready pulses; delayed capillary refill; and hypotension (with severe dehydration).

It may be possible to estimate fluid loss from capillary refill time. Capillary refill of less than 2 seconds corresponds with a fluid loss of less than 50 mL/kg; refill time of 2 to 3 seconds is associated with losses of 50 to 90 mL/kg; and refill time greater than 3 seconds occurs with losses of 100 mL/kg or more (Robson, 1992).

Laboratory Assessment

In fluid volume deficit, laboratory markers may alert the nurse to alterations in fluid volume. Blood urea nitrogen and creatinine may increase because dehydration can result in a decrease in GFR. Creatinine levels are often higher than blood urea nitrogen levels. Elevated urine specific gravity may be seen in older children, along with moderate proteinuria. These results are often absent in infants. Hemoconcentration may occur with fluid volume deficit. Characteristics of hemoconcentration include increased hematocrit, hemoglobin, and RBC levels.

Serum sodium levels indicate the relative losses of fluid and electrolytes. Even in children with hypernatremia, total body protein is usually decreased. Bicarbonate levels indicate whether the child is acidotic or alkalotic. Potassium levels are of limited value early on.

Critical Care Management

Initial therapy for the child with a fluid volume deficit is directed toward quickly expanding ECF volume to treat or prevent shock. Ringer's lactate at 10 to 20 mL/kg is usually the fluid of choice. For the child with severe dehydration, rapid fluid resuscitation with as much as 40 mL/kg may be necessary. Peripheral perfusion, heart rate, urine output, and blood pressure are monitored to determine the child's response to therapy.

Once initial resuscitation has been accomplished, therapy is directed toward definitive water and electrolyte replacement. For isotonic or hypotonic dehydration, one half of the calculated loss is replaced along with maintenance fluids over the next 8 hours, usually with 5% dextrose and 0.45 normal saline (NS) (Wetzel, 1991). The calculated loss can be determined by multiplying the assessed percentage of dehydration by the child's body weight. For example, a 10-kg child who is 10% dehydrated has lost 10% of his body weight, or 100 mL/kg, for a total fluid loss

Table 13–6. CALCULATION OF MAINTENANCE FLUID

Per Day Body Weight (kg)	Fluid Requirements/Day
<10	100 mL/kg
10–20	1000 mL + 50 mL/kg for each kg above 10
>20	1500 mL + 20 mL/kg for each kg above 20

Per Hour Body Weight (kg)	Fluid Requirements/Hour
<10	4 mL/kg
10–20	2 mL/kg for each kg above 10
>20	1 mL/kg for each kg above 20

of 1000 mL (Wetzel, 1991). Calculation of maintenance fluid is presented in Table 13–6. Potassium chloride (20 mEq/L) may be added once urine output has been established. Ongoing losses may be replaced concurrently with Ringer's lactate. The other half of the calculated loss along with maintenance fluid is replaced over the next 16 hours, usually with 5% dextrose and 0.45 NS with 20 mEq/L of potassium. The resuscitation bolus of Ringer's lactate is not included in the calculation to determine deficit and maintenance needs (Wetzel, 1991). An example of fluid replacement in a dehydrated child is presented in Table 13–7.

Fluid resuscitation described earlier is the initial treatment, if appropriate for moderate to severe dehydration. Following initial therapy, further replacement is calculated as maintenance plus estimated fluid deficit given evenly over the next 48 to 72 hours, with 5% dextrose and 0.2 NS being the fluid of choice. Fluid replacement that occurs too rapidly can cause neurologic complications, including seizures.

An additional early consideration for the child with hyponatremic dehydration is sodium replacement. If the child is severely hyponatremic (serum sodium <120 mEq/L), a 3% solution of sodium chloride (NaCl) can be rapidly given. Usually 4 mL/kg is given

Table 13–7. FLUID REPLACEMENT IN DEHYDRATION

To calculate the fluid requirements for a 20-kg child who is 10% dehydrated (serum sodium 132).

Deficit	20 kg × 10% (or 100 mL/kg) = 2000 mL
Maintenance	(10 kg × 4 mL/kg/hr) + (10 kg × 2 mL/kg/hr) = 60 mL/hr

Time	Administered Fluid
0–30 minutes	20 mL/kg Ringer's lactate
30 min–8 hours	1/2 the deficit (1000 mL)/8 hours = 125 mL/hr + maintenance fluids (60 mL/hr) or 185 mL/hr of D_5 • 45 NS + 20 mEq/L potassium
9–24 hours	1/2 the deficit (1000 mL)/16 hours = 63 mL/hr + maintenance fluids (60 mL/hr) or 123 mL/hr of D_5 • 45 NS + 20 mEq/L potassium

From Wetzel, R. C. (1996). Shock and fluid resuscitation. In D. G. Nichols, et al. (Eds.). *Golden hour: The handbook of advanced pediatric life support* (2nd ed., p. 131). St. Louis: Mosby–Year Book.

over 10 minutes to return to serum sodium to 125 mEq/L (Wetzel, 1991).

The extent of hypernatremic dehydration is more difficult to assess because water moves from the intracellular to the extracellular space, thus preserving the circulating volume. Seizures may develop before or during replacement therapy and are thought to be the result of intracellular dehydration. Long-term neurologic sequelae and death may result.

Serum Na correction in hypernatremia should take place no faster than 0.5 to 1.0 mEq/L/hour, because rapid correction of serum sodium can lead to cerebral edema. During replacement therapy, serum sodium levels are monitored every 2 to 4 hours. If serum sodium levels decrease too rapidly, the rate of hydration is decreased or the sodium content in the replacement fluid is increased. If levels decrease too slowly, the rate of hydration is increased. If the child demonstrates neurologic symptoms, cerebral edema is suspected and treated.

Fluid Volume Excess

Fluid volume excess occurs when there is (1) increased sodium concentration and water volume because of retention and/or excessive intake; (2) decreased renal excretion of water and sodium; and (3) decreased mobilization of fluid within the intracellular space (Baer, 1988). The major causes of excess fluid volume in infants and children are cardiorespiratory dysfunction, renal dysfunction, and inappropriate secretion of antidiuretic hormone, in which where serum sodium levels are decreased in the presence of fluid overload.

Clinical Assessment

The child experiencing fluid volume excess may present with weight gain, systemic and peripheral edema, puffy eyelids, increased central venous or right atrial pressure, tachypnea with increased work of breathing, hepatomegaly, and bounding pulses.

Daily weights on the same scale with notations of any items weighed with the child (i.e., endotracheal tube, arm board, dressings) are necessary to evaluate variations in observed weight. Significant variations are weight gains of 50 g/24 hours in the infant, 200 g/24 hours in the child, and 500 g/24 hours in the adolescent.

Children with fluid volume excess may have decreased urine output resulting from the underlying physiologic process (i.e., renal failure), and thus close monitoring of urine output is critical. Additional assessments include cardiac and respiratory auscultation for the development of a gallop rhythm and rales; evaluation of skin turgor and elasticity, blood pressure, and pulmonary artery wedge or left atrial pressure; and measurement of abdominal girth.

Laboratory Assessment

Laboratory assessment data may be of little significance in determining the presence of excessive

ECF volume. The following may be present: decreased hematocrit (because of hemodilution), decreased urine sodium levels, and decreased specific gravity of the urine. Normally, urine osmolality correlates well with specific gravity; hence, low urine osmolality values may be encountered. A chest radiograph may demonstrate pulmonary edema. Other changes are most closely linked to the underlying etiology of the excess fluid volume such as congestive heart failure.

Critical Care Management

The primary clinical implication of fluid volume excess, hypervolemia, is the potential for development of heart failure and pulmonary or cerebral edema, which are potentially life-threatening complications. Excessive ECF volume is usually treated by eradicating the underlying etiologies, as well as reducing the excessive volume. General fluid volume excess is treated with fluid restriction and the use of diuretics, although the overuse of diuretics can lead to volume depletion. Low-dose dopamine is useful to increase renal blood flow and promote sodium and water excretion. Sodium restriction may be used to indirectly decrease fluid retention.

Children with certain conditions, such as septic shock, may manifest signs and symptoms of pulmonary edema, despite the presence of hypovolemia. This occurs because of increased capillary permeability, which results in capillary "leak." Therefore, interventions may be required to treat the pulmonary edema, increase the ECF volume, and treat the underlying shock.

ELECTROLYTE DISORDERS

Sodium

Sodium (Na^+) is the major cation of the extracellular compartment. It regulates the voltage of action potentials in skeletal muscles, nerves, and the myocardium. The action or diffusion potential of the cell membrane occurs in response to the sodium and potassium concentration in the ECF and the ICF. Sodium plays a significant role in the maintenance of acid-base balance through combining with anions such as chloride and bicarbonate. Sodium is also responsible for the maintenance of water balance (volume) in the ECF through maintenance of the osmotic pressure (osmolality). Consequently, imbalances in water and sodium often occur together and are equated with alteration in serum osmolality. Extracellular sodium concentration is normally 135 to 145 mEq/L. The intracellular sodium concentration is usually 3 to 5 mEq/L.

Sodium is actively absorbed by the intestines and excreted by the kidneys and skin. The kidneys regulate sodium excretion primarily under the influence of the renin-angiotensin-aldosterone system. Renin is released by the kidneys in response to sodium concentration changes in the tubular fluid. The major factors that influence sodium excretion are the GFR and aldosterone. Alterations in the sodium levels in the body are often the result of clinical conditions involving fluid volume excess or deficit.

Hyponatremia

Hyponatremia, defined as a serum sodium concentration below 130 mEq/L, is a commonly encountered electrolyte disturbance occurring in about 1.5% of children hospitalized after the newborn period (Berry & Belsha, 1990). In the critically ill child, hyponatremia may occur as the result of fluid retention or sodium loss, or both. True hyponatremia must be differentiated from pseudohyponatremia. Pseudohyponatremia is a falsely low serum sodium value that may occur in patients with hyperlipemia or hyperproteinemia, or both. In children, diabetes mellitus is the most common cause of pseudohyponatremia.

Hyponatremia and hypovolemia may occur with renal or extrarenal losses. Losses may occur through diarrhea and vomiting or through other disorders such as burns or peritonitis. Other causes include excessive diuretics, osmotic diuresis, and adrenal insufficiency.

Hyponatremia and hypervolemia occurs most often in situations when the retention of water exceeds that of sodium. Causes include water intoxication, nephrotic syndrome, cardiac failure, cirrhosis, renal failure, and syndrome of inappropriate antidiuretic hormone (SIADH). In this situation, the hyponatremia is usually dilutional, so that true total body sodium is normal or even elevated.

Clinical Assessment. The severity of symptoms associated with hyponatremia depends on how quickly it develops. Central nervous system changes, such as lethargy and disorientation, are often accompanied by nausea, vomiting, and muscle cramps. Serum sodium levels of less than 120 mEq/L are associated with seizures and coma. This is related to the development of cerebral edema resulting from cellular swelling, and may be severe enough to cause cerebral herniation and death. Children who develop hyponatremia less acutely (over several days to weeks) may be asymptomatic or may develop only lethargy, nausea, and vomiting.

If hyponatremia is associated with fluid volume deficit the clinical assessment and findings will be the same as with moderate to severe dehydration. Decreased skin turgor may be seen accompanied by tachycardia; dry mucous membranes; decreased tearing or sweating; and alteration in systemic perfusion, as manifested by mottling, increased capillary refill time, and decreased central venous pressure.

Laboratory Assessment. The most helpful laboratory values for assessing the child with hyponatremia are serum sodium and serum osmolality measured simultaneously with urine electrolytes and urine specific gravity. The specific findings vary, depending upon whether the hyponatremia is associated with fluid volume deficit, fluid volume excess, or normal fluid volume.

Critical Care Management. The critical care management of a child with hyponatremia varies depending upon the relationship to fluid volume. With severe symptomatic hyponatremia with hypovolemia, serum sodium levels are rapidly elevated to 120 to 125 mEq/L by infusion of a hypertonic 3% saline solution. The amount of 3% saline necessary to raise the serum sodium level is judged to be 4 mL/kg or is calculated by the formula

$$(125 \text{ mEq/L} - \text{observed Na}^+ \text{ mEq/L}) \times \text{body weight (kg)} \times 0.6 \text{ L/kg}$$
(Paschall & Melvin, 1993)

A solution of 3% saline contains approximately 0.5 mEq Na/mL and is given over 30 minutes (Table 13–8). Serum sodium levels are monitored closely. If shock is present because of hypovolemia, 0.9% NS is given rapidly. Ongoing losses are replaced and specific treatment of the underlying cause is given.

Correction of hyponatremia with hypervolemia is directed toward treatment of the underlying cause. Administration of saline to increase sodium levels is not recommended because total body sodium may be normal and saline infusion may expand the ECF and worsen the situation. Total body water may be decreased by fluid restriction up to as much as 50% maintenance.

Table 13–8. SUGGESTED GUIDELINES FOR ADMINISTRATION OF ELECTROLYTE SOLUTIONS

Electrolyte	Administration Guidelines	Monitoring
Sodium (chloride)	• Hypertonic saline solutions (3 or 5%) may be given for severe hyponatremia (<120 mEq/L) when the patient is symptomatic. Infuse over approximately 30 minutes. The amount of hypertonic saline solution needed can be calculated by the following formula: mEq Na = (0.60) (body weight in kg) (125 − Na). Discontinue infusion when serum Na reaches 120–125 mEq/L and begin water restriction.	• Monitor serum sodium frequently. • Administer through large vein. • Maximum rate: 1 mEq/kg/h.
Potassium (chloride)	• IV push or undiluted potassium is never administered. • Recommended maximum dose is 0.5 mEq/kg/hr in children, although dosages of 0.25–1.0 mEq/kg/hr may be used for severe depletion. • Recommended maximum concentration for solution for peripheral lines is 40 mEq/L to prevent local irritation at infusion site. • Recommended maximum concentration for infusion for central lines is 1 mEq/2 mL. • Infusion rates of less than 0.3 mEq/kg/hr and concentrations of less than 60 mEq/L are usually adequate for replacement and maintenance of potassium.	• Continuous ECG monitoring is necessary during KCl intermittent infusion (≥0.5 mEq/kg/hr). • Monitor serum potassium levels frequently. • Use with caution in patients with renal impairment (avoid use if patient anuric or severely oliguric).
Calcium (chloride, gluconate)	• Administer slowly (no faster than 50 mg/min for CaCl₂; 100 mg/min for Ca gluconate) into a central line (in an emergent situation, may be given into a peripheral line if no central access is available). • May be administered by continuous infusion via peripheral intravenous line. Maximum concentration should not exceed 20 mg/mL. • Administer boluses in a dextrose or saline solution with no additives. Calcium is incompatible with many medications. Boluses are not administered in parenteral nutrition solutions or with intralipids.	• Monitor intravenous site closely. Necrosis and sloughing will occur with extravasation. • Monitor patients on digoxin who are receiving calcium supplements closely because elevated calcium levels precipitate digoxin-related arrhythmias. • Monitor for bradycardia, hypotension, and cardiac arrhythmias.
Phosphorus	• Potassium or sodium phosphate can be diluted in IV maintenance fluids; infusion rate should not exceed 0.05 mmol/kg/hr. The usual dose for both is 0.15–0.33 mmol/kg/dose IV over 6 hours.	• Side effects associated with rapid administration include hypotension.
Magnesium (sulfate)	• Administration by IV push is not recommended but in emergent situations may be diluted to 10 mg/mL and given slowly over 3–5 minutes. Dose should not exceed 150 mg/min. ECG should be monitored during administration. • Infusions are recommended to be diluted to <10 mg/mL and infused over at least 15–30 minutes. Maximum concentration is 200 mg/mL.	• Monitor patient closely for signs of hypermagnesemia. Cardiac arrest may occur with magnesium levels of 12–15 mEq/L.

Hypernatremia

Hypernatremia is defined as an excess of sodium in the ECF. It exists when serum sodium levels exceed 150 mEq/L (Conley, 1990). Severe clinical consequences are often encountered when serum sodium levels exceed 160 mEq/L (Paneth, 1980). Pure sodium excess is unusual, but has been reported as a result of feeding improperly mixed high-sodium rehydration solutions or formulas to infants or to older children who cannot gain water for some reason (Conley, 1990). Hypernatremia may also occur as the result of excessive administration of sodium bicarbonate during resuscitation endeavors.

In addition to an actual increase in sodium, hypernatremia can result from losses of water or from water deficit in excess of sodium deficit (Thelan et al., 1990). Conditions that produce fluid deficit and hypernatremia include diabetes insipidus, diabetes mellitus, excess sweating, increased insensible water loss, diarrhea, dehydration, and lack of thirst (Conley, 1990).

Clinical Assessment. The child with hypernatremia may manifest many of the same clinical signs and symptoms as those seen with dehydration. Loss of body weight greater than 10% or sodium levels above 150 mEq/L are accompanied by decreased skin turgor, and there is a characteristic "doughy" texture to the skin over the abdomen when it is pinched (Conley, 1990). The child may also be irritable, and a high-pitched cry is common. Periods of lethargy may alternate with the irritability. If the hypernatremia is allowed to progress without correction, increased muscle tone, coma, and seizures may result.

Central nervous system dysfunction often accompanies serum sodium concentrations over 158 mEq/L (Paneth, 1980). The central nervous system changes are thought to be the result of intracellular dehydration; shift of fluid from brain cells to cerebral vessels leading to subdural, subarachnoid, and intracerebral bleeding; decreased microvascular perfusion related to increased blood viscosity caused by increased plasma osmolarity; and intracranial bleeding caused by damage to the bridging veins as brain content contracts away from the skull (Barbero, 1992; Paschall & Melvin, 1993). Symptoms progress from restlessness and irritability through ataxia and tremulousness, tonic jerks, seizures, and eventually to death if uncorrected (Conley, 1990). Although the severity of the symptoms is directly related to the level of excess sodium, recovery from the central nervous system dysfunction appears unrelated, and neurologic sequelae are common (Paneth, 1980).

Laboratory Assessment. Serum sodium levels remain the best laboratory confirmation of hypernatremia. Urine osmolality also provides useful information on the degree of water loss associated with the excess sodium levels. If hypernatremia is merely believed to be an observed finding associated with an underlying disease state, diagnostic testing related to the suspected condition is also undertaken. In the child suspected of diabetes mellitus, glucose screen-

ing and glucose tolerance testing may be indicated. Similarly, culture sampling is indicated in cases when an infectious process appears to be the underlying etiology for the hypernatremia.

Critical Care Management. Hypernatremia may produce serious problems related to central nervous system dysfunction. The severity of the initial clinical signs is not predictive of the degree of residual neurologic impairment. Therefore, although careful attention must be directed at monitoring the child with hypernatremia, it is even more important to evaluate children at risk for hypernatremia to prevent this disturbance.

Treatment of hypernatremia is directed toward removal of excess sodium, if present, and correction of the underlying disorder. If fluid volume deficit is severe and shock is present or imminent, volume expansion must be undertaken, regardless of sodium levels. Isotonic solutions such as normal saline or lactated Ringer's solution are used in initial treatment. After initial stabilization and blood pressure recovery, hypotonic fluids may be administered to bring sodium levels down at the rate of 0.5 mEq/L/hour (Conley, 1990). More rapid reduction is associated with neurologic morbidity and mortality. Administration of fluid without sodium is never indicated, even during correction.

Children with hypernatremia and fluid volume deficit are at significant risk for cerebral edema and seizures with rapid correction of fluid deficit. Volume deficits are replaced over 48 to 72 hours after initial intervention to prevent shock.

For children with increased total body sodium and overhydration, excess sodium may be removed through the use of diuretics and decreased sodium administration if renal function is intact. If renal function is not intact, dialysis may be required (Wood & Lynch, 1992).

Potassium

Potassium has four major roles in the body. As the primary intracellular cation, potassium plays an important role in the action potentials in the nervous system, skin and smooth muscles, and the heart (myocardial electrical pacing). Acid-base balance is enhanced through the maintenance of electroneutrality of the body fluids. In cell anabolism, potassium is released from cells when the body relies on cell catabolism for energy. The biochemical reactions related to carbohydrate metabolism and synthesis of proteins require potassium also. Maintenance of intracellular osmolarity is accomplished through the "sodium-potassium" (active transport) pump (see Fig. 13–8). The normal range of serum potassium is 3.5 to 5.5 mEq/L with a concentration of 160 mEq/L inside the cell.

Potassium excretion is enhanced by aldosterone, an increase in cellular potassium, and increased activity of the distal portion of the nephron. Aldosterone is the primary controller of potassium secretion by the kidneys. Aldosterone controls the potassium concentration exactly, despite the daily fluctuations in potassium intake.

Hypokalemia

Hypokalemia is defined as a potassium deficit in the ECF: a serum potassium concentration less than 3.5 mEq/L. Potassium deficit in children is related to metabolic alkalosis; decreased potassium intake; external losses, such as those that may accompany vomiting, diarrhea, gastric suction, diuretic therapy, certain medications, or renal disease; and redistribution of extracellular potassium into the intracellular space (Brem, 1990; Feld et al., 1988; Thelan et al., 1990).

Clinical Assessment. Clinical symptoms are most common in the child experiencing acute potassium loss and may include muscle weakness, abdominal distension, and paralytic ileus. Other symptoms include lethargy, irritability, hyporeflexia, tetany, nausea, and vomiting.

Electrocardiographic changes may also be seen in the child with hypokalemia. These changes include flattened, inverted T waves and the presence of U waves following the QRS complex. Additional arrhythmias may be found in children with hypokalemia who have been treated with digitalis preparations (Brem, 1990).

Hyperglycemia develops with hypokalemia because insulin release is impaired (Clive & Stoff, 1984). Glucose homeostasis is impaired because of the altered insulin release.

Because potassium ions shift into the vascular space when acidosis develops, a mild elevation in serum potassium is seen with acidosis, which can be life-threatening in the critically ill child. A decline in serum potassium accompanies metabolic alkalosis, because potassium ions move into the cells to maintain the transmembrane electrical potential. The direction of the change in pH is opposite the change in serum potassium values.

Laboratory Assessment. Laboratory assessment of the child experiencing hypokalemia is accomplished through measurement of serum potassium levels. Bicarbonate levels and serum pH may be useful in determining whether an underlying acid-base disturbance has occurred.

Critical Care Management. The most significant problems caused by hypokalemia are related to cardiac dysfunction and muscle paralysis, including paralytic ileus. Treatment of hypokalemia is indicated whenever the serum potassium level falls below 3 mEq/L or the child exhibits symptoms related to hypokalemia (Paschall & Melvin, 1993). The speed of correction is related to the severity of the symptoms and the serum potassium level because too-rapid correction may cause hyperkalemia. Oral replacement is preferred if time and the child's condition permit. A dose of 0.5 to 1.0 mEq/kg (maximum 20 mEq) usually corrects the hypokalemia if ongoing losses are controlled (Paschall & Melvin, 1993). This dose

may be repeated every 4 to 8 hours. If intravenous replacement is required, concentrations up to 40 mEq/L are considered safe. Some recommend electrocardiogram (ECG) monitoring for concentrations higher than 40 mEq/L. The underlying cause of the hypokalemia is considered and treated.

In severe cases of potassium depletion, in which serum potassium levels are below 2.5 mEq/L, intravenous potassium replacement is used. Dosages of 0.25 mEq/kg/hour to 1.0 mEq/kg/hour may be used to correct severe depletion. Table 13–8 gives additional recommendations for administration. Continuous ECG monitoring for arrhythmias and frequent assessment and determination of serum potassium levels are critical to avoid complications associated with hyperkalemia.

If the child has alkalosis, potassium is replaced as the chloride salt because chloride depletion often accompanies hypokalemia (Perkin & Levin, 1990). If the child has hypokalemia and acidosis, serum potassium levels at a normal pH are lower, and thus correcting the pH before the hypokalemia can make the serum potassium level dangerously low (Perkin & Levin, 1990).

Hyperkalemia

Hyperkalemia is an excess of potassium in the extracellular fluid, existing when the plasma potassium level exceeds 5.5 to 6.0 mEq/L (Brem, 1990; Feld et al., 1988). There are four general categories of etiologies of hyperkalemia: altered renal excretion, impaired extrarenal regulation, shift from the intracellular to extracellular fluid, and increased potassium intake (Brem, 1990). Pseudohyperkalemia is relatively common and may be produced by conditions such as an increased WBC count above 100,000/mm^3 or a platelet count greater than 750,000/mm^3. A release of intracellular potassium during the clotting process results in the abnormal serum potassium level seen in that circumstance (Feld et al., 1988).

Conditions associated with altered renal excretion include renal dysfunction and the administration of potassium-sparing diuretics such as spironolactone and triamterene (Baer, 1988; Brem, 1990). Children with longstanding or congenital urologic abnormalities are likely to demonstrate subtly impaired renal potassium excretion. Reflux nephropathy, prune belly syndrome, and obstructions associated with bilateral hydronephrosis are likely to be associated with dysfunction of tubular epithelium leading to abnormalities of potassium excretion (Brem, 1990).

Impaired extrarenal regulation may be produced by such conditions as diabetes mellitus and adrenocortical insufficiencies, or administration of drugs such as heparin, beta-blocking agents, and angiotensin-converting enzyme (ACE) inhibitors (Brem, 1990). The absence of insulin limits the uptake of potassium from the ECF (Clark, 1989). Decreased mineralocorticoid activity impairs excretion of potassium by the kidney and colon, whereas drugs such as heparin or ACE inhibitors limit aldosterone release from the adrenal gland (Brem, 1990).

The shift of potassium from intracellular to extracellular fluid may be produced by rapid cell breakdown that accompanies cancer chemotherapy, burns or trauma, severe acidosis, hypertonicity, or the administration of succinylcholine (Baer, 1988; Brem, 1990; Feld et al., 1988). In these cases there may be normal body stores of potassium despite abnormal serum levels.

Hyperkalemia may also be produced by excessive intake of potassium, usually in the form of intravenous fluids or the oral ingestion of medications or food substances high in potassium. Although hyperkalemia may occur in young children by this mechanism, excessive intake is most often linked with impaired renal function.

Clinical Assessment. Mild elevation of potassium levels may not be clinically apparent. Clinical signs and symptoms associated with moderate to severe hyperkalemia reflect alteration of bioelectric processes with depolarization of excitable cells. They include muscle weakness, confusion, ascending paralysis, alterations of gastrointestinal function, and alterations in cardiac function. Severe hyperkalemia may lead to ventricular arrhythmias, cardiac arrest, and death (Farrington, 1991).

Cardiac dysfunction caused by hyperkalemia is the most serious and potentially the most life-threatening symptom. It is manifested by ECG changes. Initially there are tall peaked T waves present in precordial leads. This is followed by decreased amplitude of the R wave, widened QRS complex, prolonged PR interval, and disappearance of the P wave. Finally, there is blending of the QRS complex into the T wave, forming the classic sine wave of hyperkalemia. Although the sequence of ECG changes usually follows a pattern, the potassium levels at which the changes are seen varies between children.

Laboratory Assessment. Serum potassium levels provide the most useful information in the recognition of hyperkalemia. Bicarbonate levels and pH may be useful in evaluating underlying acid-base disorders. Care is taken to ensure that phlebotomy or heelstick techniques for laboratory testing are performed in such a way as to prevent falsely high values associated with hemolysis.

Critical Care Management. Treatment of hyperkalemia depends upon the clinical presentation. Potassium levels less than 6.5 mEq/L may require only discontinuation of fluids containing potassium along with close monitoring of serum potassium levels. Increasing potassium excretion with sodium polystyrene sulfonate (Kayexalate), especially in patients with diminished renal function, also helps to decrease potassium levels. Kayexalate, 1 to 2 g/kg, is given orally (PO), by nasogastric (NG) tube, or by rectum in a dextrose or sorbitol solution (by rectum is the preferred route). It can be given every 6 hours orally or enterally, or every 2 to 6 hours rectally. Because Kayexalate may bind calcium and magnesium, symptoms related to deficiencies in these electrolytes may occur.

Potassium levels higher than 6.5 mEq/L or those producing ECG changes are treated immediately. In the presence of life-threatening arrhythmias, calcium gluconate at 100 mg/kg or calcium chloride at 20 mg/kg may be given to reduce the cardiac toxicity associated with hyperkalemia (Farrington, 1991). Calcium increases the cardiac threshold potential, thereby reducing membrane depolarization and reestablishing a more normal relationship between resting membrane potential and firing threshold (Farrington, 1991). The onset of action of calcium is within minutes and the effects last for about 30 minutes.

Redistribution of potassium from the ECF to ICF decreases the elevated serum potassium level. This is accomplished by the administration of sodium bicarbonate, 1 to 2 mEq/kg, injected intravenously over 3 to 5 minutes. Sodium bicarbonate lowers the serum potassium level within 30 to 60 minutes, with the effects lasting several hours. Blood pH is monitored in children receiving this therapy. Children with respiratory failure are carefully evaluated, because sodium bicarbonate increases carbon dioxide (CO_2) production and may worsen respiratory acidosis if CO_2 cannot be excreted by the lungs.

Glucose, 0.5 g/kg, accompanied by regular insulin, 0.1 unit/kg, may also be used to shift potassium into the ICF. Cellular uptake of potassium from the ECF is enhanced with the glucose and insulin administration. The alteration in potassium level obtained with glucose and insulin therapy may last several hours (Farrington, 1991; Feld et al., 1988)

The diuretic furosemide (Lasix) may also be used to aid in children with adequate renal function. However, the amount of potassium removed is unpredictable. Therefore, diuretics are used only as an additional treatment modality.

The most effective mechanism for potassium removal is hemodialysis. It is the treatment modality of choice in cases of life-threatening hyperkalemia (Farrington, 1991). Although peritoneal dialysis may be used, it must be started early to be effective.

Calcium

Calcium, along with magnesium and phosphorus, plays a critical role in nerve transmission, bone composition, and regulation of enzymatic processes. Balance of these three electrolytes is maintained through intestinal absorption and renal excretion. The majority of calcium (98%–99%) is stored in the skeleton and teeth and the remainder is found in soft tissue and serum. Approximately 50% of serum calcium is ionized; the rest is bound to protein or anions. Only ionized calcium is used by the body for essential processes such as cardiac function, muscular contraction, nerve impulse transmission, and clotting. Therefore, the ionized calcium level is of greatest physiologic significance. Because ionized calcium level has little relationship to total serum calcium, direct measurement of ionized calcium is critical whenever a clinically important situation exists in which calcium levels may play a role. Total serum calcium levels range between 9.0 and 11.0 mg/dL; ionized calcium levels range between 4.4 and 5.4 mg/dL.

The roles of calcium in the body are conduction of electrical impulses in cardiac and skeletal muscles, activation of clotting mechanisms, involvement in the coagulation process, formation of bones and teeth, and mediation of hormonal production. Calcium also activates serum complement, a major factor in the function of the immune system. Calcium lines the pores of all cells and, with its positive charge, controls the ability of sodium to enter during depolarization because like charges repel each other. Consequently, calcium aids in the maintenance of cellular permeability.

Approximately 40% of the total serum calcium is bound to protein. Changes in plasma protein levels affect total serum calcium levels. Hypoalbuminemia decreases total serum calcium and increased albumin levels has the opposite effect. The binding of calcium to protein is affected by pH. If the pH is normal, approximately 40% of the total plasma calcium is bound to the serum albumin. A decrease in serum pH as seen with acidosis increases ionized calcium. In this situation, more calcium is removed from protein binding sites and is available for participation in chemical reactions. An increase in pH as seen with alkalosis increases binding and decreases ionized calcium. Even though the ionized calcium level is changed, total serum calcium levels may be unchanged.

Calcium regulation takes place through a number of different factors. Vitamin $D_{1,25}$ controls the intestinal absorption of calcium. Parathyroid hormone (PTH) regulates renal excretion of calcium. PTH secretion varies inversely with ionized calcium levels and is inhibited by hypomagnesemia and vitamin $D_{1,25}$ (Allen, 1992). Vitamin D, PTH, and serum phosphate levels control bone deposition and resorption of calcium.

Normally, because of the constant activity of bone deposition and resorption, there is little net change in serum calcium. However, when this activity is disturbed, bone is a reservoir to balance serum calcium levels. PTH, along with vitamin D-1,25, can change the degree of bone resorption. With increased levels of PTH, release of calcium from the bone is increased.

As mentioned earlier, renal calcium regulation is controlled by PTH in the distal nephron. Renal calcium reabsorption increases with increases in serum PTH.

Hypocalcemia

Hypocalcemia is a decrease of calcium in the extracellular fluid and exists when serum calcium levels are below 8 mg/dL in full-term infants and older children, and when ionized calcium levels are below 4 mg/dL. Though the definition of hypocalcemia re-

Table 13–9. CAUSES OF HYPOCALCEMIA

Disturbance in parathyroid hormone metabolism
Decreased production: hypoparathyroidism (surgical, infiltrative, idiopathic)
Hypomagnesemia
Hyperphosphatemia
Disturbance in vitamin D metabolism
Decreased intake: nutritional malabsorption
Protein malnutrition
Parenchymal liver disease
Anticonvulsant therapy
Nephrotic syndrome
Renal failure
Acute pancreatitis
Burns
Sepsis
Chemotherapy
Transfusion with citrate-preserved blood
Certain medications: aminoglycosides, glucagon, phenobarbital, phenytoin

Adapted from Agus, Z.S., & Goldfarb, S. (1985). In A.I. Arieff & R.A. DeFronzo (Eds.). *Fluid, electrolyte, and acid-base disorders* (Vol. 1, p. 516). New York: Churchill Livingstone.

flects a deficit in extracellular fluid concentration, the vast majority of calcium is bound either to bone or to protein. Since serum stores are replaced through the action of parathyroid hormone, most discussions of hypocalcemia are related to parathyroid function. In addition, absorption of calcium from the intestinal tract, excretion from the kidneys, and bone rebuilding help regulate the available stores (Thelan et al., 1990).

Hypocalcemia in children may be related to protein malnutrition, since decreased albumin for binding leads to decreased calcium levels. Other etiologies are listed in Table 13–9. Alterations in acid-base balance may also result in hypocalcemia.

Clinical Assessment. The child experiencing hypocalcemia may be asymptomatic or may present with signs and symptoms because of increased neuromuscular excitability. Tingling may be noted around the mouth, or in the fingertips and hands. Facial twitching caused by tapping on the facial nerve anterior to the ear (Chvostek sign) or carpopedal spasm caused by prolonged inflation of a blood pressure cuff (longer than 2–3 minutes) (Trousseau sign) may be noted. Muscle cramps, tetany, seizures, and laryngospasm may also occur (Lynch, 1990). Decreased myocardial contractility, hypotension, and a prolonged QT segment are potentially significant cardiovascular symptoms seen with hypocalcemia.

Laboratory Assessment. The total serum calcium level and the serum ionized calcium are the most useful laboratory tests in identifying hypocalcemia. Magnesium and phosphate samples are also taken. Arterial blood gases may demonstrate respiratory alkalosis as a cause of hypocalcemia. Because hypocalcemia may be linked to parathyroid dysfunction, complete evaluation may include analysis of levels of PTH. In addition, because hypocalcemia is associated with hypoproteinemia, plasma protein levels may be evaluated (Table 13–10).

Table 13-10. NORMAL LABORATORY VALUES IN ASSESSMENT OF CALCIUM ALTERATIONS

Test	Normal Values
Calcium (total)	
Infant	7.0–12.0 mg/dL
Child	8.0–11.0 mg/dL
Adolescent	8.5–11.0 mg/dL
Calcium (ionized)	4.4–5.4 mg/dL
Plasma protein (total)	
Infant (1–3 mo)	4.7–7.4 g/dL
Infant (3–12 mo)	5.0–7.5 g/dL
Child (1–15 yr)	6.5–8.6 g/dL
Serum parathyroid hormone (PTH)	
C-terminal	400–900 pg/mL
N-terminal	200–600 pg/mL

Critical Care Management. Two major areas of concern in the child experiencing hypocalcemia are neuromuscular dysfunction and alteration of cardiac function. Treatment of hypocalcemia is directed at both identification of the underlying etiology and correction of the alteration. Treatment of underlying conditions that are causing hypocalcemia is considered. Respiratory alkalosis is readily treatable. If hyperphosphatemia exists, correction should take place because administration of calcium may cause deposition of calcium-phosphate salts. A calcium phosphate product in a dose higher (total serum calcium × phosphate) than 80 mg/dL is avoided (Paschall & Melvin, 1993). Because hypomagnesemia affects PTH release and correction of hypocalcemia, this complication is considered and treated if hypocalcemia is severe or persistent. Any other underlying conditions, such as renal disease or hypoproteinemia, are also treated.

Acute hypocalcemia, especially in the child with impending neuromuscular or cardiovascular collapse, requires restoration of the serum ionized calcium level. Treatment is provided by intravenous administration of either calcium gluconate (9 mg elemental calcium/mL) or calcium chloride (36 mg elemental calcium/mL). The dosage for calcium gluconate is 100 mg/kg; the dose for calcium chloride is 10 to 20 mg/kg. Less thrombophlebitis and tissue necrosis with extravasation is noted with calcium gluconate, although all solutions with calcium salts are capable of causing tissue damage with extravasation. For this reason, calcium salts are administered through a central vein. Calcium is used cautiously in the digitalized child, because calcium may potentiate digoxin toxicity. Rapid administration of calcium may cause bradycardia and asystole, and thus ECG monitoring and slow administration (50 mg/minute for $CaCl_2$; 100 mg/min for Ca gluconate) is indicated (see Table 13–8).

Hypercalcemia

Hypercalcemia is an excess of calcium in the ECF and exists when the total serum calcium level exceeds 10.5 to 11 mg/dL (Mimouni & Tsang, 1987).

However, symptoms are not usually noted until the serum calcium level is higher than 12 mg/dL. Levels higher than 15 mg/dL may be life-threatening. Hypercalcemia may be caused by iatrogenic overtreatment of hypocalcemia, malignancies, immobility, hypophosphatemia, hyperparathyroidism, hyperthyroidism, vitamin D intoxication, subcutaneous fat necrosis, hypophosphatasia, and familial hypercalcemia. It is seen most commonly in the critically ill child concurrently with hyponatremia and hyperkalemia and as chronic renal failure resolves.

Clinical Assessment. Central nervous system symptoms occur most often and include lethargy, stupor, and coma (Paschall & Melvin, 1993). Seizures may also occur. Anorexia, nausea, and vomiting may ensue. A shortened QT interval on ECG may appear (DiGeorge, 1987). With severe, chronic hypercalcemia, calcification of the cornea, blood vessels, and kidneys may occur (Paschall & Melvin, 1993).

Laboratory Assessment. Laboratory assessment includes serum calcium, ionized calcium, plasma protein levels, and parathyroid hormone concentration (see Table 13–10). Changes in serum albumin levels affect calcium. For every 1.0 mg/dL change in albumin from the normal value, there is a corresponding 0.8 mg/dL change in ionized calcium (Baer, 1988).

Critical Care Management. Because serum calcium levels above 15 mg/dL may be life-threatening, immediate attention must be directed at reducing the amount of calcium in the ECF in addition to treating the underlying disorder. This is accomplished by administration of intravenous fluids to dilute the calcium in the ECF. "Loop" diuretics, such as furosemide, may also be used to enhance calcium excretion (Thelan et al., 1990). These therapies can also produce losses of sodium, potassium, magnesium, and phosphate (Allen, 1992). Thiazide diuretics restrict calcium excretion and are therefore contraindicated in the management of hypercalcemia (Levine & Kleeman, 1987). Vitamin D and antacids with calcium are not administered.

Additional therapies may be used to treat the underlying disorder. If excessive bone resorption because of malignancy or immobility is a problem, calcitonin (10 units/kg intravenously [IV] every 4–6 hours), mithramycin (25 μg/kg IV over 4 hours), prednisone (1–2 mg/kg/day IV divided into four doses), and indomethacin (1 mg/kg/day) may inhibit the process (Allen, 1992). Calcitonin is the least toxic and works by impeding PTH-induced bone resorption. It peaks at about 1 hour after administration.

Mithramycin is a toxic antibiotic that inhibits osteoclastic activity, but it depresses liver, kidney, and bone marrow function. Prednisone inhibits osteoclastic activity and intestinal absorption of calcium. Indomethacin acts only when bone resorption is the result of prostaglandin-secreting tumors, which are rare. Intravenous or oral phosphorus preparations may be used to increase bone deposition of calcium, although they should not be used in patients with hyperphosphatemia or renal failure because of the risk of calcification in the soft tissues.

Chloride

Chloride is the most abundant anion found in the ECF. Its major role is as a buffer in the maintenance of acid-base balance. Chloride, with sodium, also maintains serum osmolality. Chloride competes with bicarbonate for the cations in ECF to establish electrical neutrality. Passively attracted to positively charged cations, chloride ions balance the positively charged electrolytes in ECF and create sodium chloride (NaCl), hydrochloric acid (HCl), potassium chloride (KCl), and calcium chloride ($CaCl_2$).

Because chloride is usually combined with one of the major cations in the body, changes in serum chloride levels are usually indicative of changes in other electrolytes or in acid-base balance (Thelan et al, 1990).

Chloride ions are highly concentrated in gastric secretions and perspiration. Factors influencing excretion are acidosis and alkalosis because, as serum levels of bicarbonate change from the secretion of hydrogen ions, reciprocal changes in the serum chloride commonly occur (Robson, 1992). Normal serum chloride levels in children are 95 to 108 mEq/L.

Hypochloremia

Hypochloremia is a deficit of chloride in the ECF, which exists when serum chloride levels are below 95 mEq/L. Hypochloremia is typically seen with metabolic alkalosis because the retention of bicarbonate leads to excretion of chloride ions. Hypochloremia may also occur when the loss of chloride from the body exceeds sodium losses. It may be caused by excessive loss of gastric secretions or prolonged diarrhea. It may also occur as a consequence of excessive use of potent diuretics. Urinary losses of chloride may exceed sodium losses during correction of metabolic acidosis and during potassium deficiency (Barbero, 1992). Hypochloremia may occur as the result of limitation of chloride intake, which might accompany salt restricted diets, and excessive sweating such as that seen with the febrile child.

Clinical Assessment. The clinical findings in children with hypochloremia result mostly from the loss of sodium, potassium, and ionized calcium rather than chloride loss (Plumer & Cosentino, 1987). In a child with chloride loss that is disproportionate to sodium loss, clinical findings may include hyperirritability or agitation, muscle weakness or tetany, and slow shallow respirations. When there has been proportionate loss of sodium and chloride, clinical findings are characteristic of those found in hyponatremia and/or fluid volume deficit.

Laboratory Assessment. Laboratory assessment includes serum chloride, serum sodium, and bicarbonate levels, and pH. The pattern characteristic of hypochloremia is a decreased serum chloride, decreased serum sodium, and increased pH and bicarbonate levels (Baer, 1988).

Critical Care Management. Treatment for hypochloremia includes treating the primary underlying etiology while correcting the imbalance. The imbalance is usually corrected through the administration of sodium chloride, potassium chloride, or ammonium chloride. Three fourths of the imbalance is often replaced with sodium chloride and the remaining one fourth is replaced with potassium chloride. Ammonium chloride is used instead of potassium chloride if serum potassium levels are elevated (Baer, 1988). A 0.9% solution of sodium chloride is used to correct chloride imbalance. The dose varies, based on the child's normal fluid volume requirements. Usually potassium chloride is given in a dose of 0.5 to 1.0 mEq/kg over a 1- to 2-hour period. The dosage of ammonium chloride is calculated by multiplying the serum chloride deficit by the ECF volume (approximately 20% of body weight in kilograms) (Alfaro-LeFevre et al., 1992).

Hyperchloremia

Hyperchloremia is an excess of chloride in the ECF and exists when serum chloride levels exceed 108 mEq/L. Etiologies of hyperchloremia include excessive chloride intake, usually associated with medication administration, and conditions that lead to metabolic acidosis with excessive loss of bicarbonate ions, such as diarrhea, renal failure, and administration of isotonic saline solution (Thelan et al., 1990). As with hypochloremia, chloride excess may occur proportionately to increased sodium level, or chloride excess may be disproportionate to sodium excess. If the chloride increase is not proportionate to the sodium increase, hyperchloremic acidosis can result because of decreased hydrogen ion secretion in the proximal tubules (Baer, 1988).

Clinical Assessment. In the child experiencing chloride excess that is disproportionate to sodium excess, the following clinical findings may be present: muscle weakness, decreased level of consciousness, lethargy, and deep, rapid respirations (Baer, 1988; Thelan et al., 1990). When chloride excess occurs proportionately to sodium excess, the signs and symptoms associated with hypernatremia and/or fluid volume deficit predominate.

Laboratory Assessment. Laboratory assessment includes serum chloride, sodium, and bicarbonate levels, and pH. The pattern of laboratory values seen in hyperchloremia includes elevated serum chloride and sodium and decreased bicarbonate and pH levels. If urine pH is recorded, an increased value may be seen; however, this finding is unreliable. The changes in pH and bicarbonate levels are reflective of the acid-base disturbance that accompanies hyperchloremia, rather than the hyperchloremia itself.

Critical Care Management. The treatment of hyperchloremia is directed at identification of the underlying etiology and correction of acid-base disturbances and electrolyte and fluid imbalances. Fluids (either oral or intravenous) may be increased to dilute the excess chloride. Sodium bicarbonate may be indicated to correct the underlying metabolic acidosis. Diuretics may be used to eliminate chloride as well as sodium.

Phosphate

Phosphate, like calcium, is present in large quantities in bone. Eighty-five percent of phosphorus is held in the bone with calcium. Ten percent of phosphorus is found in the ECF. Phosphorus is also found in the teeth and soft tissues, and 5% of the total level is in the ICF. Phosphorus, the primary intracellular anion, exists in a variety of forms as phosphate and elemental phosphorus. Phosphates (components of phosphoproteins and phospholipids) play a significant role in intracellular energy-producing reactions. In addition, tissue oxygenation, central nervous system function, carbohydrate utilization, and leukocyte function are influenced by phosphates. Tissue oxygenation is dependent on the red cell's ability to transport oxygen to the tissues and on 2,3-diphosphoglycerate (2,3-DPG), an organic phosphate in RBCs that binds hemoglobin and decreases its affinity for oxygen. The kidney plays the major role in phosphorus homeostasis. More than 90% of plasma phosphate is filtered at the kidney and most reabsorption occurs in the proximal tubule.

The normal serum phosphate level may be as high as 6 mg/dL in infants and children compared with levels of 2.5 to 4.5 mg/dL in adults. Serum phosphorus levels are higher in the pediatric population because of the high rate of skeletal growth.

Hypophosphatemia

Hypophosphatemia is defined as an abnormally low concentration of inorganic phosphorus in serum. In children, levels below 3 mg/dL are usually defined as hypophosphatemia, although symptoms may not be present until the level is below 2 mg/dL (Fitzgerald, 1978). Levels lower than 1 mg/dL may be life-threatening.

The major causes of phosphate deficiency are severely limited intake, intestinal defects that prevent absorption, and renal tubular leaks (Masiak, 1985). Limited intake of phosphate is related to vomiting or long-term starvation, because phosphorus is abundant in normally consumed foods and beverages. Intestinal malabsorption of phosphate may occur because of excessive use of antacids, which bind phosphorus in the gastrointestinal tract, and malabsorption syndromes in which watery stools result, such as Crohn's disease or ulcerative colitis (Masiak, 1985). Malabsorption of phosphate also occurs in the presence of increased calcium levels. Renal tubular leaks, resulting in excess loss of phosphate, occur with rapid catabolism and destruction of body tissue. Metabolic acidosis is the predominant finding when this mechanism of phosphate loss is present. In children, burns may also produce hypophosphatemia as a result of renal wasting (Baker, 1985). In addition,

diuretic administration may lead to renal tubular leaks.

Hypophosphatemia is also seen in children with diabetic ketoacidosis (because of renal wasting), as a concurrent finding with administration of cytotoxic agents for treatment of tumors, with phosphate-poor parenteral hyperalimentation, and when low phosphate diets are used to treat renal failure (Thelan et al., 1990).

Clinical Assessment. Severe hypophosphatemia can affect multiple body systems, including the central nervous system and the hematologic, cardiac, and respiratory systems. Central nervous system dysfunction may be manifested by irritability, apprehension, disorientation, and altered level of consciousness. In severe hypophosphatemia, coma may occur. Neuromuscular findings may include tremors and seizures. These findings are most closely linked to the diminished intracellular ATP production and tissue hypoxia (Masiak, 1985).

Hematologic changes are also commonly encountered with hypophosphatemia. Hemolytic anemia may result from inadequate ATP for maintenance of the red cell membrane. Oxygen-hemoglobin binding capacity drops as a result of reduced availability of 2,3-DPG (Masiak, 1985). Leukocytes demonstrate decreased phagocytosis, and platelet abnormalities are also seen. The platelet abnormalities may account for increased epistaxis and gastrointestinal bleeding in children with hypophosphatemia (Masiak, 1985).

Cardiac and respiratory dysfunction occur as a result of altered electrical conduction and diminished levels of ATP. Cardiac findings in the critically ill child include premature ectopic beats and depressed myocardial function. Respiratory failure may result from respiratory muscle dysfunction associated with hypophosphatemia. Reduced activity level and fatigue are also encountered as a result of the cardiac and respiratory dysfunction.

Laboratory Assessment. The serum phosphorus level is of the greatest use in identification of hypophosphatemia. Because metabolic acidosis may also occur in hypophosphatemia, pH and bicarbonate levels yield useful information.

Critical Care Management. As with all electrolyte imbalances, the first step in the treatment process is to identify the underlying etiology and take steps to correct it. Then, replacement of phosphorus is undertaken. Replacement is generally done very slowly, because the actual serum level may not reflect a deficit in the intracellular compartment. Unless acute symptoms are present, phosphate depletion is treated by enteral administration of phosphorus 10 to 20 mg/kg/day divided into several doses to minimize diarrhea (Paschall & Melvin, 1993). Parenteral administration of phosphates is usually restricted to children with levels below 1 mg/dL (Baker, 1985). The dose generally recommended is 0.15 to 0.33 mmol/kg given as a continuous infusion over at least 6 hours (see Table 13–8). Subsequent dosages are based on the response to the initial dose. Either potassium or sodium phosphate may be used, with the potential complications associated with hyperkalemia or hypernatremia. Other adverse effects of phosphate administration include hyperphosphatemia, which may result in hypocalcemia, and hypotension. Care must be exercised in the administration of parenteral phosphorus. It must be well diluted to avoid irritation of the blood vessels, extravasation, and/or infiltration leading to tissue necrosis. Administration of large quantities of phosphorus may lead to precipitation with calcium if levels are not carefully monitored (Thelan et al., 1990).

Hyperphosphatemia

Hyperphosphatemia is defined as an excess of phosphate in the ECF and exists when phosphate levels exceed 4.5 mg/dL. Hyperphosphatemia may be produced by chronic renal failure, rapid cell catabolism, excessive intake of phosphates, neoplastic diseases, hyperparathyroidism, and excess consumption of vitamin D metabolites (Baer, 1988; Thelan et al., 1990). Elevated phosphate levels seldom become a concern unless renal excretion of phosphorus is impaired.

In chronic renal failure the renal tubules no longer excrete phosphorus, despite continued uptake in the gastrointestinal system. The disruption in renal function accompanied by decreased glomerular filtration rate leads to impaired phosphate elimination.

Rapid cell catabolism leads to the release of the cellular phosphorus stores into the ECF. Children being treated with chemotherapy for neoplastic disease of lymphatic origin may also develop hyperphosphatemia because of leakage of phosphates into the circulation as a result of cytolysis of cells (Masiak, 1985).

Hyperphosphatemia may also be seen in children at times of rapid growth, because serum phosphate levels may reach 6.0 mg/dL during periods of rapid growth. Vitamin D, which increases absorption of phosphorus in the gastrointestinal tract, may be helpful in providing phosphorus for bone growth and cellular function.

Clinical Assessment. An inverse relationship exists between phosphorus and calcium in the ECF. Therefore, in conditions producing hyperphosphatemia, hypocalcemia also exists. The relationship between these two imbalances accounts for the fact that the clinical signs and symptoms associated with hyperphosphatemia are the same as those found in the child experiencing hypocalcemia. Clinical findings include tachycardia, hyperreflexia, abdominal cramps, nausea, and diarrhea. Muscle tetany and soft-tissue calcifications are the more prominent findings in hyperphosphatemia (Kurokawa, 1985).

Laboratory Assessment. Laboratory testing in children suspected of having hyperphosphatemia includes serum phosphate levels as well as serum calcium levels. An elevated phosphate level is seen in conjunction with a clinically significant decreased serum calcium value.

Critical Care Management. Treatment should be directed both at determining the underlying etiology and correcting the imbalance. Hyperphosphatemia may be treated using dietary restrictions of phosphorus. If this does not result in lowered phosphate levels, aluminum antacids may be used. The antacids bind with the phosphate in the intestines and thus facilitate elimination. Adequate hydration and correction of hypocalcemia also enhance phosphate elimination. For the child with life-threatening symptoms, fluids to increase renal phosphate losses, treatment of hypocalcemia, and/or dialysis may be indicated.

Magnesium

Magnesium is the second most abundant intracellular cation. The distribution of magnesium is similar to that of potassium and is approximately 60% in the mineral component of bone, 40% in the body cells, and less than 1% in the ECF. The major roles of magnesium can be divided into three areas: enzyme and biochemical activation, mediation of skeletal muscle tension, and inhibition of electrical activity at the neuromuscular junction. Magnesium serves as a cofactor in numerous enzyme reactions that involve transfer of a phosphate group: metabolism of glucose, pyruvic acid, and ATP. Magnesium has a similar role to calcium as an inhibitor of electrical activity in neuromuscular function. Magnesium acts directly on the myoneural junction, affecting neuromuscular irritability and contractility of cardiac and skeletal smooth muscle (Innerarity & Stark, 1990).

The serum magnesium concentration is regulated primarily by the kidney. The kidneys have an extraordinary ability to conserve magnesium and with decreased intake of magnesium excrete less than 1 mEq/day. When the concentration of magnesium in the glomerular filtrate exceeds certain limits, large quantities of magnesium are lost in the urine (Masiak, 1985). Reabsorption occurs in the ascending limb of the loop of Henle and is modulated by the serum concentration of ionized magnesium.

Serum magnesium levels provide an imprecise measure of body magnesium stores because less than 1% of total body magnesium exists in the serum. Normal magnesium levels in the child are 1.5 to 2.5 mEq/L. Magnesium levels show small variations, correlating directly with changes in serum calcium and inversely with phosphorus (Kliegman & Wald, 1986). About 35% of the available magnesium is bound to protein.

Hypomagnesemia

Hypomagnesemia is the deficit of magnesium in ECF. Hypomagnesemia generally exists when the serum magnesium level is less than 1.4 mEq/L. There are three principal etiologies of decreased magnesium in the ECF: decreased intake, decreased intestinal absorption, and excessive loss of body fluids

(Baer, 1988). In younger children, hypomagnesemia is most often related to lack of magnesium administration during the time the child is NPO, or in malnutrition (decreased intake), severe diarrhea (decreased intestinal absorption), or severe dehydration (excessive loss of body fluids). Excessive use of diuretics (excessive loss of body fluids) and laxatives (decreased intestinal absorption) may also result in hypomagnesemia in the adolescent. Aminoglycoside antibiotics and antineoplastic agents may induce hypomagnesemia in children of any age because these drugs induce renal magnesium wasting (Innerarity, 1990).

Other imbalances seen with hypomagnesemia are hyponatremia, hypokalemia, hypophosphatemia, and distal renal tubular acidosis. Hypomagnesemia may damage the ATP-dependent sodium, potassium, phosphate, and hydrogen pumps, which will cause excess urinary losses of these electrolytes (Weigle & Tobin, 1992).

Clinical Assessment. The signs and symptoms of hypomagnesemia are similar to those of hypocalcemia and include neuromuscular excitability, tetany, and cardiac dysrhythmias (Thelan et al., 1990). Cardiac rhythm disturbances include premature ventricular beats and ventricular tachycardia and fibrillation (Wood & Lynch, 1992). Despite generalized neuromuscular excitability, respiratory muscle depression may occur, creating a need for mechanical ventilation (Flink, 1987).

Clinically, the child may appear to be confused, and may complain of dizziness or have hallucinations. Seizures may develop with progression to coma (Innerarity, 1990). In addition, the child may present with many of the same clinical signs that are found with hypocalcemia. The signs and symptoms of hypomagnesemia are often compounded by the coexistence of hypocalcemia and hypokalemia. When these electrolyte disturbances are persistent, hypomagnesemia may exist. Table 13–11 presents the relationships between signs and symptoms of these three electrolyte disturbances.

Laboratory Assessment. Laboratory testing includes serum magnesium, potassium, and calcium. Urine testing for magnesium and calcium may be useful, although it is not necessarily required to confirm the abnormality. Decreased serum magnesium levels are accompanied by decreased potassium levels in 50% of children evaluated (Innerarity, 1990). Urine magnesium levels are also decreased.

Critical Care Management. Treatment of hypomagnesemia is directed at identification of the underlying etiology as well as correction of the imbalance. With severe magnesium deficiency resulting in symptoms such as ventricular arrhythmias and/or seizures, intravenous magnesium sulfate may be diluted to 10 mg/mL and given slowly over 3 to 5 minutes. Subsequent doses may be repeated if necessary, based on the child's response and serum magnesium levels. Adequate renal function must be assured before treatment is undertaken, because if function is diminished hypermagnesemia will result (Thelan et al., 1990). Other complications of parenteral magnesium administration include neuromuscular and respiratory depression, hypotension, and malignant arrhythmias.

Although oral and intramuscular magnesium administration may be more easily accomplished, neither can be relied upon to correct a serious deficit. Intramuscular magnesium absorption is erratic, based on the amount of subcutaneous fat tissue. Intestinal absorption of oral magnesium is extremely variable. If either intramuscular or oral replacement is chosen, careful attention must be directed at monitoring serum levels.

Hypermagnesemia

Hypermagnesemia is defined as an excess of magnesium in the ECF. Hypermagnesemia exists when the serum magnesium level exceeds 2.5 mEq/L. This condition most often occurs as the result of underlying chronic renal disease. Transient increases in serum magnesium levels may accompany ECF deficit or excessive administration of magnesium-containing drugs (Metheny, 1987).

Clinical Assessment. The child with hypermagnesemia demonstrates profound clinical signs and symptoms associated with central nervous system depression. The findings may include lethargy, mus-

Table 13–11. CLINICAL PICTURE OF MAGNESIUM DEFICIENCY AND ASSOCIATED ABNORMALITIES OF CALCIUM AND POTASSIUM

Cerebellar	Mental	Hypocalcemia and Hypokalemia	
		Neuromuscular	Cardiac
Vertigo	Delirium	Muscle tremor	Increased QT interval
Ataxia	Apathy	Twitching	Decreased ST segment
Nystagmus	Depression	Weakness	Broad, flat T waves
Athetoid and choreiform movements	Personality changes	Hyperreflexia	Digitalis toxicity
	Coma	Chvostek sign	Arrhythmias
	Irritability	Carpopedal spasm	
		Tetany and seizures	

From Lau, K. (1985). Magnesium metabolism: Normal and abnormal. In A.I. Arieff & R.A. DeFronzo (Eds.). *Fluid, electrolyte and acid-base disorders* (Vol. 1, p. 610). New York: Churchill Livingstone.

cle weakness, inability to swallow, diminished gag reflex, generalized hyporeflexia, hypotension, bradycardia, and ECG changes (prolonged PR, QRS, and QT intervals, AV block) (Thelan et al., 1990). Severe hypermagnesemia may lead to coma or cardiac arrest.

Laboratory Assessment. Laboratory assessment of hypermagnesemia is performed by evaluating serum magnesium level. However, because hypermagnesemia is most often associated with chronic renal disease, renal function tests including blood urea nitrogen (BUN) and serum creatinine may be useful in identifying the underlying etiology.

Critical Care Management. Treatment of hypermagnesemia is directed at both correction of the imbalance and identification and treatment of the underlying etiology. Calcium gluconate or other calcium salts may be administered because calcium is an antagonist to magnesium and often reverses the cardiac manifestations of hypermagnesemia. Intravenous hydration facilitates renal excretion of excess magnesium in the presence of normal renal function. If renal dysfunction is apparent, dialysis may be indicated.

SUMMARY

This chapter has presented the regulation and assessment of fluid and electrolyte balance in critically ill children. Care of the critically ill child depends on accurate assessment and complete understanding of the unique interrelationships of these substances. Minor deviations in electrolyte and fluid balance may produce profound complications in children. Therefore, careful attention to signs and symptoms, and appropriate intervention to alleviate the abnormality and correct the underlying etiology, may reduce the severity and length of time of critical illness.

References

Alfaro-LeFevre, R., et al. (1992). *Drug handbook: A nursing process approach.* Redwood City, Ca: Addison-Wesley Nursing, The Benjamin/Cummings Publishing.

Allen, D.B. (1992). Disorders of the endocrine system relevant to pediatric critical illness. In B.P. Fuhrman & J.J. Zimmerman (Eds.). *Pediatric critical care* (pp. 781–796). St. Louis: Mosby–Year Book.

Andrews, M., & Mooney, K. (1990) Alteration of renal and urinary tract function in children. In K. McCance & S. Huether (Eds.). *Pathophysiology: The biologic basis for disease in adults and children* (pp. 1160–1171). St. Louis: C.V. Mosby.

Baer, C. (1988). Regulation and assessment of fluid and electrolyte balance. In M. Kinney, D. Packa, & S. Dunbar (Eds). *AACN Clinical Reference for Critical-Care Nursing* (2nd ed., pp. 193–236). New York: McGraw-Hill.

Baker, W. (1985). Hypophosphatemia. *American Journal of Nursing,* 22(4):999.

Barbero, G.J. (1992). General considerations in the care of sick children. In R.E. Behrman (Ed.). *Nelson textbook of pediatrics* (14th ed., pp. 171–211). Philadelphia: W.B. Saunders.

Berry, P., & Belsha, C. (1990). Hyponatremia. *Pediatric Clinics of North America,* 37(2):351–363.

Boineau, F., & Lewy, J. (1990). *Nelson essentials of pediatrics.* Philadelphia: W.B. Saunders.

Brem, A. (1990). Disorders of potassium homeostasis. *Pediatric Clinics of North America,* 37(2):419–427.

Clark, D. (1989). Potassium disorders. In J. Abuelo (Ed.). *Renal pathophysiology: The essentials* (pp. 116–133). Baltimore: Williams & Wilkins.

Clive, D., & Stoff, J. (1984). Renal syndromes associated with nonsteroidal inflammatory drugs. *New England Journal of Medicine,* 310:563–572.

Conley, S. (1990). Hypernatremia. *Pediatric Clinics of North America,* 37(2):365–372.

Costarino, A., & Baumgart, S. (1986). Modern fluid and electrolyte management of the critically ill premature infant. *Pediatric Clinics of North America,* 33(1):153–178.

DiGeorge, A. (1992). Disorders of the parathyroid glands. In R. Behrman (Ed.). *Nelson's textbook of pediatrics* (14th ed., pp. 1431–1435). Philadelphia: W.B. Saunders.

Engle, W. (1986). Evaluation of renal function and acute renal failure in the neonate. *Pediatric Clinics of North America,* 33(1):129–151.

Farrington, E. (1991). Treatment of hyperkalemia. *Pediatric Nursing,* 17(2):190–192.

Feld, L., Kaskel, F., & Schoeneman, M.J. (1988). The approach to fluid and electrolyte therapy in pediatrics. *Advances in Pediatrics,* 35:497–536.

Fitzgerald, F. (1978). Clinical hypophosphatemia. *Annual Reviews in Medicine,* 29:177.

Flink, E. (1987). Magnesium deficiency. *Hospital Practice,* 15:1161.

Goldberger, E. (1986). *Primer of water, electrolyte and acid-base syndromes.* Philadelphia: Lea & Febiger.

Guyton, A. (1991). *Textbook of medical physiology* (8th ed.) Philadelphia: W.B. Saunders.

Innerarity, S. (1990). Electrolyte emergencies in the critically ill renal patient. *Critical Care Nursing Clinics of North America,* 2(1):89–99.

Innerarity, S., & Stark, J. (1990). *Fluid and electrolytes.* Springhouse, PA: Springhouse Publications.

Kliegman, R., & Wald, M. (1986). Problems in metabolic adaptation: Glucose, calcium, and magnesium. In M. Klaus & A. Fanaroff (Eds.). *Care of the high risk newborn* (3rd ed., pp. 220–238). Philadelphia: W.B. Saunders.

Kurokawa, K., et al. (1985). Physiology of phosphorus metabolism and pathophysiology of hypophosphatemia and hyperphosphatemia. In A. Arieff & R. DeFronzo (Eds.). *Fluid, electrolyte and acid-base disorders* (Vol. 1, pp. 625–660). New York: Churchill Livingstone.

Levine, M., & Kleeman, C. (1987). Hypercalcemia: Pathophysiology and treatment. *Hospital Practice,* 22(7):93.

Lynch, R. (1990). Ionized calcium. *Pediatric Clinics of North America,* 37(2):373–389.

Masiak, M. (1985). Potassium, magnesium, phosphorus, and calcium imbalances. In M. Masiak, M. Naylor, & L. Hayman (Eds.). *Fluids and electrolytes through the life cycle* (pp. 67–84). Norwalk, CT: Appleton-Century-Crofts.

Metheny, N. (1987). *Fluid and electrolyte balance: Nursing considerations.* Philadelphia: J.B. Lippincott.

Mimouni, F., & Tsang, R. (1987). Disorders of calcium and magnesium metabolism. In A. Fanaroff & R. Martin (Eds.). *Neonatal-perinatal medicine* (pp. 1077–1092). St. Louis: C.V. Mosby.

Moore, K.L. (1983). *Before we are born: Basic embryology and birth defects* (2nd ed., pp. 170–189). Philadelphia: W.B. Saunders.

Naylor, M. (1985). Interruptions in water and sodium balance. In M. Masiak, M. Naylor, & L. Hayman (Eds.). *Fluid and electrolytes through the life cycle* (pp. 41–66). Norwalk, CT: Appleton-Century-Crofts.

Paneth, N. (1980). Hypernatremic dehydration in infancy: An epidemiologic review. *American Journal of Diseases of Childhood,* 134:785–792.

Paschall, J.A., & Melvin, T. (1993). Fluid and electrolyte therapy. In P.R. Holbrook (Ed.). *Textbook of pediatric critical care* (pp. 653–702). Philadelphia: W.B. Saunders.

Perkin, R.M., & Levin, D.L. (1990). Mineral and glucose requirements and abnormalities. In D.L. Levin & F.C. Morriss (Eds.). *Essentials of pediatric intensive care* (pp. 121–136). St. Louis: Quality Medical Publishing.

Plumer, A., & Cosentino, F. (1987). *Principles and practice of intravenous therapy*. Boston: Little, Brown.

Robson, A. (1992). Parenteral fluid therapy. In R. Behrman (Ed.). *Nelson textbook of pediatrics* (14th ed., pp. 171–211). Philadelphia: W.B. Saunders.

Schwartz, G., et al. (1976). A simple estimate of glomerular filtration rate in children derived from body length and plasma creatinine. *Pediatrics*, 58:259–263.

Schwartz, G., et al. (1984). A simple estimate of GFR in children. *Journal of Pediatrics*, 104:849–854.

Sherry, S., & Kramer, I. (1955). The time to passage of the first stool and first urine in the newborn infant. *Journal of Pediatrics*, 46:158–159.

Thelan, L., Davie, J, & Urden, L. (1990). *Textbook of critical care nursing: Diagnosis and management*. St. Louis: Mosby–Year Book.

Tisher, C., & Madsen, K. (1991). Anatomy of the kidney. In B. Brenner & F. Rector (Eds.). *The kidney* (4th ed., pp. 5–7). Philadelphia: W.B. Saunders.

Walker, W.A., & Hendricks, K.M. (1985). *Manual of pediatric nutrition*. Philadelphia: W.B. Saunders.

Weigle, C.G.M., & Tobin, J.R. (1992). Metabolic and endocrine disease in pediatric intensive care. In M.C. Rogers (Ed.). *Textbook of pediatric intensive care* (2nd ed., Vol. 2, pp. 1235–1289). Baltimore: Williams & Wilkins.

Wetzel, R.C. (1991). Shock and fluid resuscitation. In D.G. Nichols et al. (Eds.). *Golden hour: The handbook of advanced pediatric life support* (pp. 81–104). St. Louis: Mosby–Year Book.

Wood, E.G., & Lynch, R.E. (1992). Fluid and electrolyte balance. In B.P. Fuhrman & J.J. Zimmerman (Eds.). *Pediatric critical care* (pp. 671–688). St. Louis: Mosby–Year Book.

Wood, R., Boat, T., & Doershuk, C. (1975). Cystic fibrosis. In J. Murray (Ed.). *Lung disease, state of the art*. New York: American Lung Association.

Suggested Readings

Chenevey, B. (1987). Overview of fluids and electrolytes. *Nursing Clinics of North America*, 22(4):749–759.

Graves, L. (1990). Disorders of calcium, phosphorus, and magnesium. *Critical care nursing quarterly*, 13(3):3–13.

Hazinski, M. (1988). Understanding fluid balance in the critically ill child. *Pediatric Nursing*, 14(3):231–236.

Lancaster, L. (1987). Renal and endocrine regulation of water and electrolyte balance. *Nursing Clinics of North America*, 22(4):761–779.

CHAPTER *14*

Nutrition

JUDY VERGER

During an acute physiologic crisis, the attention of the healthcare team is on stabilizing the condition of the patient. Thus, nutritional support is often not a priority, even though it is accepted that nutritional interventions can improve patient recovery and survival (A.S.P.E.N. Board of Directors, 1993). Both an acquired and a preexisting tendency toward protein-energy malnutrition (PEM) have been documented in hospitalized children (Cooper et al., 1981, Cooper et al., 1982; LeLeiko & Benkov, 1986; Merritt & Suskind, 1979; Parsons et al., 1980; Pollack et al., 1981; Pollack et al., 1982). Previous work by Pollack and associates (1981, 1982) found that 16% to 19% of PICU patients were malnourished. Those children at risk for serious nutritional deficiencies were younger than 2 years of age and had medical problems rather than surgical problems. Acute PEM has been linked to higher mortality and increased physiologic instability (Pollack, Ruttimann, & Wiley, 1985).

The risk of malnutrition for critically ill children is increased by their higher metabolic needs and by other associated conditions common to the pediatric intensive care population. Congenital heart disease, bronchopulmonary dysplasia, gastrointestinal reflux, and other chronic conditions commonly lead to feeding difficulties and can predispose critically ill children to undernutrition and growth failure (Huddleston et al., 1993; Quinn & Askanazi, 1987; Rosenthal,

1993; Shepard et al., 1987). Children have larger obligate energy needs because the major metabolic organs make up a larger proportion of body weight. These higher energy requirements combined with lower macronutrient stores make children less able to withstand nutritional deprivation (Pollack et al., 1982).

Protein-calorie malnutrition has a detrimental effect on a number of major body systems (Table 14–1). Malnutrition causes mobilization of muscle protein stores and negative nitrogen balance (Steffee, 1980). Malnutrition may be a cofactor in morbidity and death in patients with hypermetabolism and organ dysfunction (Cerra, 1986; Lehmann, 1993; Quinn & Askanazi, 1987). According to Jeejeebhoy (1994), nutrition changes muscle performance before affecting body composition, and patient outcomes correlate with these functional changes. Protein and calorie depletion dramatically compromises immunocompetence, resulting in an increased risk of infection with altered cell-mediated immunity, altered antibody responses, and impaired wound healing (Irvin & Hunt, 1974; Konstantinides & Lehmann, 1993; Lehmann, 1993; Sorensen, Leiva, & Kuvibidila, 1993). Low albumin may negatively affect oxygen diffusion and the ability of neutrophils to kill bacteria. Protein, carbohydrates, fats, and various vitamins and minerals are responsible for synthesis and collagen

Table 14-1. SELECTED EFFECTS OF MALNUTRITION ON BODY SYSTEMS

Organ System	Pathophysiology	Nursing Diagnosis
Immunologic/hematologic	Stem cell failure Decreased erythropoietin synthesis Decreased lymphocytic production Altered antibody response/cell-mediated immunity	Fatigue related to anemia Potential for infection Alteration in tissue perfusion Alteration in skin integrity
Metabolic	Mobilization of skeletal muscle Decreased visceral protein synthesis Reduced vascular osmotic gradient Negative nitrogen balance	Alteration in nutrition; protein less than body requirements Potential fluid volume deficit related to decreased intake, excessive losses Potential for injury and impaired physical mobility Alteration in skin integrity
Respiratory	Decreased ventilatory drive Decreased surfactant Decreased respiratory muscle mass Decreased vital capacity Decreased functional residual capacity	Potential for hypoxia Impaired gas exchange
Cardiac	Decreased cardiac output, stroke volume, contractility Preload intolerance Dysrhythmias	Alteration in tissue perfusion
Gastrointestinal	Depressed enzymatic activity Reduced absorptive surface area Intestinal bacterial overgrowth Impaired motility Decreased pancreatic function	Alteration in bowel elimination

Adapted from Lehmann, S. (1993). Nutrition support in the hypermetabolic patient. *Critical Care Nursing Clinics of North America,* 5(1), 97–103.

strength and therefore wound integrity. The incidence of mortality is increased with malnutrition severe enough to depress cell-mediated immunity (Meakins et al., 1977; Meyer et al., 1994).

Malnutrition has a widespread effect on the heart and lungs, predisposing the patient to cardiopulmonary failure (Murphy & Conforti, 1993; Rothkopf et al., 1989; Weissman & Hyman, 1987). These muscles, like other muscles in the body, require sufficient protein and calories to perform their physiologic activities. Without adequate protein and energy support, the pediatric patient can experience a decrease in ventilatory drive and respiratory efficiency, decrease in surfactant resulting in a change in pulmonary compliance, decrease in diaphragm mass and muscle atrophy, decrease in vital capacity, and decrease in clearance of bacteria by the lungs (Arora & Rochester, 1982; Doekel et al., 1976; Kelly et al., 1984; Schlichtig & Sargent, 1990; Weissman et al., 1983; Whittaker et al., 1990). Weaning from mechanical ventilation may be inhibited (Bassili & Deitel, 1981). Hypomagnesemia and hypophosphatemia may specifically contribute to respiratory muscle depletion (Agusti et al., 1984; Dhingra et al., 1984). Structural and functional effects on the cardiac muscle have been demonstrated as a response to malnutrition (Murphy & Conforti, 1993). A decrease in heart volume proportional to a decrease in body weight has been found (Heymsfield et al., 1978). Also, a decrease in cardiac output and stroke volume, hypotension, and bradycardia have been demonstrated (Viart,

1977). Electrocardiographic changes may also occur. Vitamin and trace element deficiencies may affect cardiac performance (Pollack, 1993).

Other physiologic conditions associated with malnutrition include the gastrointestinal changes of gut mucosal atrophy, decreased intestinal motility, malabsorption, and decreased pancreatic function (Pollack, 1993; Suskind, 1975). Malnutrition may also depress fibronectin and other proteins (Scott et al., 1982).

This chapter focuses on nutritional support for the critically ill child. Discussion of embryology and anatomy and physiology of the pediatric gastrointestinal system provides the background for understanding how nutritional support can be most effective. Nutritional assessment and nutritional management in the pediatric intensive care unit (ICU) is presented along with appropriate interventions.

EMBRYOLOGY

The digestive tract and biliary passages develop from the primitive gut (Moore, 1993). As early as the third week of gestation the primitive gut can be differentiated into the foregut, the midgut, and the hindgut. The pharynx, esophagus, stomach, duodenum (proximal to the opening of the bile duct), liver, pancreas, and bile duct system develop from the foregut. The duodenum distal to the opening of the bile duct, jejunum, ileum, cecum, appendix, ascending colon, and proximal part of the transverse colon are derived from the midgut. Other parts of colon including the left one third to one half of the transverse colon, the rectum, and the superior part of the anal canal originate from the hindgut.

The esophagus and trachea are one tube until the fourth week of gestation, when the tracheoesophageal septum forms to separate the laryngotracheal tube and the esophagus. The esophagus is almost occluded by the proliferating epithelium during the fifth to sixth week of gestation. At about 7 weeks the esophagus elongates and reaches its final length. By the end of the embryonic period the esophagus hollows (recanalizes).

The stomach is first distinguished as a dilatation of the gut during the fourth to fifth week of embryonic development. The stomach rotates clockwise longitudinally and moves from the neck region into the abdomen. The growth rate of the stomach wall varies, forming lesser and greater curvatures and giving the stomach its asymmetric appearance.

The liver, gallbladder, and biliary duct system begin development during the fourth to fifth week of gestation from the hepatic diverticulum. The liver grows rapidly and soon fills most of the abdominal cavity. In the sixth week of gestation hemopoiesis begins, giving the liver a bright red appearance. By the end of gestation hemopoietic activity subsides, liver growth slows, and its size relative to body weight is reduced. The biliary apparatus is functional by the thirteenth to sixteenth week.

Bile formation by the hepatic cells begins during the twelfth week. Bilirubin (bile pigments) begins to form and enter the duodenum during the thirteenth to sixteenth week of development. Bilirubin gives duodenal contents a dark green or meconium color. The biliary apparatus is functional at 13 to 16 weeks of gestation.

The pancreas is created from ventral and dorsal buds and fuse in its final form during the seventh week of gestation. Somatostatin, glucagon, insulin, and pancreatic polypeptide-containing cells appear at or before the tenth week of gestation. Insulin secretion begins at about 20 weeks.

The duodenum begins to develop early in the fourth week of gestation, originating from the foregut and midgut. The duodenum rotates with the stomach. During the fifth and sixth weeks, the lumen of the duodenum narrows and may be occluded by epithelial cells. By approximately the sixth week, the gut lengthens rapidly and causes a U-shaped region of the future jejunum and the entire transverse colon to transiently herniate into the umbilical cord. The intestines continue to develop within the umbilical cord. At the tenth to twelfth week of gestation, while the intestines rotate counterclockwise 270 degrees, reentry of the intestines occurs. By the end of the embryonic period, the lumen hollows. Further positioning of the small intestine, appendix, and transverse and sigmoid colon continues until the gastrointestinal tract assumes its final anatomic position at 20 weeks of gestation and becomes fixed to the posterior abdominal wall.

The colon is formed at the sixth week of gestation by division of the rectum and upper anal canal from the urogenital sinus. The rectum and the superior part of the anal canal are also separated from the exterior by the cloacal (anal) membrane. This anal membrane normally breaks down by the seventh to eighth week forming the anal canal.

ESSENTIAL ANATOMY AND PHYSIOLOGY

Growth and maintenance of the human body is dependent on the digestion and absorption of nutrients and water. This process begins in the oral cavity and ends at the anal sphincter. Supported by a rich blood supply, the lymphatic system, and intrinsic and autonomic nervous innervation, the gastrointestinal tract allows for food to be moved through the body, where it is exposed to and absorbed by a large surface area.

The oral cavity is composed of the lips, tongue, cheeks, teeth, taste buds, and salivary glands. These structures decrease the size of food, stimulate saliva secretion, and move food in position for swallowing.

The pharynx provides for the movement of food into the esophagus. Food passes through the pharynx to the esophagus in approximately 1 second.

The esophagus is a channel for the passage of food from the pharynx to the stomach. Along the length of the esophagus are glands that secrete mucus to provide lubrication for the passage of food. The lower gastroesophageal sphincter is located at the distal 2 to 5 cm of the esophagus. This sphincter surrounds the opening of the stomach with increased amounts of muscle and remains narrowed until a wave of peristalsis moves through it.

The stomach is a pear-shaped organ with the esophagus at the top end and the duodenum at the lower end. The stomach is the most dilated part of the gastrointestinal tract and is an easily distensible reservoir for food. In infancy, the stomach usually is transverse. By approximately age 7, it is the shape and position of the adult stomach. At birth the stomach has the capacity to hold approximately 10 to 20 mL. By 3 months the stomach's capacity is 150 to 200 mL, and by age 10 it is about 750 to 900 mL. Stomach capacity is important to consider when providing enteral feedings for the critically ill infant. The lining of the stomach is made up of mucosal folds called rugae. Within these folds are chief, parietal and mucous neck cells that secrete various elements of digestive juice. The newborn stomach mucosal wall is thinner than that of an adult.

The liver and pancreas empty into the small intestine. The pancreas lies parallel to and beneath the stomach and has the internal structure identical to that of the salivary gland. The major function of the pancreas is digestion and utilization of dietary nutrients. The liver assists with digestion by synthesizing bile acid.

The small intestine consists of the duodenum,

jejunum, and ileum and extends from the pyloric sphincter at the bottom of the stomach to the ileocecal valve. The lining of the small intestine consists of folds called villi that project into the intestinal lumen. Microvilli cover the membranes of mature epithelial cells that make up the villus tip and form the brush border region. The brush border contains digestive enzymes and contributes to the transfer of nutrients and electrolytes. This area is highly specialized for absorption. Pit-like structures exist between villi called the "crypts of Lieberkühn" and are composed of absorptive cells and goblet cells that produce mucus. Three sets of lymph nodes also exist along the bowel.

The large intestine begins with the ileocecal valve at the cecum. It includes the appendix and extends through the ascending, transverse, and descending colon and ends at the rectum and anal canal. The internal and external sphincters are made up of the anorectal ring. In the large intestine there is an increase in the number of goblet cells.

An infant's intestinal length is proportionately larger than that of an adult. This proportional increase allows for larger amounts of fluid to be lost by the infant.

The physiologic and biochemical functions of the gastrointestinal tract are dependent on motility, secretion, digestion, and absorption. At birth, most of these functions are present although some developmental differences in absorption, membrane permeability, and types of gastric secretions do exist (Table 14–2).

Motility

Movement within the gastrointestinal tract is initiated by muscle contraction and is influenced by the nervous system, blood flow, temperature, and hormones (Bullock & Rosendahl, 1992; Hyman & DiLorenzo, 1993). The intestinal tract is stimulated by distension, most often from the presence of food. Peristalsis, the basic propulsive movement, is initiated. A ring of muscle around the gut contracts and moves through the alimentary tract.

During swallowing, food is transported from the posterior part of the mouth to the stomach. The process of swallowing is initiated by the central nervous system. Stimulation of receptors around the opening of the pharynx elicit the swallowing reflex and protect the trachea. The act of swallowing is primarily an automatic reflex for the first 3 months of life. Swallowing starts to become voluntary beginning at 6 weeks and by 6 months is fully voluntary. The primary peristaltic wave spreads into the stomach in 8 to 10 seconds. If this primary peristaltic wave does not move all the food to the stomach, secondary waves are initiated. During peristaltic contractions the stomach and duodenum become relaxed and fill.

When the stomach is distended, peristaltic waves act to mix the food. During this time the pylorus remains almost closed allowing only water and other fluid to empty. Periodically the waves of peristalsis become markedly stronger. The stronger pressure gradient results in the semiliquid food called "chyme" to move into the duodenum. The rate of gastric emptying is influenced by the osmolarity and volume of the food. Hypertonic feeds and high fat content delay emptying. Once peristalsis has developed in the newborn, the stomach empties in approximately 2 hours. The rapid transit time and small stomach capacity contribute to the frequency and amount of feeding and stools in infants. Human milk moves through the stomach faster than cow's milk (Cavelli, 1981). In older infants and children stomach emptying takes place in 3 to 6 hours.

As chyme enters the small intestine, contractions similar to those in the stomach occur. These peristaltic waves are weak and function to move some of the chyme toward the colon, spreading it along the intestine. Most of the chyme will stay in the duodenum until additional food is eaten and a new gastroenteric reflex intensifies peristalsis.

When chyme reaches the colon, contractions are poorly coordinated. These sluggish but persistent movements may occur several times each day. The result is a delay of 8 to 15 hours to move chyme from the ileocecal valve to the transverse colon.

Defecation is stimulated when feces enter the rectum. Peristaltic waves in the descending colon, sigmoid, and rectum are initiated. Relaxation of the internal sphincter results in contraction of the external sphincter. Voluntary control of the external sphincter allows a person to inhibit sphincter contraction, permitting defecation. Voluntary control of the external sphincter also allows for keeping the sphincter contracted.

Secretion

Throughout the gastrointestinal tract, glands secrete enzymes and hormones used in digestion (Table 14–3). Mucus is also secreted to lubricate and protect the alimentary tract. The presence of food usually stimulates the glands in the region of the food and the surrounding areas to secrete digestive juices. The secretion of saliva by the parotid, submandibular, and sublingual glands begins the process of digestion and absorption. Gastric secretion is regulated by the parasympathetic fibers of the nervous system and by

Table 14–2. DEVELOPMENTAL DIFFERENCES OF INFANT'S GASTROINTESTINAL TRACT

Decreased pool of bile acid
Increased permeability to whole proteins
Increased gastrin and cholecystokinin level
Mucosal wall is proportionally longer
Immature pancreatic secretory function
Lower trypsin, chymotrypsin, and carboxypeptidase B levels

Data from Motil, K. (1993). Development of the gastrointestinal tract. In R. Wyllie & J. Hyams (Eds.). *Pediatric gastrointestinal disease* (pp. 3–16). Philadelphia: W. B. Saunders.

Table 14–3. SELECTED GASTROINTESTINAL ENZYMES AND HORMONES

Organ	Enzyme	Action
Salivary glands	Ptyalin	Starch to smaller carbohydrates
Stomach	Pepsin (chief cells) intrinsic factor	Protein to polypeptides
	Gastric lipase	Triglycerides to glycerides and fatty acids
	Gastrin	Stimulates gastric acid secretion in the presence of stomach distension
	Somatostatin*	Inhibits various hormones, secretions, and motor effects
Pancreas	Elastase	Protein to amino acid
	Trypsin	Protein and polypeptides to amino acids
	Chymotrypsin	Proteins and polypeptides to amino acids
	Nuclease	Nucleic acids to nucleotides
	Carboxypeptidase A & B	Polypeptides to smaller polypeptides
	Pancreatic lipase	Lipids to glycerol, glycerides, free fatty acids
	Pancreatic amylase	Starch to two disaccharide units (maltose)
	Cholesterol esterase	Hydrolysis of ester bonds in cholesterol and vitamins A, D, & E
	Phospholipase A_2	Phospholipid digestion
Intestines	Enteroglucagon	Inhibits gastric function
	Aminopolypeptidase	Polypeptides to smaller peptides
	Dipeptidase	Dipeptides to amino acids
	Maltase	Maltose to glucose
	Lactase	Lactose to glucose, galactose
	Sucrase	Sucrose, glucose, fructose
	Intestinal lipase	Fats to glycerides, glycerol, fatty acids
	Gastone	Inhibits gastric secretion in presence of fats, sugars, and acids
	Secretin	Stimulates hepatic bile and pancreatic electrolyte and fluid secretion in the presence of polypeptides and acids
	Cholecystokinin-pancreozymin (CCK-PZ)	Stimulates pancreatic enzyme secretion and gallbladder contraction to release bile in the presence of fats

*Also found in the pancreas and small and large intestine.

hormonal mechanisms. In the stomach, gastric pepsin initiates protein digestion. Gastric lipase affects fat hydrolysis.

Pancreatic juice is released into the duodenum mainly in response to the presence of chyme. The characteristics of the pancreatic juice are determined by the type of food. Large volumes of bicarbonate ions neutralize the acid from the stomach. Also contained in pancreatic juice are various enzymes that act on proteins, carbohydrates, and fat. Pancreatic secretion, like gastric secretion, is regulated by neural and hormonal mechanisms. Bile and bile salts are also released into the duodenum by way of the bile duct apparatus. Bile and bile salts are secreted by liver cells and act to digest fat. Intestinal glands are stimulated by tactile stimulation, chemical irritation, distension, or motility within the gut.

Brunner glands and other cells of the intestinal mucosa secrete mucus. The crypts of Lieberkühn secrete pure extracellular fluid, supplying a vehicle for absorption of substances from chyme. The large intestine is lined with mucous cells that secrete only mucus.

Digestion and Absorption

Digestion and absorption by the gastrointestinal tract provide the organic molecules of fat, carbohydrates, and protein to provide energy for the body to function. The gut prepares food by chemical and mechanical means so it can be absorbed through the mucosal lining into the blood and lymph.

Chewing of food is important for digestion of all foods, but it is particularly necessary for raw vegetables. Cellulose membranes are undigestible unless broken down. The child with teeth can therefore change from a soft food diet to a diet that includes foods requiring biting and chewing.

All major nutrients are absorbed in the small intestine. Bile salts and vitamin B_{12} are absorbed only in the terminal ileum. The large intestine is primarily concerned with the absorption of water and electrolytes and functions in the synthesis of vitamin K and some B complex vitamins. The resultant feces usually consist of three-fourths water. The remaining one fourth is solid material, of which approximately 30% is dead bacteria. The brown color is the result of breakdown products of bilirubin called stercobilin and urobilin. The odor is caused primarily by the end-products of bacterial action. Table 14–4 lists the nutrients obtained through food and their site of absorption.

Carbohydrate digestion begins in the mouth where food mixes with ptyalin, an enzyme contained in saliva. Ptyalin hydrolyzes starch into maltose and other small glucose polymers. Pancreatic amylase and various other enzymes from the brush border of the intestinal epithelium are responsible for further digestion of carbohydrates in the small intestine.

Carbohydrates are absorbed mostly in the form of a monosaccharide such as glucose, galactose, and fructose. Glucose transport is related to the sodium-coupled glucose transport system. Glycerides move across the small intestinal wall by diffusion and by active transport against a concentration gradient. The glucose and galactose transport rate in infants is low compared with that in adults and apparently increases during the first year of life. The digested products are absorbed into the portal blood. Most of the carbohydrates are used for energy, although some excess glucose is stored as glycogen in the liver. Additional carbohydrates are changed into fat and stored as triglyceride.

The digestion of protein begins in the stomach with gastric acid secretion. These acids denature complex proteins, making them more conducive to the actions of proteolytic enzymes. Pepsin begins the digestion of protein in the stomach, providing approximately 10% to 30% of total protein digestion. Protein digestion continues in the small intestine under the influence of the pancreatic enzymes and mucosal enzymes. Protein absorption occurs mostly in the duodenum and jejunum in the form of amino acids. As with glucose transport, the sodium transport mechanism probably provides for amino acid transport. Amino acids are used in production of enzymes, in synthesis of plasma proteins, as components in liver structural proteins, in the gut, and in other organs and muscles. In certain conditions, amino acids are used in glyconeogenesis to make glucose when glycogen stores cannot meet the body's caloric needs. Valine, leucine, isoleucine, lysine, threonine, tryptophan, phenylalanine, and methionine are essential amino acids. Tyrosine and cysteine are semi-essential because they can be synthesized only from essential precursors.

Newborn proteolytic activity and absorptive function is not fully developed. Intestinal permeability to whole proteins is increased in infants (Udall & Walker, 1982). The increased permeability allows for cow's milk proteins and other allergens to traverse the intestinal wall. This may increase the infant's susceptibility to gastrointestinal allergies.

Appropriate fat digestion and absorption depends on the proper functioning of the pancreas hepatobiliary system and the absorptive sites within the jejunum, ileum, and lymph nodes. Long-chain triglycerides make up 98% of natural fats. Smaller quantities of other fats including phospholipids, cholesterol, and cholesterol esters are also used by the body. Most digestion and absorption of fat occur in the small intestine, with the majority of fat absorbed by the middle one third of the jejunum. Lipolysis is dependent on the presence of bile acid, phospholipase A_2, and pancreatic lipases. Triglycerides are broken down to fatty acids and glycerol. Phospholipid envelops the triglyceride. Bile salts and fatty acids form micelles and attach themselves to the surface of epithelial cells. Fatty acids then diffuse into the cell and re-form to triglyceride molecules, which are released into the lymphatics and then to the systemic circulation. Medium-chain triglycerides are digested and transported through the intestinal lumen faster than long-chain triglycerides. Medium-chain triglycerides do not require bile salts and pancreatic lipase for digestion.

In infants younger than 1 year of age only 80% to 95% of triglycerides are absorbed (Heubi et al., 1982). A smaller pool of bile acid results in the inefficient absorption of fat. To minimize fat malabsorption, infants use alternative mechanisms to facilitate fat digestion.

Water absorption is dependent on movement of electrolytes. By diffusion water follows electrolytes across the intestinal membrane by passing through membrane pores. When chyme is dilute, water is absorbed through the intestinal mucosa into the blood. The greatest proportion of water absorption is in the jejunum and proximal part of the large intestine.

The information available regarding mineral, vitamin, and trace element absorption is limited. Electrolytes, like water, are absorbed through membrane pores or by transport into the blood. Greater absorption occurs in the proximal rather than the distal portion of the small intestine. Electrolytes are also absorbed in the large intestine. Sodium, chloride, potassium, and bicarbonate are more easily absorbed because they are monovalent, whereas polyvalent electrolytes such as calcium and magnesium are more difficult to absorb. Absorption of calcium occurs by active transport primarily in the duodenum, whereas phosphorus absorption takes place mostly in the jejunum. Calcium and phosphorus intake greatly affects phosphorus absorption. The absorption of trace elements is dependent on the milk source. Breastfed infants are more efficient in absorbing trace elements than infants fed cow's milk–based formulas (Motil, 1993).

NUTRITIONAL ASSESSMENT

The nutritional assessment of a critically ill child requires various methods and tests. No single clinical, biochemical, or growth measurement gives a

Table 14–4. NUTRIENT SITE OF ABSORPTION

Nutrient	Primary Sites of Absorption
Glucose	Duodenum, upper jejunum
Sucrose	Jejunum, ileum
Lactose	Jejunum, upper ileum
Amino acids	Duodenum, jejunum
Fats	Duodenum, upper jejunum
Sodium	Jejunum, ileum
Potassium	Jejunum, ileum
Calcium	Duodenum
Magnesium	Duodenum
Iron	Duodenum
Vitamin D	Jejunum, ileum
Vitamin B_{12}	Terminal ileum
Water	Stomach, small and large intestine

complete picture of a child's nutritional status. The process must be dynamic and allow for selection of different assessment methods during the child's ICU stay.

The purpose of the nutritional assessment is to identify the presence or absence of malnutrition, determine the child's nutritional requirements and preferred alimentation method, and assess the effects of any nutritional intervention. A systematic review and interpretation of the child's history and physical examination results with accurate anthropometric and laboratory measurements are required.

Nursing History

A reliable and complete nursing history is the first step in completing a nutritional assessment (Table 14–5). These data aid in providing a basis for subsequent assessment parameters. Prenatal events including gestational age, birth weight, and length give important baseline information when assessing growth patterns. Data such as feeding history, including type, frequency, amount of intake, and questions concerning who feeds the child and how the food is prepared, are important. Obtaining information about the child's frequency of regurgitation, vomiting, bowel pattern (constipation or diarrhea), and weight loss or gain including the timeframe in which it occurred is recommended. Also important to note are those factors that may influence intake such

as ability to suck; general appetite; recent trauma or infection; surgery; underlying chronic illness or other diseases; level of gastrointestinal function; and feeding abnormalities, allergies, and intolerances. Review of the child's medications is important because of the possible effect of these medications on the gastrointestinal tract and their potential for causing nutritional disturbances. A family history must be a component of the nutritional assessment. Socioeconomic status, hygiene practices, and stress within the family can affect the child's diet and how the child uses and relates to food.

Dietary History

The child's diet history and an analysis of the child's current diet to determine nutritional composition and quantity are important. Knowledge of the child's preadmission intake may be particularly helpful for the chronically ill child in the ICU. To collect information regarding the child's preadmission diet, parents can be asked to recall all the child has eaten in the past 24 to 48 hours. Calorie count is the best method to document a child's current diet. The child's enteral and intravenous intake for a 24-hour period can be recorded and analyzed.

Physical Assessment

A careful physical examination is performed with a specific interest in uncovering subtle signs of deficiencies in macronutrients (protein, energy) and micronutrients (vitamins, minerals, and trace elements) (Table 14–6). Most critically ill children do not display overt signs of malnutrition. Among the clinical signs that may provide evidence suggesting nutritional deficiencies are the child's general appearance; muscular development and tone; skeletal structure; and condition of the gums, teeth, hair, skin, and eyes. Commonly seen in malnutrition is hair that lacks shine and is dry; lips that are red or swollen; a tongue that is smooth and swollen; spongy and easily bleeding gums; and skin that is dry, thin, and wrinkled. The child may also have diarrhea, constipation, or vomiting. Because the origin of these signs may not be nutritional, further testing is necessary to determine the cause.

Anthropometric Measurements

Assessment of growth is important for critically ill children. Anthropometric measurements including weight, height, length, head circumference, triceps skin fold, and midarm circumference are noninvasive and easily taken. Weight, length, height, and head circumference are traditionally considered to be convenient clinical measurements and can serve as minimum standards for the average ICU patient.

Plotting weight, stature, and head circumference

Table 14–5. NUTRITIONAL ASSESSMENT OF A CRITICALLY ILL CHILD

NURSING HISTORY
Birth data and prenatal history
  Gestational age
  Birth weight, length, head circumference
  Maternal nutrition
Chronic illnesses
Congenital/chromosomal abnormalities
Relevant trauma, illness, surgery
Level of gastrointestinal function
  Oral feedings
  Tube feedings
  Parenteral nutrition
Feeding history
  Ability to suck
  Frequency and amount of intake
  Vomiting/spitting-up
  General appetite
  Food preparation
  Who feeds child
Bowel pattern (diarrhea, constipation)
Weight loss or gain
Medications
Family/lifestyle factors
Socioeconomic status
Travel
Hygiene practices
Stress within family

Data from Hobenbrink, K. (1987). The pediatric patient. In C. Lang (Ed.). *Nutritional support in critical illness* (pp. 33–59). Gaithersburg, MD: Aspen Publication.

Table 14–6. SELECTED CLINICAL FINDINGS ASSOCIATED WITH NUTRITIONAL DEFICIENCIES/EXCESSES

Organ	Finding	Nutritional Deficiency/Excesses to be Considered
General	Underweight, short stature	Calories
	Overweight	Excess calories
	Edematous, decreased activity level	Protein
Subcutaneous tissue	Decreased fat fold	Calories
	Increased fat fold	Excess calories
	Edema	Protein, thiamine
Face	Moon face, diffuse depigmentation	Protein
Mucous membranes	Pale	Anemia
Hair	Lack of curl, dull altered texture, depigmented, easily plucked, thin	Protein
	Hair loss	Zinc, biotin, essential fatty acids
	Coiled, corkscrew-like	Vitamin A, ascorbic acid
Lips	Angular stomatitis	Riboflavin
Gums	Swollen, bleeding	Ascorbic acid
Teeth	Caries	Fluoride
	Mottled, pitted enamel	Excess fluoride
Tongue	Smooth, pale, atrophic	Anemia
	Red, painful, denuded, edema	Niacin, riboflavin, vitamin B_{12}
Nails	Spoon-shaped, koilonychia	Iron
Muscles	Decreased muscle mass (wasting)	Protein, calories
Neurologic	Ataxia, sensory loss, motor weakness	Vitamin B_{12}, vitamin E
	Psychomotor change, confusion, irritable	Protein
	Loss of vibratory sense, deep tendon reflexes	Thiamine, vitamin B_{12}
	Sensory loss, motor weakness	Thiamine
	Peripheral neuropathy	Pyridoxine
Skin	Generalized dermatitis	Zinc, biotin, essential fatty acids
	Symmetric dermatitis of skin exposed to sunlight, thickened pressure points, trauma	Niacin
	Petechiae, purpura, ecchymosis	Ascorbic acid, vitamin K
	Scrotal, vulval dermatitis	Riboflavin
Eyes	Dry (xerosis) conjunctiva	Vitamin A
	Photophobia	Zinc
	Conjunctival pallor	Anemia
Skeletal	Costochondral beading, pigeon chest	Vitamin D
	Harrison's groove, knock-kneed or bowed legs, craniotabes, frontal and parietal bossing, open anterior fontanelle	
	Epiphyseal enlargement	Vitamin D, ascorbic acid
	Bone tenderness, hemorrhages	Ascorbic acid
Gastrointestinal	Hepatomegaly (fatty infiltration)	Protein
Cardiovascular	Tachycardia, cardiomegaly, congestive heart failure	Thiamine
	Cardiomyopathy	Selenium
Endocrine	Hypothyroidism, goiter	Iodine
	Glucose intolerance	Chromium
Other	Altered taste	Zinc
	Delayed wound healing	Zinc, ascorbic acid, protein
	Parotid enlargement	Protein

Adapted from Figueroa-Colon, R. (1993). Clinical and laboratory assessment of the malnourished child. In R. Suskind and L. Lewinter-Suskind (Eds.). *Textbook of pediatric nutrition* (2nd ed., p. 195). New York: Raven Press.

on growth charts is essential to identify growth patterns that are indicative of acute or chronic malnutrition. Weight for age, height for age, head circumference, and weight for length and height can be plotted using National Center for Health Statistics (NCHS) charts (Cooper & Heird, 1982; Hamill et al., 1979). Standard growth charts can be found in Appendix II. Special growth charts are available for children with special health problems such as Down syndrome and prematurity.

Weight is used as a gross indicator of body fat and protein stores. For the typical ICU patient in bed, weight should be measured daily on a calibrated pan or sling scale. For those children able to stand, a platform scale can be used. The scale is accurately calibrated with whatever gown, sheet, diaper, or equipment is needed for the child. Armboards, casts, and other heavy items are estimated and then subtracted from the total weight. Ideally the child is weighed with the same scale and at the same time each day.

The child is weighed on admission as a baseline and daily as the child's acuity permits and until the child's growth pattern has stabilized. Weekly weight trends are more relevant than daily fluctuations in assessing a critically ill child's growth. An unexplained weight loss of greater than 5% of the child's admission weight places the child nutritionally at risk. The frequent changes in body water content from the occurrence of capillary leak syndrome with edema reduce the effectiveness of weight as an indicator of changes in body mass and therefore nutritional status.

Weight in relation to height is plotted as an assessment of current nutritional status. Normal childhood growth usually occurs with some expected fluctuation between the fifth and the ninety-fifth percentile. A child with a measurement of less than the fifth percentile is considered to have growth failure and warrants a complete nutritional assessment. A measurement of greater than the ninety-fifth percentile is considered overnourished.

Obtaining the child's length and height assists in estimation of ideal body weight and the monitoring of length and height variations over time. After 1 to 2 years of age, a healthy infant's height and weight normally proceed along the same percentile. Length and height are affected when undernutrition occurs chronically. In the face of malnutrition, a decrease in height velocity is slower to develop than a decrease in weight. Recumbent length measurement is typically obtained on children from birth to 2 years of age. Standing height is obtained on ambulatory children who are 2 to 18 years of age. Because most critically ill children cannot stand, several options are available. Direct measurement of a child with a tape measure will sacrifice accuracy. For children up to 36 months of age, a length board can be used. The recumbent measurement of a child up to age 5 may result in approximately 2 cm greater length than an upright height measurement. The length of a nonambulatory child age 3 to 18 years can be estimated by measuring lower leg or upper arm length (Spender et al., 1989). This technique is an estimate of linear growth in children when height and length cannot be reliably assessed using traditional means. Upper arm length is measured from the acromion to the head of the radius. Lower leg length is measured from the superior medial border of the tibia to the inferior border of the medial malleolus with the child sitting and one leg crossed over the other horizontally.

Head circumference measurement also contributes to a complete nutritional assessment. Head circumference changes with chronic malnutrition. The brain is often preferentially spared for growth during malnutrition and only slows its growth with long-term chronic malnutrition. Serious malnourishment during critical stages of brain development may cause diminished brain and head growth and impaired developmental and intellectual potentials. Measurements are obtained in children up to 36 months of age using a flexible, nonstretchable tape measure. The head is measured at the greatest circumference around the frontal bones, superior to the supraorbital ridge and over the occipital prominence. It is recommended that infants age 1 week to 15 months have a head circumference measurement each week and children age 15 months to 3 years have their head circumference measured every 3 to 4 weeks.

Triceps skinfold (TSF) and midarm circumference (MAC) assess muscle mass and body fat content,

respectively. These measurements require the use of constant tension calipers such as Lange or Holtain skinfold calipers and a nonstretchable tape measure. Because approximately 50% of the body's adipose tissue is located in the subcutaneous tissue, TSF provides an estimate of body fat stores. Skinfold calipers pinch the skin and its underlying subcutaneous tissue over the triceps midway between the shoulder (acromion) and the elbow (olecranon). To ensure accuracy, nutritionists repeat this process three times using established techniques. Midarm circumference is an estimate of skeletal muscle mass and somatic protein reserves. The diameter of the arm is determined by using a tape measure over the same area of the arm used when measuring TSF.

The child's measurements are compared with standards established by the Ten State Nutrition Study (Frinsancho, 1981). Excessive fat stores and muscle mass are indicated by a greater than ninety-fifth percentile, and depletion in fat stores and muscle mass is indicated by less than the fifth percentile. The accuracy of both TSF and MAC may be affected by fluid shifts and edema.

Biochemical Indices

Laboratory data can be used to evaluate biologic functions dependent on nutrition. Serum and urine assays provide objective information to support dietary assessments, physical findings, and anthropometric measurements. Biochemical measurements also serve to identify nutritional deficiencies not found clinically (Table 14–7).

Plasma Proteins

Identifying various proteins in assessing nutritional status has proven valuable (Church & Hill, 1987; Kuhn, 1990). As a means of quantifying a child's body protein stores, certain proteins that circulate in the body can be measured. Protein measurements, however, reflect body stores with varying degrees of precision. A number of physiologic and pathologic factors seen in critically ill children such as liver disease, renal failure, trauma, infection, and inflammation also affect body protein and make the interpretation of these measurements difficult.

Serum albumin was one of the first biochemical markers identified for malnutrition. A low level of serum albumin has been associated with a decrease in dietary protein intake and an increase in morbidity and mortality (Benjamin, 1989; Murry et al., 1988). Albumin has a half-life of 20 days and reacts very slowly to changes in protein intake. As the major protein synthesized by the liver, albumin levels are also affected by hepatic disease, as well as infection, injury, hydration of the child, renal failure, intestinal disease, ongoing protein losses from drainage tubes or wounds, and exogenous infusion of albumin. In children older than age 1 year, mild protein depletion may be indicated by serum albumin levels

Table 14-7. BIOCHEMICAL INDICES

Test	Neonate Birth–1 mo	Infant 1–12 mo	Child 1–4 yr	Child 5–8 yr	Child 9–18 yr
Protein					
Blood					
Serum albumin (g/dL)	≥2.5	≥3	≥3.5	≥3.5	≥3.5
Retinol binding protein (mg/dL)	2–3	2–3	2–3	2–3	3–6
Blood urea nitrogen (mg/dL)	7–22	7–22	7–22	7–22	7–22
Prealbumin (mg/dL)	20–50	20–50	20–50	20–50	20–50/60
Transferrin (mg/dL)	170–250	170–250	170–250	170–250	170–250
Fibronectin (mg/dL)	30–40	30–40	30–40	30–40	30–40
Urine					
Creatinine/height index	>0.9	>0.9	>0.9	>0.9	>0.9
Vitamin A					
Plasma retinol (g/dL)	≥30	≥30	≥30	≥30	≥30
Vitamin D					
25-OH-D$_3$ (ng/mL)	≥20	≥20	≥20	≥20	≥20
Riboflavin					
Red cell glutathione reductase stimulation effect (%)	<20	<20	<20	<20	<20
Folacin					
Serum folate (ng/mL)	>6	>6	>6	>6	>6
Red blood cell folate (ng/dL)	>160	>160	>160	>160	>160
Vitamin K					
Prothrombin time (seconds)	11–15	11–15	11–15	11–15	11–15
Vitamin E					
Red blood cell hemolysis test (%)	≤10	≤10	≤10	≤10	≤10
Vitamin C					
Plasma (mg/dL)	>0.2	>0.2	>0.2	>0.2	>0.2
Thiamine					
Red blood cell transketolase stimulation effect (%)	<15	<15	<15	<15	<15
Vitamin B$_{12}$					
Serum vitamin B$_{12}$ (pg/mL)	≥200	≥200	≥200	≥200	≥200
Iron					
Hematocrit (%)	31	33	36	39	36
Hemoglobin (g/dL)	12	12	13	14	13
Serum ferritin (ng/mL)	>10	>10	>10	>10	>10
Serum iron (g/dL)	>30	>40	>50	>60	>60
Serum total iron-binding capacity (g/dL)	350–400	350–400	350–400	350–400	350–400
Zinc					
Serum zinc (g/dL)	80–120	80–120	80–120	80–120	80–120

Adapted from Klish, W. (1993). Nutritional assessment. In R. Wyllie & J. Hyams (Eds.). *Pediatric gastrointestinal disease* (p. 1108). Philadelphia: W. B. Saunders.

of 2.8 to 3.5 g/dL, whereas severe depletion may be indicated by serum albumin levels less than 2.1 g/dL. The nonsensitivity and nonspecificity of albumin make it a poor indicator of acute malnutrition in a critically ill child. Its major role is in the assessment of the severity of chronic malnutrition.

Transferrin, also synthesized by the liver, is used to transport almost all the iron in the plasma. Transferrin has a half-life of approximately 8 days and therefore is more sensitive than albumin to protein deficiency. A transferrin level of 100 to 170 mg/dL may reflect moderate malnutrition, and a level of less than 100 mg/dL may indicate severe malnutrition. Transferrin is known to rise rapidly during iron deficiency and may be affected by other nonnutritional factors including nephrotic syndrome, neoplastic disease, and liver disorders.

Prealbumin is considered more sensitive to acute visceral protein changes than albumin and transferrin and may be the most helpful protein to measure in the critically ill patient (Church & Hill, 1987; Marvin, 1988). Prealbumin has a shorter half-life (2 days) and smaller body pool than albumin and transferrin. It decreases rapidly with lower than normal protein and/or energy intake and produces a significant rise with adequate protein and calorie replacement (Benjamin, 1989). Prealbumin aids in the transport of thyroxin and is affected by infection and trauma.

Retinol-binding protein relative to the other visceral proteins has a very short half-life (10–12 hr). Retinol-binding protein levels vary with protein-energy status (Figueroa-Colon, 1993). However, retinol-binding protein is not used frequently for diagnosis of malnutrition because it is present only in very small concentrations. Serum levels may rise in liver disease and be lowered in vitamin A deficiency.

Plasma fibronectin is a large glycoprotein with a half-life of about 4 to 24 hours. Fibronectin is sensitive to nutritional deprivation in stressed and non-stressed patients and to refeeding (Benjamin, 1989; Scott et al., 1982). Shock, burns, trauma, and infection lower fibronectin levels.

Somatomedin C may be a useful indicator of overall nutrition and nitrogen balance (Kuhn, 1990). Somatomedins are insulin-like growth-promoting peptides produced by the liver in response to growth hormone stimulation. Somatomedin C is thought to decrease in patients with protein-calorie malnutrition. Somatomedin C has a limited value because its levels are reduced by inflammatory and other diseases.

Urine Screening for Somatic Proteins

Although urine is sometimes difficult to collect, urine screening for creatinine and urea nitrogen can be valuable in assessing the nutritional status of the critically ill child. Creatinine height index reflects muscle mass, assuming that renal function is normal. Creatinine, the metabolic product of creatine, is stored in muscle and excreted by the kidney at a relatively constant rate. Creatinine excretion is measured in a 24-hour urine collection. The 24-hour creatinine excretion of the patient is divided by a 24-hour creatinine excretion of the same-height child and multiplied by 100 to obtain an index.

$$\frac{\text{24-hour urine creatinine excretion (mg)}}{\text{24-hour urine creatinine excretion/same-height child (mg)}} \times 100$$

In the well-nourished child the creatinine-height index (CHI) is close to 100%. Severe protein-calorie malnutrition is indicated by a CHI under 40%. Moderate depletion is indicated by a CHI of 40% to 60%, and mild depletion is indicated by a CHI of 60% to 80% (Figueroa-Colon, 1993). Creatinine excretion can be affected by hydration state and catabolic states (Benjamin, 1989).

Urea nitrogen excretion also requires 24-hour urine collection and can be used to estimate nitrogen balance and assess catabolic state. Nitrogen balance determines the state of metabolic balance or protein turnover by subtracting nitrogen excretion from nitrogen intake. Nitrogen balance is calculated as follows:

$$\left(\frac{\text{protein intake [g/24 hours]}}{6.25}\right) - \left(\text{urine urea nitrogen [g/24 hours]} + 4\right)$$

Protein intake is divided by 6.25 to determine the intake of nitrogen. This factor is the average nitrogen intake in dietary protein. A constant of 4 is added to urine urea nitrogen to account for the other body nitrogen losses (stool, skin, etc.). If the answer to the above equation is above zero, the patient is adding lean body mass and is in an anabolic state. This indicates growth or recovery from an illness. If the number is negative or below zero, the child is catabolic and losing protein or lean body mass. This state suggests the need to add protein alone or a combination of protein and calories to the diet. In addition to malnutrition a negative nitrogen balance may also

be caused by hypoperfusion, fever, sepsis, shock, and steroid therapy.

Additional Screening

As mentioned previously, protein malnutrition can cause an impaired immune response. Lymphocyte count and skin testing for energy have been used to determine the competence of the immune system. Total lymphocyte count decreases with visceral protein depletion and increases with improved nutritional status (Lehmann, 1991; McIrvine & Mannick, 1983). Delayed cutaneous hypersensitivity (DCH) is an assessment of the degree to which the body can mount an antigen-antibody response by testing of skin antigens. Serial skin tests have been done using a variety of antigens including mumps organisms, *Candida,* and streptokinase. Fever, sepsis, stress, general anesthesia, steroid therapy, surgery, trauma, and a variety of other causes have been reported to affect lymphocyte count and DCH (Marvin, 1988; Twomey et al., 1982). Randall & Blackburn (1987) also recommend that skin testing not be done for 7 to 10 days after injury. In the ICU setting these tests are impractical and are generally unreliable as an indicator of nutritional status.

Measurement of body composition is a newer type of nutritional analysis and involves the estimation of body components. Many different methods exist with varying accuracy, methodology, and applicability to the child in the ICU. Total body water is an estimate of the nonfat body mass (Lukaski & Johnson, 1985). After orally administering water labeled with an isotope, the dilution of the isotope is measured by collecting and analyzing urine or serum. Neutral fat does not bind with water, and water in lean body mass is relatively constant (73.2% water). Nonfat or lean body mass can be determined by subtraction. Overestimation of body water content may occur. The expense of this method limits its use.

Body imaging to estimate fat or muscle thickness can be obtained by radiographs, nuclear magnetic resonance imaging, ultrasound, and computed tomography. These measurements are converted using statistical and mathematical relationships. Limitations of these methods for critically ill children include the relatively high cost, the relatively time-consuming nature of many of these procedures, and the added radiation exposure.

Other methods of measuring body composition include total body potassium, neutron activation, total body electrical conductivity (TOBEC) and bioelectrical impedance (Figueroa-Colon, 1993; Fiorotto et al., 1987; Kushner & Schoeller, 1986; Lukaski et al., 1986). A total body counter is needed to measure potassium 40, which resides in the muscles of the body. Neutron activation determines the concentration of potassium, sodium, nitrogen, chloride, phosphorus, calcium, and changes in body composition. Electrical activity is used to estimate fat free body mass. Currently these methods are expensive, carry some added risk for the patient, and need further testing and design modifications to be useful to the pediatric critical care population.

Indirect Calorimetry

Indirect calorimetry is increasingly available to assist in evaluating caloric needs, determining energy expenditure, and measuring utilization of various nutrients (Chwals et al., 1988; McClave & Snider, 1992). Metabolic carts brought to the bedside measure the rate of pulmonary gas exchange (Branson, 1990). Using a sophisticated analyzer, carbon dioxide and oxygen levels in inspired air and expired air are measured and compared to determine energy expenditure. Oxygen consumption and carbon dioxide production represent valid measurements of intracellular metabolism (Ferrannini, 1988). The amount of oxygen absorbed across the lung is assumed to be equal to the amount of oxygen consumed for metabolic processes.

Metabolic carts are capable of calculating a child's respiratory quotient (RQ) or ratio of carbon dioxide molecules produced to molecules of oxygen consumed. The determination of RQ assists in evaluating substrate utilization (Elia & Livesey 1988). The RQ varies from 0.7 to 1.2 depending on the metabolite (Edes, 1991). An RQ of 1 reflects pure glucose metabolism, whereas an RQ of 0.8 suggests protein metabolism and an RQ of 0.7 suggests fat utilization (Branson, 1990). The goal is to keep the child, once fed, at an RQ of equal to or slightly lower than 0.9 (Lehmann, 1993). An increase in energy expenditure seen with hypermetabolism is associated with an RQ of approximately 0.8.

Overfeeding and nutrient utilization can also be monitored by indirect calorimetry. The administration of large glucose concentrations has been associated with increased carbon dioxide production, which may lead to an increased RQ (Askanazi et al., 1980). Edes (1991) suggests that when RQ is greater than 1, total calories may be decreased. When RQ is less than 1 but greater than 0.85, carbohydrates are being converted to fat (Lehmann, 1993). Fat calories can be substituted for carbohydrate calories when further reduction of the RQ is seen as beneficial to the child. Simply adding fat calories, however, may not benefit the child if total calories are in excess of his or her needs. Edes also suggests that patients on long-term ventilatory support or patients who will not undergo weaning for several days may not benefit from a reduction in RQ or a change in the diet to high-fat feedings.

Metabolic carts are classified according to technique of measurement. Open- and closed-circuit metabolic carts are available (McClave & Snider, 1992). When measurements are being taken, the child needs to be as quiet as possible with no interaction between patient and caregivers or visitors. Something as simple as a parent or nurse coming into the room can affect the measurement. Weissman and associates (1986) recommend that unstable patients be monitored two to three times per week, whereas in more stable patients condition can be monitored weekly.

In general, indirect calorimetry predicts energy expenditure with much higher confidence than the traditional formulas (Foster et al., 1987). However, measurements are affected by higher oxygen concentrations. The expense of the necessary equipment and the need for an experienced technician has limited the use of indirect calorimetry in many PICUs.

NUTRITIONAL MANAGEMENT

Nutritional management of critically ill children involves providing protein and calories sufficient for resolution of stress, enhancing protein and calories for growth, and supplementing vitamins and minerals. Specialized nutritional support is initiated with specific goals. During the beginning phase of critical illness, the goal of therapy is to stabilize lean body mass. After the initial hypermetabolic period, nutritional goals broaden to include provision of positive anabolic growth, improvement of visceral protein, and replenishment of muscle glycogen and mineral stores. The correction of the organ system dysfunction associated with malnutrition may take days to weeks (Pollack, 1993). The ultimate plan for nutritional support depends on the child's basal metabolic needs, the nutritional condition of the child, the metabolic response and nutrient requirements of critical illness, the child's age, and the ability to provide parenteral and enteral therapy. If adequate oral intake is not expected, children admitted to ICUs should receive nutritional support within 36 hours of their admission (Kuhn, 1990). Those children with injury or sepsis or those who are admitted to the PICU malnourished are particularly vulnerable and require the highest priority.

Basal Metabolic Rate

Basal metabolic rate (BMR) is the energy required to maintain functional cellular activities. Because metabolism affects energy needs, whatever changes metabolic response affects caloric and nutrient needs of the child. More than 60% of the child's energy needs are necessary for daily function of the heart, kidneys, and brain (Holliday, 1971). These body organs make up 16% to 17% of the body weight of a child, as compared with 5% to 6% of the body weight for adults. Basal metabolic rate per kilogram differs according to age. Infants have a higher metabolic demand per kilogram, requiring a larger percentage of calories for growth. During infancy, BMR is approximately 50 kcal/kg/day; by adolescence the caloric needs of the child have decreased by 50% to 20 kcal/kg/day (Huddleston et al., 1993). BMR is at its highest level per kilogram up to the age of 24 months. BMR is affected by a variety of factors other than age. In both starvation and obesity, BMR decreases. For every 1-degree increase in temperature,

Table 14-8. METABOLIC RESPONSE OF STRESS VERSUS STARVATION

Characteristics	Critical Illness	Starvation
Metabolic rate	+ to + + +	−
Energy requirements	+ to + + +	−
Primary fuels	Mixed	Fat
Protein breakdown	+ + +	+
Amino acid oxidation	+ + +	+
Urinary nitrogen excretion	+ + +	+
Hepatic protein synthesis	+ + +	+
Total body protein synthesis	−	−
Gluconeogenesis	+ + +	+
Ketone production	+	+ + + +
Rate of malnutrition development	+ + +	+
Respiratory quotient (RQ)	0.80	0.7

+, increased; −, decreased.

Adapted from Pollack, M. (1993). Nutritional support of children in the intensive care unit. In R. Suskind & L. Lewinter Suskind (Eds.). *Textbook of Pediatric Nutrition* (2nd ed., p. 209). New York: Raven Press; Cerra, F. (1989). Nutrition in trauma, stress and sepsis. In W. Shoemaker, S. Ayers, A. Grevnik, P. Holbrook & W. Thompson (Eds.). *Textbook of critical care* (2nd ed., p. 1118). Philadelphia: W.B. Saunders.

there is a 10% to 13% increase in metabolic rate. Drugs such as caffeine, beta blockers, and catecholamines increase BMR. Pathologic states, such as respiratory failure, increase BMR. Extreme amounts of energy may be used in the work of breathing of a child with respiratory failure (Field et al., 1982b).

Metabolic Response to Starvation Versus Stress

An understanding of the dramatic differences of the body's response to starvation and the catabolic effects of stress is important for safe and effective nutritional support of critically ill children (Table 14-8). Unlike critical illness, which results in rapid protein-energy malnutrition (PEM), starvation produces malnutrition in days to weeks (Huddleston et al., 1993). The process of starvation results from a

decrease of nutrient intake with normal nutrient use. This phenomenon essentially represents no stress to the body. Carbohydrate stores are usually consumed within 24 hours. The breakdown of amino acids from protein (gluconeogenesis) is initiated to supply glucose. If starvation continues for several weeks, the body adapts to lack of glucose. Protein utilization is reduced and there is a conservation of nutrients. Body fat becomes the major energy source. Starvation causes a decrease in the child's metabolic rate and total energy expenditure. Little or no activation of metabolic mediators occurs, and no increase in insulin resistance exists. In starvation the child's RQ is low (0.7).

The metabolic response of critical illness is very different from that of simple starvation. Normal utilization of nutrients is altered. This response is coordinated by catecholamines, cortisol, glucagon, and growth hormone and characterized by use of nutrients from all sources (Cerra, 1987; Fitzsimmons & Hadley, 1991; Huddleston et al., 1993; Lehmann, 1993). Interleukin-1 and tumor necrosis factor may be mediators for this response (Pollack, 1993).

Catecholamines released in response to the stress of injury or illness create a diabetic-like response by increasing the mobilization of glucose and resistance to insulin. Epinephrine suppresses insulin, leaving additional glucose available for energy needs. Glucagon antagonizes the anabolic effect of insulin, leading to more hyperglycemia and protein breakdown. Glucocorticoids trigger gluconeogenesis, converting amino acids to glucose. Endogenous protein breakdown is accelerated to provide glucose to meet energy needs. Much of protein degradation comes from the wasting of skeletal muscle and results in an increased loss of nitrogen through the urine (Rennie, 1985). Amino acids may supply up to 25% of the energy in the stressed patient, resulting in a higher RQ (0.85) than with starvation (Elwyn, 1989). Fat mobilization, utilization, and depletion are also increased. Cortisol acts to enhance the catecholamine effect by breaking down fat into free fatty acids (Pollack, 1993).

Table 14-9. RECOMMENDED DAILY ALLOWANCE GUIDELINES

Category	Age (yr)	Weight (kg)	Height (cm)	REE* (kcal/day)	Energy Allowance (kcal/kg)	Energy Allowance (kcal/day)
Infants	0.0–0.5	6	60	320	108	650
	0.5–1.0	9	71	500	98	850
Children	1–3	13	90	740	102	1300
	4–6	20	112	950	90	1800
	7–10	28	132	1130	70	2000
Males	11–14	45	157	1440	55	2500
	15–18	66	176	1760	45	3000
	19–24	72	177	1780	40	2900
Females	11–14	46	157	1310	47	2200
	15–18	55	163	1370	40	2200
	19–24	58	164	1350	38	2200

*Resting Energy Expenditure.

Adapted with permission from RECOMMENDED DIETARY ALLOWANCES: 10TH EDITION. Copyright 1989 by the National Academy of Sciences. Courtesy of the National Academy Press, Washington, D. C.

Infants: kcal per 24 hours = 22 + (31 × wt) + (1.2 × ht)
Males: kcal per 24 hours = 66 + (13.7 × wt) + (5 × ht) 6.8 × age)
Girls kcal per 24 hours = 655 + (9.6 × wt) + (1.8 × ht) 4.7 × age)

Wt = weight (kg); ht = height (cm); age = age in years

The metabolic response to critical illness is not preventable; however, nutritional support can minimize protein loss. The catabolic effect of breaking down cellular materials, which occurs during critical illness, precludes growth and organ development in the critically ill child. When catabolism exceeds anabolism (the synthesis of cellular materials), tissues are lost and the body loses weight. Catabolism and anabolism cannot occur simultaneously (Kinney & Elwyn, 1983). The degree of increase in energy expenditure and protein catabolism is proportionate to the severity of illness and previous nutritional status of the child (Clifton et al., 1986; Pollack, 1993; Tilden et al., 1989). For example, a child with a minor infection does not have as much energy expenditure and protein breakdown as a child with sepsis. This increase in energy expenditure plays a major role in the development of PEM in the intensive care unit.

Determining Energy Needs

Estimation of the child's energy needs is essential for the provision of nutritional support. The energy requirements of a critically ill child are highly individualized and may vary widely. Traditionally, caloric needs have been estimated by using the Recommended Dietary Allowance (RDA) guidelines or by determining basal metabolic rate (BMR) or resting energy expenditure (REE) and multiplying by activity or injury stress factors. These factors are said to adjust for increases in energy expenditure (Cerra, 1986). Indirect calorimetry, as previously discussed, may also be used to estimate caloric needs especially in cases when multiple processes are occurring simultaneously (Gebara et al., 1992).

The RDA recommendations developed by the National Research Council, Food and Nutrition Board (1989) are based on intakes associated with normal growth. The RDA provides estimates of average needs of healthy children exceeding basic energy expenditure by approximately 20% to 50% (Table 14–9). Recommended daily allowance guidelines for infants are based on ad libitum intakes associated with normal growth. Because the RDA is based on the needs of healthy children, these guidelines are not the most reliable as estimates of the energy needs for critically ill children.

Formulas like the Harris Benedict equation (top of page) (Harris Benedict, 1919; Roza & Shizgal, 1984) and a variety of other nomograms based on age, weight, and height may be used to determine basic energy needs (*Energy & Protein Requirements*, 1985; Hendricks & Walker, 1990; Marian, 1993). The Harris Benedict equation calculates basal energy expenditure (BEE) and can be used with children older than age 10 years. An equation has also been developed for infants (Caldwell & Kennedy, 1981; Lang, 1987).

To estimate the increase in metabolic needs associated with illness, researchers looking at the adult population have quantified the metabolic effect of various types of activities and degrees of stress. Routine activities common to the ICU increase oxygen consumption (Weissman et al., 1984) (Table 14–10). The greatest increase is caused by chest physiotherapy at 40% above REE. Adjustment of calories for the degree of stress has been suggested (Cerra, 1986; Wilmore, 1977) (Table 14–11). Trauma may increase energy needs by a factor of 1.25 to 1.5 (25%–50%), sepsis may increase energy expenditure by a factor of 1.3 to 1.6 (30%–60%), and severe burns or major stress may increase REE 80% to 100%.

Results from pediatric studies examining measured energy expenditure in the critically ill child have confirmed energy expenditure above REE

Table 14–10. EFFECT OF ACTIVITY ON OXYGEN CONSUMPTION

ICU Activities	Oxygen Consumption*
Chest physiotherapy	40% ↑
Chest x-ray	25% ↑
Dressing change	25% ↑
Visitation/bath	20% ↑
Moving body	20% ↑

*All percentages are approximate.
Data from Weissman, C., Kemper, M., Damask, M., Askanazi, J., Hyman, A. & Kinney, J. (1984). The effect of routine intensive care interaction on metabolic rate. *Chest*, 86, 815–818.

Table 14–11. STRESS FACTORS

Representative Stress State	Stress Factor
Simple starvation	1.0
Postoperative recovery: uncomplicated surgery	1.0
Sepsis (moderate)	1.3
Sepsis (severe)	1.5–1.6
Trauma: mild (e.g., long bone fracture)	1.2
Trauma: central nervous system (sedated)	1.3
Trauma: moderate to severe	1.5
Burns (proportionate to burn size)	up to 2.0

Pollack, M. (1993). Nutritional support of children in the intensive care unit. In R. Suskind & L. Lewinter-Suskind (Eds.). *Textbook of pediatric nutrition* (2nd ed., p. 214). New York: Raven Press.

Table 14-12. COMPARISONS OF MACRONUTRIENT NEEDS

Age	Total Calories (kcal/kg/day)	Protein (g/kg/day)	Carbohydrates (%)	Fat (%)
Preterm	120	3.0–3.5	34–39*	39–43*
Infant (≤ 12 months)	105–115	2.0–2.5	35–65	30–55
Toddler (1–2 years)	85–95	1.5–2.0	50–55	30
Preschool (3–5 years)	80–90	1.5–2.0	50–55	30
School (6–12 years)	70–80	1.0–1.5	50–55	30
Adolescent (13–18 years)	40–65	1.0	50–55	30

*Determined from amount of carbohydrate and fat found in breast milk.

Adapted from Huddleston, K., Ferraro-McDuffie, A., & Wolff-Small, T. (1993). Nutritional support of the critically ill child. *Critical Care Nursing Clinics of North America,* 5(1), 68; data from Hobenbrink, K., & Oddlesitson, N. (1989). Pediatric nutrition support. In E. Shronts (Ed.). *Nutrition support dietetics* (p. 231). Gaithersburg, MD: Aspen Publications; and Pereira, G., & Barbosa, N. (1986). Controversies in neonatal nutrition. *Pediatric Clinics of North America,* 33, 1.

(Chwals et al., 1988; Tilden et al., 1989; Winthrop et al., 1987). In practice, for the majority of critically ill children with moderate stress from trauma, sepsis, or surgery, REE can be multiplied by a factor of 1.5 or a 50% increase above REE (Zlotkin et al., 1985). Otherwise, the well-nourished child on bedrest with moderate stress may require REE times 1.3 or 30% above REE. Long-term growth failure may require an increase of 50% to 100% above REE.

Certain clinical situations may produce a decrease in energy expenditure. A decrease in energy expenditure may occur with paralysis (58%) and with sedation and pain relief (5%–10%) (Clifton et al., 1986; Swinamer et al., 1988).

Although stress factors are used routinely in estimating the caloric needs of patients with critical illness, some authors have contested these factors as too high (Koruda & Rombeau, 1986; Shanbhogue & Lloyd, 1992). Studies done using indirect calorimetry to measure REE have found energy expenditure to be lower than other research using other methods to estimate increased caloric needs (Chwals et al., 1988; Gebara et al., 1992; Major, 1988). Therefore, the currently available formulas and clinical estimates may not necessarily be adequate in predicting the amount of calories needed by the critically ill child (Weissman et al., 1986). Clinical response to feeding is the best indicator of caloric adequacy.

Although adequate nutrition is essential for the critically ill child, overnutrition cannot be overlooked as a potential complication. Overfeeding with excessive calories may cause hepatic dysfunction and congestive heart failure, may worsen respiratory insufficiency, and may increase metabolic rate (Chwals, 1994; Chwals et al., 1988; Major, 1988). The work of breathing may be affected by an increase in adipose tissue throughout the abdomen and chest. Increases in oxygen consumption and hypercapnia, which may result from overfeeding, can interfere with weaning. Elevations in the RQ can be attributed to the metabolism of an increased carbohydrate load, which may

result in an RQ of greater than 1.0 to 1.3 (Askanazi et al., 1980; Askanazi et al., 1981; Dark et al., 1985).

Nutrient Distribution

Once a child's total caloric needs are estimated, macronutrient distribution of kilocalories is determined. Appropriate amounts of vitamins, minerals, and trace elements are also added. For the critically ill child, providing a mix of energy sources is necessary (Table 14–12). Pollack (1993) suggests that dividing the nonprotein calories equally between fats and carbohydrates is a reasonable approach to nutrient distribution.

Macronutrient Needs

Protein provides amino acids for continuous tissue synthesis and repair, transport of nutrients, and maintenance of immune function. Protein requirements change, as does metabolic rate. As a child gets older and metabolic needs decrease, so will the need for protein. The RDA provides guidelines for protein intake. These recommendations are based on minimum protein intake necessary to maintain nitrogen balance (National Research Council, Food and Nutrition Board, 1989). One gram of protein equals 4 calories. Infants require 7% to 16% protein and children older than 1 year require 7% to 9% protein in the diet.

Along with providing the right dose of protein, adjusting the protein source to include branched-chain amino acids (valine, isoleucine, and leucine) may benefit children during injury or sepsis (Bower et al., 1985; Cerra, 1990; Skeie et al., 1990; Teasley & Buss, 1989). Branched-chain amino acids used with the appropriate amounts of carbohydrate and fat may increase muscle protein levels, improve nitrogen balance, reduce weight loss, and improve immune function.

The amino acids glutamine and arginine are newly considered as having an important role for the critically ill in maintaining the structure and function of the gut and for treatment in the stressed hypermetabolic patient (Lehmann, 1993). Glutamine is important in protein synthesis and may be the principal means of nitrogen transfer from the muscle to visceral organs. During hypermetabolic states, glutamine is consumed at higher concentrations by the gastrointestinal tract and may reflect an increase in metabolic need (Souba et al., 1990). The addition of glutamine to enteral and parenteral nutrition may improve nitrogen balance, enhance intestinal mucosal repair, minimize villous atrophy, and reduce bacterial translocation (Burke et al., 1989; Daly et al., 1990; Hammarquist et al., 1989; Lacey & Wilmore, 1990; O'Dwyer, 1989; Zeigler et al., 1990). Arginine may reduce protein breakdown, which may have a potent effect on depressed immunity and enhance the body's wound healing ability (Barbul, 1990; Daly et al., 1988).

To ensure maximum utilization of protein, calculating the ratio of nonprotein calories to nitrogen may be useful. The amount of nitrogen reflects protein in the diet. One gram of nitrogen is equal to 6.25 g of protein. In the typical American diet, the ratio of nonprotein calories, those from carbohydrates and fat, to grams of nitrogen is approximately 200 to 300 calories to 1 g of nitrogen. The inefficient use of amino acids along with an increase in excretion of urinary urea nitrogen by the critically ill suggests the need for higher protein intake. Lowering the ratio of nonprotein calories to nitrogen may especially benefit children with high protein needs such as burns, continuing losses through chest tube drainage, nasogastric suctioning, intractable diarrhea, and substantial blood loss (Ament et al., 1993; Cerra, 1987; Lehmann, 1993; Marvin, 1988). Nutritional support may be maximized by providing nonprotein to nitrogen ratios of approximately 80 to 100:1 for highly stressed patients (Konstantinides et al., 1984).

Nonprotein calories are provided by carbohydrates and fat. Carbohydrates ingested primarily as disaccharides, starches, and polysaccharides are the major source of energy for the body. Depending on the source, 1 g of carbohydrate equals approximately 4 calories. Excessive carbohydrate intake may contribute to respiratory failure. Hyperglycemia and hepatic steatosis may also be caused by a high glucose load (Askanazi et al., 1981). Fat is essential to cell integrity and provides a high caloric content (Huddleston et al., 1993). Fat has the highest caloric density of any nutrient with 1 g of fat equal to approximately 9 calories. In general, to avoid essential fatty acid deficiency, 4% to 8% of the total calories ingested should be from a lipid source (Pollack, 1993). Infant metabolism requires a greater dependence on fat for energy (Huddleston et al., 1993). For critically ill patients increasing the fat portion of the nonprotein energy requirement by shifting away from the carbohydrate portion may decrease hyperglycemia and prevent respiratory failure (Nordenstrom et al., 1982).

Micronutrient Needs

Micronutrients are an essential part of the critically ill child's diet. Guidelines established by the RDA for vitamins and minerals and trace elements are used as recommendations for providing micronutrients (Table 14–13). For the critically ill child, individually calculated amounts of vitamins and electrolytes are often necessary. Replacement of these elements is guided by monitoring appropriate serum levels. Deficiencies may have occurred before the child's critical illness or from inadequate replacement of current needs. If deficiencies exist, supplementation is necessary. These deficiencies may affect the metabolic processes that are necessary for recovery. Small infants also have a reduced capacity to store minerals and zinc (Huddleston et al., 1993).

COLLABORATIVE INTERVENTIONS

Delivery of nutrients to a critically ill child is often challenging. If oral intake is inadequate or not feasible, nourishment by another delivery method is necessary.

Enteral Feeding

When oral intake is insufficient in a child with adequate digestive and absorptive capacity, enteral tube feedings are initiated (A.S.P.E.N. Board of Directors, 1993). Enteral feedings provide nourishment using the gastrointestinal tract and are preferred. This mode of therapy preserves the normal sequence of nutrient delivery and is less costly and safer (Buckner, 1990; Cerra, 1990; Lehmann, 1993). Enteral nutrition is associated with reduced morbidity and mortality, decreased potential for bacterial translocation, improved host response, higher pancreatic enzymes and disaccharidase activities, and enhanced nutrient utilization as compared with parenteral therapy (Berger & Adams, 1989; Border et al., 1987; Lowry, 1990; Mochizuki et al., 1984; Moore et al., 1989; Peterson et al., 1988; Wilmore et al., 1988). Despite the common practice of withholding enteral nutrition to prevent feeding intolerances and avoid gut malfunction, early enteral feedings have significant benefits (Minard & Kudsk, 1994). Seemingly small amounts of nutrients enterally administered benefit the integrity and function of the gastrointestinal tract (Dunn et al., 1988; LeLeiko et al., 1993; Slagle & Gross, 1988). Even when nutrition is delivered parenterally, mucosal atrophy and impairment of absorptive capacity may occur when nutrients are not supplied directly to the gastrointestinal tract (Alexander, 1990; Edes, 1991; Ellis et al., 1991). In addition, wound healing may be improved with early postoperative enteral nutrition (Schroeder et al., 1991).

The few contraindications of enteral feedings include gastrointestinal obstruction involving the en-

Table 14–13. VITAMINS, MINERALS, AND TRACE ELEMENTS

	Age (yr)	Weight (kg)	Height (cm)	Fat-Soluble Vitamins				Water-Soluble Vitamins							Minerals			Trace Elements			
				Vit. A (µg)	Vit. D (µg)	Vit. E (mg)	Vit. K (µg)	Vit. C (mg)	Thiamine (mg)	Riboflavin (mg)	Niacin (mg NE)	Vit. B_6 (mg)	Folate (µg)	Vit. B_{12} (µg)	Calcium (mg)	Phos-phorus (mg)	Magne-sium (mg)	Iron (mg)	Zinc (mg)	Iodine (µg)	Selenium (µg)
Infants	0.0–0.5	6	60	375	7.5	3	5	30	0.3	0.4	5	0.3	25	0.3	400	300	40	6	5	40	10
	0.5–1.0	9	71	375	10	4	10	35	0.4	0.5	6	0.6	35	0.5	600	500	60	10	5	50	15
	1–3	13	90	400	10	6	15	40	0.7	0.8	9	1.0	50	0.7	800	800	80	10	10	70	20
	4–6	20	112	500	10	7	20	45	0.9	1.1	12	1.1	75	1.0	800	800	120	10	10	90	20
	7–10	28	132	700	10	7	30	45	1.0	1.2	13	1.4	100	1.4	800	800	170	10	10	120	30
Males	11–14	45	157	1000	10	10	45	50	1.3	1.5	17	1.7	150	2.0	1200	1200	270	12	15	150	40
	15–18	66	176	1000	10	10	65	60	1.5	1.8	20	2.0	200	2.0	1200	1200	400	12	15	150	50
	19–24	72	177	1000	10	10	70	60	1.5	1.7	19	2.0	200	2.0	1200	1200	350	10	15	150	70
Females	11–14	46	157	800	10	8	45	50	1.1	1.3	15	1.4	150	2.0	1200	1200	280	15	12	150	45
	15–18	55	163	800	10	8	55	60	1.1	1.3	15	1.5	180	2.0	1200	1200	300	15	12	150	50
	19–24	58	164	800	10	8	60	60	1.1	1.3	15	1.6	180	2.0	1200	1200	280	15	12	150	55

Adapted with permission from RECOMMENDED DIETARY ALLOWANCES: 10TH EDITION. Copyright 1989 by the National Academy of Sciences. Courtesy of the National Academy Press, Washington, D.C.

Table 14-14. BREAST MILK AND SELECTED INFANT FORMULAS

	Kcal/mL	Carbohydrate (g/100 mL)	Fat (g/100 mL)	Protein (g/100 mL)	Components
Breast milk	0.67	7.2	4	1.05	
Cow's milk					
Term protein formulas					
Similac	0.67	7.2	3.6	1.5	Lactose; soy, coconut oil; nonfat milk
Enfamil	0.67	6.9	3.8	1.5	Lactose; coconut oil, soy; nonfat milk, demineralized whey
SMA	0.67	7.2	3.6	1.5	Oleo; lactose; coconut, safflower, soy oil; nonfat milk, demineralized whey; reduced sodium
Gerber	0.67	7.3	3.7	1.5	Lactose, soy, coconut oil; nonfat milk
Good Start	0.67	7.2	3.4	1.6	Hydrolyzed whey, whey protein concentrate; lactose maltodextrins; palm oil, safflower oil, soy oil
PM 60/40	0.67	6.9	3.8	1.6	Whey, casein; coconut, oleo, soy oil; lactose; reduced sodium
Soy-based formulas					
Isomil	0.67	6.8	3.6	2.0	Corn syrup solids, sucrose; soy and coconut oil; soy protein isolate, L-methionine
ProSobee	0.67	6.9	3.6	2.0	Corn syrup solids, soy and coconut oil; soy protein isolate, L-methionine
Nursoy	0.67	6.9	3.6	2.1	Sucrose; oleo, coconut, safflower, soy oils; soy protein isolate, L-methionine
RCF	0.40	0	3.6	2.0	Soy protein isolate; soy and coconut oil; no carbohydrate
Preterm infant formulas					
Similac Special Care	0.81	8.6	4.4	2.2	Corn syrup solids, lactose; MCT oil, corn and coconut oil; nonfat milk, demineralized whey
Enfamil Premature	0.81	8.9	4.1	2.4	Same as above
"Preemie" SMA	0.81	8.6	4.4	2.0	Lactose, maltodextrine; MCT oil, coconut, oleo, soy oil; nonfat milk, demineralized whey
Specialized formulas					
Nutramigen	0.67	8.8	2.6	2.2	Sucrose, modified tapioca starch; corn oil; casein hydrolysate
Protagen	0.67	7.8	3.2	2.4	Corn syrup solids, lactose; MCT oil and corn oil; sodium caseinate
Pregestimil	0.67	9.1	2.7	1.9	Corn syrup solids, modified tapioca starch; corn oil and MCT oil; casein hydrolysate with amino acids
Alimentum	0.67	6.8	3.7	1.8	Tapioca starch, sucrose; MCT oil, safflower oil, soy oil, casein hydrolysate with amino acids

Adapted from Abad-Sinden, A., & Sutphen, J. (1993). The practical use of infant formulas. In R. Wyllie & J. Hyams (Eds.). *Pediatric gastrointestinal disease* (p. 1084). Philadelphia: W. B. Saunders; data from American Academy of Pediatrics. Committee on Nutrition (1993). *Pediatric nutrition handbook* (3rd ed.). Chicago: American Academy of Pediatrics.

tire small intestine, severe malabsorption, severe fluid restriction, high caloric requirements beyond those which safe enteral feedings can provide, and severe short bowel syndrome (A.S.P.E.N. Board of Directors, 1993). In addition, an infant at risk for developing necrotizing enterocolitis may need a delay in enteral feedings for 1 to 2 weeks.

Enteral feedings in the past have been avoided following surgery in the initial phases of critical illness because of the potential for gastric stasis. This complication, however, can be avoided by placing the feeding tube in the child's duodenum or jejunum. For this reason, the potential for gastric stasis may no longer be considered a contraindication for the initiation of enteral feedings (Bower et al., 1986).

Selection of Formulas

Human breast milk, along with a variety of formulas, is available for the enteral nutrition of infants

(Table 14-14). The selection of these enteral products is based on the child's age-related nutritional needs, underlying physiology and pathophysiology, clinical status, and gastrointestinal function.

Breast milk has long been recommended whenever possible as the ideal food for infants and should be given strong consideration for the critically ill child (American Academy of Pediatrics, 1993). Human milk provides essential immunologic properties, growth-stimulating properties, and a balance of nutrients and digestive substances (American Academy of Pediatrics, Committee on Nutrition, 1993; Report of the Dietary Guidelines Advisory Committee on the Dietary Guidelines for Americans, 1990; The Surgeon General's Report on Nutrition and Health, 1988). Human milk proteins provide amino acids for growth as well as for digestion, host defense, and possibly tissue maturation (Garza et al., 1993; Garza et al., 1987). For infants at greater risk of infection, breast milk may be especially beneficial (Sorensen et al., 1993). The decreased infection rate in breastfed infants has been attributed by some to IgA and other antimicrobial properties found in human milk (Beckholt, 1989). The fat in human breast milk is thought to be more absorbable because of the positioning of the fatty acids. Iron, zinc, and other nutrients, except possibly chloride, tend to be more bioavailable in human milk.

While the infant is in the intensive care unit, breastfeeding mothers must be supported. Mothers can use manual or electric breast pumps to express milk for their infant (Walker, 1992). Breast milk can then be stored in glass or plastic containers in the refrigerator for 24 to 48 hours or stored in the freezer compartment of refrigerators for 2 to 3 weeks or in a deep freeze of 20°C for 3 to 6 months and given to the infant as needed (American Academy of Pediatrics & American College of Obstetricians & Gynecologists, 1986; The Human Milk Banking Association of North America, 1993). Frozen milk should be thawed quickly under running water. Once the milk is defrosted, it can be refrigerated for 24 hours.

For infants for whom breast milk is not available, there are a variety of commercially prepared formulas. Standard formulas for infants younger than 12 months of age contain whole protein and require intact biliary, pancreatic, and intestinal function. Although based on breast milk, formulas tend to have higher levels of polyunsaturated fat and lower levels

of monounsaturated fat and they lack the range of complex carbohydrates found in breast milk. Infant formulas tend to have higher nutrient concentrations compared with breast milk because the bioavailability of the nutrients contained in formula is lower. For children younger than 1 year of age, standard formulas have the same caloric densities, nearly identical osmolalities (250–320 mOsm), and provide 20 calories/ounce or 0.67 calorie/mL. The type of infant formula can be selected based on the child's needs (Table 14–15). Cow's milk–based formulas for healthy full-term infants (SMA, Similac, Enfamil, and Gerber Baby Formula) contain lactose as the major carbohydrate. Soy and coconut oil blends provide fat for the majority of these formulas. Soy-based formulas (Isomil, ProSobee, Nursoy) are recommended for infants exhibiting a primary or secondary lactose intolerance. Specialized formulas are available for infants who have malabsorption problems or are intolerant of the carbohydrates, fats, or protein contained in standard infant formula. Formulas should be prepared and refrigerated when opened for no longer than 24 hours.

For children older than 1 year of age there are various formula options (Table 14–16). PediaSure is the only formula specifically designed for children 1 to 6 years of age. PediaSure provides a higher caloric value with an increase in grams of protein and carbohydrate and a decrease in fat content compared with infant formulas. Higher amounts of calcium, phos-

Table 14–15. FORMULA SELECTION FOR INFANTS (<1 year of age)

	Formula Description	Suggested Formulas
Healthy term infant	60:40 whey:casein or casein formula	Enfamil SMA Gerber Similac
	Whey hydrolyzed; hypoallergenic	Carnation Good Start
<34 weeks gestation	Premature infant formula	Similac Special Care "Preemie" SMA Enfamil Premature
Uncomplicated lactose intolerance; casein sensitive	Lactose-free soy protein Isolate formula (sucrose and corn-free also available)	ProSobee Isomil Nursoy
Organ dysfunction (e.g., renal, cardiac)	Low electrolyte Low renal solute load	SMA PM 60/40
Severe steatorrhea associated with bile acid deficiency, ileal resection, or lymphatic anomalies; fat malabsorption	Infant formula with MCT oil	Protagen Pregestimil Alimentum
Allergy to cow's milk (casein) and soy protein	Hypoallergenic casein hydrolysate	Nutramigen Pregestimil Alimentum
Abnormal nutrient absorption, digestion, and transport; generalized malabsorption; severe intractable diarrhea; protein calorie malnutrition	Hydrolyzed casein with part of fat from MCT oil (lactose-free)	Pregestimil Alimentum
Abnormal nutrient absorption and transport; malabsorption of protein and fat; intractable diarrhea; protein calorie malnutrition	Hydrolyzed casein with percentage of fat from MCT oil (lactose-free and sucrose-free)	Pregestimil

Adapted from Wilson, S.E., et al. (1987). An algorithm for pediatric enteral alimentation. *Pediatric Annals,* 16, 233; in Hendricks, K., & Walker, W. (1990). *Manual of pediatric nutrition* (2nd ed.). St. Louis: Mosby–Year Book.

Table 14–16. SELECTED PEDIATRIC AND ADULT FORMULAS

	Calories (kcal/mL)	Protein (gm/L)	Fat (gm/L)	Carbohydrate (gm/L)
Standard Formulas (1–6 years)				
PediaSure	1	30	50	110
Standard Formulas (> 6 years)				
Enrich	1.10	39.7	37.2	162
Ensure	1.06	37.2	37.2	145
Ensure Plus	1.5	54.9	53	200
Isocal	1.06	34	44	133
Jevity	1.06	44	36.8	151.7
Isotein HN	1.2	68	34	156
Magnacal	2.0	70	80	250
Meritene	0.96	57	32	110
Osmolite	1.06	37	37	145
Protagen	1	36	48	117
Precision HN	.96	29	30	144
Resource Plus	1.5	55	53	200
Ross SLD	0.7	38	0.5	137
Susta II	1.06	46	35	141
Sustacal Liquid	1.0	61	23	140
Predigested Formulas				
Criticare HN	1.06	38	3	222
Vital HN	1.0	42	10.4	185
Vivonex	1.8	38	3.0	206
Fiber Enriched Formulas				
Complete	1.07	43	37	141
Disease-Specific Formulas				
Amin-Aid	1.96	19.4	46	366
Hepatic Aid	1.78	44	36	169
Peptamen	1.0	40	39	127
Pulmocare	1.5	63	92	106
Stresstein		70	28	170
Traumacal	1.5	83	68	143
Traum-Aid HBC	1.0	56	12.4	166
Travasorb Hepatic	1.1	29	15	215
Travasorb Renal	1.35	23	18	270

Adapted from Committee on Nutrition, American Academy of Pediatrics (1993). *Pediatric nutrition handbook* (3rd ed., pp. 380–384). Elk Grove Village, IL.

phorus, and vitamin D with similar osmolarity to infant formulas (325 mOsm/kg) are also characteristic of PediaSure. For those children at the lower end of this age range who have malabsorption problems, special infant formulas may be continued while adding age-appropriate nutrient supplements. In these situations, clinicians may consider adding vitamin B_6, zinc, iron, calcium, and phosphorus to the diet.

Adult formulations are generally used in children older than 6 years of age with vitamin or mineral supplements given as indicated. These products range in caloric density from 1 to 2 kcal/mL and in general have a higher osmolarity (450–810 mOsm/L). Selection of these formulas is based on standards similar to those of infant formulas (Table 14–17). For the majority of patients, complete or standard lactose-free formulas are adequate. Standard adult formulas require the patient to have normal digestive capacity. These formulas are isotonic, providing 1 cal/mL with a relatively high carbohydrate to fat ratio and intact or almost intact protein. For patients receiving tube feedings on a long-term basis or for those patients with diarrhea or constipation, fiber-enriched formulas may be useful. These formulas are

usually isotonic to slightly hypertonic and provide 1 kcal/mL. Calorically enhanced formulas provide 1.5 to 2.0 cal/mL and may be used for patients who are on fluid restrictions or those who require a higher caloric intake.

Predigested or elemental formulas are usually hyperosmolar solutions that contain oligopeptides or amino acids as protein and oligosaccharides or disaccharides as carbohydrate. For older children and adolescents with malabsorption problems these formulas are appropriate because they require minimal digestion and are almost completely absorbed. Predigested or elemental formulas typically provide 1 cal/mL. Special disease formulas vary in amino acid and nutrition distribution.

There are several methods to increase caloric density of formula above standard (Table 14–18). Depending on the needs of the infant or child, calories and nutrient module supplements of protein, fat, and carbohydrate can be added to enteral formulas (Smith & Heymsfield, 1983). By using less free water to reconstitute formulas, calories can be increased above the formula's standard caloric concentration. In addition many infant formulas are now commer-

Table 14-17. SELECTION OF OLDER CHILD AND ADOLESCENT FORMULAS

	Formula Description	Suggested Formulas
Normal GI tract (child 1–6 yr)	Nutritionally complete for age group	PediaSure
Normal GI tract (> 6 yr) Standard meal replacement	Nutritionally complete	Ensure Sustacal Osmolite Isocal
Higher protein/calorie needs (e.g., burns)	Nutritionally complete with high protein/calorie formula	Ensure Plus Isocal HCN Sustacal HC Ensure Plus HN Resource Plus Magnacal Ensure HN Isocal HN
Significant pulmonary compromise	High-fat formulation	Pulmocare
Significant trauma requiring very high protein needs	High-protein formulation	Traumacal
Abnormal GI tract functioning	Elemental/semi-elemental formula	Criticare HN Peptamen Tolerex Vivonex TEN Vital HN

Adapted from Hendricks, K., & Walker, W. (1990). *Manual of pediatric nutrition* (2nd ed., pp. 91–92). With permission from Mosby–Year Book, Inc.

Table 14-18. METHODS FOR INCREASING CALORIC DENSITY OF INFANT FORMULAS

Method	Advantages	Disadvantages	Recommendations

Add less water to powdered/
  liquid concentrate formulas
	Simple, easy
	Maintains standard ratio of
	  protein, fat, and
	  carbohydrate
		Increases solute load
		May prolong gastric emptying,
		  especially if >24 kcal/oz
		May cause diarrhea
		May precipitate dehydration in
		  patients at risk for excessive
		  losses
			Monitor renal status
			Monitor for symptoms of reflux,
			  abdominal distension
			Monitor for symptoms of
			  dehydration

Add protein (e.g., Propac Pro-
  mix)
	Relatively easy	May increase solute load
		High caloric density
			See recommendation for other
			  additives

Add carbohydrate (e.g.,
  Polycose, Moducal)
	Relatively easy to obtain and
	  add to formula
	Relatively inexpensive
	Provides readily available
	  source of energy
	
	Polycose and Moducal are
	  easily digested
	Does not delay gastric
	  emptying
		When used in excess, may
		  increase work of breathing
		May cause osmotic diarrhea
		Base formula may fall short of
		  RDA for protein
		Overall vitamin and mineral
		  content may be below RDA
			Monitor respiratory status
			Monitor stool output, check
			  stool for reducing substances
			Monitor total daily protein
			Supplement vitamins and
			  minerals as required

Add fat (i.e., long-chain
  triglycerides [LCT], vegetable
  oils; medium-chain
  triglycerides [MCT]
  microlipids)
	LCT easy to obtain and
	  inexpensive
	MCT more rapidly digested,
	  more readily absorbed
	Microlipids are emulsified
	MCT are not emulsified
		LCT slow gastric emptying
		May aggravate reflux
		MCT very expensive
		MCT will adhere to tubing
		May cause diarrhea
		Aspiration of fat can be
		  dangerous
		Base formula may fall short of
		  RDA for protein
		Overall vitamins and minerals
		  may fall short of RDA
			Monitor for reflux, abdominal
			  distension
			Reserve MCT for fat
			  malabsorption, or delayed
			  gastric emptying
			Combination of LCT and MCT
			  may improve tolerance
			Monitor tolerance, stool output,
			  serum triglycerides
			Monitor daily protein
			Do not exceed 60% of total
			  calories from fat
			Supplement vitamins and
			  minerals

Adapted from Huddleston, K., Ferraro-McDuffie, A., & Wolff-Small, T. (1993). Nutritional support of the critically ill child. *Critical Care Nursing Clinics of North America,* 5(1), 75.

cially available in concentrations of 24 cal/oz (0.8 cal/mL) and 27 cal/oz (0.9 cal/mL). When providing concentrated formulas to an infant or child it is important to be conscious of the increasing renal solute load.

Single modular components can be added in the form of protein, fats, or carbohydrates. Protein in the form of Propac (16 cal/Tbsp) and Promix (17 cal/Tbsp) can be added to the diet to increase protein density. Fat modules, such as medium-chain triglyceride (MCT) oil (7.7 cal/mL) and microlipids (4.5 cal/mL), can be added in small volumes to existing formulas to increase caloric density. Smaller volumes avoid separation of fat in the formula and reduce the chance of overwhelming the absorptive capacity of the intestine, which may occur with a large bolus of lipid. MCTs are more easily absorbed, better utilized, smaller, and have greater water solubility. Carbohydrate modules like Moducal and Polycose provide 2 cal/mL of supplemental carbohydrates. The addition of excessive carbohydrates can increase the work of breathing. A human milk fortifier can also be used to increase the caloric content of breast milk. Two packets per 50 mL provide 24 cal/oz. Protein, calcium, phosphorus, and vitamin concentrations are also increased with human milk fortifier. A higher risk of nutrient imbalances can occur when modular units are added to the diet, and therefore extra care must be taken to adhere to the recommended nutrient distribution guidelines.

Delivery Methods

Adequate delivery of enteral feedings can be accomplished by a number of methods (Table 14–19). The route chosen for enteral nutrition is dependent on the level of gastrointestinal function, the expected duration of tube feeding, and the child's potential for aspiration (Monturo, 1990). Feeding the child into the stomach allows for gastric acid and other hormones to respond normally in the digestive process. Typically, gastric feedings enable the child to tolerate a larger osmotic load, have more flexibility in feeding schedule, greater mobility between feedings, and incur less administration expense (Fuchs, 1993). The gastric feeding site is recommended when there is minimal risk of aspiration. For children with the potential for difficulties in tolerating feeding from inadequate gastric motility or with an unacceptable risk of aspiration from gastroesophageal reflux, enteral tubes are placed in the duodenum or jejunum (Edes, 1991). Placing the tube past the pyloric sphincter reduces the risk of aspiration and is recommended with increasing regularity as the method of enteral feeding administration for critically ill children (A.S.P.E.N. Board of Directors, 1993).

For temporary enteral feedings an oro- or nasogastric or intestinal tube can be placed. Orogastric tubes are appropriate for infants younger than 4 weeks of age. The oropharynx is used to avoid potential airway obstruction in these obligate nose breathers. Naso-gastric and nasoenteric tubes are commonly placed in older infants and children. Tubes composed of soft nonreactive materials with weighted tips such as silicone (Silastic) or polyurethane are desirable. These tubes are long-lasting, pliable, and less likely to cause nose irritation. Polyvinylchloride tubes are much less desirable and should only be used to meet short-term needs. Polyvinylchloride tubes stiffen with age and exposure to acid resulting in an increased risk of perforation, lower esophageal sphincter dysfunction, gastroesophageal reflux and nose erosion. Decompression tubes should never be used for feeding children because of the risk of aspiration. With feeding, aspiration becomes more likely because the side holes of decompression tubes often lie proximal to the stomach.

Placement of a feeding tube can be accomplished with an appropriate-size tube, lubricating jelly as needed, gloves, syringe, hypoallergenic tape, and a stethoscope. The size of the feeding tube is dependent on the age and size of the patient. Appropriate nasogastric tube insertion length can be determined by measuring from the tip of the nose to the ear and from the ear to the xiphoid process. A patent naris should be selected. Viscous lidocaine on the tip of the tube and nares may help make tube placement more comfortable (LeLeiko et al., 1993). During insertion, if not contraindicated, the patient's head is slightly flexed and the head of the bed is in high Fowler's position.

Transpyloric tubes are more difficult to position. Small soft tubes require slow gradual insertion over 1 to 2 minutes. Use of a stylet will stiffen the tube but increase the risk of pneumothorax (Walsh & Banks, 1990). Spontaneous transpyloric migration and concurrent radiographic or endoscopic use are common approaches to insertion. A successful method used in the critically ill was described by Ugo and associates (1992). This technique involves placing the child on the right lateral side, inserting the tube into the gastric region, and confirming position by auscultation. Air is then injected through the tube to facilitate movement through the pylorus. The tube is advanced in 1- to 2-cm increments.

Various methods for checking feeding tube placement have been used. The traditional method of air insufflation into the tube and auscultation of a "whoosing" or "popping" sound over the mid-epigastric region or upper left quadrant of the abdomen for gastric tubes and over the upper right quadrant for intestinal tubes can no longer be recommended. This method may be misleading and dangerous to the patient. Metheny and associates (1986, 1990b) found that sounds generated by air insufflation through small-bore feeding tubes are unreliable as an indicator of tube placement. In addition, these tubes often migrate from the intended location. Also, aspiration of fluid alone does not ensure that the tube is in the correct position (Metheny, 1988). Fluid may be inadvertently aspirated from the pleural space or

Table 14-19. ENTERAL FEEDING SITES AND ROUTES

Site	Route	Advantage	Disadvantage	Indications	Contraindications
Stomach		Allows for normal digestive processes and hormonal responses Tolerance of larger osmotic loads Decreased incidence of dumping syndrome Greater mobility between feedings Greater flexibility in feeding schedule and formula choice		Usually first consideration for enteral nutrition	Delayed gastric emptying Pulmonary aspiration Gastroesophageal reflux Intractable vomiting Impaired or absent gag reflex
	Orogastric	Does not obstruct nasal passage	May increase salivary flow and make clearance more difficult	Infants <4 weeks of age Nasal passage obstruction Basilar skull fracture	Older infant or child with gag reflex
	Nasogastric	Easy intubation	Nasal, esophageal, or tracheal irritation Local skin care required Easily dislodged by a toddler Easily dislodged by a forceful cough May stimulate gag Caretaker must be well trained Limited long-term compliance in the home care setting	For short-term use	Same as for the stomach
	Gastrostomy	Allows patient greater mobility Feedings are generally well tolerated Larger diameter feeding tube lessens chances of obstructional/clogged feeding tube Does not obstruct the airway	Typically requires a surgical procedure for placement May result in increased gastroesophageal reflux Occasional leakage around the insertion site Skin irritation and infection Risk of intra-abdominal leak with peritonitis	Prolonged enteral nutritional support	Same as for the stomach
Small intestine		Can feed enterally despite poor gastric motility and persistent high gastric residuals Lessens the chances of gastric distension	Less mixing of formula with pancreatic enzymes Limited choices of feeding schedule and formula selection Greater risk of bacterial overgrowth Greater risk of bowel perforation Changes small bowel intestinal flora	Congenital upper GI anomalies Inadequate gastric motility Following upper GI surgery Patients with increased risk of aspiration	Nonfunctioning GI tract
	Nasojejunal/nasoduodenal		Requires radiographic proof of adequate placement May be difficult to place Tube is easily displaced during peristalsis	For intermediate-term nutritional support	
	Jejunostomy		Technically difficult to place	Jejunal feedings for >6 months For postoperative nutritional management of abdominal surgery while a paralytic ileus exists	Patients at operative risk

Adapted from Hendricks, R., & Walker, W. (1990). *Manual of pediatric nutrition* (2nd ed., pp. 74–75). With permission from Mosby–Year Book, Inc.

lung (Grossman et al., 1984). The aspirate's pH needs to be checked with pH paper (Metheny, 1988). An acidic pH of 1.0 to 5.5 indicates that the tube is in the stomach when gastric acid inhibitors are not used, and a highly alkaline pH of greater than 7.0 is indicative of intestinal fluid. Because of questions regarding the reliability of traditional methods for checking tube placement, an abdominal radiograph is the definitive method for confirming correct tube placement (Dorsey & Cogordon, 1985; Metheny et al., 1986; Perry & Potter, 1992).

For those children requiring a prolonged enteral delivery system, a gastrostomy or jejunostomy is indicated (DeChicco & Matarese, 1992). Traditionally, gastrostomy tubes have been placed surgically. For these children, gastrointestinal reflux becomes a common problem (Jolley et al., 1986). Gastrostomy tubes can cause skin breakdown and reduced gastric capacity. Typically, gastrostomies do not provide stabilization of the tube at the stoma and therefore tend to cause migration of the tube in and out of the abdominal cavity, causing enlargement of the stoma and inadvertent removal of the tube (Huddleston, 1989).

With the advent of percutaneous endoscopic gastrostomy (PEG) tubes, a safe nonsurgical option can now be offered to children requiring a gastrostomy (Neal & Slayton, 1992). Under endoscopic guidance, a feeding tube is placed through a wall puncture (DiLorenzo et al., 1992). The placement of a PEG tube may be done at the bedside or in the endoscopy suite with intravenous sedation or, in the case of young uncooperative children, in the operating room under general anesthesia. The PEG tube is stabilized by crossbars internally and externally in a subcutaneous fistula created between the gastric mucosa and abdominal wall. When anesthesia is not used, the intraoperative and postoperative complications are avoided. Feedings can usually be introduced within 24 hours. There is also a reduction in the cost when compared to surgical placement (Benkov et al., 1986; Gauderer, 1991).

Skin level profile and nonreflux devices such as the Button, Gastroport, and Mic-Key are now an option for children requiring long-term feeding tubes (Faller et al., 1993; Huddleston & Palmer, 1990; Steele, 1991). The Button is a type of gastrostomy that has a mushroom dome with a one-way antireflux valve in the stomach. The Button sits flush against the skin, reducing migration along the gastrointestinal tract and the risk of accidental removal (Gauderer et al., 1988; Townsend, 1990). A well-developed gastrostomy stoma is needed prior to placement of a Button. The Mic-Key can be used for both feeding and decompression. The Mic-Key operates like a foley catheter. It is held in place with a balloon and therefore does not cause any pain or trauma on insertion.

A jejunostomy can also be placed in a child with long-term nutritional support needs. This route is employed in those children who are at increased risk for gastric aspiration or who have undergone extensive gastric or duodenal surgery. Endoscopic jejunostomy is a relatively new technique of placing jejunostomy tubes and requires a similar placement method to a PEG, although it is technically more difficult (DeChicco & Matarese, 1992).

Enteral Feeding Administration

Intermittent and continuous feedings are two techniques of enteral feeding administration. Intermittent bolus feedings are usually reserved for older children or those children with no history or potential for feeding intolerance. Intermittent bolus feedings can be given only via gastric tubes because the stomach is needed as a reservoir for the large volumes of formula administered. Gastrostomy tube feedings are commonly given by the bolus method. Intermittent tube feedings are thought to mimic normal eating patterns by allowing the gut to rest. Bolus feedings do not require a feeding pump and, therefore, are less expensive and increase patient mobility.

In the acute phase of critical illness continuous feedings are often more effective than bolus feedings. Continuous feedings are typically better tolerated and decrease the risk of aspiration (Koruda et al., 1987). Infants with smaller gastric capacity and those children with the potential for gastroesophageal reflux especially benefit from continuous feedings. Continuous feedings can be delivered throughout the day or while the child is asleep. Parker and associates (1981) found better weight gain; improved absorption of fat, calcium, zinc, and copper; and a positive nitrogen balance in critically ill children who received continuous rather than intermittent enteral feedings. Infants with congenital heart disease who received continuous enteral feedings demonstrated an improvement in anthropometric measurements and significant weight gain without heart failure (Vanderhoof et al., 1982). Transpyloric and continuous feedings are preferred in head-injured patients to prevent aspiration and achieve maximum caloric intake (Zaloga, 1991). Feedings via the duodenum or jejunum require formula to be infused continuously to avoid distension of the bowel, fluid and electrolyte shifts, and diarrhea (Rombeau & Barot, 1981). A potential risk of formula contamination exists with continuous feedings because of the longer amount of time formula is at room temperature.

Implementing and Advancing Feedings

Methods for introducing feedings to the critically ill child via enteral tube feeding are varied. It is common practice to dilute formulas to one-half or one-quarter strength at the onset of enteral feedings (Hendricks & Walker, 1990). If graded feedings are necessary, increasing the concentration before volume in gastric feedings and increasing the volume before concentration in intestinal feedings has been suggested (Berger & Adams, 1989). It is reasonable, however, to administer 100% of the therapeutic goal of the appropriate formula to children who are closely monitored and not nutritionally unstable (Fuchs, 1993). Although this method is controversial to some, it is generally well tolerated and has been repeatedly demonstrated as a safe method in a variety of patient populations (Gottschlich et al., 1988; Rees et al., 1985; Zarling et al., 1986). Graded feeding has been compared with full-strength feedings by Keohane and associates (1984). Protein intake and absorption were found to be greater in the individuals receiving full-strength formula. No difference was found in the rate of abdominal cramps or nausea. Reducing the strength of feedings, however, did produce more cases of diarrhea as compared with groups given full-strength feeding.

Monitoring Enteral Therapy

Monitoring enteral feeding and evaluating feeding tolerance are very important aspects of caring for the child with enteral feedings (Table 14–20). Evaluation of tolerance of feedings can be accomplished by monitoring complications. Complications prevent the achievement of the desired goals of enteral therapy (Cataldi-Betcher et al., 1983; Murphy, 1990). Being watchful for the causes of enteral feeding complications, taking preventative steps, and intervening when appropriate are important responsibilities when caring for critically ill children during enteral feeding (Table 14–21).

Gastrointestinal complications including diarrhea, constipation, nausea, and vomiting with or without subsequent aspiration has been reported in the enterally fed patient. Diarrhea is one of the most common complications (Moore et al., 1986). Smith and colleagues (1990) reported that 63% of critically ill mechanically ventilated patients who were tube fed had associated diarrhea. Hypertonic formula, excessive volumes, and rapid infusion rates are often blamed as the cause of diarrhea (Keohane et al., 1984). Edes and associates (1990), however, concluded that formula often is not responsible for diarrhea in tube-fed patients. Hyperosmolar electrolyte replacement and drugs, especially some antibiotics when infused undiluted into the intestinal tract, can contribute to diarrhea (Niemiec et al., 1983). Sorbitol, an ingredient in many drug preparations, is often linked to diarrhea (Edes et al., 1990). Malnutrition and low serum albumin levels have been found to be associated with diarrhea in critically ill patients who receive tube feedings (Brinson et al., 1987). Other potential causes of diarrhea include lack of fiber and impaction.

Treatment for diarrhea depends on its etiology. Care must be taken to ensure that diarrhea is actually occurring and that normal stool characteristics and stool frequency are not misjudged for diarrhea. Diarrhea associated with enteral nutrition may be adequately treated by correcting dietary factors (Ca-taldi-Betcher et al., 1983). Diarrhea may be managed by eliminating or reducing problem nutrients such as fat or lactose. To evaluate the source of the diarrhea, reducing substances of the stool should be checked. Changing the delivery rate or the administration method from intermittent to continuous or adding dietary fiber to the feeding may be useful. Recognizing drugs associated with diarrhea and avoiding formula contamination may prevent diarrhea. The addition of some antidiarrheal agents to the formula has been noted to decrease loose stool (Holtzman et al., 1990).

Constipation may occur as a result of a low-fiber diet or inadequate fluid intake. Adding fiber or choosing a high-fiber formula may eliminate constipation in the critically ill child. Constipation may also be avoided by increasing dietary free water.

Vomiting and nausea occur in about 10% to 20% of patients who are tube fed (Cataldi-Betcher et al., 1983). Vomiting may have its origin in esophageal tube placement or as a consequence of delayed gastric emptying (Benya et al., 1990). Lower esophageal sphincter incompetence with gastric reflux and pulmonary aspiration may occur. Large volumes, fast rates of infusion, hyperosmolar formulas, and hypertonic medications may contribute to the risk of nausea and vomiting. Excessive air in the stomach from air spillage of positive-pressure ventilation and air flushing of feeding tubes also may lead to vomiting.

Vomiting is particularly worrisome for patients because of the risk of pulmonary aspiration. Pulmonary aspiration is the most serious common complication of enteral tube feeding (Cataldi-Betcher et al., 1983; Schlichtig & Sargent, 1990; Winterbauer et al., 1981). To reduce vomiting and the risk of aspiration, administering formula continuously rather than by the bolus method and placing the tube past the pylorus may be useful (Berger & Adams, 1989; Hindsdale et al., 1985). In critically ill children, feeding tube placement is checked on radiographs at regular intervals. Verifying tube placement and checking formula residuals is done frequently. For those children receiving bolus feedings, tube placement is checked before each feeding. For those children on continuous gastric feeding, tube placement is checked every 3 to 4 hours. Three hours of residual volume is tolerated in the stomach (Huddleston et al., 1993). Aspiration of stomach contents in excess of this amount is considered significant and may warrant delaying or reducing the feeding rate for 1 to 2 hours. When gastric residuals remain high, a different method of delivery is sought (A.S.P.E.N. Board of Directors, 1993). To detect silent aspiration, pulmonary secretions may also be checked for the presence of glucose with oxidant reagent strips or by placing a small quantity of blue food coloring in the formula (Treloar & Stechmiller, 1984; Winterbauer et al., 1981). During tube feeding, it is also important to monitor respiratory status closely. Respiratory distress may indicate aspiration or stomach distension, which may compromise chest expansion. As a safety measure, the head of

Table 14-20. ENTERAL FEEDINGS: PATIENT MONITORING GUIDELINES

Parameter	Intermittent Feedings	Continuous Feedings	Possible Complications	Therapy	Comments
Gastrointestinal					
Residuals	q feed for 48°; thereafter if minimum residual q8°	q3°–4° for 48°; thereafter if minimum residual q8°	Abdominal distension, cramping, vomiting	For intermittent feeds consider withholding if residuals are >½ previous feed; for continuous feedings withhold if residuals equal to amount of formula infused in the previous 1–3 hours	Reassess formula Volume of feed Concentration of feed For large persistent residuals consider: Reglan therapy Continuous feeds GI function
Stool					
Frequency	Each	Each	Diarrhea	Reduce the rate of feed, dilute feed, change formula, or use continuous feeds	
Hemetest	Daily until 48° if negative results; PRN thereafter	Daily until 48° if negative results; PRN thereafter	GI irritation	Same as above	
Reducing substance	Daily during advancement; PRN thereafter	Daily during advancement; PRN thereafter	Carbohydrate intolerance	Dilute feed, change formula	
pH	Daily until 48°; thereafter PRN if pH greater than 6.0	Daily until 48°; thereafter PRN if pH greater than 6.0	Carbohydrate intolerance, bacterial overgrowth	Dilute feed, change formula	
Metabolic					
Urine					
Specific gravity	q 4–8° then daily	q 4–8° then daily	Fluid imbalance	Adjust fluid intake, adjust concentration of formula	
Sugar/acetone	Daily during advancement; thereafter PRN	Daily during advancement; thereafter PRN	Glucose intolerance	Reduce feeds, give insulin, continuous, feeds	
Serum					
Electrolytes	q 24°–48° during advancement; thereafter PRN	q 24°–48° during advancement; thereafter PRN	Electrolyte imbalance		Electrolyte imbalances in tube-fed patients are usually associated with underlying medical conditions
Nutritional weight	Daily	Daily			
Nutritional profile (BUN, creat., blood sugar, Na, K, Cl, Ca, P, Mg, alk phos., Bili, LDH, SGOT, total pro., Alb., TG, CO_2)	Initially and q Monday or PRN until normalized	Initially and q Monday or PRN until normalized			
Complete nutrition assessment	Weekly	Weekly			
Technical					
Tube placement	q feed	q 3°–4°	Tube displacement	Reposition tube	
Position patient	q feed	q 3°	Aspiration	Maintain upper body position of 30 degrees during feeds and for 30–45 minutes thereafter	Especially important for children with gastroesophageal reflux and altered gastric motility

°, hours.
Adapted from Hendricks, R., & Walker, W. A. (1990). *Manual of pediatric nutrition* (2nd ed., pp. 104–105). With permission from Mosby–Year Book, Inc.

Table 14–21. COMMON COMPLICATIONS OF ENTERAL FEEDINGS

Problem	Causes	Intervention
Gastrointestinal		
Diarrhea/dumping syndrome	Rapidly delivered formula	Decrease delivery rate
	Hypertonic formula	Alter formula carbohydrate and electrolyte content
	Hypertonic medications	Recognize or avoid drugs that result in diarrhea
	Substrate intolerance	Use parenteral nutrition or elemental formula
	Bacterial contamination of formula	Recognize and reduce the cause for contamination
	Lack of fiber	Avoid lactose-containing products
	Concomitant antibiotic therapy	
	Mucosal atrophy and malnutrition	
	Impaction	
Constipation	Low fiber intake	Add fiber or choose a high-fiber formula
	Inadequate fluid intake	Increase free water intake
		Add prune juice
Vomiting, nausea, aspiration	Fat intolerance	Reevaluate tube placement
	Bowel ileus	Consider continuous or transpyloric feedings
	Swallowing excess air	Metoclopramide may be given to enhance motility
	Improper tube placement	Reduce carbohydrate content of formula
	Infusion rate too rapid	Reduce rate and/or concentration as indicated
	Large residuals	Aspirate air from feeding tube prior to feedings
	Hyperosmolar formula	Position patient on the right side
	Hypertonic medications	
	Gastroesophageal reflux	
	Gastric hypomotility	
Technical		
Clogged feeding tube	Failure to irrigate feeding tube regularly	Flush tubing with water
	Formula too viscous for diameter of feeding tube	Replace tubing
	Administration of medications via feeding tube	Follow manufacturer's recommendations for tube size
Perforation of the intestine	Improper tube placement	Stop feedings
Nasal and pharyngeal irritation	Improper skin care	Use polyurethane or Silastic feeding tubes
	Extended use of polyvinyl tubes	Periodically change nares used for feeding tube
Metabolic Disturbances		
Fluid and electrolyte imbalance	Cardiac and/or renal insufficiency	Evaluate cause and treat
	Hypertonic medications	Increase fluid intake as indicated
	Severe protein-calorie malnutrition	Decrease formula concentration
	Malabsorption	
	Inadequate fluid intake	
Hyperglycemia	Insufficient insulin production or utilization	Give insulin
	Trauma or sepsis	Reduce flow rate
	Excessive carbohydrate intake	Reduce carbohydrate content of the formula
Azotemia	High protein intake	Decrease protein content of the feeding
	Renal immaturity or dysfunction	
	Liver disease	
	Metabolic dysfunction (e.g., inborn errors of metabolism)	
Infection	Inadequate mouth care	Routine mouth care
	Improper formula-mixing technique	Use clean technique when mixing formula
	Use of contaminated equipment or supplies	Change delivery set ups every 24–48 hours
	Long hang time of formula	Hang formula for 4–8 hours only
Oral Aversion	Negative oral experiences (e.g., traumatic tube intubation)	Provide pacifier for non-nutritive sucking
	No positive oral experiences (e.g., thumb-sucking, nipple feeding)	Implement oral stimulation program

Adapted from Hendricks, K., & Walker, W. (1990). *Manual of pediatric nutrition* (2nd ed., pp. 106–107). With permission from Mosby–Year Book, Inc.

the bed may be elevated 30 to 45 degrees during feeding and for a period after feeding. For those children with cuffed endotracheal tubes, inflation of the cuffs may reduce the likelihood of aspiration (Taylor, 1992). A gastric emptying agent such as metoclopramide (Reglan) may be given to assist in gastric motility and improve gastric emptying (Koruda et al., 1987; Huddleston et al., 1993).

Nasal and pharyngeal irritation and tube occlusion are among the common technical complications of feeding tubes (Bohnker et al., 1985; Cataldi-Betcher et al., 1983). Maintaining skin integrity is critical to preventing nasopharyngeal erosion. When using polyvinylchloride tubes, changing the tube every 3 days and alternating nares become especially important. Polyurethane and Silastic pediatric tubes allow for longer use of each tube and reduced rate of tissue irritation and erosion (A.S.P.E.N. Board of

Directors, 1993). Frequent assessment of the naris is essential to note if breakdown is occurring. Routine skin care of the area is recommended. Nasoenteric tubes may also cause sinusitis, otitis media, gagging, esophagitis, esophageal fistulae, rupture of esophageal varices, and perforation of the pharynx or lung tissue and gastrointestinal tract (Bernard & Forlaw, 1984; Eldar & Meguid, 1984; Valentine & Turner, 1985).

Clogging of the feeding tube may occur, especially when using tubes with small diameters. Thick formula remaining in the tube and highly viscous medications increase the likelihood of this type of complication. To ensure enteral tube patency and prevent tube occlusion, water or air may be flushed through the tube. For bolus feedings, the tube may be flushed following each feeding, and for continuous feedings the tube may be flushed every 8 hours.

Preventing enteral feeding–related infection is a necessary aspect of the care of a child on tube feedings. A child who is receiving enteral feedings and nothing by mouth needs routine mouth care with saline or an antimicrobial mouthwash. This important aspect of care provides comfort and prevents infection in the oral cavity. Tube feeding is an almost perfect medium for bacterial growth. Contamination can occur while the feeding is mixed or during administration of the formula. To reduce the risk of infection and prevent formula contamination, feeding bags and delivery sets are changed every 24 to 48 hours. A supply of formula lasting no more than 4 to 8 hours is to be hung at one time. Adding new formula to remaining formula is to be avoided (Anderson et al., 1984; Kuhn, 1990).

Close metabolic monitoring to prevent electrolyte and other nutrient imbalances is essential for patients on nutritional support. Children receiving high-caloric formulas require frequent monitoring of urine specific gravity, sugar, and acetone. A serum profile including sodium, potassium, chloride, calcium, phosphorus, magnesium, alkaline phosphate, bilirubin, lactic dehydrogenase (LDH), serum glutamic oxaloacetic transaminase (SGOT), total protein, albumin, glucose, triglycerides, carbon dioxide (CO_2), blood urea nitrogen (BUN), and creatinine should be done routinely. Use of high-caloric formulas can lead to increased renal solute load and potential dehydration. Hyperkalemia and hyponatremia occur more frequently than many other metabolic complications. Hypo- and hyperglycemia may also occur.

A critical component in the care of any child who is enterally fed is the promotion of the suck-swallow reflex. Children who have few positive oral experiences often develop an oral aversion. This is particularly common in the medically fragile patients who are technology-dependent. Non-nutritive sucking appears to enhance physical growth and assist the child in the transition from tube feedings to oral feedings. Non-nutritive sucking is believed to increase nutrient absorption from the gut (Gill et al., 1992; Miller & Anderson, 1993; Woodson & Hamilton, 1988). Studies involving premature infants demonstrated earlier weaning from gavage feeding when the infant was provided with opportunities for non-nutritive sucking (Bernbaum et al., 1983; Field et al., 1982a). To encourage the transition to oral feedings, these early pleasurable feeding experiences assist in reducing the risk of food aversions (Bazyk, 1990). For the child on chronic enteral feedings, an oromotor stimulation program is an especially important adjunct to tube feeding. Although it may take months to years for some children to achieve the transition, it is important to always keep in mind the goal of weaning the child from tube feedings to oral feedings.

Enterostomy tubes carry the additional potential complications of wound infection or dehiscence, skin irritation from leakage of gastric contents around the tube site, inadvertent traumatic removal of the tube, obstruction of the pylorus, and small intestine adhesion (Fuchs, 1993). The gastrostomy site is inspected daily for redness, swelling, and drainage. The site is cleaned with soap and water, or hydrogen peroxide and water for a stoma with debris. Bacitracin ointment may be applied and the site dressed (DiLorenzo et al., 1992). A stomadhesive or skin barrier can be used to protect the skin. For the child with a button, the button is rotated in a full circle during cleaning (Steele, 1991).

Enterally administered medications and drug-nutrient interactions can cause difficulty for the enterally fed critically ill child (Miyagawa, 1993; Seshadri & Meyer-Tehambel, 1993). Administration of hypertonic medications may cause gastric distension, nausea, vomiting, and diarrhea (Edes et al., 1990). Drug absorption is affected by the presence of food in the stomach (Miller, 1993) (Table 14–22). Tube placement can affect absorption and bioavailability of medications. Hypertonic preparations (potassium chloride elixir, hyperosmolar antibiotic suspension) need to be administered in the stomach to avoid gastrointestinal intolerance. Carbohydrate intake increases theophylline levels, whereas protein causes a decrease in theophylline levels. Absorption of phenytoin (Dilantin) may be impaired when it is mixed with enteral products. There appears to be an interaction between phenytoin and the sodium, calcium caseinates, and calcium chloride found in many formulas. General recommendations for administering drugs through a feeding tube include flushing the feeding tube with a bolus of water before and after administering the drug, preventing the mixing of drugs before administration, diluting hyperosmolar or irritant medications, giving liquid medications when possible, and crushing tablets to a fine powder before administration (Berger & Adams, 1989).

Parenteral Nutrition

Total parenteral nutrition (TPN) is composed of a hypertonic solution of water, glucose, amino acids, vitamins, minerals, trace elements, and an isotonic lipid emulsion. When the critically ill child's gastroin-

Table 14–22. EFFECTS OF NUTRIENTS ON ABSORPTION OF SELECTED DRUGS

Decreased Drug Absorption With Food in the Stomach	Delayed Drug Absorption With Food in the Stomach	Enhanced Drug Absorption With Food in the Stomach
Ampicillin	Acetaminophen	Chlorothiazide
Aspirin	Aspirin	Diazepam
Captopril	Cefaclor capsules	Erythromycin estolate
Cephalexin suspension	Cephalexin capsules	Erythromycin
Tetracycline	Sulfonamides	ethylsuccinate
Erythromycin stearate	Cimetidine	suspension
Hydrochlorothiazide	Digoxin	Hydralazine
Nafcillin	Furosemide	Propranolol
Penicillin G or V	Quinidine	Spironolactone
Phenobarbital		
Rifampin		

Adapted from Miller, M. (1993). Nutrient-drug interactions in children. In R. Suskind & L. Lewinter-Suskind (Eds.). *Textbook of pediatric nutrition* (p. 254). New York: Raven Press.

testinal tract is unable to absorb nutrients or when the enteral route cannot be used for a prolonged period of time, parenteral nutrition can greatly benefit the child (Pillar et al., 1990) (Table 14–23).

Selection of Route

Hyperalimentation may be given via the peripheral or central route. The hypertonic fluids of parenteral nutrition require a large-diameter, high-flow vein, with a dedicated port. The choice between peripheral and central routes is based on the child's nutritional needs, clinical condition, and expected duration of illness. Different types of equipment and varying levels of expertise are required for insertion of peripheral and central venous access devices. The peripheral route is designed to supplement oral intake or to meet short-term nutritional needs without high nutritional requirements. The peripheral route is limited by the glucose content of the fluid and is restricted to 10% to 12.5% dextrose and 2% amino acid solutions. The central route provides a larger, more stable vein that will tolerate higher intravenous glucose concentrations.

To administer parenteral nutrition centrally, a catheter is typically placed in the superior vena cava, via the internal or external jugular vein or subclavian with the catheter tip just at the right atrium. A vein in the antecubital fossa or the inferior vena cava via the femoral vein may also be used. The femoral vein is usually avoided, however, because of the increased risk of contamination. Another alternative to percutaneous central line access is peripherally inserted central catheters (PICC) (Roundtree, 1991). A PICC is a long, flexible silicone catheter designed to be inserted into the median basilic or cephalic vein via the antecubital space. The catheter is threaded until it reaches in the axillary or subclavian vein or the superior vena cava (DeChicco & Matarese, 1992). This type of catheter may also be placed in the femoral vein and advanced to the inferior vena cava.

For those patients who require long-term parenteral nutrition, catheters can be placed surgically. The Broviac catheter was the first long-term, small-lumen, flexible catheter. The Hickman catheter was introduced shortly thereafter, followed by the development of various other single- and multilumen long-term catheters (Marcoux et al., 1990). Implantable ports are also considered for long-term access and may offer less risk of infection. A subcutaneous pocket, usually on the chest, is created to implant the device. All central catheters require radiographic confirmation of catheter placement before infusing parenteral nutrition.

Composition of Formula

The parenteral nutrition formula is tailored to meet the critically ill child's nutritional and fluid requirements (Table 14–24). Children with special nutritional needs resulting from renal disease, hepatic disease, and other conditions may require modified formulations.

Dextrose is the principal form of carbohydrate supplied and the most common energy source of most parenteral regimens. Calories from carbohydrates may provide as much as 40% to 60% of the diet. In parenteral solution, unlike enteral formulas, dextrose provides 3.4 cal/g, with 10% dextrose providing 0.34 kcal/mL and 20% dextrose providing 0.68 cal/mL. The concentration of dextrose is often started at a 10% dextrose concentration and then gradually

Table 14–23. INDICATIONS FOR PARENTERAL NUTRITION

Indications	Selected Examples
Severe catabolic state	Hypermetabolic state (e.g., burns, multisystem organ failure, sepsis)
NPO for 2–5 days with suboptimal nutrition status and inability to use enteral route	Enterocutaneous fistula Anastomotic leak Paralytic ileus Transplantation
Intractable vomiting	Enteral feeding intolerance Severe acute pancreatitis
Diarrhea	Severe acute flare of inflammatory bowel disease Chemotherapy
Paralytic ileus	Trauma/abdominal surgery when adequate enteral diet is not expected to resume within 3–7 days
Small bowel obstruction	Adhesions Intestinal atresia Intestinal pseudo-obstruction
Malabsorption	Severe mucosal injury Short bowel syndrome Radiation enteritis Protein-losing enteropathy

Adapted from Ament, M., Reyen, L., & Guss, W. (1993). Parenteral nutrition in infants and children. In R. Wyllie & J. Hyams (Eds.). *Pediatric gastrointestinal disease* (pp. 1140–1156). Philadelphia: W. B. Saunders.

Table 14–24. FORMULATING A TOTAL PARENTERAL NUTRITION SOLUTION

Nutrient	Infant			Child		
	Begin	Advance	Maximum	Begin	Advance	Maximum
Carbohydrate						
(mg/kg/min)	4–6	2–3	10–12	4–6	2–4	10–12
(g/kg)	5–9	3–4	14–17	5–9	3–6	14–17
Fat						
20% concentration						
(g/kg)	0.5–1	0.5–1	3–4	1–2	1	4
Protein						
(g/kg)	2–2.5		3	1.0–2		2.5

Note: Monitor nutritional parameters and tolerance and advance as indicated.
Adapted from Huddleston, K., Ferraro-McDuffie, A., & Wolff-Small, T. (1993). Nutritional support of the critically ill child. *Critical Care Clinics of North America, 5* (1), 72.

increased over 2 days or as tolerated. With gradual increases in the dextrose concentration, the pancreas is given time to increase its insulin response and avoid hyperglycemia and glucosuria with a secondary osmotic diuresis (Kalhan et al., 1986; Kuhn, 1990).

Parenteral protein is supplied in the form of synthetic crystalline amino acids. Protein provides 4 kcal/g. The type of formulation chosen is based on the child's age and disease state (Table 14–25). The selection of the type of amino acid solution may affect the protein utilization, patient tolerance, and ability to avoid deficiencies. Trophamine has a similar amino acid pattern to breast milk and is designed for children younger than 6 months of age. Trophamine has higher amounts of tyrosine and histidine, which

are essential for infants. Novamine provides essential and nonessential amino acids appropriate for children older than 6 months of age. Special amino acid solutions for children with special needs are also available. Glutamine added to parenteral formulations may decrease the degree of intestinal atrophy when enteral feedings are not administered (Hwang et al., 1986). The usual recommendation of parenteral amino acids is 2 to 3 g protein for infants, 2 to 2.5 g/kg daily of protein for older children, and for adolescents 1 to 1.5 g/kg of protein daily (Huddleston et al., 1993). Nitrogen retention is reduced when protein is supplied parenterally. Therefore, when administering protein parenterally amino acids are supplied in a higher concentration (Heird et al.,

Table 14–25. REPRESENTATIVE PARENTERAL AMINO ACID SOLUTIONS

Preparations	Concentrations Available (%)	Nitrogen (g/100 mL)	Essential Amino Acid (%)	Special Characteristics
Aminosyn	3.5	0.55	46	Premature infant formulas available that contain taurine
	5.0	0.79		
	7.0	1.1		
	8.5	1.34		
	10.0	1.57		
Aminess	5.2	0.66	100	Only essential amino acids; used predominantly for renal failure
BranchAmin	4.0	0.44	100	Only components isoleucine, leucine, valine
FreAminee	3.0	0.46	49.1	High branched-chain formulations available
	6.9	0.97		
	8.5	1.3		
	10.0	1.53		
HepatAmine	8.0	1.2	55	Increased amount of branched-chain amino acids
Nephramine	5.4	0.64	99.6	Almost exclusively essential amino acids
Novamine	11.4	1.8	50.7	Highest protein concentration available
	15.0	2.37		
Renamin	6.5	1.0	66.5	
Travasol	2.75	0.46	45.3	Alanine and glycine predominant nonessential amino acids
	3.5	0.59		
	4.25	0.71		
	5.5	0.93		
	8.5	1.43		
	10.0	1.65		
TrophAmine	6.0	0.93	57.3	Contains taurine
	10.0	1.55		

Note: Percentages and values given are approximate; manufacturer's labeling should be consulted for exact values.
Adapted from Ament, M., Reyen, L., & Guss, W. (1993). Parenteral nutrition in infants and children. In R. Wyllie & J. Hyams (Eds.). *Pediatric gastrointestinal disease* (p. 1143). Philadelphia: W. B. Saunders.

1987). Children who are well hydrated with normal renal function can receive the full amount of protein recommended at the outset of therapy. When advancing amino acid concentration is necessary, daily increases of 0.5 g/kg are recommended for neonates, whereas 1 g/kg daily is recommended for older infants and children (Ament et al., 1993). Care must be taken not to administer greater amounts of protein than recommended because azotemia, hyperammonemia, and an increase in minute ventilation and oxygen consumption may occur (Rothkopf et al., 1989).

Fat is supplied in the form of a lipid solution produced from either soybean oil alone or a mixture of safflower and soybean oils (Table 14–26). These lipids are stable for a moderate period of time at room temperature. The use of intravenous fats provides a concentrated source of energy while preventing essential fatty acid deficiency (Hendricks & Walker, 1988). To achieve this goal, at least 4% to 8% of the child's diet must be from fat. The percentage of fat in the diet, however, should not exceed 50% of the total calories, or 3 to 4 g/kg daily. Fat intolerance, as indicated by elevated serum triglycerides, may interfere with immune function and should be avoided (Zlotkin et al., 1985).

A suggested method of introducing and advancing parenteral nutrition is to begin on day 1 with 2 g/kg of lipid emulsion and 10% dextrose and then on day 2 to advance the lipids to 3 g/kg daily along with the dextrose. Ten percent fat emulsion (11 cal/mL) has been used as the standard for children; however, the use of 20% lipid emulsion (20 cal/mL) is becoming increasingly popular. Twenty percent lipids provide the same calories at less volume. Haumont and co-workers (1989) suggest that infants hydrolyze 20% lipid emulsion better than 10% emulsion. In general, higher fat emulsions allow for a decrease in carbohydrate administration and may reduce the child's carbon dioxide production and respiratory quotient. Fat emulsions have traditionally been administered separately to prevent clogging of the intravenous catheter; however, modern lipids can be mixed into triple-mixed total nutrient admixtures (Messing et al., 1982; Wroblewski & Young, 1991). When administering lipids, an inline filter is never used with lipid emulsion because the particles are too large.

Electrolytes, vitamins, and minerals must be added to parenteral solutions to provide nutrients

Table 14–27. COMPOSITION OF INTRAVENOUS MULTIVITAMIN PREPARATIONS

	MVI-12 (per 5 mL)	MVI-Pediatric (per 10 mL)
Fat-soluble		
A (mg)	1 (3300 USP units)	0.7
D (phytonadione)	5 (200 USP units)	10
E (mg)	10 (10 USP units)	7
K (μg)	—	200
Water-soluble		
Ascorbic acid (C) (mg)	100	80
Thiamine (B_1) (mg)	3	1.2
Riboflavin (B_2) (mg)	3.6	1.4
Pyridoxine (B_6) (mg)	4	1
Niacin (as niacinamide) (mg)	40	17
Pantothenate (as dexpanthenol) (mg)	15	5
Biotin (μg)	60	20
Folate (μg)	400	140
Vitamin B_{12} (μg)	5	1

Note: Values given are approximate. Consult manufacturer's labeling for exact values.

Adapted from Ament, M., Reyen, L., & Guss, W. (1993). Parenteral nutrition in infants and children. In R. Wyllie & J. Hyams (Eds.). *Pediatric gastrointestinal disease* (p. 1145). Philadelphia: W. B. Saunders.

essential for metabolism and cellular function (Table 14–27). Pediatric and adult multiple vitamin preparations are available. Sodium, potassium, calcium, phosphorus, and magnesium are added separately to parenteral nutrition preparations. Zinc, copper, chromium, and manganese are added as trace elements. Intravenous iron is administered to children not receiving iron by enteral means. In children with renal failure, calcium amounts are decreased and magnesium, phosphorus, and potassium are eliminated.

There is not much definitive information concerning the parenteral requirements of vitamins or minerals available for critically ill children (Greene et al., 1988). Current guidelines reflect the needs of children who are healthy and are fed orally. The pediatric multivitamin solution used for infants and children younger than 11 years includes vitamin K, lower amounts of the B vitamins, and larger amounts of vitamin D. The adult formulation MVI-12 is used for children older than 11 years. The dextrose–amino acid component of TPN is stable for up to 30 days; however, with the addition of vitamins and minerals, the solution becomes highly unstable. Refrigeration in a dark place is required, and the solution should be used within 24 hours (Goldman et al., 1973).

Water is also an essential part of parenteral nutrition. Typically, fluid requirements are calculated by body weight (see p. 396). Fluid requirements may be adjusted according to the child's fluid needs. For example, a child with high insensible water loss through a drainage tube, diarrhea, respiratory failure, infection, or elevated temperature may require increased fluids, whereas a child under a radiant warmer or with cardiac disease may require fluid restriction.

Table 14–26. FAT EMULSIONS FOR PARENTERAL NUTRITION

	Base	Concentration (%)	Grams/L	Calories/mL
Intralipid	Soybean oil	10	100	1.1
		20	200	2.0
Liposyn	Safflower oil	10	100	1.1
		20	200	2.0
Travemulsion	Soybean oil	10	100	1.1
		20	200	2.0

Adapted from Ament, M., Reyen, L., & Guss, W. (1993). Parenteral nutrition in infants and children. In R. Wyllie & J. Hyams (Eds.). *Pediatric gastrointestinal disease* (pp. 1040–1056). Philadelphia: W. B. Saunders.

Medications can also be mixed or added to TPN to decrease cost, restrict fluids, decrease time, and reduce the risk of potential contamination of the parenteral nutrition (Miyagawa, 1993). Drug compatibility varies (Table 14–28). Parenteral nutrition solutions can inactivate or reduce drug potency and cause precipitation of electrolytes and medications. Drug compatibility must be assessed for pharmacokinetics and physical stability. Well-versed pharmacists can be very helpful in determining compatibility.

The success of parenteral nutrition is ensured by effective administration; evaluation of the child's response to therapy; and close, frequent monitoring of complications (Table 14–29). All parenteral nutrition should be administered by maintaining a constant rate via an infusion pump or controller. To establish a baseline of comparison, initial monitoring of the patient on parenteral nutrition should include complete laboratory assessment of fluid and electrolytes, acid-base, renal, hepatic, and nutritional status. During the initial stages of administration, parenteral nutrition requires daily monitoring of many laboratory values. As changes in parenteral solutions become unnecessary and as the disease acuity permits, less frequent monitoring is needed. Hourly accurate intake and output and frequent assessment of fluid requirements are also indicated.

Parenteral nutrition is fraught with many complications including those related to technical, infectious, and metabolic causes (Table 14–30). The major catheter-related complication is infection. Local as well as systemic infections can occur. The most common infections result from *Staphylococcus aureus* and *Candida albicans* (Berger & Adams, 1989). Fat emulsions provide an excellent medium for gram-positive, gram-negative, and fungal growth, whereas crystalline amino acid and dextrose solutions primar-

ily support fungal infections (Thompson & Robinson, 1991). More susceptibility to catheter infection has been observed with peripheral versus central lines, lower limb catheterization versus upper limb, and catheters exiting the neck (internal jugular) versus those exiting the upper chest (subclavian) (Early et al., 1990; McCarthy et al., 1987; Pemberton et al., 1986; Plit et al., 1988; Wolfe et al., 1986). Multilumen catheters have led to higher infection rates than those of single-lumen catheters in some studies, although other authors argue that the use of multilumen catheters need not increase the rate of infection (Gil et al., 1989). Sepsis related to TPN may result from contamination at the insertion site and migration of bacteria along the catheter (Murphy & Conforti, 1993). Patients who are mechanically ventilated via artificial airways seem to be at increased risk for infection. The bacterial colonization associated with mechanical ventilation may contribute to this increased risk (Holtzman et al., 1990).

Preventing catheter-related infection is one of the biggest challenges in caring for the child with parenteral nutrition. Adherence to regular and meticulous care of the catheter and site is essential. Strict aseptic technique, a topical defatting solution, an antiseptic agent, and an antiseptic ointment may be used to clean and maintain the site (Heird, 1993). An occlusive or semiocclusive dressing is then placed over the insertion site and changed at least three times a week or when soiled (Marvin, 1988; Robertson, 1991). Daily monitoring of local and systemic signs of infection is important, including redness, pain, swelling, and exudate at the site; fever; and chills (Kuhn, 1990; Wickham et al., 1992). Periodic guidewire replacement of catheters has been shown to be a safe means of minimizing catheter-related infections (Bozzetti et al., 1983). Tunneling of the catheter through the subcutaneous tissue prior to entering the vein may reduce the risk of infection (Marvin, 1988). Unnecessary use of the catheter for blood transfusions or blood sampling is discouraged (McCarthy et al., 1987). An inline 0.22 μm filter between the catheter and the administration tubing is advocated by some clinicians to reduce the potential for systemic infection from contamination of parenteral solution (Baumgartner & Schmidt, 1985). To assure sterility during infusion of TPN, a 24-hour expiration period is recommended from time of hanging the fluid. Tubing is changed daily or with every new bottle or bag.

Whenever catheter-related septicemia is suspected, taking blood culture samples is a reasonable recommendation. If the child develops a fever, blood cultures are drawn from the central line and peripheral vein, and antibiotics are started. Cultures are repeated if the initial blood culture result is positive and continued until culture results are negative.

The metabolic complications of parenteral nutrition usually are related to the nutrient components of the parenteral solution. Inaccurate assessment of the child's current and ongoing needs may result in nutrient disorders. Electrolyte and vitamin disorders may occur. Hyperglycemia is the most common meta-

Table 14–28. COMPATIBILITY OF SELECTED DRUGS WITH PARENTERAL NUTRITION

Drugs	Visual Compatibility	Microbiologic Compatibility
Amikacin	Incompatible	Incompatible
Amphotericin B	Incompatible	—
Ampicillin	Incompatible	Incompatible
Cefazolin	Compatible	—
Cephalothin	Compatible	Compatible
Chloramphenicol	Compatible	Compatible
Clindamycin	Compatible	Compatible
Corticosteroids	Compatible	—
Digoxin	Compatible	Compatible
Gentamicin	Compatible	Compatible
Imipenem-cilastatin	Incompatible	Incompatible
Metoclopramide	Compatible	Compatible
Oxacillin	Compatible	—
Penicillin	Compatible	Compatible
Tetracycline	Incompatible	Incompatible
Ticarcillin	Compatible	—
Tobramycin	Compatible	Compatible
Vancomycin	Compatible	Compatible

Reprinted with permission of Miyagawa, C. (1993). Drug-nutrient interactions in critically ill patients. CRITICAL CARE NURSE®, 13 (5), 69–90.

Table 14–29. MONITORING PARAMETERS FOR PARENTERAL NUTRITION SUPPORT

Variable	Admission	q1 Hour	q8 Hours	Daily	Weekly	As Indicated
Growth						
Weight	X			X		
Height	X					X (monthly)
Head circumference (<3 yr)	X					X (monthly)
Skinfold thickness	X					X (monthly)
Midarm circumference	X					X (monthly)
Fluid balance (I & O)	X	X				
Temperature				X		
Vital signs	X					X
Urine glucose/acetone			X			
Catheter site/function		X				
Biochemical Indices						
Sodium	X				X (2–4x/wk initially)	
Potassium	X				X (2–4x/wk initially)	
Chloride	X				X (2–4x/wk initially)	
CO_2	X				X (2–4x/wk initially)	
Glucose	X				X (2–4x/wk initially)	
BUN	X				X	
Creatinine	X				X	
Triglycerides	X				X (2–4x/wk initially)	
Calcium	X				X (2–4x/wk initially)	
Magnesium	X				X (2–4x/wk initially)	
Phosphorus	X				X (2–4x/wk initially)	
Albumin	X				X	
ALT	X				X	
Alkaline phosphatase	X				X	
Total and direct bilirubin	X				X (2x/wk initially)	
Iron						X (monthly)
Copper						X (monthly)
Zinc						X (monthly)
Selenium carnitine					X	
Ammonia						X

Data from Heird, W. (1993). Parenteral support of the hospitalized patient. In R. Suskind & L. Lewinter-Suskind (Eds.). *Textbook of pediatric nutrition* (pp. 225–238). New York: Raven Press; adapted from *The TPN handbook* (5th ed.) (1993). Boston Nutrition Support Service, Children's Hospital, Boston.

bolic complication (Orr, 1992). Avoiding hyperglycemia is a prime consideration when increasing the amount of dextrose. Frequent monitoring of glucose metabolism by serum and urine glucose levels is helpful in evaluating hyperglycemia. Hypoglycemia may be seen when dextrose is abruptly stopped. Administering 10% dextrose solution is recommended if the catheter becomes plugged or must be discontinued (Marvin, 1988). Hypercholesterolemia, phospholipidemia, and hypertriglycemia may occur especially when increasing the amount of lipids administered. Monitoring lipid clearance by routinely checking triglyceride levels becomes important. Appropriate adjustments of nutrients in the infusion may prevent or correct complications.

Other catheter-related complications include the technical complications associated with catheter insertion and use of a venous access system. Technical complications associated with insertion include pneumothorax, hemothorax, cardiac perforation, nerve injuries, and hematoma. Air embolism and extravasation may occur during a break in the system (Gemlo et al., 1988; Reed et al., 1985; Wickham et al., 1992). Use of Luer-Lok connections, along with having the patient lie flat during discontinuation of

tubing, can prevent air embolism (Marvin, 1988). Catheter malposition, dislodgement, and thrombosis may also occur during use of a venous access system. Clotting within the catheter may be related to the frequency of blood drawing (Marvin, 1988). Facial swelling, edema of the neck and chest, difficulty with the infusion of fluid, and neck pain are all signs of potential catheter thrombosis (Beers et al., 1990; Wickham et al., 1992). These signs and symptoms of thrombosis may be subtle and delayed until complete occlusion of the vein occurs (Brown-Smith et al., 1990; Moss et al., 1989). Thrombolytic agents can be used to prolong catheter life and reestablish catheter patency. Streptokinase and urokinase dissolve clots by triggering the body's own fibrinolytic system (Brown-Smith et al., 1990).

SUMMARY

Nutritional needs of critically ill children are often underestimated. Children in intensive care units have demonstrated both an acquired and preexisting tendency toward protein-energy malnutrition. The changes in metabolic demands generated from injury

Table 14-30. COMPLICATIONS OF PARENTERAL NUTRITION

	Etiology	Intervention
Infection	Contamination at insertion site	Regular and meticulous site care
	Contamination of infusate	Use an in-line filter
	Equipment contamination	24-hour hang time for parenteral nutrition solutions
		Refrigerate solutions until used
		Change tubing every 24 hours or with each bottle
Metabolic		
Hyperglycemia	Excessive intake 2° to hyperosmolarity or high infusion rate	Monitor infusion hourly
		Monitor serum and urine glucose
		Decrease infusion rates
Hypoglycemia	Abrupt cessation of infusion	If parenteral stopped suddenly infuse 10% dextrose solution
Azotemia	Excessive amino acid intake	Decrease protein content of parenteral solution
Electrolyte, vitamin disorders	Excessive or inadequate intake	Correct composition of parenteral solution
Hypercholesterolemia/phospholipidemia	Character of or excessive use of lipid emulsion	Reduce lipid rate and monitor
Hypertriglyceridemia		Extend length of infusion
Fatty acid deficiency	Limited fat intake	Provide 4%–8% linoleic acid
Hepatic disorders		Avoid excessive calories as protein
Technical		
Infiltrations, phlebitis	High osmolarity of infusate	Check site q 30 min to 1 hour and move peripheral IV as necessary
	Prolonged use of single vein	
Thrombosis	Frequent blood drawing	Change catheter sites routinely
	Prolonged use of single vein	Monitor sites hourly
		Streptokinase/urokinase as indicated
Air embolism	Break in system	Immediately clamp catheter
		Place patient in Trendelenburg position
Extravasation	Break in system	Clamp catheter
		Use Luer-Lok connections
Breakage of catheter	Prolonged catheter use, defective, inadvertent puncture	Clamp catheter and repair

and sepsis make these children's nutritional needs very complex. Nutritional support can positively affect the recovery and survival of hospitalized patients. The nutrition received in childhood may have significant consequences as the child grows, making further work in the area imperative. When caring for a critically ill child, understanding and advocating for the child's metabolic needs is essential.

References

American Society of Parenteral and Enteral Nutrition. Board of Directors (1993). Guidelines for the use of parenteral and enteral nutrition in adult and pediatric patients. *Journal of Parenteral and Enteral Nutrition,* 17 ([Suppl] 4).

Abad-Sinden, A., & Sutphen, J. (1993). The practical use of infant formulas. In R. Suskind & L. Lewinter-Suskind (Eds.). *Textbook of pediatric nutrition* (pp. 1081–1089). New York: Raven Press.

Agusti, A., Torres, A., Estopa, R., & Agustivdal, A. (1984). Hypophosphatemia as a cause of failed weaning: The importance of metabolic factors. *Critical Care Medicine,* 12, 142–143.

Alexander, J. (1990). Nutrition and translocation. *Journal of Parenteral and Enteral Nutrition,* 14, 170s–174s.

Ament, M., Reyen, L., & Guss, W. (1993). Parenteral nutrition in infants and children. In R. Wyllie & J. Hyams (Eds.). *Pediatric gastrointestinal disease* (pp. 1140–1156). Philadelphia: W.B. Saunders.

American Academy of Pediatrics, Committee on Nutrition (1993). *Pediatric nutrition handbook* (3rd ed.). Chicago: American Academy of Pediatrics.

American Academy of Pediatrics and American College of Obstetricians and Gynecologists (1986). *Guidelines for perinatal care* (3rd ed.).

Anderson, K., Norris, D., Godfrey, L., Kirk Avent, C., & Butterworth, C. (1984). Bacterial contamination of tube-feeding formulas. *Journal of Parenteral and Enteral Nutrition,* 8, 673–678.

Arora, N., & Rochester, D. (1982). Respiratory muscle strength and maximal voluntary ventilation in undernourished patients. *American Review of Respiratory Disease,* 126, 5–8.

Askanazi, J., Nordenstrom, J., Rosenbaum, S., Elwyn, D., Hyman, A., Carpentier, Y., & Kinney, J. (1981). Nutrition for the patient with respiratory failure: Glucose vs fat. *Anesthesiology,* 54(5), 373–377.

Askanazi, J., Rosenbaum, S., Hyman, A., Silverberg, P., Milic-Emili, J., & Kinney, J. (1980). Respiratory changes induced by the large glucose loads of total parenteral nutrition. *Journal of the American Medical Association,* 243, 1444–1447.

Barbul, A. (1990). Arginine and immune function. *Nutrition,* 6, 53–58.

Barton, R., & Cerra, F. (1989). The hypermetabolism. Multiple organ failure syndrome. *Chest,* 96, 1153–1160.

Bassili, H., & Deitel, M. (1981). Effects of nutritional support on weaning patients off ventilators. *Journal of Parenteral and Enteral Nutrition,* 5(2), 161–163.

Baumgartner, T., & Schmidt, L. (1985). Filters and their implications in healthcare. *Nutrition Support and Service,* 5, 7–14.

Bazyk, S. (1990). Factors associated with the transition to oral feeding in infants fed by nasogastric tubes. *The American Journal of Occupational Therapy,* 44(12), 1070–1078.

Beckholt, A. (1989). Breast milk for infants who cannot breastfeed. *Journal of Obstetric, Gynecologic and Neonatal Nursing,* 19(3), 216–220.

Beers, T., Burnes, J., & Fleming, C. (1990). Superior vena caval obstruction in patients with gut failure receiving home parenteral nutrition. *Journal of Parenteral and Enteral Nutrition,* 14, 474–479.

Benjamin, D. (1989). Laboratory tests and nutritional assessment, protein-energy status. *Pediatric Clinics of North America,* 36, 139–161.

Benkov, K., Kazlow, P., Waye, J., & LeLeiko, N. (1986). Percutaneous endoscopic gastrostomies in children. *Pediatrics,* 77, 248–250.

Benya, R., Langer, S., & Mobarhan, S. (1990). Flexible nasogastric feeding tube tip malposition immediately after placement. *Journal of Parenteral and Enteral Nutrition,* 14, 108–109.

Berger, R., & Adams, L. (1989). Nutritional support in the critical care setting (Part 2). *Chest,* 96(2), 372–380.

Bernard, M., & Forlaw, L. (1984). Complications and their prevention. In J. Rombeau & M. Caldwell (Eds.). *Clinical Nutrition* (Vol. 1, pp. 542–569). Philadelphia: W.B. Saunders.

Bernbaum, J., Pereira, G., Watkins, J., & Peckham, G. (1983). Nonnutritional sucking during gavage feeding enhances growth and maturation in premature infants. *Pediatrics,* 71, 41–45.

Bohnker, B., Artman, L., & Hoskins, W. (1985). Intranasal retraction of nasogastric feeding tube: Case reports and suggestion for design modification. *Journal of Parenteral and Enteral Nutrition,* 9, 53–54.

Border, J., Hassett, J., LaDuca, J., Seibel, R., Steinberg, S., Mills, B., Losi, P., & Border, D. (1987). The gut origin septic states in blunt trauma in the ICU. *Annals of Surgery,* 206, 427–448.

Bower, R., Kern, K., & Fischer, J. (1985). Use of branched chain amino acid enriched solutions in patients under metabolic stress. *The American Journal of Surgery,* 149, 266–270.

Bower, R., Talamini, M., Sax, H., Hamilton, F., & Fischer, J. (1986). Postoperative enteral vs parenteral nutrition: A randomized controlled study. *Archives of Surgery,* 121, 1040–1045.

Bozzetti, F., Terno, G., Bonfanti, G., Scarpa, D., Scotti, A., Ammatuna, M., & Bonalum, M. (1983). Prevention and treatment of central venous catheter sepsis by exchange via a guidewire. A prospective controlled trial. *Annals of Surgery,* 198, 48–52.

Branson, R. (1990). The measurement of energy expenditure: Instrumentation, practical considerations and clinical application. *Respiratory Care,* 35, 640–659.

Brinson, R., Curtis, W., & Singh, M. (1987). Diarrhea in the intensive care unit: The role of hypoalbuminemia and the response to a chemically defined diet (case reports and review of the literature). *Journal of the American College of Nutrition,* 6, 517–523.

Brown-Smith, J., Stoner, M., & Barley, Z. (1990). Tunneled catheter thrombosis: Factors related to incidence. *Oncology Nursing Forum,* 17, 543–549.

Buckner, M. (1990). Perioperative nutritional problems. *Critical Care Nursing Clinics of North America,* 2, 559–566.

Bullock, B., & Rosendahl, P. (1992). *Pathophysiology adaptations and alterations in function* (3rd ed.). Philadelphia: J.B. Lippincott.

Burke, D., Alverdy, J., Aoys, E., & Moss, G. (1989). Glutamine-supplemented total parenteral nutrition improves gut immune function. *Archives of Surgery,* 124, 1396–1399.

Caldwell, M., & Kennedy, C. (1981). Normal nutritional requirements. *Surgical Clinics of North America,* 61, 489–507.

Cataldi-Betcher, E., Seltzer, M., Slocum, B., & Jones, K. (1983). Complications occurring during enteral nutrition support: A prospective study. *Journal of Parenteral and Enteral Nutrition,* 7, 546–552.

Cavelli, B. (1981). Gastric emptying in infants fed human milk or infant formula. *Acta Paediatric Scandinavia,* 70, 639–641.

Cerra, F. (1986). The role of nutrition in the management of metabolic stress. *Critical Care Clinics,* 2, 807–819.

Cerra, F. (1987). Hypermetabolism, organ failure and metabolic support. *Surgery,* 101, 1–14.

Cerra, F. (1990). How nutrition intervention changes what getting sick means. *Journal of Parenteral and Enteral Nutrition,* 14, 164S–169S.

Church, J., & Hill, G. (1987). Assessing the efficacy of intravenous nutrition in general surgical patients: Dynamic nutritional assessment with plasma proteins. *Journal of Parenteral and Enteral Nutrition,* 11, 135–139.

Chwals, W. (1994). Overfeeding the critically ill child: Fact or fiction. *New Horizons,* 2, 147–155.

Chwals, W., Lally, K., Woolley, M., & Hossein Mahour, G. (1988). Measured energy expenditure in critically ill infants and young children. *Journal of Surgical Research,* 44, 467–472.

Clifton, G., Robertson, C., & Choi, S. (1986). Assessment of nutrition status of head injured patients. *Journal of Neurosurgery,* 64, 895–901.

Cooper, A., & Heird, W. (1982). Nutritional assessment of the pediatric patient including the low birthweight infant. *The American Journal of Clinical Nutrition,* 35, 1132–1141.

Cooper, A., Jakobowski, D., Spiker, J., Floyd, T., Ziegler, M., & Koop, C. (1981). Nutritional assessment: An integral part of the perioperative pediatric surgical evaluation. *Journal of Pediatric Surgery,* 16, 554–561.

Daly, J., Reynolds, J., Sigal, R., Shou, J., & Liberman, M. (1990). Effect of dietary protein and amino acids on immune function. *Critical Care Medicine,* 18, S86–S92.

Daly, J., Reynolds, J., Thom, A., Kinsley, L., Dietrick-Gallagher, M., Shou, J., & Ruggieri, B. (1988). Immune and metabolic effects of arginine in the surgical patient. *Annals of Surgery,* 208, 512–523.

Dark, D., Pingleton, S., & Kerby, G. (1985). Hypercapnia during weaning. A complication of nutritional support. *Chest,* 88(1), 41–43.

DeChicco, R., & Matarese, L. (1992). Selection of nutrition support regimens. *Nutrition in Clinical Practice,* 7, 239–245.

Dhingra, S., Solven, F., Wilson, A., & McCarthy, D. (1984). Hypomagnesemia and respiratory muscle power. *American Review of Respiratory Disease,* 129, 497–498.

DiLorenzo, J., Dalton, B., & Miskovitz, P. (1992). Percutaneous endoscopic gastrostomy. *Postgraduate Medicine,* 91(1), 277–296.

Doekel, R., Zwillich, C., Scoggin, C., Krygen, M., & Weil, J. (1976). Clinical semistarvation. Depression of hypoxic ventilatory response. *New England Journal of Medicine,* 295(7), 358–361.

Dorsey, J., & Cogordon, J. (1985). Nasotracheal intubation and pulmonary parenchymal perforation. *Chest,* 87, 131–132.

Dunn, L., Hulman, S., Weiner, J., & Kliegman, R. (1988). Beneficial effects of early hypocaloric enteral feeding on neonatal gastrointestinal function: Preliminary report of a randomized trial. *Journal of Pediatrics,* 112, 622–629.

Early, T., Gregory, R., Wheeler, J., Snyder, S., & Gayle, R. (1990). Increased infection rate in double lumen versus single lumen Hickman catheters in cancer patients. *Southern Medical Journal,* 83, 34–36.

Edes, T. (1991). Nutrition support of critically ill patients. *Postgraduate Medicine,* 89(5), 193–238.

Edes, T., Walk, B., & Austin, J. (1990). Diarrhea in tube-fed patients: Feeding formulas not necessarily the cause. *The American Journal of Medicine,* 88, 91–93.

Eldar, S., & Meguid, M. (1984). Pneumothorax following attempted nasogastric intubation for nutritional support. *Journal of Parenteral and Enteral Nutrition,* 8, 450–452.

Elia, M., & Livesey, G. (1988). Theory and validity of the direct calorimetry during net lipid synthesis. *The American Journal of Clinical Nutrition,* 47(4), 591–607.

Ellis, L., Copeland, E., & Souba, W. (1991). Perioperative nutritional support. *Surgical Clinics of North America,* 71(3), 493–507.

Elwyn, D. (1989). Nutritional recommendations of stressed patients. In W. Shoemaker (Ed.). *Textbook of Critical Care* (2nd ed., pp. 1085–1092). Philadelphia: W.B. Saunders.

Energy and Protein Requirements (1985). FAO/WHO/UUN, Expert Consultation. Geneva: World Health Organization.

Faller, N., Lawrence, K., & Ferraro, C. (1993). Gastrostomy, replacement, feeding tubes: The long and short of it . . . *Ostomy/Wound Management,* 39(1), 26–33.

Ferrannini, E. (1988). The theoretical bases of indirect calorimetry: A review. *Metabolism,* 37, 287–301.

Field, S., Kelly, S., & MacKlem, P. (1982a). The oxygen cost of breathing in patients with cardiorespiratory disease. *American Review of Respiratory Disease,* 126, 9–13.

Field, T., Ignatoff, E., Stringer, S., Brennan, J., Greenberg, R., Widmayer, S., & Anderson, G. (1982b). Nonnutritive sucking during tube feedings: Effect on preterm neonates in an intensive care unit. *Pediatrics,* 70, 381–384.

Figueroa-Colon, R. (1993). Clinical and laboratory assessment of the malnourished child. In R. Suskind & L. Lewinter-Suskind

(Eds.). *Textbook of pediatric nutrition* (pp. 207–216). Philadelphia: W.B. Saunders.

Fiorotto, M., Cochran, W., Funk, C., Sheng, H., & Klish, W. (1987). Total body electrical conductivity measurements: Effects of body composition and geometry. *American Journal of Physiology, 252,* R794–R800.

Fitzsimmons, L., & Hadley, S. (1991). The metabolic response to injury in the surgical/trauma patient. *Dimensions in Critical Care Nursing,* 10, 4–12.

Foster, G., Knox, L., Dempsey, D., & Mullen, J. (1987). Caloric requirements in total parenteral nutrition. *Journal of the American College of Nutrition,* 6, 231–253.

Frisancho, A. (1981). New norms of upper limb fat and muscle areas for assessment of nutritional status. *The American Journal of Clinical Nutrition,* 34, 2540–2545.

Fuchs, G. (1993). Enteral support of the hospitalized child. In R. Suskind & L. Lewinter-Suskind (Eds.). *Textbook of Pediatric Nutrition* (pp. 239–246). New York: Raven Press.

Garza, C., Butt, N., & Goldman, A. (1993). Human milk and infant formula. In R. Suskind & L. Lewinter-Suskind (Eds.). *Textbook of pediatric nutrition* (2nd ed.). (pp. 33–42). New York: Raven Press.

Garza, C., Schanler, R., Butte, N., & Motil, K. (1987). Special properties of human milk. *Clinics in Perinatology,* 14, 32.

Gauderer, M. (1991). Percutaneous endoscopic gastrostomy: A ten year experience with 220 children. *Journal of Pediatric Surgery,* 26, 288–292.

Gauderer, M., Olsen, M., Stellato, T., & Dokler, M. (1988). Feeding gastrostomy button: Experience and recommendations. *Journal of Pediatric Surgery,* 23, 24–28.

Gebara, B. Gelmini, M., & Sarnaik, A. (1992). Oxygen consumption, energy expenditure and substrate utilization after cardiac surgery in children. *Critical Care Medicine,* 20, 1550–1554.

Gemlo, B., Rayner, A., Swanson, R., Young, J., Homann, J., & Hohn, P. (1988). Extravasation. A serious complication of the split sheath introducer technique for venous access. *Archives of Surgery,* 123, 490–492.

Getchell, E. (1983). Estimating energy and protein needs for the hospitalized child. *The American Journal of Intravenous Therapy and Clinical Nutrition,* 10, 4–15.

Gil, R., Kruse, J., Thill-Baharozian, M., & Carlson, R. (1989). Triple versus single lumen central venous catheters: A prospective study in a critically ill population. *Archives of Internal Medicine,* 149, 1139–1143.

Gill, N., Behnke, M., Conlon, M., & Anderson, G. (1992). Nonnutritive sucking modulates behavioral state for preterm infants before feeding. *Scandinavian Journal of Caring Science,* 6, 3–7.

Goldman, D., Martin, T., & Worthington, W. (1973). Growth of bacteria and fungi in total parenteral nutrition. *The American Journal of Surgery,* 128, 314–318.

Gottschlich, M., Warden, G., Michel, M., Havens, P., Kopcha, R., Jenkins, M., & Alexander, J. (1988). Diarrhea in tube-fed burn patients: Incidence, etiology, nutritional impact and prevention. *Journal of Parenteral and Enteral Nutrition,* 12, 338–345.

Greene, H., Hambidge, K., Schanler, R., & Tsang, R. (1988). Guidelines for the use of vitamins, trace elements, calcium, magnesium, phosphorus in infants receiving total parenteral nutrition: Report of the subcommittee on clinical practice issues of the American Society of Clinical Nutrition. *The American Journal of Clinical Nutrition,* 48, 1324–1342.

Grossman, T., Duncavage, J., Dennison, B., Kay, J., & Toohill, R. (1984). Complications associated with narrow-bore nasogastric tube. *Annals of Otology, Rhinology and Laryngology,* 93, 460–463.

Hamill, P., Drizd, T., Johnson, C., Reed, R., Roche, A., & Moore, W. (1979). Physical growth: National Center for Health Statistics percentiles. *The American Journal of Clinical Nutrition,* 23, 607–629.

Hammarquist, F., Wernerman, J., Rustom, A., Ali, R., Vonderdecken, A., & Vinnars, E. (1989). Addition of glutamine to total parenteral nutrition after elective abdominal surgery spares free glutamine in muscle, counteracts the fall in muscle protein synthesis, and improves nitrogen balance. *Annals of Surgery,* 209, 455–461.

Harris Benedict, F. (1919). *A biometric study of basal metabolism in man* (p. 279). Washington, D.C.: Carnegie Institute Washington Publications.

Haumont, D., Deckelbaum, R., Richelle, M., Dahlan, W., Coussaert, E., Bihain, B., & Carpentier, Y. (1989). Plasma lipid and plasma lipoprotein concentrations in low birthweight infants given parenteral nutrition with twenty and ten percent lipid emulsion. *Journal of Pediatrics,* 115, 787–793.

Heird, W. (1993). Parenteral support of the hospitalized patient. In R. Suskind & L. Lewinter-Suskind (Eds.). *Textbook of pediatric nutrition* (pp. 225–238). New York: Raven Press.

Heird, W., Dell, R., Helms, R., Greene, H., Ament, M., Karna, P., & Storm, M. (1987). Amino acid mixture designed to maintain normal plasma amino acid patterns in infants and children requiring parenteral nutrition. *Pediatrics,* 80, 401–408.

Hendricks, K., & Walker, W. (1990). *Manual of pediatric nutrition* (2nd ed.). Philadelphia: B.C. Decker.

Heubi, J., Balistreri, W., & Suchy, F. (1982). Bile salt metabolism in the first year of life. *Journal of Laboratory and Clinical Medicine,* 100, 127–136.

Heymsfield, S., Bethel, R., Ansley, J., Gibbs, D., Felner, J., & Nutter, D. (1978). Cardiac abnormalities in cachectic patients before and during nutritional repletion. *American Heart Journal,* 95, 584–594.

Hindsdale, J., Lipkowitz, G., Pollack, T., Hoover, E., & Jaffe, B. (1985). Prolonged enteral nutrition in malnourished patients with nonelemental feeding. *The American Journal of Surgery,* 149, 334–338.

Holliday, M. (1971). Metabolic rate and organ size during growth from infancy to maturity and during late gestation and early infancy. *Pediatrics,* 47, 169–179.

Holtzman, G., Warner, S., Melnik, G., & Beer, W. (1990). Nutritional support of pulmonary patients: A multidisciplinary approach. *AACN Clinical Issues,* 1(2), 300–312.

Huddleston, K. (1989). MIC or foley: Comparing gastrostomy tubes. *Maternal and Child Nursing,* 14, 20–23.

Huddleston, K., & Palmer, K. (1990). A button for gastrostomy feedings. *Maternal and Child Nursing,* 15, 315–319.

Huddleston, K., Ferraro-McDuffie, A., & Wolff-Small, T. (1993). Nutritional support of the critically ill child. *Critical Care Nursing Clinics of North America,* 5(1), 65–78.

Hwang, T., O'Dwyer, S., Smith, R., & Wilmore, D. (1986). Preservation of small bowel mucosa using glutamine enriched parenteral nutrition. *Surgical Forum,* 38, 56–58.

Hyman, P., & DiLorenzo, C. (1993). Gastrointestinal motility. In R. Wyllie & J. Hyams (Eds.). *Pediatric gastrointestinal disease* (pp. 53–63). Philadelphia: W.B. Saunders.

Irvin, T., & Hunt, T. (1974). Effect of malnutrition colonic healing. *Annals of Surgery,* 186, 765–772.

Jeejeebhoy, K. (1994). How should we monitor nutritional support: Structure and function? *New Horizons,* 2, 131–138.

Jolley, S., Tunell, W., Hoelzer, D., Thomas, S., & Smith, E. (1986). Lower esophageal pressure changes with tube gastrostomy: A causative factor of gastroesophageal reflux in children? *Journal of Pediatric Surgery,* 21, 624–677.

Kalhan, S., Oliven, A., King, K., & Lucero, C. (1986). Role of glucose regulation of endogenous glucose production in human newborn. *Pediatric Research,* 20, 49–52.

Kelly, S., Rosa, A., Fields, S., Coughlin, M., Shizgal, H., & MacKlem, P. (1984). Inspiratory muscle strength and body composition in patients receiving total parenteral nutrition therapy. *American Review of Respiratory Disease,* 130, 33–37.

Keohane, P., Attrill, H., Love, M., Frost, P., & Silk, D. (1984). Relation between osmolality of diet and gastrointestinal side effects in enteral nutrition. *British Medical Journal,* 288, 678–680.

Kinney, J., & Elwyn, D. (1983). Protein metabolism and injury. *Annual Review of Nutrition,* 3, 433–466.

Konstantinides, N., & Lehmann, S. (1993). The impact of nutrition on wound healing. *Critical Care Nurse,* 13(5), 25–33.

Konstantinides, N., Teasley, K., Lysne, J., Shronts, E., Olson, G., & Cerra, F. (1984). Nutritional requirements of the hypermetabolic patient. *Nutrition Support Service,* 4, 41–50.

Koruda, M., & Rombeau, J. (1986). Clinical studies of energy metabolism. *England Biomedical,* 1, 19–24.

Koruda, M., Guenter, P., & Rombeau, J. (1987). Enteral nutrition in the critically ill. *Critical Care Clinics,* 3, 133–153.

Kuhn, M. (1990). Nutritional support for the shock patient. *Critical Care Clinics of North America,* 2, 201–220.

Kushner, R., & Schoeller, D. (1986). Estimation of total body water by biochemical impedance analysis. *The American Journal of Clinical Nutrition,* 44, 417–424.

Lacey, J., & Wilmore, D. (1990). Is glutamine a conditionally essential amino acid? *Nutrition Reviews,* 48, 297–309.

Lang, C. (1987). *Nutritional support in critical care.* Gaithersburg, MD: Aspen Publishers.

Lehmann, S. (1991). Immune function and nutrition. *Journal of Intravenous Nursing,* 14, 406–418.

Lehmann, S. (1993). Nutrition support in the hypermetabolic patient. *Critical Care Nursing Clinics of North America,* 5(1), 97–103.

LeLeiko, S., & Benkov, K. (1986). Nutritional support for hospitalized children. *Hospital Practice,* 21, 179–190.

LeLeiko, N., Burke, P., & Chao, C. (1993). Enteral nutrition. In R. Wyllie & J. Hyams (Eds.). *Pediatric gastrointestinal disease* (pp. 1124–1139). New York: Raven Press.

LeLeiko, N., Luder, E., Fridman, M., Fersel, J., & Benkov, K. (1986). Nutritional assessment of pediatric patients admitted to an acute-care pediatric service utilizing anthropometric measurements. *Journal of Parenteral and Enteral Nutrition,* 10, 166–168.

Lowry, S. (1990). The route of feeding influences injury responses. *Journal of Trauma,* 30, S10–S15.

Lukaski, H., & Johnson, P. (1985). A simple inexpensive method of determining total body water using a tracer dose of D_{20} and infrared absorption of biological fluids. *The American Journal of Clinical Nutrition,* 41, 972–973.

Lukaski, H., Bolonchuk, W., Hall, C., & Siders, W. (1986). Validation of tetra polar bioelectrical impedance method to assess human body composition. *Journal of Applied Physiology,* 60, 1327–1332.

McCarthy, M., Shives, J., Robinson, R., & Broadie, T. (1987). Prospective evaluation of single and triple lumen catheter in total parenteral nutrition. *Journal of Parenteral and Enteral Nutrition,* 11, 259–262.

McClave, A., & Snider, H. (1992). Use of indirect calorimetry in clinical nutrition. *Nutrition in Clinical Practice,* 7, 207–221.

McIrvine, A., & Mannick, J. (1983). Lymphocyte function in the critically ill surgical patient. *Surgical Clinics of North America,* 63, 245–261.

Major, M. (1988). Nutritional support of the mechanically ventilated patient. *Critical Care Nursing Quarterly,* 11(3), 50–61.

Marcoux, C., Fisher, S., & Wong, D. (1990). Central venous access devices in children. *Pediatric Nursing,* 16(2), 123–133.

Marian, M. (1993). Pediatric nutrition support. *Nutrition in Clinical Practice,* 8(5), 199–209.

Marvin, J. (1988). Nutritional support of the critically injured patient. *Critical Care Nursing Quarterly,* 11, 21–34.

Meakins, J., Pietsch, J., Bubenick, O., Kelly, R., Rode, H., Gordon, J., & MacLean, L. (1977). Delayed hypersensitivity: Indicator of acquired failure of the host defenses in sepsis and trauma. *Annals of Surgery,* 186, 241–250.

Merritt, R., & Suskind, R. (1979). Nutritional survey of hospitalized pediatric patients. *The American Journal of Clinical Nutrition,* 32, 1320–1325.

Messing, B., Beliah, M., Girard-Pipau, F., Leleve, D., & Bermer, J. (1982). Technical hazards of using nutritive mixtures in bags for cyclical intravenous nutrition in 48 gastroenterological patients. *Gut,* 23, 297–303.

Metheny, N. (1988). Measures to test placement of nasogastric and nasointestinal feeding tubes: A review. *Nursing Research,* 37(6), 324–329.

Metheny, N., Hampton, K., & Williams, P. (1990a). Detection of inadvertent respiratory placement of small-bore feeding tubes: A report of 10 cases. *Heart & Lung,* 19(6), 631–638.

Metheny, N., McSweeney, M., Wehrle, M., & Wiersema, L. (1990b). Effectiveness of the auscultatory method in predicting feeding tube placement. *Nursing Research,* 39, 262–267.

Metheny, N., Spies, M., & Eisenberg, P. (1986). Frequency of nasoenteral tube displacement and associated risk factors. *Research in Nursing Health,* 9, 241–247.

Meyer, N., Muller, M., & Herdon, D. (1994). Nutrition support of the healing wound. *New Horizons,* 2, 202–214.

Miller, H., & Anderson, G. (1993). Nonnutritive sucking: Effects on crying and heart rate in intubated infants requiring assisted mechanical ventilation. *Nursing Research,* 42(5), 305–307.

Minard, G., & Kudsk, K. (1994). Is early feeding beneficial? How early is early? *New Horizons,* 2, 156–163.

Miyagawa, C. (1993). Drug-nutrient interactions in critically ill patients. *Critical Care Nurse,* 13(5), 69–90.

Mochizuki, H., Trocki, O., Dominioni, L., Brackett, K., Joffe, S., & Alexander, J. (1984). Mechanism of prevention of postburn hypermetabolism and catabolism by early enteral feeding. *Annals of Surgery,* 200, 297–310.

Monturo, C. (1990). Enteral access device selection. *Nutrition in Clinical Practice,* 5, 207–213.

Moore, K. (1993). *The developing human* (5th ed.). Philadelphia: W.B. Saunders.

Moore, M., Guenter, P., & Bender, J. (1986). Nutrition related nursing research. *Image, Journal of Nursing Scholarship,* 18(1), 18–21.

Moore, R., Moore, E., Jones, T., McCroskey, R., & Peterson, V. (1989). TEN versus TPN following abdominal trauma—reduced septic morbidity. *The Journal of Trauma,* 29, 916–923.

Moss, J., Wagman, L., Riihimaki, D., & Terz, J. (1989). Central venous thrombosis related to silastic Hickman-Brovica catheter in oncologic population. *Journal of Parenteral and Enteral Nutrition,* 13, 397–400.

Motil, K. (1993). Development of the gastrointestinal tract. In R. Wyllie & J. Hyams (Eds.). *Pediatric gastrointestinal disease* (pp. 3–16). Philadelphia: W.B. Saunders.

Murphy, J. (1990). Tube feeding problems and solutions. *Advancing Clinical Care,* 5, 7–11.

Murphy, L., & Conforti, C. (1993). Nutritional support of the cardiopulmonary patient. *Critical Care Nursing Clinics of North American,* 5(1), 57–64.

Murry, M., Marsh, M., Wochos, D., Moxness, K., Offord, K., & Callaway, C. (1988). Nutritional assessment of intensive care unit patients. *Mayo Clin Proceedings,* 63, 1106–1115.

National Research Council, Food and Nutrition Board (1989). *Recommended dietary allowance* (10th ed.). Washington, D.C.: National Academy Press.

Neal, J., & Slayton, D. (1992). Neonatal and pediatric PEG tubes. *Maternal and Child Nursing,* 17, 184–191.

Niemiec, P., Vanderveen, T., Morrison, J., & Hohenwarter, M. (1983). Gastrointestinal disorders caused by medication and electrolyte solution osmolality during enteral nutrition. *Journal of Parenteral and Enteral Nutrition,* 7, 387–389.

Nordenstrom, J., Carpentier, Y., Askanazi, J., Robin, A., Elwyn, D., Hensle, T., & Kinney, J. (1982). Metabolic utilization of intravenous fat emulsion during total parenteral nutrition. *Annals of Surgery,* 196, 221–231.

O'Dwyer, S., Smith, R., Hwang, T., & Wilmore, D. (1989). Maintenance of small bowel mucosa with glutamine-enriched parenteral nutrition. *Journal of Parenteral and Enteral Nutrition,* 13, 579–585.

Orr, M. (1992). Hyperglycemia during nutrition support. *Critical Care Nurse,* 12, 64–70.

Parker, D., Stroops, S., & Greene, H. (1981). A controlled comparison of continuous versus intermittent feeding in the treatment of infants with intestinal disease. *Journal of Pediatrics,* 99, 360–364.

Parsons, H., Francoeur, T., Howland, P., Spengler, R., & Pencharz, P. (1980). The nutritional status of hospitalized children. *American Journal of Clinical Nutrition,* 33, 1140–1146.

Pemberton, L., Lyman, B., Lander, V., & Covinskey, J. (1986). Sepsis from triple and single lumen catheters during total parenteral nutrition in surgical or critically ill patients. *Archives of Surgery,* 121, 591–594.

Perry, A., & Potter, P. (1992). *Clinical nursing skills and techniques.* St. Louis: C.V. Mosby.

Peterson, V., Moore, E., Jones, T., Rundus, C., Emmett, M., Moore, F., McCroskey, B., Haddix, T., & Parsons, P. (1988). Total enteral nutrition versus total parenteral nutrition after major torso injury: Attenuation of hepatic protein reprioritization. *Surgery,* 104, 199–207.

Pillar, B., Perry, S., & Radany, M. (1990). The appropriate use of high cost, high risk technologies: The case of total parenteral nutrition. *Quality Review Bulletin,* 16, 214–217.

Plit, M., Lipman, J., Eidelman, J., & Gavaudan, J. (1988). Catheter related infection. A plea for consensus with review and guidelines. *Intensive Care Medicine,* 14, 503–509.

Pollack, M. (1993). Nutritional support of children in the intensive care unit. In R. Suskind & L. Lewinter-Suskind (Eds.). *Textbook of pediatric nutrition* (2nd ed., pp. 201–216). New York: Raven Press.

Pollack, M., Ruttimann, U., & Wiley, J. (1985). Nutritional depletion in critically ill children: Association with physiologic instability and increased quality of care. *Journal of Parenteral and Enteral Nutrition,* 9, 309–313.

Pollack, M., Wiley, J., & Holbrook, P. (1981). Early nutritional depletion in critically ill children. *Critical Care Medicine,* 9, 580–583.

Pollack, M., Wiley, J., Kanter, R., & Holbrook, P. (1982). Malnutrition in critically ill infants and children. *Journal of Parenteral and Enteral Nutrition,* 6, 20–24.

Quinn, T., & Askanazi, J. (1987). Nutrition and cardiac disease. *Critical Care Clinics,* 3, 167–184.

Randall, S., & Blackburn, G. (1987). Nutritional therapy in trauma and sepsis. In J. Seigel (Ed.). *Trauma, emergency surgery, and critical care* (pp. 543–562). New York: Churchill Livingstone.

Reed, W., Newman, K., Applefeld, M., & Sutton, F. (1985). Drug extravasation as a complication of venous access ports. *Annals of Internal Medicine,* 102, 788–790.

Rees, R., Keohane, P., Grimble, G., Frost, P., Attrill, H., & Sik, D. (1985). Tolerance of elemental diet administered without starter regimen. *British Medical Journal,* 290, 1869–1870.

Rennie, M. (1985). Muscle protein turnover and the wasting due to injury and disease. *British Medical Bulletin,* 41, 257–264.

Report of the Dietary Guidelines Advisory Committee on the Dietary Guidelines for Americans (1990). Hyattsville, MD: US Department of Agriculture.

Robertson, J. (1991). Changing central venous catheter lines: Evaluation of a modification to clinical practice. *Journal of Pediatric Oncology Nursing,* 8, 173–179.

Rombeau, J., & Barot, L. (1981). Enteral nutrition therapy. *Surgical Clinics of North America,* 61, 605–620.

Rosenthal, A. (1993). Nutritional considerations in the prognosis and treatment of children with congenital heart disease. In R. Suskind & L. Lewinter-Suskind (Eds.). *Textbook of pediatric nutrition* (pp. 383–391). New York: Raven Press.

Rothkopf, M., Stanislaus, G., Haverstick, L., Kretan, V., & Askanazi, J. (1989). Nutritional support in respiratory failure. *Nutrition in Clinical Practice,* 4, 166–172.

Roundtree, D. (1991). The PIC catheter: A different approach. *American Journal of Nursing,* 91(8), 22–26.

Roza, A., & Shizgal, H. (1984). The Harris-Benedict equation reevaluated: Resting energy requirements and the body cell mass. *The American Journal of Clinical Nutrition,* 40, 168–182.

Schlichtig, R., & Sargent, S. (1990). Nutritional support of the mechanically ventilated patient. *Critical Care Clinics,* 6, 767–784.

Schroeder, D., Gillanders, L., Mahr, K., & Hill, G. (1991). Effects of immediate postoperative enteral nutrition on body composition, muscle function and wound healing. *Journal of Parenteral and Enteral Nutrition,* 15(4), 376–383.

Scott, R., Sohmer, P., & MacDonald, M. (1982). The effect of starvation and repletion on plasma fibronectin in man. *Journal of the American Medical Association,* 248, 2025–2027.

Seshadri, V., & Meyer-Tehambel, O. (1993). Electrolyte and drug management in nutritional support. *Critical Care Nursing Clinics of North America,* 5(1), 31–36.

Shanbhogue, R., & Lloyd, D. (1992). Absence of hypermetabolism after operation in the newborn infant. *Journal of Parenteral and Enteral Nutrition,* 16, 333–336.

Shepard, R., Wren, J., Evans, S., Landen, M., & Ong, T. (1987). Gastroesophageal reflux in children. Clinical profile, course and outcome with active therapy in 126 cases. *Clinical Pediatrics,* 26, 55–60.

Skeie, B., Kvetan, V., Gil, K., Rothkopf, M., Newsholme, E., & Askanazi, J. (1990). Branched chain amino acids: Their metabolism and clinical utility. *Critical Care Medicine,* 18, 549–571.

Slagle, T., & Gross, S. (1988). Effect of early low-volume enteral

substrate on subsequent feeding tolerance in very low birth weight infants. *Journal of Pediatrics,* 113, 526–531.

Smith, C., Manrie, L., Brogdon, C., Faust-Wilson, P., Lohr, G., Gerala, K., & Pingleton, S. (1990). Diarrhea associated with tube feeding in mechanically ventilated critically ill patients. *Nursing Research,* 39, 148–152.

Smith, J., & Heymsfield, S. (1983). Enteral nutrition support: Formula preparation from modular ingredients. *Journal of Parenteral and Enteral Nutrition,* 7, 280–288.

Sorensen, R., Leiva, L., & Kuvibidila, S. (1993). Malnutrition and the immune response. In R. Suskind & L. Lewinter-Suskind (Eds.). *Textbook of pediatric nutrition* (2nd ed., pp. 141–160). New York: Raven Press.

Souba, W., Herskovitz, D., Austgen, T., Chen, M., & Salloum, R. (1990). Glutamine nutrition: Theoretical considerations and therapeutic impact. *Journal of Parenteral and Enteral Nutrition,* 14, 237S–243S.

Spender, Q., Cronk, C., Charney, E., & Stallings, V. (1989). Assessment of linear growth of children with cerebral palsy: Use of alternative measures to height and length. *Developmental Medicine Child Neurology,* 31, 206–214.

Steele, N. (1991). The button: Replacement of gastrostomy device. *Journal of Pediatric Nursing,* 6(6), 421–424.

Steffee, W. (1980). Malnutrition in hospitalized patients. *Journal of the American Medical Association,* 244, 2630–2635.

Suskind, R. (1975). Gastrointestinal changes in the malnourished child. *Pediatric Clinics of North America,* 22, 873–883.

Swinamer, D., Prang, P., Jones, R., Grace, M., & Garner King, E. (1988). Effect of routine administration of analgesia on energy expenditure in critically ill patients. *Chest,* 92, 4–10.

Taylor, T. (1992). Comparison of two methods of nasogastric tube feeding. *Neurology Nurse,* 14, 49–55.

Teasley, K., & Buss, R. (1989). Do parenteral nutrition solutions with high concentrations of branched-chain amino acids offer significant benefits to stressed patients? *DICP, The Annals of Pharmacotherapy,* 23, 411–416.

The Human Milk Banking Association of North America (1993). *Recommendations for collection, storage, and handling of a mother's milk for her own infant in the hospital setting.* West Hartford, CT: The Human Milk Banking Association of North America, Inc.

The Surgeon General's Report on Nutrition and Health (1988). Washington, D.C.: US Department of Health and Human Services.

Thompson, B., & Robinson, L. (1991). Infection control of parenteral nutrition solutions. *Nutrition in Clinical Practice,* 6, 49–54.

Tilden, S., Watkins, S., Tong, T., & Jeevanandam, M. (1989). Measured energy expenditure in pediatric intensive care patients. *American Journal of Disabled Children,* 143, 490–492.

Townsend, L. (1990). Practical considerations of the gastrostomy button. *Gastroenterology Nursing,* 14, 18–26.

Treloar, D., & Stechmiller, J. (1984). Pulmonary aspiration in tube-fed patients with artificial airways. *Heart & Lung,* 13, 667–671.

Twomey, P., Zeigler, D., & Rombeau, J. (1982). Utility of skin testing in nutritional assessment. A critical review. *Journal of Parenteral and Enteral Nutrition,* 6, 50–58.

Udall, J., & Walker, W. (1982). The physiologic and pathologic basis for the transport of macromolecules across the intestinal tract. *Journal of Pediatric Gastroenterology,* 1, 295–301.

Ugo, P., Mohler, P., & Wilson, G. (1992). Bedside post-pyloric placement of weighted feeding tubes. *Nutrition in Clinical Practice,* 7, 284–287.

Valentine, R., & Turner, W. (1985). Pleural complications of nasoenteric feeding tubes. *Journal of Parenteral and Enteral Nutrition,* 9, 605–607.

Vanderhoof, J., Hofschire, P., Baloff, M., Guest, J., Murray, N., Pinsky, W., Kuglen, J., & Antonsan, D. (1982). Continuous enteral feedings an important adjunct to the management of complex congenital heart disease. *American Journal of Disabled Children,* 136, 825–827.

Viart, P. (1977). Hemodynamic findings in severe protein calorie malnutrition. *The American Journal of Clinical Nutrition,* 30, 334–348.

Walker, M. (1992). Breastfeeding in the preterm infant. *NAACOG Clinical Issues, 3,* 620–633.

Walsh, S., & Banks, L. (1990). How to insert a small-bore feeding tube safely. *Nursing90,* 55–59.

Weissman, C., & Hyman, A. (1987). Nutritional care of the critically ill patient in respiratory failure. *Critical Care Clinics, 3,* 185–203.

Weissman, C., Askanazi, J., Rosenbaum, S., Hyman, A., Milic-Emili, J., & Kinney, J. (1983). Amino acids and respiration. *Annals of Internal Medicine, 98,* 41–44.

Weissman, C., Kemper, M., Askanazi, J., Hyman, A., & Kinney, J. (1986). Resting metabolic rate of the critically ill patient. Measured versus predicted. *Anesthesiology, 64,* 673–679.

Weissman, C., Kemper, M., Damask, M., Askanazi, J., Hyman, A., & Kinney, J. (1984). The effect of routine intensive care interaction of metabolic rate. *Chest, 86,* 815–818.

Whittaker, J., Ryan, C., Buckley, P., & Road, J. (1990). The effects of refeeding on peripheral and respiratory muscle function in malnourished chronic obstructive pulmonary disease patients. *American Review of Respiratory Disease, 142,* 283–288.

Wickham, R., Purl, S., & Welker, D. (1992). Long term central venous catheters: Issues for care. *Seminars in Oncology Nursing, 8*(2), 133–147.

Wilmore, D. (1977). *The metabolic management of the critically ill.* New York: Plenum Publishing.

Wilmore, D., Smith, R., O'Dwyer, S., Jacobs, D., Ziegler, T., & Wang, X. (1988). The gut: A central organ after surgical stress. *Surgery, 104,* 917–923.

Winterbauer, R., Durning, R., Barron, E., & McFadden, M. (1981). Aspirated nasogastric feeding solution detected by glucose strips. *Annals of Internal Medicine, 95,* 67–68.

Winthrop, A., Wesson, D., Penharz, P., Jacobs, D., Heim, T., & Filler, R. (1987). Injury severity, whole body protein turnover and energy expenditure in pediatric trauma. *Journal of Pediatrics, 22,* 534–537.

Wolfe, B., Ryder, M., Nishikawa, R., Halsted, C., & Schmidt, B. (1986). Complications of parenteral nutrition. *The American Journal of Surgery, 152,* 93–99.

Woodson, R., & Hamilton, C. (1988). Heart rate estimates of motor activity in preterm infants. *Infant Behavior and Development, 9,* 283–290.

Wroblewski, B., & Young, L. (1991). Topics in parenteral nutrition for the 1990's. *Focus on Critical Care, 118*(4), 276–285.

Zaloga, G. (1991). Bedside method of placing small bowel feeding tube in critically ill patients. A prospective study. *Chest, 100,* 1643–1646.

Zarling, E., Parmar, J., Mobarhan, S., & Clapper, M. (1986). Effect of enteral formula infusion rate, osmolality and chemical composition upon clinical tolerance and carbohydrate absorption in normal subjects. *Journal of Parenteral and Enteral Nutrition, 10,* 588–590.

Zeigler, T., Benfell, K., Smith, R., Young, L., Brown, E., Ferrari-Baliviera, E., Lowe, D., & Wilmore, D. (1990). Safety and metabolic effects of L-glutamine administration in humans. *Journal of Parenteral and Enteral Nutrition, 14,* 137S–146S.

Zlotkin, S., Stallings, V., & Pencharz, P. (1985). Total parenteral nutrition in children. *Pediatric Clinics of North America, 32,* 381–400.

CHAPTER 15

Thermal Regulation

ARTHUR J. ENGLER
CINDY HYLTON RUSHTON

**ESSENTIAL PHYSIOLOGY OF
   TEMPERATURE REGULATION**
Physiologic Control of Body Temperature
Behavioral Control of Body Temperature
Mechanisms of Thermoregulation
**NURSING INTERVENTIONS TO MAINTAIN
   NORMOTHERMIA**
Assessment and Maintenance of Normal Body
   Temperature
Assessment of Temperature Imbalance
Thermoregulation Devices

**ABNORMALITIES OF BODY TEMPERATURE
   REGULATION**
Hyperthermia
Drug Fever
Malignant Hyperthermia
Nursing Care of Patients With Elevated Body
   Temperature
Hypothermia
Nursing Care of Patients With Decreased Body
   Temperature
SUMMARY

Heat is a natural byproduct of metabolism. It is constantly produced and continuously lost to the environment. When the quantity of heat produced is equal to the amount lost, homeostasis exists. If heat production and heat loss are not in balance, body temperature will rise or fall.

Normal thermoregulatory function serves to maintain body temperature within a narrow range. Both environmental and maturational factors can cause or contribute to *ineffective thermoregulation:* the inability to maintain normal body temperature in the presence of changing environmental factors (Carpenito, 1989). Critically ill infants and children are at high risk for ineffective thermoregulation resulting from both environmental and maturational factors (Table 15–1). Critical care nurses play an essential role in protecting patients from adverse environmental factors and in identifying patients at risk from maturational factors that may impair effective thermoregulation.

Many patients in the pediatric intensive care unit (PICU) experience *altered body temperature:* the inability to maintain normal body temperature because of internal factors (Carpenito, 1989). Abnormal body temperature may be the result of illness (such as infection, surgery, or shock) or its therapy.

Internal factors that contribute to, or are risk fac-

tors for, altered body temperature include pathophysiologic and treatment-related factors. For example, traumatic brain injury or congenital central nervous system (CNS) malformations may produce recurrent, transient elevations in body temperature. In contrast, certain hypothalamic lesions produced by cerebrovascular hemorrhage, neurosurgical procedures, or tumors may result in low body temperature resulting from decreased ability to produce heat. Furthermore, a depressed or injured CNS results in a diminished response to cold and minimizes shivering as a means of generating heat.

Table 15–1. FACTORS RELATED TO INEFFECTIVE
THERMOREGULATION

Environmental	Maturational
Changing environmental temperature	Extremes of age
Insufficient heating or humidification	Large ratio of body surface area to body mass
Physical contact with or proximity to cold or warm objects	Metabolic immaturity and decreased heat production
Wet or exposed body surfaces	Rapid metabolic rate
Excessive or insufficient clothing or coverings	Thin layer of subcutaneous fat

Shock states limit peripheral perfusion in response to hypotension and endogenous catecholamine-mediated subcutaneous vasoconstriction. These responses reduce peripheral blood flow, thereby diminishing heat dissipation and resulting in increased core temperature.

Treatment-related factors leading to alterations in body temperature include medications (e.g., vasopressors or sedatives), parenteral fluids or blood transfusions, renal dialysis, anesthesia, and surgery. For instance, anesthesia inhibits most of the body's heat-producing and heat-conserving mechanisms. When infants or children are unconscious or paralyzed (either pharmacologically or nonpharmacologically), postural changes are no longer possible because muscular activity is obliterated. Anesthetic agents may also depress the hypothalamic thermoregulatory center, causing vasodilatation and depression of the metabolic rate, thereby reducing heat production and increasing heat loss (Bissonnette & Sessler, 1992; Gauntlett et al., 1985). Induced hypothermia for extracorporeal circulation, exposure to cold ambient temperature, and exposure of the thoracic cavity during open heart surgery are specific treatment-related risk factors for infants and children. The consequences of intraoperative hypothermia are often not manifested until the postoperative phase. Small incremental drops in temperature markedly increase oxygen consumption at a time when oxygen supply to tissues is marginal, resulting in hypoxemia (Gauntlett et al., 1985).

Pediatric critical care nurses are in a position to appreciate a variety of environmental, situational, and individual factors that can result in either altered body temperature or ineffective thermal regulation in patients in the PICU. Care of infants and children based on an understanding of the dynamic interface between the patient and the environment can maximize the ability of nurses to assist patients to maintain a normal body temperature despite the stress of illness.

ESSENTIAL PHYSIOLOGY OF TEMPERATURE REGULATION

Physiologic Control of Body Temperature

Heat production and heat loss are controlled in two states. First, the transfer of heat to the body skin surface from the central core establishes an internal thermal gradient. Second, heat is dissipated from the skin surface to the surrounding environment. This balance is critical to normal thermoregulatory function and is summarized in Figure 15–1.

Body temperature regulation is controlled almost exclusively by intricate nervous system feedback mechanisms located in the hypothalamus. Heat-sensitive neurons located in the preoptic area of the hypothalamus are the body's most influential temperature receptors. These receptors respond to rising temperature by increasing their impulse output and to falling temperature by decreasing their output.

Additional temperature receptors are found in the skin. These consist of both warmth and cold receptors. There are four to 10 times as many cold as warmth receptors. These receptors convey nerve impulses to the hypothalamus where the information is used to regulate body temperature. Receptors in the spinal cord itself, the abdomen, and other internal body structures also transmit signals, primarily cold signals, to the CNS to help in temperature control. Peripheral thermoreceptors dispatch signals to the posterior hypothalamus where they are integrated to control heat loss and heat production (Guyton, 1987). This "hypothalamic thermostat" is the primary temperature control mechanism in the body.

The Body's Response to Heat

Overheating of the hypothalamic thermostatic area increases the pace of heat loss by two essential processes. The first prompts the sweat glands to

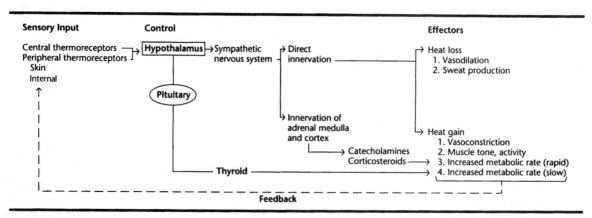

Figure 15–1 ● ● ● ● ● ●

Thermoregulation. (Reprinted by permission of Neonatal Network, Vol. 13, Number 2, 1994, p. 15, Fig. 1.)

boost evaporative heat loss from the body. The second inhibits sympathetic centers in the posterior hypothalamus. This allows vasodilatation and, consequently, increased heat loss from the skin (Guyton, 1987).

The Body's Response to Cold

When the body cools down to a normal temperature (37°C), several mechanisms reduce heat loss and escalate heat production. Vasoconstriction of the epidermal vessels is one of the body's earliest efforts to enhance heat conservation. The posterior hypothalamus mobilizes the sympathetic nervous system and initiates powerful vasoconstriction throughout the body. This decreases conduction of heat from the internal core to the skin. When vasoconstriction develops, the only heat loss that persists is that via the fat insulators of the skin. Vasoconstriction can diminish heat loss eight-fold and can very forcefully conserve heat. When the temperature of the hypothalamic thermostat falls below normal body temperature, the elimination of sweating is absolute. This arrests evaporative cooling except for insensible evaporation (e.g., from the respiratory tract) (Guyton, 1987).

The body also increases heat production in the event of cold stress. This occurs in three distinct ways when body temperature drops below 37°C. First, hypothalamic stimulation of shivering occurs. The primary motor center for shivering is located in the posterior hypothalamus. Cold stress stimulates and heat inhibits this nerve center. When muscle tone is increased to a critical level in response to cold stress, shivering begins. As a result, heat production can increase four to five times the normal amount.

Second, chemical thermogenesis commences. The rate of cellular metabolism increases as a result of sympathetic stimulation or circulating epinephrine. In the adult, this generally accounts for an increase in heat production of no more than 10% to 15%. In infants, however, chemical thermogenesis can increase the rate of heat production as much as 100% and is a crucial mechanism (Guyton, 1987).

Thermogenesis in infants is different than in older children or adults. In infants, brown fat is the biochemical substance used in chemical thermogenesis. Brown fat cells are approximately one half the size of white fat cells. Brown fat is found in the subcutaneous tissue, adjacent to the major blood vessels of the neck, abdomen, and thorax, between the scapulae, and in large quantities in the suprarenal areas. At birth 1% to 6% of the infant's body weight consists of brown fat (Elder, 1989). Brown fat cells contain finely scattered lipid droplets and are cytoplasm-rich in mitochondria, which facilitates energy transformation and heat production.

Cold stress produces a release of norepinephrine and thyroid hormones. This response in turn triggers a lipolytic process in the brown fat stores. Triglycerides in the fat are broken down into fatty acids and glycerol. These fatty acids then enter the thermogenic pathways that produce the common pool of metabolic acids. Besides thermogenesis, glycolysis may be stimulated, resulting in a transient increase in serum glucose levels. Because infants are unable to shiver or actively alter their environment, they depend on nonshivering (chemical) thermogenesis, that is, use of brown fat, to increase heat production (Perlstein, 1992).

If cold stress is sustained, increased thyroxine production results in an elevated rate of cellular metabolism throughout the body. This mechanism requires several weeks to become operative, and thus it cannot be considered a primary response to cold stress (Guyton, 1987). (See Fig. 15–2 for a summary of physiologic consequences of cold stress.)

Behavioral Control of Body Temperature

One of the most useful mechanisms governing body temperature in older children involves the perception of heat or cold and the child's response to that perception (Prosser & Nelson, 1981). When the temperature of the preoptic area of the hypothalamus rises, this produces the sense of being warm; cooling of the skin and possibly other receptors produces the awareness of being cold. Older children and adolescents who experience either of these sensations usually take steps to reestablish a feeling of comfort.

Effective behavioral control of temperature depends on both an intact sensory-motor system and

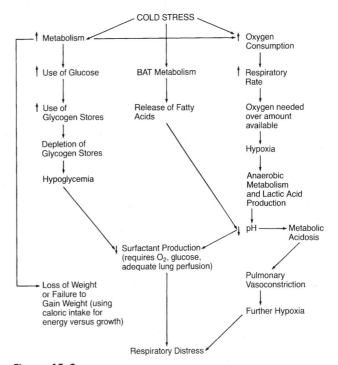

Figure 15–2 ● ● ● ● ● ●
Physiologic consequences of cold stress in infants. BAT, brown adipose tissue. (From Blackburn S.T., & Loper D.L. (1992). *Maternal, fetal, and neonatal physiology* (p. 692). Philadelphia: W.B. Saunders.)

an ability to communicate perceptions. For example, regulation of body temperature is inadequate below the level at which the sympathetic nerves leave the cord in spinal cord transection. This occurs because the hypothalamus can no longer control skin blood flow or the degree to which sweating is possible. To maintain thermal homeostasis, the affected person needs to rely on responses to cold and hot sensations in the region of the head to make suitable behavioral and environmental adaptations (Guyton, 1987).

Critically ill infants and children have a limited ability to alter their environment in response to their perception of temperature variations. Moreover, their ability to communicate their perceptions is often limited by their developmental stage and the severity of their illness.

Mechanisms of Thermoregulation

Thermoregulation allows conservation of body temperature within a very fine range. The range of normal body temperature measured orally is 37.5 ± 2°C, with the rectal temperature being 1°C higher (Casella et al., 1987) (Table 15–2). The core body temperature varies 1.1°C during the day, with the highest temperature occurring in late afternoon or evening and the lowest occurring around 4 AM. Presumably, this holds true in critically ill infants and children. Once thought to be the result of exogenous factors such as muscular exercise or feeding activity, it is now clear that these periodic fluctuations in temperature are the result of the operation of an endogenous system (Matusik, 1985). Despite the influence of certain conditions that alter the regulation of body temperature, among them fever, the human organism is capable of immense thermoregulatory adaptations and changes.

Circadian cycles influence childhood temperature. Temperature variation is one of the earliest rhythms to develop in infants and begins to appear after the first week of life. These rhythm changes develop progressively until age 5 years, when the adult pattern is present (Matusik, 1985).

The stability of body temperature varies inversely with the size of the body. This means that in infants with a rapid metabolic rate and somewhat large body surface area, the oral and rectal temperature may

Table 15–2. COMPARABLE CLINICAL TEMPERATURES IN A RESTING AFEBRILE SUBJECT WITH RECTAL TEMPERATURE AS A REFERENCE

Rectal approximately 37°C
Oral 0.3–0.5°C lower than rectal
Esophageal 0.2°C lower than rectal
Pulmonary artery 0.2–0.3°C lower than rectal
Tympanic membrane 0.05–0.25°C lower than rectal
Bladder temperature 0.1–0.2°C lower than rectal
Axillary temperature 0.6–0.8°C lower than rectal

From *AACN Clinical Issues,* 4 (1), 49, 1993.

vary through a range perhaps twice that of adults (Livingston, 1985). Because of the infant's small size, increased ratio of body surface area to mass, and elevated thermal conduction rate, the thermoregulatory ability of infants is restricted and easily overwhelmed by the environment (Davis, 1990). Conversely, adults exhibit very stable body temperature mechanisms.

Heat Loss

The amount of heat loss that occurs varies according to atmospheric conditions, such as the speed of air currents passing over the body and the relative humidity of the air. The common modes of heat loss are via (1) radiation, conduction, and convection from the skin; (2) evaporation of sweat and insensible perspiration; (3) warming and humidifying of inspired air; and (4) urine and stool. Only the first two are under direct physiologic control. Of the sources under direct control, radiation accounts for approximately 50% of the total heat loss and convection about 15%. Most of the remainder (about 30%) occurs through evaporation of water (Livingston, 1985).

Radiation is the loss of heat that radiates from the body to surroundings that are cooler than the body itself. It involves the transfer of heat between two objects, independent of the environmental temperature. The difference in temperature between the body and objects in the environment directly affects the rate at which a body cools via radiation (Livingston, 1985). For example, radiative heat losses can occur even when nude infants are in warm but transparent, single-walled incubators, particularly when near a cold wall or window. The total radiating surface of infants or children also influences heat loss. In fact, radiative heat loss is proportionally greater in smaller infants and children and represents the most serious source of heat loss for this group (Davis, 1990).

Conductive heat loss involves the transfer of heat between two surfaces that are in direct contact with each other. The intensity of conductive heat loss depends on the temperature gradient between the body and the surface with which it is in contact, the total body surface area, and the conductivity of the material contacting the body. In addition, physiologic factors influencing conductive heat loss are the velocity of cutaneous blood flow and the thickness of the body's subcutaneous insulating tissue (Davis, 1990).

Convection is simply the movement of air. Heat loss by convection refers to heat conducted to the air and then carried away by convection currents. Insignificant amounts of convection always occur because heated air naturally rises away from the body. The degree of convective heat loss depends on several conditions, including the temperature of the air, volume of airflow, and the specific heat of the flowing air. Exposure of infants or children to drafts or increased airflow causes convective heat loss and is a stimulus for increased oxygen consumption.

Evaporative losses, primarily through the skin and

lungs, account for a significant portion of heat loss. Infants are particularly vulnerable because their skin is thinner than that of older children, which increases evaporative losses. When water evaporates from the skin, 0.58 calories of heat are lost for every gram of water that evaporates. Under normal conditions, nearly 20% of the total body heat loss occurs from evaporation. Little can be done about this in terms of body temperature regulation because evaporative heat loss results from continuous diffusion of water molecules at any body temperature. However, excessive evaporative loss can be controlled by regulation of sweating, primarily by environmental manipulation.

Besides transepidermal evaporation, the respiratory system also serves as a route of evaporative heat loss. Evaporative losses via the respiratory tract are higher in infants as a result of their higher minute ventilation (the product of respiratory rate and tidal volume) in relation to body weight. Adequate environmental humidity minimizes evaporative losses from the lungs and skin surfaces. Physical factors affecting the rate of evaporation include relative humidity, velocity of airflow, and minute ventilation. Physiologic factors include the infants' ability to sweat and their rate of minute ventilation (Davis, 1990).

The neutral thermal zone of infants is the range of ambient temperatures at which the metabolic rate is minimal and temperature regulation is achieved by nonevaporative physical processes (Davis, 1990). The neutral thermal environment (NTE) is further described as the ambient temperature and humidity in which the control of body temperature is achieved by vasomotor adjustments, with minimal oxygen consumption and heat production. This narrow range of temperatures in infants varies with gestational age, postnatal age, weight, and clothing. With increasing age and weight, the NTE widens and lower environmental temperatures are tolerated (Gauntlett et al., 1985).

Sweating

Sweating is an important means of controlling heat balance. Full-term infants, for example, begin to sweat with rectal temperatures of 37.5 to 37.9°C and an ambient temperature higher than 35°C. As body temperature rises, the anterior part of the hypothalamus is stimulated. The impulses from this area are transmitted through the anatomic pathways to the spinal cord and through the sympathetic outflow to the sweat glands in the skin everywhere in the body (Guyton, 1987). When the body temperature increases as little as 1°C, the sweat glands secrete large amounts of sweat to the skin surface (Quinton, 1983). This produces rapid evaporative cooling of the body. The rate of sweating varies according to environmental factors.

Excessive sweating can deplete extracellular fluid levels of electrolytes, particularly sodium and chloride. Cholinergic sympathetic nerve fibers ending on or near the glandular sweat cells elicit the secretions, which contain large amounts of sodium chloride. Similar to its effect on the renal tubules, aldosterone works in the sweat glands by augmenting the rate of active reabsorption of sodium by the ducts. This process also carries chloride with it because of the electrical gradient that develops across the epithelium with the reabsorption of sodium. Aldosterone can minimize the loss of sodium chloride in sweat when the plasma concentration is already low. Becoming acclimatized to the heat can diminish this loss because of increased aldosterone production resulting from decreased salt reserves in the body (Guyton, 1987).

NURSING INTERVENTIONS TO MAINTAIN NORMOTHERMIA

Nurses can help to maintain the body temperature of critically ill infants and children within normal limits primarily by managing external factors. The environment may be manipulated based on the principles of conduction, convection, radiation, evaporation, and the impact of each on body temperature (Table 15–3). Factors such as ambient air temperature, humidity, airflow velocity, and the temperature of objects in direct contact with children's skin are all considered part of the environment. Each of these factors should be considered when making alterations to support an NTE.

Evaporative losses can be minimized by keeping infants and children (especially their heads), clothing, and bed linens dry. Evaporative and conductive losses from respiratory mucosa can be minimized by humidifying and warming inspired gases. In contrast, gases may be humidified and cooled when infants or children are hyperthermic. High humidity tends to reduce insensible water losses and evaporative losses; however, it also encourages the growth of gram-negative bacilli on the skin, including *Escherichia coli* and *Pseudomonas aeruginosa*. Hence, a relative level of humidity, approximately 50%, provides optimal conditions for infants (Frigoletto & Little, 1988).

Conductive heat losses can be reduced by assuring that cold surfaces are not in direct contact with children's skin and by using various types of thermal insulation such as blankets and head coverings. Nurses can position children to avoid drafts and maintain the environmental temperature within the neutral thermal zone to avoid convective losses. Radiant heat loss can be minimized by increasing the room temperature, using external heating devices, and applying thermal insulators such as plastic or aluminized plastic sheeting.

Assessment and Maintenance of Normal Body Temperature

The medical and surgical treatment of critically ill or injured infants and children often aggravates heat

Table 15–3. PREVENTION OF HEAT LOSS AND OVERHEATING IN THE NEONATE

Mechanisms	Sources of Heat Loss/Overheating	Interventions
Conduction	Cool mattress, blanket, scale, table, x-ray plate, or clothing	Place warm blankets on scales, x-ray plates, other surfaces in contact with the infant
		Warm blankets and clothing before use
		Preheat incubators, radiant warmers, heat shields
	Heating pads, hot water bottles, chemical bags	Avoid placing infant on any surface or object that is warmer than the infant
Convection	Cool room, corridors, or outside air	Maintain room temperature at levels adequate to provide a safe thermal environment for infants (72 to 76°F)
		Transport infants in enclosed, warmed incubators through internal hallways and between external environments (e.g., ambulance to nursery)
		Open incubator portholes only when necessary and for brief periods
		Use plastic sleeves on portholes
		Swaddle with warm blankets (unless under radiant warmer) or stretch transparent plastic across infant between radiant warmer side guards; use caps with adequate insulation quality or hooded blankets
	Convective air flow incubator	Monitor incubator temperature to avoid temperatures warmer than infant's body temperature
	Drafts from air vents, windows, doors, heaters, fans, air conditioners	Place infants away from air vents, drafts, and other sources of moving air particles
		Use side guards on radiant warmers to decrease cross current air flow across infant; stretch transparent plastic across infant between radiant warmer side guards
	Cold oxygen flow (especially near facial thermal receptors)	Warm oxygen and monitor temperature inside oxygen hood
Evaporation	Wet body surface and hair in delivery room or with bathing	Dry infant, especially head, immediately after birth with a warm blanket or towel
		Use caps with adequate insulation quality or hooded blankets
		Replace wet blankets with dry, warm ones and place in warm environment
		Delay initial bath until temperature has stabilized then give sponge bath
		Bathe in warm, draft-free environment and place on warmed towels and dry immediately; bathe under a radiant warmer
	Application of lotions, solutions, wet packs, or soaks to infant	Prewarm solutions and soaks; maintain warmth during use
		Avoid overheating solutions and soaks
	Water loss from lungs	Warm and humidify oxygen
	Increased insensible water loss in VLBW or ill infants	Increased incubator humidity levels may be necessary, especially in dry climates or with VLBW infants
Radiation	Placement near cold or hot external windows or walls, placement in direct sunlight	Place incubators, cribs, and radiant warmers away from external walls and windows, direct sunlight
		Use thermal shades on external windows
		Line incubator with aluminum foil
	Cold incubator walls	Use double-walled incubators or heat shields or cover with plastic film
		Prewarm incubators, radiant warmers, heat shields
	Heat lamps	Avoid use whenever possible; if used, monitor temperature every 10 to 15 minutes to avoid burns

From Blackburn S.T., Loper D.L. (Eds.) (1992). *Maternal, fetal, and neonatal physiology: A clinical perspective* (p. 681). Philadelphia: W.B. Saunders. VLBW, very low birth weight.

loss through skin and body cavity exposure, administration of cold intravenous fluids and blood products, and anesthetic administration. Hypothermia may contribute to inaccuracies in patient assessment and may complicate resuscitation of injured infants or children. Because the risk for alterations in body temperature are greater for critically ill infants and children, assessment of temperature and the body's thermoregulatory capabilities must be accurate and ongoing.

Frequent monitoring of critically ill infants' or children's body temperature is needed to establish baseline parameters and guide nursing interventions. Temperature should be measured at recommended intervals for age and condition. Various techniques are used to measure core, regional, and skin temperatures in critically ill infants and children. Each is evaluated based on their relative advantages and disadvantages. The method selected is based on individual patient needs and the net balance of advantages and disadvantages of the system accurately monitoring body temperature. The site selected for estimating infants' or children's temperature should be recorded and used consistently in serial measurements. Moreover, because of the inaccuracy of many thermometers in clinical use, the same thermometer should be used consistently for an individual patient.

Central Temperature Monitoring

The core or central temperature is the temperature sensed by the temperature-regulating center of the hypothalamus. This temperature reflects the temperature of the blood flowing through the branches of the carotid arteries to the hypothalamus. Pulmonary artery catheters and esophageal, tympanic, or nasopharyngeal temperature probes monitor the temperature of blood, which approximates the temperature of the carotid artery and may be used for continuous assessment of central or core temperature (Vacanti & Ryan, 1986). Although useful, esophageal and nasopharyngeal temperature probes are not routinely used in PICU settings. Urinary bladder temperature (UBT), using a urinary catheter with an indwelling temperature-sensing element, may also be measured. In fact, several researchers have found that the UBT is the most accurate measure of core temperature in adults (Ramsay et al., 1985; Moorthy et al., 1985).

Core temperature may also be measured by central venous catheters. A pulmonary artery catheter with a distal tip thermistor accurately reflects pulmonary blood temperature. Because of its invasive nature, it is only used for critically ill infants and children who also require advanced hemodynamic monitoring. Hypotension and endogenous catecholamine-mediated subcutaneous vasoconstriction reduce skin blood flow, thereby diminishing heat dissipation. Moreover, shock states increase cardiac and respiratory muscle contraction, thereby increasing heat production and core temperature and creating a disparity between regional temperature readings and actual core temperature. In such cases, it may be prudent to use core temperature measurements to detect such disparities before deleterious effects occur (Buck & Zaritsky, 1989).

Peripheral Temperature Monitoring

Noncentral temperature measurement does not reflect core temperature but rather regional temperature. Regional temperature is affected by a variety of factors that may affect regional blood flow such as intravascular volume, vascular tone, or environmental conditions. These methods are convenient and useful in monitoring changes and trends in temperature but lack the accuracy of most core temperature techniques. In contrast to core temperature reading techniques, regional temperature monitoring can detect physiologic decompensation in response to persistent hypothermia or hyperthermia. When hypothermia persists, for example, children's increased metabolism fails to compensate for the body cooling and results in regional blood flow shifts causing metabolic acidosis and eventually apnea (Vacanti & Ryan, 1986).

Generally, regional temperatures are measured us-

ing electronic thermometers. Temperature measuring sites include the oral, rectal, and axillary locations. In the critical care setting, the oral route is infrequently used, whereas rectal or axillary routes predominate. Measuring rectal temperature is generally unnecessary. The risk of rectal perforation and the repeated invasiveness of the procedure are probably not warranted, particularly in young infants (Whaley & Wong, 1991). Rectal temperature probes can be influenced by the presence of stool in the rectum, which can act as an insulator and produce markedly delayed responses to core temperature changes (Davis, 1990). In addition, relying solely on rectal temperature measurements that may not reflect rapid changes in core temperature may lead to delayed recognition of temperature extremes. Rectal probes and temperatures are always avoided in infants and children with inflammatory bowel disease, absolute neutropenia, or evidence of coagulation disorders or thrombocytopenia. Axillary temperature has been shown to reflect rectal temperature, when measured properly, and is less hazardous (Frigoletto & Little, 1988). When temperature is measured, the relationship to environmental temperature should be determined.

Skin temperature may be measured either by electronic thermometers or by electronic skin temperature thermistor probes that provide continuous assessment of temperature. They are a useful adjunct to other standard temperature-measuring devices but can be affected by poor perfusion, equipment dysfunction, or improper application. Critically ill patients who require the use of overbed warmers or warming blankets are continuously monitored for skin temperature with appropriate alarms for under- or overheating. When skin temperature is continuously monitored, temperature is also measured periodically with an electronic thermometer.

For critically ill infants or children, a combination of temperature measuring techniques is often indicated. This is necessary to detect variations in temperature that occur in response to physiologic dysfunction associated with critical illness or injury. Because there may be significant differences between peripheral and core temperatures, critical care nurses must become skilled in interpreting the implications of these differences in light of the patient's physiologic status. They must institute the proper interventions to avoid untoward effects.

Assessment of Temperature Imbalance

Wide variations in temperature produce alterations in cardiac output, oxygen consumption, and insensible water losses. With hyperthermia, heart rate increases, whereas with hypothermia, heart rate commonly decreases. Blood pressure can also be affected. For instance, blood pressure and cardiac output drop precipitously as hypothermia becomes more severe. Cardiac dysrhythmias, such as conduction delays and abnormal atrial and ventricular rhythms, may be evident. Respiratory rates may also vary. Hypothermic infants, for example, may experience periods of apnea or shallow breathing. In contrast, infants or children with fever or hyperthermia may become tachypneic.

Neurologic function may be impaired when infants or children experience temperature imbalance. For example, severe hypothermia (a core temperature lower than 35°C) may complicate neurologic assessment as pupils dilate, level of consciousness declines, reflexes and respirations diminish, and varying degrees of amnesia occur. Cerebral blood flow has been estimated to decrease 6% to 7% for every 1°C decrease in body temperature (Reuler, 1978). This is of particular concern for infants or children who have experienced multiple trauma or multisystem organ failure. All patients with hypothermia are monitored for changes in level of consciousness, signs of irritability or lethargy, diminished ability to arouse, and changes in muscle tone. Hence, measures to promote thermal neutrality are instituted as early as possible to ensure accurate neurologic assessment. Seizures may occur following periods of hypothermia as a result of ischemic brain injury and cerebral edema and are routinely assessed.

Oxygen consumption and tissue perfusion are important assessment parameters. Oxygen saturation using arterial or mixed venous blood can provide an important indicator of oxygen consumption. Often oxygen saturation of mixed venous blood indicates changes in physiologic status before changes in heart rate, pulmonary capillary wedge pressure (PCWP), or blood pressure are evident (Earp, 1989). Supplemental oxygen may be necessary to combat hypoxemia, particularly in hypothermic infants and children.

Tissue perfusion, assessed from skin color, temperature, and capillary refill, needs to be routinely monitored. Pale, cool skin is an early manifestation of the vasoconstrictive response to cold stress or a decrease in core temperature. With hyperthermia, the skin may appear flushed as vasodilatation occurs. Flushing may also occur because oxygen is not liberated from hemoglobin as readily when either low temperatures or overheating occurs (Merenstein et al., 1985). Evidence of sweating should be monitored in hyperthermic children.

Increased muscle activity is associated with heat production, whereas diminished muscle activity is often indicative of reduced heat production. Infants and children who are experiencing either elevated or reduced temperature may manifest changes in motor activity and therefore are monitored for such changes and the findings documented.

Routine assessment for the presence of shivering permits early detection and intervention. Shivering develops in a predictable fashion. It begins with masseter contractions and then proceeds to contractions of the trunk and long muscle groups. It culminates with generalized body-shaking and teeth-chattering (Holtzclaw, 1985). Assessment for the presence of shivering includes palpation of the mandible for vibration and close inspection of facial, neck, and chest muscles for fasciculation. Central and peripheral temperatures are routinely assessed and compared. Assessment for shivering is continued until central and peripheral temperatures are normal (Earp, 1989).

Fluid balance and renal function must be carefully monitored when body temperature becomes deranged. Because the rate of fluid loss increases as a result of hyperthermia, adequate hydration must be maintained. Adequate hydration prevents the complications of dehydration and promotes heat dissipation. When infants and children are hypothermic and peripherally vasoconstricted, fluids are carefully regulated during rewarming. When patients have vasoconstriction, fluid requirements are diminished; as warming occurs the intravascular space expands, thereby increasing fluid requirements to maintain cardiac output. Infants' and children's ability to concentrate urine is impaired as hypothermia worsens. Acute tubular necrosis may occur as a result of diminished cardiac output and renal perfusion and myoglobinuria. Measurement of fluid balance enables nurses to prevent fluid overload or deficit. Fluid deficit following a period of hypothermia is often the result of increased insensible water loss during rewarming.

Laboratory data are routinely monitored to detect metabolic, biochemical, and hematologic derangements frequently associated with thermal instability. For example, excessive sweating can deplete extracellular fluid levels of electrolytes, particularly sodium and chloride. Serum electrolytes, blood urea nitrogen, creatinine, measures of acid-base balance, serum and urine osmolarity, hemoglobin, hematocrit, platelets, and other specific biochemical determinations are assessed regularly.

Hypothermia may cause metabolic acidosis. Acidosis coupled with hypothermia results in a left shift in the oxyhemoglobin dissociation curve, thereby impairing oxygen release at the tissue level. Arterial blood gases are monitored closely and measures instituted to prevent episodes of hypoxemia and acidosis. Hyperthermia can cause biochemical changes, depending on the underlying cause.

Hypoglycemia is another common finding in infants who experience alterations in temperature. It results from depletion of glycogen stores in the attempt to maintain core temperature in the normal range. In contrast, a transient hyperglycemic response is a common finding in older infants and children with alterations in temperature. This occurs as part of the body's response to stress, which liberates glucose to fuel the response.

Laboratory studies used in the determining the source of fever or hyperthermia may include indirect and direct studies. Indirect studies, such as the white blood count and the erythrocyte sedimentation rate, reflect the body's response to infection. Indirect tests may serve as screening devices for identifying subgroups of infants and children at high risk of occult bacteremia (Table 15–4). Direct studies include blood and urine culture and sensitivity, and rapid tests for detection of bacterial antigen (e.g., the Wellcogen). Direct tests allow detection of the specific causative organism (Kline & Lorin, 1990).

Other diagnostic tests may include cerebrospinal fluid examination or urinalysis. In addition, examinations such as radiographs; ultrasounds and computerized tomographic (CT) scans; magnetic resonance imaging (MRI); or other nuclear medicine studies of the lungs, abdomen, and other organs, may be indicated to determine the underlying cause of the temperature derangement.

Thermoregulation Devices

Maintaining an NTE and a normothermic body temperature are common nursing goals when caring for critically ill infants and children. Various thermoregulation devices are regularly used in the critical care setting. This area is particularly crucial when transferring infants or children to other units within the hospital or another facility (Table 15–5).

Warming Devices

In addition to manipulating environmental conditions to alter the ambient temperature, specialized equipment is often necessary to maintain an NTE. Various types of devices are used for this purpose. For infants, some type of closed warming device is commonly used, such as single- or double-walled incubators. These convection-warmed devices are used for thermal regulation of the infant's ambient air. Standard closed incubators control infant temperature by recirculation of warmed and humidified air. The temperature of the air in the incubator is determined by infant size, gestational age, and postnatal age (Frigoletto & Little, 1988). Plastic blankets or heat shields inside the incubator also reduce convective and evaporative losses. Disadvantages of this type of device include heat losses when the incubator is entered, potential variations in both incubator and

Table 15–4. RISK OF OCCULT BACTEREMIA

	Low Risk	High Risk
Age	>3 yr	<2 yr
Temperature	<39.4°C	>40°C
WBC (per mm²)	>5000	<15,000
Observational variables	Normal	Abnormal
		History of contact with *Haemophilus influenzae* or *Neisseria meningitidis*
		History of bacteremia
		Immunologic impairment

From Kline M.W., & Lorin M.I. (1990). Fever without localizing signs. In F.A. Oski, C.D. DeAngelis, R.D. Feigin, & J.B. Warshaw (Eds.). *Principles and practice of pediatrics* (p. 1023). Philadelphia: J.B. Lippincott.

Table 15–5. PREVENTION OF THERMAL INSTABILITY DURING INTRA- AND INTERHOSPITAL TRANSFERS

Factor	Intervention
Ambient temperature	Maintain within age-appropriate thermoneutral zone. Operating rooms might need to be as warm as 26°C for preterm infants and small children (Bissonnette & Sessler, 1992)
Warming/ cooling devices	Many passive and active skin-surface devices are available, including heating lamps, circulating warm or cool water blankets, infrared radiant heaters, and convection heaters (Meyer-Pahoulis et al., 1993)
	Passive insulators, such as plastic wrap and insulated blankets, are useful in controlling heat loss, especially when outside
Airway humidification	Heat and humidity can be actively regulated in inspired gases to promote normothermia
Adequate oxygenation	Monitor oxygen requirements via pulse oximetry and provide supplemental oxygen as needed (Meyer-Pahoulis et al.)
Parenteral fluid temperature	Fluid warmers may be effectively used for hypothermic patients, especially when the device is close to the intravenous insertion site

infant temperatures during heating cycles, and diminished accessibility of infants for assessment and treatment (Morriss et al., 1984).

Open radiant warmers are useful to regulate temperature, particularly when infants require frequent monitoring and medical and nursing interventions. A radiant warmer consists of an electrically heated element that emits radiation within the infrared region of the electromagnetic spectrum. Radiation within this range allows optimal absorption of the energy by the skin. Heating of the skin causes vasodilatation and increased blood flow to the skin. Moreover, it provides an avenue for heat transfer from the skin surface to the blood and eventually to deeper structures.

The advantages of radiant warmers include a superior servo-control mechanism, greater consistency in surface temperature, improved patient access, and easier cleaning. The disadvantages associated with infrared radiation used in radiant warmers include risk of cataracts, flash burns of the skin, and heat stress (Morriss et al., 1984). In addition, radiant warmers promote insensible water loss, increase oxygen consumption, and slightly increase metabolic rate, depending on infant weight and gestational age. Fluid requirements may be increased by 10% to 20%, particularly when radiant warmers are used in conjunction with phototherapy. Hence, fluid requirements are adjusted depending on clinical and biochemical data. Radiant warmers are generally used in the servo-control mode with the abdominal temperature maintained at 36.5 to 37°C (Frigoletto & Little, 1988).

Servo-controlled devices automatically adjust heat output in response to changes in patients' skin temperature to maintain the temperature at a predetermined level. Some use an anterior abdominal wall temperature servo-control mechanism to regulate skin temperature within a thermal-neutral range (36.5–37°C) by automatic air temperature control. Core temperature is measured frequently when servo-control is used to avoid overheating if the skin sensor loosens. In addition, accurate assessment of the infant's temperature may be compromised when a servo-control device is used because the temperature is regulated to maintain it at the predetermined level.

For older children, external heat sources such as radiant warmers or heating blankets are often used. Radiant warmers are external heat sources that are portable units that can be placed above infants or children or units affixed to infant bassinets. These units warm the air above the patient's body and contribute to raising the surface temperature. These devices are available with servo-controlled or manual heating systems.

Circulating water mattresses may be used to raise a patient's temperature and reduce conductive heat losses. Warming mattresses set at 40°C covered with two layers of cotton blankets have been shown to be effective in heat conservation (Goudsouzian et al., 1973). However, these devices are useful only in infants and children weighing less than 10 kg. Above this weight the ratio of body surface area to body mass is insufficient to achieve reasonable benefit. Heating blankets should be used judiciously in infants and children, because when children are cold and peripherally vasoconstricted the ability of surface capillaries to dissipate heat is diminished, increasing the risk for burns from external heat sources. Hence, continuous monitoring of temperature and assessment of responses to interventions for rewarming are crucial to avoid tissue injury. It is recommended that the fluid temperature in the heating blanket never exceed 39°C to avoid burns (Dedrick & Cote, 1986).

When rapid rewarming is necessary, cardiopulmonary bypass may be used. This allows direct perfusion of the central circulation with warmed blood, reducing cardiac irritability and the risk of ventricular fibrillation and cardiac arrest. Alternatively, body cavities such as the chest, peritoneum, or gastrointestinal tract may be irrigated with warmed fluids.

Cooling Devices

When infants or children become hyperthermic, surface cooling techniques such as removing heat-conserving clothing or blankets or packing in ice may be used. Most commonly, external cooling blankets are applied. Whatever method is used for surface cooling, the patient's vital signs, perfusion, and skin integrity are assessed frequently. If additional temperature reduction is needed, body temperature can be reduced by core cooling. This can be achieved by lavage of gastric or peritoneal cavities and the administration of iced intravenous fluids.

Extreme variation in temperature, hypo- or hyperthermia, can result in death or serious injury, and thus alarm systems and range controls of all equipment used to regulate temperature require regular testing.

ABNORMALITIES OF BODY TEMPERATURE REGULATION

Hyperthermia

Hyperthermia is a state in which a person has a sustained elevation in body temperature (more than 37.8°C orally or 38.8°C rectally) because of internal or external factors (Carpenito, 1989). Internal factors such as fever, malignant hyperthermia, or heat-related illnesses, and external factors such as extreme environmental conditions or accidental overheating contribute to the development of hyperthermia. Diagnostic characteristics of hyperthermia are shown in Table 15–6. The most common cause of hyperthermia is fever. Although relatively uncommon, malignant hyperthermia may also necessitate a patient's admission to a critical care unit.

Fever must be distinguished from other types of elevations in body temperature. First, the "set-point" is that temperature around which body temperature is regulated by the thermostat-like mechanism in the hypothalamus. "Hyperthermia" is that situation in which body temperature exceeds the set-point. This usually results from conditions producing more heat than the body can dissipate (e.g., in heat stroke, aspirin toxicity, or hyperthyroidism). "Fever" is an elevation in the set-point such that body temperature is regulated at a higher level (Whaley & Wong, 1991). In any discussion of fever, it is important to remember that fever is a *symptom*, not a disease, and should be viewed as reflecting an underlying disorder.

Fever may result from abnormalities in the brain

Table 15–6. DIAGNOSTIC CHARACTERISTICS OF HYPERTHERMIA

Major
Oral temperature of >37.8°C or rectal temperature of >38.8°C
Minor (may or may not be present)
　Flushed skin
　Skin that is warm to the touch
　Tachycardia
　Tachypnea
　Shivering
　"Goose bumps"
　Dehydration
　Specific or generalized aches and/or pains
　Malaise
　Fatigue
　Weakness
　Loss of appetite

Data from Carpenito, L.J. (1989). *Nursing diagnosis: Application to clinical practice* (3rd ed., p. 150). Philadelphia: J.B. Lippincott.

Table 15-7. PATHOPHYSIOLOGIC BASES OF FEVER

Pathophysiology	Etiology
High set-point	Infection, collagen-vascular disease, malignancy
Excess heat production	Salicylate overdose, hyperthyroidism, excessive environmental temperature, malignant hyperthermia
Defective heat loss	Ectodermal dysplasia, heat stroke, anticholinergic drugs

From Lovejoy, Jr., F.H. (1989). *The etiology and treatment of fever: Current concepts*. Pediatric Update: New Developments in Fever Management. Fort Washington, PA: McNeil Consumer Products.

itself, the presence of toxins that affect the brain's temperature control areas, infection, dehydration, or other causes (Guyton, 1987). Generally, fever results from a pyrogen-mediated elevation in the hypothalamic set-point. The major problems resulting in fever include an increase in the hypothalamic thermoregulatory set-point, excess heat production, and defective heat loss (Lovejoy, Jr., 1989) (Table 15-7).

Instrumental in resetting the hypothalamic thermostat are pyrogens, substances that cause the set-point to be increased. These pyrogens may be proteins, breakdown products of proteins, or certain other substances (e.g., lipopolysaccharide toxins secreted by bacteria). Pyrogens may be present during disease states. When the set-point is elevated, all the body's efforts turn to decreasing heat loss and increasing heat production. Heat production is increased via increased muscle tone, activity, and metabolic rate and decreased heat loss, especially through peripheral vasoconstriction (Lorin, 1990). These changes help the body to reach its new temperature within hours (Guyton, 1987).

The pathophysiologic mechanism of fever includes the production of hormone-like mediators by macrophages and cells of the reticuloendothelial system. This results in (1) an increase in CNS production of prostaglandin E_2, which increases the hypothalamic set-point and temperature; (2) an increase in neutrophil release from the bone marrow; (3) a decrease in serum iron and zinc; (4) a change in hepatic protein production; and (5) an increased T-lymphocyte proliferation. Interleukin-1 (IL-1) is a substance common to these pathways (Littlefield, 1987). Undesirable effects of fever are listed in Table 15-8.

For normal healthy infants and children, these demands pose no particular threat. For those with underlying disease, especially that involving the heart or lungs, the increased demands are potentially harmful, or even fatal. In susceptible infants and children 6 months to 5 years old, fever can precipitate seizures. Generally, these seizures are benign but they are very upsetting to both parents and children and may result in invasive, expensive, and probably unnecessary procedures (Lorin, 1990).

Febrile conditions share several characteristics. Chills occur when the hypothalamic set-point abruptly rises to a higher-than-normal level because of tissue destruction, presence of pyrogenic substances, or dehydration. As the body attempts to attain its new temperature setting, the blood temperature is lower than the set-point temperature for several hours. Autonomic responses to increased body temperature occur, such as chills, vasoconstriction, and shivering. When the blood temperature reaches the set-point temperature, the person feels neither hot nor cold. As long as the factor producing the fever continues, the body temperature is regulated normally, but at a higher level. If the factor producing the fever is suddenly removed, the set-point abruptly decreases to its normal lower level. The body then feels "overheated" and reacts with intense sweating and hot skin resulting from a general vasodilatation caused to dissipate heat more quickly. This is known as the "crisis" or "flush" (Guyton, 1987).

Fever has several other causes. Traumatic brain injury or congenital CNS malformations can produce recurrent, transient elevations in body temperature. Other noninfectious causes of fever are (1) iatrogenic (e.g., heavy blankets, overdressing, mechanical); (2) thrombophlebitis resulting from intravenous catheterization; (3) infusions of irritating fluids; and (4) endocrine disorders. Certain hypothalamic lesions produced by cerebrovascular hemorrhage, neurosurgical procedures, or tumors may produce decreased thermoregulatory ability. Drugs that produce fever (in toxic doses) include lysergic acid diethylamide (LSD), cocaine, amphetamines, salicylates, anticholinergics, prostaglandin E_1 and tricyclic antidepressants (Littlefield, 1987).

Treatment of Fever

The decision to treat fever can be difficult. An important principle is that not all fevers *need* to be treated; body temperature does not always need to be completely normal. Recommendations for treatment include (1) high fever (40°C or above); (2) fever in infants and children at risk for febrile seizures, (3) fever in infants and children with underlying neurologic or cardiopulmonary disease; or (4) fever in any situation in which heat illness (e.g., heatstroke) is suspected. If the only reason to treat a fever is patient comfort, the recommendation is not to treat (Lorin, 1990).

Once the decision to treat a fever has been made, the choice of a specific modality is based on a number of considerations. Because fever is the result of an

Table 15-8. UNDESIRABLE EFFECTS OF FEVER

Patient discomfort
Increased metabolic rate
Elevated oxygen consumption
Increased carbon dioxide production
Increased cardiovascular and pulmonary system demands

Data from Lorin, M.I. (1990). Pathogenesis of fever and its treatment. In F.A. Oski, C.D. DeAngelis, R.D. Feigin, & J.B. Warshaw (Eds.). *Principles and practice of pediatrics* (pp. 1019-1021). Philadelphia: J.B. Lippincott.

elevated hypothalamic set-point, the most logical means of treating the fever is by restoring the setpoint to a normal level. Aspirin, acetaminophen, ibuprofen, and naproxen all work in this way. Aspirin and acetaminophen are equally effective at similar doses. Ibuprofen and naproxen are newer drugs and appear to be about as effective as aspirin and acetaminophen (Table 15–9). Questions remaining for these newer drugs regard their effectiveness at lower dosages and their longer duration of action (Lorin, 1990).

In therapeutic doses, aspirin is the most toxic of the choices. Potentially serious side effects are gastritis, gastrointestinal bleeding, diminished platelet functioning, decreased urinary sodium excretion, and lowered immune response. These effects are seen frequently with aspirin, less often with ibuprofen and naproxen, and not at all with acetaminophen. In fact, acetaminophen has no side effects at therapeutic levels. Aspirin, and possibly ibuprofen and naproxen, because of their pharmacologic similarity, has been implicated in the development of Reye's syndrome (Lorin, 1990).

Another method of fever reduction is external cooling, generally by sponging with tepid water. This may be used with or without the administration of antipyretic medications. External cooling is the treatment of choice for heat-related illnesses. Its use in fever is generally recommended only if a heat-related illness may be the partial or total cause of the elevated body temperature (Table 15–10) (Lorin, 1990).

Sponging as a method of fever reduction usually adds nothing other than discomfort when used with previously well infants or children with non–lifethreatening fever. Used with aspirin or acetaminophen, it is only slightly more effective than either drug used alone. When ice water is used, cooling is more rapid and more uncomfortable; ice water should be used only in the case of heat illness. Sponging is useful in infants or children with neurologic disorders because many have abnormal temperature con-

Table 15–9. RECOMMENDED ANTIPYRETIC DOSAGES*

Acetaminophen Ibuprofen	15 mg/kg every 4 hr
Pediaprofen	Children 6 mo to 12 yr: 5–10 mg/kg/dose every 6–8 hr, not to exceed 40 mg/kg/day
	Children older than 12 yr: 200–400 mg/kg/dose every 6–8 hr, not to exceed 40 mg/kg/day for fever
Children's Advil	Children 12 mo or older: 5–10 mg/kg/dose every 6–8 hr, not to exceed 40 mg/kg/day for fever
Naproxen	Children 2 yr or older: 10 mg/kg/day in 2 doses

*The half-life of these drugs is significantly longer in the newborn and young infant. They should be used with caution and in lower dosages.
Data from Lorin, M.I. (1990). Pathogenesis of fever and its treatment. In F.A. Oski, C.D. DeAngelis, R.D. Feigin, & J.B. Warshaw (Eds.). *Principles and practice of pediatrics* (p. 1020). Philadelphia: J.B. Lippincott; and Whaley, L.F., & Wong, D.L. (1991). *Nursing care of infants and children* (p. 1154). St. Louis: Mosby–Year Book.

Table 15–10. USE OF EXTERNAL COOLING METHODS FOR TREATING ELEVATED TEMPERATURE

Cooling Method	Indications
Tepid sponging **instead of** antipyretic drugs	Very young infants
	Severe liver disease
	History of hypersensitivity to antipyretic drugs
Tepid sponging **plus** antipyretic drugs	High fever (>40°C)
	History of febrile seizures, neurologic disorders, or brain damage
	Infection plus suspicion of overheating
	Septic shock*
Cold sponging **alone**	Heat illness

*May require cold sponging.
From Lorin, M.I. (1990). Pathogenesis of fever and its treatment. In F.A. Oski, C.D. DeAngelis, R.D. Feigin, & J.B. Warshaw (Eds.). *Principles and practice of pediatrics* (p. 1021). Philadelphia: J.B. Lippincott.

trol mechanisms and respond poorly to antipyretics. It is preferable to use sponging in infants and children with demonstrated hypersensitivity to antipyretics or in those who have liver disease. Sponging should normally be done with tepid water (approximately 30°C). Alcohol should not be used because the fumes may be absorbed through the lungs, and possibly skin, and may produce alcohol intoxication (Lorin, 1990). External cooling devices may also be effective in reducing body temperature.

Treatment of fever associated with suspected bacteremia generally includes antibiotics. Specific antibiotic recommendations are directed at the most common bacterial pathogens. In any case, the patient is followed carefully to monitor the effectiveness of the treatment regimen. When infants and children are critically ill and febrile, parenteral antibiotic therapy may be initiated in tandem with the diagnostic workup. Infants and children with underlying disorders that predispose them to serious bacterial infections, such as immunodeficiency states, sickle cell disease, and others, are generally aggressively treated with antibiotics to forestall the development of an overwhelming sepsis (Kline & Lorin, 1990). Moreover, if the source of the fever is determined to be infectious in nature, proper infection control and therapeutic measures should be initiated.

Drug Fever

Fever may be a complication of drug therapy; the drugs themselves produce this fever. Drug fever might be the result of a hypersensitivity reaction to any number of drugs, particularly antibiotics. Drug fever is considered if a clinically improved patient develops an unexplained fever after receiving drugs known to produce febrile reactions 7 to 10 days after their institution. Drugs that raise the basal metabolic rate, produce increased skeletal muscle activity, or lower cutaneous blood flow may produce an increase in body temperature that will normalize after the drug is stopped (Littlefield, 1987).

Malignant Hyperthermia

Malignant hyperthermia (MH) is a hypermetabolic crisis triggered by the administration of a certain quantity of potent volatile anesthetic agents or by the depolarizing muscle relaxant succinylcholine (SCH) or other drug (Muldoon et al., 1989). Halogenated anesthetic agents (e.g., enfluorane and halothane) are most often implicated in the development of MH.

Malignant hyperthermia is an autosomally dominant, pharmacogenetically transmitted disease of the musculoskeletal system caused by a defect in metabolism. Factors implicated in the development of an MH crisis are stress, the presence of a mild infection, muscle injury, and exercise (Fraulini, 1977; Gronert et al., 1980).

In non-MH susceptible infants and children, anesthesia causes the thermoregulatory system to lose effectiveness so that body temperature eventually reflects ambient environmental temperature (Wlody, 1989). This does not happen in MH. The incidence of MH ranges from one in 15,000 pediatric patients to one in 150,000 adult patients. The apparently higher incidence in infants and children is probably the result of the more common use of mask induction of anesthesia with halothane in this age group, often followed by intravenous or intramuscular SCH. Intravenous induction is the preferred route in adults (Harris, 1990). The population at the greatest risk for the development of MH is young males (Muldoon et al., 1989).

The site of the primary lesion implicated in the pathogenesis of MH is skeletal muscle and is related to disturbed calcium metabolism (Kozak-Reiss et al., 1988; Muldoon et al., 1989; Nelson & Flewellen, 1983). One theory is that a defect in the muscle cell membrane causes loss of control of intracellular ionized calcium levels, leading to an increase in calcium in skeletal muscle and abnormal muscle activity. This produces an increased metabolic rate resulting in increased oxygen consumption and metabolic acidosis. These conditions create a tremendous strain on the cardiopulmonary system (Wlody, 1989). As hyperthermia continues, the myoplasmic calcium concentration remains elevated, producing continued muscle contraction and heat production (Forestner, 1981).

Initially there is an anesthetic-induced increase in aerobic and anaerobic metabolism manifested by massive production of heat, carbon dioxide, and lactic acid. This results in respiratory and metabolic acidosis along with a rapid increase in temperature. Tachycardia is accompanied by other signs of circulatory and metabolic stress. Abnormal muscle activity develops, which may progress to whole-body rigidity. An increase in muscle permeability produces increased serum levels of potassium, phosphorus, calcium, sodium, and creatine phosphokinase (CPK). Muscle edema develops and an excessive release of myoglobin from muscle results in gross myoglobinemia. Disseminated intravascular coagulopathy and cardiac or renal failure may develop. Death may result from a combination of gross electrolyte disturbances, especially hyperkalemia, leading to cardiac failure (Muldoon et al., 1989).

The clinical course of MH is extremely variable. It can be fulminant, rapidly progressing to metabolic acidosis and death if not diagnosed and treated promptly. The sequence and severity of clinical events depend on (1) the types and concentrations of anesthetics involved; (2) the nature and extent of underlying myopathy; and (3) the promptness of diagnosis and initiation of appropriate treatment. MH is potentially fatal if not treated immediately with dantrolene sodium (Wlody, 1989). Before the development of this drug, mortality was 70%; now it is estimated to range from 10% to more than 50%, but is still considerably higher if MH occurs outside the surgical suite (Marchildon, 1982; Muldoon et al., 1989; Ording, 1985; Rogers & Sturgeon, 1985).

Tachycardia is the first sign seen if end-expiratory carbon dioxide is not measured (Table 15–11). Tachycardia occurs in 96% of all patients with MH within 30 minutes of anesthesia induction (Henschel, 1987). Rapid ventricular arrhythmias (e.g., bigeminy and ventricular tachycardia) may occur (Wlody, 1989). Tachycardia and/or dysrhythmias usually occur before fever, and thus MH should be suspected when these signs occur unless there are other obvious causes for them. Cardiac arrhythmias result from the stress of MH on the myocardium, probably resulting from the hypermetabolic state. The electrocardiographic tracing shows tall, peaked T waves and/or ST-segment depression (Wlody, 1989).

Muscle rigidity may or may not occur. If seen, it usually occurs first in the muscles of the jaw, extremities, or chest, usually before the administration of SCH. Instead of relaxing, the jaw tightens, making intubation difficult or impossible. There may be facial

Table 15–11. CLINICAL PRESENTATION OF MALIGNANT HYPERTHERMIA

Clinical Findings	Laboratory Findings
Tachycardia	Marked elevation of end-tidal carbon dioxide
Tachypnea—spontaneous ventilation	Hypercarbia—central venous and arterial
Unstable blood pressure	
Fever—rapid rise (1°F/15 min) Sustained rise (to 42°C)	Acidosis—respiratory and metabolic
Rigidity—especially trismus	Central venous and arterial desaturation
Cyanosis—dark blood in surgical field, mottling of skin	Hyperkalemia
Profuse sweating	Elevated creatinine phosphokinase (CPK), myoglobinemia

From Muldoon, S.M., Boggs, S.D., Freas, W. (1989). Malignant hyperthermia. In W.C. Shoemaker, S. Ayres, A. Grenvick, P.R. Holbrook, & W.L. Thompson (Eds.). *Textbook of critical care* (2nd ed., vol. 2, p. 110). Philadelphia: W.B. Saunders.

muscle fasciculation. Rigidity then travels through other skeletal muscles. There is an increased risk among patients with muscle injury just before anesthesia induction (e.g., trauma victims). Approximately 20% of patients with MH have no increase in muscle tone (Wlody, 1989).

Fever is the clinical hallmark of MH and results from many biochemical derangements. It is a somewhat late sign and may not occur at all if dantrolene is promptly administered (Wlody, 1989). Without treatment, the body temperature can rise 1°C every 5 minutes (Nelson & Flewellen, 1983). The risk of mortality from MH is related to the maximum body temperature reached, although patients with temperatures of 44°C have survived.

Patients undergoing anesthesia should be observed for evidence of fever. Signs of fever during surgery include hot, flushed skin; a hot anesthetic rebreathing bag; and hot tissue around the operative site. A change in skin color may accompany the development of MH. Flushed, rosy skin (similar to the familiar "atropine flush") may occur from the increased production of body heat. To dissipate the heat, vasodilatation occurs. The flushed skin subsequently becomes mottled, then cyanotic. Simultaneously, the surgeon notes dark blood at the operative site (Wlody, 1989).

Other clinical features of MH may occur following discontinuation of anesthesia (Table 15–12). Minimal preanesthetic screening should include measurement of serum creatine phosphokinase (CPK) in first-degree relatives of a known MH-susceptible person. If elevated, it is considered reliable evidence that the person is also MH susceptible. In general, random screening of CPK is not useful (Muldoon et al., 1989).

Treatment of MH includes discontinuating the anesthetic, cooling, hyperventilation, restoration of acid-base balance, and administration of medications to treat dysrhythmias and relax skeletal muscle con-

tractions. All interventions are carried out simultaneously. In addition, dantrolene sodium is administered without delay (Wlody, 1989). Dantrolene is a lipid-soluble hydantoin derivative with direct effects on skeletal muscle. It is given intravenously, initially 2.5 mg/kg, increasing to a total of 10 mg/kg (Muldoon et al., 1989).

Nursing Care of Patients With Elevated Body Temperature

Hyperthermia may be treatable by nursing intervention alone (e.g., by correcting external causes such as inappropriate clothing for environmental conditions, exposure to the elements, or dehydration). In other cases, such as malignant hyperthermia, nursing intervention alone is insufficient, and medical and other interventions may be necessary.

The impact of core hyperthermia on an already compromised patient can be deleterious. Oxygen consumption rises 10% to 12% for every 1°C temperature elevation (Buran, 1987). The increased metabolic demand in response to hyperthermia may produce progressive metabolic acidosis as oxygen delivery to the tissues is compromised (Buck & Zaritsky, 1989). Arterial blood gases and biochemical balance are monitored closely to detect acid-base imbalances and hypoxemia. Proper treatment of acidosis is promptly instituted to prevent untoward effects.

Sustained tachycardia in hyperthermic infants and children may compromise myocardial perfusion and diastolic filling, and may lead to greater stress on an already compromised heart. Moreover, infants or children experiencing hyperthermia should be observed for sweating and peripheral vasodilatation, both of which greatly increase loss of heat from the skin.

Regardless of the measures instituted to reduce temperature, shivering must not be stimulated. Shivering is a normal compensatory response to heat loss, but in the hemodynamically compromised patient, the effects can be deleterious. Shivering increases metabolic rate, carbon dioxide production, and myocardial oxygen consumption, all of which eventually result in increasing the myocardial workload. Arterial oxygen saturation decreases and systemic vascular resistance and heart rate increase with shivering. In addition, oxygen consumption increases 500% (Pflug et al., 1978), and the production and accumulation of lactic acid accelerate, which may culminate in lactic acidosis (Earp, 1989).

Nurses, therefore, focus on determining the proper combination of interventions to reduce temperature and avoid shivering. If shivering develops, measures are instituted to avoid the metabolic and hemodynamic consequences. Appropriate nursing interventions for shivering modify the rate of heat loss from the skin and interfere with the body's determination of heat loss (Holtzclaw, 1990). Various techniques have been suggested. Intravenous narcotics have been used to suppress shivering but may also pro-

Table 15–12. Associated Features of Maligant Hyperthermia

Clinical findings
Persistent coma
Acute cerebral edema
Unstable blood pressure
Acute pulmonary edema
Acute tubular necrosis
Decreased coagulation
Laboratory findings
Increased $PaCO_2$
Decreased PaO_2
Increased serum calcium
Increased potassium
Increased magnesium
Increased blood urea nitrogen
Increased glucose
Increased creatine phosphokinase
Increased serum glutamic oxaloacetic transaminase
Increased creatinine
Decrease in all clotting factors

Adapted with permission from *AORN Journal* 50 (2), August 1989, page 290. Copyright © AORN Inc., 2170 S Parker Road, Suite 300, Denver, CO 80231.

Table 15–13. LEVELS OF CLINICAL HYPOTHERMIA

Level	Temperature (°C)
Normothermia	36.6–37.5
Mild hypothermia	34–36.5
Moderate hypothermia	28–33.5
Deep hypothermia	17–27.5
Profound hypothermia	4–16.5

Data from Elder, P.T. (1989). Accidental hypothermia. In W.C. Shoemaker, S. Ayres, A. Grenvik, P.R. Holbrook, & W.L. Thompson (Eds.). *Textbook of critical care* (2nd ed., vol. 2, pp. 101–109). Philadelphia: W.B. Saunders.

duce side effects such as nausea or hypotension (Jaffe & Martin, 1980). An alternative is wrapping the extremities with towels during surface cooling with a hypothermia blanket (Holtzclaw, 1990).

Psychological support is particularly important when dealing with critically ill infants and children who are further distressed by both the discomfort of fever and its treatment. Interventions are based on the developmental stage and cognitive ability of the patient.

Hypothermia

Hypothermia is defined as any core body temperature less than 35°C. Degrees of hypothermia are detailed in Table 15–13. At low body temperatures (below 34°C), the hypothalamus functions minimally, and below 29°C cannot regulate temperature at all. Loss of temperature-regulating capability produces a rapid decrease in body temperature and eventually results in death (Guyton, 1987). When temperature drops low enough to trigger thermoregulatory control mechanisms, shivering thermogenesis and a generalized catecholamine release occur. Responses of the sympathetic nervous system prompt many other physiologic responses to produce the diagnostic characteristics of hypothermia (Table 15–14).

Infants and children are among high-risk groups for hypothermia, especially if unconscious, immobile, sedated, or malnourished. Mild hypothermia can frequently be observed in infants and children admitted to critical care units because of cold ambient temperatures. Table 15–15 outlines predisposing factors.

Table 15–14. DIAGNOSTIC CHARACTERISTICS OF HYPOTHERMIA

Major (present in 80–100% of cases)
  Oral temperature of <35°C or a rectal temperature of <35.5°C
  Cool skin
  Pallor (moderate)
  Shivering (mild)
Minor (present in 50–79% of cases)
  Mental confusion, drowsiness, restlessness
  Bradycardia and bradypnea
  Cachexia, malnutrition

Data from Carpenito, L.J. (1989). *Nursing diagnosis: Application to clinical practice* (3rd ed., p. 153). Philadelphia: J.B. Lippincott.

Table 15–15. FACTORS PREDISPOSING INFANTS AND CHILDREN TO THERMAL INSTABILITY

Relatively large body surface area
Relatively limited nutritional reserve
Impaired cardiac, renal, hepatic, or endocrine function
Impaired behavioral, neural, and endocrine responses (from underlying physical and physiologic states)
Impaired neuroendocrine response (from pharmacologic agents)
Cardiopulmonary resuscitation, anesthesia, and/or extended radiographic procedures

Data from Brink, L. W. (1990). Abnormalities in temperature regulation. In D.L. Levin & F.C. Morris (Eds.). *Essentials of pediatric intensive care* (pp. 175–185). St. Louis: Quality Medical Publishing; and Elder, P.T. (1989). Accidental hypothermia. In W.C. Shoemaker, S. Ayres, A. Grenvik, P.R. Holbrook, & W.L. Thompson (Eds.). *Textbook of critical care* (2nd ed., vol. 2, pp. 101–109). Philadelphia: W.B. Saunders.

Moderate to severe hypothermia is often present in patients who have suffered trauma, exposure, drowning, ingestion of poisons, or shock. Infants or children with unexplained altered responsiveness should be evaluated for hypothermia by measuring core temperature (Brink, 1990).

There are many pharmacologic agents that may contribute to hypothermia. Phenothiazines and barbiturates exert a direct effect on the anterior hypothalamus, decreasing its responsiveness to cold. Neuromuscular blocking agents and phenothiazines decrease the body's ability to engage in shivering thermogenesis. Vasodilators inhibit the peripheral vascular vasoconstrictor response and increase heat loss, thus decreasing temperature stability. Long-term use of vasopressors depletes catecholamine reserves and alters receptor function, thus impairing the peripheral vascular response to cold stress (Brink, 1990).

One clinical phenomenon that may produce severe hypothermia is cold water drowning (i.e., drowning in freezing water). Even in warm climates, however, the temperature of pool water can be significantly lower than air temperature. Even moderate water temperatures are lower than body temperature. The relatively large body surface area of infants and children predisposes them to rapid heat loss in water. As a consequence, small infants or children can become hypothermic even in relatively warm pool water in a moderate climate (Rogers, 1987).

Therapeutic, or induced, hypothermia is used to reduce metabolic demands during cardiac surgery. Induced hypothermia for cardiac surgery involves both systemic and cardiac cooling. Systemic hypothermia is achieved by cooling the blood as it is circulated through the heat exchanger of the cardiopulmonary bypass pump. Cardiac hypothermia is achieved by injection of a cooled pharmacologic cardioplegic solution into the aortic root. Initially a regional temperature gradient occurs because the core (heart and brain) is cooled first and the peripheral tissues remain warm. Gradually the skin temperature drops and eventually approximates the core temperature as heat is dissipated. During this time, the body's inherent thermoregulatory mechanisms cease, resulting in profound hypothermia (Earp, 1989). Rewarming is initiated by warming the blood circulated through the body and discontinuing extracorporeal circulation. During this phase, the core is warmed first and the regional and peripheral areas (rectum, bladder, skin) remain cooler, creating another temperature gradient. As the patient's thermoregulatory function returns, the patient is vulnerable to shivering.

Nursing Care of Patients With Decreased Body Temperature

Once the diagnosis of hypothermia is made, continuous core body temperature measurement is initiated and a thorough evaluation is made for risk factors (Table 15–16) and potential complications. Important assessments following the diagnosis of hypothermia include (1) electrocardiographic monitoring (significant arrhythmias may occur because of

Table 15–16. RISK FACTORS FOR HYPOTHERMIA

Etiology	Mechanism
Exposure Trauma Drowning	Increased heat loss, especially conductive heat loss (wet clothes or immersion) or convective losses (wind)
CNS depression Head injury Cerebral hemorrhage, tumor, or infection	Direct central effect on thalamic temperature center
Drug-induced Narcotics Barbiturates Phenothiazines Alcohol	CNS depression and vasodilatation CNS depression α-Adrenergic block, impaired shivering thermogenesis, lowered set-point CNS depression (and associated trauma, exposure, and impaired behavioral responses)
Endocrine abnormalities Hypoglycemia Hypothyroidism Hypopituitarism	Impaired thermogenesis, limited metabolic response to cold Impaired hypothalamic response to cold
Spinal cord transection	Interrupted sensory afferent Inability to sense cold Impaired central reflex and behavioral responses
Skin disorders Erythrodermas Burns	Increased transdermal water and heat losses
Therapeutic Treatment of Reye's syndrome Cardiopulmonary bypass	CNS depression

Data from Brink, L.W. (1990). Abnormalities in temperature regulation. In D.L. Levin & F.C. Morris (Eds.). *Essentials of pediatric intensive care* (pp. 175–185). St. Louis: Quality Medical Publishing; and Elder, P.T. (1989). Accidental hypothermia. In W.C. Shoemaker, S. Ayres, A. Grenvik, P.R. Holbrook, & W.L. Thompson (Eds.). *Textbook of critical care* (2nd ed., vol. 2, pp. 101–109). Philadelphia: W.B. Saunders.

myocardial irritability); (2) arterial blood pressure monitoring; and (3) frequent evaluation of acid-base status and serum electrolytes and blood glucose levels. External and/or core rewarming is instituted promptly.

Interpretation of arterial blood gas results in the hypothermic patient may necessitate the use of correction curves or values on rewarmed specimens. This is recommended because low temperatures cause carbon dioxide solubility to change, forcing the oxygen dissociation curve to shift to the left. When a specimen is drawn from a hypothermic patient and warmed to 37°C, the solubility of carbon dioxide decreases, resulting in a higher $PaCO_2$ and lower pH than exists in the patient. PaO_2 values should be corrected for temperature because warming the blood increases the solubility of oxygen and results in PaO_2 values significantly higher than in the patient (Brink, 1990). According to Shapiro and Cane (1989), however, if the patient's temperature is 35 to 39°C, there is little to be gained in correcting blood gas values. If the patient's temperature falls outside this range, it may be clinically useful to correct blood gas values with an uncorrected PaO_2 less than 60 torr, or an uncorrected $PaCO_2$ less than 30 torr, since these values may be higher than actual measurements.

Shivering thermogenesis begins at temperatures of 30 to 35°C. This results in a small increase in heat production, whereas oxygen consumption and metabolic rate increase significantly. Transient hyperglycemia may result from glycogenolysis in the liver and muscles. The catabolism of fat can produce ketosis. Lactate production ends in metabolic acidosis, and compensatory respiratory alkalosis follows. These changes peak at 34 to 35°C.

As hypothermia deepens, shivering thermogenesis ceases. Nonshivering thermogenesis occurs until the core temperature falls below 30°C. Heat production and metabolic rate both fall below baseline requirements at this point (Brink, 1990; Elder, 1989). Total oxygen consumption is proportionately decreased. There is a 6% fall in oxygen consumption for every degree Celsius the core temperature decreases. However, the extent of reduction of metabolism varies in each organ system (Brink 1990). When the temperature is normal, oxygen consumption is highest in the kidney, which is the organ most rapidly affected by hypothermia.

"Cold diuresis" is a term used to describe the renal response to cold. This denotes adequate urine output despite a significant impairment in renal blood flow and glomerular filtration rate. Diuresis may continue despite systemic hypotension, dehydration, and hyperosmolarity, presumably because of a defect in renal tubular reabsorption of water (Brink, 1990).

Changes in the cardiovascular system occur with hypothermia. The initial catecholamine-induced tachycardia is transient. During the phase of shivering thermogenesis, there is a decrease in cardiac conductivity and automaticity and an increase in the refractory period (Brink, 1990). Table 15–17 outlines the characteristic cardiac effects of various levels of hy-

Table 15–17. CARDIAC DYSRHYTHMIAS IN HYPOTHERMIA

Core Temperature	Arrhythmia
<34°C	Atrial fibrillation (more severe bradydysrhythmias noted with cooling)
<30°C	First-degree atrioventricular block
<20°C	Third-degree atrioventricular block

Data from Brink, L.W. (1990). Abnormalities in temperature regulation. In D.L. Levin & F.C. Morris (Eds.). *Essentials of pediatric intensive care* (p. 180). St. Louis: Quality Medical Publishing.

pothermia. These arrhythmias may not be treatable until core rewarming occurs. However, electrocardiographic monitoring may be useful in identifying the severity of hypothermia. The J-point elevation, for example, is potentially useful in diagnosing the severity of hypothermia (Brink, 1990).

Another significant effect of hypothermia is hemodynamic. Both myocardial contractility and vasomotor tone are impaired by hypothermia. This may produce profound hemodynamic collapse. During rewarming, significant hypotension may occur in response to peripheral vasodilation. Severe hypothermia may make cardiac resuscitation impossible, and thus rewarming should continue during resuscitation (Rogers, 1987). Elder (1989) suggests that resuscitation be continued until a core temperature of 32 to 33°C has been obtained, particularly if the primary cause of the cardiac arrest is hypothermia. However, resuscitation efforts are applied thoughtfully in the severely hypothermic child. Core temperature below 28°C places the child at high risk for ventricular fibrillation, which may be induced by cardiac compression. If the child presents with a nonarrest cardiac rhythm, chest compression is not implemented even in the face of severe bradycardia (Bolte et al., 1988). Chest compression is necessitated in patients with asystole or ventricular fibrillation.

The respiratory system shows less uniform effects. Initially, cold stimulates tachypnea. Shivering thermogenesis may produce compensatory alkalosis; however, below 30°C, hypoventilation is frequently seen. Central apnea occurs as hypothermia progresses (Brink, 1990). In addition, oxygen consumption rises and may produce hypoxia.

The CNS response varies with the degree of hypothermia. Mild to moderate hypothermia can produce confusion and behavioral changes. As the core temperature continues to drop, stupor worsens and coma results. Below 26°C, unresponsiveness; flaccidity; and fixed, dilated pupils follow. The CNS can benefit from the reduced metabolic and oxygen demands that result from hypothermia. Factors that determine the degree of benefit include (1) degree and duration of hypothermia; (2) underlying disease processes; (3) cardiorespiratory status; and (4) prior or concomitant medication usage (Brink, 1990). Because the effects of hypothermia on the CNS may be profound, rewarming to a temperature higher than 35°C is recommended before evaluation of brain death is undertaken (Brink, 1990; Rogers, 1987).

Pharmacologic effects of hypothermia are varied. Moderate to severe hypothermia produces such a serious decrease in metabolic rate that oxygen consumption and the rate of biochemical reactions slow considerably. As a result, drug levels and effects are difficult to evaluate in hypothermic patients. Decreased cardiac output, dehydration, slowed hepatic metabolism, impaired glomerular filtration, and abnormal renal tubular filtration and reabsorption can all result in reduced drug clearance (Brink, 1990). Hypothermia, for example, elevates the toxic dose of digitalis, whereas it decreases the inotropic dose. Potassium- and calcium-induced cardiac arrhythmias are possible because of increased myocardial sensitivity during hypothermia. Finally, temperatures below 26°C depress the cardiotonic effects of catecholamines; mild to moderate hypothermia, however, enhances their effects (Brink, 1990). Other pharmacologic effects include heightened sensitivity to anesthetic agents and barbiturates. Both barbiturates (because of their depressant effect) and phenothiazines (because of their alpha-adrenergic blocking effects) potentiate hypothermia.

With body temperature below 30°C, hyperviscosity and hypercoagulability of the blood may occur. This results from a rising hematocrit resulting from the cold diuresis that accompanies hypothermia. Infection is also a danger as a result of neutropenia, and coagulopathies can be accentuated because of thrombocytopenia (Brink, 1990).

Nursing Interventions

Generally, external warming devices are used to return the patient's temperature to the normal range in the case of mild to moderate hypothermia (i.e., core temperature 30–35°C). Radiant warmers, heating blankets or pads, warmed blankets, and head coverings are commonly used. Reflective blankets (lightweight metallic blankets that reflect up to 80% of radiant heat to the body) (Crayne & Miner, 1988) and buntings insulated with Thinsulate (Holtzman, 1985) have been recommended. A combination of modalities may be superior to a single rewarming technique (Topper & Stewart, 1984).

When instituting such measures, nurses are vigilant in their assessment of the patient's responses to the treatments. Radiant warmers are used only with the servo-control option to avoid thermal injury to the skin. Heating pads and blankets and other warming devices must be used with caution. Critically ill infants or children are not likely to be able to perceive a thermal injury or communicate it to nurses.

Severe hypothermia (core temperature lower than 30°C), for example, as a result of cold-water submersion, often requires active internal warming methods in addition to external warming measures. In such circumstances, measures such as heated humidified air, warmed intravenous fluids, and gastric or colonic lavage with warmed solutions or peritoneal dialysis may be implemented. Extracorporeal rewarming (ECR) may be required in the most severe circumstances (Bolte et al., 1988). ECR has been advocated as a rewarming technique in hypothermic patients to reduce the problems of rewarming shock, dysrhythmias, and thermal injury associated with external warming devices (Feldman et al., 1985; Reuler, 1978).

ECR diverts a significant portion of the patient's cardiac output through the extracorporeal membrane oxygenator and blood warmer. Gradual rewarming is facilitated by maintaining a warming gradient of approximately 10°C between the perfusate in the extracorporeal circuit and the patient's core temperature until body temperature reaches a normal range (Bolte et al., 1988). Slow rewarming avoids the sudden recirculation of cold, acidotic blood from the vasoconstricted peripheral vascular beds to the central circulation. This phenomenon, referred to as "rewarming shock" or "afterdrop," is manifested by a fall in core temperature and serum pH. Because rapid rewarming increases the risk of ventricular fibrillation, gradual rewarming is the goal in any severely hypothermic patient, regardless of the intervention selected. Throughout the rewarming phase, the patient is closely monitored for cardiac dysrhythmias and coagulopathies resulting from systemic heparinization if ECR is used.

During rewarming following induced hypothermia for extracorporeal circulation, afterdrop may also develop (Earp, 1989). Therefore, cardiovascular and hemodynamic monitoring must accompany temperature measurement during the rewarming phase.

SUMMARY

The incidence of altered body temperature and ineffective thermoregulation is significant among patients in the PICU. The risks to physiologic stability in critically ill infants and children are high. Critical care nursing practice can correct environmental factors leading to altered body temperature, support thermoregulatory processes, provide physical comfort during interventions to normalize body temperature, and ensure physiologic stability in patients with altered body temperature or ineffective thermoregulation.

References

Bissonnette, B., & Sessler, D.I. (1992). Thermoregulatory thresholds for vasoconstriction in pediatric patients anesthetized with halothane or halothane and caudal bupivacaine. *Anesthesiology, 76,* 387–392.

Bolte, R.G., Black, P.G., Bowers, R.S., Thorne, J.K., & Corneli, H.M. (1988). The use of extracorporeal rewarming in a child submerged for 66 minutes. *Journal of the American Medical Association, 260,* 377–379.

Brink, L.W. (1990). Abnormalities in temperature regulation. In D.L. Levin & F.C. Morriss (Eds.). *Essentials of pediatric intensive care* (pp. 175–185). St. Louis: Quality Medical Publishing.

Buck, S.H., & Zaritsky, A.L. (1989). Occult core hyperthermia complicating cardiogenic shock. *Pediatrics, 83,* 782–784.

Buran, N.J. (1987). Oxygen consumption. In M.R. Pinsky & J.V.

Snider (Eds.). *Oxygen transport in the critically ill* (pp. 16–21). Chicago: Year Book Medical Publishers.

Carpenito, L.J. (1989). *Nursing diagnosis: Application to clinical practice* (3rd ed., pp. 143–161). Philadelphia: J.B. Lippincott.

Casella, E.S., Rogers, M.C., & Zahka, K.G. (1987). Developmental physiology of the cardiovascular system. In M.C. Rogers (Ed.). *Textbook of pediatric intensive care* (pp. 329–365). Baltimore: Williams & Wilkins.

Crayne, H.L., & Miner, D.G. (1988). Thermo-resuscitation for postoperative hypothermia using reflective blankets. *AORN Journal, 47,* 222–227.

Davis, P.J. (1990). Temperature regulation in infants and children. In E.K. Motoyama & P.J. Davis (Eds.). *Smith's anesthesia for infants and children* (pp. 143–156). Baltimore: C.V. Mosby.

Dedrick, D.F., & Cote, C.J. (1986). Pediatric equipment. In J.F. Ryan, I.D. Todres, C.J. Cote, & N.G. Goudsouzian (Eds.). *A practice of anesthesia for infants and children* (pp. 271–281). Orlando, FL: Grune & Stratton.

Earp, J.K. (1989). Thermal gradients and shivering following open heart surgery. *Dimensions of Critical Care Nursing, 8,* 266–273.

Elder, P.T. (1989). Accidental hypothermia. In W.C. Shoemaker, S. Ayres, A. Grenvik, P.R. Holbrook, & W.L. Thompson (Eds.). *Textbook of critical care* (2nd ed., 2 vols., pp. 101–109). Philadelphia: W.B. Saunders.

Feldman, K.W., Morray, J.P., & Schallar, R.T. (1985). Thermal injury caused by hot pack application in hypothermic children. *American Journal of Emergency Medicine, 3,* 38–41.

Forestner, J.E. (1981). Complications of anesthesia. In J.D. Hardy (Ed.). *Complications in surgery and their management* (4th ed., pp. 209–211). Philadelphia: W.B. Saunders.

Fraulini, K.E. (1977). *After anesthesia.* East Norwalk, CT: Appleton & Lange.

Frigoletto, F.D., & Little, G.A. (Eds.). (1988). *Guidelines for Perinatal Care* (2nd ed., pp. 274–281). Elk Grove Village, IL/Washington, DC: American Academy of Pediatrics/American College of Obstetricians and Gynecologists.

Gauntlett, I., Barnes, J., Brown, T., & Bell, B. (1985). Temperature maintenance in infants undergoing anaesthesia and surgery. *Anaesthesia and Intensive Care, 13,* 300–304.

Goudsouzian, N.G., Morris, R.H., & Ryan, J.F. (1973). The effects of a warming blanket on the maintenance of body temperature in anesthetized infants and children. *Anesthesiology, 39,* 351–353.

Gronert, G.A., Thompson, R.L., & Onofrio, B.M. (1980). Human malignant hyperthermia: Awake episodes and correction by dantrolene. *Anesthesia and Analgesia, 59,* 377–378.

Guyton, A.C. (1987). *Human physiology and mechanisms of disease* (4th ed., pp. 545–552). Philadelphia: W.B. Saunders.

Harris, M.F. (1990). Malignant hyperthermia. In D.L. Levin & F.C. Morriss (Eds.). *Essentials of pediatric intensive care* (pp. 453–458). St. Louis: Quality Medical Publishing.

Henschel, E.O. (Ed.). (1987). *Malignant hyperthermia: Current concepts.* New York: Appleton-Century-Crofts.

Holtzclaw, B.J. (1985). Postoperative shivering after cardiac surgery: A review. *Heart & Lung, 15,* 292–299.

Holtzclaw, B.J. (1990). Control of febrile shivering during amphotericin B therapy. *Oncology Nursing Forum, 17,* 521–522.

Holtzman, I.R. (1985). A method to maintain infant temperature. *American Journal of Diseases in Childhood, 139,* 390–392.

Horvath, S.M., Spurr, G.B., Hutt, B.K., & Hamilton, L.H. (1956). The metabolic cost of shivering. *Journal of Applied Physiology, 8,* 595–602.

Jaffe, J.H., & Martin, W.R. (1980). Opioid analgesics and their antagonists. In A.G. Gilman & L.S. Goodman (Eds.). *The pharmacologic basis of therapeutics* (pp. 494–534). New York: Macmillan.

Kline, M.W., & Lorin, M.I. (1990). Fever without localizing signs. In F.A. Oski, C.D. DeAngelis, R.D. Feigin, & J.B. Warshaw (Eds.). *Principles and practice of pediatrics* (pp. 1021–1023). Philadelphia: J.B. Lippincott.

Kozak-Reiss, G., Gascard, J.P., Herve P., Jehanson, P., & Syrota, A. (1988). Malignant and exercise hyperthermia: Investigation of 73 subjects by contracture tests and P31 NMR spectroscopy. *Anesthesiology, 69* (3A [Suppl.]), A415.

Littlefield, L.C. (1987). Management of fever. In R.A. Hoekelman,

S. Blatman, S.B. Friedman, N.M. Nelson, & H.M. Seidel (Eds.). *Primary pediatric care* (pp. 273–277). St Louis: C.V. Mosby.

Livingston, R.B. (1985). Neurophysiology. In J.B. West (Ed.). *Best and Taylor's physiological basis of medical practice* (pp. 970–1312). Baltimore: Williams & Wilkins.

Lorin, M.I. (1990). Pathogenesis of fever and its treatment. In F.A. Oski, C.D. DeAngelis, R.D. Feigin, & J.B. Warshaw (Eds.). *Principles and practice of pediatrics* (pp. 1019–1021). Philadelphia: J.B. Lippincott.

Lovejoy, Jr., F.H. (1989). The etiology and treatment of fever: Current concepts. *Pediatric update: New developments in fever management.* (Available from Department of Medical Affairs, MacNeil Consumer Products, Camp Hill Rd., Fort Washington, PA 19034.)

Marchildon, M.B. (1982). Malignant hyperthermia: Current concepts. *Archives of Surgery, 117,* 349–351.

Matusik, M.C. (1985). Chronobiology. In A.R. Colon & M. Ziai (Eds.). *Pediatric pathophysiology* (pp. 471–484). Boston: Little, Brown.

Merenstein, G.B., Gardner, S.L., & Blake, W.W. (1985). Heat balance. In G.B. Merenstein & S.L. Gardner (Eds.). *Handbook of Neonatal Intensive Care* (pp. 85–96). St. Louis: C.V. Mosby.

Moorthy, S.S., Winn, B.A., Jallard, M.S., Edwards, K., & Smith, N.D. (1985). Monitoring urinary bladder temperature. *Heart & Lung, 14,* 90–93.

Morriss, F.C., Grandy, M.E., & Johnson, L.T. (1984). Radiant warming devices. In D.L. Levin (Ed.). *A practical guide to pediatric intensive care* (pp. 485–487). St. Louis: C.V. Mosby.

Muldoon, S.M., Boggs, S.D., & Freas, W. (1989). Malignant hyperthermia. In W.C. Shoemaker, S. Ayres, A. Grenvik, P.R. Holbrook, & W.L. Thompson (Eds.). *Textbook of critical care* (2nd ed., 2 vols., pp. 109–113). Philadelphia: W.B. Saunders.

Nelson, T.E., & Flewellen, E.H. (1983). The malignant hyperthermia syndrome. *New England Journal of Medicine, 309,* 416–418.

Ording, H. (1985). Incidence of malignant hyperthermia in Denmark. *Anesthesia and Analgesia, 64,* 700–704.

Perlstein, P. (1992). Physical environment. In A.A. Fanaroff & R.J. Martin (Eds.). *Neonatal-perinatal medicine: Diseases of the fetus and infant* (5th ed., pp. 401–419). St. Louis: C.V. Mosby.

Pflug, A.E., Aasheim, G.M., & Foster, C. (1978). Prevention of post-anesthesia shivering. *Canadian Anesthesiology Society Journal, 25,* 43–49.

Prosser, C.L., & Nelson, D.O. (1981). The role of nervous systems in temperature adaptation of poikilotherms. *Annual Review of Physiology, 43,* 281–300.

Quinton, P.M. (1983). Sweating and its disorders. *Annual Review of Physiology, 34,* 429–452.

Ramsay J.G., Ralley, F.E., Whalley D.G., Delli Colli, P., & Wynands, J.E. (1985). Site of temperature monitoring and prediction of afterdrop after open heart surgery. *Canadian Anesthesiology Society Journal, 32,* 607–612.

Reuler, J.B. (1978). Pathophysiology, clinical settings and management. *Annals of Internal Medicine, 89,* 519–527.

Rogers, A., & Sturgeon, L. (1985). Malignant hyperthermia: A perioperative emergency. *AORN Journal, 41,* 369–374.

Rogers, M.C. (1987). *Textbook of pediatric intensive care* (Vols. 1, 2). Baltimore: Williams & Wilkins.

Shapiro, B.A., & Cane, R.D. (1989). Interpretation of blood gases. In W.C. Shoemaker, S. Ayres, A. Grenvik, P.R. Holbrook, & W.L. Thompson (Eds.). *Textbook of critical care* (2nd ed., 2 vols., pp. 305–311). Philadelphia: W.B. Saunders.

Topper, W.H., & Stewart, T.P. (1984). Thermal support of the very-low-birth-weight infant: Role of supplemental conductive heat. *Journal of Pediatrics, 105,* 810–814.

Vacanti, F.X., & Ryan, J.F. (1986). Temperature regulation. In J.F. Ryan, I.D. Todres, C.J. Cote, N.G. Goudsouzian (Eds.). *A practice of anesthesia for infants and children* (pp. 19–23). Orlando, FL: Grune & Stratton.

Whaley, L.F., & Wong, D.L. (1991). *Nursing care of infants and children.* St. Louis: C.V. Mosby.

Wlody, G.S. (1989). Malignant hyperthermia: Potential crisis in patient care. *AORN Journal, 50(2),* 286–298.

CHAPTER 16

Host Defenses

CATHY ROSENTHAL-DICHTER
MARY ALLEN

Host defenses are of considerable importance to the pediatric critical care nurse because of the age and vulnerability of the patient population and the complexities of critical care illness and the critical care environment. Host defenses may be altered because of developmental, situational, or congenital stressors. Whatever the process or mechanism of alteration, outcome of altered host defenses ranges from hyperactivity of the immune system, manifested clinically as hypersensitivity (allergies or autoimmune disease), to hypoactivity of the immune system, manifested as an increased susceptibility to infection. This chapter will focus on hypoactivity as the most common alteration in host defenses in the pediatric critical care patient.

THE IMMUNE SYSTEM

Functions of the Immune System

The most notable function of the immune system is host defense, or the active protection of the host from invading microorganisms (Grady, 1988). The other functions of the immune system are related to host defense, but in the role of proactive maintenance. Homeostasis, the second function of the im-

mune system, is the process in which the immune system maintains a balance between the old and new immune cells as a part of normal physiologic functioning. Homeostasis is the removal of old cells and debris resulting from normal catabolism, growth, and injury. Homeostasis keeps the body's internal environment clean and easy to survey. The third function of the immune system, surveillance, is the process in which the immune cells differentiate self from mutated self cells (nonself).

Nonspecific Versus Specific Immunity

Every person, whether healthy or immunocompromised, is in contact with millions of actual and potential microorganisms on a daily basis. The well orchestrated, complex, and efficient cadre of defenses provided through the immune system is a barrier to these invaders. Host defenses can be classified as nonspecific or specific. Nonspecific defenses are generic host responses to a foreign agent. These responses are not tailored to an individual agent but are the same responses to any agent at any time. Nonspecific host defenses include first and second lines of defense, the natural barriers and the inflammatory responses, respectively. In contrast, specific defenses depend on the exposure to a foreign agent, recognition of the agent as foreign, and the host's individual reaction to that agent. The specific immune responses of the host include the third line of defense and include humoral immunity (immunoglobulin) and cell-mediated immunity.

Concept of Human Defense

Normal immune defense is maintained through the protection of self and the destruction of nonself. To perform host defense, yet maintain the integrity of self, a genetic blueprint (deoxyribonucleic acid [DNA] code) at the molecular level assists the immune system in discriminating self from nonself or altered self. Nonself is comprised of foreign or alien molecular structure and is referred to as antigenic, or as an antigen.

The specific immune system discriminates between self and nonself through the major histocompatibility complex (MHC) molecules for each species. The MHC molecules specific to the human species are human leukocyte antigens (HLA). HLA antigens are inherited according to mendelian laws, with a genotype determined by one paternal and one maternal haplotype. Close relatives share some of the these antigens, whereas identical twins share all of these antigens. Figure 16–1 reflects the diagrammatic representation of inheritance of the HLA antigens in a family.

Although first discovered on white blood cells and coined "human leukocyte antigens," HLA antigens are actually located on the surfaces of most nucleated cells in the body, as well as platelets. HLA antigens of the MHC are divided into two classes (class I and II) based on function, types of cell antigens expressed on the cell membrane surfaces, and structure. Class I includes HLA-A, -B, and -C antigens and is found on all nucleated cell surfaces and platelets. Class II includes HLA-D and HLA-DR antigens and is located nearly exclusively on the surfaces of certain immune cells (macrophages and B lymphocytes).

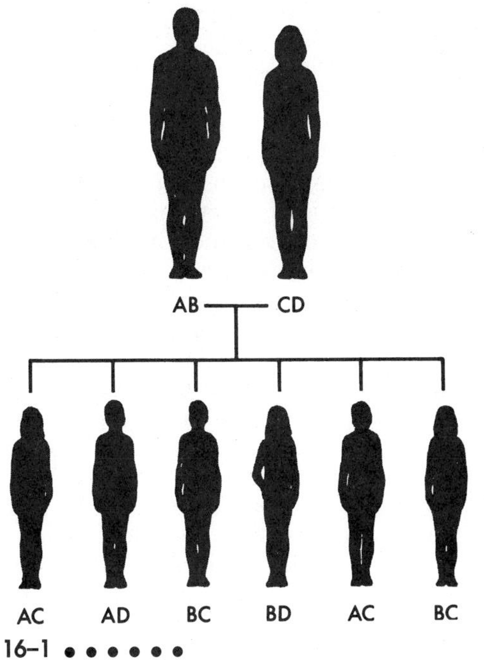

Once thought to be important only in the transplantation process, HLA antigens are now known to play a comprehensive role in determining self versus nonself and in autoimmune disease processes. Class I antigens serve as identification markers of self and assist in the elimination of cells infected with intracellular microorganisms, mutated or malignant cells, or rejection of tissue grafts. Class II antigens serve as identification markers of exogenous antigens and assist in the elimination of extracellular microorganisms.

Self cells normally do not evoke an immune response due to their display of recognizable HLA antigens. Nonself describes an entity which is different in structure and evokes an immune response. To stimulate an immune response, a nonself molecule is generally at least a molecular weight greater than 10,000 daltons. Smaller nonself molecules do not elicit an immune response, unless combined with a carrier molecule, and are referred to as haptens. A clinical example is a drug molecule that is adsorbed onto a red blood cell (RBC) to result in an immune hemolytic anemia reaction.

Figure 16–1 ● ● ● ● ● ●

HLA antigens are inherited from parents: one set of HLA antigens is inherited from the mother, and the second set from the father. Each set of inherited antigens is co-dominant (i.e., each set is co-expressed on the surfaces of the pertinent body cells. (From Smith, S. L. (1990). *Tissue and organ transplantation: Implications for professional nursing practice* (p. 25). St. Louis: Mosby–Year Book.)

Cells of Host Defense

White Blood Cells

White blood cells (WBCs) or leukocytes are the mobile units of the immune system and are colorless blood cells that defend the body against infection. These cells are categorized as granulocytes, monocytes/macrophages, and lymphocytes. Granulocytes are critical in engulfing and phagocytizing microorganisms and are nonspecific in nature. They are further categorized as neutrophils, eosinophils, and basophils. Monocytes/macrophages also engulf microorganisms, but more importantly are a link between the nonspecific and specific immune responses. Lymphocytes (B and T cells) are the key players in specific, acquired response. Table 16–1 reviews the normal values for each of the WBCs. Each WBC is discussed separately.

Neutrophils. Neutrophils account for approximately 60% to 70% of the total circulating WBC count. In addition to neutrophils in the circulation, there is a large population of neutrophils stored in the bone marrow and available to replenish the bloodstream. An equivalent portion of neutrophils are also temporarily stored in small vessels or adhered to the walls of large blood vessels. These neu-

Table 16-1. NORMAL WHITE BLOOD CELL VALUES

Cell Type	Differential (%)	Absolute Number (mm³)
Total WBC Count		
Birth	100	9000–30,000
24 hours		9400–34,000
1 month		5000–19,500
1–3 years		6000–17,500
4–7 years		5500–15,500
8–13 years		4500–11,000
>13 years		5000–10,000
Granulocytes		
Neutrophils	60–70	3000–7000
Segmented	56	2800–5600
Bands	3–6	150–600
Eosinophils	2–5	50–400
Basophils	<1	25–100
Monocytes	2–8	100–800
Lymphocytes	20–40	1000–4000
T cells	60–88*	600–2200
B cells	3–21*	100–400
NK cells	5–10*	50–400

*Percentage of total lymphocyte count rather than percentage of total WBC count.

Modified from D. Tribett (1989). Immune system function: Implications for critical care nursing practice. *Critical Care Nursing Clinics of North America,* 1(4):727; Behrman, R.E., & Vaughn, V.C. III (eds). *Nelson textbook of pediatrics* (13th ed.) Philadelphia: W.B. Saunders.

trophils are referred to as the *marginal pool.* Neutrophils in the intravascular space are composed of the circulating and marginal pools. Neutrophils are also plentiful in the body's tissues. In fact, there are twice as many neutrophils in the tissues as in the intravascular space.

Neutrophils develop and mature in the bone marrow for approximately 10 days. They spend approximately 12 hours in the circulation before migrating to the tissues, where they live for only a few days. The primary function of neutrophils is to move to the site of invasion and destroy microorganisms through the process of phagocytosis. Neutrophils are the first WBCs to respond and the most numerous WBCs found at the site of tissue injury.

A mature neutrophil is described as a polymorphonuclear leukocyte (PMNL) or segmented neutrophil because of the appearance of the nucleus. Normally, segmented neutrophils or "segs" constitute the majority of circulating neutrophils. The nucleus of the immature neutrophil is not segmented, and is therefore referred to as a "band" or "stab." The presence of greater than normal numbers of immature neutrophils in the circulation *(neutrophilia)* is clinically significant because the immature neutrophil's ability to phagocytize is less effective than that of a mature neutrophil, and more importantly may signify that there is a problem.

Neutrophilia, an increased number of circulating neutrophils, is often accompanied by an increase in the number of bands, because the bone marrow releases a supply of neutrophils in response to the body's demands without regard to the cell's maturity or readiness for release. Neutrophilia is also observed in situations that stimulate secretion of epinephrine, adrenocorticotrophic hormone (ACTH), or adrenal corticosteroids and/or cause increases in cardiac output. Therefore, neutrophilia is observed in patients experiencing infection; stress response from surgery, hemorrhage, or emotional distress; and metabolic disorders such as diabetes.

Neutropenia, a decreased number of circulating neutrophils, is often associated with a pathologic or malignant condition. Conditions such as aplastic anemia or treatment with cytotoxic agents result in neutropenia. Neutropenia is technically defined as less than 3,000 cells/mm³ of absolute neutrophils.

Eosinophils. Eosinophils account for approximately 2% to 5% of the circulating WBCs in healthy, nonallergic individuals, but up to 50% in patients with parasitic infections or (less often) allergic conditions (Jett & Lancaster, 1983). Following maturation in the bone marrow, the eosinophil is released into the circulation and remains there for a brief time before migrating to the tissues. Unlike other cells, eosinophils can recirculate back and forth from the circulation to the tissues. Their time in the tissues is approximately 12 days. Although eosinophils have the ability to phagocytize, the process is less efficient than that of the neutrophil. The eosinophil's role in host defense is not exactly known, but is believed to be involved in the "turning off" of the immune response because it arrives last to the site of infection.

Eosinophils, like neutrophils, basophils, and mast cells, can be triggered to degranulate. Degranulation is the process in which intracellular granules fuse with the target cell's plasma membrane and cellular contents are released to the outside of the cell (Lydyard & Grossi, 1989a). If the target is too large to phagocytize, the eosinophils can shower the target with toxins located in their granules.

As previously mentioned, eosinophilia, an increased number of circulating eosinophils, is observed in patients with parasitic infection and allergic conditions. It is also observed in patients with chronic skin infections, gastrointestinal conditions such as ulcerative colitis and Crohn's disease, and rare conditions such as hypereosinophilia. Eosinopenia, a decreased number of circulating eosinophils, is observed in patients with acute mononucleosis and other acute infections, as well as conditions or therapies stimulating adrenal steroid production.

Basophils and Mast Cells. Basophils represent the smallest proportion of granulocytes in the circulation, usually less than 1% of circulating WBCs. The basophil's production, distribution, and lifespan are not thoroughly understood. Basophils possess granules containing heparin, histamine, and other mediators, which can degranulate with the proper stimulus. Basophilia, an increased number of circulating basophils, is seen in leukemia, and less frequently with allergies and infectious diseases such as tuberculosis, influenza, and chicken pox. A decreased basophil count is observed in patients with allergic reactions or in those who are receiving prolonged steroid therapy.

The mast cell is often indistinguishable from the basophil, but the two cells do differ. Mast cells do not circulate in the bloodstream, but instead are found throughout the body's tissues, particularly the skin and mucosal linings of the respiratory and gastrointestinal tracts. Like the basophil, mast cells store granules with histamine and other potent mediators that are important in the inflammatory response and tissue repair. When the mast cell or basophil is inappropriately activated, these granules may lead to an allergic response. Because mast cells do not circulate, the suffixes "-philia" and "-penia" are not usually used to refer to abnormal numbers of mast cells. An abnormal accumulation of mast cells is termed "mastocytosis," and can range from benign skin lesions to organ infiltration resulting in organ dysfunction and death.

Monocytes and Macrophages. Like neutrophils, monocytes (in the circulatory system) and macrophages (free and fixed, but usually in various tissues) have the ability to phagocytize. Monocytes are large, nongranular leukocytes with kidney-shaped nuclei. They comprise 2% to 8% of total circulating WBCs. Following release from the bone marrow, monocytes spend only a brief time in the circulatory system (1–2 days) before they migrate to their primary site of action, the tissues. Following migration into the tissue, monocytes undergo differentiation into macrophages.

Because monocytes are circulating WBCs, they can be quantified in the differential WBC count. Monocytosis, an increase in the number of circulating monocytes, is observed in patients with viral, parasitic, or rickettsial infections, although this finding may indicate a recovery phase and may be a favorable sign. A decrease in the circulating monocyte count, monocytopenia, is not clinically significant, but may be observed in patients with human immunodeficiency virus (HIV) infection or in patients receiving prednisone therapy.

The macrophage is capable of phagocytizing larger and greater numbers of particles than the neutrophil. It has a primary role in nonspecific defense through its phagocytic activities, but also in specific defense by its processing and presentation of the antigen to the helper T cell. Thus, the macrophage serves as a link between the nonspecific and specific host defenses. The macrophage is also involved in the production and release of cytokines. It produces interleukin-1 (IL-1), a known pyrogen and mediator of the inflammatory response. The macrophage also produces interferon in the presence of viral invasion.

Lymphocytes. The lymphocyte is a small, mononuclear cell that comprises 20% to 40% of the circulating WBCs. The lymphocyte is produced in the bone marrow and migrates to other parts of the body for differentiation and maturation into several distinct subsets of lymphocytes. Lymphocyte subsets include B cells, T cells, and natural killer (NK) cells based on differences in their immune function and surface molecules (phenotypic markers) (Wood & Sampson, 1989).

Although these cells are normally measured in the periphery, lymphocytes circulate through a network of interconnected passages referred to as the recirculating pathway. In the recirculating pathway, lymphocytes survey the body for invading organisms or antigens by traveling between the blood, lymphatic vessels, lymphoid tissue, bone marrow, and back to the blood. Lymphocytes can also be found in specialized tissue collections, spleen, thymus, the mucosa of the gastrointestinal tract, and many other body tissues.

Lymphocytosis, an increase in the number of circulating lymphocytes, is seen in patients with viral infections, such as infectious mononucleosis and infectious hepatitis; lymphocytic leukemia; and lymphoma. Lymphopenia, a decrease in the number of lymphocytes, is commonly seen in patients with congenital immunodeficiencies, acquired immunodeficiency syndrome (AIDS), uremia, or Cushing's disease or following the administration of cortisol or ACTH.

B Cells. B cells make up approximately 10% to 15% of the total lymphocyte count, with alterations in the number of B cells considered clinically significant (Table 16–2). The B cell is primarily responsible for humoral immunity (HI) through its transformation into a plasma cell that secretes immunoglobulin. HI primarily protects the host from bacterial infection and viral invasion.

The term "immunoglobulin" refers to a group of serum proteins that are composed of antibody molecules. Immunoglobulins are specialized molecules synthesized by plasma cells serving as flexible adapters connecting immune cells and antigens. "Antibody" is the term reserved for an individual immunoglobulin molecule, one for which the "destiny" antigen is known. The primary purpose of antibody is to bind to its "destiny" or predetermined antigen and either neutralize it or enable the cells of the immune system to destroy it.

Immunoglobulins are composed of polypeptides (chains of amino acids) formed into a basic Y-shaped structure. The basic immunoglobulin molecule consists of two identical long (heavy) chains and two identical short (light) chains held together by chemical bonds (Fig. 16–2). Both the heavy and the light chains have a variable segment at one end of the molecule and a constant segment at the other end of the molecule. The variable segment binds to the antigen for which it was made, and is referred to as the antigen binding fragment (Fab) (Grady, 1988; Roitt, 1988). Although the variable segment is unique, the sequence of amino acids that comprises the constant segment of the immunoglobulin molecule remains identical within each class of immunoglobulin and is thus referred to as the constant fragment (Fc).

Human immunoglobulin molecules are divided into five classes based on the structure of their constant segments: IgG, IgA, IgM, IgE, and IgD. Phagocytes and other immune cells have receptors on their surfaces into which the Fc portion of the Ig molecule fits. This receptor is termed an "Fc receptor." Table

Table 16–2. LYMPHOCYTES: LABORATORY ANALYSIS AND CLINICAL SIGNIFICANCE OF ALTERATIONS

Cell Type	Total Lymphocyte Count (%)	Absolute Count (per mm³)*	Clinical Significance of Alterations
T cells	60–88	600–2200	Decreased: Malignant disease AIDS Post-viral infection (temporary) Severe combined immunodeficiency DiGeorge syndrome Nezelof's syndrome Increased: Graves' disease
Helper T	34–67	493–1191	Decreased: AIDS
Cytotoxic-suppressor T	10–49	182–785	Decreased: Overall lymphopenia
B cells	3–21	100–400	Decreased: X-linked hypogammaglobulinemia Selective deficiency of IgG/IgA/IgM Lymphoma Multiple myeloma Nephrotic syndrome
NK cells	5–10	50–400	Increased: Lymphocytic leukemia Lupus erythematosus

*These values most accurately reflect the older child/adolescent. Recent evidence reveals that absolute lymphocyte counts may be higher in the infant and young child.

Data from F.T. Fischbach, 1992. *A manual of laboratory and diagnostic tests* (4th ed). Philadelphia: J.B. Lippincott; D. Tribett, 1989. Immune system function: Implications for critical care nursing practice. *Critical Care Nursing Clinics of North America,* 1(4):727.

16–3 is a review of the major classes of human immunoglobulin with their respective serum levels, mechanisms of action, and location.

T Cells. Following production in the bone marrow, T cells differentiate in the thymus and are re-released into the circulation where they comprise 80% of all lymphocytes. In general, T cells are responsible for cell-mediated immunity (CMI), which protects the host from infections with intracellular organisms, such as viruses, fungi, protozoa, and helminth parasites. T cells are also involved in the elimination of mutant or tumor cells and are involved in the immune response triggered during tissue graft or organ transplant rejection.

During differentiation in the thymus, T cells develop into one of four distinct subclasses: helper T cell, suppressor T cell, cytotoxic T cell, or memory T cell. Mature T cells have specialized molecules on their surface, which are referred to as clusters of differentiation (CD). Helper T cells have a cluster of differentiation 4 (abbreviated CD4 or T4). Cytotoxic and suppressor T cells have a cluster of differentia-

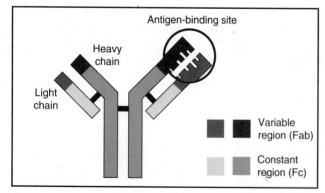

Figure 16–2 ● ● ● ● ● ●

The structure of an immunoglobulin molecule. The Fab segment is variable and attaches to its destiny or predetermined antigen. The Fc segment can attach to any cell that has an Fc receptor. (From Schindler, L. W. (1992). *The immune system—How it works.* United States Department of Health and Human Services, Bethesda, MD. NIH publication number 92-3229, p. 6.)

Table 16–3. HUMAN IMMUNOGLOBULINS

Ig	% in Serum	Location	Activity and Function
IgG	75	Intravascular, extravascular	Opsonization Neutralization Complement fixation
IgA	15	Found in mucous membrane secretions, intravascular	Neutralization Prevention of surface attachment
IgM	10	Intravascular	Agglutination Complement fixation
IgE	0.1	Bound to mast cells and basophils	Release of histamine and other mediators from mast cells and basophils
IgD	<1	Located on surface of B cells	Function not yet defined May be important to B cell differentiation

Adapted from Grady, C. (1988). Host defense mechanisms: An overview. *Seminars in Oncology Nursing,* 4(2):92.

tion 8 (abbreviated CD8 or T8). Memory T cells have CD corresponding to the distinct subclass of memory cell: helper, cytotoxic, or suppressor.

Helper T cells have many functions such as producing lymphokines, which then stimulate the cloning and differentiation of B cells. Helper T cells are also active in several nonspecific host responses such as attracting macrophages and neutrophils. Following helper T cell activation and the production of lymphokines, suppressor T cells are activated. Suppressor T cells curb the immune response. Cytotoxic T cells (effector cells) are responsible for direct destruction of target cells in the specific immune response. Memory cells are formed with the initial antigen contact and are involved in subsequent contacts with the antigen.

Because helper T cells orchestrate the entire immune response, it is essential to have adequate numbers of these cells. Normally, there are twice as many helper T cells as there are cytotoxic/suppressor T cells. Although some clinicians measure the ratio of helper T cells to cytotoxic/suppressor T cells, this is less clinically useful than absolute numbers or percentages of the T cell subclasses. Alterations in the numbers of T cells and/or their subclasses are considered clinically significant (see Table 16–2).

Natural Killer Cells. Natural killer (NK) cells comprise approximately 5% to 10% of the total lymphocyte count. A number of terms are used to describe the NK cell; it is often referred to as "null," "blank," or "non T non B cell" because of the lack of T or B cell identification markers. The NK cell is a member of a group of large, granular lymphocytes (LGLs) with nonspecific cytotoxic abilities. The target cell for the NK cell is the tumor cell or virally infected cell. The NK cell's cytotoxic abilities are nonspecific in nature, because the cell can destroy its target without prior sensitization.

LGLs may be stimulated in the laboratory with interleukin-2 to become lymphokine-activated killer (LAK) cells. Although these cells remain nonspecific, they respond to a greater diversity of targets than the NK cell. Protocols employing LAK cells are undergoing clinical trials in the treatment of many malignancies.

Cell Counts

Total WBC Count. The normal total WBC count is 5000 to 10,000 cells/mm³ and may vary, depending on the time of day. However, total WBC count varies with the age of the infant and young child. The WBC count only reflects the circulating WBCs, not those WBCs marginated to vessel walls, circulating in the lymphatic system, or sequestered in body tissues. As a general screening test for immune function, the total WBC count serves as an indicator of the inflammatory response or disease states, presence of an infection, and response to therapy.

Increases and decreases in the total WBC count from normal levels are referred to as "leukocytosis" and "leukopenia," respectively. Leukocytosis is usu-

ally the result of an increase in one type of WBC rather than a proportional increase in all types of WBCs and is commonly indicative of the presence of infection. Leukocytosis can be the result of release of additional WBCs from the bone marrow in response to infection, trauma, and physical or emotional stress, but also can be the result of increased production of abnormal WBCs, as in leukemia. Any condition that increases blood flow or cardiac output will result in the recruitment of WBCs into the circulation from the marginating pool. Leukopenia, on the other hand, is associated with conditions that either depress the bone marrow's hematopoietic function or stress the bone marrow by exceeding bone marrow supplies or ability to replenish supplies.

Differential WBC Count. The differential WBC count is a report of the five different types of WBCs (neutrophils, basophils, eosinophils, monocytes, and lymphocytes) as a percentage of the total WBC count. The reported percentage for each cell type determines the number of mature circulating WBCs and the absolute number of the various types of WBCs. The differential count evaluates the bone marrow's ability to produce those particular cells. The differential WBC count also reflects the morphology of cells, such as the presence of abnormal WBCs or atypical lymphocytes. Lymphocyte subclasses are not a component of the differential WBC count and are not routinely quantified because the process requires specialized equipment. However, the acquired immunodeficiency syndrome (AIDS) epidemic has increased the availability of lymphocyte subclass measurements, since these measurements are integral to treatment decisions in these patients.

Under certain clinical conditions, the WBC differential may reveal an excess of immature WBCs or an excess of aged WBCs. These alterations are often referred to as "shifts." The presence of an excess number of immature cells (bands) is referred to as a "shift to the left." It is usually an indication of the presence of severe infection in which an increased quantity of immature neutrophils is released from the bone marrow. The more severe the infection, the greater the shift to the left noted in the differential count. A "right shift" usually refers to an increased number of circulating mature neutrophils, which can be observed in patients experiencing pernicious anemia, morphine addiction, or vitamin deficiency (folate or B_{12}).

On the other hand, some clinicians use the term "right shift" in a different context. Instead of viewing a shift as a reflection of the developmental stage of neutrophils (immature versus mature), a shift is viewed as the type of cell excessively prominent. In this context, a "right shift" indicates lymphocytosis seen in viral infections. Considering the different meanings, it is important and accurate to describe the laboratory observation rather than merely stating "shift to the right" or "shift to the left."

Absolute Neutrophil Count (ANC). The ANC quantifies the total number of circulating neutrophils per cubic millimeter. The ANC includes mature neutrophils ("polys" and "segs") as well as immature neutrophils ("bands"). The ANC serves as a reliable barometer of the patient's degree of risk of infection in that the lower the cell count and the longer the time the patient experiences the neutropenic state the higher the patient's risk of infection. In general, the risk of infection significantly increases if the ANC falls to certain levels (slightly increased with an ANC of 1500/mm^3, moderately increased with an ANC of 1000/mm^3, and greatly increased with an ANC of 500/mm^3). However, the patient's primary disease process also influences the risk of infection. Patients with a low ANC are at high risk of infection from their own gastrointestinal flora in addition to exogenous gram-negative bacteria, gram-positive bacteria, such as *Staphylococcus aureus* and *S. epidermitis,* and fungal infections, such as from *Candida* and *Aspergillus.* To calculate an ANC, see Table 16–4. The absolute cell count may be determined for any cell type using the same process shown in Table 16–4.

Absolute Lymphocyte Count and Lymphocyte Subsets. Although lymphocyte counts were once thought to be comparable in patients of all ages, there is recent evidence to refute this belief. This is exemplified in the change in prophylaxis of *Pneumocystis carinii* pneumonia in infants and children with HIV infection. Prophylaxis in young children is no longer started at lymphocyte counts below 200 cells/mm^3, but rather at higher and more age-appropriate levels. It appears that although the total lymphocyte count and lymphocyte subsets are an equivalent percentage of the total WBC count in all ages of patients, the infant and young child's higher WBC count yields greater absolute numbers of lymphocytes and subsets of lymphocytes. Therefore, age is an important consideration in the interpretation of the total lymphocyte count and subsets of lymphocytes, especially in children with HIV infection (Denny et al., 1992; Kotylo et al., 1993).

Tissues of Host Defense

The lymphoid system is composed of tissues, organs, and interconnecting vessels and is responsible for the production, maturation, storage, and activation of host defense cells, particularly the lymphocytes. The lymphoid system is divided into primary or secondary lymphoid tissues. Primary (central) lymphoid tissue or organs are sites for lymphopoiesis (development and maturation of B cells and T cells), whereas secondary (peripheral) lymphoid tissues and organs are the environment in which immune cells are activated to conduct host defense.

Although traditionally, primary and secondary lymphoid tissue is categorized as two discrete groups, there are exceptions to this approach. For instance, the bone marrow, although thought of as a primary lymphoid organ, is also considered a secondary lymphoid organ because it stores lymphocytes. Conversely, the spleen and liver, usually categorized as secondary organs, can serve as primary organs. In the face of bone marrow failure, the spleen and liver can become the centers of hematopoiesis (Rhoades & Pflanzer, 1992).

Primary Lymphoid Tissue and Organs

The primary (central) lymphoid tissues include the thymus and the bone marrow. The thymus gland is an encapsulated structure located in the anterior mediastinum directly behind the sternum. The thymus is very large relative to fetal body size at birth (10–15 g), reaches peak mass at puberty (30–40 g), then begins and continues to involute throughout adult life (Cooper & Buckley, 1982; Bellanti & Kadlec, 1985). The primary function of the thymus is the maturation and differentiation of T cells. In addition, the production and secretion of thymosin and other thymic hormones influence lymphopoiesis and the maturation and differentiation of the various subsets of T cells.

The human bone marrow is the location for hematopoiesis, a series of events that begins with the pluripotent stem cell and progresses to the development of a full line of functional blood cells. Through hematopoiesis, the pluripotent stem cell is capable of creating all lines of differentiated cells, including erythrocytes, granulocytes, monocytes and macrophages, lymphocytes, and platelets. In adults, hematopoiesis occurs in red bone marrow contained primarily in the flat bones, such as the sternum, ribs, skull, iliac crest, and proximal ends of long bones. However, in infancy, hematopoiesis occurs in nearly all bones. The bone marrow is also the location for B cell maturation and differentiation.

The bone marrow and associated hematopoietic function may be altered by many diseases and treat-

Table 16–4. CALCULATION OF ABSOLUTE NEUTROPHIL COUNT (ANC)

1. Obtain patient's total WBC count.	WBC = 5 k/mm^3
2. Translate the total WBC count into an absolute number ("k" means 1000 cells).	5 × 1000 = 5000 Absolute WBC count = 5000/mm^3
3. Obtain WBC differential* and add the percentages of "polys" plus "bands."†	Polys = 60% Bands = 10% 60% + 10% = 70%
4. Translate the percentage of "polys" plus "bands" into an absolute number by dividing by 100.	70% ÷ 100 = 0.7
5. Multiply the absolute WBC count by the absolute "poly" plus "band" count.	5000 × 0.7 = 3500 ANC = 3500/mm^3

*Generally, the WBC differential count is based on a sample of 100 cells. In persons with severe leukopenia, the differential count may be based on a sample of 50 cells. Conversely, in persons with leukocytosis, the differential count may be based on a sample of 200 cells. Regardless of the number of cells used for the count, the individual cells will represent an overall percentage of the total, and the same procedure outlined above is used to determine an ANC.

†Although bands are immature neutrophils, they are included in the ANC since they are relatively functional.

ments. Malignancies can have a direct impact through bone marrow infiltration by malignant cells or an indirect impact through the side effects of cytotoxic agents. Other diseases affect hematopoiesis through destruction of an individual cell line, such as that which occurs in AIDS (helper T cell) or all cell lines such as those in aplastic anemia (pluripotent stem cell). Bone marrow aspiration and biopsy provide quantitative and qualitative information regarding bone marrow function.

Secondary Lymphoid Tissue and Organs

The secondary organs include the lymph system, spleen, liver, and the mucosa-associated lymphoid tissues (MALT), including the tonsils and Peyer's patches of the gut. The secondary tissues and organs serve as the environment in which the WBCs, specifically the lymphocytes, travel to and enter any part of the body to perform their host defense functions. Lymphocyte storage and activation occur in the secondary lymphoid tissues. Bone marrow, in addition to being a primary lymphoid organ, is also a secondary lymphoid organ.

Lymphatic System. The lymphatic system is comprised of nodes, lymphatic fluid (lymph), and lymphatic vessels, and is an accessory route by which fluids can flow from the interstitial spaces into the blood. The lymphatic vessels parallel the venous system and drain into either the thoracic duct or the right lymphatic duct and eventually into the central venous circulation.

The amount of fluid or lymph collected and transported through the lymphatic system is approximately 120 mL/hour (Guyton, 1986a). As the lymph is transported through this network, it also travels through lymph nodes. Lymph nodes are strategically located at junctions of lymphatic vessels and are usually kidney-shaped, bean-sized organs. The lymph node serves as a filtering station for the WBCs to identify, process, and remove particulate matter or antigens. The lymph node also adds lymphocytes to the lymph fluid to increase the numbers of circulating lymphocytes. A lymph node biopsy and/or lymphangiography reveals information on the function of the lymphatic system.

Spleen. The spleen is the largest lymphoid organ and lies in the upper left quadrant of the child's abdomen. It is comprised of two types of tissue: red pulp and white pulp. The red pulp, containing venous sinusoid areas, is primarily concerned with the destruction and removal of old or damaged erythrocytes, whereas the white pulp contains lymphoid tissue. The function of the spleen is to filter the blood as it travels through the splenic tissue. Antigens are trapped in the filtering mechanisms, where resident B cells and T cells are activated and destroy the antigen.

Following loss of the spleen (surgical splenectomy or autosplenectomy resulting from sickle cell anemia), patients experience an increased risk of overwhelming postsplenectomy infection (OPSI), predominantly from encapsulated bacteria. In the asplenic pediatric patient, this risk is exacerbated because of other immunologic deficits, such as diminished phagocytic and complement function, and reduced immunoglobulin levels. In the asplenic patient, the liver assumes the spleen's role in clearing mature and damaged RBCs (Rhoades & Pflanzer, 1992).

Liver. Located in the upper right quadrant of the abdomen, the liver serves as a filtering organ for the blood returning from the gastrointestinal (GI) tract. Venous sinusoids within the liver are lined with large, fixed macrophages, referred to as Kupffer cells, which are highly phagocytic. Because venous portal blood has drained from the intestines, it usually contains considerable quantities of particulate matter and bacteria. Kupffer cells are capable of removing more than 99% of all particulate matter in the portal venous blood before the blood completes its course through the entire sinusoidal passages (Guyton, 1986b).

Laboratory tests, such as for hepatic enzymes and bilirubin, can indicate the quality of liver function. A liver biopsy or noninvasive procedures, such as computerized tomography (CT) or magnetic resonance imaging (MRI), provide information on the structure and function of the liver.

Mucosa Associated Lymphoid Tissues (MALT). Throughout the body there are dispersed aggregates of nonencapsulated lymphoid tissues. These tissues are referred to as mucosa associated lymphoid tissues (MALT) and are found in a variety of places, but especially in the submucosal areas of the gastrointestinal (Peyer's patches, tonsils), respiratory, and urogenital tracts (Lydyard & Grossi, 1989b). These tissues function like other secondary lymphoid tissues, but are strategically placed close to potential sites of invasion. Both macrophages and lymphocytes are present to allow nonspecific and specific activity, respectively, to occur as needed.

DEVELOPMENTAL ANATOMY AND PHYSIOLOGY OF HOST DEFENSES

First Line of Defense

The most primitive defense mechanisms of any host, healthy or compromised, are the natural barriers that provide protection from the environment. These barriers include epithelial surfaces with their unique physical, chemical, and mechanical capacities that impede the entrance of microorganisms. The major components of the first line of defense include the phenomena of colonization and bacterial interference, and the unique functions of each of the following tissues and organ systems: integumentary, respiratory, GI, genitourinary, and ophthalmologic. The structure and function of each of these barriers vary, therefore each will be discussed separately, followed by the developmental alterations noted in the infant

Table 16–5. BARRIERS: THE FIRST LINE OF DEFENSE

Integumentary	Intact skin
	Intact mucous membranes
	Acidic pH
	Bacterial interference
	Sweat glands—lysozyme
	Sebaceous glands—sebum/fatty acids
Respiratory	Intact mucous membranes
	Aerodynamic filtration
	Humidification
	Mucociliary transport system
	Bacterial interference
	Alveolar macrophages
	Lysozyme
	Secretory IgA
	Sneeze, cough, gag reflexes
Gastrointestinal	Intact mucous membranes
	Gastric acidity
	Pancreatic and intestinal secretions
	Intestinal motility
	Bacterial interference
	Secretory IgA
	Phagocytic cells
	Breast milk (lactating females)
Genitourinary	Flushing action of urination
	Acidic pH of urine
	Length of urethra (male)
	Prostatic secretions (male)
	Acidic pH of vagina (female)
	Secretory IgA
	Bacterial interference
Eye	Flushing action of tearing
	Lysozyme
	Secretory IgA
	Blink reflex

Adapted from Adams, A. (1985). External barriers to infection. *Nursing Clinics of North America, 20*(1):146.

and young child. Barriers and their unique characteristics are summarized in Table 16–5.

Colonization and Bacterial Interference

All body tissue and organ systems exposed to the external environment are composed of epithelial cell surfaces. These epithelial surfaces are normally colonized by indigenous bacterial flora that aid in the process of host defense and the prevention of infection. Colonization, the residence of microorganisms, is influenced by a variety of environmental factors including dietary intake, sanitary conditions, air pollution, and hygienic habits (Tramont, 1990). There are generally two types of flora harbored by a host: normal resident (indigenous) flora that, if disturbed, reestablishes residency easily, and transient flora that may colonize the host for varying periods of time, from hours to weeks, without taking up permanent residence.

It is thought that the presence of indigenous bacterial flora prevents or retards colonization by other potentially harmful organisms through a variety of mechanisms, but the exact phenomenon of bacterial interference is not completely understood. Known mechanisms of indigenous flora that prevent or re-

tard colonization by other organisms include competition for the same nutrients, competition for the same receptors on host cells, and production of products that are toxic to other organisms. In addition, indigenous flora provides continuous stimulation and keeps the immune system alert to respond (Adams, 1985; Tramont, 1990).

Although the newborn's skin is essentially sterile at birth (Donowitz, 1988), the acquisition and maintenance of normal epithelial flora contribute to the newborn's development of the first line defense. Within 48 hours, the newborn begins to colonize organisms that are easily obtained from the environment, nursery personnel, and family. Within approximately 6 weeks of age, the newborn's skin flora is quantitatively comparable to that of older children and adults (Leyden, 1982).

Integumentary: Skin and Mucous Membranes

The intact skin is an effective physical barrier to the penetration of microorganisms. Few organisms can directly and effectively penetrate the skin; instead they must rely on a vector (an organism that will transmit infection), a primary lesion, or a (synthetic) device for entrance (Tramont, 1990). Few organisms find the skin conducive for growth because the skin is a generally dry, mildly acidic (pH 5–6) environment. In addition, desquamation, or the natural sloughing process, hampers residence on epithelial surfaces.

The skin serves as a chemical as well as a physical barrier for the body's internal environment through the secretion of lysozyme and sebum. Secreted by the sweat gland, lysozyme can attack and lyse the cell membranes of gram-positive and gram-negative bacteria. Sebum, secreted by the sebaceous glands, is an oily substance that has been postulated to have antifungal and antibacterial properties, although none of these claims have been substantiated (Holbrook & Sybert, 1988).

The external epithelial surfaces are not the only ones with these physical and chemical properties. Mucous membranes and the internal epithelial surfaces are colonized with numerous organisms that assist with the phenomenon of bacterial interference. Virtually all secretions of mucous membranes contain lysozyme as well as immunoglobulins IgA and IgG, and significant amounts of iron-binding proteins, such as lactoferrin. Lactoferrin, among other iron-binding proteins, maintains the level of free iron below the level in which bacteria flourish.

The newborn's skin is about 1 mm thick at birth and increases to approximately twice that thickness at maturity. The newborn has scant amounts of stratum corneum, the barrier component of the skin, resulting in increased skin permeability (Malloy & Perez-Woods, 1991). The stratum corneum develops quickly and is considered an adequate barrier at 2 weeks of age (Harpin & Eutter, 1983). It is similar to that of the adult by about 4 months of age (Fairley & Rasmussen, 1983).

The sebaceous glands at birth are well developed and are active during the neonatal period under the influence of maternal androgens acquired transplacentally (Ramasastry et al., 1970). Following the neonatal period, the sebaceous glands involute and produce only small amounts of sebum until puberty (Holbrook, 1982).

The sweat glands are formed with associated patent ducts by the end of the second trimester of gestation (Hashimoto et al., 1965), although sweating has a delayed onset of several days in the newborn. Sweating is noted first on the face, then on the palms of the hands and feet, and later on the remainder of the body (Holbrook, 1982). The differences noted in sweating may be related to the immaturity of autonomic (sympathetic) control of sweating rather than the structural immaturity of the glands. Complete neural control of sweat glands is noted between 2 and 3 years of age. Diminished sweat production may result in lower quantities of bactericidal and fungicidal substances and, in some, alteration in the physical barrier of the infant/young child's skin.

Respiratory System

The respiratory tract has numerous nonspecific and specific defense mechanisms. The nonspecific mechanisms are comprised of the aerodynamic filtration; the mucociliary transport system; sneeze, cough, and gag mechanisms; and alveolar macrophages. Many foreign particles come into contact with the mucous membranes of the respiratory tract because of the turbulent airflow that is characteristic of the upper airway and tracheobronchial tree. Most particles escaping this filtration system are eliminated by the mucociliary transport system, by being entrapped in mucus and swept upward by the cilia and then expectorated or swallowed. These mechanisms are normally efficient and eliminate approximately 90% of inhaled particles.

Another major function of the upper respiratory tract, humidification, aids the filtration capacities of the lung. Small hydroscopic organisms or particles absorb water from the moist respiratory tract, enlarge in size, and are more easily phagocytized (Tramont, 1990). The respiratory tract has detoxification defenses that include diluting substances with bronchial secretions and alveolar fluids and phagocytizing substances by the alveolar macrophages (Bellanti & Kadlec, 1990).

The small airways of the infant and young child make a significantly greater contribution to airway resistance compared with those in the adult (Bellanti & Kadlec, 1990). This increase in resistance to flow places the child at greater risk for airway occlusion resulting from edema or inflammatory exudate. Normal defense mechanisms of the respiratory tract may be disrupted by such narrowing or obstruction.

Gastrointestinal System

Defense mechanisms of the GI tract include saliva; antibacterial effect of gastric acid, digestive enzymes, pancreatic secretions, intestinal secretions, and bile; intestinal motility; and indigenous flora (Adams, 1985; Bousvaros & Walker, 1990; Tramont, 1990). Most organisms enter the GI tract through the mouth and are readily destroyed either in the mouth by saliva containing antimicrobial factors, such as lysozyme and immunoglobulin A (IgA), or in the stomach by the highly acidic (normal gastric pH <4) environment. Organisms in partially digested food particles encounter both a thick intestinal mucous layer and an intact mucosal epithelium as deterrents to their viability (Adams, 1985; Bousvaros & Walker, 1990). Mucin released by goblet cells serves several purposes in the prevention of microorganism adhesion to mucosal surfaces. Goblet cell mucin contains glycoproteins that not only compete with bacteria and antigens for gut surface binding sites, but also provide a site for secretory IgA to attach and successfully bind with antigens (Bousvaros & Walker, 1990).

Pathogen attachment to mucosal epithelium is also discouraged through peristalsis. Peristalsis propels the antigen through the GI tract, decreasing the opportunity for the antigen to settle and attach. The continual shedding of epithelial cells in the intestinal tract also limits the efficacy of an infectious process.

Secretory IgA, a component of the third line of defense (specific immune response), is the predominant immunoglobulin on all mucosal surfaces. It assists in the prevention of attachment and invasion of microorganisms and in the limitation of the amount of food antigen that enters the systemic circulation from the GI mucosa (Silverman & Roy, 1983).

Secretory IgA is a form of antibody that is particularly adapted to the unique needs of the GI tract. It has three unique features: it is a double molecule, it resists digestion, and it does not activate complement. Serum IgA molecules have two antigen binding sites by which to attach to a microorganism. In contrast, the secretory IgA molecule is a "dimer" or double molecule, meaning that it is composed of two Y-shaped immunoglobulin molecules joined together at their constant segments. Thus, secretory IgA has four antigen binding sites and consequently has a greater ability to trap microorganisms and prevent attachment to and colonization of the GI tract. The epithelial cells of the GI tract provide secretory IgA with a molecule termed the "secretory piece." It is the secretory characteristic that prevents secretory IgA from being easily destroyed by the various digestive secretions and enzymes. Enzymes that microorganisms use to destroy serum IgA are often ineffective at destroying secretory IgA. Secretory IgA does not activate the complement cascade, thus preventing the triggering of an inflammatory response.

At birth, newborn saliva contains no secretory IgA, although half of infants have detectable secretory IgA levels by 28 days of age (Selner et al., 1968). Mellander and coworkers (1985) have found that levels of secretory IgA can increase toward adult levels within a few weeks of life if the host is subjected to intense exposure to microbes. Secretory IgA concentrations rise more quickly than serum IgA concentrations. There is some evidence indicating that there are only a few secretory IgA–producing cells in the submucosa of the GI tract at birth and that breast feeding may be required to obtain optimal levels of secretory IgA in that area (Goldman, Ham-Pong, & Goldblum, 1985).

Young children's serum level of IgA remains low for months, and they are dependent on an exogenous source of IgA. Breast milk provides this exogenous source of IgA as well as lactoferrin, lysozyme, and lymphocytes (Bousvaros & Walker, 1990). Breast milk can offer as much as 0.5 to 1 g of secretory IgA antibodies to the fully breastfed infant daily (Hanson et al., 1990). This amount of secretory IgA is equivalent to approximately one-third that normally produced by an average adult for defense.

Breast milk, with its many components, may aid the infant's mucosal defenses, but the exact role that each of these components plays is still undefined (Hanson et al., 1990). It is generally accepted that breast milk provides the GI tract some protection from food allergies and microorganisms until the infant's mucosal immune system matures. Lymphocytes provided in breast milk may actually attach in the lamina propria of the infant's intestinal tract (Silverman & Roy, 1983).

An additional chemical property of the GI tract is the acidity of the stomach. At birth, the gastric pH is approximately 6, but normally reaches a pH of 2 to 3 within the first 24 hours of life (Ebers et al., 1956; Grand et al., 1976). Acidity of the stomach gradually increases through childhood, then it plateaus to adult levels at 10 years of age.

The presence and function of mucin are also different in infants. Although comparative studies of mucin in human newborns and adults are not extensive, animal data suggest that newborn mucin may have a decreased ability to serve as a competitive inhibitor to certain organisms, such as *Vibrio cholerae* (cholera) (Bousvaros & Walker, 1990).

Peristaltic motion is intact at birth, with evidence that even the newborn's peristaltic contractions occur at the same frequency as the adult's (Morriss et al., 1986). However, unlike the adult's, the newborn's intestinal epithelium allows certain molecules to pass into the systemic circulation. The maturation of the intestinal epithelium is thought to occur in response to hormones and a variety of growth factors, but the specific mechanisms are unknown (Bousvaros & Walker, 1990).

Genitourinary Tract

Organisms in the lower urinary tract are normally eliminated during urinary evacuation. In addition, normally acidic urine maintains the sterility of urine. In the male, the length of the urethra provides a physical protective barrier to pathogens. Antimicro-bial substances, such as prostatic fluid secretions and secretory IgA, also assist in urinary tract defenses.

The female's vagina supports a large amount of indigenous microorganisms, primarily lactobacilli. The epithelial surfaces of the vagina contain increased amounts of glycogen, which is then metabolized into lactic acid by the bacterial flora. This creates an acidic and unfavorable environment for most potential pathogens.

Urine levels of secretory IgA may be an indication of the degree of risk for urinary tract infection (UTI). Fliedner and coworkers (1986) found that girls with a history of a UTI have lower levels of secretory IgA in the urine during noninfected periods than girls without previous UTIs. It has also been reported that urine levels of secretory IgA are elevated in children with symptomatic UTIs compared with children without infection (Svanborg Eden et al., 1985).

Ophthalmologic Defenses

The eye is equipped with eyelashes and the blink reflex to mechanically augment defenses. Tearing is the major external defense for the eye. Tears drain through the lacrimal duct and deposit organisms into the nasopharynx for the mucociliary transport system to eliminate. Tears contain high concentrations of lysozyme.

Tearing is present by approximately 6 weeks of age, and lysozyme levels in the normal infant and the adult are comparable. Stiehm and coworkers (1971) found that infant tears had a mean lysozyme level of 0.62 mg/mL compared with adult tears with a mean of 2 mg/mL. The biologic or clinical significance of these findings remains unclear.

Second Line of Defense

Penetration of microorganisms into the internal environment signifies a breach of the first line of defense. Once the internal environment is threatened through an extrinsic insult (vascular access, Foley catheter, burn, trauma, etc.) or an intrinsic insult (thrombosis, malignancy, etc.), the second line of defense is triggered. These secondary defenses, like first line defenses, are nonspecific and occur immediately and independently of the body recognizing the specific antigen. Preexisting cell types and chemical mediators form the second line of defense. This line of defense consists of inflammation, phagocytosis, and complement activation.

Inflammation

The goals of the inflammatory response are distinct and are consistently well described in the literature: the goals are to localize, dilute, and destroy the offending antigen (if present), to maintain vascular integrity and minimize tissue damage, and to transport cells and substances to the area requiring tissue repair. The inflammatory process is triggered by any cell or tissue injury. The hallmark of the inflammatory response is the release of chemical mediators, such as histamine, bradykinin (and other kinins), serotonin, and prostaglandins. The process generally begins as a localized response accompanied by classic symptoms that include erythema, edema, warmth, and pain. The systemic response marks the inability of the local response to fulfill the goals of containment and is manifested by leukocytosis, neutrophilia, fever, and others. The mechanisms of the localized inflammatory response are described first.

The immediate response to injury is vasoconstriction so that the formation of the fibrin plug and margination of leukocytes, erythrocytes, and platelets can begin. The brief period of vasoconstriction is followed by a longer period of vasodilation, manifested by redness, heat, and increased capillary permeability. Increased capillary permeability allows plasma and cells to leak out of the vascular space and attend to the tissue injury. The result of this plasma and cell movement into the tissue is interstitial swelling (edema) and the formation of an inflammatory exudate. Although the development of swelling may be physically restricting in the inflamed area, the inflammatory exudate ultimately assists in accomplishing the previously stated goals of inflammation. Pain of the inflammatory site is the result of various events, but predominant is the release of kinins and swelling or restriction of the site.

In response to the inflammation, leukocytes are released from the bone marrow and marginating pool into the circulation. Leukocytosis is indicated by an increase in WBC count from a normal count up to 30,000 cells/mm^3. The cells and/or bacteria at the site of cellular or tissue injury release substances that attract neutrophils to the site within minutes of the initial insult. The neutrophil response in inflammation predominates for the initial 24 to 48 hours. Monocytes are subsequently attracted to the site to augment the neutrophil's phagocytic activity.

Once in the general area of the inflamed tissue, the neutrophil will line up against the blood vessel wall (pavement) and migrate through the epithelial gaps of the vessel into the interstitial space by a process referred to as "diapedesis." Once in the injured tissue, the neutrophil and other phagocytes continue their purposeful movement, referred to as "chemotaxis," to the site of inflammation. Chemotactic substances are chemical substances that attract or move phagocytes to necessary sites.

Following the initial neutrophil response to inflammation, the monocyte/macrophage response predominates. This phase of the inflammatory process varies, depending on several factors. If a virus is present, the monocyte arrives and produces alpha interferon which has anti-viral properties. The monocyte may also migrate into the tissue to further differentiate into a macrophage and efficiently phagocytize bacteria, cellular debris, and dead neutrophils. The activated macrophage may then release the cytokine IL-1 to act as an endogenous pyrogen that

causes fever and inhibits further microorganism growth. The monocyte/macrophage response is a vital link between the nonspecific and specific immune responses. The response signifies the need for specific cells to enter the inflammatory response.

If the amount or virulence of a microorganism is overwhelming, or the injury is extensive, signs of a systemic inflammatory process can be seen (leukocytosis, neutrophilia, malaise, inability to gain weight or weight loss, and fever). In contrast to clear descriptions of the local inflammatory response, the description and categorization of the systemic inflammatory response have been inconsistent and unclear (Bone, 1991). Recently, the American College of Chest Physicians (ACCP) and the Society of Critical Care Medicine (SCCM) consensus conference was held to provide a conceptual and practical framework to various clinical syndromes (bacteremia, sepsis, trauma, etc.) involving a systemic inflammatory response (ACCP-SCCM, 1992). The proposed terminology recognizes that the host is an active participant in the immune response to both infectious and noninfectious insults. Although the details of the proposed terminology can be found elsewhere (ACCP-SCCM, 1992; Hazinski et al., 1993), the term *systemic inflammatory response syndrome* (SIRS) is the most applicable to this chapter. SIRS is defined as a systemic or nonlocalized response to a variety of infectious, but also noninfectious, insults (ACCP-SCCM, 1992). SIRS is manifested by two or more proposed observable and objective clinical criteria; these criteria are included in the assessment portion of this chapter.

The classic signs of the local inflammatory process may not be obvious in infants and young children, because they are less able to localize infection. Signs of a systemic inflammatory process also may be developmentally different. As noted, the normal systemic response to the inflammation is leukocytosis. However, neutropenia, rather than neutrophilia, is a common observation noted in septic newborns and young infants. This observation is most likely the result of several mechanisms including depletion of a relatively small neutrophil storage pool, a disturbed regulation of bone marrow release, and an inability of the stem cell to proliferate at a faster rate (Polin & St. Geme, 1992).

Although the quantity of peripherally circulating neutrophils is similar in the infant and the adult, the infant has considerably smaller numbers of stored neutrophils per kilogram of body weight than the adult. It is uncertain at what age the infant storage pool achieves normal adult size (Abramson et al., 1989). Because of the infant's smaller neutrophil storage pool, there is less ability to repeatedly replace the number of circulating neutrophils. Therefore, the infant's neutrophils can easily be depleted in the face of an infection, leading to neutropenia (Christensen et al., 1982).

The storage pool of neutrophils also contains various stages of developing neutrophils that are released at a time of need (Christensen et al., 1982). This may result in the release of neutrophils that are too immature to effectively function during times of increased demand or diminished supply. Release of immature neutrophils can be observed in all patients, but animal data suggest that it may be exaggerated in the infant and young child (Christensen & Rothstein, 1980).

Another developmental difference noted in the inflammatory response is the movement and mobility of phagocytic cells, particularly the neutrophil. Data suggest that the newborn's neutrophil chemotaxis is altered (Anderson et al., 1983; Masuda et al., 1989). In addition, neutrophil chemotactic activity remains unchanged for the first 24 months of life and may not reach adult activity until approximately 16 years of age (Klein et al., 1977). Monocyte chemotactic activity in infants and children is less well understood. Klein and coworkers (1977) found that monocyte chemotaxis in the infant and young child under the age of 6 years was extremely poor and significantly less than that of older children and adults. However, both deficient (Klein et al., 1977) and normal (Pahwa et al., 1977) monocyte chemotaxis have been reported.

The infant's neutrophils have less ability to aggregate and are less deformable than the adult's (Miller, 1983). The phagocyte's capacity for deformability is essential for chemotaxis and for movement through small intercellular spaces (Snyderman & Pike, 1977). The infant's neutrophil surface is more rigid, which may impair the neutrophil's movements though capillary walls and bone marrow sinusoids. This may partially explain impaired chemotaxis and, thus, the inability to localize infection.

The infant displays a much slower and less intense shift to a mononuclear cell response (Bullock et al., 1969). This is different from the mature response to inflammation with a shift from a predominantly granulocytic (neutrophil) to a predominantly mononuclear (monocyte) response occurring in approximately 24 to 48 hours. The clinical implication of this phenomenon is unclear.

Phagocytosis

The primary role of phagocytic cells is to destroy foreign substances or microorganisms. Once phagocytes are mobilized, the process of phagocytosis may begin. Phagocytosis is multiphasic. Neutrophils (and other white cells) recognize the target to be ingested, attach, ingest, and finally digest the target through a variety of intracellular antimicrobial mechanisms (Bellanti & Kadlec, 1985). Figure 16–3 presents a schematic representation of phagocytosis.

To function effectively, the neutrophil and other phagocytes must be able to migrate to the site of inflammation, then ingest and kill the target cell through bactericidal activity. The quality of the newborn's neutrophil phagocytic activity is not clearly understood. Some evidence indicates that phagocytosis in the newborn is deficient (Goldman et al., 1985), whereas others report that phagocytic activity is normal (Abramson et al., 1989; Miller, 1980). These inconsistencies are perhaps related to the experimental design and the sensitivity of the methods of measuring phagocytic activity (Miller, 1989). Phagocytic activity may change, depending on the medium within which the neutrophil functions (Miller, 1969). For instance, Dossett and coworkers (1969) found that the phagocytic activity of the neonatal neutrophil in the presence of adult sera was normal, but function was abnormal in the presence of neonatal sera. It is important to note that the contact between the phagocyte and the target cell is mediated by opsonins, and phagocytosis of these target cells may be diminished because of the reduced quantities of circulating opsonins, such as complement proteins or immunoglobulins. Although bactericidal activity of the newborn phagocyte has been reported as normal or equal to adult bactericidal activity, there is strong evidence that bactericidal activity is diminished in the presence of stress or secondary illness, such as respiratory distress syn-

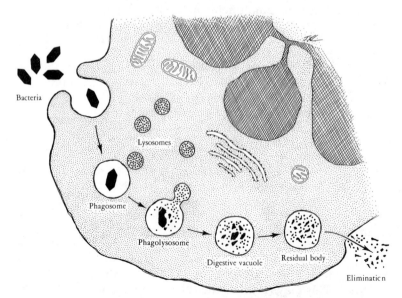

Figure 16–3 ● ● ● ● ● ●

Schematic representation of phagocytosis showing ingestion process and intracellular digestion. (From Bellanti, J. A., Kadlec, J. V. (1985). General immunobiology. In J. A. Bellanti (Ed.). *Immunology III*, p. 18. Philadelphia: W. B. Saunders.)

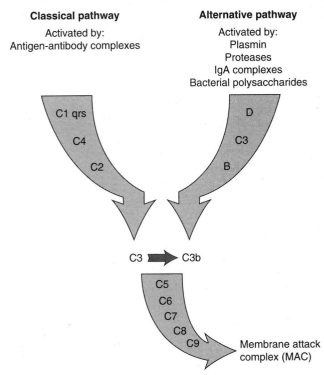

Classical pathway

Activated by:
Antigen-antibody complexes

Alternative pathway

Activated by:
Plasmin
Proteases
IgA complexes
Bacterial polysaccharides

C1 qrs
C4
C2

D
C3
B

C3 → C3b

C5
C6
C7
C8
C9

Membrane attack
complex (MAC)

Figure 16–4 ● ● ● ● ● ●

The complement system consists of two separate but interrelated enzyme cascades: the classical and alternative pathways. Each is activated by different stimuli, but the result is a final common pathway leading to enhancement of inflammation, assistance in chemotaxis, mediation of opsonization, and target membrane rupture. (Adapted from Frank, M. M. (1994). Complement and kinin. In Stites, D. P., Terr, A. I., Parslow, T. G. (Eds.). *Basic and clinical immunology*, 8th ed., p. 125. Norwalk, CT: Appleton & Lange.)

drome or sepsis (Anderson et al., 1983; Wright et al., 1975).

Impaired phagocyte function increases the infant and young child's risk of infection and impairs their ability to localize infection. The clinical consequence is a higher incidence of severe recurrent bacterial infections.

Complement System

The complement system is a complex group of more than 20 interacting proteolytic enzymes and regulating proteins that are found in plasma and extracellular fluids. The complement system, like the coagulation system, reacts sequentially in a series of enzymatic reactions in a cascading manner (Fig. 16–4).

Complement may be activated by several factors, such as the release of plasmin or protease from damaged cells or microorganisms, the formation of antigen-antibody complexes, the presence of viruses or bacteria in the circulation, the release of endotoxin by gram-negative bacteria, or the aggregation of immunoglobulins or platelets. The complement system consists of two separate but interrelated enzyme cascades: the classical pathway and the alternative pathway. Both pathways lead to the generation of C3

and C3b and a final common pathway. Activation of the classical pathway is only initiated by antibody-antigen complexes, whereas the alternative pathway does not have an absolute requirement for antibody for activation (Frank, 1994).

Activation of either pathway of the complement cascade leads to enhancement of inflammation, mediation in the opsonization process (the process of coating an organism with antibodies or proteins to increase its palatability to phagocytes), mediation of lytic destruction of cells, and assistance in chemotaxis (Wood & Sampson, 1989).

Of all of the mediators in the inflammatory response, only the complement system has been extensively investigated in the newborn (Miller, 1983). Complement synthesis by the fetus is present in the first gestational month (Goldman et al., 1985) with no evidence of placental transfer (Berger & Frank, 1989). Complement proteins gradually increase to 60% to 80% of normal adult levels at birth for the classical pathway and lower percentages for the alternative pathway (Berger & Frank, 1989; Goldman et al., 1985), but it is not until about 3 to 6 months of age that serum complement levels are within normal adult range (Goldman et al., 1985).

The young child normally possesses each component of the complement cascade, but the levels are low and may lead to a relative and subtle deficiency in complement system function. Serum complement plays a significant role in the opsonization of bacteria. The complement system also has a pivotal role in the chemotaxis of phagocytes toward the site of injury or infection. The newborn's complement system reveals diminished opsonic and chemotactic activity, especially in the alternative pathway of complement activation (Goldman et al., 1985; McCracken & Eichenwald, 1971; Polin & St. Geme, 1992). Low complement levels at birth may contribute to the newborn's afebrile and absent leukocytic response to infection (Berger & Frank, 1989).

Third Line of Defense

If nonspecific defenses fail, a specific acquired response is triggered. The specific immune response is complex and still not fully understood. Specific immunity is comprised of two different mechanisms; humoral immunity (HI), primarily involving the B cell, and cell-mediated immunity (CMI), primarily involving the T cell. Each of these two forms of immunity involves different cells, mediators, and means of function, but there is significant interaction and interdependence between the two immunities.

The distinguishing features of an acquired immune response are specificity, heterogeneity, and memory. Specificity refers to the characteristic by which an individual lymphocyte responds to its destiny or predetermined antigen. Specific immunity is also characterized by heterogeneity. Heterogeneity is the involvement of a variety of different cells and cell products that work together in diverse ways to pro-

Table 16–6. COMPARISON OF PASSIVE AND ACTIVE IMMUNITY

	Passive	Active
Genesis	No participation of the host. A transfer of preformed substances or sensitized cells from an immunized host to a nonimmune host.	Active participation of host following exposure to antigen either naturally (subclinical or clinical disease) or by immunization (vaccination).
Components of humoral and cell-mediated immunity	Cells and their products (immunoglobulin and cytokines)	Effector cells (helper T cells, cytotoxic T cells, B cells) and memory cells and their respective products.
Onset of action	Immediate	Delayed, following recognition and preparation phase of acquired immunity.
Duration	Temporary	Long-lived
Clinical application	IVIg in immune deficiency states. Prophylaxis, such as hepatitis B immunoglobulin, VZV* immunoglobulin	Vaccination

*VZV = varicella zoster virus

Modified from Herscowitz, H.B. (1985). Immunophysiology: Cell function and cellular interactions in antibody formation, p. 117. In J. Bellanti (Ed.). *Immunology III*. Philadelphia: W.B. Saunders.

tect the host. Memory, an attribute acquired by lymphocytes while participating in a first immune response with an antigen, enables lymphocytes to recall subsequent exposures to their destiny antigen. This first encounter with an antigen triggers a primary immune response. A second or subsequent exposure to an antigen, occurring months to years later, will stimulate an accelerated and augmented response because of the immunologic memory of lymphocytes.

Acquisition of Specific Immunity

Specific immunity may be "acquired" either actively or passively. Specific immunity is acquired actively when the body is exposed to a particular antigen, mounts an immune response to that antigen, and results in the formation of immunologic effector and memory cells. Contracting mumps or receiving a vaccine is an example of actively acquiring specific immunity. Specific immunity also may be acquired passively through the transfer of sensitized cells or their products (i.e., immunoglobulin) from one person to another. Maternal transfer of antibody across the placenta to the fetus is an example of passively acquiring specific immunity. The characteristics of passive and active specific immunity are contrasted in Table 16–6.

Components of Acquired Immunity

The specific immune response (Fig. 16–5) is often divided into three phases or limbs: afferent, central, and efferent. The afferent limb involves the recognition and presentation of an antigen to the B cell or T cell. The central limb involves the cloning and differentiation of activated cells as well as the production and release of cytokines. The efferent limb involves the actual elimination of the target cell or antigen. Memory cells are developed during the central and efferent limbs of the specific immune response.

Recognition Phase (Afferent Limb). The first phase of the specific immune response involves the recognition and processing of the antigen. Each lymphocyte (B cell, helper T cell, and cytotoxic T cell) requires the formation of a complex with the antigen-presenting cell and antigen to recognize the antigen as foreign and begin the activation process. The manner in which a B cell and a T cell recognize an antigen is different.

A B cell recognizes its destiny antigen when the antigen contacts the immunoglobulin projecting from the B cell's surface. Although most B cell recognition of antigens occurs with great assistance from the T cells, certain antigens can trigger B cells with little T cell assistance. This is sometimes referred to as "T cell independent" activation and occurs most often with exposure to encapsulated bacteria, such as *Haemophilus influenzae* and *Streptococcus pneumoniae*. B cells activated in this manner do not form memory cells to protect against future exposure to the microbe; in addition, these B cells can only produce the IgM class of antibody.

In contrast to the B cell, T cells recognize antigen only when the antigen is combined with HLA antigens. Class II HLA antigens are required for helper T cell activation, whereas class I HLA antigens are required for cytotoxic T cell activation.

Helper T cell antigen recognition begins with a macrophage ingesting an antigen, and converting (processing) the antigen into a form that is easily recognized by the helper T cell. The macrophage re-expresses the antigen on its cell membrane along with the class II HLA-DR antigen. The antigen-HLA complex is then presented to the unprimed helper T cell and combines with the T cell destiny antigen receptor. Helper T cell antigen recognition is also facilitated by numerous cytokines, such as IL-1, which is produced by the macrophage during its processing of the antigen. Other signals may be required for helper T cell activation, and are the focus of intense research.

Cytotoxic T cells require antigen to be combined with class I HLA antigens. For example, a cell infected with a virus projects viral antigens on its sur-

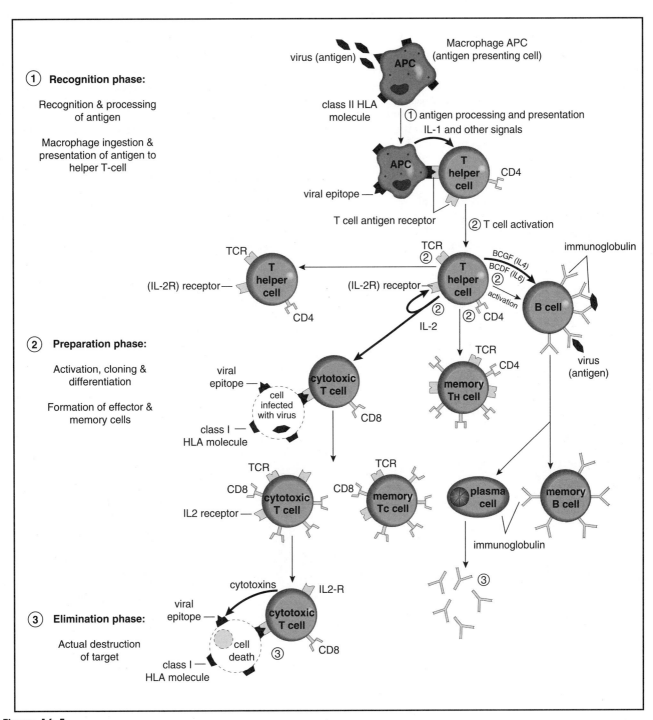

Figure 16–5 ● ● ● ● ● ●

The grand scheme of specific, acquired immunity is comprised of humoral (immunoglobulin) immunity (HI), orchestrated by the B cell, and cell-mediated immunity (CMI), orchestrated by the T cell. Note the interdependence between the B and T cells. The three phases of the specific immune response are indicated by numbers in the figure: (1) recognition phase, (2) preparation phase, and (3) elimination phase. (Adapted from Goodman, J. W. (1994). The immune response. In Stites, D. P., Terr, A. I., Parslow, T. G. (Eds.). *Basic and clinical immunology*, 8th ed., p. 43. Norwalk, CT: Appleton & Lange.)

face in combination with the cell's class I HLA antigens. The antigen-HLA complex is then presented to the appropriate, unprimed cytotoxic T cell and combines with the T cell destiny antigen receptor. IL-2, produced by the helper T cell, serves as a second signal for the cytotoxic T cell.

In utero, maternal host defense mechanisms shield the fetus from exposure to environmental antigens, and the placenta provides a shield from maternal host defenses. Although the infant is born with the capacity to perform nonspecific host defenses, the product of immunologic experience (specific host defense) is acquired (Vogler & Lawton, 1985).

At birth, the newborn is capable of recognizing self from nonself; however, there are several developmental differences regarding the presentation of the antigen to the helper T cell. Research in animals reveals marked differences in the antigen-presenting ability of immune cells between various age groups. For example, the young animal's macrophage is less able to present antigens to the helper T cell. This may be the result of the lack of the neonate's macrophage expression of HLA-DR on its cell surface (Lu & Unanue, 1985; Tweady et al., 1982). In human inves-

tigations, diminished numbers of HLA-DR monocytes have been reported in the neonate. For instance, only 10% to 25% of neonate monocytes revealed HLA-DR antigens as compared with 75% to 95% of adult monocytes (Lu & Unanue, 1985; Tweady et al., 1982). With less assistance from antigen-presenting cells, the young child's T cells may be less able to recognize antigens. This finding may influence the effectiveness of the specific immune response in the young child because recognition is the first and more important step in specific immunity.

Preparation Phase (Central Limb). Once an antigen is presented to the unprimed lymphocyte, the second phase of the specific immune response, the preparation phase, begins. During this phase lymphocytes undergo activation, cloning, and differentiation to form effector cells and memory cells. (The cloning of lymphocytes during the preparation phase accounts for the lymphadenopathy that accompanies infection. The lymph nodes are swollen because of the extensive cloning of the activated B and T cells.) Figure 16–6 is a review of the primary and secondary clonal expansion of lymphocytes in response to an antigen.

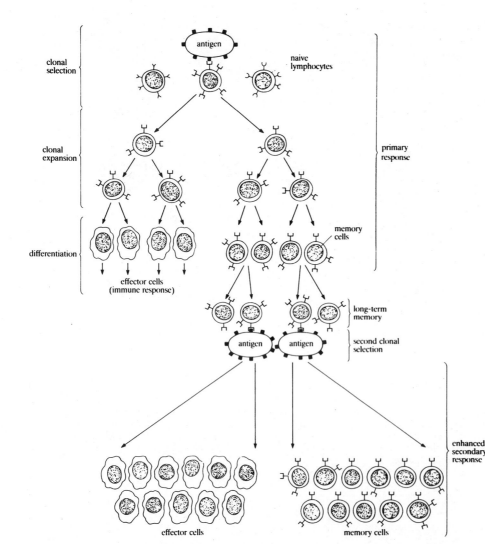

Figure 16–6 ● ● ● ● ● ●

T and B cells carrying specific antigen receptors are produced in the primary lymphoid organs and from the unprimed lymphocyte pool. Following activation by their destiny antigens (labeled antigen A in figure), lymphocytes clone and differentiate into either effector cells (e.g., cytotoxic T cells, helper T cells, or antibody-secreting plasma cells) or memory cells. This cellular proliferation constitutes the primary response. When the memory cells are again stimulated by their destiny antigens (labeled antigen A in figure), they will clone also (the secondary response). Some of these memory cells mature into effector cells, whereas other memory cells remain as memory cells, thus increasing the size of both the effector and memory cell pools. (From Davey, B. (1990). *Immunology: A foundation text*, p. 23. Englewood Cliffs, NJ: Prentice Hall.)

Table 16-7. SELECTED CYTOKINES: TARGET CELLS AND FUNCTION

Cytokine	Target Cell	Function
IL-1 (Endogenous pyrogen)	T cell, B cell, macrophage, endothelium, tissue cell	Enhances T cell growth and function Stimulates macrophages Immunoaugmentation
IL-2 (T-cell growth factor)	T cells	Promotes T cell and B cell growth Activates T cell Enhances NK activity
BCGF (IL-4)	T cells	Enhances B cell growth and function
BCDF (IL-6)	T cells	Enhances B cell growth and function
Tumor necrosis factor (TNF)	Macrophages, T cells, and others	Enhances destruction of tumor cells

Adapted from Grady, C. (1988). Host defense mechanisms: An overview. *Seminars in Oncology Nursing,* 4(2):93.

Produced by activated lymphocytes, cytokines function as regulators of the immune response. They serve as intercellular signals to support the growth and differentiation of various immune cells, the cytotoxic mechanisms of killer cells, and other effector cell functions. Table 16–7 is a review of a select number of cytokines, target cells, and their respective functions. Refer to the biotherapy section of this chapter for a discussion of cytokines and other forms of biotherapy (see p. 499).

In the past, certain cytokines were believed to be produced only by the lymphocytes; these were referred to as "lymphokines." Others were believed to be produced only by monocytes or macrophages and were referred to as "monokines." It is now known that lymphokines and monokines are actually produced by many classes of cells; hence, the term "cytokines" is the most accurate. However, the terms "lymphokine" and "monokine" continue to be commonly employed.

Effector cells are immune cells that produce the expected result of antigen destruction. Effector cells include helper T cells, which augment the entire immune response; B cells, which indirectly attack the invader through the secretion of antibody from plasma cells; and cytotoxic T cells, which directly attack the invader. The preparation phase culminates with the creation of effector cells for effective and efficient elimination of the target. Memory cells produced following activation circulate throughout the body to survey for subsequent encounters with that antigen.

Activation of helper T cells occurs early in the immune response because of their pivotal role in the orchestration of many other immunologic events. For instance, activated helper T cells secrete IL-2, which assists in the cloning and differentiation of themselves, other helper T cells, and cytotoxic T cells. Activated helper T cells also play a key role in B cell activation through the secretion of B cell growth factor (BCGF) and B cell differentiation factor (BCDF), and other cytokines.

Two communication signals are required for activation of the helper T cell. One signal is completed through the binding of the helper T cell with the macrophage. The second signal is obtained through the secretion of IL-1, which is produced during macrophage processing of the antigen. These two signals result in helper T cell expression of IL-2 receptors on its surface membrane and the production of IL-2. The primary function of IL-2 is to amplify the response initiated by the binding of the helper T cell and macrophage, and to amplify the growth of additional helper T cells expressing IL-2 receptors (Fig. 16–7).

Most frequently, activation of the B cell requires three signals: one signal from the antigen and two (or more) signals from the activated helper T cell. Following the binding of the B cell with its destiny antigen, B cell growth factor (BCGF, IL-4) stimulates proliferation of the B cell. B cell differentiation factor (BCDF, IL-6) induces the activated B cell to differentiate into antibody-secreting plasma cells. A number of B cells do not differentiate into plasma cells, but form a pool of memory cells. There is speculation that these memory cells receive insufficient amounts of BCDF to become antibody-secreting plasma cells (Goodman, 1994) (Fig. 16–8).

Activation of the cytotoxic T cell, like that of the helper T cell, requires two signals (Fig. 16–9). The first signal is the binding of the cytotoxic T cell receptor with the class I-antigen complex; the second signal results from the IL-2 produced following helper T cell activation.

Developmental alterations of the central limb are primarily noted in the development of lymphoid cell lines and their respective function. Cytokine production and release (IL-1, IL-2, BCGF, and BCDF) necessary for activation, differentiation, and cloning of lymphocytes are intact and effective.

By the ninth gestational week, the thymus has begun to develop and becomes populated with precursor T cells, referred to as "thymocytes." It is thought that direct contact with the various regions of the thymus epithelium is required for development of mature T cells (Lawton & Cooper, 1989). The thymocytes mature as they progress from the outer to inner regions of the thymus. Within the thymus, there are three distinct stages of thymocyte differentiation, described according to their surface markers (Bellanti & Kadlec, 1985; Wilson, 1985). The most immature thymocytes are found in the periphery of the cortex. Mature thymocytes are found in the thymic medulla and express either the CD4 or the CD8 surface marker. These cells also express Class I HLA antigens (Bellanti & Kadlec, 1985; Lawton & Cooper, 1989; Wilson, 1985). Figure 16–10 shows a pictorial representation of thymus gland changes with age.

Over 90% of the thymocytes that migrate to the thymus are destroyed within the thymus during maturation. It is theorized that these thymocytes recognize self molecules as foreign, and thus are destroyed to prevent them from attacking self tissue upon release to the periphery.

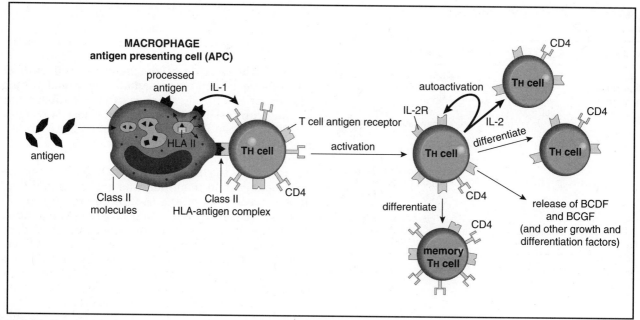

Figure 16–7 ● ● ● ● ● ●

Following the uptake and processing of the antigen by the macrophage, the antigen is reexpressed on the surface of the macrophage. The macrophage presents the Class II HLA-antigen complex to the helper T cell. Two signals are needed for helper T cell activation. The first signal is the binding of the helper T cell receptor with the Class II-antigen complex; the second signal results from the IL-1 produced during macrophage presentation of the antigen. Other signals may be needed.

The activated helper T cell expresses IL-2 receptors and produces IL-2, which triggers the cloning of helper T cells and the production of cytokines, such as BCDF (IL-4) and BCGF (IL-6). (Adapted from Goodman, J. W. (1994). The immune response. In Stites, D. P., Terr, A. I., Parslow, T. G. (Eds.). *Basic and clinical immunology*, 8th ed., p. 45. Norwalk, CT: Appleton & Lange.)

The numbers of mature T cells gradually increase in the fetal circulation with gestational age. However, the numbers of T cells present at birth vary and may be dependent on the method used for measurement. Sources reporting slightly elevated levels compared with the adult state that this finding is related to the increased numbers of suppressor T cells found in the newborn (Cooper & Buckley, 1982; Goldman et al., 1985). Other sources report significantly lower percentages than those found in the adult (Miller, 1989).

Alterations in T cell response are intertwined with alterations in monocyte/macrophage function and B cell function. Deficiencies in T cell function are multi-

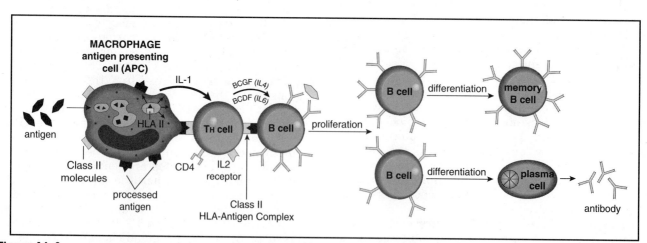

Figure 16–8 ● ● ● ● ● ●

Following the uptake and processing of the antigen by the macrophage, the antigen is reexpressed on the surface of the macrophage surface. The macrophage presents the Class II HLA-antigen complex to the helper T cell. B cell activation usually requires three signals. Following the binding of the B cell with its destiny antigen (first signal), BCGF (second signal) stimulates proliferation of the B cell. BCDF (third signal) induces differentiation. Some B cells progress to antibody-secreting plasma cells, whereas others form a pool of memory B cells. (Adapted from Goodman, J. W. (1994). The immune response. In Stites, D. P., Terr, A. I., Parslow, T. G. (Eds.). *Basic and clinical immunology*, 8th ed., p. 45. Norwalk, CT: Appleton & Lange.)

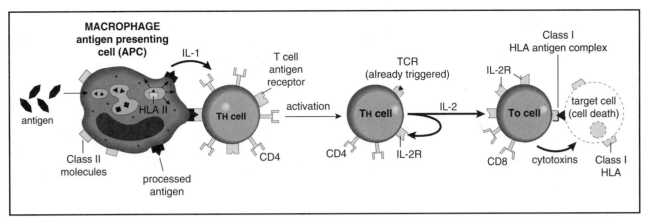

Figure 16–9 ● ● ● ● ● ●
Following the uptake and processing of the antigen by the macrophage, the antigen is reexpressed on the surface of the macrophage surface. The macrophage presents the class II HLA-antigen complex to the helper T cell. Two signals are needed for cytotoxic T cell activation. The first signal is the binding of the cytotoxic T cell receptor with the class I–HLA-antigen complex. A cell infected by a microorganism will project the invader's antigens on its surface in combination with this cell's own class I antigens. The second signal results from the IL-2 produced following helper T cell activation.

The activated cytotoxic T cell secretes toxins that eliminate the target cell. (Adapted from Goodman, J. W. (1994). The immune response. In Stites, D. P., Terr, A. I., Parslow, T. G. (Eds.). *Basic and clinical immunology*, 8th ed., p. 46. Norwalk, CT: Appleton & Lange.)

factorial, but may be the result of fewer precursors to effector T cells or a deficiency in the ability of antigen-presenting cells to activate T cells (Kamani & Douglas, 1991).

Alterations in T cell response can be illustrated by delayed hypersensitivity (DH) skin testing in which the infant and young child may not react to certain intradermal antigens. The slow maturation of skin reactivity in children may occur as a consequence of the monocyte's diminished chemotactic response

(Klein et al., 1977). On the other hand, this response may be the result of a lack of memory T cells (because of lack of antigen exposure) or overall reduced helper T cell activity, which forms the basis of the DH response.

Altered helper T cell response may also be illustrated clinically by altered B cell production of immunoglobulin. Because helper T cells play a key role in influencing the class of immunoglobulin that is made, a deficiency in helper T cells (number or function) can

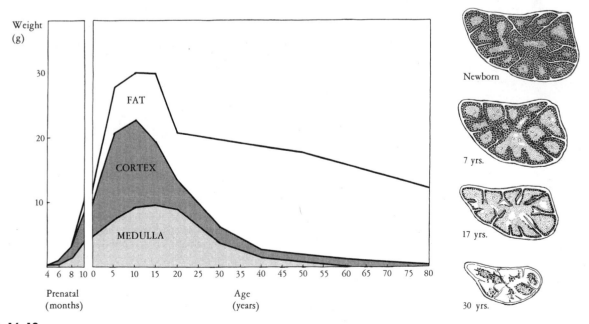

Figure 16–10 ● ● ● ● ● ●
Schematic representation of the changes in weight and composition of the thymus gland with maturation, showing involution of the gland with age. (From Bellanti, J. A., Kadlec, J. V. (1985). General immunobiology. In Bellanti, J. (Ed.). *Immunology III*, p. 44. Philadelphia: W. B. Saunders.)

result in an alteration in the type of immunoglobulin produced by B cells. A normal mature response is the elicitation of an IgM antibody response followed by an IgG antibody response within 6 to 7 days. In the newborn, the IgM response can last for 20 to 30 days with no subsequent IgG response (Douglas et al., 1989). It was previously thought that this diminished reaction was solely the result of lack of previous antigen exposure; however, the reduced number and function of helper T cells also contribute.

B cell differentiation is a discontinuous process that occurs in two distinct stages: antigen-independent and antigen-dependent phases. The first stage, which is genetically predetermined, involves the differentiation of stem cells into pre-B cells. Although the first stage of B cell differentiation begins in the fetal liver, further B cell differentiation occurs in the bone marrow when that location becomes the primary site of hematopoiesis (at 20 weeks' gestation) (Lawton & Cooper, 1989). The earliest cells committed to antibody production are termed pre-B cells, and they lack surface immunoglobulins (Vogler & Lawton, 1985). B cells with surface immunoglobulin are found in the fetal peripheral blood, bone marrow, and spleen by the 11th week of gestation (Cooper & Buckley, 1982; Lawton & Cooper, 1989) but are generally restricted to the IgM class (Abney et al., 1978; Gathings et al., 1977). As development continues, the remaining classes and subclasses of immunoglobulin appear on the surface of the mature B cell clones.

The second stage of B cell differentiation is initiated by the binding of an antigen to the unprimed, resting B cell (Lawton & Cooper, 1989). Following contact with antigen, activated B cells clone and differentiate into plasma cells to secrete antibody from a single immunoglobulin class or into memory B cells. Figure 16–11 presents B cell differentiation.

Table 16–8. SERUM IMMUNOGLOBULINS IN THE FETUS, AT BIRTH, AND AGE WITH MATURE LEVELS

Ig	Synthesis by Fetus (Gestation-Weeks)	% of Adult Levels at Birth	Age at Which Adult Levels Are Achieved
IgM	10.5 weeks	10%	1–2 years
IgD	14.0 weeks	small amt	1 year
IgG*	12.0 weeks	110%**	4–10 years
IgA	30.0 weeks	small amt or none	6–15 years
IgE	10.5 weeks	small amt	6–15 years

*Crosses placenta
**Greater than or equal to maternal level
From Rosenthal, C.H. (1989). Immunosuppression in the pediatric critical care patient. *Critical Care Nursing Clinics of North America*, 1(4):775.

Despite early differentiation of the B cell population, the infant's B cells are deficient in producing comparable adult levels and subclasses of immunoglobulins. Serum Ig levels and degree of synthesis at birth and the age in which the levels are comparable to the adult are reflected in Table 16–8. Although the IgG level seems comparable in the newborn and adult, the level reflects the transplacental acquisition of maternal antibody during, primarily, the third trimester of gestation (Wilson, 1985). The infant is lowest in immunoglobulin concentrations at about 4 to 5 months of age when maternal IgG begins to decrease through natural catabolism and when infant synthesis of immunoglobulin is low (Cooper & Buckley, 1982). This period is referred to as one of physiologic hypogammaglobulinemia (Griffin, 1986), and during this time, the infant is most susceptible to infections caused by viruses, *Candida*, and acute inflammatory bacteria (*S. aureus, S. haemolyticus, S. pneumoniae, H. influenzae* type B, *N. meningitidis*) (Pabst &

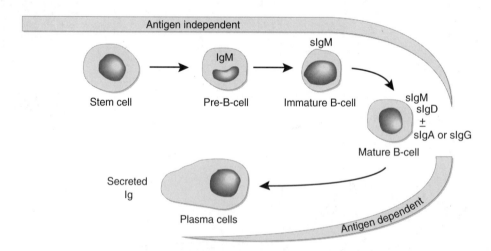

Figure 16–11 ● ● ● ● ● ●

Developmental stages of B cells. The diagram depicts the discontinuous stages of development: antigen independent and antigen dependent. The earliest cells are termed pre-B cells and contain immunoglobulin (IgM) in their cytoplasm. Immature B cells contain IgM on their surface (depicted as sIgM in the figure). As development continues, the remaining classes of immunoglobulin appear on the surface of the mature B cell clones (also depicted in the figure with an s prior to the Ig). The antigen dependent phase begins antigen binding to the unprimed mature B cell, which then differentiates into plasma cells and memory cells (not depicted in figure). (Redrawn from Lawton, A. R. (1982). In Twomey, J. J. (Ed.). *The pathophysiology of human immunologic disorders.* 11–28. Baltimore: Urban & Schwarzenberg.)

Kreth, 1980). This state can range in duration from patient to patient, and can be prolonged to such an extent that the young child suffers from recurrent and severe infections.

There are numerous explanations for minimal synthesis of fetal and newborn immunoglobulin. The rare numbers of plasma cells and small amount of immunoglobulin synthesized by the fetus are thought to reflect the normally sterile intrauterine environment and lack of antigenic exposure in utero (Miller, 1989). Maternal antibodies in the newborn's circulation may exert a strong immunosuppressive effect on the infant's ability to mount an independent immune response and to subsequently produce antibodies (Miller, 1980). In addition, the dominance of newborn suppressor T cells (Goldman et al., 1985) and bilirubin levels higher than 15 mg/dL (Nejedla, 1970) have also been implicated in the increased numbers of newborn immature B cells and decreased Ig production.

As the infant's exposure to antigen increases, a repertoire of antibodies to antigens is developed and the memory component to humoral immunity is heightened through the development of the various IgG subclasses. Intrauterine infection may also accelerate the fetus' immunoglobulin production dramatically. Following intrauterine infection and the experience with such intense antigenic stimulation, the infant may be born with adult levels of IgM and increased levels of IgG and IgA (Lawton & Cooper, 1989).

Elimination Phase (Efferent Limb). The actual elimination of the target cell or antigen occurs in the efferent limb of the specific immune response. To ensure effective destruction of the antigen, the efferent limb usually consists of a dual response by circulating antibody (HI) and effector T cells (CMI). Specific immunity elimination of the antigen occurs through the mechanisms of immunoregulation, cytotoxicity, and memory.

Immunoregulation. Immunoregulation is not well understood, but appears to be the fine balance and feedback that occur between the helper T cells and suppressor T cells. When properly balanced, there is just enough of an immune response to eliminate the invading organism, but not enough to cause host injury.

Data on the immunoregulatory function of pediatric T cells are complex. Investigators note that adult T cells are better equipped than newborn T cells at helping B cells synthesize immunoglobulin (Hayward & Lawton, 1977). Newborn T cells exhibit more suppressor activity compared with adults (Rodriguez et al., 1981). Controversy exists regarding the basis of these findings. These findings may be partly related to newborn helper T cells being less functional (see Cytotoxicity), whereas other investigators suspect an intrinsically more functional suppressor T cell or enhanced suppressor T cell function as a remnant of fetal life. Altman and coworkers (1984) suggest that the fetus has increased suppressor T cell activity to prevent maternal rejection, but this in-

creased suppressor activity remains apparent after birth. In summary, this question remains: is increased newborn suppressor T cell activity (1) the result of the immaturity of newborn helper T cells; (2) related to newborn suppressor T cells being intrinsically more active than those of adults; or (3) a remnant of fetal life to prevent maternal rejection?

Cytotoxicity. The actual killing of antigen is accomplished through cytotoxic T cell activity and is sometimes referred to as cell-mediated cytotoxicity. Cell-mediated cytotoxicity includes three basic yet distinct phases: (1) the effector cell binds to the target or antigen; (2) it degranulates, showering the target cell membrane with toxins that destroy the antigen; and (3) certain cytokines are released by activated cytotoxic T cells (i.e., tumor necrosis factor and gamma interferon), which can, by themselves, cause direct cytotoxic effects and death of the targeted cell (Rook, 1991).

The NK cell is another immune cell that is involved in cytotoxicity through a mechanism of action that is similar to that of cytotoxic T cells. It is thought that whether the killing of the antigen is the result of cytotoxic T cell or NK cell activity, the mechanisms are similar. Although both cells have similar cytotoxic mechanisms, only cytotoxic T cell activity is considered to be a third line of defense, because it is specific in nature.

Cytotoxicity is diminished in the newborn period (Miller, 1989), whether the elimination of the target is through the activity of the cytotoxic T cell, natural killer (NK) cell, or antibody-dependent cellular cytotoxicity (ADCC) (see the section on antibody-antigen interaction below). The reason for this finding is unknown, but may be related to the newborn T cell's diminished ability to produce cytokines, such as gamma-interferon and IL-4 (Lawton & Cooper, 1989; Parkman, 1991). Reduced gamma-interferon appears to be related to the reduced numbers of memory T cells. As previously reviewed, once the macrophage presents the antigen to the helper T cell, the activated T cell secretes gamma-interferon and IL-2. Gamma-interferon subsequently activates the macrophages to ingest and kill the invading intracellular pathogen. Macrophages that are not gamma-interferon activated do not kill as efficiently (Lu & Unanue, 1985). The clinical consequence of this phenomenon is a diminution of macrophage antiviral properties (Bryson et al., 1980; Cooper & Buckley, 1982) and may contribute to the severity of viral illness seen in many newborns (Parkman, 1991).

Although NK cell activity is diminished, cytotoxic activity from lymphokine-activated killer (LAK) cells is not diminished. The addition of IL-2 in vitro to nonspecific lymphocytes results in the recruitment of cells that display strong nonspecific cytotoxic activity. Newborns have been found to have an equivalent, if not a heightened, degree of LAK cell cytotoxic activity (Sancho et al., 1986).

Antibody-Antigen Interaction. There are six major antibody-antigen interactions: neutralization, agglutination, precipitation, opsonization, complement fixation, and lysis. When antibody "neutralizes" a microorganism, it renders the microorganism ineffective or incapable of action. Thus, when enough antibody molecules bind to a microorganism, it may no longer pose risk to a host cell. Antibody may also bind to toxins, thus preventing the toxin from attaching to and poisoning a host cell. Antibody can also agglutinate or precipitate an antigen, rendering it inactive by causing it to form clumps or solidify, respectively.

Antibody greatly enhances nonspecific immune responses. For instance, opsonization, the process in which antibody coats the antigen, greatly enhances the ability of phagocytes to engulf the foreign particle. The binding of antibody to antigen may also lead to activation of the complement cascade. Certain complement components produced in this process are tremendously important in enhancing phagocytosis through opsonization, attracting phagocytes through chemotaxis, and lysing bacteria.

Antibody molecules can be instrumental in destroying an antigen through a process called *antibody-dependent cellular cytotoxicity* (ADCC). During ADCC, the variable segment (Fab) of the antibody molecule attaches to an antigen while the constant segment (Fc) fits into the Fc receptor on a monocyte, neutrophil, eosinophil, NK cell, or cytotoxic T cell. This antibody-Fc receptor connection stimulates the involved immune cell (monocyte, neutrophil, eosinophil, NK cell, or cytotoxic T cell) to release poisonous chemicals to destroy the antigen by lysis.

As previously mentioned, ADCC depends on antibody (immunoglobulin). The diminished ability of newborns to destroy target cells via ADCC is related to reduced levels of antibody or reduced B cell production of immunoglobulin. Clinical ramifications of this finding include the increased number of bacterial infections noted in infants (Pabst & Kreth, 1980).

Memory. Memory cells reside in the host to await subsequent exposures to their destiny antigen. The memory cell reacts in subsequent exposures to that antigen by producing an augmented response, as compared with the primary exposure.

The secondary response to an antigen characteristically differs from the primary response in that there is a shorter latent period, a more rapid rate of antibody synthesis, and a higher peak titer of antibody that persists for a longer period of time (Davey, 1990). In addition, the dose of the antigen required to elicit a secondary response is normally much less than that required to initiate a primary response (Davey, 1990). These differences are directly related to the number of antigen-sensitive cells called memory cells.

The infant and young child have fewer memory cells. The reduced secondary immune response in these patients may be the result of either the reduced numbers of memory cells, or a reduced effectiveness of these cells during secondary immune response.

STRESSORS OF HOST DEFENSE

There are many stressors that impair host defenses. Situational stressors can be divided into three categories: (1) iatrogenic stressors, (2) transient immune dysfunctions, and (3) acquired or primary immunodeficiencies.

Based on the cause, the duration, and the reversibility of the stressor, the infant or young child's condition can be referred to as immunosuppressed or immunodeficient. Immunosuppression is a diminution in a previously competent immune system that can be intentional (as in the transplantation process or during chemotherapy) or unintentional (as the result of malnutrition). It is usually temporary. Immunodeficiency refers to a permanent immunologic state that is usually genetic or congenital in origin. Regardless of the immunologic stressor, the final common pathway of immunosuppression and immunodeficiency is the same: altered host defense, impaired immune function, and an increased susceptibility to infection. *Immunocompromise* is a global term that encompasses the terms immunosuppression and immunodeficiency and describes the patient with a less than optimal immune function and host defense. The immunocompromised patient is also at increased risk for certain types of malignancies (leukemia and lymphoma).

Iatrogenic Stressors

The critically ill child often experiences iatrogenic interference to host defenses. Common PICU diagnostic and therapeutic interventions interfering with host defense and immunologic function include anesthesia procedures (Blackburn & Menkes, 1983; Tsuda & Kahan, 1983); pharmacologic interventions such as neuromuscular blockers, narcotics, sedatives, and barbiturates; immunosuppressive therapies such as chemotherapy, radiation, and corticosteroids; and extensive blood component administration (Schot & Schuurman, 1986). The child is also subjected to numerous invasive procedures in the PICU such as tracheal intubation, and catheterization or cannulation of body orifices and cavities. Each of these stressors disrupts the child's physical, mechanical, and chemical barriers and increases the risk of nosocomial infection. Common stressors to the critically ill child's first line of defense will be explored individually.

Endotracheal tube (ETT) intubation directly bypasses the respiratory tract's local host defenses, increases the incidence of bacterial colonization, and acts as a foreign object in the airway. In bypassing the upper respiratory tract, the ETT facilitates direct access of microorganisms to the lower respiratory tract. The presence of the ETT decreases the effectiveness of the cough reflex by interfering with glottic closure. Local mucosal irritation and trauma and repeated introduction of suction catheters impede the function of the mucociliary transport (Gal, 1988).

Respiratory secretions and the endotracheal tube itself can act as reservoirs for bacteria, specifically *Pseudomonas aeruginosa* (Ramphal et al., 1987; Sheth et al., 1983; Sottile et al., 1986). Proliferation of bacteria occurs because the ETT serves as a haven for bacteria growth and is sequestered from host defenses and antibiotics (Stamm, 1978). Colonization of the child's airway occurs within 72 hours of intubation (Riggs & Lister, 1987).

The mere presence of the ETT can lead to increased mucus secretion, stagnation of mucus, airway inflammation, and tracheal mucosal injury (Levine & Niederman, 1991). As a reflex to any foreign object in the airway, secretion of mucus is increased and results in stagnation and pooling. The tracheal mucosa may be traumatized by the piston-like motion of the ETT tip along the tract of tube insertion during breathing as well as by cuff injury (in the older child) to the tracheal wall. This mechanical trauma evokes an inflammatory response and bacterial colonization (Levine & Niederman, 1991; Steen, 1988). Piston-like motion may be increased in the younger critically ill child because of the use of an uncuffed endotracheal tube.

Aspiration of bacteria from a previously colonized oropharynx or tracheobronchial tree constitutes the cause of the majority of nosocomial pneumonias. Despite inflation of the cuff, aspiration around an ETT cuff can occur (Levine & Niederman, 1991). With the use of uncuffed endotracheal tubes in the pediatric population, the incidence of aspiration can be assumed to be frequent. One survey reports aspiration in up to 70% in intubated infants and children (Browning & Graves, 1983).

Intravascular lines, specifically arterial, central venous, pulmonary artery, and peripheral intravenous catheters, are frequently used within the pediatric critical care setting. The presence and duration of use significantly increase the child's risk to bacteremia and, subsequently, nosocomial infection. All catheters must pass through the first line of defense, the epithelial surface, either through direct percutaneous or surgical cutdown insertion. With the passage of the catheter through the skin surface, the catheter has the potential to become colonized with indigenous or hospital-acquired flora. In addition, a fibrin sheath soon forms around the inserted catheter and provides an environment for bacterial growth and migration down the catheter and toward the bloodstream. These catheters may also become contaminated through infusate solution or entry sites, such as stopcocks and injection ports, and by microorganisms from other infected sites in the body (Merritt, 1992).

Many critically ill children require nasogastric tube (NG) placement, and the result of placement to host defense is essentially the same in all patients, regardless of age. The presence of the tube is thought to hinder the closure of the esophageal sphincter and to promote the reflux of gastric contents leading to a risk of aspiration pneumonia (Riggs & Lister, 1987). Because 25% to 35% of children younger than 6 months of age are thought to experience some degree of reflux without the placement of a gastric tube (Browning & Graves, 1983), the placement of a gastric tube significantly increases this risk. Pediatric

NG tubes also have small lumens and therefore have a propensity to become obstructed and are thus limited in the removal of gastric secretions.

Urinary tract infections (UTIs) are *not* the most common nosocomial infection in the pediatric population, as they are in the adult population (Hoyt, 1989; Warren, 1991), but are second to upper respiratory infections. UTIs represent only 10% of all hospital-acquired infections in children in the National Nosocomial Infection Surveillance (NNIS) Survey (Horan et al., 1986), although the incidence is higher in the critically ill child.

A urinary catheter attached to a closed urinary drainage system facilitates bacteremia in the host in a variety of ways. During placement, the catheter will "push" or "drag" urethral organisms into the bladder, and the indwelling catheter enhances bladder colonization by serving as a conduit for organism growth and movement (Warren, 1991). Urine can no longer flow through the urethra and flush microorganisms from the body.

Diagnosis of a UTI may be challenging because the infant or young child is often unable to communicate the presence of symptoms. In addition, the child in the PICU may often have multiple reasons for a fever or abdominal pain (Cobb & Danner, 1993). Children often present with age-specific signs and symptoms of urinary tract infections (Sherbotie & Cornfeld, 1991) and experience more asymptomatic bacteriuria than adults (Stull & LiPuma, 1991). These findings pose an increased risk of delayed recognition and treatment of UTI in children.

Chest tube placement offers resistance to chest wall movement because of pain and immobility (Hoyt, 1989), which results in poor clearance of respiratory secretions, decreased compliance with pulmonary toilet exercises, and thus increased incidence of pneumonias. Pediatric chest trocars, like other types of pediatric catheters, have small lumens and have a propensity to clot in the presence of blood. This leads to pooling of drainage and the risk of colonization and microorganism growth.

The incidence of nosocomial infection reflects the numerous invasions of the child's natural barriers (first line of defense). Although pediatric critical care–related nosocomial infections are not as extensively described as those in other settings, there are some reports in the literature. In addition, extrapolation and comparison of adult versus pediatric as well as ICU versus acute care patient populations are helpful. Several studies of nosocomial infections in hospitalized patients suggest that infection rates are actually lower in the pediatric patient population compared with the adult (Horan et al., 1986; Donowitz et al., 1982; Wenzel et al., 1983; Brown et al., 1985). Developmental differences must be considered when interpreting this data. For example, only 5% of adult nosocomial infections are viral in origin, whereas in children, 23% to 27% of infections are viral in origin (Ford-Jones et al., 1989; Haley et al., 1986; Welliver & McLaughlin, 1984; Valenti et al., 1980). Children also have a higher incidence of GI and upper respiratory tract infections and lower rates of urinary tract infections (Ford-Jones et al., 1989; Welliver & McLaughlin, 1984; Brown et al., 1985). Investigators considering these developmental differences report pediatric nosocomial infection rates ranging from 4.1% to 6.0% (Ford-Jones et al., 1989; Welliver & McLaughlin, 1984), which is similar to the 4.1% rate reported for hospitalized patients as a whole by the National Nosocomial Infection Surveillance (NNIS) survey of large teaching hospitals, an adult-oriented database (Horan et al., 1986). Therefore, the incidence between general pediatric and adult nosocomial infections is comparable with distinct qualitative differences.

Intensive care unit patients, regardless of age, have hospital-acquired infection rates that are two to five times higher than patients on general inpatient units (Donowitz et al., 1982; Donowitz, 1986; Wenzel et al., 1983). Mere presence in the ICU dictates the severity of illness and the need for invasive diagnostic and therapeutic interventions that place the patient at risk for nosocomial infection. It has been reported that the risk of nosocomial infection in a PICU generally rises with increasing length of stay and duration of arterial and central venous catheterization, endotracheal intubation, mechanical ventilation, intracranial pressure monitoring, and neuromuscular blockade (Milliken et al., 1988). In addition, the younger the child in the PICU, the higher the risk for infection. Infants 1 month old or younger have a two to three times higher risk for infection than patients who were at least 2 years old (Milliken et al., 1988).

Transient Immune Dysfunction

Transient immune dysfunction may result indirectly from the cause for the child's admission to the PICU. Severe musculoskeletal trauma, thermal injury, or major surgery are examples of overwhelming tissue injuries that can produce transient immunocompromise. Regardless of the type of tissue injury (trauma versus thermal injury), the resultant immunocompromise is similar and involves all components of the immune system. Infection is the most frequent fatal complication after major tissue injury (Howard, 1979; Hauser & Holbrook, 1988); the more severe the injury, the greater the immune system dysfunction, and the higher the risk of sepsis and death (Hauser & Holbrook, 1988). Every investigated component of the immune system has revealed an alteration in function following major tissue injury.

Malnutrition leads to a mosaic of changes affecting both nonspecific and specific host defenses (Gershwin et al., 1985; Chandra, 1983). Studies of infant and child mortality show the influence of nutritional state on susceptibility to infection (Scrimshaw et al., 1968). In one inter-American study of mortality in children younger than 5 years of age, nutritional deficiency was the primary or associated cause of death in 57% of cases (Scrimshaw et al., 1968).

Factors that interfere with adequate tissue perfusion and oxygen delivery, such as hypoxemia, shock, and hypothermia, affect inflammatory response, phagocytosis, and wound healing. The efficiency of neutrophils in killing bacteria is related to a level of oxygen in the tissues, not just in the circulation. For example, because an activated phagocyte's oxygen consumption increases 10 to 20 times over its resting metabolism (Hotter, 1990), it must have access to adequate oxygen to perform its phagocytic functions.

Shock produces a maldistribution of blood flow and significantly reduces the availability of oxygen to the tissues. Therefore, the immunologic effects seen in states of shock and hypoxemia are similar. In addition, animal studies indicate that hemorrhagic shock causes depression in phagocytosis (Kaplan & Saba, 1976), chemotaxis (Davis et al., 1983), and lymphocyte proliferation (Abraham & Regan, 1985).

Induced hypothermia has also been associated with an increased risk for bacterial infection (Hauser & Holbrook, 1988; Bohn et al., 1986). Laboratory studies reveal that the increased risk of infection may be a result of depressed neutrophil migration in low temperature states (Lewin, Brettman, & Holzman, 1981).

All patients with chronic renal failure, regardless of age, experience a high incidence of infection, with approximately 40% of patients dying of an infectious complication (Slavin, 1990). Although data are inconclusive and often contradictory, it is generally believed that there are many factors in the patient with renal failure that contribute to altered host defenses and increased susceptibility to infection.

The primary immune abnormality seen in patients with both acute and chronic renal failure is lymphocytopenia and a sequestration of lymphocytes to the bone marrow (Slavin, 1990). It appears that the uremic state and its effect on the blood sera is responsible for the defects seen in cellular immunity. Washed uremic lymphocytes incubated in normal blood sera respond normally as opposed to lymphocytes in uremic blood sera (Slavin, 1990).

Cardiopulmonary bypass can be viewed as an iatrogenic cause of immune dysfunction. The movement of the immune cells and proteins through the heart-lung bypass machine causes cellular destruction, complement activation, and other changes that result in impaired immune function (Hauser & Holbrook, 1988). It has been reported in animals and adults that the rapid flow through the bypass machine results in decreased complement levels, decreased immunoglobulin levels, increased leukocyte adherence, depressed phagocytosis, and a transient neutropenia (Utley, 1982). Similar findings are reported in children following cardiac surgery (Hauser et al., 1991). Depressed complement levels have been noted postoperatively in children and were still observed 24 hours following surgery (Hauser et al., 1991). This finding is in contrast to the observation in adults of a return to preoperative complement levels within 4 hours postoperatively (Chiu & Samson, 1984). Other immunologic findings following pediatric cardiac surgery include lymphopenia, decreased helper T cells, and decreased levels of IgG and IgM (Hauser et al., 1991). Minimal information is available on the effect of extracorporeal membrane oxygenation (ECMO) or cardiac assist devices on host defenses.

Acquired or Primary Immunodeficiencies

Acquired Immunodeficiency Syndrome (AIDS)

Children are most often infected by HIV by being born to mothers who are infected with the virus, but they also are infected during transfusions of blood components (i.e., factor VIII), and at times, through sexual abuse (Cooper et al., 1988). Pediatric patients with AIDS experience immunocompromise through profound defects in various components of the immune system, especially defects in the helper T cell and B cell functions (Albano & Pizzo, 1988). Whereas the adult AIDS patient typically experiences a preponderance of opportunistic infections, the pediatric AIDS patient typically experiences a higher incidence of bacterial infections. It is thought that bacterial infections are more common in the child because of the greater degree and the earlier onset of B cell abnormalities (Albano & Pizzo, 1988). Chapter 28 provides discussion of the critically ill child with HIV infection.

Primary Immunodeficiency

Unlike AIDS, primary immunodeficiency syndromes are rare and infrequently recognized (Rotrosen & Gallin, 1990). Approximately 400 new cases of immunodeficiency are reported in the United States each year (Stiehm, 1989) and the relative distribution of immunodeficiencies is shown in Figure 16–12. Primary immunodeficiencies are conventionally divided into disorders involving B cells, T cells, phagocytes, complement, or a combination.

B Cell Disorders. Unlike the growing number of patients with T cell disorders, the number of patients with B cell disorders is stable (Heinzel, 1989). Antibody deficiencies are the most common B cell disorders and are present in approximately one-half of the patients with primary immunodeficiency (Rotrosen & Gallin, 1990; Wood & Sampson, 1989). Patients with B cell disorders have a diminished ability to form immunoglobulins and consequently are unable to generate effective antibody-antigen interactions (Heinzel, 1989).

B cell disorders are a diverse group of immunodeficiencies, and may be manifested as a deficiency in all classes of immunoglobulins (panhypogammaglobulinemia), a deficiency in only one class of immunoglobulin, or a combination of deficiencies in some classes with overproduction of immunoglobulin in another class. In most articles, discussions of B cell deficiencies are separated from those of T cell defi-

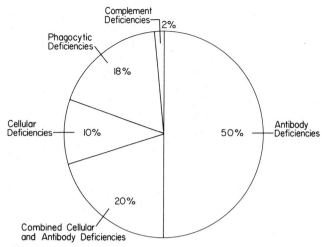

Figure 16–12 ● ● ● ● ● ●

Relative distribution of the primary immunodeficiencies. (From Stiehm, E. R. (1989). Immunodeficiency disorders: General considerations. In Stiehm, E. R. (Ed.). *Immunological disorders in infants and children*, 3rd ed., p. 158. Philadelphia: W. B. Saunders.)

ciencies, when in fact the B cell deficiencies are frequently intertwined with T cell dysfunction. In addition, the literature contains commonly used terms that are not accurate or current with recent advances in immunology. For example, the child with X-linked "agammaglobulinemia" actually has measurable levels of antibody; however, levels are so low as to be clinically insignificant. Consequently, it is more accurate to refer to the child as having panhypogammaglobulinemia.

The pattern of infection associated with B cell disorders is characteristically recurrent sinopulmonary tract infections with encapsulated bacteria and, less frequently, gram-negative organisms (Heinzel, 1989). Pyogenic bacteria, such as pneumococci, meningococci, streptococci, *H. influenzae*, and enteroviruses are common etiologic organisms. Because of the deficiency in the ability to form antibodies from mature plasma cells, reinfection from the same organism is common, even following normal childhood immunization.

T Cell Disorders. T cell disorders are present in approximately 40% of patients with primary immunodeficiencies (Rotrosen & Gallin, 1990); however, 75% of these cases are associated concomitantly with antibody deficiencies. Patients with T cell disorders have a limited ability to produce mature T cells and therefore are unable to assist with the activation of the immune response. This results in the survival and replication of intracellular organisms inside host immune cells. The microorganisms associated with T cell disorders are characteristically viruses, fungi, protozoa, and intracellular bacteria (Wood & Sampson, 1989; Young, 1989). Patients with T cell disorders also experience an increased incidence of certain malignancies (such as leukemia or lymphoma), possibly because there may be uncontrolled T cell regulation of B cell growth (Wood & Sampson, 1989).

Phagocytic Disorders. Patients who have phagocytic disorders have either an insufficient number or inadequate function of neutrophils and monocytes and/or macrophages. Impaired phagocytic function may be further classified as chemotactic, opsonic, ingestion, or killing defects. Infection patterns are similar to those seen in patients with B cell disorders, although the severity of infection often equals or surpasses that of B cell disorders (Cooper & Buckley, 1982). Patients with phagocytic disorders involving inadequate functioning are considered at risk for infection despite a "normal" WBC count.

Complement Deficiencies. Deficiencies have been described for each of the key components of complement; however, an increase in the susceptibility to infection is commonly noted for deficiencies in C2, C3, C5, C6, C7, and C8 (Cooper & Buckley, 1982). Infection patterns vary depending on which component of complement is deficient. For instance, infections in a child with deficiencies of C2 and C3 are similar to those in a child with a B cell disorder. The child with a complement deficiency in terminal complement components (C5 through C8) has infections from meningococcal or gonococcal organisms (Cooper & Buckley, 1982).

Combined Immunodeficiencies. There are several rare disorders that are based on a combined immunodeficiency of both HI and CMI. These disorders are the most severe of all the immunodeficiencies because the child is unable to form antibody and lacks T cells to orchestrate the immune response and to destroy cells infected with intracellular microorganisms. Persons with combined B and T cell disorders suffer from multiple severe infections (bacterial, fungal, viral, and protozoal); diarrhea; and muscle wasting.

A well-known example of a combined B and T cell disorders is severe combined immunodeficiency disease (SCID). SCID is a rare inherited disorder occurring in only one in 1 million live births in the United States. SCID may be caused by several immunologic abnormalities, but all result in the lack of development or function in B cells and T cells. One form of SCID occurs as a consequence of adenosine deaminase deficiency (ADA). B and T cells produce chemicals that can accumulate to toxic levels within these cells. Normally, these cells produce an enzyme (ADA) that destroys the excess amount of the toxins. In the child with ADA deficiency, this key "detoxifying enzyme" is missing, resulting in the accumulation of this toxin and the poisoning of the B and T cells.

COLLABORATIVE MANAGEMENT OF ALTERED HOST DEFENSES

Patients with actual or potential impaired host defenses require a collaborative approach to management. Comprehensive patient assessment is an integral component to collaborative management. Interventions for the child with or at risk for impaired host defenses can be categorized into three therapeutic collaborative goals: (1) augmentation of the host immune response; (2) prevention of infection; and (3) treatment of infections.

Assessment of the Patient

It is imperative that comprehensive assessments of the critically ill child include an immunologic component. Assessing the patient's host defenses begins with the identification of risk factors. The critically ill child presents with many factors that are known to impair host defense or immune function. These risk factors include young age; presenting illness and associated interventions; poor nutritional status; and past medical history including immunization, childhood diseases, and stress. Although these factors and their associated effects are reviewed in other sections of this chapter, it is imperative that they be assessed as a part of the patient history and addressed in the patient's plan of care.

Assessment of childhood immunizations, in addition to immunizations received for foreign travel, should be included in the patient's history. With the discovery and use of vaccinations, the incidence of several childhood infectious diseases has been greatly reduced, and in some cases, eradicated (Slota, 1993). Compliance with immunization schedules is to the credit of many school systems, who mandate up-to-date immunization records for matriculated children. However, many young children not yet enrolled in school may lack immunizations.

The results of recent tuberculosis screening, either through skin testing or chest radiographs should be included in the patient's history. Blood component transfusion history includes the patient's experience with and total number of past transfusions, and the year in which these transfusions occurred. These data help identify patients who may have developed antibodies to cells or substances in blood components as well as the patient who is at risk for blood-borne infections, such as hepatitis B or C, cytomegalovirus (CMV), and HIV.

The adolescent and young adult should also have a sexual history completed. Sexual activity is a risk factor for impaired immune function. Unprotected sexual intercourse increases the likelihood of exposure to and acquisition of HIV infection and other sexually transmitted diseases. This risk is increased with intercourse involving multiple, homosexual, or intravenous drug–abusing partners.

The child's past medical history should also include details of chronic or recurrent infections. A careful, detailed history assists in separating the immunologically competent child from the child with "too many infections." A healthy young child may experience six to eight respiratory infections per year and more than eight if the child is exposed to siblings or other children in day care settings (Wood & Sampson, 1989). Cues, such as repeated infections without a symptom-free interval, increased dependency on antibiotics, unexpected or severe complications to infection, or infection with an unusual or opportunistic organism, are often a significant part of the history of a child with primary immunodeficiency.

Although a primary immunodeficiency may be suspected in the young child who presents with a life-threatening infection in the first year of life or with a history of chronic or recurrent infections, it is also important to consider nonimmunologic causes of "too many infections" (Stiehm, 1989).

In addition to exploring the past medical history of the patient, a comprehensive family history is helpful. Primary immunodeficiencies, in particular, may have a clear pattern of inheritance (Wood & Sampson, 1989).

Physical and Laboratory Assessment

Comprehensive assessment and monitoring of immune cells, tissues, and organ systems, followed by observation of the first, second, and third line of defense, are imperative.

First Line of Defense. Any sign of a disruption in host defense or an infectious process should be noted, documented, and addressed in the patient's plan of care. Table 16–9 reflects physical assessment findings from the immunologic perspective. Pediatric critical care nurses can easily incorporate an immunologic assessment into a routine nursing assessment.

Laboratory assessment of the first line of defense includes cultures of sputum, wound, stool, urine, and other body fluids. Bedside analysis of gastric and urinary pH assists in determining the status of the child's chemical barriers.

Table 16–9. IMMUNOLOGIC PHYSICAL ASSESSMENT FINDINGS

Category/System	Assessment Findings
Skin/hygiene	Altered temperature, diminished turgor, dehydration, signs of infection, oral lesions, breaks in integrity, purpura, palpable lymph nodes, rhinitis, dermatitis, urticaria, eczema
Mobility/comfort	Decrease in level of activity, muscle weakness, fever, chills, joint swelling or tenderness
Respiratory	Altered rate/depth of respirations, wheezing, crackles, bronchospasm, cough, hypoxemia
Cardiovascular	Vasculitis, pale skin and mucous membranes
Gastrointestinal	Altered bowel sounds, vomiting, chronic diarrhea, hepatosplenomegaly, protuberant abdomen (not age appropriate)
Neurologic	Altered level of consciousness, deficits in sensory and/or motor function, diminished cranial nerve function (blink, tear, cough, swallow, and gag)

Modified from C.H. Rosenthal (1989). Immunosuppression in the pediatric critical care patient. *Critical Care Nursing Clinics of North America*, 1(4):781.

Second Line of Defense. The presence or absence of the inflammatory response is directly assessed by the nurse, with phagocytosis and complement activation indirectly demonstrated by pus formation and fever. All disruptions in epithelial surfaces are assessed for the cardinal signs and symptoms of the inflammatory response. It is important to note those situations in which the cardinal signs of the local inflammatory response (redness, inflammation, induration, and drainage) may be diminished or absent—in the newborn infant, neutropenic patients, or patients receiving medications suppressing the inflammatory response. In addition, the newborn may have a delayed or limited ability to localize infection. In these patients, the most reliable sign of local inflammatory response is often pain at the site of infection.

Signs of diffuse inflammatory response must also be noted. As previously mentioned, the ACCP-SCCM consensus conference has proposed objective criteria characterizing the systemic inflammatory response syndrome (SIRS). The patient is classified as experiencing SIRS with acute development of more than one of the following criteria (ACCP-SCCM, 1992):

- Fever (temperature >38°C) or hypothermia (temperature <36°)
- Tachycardia (heart rate >90 beats/minute)
- Tachypnea (respiratory rate >20 breaths/minute) or Pa_{CO_2}< 32 torr
- Leukocytosis (WBC count >12,000 cells/mm^3), leukopenia (WBC <4,000 cells/mm^3), or >10% bands (immature neutrophils)

Although criteria were developed from an adult patient perspective, they are easily translated into age-appropriate criteria. Given that alterations in temperature and WBC counts are similar in patients, regardless of age, only heart rate and respiratory rate criteria require age-appropriate modification. A systemic inflammatory response is also characterized by weight loss, fatigue, malaise, and change in eating or feeding behaviors.

In critical care patients, as well as in neutropenic patients, fever is the most reliable sign of systemic inflammation. Fever is caused by pyrogens, exogenous or endogenous substances that cause the hypothalamus to adjust the temperature set-point upward. Exogenous pyrogens are derived outside of the host and are commonly microbial products, toxins, or the microbes themselves. The lipopolysaccharide produced by gram-negative bacteria is an example of an exogenous pyrogen and is commonly referred to as "endotoxin." Endogenous pyrogens are polypeptides that are produced by host immune cells, most commonly IL-1 produced by the monocyte and macrophage. Numerous other cytokines, including tumor necrosis factor (TNF), alpha-interferon, and IL-6, are also pyrogenic.

Temperatures above 39°C can contribute to host defense by augmenting T cell and B cell activity, and leading to cytotoxic T cell generation and immunoglobulin synthesis. In addition, in vitro microbial growth is suppressed at elevated temperatures. Despite these advantages in host defense, fever is often treated with antipyretics and other measures. This is especially true in the critically ill child because fever increases the child's already high metabolic rate. It is controversial as to whether reducing an elevated temperature adversely affects the outcome of patients with fever (Dinarello & Wolff, 1990).

The chest radiograph is another tool for assessing the second line of defense. However, just as other signs and symptoms of infection are masked during neutropenia, the chest radiograph may be unreliable in revealing pneumonia in the immunocompromised child, particularly the child with neutropenia. The immune response in the neutropenic child may be so diminished that even in a child with a fulminant pneumonia, the chest film may appear normal. In this patient population, once the neutrophil count begins to increase to a near-normal level, the chest x-ray appearance may often worsen, revealing the existing pneumonia.

The erythrocyte sedimentation rate (ESR) is a laboratory test that is a nonspecific indicator of systemic inflammation. In many cases, the ESR is so nonspecific that it has little clinical utility. However, in the immunocompromised child, it may be one of the few objective measurements of response to therapy or relapse. Normal values range from 0 to 25 mm/hour for males and 0 to 42 mm/hour for females.

The complement system is sometimes evaluated because of the pivotal role these proteins play in the inflammatory response and in humoral immunity. To test the integrity of the entire complement system, a total hemolytic complement (CH_{50}) level is measured, with normal values ranging from 25 to 70 units/mL (Fishbach, 1992).

Individual complement proteins, such as C3 and C4, can be quantified and the function of certain complement components evaluated. Levels of C3, the complement protein common to both pathways, normally measure 100 to 200 mg/dL. C4 levels are critical to the function of the classical pathway, with

normal serum levels ranging from 10 to 30 mg/dL. A reduction of levels of individual complement proteins or CH_{50} can be the result of either underproduction of complement or excess complement activation, or both. Therefore, additional complement function testing may be needed to identify the exact nature of the presenting patient problem.

Third Line of Defense. The third line of defense, specific immunity, is assessed through a comprehensive examination of the patient's history, clinical course, and data from laboratory testing. Laboratory testing is an attempt to reveal the immune system's ability to recognize and process foreign antigens, recall previous exposure to antigens, and produce normal amounts of effector cells to the antigens. The laboratory tests also evaluate the competence of these effector cells to antigens. Testing is often categorized into those tests that measure individual elements of the immune system (quantitative) and those tests that measure the immune response to an antigen (qualitative).

The most common quantitative tests to evaluate overall immune function include the complete blood count (CBC), total WBC count, differential WBC count, and immunoglobulin levels. Many laboratories also measure lymphocyte subclasses, T cells, and T cell subclasses.

The total immunoglobulin (Ig) level and levels for the various classes and subclasses can be determined. Normal Ig levels vary with age; therefore, it is imperative that age-adjusted values be used for all comparisons (Table 16–10 gives levels for serum Ig according to age). Ig levels can be diagnostic for congenital primary immunodeficiencies. However, if Ig levels are normal in spite of suspected immunodeficiency, an examination of the function and effectiveness of the immunoglobulin to an antigen may be indicated (qualitative testing).

Serologic testing for either antibodies or antigens can also be performed to detect current or past infection (bacterial, viral, fungal, or parasitic). A well known example of serologic testing is the enzyme-linked immunoabsorbent assay (ELISA) that is used

Table 16–10. LEVELS OF SERUM IMMUNOGLOBULINS IN NORMAL SUBJECTS AT DIFFERENT AGES

Age	Total Ig (mg/dL) Range	IgG (mg/dL) Range	IgM (mg/dL) Range	IgA (mg/dL) Range
Newborn	660–1,439	645–1,244	5–30	0–11
1–3 mos	324–699	272–762	16–67	6–56
4–6 mos	228–1,232	206–1,125	10–83	8–93
7–12 mos	327–1,687	279–1,533	22–147	16–98
13–24 mos	398–1,586	258–1,393	14–114	19–119
25–36 mos	499–1,418	419–1,274	28–113	19–235
3–5 yrs	730–1,771	569–1,597	22–100	55–152
6–8 yrs	640–1,725	559–1,492	27–118	54–221
9–11 yrs	966–1,639	779–1,456	35–132	12–208
12–16 yrs	833–1,284	726–1,085	35–72	70–229
Adult	730–2,365	569–1,919	47–147	61–330

From Stiehm, E.R., & Fudenberg, H.H. (1966). Serum levels of immune globulins in health and disease: A survey. *Pediatrics, 37*(5):717. Reprinted by permission of *Pediatrics*.

to screen blood products for, and identify persons infected with, HIV. The presence of antigens of a particular organism is an indication that the patient is currently infected with that organism. For example, the presence of *Clostridium difficile* toxin in the stool indicates the child is infected with *C. difficile*.

The presence of antibodies to a microorganism indicates an infection; the particular class of antibody can indicate if the infection occurred in the past, is occurring acutely, or is chronic. During an acute infection the initial manufactured Ig is IgM. If the infection is particularly severe, the microorganism's antigens may overwhelm and exceed the neutralizing capacity of antibody, resulting in the presence of measurable antigen in the serum. Later, the main Ig manufactured is IgG, and the antigen will no longer be measurable because the immune response successfully eradicated the infection. A child with an acute CMV infection will have anti-CMV IgM, whereas anti-CMV IgG would indicate past CMV infection. During chronic infections, the serum may contain both IgG and IgM antibodies to the microorganism as well as antigens of the microorganism.

Cell-mediated immune function (T cell responsiveness) is evaluated by using delayed hypersensitivity (DH) skin testing. DH skin testing involves the intradermal administration of antigens. The premise of DH skin testing is that if sensitized T cells to that antigen are present, the injection will cause the body to mount an inflammatory response. Because DH response depends on the T cell's prior exposure to the specific antigen as well as normal cellular chemotaxis, it is imperative to remember developmental differences in the infant and young child. The child may lack previous exposure to antigens and thus may not recognize the antigen as foreign and may not mount an immune response (Miller, 1977).

DH skin testing is performed by using one or more of the following widely accepted antigens; intermediate strength *Candida, Trichophyton*, tetanus, or mumps antigen. One or more of these antigens is injected intradermally with the dermal reaction evaluated at 24, 36, and 48 hours after application. A positive reaction is manifested by induration (hardened swelling), not erythema, and indicates intact cell-mediated immunity. The lack of dermal response indicates anergy, a lack of cell-mediated immunity, to the antigen. For example, intermediate strength purified protein derivative (PPD) is used to evaluate past exposure to tuberculosis. A positive response indicates that the child has been infected by *Mycobacterium tuberculosis*. A negative response may indicate that the child is not infected, but would also occur if the child was anergic.

In contrast to DH skin testing, immediate hypersensitivity testing determines a patient's sensitivity to allergens such as dust, animal hair, and others. DH and immediate hypersensitivity skin testing differ in purpose, immune cells involved, antigens used, the technique of administration, and the time that the tests are read.

Collaborative Interventions

Augmentation of Host Defenses

The PICU has a high incidence of nosocomial infections that are the result of impaired host defenses, rather than the virulence and numbers of microbes in the pediatric critical care environment (Espersen, 1986). Therefore, infection control procedures alone are inadequate to protect host defenses in critically ill infants and children. Instead, host defense must be supported through a systematic nursing framework. A framework modified from one proposed by Espersen (1986) is used for providing support to host defenses and includes the following five interventions:

- Maintain external barriers
- Provide nutritional support
- Reduce stress
- Optimize patient comfort
- Manipulate and augment immunologic function

Maintain External Barriers. Intact skin and mucous membranes can be preserved by maintaining adequate perfusion and oxygenation and accurate fluid intake (including modification for fever and daily insensible water losses). In addition, the promotion of active or passive range of motion will help in the preservation of skin integrity. The PICU nurse most often performs a complete assessment of the child's skin integrity during the daily bath and associated activities. Any sign of redness or disruption in the skin should be monitored. Adding small measures to routine nursing care can contribute significantly to host defense. For example, using a nonacetone adhesive remover when loosening tape or electrodes (assuring that this solution is removed) and skin preparation solutions before applying dressings can preserve the outer layers of the child's epidermis. Routine and careful mouth, eye, and perineal care may protect the child's mucous membranes and body orifices.

Promoting the evacuation and cleansing of organ systems such as the respiratory, GI, and genitourinary tracts is vital. Each of these epithelial-lined tracts is protected with a combination of secretory IgA, lactoferrin, lysozyme, and acidic lipid secretions that decrease pathogen takeover. Recognizing the importance of pulmonary, gut, bowel, and urinary evacuation in limiting the growth of enteric flora can diminish the child's risk of infection (Espersen, 1986; Griffin, 1986; Massanari, 1989). Nursing interventions may include implementing pulmonary toilet, maintaining adequate hydration, monitoring bowel activity, establishing a bowel routine, and facilitating the patency and functioning of the gastrointestinal or urinary drainage systems.

Provide Nutritional Support. The link between nutritional status and immunocompetence has been established (Cooper & Buckley, 1982). The PICU nurse has an active role in determining the timing, route, and tolerance of nutritional support. In the critically ill child, the GI tract should be used to provide nutritional support, if appropriate. It is well documented that use of the GI tract for enteral feeding, rather than parenteral nutrition, is advantageous because it will decrease the incidence of bacterial translocation across the gut lining (Mainous et al., 1994). In addition, infants with lactating mothers should be given breast milk as a component of their nutrition support because of the many advantages of breast milk in mucosal immunity.

If the child is able to take nutrition by mouth, encouragement of the child's food and fluid intake should take into consideration the child's likes and dislikes, the manner in which the child prefers food (fried versus boiled), and the time at which the child is accustomed to eating. The PICU nurse should ensure that the child has a "safe time" to eat without actual or perceived interruption, threat, or invasion. The child's developmental needs are especially important to consider in the promotion of nutritional intake.

Reduce Stress. Investigators of psychoneuroimmunology, the exploration of the interactions between the brain and the immune system and the influence on health, suggests that stress adversely affects immune function (Locke, 1982; Sternberg, 1992). The immune system and nervous system are interconnected by a complex system of chemical signals in the form of cytokines and hormones. Through these signals, each system communicates with and influences the functioning of the other system. The immune system communicates with the nervous system through cytokines released by activated immune cells. The nervous system influences immune system functioning through the action of hormones such as ACTH released from the pituitary (under the influence of the hypothalamus), norepinephrine released from the sympathetic nerves, epinephrine released by the adrenal medulla, and glucocorticoids released by the adrenal cortex (Sternberg, 1992).

Data from animal studies suggest that stress, unaccompanied by injury, depresses CMI (Hauser & Holbrook, 1988). The individual's cognitive, behavioral, and physical response to stress may also modulate or amplify the effect of stress on the immune system. In other words, stress alone may not be as immunosuppressive as is maladaptive coping to stress (Locke, 1982). The young child is particularly vulnerable to psychological stress because of limited or immature cognitive and developmental levels and lack of understanding of the critical care environment and interventions (Rosenthal, 1989).

Reducing stress in the critically ill child can be a challenge. Recognizing the child's cognitive as well as physical age and the associated developmental tasks and fears is the first step in planning stress reduction for the child. A basic stress reduction intervention includes respecting the child as an individual and respecting the right to privacy and personal body space. Recognizing and accepting the child's need for regression while providing as calm, caring, and

reassuring an environment as possible is vital to the coping of the critically ill child and family. Reducing the stress of parents and siblings has an indirect but beneficial effect on the child and should be incorporated into the child's plan of care.

Optimize Patient Comfort. Striving for and establishing comfort in the pediatric critical care patient is important not only because of the body-mind link of psychoneuroimmunology, but also in assisting the child's relative degree of cooperation with the environment, staff, and nursing and medical regimens. Nurses often play a pivotal role in the determination of the need for and the adequacy of analgesic and sedative medication. Administration of analgesics, sedatives, and narcotics (opiates) aids in comforting the child during physically and psychologically painful experiences. However, long-term use of these medications may also alter immune function and host defenses. The PICU nurse must maintain the balance between enhanced child comfort and overmedicating, which may reduce immune function.

Manipulate and Augment Immunologic Function. A rapidly changing frontier in the field of immunology is the practice of manipulating and augmenting the immune system. Although the details of these methods are beyond the scope of this chapter, intravenous immunoglobulin and the various forms of biotherapy are discussed.

Intravenous immunoglobulin (IVIg) is a solution of immunoglobulin containing many antibodies normally present in adult human blood. It is obtained from plasma-pooled whole blood of thousands of diverse adult donors, ensuring a broad spectrum of antibodies. More than 90% of IVIg solution consists of IgG immunoglobulin. The manufacturing process ensures that the levels of IgA and IgM are low to reduce the rare incidence of anaphylaxis (predominantly resulting from anti-IgA antibodies) and hemolytic transfusion reaction (predominantly resulting from IgM antibodies of the ABO and Rh blood system).

IVIg has many clinical applications, but the mechanism of action may vary related to the disease state for which the IVIg is given. Table 16–11 illustrates the various disease states and clinical conditions for which IVIg has been administered; however, the efficacy in many of these states remains unclear (NIH Consensus Conference, 1990). It was initially developed to provide passive immunity and prevent infections in persons with primary immunodeficiencies who were unable to produce or maintain adequate levels of IgG.

IVIg may be administered to persons who have been exposed to an infectious disease in which a protective vaccine is not available. It may also be administered to reduce the number or severity of infections, such as for the child with AIDS, a child undergoing bone marrow transplantation, and a low birthweight infant.

IVIg is used in many other clinical conditions because it has immunomodulatory effects that are not well characterized but are the focus of intense re-

Table 16–11. CONDITIONS IN WHICH IVIg HAS BEEN USED

Primary immunodeficiency
Hypogammaglobulinemia
Common variable immunodeficiency
Severe combined immunodeficiency
Wiskott-Aldrich syndrome
Secondary immunodeficiency
Pediatric acquired immunodeficiency syndrome (AIDS)
Bone marrow transplantation
**Inflammatory or autoimmune disorders
  (immunomodulatory)**
Kawasaki syndrome
Guillain-Barré syndrome
Immune hemolytic anemia
Immune neutropenia
Idiopathic thrombocytopenic purpura (ITP)
Condition with increased risk of infection
Low birth weight

Adapted from NIH Consensus Conference (1990). Intravenous immuno-globulin: Prevention and treatment of disease. *JAMA*, 264(24):3189–3193.

search. Evidence of these immunomodulatory effects has led to the use of IVIg in the treatment of inflammatory or autoimmune conditions such as Kawasaki syndrome or idiopathic thrombocytopenic purpura (ITP).

Compared with the first immunoglobulin used in 1952 as an intramuscular preparation, there have been many improvements in preparations of IVIg. There are several brands of IVIg available in the United States; all are purified and processed to remove or inactivate HIV, hepatitis B virus, and other microorganisms. Dosages for IVIg may vary ten-fold depending on the disorder for which it is being administered. People metabolize IVIg at unique individual rates, therefore, IVIg dosage and interval must be tailored to each patient. Table 16–12 is a review of nursing considerations in administering IVIg to the pediatric critical care patient.

Biotherapy is a broad term used to refer to various biologic treatment modalities employed to augment, restore, or modify the immune response or hematopoiesis. Through advanced biotechnologic methods, such as recombinant engineering techniques, many naturally occurring immunologic substances in the body are produced in sufficiently large quantities for clinical trials and therapeutic application (Haeuber, 1991; Johnson, 1991). Biotherapy may be used to augment or restore the immune system in the treatment of cancer, immunodeficiencies, HIV disease, and septic shock. Biotherapy is also employed to suppress or restrict the immune response such as in the prevention, diagnosis, or treatment of graft rejection or graft versus host disease, or in the treatment of autoimmune disease. Biotherapy has also become a new tool to reverse drug toxicity. Certain forms of biotherapy have nonclinical uses; they are used in the laboratory to diagnose diseases or infections, determine blood and tissue types, and differentiate between B cells and T cells.

An important nursing consideration for the use of biotherapy, because often it is an investigational therapy, is to ensure that the informed consent process is complete. In addition to the parents' or

Table 16–12. NURSING CONSIDERATIONS IN THE ADMINISTRATION OF IVIg

Dose	Doses range from 200 to 1000 mg/kg/day depending on the indications. Doses up to 2000 mg/kg are being investigated. Dosage frequency also varies for each clinical condition.
Infusion rate	5% begin at 0.5 mL/kg/hour for 30 minutes, then increase up to a maximum of 4 mL/kg/hour
Gammagard	10% begin at 0.5 mL/kg/hour for 30 minutes, then gradually increase up to 8 mL/kg/hour
Sandoglobulin	3% begin at 30–60 mL/hour for 15 minutes, then increase to 90 to 150 mL/hour
	6% begin at 60–90 mL/hour for 15 minutes, then increase to 120–150 mL/hour
	9% and 12% solutions have been used safely
Side effects	IVIg may cause several side effects; most are minor and tend to be related to the rate of infusion. If the infusion is slowed or temporarily stopped, the side effects will subside and then infusion can be resumed.
	Fever, chills, myalgia, nausea, vomiting, dizziness, diaphoresis, dyspnea, urticaria, flushing, chest tightening, headache, backache, hypotension, or elevation in blood pressure
	IVIg solution is frequently reconstituted as a 5% solution. The child receiving large doses is subjected to the administration of a large fluid volume. Monitor for fluid overload.
Adverse reactions	IVIg has the potential to cause immediate hypersensitivity or anaphylactic reactions. This reaction is rarely seen.
Nursing implications	Avoid administration concurrently with blood components or amphotericin so that if a reaction occurs, the product causing the reaction may be determined.
	Be prepared for immediate hypersensitivity or anaphylactic reaction:
	1. Properly functioning emergency equipment and epinephrine at the bedside
	2. Remain with the patient for the first 5 minutes of the infusion
	3. Obtain vital signs before infusion, 15 minutes after the start of the infusion, and every hour during the infusion.
	If the patient exhibits symptoms of anaphylaxis, immediately stop the infusion, keep the IV patent, infuse 0.9% sodium chloride, obtain vital signs, notify physician immediately. Anticipate the administration of subcutaneous epinephrine (1:1000 dilution rather than 1:10,000 dilution).
	If the child experiences an adverse reaction, note the lot number of the IVIg (often requires contact with Pharmacy Department). Because there is lot-to-lot variability in IVIg preparations, an individual patient may tolerate a preparation from a particular lot number better than preparations from other lot numbers.

guardians' consent, it is important to obtain the child's assent, when appropriate, to participate in the research process and protocol.

Another significant nursing implication in caring for the child receiving biotherapy is knowledge about the contraindications, complications, and side effects. In general, the long-term effects of biotherapy are unknown; hence, this therapy is used only when clearly indicated or when administered as part of a research protocol. Complications of therapy are variable and may be acute or chronic, nearly universal, or rare. Each biotherapy agent has unique side effects, but most agents are associated with a flu-like syndrome of fever, chills, myalgia, headache, and fatigue.

Biotherapy generally involves the administration of one form or a combination of the following: (1) biological response modifiers (BRMs or cytokines), such as colony stimulating factors (CSFs), interferons, or interleukins; (2) monoclonal antibodies (MoAbs); (3) genetically engineered enzymes; (4) autologous activated immune cells (tumor infiltrating lymphocytes [TILs] and lymphokine activated killer cells [LAK]); and (5) gene transfer therapy. In addition, the administration of IVIg (see p. 498) as an immunoregulatory substance (rather than as replacement in antibody deficient states) may be considered biotherapy. Each category of biotherapy is discussed individually, but as with all other immunologic events, these substances do not act independently or in isolation.

BRMs are soluble substances produced primarily by cells of the immune system that act as powerful communication signals between cells. In this sense, BRMs function much like hormones or neurotransmitters. BRMs regulate or influence the immune response by affecting a variety of cellular activities, especially in regard to HI and CMI. Like antibodies, BRMs are generally released in response to the presence of antigen (Herberman, 1989). However, unlike antibodies, BRMs are "nonspecific" (not specific to a "destiny" antigen).

BRMs can be categorized as colony stimulating factors (CSFs), interferons, and interleukins. Other BRMs, such as tumor necrosis factor (TNF, alpha), lymphotoxin (TNF, beta), and IL-1, have unique effects that defy categorization. They are referred to as "toxic" cytokines.

CSFs are a group of glycoproteins that are extensively involved in hematopoiesis, the process by which blood cells proliferate, differentiate, and mature (Haeuber & DiJulio, 1989). Each CSF binds to and activates the corresponding receptors found on the surface of its target cell (each CSF may have a variety of target cells) (Haeuber & DiJulio, 1989). Upon the binding to its receptor membrane, the CSF signals that target cell to initiate particular intracellular processes such as protein synthesis and replication of genetic material. That leads to differentiation, cloning, maturation, and in some cases, functional activation of that target hematopoietic cell (Haeuber & DiJulio, 1989).

Recombinant CSFs, produced by genetic engineering, have three major therapeutic applications. Two applications are to restore hematopoietic function by raising cell counts from suppressed levels, and to augment host defense against infection by enhancing the sensitivity and function of immune cells. The third application is their indirect role in containing or eliminating malignant cells. By far the most common application of CSFs is to reverse anemia, thrombocytopenia, and neutropenia following cytotoxic and radiation therapy during the treatment of cancer. Bone marrow suppression, with its consequent risks of life-threatening infection or bleeding, is the primary dose-limiting factor of cytotoxic drugs for the treatment of cancer. CSFs accelerate bone marrow recovery, which reduces the period of severe neutropenia and thrombocytopenia, thereby permitting higher doses of chemotherapy and possibly higher rates of remission or cure. Research is ongoing in using various CSFs for these multiple purposes.

There are five major endogenous human CSFs: granulocyte-CSF (G-CSF), granulocyte-macrophage-CSF (GM-CSF), macrophage-CSF (M-CSF), interleukin-3 (IL-3), and erythropoietin. Table 16–13 is a review of individual CSFs and their cellular source, action, and therapeutic application.

Interferons are substances produced by the immune cells primarily in response to viral infection. All of the interferons are antiviral, antiproliferative (cloning), and immune-modulating, but the different types of interferons may vary in efficacy in exerting these effects. Like other BRMs, interferons cause a flu-like syndrome (Figlin, 1987; Roth & Foon, 1987). Table 16–14 lists the various interferons with their respective cellular sources, actions, and therapeutic applications in pediatric critical care.

Interleukins are a form of BRMs that have received much attention. There are more than 12 identified interleukins and their unique function and contribution to the immune response are not completely understood. IL-2, the most commonly administered interleukin, increases lymphocyte proliferation (cloning) and NK cell activity (Byram, 1989; Jassak & Sticklin, 1986; Padavic-Shaller, 1988).

Most frequently, research has focused on the use of IL-2 in combination with other forms of biotherapy, such as IL-2 and LAK or IL-2 and alpha-interferon. The most notable feature of IL-2 is its adverse effect of capillary leak syndrome characterized by profound hypotension and edema. This is usually accompanied by fever, decreased systemic perfusion, and organ dysfunction such as that of the kidney and liver (Byram, 1989; Jassak & Sticklin, 1986; Padavic-Shaller, 1988). Table 16–7 provides additional information about interleukins.

Monoclonal antibodies (MoAbs) are laboratory-produced antibodies for a single "destiny" antigen. The process in which MoAbs are produced in the laboratory is reflected in Figure 16–13. MoAbs are used to prevent, diagnose, and treat graft rejection and graft versus host disease (GVHD); perform diagnostic testing; treat disease (e.g., cancer, autoimmune disease);

Table 16-13. SELECTED COLONY STIMULATING FACTORS (CSFs)

CSF	Cellular Source	Action	Therapeutic Application
Erythropoietin (EPO)	Renal cells	Stimulates production and speeds maturation of erythrocytes	Reverse anemia related to: • Chronic renal failure • HIV disease • Zidovidine therapy for HIV
IL-3 (Multi-CSF)	T cells	Stimulates growth of precursors to granulocytes, macrophages, RBCs, platelets, and mast cells	Reverse thrombocytopenia related to: • Cancer therapy
G-CSF*	Monocytes Macrophages Endothelial cells Fibroblasts	Stimulates growth and activation of neutrophils	Reverse neutropenia related to: • Cytotoxic therapy • Radiation therapy • HIV disease • Congenital neutropenia • Cyclic neutropenia
M-CSF	Monocytes Macrophages Endothelial cells Fibroblasts	Stimulates growth and activation of monocytes	Expedite bone marrow recovery following autologous bone marrow transplant
GM-CSF	T cells Endothelial cells Fibroblasts	Stimulates the growth and activation of neutrophils, eosinophils, and macrophages Enhances ability of macrophages and neutrophils to ingest bacteria and kill antibody-coated tumor cells	Expedite bone marrow recovery following autologous bone marrow transplant

*It is relatively easy to transfuse RBCs to reverse anemia or platelets to reverse thrombocytopenia. In contrast, granulocyte transfusions to reverse neutropenia are logistically difficult to perform. In addition, their therapeutic efficacy has not been reliably established.
Data from Herberman, R.B. (Ed.) (1989). Cetus immunoprimer series: Part 3: Cytokines. Cetus Corporation: Emoryville, CA.

and monitor response to treatment to eliminate toxins and reverse drug toxicity. Each therapeutic application of MoAbs is discussed separately.

Anti-T cell MoAbs, such as OKT3, are effective agents widely used in heart, liver, pancreas, and bone marrow transplants to prevent, diagnose, or treat graft rejection or GVHD. To prevent graft rejection, OKT3 is administered to prevent the child's mature T cells from rejecting the grafted or transplanted organ. To prevent GVHD in bone marrow transplant patients, the donor marrow is incubated with anti-T cell MoAbs before the marrow is infused into the recipient to purge the donor marrow of immunocompetent T cells. MoAbs can also be used to monitor subsets of T cells at the site of organ graft to assist in the diagnosis or monitoring of graft rejection (Mahon, 1991; Shaefer & Willis, 1991).

MoAbs may also be used on serum, urine, and stool samples (among others) to diagnose infections with microorganisms such as herpes simplex virus, strep-

Table 16-14. SELECTED INTERFERONS

Agent	Cellular Source	Action	Pediatric Critical Care Therapeutic Application
Alpha-interferon	T, B, NK cells Macrophages Fibroblasts Epithelial cells	Enhance NK activity Anti-viral Induces HLA-I antigen expression Induces fever Generates cytotoxic T-cells Induces macrophage killing of tumor cells	Non-Hodgkin's lymphoma Hepatitis B HIV disease Under investigation in: Hepatitis B or C
Beta-interferon	Fibroblasts Macrophages Epithelial cells	See alpha-interferon actions	Multiple sclerosis

Gamma-interferon	T and NK cells	Antiviral
		Induces HLA-1 antigen expression
		Induces microorganism and tumor cell killing of macrophages
		Regulates action of certain cytokines
		Increases NK cell activity
		Induces production of T cell suppressor factor
		Increases expression of Fc receptor
			Chronic granulomatous disease
			Under investigation in:
			  HIV disease
			  Rheumatoid arthritis
			  Chronic mycobacterial infections *(M. avium)*

Data from Herberman, R.B. (Ed.) (1989). Cetus immunoprimer series: Part 3: Cytokines. Cetus Corporation, Emoryville, CA.

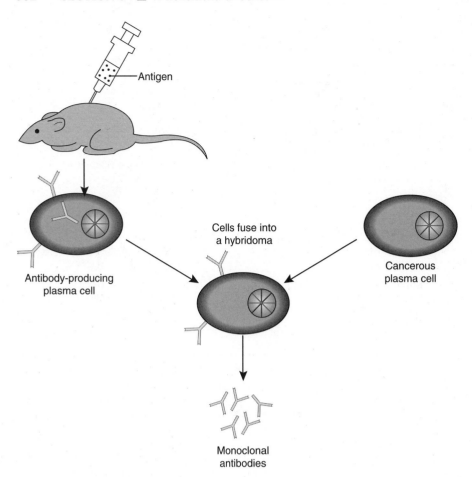

Cells fuse into
a hybridoma

Antibody-producing
plasma cell

Cancerous
plasma cell

Monoclonal
antibodies

Figure 16–13 ● ● ● ● ● ●
The target antigen is injected into a mouse stimulating the mouse plasma cells to produce antibodies to that destiny antigen. The mouse plasma cells are then harvested and fused with an immortal laboratory-grown plasma cell. These cells are then cloned and referred to as hybridomas. This hybridoma will secrete the "made to order" antibody for an indefinite period of time. Through this process, research has mimicked the immune system's humoral immunity. (Adapted from Schindler, L. W. (1992). *The immune system—How it works.* United States Department of Health and Human Services, Bethesda, MD. NIH publication number 92-3229, p. 22.)

tococci, and *Chlamydia*. In addition, MoAbs assist in the identification of cells and tissues (e.g., B cell and T cell differentiation, or HLA or blood typing).

MoAbs to various tumor antigens or tumor products can be used to confirm the diagnosis of certain types of cancers (glioma, cancer of the pancreas, lung, kidney, and others). A radioactive tracer can be attached to MoAbs so that after the MoAbs are administered, a body scan will reveal where the cancer is located within the body.

Anti-tumor MoAbs can also be used therapeutically. They attach to tumor cells, opsonizing these cells, and enhancing the tumor cells' destruction via ADCC. Anti-tumor antigen MoAbs that are attached to toxins are referred to as "conjugated" MoAbs. Often these conjugated MoAbs are combined with radioactive or other agents to assist in the treatment of various cancers, such as acute lymphocytic leukemia. In theory, these will attach solely to the tumor cells, rather than harming healthy cells and tissues (DiJulio, 1988).

More commonly in the PICU, MoAbs are used to reverse drug toxicity or minimize toxic effects. For example, in a child experiencing digoxin toxicity, the MoAb Digibind "binds" to the excess digoxin, preventing it from exerting its toxic effects. MoAbs to microbe toxins have been developed and have been used in clinical trials to determine their usefulness in reversing or ameliorating sepsis and septic shock.

The data available from these trials does not yet support the widespread use of these agents (Saez-Llorens & MacCracken, 1993; Van Dervort & Danner, 1994).

Some diseases affecting children occur as a consequence of genetic defects that result in the lack of one or more key enzymes for cell growth and metabolism. For such diseases, genetically engineered enzyme replacement therapy may halt the disease process. This involves administering the missing enzyme in adequate amounts. Because such endogenously administered enzymes may last only a short time within the body, molecules such as *polyethylene glycol* (PEG) can be attached to the enzyme to prolong its half-life (Hershfield, 1989).

This therapy is best exemplified by the treatment of ADA deficiency, a form of SCID. To treat the disease, ADA is produced in the laboratory and combined with molecules of PEG. The resultant PEG-ADA is administered to children with ADA deficiency, and in most cases has resulted in marked improvement (Hershfield, 1989).

Lymphokine activated killer cells (LAK) and tumor infiltrating lymphocytes (TILs) are forms of biotherapy that are undergoing investigation as a treatment of cancer. In some clinical trials, the cells have effectively produced tumor regression in cancers that were unresponsive to conventional therapy. Both forms of therapy involve removing lymphocytes from a person with cancer, activating these cells with IL-2, and then returning the activated cells to the patient. Theoretically, either type of activated cell would be expected to lyse tumor cells while sparing normal cells.

In LAK cell therapy, the patient is first given IL-2, then undergoes pheresis in which lymphocytes are removed. These lymphocytes are incubated with IL-2, then returned to the patient in the hope that these cells will attack the tumor. TILs are normal lymphocytes that are harvested directly from the patient's malignant tumor. Thus, in contrast to LAK cells, TILs are theoretically "programmed" against the tumor cells from which they are found. TILs are also incubated with IL-2, stimulated to clone, harvested, and reinfused into the patient (Brogley & Sharp, 1990; Corey & Collins, 1986).

Gene transfer therapy is a revolutionary means of actually replacing defective genes within the body (Carr, 1992). This highly experimental procedure was first used in children with SCID related to ADA deficiency (in whom PEG-ADA had limited success) (Blaese, 1992), and in familial hyperlipoproteinemia, a lipid disorder. Like the administration of LAK and TILs, one method of gene transfer therapy is a multistep treatment that requires the removal of specific cells from the patient, modification of these cells in the laboratory, and return of the modified cells to the patient (Antoine, 1990; Garnett, 1990). Gene transfer therapy shows tremendous potential in the cure of other diseases that are the result of a defective gene, such as cystic fibrosis (Wallace, Hall, & Kuhn, 1993).

Prevention of Infection

A second therapeutic goal in caring for the child at risk for impaired host defenses is the prevention of infection. The following three general interventions assist in meeting this goal:

- Limit exposure to reservoirs
- Prevent antigen exposure
- Consider the cost-benefit ratio of invasive techniques

Limit Exposure to Reservoirs. Prevention of infection can be facilitated by limiting the child's exposure to reservoirs, which are environments in which organisms replicate and persist. Reservoirs can be either exogenous or endogenous to the patient (Massanari, 1989). Minimizing contact with unnecessary exogenous reservoirs includes maintaining a clean PICU environment, maintaining sterile or aseptic medical equipment and supplies, and limiting exposure to infected healthcare workers and/or visitors (Massanari, 1989).

The child's room and bedside area should be damp-dusted (Griffin, 1986) and the floor mopped (Donowitz, 1988) every 24 hours and monitored for standing collections of water or other liquids (Griffin, 1986). All containers of normal saline or sterile water for irrigation purposes should be labeled with date and time opened and replaced every 24 hours. It is also important to avoid contamination of these solutions during use. The PICU environment should also provide some humidity for the benefit of the infant and child's small airways and for reduction of organisms that thrive in dry environments (Griffin, 1986). Medical equipment and supplies that must be kept sterile or aseptic include medications, total parenteral and enteral nutrition, humidifiers, face masks, manual resuscitation bags, large-bore suction catheters, suction tubing, and canisters (Griffin, 1986; Massanari, 1989). Other potential reservoirs include hand lotions (Massanari, 1989), baby oil and bath supplies, nonprescription ointments, and children's toys.

In addition to the environment, supplies, and equipment, healthcare workers, parents, siblings, and other visitors within the critical care environment are potential exogenous reservoirs. Some 15% to 20% of healthy individuals are carriers of *S. aureus* in the nasal antrum and could potentially shed these organisms into the environment (Massanari, 1989). Healthcare workers and visitors may be also infectious with other bacterial or viral organisms.

Visiting policies and traffic control measures should limit unnecessary visitors and limit the PICU environment to essential staff, patient family members, and significant others. All persons entering the PICU (including pediatric visitors) should adhere to strict handwashing procedures before and after patient visitation (Donowitz, 1988). Thorough, frequent handwashing remains the most important method of preventing the transmission of pathogens between patient and health team member or visitor (Donowitz, 1988; Griffin, 1986; Massanari, 1989). A recent study documented a 70% failure rate of healthcare members to wash their hands after contact with PICU patients or patient-related equipment (Donowitz, 1987).

A well-designed, comprehensive employee health program should be in place to minimize the spread of illness to caregivers (Rhinehart, 1989) as well as to patients. Pre-employment and yearly physical examinations to review the healthcare worker's history of communicable disease, immunization status, and immunity screening results for varicella, measles, and tuberculosis are important. Comprehensive employee health programs offer hepatitis B and yearly influenza vaccines.

A comprehensive employee health program does not replace sound judgment in determining exposure of infectious persons to critically ill infants and children. The nurse has an active and vital role in patient advocacy and carefully monitors self, team members, and visitors for evidence of an infectious process. Patients with altered host defenses should not be cared for or visited by infectious persons without appropriate safety precautions. Guiding infectious persons in delaying their visit or handwashing and using disposable masks in the child's room may lower the risk of transmission.

Unlike exogenous reservoirs, which are often identified, disinfected, or eliminated, little can be done to eradicate pathogens from the endogenous reservoir, the patient (Massanari, 1989). Many opportunistic organisms are present in a patient's system and may cause infection in a patient in a compromised state (Halliburton, 1986; Massanari, 1989). Many therapies focus on the reduction of risk of infection from endogenous GI organisms. A few examples of therapies under investigation include the effect of gut sterilization (Koruda, 1993) or selective decontamination of the gut (Bion et al., 1994; Hammond et al., 1994) and the effect of the presence or absence and type of feedings (Heyland et al., 1992; Mainous et al., 1994; Montecalvo et al., 1992) on gastric colonization and pH and the incidence of nosocomial sepsis.

Prevent Antigen Exposure. In addition to identifying the known allergies of the infant or young child, recognition of the numerous substances the child is exposed to on a daily basis in the PICU and identification of potential or actual antigens is critical. Most critical care units minimize the presence of flowers, plants, and pets in the unit, and encourage other age-appropriate sources of pleasure such as mobiles, radios, and tape players. Flexibility and exceptions are frequent in the PICU environment and are evident by the use of closed terrariums rather than potted plants, changing water in flower vases every 8 hours, or showing videotapes or photographs of pets in between the planned visits by pets. Recognizing the presence of potential antigens and vectors of infection is important. Awareness of their impact on the child and other patients in the unit and planning interventions accordingly are vital.

Consider the Cost-benefit Ratio of Invasive Techniques. Exposure to invasive medical devices or procedures represents a significant risk for nosocomial infection. Despite the risks, these devices and procedures are an integral part of the pediatric critical care environment, and will continue to be in the future. Assisting in the careful comparison of the benefits versus the risks of these invasive techniques is important, because most preventable infections are related to the use of invasive devices or procedures. Once it has been decided that the benefit outweighs the risk, care should be taken to follow institution-specific standards for invasive techniques and procedures, and the care and maintenance of the invasive devices.

Treatment of Infection

Even with host augmentation and prevention measures, the critically ill child may develop an infection. The nurse plays a major role in the identification of the infection and collaborates with the healthcare team to provide treatment.

Survey for and Identify Infection. It is imperative for the nurse to monitor fever patterns, which may assist in the identification of the cause of infection. With the exception of the newborn and young infant, the body's ability to mount a febrile response usually remains intact and, therefore, is the best indicator of infection (Rostad, 1991). Gram-negative sepsis is often accompanied by a pattern of intermittent fevers, whereas a slowly rising, but steady, fever may indicate the presence of a fungal infection (Rostad, 1991). Fever may also be a manifestation of a reaction to certain medications, such as antibiotics. In this situation, fever closely follows the medication administration and the medication *may* temporarily be discontinued to evaluate whether the fever resolves. Close attention to the proper use, method, and care of the temperature-taking device is prudent because treatment decisions are made with the data obtained from temperature taking.

Identification of the source of infection becomes a primary concern in the presence of a febrile patient. Particular attention is targeted towards the lungs and the skin (especially sites of intravenous insertion access, and perioral and perirectal areas) (Pizzo, 1989). All indwelling catheters, whether suspected or not, are sampled for culture. In addition, two peripheral blood samples are obtained from separate venipuncture sites. Other cultures the nurse may anticipate include routine urinalysis and urine culture, a stool examination and culture (if diarrhea is present), and a chest radiograph. In the febrile neutropenic patient, these cultures and diagnostic tests are anticipated, despite the absence of other clinical symptoms (Pizzo, 1989).

Treatment of Infection. Antibiotic therapy is anticipated in a critically ill child with signs and symptoms of infection. Recognition of the goal of antibiotic therapy by all members of the healthcare team is important. This includes knowledge of whether the drug is empiric or definitive therapy for a suspected or an established infection (Crawford, 1992). The properties of an ideal antibiotic are: demonstrated efficacy through controlled clinical trials, nontoxic, no alteration in normal patient or environmental flora, facilitation of rapid discharge of the patient from the hospital, and inexpensive. The antibiotic should improve the outcome of the illness through its activity against the suspected or identified organism. Because all of these properties are rarely present, the result is a compromise of one or some of these properties.

Antibiotic selection is an ongoing process with continual evaluation of the indications for antibiotic therapy, the patient's response, and laboratory data (Crawford, 1992). It is during the course of therapy that additional information is used to adjust the antibiotic regimen to ensure coverage against all suspected or identified microorganisms. The patient's response or lack of response and side effects may lead to the adjustment of the antibiotic regimen. This may result in an antibiotic that has more or all the properties of an optimal antibiotic.

Broad-spectrum antibiotics are usually begun immediately after careful initial examination and collection of specimens for culture and sensitivity testing. Selection of broad-spectrum antibiotics is often based on organisms typically found in a particular institution, whether the patient is neutropenic and the duration of the neutropenia, organisms associated with unique patient populations, and the underlying pathophysiology (e.g., renal failure). Broad-spectrum antibiotic therapy is never a substitute for the careful evaluation of the suspected infection. Pretreatment specimens are always desirable to determine the infectious organism; therefore, all desired cultures should be accurately obtained in a timely fashion (Crawford, 1992).

Once the appropriate antibiotic regimen is chosen, it is imperative that the medication be administered as soon as possible. Regardless of the method of antibiotic delivery (slow intravenous push, metered chamber, retrograde, or syringe pump), close attention to the rate of the administration, location of administration, and the deadspace of the intravenous tubing ensures that the child receives the drug completely and consistently.

An antibiotic serum drug concentration (SDC) should be obtained, when appropriate. These are often ordered by the physician as peak and trough drug levels. Results are used to adjust drug doses to maximize therapeutic efficacy (ablate microorganism growth) while minimizing or avoiding toxicity. The determination of when a serum drug concentration is obtained is based on the underlying condition of the patient and the point at which the drug reaches a steady-state condition. In the clinical setting, this is often defined according to a specific drug regimen (i.e., following the third administered dose of gentamicin). However, in the critically ill child or the child with organ dysfunction resulting in altered elimination of that drug, SDC may be obtained after the first administered dose. In order to reach and maintain a therapeutic SDC, it is imperative that all antibiotic doses be given on schedule, regardless of other scheduled diagnostic procedures or regimens.

SDC specimens must be accurately collected and labeled to ensure that the derived data are accurate. The actual time the specimen was drawn as well as the antibiotic infusion start and completion times should be noted directly on the laboratory specimens. Administration techniques can produce misleading SDC results if the delivery time is miscalculated (Gilman, 1990). The administration time, administration method, infusion duration, specimen collection container, collection time, and concomitant administered medications influence the SDC obtained.

Trough levels are always obtained before administration of an antibiotic dose. Peak levels vary depending on the class of antibiotic; aminoglycoside peak concentrations are obtained from 30 to 60 minutes after a 30-minute infusion, whereas vancomycin peak concentrations are obtained 60 minutes after a 60-minute infusion. If toxicity is suspected, SDCs may be obtained at any time in the dosing schedule.

SUMMARY

Knowledge of immunology is increasingly important for the pediatric critical care nurse for two reasons. All PICU patients experience altered host defenses; most commonly, these are changes in the structure and function of the first line of defense. In addition, the pediatric critical care nurse's knowledge of the immune system is often limited. With increasing technology and expanding knowledge of the intricacies of immunologic events, expertise in the field of immunology is imperative.

Caring for the child with altered host defenses is a challenge. This chapter has presented that children in the PICU are at risk developmentally and situationally for altered host defense. Recognition of this provides the basis for a thorough immunologic assessment, which will further identify the child at risk. Many of the interventions, including medical efforts, involve expert nursing care to promote the best possible outcome for the child.

References

Abney, E.R., Cooper, M.D., Kearney, J.F., Lawton, A.R., & Parkhouse, R.M.E. (1978). Sequential expression of immunoglobulin on developing mouse B lymphocytes: A systematic survey that suggests a model for the generation of immunoglobulin isotype diversity. *The Journal of Immunology,* 120(6):2041–2049.

Abraham, E., & Regan, R.F. (1985). The effects of hemorrhage and trauma on interleukin 2 production. *Archives of Surgery,* 120 (12):1341.

Abramson, J.S., Wheeler, J.G., & Quie, P.G. (1989). The polymorphonuclear phagocytic system. In E.R. Stiehm (Ed.). *Immunologic disorders in infants and children* (3rd ed., pp. 68–80). Philadelphia: W.B. Saunders.

ACCP-SCCM Consensus conference: Definitions for sepsis and organ failure and guidelines for the use of innovative therapies in sepsis. *Critical Care Medicine,* 20(6):864–874.

Adams, A. (1985). External barriers to infection. *Nursing Clinics of North America,* 20(1):145–149.

Albano, E.A., & Pizzo, P.A. (1988). The evolving population of immunocompromised children. *Pediatric Infectious Disease Journal,* 7(5):s79–s86.

Altman, Y., Handzel, Z.T., & Levin, S. (1984). Suppressor T-cell activity in newborns and mothers. *Pediatric Research,* 18(2):123–126.

Anderson, D.C., Hughes, B.J., Edwards, M.S., Buffone, G.J., & Baker, C.J. (1983). Impaired chemotaxigenesis by type III group B streptococci in neonatal sera: Relationship to specific anticapsular antibody and abnormalities of serum complement. *Pediatric Research,* 17(6):496–502.

Antoine, F.S. (1990). Landmark gene therapy trial progresses. *NIH Record,* XLII (18). Bethesda, MD: The National Institutes of Health.

Bellanti, J.A., & Kadlec, J.V. (1985). General immunobiology. In J.A. Bellanti (Ed.). *Immunology III* (pp. 16–53). Philadelphia: W.B. Saunders.

Bellanti, J.A., & Kadlec, J.V. (1990). Host defense mechanisms. In V. Chernick & E.L. Kendig (Eds.). *Kernig's disorders of the respiratory tract in children* (5th ed., pp. 182–201). Philadelphia: W.B. Saunders.

Berger, M., & Frank, M.M. (1989). The serum complement system. In E.R. Stiehm (Ed.). *Immunologic disorders in infants and children* (3rd ed., pp. 97–115). Philadelphia: W.B. Saunders.

Bion, J.F., Badger, I., Crosby, H.A., Hutchings, P., Kong, K.-L., Baker, J., Hutton, P., McMaster, P., Buckels, J.A., Elliot, T.S.J. (1994). Selective decontamination of the digestive tract reduces Gram-negative pulmonary colonization but not systemic endotoxemia in patients undergoing elective liver transplantation. *Critical Care Medicine,* 22(1):40–49.

Blackburn, G.L., & Menkes, E. (1983). Surgical immunology. In R.K. Chandra (Ed.). *Primary and secondary immunodeficiency disorders* (pp. 263–271). New York: Churchill Livingstone.

Blaese, R.M. (1992). Development of gene therapy for immunodeficiency: Adenosine deaminase deficiency. *Pediatric Research,* 33[Suppl.](1):s49–s53.

Bohn, D.J., Biggar, W.D., Smith, C.R., Conn, A.W., & Barker, G.A. (1986). Influence of hypothermia, barbiturate therapy, and intracranial pressure monitoring on morbidity and mortality after near-drowning. *Critical Care Medicine,* 14(6):529–534.

Bone, R.C. (1991). Let's agree on terminology: Definitions of sepsis. *Critical Care Medicine,* 19:973–976.

Bousvaros, A., & Walker, W.A. (1990). Development and function of the intestinal mucosal barrier. In T. MacDonald (Ed.). *Ontogeny of the immune system of the gut* (pp. 2–16). Boca Raton: CRC Press.

Brogley, J.L., & Sharp, E.J. (1990). Nursing care of patients receiving activated lymphocytes. *Oncology Nursing Forum,* 17(2):187–193.

Brown, R.B., Hosmer, D., Chen, H.C., Teres, D., Sands, M., Bradley, S., Opitz, E., Szwedzinski, D., & Opalenik, D. (1985). A comparison of infections in different ICUs within the same hospital. *Critical Care Medicine,* 13(6):472–476.

Browning, D.H., & Graves, S.A. (1983). Incidence of aspiration with endotracheal tubes in children. *Journal of Pediatrics,* 102(4):582–584.

Bryson, Y.J., Winter, H.S., Gard, S.E., Fischer, T.J., & Stiehm, E.R. (1980). Deficiency of immune interferon production by leukocytes of normal newborns. *Cellular Immunology,* 55(1):191–200.

Bullock, J.D., Robertson, A.F., Bodenbender, M.T., Kontras, S.B., & Miller, C.E. (1969). Inflammatory response in the neonate reexamined. *Pediatrics,* 44(1):58–61.

Byram, D.A. (1989). The immunocompromised patient: Future experiences for critical care nurses: Competence in immunotherapy. *Critical Care Nursing Clinics of North America,* 1(4):707–806.

Carr, E. (1992). Commentary on genes in a bottle. *ONS Nursing Scan in Oncology,* 1(1):16.

Chandra, R.K. (1983). Malnutrition. In R.K. Chandra (Ed.). *Primary and secondary immunodeficiency disorders* (pp. 187–203). New York: Churchill Livingstone.

Chiu, R.C.J., & Samson, R. (1984). Complement (C3, C4) consumption in cardiopulmonary bypass, cardioplegia, and protamine administration. *Annals of Thoracic Surgery,* 37(3):229–232.

Christensen, R.D., Rothstein, G., Anstall, M.D., & Bybee, B. (1982). Granulocyte transfusion in neonates with bacterial infection, neutropenia, and depletion of mature marrow neutrophils. *Pediatrics,* 70(1):1–6.

Christensen, R.D., & Rothstein, G. (1980). Efficiency of neutrophil migration in the neonate. *Pediatric Research,* 14:1147–1149.

Cobb, J.P., & Danner, R.L. (1993). Nosocomial infections in the practice of pediatric critical care. In P.R. Holbrook (Ed.). *Textbook of pediatric critical care.* Philadelphia: W.B. Saunders.

Cooper, E.R., Pelton, S.I., & LeMay, M. (1988). Acquired immunodeficiency syndrome: A new population of children. *The Pediatric Clinics of North America,* 35(6):1365–1387.

Cooper, M.D., & Buckley, R.H. (1982). Developmental immunology and the immunodeficiency diseases. *JAMA,* 248(20):2658–2669.

Corey, B.S., & Collins, J.L. (1986). Implementation of an RIL-2/LAK cell clinical trial: A nursing perspective. *Oncology Nursing Forum,* 13(6):31–36.

Crawford, G.E. (1992). Empiric selection of antibiotics. *Problems in Critical Care,* 6(1):1–20.

Critical Care/Heart, Lung, Blood Nursing Service, Clinical Center, National Institutes of Health, Bethesda, Maryland.

Davey, B. (1990). *Immunology: A foundation text.* Englewood Cliffs, NJ: Prentice-Hall.

Davis, J.H., Stevens, J.M., Peitzman, A., Corbett, W.A., Illner, H., Shires, G.T., & Shires, G.T., (1983). Neutrophil migratory activity in severe hemorrhagic shock. *Circulatory Shock,* 10(3):199–204.

Denny, T., Yogev, R., Gelman, R., Skuza, C., Oleske, J., Chadwick, E., Cheng, S.C., & Connor, E. (1992). Lymphocyte subsets in healthy children during the first 5 years of life. *JAMA,* 267(11):1484–1488.

DiJulio, J.E. (1988). Treatment of B-cell and T-cell lymphomas with monoclonal antibodies. *Oncology Nursing Forum,* 4(2):102–106.

Dinarello, C.A., & Wolff, S.M. (1990). Pathogenesis of fever. In G.L. Mandell, R.G. Douglas & J.E. Bennett (Eds.). *Principles and practice of infectious disease* (3rd ed., pp. 462–467). New York: Churchill Livingstone.

Donowitz, L.G. (1986). High risk of nosocomial infection in the pediatric critical care patient. *Critical Care Medicine,* 14(1):26–28.

Donowitz, L.G. (1987). Handwashing techniques in a pediatric intensive care unit. *American Journal of Diseases of Children,* 141(6):683–685.

Donowitz, L.G. (1988). The critical care patient. In L.G. Donowitz (Ed.). *Hospital acquired infection in the pediatric patient* (pp. 323–327). Baltimore: Williams & Wilkins.

Donowitz, L.G., Wenzel, R.P., & Hoyt, J.W. (1982). High risk of hospital-acquired infection in the ICU patient. *Critical Care Medicine,* 10(6):355–357.

Dossett, J.H., Williams, R.C., & Quie, P.G. (1969). Studies in interaction of bacteria, serum factors, and polymorphonuclear leukocytes in mothers and newborns. *Pediatrics,* 44(1):49–57.

Douglas, S.D., Hasson, W.F., & Blaese, R.M. (1989). The mononuclear phagocytic system. In E.R. Stiehm (Ed.). *Immunologic disorders in infants and children* (3rd ed., pp. 81–96). Philadelphia: W.B. Saunders.

Ebers, D.W., Smith, D.I., & Gibbs, G.E. (1956). Gastric acid in the first day of life. *Pediatrics,* 18(5):800.

Espersen, S. (1986). Nursing support of host defenses. *Critical Care Quarterly,* 9(1):51–56.

Fairley, J.A., & Rasmussen, J.E. (1983). Comparison of stratum corneum thickness in the children and adults. *Journal of the American Academy of Dermatology,* 8(5):652–654.

Figlin, R.A. (1987). Biotherapy with interferon in solid tumors. *Oncology Nursing Forum,* 14(6)[Suppl.]:23–26.

Fischbach, F.T. (1992). *A manual of laboratory and diagnostic tests* (4th ed.). Philadelphia: J.B. Lippincott.

Fliedner, M., Mehls, O., Rauterberg, E., & Ritz, E. (1986). Urinary sIgA in children with urinary tract infection. *Journal of Pediatrics,* 109(3):416–421.

Ford-Jones, E.L., Mindorff, C.M., Langley, J.M., Allen, U., Navas, L., Patrick, M.L., Milner, R., & Gold, R. (1989). Epidemiologic study of 4684 hospital-acquired infections in pediatric patients. *Pediatric Infectious Disease Journal,* 8(10):668–675.

Frank, M.M. (1994). Complement and kinin. In D.P. Stites, A.I. Terr & T.G. Parslow (Eds.). *Basic and clinical immunology* (8th ed., p. 124). Norwalk, CT: Appleton & Lange.

Frank, M.M. (1991). Complement and kinin. In D.P. Stites & A.I. Terr (Eds.). *Basic and clinical immunology* (7th ed., pp. 161–174). Norwalk, CT: Appleton & Lange.

Gal, T.J. (1988). How does tracheal intubation alter respiratory mechanics? *Problems in Anesthesia,* 2(2):191–200.

Garnett, C. (1990). First human gene therapy trial debuts at NIH. *NIH Record,* XLII (20). Bethesda, MD: The National Institutes of Health.

Gathings, W.E., Lawton, A.R., & Cooper, M.D. (1977). Immunofluorescent studies of the development of pre-B cells, B-lymphocytes and immunoglobulin isotype diversity in humans. *European Journal of Immunology,* 7(11):804–810.

Gershwin, M.E., Beach, R.S., & Hurley, L.S. (1985). *Nutrition and immunity.* Orlando: Academic Press.

Gilman, J.T. (1990). Therapeutic drug monitoring in the neonate and paediatric age group: Problems and clinical pharmacokinetic implications. *Clinical Pharmacokinetics,* 19(1):1–10.

Goldman, A.S., Ham-Pong, A.J., & Goldblum, R.M. (1985). Host defenses: Development and maternal contributions. *Advances in Pediatrics,* 32:71–100.

Goodman, J.W. (1994). The immune response. In D.P. Stites, A.I. Terr & T.G. Parslow (Eds.). *Basic and clinical immunology* (8th ed, pp. 44–48). Norwalk, CT: Appleton & Lange.

Grady, C. (1988). Host defense mechanisms: An overview. *Seminars in Oncology Nursing,* 4(2):86–94.

Grand, R.J., Watkins, J.B., & Torti, F.M. (1976). Development of the human gastrointestinal tract: A review. *Gastroenterology,* 70(5):790–810.

Griffin, J.P. (1986). Nursing care of the critically ill immunocompromised patient. *Critical Care Quarterly,* 9(1):25–34.

Guyton, A. (1986a). The lymphatic system, interstitial fluid dynamics, edema, and pulmonary fluid. *Textbook of medical physiology* (7th ed., pp. 361–373). Philadelphia: W.B. Saunders.

Guyton, A. (1986b). The protein metabolism. *Textbook of medical physiology* (7th ed., pp. 829–840). Philadelphia: W.B. Saunders.

Haeuber, D. (1991). Future Strategies in the Control of Myelosuppression: The use of colony-stimulating factors. *Oncology Nursing Forum*, 18(2):16–21.

Haeuber, D., & DiJulio, J.E. (1989). Hemopoietic colony stimulating factors: An overview. *Oncology Nursing Forum*, 16(6):247–255.

Haley, R.W., Culver, D.H., White, J.W., Morgan, W.M. & Emori, T.G. (1985). The nationwide nosocomial infection rate: A new need for vital statistics. *American Journal of Epidemiology*, 121(2):159–167.

Halliburton, P. (1986). Impaired immunocompetence. In V.K. Carrieri, A.M. Lindsey & C.M. West (Eds.). *Pathophysiological phenomena in nursing: Human responses to illness* (pp. 319–342). Philadelphia: W.B. Saunders.

Hammond, J.M., Potgeiter, P.D., & Saunders, G.L. (1994). Selective decontamination of the digestive tract in multiple trauma patients—Is there a role? Results of a prospective, double-blind, randomized trial. *Critical Care Medicine*, 22(1):33–39.

Hanson, L.A., Adlerberth, I., Carlsson, B., Zaman, S., Hahn-Zoric, M., & Jalil, F. (1990). Antibody-mediated immunity in the neonate. *Padiatrie und Padologie*, 25(5):371–376.

Hanson, L.A., & Brandtzaeg, P. (1989). The mucosal defense systems. In E.R. Stiehm (Ed.). *Immunologic disorders in infants and children* (3rd ed., pp. 40–66). Philadelphia: W.B. Saunders.

Harpin, V.A., & Eutter, N. (1983). Barrier properties of the newborn infant's skin. *Journal of Pediatrics*, 102(3):419–425.

Hashimoto, K., Gross, B.G., & Lever, W.F. (1965). The ultrastructure of the skin of human embryos: The intraepidermal eccrine sweat duct. *Journal of Investigative Dermatology*, 45(3):139–151.

Hauser, G.J., Chan, M.M., Casey, W.F., Midgley, F.M., & Holbrook, P.R. (1991). Immune dysfunction in children after corrective surgery for congenital heart disease. *Critical Care Medicine*, 19(7):874–880.

Hauser, G.J. & Holbrook, P.R. (1988). Immune dysfunction in the critically ill infant and child. *Critical Care Clinics*, 4(4):711–732.

Hayward, A.R., & Lawton, A.R. (1977). Induction of plasma cell differentiation of human fetal lymphocytes: Evidence for functional immaturity of T and B cells. *Journal of Immunology*, 119(4):1213–1217.

Hayward, A.R., & Malmberg, S. (1984). Response of human newborn lymphocytes to alloantigen: Lack of evidence for suppression induction. *Pediatric Research*, 18(5):414–419.

Hayward, A.R., & Merrill, D. (1981). Requirement for OKT8 suppressor cell proliferation for suppression by human newborn T-cells. *Clinical Experimental Immunology*, 45(3):468–474.

Hazinski, M.F., Iberti, T.J., MacIntyre, N.R., Parker M.M., Tribett, D., Prion, S., & Chmel, H. (1993). Epidemiology, pathophysiology, and clinical presentation of gram negative sepsis. *American Journal of Critical Care*, 2(3):224–235.

Heinzel, F.P. (1989). Infections in patients with humoral immunodeficiency. *Hospital Practice*, 24(9):99–130.

Herberman, R.B. (Ed.) (1989). Cetus immunoprimer series: Part 3: Cytokines. Cetus Corporation, Emoryville, CA.

Hershfield, M.S. (1989). Enzyme therapy for an inherited immunodeficiency disease. *Immune Deficiency Foundation Newsletter*, September. Columbia, MD: Immune Deficiency Foundation.

Heyland, D., Bradley, C., & Mandell, L.A. (1992). Effect of acidified enteral feedings on gastric colonization in the critically ill patient. *Critical Care Medicine*, 20(10):1388–1394.

Holbrook, K.A., & Sybert, V. (1988). Basic science. In L.A. Schachner & R.C. Hansen (Eds.). *Pediatric dermatology* (pp. 3–75). New York: Churchill Livingstone.

Holbrook, K.A. (1982). A histologic comparison of infant and adult skin. In H.I. Maibach & E.K. Boisits (Eds.). *Neonatal skin: Structure and function* (pp. 3–34). New York: Marcel Dekker.

Horan, T.C., White, J.W., Jarvis, W.R., Emori, T.G., Culver, D.H., Munn, V.P., Thornsberry, C., Olson, D.R., & Hughes, J.M. (1986). Nosocomial infection surveillance, 1984. *Centers of Disease Control Surveillance Summaries*, 35(1ss):17ss–29ss.

Hotter, A.N. (1990). Wound healing and immunocompromise. *Nursing Clinics of North America*, 25(1):193–203.

Howard, R.J. (1979). Effect of burn injury, mechanical trauma, and operation on immune defenses. *Surgical Clinics of North America*, 59(2):199–211.

Hoyt, N.J. (1989). Host defense mechanisms and compromises in the trauma patient. *Critical Care Nursing Clinics of North America*, 1(4):753–765.

Jassak, P.F., & Sticklin, L.A. (1986). Interleukin-2: An overview. *Oncology Nursing Forum*, 13(6):17–22.

Jett, M.R., & Lancaster, L.E. (1983). The inflammatory-immune response: The body's defense against invasion. *Critical Care Nurse*, 3(5):64–86.

Johnson, J. (1991). Introduction. *Oncology Nursing Forum*, 18(2[Suppl.]):2.

Kamani, N.R., & Douglas, S.D. (1991). Structure and development of the immune system. In D.P. Stites & A.I. Terr (Eds.). *Basic and clinical immunology* (7th ed., pp. 9–33). Norwalk, CT: Appleton & Lange.

Kaplan, J.E., & Saba, T.M. (1976). Humoral deficiency and reticuloendothelial depression after traumatic shock. *American Journal of Physiology*, 230(1):7–14.

Klein, R.B., Fischer, T.J., Gard, S.E., Biberstein, B.S., Rich, K.C., & Stiehm, E.R. (1977). Decreased mononuclear and polymorphonuclear chemotaxis in human newborns, infants, and young children. *Pediatrics*, 60(4):467–472.

Koruda, M. (1993). Gut sterilization to prevent nosocomial infection. *New Horizons: The Science and Practice of Acute Medicine*, 1(2):194–201.

Kotylo, P.K., Fineberg, N.S., Freeman, K.S., Redmond, N.L., & Charland, C. (1993). Reference ranges for lymphocyte subsets in pediatric patients. *American Journal of Clinical Pathology*, 100(2):111–115.

Lancaster, L.E. (1991). *Core curriculum for nephrology nursing* (2nd ed.). Pitman, NJ: American Nephrology Nurses' Association.

Lawton, A.R., & Cooper, M.D. (1989). Ontogeny of immunity. In E.R. Stiehm (Ed.). *Immunologic disorders in infants and children* (3rd ed., pp. 1–14). Philadelphia: W.B. Saunders.

Levine, S.A., & Niederman, M.S. (1991). The impact of tracheal intubation on host defenses and risks for nosocomial pneumonia. *Clinics in Chest Medicine*, 12(3):523–543.

Lewin, S., Brettman, L.R., & Holzman, R.S. (1981). Infections in hypothermic patients. *Archives of Internal Medicine*, 141(7):920–925.

Leyden, J.J. (1982). Bacteriology of newborn skin. In H.I. Maibach & E.K. Boisits (Eds.). *Neonatal skin: Structure and function* (pp. 167–181). New York: Marcel Dekker.

Locke, S.E. (1982). Stress, adaption and immunity: Studies in humans. *General Hospital Psychiatry*, 4(1):49–58.

Lu, C.Y., & Unanue, E.R. (1985). Macrophage ontogeny: Implications for host defense, T-lymphocyte differentiation, and the acquisition of self-tolerance. *Clinics in Immunology and Allergy*, 5(2):253–269.

Lydyard, P., & Grossi, C. (1989a). Cells involved in the immune response. In I.M. Roitt, J. Brostoff & D.K. Male (Eds.). *Immunology* (2nd ed., pp. 2.1–2.18). Philadelphia: J.B. Lippincott.

Lydyard, P., & Grossi, C. (1989b). The lymphoid system. In I.M. Roitt, J. Brostoff & D.K. Male (Eds.). *Immunology* (2nd ed., pp. 3.1–3.9). Philadelphia: J.B. Lippincott.

Mahon, P.M. (1991). Orthoclone OKT3 and cardiac transplantation: An overview. *Critical Care Nurse*, 11(8):42–50.

Mainous, M.R., Block, E.F., & Deitch, E.A. (1994). Nutritional support of the gut: How and why. *New Horizons: The Science and Practice of Acute Medicine.* 2(2):193–201.

Malloy, M.B., & Perez-Woods, R.C. (1991). Neonatal skin care: Prevention of skin breakdown. *Pediatric Nursing*, 17(1):41–48.

Massanari, R.M. (1989). Nosocomial infections in critical care units: Causation and prevention. *Critical Care Nursing Quarterly*, 11(4):45–57.

Masuda, K., Kinoshita, Y., & Kobayashi, Y. (1989). Heterogeneity of Fc receptor expression in chemotaxis and adherence of neonatal neutrophils. *Pediatric Research*, 25(1):6–10.

McCracken, G.H., & Eichenwald, H.F. (1971). Leukocyte function and development of opsonic and complement activity in the neonate. *American Journal of Diseases of Children*, 121(2):120–126.

Mellander, L., et al. (1985). Secretory IgA antibody response against *Escherichia coli* antigen in infants in relation to exposure. *Journal of Pediatrics,* 107(3):430–433.

Merritt, W.T. (1992). Nosocomial infections in the pediatric intensive care unit. In M.C. Rogers (Ed.). *Textbook of pediatric intensive care* (2nd ed., pp. 976–1008). Baltimore: Williams & Wilkins.

Miller, M.E. (1969). Phagocytosis in the newborn infant: Humoral and cellular factors. *Journal of Pediatrics,* 74(2):255–259.

Miller, M.E. (1977). Host defenses in the human neonate. *Pediatric Clinics of North America,* 24(2):413–423.

Miller, M.E. (1980). The inflammatory and natural defense systems. In E.R. Stiehm (Ed.). *Immunologic disorders in infants and children* (2nd ed., pp. 165–180). Philadelphia: W.B. Saunders.

Miller, M.E. (1983). Immunocompetence of the newborn. In R.K. Chandra (Ed.). *Primary and secondary immunodeficiency disorders* (pp. 157–164). New York: Churchill Livingstone.

Miller, M.E. (1989). Immunodeficiencies of immaturity. In E.R. Stiehm (Ed.). *Immunologic disorders in infants and children* (3rd ed., pp. 196–225). Philadelphia: W.B. Saunders.

Milliken, J., Tait, G.A., Ford-Jones, E.L., Mindorff, C.M., Gold, R., & Mullins, G. (1988). Nosocomial infections in a pediatric intensive care unit. *Critical Care Medicine,* 16(3):233–237.

Montecalvo, M.A., Steger, K.A., Farber, H.W., Smith, B.F., Dennis, R.C., Fitzpatrick, G.F., Pollack, S.D., Korsberg, T.Z., Birkett, D.H., Hirsh, E.F., Craven, D.E., & Critical Care Research Team (1992). Nutritional outcome and pneumonia in critical care patients randomized to gastric versus jejunal tube feedings. *Critical Care Medicine,* 20(10):1377–1378.

Morriss, F.H., Moore, M., Weisbrodt, N.W., & West, M.S. (1986). Ontogenic development of gastrointestinal motility: Duodenal contractions in preterm infants. *Pediatrics,* 78(6):1106–1113.

Nejedla, Z. (1970). The development of immunological factors in infants with hyperbilirubinemia. *Pediatrics,* 45(1):102–104.

NIH Consensus Conference. (1990). Intravenous immunoglobulin: Prevention and treatment of disease. *JAMA,* 264(24):3189–3193.

Padavic-Shaller, K. (1988). IL-2: Nursing applications in a developing science. *Oncology Nursing Forum,* 4(2):142–150.

Pahwa, S.G., Pahwa, R., Grimes, E., & Smithwick, E. (1977). Cellular and humoral components of monocyte and neutrophil chemotaxis in cord blood. *Pediatric Research,* 11(5):677–680.

Parkman, R. (1991). Cytokines and T-lymphocytes in pediatrics. *The Journal of Pediatrics,* 118(3):s21–s23.

Paul, W.E. (1989). The immune system: An introduction. In W.E. Paul (Ed.). *Fundamental immunology* (2nd ed.). New York: Raven Press.

Pizzo, P.A. (1989). Combating infections in neutropenic patients. *Hospital Practice,* 24(7):93–110.

Polin, R.A., & St. Geme, J.W. (1992). Neonatal sepsis. *Advances in Pediatric Infectious Disease,* 7:25–61.

Ramasastry, P., Downing, D.T., Pochi, P.E., & Strauss, J.S. (1970). Chemical composition of human skin surface lipids from birth to puberty. *Journal of Investigative Dermatology,* 54(2):139–144.

Ramphal, R., Guay, P., & Pier, G. (1987). *Pseudomonas aeruginosa* adhesions for tracheobronchial mucin. *Infection and Immunity,* 55(3):600–603.

Rhinehart, E. (1989). Employee health for critical care duty. *Critical Care Nursing Quarterly,* 11(4):66–74.

Rhoades, R., & Pflanzer, R. (1992). *Human physiology* (2nd ed.). Philadelphia; Saunders College Publishing.

Riggs, C.D., & Lister, G. (1987). Adverse occurrences in the pediatric intensive care unit. *Pediatric Clinics of North America,* 34(1):93–117.

Rodriguez, M.A., Bankhurst, A.D., Ceuppens, C.B., & Williams, R.C. (1981). Characterization of the suppressor cell activity in human cord blood lymphocytes. *Journal of Clinical Investigations,* 68(6):1577–1585.

Roitt, I. (1988). *Essential immunology,* (6th ed.). Oxford, London: Blackwell Scientific Publications.

Rook, G. (1991). Cell-mediated immune responses. In I.M. Roitt, J. Brostoff & D. Male (Eds.). *Immunology* (2nd ed., pp. 9.1–9.14). Philadelphia: J.B. Lippincott.

Rosenthal, C.H. (1989). Immunosuppression in the pediatric critical care patient. *Critical Care Nursing Clinics of North America,* 1(4):775–785.

Rostad, M.E. (1991). Current strategies for managing myelosuppression in patients with cancer. *Oncology Nursing Forum,* 18(2[Suppl.]):7–15.

Roth, M.S., & Foon, K.A. (1987). Biotherapy with interferon in hematologic malignancies. *Oncology Nursing Forum,* 14(6[Suppl.]):16–22.

Rotrosen, D., & Gallin, J.I. (1990). Evaluation of the patient with suspected immunodeficiency. In G.L. Mandell, R.G. Douglas & J.E. Bennett (Eds.). *Principles and practice of infectious disease* (3rd ed., pp. 139–147). New York: Churchill Livingstone.

Royce, C. (1992). Outcome standard: Immunocompromised patient. Adult/Pediatric Intensive Care Unit, Critical Care Nursing Service, Department of Nursing, Clinical Center, National Institutes of Health, Bethesda, MD.

Saez-Llorens, X., & MacCracken, G.H. (1993). Sepsis syndrome and septic shock in pediatrics: Current concepts of terminology, pathophysiology, and management. *Journal of Pediatrics,* 123(4):497–508.

Sancho, L., Martinez-A, C., Nogales, A., & de la Hera, A. (1986). Reconstitution of natural-killer-cell activity in the newborn by interleukin-2. *New England Journal of Medicine.* 314(1):57–58.

Schindler, L.W. (1992). *The immune system—How it works* (p. 6). United States Department of Health and Human Services, Bethesda, MD., NIH publication number 92-3229.

Schot, J.D.L., & Schuurman, R.K.B. (1986). Blood transfusion suppresses cutaneous cell-mediated immunity. *Clinical Experimental Immunology,* 65(2):336–344.

Scrimshaw, N.S., Taylor, C.E., & Gordon, J.E. (1968). World Health Organization Monograph. Serial Number 57. Geneva, WHO.

Selekman, J. (1990). The multiple faces of immune deficiency in children. *Pediatric Nursing,* 16(4):351–361.

Selner, J.C., Merrill, D.A., & Claman, H.N. (1968). Salivary immunoglobulin and albumin: Development during the newborn period. *Journal of Pediatrics,* 72(5):685–689.

Shaefer, M., & Willis, L. (1991). Nursing implications of immunosuppression in transplantation: Update on drug intervention. *Nursing Clinics of North America,* 26(2):291–314.

Sherbotie, J.R., & Cornfeld, D. (1991). Management of urinary tract infections in children. *Medical Clinics of North America* 75(2):327–338.

Sheth, N.K., Franson, T.R., Rose, H.D., Buckmire, F.L.A., Cooper, J.A., & Sohnle, P.G. (1983). Colonization of bacteria on polyvinyl chloride and Teflon intravascular catheters in hospitalized patients. *Journal of Clinical Microbiology,* 18(5):1061–1063.

Silverman, A., & Roy, C.C. (1983). Immune homeostasis and the gut. In A. Silverman & C.C. Roy (Eds.). *Pediatric clinical gastroenterology* (3rd ed., pp. 324–336). St. Louis: C.V. Mosby.

Slavin, R.G. (1990). Immunologic effects of uremia (pp. 198–199). In Physiological and environmental influences on the immune system. In D.P. Stites & A.I. Terr (Eds.). *Basic and clinical immunology* (7th ed., pp. 187–200). Norwalk, CT: Appleton & Lange.

Slota, M.C. (1993). The cutting edge of pediatric critical care. *Critical Care Nurse,* June[Suppl.]:22–23.

Snyderman, R., & Pike, M.C. (1977). Disorders of leukocyte chemotaxis. *Pediatric Clinics of North America,* 24(2):377–393.

Sottile, F.D., Marrie, T.J., Prough, D.S., Hobgood, C.D., Gower, D.J., Webb, L.X., Costerton, J.W., & Gristina, A.G. (1986). Nosocomial pulmonary infection: Possible etiologic significance of bacterial adhesion to endotracheal tubes. *Critical Care Medicine,* 14(4):265–270.

Stamm, W.E. (1978). Infections related to medical devices. *Annals of Internal Medicine,* 89(5, part 2):764–769.

Steen, J.A. (1988). Impact of tube design and material on complications of tracheal intubation. *Problems in Anesthesia,* 2(2):211–224.

Sternberg, E.M., Moderator (1992). The stress response and the regulation of inflammatory disease. *Annals of Internal Medicine,* 117(10):854–866.

Stiehm, E.R. (1989). Immunodeficiency disorders: General considerations. In E.R. Stiehm (Ed.). *Immunological disorders in infants and children* (3rd ed., pp. 157–195). Philadelphia: W.B. Saunders.

Stiehm, E.R., Miller, A., Zelter, P.M., Katz, R.M., & Sapse, A.T. (1971). Secretory-defense system (SDSO) in health and disease (abstr). *Pediatric Research,* 5:381.

Stiehm, E.R., & Fudenberg, H.H. (1966). Serum levels of immune globulins in health and disease: A survey. *Pediatrics*, 37(5):715–727.

Stull, T.L., & LiPuma, J.J. (1991). Epidemiology and natural history of UTI in children. *Medical Clinics of North America*, 75(2):287–297.

Svanborg Eden, C., Kulhavy, R., Marild, S., Prince, S.J., & Mestecky, J. (1985). Urinary immunoglobulin in healthy individuals and children with acute pyelonephritis. *Scandinavian Journal of Immunology*, 21(4):305–313.

Tramont, E.C. (1990). General or nonspecific host defense mechanisms. In G.L. Mandell, R.G. Douglas & J.E. Bennett (Eds.). *Principles and practice of infectious disease* (3rd ed., pp. 33–41). New York: Churchill Livingstone.

Tribett, D. (1989). Immune system function: Implications for critical care nursing practice. *Critical Care Nursing Clinics of North America*, 1(4):727.

Tsuda, T., & Kahan, B.D. (1983). The effects of anesthesia on the immune response. In R.K. Chandra (Ed.). *Primary and secondary immunodeficiency disorders* (pp. 253–262). New York: Churchill Livingstone.

Tweady, D.J., Baley, J.E., Schachter, B.Z., & Ellner, J.J. (1982). Decreased surface expression of HLA-DR antigen on human neonatal cord blood monocytes. *Clinical Research*, 30(2):359a.

Utley, J.R. (1982). The immune response to cardiopulmonary bypass. In J.R. Utley (Ed.). *Pathophysiology and techniques of cardiopulmonary bypass* (Vol. I, pp. 132–144). Baltimore, MD: Williams & Wilkins.

Valenti, W.M., Menegus, M.A., Hall, C.B., Pincus, P.H., & Douglas, R.G. (1980). Nosocomial viral infections: I. Epidemiology and significance. *Infection Control*, 1(1):33–37.

Van Dervort, A.L., & Danner, R.L. (1994). Antiendotoxin approaches to septic shock therapy. *Critical Care Medicine*, 22(4):539–541.

Vogler, L.B., & Lawton, A.R. (1985). Ontogeny of B cells and humoral immune functions. *Clinics in Immunology and Allergy*, 5(2):235–252.

Wallace, C.S., Hall, M., & Kuhn, R.J. (1993). Pharmacologic management of cystic fibrosis. *Clinical Pharmacy,* 12(9):657–674.

Warren, J.W. (1991). The catheter and urinary tract infection. *Medical Clinics of North America*, 75(2):481–493.

Welliver, R.C., & McLaughlin, S. (1984). Unique epidemiology of nosocomial infection in a children's hospital. *American Journal of Diseases in Children*, 138(2):131–135.

Wenzel, R.P., Thompson, R.L., Landry, S.M., Russell, B.S., Miller, P.J., Ponce de Leon, S., & Miller, G.B. (1983). Hospital-acquired infections in intensive care unit patients: An overview with emphasis on epidemics. *Infection Control*, 4(5):371–375.

Wilson, M. (1985). Immunology of the fetus and newborn: Lymphocyte phenotype and function. *Clinics in Immunology and Allergy*, 5(2):271–286.

Wong, D.L., & Whaley, L.F. (1990). *Clinical manual of pediatric nursing*. St. Louis: C.V. Mosby.

Wood, R.A., & Sampson, H.A. (1989). The child with frequent infections. *Current Problems in Pediatrics*, 19(5):234–281.

Wright, W.C., Ank, B.J., Herbert, J., & Stiehm, E.R. (1975). Decreased bactericidal activity of leukocytes of stressed newborn infants. *Pediatrics*, 56(4):579–584.

Young, L.S. (1989). Infections in patients with cellular immunodeficiency. *Hospital Practice*, 24(8):191–212.

CHAPTER *17*

Skin Integrity

NANCY HAGELGANS
DARLENE WHITNEY

Bumps, scrapes, and bruises are a part of the lives of active children. The comfort of a loving parent and a BandAid heal such wounds. However, infants and children who require critical care are at risk to develop wounds that will not heal with a hug and the application of a cartoon character bandage. Rather, critical illness and intensive care significantly threaten the integrity of the body's external barrier: the skin.

The skin is the largest organ of the body. Any loss of the protective barrier provided by the skin can produce a life-threatening situation during critical illness. An insult to the first line of defense against invading microorganisms places critically ill infants and children at greater risk for complications of their illness. Maintenance of skin integrity and promotion of wound healing are significant aspects of the recovery of critically ill patients of any age. Decreasing risk factors that threaten skin integrity and optimizing wound healing are integral parts of preventing complications, which increase hospital morbidity and mortality, length of stay, resource consumption, and costs. It is crucial that critical care nurses plan and assess skin care measures that result in positive patient outcomes.

The challenges nurses face in protecting patients' skin are not easily overcome. Effective intervention necessitates an understanding of skin anatomy and physiology and the maturational characteristics of skin. This chapter presents that information, as well as a discussion of wound healing and the impact of critical illness and multiple system dysfunction on skin integrity and the healing process. Guidelines for the assessment, prevention, and treatment of wounds sustained by patients in the pediatric critical care environment are also presented.

INTEGUMENTARY STRUCTURE AND FUNCTION

The skin consists of three distinct anatomic layers. These layers include the epidermis, the dermis, and subcutaneous tissue.

The epidermis, or outer avascular layer, is a five-layered wall that provides a skin barrier against microorganisms and irritating chemicals. It also impedes the exchange of fluids and electrolytes between the body and the environment. The epidermis consists of two important cell populations: keratinocytes and melanocytes. The stratum corneum, or the horny outer layer, is composed mostly of keratinocytes. Keratinocytes are flat cells that lack a nucleus and cytoplasm and consequently have a low water content. Unlike underlying cells that are moist, the stratum corneum is dry and waterproof. This offers the underlying dermal cells protection from desiccation. The second group of cells found in the epidermis are the melanocytes. They are housed in the basal layer of the epidermis. Each epidermal melanocyte has dendritic cytoplasmic extensions that make contact with 35 to 45 epidermal cells. This melanocyte-keratinocyte unit is responsible for pigmentation. Another function of the melanin is to provide some but not complete protection from ultraviolet rays.

Although the epidermal layer is only 0.05 mm to 0.1 mm thick, the barrier function of the skin resides in the stratum corneum. The keratinization or shedding of one to two cell layers of the stratum corneum prevents excessive colonization of the skin surface. In addition to continuous shedding, the flattened stratum corneum cells are tightly adherent to each other. To obtain entrance into the lower epidermis and dermis, chemicals or microorganisms must pass between tightly compacted epidermal cells.

The newborn infant's epidermal layer does not have the same protective barrier properties as that of an older child or adult. During the first week of life, infants are at risk for higher levels of water loss and a higher permeability of drug absorption. Neonates are therefore at risk for exhibiting the toxic effects of drugs through topical absorption. By the age of 2 weeks, however, the stratum corneum of even preterm infants shows considerable maturation in terms of thickness and keratin production (Harpin & Rutter, 1983). The stimulus for this rapid postnatal maturation is thought to be the change from the immersion in amniotic fluid to exposure to air, but how this is mediated is unknown.

The dermis is the second layer of skin. The dermis is 0.5 mm to 2.5 mm thick and is the principal mass of the skin. The dermis contains connective tissue, which is comprised of collagenous and elastic fibers. Embedded in the dermis are blood vessels, lymphatics, nerve endings, and hair follicles. Fibroblasts and macrophages are the predominant cells in the dermis and are responsible for the production of collagen (Bryant, 1987). The importance of the fibroblasts and macrophages to wound healing is delineated in the section Phases of Healing.

The dermis gives the skin substance, mechanical strength, and elasticity, allowing the skin to withstand severe frictional stress, yet still be extensible over joints. The dermal thickness remains constant in the first year of life, increases between years 1 and 3, then doubles between ages 3 and 7.

Beneath the dermis is the subcutaneous layer or hypodermis. This third layer varies in depth and is composed primarily of adipose tissue. It contains all the structures and appendages found in the dermis. It serves as a cushion to trauma, a heat insulator, and an important source of energy metabolism. Premature infants have poorly developed subcutaneous tissue, contributing to thermal instability and metabolic differences.

IMPAIRED SKIN INTEGRITY

Members of the North American Nursing Diagnosis Association (NANDA) (1989) define impaired skin integrity as the state in which a person's skin is adversely altered or at risk for being adversely altered. The clinical manifestations of impaired skin integrity in infants and children are varied. Rashes, from diaper area excoriation to the red itchy welts of hypersensitivity reactions to the lesions of varicella, are common throughout childhood. Tissue trauma of varying degrees may include burns, blisters, incisions, abrasions, punctures, swelling, bruises, and erythema. Critically ill infants and children may exhibit disrupted skin integrity as surgical wounds, fissures, pressure ulcers, blackened ischemic tissue, dry or cracked mucous membranes, and dry or abraded corneal surfaces. Changes in pigmentation and elasticity can also be seen in some children with chronic diseases such as graft-versus-host disease following bone marrow transplantation.

Risk Factors

There are many factors that place critically ill infants and children at particular risk for developing compromised skin integrity. Major categories include impaired physical mobility, alterations in nutrition, fluid volume deficit, decreased cardiac output, hypoxemia, and immunosuppression.

Impaired Physical Mobility

Impaired physical mobility often accompanies serious illness and can predispose areas of skin to prolonged or excessive pressure. Pressure, especially over bony prominences, compresses capillary beds supplying blood to the skin and underlying soft tissue. Oxygen and nutrient deprivation, along with a buildup of metabolic waste, results in cellular necrosis and soft tissue infarction, which appear as a pressure ulcer (Fig. 17–1).

The most common locations for excessive pressure include the occiput in infants and children and the sacrum in older children ages 10 to 14 years (Solis et al., 1988). Children with baseline sensory motor deficits, a decreased level of consciousness, or significant activity intolerance are often unable to detect or respond to prolonged pressure. Other children at added risk for developing pressure ulcers include

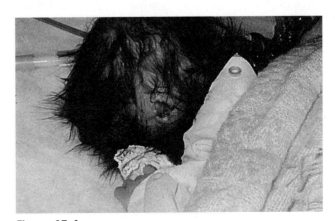

Figure 17–1 ● ● ● ● ● ●
Pressure ulcer—occiput.

those who are physically or chemically restrained, are significantly over- or underweight, or require strict bedrest for a prolonged period of time.

Impaired Nutrition: Less Than Body Requirements

Suboptimal nutrition is another factor that places critically ill infants and children at risk for skin breakdown and delayed wound healing (Stotts, 1990). Inadequate caloric intake results in gluconeogenesis, which depletes protein stores and the amino acids necessary for cell membrane integrity. An adequate intake of carbohydrates and fats is necessary to meet cellular energy requirements and support cell proliferation and phagocytosis. Insufficient protein intake results in a negative nitrogen balance and delay in wound healing by impeding neovascularization, lymphatic formation, fibroblast proliferation, and collagen synthesis (Young, 1988). Hypoalbuminemia results in interstitial edema, which slows the cellular exchange of metabolites. Sufficient intake of vitamins A and C is needed for collagen synthesis. Vitamin A also plays a role in the epithelialization of cell membranes, and vitamin C is needed to prevent capillary fragility (Young, 1988). Inadequate mineral intake, particularly of zinc, impedes cell proliferation and collagen synthesis (Ruberg, 1984).

An inadequate nutritional state can develop if intake is poor or if metabolic demands are escalated without a concomitant increase in caloric intake. Children may be unable to eat because of nausea, impaired neurologic function, respiratory distress, or orofacial trauma. They may be unable to tolerate enteral feeds because of decreased gastrointestinal motility, malabsorption, gastroesophageal reflux, congenital gastrointestinal anomalies, or surgical repairs. Even parenteral supplementation may be insufficient if fluid intake is severely restricted or intravenous access limited.

Critically ill children also encounter many stressors that escalate their metabolic needs. Stressors that place children at greatest risk include multiple trauma, burns, surgery, increased work of breathing, infection, alterations in temperature, and cancer. Children with inborn errors of metabolism and diseases such as diabetes mellitus, liver failure, and renal failure have altered metabolic states that increase their risk for inadequate nutrition (Piloian, 1992).

Fluid Volume Deficit

Because of a proportionally higher body composition of water, infants and children exhibit the negative effects of dehydration more readily than adults. Mild to moderate fluid volume deficit results in poor skin turgor and dry, cracked epithelium and mucous membrane surfaces. Severe dehydration compromises cardiac output and systemic perfusion and causes compensatory peripheral vasoconstriction. This reduces the cellular exchange of metabolites and creates a metabolic acidosis. Hypovolemia also results in low tissue oxygenation despite adequate arterial oxygenation (Chang et al., 1983). These conditions place the skin at risk for necrosis and delayed wound healing.

Dehydration may result from fluid losses resulting from diarrhea, ileostomy or jejunostomy drainage, and vomiting or nasogastric drainage. Infants and children are also particularly sensitive to insensible fluid losses because they have a proportionally greater body surface area than adults. Losses from fever, tachypnea, diaphoresis, open wounds, and use of radiant warmers, phototherapy, and extracorporeal membrane oxygen support can significantly deplete body fluid.

Decreased Cardiac Output

Decreased cardiac output predictably has negative multisystem effects regardless of etiology. For the skin, low cardiac output results in vasoconstriction of the skin's microcirculation, along with hypoperfusion. This deprives skin cells of the nutrients, oxygen, and waste removal necessary for their existence. The result is metabolic acidosis, ischemia, necrosis, and delayed wound healing. Venous stasis, a result of hypoperfusion, may develop and contribute to interstitial edema. This further impedes the exchange of cellular metabolites and increases the skin's fragility by stretching collagen fibers (Mechanic & Perkins, 1988). Children likely to experience impaired cardiac output include those with severe dehydration, electrolyte imbalance, sepsis, structural or conductive cardiac anomalies, acidosis, and hypoxemia.

Hypoxemia

Structural immaturity of the pulmonary system places infants and children at greater risk for respiratory distress. Hypoxemia results in inadequate tissue oxygenation. Accompanied by compensatory peripheral vasoconstriction, hypoxemia can result in tissue ischemia and lactic acidosis, placing the skin at risk for breakdown and delayed wound healing. Children with chronic hypoxemia may also develop polycythemia. The increased blood viscosity increases the potential of thrombus formation. Small clots have the potential to obstruct the skin's microcirculation, leading to localized areas of infarction. Children with significant, prolonged respiratory impairment and those with cyanotic heart disease are at high risk of developing skin impairment from hypoxemia.

Immunosuppression

An immature immune system also affects the integumentary system. A child whose immune system is already taxed by serious illness may not have the capacity to fight a secondary infection. This places both intact and impaired skin at risk for opportunistic infections such as from *Candida,* fungus, and

Staphylococcus. Infectious agents then compete with fibroblasts, macrophages, and healthy skin cells for nutrition (Bryant, 1987). At least one study has shown that the presence of infection, in particular systemic infection, is predictive of increased skin breakdown risk (Piloian, 1992).

The side effects of immunosuppressive therapy are also detrimental to skin integrity. Side effects include obesity, avascular necrosis, gingival hypertrophy, increased skin fragility, decreased elasticity, and delayed wound healing. Steroids also interfere with the inflammatory stage of wound healing and epithelialization (Bryant, 1987; Doughty, 1990). Children at greatest risk for suffering the ill effects of compromised immune defenses include those with primary immune dysfunctions, overwhelming sepsis, solid organ and bone marrow transplantation, and prematurity. Children with cancer undergoing chemotherapy or radiation therapy are also at high risk.

Prevention

The most important nursing intervention in preventing skin breakdown in critically ill infants and children is the early identification of risk factors (Goodrich & March, 1992). Ideally, a pediatric-specific impaired skin integrity prediction tool could be used to identify patients at high risk. At present, however, predictive tools are available only for adult patients. These tools include the Braden scale and the Norton scale (Bergstrom et al., 1987; Norton et al., 1962). Studies have not been done to support the use of these tools as valid predictors of skin breakdown in infants and children.

Modify Risk

Once a child at high risk has been clearly identified, a management plan is developed to eliminate or modify risks. Mobility can be improved by providing optimal comfort and minimizing the use of physical restraints. Consultation with physical therapists is helpful in deciding how best to facilitate the highest degree of mobility possible for each child, for example, using active and passive range of motion activities.

Nutritional assessment on admission is essential to ensure continued optimal nutrition. Consultation with nutrition support is helpful in determining whether specialized enteral feedings or vitamin and mineral supplements would be beneficial. Central parenteral nutrition is considered if a previously healthy child is expected to be unable to tolerate enteral feeding for longer than 5 days (see Chapter 14).

Fluid and electrolyte replacement is established to provide optimal hydration within the fluid constraints of the child's condition. Accurate measurements of fluid losses from diarrhea, wound drainage, stomas, emesis, and nasogastric and gastrostomy tubes are included in output totals. Losses are replaced with appropriate enteral or intravenous fluids. Insensible fluid losses from warmers, tachypnea, and fever are assessed and added into baseline fluid requirements.

The cardiac output of children at risk for poor perfusion is optimized by correcting hypoxemia, acidosis, electrolyte abnormalities, hypoglycemia, and hypovolemia. Measures are instituted to keep the child normothermic. Cardiac workload is decreased by providing scheduled rest periods, reducing stress, and promoting comfort. Inotropic agents, afterload reducers, and antidysrhythmic agents are titrated collaboratively with the physician.

For children at risk for hypoxemia, a plan is developed to optimize gas exchange. Supplementary oxygen and frequent rest periods are provided as needed. Deep breathing, coughing, and positioning are encouraged to best support oxygenation. Chest physical therapy, postural drainage, vibration, and suctioning are also provided when indicated. The hematocrit is maintained within normal limits, and bronchodilators and diuretics are administered collaboratively with the physician. Gas exchange is supported as needed with continuous positive airway pressure, manual controlled bagging, and mechanical ventilation collaboratively with the physician and respiratory therapist.

Nurses must identify immunosuppressed infants and children at high risk for infection. A plan of care that minimizes their potential for infection is developed. Appropriate precautions, which may include gowns, gloves, masks, or reverse isolation, are instituted. Good handwashing techniques are maintained, and the number of caregivers is limited. All infusion lines and dressings are aseptically changed following the Centers for Disease Control and Prevention guidelines. Prophylactic and therapeutic antibiotic, antifungal, and antiviral agents are administered collaboratively with the physician.

Vigilant Care

For all infants and children, skin conditions are assessed and recorded at each shift. Breakdown is prevented by keeping skin clean and dry. Daily baths using water and a mild soap are followed by thorough, gentle drying using patting motions. Moisturizer is used only on overly dry areas of skin. The use of products with perfumes, alcohols, and additives, including many disposable diaper wipe products, is avoided. Diapers and underpads are checked and changed frequently. Sheets and other linen are also kept dry and wrinkle free.

Nurses identify and protect areas prone to breakdown from wetness and acidic drainage. The use of protective ointments routinely on the intact skin of infants at risk has been shown to significantly reduce diaper area breakdown (Kramer & Honig, 1988).

The number of protective skin moisture barrier products on the market are plentiful. They can be found in a variety of forms (i.e., sprays, wipes, creams, and ointments). When selecting a barrier there are a few simple principles to consider: (1) ease of application—some products have a two- and three-step application process, which can be time-consuming and impractical; (2) cost—hospital charges for specialty barriers can be expensive. Furthermore, if the family wishes to continue the product's use after discharge from the hospital, it may be difficult to obtain; (3) ingredients—alcohol and perfumes are irritating and drying; and (4) ease of removal—if the barrier cakes or hardens, its removal can cause trauma to the skin. The barrier should provide moisture to the skin while protecting it from continued wetness or acidic drainage. Products as simple as Vaseline, A&D, or Desitin ointment may be sufficient to protect the infant or child's skin.

When the skin is denuded and the perineum becomes soiled, it is not necessary to remove all of the protective barrier. Each time the skin is cleansed, by taking the barrier completely off, there is a high likelihood that new epithelial growth can be disrupted. Therefore, removing only that portion of the protective barrier that is soiled is advised, along with new application of the barrier.

The use of Stomadhesive barrier and Duoderm (Convatec, Bristol-Myers Squibb Co., Princeton, NJ) over the buttocks is not advised. Stool tends to accumulate around the edges of the wafer, it does not always adhere to the child's contour, and the "melt down" it produces within the closed moist environment of a diaper can cause further trauma to the skin when it is removed. Often the area of most severe breakdown is in the gluteal crease, and the barrier wafer cannot be applied to that area. The use of heat lamps is avoided because they can burn a child.

To prevent skin irritation and epidermal stripping, adhesive use on sensitive skin is limited. Whenever possible, alternatives to tape to secure lines, tubes, and dressings are used. Good substitutes include Velcro ties, Montgomery straps, and Stockinette (Fig. 17–2). When tape is needed, consider using Transpore tape (3M Health Care, St. Paul, MN) or OpSite (Smith and Nephew Medical Limited, Hull, England)

instead of cloth tape. A protective barrier such as Stomadhesive or HolliHesive (Hollister Incorporated, Libertyville, IL) can be used under adhesives to protect sensitive areas of skin. Benzoin should be used sparingly under adhesive tape and limited to use in children older than 1 month of age. Patients will require individual assessment of possibly irritating effects of benzoin. When removing adhesives, gentle traction is applied to the skin and plenty of water or an adhesive tape remover is used to aid removal. If a tape remover product is used, the affected skin is immediately washed thoroughly with soap and water to prevent chemical irritation. The fewest number of cardiac electrodes possible should be used. The placement of all electrodes and oxygen saturation and transcutaneous probes should be changed on a basis recommended by the manufacturer and tolerated by the individual patient.

Damage from excessive or prolonged pressure is prevented with frequent position changes. Patients unable to shift their own weight are turned at least every 2 hours. A draw sheet is used in older children to prevent shearing injuries.

Bony prominences are padded or lifted off bed surfaces with pillows or soft rolls. Devices such as splints, ankle-foot orthoses, and hand rolls are padded and removed frequently to assess for erythema at pressure points. Stockinette can be used under these devices to prevent maceration from perspiration and breakdown from friction. Soft heel and elbow pads can be placed over these bony prominences to protect skin from friction damage. Hydrocolloidal adhesive dressings, such as DuoDerm Extra Thin (Convatec, Bristol-Myers Squibb Co, Princeton, NJ), can also be used over areas of intact skin at risk for breakdown to maintain integrity and over areas of existing breakdown to prevent further damage and aid healing (Ching & Mell, 1990). Routine skin massage also helps to stimulate blood flow to the skin over nonreddened bony prominences, although there has been no research to support benefits from this practice (Maklebust, 1987). The use of genuine sheepskin padding also helps to prevent pressure ulcers by reducing friction and shear (Marchand & Lidowski, 1993).

Frequent *mouth care* is also essential in maintaining optimal skin integrity. Children with teeth are assisted in using a soft bristle brush to brush their teeth. A piece of gauze can be used to clean the teeth of infants or children with sensitive or bleeding gums. Older children are assisted in flossing as tolerated. Oral mucosa is kept moist with frequent nonalcoholic and nonsweetened mouthwash or water rinses. For children unable to safely rinse, moistened Toothettes or swabs are used to keep the oral cavity from drying.

Petroleum jelly protects lips from cracking. When retaping oral endotracheal tubes, the tube is repositioned to the alternate side of the mouth to prevent pressure breakdown. For children who cannot swallow, pooled oral secretions that can foster infection and circumoral skin breakdown are suctioned. If a

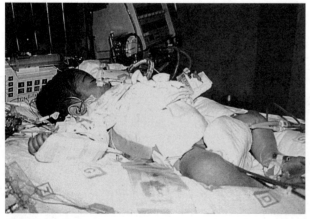

Figure 17–2 ● ● ● ● ● ●

Montgomery straps on a liver transplant patient.

child's tongue is swollen and exposed, drying injuries are prevented by covering the exposed tongue with petroleum gauze. If tongue edema is significant, a dental consultation may be considered to evaluate the benefit of using a mouth guard or props to relieve dental pressure. If oral appliances are used, a routine schedule for their removal and cleaning is implemented.

Scheduled *eye care* is also included for those infants and children lacking the sensory and/or motor abilities to protect their eyes from iatrogenic damage. Eyes are kept moist, free of debris, and protected from abrasion at all times. Lacri-lube (Allergan Pharmaceuticals, Allergan Inc., Irvine, CA) is applied from the inner to outer canthus of the eye on a set schedule and as needed to provide a moist environment. Eyes can be rinsed with sterile normal saline or artificial tears to remove debris. For children whose sclera are edematous or whose lids cannot close completely, an occlusive nonadhesive cover such as plastic wrap is cut to cover the gap between the top and bottom lids and is placed over an ample application of Lacri-lube.

Tracheostomy sites can be kept clean with half-strength hydrogen peroxide and normal saline cleansing. Split gauze sponges are placed under tracheostomy tubes to keep moisture off the neck. Soft foam Velcro ties (Dale Medical Products, Inc., Plainville, MA; Posey Co., Arcadia, CA) provide an alternative to tracheostomy tape. Ties are routinely assessed and changed promptly when wet. Velcro ties can be washed, dried, and reused.

Pressure dispersing devices are considered for infants and children with several risk factors or existing breakdown. Pressure reduction devices are products that reduce the pressures placed on tissues but do not consistently maintain pressures less than capillary closing pressures. Therefore, to be used safely, patients using these devices should be able to sense pressure and shift their own weight or be able to tolerate frequent position changes. A convoluted foam or "egg crate" mattress cut at least 2 to 4 inches thick is an effective pressure-reducing device and has been shown to prevent occiput breakdown and reduce sacrococcygeal area pressure in children (Solis et al., 1988). Gel mattresses are also very effective pressure reducers (Berjian et al., 1983). Smaller gel pads, such as Spenco Gel Skin Care pads (Spenco Medical Corporation, Waco, TX), are good for relieving pressure under specific discrete areas prone to breakdown, such as the ear or an infant's occiput. Other pressure-reducing products include water mattresses and mattress overlays that use air in a variety of ways to disperse and alternate pressure (Table 17–1).

Table 17–1. PRESSURE REDUCTION/RELIEF DEVICES

Description	Advantages	Disadvantages	Examples
Overlay: a device that is made to fit over a regular hospital mattress.			
1. **Foam:** varying density; 2–4 inch convoluted and nonconvoluted.	Primarily pressure reduction although in children may have pressure relief advantages; can be cut to fit cribs.	Can soil with incontinent patient; inability to reduce skin moisture due to lack of air flow.	Aerofoam, BioGard, DuraPedic, GeoMatt, Ultra Form Pediatric.
2. **Gel/Water Filled:** pressure reduction; water or gel conforms to patient's contours.	One time charge; low cost for water; gels are expensive.	Gravity displacement can lead to inadequate flotation; potential for leaks; heavy; question safety indications for CPR.	Aqua-Pedics (water and gel), Tender Gel and Water, Theracare (water and gel).
3. **Alternating Pressure Mattress:** an overlay with rows of air cells and pump. Pump cycles air to provide inflation and deflation over pressure points.	Constant low volume air flow; manages excess skin moisture.	Cost of pump rental; on-going monitor and maintenance of equipment; some complain pumps are noisy.	AeroPulse, AlphaBed, AlphaCare, BetaBed, Bio Flote, Dyna-CARE, Lapidus, PCA Systems, Pillo-Pump, Tenderair.
4. **Static Air:** designed with interlocking air cells that provide dry flotation. Inflated with a blower.	May be more effective than foam; easy to clean; has been documented in adult studies to reduce pressure.	Inflation level must be checked frequently by caregiver in order to maintain therapeutic levels; may cause increased perspiration due to plastic surface.	DermaGard, K-Soft, KoalaKair, Roho, Sof-Care, Tenderair.
5. **Specialty Mattress Overlay:** Fitted air-filled cushions placed over entire bed; pressures can be set and controlled by a pump.	Surface materials are constructed to reduce friction and shear and to eliminate moisture; pressure relief; can be used for prevention and/or treatment of ulcers.	Surface mattress and pump are a rental item; not available for cribs. Side rails on some beds may not adequately contain large patients.	ACUCAIR, BioTherapy, Clini-Care, CRS 4000, RibCor Therapeutic Mattress Pad.

Reprinted from *Pediatric Nursing*, 1993, Volume 19, Number 5, p. 504. Reprinted with permission of the publisher, Jannetti Publications, Inc., East Holly Avenue Box 56, Pitman, NJ 08071-0056; Phone (609) 256-2300; FAX (609) 589-7463.

Therapeutic Beds

Pressure-relieving devices differ from pressure reduction devices in that they consistently maintain pressures less than capillary closing pressures, allowing blood to flow unimpeded through the skin's microcirculation. Specialized therapeutic beds are the largest and most sophisticated group of pressure-relieving devices available. They are also designed to reduce or eliminate damage from shear, friction, and maceration on a short-term basis. Unfortunately, specialty beds are an expensive care option, and most institutions have limited resources available for bed rentals. The use of therapeutic beds is reserved for those patients at high risk for skin breakdown despite optimal nursing care. Children that frequently warrant and can benefit most from this level of intervention include those with severe pulmonary disease who require long-term high-pressure ventilation or extracorporeal membrane oxygenation support, cardiovascular instability that prohibits position changes, meningococcemia, chronic debilitation or malnutrition, and skin grafts or extensive skin breakdown already present (including burns, traumatic injury, purpura fulminans, and pressure sores).

Several types of specialty beds are currently available (Table 17–2). When deciding which bed is most appropriate for children, it is important to have a clear understanding of their present risk factors, treatment goals, and projected illness trajectory. Static low-air-loss beds consist of independently inflated air-filled cushions that provide pressure relief. They can adjust manually to a variety of positions and they are available in small and crib sizes. Most are covered with nonabsorbent nonstick sheets, and some have special features such as built-in scales. Disadvantages of these beds include cost and bulky size, the fact that the bed does not actively change the patient's position, and that the bed does not absorb fluids, which may lead to maceration, infection, and delayed wound healing. Children most likely to benefit from this type of bed are those at high risk for developing skin breakdown, those who tolerate some movement, and those who do not have extensive wounds and in whom the primary treatment goal is to prevent pressure breakdown until their underlying condition has improved.

Kinetic therapy beds are a group of beds that can be programmed to rotate a patient's position at set intervals. Rotation beds are a type of kinetic bed in which the entire bed frame moves to rotate the patient. They are often made of flat, firm foam surfaces with foam support cushions and straps. These beds are optimal for treating patients with unstable trau-

Table 17–2. SPECIALTY BEDS*

Description	Advantages	Disadvantages	Examples
Specialty beds are "high-tech" beds used in place of the standard hospital bed, are usually used on a rental basis, and are intended for short-term use. They provide pressure relief and eliminate shear, friction, and maceration, and in some cases provide lateral rotation and chest physiotherapy.			
1. Low-Air-Loss Beds: surface consists of inflated air cushions, each zone is adjusted for optimal pressure relief for patients' body size; some models have built-in scales.	Provides pressure relief in any position; treatment for Stages II-IV pressure ulcers; available in pediatric crib sizes. Ideal for treatment of heel and occipital pressure sores.	Difficult for the patient to move around in bed.	FlexiCair, Air Plus, KinAir, Mediscus; Cribs: Pedcare, PediKair, PNEU-CARE/Pedi.
2. Air Fluidized Beds: air is blown through silicone beads to "float" patient.	Treatment for deep pressure sores, burns, posterior flaps; draws fluid away from patient.	Airflow may dry out wound if latex sheet not used. Bed weights 1500 lbs. Difficult to transfer patient.	CLINITRON, FluidAir Plus, Skytron
3. Continuous Lateral Rotation Beds. *Cushion Beds:* Microprocessor-controlled low-air-loss bed inflates and deflates cushions to achieve lateral rotation. Some models include percussion, vibration, pulsation. Some raise patient high enough for ECMO support. *Table based:* Without low-air-loss cushions, achieves lateral rotation by turning complete bed frame.	Indicated for patients with a high degree of immobility, severe respiratory distress, and who are hemodynamically unstable when moved. Must have stable spine. Table based—same as above and suitable for some patients without a stable spine.	Cost	*Cushion Based:* RESTCUE, BioDyne, *Table Based:* RotoRest, Keane Mobility

*This list is a representative sampling of products, which is not intended to be all inclusive. No endorsement of any product is intended. Within each category, products must be individually evaluated on their efficacy as comfort, pressure-reducing, or pressure-relieving devices. All products within a category do not necessarily perform equally. Data from Doughty (1990), Glavis & Barbour (1990), Krasner (1991).

Reprinted from *Pediatric Nursing*, 1993, Volume 19, Number 5, p. 504. Reprinted with permission of the publisher, Jannetti Publications, Inc., East Holly Avenue Box 56, Pitman, NJ 08071-0056; Phone (609) 256-2300; FAX (609) 589-7463.

matic injury in whom the treatment goals are to prevent pressure breakdown, mobilize pulmonary secretions, and stimulate gastrointestinal mobility. Disadvantages of these beds include cost, size, waterproof cushions that may promote sweating and fluid contact with skin, and the risk of shearing injury with movement. These beds are used only until patients' initial traumatic injury has been stabilized and they can be safely moved to a bed with less risk of shearing or maceration injury.

Another subgroup of kinetic therapy beds is the active low-air-loss bed. These beds consist of independently inflated air-filled cushions that either pulsate or rotate the patient from side to side. The advantages that these beds offer include selected pressure relief, a variety of bed positions, cushions that dry quickly, and bed movement that may stimulate capillary blood flow and loosen pulmonary secretions (Lovell & Anderson, 1990). Disadvantages include cost, size, and bed movement that is relatively limited when compared to manual turning. Children who benefit most from active low-air-loss beds include those at high risk for skin breakdown who also have significant pulmonary compromise or congestive heart failure, edema, or cardiovascular instability in whom manual turning is not tolerated but in whom repositioning is essential in the care of their underlying illness.

Air fluidized or static high-air-loss beds have absorptive ceramic beads that are blown by warm air to create a fluid-like motion. The beads are contained within a thin filter sheet. The beads absorb fluid and keep both the sheet and patient continually dry. The filter sheet and chemical makeup of the beads also help to reduce the risk of infection. The fluid movement of these beds is superior to air cushions in placing minimal pressure on tissues. Temperature regulation of the bed's airflow can be manipulated to meet patient care needs. Disadvantages include cost, size, weight, inability to adjust bed height, limited bed positions, and the bed's drying effect, which may overly dry open wounds and thicken pulmonary secretions. These beds are used when the primary objective is optimal wound healing in infants and children with severe skin disorders, extensive skin breakdown, heavily draining or large open wounds, or large grafted areas.

WOUND HEALING

All critically ill patients have one thing in common, namely, the presence of a wound—defined as an interruption in the continuity of body tissue. The wound may be traumatic in origin, such as a burn or a fracture, or may be produced by placement of an intravascular line or a surgical incision. Whatever the etiology, a wound is a potential source of considerable morbidity and mortality. A major goal of intensive care management is to promote healing. A common error in the intensive care unit setting, however, is to separate wound care and wound healing from the remainder of intensive care management. Wound healing affects and is affected by critical care management decisions. Because of its importance in determining patient outcomes, knowledge of the process of wound healing is essential to critical care providers.

Orgill and Demling (1988) define wound healing as a process whereby injured tissue is repaired, resulting in the regeneration of cell lining of tissue with a reorganization of mesodermal tissue derivatives into scar. Wound healing can be categorized, in clinical terms, into first, second, and third intention healing (Fig. 17–3). Most surgical wounds are closed by first (primary) intention, wherein the edges of the wound are approximated by sutures, staples, or tape. These are wounds without significant tissue loss, and they heal without visible granulation tissue and with minimal scarring.

Healing by secondary intention takes place when a large amount of tissue is lost, when significant necrotic debris, inflammation, or exudate is present, or when wound edges do not meet. These wounds heal by granulation, epithelialization, and contraction (Wysocki, 1989).

Tertiary wound healing (delayed primary closure) occurs when a contaminated wound is left open to heal by granulation. These wounds may be loosely packed and after 3 to 7 days, when no evidence of infection is found, they are sutured closed and go on to heal by primary closure.

Phases of Healing

The cellular process of wound healing can be divided into three phases: the inflammatory or exudate phase, the proliferative or fibroblastic phase, and the remodeling or maturation phase (Table 17–3). Although these phases overlap and intertwine, each has a predictable sequence of events that distinguishes it (Hudson-Goodman et al., 1990; Sieggreen, 1987; Wysocki, 1989; Carrico et al., 1984; Orgill & Demling, 1988).

Inflammatory Phase

The first of the three phases of wound healing is the inflammatory phase. Clinically, this is characterized by erythema, warmth, edema, and pain. The function of this phase is to clear away dead cells and bacteria and stimulate the healing process. The inflammatory phase begins as soon as the injury occurs. The injury, for example, can be a surgical incision, laceration, burn, an intravenous drug infiltrate, or the consequence of prolonged pressure over a bony prominence. Whatever the initial insult, a cascade of interdependent reactions is initiated.

Immediately after the injury, a short period of vasoconstriction lasting 5 to 10 minutes occurs, slowing blood flow through the area to aid hemostasis (Alvarez et al., 1987). Vasoconstriction is followed by active vasodilation induced by the release of bradyki-

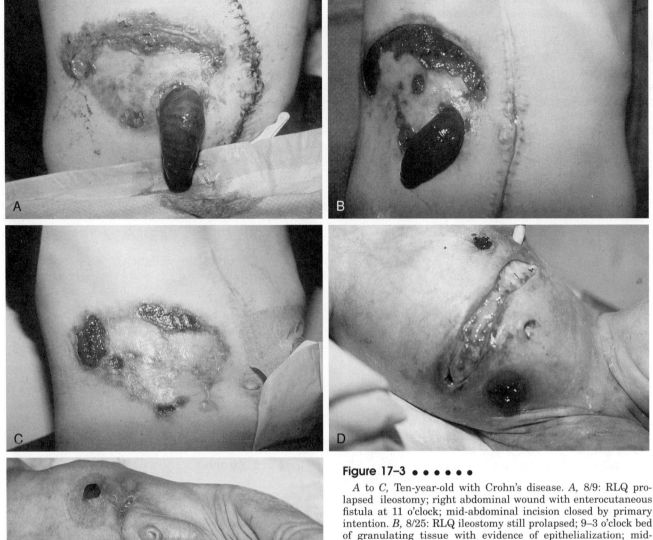

Figure 17–3 ● ● ● ● ● ●

A to *C,* Ten-year-old with Crohn's disease. *A,* 8/9: RLQ prolapsed ileostomy; right abdominal wound with enterocutaneous
fistula at 11 o'clock; mid-abdominal incision closed by primary
intention. *B,* 8/25: RLQ ileostomy still prolapsed; 9–3 o'clock bed
of granulating tissue with evidence of epithelialization; mid-
abdominal incision healed—wound edges well approximated. *C,*
10/24: RLQ ileostomy relocated to LLQ secondary to persistent
enterocutaneous secondary fistula; continued granulation and
re-epithelialization of right abdominal wound. *D* and *E,* Newborn
with necrotizing enterocolitis (NEC) status post bowel resection
with RLQ ileostomy and LUQ gastrostomy. *D,* Mid-abdominal
wound dehiscence with necrotic non-viable tissue; fascia intact.
E, Wound healed by debridement of non-viable tissue via moist
wound healing over 14 days, then surgically closed by tertiary
intention. (*A* to *E,* Courtesy of Sandy Quigley, RN, CETN,
Children's Hospital, Boston.)

nin and histamine (Orgill & Demling, 1988). During
this period, vessel walls become lined with leukocytes, platelets, and erythrocytes, which migrate into
the wound to begin the debriding process. Simultaneously, vascular permeability increases, allowing serum to gain entry into the wound. Fluid, protein,
and enzymes normally found in the intravascular
compartment leak through the vessel walls into the
extracellular space, causing edema and erythema
(Hotter, 1982).

Leukocytes migrate to the wound and provide resistance to infection. Two types of leukocytes, polymorphonuclear (PMN) granulocytes and mononuclear granulocytes, begin to digest bacteria. The
neutrophils are short-lived (2–3 days) and become
part of the wound exudate. The monocytes, which
differentiate into macrophages, become the predominant cell in the injured tissue. Their presence persists for weeks as they digest foreign material and
release a protein that stimulates the formation of
fibroblasts. This protein, along with platelet growth
factor, stimulates growth of local venular endothelial
cells that give rise to new vessels (Hunt & Halliday,
1980).

Table 17-3. PHASES OF WOUND HEALING

Phase	Clinical Observation	Cellular Activities
Inflammatory phase Typically begins at time of injury and lasts approximately 3 days	Erythema, warmth, edema, and pain	*Vasoconstriction:* platelets form along injured blood vessels; platelets release vasoconstrictive substances and promote fibrin clot to prevent hemorrhage *Vasodilation:* vasodilatory substances allow leakage of plasma into wound Leukocytes migrate through vessel walls to phagocytose bacteria and foreign materials Monocytes differentiate into macrophages, which give rise to tissue repair process
Proliferative phase Overlaps with inflammatory phase and continues until wound is healed	Beefy, red granulation tissue	*Macrophages* secrete growth-promoting substances that mediate granulation tissue and epithelialization *Collagen synthesis:* performed by fibroblasts; provides tensile strength to wound *Angiogenesis:* regeneration of a vascular network to restore capillary system to dermis
	Thin, silvery, epithelial layer surrounding granulation tissue Wound shrinkage	*Epithelialization:* cell migration across a wound *Contraction:* myofibroblasts migrate through tissue to facilitate closing the wound
Maturation phase Begins 3 weeks after wounding and may continue for several years	Shrinking, thinning, paling of scar	Remodeling of tissue matrix as fibroblasts migrate away from the wound while fibrous bundles of collagen increase the tensile strength of the scar

Anti-inflammatory agents, particularly corticosteroids, given before the wounding or during the critical 1- to 3-day inflammatory phase can markedly attenuate the inflammatory response (Orgill & Demling, 1988). Vitamin A has been found to counteract the anti-inflammatory response of corticosteroids; but when given systemically, can also attenuate the anticipated systemic steroid effect. A persistent decrease in wound blood flow as seen in dehydration or impaired cardiac output can also delay the onset of inflammation.

Proliferative Phase

The proliferative phase, also known as the fibroblastic phase, is primarily a phase of cell regeneration. This phase lasts approximately 4 to 20 days after the injury. The major processes occurring during this phase include macrophage arrival and replication, fibroblast production, collagen synthesis, angiogenesis, epithelialization, and wound contraction. The clinical observations are a moist, beefy red, granulation tissue resulting from the newly formed collagen and blood vessels. A thin, silvery, epithelial layer circumscribes the granulation tissue and finally wound shrinkage.

The macrophages and platelets seen in the inflammatory phase trigger many of the events that occur in the proliferative phase (Hunt & Eriksson, 1986; Bryant, 1987). Therefore, macrophage activity is essential to wound repair. The stimulus for fibroblast mitosis and proliferation and subsequent collagen synthesis appears to be growth factors from platelets, macrophages, lactic acid, and ascorbate (Orgill & Demling, 1988; Bryant, 1987). The fibroblasts migrate into the wound along local fibrin strands from the initial wound coagulation as well as remaining collagen strands. Collagen synthesis is the major function of fibroblasts. The fibroblasts, being metabolically active, depend upon the adequacy of local oxygen supply and neovascularization for continued proliferation. Therefore, impaired perfusion, tissue hypoxia, and the lack of nutrients such as vitamin C, zinc, magnesium, and other amino acids retard the angiogenesis process (Sieggreen 1987; Orgill & Demling, 1988; Bryant, 1987; Wysocki, 1989).

Angiogenesis, or the development of new blood vessels, takes place just behind the advancing edges of fibroblasts. The immature collagen produced by fibroblasts provides vital structural support for new friable capillaries. Peak collagen synthesis occurs from 5 to 7 days in primary healing wounds, and may continue for more than a year in chronic wounds (Wysocki, 1989). Without the collagen support, these new blood vessels would not be able to withstand the pressure of arterial blood flow.

The changes in the wound thus far are visible to the naked eye and are labeled granulation tissue (Fig. 17-4). The wound is beefy red, moist, friable, and has a shiny, cobblestone appearance. Over this granulation tissue, epithelialization takes place. Epi-

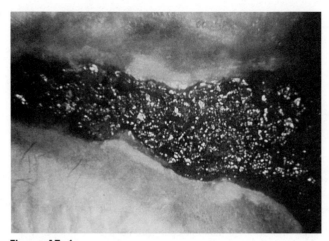

Figure 17-4 ● ● ● ● ● ●

Granulation tissue—red, beefy, and shiny appearance without evidence of infection.

thelialization is the migration of epithelial cells across a wound. Normally, new cells form from the basal layer and migrate vertically. However, when there is loss of epidermal tissue, adjacent basal cells become reprogrammed. They appear to detach from their basement membrane, divide, and migrate toward and across the wound forming a sheet of epithelium (Orgill & Demling, 1988). Once a single layer develops, additional layers develop from mitotic division of these epidermal cells. If there are any hair follicles present in the center of the wound, the epithelial tissue around them will reproduce and form islands of pink epithelial tissue that migrate toward other islands (Pollack, 1979).

The re-epithelialization process can be rapid (i.e., 3–5 days in a superficial injury) or may require several months depending upon the size of the wound, nutrient supply, and the wound environment. Optimal environmental conditions for epithelial migration are a moist, protected wound free from necrotic tissue. Non-viable tissue at the surface of the wound slows epithelialization as the repopulation of cells is retarded until lysis of necrotic tissue is complete. A surface barrier that is permeable to water vapor and oxygen and absorbs wound exudate while allowing for cell migration has been demonstrated to improve wound healing (Winter, 1965). This is the premise for many of the wound dressings that will be discussed later in the chapter.

Wound contraction is the final process that transpires during the proliferative phase. Contraction is the process by which a large wound with tissue loss is reduced in area by the inward migration of normal tissue (Bryant, 1987). The mechanism of contraction, which shrinks the wound, is the generation of cellular forces in the contractile elements of myofibroblasts. Wound contraction decreases the amount of surface area that needs to be filled by granulation and epithelialization. However, it can only occur if the surrounding tissue is pliable enough to allow movement (Hunt & VanWinkle, 1979). Wound con-

traction is exemplified by the closure of a tracheostomy, gastrostomy, or cutaneous fistula. If the loss of tissue is too great and the defect is not closed by contraction, surgical intervention may be required.

Remodeling and Maturation Phase

This third phase of healing begins approximately 20 days after the injury and extends beyond 1 year. Its primary purpose is to restore the wound to its greatest strength. This is accomplished by the maturation of collagen, the protein that provides structural strength and integrity to body tissue. Tensile strength, the maximum amount of pressure that can be applied to an object, in this case a wound, without rupture, is established by collagen (Bryant, 1987). During this phase the collagen synthesis is more mature, highly organized, and consequently stronger. In the first 2 weeks of healing, a wound can regain 30% to 50% of its original strength. By 3 months, the tensile strength of the wound nears 80%. However, a wound will never regain more than 80% of its original strength (Hunt & VanWinkle, 1979). The clinical observations of this phase include shrinking, thinning, and paling of the wound scar.

WOUND CARE

Despite optimal efforts to protect skin integrity, many critically ill children experience some form of skin breakdown during their hospitalization. Particular challenges for pediatric critical care often include perineal skin breakdown, pressure wounds, surgical wounds, ostomy care, and intravenous infiltrate injuries.

Perineal Skin Breakdown

The surface pH of the skin ranges from 4.2 to 5.6. This "acid mantle" is thought to be the skin's first defense against the penetration by undesirable agents (Bryant, 1987). The balance in the skin flora is modulated by the acid environment. Consequently, the natural defenses provided by the intact skin are lost when the integrity of the skin is disrupted.

Some common causes for children at risk for perineal breakdown include increased moisture resulting from urinary incontinence and friction forces; children with short gut syndrome, changes in bowel flora resulting in loose, watery stools; and the gut's adjustment to enteral feeding. The initial impact of stool on the perineum as a result of closure of an ileostomy or colostomy can also produce skin breakdown. The resultant "diaper dermatitis" manifests itself in a variety of ways. The most common appearance is a red, scaly, chafing epidermis where the diaper touches the skin. It can also be seen as defined, bright red areas involving the skin folds. The more severe forms include ulcerations scattered throughout the perineal area sometimes including the genitals. It is at this phase that nerve endings are exposed and the child experiences pain. When the dermatitis is complicated by a yeast infection, the skin folds become beefy red with lesions scattered at the edges of the rash.

Recognizing infants and children at risk for perineal skin breakdown is important for prevention. Kramer and Honig (1988) showed that when one applies a protective ointment to intact skin of children at risk, only 6% developed diaper dermatitis. Treatment can vary widely; however, two goals should be maintained: (1) preventing skin breakdown by promoting evaporation of moisture and keeping the skin dry, and (2) protecting the skin from further damaging effects of urine and stool while the skin heals.

In the area of prevention, the diaper is changed as soon as it is wet or soiled. The perineum can be cleaned gently with a nonperfumed diaper wipe product or nonperfumed soap and water. Caution is taken with the frequent use of water and the friction motion of cleansing because this action can irritate the skin (Zimmerman et al., 1986). A protective ointment should be applied with each diaper change. The use of diaper wipes is avoided on infants and children with known sensitivities, fair sensitive skin, or skin breakdown. For the management of mild erythema, the diaper is changed after voiding or stooling or every 2 hours as needed. Cleansing can be done either with a moisture cream or mineral oil. The application of a protective ointment always follows the cleansing procedure.

When the skin has become denuded (ulcerations), cleaning can be accomplished as indicated previously with cream or mineral oil. Because of the oozing effect of open skin, a protective ointment may not adhere. A pectin-methylcellulose powder, the type often used with ostomy care, can be sprinkled over the skin followed by a liberal application of a protective ointment. The powder helps to absorb the fluid, which then allows the ointment to adhere to the skin. During the cleansing process, only the protective ointment that has been soiled is wiped off with the reapplication of powder and ointment. This minimizes trauma to an already irritated skin area. When a monilial infection is present, an antifungal powder or cream can be applied under a protective ointment, using the same process as for cleansing.

Daily assessment of the skin is documented with an evaluation on the outcome of the intervention. Consistency is the key to a successful skin care program. Changing the regimen with every nursing shift only diminishes the effectiveness of the program. Severe perineal skin breakdown often does not show signs of healing for several days. Therefore, changes to a skin care program are not initiated until after 3 to 4 days.

The practice of leaving the diaper open to air or blowing oxygen onto the skin is not supported in research. Researchers do know, however, that the systemic circulation of oxygen is critical to wound healing. Furthermore, wounds heal more readily in a moist environment rather than a dry one. Leaving the diaper open to air only facilitates the recognition of when a patient stools.

Pressure Wounds

Many factors within the critical care environment affect how wounds occur. The physiologic structure of the infant or child's skin has the greatest impact on developing pressure wounds. The epidermis in children is far more friable than in adults because of the immature tissue structure of the dermal layer. Pressure applied externally is the major factor that compromises oxygen and nutrients supplied to the tissue.

Contributing factors in tissue compromise include immobility, altered level of consciousness, impaired sensation, alteration in temperature, altered tissue perfusion, buildup of interstitial fluid, shearing, or friction. External devices that can limit mobility and add the risk of increased pressure include oxygen delivery devices such as face masks, nasal cannulas, endotracheal tubes, negative pressure poncho, and inflation devices such as Dinamapp cuffs, abdominal binders, limb restraints, and plaster or fiberglass casts.

Continued pressure on tissues compresses capillary blood flow resulting in tissue ischemia with eventual necrosis to the skin area. When pressure is being considered as a possible cause of skin breakdown it is important to keep in mind that there is an inverse relationship between tissue pressure and time tolerance. Therefore, if the pressure applied is of a high degree, the time tolerance should be short. However, low pressure can be tolerated over longer periods of time.

A pressure ulcer is defined as a localized area of cellular necrosis that tends to develop when soft tissue is compressed between a bony prominence and firm surface for a long period of time (Maklebust, 1987). Early identification of children at risk for pressure breakdown appears to be critical to prevention. As mentioned previously, there are no predictive assessment tools available for the pediatric population. Consequently, most preventive and therapeutic measures are based on the adult literature. Future research in the pediatric population should be directed toward assessment tools to identify risk factors, the effective use of pressure relief and pressure reduction devices, and the application of various skin care products.

Despite the implementation of preventive skin care measures, pressure ulcers may be difficult to prevent and heal because of underlying conditions such as poor nutrition, poor tissue oxygenation, and infection. When there is a break in the integrity of the skin, selecting a treatment is often confusing for the bedside nurse. The staging of pressure ulcers (Table 17–4) recommended by the combined efforts of the International Association for Enterostomal Therapy (IAET) and the National Pressure Ulcer Advisory

Table 17–4. STAGING OF PRESSURE ULCERS

Stage I	Nonblanchable erythema of intact skin; the heralding lesion of skin ulceration. Discoloration of skin, warmth, or hardness also may be indicators. *Note:* Reactive hyperemia can normally be expected to be present for one-half to three-fourths as long as the pressure occluded blood flow to the area; it should not be confused with a stage I pressure ulcer.
Stage II	Partial thickness skin loss involving epidermis and/or dermis. The ulcer is superficial and presents clinically as an abrasion, blister, or shallow crater.
Stage III	Full thickness skin loss involving damage or necrosis of subcutaneous tissue that may extend down to but not through underlying fascia. The ulcer presents clinically as a deep crater with or without undermining of adjacent tissue.
Stage IV	Full-thickness skin loss with extensive destruction, tissue necrosis, or damage to muscle, bone, or supporting structures (for example, tendon or joint capsule). *Note:* Undermining and sinus tracts may also be associated with stage IV pressure ulcers.

Recommendations of the National Pressure Ulcer Advisory Panel (NPUAP, 1989 Consensus Conference).

Panel (NPUAP) classifies the degree of tissue damage observed. These stages act as guidelines for assessment as well as for treatment options. However, a wound cannot be staged if there is eschar or necrotic tissue present.

When choosing a dressing, there are seven basic principles that facilitate healing by creating an optimal microenvironment. These principles include (1) remove necrotic tissue, which can be accomplished by mechanical, chemical, or autolytic methods; (2) eradicate infection—all wounds are contaminated but not all wounds are infected. Indications for culture and sensitivity sampling include signs of local or systemic infection or evidence of bone involvement; (3) absorb excess exudate; (4) obliterate dead space; (5) maintain a moist wound surface, which facilitates cellular migration; (6) insulate the wound; and (7) protect the wound from further trauma and bacteria. Tables 17–5 and 7–6 provide information on products that meet these principles.

Surgical Wounds

As previously discussed, wound closure occurs by primary, secondary, and delayed primary or tertiary intention (Wysocki, 1989). Those healing by primary intention are surgical wounds that are approximated by sutures, staples, or tape. Wounds closed by secondary or delayed primary (tertiary) intention are usually contaminated with bacteria. Secondary intention wounds heal through the formation of new blood vessels and scar formation, whereas the tertiary wounds are often traumatic in nature, grossly contaminated, and left open to facilitate drainage. These

wounds may be loosely packed and then resutured at a later date (Meehan, 1992).

Wounds closed by suture, staples, or tape are usually dressed with gauze and a transparent dressing. This dressing can be removed in 2 to 3 days. The suture line is kept clean and protected. The size, type, and location of the wound as well as surgeon preference determine if additional dressings or routine cleansing is needed after the primary dressing has been removed. Dilute solutions of betadine, hydrogen peroxide, normal saline, or antibacterial preparations may be used. Once staples and sutures are removed, usually after 7 to 10 days, the wound is left open to air but protected from trauma. If Steristrips are used to approximate wound edges, they are left undisturbed until they peel off. Those incisions that include a Penrose drain may require frequent dressing changes using sterile technique and absorbent gauze. The use of Montgomery straps is helpful in this situation to reduce the incidence of tape irritation with frequent dressing changes.

Delayed surgical closure of some wounds not contaminated by bacteria may be desirable if significant edema is expected or if primary closure would result in increased pressure on internal organs leading to systemic compromise. Infants having undergone open-heart surgery may have delayed closure of chest wounds to alleviate cardiac compromise and aid excess fluid removal. A mesh covering is sutured to the wound edges with several chest tube drains inserted into the wound edges. Prevention of infection is of utmost importance. Dressings are changed when saturated using strict sterile technique. Dressings usually consist of absorbent gauze and may be moistened with an antibacterial ointment or solution. Open chest dressings can be gently secured with a Stockinette wrap to limit skin breakdown from repeated adhesive tape removal (Fig. 17–5).

Children undergoing surgical repair of large abdominal defects such as gastroschisis or omphalocele may also require delayed wound closure to prevent respiratory compromise or impaired organ perfusion. Staged abdominal wound closures often include the use of a Silastic pouch, which is sutured to the edges of the wound. The protruding bowel is placed in the pouch and tension is applied to the pouch to support the intestinal weight. On a daily basis the tension on the pouch is lessened and the bowel is lowered into the abdominal cavity as tolerated. Wound management considerations in caring for a child with a Silastic pouch include preventing infection through strict adherence to sterile technique, keeping the bowel moist with frequent warmed irrigations, preventing changes in pouch tension, and assessing and maintaining bowel perfusion.

Open draining wounds are often more of a challenge than closed defects and require diligent effort toward the prevention of cross-contamination from other wound sites and maintenance of surrounding intact skin. Using universal precautions and adhering to the institution's protocol for changing dressings is imperative to reducing further bacterial contamination.

If wounds have excessive 1drainage, such as that seen with a fistula, a closed drainage and suction system may be necessary. This requires the insertion of suction catheters at the wound skin edge. These catheters should not come in contact with or lie on exposed viscera. Another alternative to collecting excessive drainage is to use a pouching technique similar to that for an ostomy. The skin barrier is cut to fit the wound opening, thereby protecting intact skin. The pouch, either a one- or two-piece system, can then be applied. Applying a thin layer of barrier paste to the edges of the wound may

Table 17–5. PROPERTIES OF COMMONLY USED DRESSING MATERIALS

Dressing Categories	Examples	Indications	Advantages	Disadvantages	Considerations
Dry gauze/fine mesh gauze		Stage III, IV	Absorb wound exudate, protect wound, effective delivery of topical solutions if kept moist.	When left to dry in the wound, it may remove viable tissue; labor intensive.	Helps to physically debride necrotic tissue; excellent for packing and undermining; use rolled gauze for packing large wounds; pack loosely; use wide mesh gauze for debriding; do not use cotton-filled materials on wound surface.
Moisture vapor permeable membranes (MVP films)	Acuderm, Bio-clusive, Blister Film, Clear Skin, Ensure It, Op Site, Tegaderm, Omiderm, Polyskin	Intravenous sites; superficial abrasions; blisters; minor burns; donor sites; stage I, II, or III pressure ulcers	Maintains physiologic environment; provides bacterial barrier; transparent; conforms to wound; waterproof; reduces pain; can be used with gauze to absorb leakage.	Adhesive can damage new wound surface epithelium upon dressing removal; nonabsorbent; some products difficult to apply; can promote wound infection.	Protect friable wound margins; avoid in wounds with infection, copious drainage, or tracts; change only if dressing leaks. Stretch and "lift off" wound bed.
Hydrocolloids	Cutinova Hydro; Confeel; DuoDerm; Restore; Hydra Pad; Intact; IntraSite; Sween-a-Peel; Tegasorb; Ultec; Replicare	Stage I, II, or III pressure ulcers; dermal ulcers; donor sites; second degree burns; abrasions	Creates a moist environment by interacting with wound fluid; provides barrier to external bacteria; protects from re-injury; fosters autolytic debridement; waterproof; reduces pain; absorbent; nonadhesive to healing tissue; easy to apply; flexible to mold over difficult areas.	May soften and lose shape with heat and friction; the interaction between wound exudate and barrier material produces a yellow to brown drainage which can be confused for purulent drainage.	Frequency of changes depends on amount of exudate (change as needed for leakage); avoid in wounds with infection or in sinus tracts; may cause peri-wound trauma when removed.
Hydrogels	Elasto GEL; Geliperm; Spenco; Vigilon; Gel-Site; NU-GEL; Clearsite; Royal Derm	Stage I, II, or III pressure ulcers; dermal ulcers; donor sites; second degree burns; abrasions; blisters; lacerations.	Nonadherent to wound. Maintains physiologic wound environment (except when dry); relieves pain; can be refrigerated and applied, which helps reduce pain secondary to radiation burns; translucent; nonadhesive.	Because dressing consists of 90% water it can macerate surrounding skin; requires a cover dressing to secure in place; expensive.	Avoid in infected wounds; change when gel becomes dehydrated or perineal skin macerated; varying absorption capabilities.

Table continued on following page

Table 17–5. PROPERTIES OF COMMONLY USED DRESSING MATERIALS *Continued*

Dressing Categories	Examples	Indications	Advantages	Disadvantages	Considerations
Foam dressings Polymeric and composite polymeric dressing	Allevyn, BioBrane, Epi-Lock; Kontour; Lyofoam; Primaderm; Synthaderm; Viasorb; Mitraflex	Stage I, II, or III pressure ulcers; dermal ulcers; donor sites; burns; abrasions; lacerations; partial-thickness wounds; graft sites; highly exudative chronic wounds; dressing for tracheostomy drain sites.	Insulates wound; provides some padding; maintains physiologic environment; reduces pain; permits some autolytic debridement; nonadherent to wound.	Poor barrier; nontransparent; requires taping of edges.	One layer usually absorbs or wicks exudate while another layer maintains moist environment while adhering to skin; change every 24 hours or when leaking occurs.
Wound exudate absorbers; powders; pastes	Bard Absorption Dressing; Comfeel Ulcer Powder; DuoDerm Granules; Comfeel Paste; DuoDerm paste granules; Hollister wound exudate absorber; Pharmaseal; HydraGram; Envisan	Hydrophilic compounds that attract bacteria, exudate debris through osmotic forces in wound. Heavily draining chronic wounds; autolytic debridement.	Absorbs in varying degrees; maintains moist environment; facilitates debridement. Decreases number of dressing changes required.	Can cause pain with application; requires cover dressing; materials leak from dressing edges if not well taped; difficult to remove from tracts and deep pockets.	Partially fill wound to allow for expansion of materials; not for wounds with fistulas/tracts that prevent/hinder removal; monitor electrolytes if copious drainage; may increase wound pH.
Wound gels	Carrington Gel; Geliperm; Intrasite; Spand-Gel; Dermal wound gel; Biolex	Stage I, II, or III ulcers.	Good "filler" for small deep wounds; easy to apply; maintains moist environment; helps to soften or slough eschar in necrotic wound.	Requires a cover dressing; variable absorbency.	Avoid in infected wounds; change every eight hours.
Calcium alginates	Kaltostat; Sorbsan; Curasorb; Algosteril; Algiderm	Highly exudating wounds	Nonadherent to wound; absorbent dressing made from seaweed; may be used with infected wounds; nonwoven fiber dressings that convert to a firm gel/fiber mat when mixed with wound exudate.	Requires less frequent dressing changes; highly absorbent; excellent for packing and undermining; requires cover dressing; characteristic odor to dressing when removed.	

Reprinted from *Pediatric Nursing*, 1993, Volume 19, Number 5, p. 504. Reprinted with permission of the publisher, Jannetti Publications, Inc., East Holly Avenue Box 56, Pitman, NJ 08071-0056; Phone (609) 256-2300; FAX (609) 589-7463.

help to seal the barrier and prevent leakage. The catheter drainage system and pouch both prevent cross-contamination and facilitate accurate measurement of all drainage.

Ostomy Care

An ostomy is described as a surgically formed opening that serves as an exit site between the gastrointestinal system or the urinary tract to the out-side of the body. The pediatric patient may have a gastrointestinal or urinary diversion for a variety of reasons. Urinary ostomies, however, are an infrequent occurrence for the patient in the critical care unit. Therefore, the remainder of this section will discuss the care of fecal ostomies.

Fecal ostomies may consist of an ileostomy or colostomy. The stoma is constructed by bringing the bowel through the rectus muscle to the abdominal wall. The stoma should protrude about 2 cm, allowing for easier stoma management and less likelihood of skin

Table 17-6. TOPICAL AGENTS USED FOR WOUND CARE

Category	Examples	Considerations	Nursing Intervention
Isotonic solutions	Normal saline	Nontoxic to healing tissue; readily available.	Used for rinsing, irrigating, and packing; used to cleanse wound before obtaining a culture.
Antiseptic solutions	Acetic acid .25%	Cytotoxic to fibroblasts; effective against *Pseudomonas*.	Use as 0.25% solution for irrigating or continuous moist packing; discontinue use as soon as granulation tissue is noted.
	Hydrogen peroxide 3%	Cytotoxic to fibroblasts; potential for air emboli when used as an irrigant under pressure.	Avoid using as irrigant in deep wounds or wounds with tunneling; limit use to removing dried blood; dilute to ½ strength.
	Povidone iodine 1%	Cytotoxic especially in detergent form; when used at .001% concentration, it has a bactericidal and noncytotoxic effect. Absorbed by RBCs, therefore potentially causes metabolic acidosis, renal problems, cardiac instability if used in large wounds over a period of time.	Use in concentration of 10% or less if used for packing; change dressing frequently to maintain activity; discontinue when wound is clean and granulating.
	Sodium hypochloride 0.2% (Dakin's solution)	Cytotoxic to fibroblasts at full strength; used at .005% concentration it has a bactericidal with no cytotoxic effect.	If used as packing, moisten frequently to maintain activity; discontinue use when wound is clean and granulating; reduce concentration if patient complains of stinging.

Reprinted from *Pediatric Nursing*, 1993, Volume 19, Number 5, p. 504. Reprinted with permission of the publisher, Jannetti Publications, Inc., East Holly Avenue Box 56, Pitman, NJ 08071-0056; Phone (609) 256-2300; FAX (609) 589-7463.

complications. Ileostomy stomas are always pouched regardless of patient age because of the caustic contents of the effluent. A colostomy, on the other hand, can often be left without an appliance, and stool can be collected in a diaper, especially for the infant and toddler. However, in the intensive care unit this may not be feasible because of the risk for infecting invasive lines, incisions, or open wound sites.

Management of the pediatric stoma and skin requires special considerations. The first of these is selection of a stoma site. In the neonate or trauma victim, the surgery is often emergent with no time for assessment of the abdomen. In addition, it is difficult to predict physical growth in a baby; therefore, selection of the stoma site is rarely performed. Ideally, the stoma should be placed away from the umbilical cord in newborns, below the belt line in the older child, and away from creases, incisions, or old scars. A stoma placed in any one of these areas can make pouching adherence more difficult.

The second consideration is the postoperative assessment of the stoma. Healthy mucosa is moist pink or red in color. Ischemia (evidenced by deep red, purple, or black bowel tissue) or excessive bleeding is reported to the surgeon. Measurement of abdominal girth at the umbilicus, auscultation of bowel sounds, and measurement of stool output is part of an every-8-hour assessment. A clear pouch over the stoma allows for easy assessment of bowel mucosa.

The third consideration is the pouch system. The advantages of pouching include: (1) protection of the peristomal skin, (2) containment of drainage, (3) elimination of odor, and (4) cost containment (Boarini, 1989). The components of a pouching system include a skin barrier and a drainage pouch. There are a few pediatric products available, and these are listed in Table 17-7. One- and two-piece systems are available with either a precut opening or a cut-to-fit starter hole. A cut-to-fit appliance offers the best fit for those stomas that are not perfectly round. It also allows for adjustments to be made as the stoma changes in size. The one-piece appliance has the skin barrier attached to the pouch, whereas the two-piece system has a separate wafer with a flange (faceplate) and a snap-on pouch. Fecal pouches are the drainable type and have a tail closure device, either separate from or attached to the pouch.

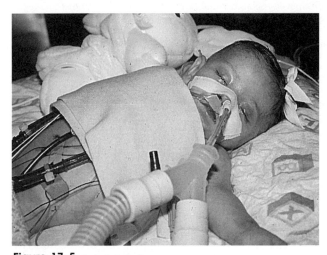

Figure 17-5 ● ● ● ● ● ●
Open chest with Stockinette.

Table 17-7. OSTOMY AND SKIN CARE PRODUCTS

Type of Product	Indications	Considerations	Examples
A. Skin barriers: *used to protect skin from stomal effluent; to treat irritated skin allowing it to heal.*			
	Solid wafer: protects skin; fits to base of stoma; adheres to irritated skin; increases pouch seal due to added firmness to the faceplate	Duoderm is used on irritated skin; Durahesive is made for urinary stomas and difficult-to-pouch stomas ($$$); remainder of solid wafers are used with intact skin	Convatec: Stomahesive Duoderm Durahesive Hollister: Premium Skin Barrier HolliHesive United: Soft & Secure Coloplast: Comfeel
	Paste: fill in folds and creases making a smooth pouching area; protect inner pouch seal around stoma increasing pouch system wearing time	All pastes must dry before pouching; contains alcohol and will "sting" when applied to irritated skin	Convatec: Stomahesive Paste Hollister: Karaya Paste
	Powder: absorbs fluid from denuded skin thus allowing better adherence of the ostomy appliance to the skin; can be used in conjunction with other barriers	Lightly sprinkle over irritated skin	Convatec: Stomahesive Powder Hollister: Karaya Powder
B. Skin sealant: *a liquid copolymer that provides a protective layer to the skin surface by protecting the skin from the shearing force of removing tapes and adhesives.*			
	Use under adhesive tape and adhesive portion of ostomy faceplate; is not necessary under solid wafer barrier; should not be used on premature infant or fragile skin	Most contain alcohol and will "sting" irritated skin; compound tincture of Benzoin contains allergens which can cause irritation; the bound formed between Benzoin and the tape is stronger than the underlying epidermal/dermal bond; therefore when tape is removed from the skin of a premature infant where Benzoin is used, it can cause epidermal stripping; available in wipes and liquid form	Convatec: AllKare United: Skin Prep, Benzoin preparations Mentor: Skin Shield Bard: Protective Barrier
C. Ostomy pouch: *used to collect effluent.*			
	One piece: pre-cut and cut-to-fit; urinary and fecal drainage	Usually have flexible barrier which is excellent for pouching stomas in a crease or fold; most are odorproof	Convatec: Little Ones* Active Life Dansac* Hollister: Coloplast Bard: Fistula Pouch (Fecal Only)
	Two piece: pre-cut and cut-to-fit; urinary and fecal drainage; snap-on pouch to flange wafer	Good for flat pouching surface; pouch can be removed/replaced while faceplate remains intact; wafer flange and pouch flange must match; snap-on system may be painful for immediate post-op; however, pouch and wafer can be applied as one unit; odorproof	Convatec: Little Ones* SurFit Hollister Coloplast United

*Made specifically for infants and young children.

Reprinted from *Pediatric Nursing,* 1994, Volume 20, Number 1, p. 72–73. Reprinted with permission of the publisher, Jannetti Publications, Inc., East Holly Avenue Box 56, Pitman, NJ 08071-0056; Phone (609) 256-2300; FAX (609) 589-7463.

The manufacturing of a pediatric appliance has made pouching easier, but often these specialized pouches can be too big for the abdomen of a small infant. An alternative is to use a pediatric fistula pouch that has a smaller pouching diameter. Most fistula pouches have an adhesive backing; therefore, a wafer barrier must be cut to fit the adhesive portion of the pouch before applying it to the infant's skin.

The proper application of the pouch is another consideration that can influence adherence and decrease the risk of skin breakdown. The appliance requires changing as soon as effluent leaks from under the barrier. Taping a leaking pouch to reinforce the seal only traps stool under the barrier, which leads to skin breakdown. Ideally, the process used to pouch a stoma allows the appliance to remain in place for several days and up to 1 week. However, the activity of the child, the consistency of the effluent, stomal placement, and the condition of the peristomal skin are just a few examples of factors that can influence the wearing time.

The appliance is removed carefully. Warm water and a soft cloth or gauze can be used to facilitate its removal. Adhesive removers are also helpful but are limited to use in full-term infants and children with intact skin. The peristomal skin is inspected for breakdown and the stoma assessed for physical changes. The skin can be cleansed with mild soap and water and is dried thoroughly before the application of a new appliance. It is normal to have a small amount of bleeding from the stoma from the manipulation of the appliance around the vascular stomal tissue. Persistent bleeding is referred to the physician for further evaluation.

The diameter of the child's stoma is measured and a pattern made, especially for an irregularly shaped stoma. The internal diameter of the barrier should be $\frac{1}{16}$th to $\frac{1}{8}$th inch larger than the stoma (Adams & Selekof, 1986). The barrier should fit snugly but not so tight that it constricts the stoma. Warming the skin barrier between the nurse's hands for 1 to 2 minutes allows for better adherence to the skin. A barrier paste (see Table 17–7) can be applied to the peristomal skin to fill in any irregular edges or creases to make a smooth pouching surface. Most preparations contain alcohol and burn when applied to irritated skin. The paste is sticky and sometimes difficult to control. Placing a small amount of paste into a syringe allows for a more precise application (Embon, 1990). A moistened cotton-tipped applicator can help to shape the paste around the stoma. When applying the pouching system, the tail of the bag is directed in a downward position to facilitate emptying. The pouch is emptied when it is one-third to one-half full to decrease the amount of weight the appliance must support.

The fifth concern when managing pediatric stomas is the peristomal skin. The suggestions previously stated regarding the appropriate pouch selection, and application techniques, can reduce the incidence of skin irritation. Despite meticulous techniques, skin breakdown may still occur. The following are two of the more common peristomal skin complications seen in the intensive care unit, their clinical features, and possible interventions.

Irritant Dermatitis

Inflammation of the skin resulting from contact with a chronic irritant may be caused by poor stomal construction, causing effluent to be in constant contact with the skin, poor technique in appliance care, or too many products used on the skin. When multiple products are used, there is the chance that the interaction of these ingredients can increase the skin's sensitivity. The cutaneous manifestations can vary in severity from erythema and swelling to ulceration and bleeding. It may be necessary to do a patch 'or skin test of the products to determine the cause.

A topical steroid may be needed to reduce the inflammation, pain, and itching. Resizing the pouch and changing it as soon as leakage occurs are other interventions.

Candidiasis

Fungal or yeast infection (*Candida albicans*) may be caused by moisture around or under the appliance, the use of systemic antibiotic therapy that alters the flora of the body, immunosuppressive medications, or chemotherapy. The clinical features include erythema and maceration of the skin, papules and/or pustules, and satellite lesions. Possible interventions include resizing the appliance to fit properly or dusting the skin with an antifungal powder, such as Mycostatin (Westwood Squibb Pharmaceuticals, Buffalo, NY), prior to applying the barrier.

Intravenous Infiltrate Injury

Virtually all critically ill pediatric patients have some type of intravascular access device in place during their acute treatment. Critical care nurses routinely care for patients with a wide variety of intravenous catheters and intravenous medication needs. Among the many well-known risks of intravenous therapy, extravasation is a complication that has the potential to cause serious morbidity through direct skin and tissue damage (Fig. 17–6).

Extravasation or infiltration is the leakage of intravenous fluid and/or medication into interstitial tissues. This leakage can occur from cannula dislodgment, punctures in the venous wall, seepage around the insertion site resulting from elevated venous pressures, or drainage through damaged endothelium that has become permeable to the infusate. The extent of tissue damage sustained from an extravasation is dependent on the physicochemical nature of the infusate, the volume infiltrated, and the patient's

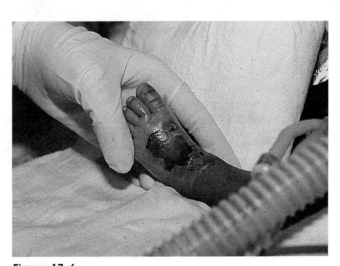

Figure 17–6 ● ● ● ● ● ●
Extravasation injury.

clinical condition and skin integrity at the time of the injury (Flemmer & Chan, 1993; Millam, 1988). Damage can range from mild erythema and edema, which resolve spontaneously within several days, to extensive full-tissue necrosis and sloughing, which requires aggressive, invasive, and often painful treatments over an extended period of time. Severe extravasation injuries can result in serious infection, which may be life-threatening to an already compromised child. Other results may be loss of limb function from nerve or ligament damage and amputation.

Infusates that have the potential to cause the most significant injury if extravasation occurs include those that are hyperosmolar, vasoconstrictive, alkaline, poorly water-soluble, or directly cytotoxic (Mac-Cara, 1983). Hyperosmolar agents are substances that have a higher osmolality than that of serum. Higher osmolality fluids are irritating to venous endothelium and can induce inflammation and capillary leak. As hyperosmolar fluids leak into the interstitial space, they cause edema, vasoconstriction, and ischemia, which may result in cellular necrosis. Hyperosmolar solutions include dextrose concentrations of 10% or greater and those with high amino acid or electrolyte concentrations. Undiluted electrolytes such as potassium, calcium, and bicarbonate also have extremely high osmolalities.

Infiltrated vasoconstrictive drugs cause tissue damage by severely reducing blood flow to the affected area, resulting in localized tissue ischemia. Commonly used vasopressors such as dopamine, dobutamine, epinephrine, and norepinephrine all have the potential to cause this vasoconstrictive damage. Highly alkaline medications such as sodium bicarbonate and sodium thiopental can cause direct cellular injury if infiltrated. Drugs with low water solubility such as lorazepam, diazepam, phenytoin, digoxin, and nitroglycerin have the potential to form cytotoxic precipitates if they are introduced into interstitial tissue undiluted (MacCara, 1983). Other cytotoxic drugs include most of the antineoplastic agents. Among them, the vesicants, such as doxorubicin (Adriamycin), daunorubicin, dactinomycin, nitrogen mustard, vincristine, and vinblastine, are likely to cause the most extensive tissue damage (Millam, 1988).

Preventing severe extravasation tissue injury begins with vigilant assessment of the intravenous site. Once an infusion is in place, the site is reassessed on a routine basis to detect any early signs of infiltration and prevent large volume infiltrates. Signs to watch for include swelling, blanching, coolness, firmness, leakage around the insertion site, decreased flow rate, or increased resistance with flushing. It is not appropriate to rely on patient-reported discomfort to detect intravenous extravasation. Children have relatively loose subcutaneous tissue that can hold a significant amount of infiltrated fluid before becoming painful, and many critically ill children are simply too young, too sick, or too sedated to alert the nurse to a potential extravasation. To aid frequent observation, do not obscure the intravenous site with excessive tape, gauze wrap, "welcome" sleeves, or protective covers.

When placing intravenous access devices, the nurse should try to use a location that will minimize the risk of dislodgment resulting from movement. In general, avoid joint spaces. Restraining a limb with a board will limit flexion but it will not prevent rotation, which can also cause the cannula tip to slip out of the vein. When choosing an optimal site for placement of a catheter, each child's individual needs must be assessed. The hand that a child writes with or likes to suck is not used. The feet of a child who frequently kicks or is able to stand are not used. When choosing a catheter, soft plastic cannulas are better choices than rigid steel needles, which have been shown to increase the risk of infiltration (Tully et al., 1981). When an infusion pump is used to deliver solutions peripherally, a volumetric cassette pump is the best choice with a maximum delivery pressure of less than 20 pounds per square inch (MacCara, 1983). Syringe pumps must be used cautiously because they often have higher flow pressures.

When administering medications peripherally, they are diluted in the largest volume of fluid possible and infused slowly. To reduce the chance for caustic extravasations to occur, nurses may advocate central venous access device placement in those children who will require high-concentration parenteral nutrition, frequent electrolyte replacement, pressor support, or chemotherapy. In most cases, unless an acute emergency situation warrants peripheral administration, vasopressor drips and boluses of highly irritating drugs are administered via a central venous line.

The goal of treatment following the identification of an extravasation is to limit the extent of skin and tissue damage incurred. In all cases, the first intervention is to stop the infusion. The infusion is disconnected and an attempt is made to aspirate some of the infiltrated fluid from the tissues through the intact cannula. The cannula is left in place and the nurse consults with a physician about whether the administration of an antidote is warranted. At this time, staging the infiltrate (Table 17–8) is helpful. Any site that fits the characteristics of a stage III or IV infiltrate will require immediate and aggressive intervention because there is a high risk for extensive deep tissue damage (Flemmer & Chan, 1993). It is also important to keep in mind that some infusates continue to cause progressive damage over a period of hours to days. The extent of this damage potential is not evident on initial assessment. Drugs that may cause delayed injury include dopamine, Levophed, calcium, potassium, sodium bicarbonate, vancomycin, amphotericin B, dextrose concentrations of 20% and higher, and most chemotherapeutic agents (Millam, 1988).

There are several substances that have been found to be useful in limiting the extent of tissue injury associated with the extravasation of certain infusates (Brusko, 1990; Dorr, 1990; Larsen, 1982). These anti-

Table 17–8. STAGING OF INTRAVENOUS INFILTRATES

Stage	Characteristics
I	Painful IV site No erythema No swelling
II	Painful IV site Slight swelling (0%–20%) No blanching Good pulse below infiltration site Brisk capillary refill below infiltration site
III	Painful IV site Marked swelling (30%–50%) Blanching Skin cool to the touch Good pulse below infiltration site Brisk capillary refill below infiltration site
IV	Painful IV site Extensive swelling (>50%) Blanching Skin cool to the touch Decreased or absent pulse* Capillary refill >4 seconds* Skin breakdown or necrosis*

*The presence of any one of these characteristics constitutes a stage IV infiltrate (Millam, 1988).

Reprinted from *Pediatric Nursing*, 1993, Volume 19, Number 4, p. 424. Reprinted with permission of the publisher, Jannetti Publications, Inc., East Holly Avenue Box 56, Pitman, NJ 08071-0056; Phone (609) 256-2300; FAX (609) 589-7463.

dotes are administered via the infiltrated catheter or through multiple subcutaneous injections or topically. Hyaluronidase is useful in treating most irritating but nonvasopressor infiltrates. Hyaluronidase works by temporarily dissolving normal interstitial barriers, allowing the infiltrated solution to diffuse over a greater area. In effect, the solution becomes diluted, allowing for faster absorption. The usual dosage is a concentration of 15 units per mL administered by five subcutaneous injections of 0.2 mL each into the affected area (Zenk, 1981). Hyaluronidase is most effective if administered within 2 hours after the infiltrate has been identified, but it may be beneficial if given up to 12 hours after extravasation (Young et al., 1991). Hyaluronidase has few known side effects, but may rarely cause urticaria.

Phentolamine is a helpful antidote for vasopressor infiltrates because it is an alpha-adrenergic blocker that directly reverses the vasoconstrictive effects that can cause tissue ischemia and necrosis. The dosage range is 5 mg to 10 mg diluted in 10 mL of normal saline administered by multiple subcutaneous injections of 0.5 mg each into the affected area. Phentolamine is most effective if given within 12 hours of the extravasation. Careful assessment needs to be made before treating a child with phentolamine because it has the potential to cause acute prolonged hypotension from vascular smooth muscle relaxation. Phentolamine can also cause tachycardia and dysrhythmias.

Glyceryl trinitrate in the form of transdermal nitroglycerin patches or ointment may be a safer and less invasive treatment option than injections of hy-

aluronidase or phentolamine in the treatment of extravasations that result in ischemia. The beneficial effects of topical nitroglycerin have been demonstrated in the treatment of children with vasopressor extravasations (Denkler & Cohen, 1989; Wong et al., 1992), parenteral nutrition extravasations (O'Reilly et al., 1988), and purpura fulminans (Irazuzta & McManus, 1990). Nitroglycerin is a nonspecific vascular smooth muscle relaxant that can improve collateral circulation to localized areas of peripheral ischemia. The recommended dosage is 4 mm of 2% nitroglycerin ointment per kilogram of body weight applied topically over the affected area every 8 hours until perfusion is restored (Wong et al., 1992). Local vasodilation effects occur within 15 to 30 minutes. To minimize the potential for systemic hypotension, caution is taken in using topical nitroglycerin on infants younger than 21 days old and in children with existing skin breakdown because absorption may be increased.

Other medications that may be used to counteract or mitigate the damaging effects of some infiltrates include hydrocortisone or dexamethasone to decrease inflammation. Case reports also suggest that sodium thiosulfate, sodium bicarbonate, ascorbic acid, and sodium edetate may be beneficial in treating some extravasation injuries (MacCara, 1983). It is thought that these drugs help to inactivate some infiltrated drugs or decrease their binding to cellular deoxiribonucleic acid (DNA).

Once an appropriate antidote has been administered (Table 17–9) or the decision to treat conservatively has been made, the cannula is removed and the site elevated to decrease edema. Warm compresses are applied to infiltration sites of noncaustic solutions regardless of osmolarity (Hastings-Tolsma et al., 1993). Warmth improves circulation to the affected area and increases the rate of fluid absorption. Cool to cold compresses are applied to caustic, highly irritating extravasations to reduce ulceration (Hastings-Tolsma et al., 1993).

Despite aggressive treatment, some extravasation injuries result in tissue damage that requires surgical intervention and wound care. For all serious infiltrations, the nurse should encourage a plastic surgery consultation to address physical, functional, and cosmetic issues promptly. For all extravasations, careful and frequent assessment of the site includes circulatory, sensory, and motor functions. Accurate documentation of the site's condition is done daily until the tissue damage has healed.

SUMMARY

This chapter has presented information about the pediatric integumentary system and wound healing as they relate to the critically ill child. The concepts are an essential part of every critical care nurse's knowledge base in providing quality patient care. Although nurses may not have control over many of the factors that place critically ill infants and children at

Table 17–9. ANTIDOTES

Medication	Antidote	Dose
Acyclovir	Hyaluronidase 15 μ/mL	0.2 mL × 5 doses SQ
Aminophylline	Hyaluronidase 15 μ/mL	0.2 mL × 5 doses SQ
Amphotericin	Hyaluronidase 15 μ/mL	0.2 mL × 5 doses SQ
Calcium salts	Hyaluronidase 15 μ/mL	0.2 mL × 5 doses SQ
Carmustine	Sodium bicarbonate 8.4%	5 mL SQ
Chloramphenicol	Hyaluronidase 15 μ/mL	0.2 mL × 5 doses SQ
Cisplatin	Sodium thiosulfate—1/6 M solution (4 mL of 10% sodium thiosulfate (1000 mg/10 mL) mixed with 6 mL of sterile water)	Inject 2 mL of this 1/6 M solution for each 100 mg of cisplatin
Dacarbazine	Sodium thiosulfate (dilute as with cisplatin)	Multiple SQ injections for a total of 4–5 mL
Dactinomycin (actinomycin D)	Sodium thiosulfate (dilute as with cisplatin)	Multiple SQ injections for a total of 4–5 mL
	Ascorbic acid	50 mg SQ
	Cold compress or hydrocortisone sodium succinate	50–200 mg SQ
Daunorubicin	Sodium bicarbonate 8.4% +	5 mL SQ
	Dexamethasone	4 mg SQ
	Cold compress	
Dextrose 10%	Hyaluronidase 15 μ/mL or nitroglycerin ointment 2%	0.2 mL × 5 SQ
		4 mm per kg
	Cold compress	q8 hours until perfusion restored
Diazepam	Hyaluronidase 15 μ/mL	0.2 mL × 5 doses SQ
Dobutamine	Phentolamine 5 mg to 10 mg in 10 mL saline or nitroglycerin ointment 2%	Multiple 0.5 mg doses SQ up to 10 mg
		4 mm per kg q8 h
Dopamine	Phentolamine 5 mg to 10 mg in 10 mL saline or nitroglycerin ointment 2%	Multiple 0.5 mg doses SQ up to 10 mg
		4 mm per kg q8 h
Doxorubicin (Adriamycin)	Hydrocortisone sodium succinate	50–200 mg SQ
	Hydrocortisone cream 1% or	Apply BID
	Sodium bicarbonate 8.4% +	5 mL SQ
	Dexamethasone	4 mg SQ
	Cold compress	
Epinephrine	Phentolamine 5 mg to 10 mg in 10 mL saline or nitroglycerin ointment 2%	Multiple 0.5 mg doses SQ up to 10 mg
		4 mm per kg
Etoposide (VP-16)	Hyaluronidase 150 μ/mL	1 mL to 6 mL SQ via multiple injections; repeat over several hours
	Warm compress	
Gentamicin	Hyaluronidase 15 μ/mL	0.2 mL × 5 doses SQ
Mannitol	Hyaluronidase 15 μ/mL	0.2 mL × 5 doses SQ
Mechlorethamine (nitrogen mustard)	Sodium thiosulfate (dilute as with cisplatin)	Inject 2 mL of this 1/6 M solution for each mg of mechlorethamine
	Cold compress	
Metaraminol	Phentolamine 5 mg to 10 mg in 10 mL saline	Multiple 0.5 mg doses SQ up to 10 mg
Mitomycin	Sodium thiosulfate (dilute as with cisplatin)	Multiple SQ injections for a total of 4–5 mL
Nafcillin	Hyaluronidase 15 μ/mL	0.2 mL × 5 doses SQ
Norepinephrine	Phentolamine 5 mg to 10 mg in 10 mL saline or nitroglycerin ointment 2%	Multiple 0.5-mL doses SQ up to 10 mg
		4 mm per kg q8 h
Oxacillin	Hyaluronidase 15 μ/mL	0.2 mL × 5 doses SQ
Parenteral nutrition	Hyaluronidase 15 μ/mL	0.2 mL × 5 doses SQ
	Nitroglycerin ointment 2%	4 mm per kg q8 h
Penicillin G	Hyaluronidase 15 μ/mL	0.2 mL × 5 doses SQ
Phenytoin	Hyaluronidase 15 μ/mL	0.2 mL × 5 doses SQ
Piperacillin	Hyaluronidase 15 μ/mL	0.2 mL × 5 doses SQ
Potassium salts	Hyaluronidase 15 μ/mL	0.2 mL × 5 doses SQ
	Cold compress	
Radiocontrast dye	Hyaluronidase 15 μ/mL	0.2 mL × 5 doses SQ
Sodium bicarbonate	Hyaluronidase 15 μ/mL	0.2 mL × 5 doses SQ
Teniposide (VM-26)	Hyaluronidase 150 μ/mL	1–6 mL SQ via multiple injections; repeat over several hours
	Warm compress	
Tromethamine	Hyaluronidase 15 μ/mL	0.2 mL × 5 doses SQ
Vancomycin	Hyaluronidase 15 μ/mL	0.2 mL × 5 doses SQ
Vinblastine	Hyaluronidase 150 μ/mL or	1–6 mL SQ via multiple injections; repeat over several hours
	Sodium bicarbonate 8.4%	5 mL SQ
	Warm compress	
Vincristine	Hyaluronidase 150 μ/mL	1–6 mL SQ via multiple injections; repeat over several hours
	Warm compress	

Courtesy of Patricia A Berry R.N.; Staff Nurse II; MICU. Darlene Whitney R.N., B.S.N., CCRN; Staff Nurse II; MICU. Kathleen Gura B.S., R.Ph; Clinical Pharmacist. Lorena Klaes, R.Ph; Clinical Pharmacist; MICU. Children's Hospital, Boston.

Data from: Black, 1988; Brusko, 1990; Denkler & Cohen, 1989; Dorr, 1990; Drug Facts and Comparisons, 1994; Flemmer & Chan, 1993; Hastings-Tolsma et al., 1993; Ignoffo & Friedman, 1980; Irazuzta & McManus, 1990; Larsen, 1982; MacCara 1983; Wong et al., 1992; Young & Mangum, 1991.

risk for skin breakdown and delayed wound healing, nurses do have the ability to positively influence patient care outcomes through knowledgeable assessment, prevention, treatment, and evaluation.

References

Adams, D.A., & Selekof, J.L. (1986). Children with ostomies: Comprehensive care planning. *Pediatric Nursing, 12,* 429–433.

Alvarez, O.M., Goslen, J.B., Eaglstein, W.H., Welgers, H.G., & Strecklin, G.P. (1987). Wound healing. In T.B. Fitzpatrick, A.Z. Eisen, K. Wolff, I.M. Freedberg & K.F. Susten (Eds.). *Dermatology in general medicine* (3rd ed., pp. 321–336). New York: McGraw-Hill.

Bergstrom, N., Demuth, P.J., & Braden, B.J. (1987). A clinical trial of the Braden scale for predicting pressure sore risk. *Nursing Clinics of North America, 22,* 417–428.

Berjian, R.A., Douglass, H.O. Jr., Holyoke, E.D. (1983). Skin pressure measurements on various mattress surfaces in cancer patients. *American Journal of Physical Medicine, 62*(5), 217–226.

Black, R. (1988). Vein extravasation: A severe complication of IV therapy. *Parenterals, 6,* 1–7.

Boarini, J.H. (1989). Principles of stoma care for infants. *Journal of Enterostomal Therapy, 16*(1), 21–25.

Brusko, C. (1990). Treatment of extravasation caused by intravenous drugs. *Clinical Trends in Hospital Pharmacy, 4,* 39–43.

Bryant, R. (1987). Wound repair: A review. *Journal of Enterostomal Therapy, 14*(6), 262–266.

Carrico, T.J., Mehrhof, A., & Cohen, I.K. (1984). Biology of wound healing. *Surgical Clinics of North America, 64*(4), 721–733.

Chang, N., Goodson, W.H., Grottup, F., & Hunt, T.K. (1983). Direct measurement of wound and tissue oxygen tension in postoperative patients. *Annals of Surgery, 197,* 470–478.

Ching, D., & Mell, D.L. (1990). Use of adhesive dressings in skin care: DuoDERM Extra Thin. *Journal of Pediatric Health Care, 4*(3), 155–156.

Denkler, K.A., & Cohen, B.E. (1989). Reversal of dopamine extravasation injury with topical nitroglycerin ointment. *Plastic and Reconstructive Surgery, 84*(5), 811–813.

Dorr, R.T. (1990). Antidotes to vesicant chemotherapy extravasation. *Blood Review, 4*(1), 41–60.

Doughty, D. (1990). The process of wound healing: A nursing perspective. *Progressions, 2*(1), 3–12.

Embon, C. (1990). Ostomy care for the infant with necrotizing enterocolitis: Nursing considerations. *Journal of Perinatal and Neonatal Nursing, 4*(3), 56–63.

Flemmer, L., & Chan, J.S. (1993). A pediatric protocol for management of extravasation injuries. *Pediatric Nursing, 19*(4), 355–358, 424.

Glavis, C., & Barbour, S. (1990). Pressure ulcer prevention in critical care: State of the art. *AACN, 1*(3), 602–613.

Goodrich, C., & March, K. (1992). From ED to ICU: A focus on prevention of skin breakdown. *Critical Care Nursing Quarterly, 15*(1), 1–13.

Harpin, V.A., & Rutter, N. (1983). Barrier properties of the newborn infant's skin. *The Journal of Pediatrics, 102*(3), 419–425.

Hastings-Tolsma, M.T., Yucha, C.B., Tompkins, J., Robson, L., & Szeverenyi, N. (1993). Effect of warm and cold applications on the resolution of IV infiltrations. *Research in Nursing and Health, 16,* 171–178.

Hotter, A. (1982). Physiologic aspects and clinical implications of wound healing. *Heart & Lung, 11*(6), 522–530.

Hudson-Goodman, P., Girard, N., & Brewer-Jones, M. (1990). Wound repair and the potential use of growth factors. *Heart & Lung, 19*(4), 379–384.

Hunt, A., & Eriksson, E. (1986). Management of burn wound. *Clinics in Plastic Surgery, 13*(1), 57–67.

Hunt, T.K., & Halliday, B. (1980). Inflammation in wounds. From "laudable pus" to primary repair and beyond. In T.K. Hunt (Ed.) *Wound healing and wound infection: Theory and surgical practice* (pp. 281–293). New York: Appleton-Century-Crofts.

Hunt, T.K., & VanWinkle, W. (1979). Normal repair. In T.K Hunt & J.E. Dunphy (Eds.). *Fundamentals of wound management* (pp. 2–67). New York: Appleton-Century-Crofts.

Ignoffo, R.J., & Friedman, M.A. (1980). Therapy of local toxicities carried by extravasation of cancer chemotherapeutic drugs. *Cancer Treatment Reviews, 7,* 17–27.

Irazuzta, J., & McManus, M.L. (1990). Use of topically applied nitroglycerin in the treatment of purpura fulminans. *Journal of Pediatrics, 117,* 993–995.

Kramer, D., & Honig, P.J. (1988). Diaper dermatitis in the hospitalized child. *Journal of Enterostomal Therapy, 15*(4), 167–170.

Krasner, D. (1991). Patient support surfaces. *Ostomy/Wound Management, 33,* 57–60.

Larsen, D.L. (1982). Treatment of tissue extravasation by antitumor agents. *Cancer, 49,* 1796–1799.

Lovell, H.W., & Anderson, C.L. (1990). Put your patient on the right bed. *RN,* (May), 66–72.

MacCara, M.E. (1983). Extravasation: A hazard of intravenous therapy. *Drug Intelligence and Clinical Pharmacy, 17,* 713–717.

Maklebust, J. (1987). Pressure ulcers: Etiology and prevention. *Nursing Clinics of North America, 22,* 359–377.

Marchand, A.C., & Lidowski, H. (1993). Reassessment of the use of genuine sheepskin for pressure ulcer prevention and treatment. *Decubitus, 6*(1), 44–47.

Mechanic, H.F., & Perkins, B.A. (1988). Preventing tissue trauma. *Dimensions of Critical Care Nursing, 7*(4), 210–218.

Meehan, P.A. (1992). Open abdominal wounds: A creative approach to a challenging problem. *Progressions, 4*(2), 3–11.

Millam, D.A. (1988). Managing complications of IV therapy. *Nursing88, 18*(3), 34–42.

North American Nursing Diagnosis Association (1989). Taxonomy I: With official diagnostic categories (revised 1989). St. Louis.

Norton, D., McLaren, R., & Exton-Smith, A.N. (1962). *An investigation of geriatric nursing problems in hospitals.* London: National Corporation for the Care of Old People, 197.

Olin, B.R. (Ed.). *Drug facts and comparisons.* (1994). St. Louis: Wolters Kluwer.

O'Reilly, C., McKay, F.M., Duffty, P., & Lloyd, D.J. (1988). Glyceryl trinitrate in skin necrosis caused by extravasation of parenteral nutrition [letter]. *Lancet, 2*(8610), 565–566.

Orgill, D., & Demling, R.H. (1988). Current concepts and approaches to wound healing. *Critical Care Medicine, 16*(9), 899–908.

Piloian, B.B. (1992). Defining characteristics of the nursing diagnosis "high risk for impaired skin integrity." *Decubitus, 5*(5), 32–47.

Pollock, S.V. (1979). Wound healing: A review of the biology of wound healing. *Journal of Dermatologic Surgery and Oncology, 5,* 389–392.

Ruberg, R.L. (1984). Role of nutrition in wound healing. *Surgical Clinics of North America, 64*(4), 705–713.

Sieggreen, M.Y. (1987). Healing of physical wounds. *Nursing Clinics of North America, 22,* 2, 439–447.

Solis, S., Krouskop, T., Trainer, N., & Marburger, R. (1988). Supine interface pressure in children. *Archives in Physical and Medical Rehabilitation, 69,* 524–526.

Stotts, N.A. (1990). Nutrition: A critical component of wound healing. *AACN Clinical Issues, 1,* 585–594.

Tully, J.L., Friedland, G.H., Baldini, L.M., & Goldman, D.A. (1981). Complications of intravenous therapy with steel needles and Teflon catheters. A comparative study. *American Journal of Medicine, 70*(3), 702–706.

Winter, G.D. (1965). A note on wound healing under dressings with special reference to perforated film dressing. *Journal of Investigative Dermatology, 45,* 299.

Wong, A.F., McCulloch, L.M., & Sola, A. (1992). Treatment of peripheral tissue ischemia with topical nitroglycerin ointment in neonates. *Journal of Pediatrics, 121*(6), 980–983.

Wysocki, A. (1989). Surgical wound healing. *AORN Journal, 49*(2), 502–518.

Young, M.E. (1988). Malnutrition and wound healing. *Heart & Lung, 17*(1), 60–67.

Young, T.E., & Mangum, O.B. (1991). *Neofax, a manual of drugs used in neonatal care* (4th ed.). Columbus, OH: Ross Laboratories.

Zenk, K. (1981). Management of intravenous extravasations. *Infusion, 5,* 77–79.

Zimmerman, R., Lawson, K., & Calvert, C. (1986). The effects of wearing diapers on skin. *Journal of Pediatrics, 101,* 721–723.

CHAPTER *18*

Pain and Aversive Stimuli

CAROL J. HOWE
KIMBERLY MASON
PEGGY C. GORDIN

Pain is an elusive phenomenon in any clinical setting, but in the pediatric intensive care unit (PICU) its accurate identification and effective management pose special challenges to caregivers. Pain has been defined as "an unpleasant sensory and emotional experience associated with actual or potential tissue damage, or described in terms of such damage" (IASP, 1979). McCaffery (1972) defines pain as "whatever the experiencing person says it is, existing whenever the experiencing person says it does." It is implicit that pain is both an emotional and physical experience.

For children, a stay in a PICU may be filled with many experiences of pain, discomfort, distress, and suffering. Surgery, trauma, or invasive procedures may produce tissue damage and cause a significant amount of pain and distress in the critically ill child. Less obvious sources of painful and distressing stimuli include the many tubes that twist and pull with any movement, airway suctioning, removal of tape and electrodes, procedures such as chest tube insertion, intravenous (IV) catheter insertion, venous and arterial blood sampling, and heel sticks. In addition, aspects of the PICU environment such as continuous bright lights, loud noises, and unpredictable caregiving events are all potential sources of aversive stimulation that can affect patients physiologically and behaviorally.

Until recently, pain and pain management in children had received little attention in research or clinical practice. Numerous studies have demonstrated that pain is consistently undertreated in the pediatric population when compared with adults who are undergoing medical treatment for similar problems (Eland & Anderson, 1977; Beyer, 1983; Schecter et al., 1986). The reasons for this phenomenon are many. Healthcare providers have a number of misconceptions and biases toward pain and pain management. These beliefs dictate intervention or, in this case, the lack of intervention. However, challenges to these beliefs and misconceptions are slowly changing clinical practice related to pain management.

OBSTACLES TO EFFECTIVE PAIN MANAGEMENT IN CHILDREN

Historically, research from the 1940s (McGraw, 1941) supported the idea that children are incapable of perceiving and responding to pain to the same degree as adults because of neurologic immaturity. Specifically, incomplete myelinization of peripheral sensory nerves was thought to mean that babies could not feel much pain, and therefore justified performing procedures ranging from circumcision to major surgery without anesthesia in newborns (Shearer, 1986). These ideas were widely accepted and incorporated into medical textbooks. In recent years this notion has been refuted in both the lay and professional literature, but there are clinicians who continue to believe that pain is not a major problem requiring treatment in infants and young children.

Healthcare professionals may cite the "resiliency" of children or their ability to "bounce back" as indicators that children do not feel pain as adults do. In fact, children's ability to cope with distress through active behaviors such as play represent positive coping mechanisms. Because of misinterpretation of observed behaviors, caregivers may withhold pharmacologic support for children who are experiencing severe pain.

Physicians and nurses may also believe that children have no memory of painful experiences so that potent analgesics are unnecessary. Although children who experienced painful procedures as infants do not describe detailed memories of those events, many parents of former PICU patients report unusual behavior and fears in their children that they associate with the PICU stay. Older children often cite invasive procedures—injections, chest tube insertions, bone marrow aspirates, lumbar punctures, IV sticks—as the worst experiences of a hospital stay.

In addition, there is concern regarding the administration of narcotics to infants and children, who seem to metabolize and respond to opiates differently than adults. There are some differences in narcotic pharmacodynamics and pharmacokinetics in infants younger than 6 months of age, but adequate analgesia can still be provided safely with appropriate dosages and intervals for drug administration (Anand & Shapiro, 1993). Children have not been found to be any more sensitive than adults to the respiratory depressant effects of morphine (Schecter, 1989). Most of the cases of respiratory arrest following narcotic administration to children probably can be traced to inappropriate administration technique (rapid IV bolus) or to overdoses.

Other obstacles to the recognition and treatment of pain are the personal, professional, and societal attitudes toward pain that all health professionals possess as a part of their value system. Many clinicians still adhere to the philosophy that there is a specific, correct amount of pain for a given stimulus. This "amount" of pain may be based upon the caregiver's own experience, or upon what has been taught as conventional wisdom during professional training. For example, a nurse caring for a multiple trauma patient may assert that after fractures are set, the patient should not have much pain.

Cultural expectations of caregivers influence their clinical judgment of and responses to patients in pain. In Western cultures the ability to tolerate pain is seen as a sign of strong character and, hence, painful experiences are thought to be "character-building." Bravery is a greatly admired personality trait, and even parents may encourage children to suppress their expression of pain and "be brave." In addition, some people view pain and suffering in the context of their religion, as a penance or punishment for some moral failure. These attitudes may subtly influence decision-making regarding the use of analgesics for patients.

ANATOMY AND PHYSIOLOGY

Pain recruits a tremendous response on many levels: the peripheral nervous system, the autonomic and skeletal motor systems, and the central nervous system are all involved. A "hard-wire" model is often used to describe pain transmission and pain perception. Although this model is useful for learning and understanding, it must be remembered that pain remains somewhat elusive in its complexity. How individuals respond to pain often defies straightforward anatomic and physiologic explanation. There is not a one-to-one relationship between a noxious stimulus and an individual's response to the pain.

Peripheral Nervous System

With tissue damage from injury, mediator molecules are released by or leak out from damaged cells. These mediators sensitize or depolarize the nociceptors, initiating the pain impulse. Identified mediators include substance P, prostaglandin E, bradykinin, histamine, and potassium. More specifically, substance P is a possible excitatory neurotransmitter that activates ascending spinal tracts. Prostaglandin E sensitizes tissues to bradykinin. Histamine, potassium, and bradykinin are released from mast cells and are actively involved in the inflammatory response seen with painful injuries. Peripherally acting agents such as aspirin, acetaminophen, and nonsteroidal anti-inflammatory agents inhibit prostaglandin synthesis and activation of the nociceptor.

Peripheral afferent nerve fibers primarily responsible for nociception are of two main types: the A-delta fibers and the C-polymodal fibers. The A-delta fibers are thinly myelinated neurons. They conduct impulses at rapid velocity and have a low threshold for firing. Once activated, these fibers are associated with what is described as "first pain": a sharp, intense, and well-localized sensation. The C-polymodal fibers are unmyelinated; they conduct impulses at a slower speed and have a relatively high firing threshold. They are associated with a later onset or "second pain," which is described as a poorly localized, dull, burning, prolonged sensation.

Both A-delta and C-polymodal fibers share the property of sensitization, which has clinical implications. Both nociceptors become more sensitive and more reactive with repeated episodes of noxious stimulation. Injuries such as burns, bruises, and abrasions are often accompanied by hyperesthesia (increased sensitivity to mild stimuli) or hyperalgesia (increased sensitivity to painful stimuli). The threshold to sensory stimulation is decreased, and even commonly innocuous stimulation is experienced as painful.

Peripheral nociceptors remain unmyelinated or thinly myelinated throughout the life cycle from infancy to adulthood. Lack of myelination does not imply lack of conduction and perception, but, rather, slower conduction. Therefore, the lack of myelination of peripheral nerves in the infant does not support the assertion that infants cannot appreciate pain. Moreover, the slower conduction velocity characteristic of unmyelinated nerves may well be offset by the shorter distances that the nerve impulse travels in a small infant (Anand & Hickey, 1987).

Spinal Cord

Nociceptors and other sensory fibers travel to and converge on cells within the dorsal horn of the spinal cord. The dorsal horn cells activate several central mechanisms involved in the appreciation and response to painful stimuli. Some dorsal root neurons initiate a protective, spinal reflex in response to pain; for example, pulling one's hand away from a hot stove even before the heat and burning are consciously realized. Some dorsal horn cells are involved with inhibition of further incoming nociceptive input. When these cells become damaged from nerve injury and inhibition is removed, pain sensation increases. Most importantly, dorsal horn cells activate central transmission tracts that relay peripheral input to higher brain centers.

Central Nervous System

The spinothalamic and the spinoreticular tracts are the main central pathways of pain impulse transmission. These tracts synapse in different areas of the thalamus and then continue and ultimately terminate in various areas of the cortex.

The spinothalamic tract travels to and synapses in the lateral thalamus. From here the tract continues to and terminates in the somatosensory cortex. The spinothalamic tracts "map" information onto the somatosensory cortex so that individuals are able to identify and localize pain.

The spinoreticular pathway ascends to the brainstem reticular formation. Some of these communications continue to the lateral thalamus and onward to the somatosensory cortex. Others travel to the medial thalamus, which continues to the association cortex or, more specifically, to the limbic system and the frontal cortex. These higher cortical areas recruit a sophisticated response to pain, which involves the appreciation of pain intensity, the desire to escape from pain, and the anxiety that accompanies the need to be rid of painful stimuli. It dictates how emotions, personality, culture, gender, past experience with pain, and the meaning of the pain contribute to an individual's perception and response to pain.

The spinothalamic and the spinoreticular tracts are completely myelinated by 30 weeks of gestation (Anand & Carr, 1989). Maturation of nerve pathways that interconnect the various central structures involved in pain, such as the limbic system, sensory cortex, thalamus, brainstem, hypothalamus, and associative areas of the cerebral cortex, has not been studied. It is proposed that these links may occur during early infancy and childhood.

In addition to receiving and interpreting information from peripheral input, the central nervous system acts as a sensory modulation system. This modulation system involves the endogenous opiates (short-chain enkephalins and long-chain endorphins) and their action at opiate receptors. The endogenous compounds are identical pharmacologically to morphine in their action on opiate receptors. Opiate receptors are present throughout the body and are widely distributed in the central nervous system with greater concentrations in the dorsal horn and the periaqueductal gray matter. Action of endogenous opiates and opioid analgesics on these central receptors is thought to provide analgesia. Opiate receptors are also present in many tissues that are not involved in analgesia. Action of opioids on these receptors is responsible for many of the side effects and complications seen with opioid administration (i.e., respiratory depression, pupillary constriction, and decreased gut motility).

Gate Control Theory

The *gate control theory* was developed by Melzack and Wall in 1965 and is the most widely accepted theory of pain today. This theory postulates that pain is not a function of any one part of the nervous system but is the result of interactions between physical, cognitive, and experiential components. The premise of this theory is the existence of a "gate" in the spinal cord that modulates the perception of pain.

In brief, painful stimuli activate nerve impulses that are transmitted to three spinal cord systems: the cells of the substantia gelatinosa (the gate), the

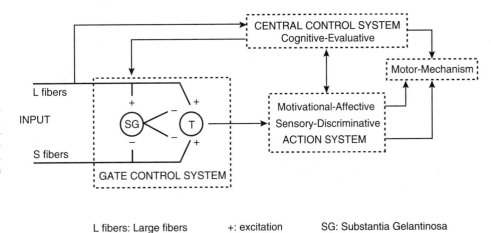

Figure 18–1 ● ● ● ● ● ●
Schematic diagram of the gate control theory of pain mechanism. (Based on Melzack & Wall, and Melzack & Casey. Reprinted from Advances in Nursing Science, Vol. 2, No. 2, p. 146, with permission of Aspen Publishers, Inc., © 1980).

L fibers: Large fibers   +: excitation   SG: Substantia Gelantinosa
S fibers: Small fibers   −: Inhibition   T: Transmission cells

dorsal column fibers, and the central transmission cells (T-cells) (Fig. 18–1). The cells of the substantia gelatinosa in the dorsal horn form the gate control system. Pain perception is modulated by the gate as it opens or closes, depending on neural input. To inhibit pain, the gate maintains a naturally closed position; the A-beta fibers, which respond to touch, "close" the gate by increasing the gate's inhibitory activity. Nociceptive impulses from the A-delta and C-fibers "open" the gate by decreasing its inhibitory activity, which increases pain perception.

Impulses to the dorsal column fibers of the spinal cord bypass the gate mechanism to proceed directly to the central control system in the brain. Selective brain centers, the cerebral cortex and reticular formation in the thalamus, are activated. These cortical functions identify, evaluate, and selectively modify sensory input.

The central transmission cells or T-cells, thought of as the "action" system, compile information from the large and small fibers and from the descending pathways. When the information exceeds a critical level, the T-cells activate neural mechanisms that are responsible for the perception of and response to pain. As conceptualized, the gate control theory explains the physical aspects of pain as well as how psychological factors influence a patient's experience of pain.

TYPES OF PAIN

Acute pain is characterized by a sudden onset of pain, usually with a demonstrable cause. Although the duration may vary, it generally has a limited and predictable course. Acute pain may function as a warning system by directing the individual's attention to injury or disease. The treatment approach tends to be simple, with a bias towards pharmacologic management.

Definitions of chronic pain tend to focus on duration of the pain, with 3 to 6 months cited commonly as the time period. Chronic pain may mean any pain

that persists beyond the usual course of a disease or injury. Unlike acute pain, chronic pain has a major impact on the family system as the child's pain and care become incorporated into the daily routine of the child and family. Children with chronic pain may become depressed and may learn a helpless attitude toward the pain. Chronic pain treatment plans are complex and an interdisciplinary team approach that incorporates pharmacologic and psychological support may produce the most effective management plan.

Procedural pain may be the most difficult for children to endure during their PICU stay. Unfortunately, painful procedures are often necessary for diagnostic and treatment purposes. Repeated procedures cause children physical pain as well as immeasurable suffering. The fear, anxiety, and loss of control can be overwhelming for children and their parents.

CHILDREN'S RESPONSES TO PAIN

Children's developmental level, culture, and personality traits, as well as past experiences with pain, the meaning of the present pain, and parental presence all influence the response to pain. Several authors (Pridham et al., 1987; Gaffney & Dunne, 1987) have described the influence of cognitive development on children's concept of pain. Piaget's developmental theory provides the framework. During the sensorimotor period of development, infants are learning about the world through sensory experiences. Although the sensory system may be quite well developed, infants' motor responses are immature. Responses to pain are generalized and difficult to distinguish from responses to other distress-causing stimuli. For example, crying and agitation may be the result of hunger, separation anxiety, respiratory insufficiency, or pain. Because the response to pain is not well-differentiated, caregivers need to be particularly careful to interpret an infant's behavior correctly and plan appropriate intervention.

Children age 2 to 7 years are in the preoperational stage of development. Children in this age group are very egocentric in their thinking and believe that all events and sensations originate from their internal world. They have little understanding of cause-and-effect relationships, and thus unrelated events may become linked. Because of inaccurate assignment of cause and effect, children this age often misconstrue the meaning and cause of pain. They may view pain as a punishment for past misdeeds or bad thoughts. Young children need to be repeatedly reassured that procedures and/or painful experiences are not punishments.

Young children focus on external physical cues such as blood or needles to define pain. Children who have an endotracheal tube, nasogastric tube, foley catheter, IV lines, and monitor hookups may associate these attachments with discomfort and pain. When they are removed, they feel much better. Because of their fears of bodily injury and mutilation, breakdowns in skin integrity from cuts, abrasions, or incisions are extremely threatening to children. They believe that all of their body and blood will leak out. BandAids and dressings hold a special power for children as they fix the "leak" and hold the body in.

Children 7 to 12 years old, who are in the concrete operational stage, become more logical and reasonable in their thinking. They are in the process of gaining greater command over their world and tend to be achievement-oriented. Because these children are often organized by "rules," they respond well to rituals to cope with painful events. Once these rituals and routines are established, they must be followed consistently to be effective.

Adolescents, in the formal operations stage, are capable of abstract thinking and have an understanding of "if-then" relationships. Although capable of adult-level problem-solving, adolescents lack the life experiences that facilitate consistent mature responses. During stressful situations, adolescents may vacillate between adult responses and regression to immature behaviors.

Children's past experiences with pain, how pain was managed, and how they were able to cope all influence their responses to current pain sensations. Children who have had painful experiences in the past may use this information to cope successfully with the present situation. On the other hand, memories of pain and how difficult or frightening the situation was may increase anxiety and exacerbate pain. There may be lingering fear of being unable to cope. Children with little pain experience may have developed coping skills in response to other stressful events. Nurses should discuss with children, or their parents, coping responses to stress, distress, emotional upset, and worry. These skills may be generalized to help children cope with pain.

Cultural expectations of how a person should respond to pain are learned early in life and have been shown to be consistent through second- and third-generation immigrants (Johnson & Eland, 1988). Cultural background dictates how much pain is ac-

Table 18–1. USEFUL MNEMONIC TO OBTAIN A PAIN HISTORY

P	Palliative and provocative factors	What makes the pain better? (e.g., hot/cold packs, imobilizing painful body part, repositioning, sleeping) What makes the pain worse? (e.g., eating, fatigue, movement)
Q	Quality	What does the pain feel like? (e.g., shooting, throbbing, stabbing, pulsing, burning, tingling)
R	Region and radiation	Where is the pain? Does it spread anywhere else?
S	Severity	How bad is the pain? Use pain rating scales to aid communication of pain intensity
T	Timing	When did the pain start? How long have you had the pain? Is the pain constant or intermittent?

ceptable and how much emotion may be shown. Because a child is exposed to a variety of cultural influences, including television, no cultural stereotype should be thought of as descriptive of all patients, but individual cultural expression should be considered during pain assessment.

PAIN ASSESSMENT

There are many factors to consider when assessing for pain in a critically ill infant or child. The age of the child, the cognitive and social development, and the illness and its treatment all influence a child's ability to communicate pain. In children who are able to communicate and can describe their discomforts directly, pain assessment is often easier; however, fear, confusion, and developmental immaturity hinder children's ability to communicate with caregivers. Critically ill children who are unconscious, sedated, mechanically ventilated, and/or paralyzed may be experiencing severe pain, but are unable to communicate this to others.

Because there is no single indicator of pain, a multidimensional approach to pain assessment is necessary. Consideration of the clinical situation or context, observations of physiologic and behavioral changes, and the patient's self-report all provide information about a patient's pain. From a synthesis of this information, the clinician formulates a clinical judgment of the child's pain and a plan for intervention.

Self-report

Children are quite capable of describing many aspects of their pain. Through a brief but comprehensive interview, the caregiver may learn much about the patient's pain. A useful mnemonic is "PQRST" (Table 18–1), which may help to organize questions regarding the pain's intensity, location, duration, precipitating factors, and quality.

In many instances, such as postoperatively, one may infer a pain history from the situational context, and information regarding pain intensity becomes the most useful variable. However, information regarding other aspects of the pain (PQRST) will help to delineate the problem so that management can be more effective. For example, following bowel surgery, a child may experience incisional pain as well as gas pain. It is important to differentiate between the two because incisional pain responds best to narcotics, whereas gas pain worsens with narcotics and responds to increased activity and movement by the patient.

Many pain assessment tools are available for use in clinical practice. The easiest and most accessible method to assess pain intensity is a verbal 0 to 10 scale. The scale should be anchored on each end with 0 meaning no pain or hurt and 10 the worst pain or hurt you could ever imagine. To use the numeric scale, the child must be able to count to 10 and

Figure 18–3 ● ● ● ● ● ●

Faces rating scale. Explain to the child that each face is for a person who feels happy because he has no pain (hurt) or sad because he has some or a lot of pain. Face 0 is very happy because he doesn't hurt at all. Face 1 hurts just a little bit. Face 2 hurts a little more. Face 3 hurts even more. Face 4 hurts a whole lot, but Face 5 hurts as much as you can imagine, although you don't have to be crying to feel this bad. Ask child to choose the face that best describes how he/she is feeling. Rating scale is recommended for persons age 3 years and older. (From Whaley, L., & Wong, D. (1991). *Nursing care of infants and children* (ed. 5, 1995.) Copyrighted by Mosby-Year Book, Inc. Reprinted by permission. The Wong-Baker Faces Pain Scale may be reproduced for clinical and research use, provided the copyright information is retained with the scale.)

understand the principles of rank and order. Some young children may be able to recite numbers but have little understanding of increasing levels of pain using the scale. These children tend to give extreme scores; it either does not hurt with a score of 0 or it hurts with a score of 10. For these children, a scale better suited to their cognitive ability may be more useful.

The visual analogue scale (VAS) is a 10-cm line, aligned horizontally or vertically. It may be delineated with numbers 0 to 10 at 1-cm intervals or with word modifiers such as no pain, moderate pain, and extreme pain. With the scale anchored on each end, the child is asked to place a mark on the line that represents how much pain they feel. The VAS may be used to rate other discomforts as well, such as nausea and fatigue.

Several faces scales have been developed for younger children to rate pain intensity (Fig. 18–2, 18–3). They present faces ranging from happy, not hurting to sad, hurting arranged linearly along a vertical or horizontal line. Some have corresponding numbers to aid caregivers in identifying and communicating the child's pain intensity.

The original poker chip tool uses four red chips to indicate "pieces of hurt" (Hester, 1979). The tool was later modified by adding a white poker chip to represent "no hurt" (Molsberry, 1979). The child is presented with the poker chips and is instructed to pick up the chip or chips that represent how many pieces of hurt they are experiencing.

The Eland color scale is unique in that it addresses both pain location and intensity (Fig. 18–4). The child is presented with back and front views of a body outline and is asked to choose four color crayons to represent different levels of pain. The location of the pain may be marked directly on the body parts affected. Pain intensity is indicated by the color that the child chooses to color or mark the painful part. The Eland tool has been shown numerous times to be a very sensitive tool for identifying painful locations. Some children have located metastasis from cancer

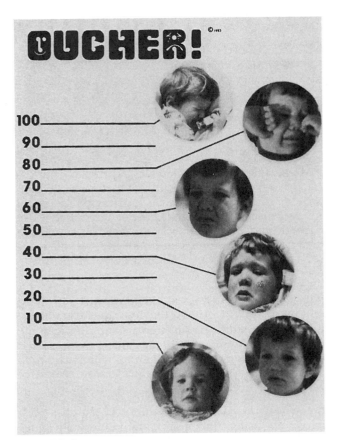

Figure 18–2 ● ● ● ● ● ●

The Oucher was developed and copyrighted by Judith E. Beyer, RN, PhD, 1983. New versions for African-American and Hispanic patients are also available. (For copies and information, contact: Judith E. Beyer, RN, PhD, University of Colorado Health Sciences Center, School of Nursing, Campus Box C-288, 4200 East 9th Avenue, Denver, Colorado 80262.)

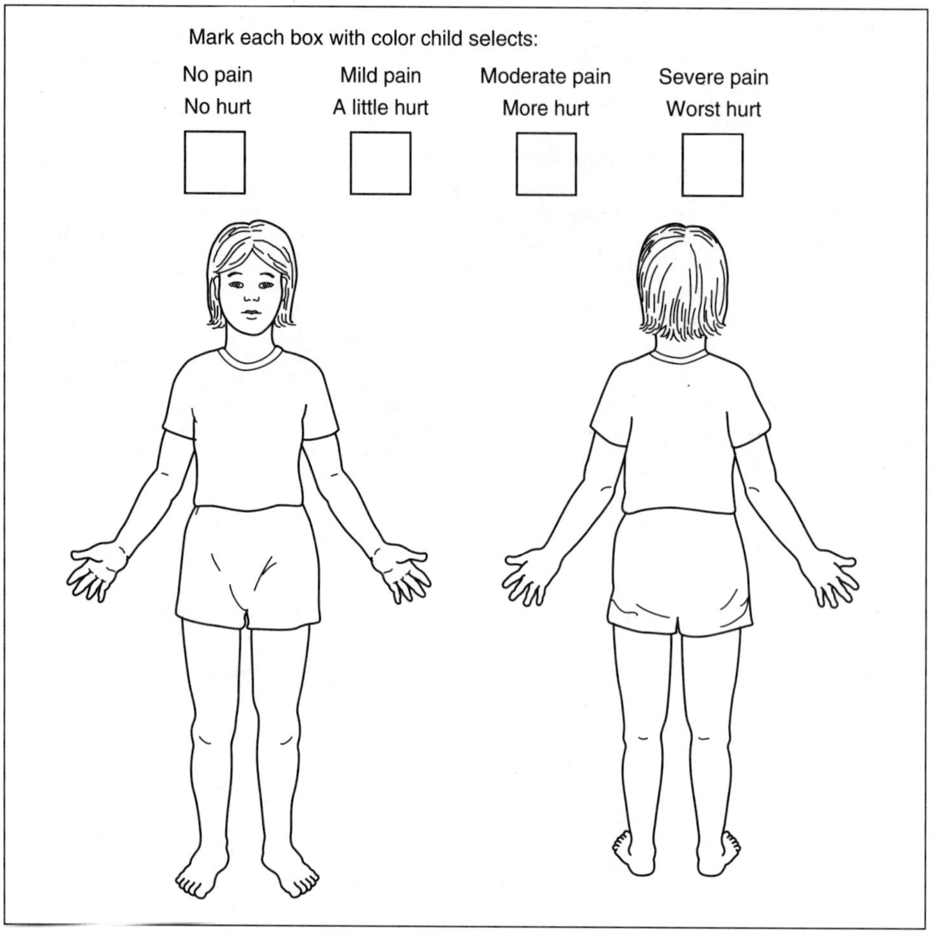

Mark each box with color child selects:

| No pain | Mild pain | Moderate pain | Severe pain |
| No hurt | A little hurt | More hurt | Worst hurt |

Figure 18–4 ● ● ● ● ●
Eland color scale. Redrawn with permission of the author, who also gives permission for this to be duplicated for use in clinical practice. (Permission from Joann M. Eland.)

before objective evidence has been detected (Eland, 1986).

Pain intensity scales provide a means for communication between child and caregiver as well as between caregivers. Understanding how a child is rating pain intensity over a continuum of time and activities gives more information about the child's experience. Changes in therapy may be geared to meeting the deficiencies in pain coverage. For example, the child may rate the pain as 1 out of 10 while at rest, but it escalates to 8 out of 10 with movement. Greater emphasis may be placed on relieving pain during periods of activity and decreasing analgesia while the child is at rest.

Physiologic Indicators

The physiologic response to acute pain is generalized system activation. Children in acute pain most often have an elevated heart rate, respiratory rate, and blood pressure. The cardiovascular and respiratory responses are a result of the release of catecholamines from the adrenal medulla in the body's preparation for "fight or flight." Young infants may respond somewhat differently with an increase or decrease in heart rate (Johnston & Strada, 1986). The magnitude and intensity of the change in heart rate are related to the duration and intensity of the stimulus and the temperament of the individual infant. Other physical signs of pain are also the result of the "fight or flight" or stress response: diaphoresis, skin color changes, and increased muscle tension. Increased pulmonary vascular resistance, increased intracranial pressure, and decreased PaO_2 may also occur (Anand, 1989).

The hormonal and endocrine responses to pain include the release of corticosteroids, growth hormone, and catecholamines as well as a decrease in insulin secretion. This leads to hyperglycemia and a breakdown of carbohydrate and fat stores. Utilization of fat for energy may cause metabolic acidosis resulting from an increase in blood lactate, pyruvate, ketone bodies, and nonesterified fatty acids (Anand, 1989). If allowed to continue, this catabolic process results in a poor environment for healing. Currently, these responses are measured in clinical research but remain impractical for use in the clinical setting.

The body cannot sustain the stress response for extended periods. Physiologic adaptation will occur, sometimes within minutes of the painful stimulus. Vital signs will return to normal and other physical parameters associated with acute pain, such as sweating and pupillary dilatation, will cease. A nurse assessing a child for pain may be misled by the presence of "normal" physiologic parameters. It is important to remember that physiologic changes are neither sensitive nor specific parameters for pain.

Behavioral Indicators

In critically ill infants or children who present with signs of the physiologic stress response and who are not able to communicate, behavioral cues of pain are crucial. Learning each individual's response to pain requires awareness and time to get to know the patient. The nurse is then able to make pain assessments that incorporate the individual patient's behavioral responses to discomfort.

Common behavioral responses to pain have been well described. Specific facial expressions have been identified. In the infant, the typical facial expression of pain consists of brow lowered and drawn together; bulging forehead with vertical furrows between the brows; a broadened nasal root; eyes tightly closed; and an angular, squarish mouth with taut tongue (Johnston & Strada, 1986). In the older child, facial expressions associated with pain are more varied: any distortion may indicate pain. A wrinkled, squeezed forehead; tightly shut or widely opened eyes; or tightly shut or widely opened mouth may all express pain (McCaffery & Beebe, 1989).

Vocalizations and body movements provide the crux of nonverbal communication about how a person is feeling. Crying, groaning, moaning, grunting, and screaming are powerful communications. Rigid posturing, guarding a particular body part, refusal to move, head rocking, and general fidgeting may all be signs of pain. Infants, less organized in their response to pain and distress, may demonstrate a Moro response, flailing extremities, and crying.

Behaviors seen with chronic pain may differ dramatically from those seen in children suffering from acute pain episodes. Children suffering from chronic pain may not demonstrate an overt behavioral manifestation of pain such as crying, but other behavioral changes may occur. The child may sleep more, have a decrease in appetite, and appear depressed and withdrawn.

Interpretation of behaviors presents several problems. Pain estimates may vary, depending on the behavioral criteria used by each observer to infer pain. Although one health professional may believe that a patient's behaviors indicate pain, another may interpret the behaviors as signs of anxiety or emotional distress. Several behavioral observation pain scales have been developed to help caregivers be more objective, systematic, and consistent in their assessment of pain behaviors. McGrath and coworkers (1985) developed the Children's Hospital of Eastern Ontario Pain Scale (CHEOPS), a behavioral scale used to assess postoperative pain in infants and children (Table 18–2). Initial reliability and validity statistics have been reported for use of this scale in the postanesthesia care unit. The CHEOPS is used for acute pain experiences only. The Attia scale (Attia, 1987) is a similar behavioral observation scale developed for newborns experiencing acute pain (Table 18–3). Initial reliability and validity studies are currently being conducted.

When the infant or child is unable to communicate information directly regarding their pain, caregivers often must rely solely on physiologic and behavioral changes for assessment. However, these signs may indicate another source of distress or stress; it is important to examine the context or situation in which changes in physiologic and behavioral signs are observed. Given the infant's or child's diagnosis and treatments, is it reasonable to infer that this patient is experiencing pain? Do these physiologic or behavioral changes respond to analgesics? What other factors may be contributing to the patient's distress?

The next section addresses the need to consider the patient's overall condition to delineate and rule out all causative factors that contribute to distress, pain, and agitation in the PICU patient.

ASSESSMENT OF AGITATION

Agitation is a particularly common problem in the PICU. The critically ill child can rarely tolerate the physiologic stress and consumption of calories from agitation. In addition, agitated patients consume much nursing time, increasing the impact of the already stressful PICU environment on caregivers.

Agitation is a form of behavioral communication for patients who are unable to communicate verbally because of age, illness, neurologic status, or intubation. Agitation is not a diagnosis; it is simply a sign that something is wrong. Agitation may be the result of internal pathophysiologic causes, internal sensations (pain), or external stimuli that are causing either pain or emotional distress. Effective nursing management requires a calm, systematic approach to determine the cause of the behavior (Fig. 18–5).

One of the most common causes of agitation in the ventilator-dependent PICU patient is impaired gas exchange, which can occur for a variety of reasons. Airway obstruction should always be ruled out immediately by manual ventilation, auscultation of breath sounds, capnography, and suctioning as necessary. If there is any doubt regarding airway patency, the patient should be reintubated or have the tracheostomy tube changed.

Inadequate ventilator support is another common cause of agitation in the critically ill child. Patients often require a higher level of support when oxygen demands are increased by activity, anxiety, or the stress of caregiving procedures.

Impaired gas exchange can also occur as a result of large or small airway disease. Tracheobronchomalacia (TBM) has been increasingly recognized as a cause of agitation and cyanotic episodes in chronically ventilated infants. In this disorder, the cartilage that provides rigidity to the large airways is either damaged (acquired form) or fails to develop properly (congenital form), so that the airway collapses whenever intrathoracic pressure is increased or airway pressure is decreased. Infants with TBM often become agitated during bowel movements, crying, or suctioning. Auscultation of breath sounds during an episode of agitation reveals severely diminished air movement during both inspiration and expiration.

Table 18–2. CHEOPS

Item	Behavior	Rating	Definition
Cry	No crying	1	Child is not crying
	Moaning	2	Child is moaning or quietly vocalizing silent cry
	Crying	2	Child is crying, but the cry is gentle or whimpering
	Scream	3	Child is in a full-lunged cry; sobbing may be scored with complaint or without complaint
Facial	Composed	1	Neutral facial expression
	Grimace	2	Score only if definite negative facial expression
	Smiling	0	Score only if definite positive facial expression
Child verbal	None	1	Child not talking
	Other complaints	1	Child complains but not about pain e.g. "I want to see mommy" or "I am thirsty"
	Pain complaints	2	Child complains of pain
	Both complaints	2	Child complains about pain and other things, e.g., "It hurts, I want mommy"
	Positive	0	Child makes any positive statement or talks about other things without complaint
Torso	Neutral	1	Body (not limbs) is at rest; torso is inactive
	Shifting	2	Body is in motion in a shifting or serpentine fashion
	Tense	2	Body is arched or rigid
	Shivering	2	Body is shuddering or shaking involuntarily
	Upright	2	Child is in a vertical or upright position
	Restrained	2	Body is restrained
Touch	Not touching	1	Child is not touching or grabbing at wound
	Reach	2	Child is reaching for but not touching wound
	Grab	2	Child is grabbing vigorously at wound
	Restrained	2	Child's arms are restrained
Legs	Neutral	1	Legs may be in any position but are relaxed; includes gentle swimming or serpentine-like movements
	Squirming/kicking	2	Definitive uneasy or restless movements in the legs and/or striking out with foot or feet
	Drawn up/tensed	2	Legs tensed and/or pulled up tightly to body and kept there
	Standing	2	Standing, crouching, or kneeling
	Restrained	2	Child's legs are being held down

From McGrath P., et al (1985). *Advances in pain research and therapy/the CHEOPS: A behavioral scale to measure postoperative pain in children* (pp. 395–402). New York: Raven Press.

Hypercarbia and hypoxemia are also present. Manual ventilation usually relieves the episode. Using a slower respiratory rate and higher peak inflating and end-expiratory pressures is recommended. Often these "spells" can be controlled by increasing the patient's baseline end-expiratory pressure (PEEP) to a higher level so that the airway is stinted open by the positive pressure. The exact level of PEEP needed

Table 18–3. POSTOPERATIVE COMFORT SCORE

	0	1	2
1. Sleep during preceding hour	None	Short naps: between 5 and 10 minutes	Longer naps: ≥10 minutes
2. Facial expression of pain	Marked, constant	Less marked, intermittent	Calm, relaxed
3. Quality of cry	Screaming, painful, high pitched	Modulated i.e., can be distracted by normal sound	No cry
4. Spontaneous motor activity	Thrashing around, incessant agitation	Moderate agitation	Normal
5. Spontaneous excitability and responsiveness to ambient stimulation	Tremulous, clonic movements, spontaneous Moro reflexes	Excessive reactivity (to any stimulation)	Quiet
6. Constant and excessive flexion of fingers and toes	Very pronounced, marked and constant	Less marked, intermittent	Absent
7. Sucking	Absent or disorganized sucking	Intermittent (3 or 4) and stops with crying	Strong, rhythmic, with pacifying effect
8. Global evaluation of tone	Strong hypertonicity	Moderate hypertonicity	Normal for the age
9. Consolability	None after 2 minutes	Quiet after 1 minute of effort	Calm before 1 minute
10. Sociability (eye contact) Response to voice, smile Real interest in face	Absent	Difficult to obtain	Easy and prolonged

From Attia I. et al.: Measurement of postoperative pain and narcotic administration in infants using a new clinical scoring system. *Anesthesiology* 67(3a), September 1987, p. a532.

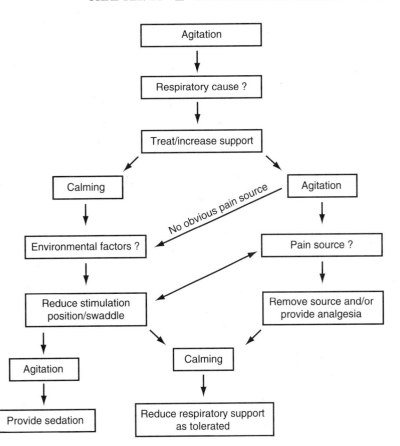

Figure 18–5 ● ● ● ● ● ●

A decision flow chart for the assessment and management of agitated infants.

may be determined by either pulmonary function testing, airway fluoroscopy, or bedside bronchoscopy under sedation.

Bronchospasm is another common cause of impaired gas exchange in the ventilated PICU patient; it can result in agitation and cyanotic episodes. Differentiation from TBM is sometimes difficult, but usually patients with bronchospasm have a more gradual onset to their distress, with wheezing that is more predominant on exhalation, at least in the early stages. The chest radiograph of a patient with bronchospasm is more likely to show air-trapping than that of a patient with TBM. Patients with bronchospasm do not recover quickly with manual ventilation. The problem is usually more effectively controlled through the use of bronchodilating agents.

Another cause of agitation in the critically ill child can be poor tissue perfusion. Causes of decreased tissue perfusion include septic shock; decreased myocardial contractility; hypovolemic shock; anatomic cardiovascular defects such as critical coarctation or aortic stenosis, which obstruct systemic blood flow; and cardiovascular alterations in which the balance between pulmonary and systemic blood flow is disturbed, such as in pulmonary hypertension or in patients with large aortopulmonary shunts. In these patients, the decreased tissue perfusion results in tissue hypoxia, conversion to anaerobic metabolism, and lactic acidosis. Metabolic acidosis stimulates the physiologic stress response.

Pain is another major cause for agitation in the PICU. Nurses must constantly review a mental

"checklist" of possible causes for discomfort in their patients. Some sources of more severe pain are easily recognized: surgical incisions, chest tubes, major skin breakdown, or traumatic injuries. However, other possible sources of moderate-to-severe pain are less obvious and require caregivers to have a high level of suspicion for detection. Examples of this may be stress ulcers or bowel obstruction in a patient recovering from surgery or an infiltrated IV line. In general, pain should always be considered and ruled out as a contributing factor in a patient with repeated episodes of agitation. A trial of analgesics, even in the absence of a clear pain source, is appropriate and should be standard in the systematic approach to managing agitation in a critically ill child.

PHARMACOLOGIC MANAGEMENT OF PAIN AND AGITATION

The following discussion concerns both pharmacologic and nonpharmacologic management of patients with pain and agitation. Although each topic is discussed separately for organizational clarity, it is important to recognize that the best management involves an integrated approach that considers both pharmacologic and nonpharmacologic strategies with the overall goal to provide comfort. Medications, delivery systems, and general concepts for pain management will first be reviewed, followed by a discussion of sedatives for agitation management. Table 18–4 contains information on dosage, routes of ad-

Table 18-4. PHARMACOLOGIC MANAGEMENT OF PAIN AND AGITATION

Drug	Dosage	Approximate Equianalgesic Dose	Route	Onset of Action	Duration of Action
Narcotic Analgesics					
Morphine	Neonates & infants: (0.03 mg/kg) Children: 0.1 mg/kg Continuous infusion: Neonates & infants: 15 mcg/kg/hr Children: 20 mcg/kg/hr Epidural: 0.03–0.05 mg/kg q 6–12 hr infusion 3 mcg/kg/hr	10 mg q 3–4 hr	IV, IM, SC	IV: 10–15 min IM: 20–30 min	4 hr
Fentanyl	1–5 mcg/kg Continuous infusion: 1–3 mcg/kg/hr	0.1 mg (100 mcg)	IV, IM	3–5 min	30–60 min
Sufentanil	0.1–0.5 mcg/kg Continuous infusion: 0.1–0.3 mcg/kg/hr	0.01–0.02 mg (10–20 mcg)	IV	Immediate	30–60 min
Methadone	0.1 mg/kg	10 mg q 6–8 hr	PO, IM, SC	1 hr	IM: 3–4 hr PO: 6–12 hr
Codiene	0.6–1.0 mg/kg	75–90 mg q 3–4 hr	PO	1 hr	4–6 hr
Meperidine	1 mg/kg	100 mg q 3 hr	IV, IM, SC, PO	IV: 10 min IM: 15–20 min PO: 20 min	2–4 hr 3 hr
Benzodiazepines					
Diazepam	0.1–0.2 mg/kg	NA	IV, PO	IV: 15 min PO: 30–60 min	IV: 4–6 hr PO: 6–8 hr
Lorazepam	0.05–0.1 mg/kg	NA	IV, IM, PO	IV: 15 min PO: 30–60 min	8–12 hr
Midazolam	0.05–0.1 mg/kg	NA	IV, IM, PO	IV: 2–5 min IM: 20–30 min PO: 10–30 min	2 hr
Barbiturates					
Phenobarbital	2–5 mg/kg	NA	IV, PO	IV: 5 min PO: 20–60 min	8–12 hr
Pentobarbital	2 mg/kg	NA	IV, IM, PO, PR	IV: <5 min IM: <20 min PO: 20–60 min PR: 20–60 min	4–6 hr
Sodium thiopental	4 mg/kg	NA	IV	30–60 sec	5–10 mm
Hyponotic					
Chloral hydrate	Sedative: 25–50 mg/kg Hyponotic: 75–100 mg/kg	NA	PO, PR	30–60 min	6–8 hr
General Anesthetic & Analgesic					
Ketamine	Single dose: 5 mg/kg IM 1–2 mg/kg IV		IV, IM	IM: 3–10 min IV: 30 sec	12–60 min 5–20 min

NA, not applicable. Anxiolytics, sedatives do not provide analgesia.

ministration, and onset and duration of action for pharmacologic control of pain and agitation. A section on nonpharmacologic strategies that emphasizes nursing interventions appropriate for patients experiencing pain, distress, or both is included.

Pain Management: Nonopioids

For mild-to-moderate pain, a nonopioid drug is recommended. This includes acetaminophen and the nonsteroidal anti-inflammatory drugs (NSAIDs) such as aspirin, ibuprofen, Naprosyn, and ketoprofen. These agents inhibit prostanglandin synthesis and action. When used aggressively, such as on an around-the-clock regimen, these analgesics provide powerful pain relief. For example, 650 mg of acetaminophen is equianalgesic to 30 mg of codeine (Beaver, 1984). Because peripherally acting agents inhibit pain pathways differently than narcotics, these agents yield an additive analgesic effect when combined with narcotics. However, they do exhibit a ceiling effect, which means that a maximum level of analgesia is eventually achieved, despite increased doses.

There are many oral NSAIDs available; ketorolac tromethamine is the first injectable NSAID. Ketorolac is a promising analgesic for critically ill patients. It provides powerful analgesia without the side effects seen with narcotics. Currently, ketorolac has not been approved for use in children. However, several studies are being conducted to evaluate the pharmacokinetics and pharmacodynamics of ketorolac in pediatric populations. In the meantime, many pediatric institutions use ketorolac routinely. Although it is marketed as an intramuscularly administered agent, many institutions give ketorolac intravenously (Cohen, D.E. Personal communication, November 1995).

From comparison studies, ketorolac offers analgesia similar to many of the opioids without the problematic side effects such as respiratory depression and sedation. Equianalgesic doses are cited as 30 mg ketorolac IM or IV equivalent to 12 mg morphine IM or IV (O'Hara et al., 1987). When combined with a narcotic, ketorolac lowers the overall narcotic requirement. For patients with severe pain who require significant doses of narcotic to control their pain and who are experiencing many troublesome side effects, the addition of ketorolac to the pharmacologic regimen may be very useful. Ketorolac does have its own side effects, which are similar to those of other NSAIDs. Nurses should monitor patients for signs and symptoms of stomach upset, ulcers, and platelet functioning. Ketorolac should not be used in patients at risk for bleeding and should be limited to use of less than 1 week.

Pain Management: Opioids

Morphine

Morphine sulfate is a naturally occurring substance derived from opium. Considered the "gold standard" of narcotics, morphine is used as the standard of comparison for all narcotics. Morphine is used as an example to describe principles of narcotic titration and the general use of opioids for pain management.

For all narcotic analgesics, there are recommended initial doses (see Table 18–4). Although these are recommended starting doses, they are not rigid standards. Because individual patients vary in their response to narcotics, the dose must be adjusted for each. The ideal dose of narcotic is that which produces adequate analgesia with manageable side effects for a particular patient. To titrate morphine safely, it is necessary to understand its pharmacokinetics and pharmacodynamics. Intravenously administered morphine crosses the blood-brain barrier and peak action occurs at 6 to 10 minutes. Evaluation of the patient for maximal analgesic effect and side effects should coincide with the time of peak action.

Further titration of morphine depends on the child's response to the initial dose of morphine. The evaluation of responses to narcotics provides valuable information. For children who remain alert and are still complaining of pain, it is safe to titrate further doses of morphine, using doses equivalent to half the initial dose. No additional dose of morphine should be given to children who are somewhat sedated but have no signs of respiratory compromise after their initial dose. They should be assessed frequently for break-through pain and further need for analgesia. Children with excessive sedation and signs of respiratory depression who continue to ventilate well should be physically stimulated and instructed to take deep breaths. If their respiratory status becomes significantly compromised, emergency administration of a narcotic antagonist such as naloxone should be considered.

Naloxone is used to reverse complications of narcotic agonists. Naloxone administration must be considered carefully, because it is not a benign medication. When given, it reverses analgesia and may result in vomiting, significant hypertension, and pulmonary edema. In most references, the naloxone dose for narcotic reversal is 100 mcg/kg/dose (0.1 mg/kg). Recently, pain experts have recommended a gentler titration of naloxone when the clinical situation permits (Cohen, D.E. Personal communication, November 14, 1995). For children with a medical history including recently administered narcotics, naloxone may be titrated conservatively in doses of 1 mcg/kg every 30 to 60 seconds until the child is responsive. Aggressive titration of naloxone remains appropriate for those children seen in emergency rooms in respiratory or cardiac arrest from a narcotic overdose. Because the half-life for naloxone is significantly shorter than that of a narcotic, approximately 20 minutes, the child should be frequently assessed for the need for subsequent doses or an infusion of naloxone.

Assuming that initial pain control is achieved, a plan for a narcotic administration regimen should be developed. The dosing schedule for future narcotic doses depends on the nature of the patient's pain. Traditional as-necessary (prn) scheduling of narcotics works on the premise that the return of pain dictates the need for additional narcotic doses. A prn schedule is appropriate for children who have intermittent, unpredictable pain or who have pain related to specific activities. For example, the child may be comfortable at rest but the pain increases dramatically with physical therapy. Planning for pain management prior to physical therapy allows the child to participate more fully.

For children experiencing constant pain, a prn schedule is not recommended. Nurses may anticipate and prevent the return of pain by administering narcotics on an around-the-clock schedule. With an around-the-clock schedule, there is less fluctuation in plasma narcotic concentration, and thus smoother pain control is achieved.

Patients who have severe, ongoing pain may be started on a continuous morphine infusion. The advantage of an infusion is that the patient's pain management may be smoother with fewer peaks and troughs. However, several problems should be anticipated. A continuous infusion of morphine does not reach steady state for 8 to 12 hours. How a child will respond to a change in the dose of the infusion will not be apparent for a lengthy period of time. The child's pain also may change at any time, but the narcotic will infuse at the same rate despite changes in the pain. This is potentially problematic because the child's response to a narcotic infusion is dependent upon the child's pain state and the metabolism of the medication that results. If the pain state changes, the child's response to the infusion may change. With these considerations in mind, a reasonable recommendation for an initial infusion rate is 0.02 mg/kg/hr following a loading dose of 0.1 mg/kg. Rescue doses of 0.02 mg/kg/dose may be given on a prn basis.

Special considerations are necessary when giving narcotics to young infants. Generally, morphine given to infants younger than 6 months of age tends to have a longer elimination half-life and a lower clearance rate (Koren et al., 1985; Lynn & Slattery, 1987; Purcell-Jones et al., 1987). The duration of action of morphine is highly variable among infants in this age group. Because of the unpredictability in response, narcotic titration in young infants must be conservative with a recommended morphine starting dose of 0.03 mg/kg. Initiating a narcotic infusion should be dictated by conservative estimates of starting dose. The infant's response to a narcotic dose should be assessed carefully. Once the infants's response is known, it becomes easier to titrate further doses of narcotic. Infants older than 6 months become more predictable in their response to morphine, with the elimination half-life approaching the 2- to 3-hour timeframe typical of older children and adults.

Meperidine

Although meperidine is a commonly used analgesic, it is not the drug of choice for pain management. Meperidine has a rapid bolus effect and is shorter acting than generally thought, especially in young children. Repeated intramuscular (IM) injections of meperidine are painful and irritating to muscle tissue and may precipitate muscle fibrosis (Jaffe & Martin, 1985). Meperidine has been associated with central nervous system (CNS) alterations from the accumulation of an active metabolite, normeperidine. Normeperidine is a CNS stimulant and may cause moodiness, tremors, twitches, and major motor seizures. Although the half-life of meperidine is 3 to 4 hours, the half-life of normeperidine is 15 to 30 hours. Meperidine is not recommended for patients requiring ongoing pain management.

Fentanyl

Fentanyl (Sublimaze) is a synthetic opioid agonist that is 80 to 100 times more potent than morphine. Originally used intraoperatively for anesthesia, fentanyl is becoming more commonly used for pain management in critically ill patients. Its onset of action is rapid, with peak effect within minutes of IV dosing and a duration of analgesia lasting 30 to 60 minutes. Like morphine, fentanyl is metabolized in the liver and excreted primarily in urine, and should be used cautiously in patients with liver or renal dysfunction. Because fentanyl administration is not associated with histamine release, it has become a popular analgesic for critically ill patients at risk for hypotension and bronchospasm.

The most serious complication with fentanyl is chest wall rigidity, which may occur with large doses and/or rapid administration. Doses associated with chest wall rigidity are *rarely* used outside of the operating room setting. This complication may be avoided with slow administration of fentanyl. Muscle relaxants and naloxone are used to treat chest wall rigidity. Other side effects of fentanyl are similar to those seen with all narcotic analgesics: respiratory depression, pruritus, urinary retention, nausea and vomiting, and sedation.

Sufentanil (Sufenta) is five to 10 times more potent than fentanyl. Highly protein-bound and lipophilic, sufentanil has a faster onset of action and shorter duration of action than fentanyl. Sufentanil is useful when a patient requires high doses of fentanyl but must have fluid restrictions.

Methadone

Methadone is a long-acting narcotic analgesic; duration of action is two to eight times longer than morphine. Actions and side effects are similar to other narcotics. In equianalgesic doses, methadone produces analgesia and dose-related somnolence and respiratory depression, similar to morphine. The dosing of morphine and methadone is similar in single IV doses. Because methadone tends to accumulate, long-term methadone doses are smaller and less frequent and must be immediately decreased upon identification of untoward effects. Well absorbed orally, methadone is ideal for the long-term management of pain. Providing consistent baseline analgesia with methadone allows titration of high doses of shorter acting narcotics.

Nalbuphine (Nubain)

Nalbuphine is a synthetic opioid of the mixed agonist-antagonist type. It is equianalgesic to morphine and has a duration of action of 3 to 6 hours. There is speculation that nalbuphine has less smooth muscle effect on the gut and biliary tree. Some physicians prefer nalbuphine for patients with gastrointestinal or biliary dysfunction, or following bowel surgery. Unlike morphine, there is a ceiling for analgesic effect with nalbuphine. Doses higher than 0.2 mg/kg/dose do not provide increased analgesia. Because of this ceiling effect, nalbuphine is not recommended for patients requiring large doses of narcotic for pain relief. Patients who have been maintained on an opioid agonist such as morphine and are physiologically dependent cannot be switched to nalbuphine because of the risk of withdrawal symptoms.

Delivery Systems

Patient-controlled Analgesia

Patient-controlled analgesia (PCA) is a delivery system in which the patient presses a button to self-administer narcotic doses; the patient may be receiving a background continuous infusion of narcotic as well. Although the patient may push the PCA button infinitely, the PCA device will only successfully deliver a narcotic dose when the preset refractory time period has passed. For safety, a total hourly maximum setting limits the overall availability of narcotic to the patient.

Several theoretical concepts lend support to PCA use in clinical practice. Pharmacologically, PCA provides smoother pain control than other methods of delivering pain medications. Traditional intermittent IV dosing results in large fluctuations in analgesic blood concentration. Following a narcotic bolus, the analgesic blood concentration rises and the patient obtains pain relief, becomes sedated, and falls asleep. Several hours later, as the drug blood concentration drops, the patient wakes in pain. With a PCA, the patient is able to finely titrate the amount of narcotic delivered to simultaneously maximize analgesia and minimize side effects.

Patients gain an element of self-control when using PCA. They are no longer as dependent on healthcare providers to ensure pain relief. Most patients report greater satisfaction with pain relief when using PCA in comparisons with more traditional methods of pain management.

The lower age limit for potential candidates for PCA varies with individual children and their developmental level and needs. Children who are 7 to 8 years old and older can readily use PCA. Some advocate using PCA in children as young as 4 or 5 years and have reported success in this age group (Meretoja et al., 1991). PCA is thought to provide older children with a sense of self-control in a situation in which they typically hold very little power; however, it is unclear whether younger children desire this control. Whether PCA is a preferred pain management approach for the younger child requires additional clinical investigation. Children who are developmentally delayed or who have a severe learning disability may have difficulty using the PCA device, and they warrant special consideration when considering this option for pain management. Patients must be alert, oriented, and physically able to

push a button. Patients in the PICU following surgery and trauma and during cancer treatment may benefit from PCA.

Parent-controlled analgesia has recently been described in a study that evaluated the use of this technique in children with cerebral palsy undergoing various orthopedic procedures (Webb, 1991). Parents reported greater satisfaction with this mode of pain management than other methods employed during previous hospitalizations.

Potential candidates for parent-controlled analgesia should be considered carefully. Because the child's safety is paramount, caregivers should carefully evaluate parents in terms of their ability to provide parent-controlled analgesia. Parents who successfully manage the care of a chronically ill child at home may be very capable of assuming the responsibilities for parent-controlled analgesia. They may wish to retain some control over their child's care during a hospital stay and are often familiar with hospital routines. On the other hand, parents of children who are undergoing a single elective procedure may not be the best candidates to provide parent-controlled analgesia. These families are unfamiliar with the hospital routine and the care of their child after surgery.

Epidural Analgesia

Epidural analgesia is often used to manage postoperative pain and other severe pain that cannot be controlled well by other methods. The epidural space is a potential space that lies between the dura mater of the spinal cord anteriorly and the ligamentum flavum posteriorly. It extends from the cranium to the sacrum and contains nerve roots, fat, loose connective tissue, and a plexus of veins (Fig. 18–6).

When analgesics are infused in the epidural space, they move across the dura mater and subarachnoid space into the cerebral spinal fluid. The analgesic

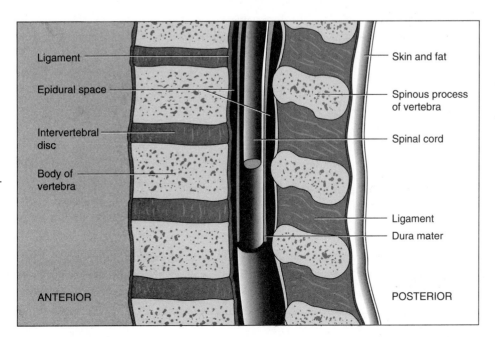

Figure 18–6 ● ● ● ● ● ●
Epidural space depicted with surrounding anatomy.

agents bind with the opioid receptors in the dorsal horn of the spinal cord to provide direct analgesic action. Narcotics and local anesthetics, alone or in combination, are typically used for epidural analgesia. Whether narcotic or local anesthetic is favored as the predominant agent is a matter of physician preference. Theoretically, the combination of narcotic and local anesthetic provides a synergistic effect so that the lowest possible dose of each agent is used for analgesia. Fentanyl, morphine, and bupivacaine are the agents most commonly used.

The decision of which narcotic to use is influenced by the level or location of the painful injury. Morphine and fentanyl hold different solubility properties; morphine is water-soluble, whereas fentanyl is lipid-soluble. Because morphine is hydrophilic, it readily diffuses and travels upward within the cerebral spinal fluid. There is a "spread" of analgesic, which is useful for patients who have high incision

sites or wounds from thoracotomies, pectus repair, or flailed chest. By contrast, fentanyl is lipophilic and tends to bind to receptors in close proximity to the injection site. Theoretically, analgesic effect is seen from the level of the epidural injection and progresses downward.

Epidural analgesia may be provided in three forms: "single shot" or single dose, intermittent boluses, or continuous epidural infusion. A single shot, given perioperatively, may provide very effective analgesia; epidural fentanyl is effective for 6 to 8 hours, whereas epidural morphine lasts from 8 to 24 hours.

The nurse must be aware of and assess for potential problems with epidural analgesia to assure safe patient care. Patients are closely monitored for drug-related complications as well as for complications related to catheter placement. This involves assessment for complications resulting from the narcotic

Table 18–5. COMPLICATIONS OF EPIDURAL ANALGESIA

	Etiology/Cause	Assessments	Treatment of Complication
Narcotic Related Side Effects			
Respiratory depression 　Early onset (2–4 hr) 　Late Onset (8–24 hr)	Systemic absorption of 　narcotic Central migration of 　narcotic	C-R monitor q 1h respiratory assessment Increase ventilator support	Turn off infusion Physical stimulation Instruct patient to breathe Increase ventilator support Naloxone administration
Pruritus	Central effects of narcotic	Patient reports itching 　around face	Nalbuphine Cool compresses
Nausea and vomiting	Central effects of narcotic	Patient report Vomiting	Antiemetics Nalbuphine Avoid strong smells
Urinary retention	Pooling of epidural narcotic/ 　local anesthetic in the 　sacral area around nerves 　innervating the bladder	Bladder distension Time of last void	Nalbuphine Urinary cathetrization Warm compress over bladder Apply gentle pressure over 　bladder
Local Anesthetic Effects/Side Effects			
Hypotension	Vasodilatation in peripheral 　vessels of lower 　extremities	Blood pressure	IV hydration
Sensory blockade	Level of blockade is dose- 　related	Determine level of sensory 　block with cold or 　pinprick, start in lower 　extremities and move 　upwards Changes in level of sensory 　loss indicates progressing 　or regressing blockade	Increase or decrease in 　epidural infusion as indicated 　by assessment
Motor blockade	Level of blockade is dose- 　related	Assess motor function, ask 　patient to wiggle toes, 　move feet, legs	Decrease infusion rate if motor 　blockade evident Assist patient during transfers 　and ambulation
Catheter Migration Complications	Catheter migration into 　vascular space	Early: tingling around the 　mouth or lips, 　tremulousness, funny 　taste in mouth, general 　feeling of unease, 　restlessness Late: hypotension, seizures, 　cardiac arrest	Stop epidural infusion Assure emergency support is 　available
	Catheter migration into 　subarachnoid space	Spinal blockade Paralysis	

C-R, cardiorespiratory.

and/or the local anesthetic. Table 18–5 outlines the most common complications of epidural analgesia and their management.

Key Concepts Related to Opioids

It is important to clarify key terms often used in relation to narcotic use: addiction, physical dependence, and physical tolerance. The misunderstanding of these phenomena perpetuates caregivers' presumptions regarding patients' responses to pain and pain management therapy. Lack of knowledge regarding the principle of equianalgesia often leads to undertreatment of pain.

Addiction is defined as the use of narcotics or other drugs for psychic effects, not for approved medical reasons. Addiction is a growing social problem that has received much recent attention in the media. Fear of "drugs" is prevalent among healthcare providers and the general public. Although this fear may be appropriate in the public domain, it may interfere with the approved medical use of narcotics for pain management. Some healthcare providers are reluctant to use narcotics for pain management because they fear "addicting" their patients. However, these fears are unwarranted; all studies show that regardless of dose or length of narcotic use for pain management, the incidence of narcotic addiction following therapeutic use is less than 1% percent (Marks & Sachar, 1973; Porter & Jick, 1980; Foley & Rogers, 1981; Twycross, 1974).

Tolerance is a pharmacologic property of opioids in which *increasing* doses are required to gain the *same* effect. Patients who require opioid management for 5 days or longer may develop tolerance to the narcotic. The first sign of tolerance to a narcotic is typically a decreased duration of action. Where a patient's narcotic dose had previously provided 4 hours of analgesia, with tolerance the patient experiences pain in 3 hours. For continued analgesia, the opioid dose needs to be increased and/or the time interval between doses decreased. There is no ceiling effect with narcotics and thus escalations in dose will continually provide the same level of pain relief. It is a common misconception that tolerance interferes with the clinical efficacy of the opioid and that eventually the opioid will no longer be able to provide analgesia. Some think that the opioid needs to be "saved" until the patient really needs it. Unfortunately, this misconception leads to the underuse of narcotics when use is warranted for severe pain. Most pain can be effectively treated with appropriate escalations in narcotic dose.

Physical dependence is also a pharmacologic property of opioids that is defined by a withdrawal syndrome following sudden discontinuation of the opioid or administration of an opioid antagonist. Many confuse the terms "physical dependence" and "addiction." Physical dependence is an expected outcome of opioid use. Generally, it is assumed that physical dependence will develop after 5 to 7 days of chronic opioid

Table 18–6. CALCULATION OF WEANING SCHEDULE FOR DISCONTINUING OPIOID

1. Calculate the total amount of opioid received in 24 hours
2. Reduce this amount by 50% by decreasing dose; maintain dosing intervals previously established, do not increase interval between doses
3. Wean subsequent doses by 10% per day as tolerated

therapy. For patients who no longer need the narcotic for pain relief, it is best to establish a weaning schedule to minimize discomforts or complications that may occur from discontinuing the medication abruptly.

Table 18–6 outlines a recommended *weaning* schedule. For some patients, the initial large drop in narcotic dose is more easily tolerated than later decreases. Patients may not experience withdrawal symptoms during the initial weaning process but may begin to experience symptoms when lower doses are reached. Should withdrawal symptoms occur, the patient may need to be maintained on a dose for a longer period of time before further decreases are initiated. Young infants who have been maintained on opioids for lengthy periods may require a slower wean, such as decreases of 5% to 10% every other day.

It is important to assess patients being weaned from narcotics for signs and symptoms of *withdrawal*. Withdrawal symptoms may not occur for 48 to 72 hours after discontinuation of the narcotic. Because of this time lag, health providers may not associate the symptoms with narcotic withdrawal. Symptoms range from yawning, tearing, rhinorrhea, sweating, restlessness, irritability, tremors, dilated pupils, and anorexia during the first day, progressing to nausea and vomiting, diarrhea, chills, muscle spasm, and increasing irritability during the second and third day following the last narcotic dose (Jaffe & Martin, 1985).

Abstinence scoring (Finnigan et al., 1975) has been used to objectively assess for the presence of iatrogenic physical withdrawal and to provide guidelines for managing narcotic weaning (Caron & Maguire, 1990). As shown in Table 18–7, each physical sign is assigned a weighted score. Scoring begins before dose reduction and continues throughout the weaning period. Narcotic weaning is held if the patient's abstinence score increases.

Equianalgesia

When changing a child's narcotic regimen, whether it is a change in delivery route or a change in type of narcotic, it is important to consider the principle of equianalgesia. Lack of knowledge about equianalgesic doses of narcotics is a potential cause of poor pain control. For example, many healthcare providers and patients may assume that better pain relief is achieved with IV delivery as compared with oral drug management. This is not true; proper dosing is more

Table 18–7. NEONATAL ABSTINENCE SCORE SHEET

System	Signs and Symptoms	Score
Central nervous system disturbances	Excessive high-pitched (or other) cry	2
	Continuous high-pitched (or other) cry	3
	Sleeps < 1 hour after feeding	3
	Sleeps < 2 hours after feeding	2
	Sleeps < 3 hours after feeding	1
	Hyperactive Moro reflex	2
	Markedly hyperactive Moro reflex	3
	Mild tremors when disturbed	1
	Moderate to severe tremors when disturbed	2
	Mild tremors when undisturbed	3
	Moderate to severe tremors when undisturbed	4
	Increased muscle tone	2
	Excoriation	1
	Myoclonic jerks	3
	Generalized convulsions	5
Metabolic and vasomotor or respiratory disturbances	Sweating	1
	Fever of 37.2°C to 38.2°C (99°F to 100.8°F)	1
	Fever > 38.4°C (101°F)	2
	Frequent yawning (more than 3 to 4 times/interval)	1
	Mottling	1
	Nasal stuffiness	1
	Sneezing (more than 3 to 4 times/interval)	1
	Nasal flaring	2
	Respiratory rate > 60/min	1
	Respiratory rate > 50/min with retractions	2
Gastrointestinal disturbances	Excessive sucking	1
	Poor feeding	2
	Regurgitation	2
	Projectile vomiting	3
	Loose stools	2
	Watery stools	3

Adapted from Finnigan L. P., Kron R. E., Cannaughton J. F., Emich J. P. A scoring system for evaluation and treatment of neonatal abstinence syndrome: A new clinical and research tool. In: Morselli P. L., Garattini S., Sereni F. (Eds.). *Basic and Therapeutic Aspects of Perinatal Pharmacology.* New York, NY: Raven Press; 1975; reprinted from the *Journal of Perinatal and Neonatal Nursing,* July 1990, p. 70.

important. For example, to change from IV to oral morphine, the dose must be tripled to obtain similar pain relief.

Patients suffering from intolerable side effects may benefit from a change in narcotic. For patients who are physically dependent on a narcotic, it is recommended that the dose of the new narcotic be based on one-half to two-thirds of the equianalgesic dose. The full equianalgesic dose should not be administered because there may be incomplete cross-tolerance to different narcotic agents. Administering the full equianalgesic dose could produce respiratory depression and excessive sedation. Vigilant pain assessment and evaluation of the patient's response to the new narcotic should guide further titration of the new narcotic.

Agitation Management: Sedatives

Sedatives are commonly used in the PICU to facilitate mechanical ventilation, decrease anxiety and agitation, normalize sleep-wake cycles, and to make procedures more tolerable. The optimal method of providing sedation for critically ill infants and children is unknown. Various medications have been used in the absence of sufficient research or rationale. Some of the more common sedatives used in PICUs include barbiturates, benzodiazepines, and chloral hydrate. In addition, opioids and neuromuscular blocking agents have also been used ostensibly to "calm" distressed and agitated patients.

Paralyzing agents are often administered to intubated patients to decrease oxygen requirements, and facilitate mechanical ventilation by preventing the patient's "competing" with the ventilator. Unfortunately, some caregivers hold the misconception that paralyzing agents and muscle relaxants, in addition to their primary effects, also provide analgesia and sedation. The use of these agents may be deceiving. They serve as a behavioral straightjacket; the child appears calm and comfortable despite discomforts or emotions that they may be feeling. Caregivers who become accustomed to the routines of PICU care may become desensitized to what and how a child is feeling. This, combined with the child's inability to "fight," may result in inadequate efforts to minimize pain and suffering. Nurses are in a crucial position to critically assess a patient for potential reasons for pain and to advocate appropriate pain management. Ideally, appropriate analgesia and sedation should be provided when paralyzing agents are used. Caregivers can assess the adequacy of analgesia and sedation by following change trends in pupil size and vital signs.

In light of the lack of solid research regarding chronic sedation in the pediatric population, healthcare providers must carefully consider the known actions and side effects of the various drugs. For example, administration of multiple sedatives do nothing to ease the distress of a patient who is in severe pain, and may make matters worse. Alternatively, placing a patient who is disoriented and combative as a result of a head injury on a high-dose narcotic infusion may also result in an undesirable outcome. A discussion of some of the specific medications and general principles regarding the use of sedation in critically ill patients follows.

Choral Hydrate

Chloral hydrate is a hypnosedative similar to the barbiturates. It has been used extensively in the sedation of infants and children. Because it has little effect on central respiratory drive, it is an ideal one-time sedative for infants and children undergoing nonpainful procedures, such as computed tomography, magnetic resonance imaging, or electroencephalography.

A survey of how agitation was managed in neonates (Franck, 1987) revealed that chloral hydrate was being used as a maintenance sedative for some critically ill neonates, particularly those infants with bronchopulmonary dysplasia. Chronic use of chloral hydrate leads to concerns about accumulation of a metabolite, trichlorethanol (Hartley et al., 1989;

Reimche, 1989). Specifically, chloral hydrate is rapidly absorbed and metabolized in the liver by alcohol dehydrogenase to trichlorethanol. Trichlorethanol is responsible for most of the sedative-hypnotic effects of the drug. Although the half-life of chloral hydrate is very short, a matter of minutes, the half-life of trichlorethanol may be very long and is dependent upon the serum concentration of the metabolite. Accumulation of trichlorethanol to toxic levels may occur within several days of use. The signs and symptoms of toxicity include CNS depression manifested as hypothermia or coma, respiratory depression (difficulty weaning from ventilator), cardiovascular effects (hypertension, atrial/ventricular dysrhythmias), or gastrointestinal effects (emesis, esophageal stricture, or gastric necrosis).

With chronic chloral hydrate therapy, there is evidence of tolerance and physical dependence. Oftentimes, an infant who receives periodic doses for agitation episodes slowly requires increasing amounts of chloral hydrate to maintain effect. The dosing schedule may become more regulated on an around-the-clock basis, and the dose may be increased. Infants who have their chloral hydrate dose held or delayed may show signs of withdrawal very similar to the delirium tremors seen in alcohol detoxification. For infants who need to be weaned from chloral hydrate, a weaning schedule similar to that used for narcotic tapering should be instituted.

Barbiturates

Historically, barbiturates were used extensively for sedation management in the PICU. Barbiturates exert a powerful central depression effect that ranges from mild sedation to deep anesthesia. The elimination half-life for the barbiturates is very long, usually longer than 24 hours. With repeated doses, as often needed for PICU management, barbiturates and their metabolites may accumulate and may delay recovery. Accordingly, the use of barbiturates tends to be discouraged in favor of the safer benzodiazepines.

Barbiturates have no analgesic effect. In fact, some reports indicate that barbiturates are hyperalgesic. In other words, pain perception may be more acute. A paradoxical excitation may result, which is manifested by restlessness, excitement, delirium, or agitation.

Benzodiazepines

The benzodiazepines are useful sedatives in the PICU setting. These agents have powerful CNS effects to induce sleep, sedation, hypnosis, anxiolysis, muscle relaxation, and most notably, anticonvulsant activity and amnesia. Benzodiazepines also have respiratory and cardiovascular effects that may result in decreased alveolar ventilation, manifested by decreased oxygen saturation and carbon dioxide accumulation, decreased blood pressure, and increased heart rate. In some patients, benzodiazepines have a paradoxical excitatory effect. Patients may become disinhibited and display bizarre behaviors. For patients with severe pain, the loss of self-control may decrease their ability to effectively cope with pain.

Several benzodiazepines are commonly used: diazepam (Valium), lorazepam (Ativan), and midazolam (Versed). Diazepam and lorazepam are both long-acting benzodiazepines that are lipid-soluble. They are very irritating to venous tissue and can cause severe thrombophlebitis. Elimination times may be prolonged in the child with compromised hepatic or renal function. Because of delayed elimination, regular dosing or a continuous infusion of a long-acting benzodiazepine may lead to accumulation of the agent and its metabolites. The duration of action of these benzodiazepines or their metabolites may cause prolonged sedation. For those children on mechanical ventilation, weaning ventilator support may be more difficult.

Midazolam, a more recently developed benzodiazepine, has a rapid onset and a short duration of action. Its elimination half-life is 2 to 4 hours after a single dose, although the half-life may be unpredictably longer in the critically ill patient. It is water-soluble and can be comfortably administered through peripheral veins. A low-dose infusion of midazolam provides for smooth sedation without the peaks and troughs seen with intermittent doses. In addition to an infusion, "rescue doses" or intermittent doses ordered for break-through agitation provide for appropriate titration of midazolam in response to a patient's changing needs for sedation.

Because midazolam is a relatively new drug, long-term effects are unknown. Some studies have found midazolam to be a safe and practical medication for sedation (Michalk et al., 1988; Silvasi et al., 1988). However, it has recently been reported that midazolam therapy may cause reversible neurologic abnormalities (Bergman et al., 1991) perhaps related to chemical withdrawal.

Benzodiazepine and Opioid Combination Therapy

Narcotics and benzodiazepines are often combined for analgesic and sedative effects. It is important to consider the motivation behind the use of each agent, alone and in combination. For agitation that is primarily related to pain, a narcotic should provide the crux of therapy. In contrast, if pain stimulus appears minimal yet the patient remains agitated, sedatives may be the appropriate approach.

When both agitation and pain are management issues, a combination of opioid and benzodiazepine therapy may be warranted. When combining these agents, there is an additive effect in both therapeutic effects and side effects or complications. When first initiating the sedation/analgesia regimen, it is important to carefully titrate each to minimize potential complications. Depending on whether agitation is primarily the result of pain or other distressing events, either a narcotic or benzodiazepene will be the first-line medication. This medication should be

Table 18–8. MONITORING AND MANAGEMENT OF PATIENTS RECEIVING SEDATION FOR PROCEDURES

Level of Sedation	Personnel	Monitoring	Equipment	Documentation
Conscious sedation	One BLS-trained individual responsible to observe the patients (PALS certification encouraged)	*Continuous pulse oximetry *Continuous HR monitoring Intermittent monitoring of BP & RR Maintain head position and airway patency	Suction apparatus Bag & mask capable of delivering >90% oxygen	Name, route, time of administration, and dosage of all medication Record VS and SaO₂ until alert
Deep sedation	One BLS-trained individual responsible to *constantly* observe the patient (PALS certification encouraged)	Continuous pulse oximetry Continuous electrocardiogram RR and BP monitored every 5 minutes Maintain head position and airway patency	Suction apparatus Bag & mask capable of delivering >90% oxygen Electrocardiogram Defibrillator Vascular access	Name, route, time of administration and dosage of all medications Record VS and SaO₂ every 5 minutes until responsive

*Optimal.
BLS, basic life support; BP, blood pressure; PALS, pediatric advanced life support; RR, respiratory rate; HR, heart rate; VS, vital signs.

titrated according to recommended guidelines (on a mg/kg basis). The second-line medication should be dosed as half the recommended guidelines. Doses may be adjusted up or down according to therapeutic effect.

Sedation and Analgesia for Distressing Procedures

In the PICU, children are likely to experience unpleasant, invasive, distressing, and painful procedures. In addition to providing emotional support and teaching to both children and their families, critical care nurses provide appropriate pharmacologic agents to make the procedure tolerable. Medications are frequently administered before procedures are performed (Curley et al, 1992). The goals of sedation in these situations are (1) to protect patients' safety; (2) to minimize physical discomfort; (3) to minimize potentially negative physiologic responses to pain and distress; (4) to control behavior; and (5) to maximize the potential for amnesia (American Academy of Pediatrics [AAP], 1992). It is especially important to provide adequate sedation to children who will undergo repeated procedures. Providing maximum treatment for pain and anxiety during the first procedure minimizes the development of anticipatory anxiety before subsequent procedures (Acute Pain Management Guidelines Panel, 1992)

Two levels of sedation have been defined (AAP, 1992). Conscious sedation is a controlled state of depressed consciousness during which the patient maintains protective reflexes and a patent airway independently and continuously. The patient responds appropriately to either physical stimulation or verbal command. Deep sedation, on the other hand, is a controlled state of depressed consciousness or unconsciousness from which the patient is not easily aroused. Loss of protective reflexes and the ability to maintain a patent airway independently and respond appropriately to physical stimulation or verbal command may accompany deep sedation. The

patient who is administered medication to achieve conscious sedation may have progressive effects into a state of deep sedation and obtundation.

The American Academy of Pediatrics has developed guidelines for the monitoring and management of children receiving sedation for diagnostic and therapeutic procedures. These recommendations are presented in Table 18–8. Critical care nurses play an important role in monitoring patients during and after procedures for which sedation is required.

NONPHARMACOLOGIC MANAGEMENT OF PAIN AND AGITATION

Providing comfort to patients experiencing pain or distress is completely within the domain of nursing practice. Still, nonpharmacologic comfort measures may be neglected as nurses focus on the technology and tasks necessary for the care of critically ill infants and children. For patients and families, comfort that nurses provide is extremely important.

Environmental Control

The PICU is a brightly lit and noisy place that often overwhelms the healthy adults who visit and work there. It is easy to imagine the impact on a small, sick child who is restrained from any purposeful response by equipment and adult caregivers. In addition, critically ill patients may have altered cerebral tissue perfusion or may be receiving medications that impair sensory processing and coping abilities. With this combination of pathophysiology and iatrogenic stress, it is not surprising that some patients become confused, agitated, or even combative.

Introducing predictability into the chaotic environment may help children cope with the many distressing experiences in the PICU. The unexpectedness of the treatments and procedures keep children in a constant state of tension and readiness. Because all interactions are potentially threatening, children may begin to generalize their distress toward all approaches by caregivers. They may become distressed and hypersensitive to seemingly benign, routine procedures of care.

Behavioral conditioning may actually occur when a seemingly non-noxious stimulus is paired with an unpleasant experience on a regular basis. Some common examples of this are the pairing of ventilator alarms with suctioning and handling of extremities before needle sticks for blood sampling or IV insertion. Some patients begin to expect that whenever they hear a ventilator alarm or feel someone touch their foot something unpleasant will happen. This can result in agitated behavior that seems to occur without any consistent pattern; the PICU environment itself is the trigger for such episodes. This is called a "conditioned aversive response" (Hyde & McCown, 1986). Sedation and careful structuring of the patient's experiences to "unlearn" these associations is necessary to treat this cause of distress. However, it is much easier to prevent this type of learning than to unlearn it after a problem develops.

General principles of individualized developmental care may be implemented by PICU nurses to prevent and manage agitation in their patients (Lawhon & Melzar, 1988). Individualized developmental care refers to a patient-specific plan of care that addresses environmental structure, positioning and handling techniques, and family involvement in caregiving. Some interventions to structure the environment include scheduling quiet times, reducing unit light levels at night and nap times, using caps on ventilator tubing to eliminate alarms sounding with suctioning or disconnections, answering monitor alarms promptly, and turning down the volume on constant noise sources such as pulse oximeters. In some instances, the use of specific sensory cues to help the child discriminate between "safe" times and "procedure" times may be necessary. For example, common procedures such as endotracheal suctioning may be anticipated for patients by alerting them with a verbal, auditory, or tactile prompt that they will soon be suctioned. At the end of suctioning, another prompt may be given that signals the end of care and the start of safe, protected time. A regular and predictable routine provides a structure for the child to interpret the cues of daily life in the PICU.

Physical Comfort Measures

Keeping children warm, applying a warm or cold pack, repositioning a painful body part, providing support with a blanket roll—the list of physical comfort measures is endless. The effects of good positioning cannot be underestimated. Normally, a person makes numerous, small, unconscious changes in body position to relieve pressure and discomfort. A critically ill child may be unable to make these movements independently. The seemingly small discom-

forts related to position can influence the child's response to care routines and painful procedures. The child should be positioned in neutral alignment, with all parts of the body supported and the joints slightly flexed. Frequent position changes are important and may be necessary more often than every 2 hours, depending on the medical status of the child. Positioning a patient so that self-calming behaviors (for example, sucking a thumb or fingers) are supported is a simple way to assist patients to cope with the stressors inherent in PICU care.

Physical treatments to reduce the painful stimulus may be effective. Application of heat or cold can affect the vascular and muscular systems as well as hormone production to provide pain relief. Transcutaneous electrical stimulation (TENS) stimulates tissue via external electrodes and produces a pleasant tingling or massaging sensation. The stimulus may increase blood flow near the electrodes, which indirectly helps the healing process or relaxes muscle spasm.

For infants and very young children, interventions are aimed at decreasing distress and the resulting behavioral disorganization that may overwhelm them. Swaddling infants to bring their extremities midline and rhythmic rocking introduce behavioral organization and calming. Some PICUs are able to use hammocks over cribs or mechanical swings to provide a constant, gentle swaying motion. Allowing the infant to suck on a pacifier takes advantage of natural self-calming behaviors.

Patient and Family Education

Patient and family teaching should include information about pain, pain assessment, and pain management. Children must be taught and given permission to tell caregivers that they are hurting. Pain assessment tools should be introduced to children and opportunities to practice encouraged as they become expert in communicating about the pain they are experiencing. Children and their families should be taught about their pain medications. Specifics include the drug name, route of administration, how it is expected to help, and what would be changed if it proves to be ineffective. Concerns about addiction should be raised and addressed directly. If patient-controlled analgesia is the treatment of choice, special efforts should be made to ensure that the child understands how to use it.

Cognitive-behavioral Techniques

Children have incredible inner resources that give them the ability to cope with distress—their imaginations, their ability to focus to the extent of being unaware of their surroundings, their ability to distract themselves through play, and their motivation to try new things. Nurses may tap into these resources and teach children systematic strategies to cope with painful events.

Distraction, visual imagery, and relaxation exercises all require children to focus or concentrate on an idea or activity so that they are less able to attend to the pain that they are experiencing. Talking, singing, listening to music, counting, reading stories aloud, playing a game, or playing with toys may give children a slight reprieve from their discomforts.

Children can be taught to use progressive muscle relaxation, guided imagery, breathing, and counting exercises. Although these methods do require instruction and practice, they can be effectively used to cope with pain. They should be introduced and practiced when the child is not agitated or distressed for optimal learning. Some children prefer to have a coach or a tape recording of their relaxation exercise, whereas others do better on their own.

Rhythmic breathing exercises or counting routines can be very successful because these activities demand a significant level of concentration. Depending on the child's ability to concentrate, a sophisticated distraction and relaxation routine can be developed that requires the child to concentrate on more and more information at one time. For example, an approach to a school-age child who is having difficulty tolerating chest physical therapy because of pain from a chest tube is to instruct the child to slowly count backward from 100 to zero while a story is told.

Depending on their illness state, some children may learn to be active participants in their care, allowing them to retain some self-control. Even young children may be assigned a small "job" such as holding the tape, pouring saline on the dressing, or pulling off the old dressing. Such tasks help to focus the child on the job at hand rather than on the accompanying distress. Choices should be offered to the child whenever possible. For example, "Should we start with the burn dressing or the central line dressing change?"

Play therapy and medical play are important for any child who is undergoing medical treatment. Through play, children gain more command and control over their hospital experience. Most patients in the PICU may not be able to actively participate in a program of medical play, but they can benefit from hearing stories or tapes about the hospital. As the child's status improves, more active play alternatives should be offered. Most children welcome a nurse's or doctor's "bag" filled with medical equipment such as syringes, IV boards, IV tubing, tourniquets, Band-Aids, and alcohol swabs. By allowing children to play with and manipulate these devices, they gain a sense of mastery over the objects and become less sensitized to the presence of these objects at their bedside. Medical play can be an important emotional outlet for children as they act out feelings that they may be unable to express otherwise. Ideally, the play is supervised, so that an experienced caregiver can help the child process feelings and explore strategies for coping with distress.

In the PICU environment, the effectiveness of parents as support for a child who is in pain, who is distressed and agitated, or who must undergo painful procedures should not be overlooked. Children view their parents as comforting figures. The familiar, soothing touch and voice of a parent are probably the most potent comfort measures available for sick children. Too often the concern in the PICU is that such activity may jeopardize a patient's unstable physiologic status. A study by Mitchell and coworkers (1985) found no change in intracranial pressure beyond the range of resting variability with a planned stroking and soothing regimen in patients with cerebral hypertension. The physiologic manifestations of pain and distress may themselves be more detrimental than the physiologic effects of parental calming and soothing. PICU nurses can advocate for and support the close presence of parents at the bedside as calming and comforting for all critically ill children.

Because children may react to their parents' fears, it is important to provide parents with adequate support so that they can be effective with their critically ill child. Parents who are especially fearful may respond well to a nurse's direction regarding specific activities that they are able to do for their child.

NURSING'S ROLE IN PAIN MANAGEMENT

Nurses have a tremendously important role in pain assessment and management. Their contributions both in direct care and institutional systems that promote pain assessment and management are significant. Direct care includes pain assessment, medication administration, reassessment, providing relaxation exercises, positioning, involving parents, teaching pain relief measures, and others; the list is potentially endless.

Nurses' participation is necessary in developing and establishing the institutional systems that promote quality care in the area of pain management. Nurses may actively decide which pain assessment tools will be used and ensure that they are readily available for staff and patients to use. For example, a selection of pain assessment tools may be compiled on a single sheet of paper, copied, and placed on every bedside clipboard. With some funding, pain assessment tools may be laminated and posted in each patient room.

Nurses can also influence patient documentation systems to include a specific section for pain assessments. By using a pain flow sheet, Stevens (1990) found that nurses had patients who were in less pain, were assessed more frequently, and received more narcotic analgesics.

In recent years, there has been extensive work in pain management guideline development with accompanying recommendations for quality improvement monitoring. In 1992, the Agency of Health Care Policy and Research published a *Quick Reference Guide for Clinicians*. This guideline provides principles and recommendations for pain assessment and management. Nurses may be actively involved with the implementation of these guidelines (Schmidt et al., 1994).

The AHCPR recommends that institutions develop quality improvement standards and monitoring to ensure continued efforts in pain assessment and treatment. The American Pain Society (APS) (1990) also proposes quality improvement methods to promote pain management practice. The American Pain Society published recommendations for patient outcomes and institutional actions to promote quality pain control (APS, 1990). A patient satisfaction survey is included that asks patients about their pain, pain score, and satisfaction with care related to pain. Nurses have used this survey to examine patients' perception of pain management (Miakowski et al., 1994). Ferrell (1991) developed a chart audit that may be used to examine nursing practice and documentation. A nursing unit or department may take a combined approach of chart audits and patient/family surveys to gather information about current practice and areas that need improvement.

SUMMARY

The needs of critically ill infants and children for accurate assessment and effective management of pain and distress are enormous. Still, healthcare providers are only beginning to understand pain and agitation and their assessment and management. Clinical and basic research are generating questions, answers, and further questions and answers about pain and distress at a very rapid pace. Nurses have been at the forefront of many clinical investigations that have led to improved assessment and treatment of pain and aversive stimulation in infants and children. The future will bring alterative strategies to help manage pain and agitation in the PICU. Critical care nurses are uniquely positioned to appreciate the complex nature of pain and distress and to promote holistic management of both.

References

Acute Pain Management Guidelines Panel (1992). *Acute pain management in infants, children, and adolescents: Operative and medical procedures. Quick reference guide for clinicians.* AHCPR Pub. No. 92-0020. Rockville, MD: Agency for Health Care Policy and Research, Public Health Service, U.S. Department of Health and Human Services.

American Academy of Pediatrics, Committee on Drugs (1992). Guidelines for monitoring and management of Pediatric patients during and after sedation for diagnostic and therapeutic procedures. *Pediatrics,* 89(6), 1110–1116.

American Pain Society Subcommittee on Quality Assurance Standards (1990). Standards for monitoring quality of analgesic treatment of acute pain and cancer pain. *Oncology Nursing Forum,* 17(6), 952–954.

Anand, K.J.S., & Carr, D.B. (1989). The neuroanatomy, neurophysiology, and neurochemistry of pain, stress, and analgesia in newborns and children. *Pediatric Clinics of North America,* 36(4), 795–821.

Anand, K.J.S., & Hickey, P.R. (1987). Pain and its effects in the human neonate and fetus. *New England Journal of Medicine,* 317, 1321–1329.

Anand K.J.S., & Shapiro B.S. (1993). Pharmacotherapy with systemic analgesics. IN K.J.S. Anand, & P.S. McGrath (Eds.). *Pain in neonates* (pp. 157–200). London: Elsevier Science Publishers.

Beaver, W.T. (1984). Combination analgesics. *American Journal of Medicine,* 38–53.

Bergman, I., et al. (1991). Reversible neurologic abnormalities associated with prolonged intravenous midazolam and fentanyl administration. *Journal of Pediatrics,* 119, 644–649.

Beyer, J.E., et al. (1983). Patterns of postoperative analgesic use with adults and children following cardiac surgery. *Pain,* 17, 71–81.

Caron, E., & Maguire, D.P. (1990). Current management of pain, sedation, and narcotic physical dependency of the infant on ECMO. *Journal of Perinatal and Neonatal Nursing,* 4(1), 63–74.

Curley, M.A.Q., McDermott, B., Berry, P., Hurley, J., Mackey, C., McAleer, D., Alsip, C. (1992). Nurses' decision making regarding the use of sedatives and analgesics in pediatric ICU. *Heart & Lung,* 21(3), 296.

Eland, J.M. (1981). Minimizing pain associated with prekindergarten intramuscular injections. *Issues in Comprehensive Pediatric Nursing,* 5, 361–372.

Eland, J.M. (1986). Pain in children. In Hockenberry, M., & Coody, D. (Eds.). *Pediatric hematology-oncology: Perspectives in care* (pp. 394–406). St Louis: C.V. Mosby.

Eland, J.M., & Anderson, J.E. (1977). The experience of pain in children. In A. Jacox, (Ed.). *Pain: A sourcebook for nurses and other health professionals* (pp. 453–473). Boston: Little, Brown.

Foley, K.M., & Rogers, A. (1981). *The management of cancer pain. The rational use of analgesics in the management of cancer pain* (Vol. 2). Nutley, NJ: Hoffmann-LaRoche, Inc.

Ferrell, B.R., Wisdom, C., Rainer, M., & Alleto, J. (1991). Pain management as a quality of care outcome. *Journal of Nursing Quality Assurance,* 5(2), 50–58.

Finnegan, L.P., Kron, R.E., Cannaughton, J.F., & Enrich, J.P. (1975). A scoring system for evaluation and treatment of neonatal abstinence syndrome: A new clinical and research tool. In: P.L. Morselli, S. Garattini, & F. Sereni (Eds.). *Basic and therapeutic aspects of perinatal pharmacology.* New York: Raven Press.

Franck, L.S. (1987). A national survey of the assessment and treatment of pain and agitation in the neonatal intensive care unit. JOGNN, 387–393.

Gaffney, A., & Dunne, E.A. (1987). Children's understanding of the causality of pain. *Pain,* 29, 91–104.

Hartley, S., Franck, L.S., Lundergan, F. (1989). Maintenance sedation of agitated infants in the neonatal intensive care unit with chloral hydrate: new concerns. *Journal of Perinatology,* 9(2), 162–164.

Hester, N.O. (1979). The preoperational child's reaction to immunization. *Nursing Research,* 29, 250–254.

Hyde, B.B., & McCown, D.E. (1986). Classical conditioning in neonatal intensive care nurseries. *Pediatric Nursing,* 12(1), 11–13.

International Association for the Study of Pain, Subcommittee on Taxonomy (1979). Pain terms: A list with definitions and notes on usage. *Pain,* 6, 249–252.

Jaffe, J.H., & Martin, W.R. (1985). Opioid analgesics and antagonists. In A.G. Gillman, et al. (Eds.). *The pharmacological basis of therapeutics* (ed 7, pp. 532–581). New York: Macmillan.

Johnson M.R., & Eland J.M. (1988). Pain. In J.M. Flynn, P.B. Heffron (Eds.). *Nursing: From Concept to Practice* (2nd ed., pp. 519–542). Norwalk, CT: Appleton & Lange.

Johnston, C.C., & Strada, M.E. (1986). Acute pain response in infants: A multidimensional description. *Pain,* 24, 373–382.

Kaiko, R.F., et al. (1983). Central nervous system excitatory effects of meperidine in cancer patients. *Annals of Neurology,* 13(2), 180–184.

Kim, S. (1980). Pain: Theory, research and nursing practice. *Advances in Nursing Science,* 2(2), 43–59.

Koren, G., et al. (1985). Postoperative morphine infusion in newborn infants: Assessment of disposition characteristics and safety. *The Journal of Pediatrics,* 107(6), 963–967.

Lawhon, G., & Melzar, A. (1988). Developmental care of the very low birth weight infant. *Journal Perinatal and Neonatal Nursing,* 2(1), 56–65.

Lynn, A.M., & Slattery, J.T. (1987). Morphine pharmacokinetics in early infancy. *Anesthesiology, 66,* 136–139.

McCaffery, M. (1972). *Nursing management of the patient with pain.* Philadelphia: J.B. Lippincott.

McCaffery, M., & Beebe, A. (1989). *Pain: clinical manual for nursing practice.* Philadelphia: C.V. Mosby.

McGrath, P., et al. (1985). CHEOPS: A behavioral scale for rating postoperative pain in children. In H.L. Felds, et al. (Eds.). *Advances in pain research and therapy* (pp. 395–402). New York: Raven Press.

McGraw, M.B. (1941). Neural maturation as exemplified in the changing reactions of the infant to a pin prick. *Child Development, 12,* 31–42.

Marks, R.D., & Sachar, E.J. (1973). Undertreatment of medical inpatients with narcotic analgesics. *Annals of Internal Medicine, 78,* 173–181.

Melzack, R., & Casey, K.L. (1968). Sensory, motivational and central control determinants of pain: A new conceptual model. In D. Kenshalo (Ed.). *The Skin Senses.* Springfield, Il: Charles C. Thomas.

Melzack, R., & Wall, P. (1965). Pain mechanisms: A new theory. *Science, 150,* 971–979.

Meretoja, O.A., Korpela, R., & Dunkel, P. (1991). Critical evaluation of PCA in children (abstract). *Journal of Pain and Symptom Management, 6*(3), 191–215.

Miaskowski C., Nicols R., Brody R., & Synold T. (1994). Assessment of patient satisfaction utilizing the American Pain Society's Quality Assurance Standards on Acute and Cancer-Related Pain. *Journal of Pain and Symptom Control, 9*(1), 5–11.

Michalk, S., et al. (1988). Midazolam infusion for basal sedation in intensive care: absence of accumulation. *Intensive Care Medicine, 15,* 37–41.

Mitchell, P.H., et al. (1985). Critically ill children: The importance of touch in a high-technology environment. *Nursing Administration Quarterly, 9*(4), 38–46.

Molsberry, D. (1979). Young children's subjective quantifications of pain following surgery. Unpublished master's thesis, University of Iowa.

O'Hara, D.A., et al. (1987). Ketorolac tromethamine as compared with morphine sulfate for treatment of postoperative pain. *Clinical Pharmacology and Therapeutics, 41*(5), 556–561.

Porter, J., & Jick, H. (1980). Addiction rare in patients treated with narcotics. *New England Journal of Medicine, 302,* 123.

Pridham, K.F., Adelson, F., & Hansen, M.F. (1987). Helping children deal with procedures in a clinic setting: A developmental approach. *Journal of Pediatric Nursing, 2*(1), 13–22.

Purcell-Jones, G., Dormon, F., & Sumner, E. (1987). The use of opioids in neonates. A retrospective study of 933 cases. *Anaesthesia, 42,* 1316–1320.

Reimche, L.D., et al. (1989). Chloral hydrate sedation in neonates and infants—clinical and pharmacologic considerations. *Developmental Pharmacology and Therapeutics, 12,* 57–64.

Schecter, N.L. (1989). The undertreatment of pain in children: An overview. *Pediatric Clinics of North America, 36*(4), 781–794.

Schecter, N.L., Allen, D.A., & Handson, K. (1986). The status of pediatric pain control: A comparison of hospital analgesic usage in children and adults. *Pediatrics, 77,* 11–15.

Schmidt K., Holida D., Kleiber C., Petersen M., & Phearman L. (1994). Implementation of the AHCPR pain guidelines for children. *Journal of Nursing Care Quality, 8*(3), 68–74.

Shearer, M.H. (1986). Surgery in the paralyzed unanesthetized newborn. *Birth, 13,* 79.

Silvasi, D.L., et al. (1988). Continuous intravenous midazolam infusion for sedation in the pediatric intensive care unit. *Anesthesia Analgesia, 67,* 286–288.

Stevens B. (1990). Development and testing of a pediatric pain management sheet. *Pediatric Nursing, 16*(6), 543–548.

Twycross, R.G. (1974). Clinical experience with diamorphine in advanced malignant disease. *International Journal or Clinical Pharmacology, 9,* 184–198.

Webb, C.J., Paarlberg, J.M., & Sussman, M. (1991). The use of a PCA device by parents or nurses for postoperative pain in children with cerebral palsy (abstract). *Journal of Pain and Symptom Management, 6*(3), 160.

Final Common Pathways

This section presents state-of-the-art nursing care for patient problems within each body system. A focus on the final common pathways of many disease states is presented so that system dysfunction is viewed broadly and addressed within a nursing framework. The etiology, incidence, and pathogenesis of specific disorders that lead to development of a final common pathway are also presented when appropriate. Critical care management, including both independent and collaborative nursing care measures, is focused broadly on the final common pathways of system dysfunction and specifically on patient care unique to a particular disorder.

CHAPTER *19*

Cardiovascular Critical Care Problems

JANIS BLOEDEL SMITH
ANNETTE L. BAKER
PAULA J. MOYNIHAN
PATRICIA LINCOLN
PATRICIA LAWRENCE KANE

Cardiovascular dysfunction necessitates admission to a critical care setting across the lifespan. The percentage of PICU patients with cardiovascular dysfunction was 13% to 38% in one multicenter study (Pollack et al., 1987) and 24% in the American Association of Critical Care Nurses role delineation study of 1989 to 1990. Cardiovascular dysfunction may be the consequence of hypovolemia, myocardial dysfunction, cardiac rhythm disturbances, increased afterload, or pericardial tamponade. It is important to note that myocardial dysfunction may be either the result of a primary cardiac problem or the final pathophysiologic consequence of a variety of other problems, most often maldistributive shock. Cardiovascular dysfunction results in a low-flow shock state and inadequate tissue perfusion.

ASSESSMENT OF PATIENTS WITH CARDIOVASCULAR DYSFUNCTION

The clinical picture of the patient with inadequate tissue perfusion can be clearly described, because low cardiac output results in characteristic attempts at physiologic compensation that are readily apparent on physical examination.

The first sign of physiologic distress in infants and children is tachycardia. Tachycardia occurs with fever, anemia, hypovolemia, dyspnea, activity, and excitement or anxiety. In fact, it is an ominous sign of cardiac dysfunction if heart rate does not increase in the face of physiologic distress. Evaluation of the significance of a rapid heart rate is aided if the tachycardia persists in sleep, because sleep rules out nonphysiologic sources of distress. In addition, it is useful to quantify the degree of elevation in heart rate (i.e., heart rate increased by ten beats per minute or 10% above baseline), and important to follow trends in the increase in heart rate across time.

Tachycardia related to physiologic distress is the result of sympathetic nervous system (SNS) stimulation. SNS stimulation also results in increased minute ventilation. Typically, the respiratory rate, and sometimes the depth of respiration, are increased.

SNS stimulation also results in peripheral vasoconstriction. As a consequence, arterial blood pressure is maintained even in situations when cardiac output is low. Vasoconstriction elevates the diastolic blood pressure and narrows the pulse pressure, maintaining mean and systolic pressure at normal levels. Peripheral vasoconstriction is evidenced by weak peripheral pulses, cool extremities, pallor or mottling, and prolonged capillary refill. These are classic early signs of low cardiac output and decreased tissue perfusion, even in the presence of "normal" blood pressure.

If increased heart rate and peripheral vasoconstriction are not sufficient to manage decreased cardiac output, continued SNS stimulation results in regional redistribution of blood flow to ensure perfusion of vital organs. Blood is shunted away from the skin, gastrointestinal tract, kidneys, and liver to maintain circulation to the heart, lungs, and brain. Decreased perfusion of the skin and subcutaneous tissue is evident in mottling and cooling of the extremities (Fig. 19–1). Inadequate perfusion of the gastrointestinal tract is often apparent first when infants or children develop feeding intolerance but may progress to the development of paralytic ileus and gastrointestinal necrosis. Decreased urine output is the consequence of inadequate renal blood flow, because the glomerular filtration rate is decreased. Acute tubular necrosis

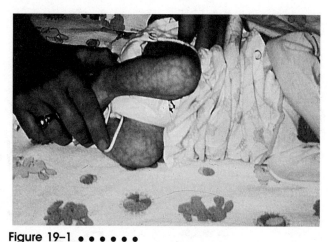

Figure 19–1 ● ● ● ● ●

Marked mottling of the skin in an infant with regional redistribution of blood flow due to congestive heart failure.

(ATN) is the eventual outcome. Impaired hepatic function is evidenced by abnormalities in coagulation, the development of jaundice, and other alterations in liver function.

Determination of electrolyte, acid-base, and substrate abnormalities is important in the care of pediatric patients with impaired tissue perfusion because of their effect on cardiac performance. These abnormalities occur as the consequence of decreased tissue perfusion and can compound cardiac dysfunction. Serum electrolytes, calcium, glucose, urea nitrogen, and creatinine are measured to establish their baseline values in patients with low cardiac output, with measurements repeated at intervals determined by the individual patient's physiologic status.

Arterial blood gases, pH, and base excess or deficit provide specific information about the adequacy of tissue perfusion and oxygenation. Metabolic acidosis develops when tissues are inadequately perfused and use anaerobic routes for metabolism. Lactic and other organic acids accumulate and require buffering by the buffer bases, resulting in utilization of the base and a base deficit. Metabolic acidosis causes decreased myocardial contractility and decreased adrenergic receptor sensitivity and predisposes to myocardial irritability and lethal cardiac rhythm disturbances.

FINAL COMMON PATHWAYS

Regardless of the cause of inadequate tissue perfusion, if cardiovascular performance cannot be restored, the outcome is similar in all. The heart, lungs, and central nervous system are inadequately perfused. The consequences are impaired cardiac performance, cardiac dysrhythmias and arrest; pulmonary edema and adult respiratory distress syndrome; and irreversible central nervous system ischemia. The clear goal is to intervene successfully before these devastating consequences occur.

PROVIDING BASELINE SUPPORT

Care of patients with inadequate tissue perfusion as a consequence of cardiovascular dysfunction is predicated on minimizing metabolic demands. Conserving energy and avoiding stress lowers oxygen demand and reduces the work of the heart. Promoting rest is of primary importance. Close monitoring of physiologic status and needed care are planned to allow periods of undisturbed rest between care and treatment. If the child is unable to rest because of irritability or extreme restlessness, a physiologic source for distress is assessed and corrected, and sedation is provided, if necessary.

The work of breathing is minimized to conserve energy and decrease metabolic demands. Cardiovascular dysfunction is characterized by pulmonary venous congestion, decreasing lung compliance, and increasing respiratory work. Increased work of breathing is often accentuated when the child is lying in a flat, supine position. In this position, fluid in the lungs is evenly distributed and is reabsorbed in greater quantities, increasing pulmonary blood volume. The best position for these children is semi-Fowler's, which promotes the pooling of both lung fluid and pulmonary blood in the dependent portions of the lungs. This maneuver limits reabsorption of pulmonary fluid, decreases pulmonary venous blood volume, and lowers pulmonary vascular resistance. Pulmonary congestion is also limited to the bases of the lung, easing respiration. The liver, often enlarged with myocardial failure, is displaced downward, which prevents it from impinging on diaphragmatic movement and permits greater thoracic expansion.

Administration of humidified oxygen may be necessary if tissue hypoxia and acidosis are noted. Mechanical ventilation can improve cardiovascular function by decreasing blood flow to the intercostal muscles and diaphragm. The respiratory muscles of the dyspneic patient consume relatively high amounts of oxygen. Oxygen delivery to other tissues, especially to the brain, liver, and the heart itself, can be increased by decreasing the metabolic demand of working to breathe (Klem, 1993).

Cardiovascular dysfunction results in exhaustion and dyspnea, which are often accentuated during feeding. Acute dysfunction, marked by tissue hypoxia and acidosis, necessitates fluid and electrolyte administration by the intravenous route. Myocardial failure often requires restriction of fluid intake. The child's needs for adequate fluid and caloric intake are carefully assessed and provided by the route that is determined to also allow for rest and conservation of energy. High-calorie formulas are often recommended for infants able to be fed, and nutritional quality rather than quantity is the emphasis for patients of all ages. Enteral intake is best offered in small amounts at fairly frequent intervals. Ensuring that blood glucose and electrolytes are in the normal range maximizes myocardial performance.

Maintenance of normal body temperature conserves energy because both hypothermia and fever result in thermal stress. Wide variations in body temperature produce alterations in cardiac output and oxygen consumption. Hyperthermia increases heart rate, while severe hypothermia can result in precipitous drops in cardiac output and blood pressure.

HEART FAILURE

Heart failure, regardless of the age of the patient, is a clinical syndrome in which the heart is unable to provide cardiac output (CO) sufficient to meet the metabolic requirements of the body, including those related to growth and development. Heart failure is encountered frequently during infancy, but is an infrequent initial occurrence in children after the age of 1 year.

Etiology

Congenital heart defects (CHDs) are usually the cause of heart failure in infancy and childhood, although the frequency is difficult to assess. In infants with heart defects, more than 80% have heart failure as a major component of their clinical presentation (Fyler et al., 1980). After infancy, the frequency of heart failure decreases sharply.

Primary myocardial disease, most often myocarditis, can cause heart failure at any age. In addition, heart failure may develop following open-heart surgical repair of a congenital heart defect. Heart failure can also be a consequence of severe cardiac dysrhythmias, rheumatic heart disease, endocarditis, and cardiomyopathy.

Heart failure may develop as a consequence of changes in pH and arterial blood gas tension that accompany asphyxia from any cause, from neonatal asphyxia through end-stage pulmonary disease from chronic disorders such as cystic fibrosis. Low PaO_2 and pH and elevated $PaCO_2$ affect the myocardium and both the systemic and pulmonary vasculature. Other infrequently encountered causes of myocardial failure include severe anemia, glycogen storage disease, vasculitis, carnitine deficiency, muscular dystrophy, cardiac tumors, and various other metabolic diseases. In addition, heart failure can be iatrogenically induced by excessively rapid infusion of fluid.

The causes of heart failure in infancy and childhood can be classified on the basis of the fundamental disturbance in myocardial performance (Talner, 1989; Table 19–1). The timing of the development of heart failure symptoms provides a valuable clue to likely diagnoses (Artman & Graham, 1982). After birth, hemodynamic changes related to the expected decrease in pulmonary vascular resistance (PVR) and closure of the ductus arteriosus are primarily responsible for the development of heart failure signs and symptoms in patients with CHD. As a consequence, heart failure most often develops in the first 6 weeks of life. Table 19–2 presents these data.

Table 19–1. CAUSES OF HEART FAILURE

> **ALTERATIONS IN WORK LOAD**
> **Volume overloading of the ventricles**
> Large left-to-right shunt
> Ventricular septal defect
> Atrioventricular septal defect
> Patent ductus arteriosus
> Valvular insufficiency
> Aortic, mitral, pulmonary
> Systemic arteriovenous fistulae
> **Pressure overloading of the ventricles**
> Obstruction to outflow
> Aortic stenosis
> Pulmonary stenosis
> Coarctation of the aorta
> Obstruction to inflow
> Mitral stenosis
> Cortriatriatum
> Tricuspid stenosis
>
> **ALTERATIONS IN INOTROPIC FUNCTION**
> Inflammatory disease
> Electrolyte disturbances
> Metabolic disease
> Coronary artery lesions
>
> **ALTERATIONS IN CHRONOTROPIC FUNCTION**
> Tachydysrhythmias
> Profound bradycardia
> Complete heart block

Pathogenesis

Determinants of Cardiac Performance

The factors that control cardiac output regardless of age are preload or diastolic volume; afterload or the ventricular wall tension developed during ventricular ejection; contractility or the inotropic state of the myocardium; and heart rate. From a developmental perspective, heart function in the newborn and very young infant is at nearly maximal levels under baseline conditions.

The newborn heart exhibits a greater resting tension for any degree of stretch, indicating decreased ventricular compliance. End-diastolic volume is high as compared with that in the adult, limiting diastolic reserve and decreasing adaptation to an increased volume load, such as a large left-to-right shunt. When stimulated to contract, the newborn heart develops less tension than the adult heart. Therefore, the response to an acute increase in afterload, such as that which might occur with coarctation of the aorta, is also impaired. The developing heart is thought to have a relative decrease in contractile mass, with a predominance of noncontractile elements.

Hemodynamic Characteristics

Heart failure in pediatric patients is characterized by two fundamental hemodynamic states. In patients with volume loading conditions, particularly large left-to-right shunts, heart failure occurs despite high CO. The pulmonary circulation receives tremendous volume at the expense of systemic blood flow. Myocar-

Table 19–2. LIKELY CAUSES OF HEART FAILURE RELATED TO THE TIMING OF ITS DEVELOPMENT

CHF at Birth or Shortly After

Heart muscle dysfunction	Structural abnormalities
Asphyxia	Tricuspid regurgitation
Sepsis	Pulmonary regurgitation
Hypoglycemia	TAPVR with obstruction
Hypocalcemia	
Myocarditis	Heart rate abnormalities
Transient myocardial	SVT
ischemia	Congenital CHB
Hematologic abnormalities	
Anemia	
Hyperviscosity syndrome (hematocrit >65%)	

CHF in the First Week of Life

Heart muscle, heart rate abnormalities
Same as above, except asphyxia less likely as a cause

Structural abnormalities	Pulmonary abnormalities
PDA	Upper airway obstruction
HLHS	BPD
AS	CNS hypoventilation
TAPVR	PPHN
Coarctation of the aorta	
Renal disorders	Endocrine disorders
Renal failure	Neonatal hyperthyroidism
Systemic hypertension	Adrenal insufficiency

CHF in Early Infancy (1–6 weeks)

Heart muscle abnormalities	Structural abnormalities
Endocardial fibroelastosis	Coarctation
Anomalous origin LCA	Ventricular shunt (VSD,
Myocarditis	AVSD, SV)
Coronary calcinosis	Aortic shunt (PDA, truncus,
	AP window)
Renal disorders	Endocrine disorders
Same as above	Hypothyroidism
	Adrenal insufficiency

CHF After Infancy

Acquired heart disease	Congenital heart disease
Cardiomyopathy	Preoperative patients
Myocarditis	Eisenmenger's syndrome
Vasculitis (Kawasaki disease)	PS (rare)
	Ebstein's anomaly with
Other	increasing TR
End-stage pulmonary disease	Aortic regurgitation
Cystic fibrosis	Mitral regurgitation
Primary PAH	With onset of tachycardia
Muscular dystrophy	
	Postoperative patients
	Ventriculotomy
	Large residual left-to-
	right shunt
	Valvular regurgitation,
	especially MR, AR
	Obstructed conduit or
	mechanical valve
	Prosthetic valve
	malfunction
	CA injury
	Ventricular dysfunction

AP, aortopulmonary; AR, aortic regurgitation; AS, aortic stenosis; AVSD, atrioventricular septal defect; BPD, bronchopulmonary dysplasia; CA, coronary artery; CHB, complete heart block; CHF, congestive heart failure; CNS, central nervous system; HLHS, hypoplastic left heart syndrome; LCA, left coronary artery; MR, mitral regurgitation; PAH, pulmonary artery hypertension; PDA, patent ductus arteriosus; PPHN, persistent pulmonary artery hypertension of the newborn; PS, pulmonary stenosis; SV, single ventricle; SVT, supraventricular tachycardia; TAPVR, total anomalous pulmonary venous return; TR, tricuspid regurgitation; VSD, ventricular septal defect

dial systolic function is usually preserved in high-output failure, demonstrated by normal to increased ejection fraction and increased fiber shortening rate. Ventricular filling pressure and chamber volume are increased, indicating impaired diastolic function. Although systemic perfusion is limited with a large left-to-right shunt, pulmonary overcirculation is the major problem.

In contrast, patients with low-output heart failure primarily show impaired systolic function. Systemic perfusion is markedly decreased. The left heart obstructive defects, myocarditis, cardiomyopathies, and tachydysrhythmias produce low-output states. Im-

paired systolic function modifies the heart's diastolic properties as well, because high end-systolic volume limits ventricular filling during diastole. Ventricular filling pressures are elevated and pulmonary congestion develops, but the major problem is low systemic perfusion and compromise of vital organ function. Figure 19–2 compares high-output with low-output heart failure.

Adaptive Mechanisms

Heart failure in infants and children is modulated by adaptive mechanisms that serve to maintain per-

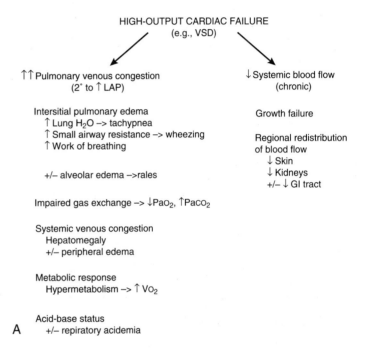

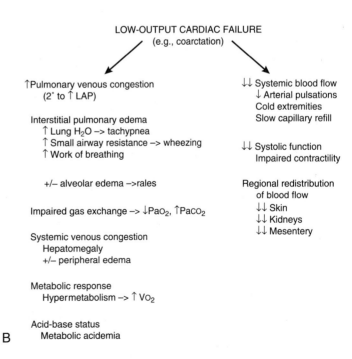

Figure 19–2 ● ● ● ● ● ●

Diagrammatic representations of high-output (*A*) and low-output (*B*) cardiac failure. VSD, ventricular septal defect; LAP, left atrial pressure.

fusion to vital organs. It is important to note that these adaptations are both beneficial and detrimental. Initial improvement is characteristic, but when heart failure is sustained, the deleterious effects of the adaptive process become evident.

Ventricular Dilatation and Hypertrophy. Ventricular dilatation is a basic response of the heart itself to the increased stress imposed by volume or pressure overload, which uses the Frank-Starling mechanism to maintain cardiac output. An increase in ventricular end-diastolic volume, even in the face of diminished fiber shortening, permits ejection of a larger stroke volume. However, chamber dilatation requires an increase in wall tension to maintain systolic pressure, increasing myocardial oxygen requirements.

Hypertrophy of the overloaded ventricle is a complex process, which, initially, is clearly compensatory. Adding new sarcomeres aids the heart in adapting to acute overload. However, chronic hypertrophy is accompanied by abnormalities at the cellular and molecular level, which, although not yet completely understood, lead to progressive myocardial damage, degeneration, fibrosis, and cell death (Katz, 1990). Chronic hypertrophy prolongs the action potential, leading to electrophysiologic abnormalities and cardiac rhythm disturbances. Hypertrophy also impairs relaxation of the heart (lusitropy), leading to diastolic dysfunction. In infants and children, removal of the abnormal workload (repair of a ventricular septal defect [VSD], relief of the coarctation) permits hypertrophy to regress.

Dilation and hypertrophy are relatively early manifestations of compromised cardiac performance. However, once evident, they signal diminished capacity to handle either further increases in mechanical load or decreases in myocardial performance.

Neurohormonal Response. A decrease in cardiac output triggers a neurohormonal response that is vital to survival in acute low-output states, such as hemorrhage. However, when sustained, the adjustments both in the peripheral circulation and in the heart that result from stimulation of the renin-angiotensin-aldosterone system (RAAS) and the sympathetic nervous system (SNS) may contribute to myocardial cell death (Katz, 1990).

RAAS stimulation causes salt and water retention, which initially augments preload. Chronic sodium and water retention results in the long-term effects of pulmonary congestion and anasarca. Vasoconstriction is the consequence of both RAAS and SNS stimulation. In the short term it serves to maintain blood pressure for perfusion of vital organs. Long-term effects are those of increased afterload: exacerbation of systolic dysfunction and increased energy requirements. In addition, SNS stimulation initially improves CO by increasing heart rate and ejection fraction. Similarly, the long-term effect is to increase energy expenditure, which hastens myocardial cell death. The increase in inotropy that results from SNS stimulation also decreases lusitropy. Figure 19–3 depicts the neurohormonal response to low CO and the consequences, which are long-term effects.

Clinical Manifestations

The signs of heart failure in infants and children are often subtle. It is useful to organize them into three general categories: signs related to impaired myocardial performance and those resulting from pulmonary and systemic venous congestion.

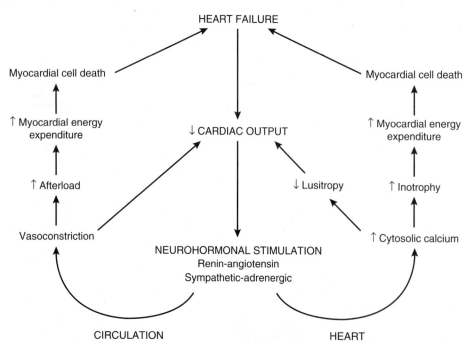

Figure 19–3 ● ● ● ● ● ●

Diagrammatic representation of the consequences of the neurohormonal response in heart failure. (Adapted from Katz, A.M. (1990). Cardiomyopathy of overload. *New England Journal of Medicine*, 322:100–110. © 1990, Massachusetts Medical Society. All rights reserved.)

Impaired Myocardial Performance

Inadequate myocardial performance results in decreased tissue perfusion. The clinical manifestations of inadequate tissue perfusion are primarily the consequence of activation of neurohormonal response to low cardiac output. In addition, cardiac failure presents additional specific symptoms related directly to poor myocardial function.

Cardiac enlargement on chest radiograph is a consistent sign of impaired function, representing ventricular dilatation and/or hypertrophy. Only in the earliest stages of heart failure is cardiac size normal. Tachycardia is commonly seen with cardiac failure and represents an adaptive mechanism to provide oxygen delivery to tissues in the face of poor systemic perfusion. An S_3 gallop rhythm is often appreciated because of rapid filling of a stiff, noncompliant ventricle. Vasoconstriction decreases peripheral perfusion, signaled by cool extremities, weak peripheral pulses, slow capillary refill, and mottling. However, with high-output heart failure, pulse pressure may be increased and the arterial pulsations bounding. Severe anemia (hemoglobin lower than 5 g/dL) causes a similar phenomenon. Vasoconstriction most often maintains blood pressure in the normal range, even when tissue perfusion is inadequate.

The increased metabolic demands of high-output heart failure, in the face of limited systemic perfusion, result in growth failure in infants. Pulmonary congestion also limits the ability of infants with heart failure to feed vigorously. Infants with cardiac failure are also noted to have increased sweating. This probably represents increased SNS activity.

Pulmonary Congestion

Signs of pulmonary congestion occur with left ventricular failure or pulmonary venous obstruction and are most often present before signs of systemic venous congestion are detected. Tachypnea that progresses to dyspnea represents the principal clinical manifestation of early interstitial pulmonary edema advancing to alveolar and bronchiolar edema. Intercostal retractions, grunting, wheezing, rales, and cough may be present as pulmonary congestion advances.

Systemic Venous Congestion

Hepatomegaly is the most consistent sign of systemic venous congestion. Enlargement of the liver reflects an increase in systemic venous volume and venous tone. Tenderness of the liver and the absence of a firm, discrete liver edge can be elicited even in older children with heart failure. Jaundice may occur with hepatic congestion.

Systemic venous congestion may be further evidenced in older children with heart failure by distention of the neck veins; however, this is a difficult sign to assess in infants. Peripheral edema is a rare finding in infants or children with cardiac failure.

Facial edema is sometimes detected, but ascites and generalized anasarca are rare, except in older children with severely compromised myocardial function or following the Fontan operation.

Diagnosis

In addition to history and physical examination findings, the diagnosis of heart failure is aided by a number of noninvasive and invasive laboratory studies. Chest radiography is necessary to assess cardiac size; it also permits assessment of pulmonary congestion. The ECG is not particularly useful, unless a dysrhythmia has precipitated the cardiac failure. Nonspecific T wave and ST segment changes are often detected. Echocardiography permits assessment of myocardial function from ventricular dimensions, fiber shortening rate, and ejection fraction. Diastolic function is evaluated from estimates of isovolumetric relaxation time, diastolic dimensions, filling time, and other parameters.

Critical Care Management

Treatment of cardiac failure necessitates careful diagnosis of the anatomic and physiologic cause, as well as attention to conditions that aggravate the problem, such as fever, anemia, agitation, and dysrhythmia. Emergent surgical intervention is necessary in a few cases, although the use of prostaglandin E_1 to maintain ductal patency permits stabilization and a more elective approach to surgery for most. Pharmacologic interventions are aimed at improving the inotropic state of the heart, decreasing the loading conditions on the heart and enhancing lusitropic function (afterload reduction), or lessening pulmonary and systemic venous congestion (diuretics). Agents to improve contractility or decrease afterload are discussed in Chapter 9. Diuretic therapy is reviewed briefly here.

Diuretic Therapy

Diuretic therapy in patients with heart failure is aimed at correcting the clinical problems of pulmonary and systemic venous congestion resulting from excessive reabsorption of sodium and water. Diuretic agents are useful to maximize sodium excretion and thereby increase the volume of urine excreted. Table 19–3 lists the various types of diuretic agents useful as adjuncts in treating patients with heart failure.

Complications of Diuretic Therapy

Because all diuretic agents increase sodium excretion, hypovolemia and hyponatremia are potential complications of their use. Acid-base imbalances can occur. Metabolic alkalosis is common with administration of the potent loop diuretics, owing to chloride depletion and volume contraction, which stimulate aldosterone production, generating the alkalosis.

Table 19–3. DIURETIC AGENTS FOR HEART FAILURE

Drug	Action
Loop Diuretics	
Furosemide	Block Na and Cl reabsorption widely at
Bumetanide	multiple medullary and cortical sites
Ethacrynic acid	Cautions: Volume contraction (free water reabsorption is blocked); hypokalemia
Cortical-diluting Segment Agents	
Thiazide diuretics	Block Na and Cl reabsorption at the
Metolazone	ascending limb; less loss of K
	Caution: volume contraction (especially with metolazone)
Potassium-sparing Agents	
Spironolactone	Aldosterone antagonist; impairs Na reabsorption and increases K and H ion secretion
	No effect on water production or reabsorption
Carbonic Anhydrase Inhibitors	
Acetazolamide	Inhibits carbonic anhydrase to decrease Na and Cl reabsorption at distal sites
	Less effect on free water production and reabsorption, but K excretion is increased
	Diuretic effects are mild only

Cl, chloride ions; H, hydrogen ions; K, potassium ions; Na, sodium ions

Metabolic acidosis is a potential complication of carbonic anhydrase inhibitors, but this usually is mild. Hypokalemia is the consequence of potassium wasting. Cardiac toxicity is possible with serum potassium less than 2 to 2.5 mEq/L. Hypokalemia can be avoided by every-other-day diuresis, administration of potassium supplements, or use of a potassium-sparing diuretic.

CYANOSIS AND HYPOXEMIA

Cyanosis and hypoxemia are commonly encountered clinical problems in pediatric patients. Cyanotic infants often present a confusing diagnostic picture. The first task is differentiating cardiac disease from pulmonary disease in these infants, followed by preparation for definitive management of those with CHD. Echocardiography is most often diagnostic, but several other clinical symptoms suggest the presence of cyanotic CHD.

Etiology and Clinical Presentation in Cyanotic Infants

CHD that produces cyanosis can be accompanied by decreased pulmonary blood flow (PBF), increased PBF, or variable PBF. Defects that result in decreased PBF are characterized by obstruction of the right heart chambers or vessels. These defects are manifested by cyanosis that is often severe following closure of the ductus arteriosus, is intensified by crying, and may be episodic. It is not relieved by the administration of oxygen, even at high concentrations. Conversely, infants with pulmonary problems

most often have amelioration of symptoms by administration of oxygen. Tachypnea not accompanied by dyspnea, retractions, grunting, or nasal flaring (which are also characteristic of pulmonary disease or edema) is indicative of a cyanotic CHD with decreased PBF.

Cardiac defects with increased PBF often result in milder cyanosis than is the case with defects that decrease PBF. However, there are two important exceptions. The first is transposition of the great arteries, and the second is total anomalous pulmonary venous return with obstructed pulmonary venous drainage. Cyanosis is severe in infants with these defects. In infants with other defects, mild to moderate cyanosis may escape detection in the neonate. Rubor or ruddiness is descriptive of the skin color associated with mild arterial oxygen desaturation. Infants with increased PBF develop signs of congestive heart failure, although signs are usually not as severe as those seen with a large left-to-right shunt. Low-output heart failure has been compared with high-output failure. The characteristic finding in low-output failure is inadequate systemic tissue perfusion.

A number of other clinical clues help to differentiate cardiac and pulmonary disease. Chest radiographs, although not always conclusive, are often helpful in detecting pulmonary disease in infants. Arterial blood gas analysis may reveal helpful differential findings. In lung disease, the $PaCO_2$ may be elevated, whereas it is normal or even decreased because of tachypnea in patients with cardiac disease. Acid-base balance is initially maintained, but inadequate tissue perfusion, which may be the consequence of ductal closure, results in lactic acidosis.

Pathogenesis

Young infants with tetralogy of Fallot are at risk for the development of sudden, severe hypoxic spells. Other cyanotic heart defects do not put infants and children at risk for acute events, but patients with heart defects may experience acute hypoxia for other reasons. Both acute hypoxia and chronic cyanosis and hypoxemia affect infants and children with heart defects uniquely.

Acute Hypoxia

Acute hypoxic episodes have the potential to occur in critically ill infants and children for various reasons, most of them pulmonary in nature. Acute hypoxia produces pulmonary hypertension, which is usually mild and rapidly reversible in healthy individuals who most often hyperventilate, becoming mildly alkalotic. In patients with heart failure and preexisting pulmonary artery hypertension, and in postoperative cardiac surgery patients, acute hypoxic episodes are potentially far more serious. In these patients, hypoxia can result in acute pulmonary vasospasm or pulmonary hypertensive crisis. This serious problem is characterized by an acute rise in pulmonary artery pressure followed by a reduction in CO and a dramatic fall in oxygen saturation. Once the crisis begins, it can be extremely difficult to interrupt the vicious cycle of right ventricular dysfunction, inadequate PBF, severe hypoxemia, and low CO. These crises may be fatal despite aggressive attempts to reverse the situation. Interventions that may be attempted include administration of fentanyl or morphine, skeletal muscle paralysis, and hyperventilation with 100% oxygen.

Chronic Hypoxia

Chronic cyanosis and hypoxemia have deleterious effects on many body systems and have been recognized for decades. These effects include changes in the following tissues and organs:

1. *Central nervous system:* Chronic hypoxia causes cerebral underperfusion and a diffuse, inflammation-like reaction. Acute cerebral insults may result, with episodes of syncope, seizures, and the possibility of death. Chronic complications include cerebral thrombosis and infarction. In addition to the risk of stroke, there is increased incidence of meningitis among young children with cyanotic CHD and brain abscess among those who are older. These can occur because venous bacteria are shunted into the systemic circulation without undergoing the normal filtering process afforded by the pulmonary macrophages.
2. *Blood:* Chronic hypoxia stimulates overproduction of red blood cells in the bone marrow, resulting in polycythemia. When polycythemia is severe, the increased viscosity of the blood impairs circulation. Thrombocytopenia and impaired platelet aggregation and reduction in the clotting factors that make up the prothrombin complex are additional complications of polycythemia. Bleeding disorders can result, primarily in older children.
3. *Heart:* Hypoxia evokes compensatory cardiac changes, including coronary vasodilation and the development of myocardial collateral circulation. Despite these changes, myocardial function is depressed, leaving older cyanotic children with a severely limited capacity for exertion. In addition, hypoxia has a deleterious effect on the conduction system, increasing the occurrence of dysrhythmias and conduction delays.
4. *Liver:* Chronic hypoxia results in depletion of the liver's glycogen stores, in addition to the clotting abnormalities described above. Hypoglycemia is the obvious consequence.
5. *Lungs:* Hypoxia and acidosis lead to increased pulmonary vascular resistance (PVR) from pulmonary vasoconstriction. Increased PVR increases right-to-left shunting, exacerbating cyanosis, hypoxia, and acidosis, and initiating a possibly vicious cycle.

Critical Care Management

Specific management of the cyanotic infant with a CHD is determined by the anatomic defect identified. Many require restoration or maintenance of ductal patency to provide either adequate systemic perfusion or sufficient PBF. Acid-base balance requires careful assessment, and metabolic acidosis is corrected by administration of sodium bicarbonate. Electrolyte balance and serum glucose level are closely monitored.

Acute hypoxic spells occur almost exclusively in infants with tetralogy of Fallot. Management of pulmonary hypertensive crisis is discussed later in this chapter.

CONGENITAL CARDIAC DEFECTS

Heart defects are classified by various taxonomies. One system that is clinically useful is based on the presence or absence of cyanosis and an estimate of the volume of PBF. These markers are determined by physical examination and chest films, permitting generation of a short list of defects in each of the categories (Table 19–4).

Acyanotic Heart Defects With Increased PBF

Congenital heart defects that produce a left-to-right shunt at varying points in the circulation lead to an increase in blood flow to the lungs. The most common lesions that create this alteration in hemo-

Table 19–4. CLASSIFICATION OF CONGENITAL CARDIAC DEFECTS

Acyanotic defects with increased PBF
Patent ductus arteriosus
Atrial septal defect
Ventricular septal defect
Atrioventricular septal defect

Acyanotic defects that obstruct flow
Coarctation of the aorta
Aortic stenosis
Pulmonic stenosis

Cyanotic defects with decreased PBF
Tricuspid atresia
Tetralogy of Fallot
Pulmonic atresia with intact ventricular septum

Cyanotic defects with increased PBF
Total anomalous pulmonary venous connection
Truncus arteriosus
Hypoplastic left heart syndrome

Cyanotic defects with variable PBF
Transposition of the great arteries
Double outlet right ventricle
Double inlet left ventricle
Single ventricle

PBF, pulmonary blood flow

Table 19–5. ACYANOTIC CONGENITAL HEART DEFECTS WITH INCREASED PULMONARY BLOOD FLOW

Defect	Cardiac Examination	Electrocardiogram	Chest Radiograph
PDA	"Machinery" murmur heard throughout systole and diastole; best heard at left upper sternal border and under left clavicle. Palpable cardiac thrill (with large PDA) at left sternal border	May be normal or demonstrate left ventricular hypertrophy	Increased pulmonary vascularity, prominent pulmonary arteries, enlargement of the left ventricle and aorta
ASD			
Ostium secundum and sinus venosus	Normal S_1. Soft systolic ejection murmur best heard at 2nd left ICS, fixed and widely split S_2	May be normal, but right axis deviation, right ventricular hypertrophy, and right BBB are detected in some	Increased pulmonary vasculature, enlargement of right atrium, right ventricle, and pulmonary artery; aorta smaller than normal
Ostium primum	Same as above	Left axis deviation, right BBB	
VSD			
Small, muscular	Loud, harsh systolic murmur localized to left sternal border. Associated cardiac thrill	Normal	Normal heart size and PBF
Moderate to large	Rumbling murmur heard best at lower left sternal border; radiates across the left chest sometimes as far as the midaxillary line. Pulmonic component of S_2 loud and widely split	Left ventricular dominance and left ventricular hypertrophy	Cardiomegaly, enlarged left atrium, enlarged left ventricle, prominent pulmonary vascular markings
Eisenmenger complex	Quieter heart murmur. P_2 loud and booming	Dominant right ventricular hypertrophy	Enlarged right atrium, right ventricle, and pulmonary artery; small distal pulmonary vessels; variability in size of left atrium and left ventricle
AVSD			
Incomplete; competent mitral valve	Same as for ASD	Same as for ostium secundum ASD	Same as for ASD
Mitral insufficiency	Systolic murmur best heard apically; radiates to the axilla	Left ventricular hypertrophy	Enlargement of left ventricle and left atrium
Complete	Combination of ASD, VSD, and atrioventricular valve insufficiency murmurs. No murmur may be present. With pulmonary artery hypertension, P_2 is loud and widely split	Left axis deviation and biventricular hypertrophy	Cardiomegaly and increased pulmonary vascular markings

ASD, atrial septal defect; AVSD, atrioventricular septal defect; BBB, bundle-branch block; ICS, intercostal space; P_2, pulmonary component of second heart sound; PBF, pulmonary blood flow; PDA, patent ductus arteriosus; S_1, first heart sound; S_2, second heart sound; VSD, ventricular septal defect

dynamics are patent ductus arteriosus, atrial septal defect, ventricular septal defect, and atrioventricular septal defect. (Table 19–5 summarizes the findings on cardiac examination, ECG, and chest radiograph of children with these defects.)

Patent Ductus Arteriosus

Patent ductus arteriosus (PDA) is a fairly common congenital heart defect, accounting for approximately 10% of the total number of cardiac defects. PDA occurs more frequently in females, and is commonly found in offspring of women who have been exposed to rubella during the first trimester of pregnancy. Approximately 15% of all children with PDA have an associated anomaly such as ventricular septal defect or coarctation of the aorta.

Etiology. The ductus arteriosus is formed during the fifth to seventh week of gestation. It connects the pulmonary artery at its bifurcation to the aorta, thereby causing blood to bypass the lungs in fetal

circulation. The ductus is approximately 1 cm in length, slightly less than 1 cm in diameter, and has a sphincter-like muscle in its wall. The ductus begins to close within 10 to 15 hours of birth, and closure is usually completed in 2 to 3 weeks. Although a ductus can close spontaneously at any time other than the newborn period, this is very unlikely after the age of 1 year because specific physiologic occurrences contribute to its closure.

At birth, concomitant with the onset of respiration, PVR decreases as the pulmonary arterioles dilate, causing a rise in PaO_2. In addition, vasoactive substances are released. The combination of the rising PaO_2 and the circulating humoral substances causes the ductus to contract. Eventually, the ductus becomes fibrous. If these processes do not occur, however, a PDA is the result. Factors known to cause a ductus to remain open are prematurity, hypoxia, and scarring of the ductus during fetal life from rubella.

Alteration in Hemodynamics. When a patent ductus arteriosus is present, alteration in normal

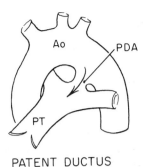

Figure 19–4 ● ● ● ● ● ●

Patent ductus arteriosus. Ao, aorta; PDA, patent ductus arteriosus; PT, pulmonary trunk. (From Perloff, J.K. (1994). *The clinical recognition of congenital heart disease*, 4th edition, p. 510. Philadelphia: W.B. Saunders.)

blood flow through the heart and lungs occurs. Because the pressure in the aorta is higher than that in the pulmonary artery, blood is shunted continuously from the aorta across the patent ductus to the pulmonary artery and the lungs, only to return again to the left heart (Fig. 19–4). This creates an increased volume load on the left side of the heart. Clinical symptoms vary directly with the amount of shunting from the aorta to the pulmonary artery.

Management. Medical management of children without serious symptoms related to PDA is conservative. Protection against infective endocarditis is necessary when dental work or a surgical procedure is performed.

Medical management of the small or premature infant with a PDA requires treating congestive heart failure (CHF) with fluid restriction, diuretics, and digitalization. If, however, CHF cannot be controlled by these measures within 48 to 72 hours, surgical intervention is recommended.

Developments in medical care have been used to treat PDA. The first method is the administration of a pharmacologic agent, indomethacin, used primarily with premature infants. Indomethacin is a prostaglandin inhibitor. Prostaglandin is known to induce active dilation of the ductus arteriosus. With the onset of birth, prostaglandin production is thought to cease. However, the exact mechanism of cessation of prostaglandin production is not yet clearly understood. Based on the theory that prostaglandins may still be working to maintain dilation of the ductus, indomethacin therapy is used to promote closure of the ductus. Indomethacin is usually given at a dose of 0.2 mg/kg orally or intravenously in a single dose and, if necessary, repeated after 8 hours and 16 hours. Because indomethacin is an acetylsalicylic acid, it cannot be given to the infant with poor renal functioning, necrotizing enterocolitis, bleeding dyscrasias, hyperbilirubinemia, or internal bleeding. When this drug is administered, close assessment for signs and symptoms of abnormal bleeding is crucial. The second method is catheter closure of the ductus. During cardiac catheterization, a "plug" is deposited in the ductus by a catheter.

Definitive Surgical Correction. Surgical correction is recommended for all infants with CHF who have not responded to medical management and for any child with a PDA over the age of 1 year. Children who do not present with any problems directly related to the PDA usually undergo surgical correction during the preschool years. The surgery is performed through a posterolateral incision in the fourth left intercostal space (ICS). In the infant, the ductus is usually ligated with heavy suture. In the older child, the ductus is divided between clamps, and the severed ends are closed by sutures. Postoperative complications are rare except in the premature infant, for whom other factors, such as respiratory distress, complicate recovery.

Atrial Septal Defect

Atrial septal defect (ASD) is a fairly common congenital heart defect, accounting for approximately 10% of the total number of cardiac defects. It occurs more frequently in females. An ASD exists when there is a communication between the left and right atrium that persists beyond the perinatal period.

Etiology. During fetal life, the atrial septum is formed during the fourth to sixth week of gestation. An opening, called the foramen ovale, persists in the atrial septum throughout intrauterine existence. This opening permits blood to bypass the lungs. After birth, with an increase in left atrial pressure (LAP), the foramen ovale closes. In the growth of the atrial septum during fetal and early perinatal life, failure of the septal layers to fuse completely results in ASD.

Alteration in Hemodynamics. Defects in the atrial septum, which can occur in different locations, are identified by where they occur. The most common site is at the center of the atrial septum at the level of the foramen ovale. This defect is called an ostium secundum ASD. If the defect occurs high in the atrial septum, it is called a sinus venosus ASD. This defect, located near the junction of the superior vena cava and the right atrium, is often associated with abnormal drainage of the right pulmonary veins. When the defect occurs low in the septum, it is identified as an ostium primum ASD (Fig. 19–5). This defect is more complex, and is often associated with abnormalities of the atrioventricular valves. Ostium primum ASDs are less common than ostium secundum or sinus venosus ASDs.

Because of higher pressure in the left atrium, and because the right atrium and right ventricle are more compliant, blood is shunted from the left atrium across the ASD into the right atrium, thereby altering normal blood flow through the heart. This creates a burden on the right side of the heart. However, significant shunting across the ASD may not occur until early childhood because of the relative noncompliance of the right atrium in infancy.

Management. Management of ASD is conservative because the majority of children are asymptomatic. Children with an ostium primum ASD with associated atrioventricular valve abnormalities who

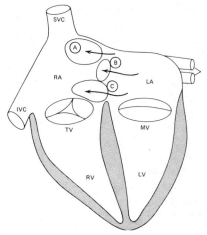

Figure 19–5 ● ● ● ● ● ●

Three locations of atrial septal defect (ASD). *A*, Sinus venosus ASD; *B*, ostium secundum ASD; *C*, ostium primum ASD. IVC, inferior vena cava; LA, left atrium; LV, left ventricle; MV, mitral valve; RA, right atrium; RV, right ventricle; SVC, superior vena cava; TV, tricuspid valve. (Reproduced by permission. *Pediatric Critical Care* by Smith. Delmar Publishers, Albany, NY, © 1985.)

present with CHF are treated with digoxin, fluid limitation, and diuretics.

Nonoperative closure of ASDs has been achieved by means of techniques performed via a cardiac catheter. A patch is folded like an umbrella or clamshell within a special catheter. It is then opened within the left atrium and drawn against the atrial septum. Transcatheter technique has been successful in a number of children.

Definitive Surgical Correction. Because most children with ASD are in a normal state of health, elective surgery is usually performed in the preschool years. Surgical correction is performed by means of a midline sternotomy incision. The child is placed on cardiopulmonary bypass. Then, either the ASD is closed by suture, or a patch of pericardium or Dacron is sutured in place. With sinus venosus ASD, the patch is placed so as to close the ASD and to direct any anomalous pulmonary venous drainage into the left atrium. Interference with cardiac conduction during surgery occurs occasionally with ostium primum ASD because the atrioventricular bundle of His is close to the area being sutured.

Ventricular Septal Defect

Ventricular septal defects are the most common congenital heart defects, accounting for 20% of the total number of cardiac defects. A ventricular septal defect (VSD) is a communication between the ventricles that permits blood to flow freely between them. This defect occurs more frequently in males; the precise etiology is unknown. VSD is seen in infants with Down's syndrome and other autosomal trisomies, and is associated with renal anomalies. VSDs are also seen in conjunction with a variety of other congenital

heart defects, especially coarctation of the aorta, PDA, and transposition of the great arteries.

Etiology. The ventricular septum is established in fetal life during the fourth to eighth week of gestation. The ventricular septum is formed from muscular and membranous tissues that fuse with the endocardial cushions and bulbous cordis. If inadequate development of these tissues occurs in fetal life, a VSD results. The size of a VSD varies from that of a pinpoint to the absence of the entire septum.

Alteration in Hemodynamics. At birth, a VSD does not alter flow of blood through the heart because pressure in the right and left ventricles is essentially equal. As the infant matures, resistance in the lungs decreases, right ventricular pressure (RVP) drops, pressure in the left ventricle becomes greater than in the right, and blood is shunted from left to right. Most often the presence of a VSD is not detected until the infant's 4- or 6-week checkup.

After the first month of life, VSD is often responsible for significant left-to-right shunting. However, the size of the shunt is determined by the size and location of the VSD, and it directly influences the child's initial clinical presentation and the effect of this excessive blood flow on the pulmonary vasculature. A sizable left-to-right shunt causes significant changes in the pulmonary vascular bed. In response to the abnormally high flow of blood that is under increased pressure, the pulmonary vessels hypertrophy and actually undergo histologic changes of the intima. As a result of these changes, an increase in PVR occurs, which further serves to increase pulmonary pressure and RVP. When pressure in the right ventricle is equal to or greater than left ventricular pressure, shunting across the VSD is eliminated or may occur in the opposite direction (Eisenmenger's complex). Figure 19–6 illustrates possible hemodynamic variations in VSD.

These hemodynamic changes are the result of pulmonary artery hypertension but do not occur in every child with VSD. Most children with VSD have small defects in the muscular portion of the ventricular septum. These are common defects that usually close spontaneously within the first 4 to 6 years of life and are not associated with large shunts. Moderate to large VSDs occur most commonly in the membranous portion of the septum, in proximity to the bundle of His and below the aortic and pulmonic valves. The size of the shunt in moderate to large VSDs varies directly with the size of the defect and the proximity of the pulmonic valve.

Management. Management of small VSDs is conservative. Because these children are asymptomatic and spontaneous closure of the defect frequently occurs, intervention is rarely necessary. Even if spontaneous closure does not occur, surgery is generally not recommended. With a small defect, life expectancy is normal, and the risk of operating is deemed greater than the risk of not operating.

Children and infants with moderate to large VSDs require close medical assessment. Their heart murmur must be evaluated frequently for an increase in

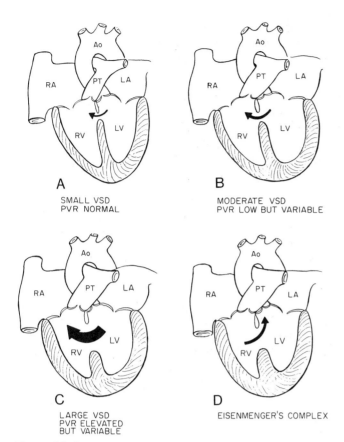

A

SMALL VSD
PVR NORMAL

B

MODERATE VSD
PVR LOW BUT VARIABLE

C

LARGE VSD
PVR ELEVATED
BUT VARIABLE

D

EISENMENGER'S COMPLEX

Figure 19–6 ● ● ● ● ● ●

A to D, Illustrations of small, moderately restrictive, and nonrestrictive (large) perimembranous ventricular septal defect. PVR, pulmonary vascular resistance; VSD, ventricular septal defect. (From Perloff, J.K. (1994). The Clinical Recognition of Congenital Heart Disease, 4th edition, p. 402. Philadelphia: W.B. Saunders.)

shunt size and for possible development of pulmonary hypertension. Signs and symptoms of pulmonary hypertension are also monitored by chest films, ECG, and echocardiogram. These children are also monitored closely for signs and symptoms of CHF, and they are often maintained on digoxin and diuretics. They are also assessed closely for signs and symptoms of pneumonia, which they are prone to develop and which can be a life-threatening illness, especially in infants. Children with large VSDs are at significant risk for the development of subacute bacterial endocarditis.

Surgical Management. In infants, surgery is necessary if CHF cannot be managed. Palliative surgery for VSD, pulmonary artery banding, decreases the volume of PBF and may be required when VSD accompanies complex CHD. This is accomplished by placing a segment of Teflon tape around the pulmonary artery. Sutures are then placed through the tape to the desired degree of constriction. This procedure is generally performed via a left posterolateral incision.

Corrective surgery is recommended for infants and children with moderate to large VSDs. The timing of surgery is dependent on the presence or absence of

complicating factors. In children who are asymptomatic, surgery is recommended in the preschool years. If growth and development are impeded by chronic respiratory infection or CHF, as well as by the presence of pulmonary hypertension, surgery is recommended during infancy. Corrective repair of VSD is achieved via a midline sternotomy incision. Cardiopulmonary bypass and deep hypothermia are required. The defect is closed by sutures or a patch. Because of the proximity of these defects to the bundle of His, extra care is taken to prevent conduction problems postoperatively.

Postoperative complications may include heart block as well as cyanosis, dyspnea, and hypotension in patients with pulmonary hypertension. Aortic insufficiency also develops in a few children, and it is identified by the presence of a widened pulse pressure and a diastolic murmur.

Atrioventricular Septal Defect

Atrioventricular septal defects (AVSDs), also called atrioventricular canal, account for approximately 5% of the total number of congenital heart defects. An AVSD exists when there is an abnormal communication between the atria or the ventricles, or when there is communication between the atria and ventricles as well as an insufficiency of the atrioventricular (AV) valves. AVSD occurs slightly more frequently in females. The precise etiology of this defect is unknown. Children with Down's syndrome, however, have a high incidence of AVSD.

Etiology. During fetal life, the endocardial cushions are responsible for the development of components of the mitral and tricuspid valves, the upper ventricular septum, and the lower atrial septum. The cushions also play a role in the placement of the atrioventricular conduction system. These developments occur between the fourth and eighth week of gestation. Inadequate development of the cushions may result in varying combinations of defects in any of these specified parts of the heart. AVSD is classified as either incomplete (partial), transitional (intermediate), or complete. The transitional form has partial fusion of the endocardial cushions, resulting in variable malformations of the AV valves, and is not discussed. The sections that follow contrast the incomplete and the complete types of AVSD.

Alteration in Hemodynamics

Incomplete AVSD. The infant or child with an incomplete AVSD presents with an ostium primum ASD as well as a variable degree of mitral valve abnormality, generally a cleft mitral valve (Fig. 19–7). If the mitral valve is competent, despite an abnormality in its structure, alteration in hemodynamics is the same as in the child with an ostium primum ASD. The presence of an insufficient mitral valve in addition to an ASD further increases the burden on the right side of the heart. If the ASD is small, however, any mitral insufficiency increases the burden on the left side of the heart.

Complete AVSD. In the complete form of AVSD,

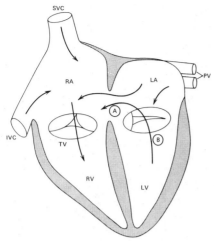

Figure 19–7 • • • • • •

Incomplete atrioventricular septal defect (AVSD). *A*, Ostium primum atrial septal defect; *B*, Cleft mitral valve. (Reproduced by permission. *Pediatric Critical Care* by Smith. Delmar Publishers, Albany, NY, © 1985.)

an ostium primum ASD, a VSD in the upper ventricular septum, and a common AV valve are present (Fig. 19–8). The end result is free communication between all chambers of the heart. Shunting occurs at the atrial and ventricular levels in a left-to-right direction. In addition, the right atrium receives blood from two other sources within the heart. During systole, the right atrium can receive blood from the left ventricle via the insufficient mitral valve and the ASD. Blood can also enter the right atrium from the right ventricle via the incompetent tricuspid valve. An excessive volume load on the right side of the heart and pulmonary vasculature is the consequence. Pulmonary hypertension is a frequent complication. The left side of the heart is also stressed by excess volume work. Factors that play an important role in determining the degree of shunting are pulmonary resistance, systemic resistance, left ventricular pressure, RVP, and the compliance of all heart chambers.

Management

Incomplete AVSD. The infant or child with an incomplete AVSD is treated in the same way as children with ASD. However, precautions against infective endocarditis are necessary because of mitral valve insufficiency. If mitral insufficiency causes CHF to develop, the child is treated with digitalization and diuretics. Close continuing assessment of these children is vital.

Complete AVSD. An infant with complete AVSD generally requires close assessment and aggressive intervention because of the frequency with which CHF occurs. Digoxin and diuretics are the treatment of choice. These children are also watched closely for signs and symptoms of pneumonia. Monitoring of heart sounds and murmurs is vital to the prognosis of these children. Auscultatory evidence of increasing pulmonary pressures is an indication of surgical intervention.

Surgical Management. Surgery is recommended immediately for those whose CHF cannot be controlled medically or when failure to thrive is present. Surgery is generally recommended before the child reaches 1 year of age, because the development of severe pulmonary vascular obstructive disease is likely thereafter. Complete intracardiac repair of complete AVSD is achieved between 6 and 12 months of age when heart failure is present and not later than 2 years of age in those without severe symptoms.

Corrective surgery is performed via a midline sternotomy incision with deep hypothermia and cardiopulmonary bypass. An incomplete AVSD is repaired with a patch of the ASD and by suturing the cleft in the mitral valve. Corrective repair of a complete AVSD involves patch repair of the ASD and VSD and repair of the mitral and tricuspid valves. The AV valves are reconstructed using available tissue from the common AV valve leaflets with the objective of achieving valve competence. Mitral valve replacement may be necessary on rare occasions. Close care is taken during suturing to prevent heart block. Postoperative complications may include heart block and persistence of atrioventricular valve insufficiency. Precautions against endocarditis are necessary both preoperatively and postoperatively.

Acyanotic Defects That Obstruct Flow

Coarctation of the aorta and aortic stenosis are two common cardiac lesions that result in increased heart work, especially affecting the left ventricle. However, because there is no abnormal connection between the systemic and pulmonary vascular systems, shunting of blood does not occur, PBF is normal, and cyanosis is absent.

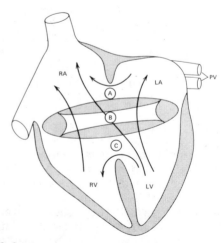

Figure 19–8 • • • • • •

Complete atrioventricular septal defect (AVSD). *A*, Ostium primum atrial septal defect; *B*, Common atrioventricular valve; *C*, Ventricular septal defect. (Reproduced by permission. *Pediatric Critical Care* by Smith. Delmar Publishers, Albany, NY, © 1985.)

Pulmonic stenosis, unless very severe, is a third common defect that does not produce either cyanosis or altered PBF despite obstruction and the increased work of the right heart. (Table 19–6 summarizes the findings on cardiac examination, ECG, and chest radiograph of children with these defects.)

Mitral stenosis—an uncommon defect—obstructs pulmonary venous return, but does not cause an al-

Table 19–6. ACYANOTIC CONGENITAL HEART DEFECTS THAT OBSTRUCT FLOW

Defect	Cardiac Examination	Electrocardiogram	Chest Radiograph
Coarctation of the aorta			
Preductal	Normal heart sounds	Right ventricular hypertrophy	Cardiomegaly
Postductal	Normal heart sounds, but S$_2$ may be accentuated with severe coarctation. With large collateral flow, continuous systolic murmurs develop	Varying degrees of left ventricular hypertrophy	Enlarged left atrium and left ventricle; dilated ascending aorta. Rib notching in children over 8 years of age with extensive collateral circulation
AS			
Valvular (Mild to moderate)	Ejection click best heard at the 4th ICS to the left of the sternum. Rough, harsh murmur best heard at base of the heart to the right of the sternal border	Left ventricular hypertrophy, or may be normal	May appear normal. Possible left ventricular enlargement and dilated ascending aorta
(Moderate to severe)	Palpable thrill best felt at the suprasternal notch and at the 2nd right ICS. Diminished S$_2$	Left ventricular hypertrophy; possible ST and T wave changes, or may be normal	Same as for mild to moderate AS. Pulmonary congestion may be seen
IHSS	Midsystolic ejection murmur best heard near the apex; palpable thrill may be present. Normal S$_2$	Left ventricular hypertrophy	Left ventricular enlargement and cardiomegaly
Subvalvular	Similar to valvular AS, with absence of ejection click	Same as for valvular AS	Similar to valvular AS, but dilation of aorta absent
Supravalvular	Normal S$_1$; absent ejection click; ejection systolic murmur; palpable thrill may be present	Same as for valvular AS	Ascending aorta smaller than normal; descending aorta normal in size
PS			
Valvular (Mild to moderate)	Ejection click after S$_1$, followed by systolic ejection murmur best heard at upper left sternal border and radiating widely. Palpable thrill at 2nd left ICS. S$_2$ widely split, with diminished pulmonic component. Right ventricular lift	Right ventricular hypertrophy	Right ventricular and main pulmonary artery enlargement. Normal left heart and pulmonary vascular markings
(Severe)	Murmur increased in duration and intensity, obscuring S$_2$. No ejection click audible	Right ventricular and right atrial hypertrophy	Same as above, with right atrial enlargement
Infundibular (Fibrous ring)	Similar to valvular PS, but no ejection click or change in intensity of S$_2$, which is widely split	Same as for valvular PS	Right ventricular enlargement. Normal pulmonary artery, left heart, and pulmonary vascular markings
(Muscular)	No ejection click. Short systolic murmur ending before S$_2$, best heard at 3rd or 4th left ICS. Palpable thrill with severe stenosis. Widely split S$_2$. Bulging of lower precordium; right ventricular heave	Same as for valvular PS	Same as for fibrous ring infundibular PS
Subinfundibular	Similar to muscular infundibular PS	Same as for muscular infundibular PS	Same as for muscular infundibular PS
Supravalvular	Systolic ejection murmur heard over sites of obstruction, radiating through pulmonary vasculature. Occasional continuous murmur. Normal S$_1$ and S$_2$; no ejection click	Variable increased right heart work	Variable enlargement of right heart chambers and main pulmonary artery. Variable changes in pulmonary vascular markings

AS, aortic stenosis; ICS, intercostal space; IHSS, idiopathic hypertrophic subaortic stenosis: PS, pulmonic stenosis; S$_1$, first heart sound; S$_2$, second heart sound

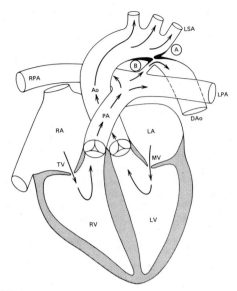

Figure 19–9 ● ● ● ● ● ●

Preductal coarctation of the aorta. *A*, Site of coarctation; *B*, Patent ductus arteriosus. (Reproduced by permission. *Pediatric Critical Care* by Smith. Delmar Publishers, Albany, NY, © 1985.)

teration in PBF or oxygen saturation, unless the valve obstructs left ventricular inflow critically. Mitral atresia or marked hypoplasia is representative of the spectrum of infants with hypoplastic left heart syndrome. Isolated mitral stenosis is not discussed here because of its rarity.

Coarctation of the Aorta

Coarctation of the aorta is a common congenital heart defect, accounting for approximately 10% of the total number of cardiac defects. It occurs more frequently in males. A coarctation, or narrowing, of the aorta usually occurs beyond the left subclavian artery at the location where the ductus arteriosus inserts. However, aortic coarctation can occur proximal or distal to the insertion of the ductus. The entire aorta may be affected, although this is infrequent. The location of the coarctation affects the entire clinical picture. Differentiation between preductal and postductal coarctation is made by the presence or absence of patency of the ductus. If the ductus remains open, the coarctation is classified as preductal; whereas, if the ductus is very small or totally obliterated, the coarctation is classified as postductal.

Other forms of CHD may occur with a coarctation. Fifty percent of children with coarctation have a bicuspid aortic valve. Preductal coarctation is often associated with other cardiac defects such as VSD. Postductal coarctation is associated with VSD and aortic stenosis, but these associated defects are seen less frequently and are generally not as severe as the defects associated with preductal coarctation.

Etiology. Between the fifth and eighth week of gestation, development of the aortic arch occurs. If the arch develops improperly, a restricted opening or lumen in the aorta results. This occurs most commonly in the area of the aorta near the site where the ductus arteriosus connects the fetal main pulmonary artery to the aorta.

Alteration in Hemodynamics

Preductal Coarctation. A preductal coarctation results in abnormal blood flow from the left and right heart. Blood leaving the left ventricle enters the ascending aorta and flows to the site of the coarctation. Below the coarctation, blood enters the descending aorta from the pulmonary artery via the ductus (Fig. 19–9). Therefore, because of the position of the coarctation, the upper half of the body is saturated by blood from the left ventricle and the lower half of the body by blood from the right ventricle. This alteration in hemodynamics causes an enlarged right ventricle, enlarged pulmonary artery, and prominent descending aorta.

Postductal Coarctation. A postductal coarctation causes alteration in normal blood flow but in a pattern entirely different from that of preductal coarctation. This coarctation is not associated with patency of the ductus and requires the development of collateral circulation to the lower half of the body (Fig. 19–10). This process begins in fetal life because the greater portion of right ventricular outflow empties into the ascending aorta via the ductus.

Because of the high pressure that develops in the ascending aorta from the narrowed portion, increased stress is placed on the left atrium and ventricle. This causes enlargement of both these chambers, although left ventricular enlargement is more pronounced.

Management. Management of a coarctation depends on the clinical presentation. The infant who presents with CHF is treated with digitalization and

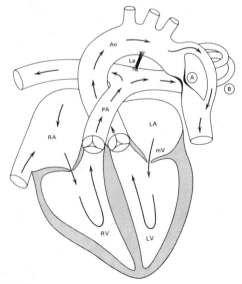

Figure 19–10 ● ● ● ● ● ●

Postductal coarctation of the aorta. *A*, Site of coarctation; *B*, Collateral circulation. (Reproduced by permission. *Pediatric Critical Care* by Smith. Delmar Publishers, Albany, NY, © 1985.)

diuretics. Circulatory collapse can occur with ductal closure.

The older child whose coarctation is detected on routine physical examination requires close assessment of blood pressure. Significant hypertension may require the use of antihypertensives preoperatively. If significant hypertension is present at rest, exercise restriction may be recommended. Antibiotic prophylaxis against bacterial endocarditis is recommended preoperatively and postoperatively because of the high risk of this serious infection in children with a bicuspid aortic valve with coarctation.

Definitive Surgical Correction. Elective surgery is recommended between the ages of 1 and 3 years in children who have postductal coarctation. During this age span, the child's aorta is good-sized, and hypertension is generally reversible. Infants with CHF and coarctation require early surgical intervention. Surgery is performed via a posterolateral thoracotomy incision. The aorta is temporarily clamped while an end-to-end anastomosis is performed. Occasionally, a graft is necessary to bridge the space made by the segment of coarcted tissue that is removed. If inadequate collateral circulation is present, hypothermia, a temporary shunt, or partial cardiopulmonary bypass is recommended to prevent ischemia to the spinal cord. If a PDA is present, as with preductal coarctation, division of the PDA is performed in addition to coarctation repair.

Subclavian-flap aortoplasty may be performed on the infant with preductal coarctation. The left subclavian artery is ligated distally. The area of coarctation is then incised to the point of origin of the subclavian artery. The subclavian artery, having been incised lengthwise to form a flap, is sutured in place over the opening created in the aorta. The advantages of this procedure are: (1) the time required for aortic cross-clamping is generally shorter, (2) the suture line is under less tension than in an end-to-end anastomosis, and (3) the flap tissue continues to grow with the child.

Postoperative complications of coarctation repair may include paraplegia, hemorrhage, and gangrenous bowel attributable to paradoxical hypertension of the abdominal arteries. These complications rarely occur, but some patients do experience abdominal pain and ileus postoperatively from paradoxical hypertension. It is important to note that hypertension does not resolve immediately after repair of a coarctation. Antihypertensives may be required for several months.

Postoperative management is aimed at controlling hypertension, because it is imperative to avoid undue stress on the suture line. This is achieved by the use of vasodilators. Sodium nitroprusside (Nipride) is the mainstay of treatment in children because of its consistent efficacy, ease of titration, and low incidence of toxicity. Some children may experience excessive tachycardia with nitroprusside, necessitating use of a beta-blocking agent such as esmolol or labetalol if cardiac contractility is not a concern. Long-term management of hypertension with propranolol (Inde-

ral) is indicated in some children, usually those who have a history of hypertension.

Maintenance of an appropriate blood pressure also requires control of postoperative pain and agitation. These interventions can be crucial in avoiding postoperative bleeding.

Aortic Stenosis

Aortic stenosis (AS) accounts for approximately 5% to 10% of the total number of congenital heart defects. It occurs more frequently in males. AS is defined as a lesion that creates obstruction of blood flow from the left ventricle. This obstruction may occur at, above, or below the aortic valve.

Etiology. The aortic valve is formed during the sixth to ninth week of gestation, when the pulmonary artery and the aorta are formed from the division of the truncus arteriosus. The cusps of the aortic valve arise from three tubercles that proliferate within the aorta. Failure of the cusps to separate, creating a fusion, causes *valvular AS*, the most common form of the defect. Most often, the valve is bicuspid. This lesion may occur with endocardial fibroelastosis, PDA, coarctation of the aorta, VSD, and pulmonic stenosis.

Stenotic muscle formation below the aortic valve results in asymmetric enlargement of the left side of the ventricular septum in idiopathic hypertrophic subaortic stenosis (IHSS). Left ventricular outflow obstruction is the consequence of septal hypertrophy and anomalous placement of the anterior leaflet of the mitral valve in the hypertrophied septum. Progressive, but variable, muscular hypertrophy occurs in this dynamic lesion. A normal aortic valve is usually present.

Discrete subvalvular AS is caused by the formation of a fibrous ring with a narrowed central orifice below the aortic valve. Aortic insufficiency is a common finding with this lesion. *Supravalvular AS* causes obstruction to left ventricular outflow by the presence of a fibrous membrane, by hypoplasia of the ascending aorta, or by an "hourglass" deformity of the aorta. This lesion is frequently found in children with Williams' syndrome, who have characteristic faces (elfin), developmental delay, and personality changes. Hypercalcemia and peripheral pulmonary stenosis may also be present. Supravalvular AS occurs less frequently than all other forms of AS (Fig. 19–11).

Alteration in Hemodynamics

Valvular AS. Obstruction at the valvular level creates increased stress on the left ventricle and ascending aorta. The left ventricle must exert increased pressure to overcome the resistance to blood flow at the stenotic valve, resulting in muscular hypertrophy. Because blood is ejected from the left ventricle under increased pressure, the turbulence of its flow stresses the ascending aorta, causing it to dilate.

IHSS. Obstruction to left ventricular outflow in this lesion occurs within the ventricle and is variable. Once again, the left ventricle must exert an increased pressure to overcome the resistance of the stenotic

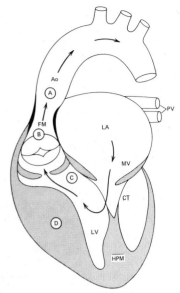

Figure 19–11 ● ● ● ● ● ●

Four locations of aortic stenosis (AS). *A,* Supravalvular AS; *B,* Valvular AS; *C,* Discrete subvalvular AS; *D,* Idiopathic hypertrophic subaortic stenosis. (Reproduced by permission. *Pediatric Critical Care* by Smith. Delmar Publishers, Albany, NY, © 1985.)

muscle. In response to this stress, the left ventricle hypertrophies. If the stress is very great, the left atrium may also enlarge to compensate for the stress occurring in the ventricle.

Discrete Subvalvular AS. Obstruction below the aortic valve creates an increased stress on the left ventricle. However, because the aortic valve is normal, no excess stress is placed on the ascending aorta. The increased stress on the left ventricle results in hypertrophy.

Supravalvular AS. This form of obstruction creates the same stress on the heart as valvular AS.

Management. The infant with critical AS who develops CHF is managed with digitalization and diuretic therapy until surgical intervention can be accomplished.

Management of AS in the older child is directed toward detection of obstruction that interferes with meeting the demands placed on the heart during exercise. It is important to note that AS is a progressive disease that requires serial evaluation.

Antibiotic prophylaxis for infective endocarditis is important for all patients with left ventricular outflow tract obstruction.

Definitive Surgical Correction. Surgical intervention is critical for the infant with severe AS, because the response to medical management of heart failure is often poor. Critically ill newborns with AS are considered to have a surgical emergency, with open valvotomy under direct vision the preferred operation.

Surgery is recommended for children with valvular AS who are symptomatic, have a left ventricular strain pattern on ECG, or have a pressure gradient of more than 70 to 80 mmHg between the left ventri-

cle and the aorta. Once the presence of severe stenosis has been established, the potential of sudden death dictates that surgical treatment not be delayed. With discrete subvalvular AS, surgery is indicated in the presence of mild to moderate stenosis because of the likelihood of both progressive obstruction and aortic insufficiency.

Supravalvular AS is amenable to operative treatment if the narrowing is discrete and can be widened with insertion of a prosthesis. When the ascending aorta is markedly hypoplastic, it is less amenable to surgical intervention.

Surgery is performed via a midline sternotomy incision. Cardiopulmonary bypass is used for all patients except the small infant with valvular AS, in whom surgery may be performed with inflow occlusion.

Valvular AS is corrected by a commissurotomy. In this procedure, the valve is dilated and the commissures of the valve are incised. In cases in which a commissurotomy would create significant aortic insufficiency, a valve replacement may be necessary. Subvalvular AS is corrected by one of two methods: the fibrous membrane may be excised, or the whole length of the fibrous area may be incised. Septal myectomy may also be performed. Supravalvular AS is surgically corrected by vertical incision of the stenosed area. A large patch is then placed in the area incised to enlarge the aortic diameter.

Potential postoperative complications include persistent stenosis, restenosis of the aortic lumen, and insufficiency of the aortic valve. Although aortic insufficiency can develop acutely in the early postoperative period, most often these problems are evidenced long after surgery, as the child matures. Aortic valve replacement may be required in adulthood.

Pulmonic Stenosis

Pulmonic stenosis (PS) is the result of an obstructive lesion that interferes with blood flow from the right ventricle. Like AS, this lesion occurs at a number of locations in the right ventricular outflow tract. PS accounts for approximately 10% of the total number of congenital heart defects. It is only slightly more common in males than in females. One variation of PS is seen with increased frequency in infants with rubella syndrome or Williams' syndrome.

Etiology. The pulmonic valve develops between the sixth and ninth weeks of gestation, at the same time as the development of the pulmonary artery and the aorta from the truncus arteriosus. It is formed by the proliferation of three tubercles within the lumen of the pulmonary artery, which later thin by tissue resorption to form the three cusps of the pulmonic valve. Failure of this process to occur results in abnormality of the valve. Such an abnormality may present as a bicuspid valve that is fused at the commissures of its two leaflets, or as a tricuspid valve with thickened leaflets that may be partially or completely fused at the commissures. In either case, *valvular PS* results, which severely restricts valve motion and impedes blood flow from the right ventricle. Valvular PS occurs in approximately 95% of the children with PS.

The infundibulum of the right ventricle is formed during the fifth to seventh week of gestation, slightly before the development of the pulmonic valve. The infundibulum develops from resorption of tissue in the bulbous cordis. If this tissue is not resorbed adequately, an area of infundibular hypertrophy results, which causes *infundibular PS*. Alternatively, abnormal bands of muscle may form within the chamber of the right ventricle. The result is *subinfundibular PS*, a rare defect. Both of these variations may be classified as *subvalvular PS*.

At approximately the same time as the development of the right ventricular infundibulum, the branch pulmonary arteries differentiate. These vessels grow to anastomose proximally with the main pulmonary artery and distally with the smaller pulmonary arteries. The development of these branch and peripheral arteries may be interfered with, and the vessels may not become sufficiently hollow. The result, *supravalvular PS*, can occur within the main pulmonary artery or within any of its branches (Fig. 19–12). Often, multiple areas of stenosis exist throughout the pulmonary vasculature. Supravalvular PS is also a rare defect.

Alteration in Hemodynamics. Regardless of the specific location of the lesion in PS, the hemodynamic result is obstruction of blood ejected from the right ventricle in systole. This obstruction places a pressure burden on the right ventricle.

Valvular PS. Obstruction to ventricular emptying and the resultant increase in RVP from valvular PS cause right ventricular and main pulmonary artery enlargement. The right ventricle enlarges as its muscular wall hypertrophies in response to the increased afterload it must overcome. The main pulmonary artery enlargement is characteristic of poststenotic dilation. However, pressure in the pulmonary trunk is normal or lower than normal, and therefore, the peripheral pulmonary vasculature and the left heart are unaffected. When severe valvular PS is present, right atrial pressure may also increase with resultant enlargement of the right atrial chamber.

Subvalvular PS. Both infundibular and subinfundibular PS are characterized by right ventricular hypertrophy that develops in response to the increased pressure in the ventricle as it pumps against an obstruction. However, the increased force is dissipated over an area of obstruction that is larger than that of valvular PS, and, as a result, the main pulmonary artery remains normal in size. Pressure in the main pulmonary artery is normal or reduced.

Supravalvular PS. Unlike the other forms of PS, supravalvular lesions produce hypertension in the main pulmonary artery as well as in the right ventricle. However, ventricular and pulmonary artery enlargement vary with the severity and location of the lesions.

Management. Children with PS are followed closely to detect, as early as possible, progression of their stenoses with growth. Although progression is less likely in children with PS than in those with AS, it is detected by changes in the murmur (increased intensity, loss of ejection click, the development of a palpable thrill), increased right ventricular hypertrophy on ECG, or increased clinical symptoms. Children with PS have a low risk of developing infective endocarditis, but antibiotic prophylaxis with dental work or other surgical procedures is generally provided.

Treatment of PS is recommended when the pressure gradient across the right ventricular outflow tract is 50 to 60 mmHg. Discrete valvular PS can be treated successfully by balloon valvoplasty in the cardiac catheterization laboratory. Exceptions are those patients with dysplastic pulmonary valves and infants that are critically ill with PS.

Definitive Surgical Correction. Surgical repair of PS is required urgently in infants with signs of heart failure. Cardiopulmonary bypass is used, and an incision is made in the pulmonary artery. Valvular stenosis is relieved by incising the fused commissures as widely as possible. The right ventricular infundibulum is palpated through the newly enlarged pulmonic valve to detect localized muscular or fibrotic obstruction. Subvalvular stenosis is excised widely by means of a right ventriculotomy.

Postoperatively, children who have had repair of valvular PS may have some degree of pulmonary regurgitation, but this is generally not significant. Patients who, before surgery, have significant right ventricular hypertension and hypertrophy may develop some degree of right-sided CHF postoperatively

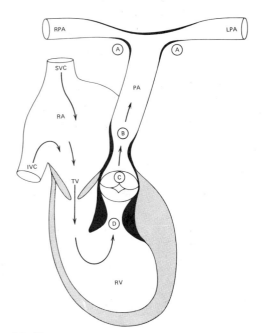

Figure 19–12 ● ● ● ● ● ●
Four locations of pulmonic stenosis (PS). *A,* Branch pulmonary artery stenosis; *B,* Discrete supravalvular PS; *C,* Valvular PS; *D,* Subvalvular PS. (Reproduced by permission. *Pediatric Critical Care* by Smith. Delmar Publishers, Albany, NY, © 1985.)

Table 19–7. CYANOTIC CONGENITAL HEART DEFECTS WITH DECREASED PULMONARY BLOOD FLOW

Defect	Cardiac Examination	Electrocardiogram	Chest Radiograph
TOF	Loud systolic murmur with palpable thrill along the entire left sternal border. Pulmonic S_2 diminished or inaudible. Prominent inferior sternum and right ventricular impulse	Right axis deviation and right ventricular hypertrophy. Occasional right atrial hypertrophy	Normal cardiac size with concavity in main pulmonary artery area. Decreased pulmonary vascular markings. Boot-shaped heart silhouette. Right aortic arch common
Pulmonary atresia with intact ventricular septum	Heart murmur may be absent; when detected, usually holosystolic blowing murmur of tricuspid regurgitation and continuous, "machinery" murmur of PDA. No pulmonic S_2	Absence of or decrease in right ventricular forces. Left ventricular dominance	Type 1: Similar to TOF. Type 2: Cardiomegaly with significant right atrial enlargement. Decreased pulmonary vascular markings
Tricuspid atresia	No tricuspid S_1. S_2 also often a single sound: no pulmonic S_2. Variable systolic (VSD and PS) murmurs or diastolic (mitral flow) murmur. Often, no murmur is audible	Left axis deviation. Left ventricular, left atrial, and right atrial hypertrophy. No right ventricular forces	Normal overall heart size with concavity in main pulmonary artery area. Right atrial, left atrial, left ventricular, and aortic enlargement. Decreased pulmonary vascular markings

PDA, patent ductus arteriosus; PS, pulmonic stenosis; S_1, first heart sound; S_2, second heart sound; TOF, tetralogy of Fallot; VSD, ventricular septal defect

and require digoxin and/or diuretic therapy for variable periods of time. Most children recover uneventfully and continue to grow and develop normally.

Cyanotic Congenital Heart Defects With Decreased PBF

Heart defects that produce cyanosis and decreased PBF are characterized by obstruction at some point in the right heart. This obstruction always results in a lower than normal flow of blood to the lungs. These obstructive defects are also associated with an abnormal opening between the pulmonary and systemic circulations or with the persistence of a fetal connection between the two systems. This permits shunting of blood from the right heart to the left heart and results in cyanosis.

Tetralogy of Fallot is the most common cyanotic CHD with decreased PBF. Pulmonary atresia with intact ventricular septum and tricuspid atresia are rare defects that result in the same alteration in hemodynamics. (Table 19–7 summarizes the findings on cardiac examination, ECG, and chest radiograph of children with these defects.)

Tetralogy of Fallot

Tetralogy of Fallot (TOF) is a fairly common congenital heart defect, accounting for 6% to 10% of the total number of cardiac defects. The child with TOF has a VSD, most often a malalignment type; PS that is usually infundibular, but may be valvular, supravalvular, or combined; right ventricular hypertrophy on ECG as a result of the increased RVP caused by the obstruction of blood flow from the ventricle; and

varying degrees of overriding (dextroposition) of the aorta (Fig. 19–13). Although these last two factors are consistently anatomically present, they do not significantly influence the physiologic alterations seen in the child with TOF. Instead, the pathophysiologic results of TOF are determined by the size of the VSD and the severity of the PS. Table 19–8 depicts the possible variations. Classic TOF, characterized by a large VSD and severe PS, is discussed here.

Etiology. Between the fourth and eighth week of

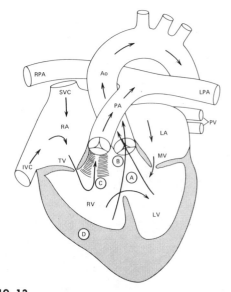

Figure 19–13 ● ● ● ● ● ●

Tetralogy of Fallot (TOF). *A*, Ventricular septal defect; *B*, Aorta overriding the ventricular septum; *C*, Pulmonic stenosis; *D*, Right ventricular hypertrophy. (Reproduced by permission. *Pediatric Critical Care* by Smith. Delmar Publishers, Albany, NY, © 1985.)

Table 19–8. VARIATIONS IN TETRALOGY OF FALLOT

Type	Characteristics
Large VSD	Mild to moderate PS ("acyanotic" tetralogy)
	Severe PS ("classic" tetralogy)
	Complete PS (tetralogy with pulmonary atresia)
Small VSD	Mild PS
	Severe PS

PS, pulmonic stenosis; VSD, ventricular septal defect

intrauterine life, the single ventricular chamber is divided in two. During the sixth to ninth week of gestation, formation of the pulmonic valve occurs, with the right ventricular infundibulum (outflow tract) developing slightly earlier than the valve. Malalignment of ventricular septation results in the variable defects seen in TOF. Sex distribution of TOF is about equal, with only slightly more males affected.

Alteration in Hemodynamics. Because of the coexisting VSD and the obstruction to blood flow from the right ventricle, blood flow to the lungs is diminished, whereas blood flow in the systemic circulation is increased because of the addition of systemic venous blood. The obstruction to right heart emptying results in increased pressure in the right ventricular chamber, permitting the right-to-left shunt.

The effect on the heart of these changes in hemodynamics includes an increase in the size and work of the right ventricle. The right atrium is usually unaffected. There is an increased volume load on the left ventricle, but this problem is generally reflected in enlargement of the aorta only, and the left ventricle remains normally compliant.

Management. Before surgical correction, children with TOF require close monitoring of their degree of hypoxia because it poses specific problems. Some children with TOF experience episodes of dramatically increased cyanosis that may progress to limpness, loss of consciousness, or seizures. These episodes are referred to by a number of designations, including "tet," cardiac, or hypoxic spells; and paroxysmal hyperpnea. These crises can lead to brain damage or even death. Tet spells are most common in the first 6 months of life and are often associated with crying, feeding, or a bowel movement, especially if these activities occur when the infant has just awakened. Spells begin with moderate but progressive dyspnea, and they culminate in hyperpnea and syncope. The precise mechanism responsible for tet spells has not been completely identified, but a vulnerable respiratory control center, tachycardia, and infundibular contraction are thought to contribute. The result is an increase in right-to-left shunting and a sharp fall in PBF, causing severely decreased levels of systemic PaO_2 and pH and a rise in the partial pressure of arterial carbon dioxide ($PaCO_2$).

Avoidance of tet spells is a primary objective. If a tet spell occurs, the infant or child is placed in a knee-chest position to mimic the squatting position spontaneously assumed by these youngsters, and ox-

ygen is immediately administered along with intravenous morphine sulfate, 0.1 mg/kg. Morphine relaxes the right ventricular infundibulum, thereby increasing PBF and decreasing the right-to-left shunt. Vital signs are monitored with care. Bradycardia, which may be associated with a tet spell, necessitates immediate intervention. Metabolic acidosis, which frequently results from the severe hypoxia characteristic of the spell, requires correction with sodium bicarbonate. Tet spells are considered to be an indication for either palliative or corrective surgery. Exercise restriction is generally not necessary for children with TOF because these youngsters tend to limit their own activity on the basis of the hypoxia.

Surgical intervention can be either a palliative procedure to increase PBF and decrease cyanosis or a definitive intracardiac repair. Indications for surgical intervention include decreased exercise tolerance, hypercyanotic spells, excessive polycythemia, and attainment of adequate size for elective repair in those with mild PS and minimal hypoxia.

Palliative Surgical Management. Palliative surgical intervention is sometimes preferred for infants who present with either severe hypoxia, hematocrit higher than 60%, tet spells, or impaired quality of life and are not considered good candidates for complete repair. The risks of total correction in these infants may be deemed greater than those associated with palliation and later corrective surgery.

A number of systemic–pulmonary artery shunt procedures have been used. The Blalock-Taussig subclavian–pulmonary artery anastomosis (Fig. 19–14) is the procedure that is generally recommended. The right or left subclavian artery is selected, depending

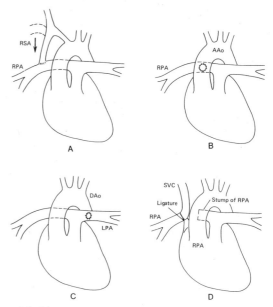

Figure 19–14 ● ● ● ● ●

Palliative shunts to increase pulmonary blood flow. *A,* Blalock-Taussig anastomosis; *B,* Waterston anastomosis; *C,* Potts-Smith-Gibson anastomosis; *D,* Glenn anastomosis. (Reproduced by permission. *Pediatric Critical Care* by Smith. Delmar Publishers, Albany, NY, © 1985.)

on the direction of the aortic arch. (The vessel on the opposite side of the arch is selected.) The artery is ligated and divided, and then turned to anastomose with the branch pulmonary artery on the same side. It is possible to construct very small shunts that are unlikely to cause pulmonary congestion but that maintain patency and successfully increase PBF. An additional advantage to the Blalock-Taussig shunt is the ease with which it is removed at the time of definitive repair. The classic Blalock-Taussig shunt is often modified: a small (3- or 4-mm) tube graft is interposed between the subclavian and pulmonary arteries.

Other palliative shunts are possible, and all serve to increase PBF: the Waterston shunt, in which the ascending aorta and right pulmonary artery are anastomosed; the Potts-Smith-Gibson operation, which consists of connecting the descending aorta and the left pulmonary artery; and the Glenn procedure, in which the right pulmonary artery is connected to the side of the superior vena cava (see Fig. 19–14). All of these procedures, however, are associated with more difficult repair at the time of corrective surgery because of significant distortion of the pulmonary artery. In addition, the Waterston and Potts shunts necessitate careful control of the size of the anastomosis. If too large, heart failure and pulmonary vascular disease may result.

Definitive Surgical Correction. Primary correction of TOF is advocated for all patients, including symptomatic young infants by some, whereas other surgical groups prefer palliation and delay of definitive repair until the infant is 6 to 8 months of age. Surgery is performed with cardiopulmonary bypass, deep hypothermia, and circulatory arrest. During corrective repair, any previously constructed palliative shunt is closed immediately before the initiation of cardiopulmonary bypass. The right ventricular outflow obstruction is excised to create an unobstructed channel to the pulmonic valve. If the pulmonic valve is also stenotic, it is incised. A patch of Dacron or pericardium may be used to enlarge the ventricular outflow tract in infants or very small children. Finally, the VSD is closed with a patch.

Postoperatively, almost all children who have had total correction of TOF demonstrate a right bundle-branch block on ECG. Some transient CHF is not uncommon, and this development requires treatment with digoxin and diuretics for several weeks or months postoperatively. If the foramen ovale is patent, right-to-left shunting persists at the atrial level in the face of CHF. Serious problems include persistent right ventricular failure and more complete forms of heart block. Pulmonic valve regurgitation occurs in some children. Antibiotic prophylaxis against endocarditis must be continued with dental work or surgical procedures. Some children continue to have limited exercise tolerance.

Pulmonary Atresia With Intact Ventricular Septum

Pulmonary atresia with intact ventricular septum (Fig. 19–15) is a rare congenital heart defect, ac-

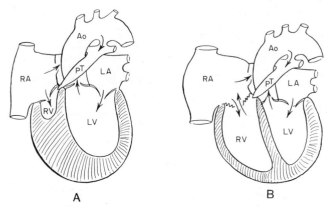

Figure 19–15 ● ● ● ● ● ●

Pulmonary atresia with intact ventricular septum. *A*, Type 1; *B*, Type 2. Ao, aorta; LA, left atrium; LV, left ventricle; PT, pulmonary trunk; RA, right atrium; RV, right ventricle. (From Perloff, J.K. (1994). *The clinical recognition of congenital heart disease*, 4th ed., p. 599. Philadelphia: W.B. Saunders.)

counting for only 1% to 3% of the total number of cardiac defects. It is the extreme form of valvular PS.

Etiology. Failure of the pulmonic valve to develop between the sixth and ninth week of gestation results in a valve that is small and imperforate. Development of the right ventricle is also affected. Children with one form of this serious defect (designated type 1) have a hypoplastic or rudimentary right ventricle, whereas others have a normal or dilated right ventricle associated with an incompetent tricuspid valve (type 2). In both types, the main and branch pulmonary arteries are usually normal in size.

Alteration in Hemodynamics. Children with type 1 pulmonary atresia have physiologic similarities with those with tricuspid atresia. Those with type 2 pulmonary atresia have slightly different hemodynamics. Systemic venous blood that enters the right atrium drains immediately into the right ventricle because of the incompetent tricuspid valve. Because no exit from the ventricle exists, it is subject to both volume and pressure overload, and blood is regurgitated into the right atrium. Pressure in the right atrium is greater than that in the left, resulting in a right-to-left shunt across the foramen ovale. Occasionally, other aortopulmonary collaterals develop as well, although this does not occur early. Therefore, blood in the left heart and the systemic circulation is a mixture of desaturated systemic venous blood and fully saturated pulmonary venous blood.

Right ventricular pressure may be systemic or suprasystemic in patients with a diminutive right ventricle. As a consequence, fistulous communications develop between the right ventricular chamber and the right, left, or, rarely, both coronary arteries. These intramyocardial sinusoids can result in retrograde coronary blood flow from the desaturated right ventricle to the aorta, resulting in both right and left ventricular ischemia and subsequent fibrosis.

Management. Management of these critically ill

infants is directed toward stabilization of their condition by control of hypoxia and correction of metabolic acidosis. CHF, when present, also requires aggressive intervention. Ductal patency is maintained by continuous IV infusion of prostaglandin E. Other supportive interventions include tracheal intubation and mechanical ventilation. Operability is dependent on the size of the right ventricle and the pulmonary arteries and the presence of sinusoids.

Surgical Management. Many surgical approaches to pulmonary atresia have been recommended, in part because of the spectrum of pathology that is seen, but also because both early and late mortality continue to occur with current interventions. Systemic–pulmonary artery shunts, open and closed pulmonary valvulotomy, combination of a shunt and valvulotomy, and right ventricular outflow tract reconstruction may be performed in infants. Regardless of the approach selected for an individual patient, the aim in all is to increase PBF to ensure the infant's survival and promote growth of the right ventricle for further palliation or repair.

When the right ventricle is near normal size, pulmonary valvulotomy alone may achieve satisfactory results. Shunt alone, usually a classic or modified Blalock-Taussig shunt, is recommended for those with a diminutive right ventricle, infundibular atresia, and high chamber pressure. Right ventricular decompression and antegrade pulmonary blood flow are unlikely with pulmonary valvulotomy in this group. Later surgical interventions are directed toward completion of a modified Fontan procedure.

Tricuspid Atresia

Tricuspid atresia occurs in 1% to 3% of children with congenital heart defects. It consists of an absent or imperforate tricuspid valve, which results in a complete right-to-left shunt at the atrial level and in variable degrees of right ventricular hypoplasia. Tricuspid atresia is slightly more common in males.

Etiology. The tricuspid valve is formed at about the fifth week of gestation as a result of the blending of endocardial cushion tissue, a portion of the ventricular septum, and ventricular muscle itself. A disruption in the formation of this valve can result in the utter lack of valve tissue and the consequent lack of a communication between the right atrium and the right ventricle.

Tricuspid atresia exists in a number of forms that vary, depending on the relationship of the great arteries (normally positioned or transposed), the nature of the ventricular septum (intact or VSD), and the nature of the pulmonic valve (normal, pulmonary atresia, or PS). These variations combine in a number of ways. Most commonly, the infant with tricuspid atresia has normally positioned great arteries; a small VSD; and a hypoplastic right ventricle, pulmonic valve, and pulmonary vessels (Fig. 19–16).

Alteration in Hemodynamics. Regardless of the various defects associated with tricuspid atresia, blood flow through the heart is essentially the same. Systemic venous return in these children flows across the atrial septum from the right to the left atrium via a patent foramen ovale or an ASD. This shunt is obligatory because there is no other exit from the right atrium, and it results in complete mixing of desaturated systemic venous blood and fully saturated pulmonary venous blood, which is then ejected by the left ventricle. Most of it flows out the aorta, where a portion shunts left to right across a PDA. Some flows through the VSD, if present, into the right ventricle, but this volume generally is small

TRICUSPID ATRESIA WITHOUT TRANSPOSITION

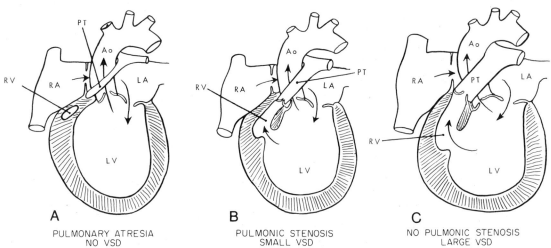

A — PULMONARY ATRESIA NO VSD

B — PULMONIC STENOSIS SMALL VSD

C — NO PULMONIC STENOSIS LARGE VSD

Figure 19–16 ● ● ● ● ● ●

Illustrations of tricuspid atresia with normally related great arteries. In all, the only outlet for right atrial (RA) blood is an interatrial communication. Variations in the ventricular septum and pulmonic valve are depicted. Ao, aorta; LA, left atrium; LV, left ventricle; PT, pulmonary trunk; RV, right ventricle. (From Perloff, J.K. (1994). *The clinical recognition of congenital heart disease*, 4th ed., p. 616. Philadelphia: W.B. Saunders.)

because of the high RVP relative to the small chamber size and because of the relative stenosis of the pulmonic valve and pulmonary vessels. Left heart work is increased as the consequence of volume overload.

Management. Before cardiac catheterization, these sick infants require stabilization of their condition and correction of acidosis. Hypoxia may be controlled or decreased by the use of IV prostaglandin E_1 to maintain ductal patency. At cardiac catheterization, balloon atrial septostomy may be necessary to maintain unrestricted flow across the atrial septum. Because some kind of palliative surgical intervention is generally necessary early on, medical care is directed toward control of hypoxia or CHF.

Surgical Management. Because the majority of children with tricuspid atresia have decreased PBF, palliative shunts to improve PBF are frequently performed in early infancy. The Blalock-Taussig shunt is the procedure of choice in young infants. After 6 months of age, the pulmonary arteries are a sufficient size and PVR is low, permitting either a classic Glenn anastomosis or a bidirectional Glenn shunt. The Glenn anastomosis avoids an increased volume load on the left ventricle and delivers 35% to 45% of the systemic venous return to the pulmonary circulation at low pressure. In infants having undergone a Blalock-Taussig shunt in early infancy, the Glenn procedure is recommended after 6 months, and the systemic arterial shunt is obliterated.

The Glenn procedure serves as a step toward complete right atrium–pulmonary artery connection with various operations that are modifications of the Fontan procedure. The Fontan procedure for repair of tricuspid atresia was first reported in 1971 (Fontan & Baudet). Later, Kreutzer and others (1973) reported their experience with repair of tricuspid atresia. Current modifications of the Fontan technique apply aspects of both Fontan's and Kreutzer's original operations.

The Fontan operation creates the state in which the force driving pulmonary blood flow is gravity. Systemic venous pressure 6 to 8 mmHg higher than ventricular end-diastolic pressure permits flow of blood through the pulmonary vasculature. A number of factors have been identified that limit success with the Fontan operation, including elevated pulmonary vascular resistance and ventricular end-diastolic pressure (i.e., heart failure).

Cyanotic Congenital Heart Defects With Increased PBF

The prenatal failure of the heart and blood vessels to differentiate into distinct systemic and pulmonary vascular systems gives rise to defects that mix arterial and venous blood. The result is cyanosis. The lack of obstruction to blood flow to the lungs results in increased PBF as PVR falls after birth in truncus arteriosus. Total anomalous pulmonary venous connection increases PBF as a consequence of abnormal venous drainage. Hypoplastic left heart syndrome (HLHS) results in increased PBF in the face of inadequate systemic output. (Table 19–9 summarizes the

Table 19–9. CYANOTIC CONGENITAL HEART DEFECTS WITH INCREASED PULMONARY BLOOD FLOW

Defect	Cardiac Examination	Electrocardiogram	Chest Radiograph
TAPVC			
With obstruction	Cardiac murmurs minimal or absent	Right ventricular hypertrophy	Increased pulmonary vascular markings. Normal-sized heart
Without obstruction	Systolic ejection murmur best heard high in the left chest. Mid-diastolic murmur best heard low in the left chest. Widely split S_2	Right axis deviation, right atrial hypertrophy, right ventricular hypertrophy	Supracardiac: "Figure-eight" or "snowman" configuration. All defects: Enlarged right atrium, right ventricle, and main pulmonary artery. Increased pulmonary vascular markings
Truncus arteriosus	Normal S_1, single S_2, ejection click. Loud, continuous (PDA type) murmur with unrestricted PBF. Murmur shortened and softened by decreasing PBF	Left ventricular hypertrophy; biventricular hypertrophy seen occasionally	Nonspecific except for alteration in pulmonary vascular markings. May detect right-sided aortic arch, and pulmonary vessels may arise abnormally high in the chest
HLHS	Dominant RV impulse, decreased impulse at apex. Single S_2 with increased intensity. Diminished peripheral pulse. Gallop rhythm in some, soft systolic murmur at LSB, mid-diastolic rumble at apex	Right ventricular hypertrophy. In some, right atrial enlargement	Cardiomegaly, increased pulmonary vascular markings

HLHS, hypoplastic left heart syndrome; LSB, left sternal border; PBF, pulmonary blood flow; PDA, patent ductus arteriosus; S_1, first heart sound; S_2, second heart sound; TAPVC, total anomalous pulmonary venous return

findings on cardiac examination, ECG, and chest radiograph of children with these defects.)

Total Anomalous Pulmonary Venous Connection

Total anomalous pulmonary venous connection (TAPVC) accounts for only approximately 1% of the total number of congenital heart defects. TAPVC is defined as a failure of pulmonary venous blood to return to the left atrium. Rather, the pulmonary veins enter either the right atrium or another site in the systemic venous system. The anomalous pathway may occur at four different levels: (1) supracardiac via the superior vena cava (Fig. 19–17A); (2) cardiac via the coronary sinus (Fig. 19–17B); (3) cardiac via direct flow to the right atrium; and (4) infradiaphragmatic via the inferior vena cava and the portal vein or ductus venosus (Fig. 19–17C). Most common is supracardiac TAPVC. An ASD, a vital component of this lesion, is always present.

TAPVC may occur with or without obstruction in the pulmonary venous pathway. TAPVC with obstruction occurs predominantly in the infradiaphragmatic type, although obstruction of supradiaphragmatic TAPVC can occur. Obstruction with infradiaphragmatic TAPVC occurs from constriction of the vein as it passes through the diaphragm or from obstruction of flow as it passes through the ductus venosus and the liver. Pulmonary venous drainage can also be obstructed by a small interatrial communication. TAPVC without obstruction occurs equally in males and females; however, TAPVC with obstruction occurs far more frequently in males.

Etiology. The pulmonary venous system develops at about the third week of gestation. The splanchnic plexus, which is connected to the umbilical vitelline veins and the cardinal veins, is in direct communication with the lung buds. The common pulmonary vein, which arises in the common atrium, grows to join the splanchnic plexus. Once the common pulmonary vein and the splanchnic plexus are joined, the cardinal veins and vitelline veins are no longer connected to the splanchnic plexus. The pulmonary veins then drain into the left atrium via the common pulmonary vein. Gradually, the common pulmonary vein is absorbed into the body of the left atrium, and four distinct pulmonary veins draining into the left atrium persist. Failure in any of these steps leading to the formation of the four pulmonary veins results in TAPVC and provides explanation of the anatomic variations seen.

Alteration in Hemodynamics

TAPVC With Obstruction. Blood from both the pulmonary and the systemic venous systems returns to the right atrium. However, because of the presence of an obstruction in the pulmonary venous pathway, the volume of blood that returns to the right atrium is not greatly increased. The right atrium remains normal in size, and the left atrium and ventricle are small. Because of higher pressure in the right than

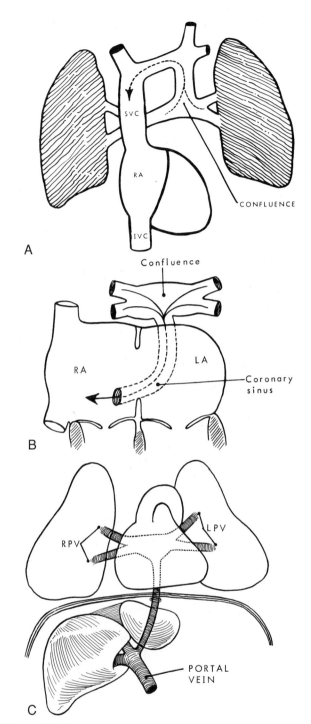

Figure 19–17 ● ● ● ● ● ●

Total anomalous pulmonary venous connection (TAPVC). *A,* Supracardiac TAPVC via a left anomalous vertical vein to the superior vena cava. *B,* Cardiac TAPVC to the coronary sinus. *C,* Infradiaphragmatic TAPVC via the portal venous system. (From Perloff, J.K. (1994). *The clinical recognition of congenital heart disease,* 4th ed., pp. 334, 336. Philadelphia: W.B. Saunders.)

in the left atrium, blood is shunted right-to-left across the ASD.

Because of the obstruction in pulmonary venous flow, pulmonary venous pressure is high, causing a rise in PVR. This leads to pulmonary artery hyper-

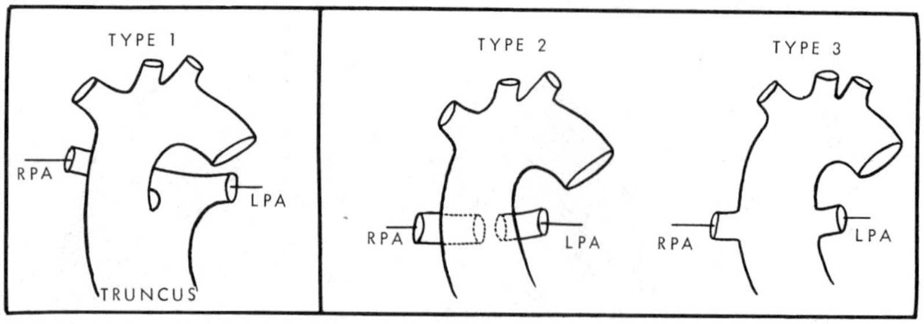

Figure 19–18 ••••••
Illustrations of the various types of truncus arteriosus. In type 1 a short main pulmonary artery arises from the truncus. In types 2 and 3 the branch pulmonary arteries arise directly from the walls of the truncus. (From Perloff, J.K. (1994). *The clinical recognition of congenital heart disease*, 4th ed., p. 688. Philadelphia: W.B. Saunders.)

tension and, in turn, puts stress on the right ventricle and may result in the fixed changes of pulmonary artery hypertension even before birth.

TAPVC Without Obstruction. Blood from both the pulmonary and the systemic venous systems returns to the right atrium, resulting in an increased volume of blood in the right heart. Blood is shunted across the ASD to the left atrium. The right atrium, right ventricle, pulmonary artery, and pulmonary vessels enlarge to compensate for the increased volume. The left atrium and ventricle may be small because of the decreased volume of blood they receive.

Management. The infant with obstructed TAPVC who presents with florid CHF, tachypnea, dyspnea, and pulmonary edema requires rapid and aggressive intervention. Stabilization of cardiovascular status is mandatory while definitive diagnosis is made. Surgery is delayed only a few hours.

Management of TAPVC without obstruction is aimed at controlling CHF and failure to thrive and treating respiratory infections. Surgery can be optimally performed at any age and is usually not delayed, because clinical improvement cannot occur with medical management alone. Untreated infants who survive to older childhood or early adulthood develop pulmonary artery hypertension. Medial hypertrophy and intimal proliferation of the pulmonary arterioles is severe by the third and fourth decades of life.

Definitive Surgical Correction. Surgical correction is performed via a midline sternotomy incision. Cardiopulmonary bypass and hypothermia are used. The common pulmonary vein is anastomosed to the left atrium. The connecting vein to the systemic venous circulation is then ligated, and the ASD is closed. In cardiac TAPVC via the coronary sinus, a patch is placed in the atrial septum to direct coronary sinus and pulmonary venous return into the left atrium. Potential postoperative complications include hemorrhage and acute pulmonary failure. TAPVC with pulmonary venous obstruction has far higher mortality from pulmonary failure.

Truncus Arteriosus

Truncus arteriosus is a rare congenital heart defect, accounting for 1% to 4% of the total number of cardiac defects. It represents failure of the primitive arterial trunk (the truncus arteriosus) to septate and

divide into a distinct aorta and pulmonary artery. Instead, a single large vessel leaves the heart, giving rise to the coronary, systemic, and pulmonary arteries, and containing only one valve. The truncus arteriosus overlies a VSD that is always seen in conjunction with this defect and is an integral part of its pathophysiology. Truncus arteriosus exists in three distinct anatomic variations. Variation occurs with respect to the size and site of origin of the pulmonary arteries. The truncus in all children with this defect features a dominant aorta. In type 1, a short pulmonary trunk arises from the truncus and divides into the branch pulmonary arteries. When the branch pulmonary arteries arise directly from the truncus, they may be close to one another (type 2) or some distance apart (type 3) (Fig. 19–18).

Etiology. The aorta and the pulmonary artery normally develop from the common truncus arteriosus at the end of the third week and during the fourth week of gestation. This occurs by virtue of the unique development of truncoconal ridges, which separate and position the great arteries. Failure of septation of the common trunk results in the persistence of a single vessel that receives blood from both the right and the left ventricles. The VSD is generally large and results from either absence or marked deficiency of the infundibular portion of the septum.

Alteration in Hemodynamics. All infants with truncus arteriosus have a common outlet for right and left ventricular blood. However, the amount of blood flow to the lungs varies, depending on the nature of the pulmonary arteries. Most have well-developed pulmonary arteries and receive several times more blood in their pulmonary circulation than is normal. Rarely, stenosis of the pulmonary arteries limits PBF. Truncal valve insufficiency is not uncommon. If severe, the additional volume load that results is added to the increased demands on the heart from excessive PBF.

Management. Management most often consists of controlling CHF with digoxin and diuretic agents. Surgery may be delayed if heart failure is successfully managed and signs of increasing PVR are not evidenced. Surgery is mandatory at an early age.

Palliative Surgical Management. In the past, for lack of a better alternative, infants with truncus arteriosus who had unrestricted PBF and CHF that was resistant to medical management were treated surgically by palliation with pulmonary artery banding. Now that reparative intervention is possible, palliative banding is no longer recommended. Children who are severely cyanotic because of decreased PBF may be helped by one of the systemic-pulmonary shunts that increase PBF.

Definitive Surgical Correction. Children with increased PBF are candidates for corrective surgical repair of truncus arteriosus. The pulmonary arteries are excised from the common truncus arteriosus and anastomosed to a valved conduit from the right ventricle. The VSD is patched in a manner that locates the truncus arteriosus to the left of the septum, where it functions as the aorta only.

With a prosthetic conduit and valve in place, these children require lifelong prophylaxis against infective endocarditis. No limitations of physical activity are necessary. Surgery is repeated if the conduit malfunctions or as it becomes inadequate in size and needs to be replaced with a larger one.

Hypoplastic Left Heart Syndrome

Hypoplastic left heart syndrome (HLHS) is a common CHD that is universally fatal without surgical intervention. In the last decade surgical reconstruction and heart transplantation have provided early positive outcomes. HLHS accounts for approximately 7% of CHDs presenting in the first year of life.

Etiology. It has been postulated that an embryonic cause of HLHS is limitation of left ventricular outflow. The left ventricle is absent or hypoplastic, and the mitral valve is atretic or hypoplastic. Aortic valve atresia or hypoplasia is a central feature in HLHS. As a result, the ascending aorta is diminutive, and flow to it is retrograde from the ductus arteriosus to the coronary arteries. In the fetus and newborn, the ductus is large and provides the pathway to perfuse the systemic circulation. An interatrial communication is needed for pulmonary venous return, and this usually is a foramen ovale (Fig. 19–19).

Alteration in Hemodynamics. Before birth, systemic perfusion and oxygenation are normal, and the fetus grows and develops normally despite the nonfunctional left ventricle. Systemic circulation is via the right ventricle through the ductus arteriosus. After birth, while ductal patency persists, systemic perfusion is maintained, although decreasing PVR results in increased PBF and impaired systemic perfusion. Cardiomegaly develops with right ventricular hypertrophy and right atrial enlargement in some.

Management. Immediate therapy is directed at restoring hemodynamic stability, correction of metabolic acidosis, and management of heart failure. Prostaglandin infusion restores or maintains ductal patency, permitting adequate systemic perfusion. Manipulation of PVR is necessary to balance pulmonary and systemic flow from the ductus, because low PVR impairs systemic perfusion (Smith & Vernon-Levett, 1993).

Surgical Management. Surgical treatment of HLHS has taken two distinctly different approaches. Heart transplantation is described as a single definitive operation that eliminates the risks of repeated

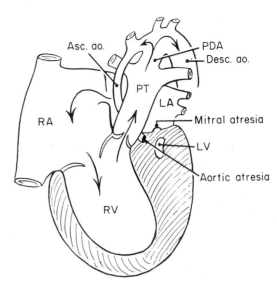

Figure 19–19 ● ● ● ● ● ●
Hypoplastic left heart syndrome (HLHS). Asc ao, ascending aorta; Desc ao, descending aorta; LA, left atrium; LV, left ventricle; PDA, patent ductus arteriosus; PT, pulmonary trunk; RA, right atrium; RV, right ventricle. (From Perloff, J.K. (1994). *The clinical recognition of congenital heart disease*, 4th ed., p. 727. Philadelphia: W.B. Saunders.)

major cardiac surgical procedures and provides the infant a structurally normal heart with two ventricles (Bailey et al., 1986; Bailey & Gundry, 1990). Reconstructive surgery in the newborn is aimed at later physiologic repair with the Fontan procedure (Norwood et al., 1983; Norwood, 1989).

Success with a staged surgical approach to HLHS was first described in 1983 (Norwood et al.). The first stage accomplishes two primary objectives: the establishment of permanent unobstructed flow from the right ventricle to the aorta and regulation of pulmonary blood flow (Fig. 19–20). The hypoplastic ascending aorta is anastomosed to the proximal transected pulmonary artery, and the aortic arch is reconstructed and augmented with a patch of pulmonary artery homograft. Unobstructed flow from the right ventricle through the native pulmonary valve and into the aorta provides systemic and coronary perfusion. PBF is provided by an aortopulmonary shunt, which provides adequate but not excessive PBF. The atrial septum is excised to ensure unimpeded pulmonary venous drainage and maximal mixing of systemic and pulmonary venous return.

Reconstructive surgery leaves the right ventricle subject to a combined pressure and volume load. When PVR is low (after age 6 months), the aortopulmonary shunt is replaced with a superior vena cava–pulmonary artery connection (modified or bidirectional Glenn procedure). Completion of reconstructive surgery is a modified Fontan procedure.

Cyanotic Congenital Heart Defects With Variable PBF

Some complex cyanotic CHDs present with a number of anatomic variations that result in alterations

Reconstructed Ascending Aorta

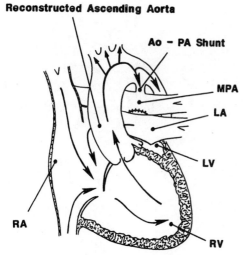

Figure 19–20 ● ● ● ● ●

Circulatory pathway after Stage I reconstructive surgery for HLHS. RA, right atrium; Ao-PA shunt, aorta pulmonary shunt; MPA, main pulmonary artery; LA, left atrium; LV, left ventricle; RV, right ventricle. (From Smith, J.B., & Vernon-Levett, P. (1993). Care of infants with HLHS. *AACN Clinical Issues in Critical Care*, 4:33.)

in the volume of PBF. Complete transposition of the great arteries is a common defect in this group, whereas all others (double outlet right ventricle, double inlet left ventricle, and single ventricle) are rare. These last defects are not discussed in this text.

Transposition of the Great Arteries

Transposition of the great arteries (TGA) accounts for approximately 5% to 7% of the total number of congenital heart defects. It occurs more frequently in males. In TGA, the great arteries are misplaced, or transposed, across the ventricular septum. The pulmonary artery arises from the left ventricle, posterior to the aorta, whereas the aorta arises from the right ventricle at a higher level than, and anterior to, the pulmonary artery (Fig. 19–21). Coexisting cardiac lesions occur in about one half of infants with TGA. The most common is VSD, followed by VSD with subpulmonic stenosis. When a coexisting lesion is present, TGA is often referred to as complicated TGA.

Complete TGA, as just described, is contrasted to *corrected transposition of the great arteries.* Corrected transposition exists when the right and left ventricles are displaced, in addition to displacement of the aorta and pulmonary artery. Because of the ventricular displacement, the pulmonary artery arises from the physiologic venous ventricle, and the aorta arises from the physiologic arterial ventricle. Therefore, systemic venous blood flows to the pulmonary artery and pulmonary venous blood to the aorta, and cyanosis is not present. Complete (i.e., uncorrected) TGA is the focus of this section.

Etiology. Between the third and fourth week of gestation, the truncus arteriosus is divided into the

pulmonary artery and the aorta. This results from spiral growth of the truncoconal ridges. Failure of the truncoconal ridges to spiral or rotate completely results in displacement of the aorta and the pulmonary artery on the ventricles.

Alteration in Hemodynamics

Uncomplicated TGA. The child with uncomplicated TGA essentially has two independent parallel circuits of circulation. Venous blood from the body flows out of the aorta to the body and returns again to the right atrium. Oxygenated blood from the lungs flows out of the pulmonary artery to the lungs and returns again to the left atrium. Intermixing of these two circuits of blood occurs at the foramen ovale and ductus arteriosus. At the level of the foramen ovale, blood is shunted from the left atrium to the right atrium or from the pulmonary circuit to the systemic circuit. Blood is shunted across the ductus arteriosus in the opposite direction from the aorta to the pulmonary artery. This alteration in hemodynamics creates a stress on the right atrium, the right ventricle, and the pulmonary vessels because of the increased volume of blood they continuously receive.

Complicated TGA. The child with TGA complicated by the presence of a VSD has two communicating circuits of circulation, which mix via the VSD. Blood from the right ventricle generally is shunted to the left ventricle because pressure in the pulmonary circuit is less than that in the systemic circuit, once the pulmonary resistance begins to fall after birth. Because an increased volume of blood is returned to the pulmonary circuit via the VSD, the left atrium receives an enlarged volume from the lungs. This causes the pressure in the left atrium to be higher than that in the right atrium. Blood, therefore, is

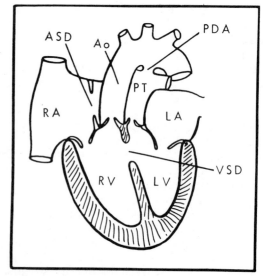

Figure 19–21 ● ● ● ● ●

Complete transposition of the great arteries. Ao, aorta; ASD, atrial septal defect; LA, left atrium; LV, left ventricle; PDA, patent ductus arteriosus; PT, pulmonary trunk; RA, right atrium; RV, right ventricle; VSD, ventricular septal defect. (From Perloff, J.K. (1994). *The clinical recognition of congenital heart disease*, 4th ed., p. 658. Philadelphia: W.B. Saunders.)

shunted from the left atrium to the right atrium via the foramen ovale. Enlargement of the right ventricle, left atrium, left ventricle, main pulmonary artery, and pulmonary vessels develops from these alterations.

The presence of subpulmonic stenosis as well as of a VSD alters the hemodynamics. Left ventricular outflow tract obstruction decreases blood flow to the lungs and increases left ventricular pressure. As a result of the increased left ventricular pressure, a greater amount of blood is shunted to the right ventricle and subsequently sent out of the aorta. Therefore, more oxygenated blood is delivered to the body. However, as the degree of obstruction increases, a substantial decrease in PBF occurs. LAP decreases, and blood is shunted from the right atrium to the left atrium. This causes further desaturation of blood delivered to the right ventricle and the aorta via the VSD and an increase in the cyanosis observed. Enlargement of the right atrium, right ventricle, and left ventricle and a decrease in size of the main pulmonary artery and the pulmonary vessels are seen. Table 19–10 summarizes the clinical findings in infants with TGA.

Management. Management in the newborn is aimed at correcting metabolic acidosis and increasing arterial oxygenation. Metabolic acidosis is corrected by the use of sodium bicarbonate. Arterial oxygenation is increased by administration of prostaglandin to maintain patency of the ductus arteriosus or by balloon atrial septostomy during cardiac catheterization. Digoxin and diuretic therapy are indicated in the infant with large intercirculatory shunts and CHF.

Surgical Management. Surgical repair of TGA is an example of progress and "change" in pediatric cardiac surgery that has occurred over the last 30 to 40 years. Some of the progress is the result of interest in "old" ideas. The first repairs of TGA were attempts at anatomic correction, placing the pulmonary artery and aorta in their normal anatomic positions. These operations, performed by Bailey in 1954 (Bailey et al., 1975) and by Kay and Cross in 1955, did not include transfer of the coronary arteries and resulted in universal mortality. Mustard and coworkers also performed an anatomic correction in 1954, with transfer of the left coronary artery, but also without success.

The focus of attempts to repair TGA then shifted from anatomic correction to "physiologic repair" by rerouting pulmonary and systemic venous return through a baffle of Dacron or pericardium, such that each atrium emptied into the opposite ventricle. First successfully applied by Senning (1959), the procedure was modified by Mustard (1964). Risk of mortality with either procedure is now low, but long-term survival of patients with these repairs has revealed late problems. Complications include systemic (right) ventricular dysfunction or failure and symptomatic arrhythmias (Turina et al., 1988).

Even before recognition of the long-term problems associated with atrial correction of TGA, attempts at developing a successful method of anatomic correction continued. Interest heightened as complications of older procedures were evidenced. Jatene and associates performed the first successful arterial switch operation (ASO) in 1975. Initially, the ASO was used only in infants diagnosed with TGA and a VSD. Use of the ASO was later expanded to include those patients with TGA and intact ventricular septum (IVS). Currently, the ASO is performed with the same low mortality expected with either atrial correction and is the operation of choice for infants with TGA. Long-term follow-up studies are in progress (Weindling, 1994).

Some infants with TGA cannot undergo ASO because of concurrent illness from premature delivery or respiratory disease, other perinatal factors, or the presence of complicating heart defects. Palliation with balloon atrial septostomy or surgical creation of an ASD; pulmonary artery banding in those with a large VSD and CHF; or systemic–pulmonary artery

Table 19–10. CYANOTIC CONGENITAL HEART DEFECTS WITH VARIABLE PULMONARY BLOOD FLOW (TGA)

Defect	Cardiac Examination	Electrocardiogram	Radiograph
TGA			
Uncomplicated	Murmur may not be present S_2 louder than normal and accentuated	Right ventricular hypertrophy, possible right atrial hypertrophy, right axis deviation. May be normal in newborn	Cardiomegaly, narrow mediastinum, increased pulmonary vascular markings. May be normal in newborn
Complicated (with VSD)	Loud S_2 Holosystolic murmur best heard at 4th ICS to left of sternum. Thrill may be present	Right ventricular hypertrophy	Cardiomegaly, narrow mediastinum, increased pulmonary vascular markings
Complicated (with VSD and sub-PS)	Loud S_2 Holosystolic murmur. Ejection systolic murmur best heard along left sternal border	Right ventricular hypertrophy	Cardiomegaly, narrow mediastinum, decreased pulmonary vascular markings

ICS, intercostal space; S_2, second heart sound; sub-PS, subvalvular pulmonic stenosis; TGA, transposition of the great arteries; VSD, ventricular septal defect

shunts in those with severe left ventricular outflow tract obstruction can often be performed with less operative risk. They permit stabilization until definitive surgery is possible.

PERIOPERATIVE MANAGEMENT OF PEDIATRIC CARDIAC SURGICAL PATIENTS

Advances in the surgical management of infants and children with congenital heart defects have significantly affected their postoperative management, as well. Broadened understanding of the anatomy and pathophysiology of various structural defects, improved understanding of neonatal physiology, use of profound hypothermia and circulatory arrest during surgery, and technologic advances in critical care instrumentation and pharmacologic intervention have combined to improve postoperative outcomes (Craig, 1991). Currently, even complex lesions are amenable to complete repair during infancy. Exceptions are defects involving single ventricle physiology.

Repair of CHD early in life can prevent or diminish the pathologic sequelae that result from prolonged abnormal hemodynamics and cyanosis. However, some unique features of the physiologic responses of the youngest cardiac surgery patients continue to challenge their postoperative management. Table 19–11 compares the advantages and disadvantages of cardiac surgery during the first month of life.

Following birth, parents of critically ill infants are often faced with the immediate transport of their infant to a center that is specifically equipped to treat the baby. Transport to a center many miles away is coupled with the stress of surgery necessary at an early age. Prenatal diagnosis permits planning to expedite the management of the infant known to have a heart defect (Sanders, 1992), as well as affording time for parental preparation and education. Parents of older infants and children are not immune to the stress of facing a major cardiac operation and may also be a distance from home and their usual sources of support.

Preoperative Preparation

An uncomplicated operative and postoperative course for cardiac surgery patients begins with preoperative assessment and preparation. All infants and children have a careful history and physical examination before surgery. The focus of the examination is to discover acute medical illnesses (upper respiratory infection, pneumonia, otitis media) that would necessitate rescheduling elective surgery, because the risk of respiratory complications is high in children who require endotracheal intubation during the course of an upper respiratory infection (Cohen & Cameron, 1991). Dental infection requires preoperative treatment to avoid the risk of subacute bacterial endocarditis, and may also necessitate rescheduling elective operations. Chronic medical problems such as diabetes, asthma, and seizure disorders, which require special management, are identified.

Routine laboratory and radiology assessments are performed. A chest radiograph is obtained in all patients. For those children having closed-heart operations of an elective nature, only a complete blood count and urinalysis are required. Seriously ill patients and those scheduled for open-heart operations generally have prothrombin time, partial thromboplastin time, platelet count, and serum electrolyte test samples obtained in addition. These laboratory tests identify problems that may require correction before surgery or special attention during the operation.

Newborn infants with severe obstructive congenital heart defects may present with severe heart failure and inadequate tissue perfusion, oliguria, and acidosis or severe cyanosis as the ductus arteriosus (DA) closes. Stabilization of the infant's condition is permitted by an intravenous infusion of prostaglandin E_1 to open the ductus and maintain its patency. Infants with severe cyanotic heart lesions are improved when ductal patency is maintained, because systemic oxygenation is significantly increased. Infants with TGA may have improved mixing and better oxygenation following balloon atrial septostomy, which is performed at cardiac catheterization. Preoperative measures to stabilize the infant's condition prevent emergency surgery in a very ill baby. Acidosis and prerenal failure resolve and cardiac failure is improved.

Perioperative Techniques

Since the introduction of the heart-lung machine nearly 40 years ago, efforts have continued toward the development of safe and reliable methods to control circulation during cardiac surgery. Refinement of these methods has improved outcomes over the past

Table 19–11. SURGICAL REPAIR OF CONGENITAL HEART DEFECTS IN THE NEONATAL PERIOD

Advantages	Disadvantages
Tolerance of hypoxia	Maintenance of BP may mask shock
CNS plasticity and resilience	Stress response to CPB may be extreme
Minimal secondary organ (i.e., heart, lung, brain) dysfunction from chronic CHF or cyanosis	Myocardial reserve (systolic and diastolic) is limited
Maximal potential for growth and development	PVR is labile
	Metabolism is fragile (glucose, acid-base balance easily disturbed)
	Nutritional reserve is limited
	Metabolic rate is high
	Liver and renal function is immature

BP, blood pressure; CHF, congestive heart failure; CNS, central nervous system; CPB, cardiopulmonary bypass; PVR, pulmonary vascular resistance

years, but cardiopulmonary bypass, hypothermia, circulatory arrest, and aortic cross-clamping can precipitate physiologic derangements in major organs during surgery, which continue into the postoperative period (Craig, 1991).

Cardiopulmonary Bypass (CPB)

CPB provides tissue perfusion and oxygenation, bypassing the patient's own heart and lungs, using a mechanical pump and oxygenator. To reroute blood, cannulas are placed in the right atrium and in the ascending aorta. Blood is removed from the right atrium, circulated through the oxygenator, and returned to the ascending aorta. Banked fresh blood is used to prime the pump circuit, and diluted to a hematocrit of about 30%. Heparin is used to provide anticoagulation, which is needed to prevent clotting of the blood in the bypass circuit.

Myocardial Protection

Bypass of the heart and lungs necessitates attention to protection of the myocardium during cardiac surgery. Both hypothermia and chemical preservation of the myocardium are currently employed.

Hypothermia and Circulatory Arrest. Moderate (20°–25°C) and deep (15°–18°C) hypothermia decreases the body's oxygen consumption, thereby protecting the brain and other vital organs during low circulatory flow with CPB. The protective effect of hypothermia is generally attributed to decreased cellular metabolic activity, reflected by both decreased oxygen consumption and glucose utilization. Core or surface cooling may be used singly or in combination. Surface cooling begins before the incision is made, and is facilitated by the environmental temperature and use of hypothermia blankets and/or ice packs. Core cooling is accomplished using the heat exchanger in the pump oxygenator. Heart rate and blood pressure decrease as body temperature falls, with asystole generally occurring between 24° and 22°C. Cooling is continued to a body temperature less than 20°C. Deep hypothermia permits circulatory arrest: the cessation of CPB. The intracardiac cannulas are removed, allowing an unobstructed field for the surgeon to perform the procedure.

Most of that which is known about morphologic changes in organ systems associated with hypothermic circulatory arrest is based on animal research. Overall, these studies indicate that the relatively short periods of hypothermic arrest required for repair of CHD are not associated with significant end-organ injury or dysfunction. Complications include renal insufficiency, necrotizing enterocolitis, liver necrosis, and atelectasis. Low-flow states in the early postoperative period or diversion of blood from visceral organs is implicated most frequently.

Impairment of the functional integrity of the brain following hypothermia and circulatory arrest has been the focus of intensive investigation since the 1960s. Experimental animal studies indicate that ce-

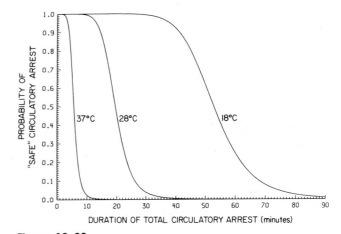

Figure 19–22 ● ● ● ● ● ●

Nomogram of probably safe circulatory arrest times in patients at various degrees of hypothermia. (From Kirklin, J.W., & Barratt-Boyes, B.G. (Eds.). (1993). *Cardiac surgery*, (2nd ed., p. 74). New York: John Wiley & Sons.)

rebral hypothermia prolongs the development of, although it cannot prevent, the metabolic and structural changes that lead to functional neurologic impairment (Mavroudis & Greene, 1992). Prolonged periods of cerebral hypothermia, without circulatory arrest, produce irreversible brain injury in animal models. Infants with adverse neurologic sequelae after periods of hypothermia and circulatory arrest demonstrate seizures, choreoathetosis, paresis, rigidity, muscular hypotonia, intellectual impairment, coma, and death (Mavroudis & Greene, 1992). A period of 35 to 45 minutes of hypothermia and circulatory arrest is judged to be "safe" (Kirklin, 1986). A nomogram can be used to estimate the probability of a "safe" circulatory arrest time (Fig. 19–22).

Aortic Cross-clamping and Chemical Myocardial Protection. When desired cooling is achieved, the heart-lung machine can be turned off, the aorta cross-clamped to prevent backflow into the left ventricle, and the heart drained to create a bloodless operating field. Myocardial protection from ischemia is achieved by decreasing metabolic and oxygen requirements with hypothermia and elective cardiac arrest. Electromechanical arrest is accomplished with injection of cold (4°C) cardioplegic solution into the aortic root. Immediate cardiac arrest and flaccidity of the heart muscle occur.

A cardioplegic solution should provide rapid and complete cardiac arrest, maintain the myocardial electrolyte environment, deliver substrates and wash out metabolites, maintain cellular pH at a protective level, and permit surgery with a bloodless operating field (Iannettoni & Bove, 1992). Although many different solutions are used in cardiac surgery today, the search for a "perfect" solution continues. Cardioplegic solutions use constituents that approximate extracellular fluid with large amounts of additional potassium to induce diastolic cardiac arrest. Potassium also prevents calcium influx, as does magnesium, a second major component of cardioplegic solutions. Magnesium also inhibits calcium release from the sarcoplasmic reticulum and reduces mitochondrial uptake of calcium. Alterations in calcium homeostasis are related to ischemic cell membrane damage and to subsequent myocardial cellular swelling and death.

Cardioplegic solutions provide significant myocardial protection, because the heart is maintained in diastole with minimal metabolic requirements, electrolyte balance is maintained, and rebeating is prevented. The operation is then performed using either a low-flow state on CPB or with the circulation arrested.

Rewarming

When the intracardiac repair is completed, surface and core warming are begun. CPB is resumed and the aortic cross-clamp removed. Spontaneous ventricular contractions usually occur at a temperature of 30° to 32°C. If the heart does not begin to beat spontaneously, electrical defibrillation may be needed. When the body temperature is nearly normal, bypass is discontinued.

Potential Postoperative Complications

The potential for complications is high following cardiac surgery in infants and children. It is necessary to maintain a high level of suspicion with regard to potential problems to detect them and intervene as early as possible.

Inadequate Tissue Perfusion

Tissue perfusion is dependent on the adequacy of cardiac output, which, in the immediate postoperative period, may change rapidly. Continuous assessment of the patient's hemodynamic status from peripheral pulses and temperature of the extremities, capillary refill, core temperature, arterial blood pressure, and filling pressures is key to the early identification of difficulty. Tissue perfusion is dependent on myocardial contractility, intravascular volume (preload), resistance to ventricular ejection (afterload), and heart rate. Low CO and impaired perfusion can be the consequence of (1) decreased intravascular volume from excessive losses, inadequate replacement, cardiac tamponade, or excessive diuresis; (2) increased systemic or pulmonary vascular resistance from vasoconstriction or hypertension; (3) decreased ventricular contractility from myocardial injury resulting from inadequate intraoperative protection, hypoxia, or CPB or from acidosis or electrolyte imbalance; (4) alteration in heart rate or rhythm; or (5) inadequate intracardiac repair with residual shunts or valve lesions. These are summarized in Table 19–12.

Inadequate Intravascular Volume. Adequate preload is essential to maintain cardiac output. Postoperatively, volume replacement may be necessary

Table 19–12. DIFFERENTIAL DIAGNOSIS OF INADEQUATE TISSUE PERFUSION

Etiology	Critical Signs*
Inadequate Preload	
Fluid Volume Deficit	Low ventricular filling pressures
Increased losses	LAP, RAP <3–5 mmHg
Inadequate replacement	CVP <5–8 mmHg
Cardiac Tamponade	Acute increase in filling pressures
Pericardial hematoma	LAP, RAP, CVP rise
Myocardial swelling	Acute decrease in chest drainage
Excessive Afterload	
Increased SVR	Normal to increased systemic
Decreased tissue	arterial pressure
perfusion	Cool, mottled extremities
SNS stimulation	Decreased peripheral pulses
Increased PVR	Acute rise in PA pressures
Hypoxia, hypercarbia	Cyanosis
Suctioning	Bradycardia
Agitation, pain	Death (a potential consequence)
Myocardial Dysfunction	
Chemical	High ventricular filling pressures
Hypothermia	LAP, RAP > 12 mmHg
Acidosis	CVP > 15–18 mmHg
Electrolyte imbalance	
Hypoxia	
Functional	
Preoperative dysfunction	
Prolonged ischemic time	
Residual hemodynamic	
problems	
Cardiac Rhythm Disturbances	ECG abnormalities

CVP, central venous pressure; ECG, electrocardiogram; LAP, left atrial pressure; RAP, right atrial pressure; SNS, sympathetic nervous system
*Seen in addition to the typical clinical signs of inadequate tissue perfusion

because of postoperative bleeding, expansion of the vascular space during rewarming, third-spacing of fluid, or diuresis. Postoperative bleeding may be the result of inadequate heparin reversal at the end of CPB or may be surgical in nature. Blood coagulation problems are assessed and corrected. Surgical bleeding is suspected when chest tube drainage is greater than 3 mL/kg/hour for over 3 hours or 5 to 10 mL/kg in any 1 hour. Volume loss of this nature is significant in light of total blood volume in infants and children (i.e., neonates 85–90 mL/kg, infants 75–80 mL/kg, children 70–75 mL/kg) and may require reoperation.

The type and amount of fluid administered when preload is inadequate is based on the patient's hematocrit and the nature of the fluid lost. Packed red blood cells are administered to patients who are bleeding or have a significantly decreased hematocrit. Fresh-frozen plasma is administered to replace clotting factors. To treat hypovolemia unrelated to bleeding, colloid or crystalloid may be infused. Boluses of fluid or blood are administered in volumes of 5 to 10 mL/kg over several minutes with filling pressures carefully assessed. Increasing LV filling pressure to a LAP greater than 14 to 16 mmHg rarely provides any additional improvement in cardiac performance.

Tamponade. Cardiac tamponade causes compression of the atria, restricting venous return to the heart and resulting in limited ventricular preload. Since early cardiac tamponade is the consequence of persistent surgical bleeding not sufficiently evacuated by the chest drains, it is essential that mediastinal or chest drainage tubes be kept patent. Evacuation of the pericardial space may be necessary if chest tube output abruptly decreases or stops and the patient becomes hemodynamically unstable. Additional signs include elevated venous or filling pressures, neck vein distension, systemic arterial hypotension, and narrow pulse pressure. The decline in arterial pressure is unresponsive to volume administration.

Cardiac tamponade necessitates prompt surgical reexploration to evacuate the pericardial hematoma and control bleeding, if excessive. If the patient's hemodynamic status is deteriorating rapidly, the sternotomy may be opened in the ICU to relieve the cardiac compression. With the situation stabilized and the circumstances less pressing, patency of the chest tubes is reestablished with aseptic manipulation of suction or thrombectomy catheters. If there is any question with regard to the diagnosis of tamponade, echocardiography can quickly demonstrate its presence or absence. Unnecessary reopening of the chest in a patient without tamponade is avoided.

Occasionally, myocardial swelling and chamber dilation prevent closing the newborn cardiac surgery patient's chest at the end of operation because of hemodynamic instability. Leaving the sternum open with the mediastinum covered with an impermeable sheet of Silastic is an option. Once myocardial swelling has subsided and both cardiac and pulmonary function have stabilized, the sternum can be closed electively in the PICU.

Excessive Afterload. Increased systemic vascular resistance (SVR) is most often the consequence of sympathetic nervous system (SNS) attempts to compensate for inadequate tissue perfusion. Increased SVR is poorly tolerated in the postoperative period when myocardial performance is most often near maximal levels. Inappropriately elevated SVR is signaled by normal to increased systemic arterial pressure accompanied by cool, mottled extremities, delayed capillary refill, and weak peripheral pulses. Metabolic acidosis may be evidenced. Treatment is aimed at reduction of afterload with vasodilator therapy.

Similarly, increases in PVR can impede pulmonary blood flow and limit left ventricular preload. Also of concern are pulmonary hypertensive crises, characterized by an acute rise in pulmonary artery pressure, which reduces cardiac output and oxygen saturation dramatically. Most often, pulmonary hypertensive crises occur in infants who have had surgical repair of a congenital cardiac defect with a large left-to-right shunt and pulmonary artery hypertension (atrioventricular canal, truncus arteriosus, unrestrictive VSD), or in infants with labile PVR (the newborn following initial reconstruction of HLHS). Pulmonary hypertension most often occurs after endotracheal tube suctioning as a result of hypoxia and hypercarbia. Hypothermia, acidosis, and alpha-adrenergic agents are also sometimes implicated, as are pain, agitation, pulmonary overinflation, increased mean airway pressure, and endotracheal tube manipulation (Backer & Mavroudis, 1993; Norris & Roland, 1994).

Once the pulmonary hypertensive crisis begins, it can be difficult to interrupt what becomes a downward spiral of hypoxemia and hypercarbia, further increases in PVR, and low CO. Sudden death during the first postoperative night after apparently successful congenital heart surgery is a documented phenomenon in patients with labile pulmonary artery hypertension (Castaneda et al., 1994), probably related to changes in the level of anesthesia, adequacy of mechanical ventilation, and interventions that distress the infant and interfere with oxygenation and ventilation. Treatment includes hyperventilation with 100% oxygen, administration of intravenous fentanyl or morphine for analgesia and calming, and paralysis with neuromuscular blocking agents.

Despite intensive attempts to reverse the pulmonary hypertensive crisis, these events may be fatal. Therefore, their prevention is vitally important. Ensuring adequate oxygenation and ventilation, minimizing noxious stimuli (especially unnecessary endotracheal suctioning), and administering sufficient sedation and analgesia for the first 24 to 48 hours following cardiac surgery are critical.

Myocardial Dysfunction. Low CO is likely the result of myocardial dysfunction when signs of inadequate tissue perfusion are accompanied by high ventricular filling pressures. Elevated ventricular end-diastolic volume and pressure are the markers of heart failure. Myocardial performance may be depressed by drugs, anesthesia, ischemia, hypoxia, and acidosis, as well as by an extensive ventriculotomy, myocardial resection, or residual hemodynamic abnormalities. Both inotropic and afterload-reducing agents are useful in improving cardiac performance. If pharmacologic therapy is ineffective, a mechanical assist device or extracorporeal membrane oxygenation may be useful.

Cardiac Rhythm Disturbances. Cardiac dysrhythmias are not uncommon after cardiac operations. Although many do not require treatment, because tissue perfusion is not compromised, treatment may be necessitated if the ventricular rate is either too slow or too rapid to maintain adequate cardiac output. In addition to specific treatment, it is important to correct electrolyte and acid-base disturbances, if present.

Critical Care Management

The primary objective of the postoperative critical care of pediatric cardiac surgery patients is the ongoing assessment and monitoring of hemodynamic status to detect common postoperative problems as early as possible, to intervene effectively, and to ensure adequate tissue perfusion. Both invasive and noninvasive methods are useful to monitor hemodynamic stability. Heart rate and rhythm, preload, afterload (both systemic and pulmonary vascular resistance), and contractility are continuously assessed. Decisions to provide pharmacologic or mechanical support are based on careful attention to hemodynamic status.

Hemodynamic Assessment

The invasive monitoring devices to be used postoperatively are established in the operating room. Invasive hemodynamic monitoring is the cornerstone of postoperative assessment. However, it is also important to recognize that the accuracy of the hemodynamic variables obtained is dependent on ensuring the systems' accuracy and that numbers have limits. The significance of simultaneous and ongoing assessment of patients after cardiac surgery by knowledgeable professional caregivers cannot be overestimated.

Heart Rate and Rhythm. A decrease or sustained increase in heart rate or variation from normal sinus rhythm has the potential to compromise CO. Heart rate and rhythm are monitored by continuous ECG. The perioperative and postoperative periods represent a time of unique physiologic stress. Heart rate is anticipated to be elevated toward the high end of the normal range. Given the limited systolic reserve characteristic of infants, tachycardia serves to maintain CO. However, sustained very high heart rate or tachydysrhythmia will reduce CO and systemic tissue perfusion.

Cardiac rhythm disturbances are not uncommon following cardiac operations. Potential causes during the operation include the surgery itself, anesthesia, cardiopulmonary bypass with or without deep hypothermia, manipulation of the conduction pathways of the heart, and high levels of endogenous and exogenous catecholamines (Castaneda et al., 1994). Additional causes during the postoperative period are metabolic and electrolyte imbalances, volume changes, hypoxemia, and hypothermia. Exogenous catecholamines, if required, predispose to rhythm disturbance, as does digoxin toxicity.

In postoperative cardiac surgery patients, ventricular dysrhythmias and atrial fibrillation are uncommon outside the older adolescent age group or in adult patients with CHD. Automatic tachycardia originating either in the atria (EAT) or at the AV junction (JET) is more common in infants following cardiac surgery than in other age groups. Conduction delay or block is associated with repair of defects near the conduction system.

There is some therapeutic value in maintaining an infant with JET at subnormal temperatures (33°–36°C). Continuous monitoring of the temperature is needed to avoid excessive hypothermia, which may precipitate ventricular dysrhythmias. When therapeutic cooling is used, cold stress and shivering are avoided by maintaining anesthesia or deep sedation and administration of skeletal muscle relaxants.

Systemic Arterial Blood Pressure. Continuous monitoring of the systemic blood pressure by means of an indwelling arterial catheter is essential. Noninvasive blood pressure measurements may not be accurate in the early postoperative period if hypothermia persists, and are not adequate in the face of potentially rapid changes in hemodynamic status. Potential for low CO and inadequate tissue perfusion is high in the early hours following cardiac surgery and may be related to a number of physiologic problems. It is important to bear in mind that infants and young children have vasoconstriction when stroke volume is decreased because of sympathetic nervous system compensatory responses. Hypotension, therefore, is most often a late sign of low CO. However, data from the systemic arterial pressure are often significant in the early detection of potential postoperative problems.

Cardiac tamponade presents with a narrowed pulse pressure as one of its classic manifestations. Other manifestations include a decrease in the mean arterial pressure, equalization and rising of the left and right atrial pressures, and abrupt cessation or marked decrease in the volume of chest tube drainage.

In contrast, a widened pulse pressure may indicate a *large aortic runoff.* For example, widened pulse pressure is a characteristic finding in a patient with PDA. As well, widened pulse pressure in a patient with a Blalock-Taussig shunt (BTS) indicates shunt patency.

In infants who have undergone a right BTS, the right radial artery is avoided as a monitoring site and noninvasive blood pressure is not measured in the right arm. Sacrifice of the right subclavian artery renders this site inaccurate. The same is true when coarctation repair is performed using a subclavian flap.

Monitoring Atrial Pressures. Central venous pressure (CVP) or right atrial pressure (RAP) provides information about systemic venous return, vascular volume, and right heart function. Transduced as a mean pressure, CVP and RAP reflect right ventricular end-diastolic pressure (RVEDP). Right ventricular failure is more common in infants than in adult patients. Elevated RAP, often as high as 15 to 18 mmHg, is sometimes noted in infants after right ventriculotomy, and is indicative of RV failure (Castaneda et al., 1994).

Although RAP is generally lower than the left atrial pressure (LAP), RV failure elevates RAP to levels greater than LAP. Following surgery to repair tetralogy of Fallot, RAP is often greater than LAP, reflecting the decreased compliance of the hypertrophied RV, as well as heart failure related to the right ventricular incision.

LAP provides information about pulmonary venous pressure, systemic volume, left ventricular (LV) preload, and LV function. Transduced as a mean pressure, it reflects LV end-diastolic pressure (LVEDP).

Low LAP, if accurate, sensitively indicates hypovolemia. In postoperative cardiac surgery patients, administration of intravascular volume to increase the LAP is indicated. If hemodynamic instability develops despite additional volume, pharmacologic support may be required.

In addition to monitoring the mean CVP or atrial pressure to determine preload and ventricular function, assessment of waveform morphology in patients following cardiac surgery yields important information postoperatively about cardiac structure and function. Large a waves result from increased resistance to ventricular filling (mitral or tricuspid stenosis, aortic or pulmonic stenosis, pulmonary hypertension, or when the atrium contracts against a closed AV valve, as occurs with nodal rhythm or AV dissociation). The a waves are absent in atrial fibrillation. Tall v waves are seen in mitral or tricuspid regurgitation, VSD, ASD, and CHF. In patients who have undergone repair of AVSD, a and v waves are carefully evaluated for evidence of tricuspid or mitral insufficiency.

Monitoring Pulmonary Artery Pressure. Pulmonary artery pressure (PAP) monitoring provides information about RV function, right ventricular outflow tract (RVOT) patency, PVR and reactivity, venous pressure in the lungs, and mean filling pressures on the left side of the heart. PAP is monitored as systolic, diastolic, and mean pressures. PA diastolic pressure corresponds to the LAP if there is no left-sided problem (e.g., mitral regurgitation). The systolic PAP is the same as the RV systolic pressure under normal circumstances.

Systemic or suprasystemic PAP in patients who have undergone cardiac surgery, usually those with a history of significant left-to-right shunting or neonates with persistent pulmonary hypertension, presents a unique problem postoperatively. Measures to avoid reflexive pulmonary vasospasm and decrease PVR are necessary. PA pressure monitoring after surgical repair of TOF provides information about residual VSD and adequacy of RVOT reconstruction. Residual VSD is suspected if PA oxygen saturations are greater than those in the RA (see below). Adequacy of RVOT reconstruction is confirmed by documenting a pressure pullback tracing as the PA line is withdrawn through the RV at the time of removal. The maximum gradient from PA to RV is measured, documented, and reported.

Monitoring Oxygenation

Systemic oxygen saturation is often monitored continuously by noninvasive pulse oximetry technique in postoperative cardiac surgery patients. Clearly, patients with complex CHD who undergo palliative reconstructive procedures are *not* anticipated to have "normal" oxygen saturation or PaO_2. However, observing trends in data from the pulse oximeter can be helpful.

Invasive monitoring of oxygen saturation also affords important data. Oxygen saturation measurements obtained from the RA line are placement-dependent. High oxygen saturation occurs in patients with high output states, left-to-right shunts, or in those in whom the catheter tip is in the superior vena cava or hepatic vein. Decreased saturation is noted in patients with low CO or those in whom the catheter tip is located in the coronary sinus or low in the inferior vena cava (Elixson, 1989).

The PA oxygen saturation is a mixed venous sample. Continuous or intermittent monitoring provides valuable information regarding oxygen supply and demand.

Simultaneous PA and RA oxygen saturations in patients receiving less than 50% inspired oxygen can help to identify residual VSD. A step up in the PA saturation from the value obtained in the RA, especially if the saturation is greater than 80%, strongly suggests the presence of a residual VSD. A PA oxygen saturation less than 80%, in the presence of normal PA pressure, virtually rules out a significant residual left-to-right shunt (Kulik, 1989).

Caring for Patients With Intracardiac Lines

Transthoracic intracardiac monitoring catheters are placed at the conclusion of surgery to guide postoperative patient assessment and management. On arrival in the PICU, chest radiographs demonstrate line location (Fig. 19–23). This information is essential in evaluating pressure and oxygen saturation data.

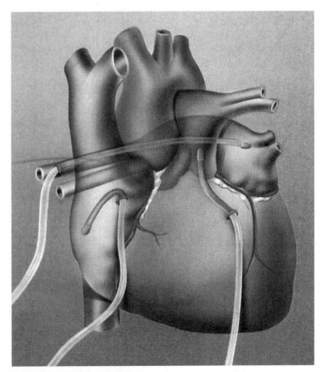

Figure 19–23 ● ● ● ● ● ●

Transthoracic, intracardiac line locations. (From Barker, S. (1993). *CV Nurse*, Second Issue 1993.)

Although RA lines may be considered for use to provide for long-term IV access, hydration, and alimentation, most intracardiac lines are reserved for hemodynamic monitoring. Maintaining a closed, sterile system is essential to prevent infection. In addition, with the left atrial catheter there are serious potential implications of an embolus in the systemic circulation. Meticulous care to avoid air emboli, in particular, is crucial, and the LA line is used only for monitoring purposes unless there is a frank emergency and no other vascular access is available.

Once intracardiac monitoring lines are no longer indicated, removal is accomplished in the PICU by specially trained nurses (Moynihan et al., 1992) or physicians. All possible data that may be needed from these lines are obtained before their removal. Examples include RA and PA oxygen saturations, an LA tracing to demonstrate elevated v waves, and PA pullback to assess for RVOT obstruction.

Complications are associated with removal of intracardiac lines. It is imperative to anticipate potential complications and, when possible, limit factors that may contribute to risk.

Bleeding and Tamponade (PA, LA). Availability of a unit of blood in the blood bank must be assured. In the case of patients with suprasystemic pulmonary artery pressure, it may be preferable to have the blood available at the bedside. Prothrombin time (PT), partial thromboplastin time (PTT), and platelet count results are obtained within the 12 hours preceding line removal. If an abnormal value is detected, treatment is provided to correct the abnormality before line removal. Patency of the patient's chest or mediastinal drains is ensured. Some physicians prescribe sedation before the removal of LA and PA lines to keep the child from crying, coughing, or performing another stimulus that may increase intravascular pressure (Backer & Mavroudis, 1993). A small amount of bleeding is not unusual, but persistent bleeding or tamponade may require evacuation. If signs of tamponade are noted, turning the patient side to side or sitting the patient up may effectively drain the collection.

Entrapment (RA, LA). Entrapment is the inability to remove an intracardiac line using the usual gentle pulling motion. Although some resistance may be felt at times, no line should ever be forcibly removed because the catheter may fragment. The line may be loosened with tension applied to it for approximately 1 hour. If this is not successful, the line is often entrapped in the fascia. The surgeon may open a portion of the sternal incision to attempt removal. If unsuccessful, cardiac catheterization or reoperation may be necessary (Gold & Castaneda, 1987).

Dysrhythmias. Rhythm abnormalities are most often noted with removal of PA lines and are most likely to occur as the line enters the right ventricle. Dysrhythmias are generally transient, but may momentarily affect the heart rate and blood pressure.

Timing. Lines are generally removed in the following order: first the PA, then the LA, and finally the RA. Optimally, the PA and LA lines are removed

before extubation to ensure an adequate airway in the event of an emergent complication. Up to 20 to 30 minutes are allowed to elapse between discontinuing each line to permit assessment for bleeding, tamponade, or hemodynamic instability.

Wound Care. Following cardiac operations, the surgical incision is routinely covered with a dry sterile dressing. After intracardiac lines and chest drainage tubes are discontinued, the dressing is usually removed and the incision left uncovered.

There is no standard technique for wound care in patients in whom sternal closure is delayed. Maintenance of sterility and protecting the patient from infection are priorities. Wound edges are cleansed with normal saline and iodophor solution, antibacterial ointment is applied to the wound edges, and the Silastic mesh is covered loosely with dry sterile dressing. If signs of tamponade occur, the incision site is assessed immediately. If the Silastic mesh appears full, immediate evacuation of the chest is indicated. When the chest is open, the water-seal chamber of the chest suction should bubble and the patient is kept clinically paralyzed and sedated. A high level of suspicion regarding subtle signs of infection is maintained and wound closure is achieved as soon as possible in the PICU or operating room.

Respiratory Care

Following cardiac surgery, most patients arrive in the PICU intubated. Report to the postoperative caregivers includes information about the patient's intubation and problems with it or with ventilatory management during the perioperative period. Initial assessment of the patient includes auscultation of the lungs to determine the appropriateness of the endotracheal tube position and the adequacy of alveolar ventilation. These clinical assessments are confirmed by chest radiographs and arterial blood gas analysis. The size and position of the tube are documented and the tube secured in place.

Initially patients are ventilated with an FiO_2 of 1.0, unless the patient has undergone palliation of single ventricle physiology with an aortopulmonary shunt. In these infants, hyperoxia decreases PVR and increases pulmonary blood flow at the expense of systemic perfusion. The FiO_2 provided to them is most often 0.25 to 0.30. FiO_2 is weaned rapidly in most patients, based on continuous pulse oximeter measurements of oxygen saturation. A volume-cycled ventilator is generally used postoperatively for cardiac surgery patients. A generous tidal volume (15–20 mL/kg) and a mechanical rate that ensures adequate ventilation and gas exchange are provided and adjusted, based on blood gas analysis. Occasionally a pressure-cycled ventilator is needed to manage very small infants.

Suctioning of the endotracheal tube is reserved for documented episodes of increased pulmonary secretions and is executed with extreme caution. Adequate ventilation and oxygenation are ensured by manual ventilation with an anesthesia bag before and after each suction passage. Maintaining 100% oxygen and mild hyperinflation and hyperventilation protects the patient from hypoxemia and hypercarbia during suctioning. However, patients with an aortopulmonary connection can develop pulmonary overcirculation in response to hyperoxia or hypocarbia. These infants receive manual ventilation with maintenance FiO_2 and the pulse oximeter is monitored throughout to ensure that pulmonary blood flow does not increase or decrease dramatically, indicated by an increase or decrease in oxygen saturation. Conversely, pulmonary vasospasm can be induced when ventilation with suctioning is inadequate, particularly in the newborn and in infants and children with pulmonary artery hypertension. Pulmonary vasospasm is potentially irreversible, resulting in death.

The length of time that cardiac surgery patients require mechanical ventilation varies, but is most often brief. It may be longer in patients with pulmonary vascular congestion from large left-to-right shunts or heart failure and in those with complex heart defects. Mechanical ventilation is continued until the patient is hemodynamically stable and able to sustain adequate respiratory function independent of the ventilator. As the patient awakens and begins to initiate respiration, the ventilator breaths are weaned. The patient's readiness for extubation is based on physical assessment and arterial blood gas analysis. The patient may be extubated when shown to be hemodynamically stable with little or no inotropic support and when alert, able to clear pulmonary secretions, and breathing comfortably on minimal mechanical ventilator support.

Patients who are unable to tolerate extubation and do not have pulmonary disease may require investigation of potential cardiac problems with echocardiogram and cardiac catheterization. Poor myocardial contractility or residual defects despite surgical repair may be responsible. Paralysis of the diaphragm from intraoperative injury to the phrenic nerve may result in inability to tolerate extubation, because infants have high reliance on the diaphragm for breathing, as compared with use of accessory or intercostal muscles. Ultrasound or fluoroscopy examination of the diaphragm assists in identifying this problem.

Vigorous diuresis in postoperative patients may result in the development of metabolic alkalosis and may delay extubation. Careful monitoring of fluid and electrolytes and appropriate electrolyte replacement can prevent difficulty. Acetazolamide (Diamox) therapy may be indicated for the ventilator-dependent patient whose total bicarbonate level approaches or exceeds 40 mEq/L, with a normal or increased respiratory rate, and in whom a trial of extubation is anticipated (Castaneda et al., 1994).

Fluid and Electrolyte Replacement

Institutional preference prevails in recommendations regarding postoperative intravenous fluids. Some restrict sodium intake for the first 24 hours, given the mild tendency for sodium retention following CPB, administering 5% dextrose in water solutions to infants and children and 10% dextrose to newborns. Solutions are changed to 5% or 10% dextrose with 0.2% normal saline after the first postoperative day. Others recommend routine use of 0.2% saline solutions on the first postoperative day to avoid hypovolemia. The volume of fluid administered is generally restricted to 50% of maintenance for patients who have required CPB for the first 24 hours and for newborns in the first 1 or 2 days of life. Fluids are increased to full maintenance thereafter. For patients not requiring CPB, full maintenance fluids are started immediately after operation. All sources of fluid intake, including flushes of intravascular and intracardiac catheters, are measured with care and included in the calculated fluid requirement.

Fluid balance is assessed from heart rate, intracardiac filling pressures, systemic arterial blood pressure, and urine output. Volume is administered to maximize the patient's CO, but with caution not to overload the circulatory system. In the immediate postoperative period rewarming results in gradual peripheral vasodilation and expansion of the vascular space, necessitating administration of blood or colloid to maintain adequate intravascular volume.

Edema is present postoperatively to some extent in all patients who undergo cardiac surgery with CPB and deep hypothermic circulatory arrest. Other contributing factors include length of the surgery, type of procedure, and amount of fluid administered intraoperatively. Total body water accumulation during cardiac surgery may be as much as 600 to 1000 mL (Vincent et al., 1984; Walsh et al., 1992; Castaneda et al., 1994). After the first postoperative night, diuretics are administered to hasten the elimination of accumulated extravascular water. Low-dose dopamine (3 mcg/kg/minute) may also be advantageous. Forced diuresis mandates attention to electrolyte balance and the possibility of acid-base disturbance.

Serum potassium levels are affected by CPB, diuretic administration, and acid-base balance. Hypokalemia is known to contribute to ventricular irritability, especially in patients administered digoxin, and can cause rhythm disturbances. Serum potassium less than 3.0 mEq/L is treated with potassium chloride supplements of 0.25 to 0.5 mEq/kg administered as a continuous infusion over 1 to 2 hours, if urine output is adequate. Care is taken to ensure that potassium supplements are not administered rapidly or in an excessively concentrated infusion, because the consequence is cardiac arrest. Hyperkalemia is rare, unless postoperative renal dysfunction is present. Treatment consists of removing all potassium from intravenous fluids and the administration of polystyrene sulfonate (1 g/kg every 4 hours) by mouth or rectum until renal function improves. Occasionally, dialysis is required.

Mild hyponatremia is common, but does not often require treatment beyond administration of diuretics and restriction of free water intake. Patients with serum sodium less than 125 mEq/L are at risk for seizures and other neurologic symptoms and require diuresis, water restriction, and cautious administration of normal saline. Hypocalcemia is seen most often in newborns and in patients transfused large volumes of blood or plasma, because blood is preserved with citrate-phosphate-dextrose, which causes precipitation of serum calcium. Administration of serum albumin may bind ionized calcium, also resulting in hypocalcemia. Stress-stimulated secretion of growth hormone increases calcium deposition in bone during infancy, increasing the occurrence of hypocalcemia. Hypocalcemia produces negative inotropy. Infants are also at risk for the development of hypoglycemia because their metabolic rate is rapid and their glycogen stores limited. Hypoglycemia depresses myocardial function and may cause seizures.

Acid-base balance is monitored with care; myocardial performance is adversely affected by acidosis. Metabolic acidosis indicates impaired tissue perfusion, usually the result of inadequate cardiac output. Treatment necessitates correction of the underlying hemodynamic problem and administration of intravenous sodium bicarbonate (1 mEq/kg/dose). Bicarbonate is usually diluted to 0.5 mEq/mL and administered slowly (no faster than 1 mEq/minute). Adequate ventilation must be ensured because the buffering action of bicarbonate results in the formation of carbon dioxide. Tromethamine (Tham) is an alternative buffering agent for patients with severe metabolic acidosis and impaired renal function or hypernatremia.

Renal Function. Urine output is a sensitive indicator of cardiac output and tissue perfusion following cardiac surgery. Urine output of 1 mL/kg/hour is anticipated in infants and young children; 0.5 mL/kg/hour (or 20–40 mL/hour) is expected urine production in older children and adults. If urine flow decreases, but physical examination and laboratory results suggest adequate CO, the diminished urine flow is most likely caused by stimulation of hormone pathways designed to retain fluid and maximize CO, which are stimulated by CPB, as well as by decreased CO and other factors. The renin-aldosterone-angiotensin system (RAAS) is stimulated by a decrease in renal blood flow, restoring CO by sodium and water retention, which increase intravascular volume. Urine output can also be diminished by the secretion of antidiuretic hormone (ADH) stimulated by CPB.

Diminished urinary output is not the sole indicator for administration of diuretics in the immediate postoperative period, although diuretics are used after the first postoperative night to hasten the elimination of accumulated extravascular water. Administration of tubular diuretics is not likely to alter the cause of vasomotor nephropathy, which may have resulted from diminished perfusion during CPB or subsequent hemodynamic instability. Acute renal failure may occur in up to 10% of infants following open-heart surgery. Serum blood urea nitrogen (BUN) and creatinine are key to assessing renal function. If, despite adequate CO, urine output remains inadequate with an upward trend in BUN and creatinine, renal replacement therapy may be indicated.

Thermal Regulation

Although induced hypothermia for cardiac surgery is reversed at the conclusion of the procedure, most often core temperature is still low and peripheral vasoconstriction persists when the patient arrives in the PICU. Hypothermia prolongs postoperative bleeding and may delay hemodynamic stabilization; may lead to acidosis, hypoglycemia, hypoxemia, increased pulmonary vascular resistance; and may induce shivering. Active rewarming is achieved with overbed warmers. Infants have a higher loss of heat via conduction, convection, radiation, and evaporation and may be slow to rewarm despite efforts to reestablish normothermia while weaning off CPB.

Establishment of a neutral thermal environment (NTE) is key to postoperative thermal regulation. Newborns and small infants are cared for in an infant warmer bed using a Servo-control mechanism. Postoperative assessment includes measurement of core temperature and the differential between core and peripheral temperatures, as well as assessment of the extremities for coolness and capillary refill. When cool extremities are noted with an elevated core temperature, low CO is suspected, resulting from redistribution of the CO away from the extremities. Loss of heat exchange capacities in the peripheral circulation results in heat retention and a high core temperature. Capillary refill is expected to be brisk when the cardiac surgery patient has been rewarmed and hemodynamic stability is achieved. In the newborn, normal refill may take 3 to 5 seconds owing to peripheral vascular adaptation. Refill time longer than 5 seconds is abnormal and reflects diminished peripheral perfusion (Monett & Moynihan, 1991).

Feeding and Nutrition

Generally, oral feedings are begun carefully soon after successful extubation. In patients who have had straightforward cardiac repairs and are recovering well, feedings can be rapidly advanced. Exceptions include newborns with umbilical artery catheters who are kept NPO because there is an association between necrotizing enterocolitis (NEC) and feeding in these infants. Patients having repair of coarctation of the aorta are not fed until hypertension is controlled and bowel sounds are active to prevent reactive mesenteric enteritis and its complications (Backer & Mavroudis, 1993). Nasogastric or transpyloric feedings are considered early for patients unable to resume oral intake within 48 to 72 hours of surgery. Because of its expense, parenteral nutrition is considered only if the gastrointestinal tract cannot be used for an extended period postoperatively. Newborns may require as much as 120 to 150 calories/kg/day for weight gain after a cardiac operation. Older

Table 19–13. TYPICAL ANTIBIOTIC REGIMEN FOR PERIOPERATIVE INFECTION PROPHYLAXIS

Amikacin (Amikin)
7.5 mg/kg/dose IV q 8–12 hr

Ampicillin
50–100 mg/kg/day IV in 3 or 4 divided doses

Ancef
15 mg/kg/dose IV q 8 hr

Gentamicin (Garamycin)*
7 days–12 years: 1.5–2 mg/kg/dose IV q 8–12 hr
>12 years: 1 mg/kg/dose IV q 8–12 hr

Oxacillin
25–50 mg/kg/dose IV q 6 hr

Vancomycin (Vancocin)**
10–15 mg/kg/dose IV q 6–8 hr

*Gentamicin is used with caution in any patient with low CO and prerenal failure
**Vancomycin is indicated in patients with penicillin allergy but is otherwise reserved for situations of true sepsis, because of the development of vancomycin-resistant organisms

infants and children are likely to have a similar increase in nutritional requirements.

Infection Prophylaxis

Broad-spectrum antibiotics, given during the perioperative period, decrease the risk of infectious complications. The invasive nature of cardiac surgery and the postoperative lines and tubes make systemic sepsis an important concern, particularly in newborns. Their relative immune incompetence necessitates antibiotic coverage for both gram-negative and staphylococcal organisms. A typical antibiotic regimen is presented in Table 19–13. Strict adherence to sterile technique both during and after the operation is also essential, as is a high level of suspicion regarding subtle symptoms that may suggest infection. Sepsis is suspected in the newborn who develops hypoglycemia, thrombocytopenia, acidosis, feeding intolerance, hemodynamic instability, hepatomegaly, hyperbilirubinemia, or elevated white blood cell count postoperatively (Backer & Mavroudis, 1993). Beyond the newborn period, fever most often heralds infectious complications. Cultures are obtained and appropriate antibiotics administered.

Central Nervous System Assessment

Neurologic complications after cardiac operations may be the consequence of cerebral ischemia, hypoxia, electrolyte imbalances, metabolic acidosis, hypoglycemia, or cerebral emboli (Barratt-Boyes, 1990). Seizure activity is the most common neurologic complication. Evaluation includes measurement of arterial blood gases and serum electrolytes, with correction of abnormalities detected. Hypoglycemia, hypocalcemia, and hypomagnesemia are causes for seizures in infants. Seizure control is necessary to avoid interference with adequate ventilation and cardiac stress.

Pain Management

Metabolic balance in postoperative cardiac surgery patients may be precarious with hypo- or hyperglycemia, metabolic acidosis, and electrolyte disturbances presenting as potential problems. Vulnerability to metabolic derangements may accentuate the detrimental effects of catabolic responses to stress triggered by major operations. The response of newborns to the stress of cardiac and noncardiac operations may be substantially greater than that of adults (Anand & Hickey, 1992). Patients with CHDs who are recovering from surgery are very sensitive to stressful interventions and have marginal organ system reserve and diminished compensatory mechanisms (Castaneda et al., 1994).

Increases in blood pressure and heart rate and decrease in arterial oxygen saturation are reliable measures of stress in critically ill infants and children, although these physiologic changes may also be caused by a number of other clinical conditions, including seizures (Walsh et al., 1992). In patients paralyzed with neuromuscular blocking agents, these physiologic signs may be the only clues available for assessment of either pain or a neurologic event (Troug & Anand, 1989; Walsh et al., 1992).

Anand and Hickey (1992) studied a group of patients in whom fentanyl anesthesia was extended into the postoperative period. Postoperative outcomes in critically ill newborns were improved by this intervention, which is theorized to minimize the hemodynamic and hormonal stress responses to surgery and postoperative care. Other approaches to postoperative analgesia are common, although intravenous narcotic analgesics are employed in most settings for at least 24 to 48 hours postoperatively. Thereafter, Tylenol with codeine, Tylenol, or nonsteroidal anti-inflammatory drugs (NSAIDs) are useful.

Other Postoperative Problems

Occasionally, infants and children develop pulmonary or renal dysfunction after cardiac operations. It is important to note that in the case of both pulmonary and renal postoperative problems, inadequate tissue perfusion and/or concomitant cardiac failure is the primary problem.

A few patients develop infectious complications. High fever should always raise the suspicion of wound infection or septicemia. Blood, tracheobronchial secretions, and urine specimens are obtained promptly for culture. Broad-spectrum antibiotic coverage is maintained or reinitiated until specific sensitivity studies are available and specific antibiotics can be administered.

ACQUIRED HEART DISEASE IN INFANTS AND CHILDREN

Acquired heart disease in pediatric patients includes a group of diseases, sometimes without known etiology, in which the central feature is involvement of the heart muscle itself. An exception is Kawasaki disease, in which the coronary arteries are involved primarily. *Idiopathic cardiomyopathy* is the term used to describe diseases involving the heart muscle that are of unknown cause. These myocardial diseases in infants and children are not the consequence of ischemic, hypertensive, congenital, valvular, or pericardial disease (Wynne & Braunwald, 1992). Specific heart muscle diseases (also called *secondary cardiomyopathy*) have a known cause and include myocarditis and Kawasaki disease. Although less common than congenital heart defects, acquired heart disease in infants and children can lead to significant cardiac dysfunction, morbidity, and mortality.

Acute Myocarditis

Myocarditis is defined as an inflammation of the myocardium that is characterized by lymphocytic infiltration and myocardial necrosis. Myocarditis can produce decreased cardiac performance, although subclinical or asymptomatic cases are common. Severe inflammation results in critical sequelae: congestive heart failure and death.

Etiology

Virtually any infectious agent can produce cardiac inflammation. Myocarditis has been described during and following a wide variety of viral, bacterial, rickettsial, fungal, and protozoal infections. The most common etiologic agents in North America are viruses, specifically Coxsackie and other enteroviruses. In addition to infectious agents, myocardial inflammation may be caused by allergic responses, medications, and systemic diseases, such as vasculitis or Kawasaki disease.

Incidence

Myocarditis is a common disease that has been documented in acute or previous infection in 25% of autopsy studies of children (Koren et al., 1986; Burch et al., 1968). However, only 0.3% of patients seen by pediatric cardiologists have clinically significant evidence of myocarditis (Moore & Soifer, 1993). A large percentage of asymptomatic or subclinical cases accounts for the discrepancy between the autopsy findings and clinical incidence.

The incidence of myocarditis is highest in children younger than 1 year of age. In one report of 228 cases of myocarditis, 41% were caused by Coxsackie virus (Woodruff, 1980). Between 5% and 12% of children infected with either influenza viruses or Coxsackie virus develop clinical myocarditis, whereas 40% of those with infectious mononucleosis have myocardial involvement, most often subclinical (Moore & Soifer, 1993).

Pathogenesis

Infectious agents cause myocardial damage by direct invasion of the myocardium, production of a myocardial toxin, or immune-related inflammation of the myocardium. Viruses injure myocardial tissue by direct destruction of the myofibrils and by cytotoxic T cell destruction of myocytes. In viral myocarditis there is strong evidence of a cell-mediated immunologic reaction as a principal mechanism of cardiac involvement. Noninfected cells may be destroyed by complement-mediated antibody action.

Clinical Manifestations

The clinical presentation of patients with myocarditis ranges from those who are asymptomatic to those with severe cardiac dysfunction progressing rapidly to fulminant CHF and death. Typically, newborns and young infants have sudden onset of symptoms and rapid progression to critical illness.

Presenting signs in young patients include lethargy, fever, and tachycardia. Respiratory distress, cyanosis, and vomiting may also be present. Older children present with fever, malaise, myalgia, gastroenteritis, pharyngitis, and meningitis, and generally are less ill appearing than are infants. In addition to tachycardia, which is out of proportion to the fever, the cardiac examination in infants and children with myocarditis reveals a thready pulse if systemic perfusion is compromised. The heart sounds are muffled if a pericardial effusion is present. With severe cardiac dysfunction a gallop rhythm and a murmur of mitral regurgitation (a high-frequency, pansystolic murmur, loudest at the apex) may be auscultated.

Diagnosis

A number of laboratory studies are indicated when myocarditis is suspected. In patients with myocarditis, the white blood cell count is elevated without a leftward shift, the sedimentation rate is elevated, liver function tests are abnormal, and lactate dehydrogenase (LDH) isoenzyme 1 and creatine phosphokinase (CPK) MB fraction are elevated. Bacterial infection is ruled out by blood culture. The nasopharynx and stool are cultured for viral isolation.

Chest radiographs demonstrate cardiac enlargement in most. Pulmonary vascularity is increased when heart failure is present. The ECG can reveal life-threatening cardiac rhythm disturbances that often accompany myocarditis. ECG also often reveals the classic electrocardiographic changes of myocarditis: low-voltage QRS complexes, low or inverted T waves, and decreased or absent Q waves in V_5 and V_6. Echocardiography is used to evaluate cardiac function and detect the presence of pericardial effusion. Most often the left ventricle is dilated, with increased left ventricular dimensions at end-systole and end-diastole. Global myocardial depression or asymmetric movement of the left ventricular free wall may be noted.

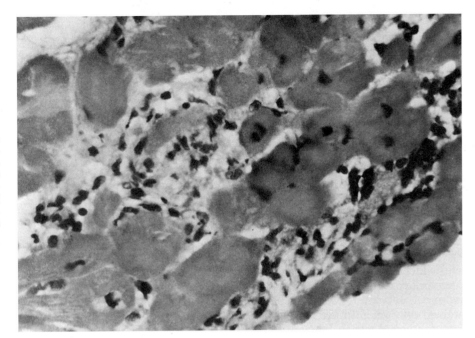

Figure 19–24 ● ● ● ● ● ●
Myocardial tissue showing focal, interstitial, lymphocytic infiltrate, and myocyte degeneration. Degenerating myocytes show closely apposed lymphocytes around it and attached to the membrane. (From Baker, A. (1994). Acquired heart disease in infants and children. *Critical Care Nursing Clinics of North America*, 6(1):183.)

Definitive diagnosis of myocarditis necessitates that myocardial biopsy, the "gold standard," demonstrate myocyte necrosis or degeneration or both, associated with an inflammatory infiltrate adjacent to the damaged myocytes (Artez, 1987). These criteria, referred to as the *Dallas criteria*, were developed after many years during which the diagnosis of myocarditis was made without standard diagnostic findings. The Dallas criteria, which define the characteristics of myocarditis from histologic examination of endomyocardial biopsy tissue obtained by cardiac catheterization (Fig. 19–24), permit accurate diagnosis and systematic investigation of myocarditis.

However, the focal and patchy nature of myocarditis, as well as the small size of tissue samples obtained at biopsy, makes it difficult to obtain a definitive diagnosis in many cases. False-negative results are common. The absence of a positive biopsy does not rule out myocarditis, and treatment is based on clinical symptoms and other diagnostic findings. Biopsy may be repeated in patients when there is a clinical suspicion of myocarditis but a nonspecific or negative biopsy result.

Critical Care Management

Management of infants and children with myocarditis remains supportive, rather than specifically aimed at a causative organism. Ensuring bedrest during the acute phase (7–14 days) is often recommended to decrease demands on the heart, but animal studies also suggest that exercise during the acute phase of myocarditis increases viral replication and worsens outcome (Cabinian et al., 1990). Administration of supplemental oxygen and/or mechanical ventilation is often necessary to maintain adequate oxygen delivery in the face of CHF. Because the potential for complete recovery of myocardial function exists even in critically ill patients with myocarditis, treatment of cardiac dysfunction is aggressive.

Anticongestive Therapy. The overall goal of treatment in patients with myocarditis is to increase CO. In the critically ill patient, early and aggressive therapy is instituted, usually combining inotropic and afterload-reducing agents. A common treatment combination is dobutamine and amrinone. Dobutamine serves as an inotrope and is especially effective in patients with refractory CHF, and amrinone has both inotropic and vasodilating properties that serve to decrease the workload of the heart. Other combinations, such as nitroprusside and dopamine, are also used. Diuretic therapy with furosemide is prescribed to reduce preload.

Vasoactive drug therapy requires frequent monitoring of central venous pressure, arterial blood pressure, and CO. Accurate hemodynamic measurements are essential in evaluating the patient's response to treatment because therapeutic decisions are based on the patient's physiologic status.

Maintenance of fluid balance is critical in this patient population. Adequate hydration to maintain critical preload and ventricular filling pressures without fluid overload is the goal of care, and accurate monitoring of intake and output and accurate daily measurement of weight are essential. Administration of diuretics and fluid restriction, necessary to decrease preload, may result in acid-base and electrolyte imbalances. Routine laboratory assessment of blood pH and electrolytes is necessary.

Some patients who recover from severe cardiac dysfunction require long-term oral anticongestive therapy. Digoxin, furosemide, and an angiotensin-converting enzyme (ACE) inhibitor are commonly employed. Digoxin is not recommended during the acute inflammatory phase, because the heart may be overly sensitive to digoxin-induced rhythm disturbances. Careful monitoring is essential when digoxin is prescribed (Moore & Soifer, 1993).

ACE inhibitors provide afterload reduction by interfering with the formation of angiotensin II (a strong vasoconstrictor). In controlled studies, the use of ACE inhibitors, such as captopril and enalapril, has been effective in slowing the course of heart failure, decreasing symptoms, and potentially prolonging survival in patients with mild to severe left ventricular dysfunction (Abramowitz, 1993; Pfeffer et al., 1992).

Dysrhythmia Management. Because cardiac rhythm disturbances can be life-threatening, aggressive therapy is instituted. Supraventricular tachycardia (SVT) is most often treated with digoxin, rather than medications that can further depress cardiac contractility. Ventricular dysrhythmias are treated with lidocaine. Second or third degree atrioventricular block can develop and is managed with temporary external pacing. Persistence beyond 2 weeks is an indication for elective placement of a permanent pacemaker (Moore & Soifer, 1993).

Anticoagulation. Anticoagulation therapy is indicated in patients with the potential for thrombus formation due to severely compromised ventricular function. Mural thrombi can potentially embolize to the cerebrovascular system, causing neurologic sequelae.

Coagulation parameters are followed closely and therapy adjusted to maintain an adequate anticoagulatory state. Because of the possibility of cerebral emboli, neurologic status is monitored closely and changes in the patient's mentation or responsiveness are evaluated immediately. Signs and symptoms of pulmonary emboli, which include acute onset of shortness of breath, tachycardia, hypoxemia, and chest pain, are assessed. The risk of systemic emboli is also present and may manifest as a change in color, temperature, or perfusion of an extremity.

Anti-inflammatory Treatment. Treatment with NSAIDs is contraindicated in patients with myocarditis. Use of more powerful anti-inflammatory agents, such as prednisone and cyclosporin, is controversial (Liu et al., 1992). Human studies have suggested a benefit, but the studies were nonrandomized and are difficult to interpret because 45% to 50% of patients with myocarditis improve spontaneously. Animal models with myocarditis suggest a poorer outcome when a steroid is administered early in the course of illness, during viral replication, suggesting that immunosuppression may enhance myocardial damage during this period (Tomioka et al., 1986). If anti-inflammatory treatment was delayed until the phase of lymphocytic infiltration, myocardial necrosis was decreased (Monrad et al., 1986; O'Connell et al., 1986), suggesting that the timing of administration may affect outcome.

A recent retrospective review of patients with myocarditis found that the use of intravenous gamma globulin was associated with improvement in recovery of left ventricular function and a trend toward improved survival in the first year after presentation (Drucker et al., 1994). Currently there are not enough data to support a specific anti-inflammatory regimen in children with myocarditis. Effective antiviral agents, immunosuppressive agents, or antilymphocytic monoclonal antibodies for treating patients with myocarditis may be options for clinical use in the future.

Mechanical Assist Devices and Extracorporeal Support. If conventional therapy is unsuccessful, other means of support may be attempted. Chang and coworkers (1992) reported the successful use of a left ventricular assist device in a patient with acute myocarditis. The use of intra-aortic balloon pump and ECMO has been reported in patients who do not respond to conventional therapy; however, experience is limited and no one therapy has been shown to alter the course of illness (Veasey et al., 1983). If cardiac function fails to improve, cardiac transplantation may be considered.

Preventing Complications. As is the case with any critically ill patient, the high potential for nosocomial infection is an important consideration. Multiple venous and arterial lines are required for the infusion of cardioactive drugs and continual invasive hemodynamic monitoring. Protecting patients from infection and vigilant assessment for early signs of localized or systemic infection are both significant.

The extensive equipment required for monitoring and mechanical support limits turning and repositioning some patients. Decreased tissue perfusion in the acutely ill patient in combination with immobility increases the potential for tissue ischemia. Skin integrity is an important concern. Attention is directed toward alleviating pressure, repositioning to whatever extent is possible on a regular basis, and employing methods to prevent skin breakdown.

Attention to the patient's nutritional requirements is extremely important to promote healing and provide a positive nitrogen balance. Because the acutely ill patient is usually not able to take food orally, adequate nutrition must be provided intravenously. Total parenteral nutrition should be instituted early in the course of illness to fulfill caloric requirements. When oral intake is resumed, high calorie supplements are provided.

Acute Rheumatic Fever

Acute rheumatic fever (ARF) is a leading cause of acquired heart disease in children in the United States. ARF is an inflammatory process affecting the heart, skin, joints, and brain that is mediated by an immune reaction to streptococcal infection. Children with ARF may experience congestive heart failure, pericarditis, or valvular heart disease that necessitates their admission to the critical care unit.

Etiology

ARF is caused by group A beta-hemolytic streptococcal pharyngitis.

Incidence

ARF had virtually disappeared in the United States, but its incidence has increased dramatically in the last 10 years (Gordis, 1985; Veasey et al., 1987). Approximately 3% of children with streptococcal pharyngitis acquire ARF, whereas one third of patients with ARF have no clear history of pharyngitis. In fact, asymptomatic streptococcal pharyngitis is common (Veasey et al., 1987). The peak incidence is in the winter and spring months. Rheumatic fever is more prevalent in population groups with poor nutrition, crowded living conditions, and limited access to healthcare. However, the recent increase in cases has included more patients from middle and upper class families without the risk factors identified. ARF is most prevalent in school-age children; incidence peaks between 6 and 16 years of age.

Pathogenesis

ARF develops from an immune-mediated reaction to a streptococcal infection, which remains to be clearly described. An inciting pharyngeal infection is followed in 1 to 4 weeks by involvement of the mesenchymal connective tissue of the heart, blood vessels, joints, and subcutaneous tissue. Vasculitis of the skin leads to erythema marginatum. In the basal ganglia and cerebellum, vasculitis causes Sydenham's chorea. Arthritis of the large joints is produced. Cardiac involvement includes valvular endocarditis, myocarditis, and pericarditis.

Cardiac involvement is diagnosed clinically in 70% of patients with ARF, but when color Doppler echocardiography is used, 90% of patients are found to have cardiac involvement (Veasey, 1987). Valvular endocarditis is the most common cardiac finding, with the mitral valve affected most frequently, followed by the aortic valve and the tricuspid valve. The pulmonary valve is rarely affected. Congestive heart failure occurs in 7% of patients with ARF. In 1960, the Cooperative Rheumatic Fever Group reported that mortality from ARF was approximately 3%, with approximately one half of patient deaths occurring several years after the acute illness because of chronic CHF from valvular lesions. No new data are currently available.

Clinical Manifestations

Manifestations of ARF are related to the structures involved. Polyarthritis is the most common finding; usually the large joints are affected and the arthritis is migratory. Lesions of erythema marginatum are seen most commonly on the trunk or inner aspects of the upper arms and thighs and are present in about 10% of patients with ARF.

Chorea is the major central nervous system manifestation. Seen more frequently in girls than in boys with ARF, there is an insidious onset of irritability, emotional lability with frequent crying, and increased clumsiness. Choreic movements and facial grimaces develop.

Table 19-14. MODIFIED JONES' CRITERIA FOR DIAGNOSIS OF ACUTE RHEUMATIC FEVER

Major	Minor
Carditis (70%)*	Previous episode of ARF (25%)
Polyarthritis (70%)	Arthralgia
Chorea (15%)	Fever (60%)
Erythema marginatum (5%)	Prolonged PR interval (40%)
Subcutaneous nodules (<5%)	Elevated ESR (95%)
	Leukocytosis
	Elevated C-reactive protein

Supporting Evidence of Streptococcal Infection

Increased titer of antistreptococcal antibodies (ASO, anti-DNAse B, streptozyme)
Recent scarlet fever
Positive throat culture for group A β-hemolytic streptococci

ARF, acute rheumatic fever; ESR, erythrocyte sedimentation rate
*Percentage of patients with specific finding

Cardiac involvement is most often detected by onset of a new heart murmur, which occurs in two thirds of patients with ARF. The most common is the murmur of mitral insufficiency, followed by aortic insufficiency. A gallop rhythm is heard in some patients who have associated CHF. ECG abnormalities are common and include bradycardia and first, second, or third degree heart block.

Diagnosis

There are no specific laboratory tests to diagnose ARF. The diagnosis is based on clinical criteria initially established in 1944 by Jones and later modified (AHA, 1984). The modified Jones criteria are divided into major and minor clinical manifestations of the disease. In addition, supporting evidence of streptococcal infection aids the diagnosis (Table 19-14). ARF is diagnosed when a patient has two of the major criteria or one major and two minor criteria and evidence of a preceding group A beta-hemolytic streptococcal infection.

The cardiac test results described above and echocardiography aid the diagnosis of ARF. An echocardiogram demonstrates a dilated left atrium when mitral insufficiency is present and can reveal the severity of the mitral regurgitation. When aortic insufficiency is present, the left ventricle may be dilated.

Critical Care Management

Management of patients with ARF who require intensive care includes the management of severe CHF, as with myocarditis. Rest to permit adequate cardiac recovery and anticongestive treatment is similar. Afterload reduction is of particular significance; it may decrease regurgitation across an incompetent mitral or aortic valve. Cardiac rhythm disturbances also require attention. Temporary external pacing may be required. In addition, eradication of the streptococcal infection to prevent immediate recurrence and prophylaxis against distant recurrences are distinct goals of therapy for patients with ARF, as is treatment of carditis and other major manifestations or acute complications.

Eradication of Infection. Eradication of group A beta-hemolytic streptococci to prevent immediate recurrence, regardless of the throat culture result at the time the patient presents for critical care or the time period from the initial infection, is key to management of patients with ARF. Penicillin G (benzylpenicillin) is the drug of choice, unless the patient is hypersensitive. In the critical care unit, penicillin G is almost always administered intravenously and is widely distributed by this route. Intramuscular administration is an alternative. Hypersensitive patients are given vancomycin intravenously or erythromycin orally.

Because of the high risk of recurrence in patients who have had ARF, antibacterial prophylaxis against streptococcal infection is essential. Prophylaxis is continued for life. Table 19–15 lists the American Heart Association recommendations for prophylaxis when patients who are at risk for the development of infectious endocarditis require procedures involving the oral mucosa, upper respiratory tract, and genitourinary or gastrointestinal tract. In addition to patients with ARF, others with CHD (before and after surgical repair) require subacute bacterial endocarditis prophylaxis.

Treatment of Carditis and Arthritis. Whether steroids or aspirin is more effective in the treatment of the carditis of ARF is controversial. Large multicenter studies reported between 1955 and 1965 did not demonstrate significant differences between the two drugs in reducing the acute cardiac inflammation. Prednisone, however, may be more effective at improving the symptoms of severe carditis (Cooperative Rheumatic Fever Study Group 1955, 1960, 1965). Neither agent has any effect on preventing chronic valvular heart disease or preventing mortality.

When arthritis is present, but carditis is mild, aspirin (100 mg/kg/day) is administered orally with doses every 4 hours for 2 to 6 weeks. The aspirin dose is then tapered to 25 mg/kg/day over 3 weeks. When carditis is moderate to severe, prednisone (2 mg/kg/day) is administered intravenously or orally for 2 weeks. It is then tapered over 3 weeks to 10 mg/day, with aspirin therapy initiated (as prescribed for mild carditis) during the second week of the steroid tapering regimen (Moore & Soifer, 1993).

Kawasaki Disease

Kawasaki disease is an acute systemic vasculitis that was first described in Japan in 1967. The acute illness itself is self-limiting, but one of five children with Kawasaki disease suffers coronary artery damage, resulting in dilation or aneurysm. Although damage can occur in any medium-sized muscular artery, the vessels most often affected are the coronary arteries. Kawasaki disease is a leading cause of acquired heart disease in children.

Etiology

The cause of Kawasaki disease is unknown. An infectious etiology is suggested. It is almost exclusively a pediatric disorder; passive immunity may develop. Geographic outbreaks occur, and there is an increase in the number of cases in the late winter and early spring. There are associations between its occurrence and recent exposure to carpet cleaning and residence near a body of stagnant water; however, cause and effect have not been established. Kawasaki disease is reported more frequently among children from higher socioeconomic groups.

Incidence

The first cases of Kawasaki disease in the United States were documented in the early 1970s. Although Japanese children have the highest incidence of this illness, regardless of where they live, Kawasaki disease occurs in all races. Blacks have the second highest rate of occurrence; white children follow. Eighty-five percent of cases occur in children under age 5, with the greatest incidence in the toddler age group (1- to 2-year-olds). Infants often present in an atypical fashion, without fulfilling diagnostic criteria; however, this age group has the highest risk of developing severe coronary artery disease. As well, chil-

Table 19–15. PROPHYLAXIS AGAINST INFECTIOUS ENDOCARDITIS

Oral and Upper Respiratory Tract Procedures
Standard
  Amoxicillin: 50 mg/kg po 1 hour before, 25 mg/kg IV 6 hours after the procedure
  Ampicillin: 50 mg/kg IV 1 hour before, 25 mg/kg IV 6 hours after the procedure

High risk
  Add gentamicin: 2 mg/kg IV 30 minutes before and 6 hours after the procedure to the IV ampicillin, above

Penicillin-allergic
  Erythromycin: 20 mg/kg po 2 hours before, 10 mg/kg po 6 hours after the procedure
  Clindamycin: 10 mg/kg IV 30 minutes before, 5 mg/kg IV 6 hours after the procedure

Genitourinary and Gastrointestinal Procedures
Low risk
  Amoxicillin: 50 mg/kg po 1 hour before, 25 mg/kg po 6 hours after the procedure

Standard
  Ampicillin: 50 mg/kg IV 30 minutes before and 8 hours after the procedure, plus
  Gentamicin: 2 mg/kg IV 30 minutes before and 8 hours after the procedure

Penicillin-allergic
  Vancomycin: 20 mg/kg IV 1 hour before and 8 hours after the procedure, plus
  Gentamicin: 2 mg/kg IV 1 hour before and 8 hours after the procedure

dren diagnosed after age 6 are also more likely to develop severe coronary artery aneurysm. Males are affected more frequently than females (1.5:1).

Pathogenesis

Kawasaki disease causes diffuse acute vasculitis of medium-sized arteries and small arterioles and venules throughout the body, with a predilection for the coronary arteries. The involvement of small peripheral blood vessels is evidenced in the inflammatory signs and symptoms that characterize this illness. During the initial acute phase, inflammation of the small arteries and venules is evident. Inflammation then progresses to involve the medium-sized muscular arteries, including the coronary arteries, with the potential development of coronary artery aneurysm. Damage to the coronary arteries is evidenced, on average, on the eleventh day after the onset of fever, although changes may be seen as early as day 7, and affected vessels may continue to enlarge for some time, reaching their maximum dimension at 28 days. In dilated vessels, the potential for thrombus exists. Over time, affected vessels heal by the process of myointimal proliferation, which can result in stenosis, especially at the distal ends of aneurysms. The myocardium is involved directly in almost all cases, with myocellular hypertrophy, degeneration of myocytes, and endocardial changes that lead to myocarditis and decreased ventricular function. Myocardial dysfunction is subclinical in most patients.

Clinical Manifestations

There is no definitive diagnostic test for Kawasaki disease. Rather, the diagnosis is based on the presence of certain clinical criteria developed by the Centers for Disease Control (Table 19–16). The presence of prolonged fever plus four of the remaining five criteria, without evidence of another known disease, is required to establish the diagnosis. In addition, there are a number of clinical and laboratory findings that support the diagnosis (Table 19–17). Clinical features include irritability, which is often extreme and may persist over the entire course of the illness.

Table 19–16. CDC CRITERIA FOR DIAGNOSIS OF KAWASAKI DISEASE

Fever >5 days unresponsive to antibiotics, and at least four of the five following physical findings with no other more reasonable explanation for the observed clinical findings:

1. Bilateral conjunctival injection
2. Oral mucosal changes (erythema of lips or oropharynx, strawberry tongue, or drying or fissuring of the lips)
3. Peripheral extremity changes (edema, erythema, or generalized or periungual desquamation)
4. Rash
5. Cervical lymphadenopathy >1.5 cm in diameter

Centers for Disease Control (1980). Kawasaki disease—New York. *Mortality and Morbidity Weekly Report,* 29:61–63.

Table 19–17. ASSOCIATED CLINICAL & LABORATORY FINDINGS IN KAWASAKI DISEASE

Elevated sedimentation rate
Leukocytosis with a left shift
Aseptic meningitis
Urethritis with sterile pyuria: microscopic examination reveals mononuclear cells
Elevated liver transaminases: commonly 2–3 times normal
Thrombocytosis: peaking 3–4 weeks after onset
Hydrops of the gallbladder
Anemia that persists until the resolution of inflammation
Irritability
Diarrhea and vomiting

Analysis of cerebrospinal fluid may demonstrate a mild aseptic meningitis. Arthritis occurs in one third of patients, usually affecting the small joints initially with progression to the large weightbearing joints. Diarrhea, nausea, and vomiting are not uncommon. Less often, enlargement (hydrops) of the gallbladder is noted.

Kawasaki disease is an acute, self-limited illness. Complete resolution of clinical symptoms and return of laboratory study results to normal often requires 6 to 8 weeks. The course of the disease is divided into three stages: acute, subacute, and convalescent phases.

The acute phase is a febrile period of 5 to 14 days, during which the clinical criteria for the diagnosis of Kawasaki disease become evident. Irritability and tachycardia are characteristic of this phase. Echocardiography is performed by the end of the first week (or earlier if clinically indicated) to evaluate cardiac function and establish a baseline for evaluation of coronary artery size and shape. Mild to moderate congestive heart failure from myocarditis, left ventricular dysfunction, and pericardial effusion may be detected. Although unusual, cardiac rhythm disturbances may occur, including first or second degree atrioventricular block, prolonged QT interval, abnormal ST segment and T wave, and low R wave amplitude.

The subacute period begins with resolution of fever, although multisystem involvement is still evident. During this stage peeling of the skin of the palms and soles begins under the fingertips and toenails. Arthritis, if present, generally affects the larger weightbearing joints in this stage. Laboratory studies reveal a hypercoagulable state with significantly elevated platelet count. A normocytic, normochromic anemia is common, and an elevated sedimentation rate persists. In those patients who develop coronary artery abnormalities, dilation or aneurysms become evident by echocardiogram in this phase.

The third stage is a convalescent phase during which the child recovers and all blood study results return to normal. Coronary aneurysms may continue to enlarge during this stage, reaching their maximum dimension approximately 28 days from the onset of illness. The only known long-term effects from

Kawasaki disease are in those children with coronary and other vessel damage. Over time, patients with coronary artery aneurysm may develop coronary stenosis.

Cardiac Findings. During the acute phase of illness, at least some degree of myocarditis is present in all children with Kawasaki disease, demonstrated by both biopsy and autopsy findings. The majority of cases are subclinical, whereas severe cases can result in CHF and cardiogenic shock. Echocardiography often reveals decreased left ventricular contractility in the acute phase. This may persist for several months, occasionally persisting 1 to 2 years before a return to normal (Newburger et al., 1989).

In the acute phase, the most common ECG changes include a prolonged PR interval and nonspecific ST and T wave changes. The dysrhythmias seen in the acute phase of Kawasaki disease are not usually life-threatening and are consistent with myocarditis. Later, abnormal ECGs may reflect myocardial infarction or ischemia in the most severely affected patients.

Valvulitis can occur in the acute phase and may result in aortic regurgitation. Late-onset aortic regurgitation is a rare finding. Mitral regurgitation is sometimes present and is thought to be the result of myocarditis in the acute stage or myocardial ischemia later.

The most important sequela from Kawasaki disease is coronary artery aneurysm. One of five untreated children develops damage to the coronary arteries in the form of aneurysms or ectasia (dilation) of one or more vessels. The duration of fever is a strong predictor of aneurysm formation: the longer the fever persists, the greater the risk of coronary aneurysm (Koren et al., 1986; Daniels et al., 1987; Ichida et al., 1987). The process of aneurysm formation and healing (regression) is dynamic. In the acute phase, damage to the coronary arteries causes weakness in the vessel wall. Over the course of subsequent weeks, the damaged vessel increases in diameter, resulting in ectasia and/or aneurysm formation. Aneurysm is defined as an internal lumen diameter greater than 3 mm in a child younger than 5 years of age or greater than 4 mm in a child 5 years or older. In addition, any segment that is 1.5 times larger than an adjacent segment is considered abnormal, as is a vessel with an obviously irregular lumen.

Coronary artery abnormalities are not often evident until the second week after the onset of fever; however, they have been detected as early as day 7 of illness. The affected vessels can continue to enlarge through the fourth week of illness, at which time their maximum dimension is generally reached. Echocardiography is highly sensitive for detection of enlargement or aneurysms in the proximal coronary arteries.

Thrombocytosis occurs during the subacute phase of illness, with platelet counts that can approach 1 million. Sluggish, swirling blood flow through enlarged coronary vessels, in combination with an elevated platelet count, increases the risk of thrombosis

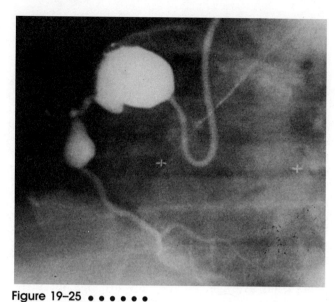

Figure 19–25 ● ● ● ● ● ●

Right coronary arteriogram demonstrating a giant proximal aneurysm and a smaller distal one.

in patients with aneurysms and places these children at risk for myocardial ischemia or infarction. At greatest risk for clot development are those with "giant aneurysms," which measure more than 8 mm in diameter (Fig. 19–25).

Over time, regression of aneurysms can occur. The majority of healing occurs during the first year or two after the onset of illness. In 50% to 66% of cases, the internal lumen diameter of aneurysmal vessels actually returns to its normal size by a process of myointimal proliferation. The amount of healing or regression in an individual patient is most closely related to the extent of damage. The larger the aneurysm, the less likely it is to return to its normal size. Regardless of the internal diameter of the coronary artery, affected vessel walls are not truly "normal" in terms of either histology or reactivity because thickening occurs in the process of healing. These vessels may be at greater risk of developing premature atherosclerotic disease.

Stenotic areas may develop in affected coronary arteries, most commonly at either the proximal or distal end of aneurysms as the vessel walls heal inward. As a consequence, blood flow to the myocardium may be impeded or occluded. If adequate collateral circulation has not developed, myocardial ischemia may result. Stenoses are not easily detectable by echocardiogram, requiring that patients be carefully monitored over time to detect myocardial ischemia by stress testing, myocardial perfusion scan, and ECG. Cardiac catheterization accurately detects stenotic areas and is generally performed a year after the onset of illness or if noninvasive testing suggests signs of decreased myocardial perfusion.

Critical Care Management

Most patients with Kawasaki disease do not require critical care. Typically, a 1- or 2-day admission is necessary, with critical care monitoring prescribed for those patients with acute ventricular dysfunction and symptoms of myocardial ischemia or infarction, and those who require systemic heparinization.

Gamma Globulin Therapy. The use of intravenous gamma globulin shortens the acute phase of Kawasaki disease and decreases the risk of coronary damage (Newburger et al., 1991). The recommended dose is 2 g/kg given intravenously in a single infusion over 8 to 12 hours (American Academy of Pediatrics, 1991). In an NIH-funded, multicenter study, gamma globulin was shown to decrease the incidence of aneurysms three- to fivefold when given within the first ten days of illness (Newburger et al., 1991).

Careful cardiac monitoring is necessary during the administration of gamma globulin. Approximately 40 mL/kg of fluid is administered with the gamma globulin over an 8- to 12-hour time period. Patients with myocardial dysfunction can experience acute CHF.

Aspirin Therapy. High doses of aspirin (20–25 mg/kg/dose every 6 hours) are used initially for anti-inflammatory effect. When the patient has been afebrile for several days, the dose is decreased to an "antiplatelet" dose (3–5 mg/kg/day). Low-dose aspirin is continued through the convalescent phase and then discontinued for those patients without coronary involvement. For patients with aneurysms, an antiplatelet dose of aspirin may be continued indefinitely.

Anticoagulation Therapy. Because of the potential for thrombosis of the coronary arteries, patients are placed on an anticoagulation regimen. Aspirin therapy alone is generally prescribed for patients with coronary aneurysms with an internal diameter less than 5 mm. When aneurysms are in the middle range (greater than 5 mm, but less than 8 mm internal diameter), dipyridamole (Persantine) may be added at a dose of 3 to 6 mg/kg/day in three doses.

If "giant" aneurysms are diagnosed, systemic heparin therapy is often instituted, especially in patients in whom the aneurysms are rapidly increasing in size. When an adequate anticoagulation state is reached, oral Coumadin is substituted and administered in addition to aspirin. A serious potential for bleeding exists when heparin or Coumadin and aspirin are administered in combination, especially for young children who are physically active. The risks and potential benefits of various anticoagulation regimens are considered on an individual basis.

Thrombolytic Therapy. Thrombolytic therapy is considered if clot formation becomes evident, through either development of myocardial infarction or detection by echocardiography. Urokinase and streptokinase have both been used to restore vessel patency (Burtt et al., 1986; Kato et al., 1987; Terai et al., 1985). The earlier thrombolytic therapy is instituted after clot formation or the onset of ischemic symptoms, the greater its efficacy. If reperfusion is obtained, systemic heparin therapy and aspirin are administered to maintain vessel patency. In addition to close assessment of laboratory measures of coagulation, assessing the patient's cardiac function is a priority. Acute myocardial dysfunction or infarction can occur.

Anticongestive Therapy. Congestive heart failure is most often a consequence of ischemic cardiomyopathy, although it may occur acutely in patients with marked myocarditis. In those rare patients, intravenous inotropes and afterload reduction may be necessary. More often, patients with CHF only require therapy with oral digoxin, diuretics, and ACE inhibitors.

Surgical Intervention. Coronary bypass surgery, although technically difficult with small vessels, has been performed in children with severe coronary artery disease. Surgery may be indicated if (1) coronary stenosis and/or occlusion is progressive, (2) collateral blood supply is not adequate, (3) the portion of myocardium to be perfused via the graft is still viable, and (4) the vessel proximal to the planned graft site is healthy (Suzuki et al., 1990). In addition to the technical difficulty of coronary artery bypass surgery in pediatric patients, children often develop collateral circulation around a coronary occlusion across time. Surgery is usually recommended only for those with life-threatening disease.

Coronary bypass surgery is contraindicated in patients with acutely inflamed or excessively small coronary vessels. Coronary artery anatomy in some also precludes bypass operation. In addition, the internal mammary arteries (most often used as graft vessels in children) may be damaged by the disease. In those patients with decreased left ventricular systolic function from ischemic heart disease who are not candidates for coronary bypass, symptom-free survival is improved by ACE inhibitors such as enalapril or captopril (Pfeffer, 1992). Patients with symptoms of congestive heart failure resulting from ischemic cardiomyopathy also receive digoxin and diuretics.

Cardiomyopathy

Cardiomyopathy is disease of the heart muscle itself, occurring in the absence of ischemia, hypertension, congenital structural defect, and valvular or pericardial disease. Cardiomyopathy may be idiopathic or primary (i.e., of unknown etiology) or secondary to a known cause or systemic disease that affects the heart muscle. Cardiomyopathy is further classified as one of three types:

1. Dilated, characterized by ventricular dilation, systolic (contractile) dysfunction, and signs and symptoms of congestive heart failure
2. Hypertrophic, usually with preserved or enhanced contractile performance, but limited diastolic function (compliance)
3. Restrictive, marked by impaired diastolic filling (Fig. 19–26).

The distinction between one category and the next is not absolute; often there is overlap. The basic characteristics of each type are outlined in Table 19–18. Restrictive cardiomyopathy is very rare in children and is not considered in the sections that follow.

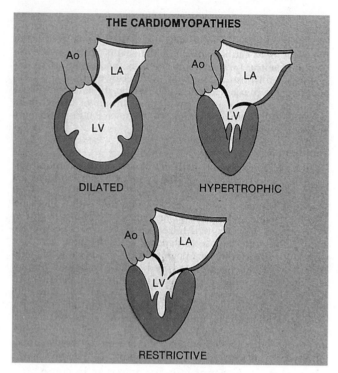

DILATED   HYPERTROPHIC

RESTRICTIVE

Figure 19–26 ● ● ● ● ● ●

Comparison of three morphologic types of cardiomyopathy. Ao, aorta; LA, left atrium; LV, left ventricle. (Modified from Roberts, W.C., Ferrans, V.J.: Pathologic anatomy of the cardiomyopathies. *Human Pathology* 6:287, 1975. In Wyngaarden, J.B., Smith, L.H., Bennett, J.C.: *Cecil textbook of medicine* 19th ed., p. 332. Philadelphia: W.B. Saunders.)

Table 19–18. CLASSIFICATION OF THE CARDIOMYOPATHIES

	Dilated	Restrictive	Hypertrophic
Symptoms	Congestive heart failure, particularly left-sided Fatigue and weakness Systemic or pulmonary emboli	Dyspnea, fatigue Right-sided congestive heart failure Signs and symptoms of systemic disease: amyloidosis, iron storage disease, etc.	Dyspnea, angina pectoris Fatigue, syncope, palpitations
Physical examination	Moderate to severe cardiomegaly; S_3 and S_4 Atrioventricular valve regurgitation, especially mitral	Mild to moderate cardiomegaly; S_3 or S_4 Atrioventricular valve regurgitation; inspiratory increase in venous pressure (Kussmaul's sign)	Mild cardiomegaly Apical systolic thrill and heave; brisk carotid upstroke S_4 common Systolic murmur that increases with Valsalva maneuver
Chest roentgenogram	Moderate to marked cardiac enlargement, especially left ventricular Pulmonary venous hypertension	Mild cardiac enlargement Pulmonary venous hypertension	Mild to moderate cardiac enlargement Left atrial enlargement
Electrocardiogram	Sinus tachycardia Atrial and ventricular arrhythmias ST segment and T wave abnormalities Intraventricular conduction defects	Low voltage Intraventricular conduction defects AV conduction defects	Left ventricular hypertrophy ST segment and T wave abnormalities Abnormal Q waves Atrial and ventricular arrhythmias
Echocardiogram	Left ventricular dilatation and dysfunction Abnormal diastolic mitral valve motion secondary to abnormal compliance and filling pressures	Increased left ventricular wall thickness and mass Small or normal-sized left ventricular cavity Normal systolic function Pericardial effusion	Asymmetric septal hypertrophy (ASH) Narrow left ventricular outflow tract Systolic anterior motion (SAM) of the mitral valve Small or normal-sized left ventricle
Cardiac catheterization	Left ventricular enlargement and dysfunction Mitral and/or tricuspid regurgitation Elevated left- and often right-sided filling pressures Diminished cardiac output	Diminished left ventricular compliance "Square root sign" in ventricular pressure recordings Preserved systolic function Elevated left- and right-sided filling pressures	Diminished left ventricular compliance Mitral regurgitation Vigorous systolic function Dynamic left ventricular outflow gradient

From Wynne J., & Braunwald E. (1992). The cardiomyopathies and myocarditides. In E. Braunwald (Ed.). *Heart Disease* (4th ed, p. 1396). Philadelphia: W. B. Saunders

Dilated Cardiomyopathy

Dilated (or congestive) cardiomyopathy is the most common cardiomyopathy in pediatric patients and results from a group of diverse disorders that cause decreased myocardial contractility and, eventually, ventricular dilation. Dilated cardiomyopathy is characterized by systolic dysfunction. Typically, the left ventricle (and sometimes the right) are enlarged, thin-walled, and poorly contractile.

Etiology. In the majority of patients, the etiology of dilated cardiomyopathy is unknown, although a link to myocarditis is often presumed. Biopsy-positive myocarditis leads to the development of dilated cardiomyopathy in as many as 50% of cases (Quigley et al., 1987). In some patients with "primary" cardiomyopathy, retrospective evidence of a postviral disorder is present in inflammatory changes on endocardial biopsy, high antibody viral titers, and others (Wynne & Braunwald, 1992). In addition, there is research evidence that patients with idiopathic cardiomyopathy have abnormalities of both cellular and humoral immunity. Antimyocardial antibodies, cytotoxic T cells, suppressor T cells, and natural killer cells have been identified in some studies (Abelman & Lorell, 1989). Possibly a prior myocarditis incorporates viral components in cardiac cells, which then serves as an antigenic source that directs the immune system to attack the myocardium.

In children, there may be genetic predisposition to develop dilated cardiomyopathy. Endocardial fibroelastosis is the second most common cause of idiopathic cardiomyopathy in children.

Secondary myocardial disease results from systemic causes in which the primary illness is extracardiac. Dilated cardiomyopathy may result from nutritional deficiencies, metabolic disorders, drug toxicity, and other systemic infections and illnesses. It is likely that dilated cardiomyopathy is the final outcome of myocardial damage that has been produced by a variety of myocardial insults that are, as yet, only incompletely understood.

Incidence. Dilated cardiomyopathy is a relatively rare illness in the pediatric population; however, its exact incidence is not known. Most patients with cardiomyopathy are 2 years of age or younger, although all ages are affected.

Pathogenesis. The precise cause of cardiac dilation and the subsequent contractile dysfunction in patients with dilated cardiomyopathy remains unclear. At postmortem examination enlargement and dilation of all four heart chambers is present, with greater ventricular than atrial dilation. Ventricular hypertrophy is sometimes seen, but the thickness of the ventricular wall is inadequate for the degree of dilation present. Small scars of the subendocardium or papillary muscles are sometimes seen in the left or right ventricle. Poor contractility permits stasis of blood, particularly in the ventricular apex, with thrombus formation.

Microscopic examination demonstrates chronic inflammation with extensive areas of fibrosis, particularly involving the left ventricular subendocardium. Myocardial cells may be hypertrophied, degenerating, or atrophied and actually necrotic.

Clinical Manifestations. Pediatric patients with dilated cardiomyopathy may be asymptomatic for months, despite ventricular dilatation. Isolated cardiac enlargement, however, is uncommon because the ability of a small patient's heart function to compensate is limited. Most present with respiratory distress or CHF. A few children are not identified until severe ventricular dysfunction occurs and cardiogenic shock with low output is present. Occasionally, ventricular ectopy or syncope may be the presenting sign.

Physical examination reveals pulmonary congestion, a quiet precordium, distant heart sounds with a prominent S_3 gallop, and hepatomegaly. If left ventricular dilation and dysfunction are severe, the murmur of mitral regurgitation may be heard at the apex. Chest radiographs reveal marked cardiomegaly and pulmonary edema (Fig. 19–27). The ECG shows nonspecific ST-T wave abnormalities and sinus tachycardia. Ventricular ectopy, low ventricular voltage, and evidence of left ventricular hypertrophy are present in many. Echocardiography shows enlargement of one or both ventricles and provides quantitative analysis of ventricular function. Shortening and ejection fraction are both decreased and, in some, regional wall motion abnormalities are detected. Mural thrombi may be evident by echocardiogram, especially in the left ventricular apex and left atrial appendage.

Diagnosis. The definitive diagnosis of dilated cardiomyopathy is aided by pathology examination of myocardial tissue obtained via cardiac catheterization. Biopsy is necessary for accurate diagnosis, because the clinical presentation and echocardiographic

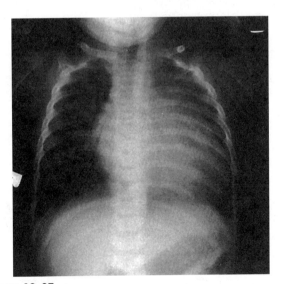

Figure 19–27 ● ● ● ● ● ●

Chest x-ray of an infant with cardiomegaly and pulmonary edema/congestive heart failure. (From Baker, A. (1994). Acquired heart disease in infants and children. *Critical Care Nursing Clinics of North America*, 6(1):182.)

findings are not substantially different in dilated cardiomyopathy, acute myocarditis, glycogen storage disease, or anomalous origin of the left coronary artery (Baker, 1994; Moore & Soifer, 1993).

Critical Care Management. Advances in supportive therapy may be able to alter the high mortality rate among children with this illness. In one study, 65% of children survived 1 year after diagnosis, but only 33% were alive at 5 years (Griffin et al., 1988). Overall survival and recovery may be higher currently (Friedman et al., 1991; Matitiau et al., 1991). Younger age at onset has been associated with better outcomes, with children younger than 2 years having a more favorable prognosis (Griffin et al., 1988).

Initial management of the patient with dilated cardiomyopathy is aimed at maximizing CO and controlling symptoms of congestive heart failure. Reduction of activity, supplemental oxygen administration, tracheal intubation, and mechanical ventilation are provided to decrease metabolic demands on the myocardium. Care is very similar to that provided to patients with acute myocarditis.

Anticoagulation therapy is instituted in patients to prevent thrombus formation in the dilated and poorly contractile heart. Management of ventricular rhythm disturbances may be necessary for some patients.

The use of beta-blockers for long-term management of pediatric patients with dilated cardiomyopathy is controversial. Early data with adult patients indicate that long-term, low-dose beta-blockade is associated with improved symptoms and left ventricular function in patients with dilated myopathy (Abramowitz, 1993).

Serial monitoring of cardiac function with echocardiography is performed to evaluate improvement or deterioration after the institution of medical management. If the patient is unresponsive to medical management or if symptoms are rapidly progressive, cardiac transplantation may be considered.

Hypertrophic Cardiomyopathy

Hypertrophic cardiomyopathy is characterized by myocardial hypertrophy, often including the ventricular septum, which is out of proportion to the hemodynamic work of the ventricle. Importantly, systemic hypertension or valvular aortic stenosis is absent in patients with hypertrophic cardiomyopathy. In some patients, a pressure gradient is present dividing the left ventricle into a high-pressure apical area and a lower-pressure subaortic area. In these individuals the terms *idiopathic hypertrophic subaortic stenosis* (IHSS) and *muscular subaortic stenosis* have been suggested. However, that terminology is inaccurate in most, who do not have obstruction to left ventricular outflow (Wynne & Braunwald, 1992).

The pathophysiologic consequence of hypertrophy of the left ventricle is abnormal relaxation or diastolic dysfunction. Diastolic dysfunction can lead to CHF, cardiac rhythm disturbances, and sudden death.

Etiology. The cause of hypertrophic cardiomyopathy is unknown. Suggested mechanisms for the pathophysiologic changes that occur include abnormal calcium kinetics, abnormal sympathetic stimulation or excessive production of catecholamines, abnormalities in dilation of the coronary arteries leading to fibrosis and compensatory hypertrophy, abnormalities of the microcirculation leading to subendocardial ischemia and diastolic stiffness, and structural abnormalities of the interventricular septum (Wynne & Braunwald, 1992). In 60% of pediatric patients with hypertrophic cardiomyopathy, there is autosomal dominant transmission of the disorder, with variable penetrance (Maron et al., 1984).

Incidence. Hypertrophic cardiomyopathy is rare in infants and children. Adolescents may develop serious cardiac rhythm disturbances and are at risk for sudden death.

Pathogenesis. The pathophysiologic process causing the cellular damage identified by endomyocardial biopsy is undefined. Microscopic findings include myocardial hypertrophy and gross disorganization of the muscle bundles, disarray in the usual cell-to-cell arrangement, and disorganization in the intracellular architecture. Fibrosis is often prominent and produces visible scars.

Impaired diastolic function and abnormal ventricular relaxation and distensibility impede diastolic filling of the ventricle. Diastolic dysfunction leads, in turn, to increased filling pressure despite a normal or small left ventricular cavity size. Increased left ventricular filling pressure leads, invariably, to elevation of the left atrial and pulmonary venous pressures.

Myocardial ischemia is common and multifactoral in hypertrophic cardiomyopathy. Major causes include impaired vasodilatory reserve (from abnormal intramural coronary arteries), increased oxygen demand (from the increased wall stress and muscle mass of the ventricle), and elevated diastolic filling pressure (with resultant subendocardial ischemia). There may be inadequate capillary density and/or systolic compression of arteries (Wynne & Braunwald, 1992).

Clinical Manifestations. The majority of people with hypertrophic cardiomyopathy are either asymptomatic or only mildly affected. Often these patients are identified during screening of relatives following the sudden death of a similarly asymptomatic person. Recognizing this disorder in children is important because of the higher mortality rate in younger patients. Death is often sudden and unexpected and has been associated, as has syncope, with competitive sports or severe exertion.

Symptomatic people most often present with dyspnea that results from impaired ventricular filling resulting from diastolic dysfunction. Infants may present with signs of CHF and a systolic heart murmur. Heart failure is rare in older children, who, in addition to dyspnea, may present with exercise intolerance, fatigue, angina, palpitations, and syncope.

Physical examination may be completely normal in asymptomatic patients. Most have a left ventricular lift, and the apical impulse is often displaced laterally and is unusually forceful. A thrill is often palpable along the left sternal border. A paradoxically split second heart sound, S_3 and S_4 gallop rhythms, and systolic murmur between the left sternal border and the apex are common. The murmur may reflect left ventricular outflow tract obstruction with a gradient or turbulent flow across the outflow tract, and concomitant mitral regurgitation. The murmur varies with the Valsalva maneuver, standing, squatting, and leg elevation.

Diagnosis. Chest radiography demonstrates cardiomegaly with normal pulmonary vascularity. The ECG is usually abnormal and demonstrates left atrial enlargement, left ventricular hypertrophy, ST segment and T wave changes, and prominent, abnormal Q waves. Cardiac rhythm disturbances are common and include sinus node and AV conduction abnormalities that may cause syncope. More often ventricular rhythm disturbances are noted, including premature ventricular contractions and episodes of nonsustained ventricular tachycardia. Supraventricular tachycardia can also occur. Because of the systolic and diastolic hemodynamic abnormalities of this disorder, cardiac rhythm disturbances are often not well tolerated.

Echocardiography demonstrates left ventricular hypertrophy: the cardinal feature of hypertrophic cardiomyopathy. Hypertrophy of the septum and the anterolateral free wall is characteristic. Narrowing of the left ventricular outflow tract is a second characteristic noted with echocardiography. With left ventricular outflow obstruction associated with a pressure gradient, abnormal motion of the mitral valve on systole is seen and mitral regurgitation, which almost always is present in the face of a pressure gradient, is demonstrated. The left ventricular chamber is small. Abnormalities of diastolic function and filling can be demonstrated in many patients. Thallium perfusion scan is becoming popular for myocardial imaging in patients with hypertrophic cardiomyopathy. Cardiac catheterization is generally reserved for those patients in whom surgical intervention is planned.

Critical Care Management. Overall management of patients with hypertrophic cardiomyopathy is directed toward alleviating symptoms, preventing complications, and reducing the risk of sudden death. Data regarding the natural history of the disorder in pediatric patients are limited. Some patients are stable without symptoms, whereas others have symptoms that rapidly progress. In one study infants who presented with congestive heart failure had poor prognosis, with most dying within a year. Asymptomatic infants had only a 50% survival rate at 1 year (Greenwood et al., 1976). Children older than 1 year of age do not usually experience heart failure, and clinical deterioration past infancy is usually slow.

Reducing the Risk of Sudden Death. Sudden death is the cause of most mortality in children with hypertrophic cardiomyopathy. Ventricular hypertrophy generally increases with somatic growth, but the extent of hypertrophy does not correlate well with the severity of symptoms. The risk of sudden death is highest in children with a history of syncope and in those with family history of sudden death from hypertrophic cardiomyopathy. The cause of sudden death is presumed to be a ventricular dysrhythmia; but in children, in whom preexisting ventricular tachycardia is less common than it is in adult patients, the precipitating event may be hemodynamic (Wynne & Braunwald, 1992). Because sudden death often occurs during exercise, strenuous exertion is avoided.

Alleviating Symptoms. Beta-blockers improve symptoms of angina, dyspnea, and presyncope in hypertrophic cardiomyopathy. The precise mechanism of action is not known with certainty, but the increase in left ventricular outflow tract obstruction that occurs with exercise is prevented, as is the chronotropic response, limiting the demand for increased oxygen. Propranolol may be given in large doses (2 mg/kg/day to a maximum of 320 mg) (Gillum, 1986).

Calcium antagonists are an alternative to beta-blockade, but there is no consensus on whether therapy should be initiated first with a beta-blocker or with a calcium antagonist. Verapamil has been used most frequently; nifedipine and diltiazem have also shown beneficial effects. Because both the hypercontractile systolic function and the abnormalities of diastolic filling may be related to abnormal calcium kinetics, blocking inward calcium transport may improve both systolic and diastolic function.

Surgical Intervention. Patients who do not respond well to medical management and are severely symptomatic may have a surgical procedure aimed at reducing the gradient across the left ventricular outflow tract. Myotomy-myectomy often relieves both the obstruction and the mitral regurgitation. Reducing left ventricular systolic pressure decreases myocardial oxygen demand and improves symptoms in 70% of patients. Perioperative mortality is low and postoperative management similar to that of other cardiac surgery patients. Patients who remain severely symptomatic following standard medical and surgical management are considered for cardiac transplantation. Figure 19–28 depicts therapeutic strategies for the management of patients with hypertrophic cardiomyopathy.

CARDIAC RHYTHM DISTURBANCES

Accurate diagnosis and definitive management of cardiac rhythm disturbances have been improved by better understanding of the mechanisms responsible for dysrhythmia production and an expanded array of treatment modalities that includes new antiarrhythmic medications, pacemaker placement, and catheter ablation of the dysrhythmic focus.

The diagnosis of dysrhythmia in an infant or child can be a relatively simple and concise procedure or a

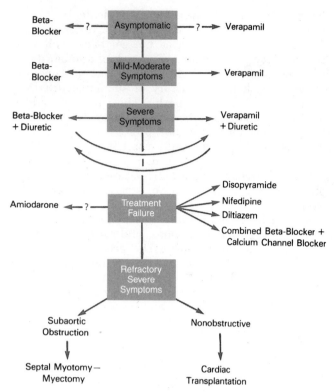

Figure 19–28 ● ● ● ● ● ●

Therapeutic strategies for patients with hypertrophic cardiomyopathy. (From Braunwald, E. (Ed.) (1989). *Heart disease: A textbook of cardiovascular medicine*, 3rd ed., Update No. 7, pp. 157–168. Philadelphia: W.B. Saunders.)

challenging and complex task. Once accurately identified, the management of abnormal heart rhythms can require routine antiarrhythmic medication or potent antiarrhythmic therapy, antitachycardia pacemaker placement, and surgical or transcatheter ablation. The sections that follow detail the diagnosis and management of cardiac rhythm disturbances in infants and children.

Etiology and Pathogenesis

A wide variety of specific cardiac disorders and systemic diseases can be the origin of a cardiac rhythm disturbance. In all, cardiac dysrhythmias are the result of abnormal impulse formation or abnormal impulse conduction, or a combination of both.

All cardiac cells are excitable. Certain cells in the sinus and AV nodes depolarize spontaneously and are designated automatic fibers. Their ability to spontaneously depolarize is called *automaticity*. The rate at which the automatic cells fire is controlled primarily by the activity of the autonomic nervous system and, secondarily, by changes in the local cellular environment (i.e., pH, Po_2, and extracellular potassium and calcium concentrations).

Abnormal impulse formation occurs when the normal sinus pacemaker is depressed or when ectopic pacemakers compete with the sinus node. For exam-

ple, sinus node automaticity may be depressed by an increase in vagal tone. Other automatic cells near the AV node or in the His-Purkinje system, which are not strongly influenced by vagal activity, can become the site of origin of the cardiac impulse. Conversely, there may be an increase in automaticity at an ectopic site. Changes in automaticity are the consequence of a local increase in SNS activity and catecholamine concentration or some local change in the cells that decreases membrane potential, such as is caused by excessive stretch, ischemia, hypokalemia, and digoxin toxicity. Ectopic impulse initiation competes with normal sinus node activity.

Abnormal impulse conduction is a second mechanism responsible for cardiac rhythm disturbances. Abnormal conduction occurs when conduction proceeds along abnormal pathways as in preexcitation (the Wolff-Parkinson-White syndrome) or other reentrant pathways, or when normal conduction is blocked as in sinoatrial block or AV conduction block.

Diagnosis

Evaluation of the infant or child with suspected or documented cardiac rhythm disturbance begins with an accurate history. Questions are targeted toward establishing (1) symptoms associated with the dysrhythmia including chest pain, fatigue, palpitations, lightheadedness, and/or syncope; (2) circumstances related to the onset and termination of the dysrhythmia; (3) past history of congenital or acquired cardiac disease; (4) history of infectious diseases; and (5) family history of cardiac rhythm disturbance or early unexplained death. The physical examination concentrates on the cardiovascular system. Cardiac auscultation reveals abnormal murmurs, clicks, and other sounds that are clues to the identification of a structural heart problem as an etiology for abnormal heart rhythm. The rate and regularity of the cardiac rhythm are assessed. Physical signs that the rhythm disturbance compromises cardiac function and/or tissue perfusion are noted.

Electrocardiogram

The surface 12- or 15-lead ECG and the cardiac rhythm strip are key for basic ECG interpretation and dysrhythmia detection, assessment, and diagnosis. However, such recordings illustrate cardiac rhythm at a single point in time and may not reveal abnormalities. The mechanism of the dysrhythmia also may remain unclear because P waves may be difficult to visualize. Recording the ECG with an esophageal electrode or from epicardial pacing wires provides additional information about electrical activity when the heart rate is very rapid or when atrial activity is difficult to distinguish from the QRS complex or T wave.

Many of the current telemetry and dysrhythmia monitoring and analysis units are helpful in caring for patients with dysrhythmias in the critical care unit. These systems recognize and store electrocardiographic strips for analysis and quantify types and numbers of specific dysrhythmias.

Echocardiography

The echocardiogram is performed to assess the structure of the heart as it is related to the etiology of a dysrhythmia and to evaluate ventricular function. Congenital heart defects often associated with cardiac rhythm disturbances are listed in Table 19–19. Decreased ventricular contractility in the face of a rhythm disturbance presents a dilemma. Has the dysrhythmia led to a poorly contractile ventricle or is a poorly functioning heart the etiology of the rhythm disturbance? Evaluation of ventricular function also is important because antidysrhythmic medications may depress function further.

Electrophysiology Study

Invasive evaluation of the conduction system is undertaken with an electrophysiology study (EPS). At cardiac catheterization, multiple catheters in the right heart are used to record the ECG from various sites (the SA node, AV node, and His bundle). Ectopic foci and accessory pathways can be located and mapped. In addition to definitive diagnosis of a rhythm disturbance, EPS permits evaluation of medication efficacy and therapeutic ablation of an ectopic focus or accessory pathway.

Sinus Dysrhythmias

Sinus bradycardia, sinus tachycardia, and sinus node dysfunction (SND) (also called sick sinus syndrome) may be seen in pediatric patients in the PICU. Both sinus bradycardia and tachycardia are fairly common, whereas SND is more common in adult patients and is usually associated with ischemic heart disease, cardiomyopathy, or age-related degenerative changes (Hanisch & Perron, 1992).

Sinus bradycardia is defined relative to the age of the patient (i.e., a heart rate less than age-related normal values). Sinus tachycardia is heart rate greater than age-related normal values (Table 19–20).

SND is manifest as sinus bradycardia or sinus arrest, or as a combination of bradydysrhythmias and tachydysrhythmias, in which the bradycardia predisposes the heart to develop ectopic beats.

Etiology and Clinical Presentation

Sinus bradycardia may be caused by hypoxia, hyperkalemia, vagal stimulation, increased intracranial pressure, hypothyroidism, sedation or anesthesia, hypothermia, or sleep. Cardiac causes include sinus node dysfunction and medication effect (e.g., digoxin or beta-blockers). Sinus tachycardia is a physiologic response to fever, sepsis, pain, anxiety, anemia, hypo-

Table 19–19. CONGENITAL HEART DEFECTS AND CARDIAC RHYTHM DISTURBANCES

UNOPERATED CONGENITAL HEART DEFECTS

Eisenmenger's syndrome (Pulmonary vascular obstructive disease)
Ventricular arrhythmias (ventricular volume and pressure overload)
Sudden death
Atrial fibrillation or flutter (AV valve regurgitation)

Pulmonary stenosis or atresia and cyanosis
SVT
Atrial flutter
Ventricular arrhythmias (especially with marked polycythemia)

Ebstein's anomaly
SVT
WPW with SVT
Atrial flutter or fibrillation
AV block
Junctional rhythm
Ventricular tachycardia and fibrillation
Sudden death

Corrected transposition of the great arteries
AV block (second or third degree)
WPW with SVT
Sudden death

Tricuspid atresia
Atrial ectopy, flutter, fibrillation
Ventricular ectopy

Aortic stenosis and coarctation of the aorta
Ventricular arrhythmias (with marked elevation of left ventricular pressure)

Tetralogy of Fallot (in older patients)
Ventricular arrhythmias
SVT

Atrial septal defects (in older patients)
Atrial flutter and fibrillation
SVT
Junctional and ectopic atrial rhythms
Sinus node dysfunction (sinus venosus ASD)
AV block (primum ASD)

POSTOPERATIVE DYSRHYTHMIAS IN CONGENITAL HEART DISEASE

Extensive atrial surgery/repairs with elevated atrial pressure (Fontan procedure, Mustard or Senning repair, total anomalous pulmonary venous return, atrial septal defect [rare])
Supraventricular dysrhythmias
    SVT*
    Atrial flutter
    Sinus node dysfunction
    Sinus bradycardia
Ventricular dysrhythmias (as patients age)

Ventricular septal surgery (Ventricular septal defect, tetralogy of Fallot, AV canal defects, subaortic stenosis)
AV conduction block
Ventricular tachycardia**

SVT, supraventricular tachycardia; WPW, Wolff-Parkinson-White syndrome; ASD, atrioseptal defect; AV, atrioventricular

*An unusual form of SVT, junctional ectopic tachycardia or accelerated junctional rhythm, is seen most commonly after repair of tetralogy of Fallot or the Fontan repair.

**Ventricular tachycardia is also noted after repair of the Ebstein anomaly, coronary artery anomalies, single-ventricle complexes with the Fontan procedure, and D-transposition of the great arteries.

volemia, thyrotoxicosis, CHF, or others, or may be caused by medication (e.g., catecholamines).

SND is most often seen in pediatric patients who have had operations for CHD. Direct trauma to the SA node or its arterial blood supply during a surgical

Table 19–20. NORMAL VALUES IN PEDIATRIC CARDIAC RHYTHM ASSESSMENT

Age Interval	Heart Rate × (range) (per minute)	P Wave Height/Duration (mm/second)	Max. PR Interval Heart Interval (rate)	(second)	QRS Duration (second)	Qt$_c$ (second)
0–24 hours	119 (94–145)	<3.0/0.06		<0.11	0.04–0.05	<0.49
1–7 days	133 (100–175)	"			"	"
8–30 days	163 (115–190)				"	"
1–3 months	154 (124–190)	<2.5/0.08	91–110	<0.14	"	"
			111–130	<0.13		
			131–150	<0.12		
			>150	<0.11		
3–6 months	140 (111–179)	"	"	"	"	"
6–9 months	140 (112–177)	"	"	"	"	<0.425
9–12 months	140 (112–177)	"	91–110	<0.15	0.05–0.06	"
			111–150	<0.14		
			>150	<0.10		
1–3 years	126 (98–163)	"	"	"	"	"
3–5 years	98 (65–132)	"		<0.16	0.06–0.08	"
5–8 years	96 (70–115)	"	<90	<0.18	"	"
			>90	<0.16		
8–12 years	79 (55–107)	"	"		0.08–0.10	"
12–16 years	75 (55–102)	"	"		"	"

Adapted from Curley, M. A. Q. (1988). Pediatric cardiac dysrhythmias. In S. V. Kelly (Ed.). *Pediatric emergency nursing.* Norwalk, CT: Appleton-Lange.

procedure or when the superior vena caval–right atrial junction is cannulated for cardiopulmonary bypass causes SND. Long-term follow-up of patients who had a Mustard or Senning repair of transposition of the great arteries revealed SND in 50% (Garson, 1990). SND or sinus bradycardia may also develop in 50% of children who undergo Fontan repair (Kugler, 1990). Also at risk for SND, although less commonly affected, are those who have operations for atrial septal defect, atrioventricular septal defect, Ebstein's anomaly, and anomalous pulmonary venous return. Infrequently, SND is seen in patients with unoperated CHDs.

Other nonsurgical causes of SND include inflammatory carditis (such as that seen with myocarditis, rheumatic fever, Kawasaki disease), cardiomyopathy, and ischemia. Increased vagal tone induces SND. Antidysrhythmic drugs (e.g., digoxin, beta-blockers, calcium channel blockers, and the type I medications) may cause SND as a side effect of their administration.

Critical Care Management

Treatment of sinus bradycardia necessitates identifying the underlying cause to remedy it. In all patients with bradycardia, assessment of the hemodynamic significance of the slow heart rhythm is essential. If possible the patient is stimulated and aroused. Acute management, if the origin of the bradycardia is cardiac or if the underlying cause cannot be corrected, for symptomatic patients is intravenous administration of atropine (0.02 to 0.04 mg/kg; minimum dose, 0.1 mg). Atropine is followed by epinephrine (0.1 to 1 mcg/kg/minute), administered by continuous infusion at a dose that maintains the desired heart rate if bradycardia recurs after one or

two doses of atropine. In infants younger than 2 months and in patients with sinus bradycardia secondary to hypoxic-ischemic insult, epinephrine is the first line drug, administered at a dose of 0.01 to 0.02 mg/kg and followed with an epinephrine infusion if necessary (Chameides, 1988).

Sinus tachycardia treatment lies in remedying the underlying cause of the physiologic response of the heart to demands for increased CO.

Most pediatric patients (70%) are asymptomatic with SND (Kugler, 1990). Infants may exhibit poor feeding, lethargy, and CHF, whereas older children experience exercise intolerance, fatigue, dizziness, and near or actual syncope. In all age groups, the clinical manifestations are related to bradycardia or limited ability to increase the heart rate with exercise. Medical management is the same as that described earlier for sinus bradycardia. Permanent pacemaker implantation is indicated for symptomatic infants and children or for those who require antidysrhythmic medications for bradycardia-tachycardia syndrome.

Atrial Dysrhythmias

Atrial dysrhythmias are the consequence of an ectopic atrial focus and are recognized by abnormal P wave morphology (i.e., size, shape, axis) when compared with the sinus node P wave. Common atrial dysrhythmias in infants and children include ectopic atrial pacemaker rhythms (e.g., coronary sinus rhythm or left atrial rhythm), premature atrial contractions (PACs), and supraventricular tachycardia (e.g., ectopic atrial tachycardia [EAT], atrial tachycardia from Wolff-Parkinson-White syndrome, and atrial flutter).

Table 19–21. TYPES OF SUPRAVENTRICULAR TACHYCARDIA

Reentry with a bypass tract
Wolff-Parkinson-White syndrome (Kent fibers)
Unidirectional accessory pathway
Permanent junctional reciprocating pathway
Lown-Ganong-Levine syndrome

Reentry without a bypass tract
Sinus node reentry
Atrial muscle reentry
Atrioventricular reentry

Ectopic focus with increased automaticity
Atrial ectopic
Junctional ectopic

Etiology and Clinical Presentation

Increased automaticity is responsible for atrial ectopic rhythms and PACs. In addition, PACs may be related to local irritation of atrial tissue from a central venous catheter within the right atrium. Both are distinguished from normal sinus rhythm by P wave morphology. Normal sinus P waves are upright in leads I, II, and AVF, with an axis of 0 to 90 degrees. Low right atrial (coronary sinus) P waves are negative in II, III, and AVF, are upright in V_6, and have an axis of 180 to 360 degrees. A left atrial rhythm produces negative P waves in II, III, AVF, and V_6 and has a P wave axis of 90 to 270 degrees. PACs are distinguished from sinus beats by the early timing of the P wave with configuration different from sinus P waves and followed by a normal QRS complex.

Accelerated atrial rhythms are caused by either increased automaticity or reentry phenomenon. EAT is caused by a single nonsinus atrial focus with abnormal automaticity. Atrial flutter is identified primarily in two groups of pediatric patients: the fetus or newborn, typically with a structurally normal heart; and more commonly, the older child with a CHD who has undergone cardiac surgery (e.g., Mustard or Senning repair, Fontan operation, Blalock-Hanlon atrial septectomy, or repair of ASD). It may also occur in patients with dilated atria, rheumatic heart disease, mitral valve prolapse, pericarditis, or cardiomyopathy (Perry, 1990).

In patients with Wolff-Parkinson-White syndrome (WPW), an accessory pathway, the bundle of Kent, connects the atria to the ventricles, placing the individual at risk for preexcitation of the ventricles and subsequent SVT. Nearly one quarter of children with SVT have WPW syndrome (Ludomirsky & Garson, 1990). WPW is seen in children with structurally normal hearts, as well as in children with CHD (Ebstein's anomaly, atrioventricular septal defect, and tricuspid atresia). Both atrial flutter and WPW are reentrant dysrhythmias. SVT may be the consequence of reentry via other bypass tracts or reentry without a bypass tract. Table 19–21 lists the types of SVT.

ECG Characteristics. Several features differentiate accelerated rhythms caused by abnormal automaticity from those that result from reentry. An automatic tachycardia is characterized by gradual "warm-up and cool-down" periods; slight variation in the R to R interval with vagal maneuvers; variations in rate that are related to body temperature and autonomic tone; and refractoriness to electrical cardioversion, overdrive pacing, and pharmacotherapy. In contrast, reentrant tachycardias are characterized by abrupt onset and termination of the rapid heart rate; unwavering regularity of the rhythm; and generally easy breaks with cardioversion, overdrive pacing, or adenosine administration. SVT must also be distinguished from sinus tachycardia. Defining characteristics of each are listed in Table 19–22.

Morphology of the P wave is abnormal, when compared with the sinus P wave, in all atrial tachycardias and may help to distinguish them from sinus tachycardia. However, P waves may be difficult to detect with rapid rhythms, necessitating evaluation of a number of leads, esophageal electrocardiogram, or atrial electrocardiogram.

The electrocardiographic appearance of atrial flutter is the characteristic "sawtooth" flutter pattern made by the rhythmic, rapid atrial activity. Atrial rates in children range from 200 to 350 beats per minute (bpm), whereas in infants rates as rapid as 350 to 600 bpm are seen. Infants and children tend to have more rapid conduction to the ventricles, but 1:1 AV conduction in atrial flutter is rare (Hanisch & Perron, 1992).

SVT resulting from WPW syndrome presents with

Table 19–22. CHARACTERISTICS OF SINUS AND SUPRAVENTRICULAR TACHYCARDIA

	Sinus Tachycardia	Supraventricular Tachycardia
History	Febrile illness, dehydration, or volume loss	Lethargy or irritability, poor feeding, pallor, diaphoresis without specific causation
Exam	Consistent with fever, dehydration, or bleeding	Signs of CHF: tachypnea, rales, dyspnea, hepatomegaly, decreased tissue perfusion
CXR	Normal heart size, clear lung fields	Cardiomegaly, pulmonary edema
ECG*	Heart rate usually >200 bpm, slight variation in R-R intervals, P waves visible, narrow QRS	Heart rate >220 bpm, regular R-R intervals, P waves may be detectable (50%), narrow QRS (>90%)
Echo	Usually normal	Ventricular dilation, dysfunction

bpm, beats per minute; CXR, chest x-ray; ECG, electrocardiogram; Echo, echocardiogram; Exam, examination; ST, sinus tachycardia
*An additional ECG finding, if the onset of the dysrhythmia is captured, is the gradual acceleration of ST as compared to the abrupt onset of SVT
Data from Hanisch, D. G., & Perron, L. (1992). Complex dysrhythmias in infants and children. *AACN Clinical Issues,* 3:255–267.

classic ECG findings: a short PR interval, a delta
wave (i.e., slurred upstroke of the PR interval into
the QRS complex), and a narrow QRS complex. SVT
in infants and children, as in adults, begins abruptly
with a rapid, monotonously regular, narrow complex
tachycardia with the rate generally greater than 220
bpm. In infants younger than 4 months of age, who
account for nearly one half of pediatric patients with
SVT, the heart rate may be 300 bpm or higher. The
P waves are visible on the ECG in 50% to 60% of
cases, whereas the QRS complex is normal in duration and morphology in 92% (Ludomirsky & Garson,
1990).

Critical Care Management

Most often PACs and ectopic atrial pacemaker dysrhythmias do not require acute intervention. They
are benign, hemodynamically insignificant rhythms;
but PACs have the potential to initiate a more significant atrial rhythm disturbance. Their presence is
noted and, if the patient's central line is implicated
in causing atrial ectopy, it is repositioned to remedy
the situation.

Management of SVT is determined by the mechanism of the dysrhythmia and the patient's clinical
status. Clinical instability is indicated by signs of
poor CO and inadequate tissue perfusion (weak peripheral pulses, prolonged capillary refill, mottling,
cool extremities, altered mental status, and hypotension). Immediate synchronized DC cardioversion is
indicated in this situation (Chameides, 1988). Table
19–23 describes the equipment, medications, and
procedure for cardioversion and defibrillation of pediatric patients.

Vagal Stimulation. In clinically stable SVT,
methods of treatment that induce strong vagal stimulation of the heart are attempted. The diving reflex
is elicited by immersing the child's face in cold water
or applying a bag of ice water to the face for 10 to 30
seconds. This technique is most effective in infants
younger than 6 months and in children older than 6
years, although it may be efficacious and is attempted in all age groups (Ludomirsky & Garson,
1990). Other vagal maneuvers include the Valsalva
(accomplished by having the child bear down or blow
against a thumb placed at the lips as if it were a
trumpet). The child may also be instructed to inspire
deeply, drink ice water, or perform a headstand for
several moments. A cough or gag may be induced if
these techniques are not successful or in children
too young to cooperatively perform vagal maneuvers.
Unilateral carotid sinus massage for 5 to 10 seconds
also induces a vagal response. Ocular pressure is
contraindicated in children because of the risk of
serious eye injury. Vagal maneuvers, with the exception of the diving reflex, are rarely successful in children younger than 4 years of age.

Pharmacotherapy. Acute management of SVT
may also include medications to disrupt the reentry
pathway. Adenosine (100–250 mcg/kg; maximum
dose 12 mg) is administered by rapid IV push and

Table 19–23. CARDIOVERSION AND DEFIBRILLATION IN PEDIATRIC PATIENTS

Indications
Synchronized cardioversion (R wave sensing assured)
   Atrial flutter or fibrillation
   Supraventricular tachycardia
   Ventricular tachycardia
   Not indicated for junctional ectopic tachycardia or chaotic
      atrial rhythm
Defibrillation (asynchronous)
   Pulseless ventricular tachycardia
   Ventricular fibrillation

Sedation (If Awake)
Midazolam: 0.10 mg/kg IV, followed by 0.05 mg/kg every 2
   minutes as needed
Diazepam: 0.2–0.5 mg/kg/dose IV every 15 minutes

Paddle Size
Infant: 4.5 cm
Child: 8 or 13 cm (assure good contact with skin)

Electrode Placement
Standard: Base at upper right chest
   Apex at left anterior axillary line
Anterior-posterior: Base on anterior chest over the heart
   Apex on the back

Energy Dose
Synchronized cardioversion: 0.5–1 watt-second (joule) per kg
   Repeat with 2 watt-second/kg if needed
Defibrillation: 2 watt-second per kg
   Repeat with 4 watt-second/kg if needed

Adapted from Perry, J. C., & Garson, A. (1989). Diagnosis and treatment
of arrhythmias. *Advances in Pediatrics*, 36:177–200.

repeated every 2 minutes to slow conduction through
the AV node. Digoxin also slows AV nodal conduction,
but requires a 12- to 24-hour period for digitalizing
the patient. Verapamil (150 mcg/kg) is also effective
for converting SVT. However, intravenous verapamil
has been associated with cardiovascular collapse (severe hypotension and cardiac arrest) in infants and
is usually not recommended for children younger
than 1 year of age. Verapamil is also contraindicated
in children with CHF and in those who are administered beta-blockers concomitantly.

Chronic pharmacologic management of SVT may
include digoxin, beta-blocking agents such as propranolol or atenolol, quinidine, encainide, flecainide,
or verapamil. Digoxin may enhance conduction
through the accessory pathway in patients with
WPW syndrome by shortening its refractory period
as it prolongs AV nodal conduction. Consequently, it
may predispose to ventricular tachycardia (VT) or
fibrillation (Perry & Garson, 1989; Moak, 1990a).
Failed medical therapy or serious side effects of potent dysrhythmic agents are indications for catheter
or surgical ablation of the reentrant pathway or ectopic focus (Crawford et al., 1990; Case et al., 1990).

Overdrive Pacing. Overdrive pacing techniques
can be used for acute management of patients with
SVT. Transesophageal pacing positions an electrode
in the esophagus behind the left atrium. The heart
is then paced at a rate 10 to 30 bpm higher than the
rate of the tachycardia for 10 to 30 seconds. After
atrial capture is achieved, the pacemaker is switched

off and the heart's normal sinus pacemaker resumes control of heart rate (Moak, 1990b).

Atrioventricular Nodal and Junctional Dysrhythmias

Atrioventricular nodal or junctional dysrhythmias are the consequence of either abnormal conduction from the SA node through the AV node, which prolongs the PR interval or produces AV dissociation, or abnormal automaticity in the AV node, which produces junctional ectopic tachycardia. Because they are similar only in terms of the location of their origin, they are considered separately.

Junctional Ectopic Tachycardia

Junctional ectopic tachycardia (JET) is an unusual form of SVT that is challenging to diagnose and treat, which, despite aggressive intervention, is associated with high mortality in infants and children (Ludomirsky & Garson, 1990).

Etiology and Pathogenesis. JET is an automatic tachycardia caused by enhanced automaticity of cells in the AV node or proximal His bundle. Most often, JET occurs acutely in infants or young children following cardiac surgery and is thought to be the consequence of trauma or edema at the bundle of His. More rarely, JET is seen as a congenital rhythm disturbance in infants with structurally normal hearts. Typically the inherent rate of the junctional pacemaker is 130 to 300 bpm.

The pathophysiologic consequences of JET are the result of both the sustained rapid heart rate associated with decreased ventricular filling time and dissociated atrial contraction. In postoperative cardiac surgery patients, profound hypotension and cardiovascular collapse may develop. Infants with congenital JET develop left ventricular dysfunction over a period of several months (Ludomirsky & Garson, 1990).

ECG Characteristics. The QRS complex in JET is narrow, making it difficult to distinguish it from an atrial tachycardia. An atrial epicardial or transesophageal ECG is most often necessary to differentiate JET from other types of SVT. These tools demonstrate an atrial rate slightly slower than the ventricular rate.

Critical Care Management. JET is most often a transient, self-limited dysrhythmia that terminates spontaneously in hours to days after onset. Hemodynamic instability demands treatment in some postoperative cardiac surgery patients and infants. The goal of management is twofold: first, to restore AV synchrony and, second, to slow the junctional tachycardia. AV synchrony is restored, provided the heart rate is less than 200 bpm, by overdrive atrial or AV sequential pacing at a rate slightly above the junctional rate. Slowing the junctional rate is best achieved by lowering the body temperature to about 34°C, using either a cooling mattress or peritoneal

lavage with cool solution (Ruggerie, 1990). Hypothermia necessitates sedation and paralysis to prevent shivering, with concomitant intubation and mechanical ventilation.

Pharmacologic therapy of JET is difficult. Procainamide in combination with hypothermia has been effective. If additional medications are required for control, a beta-blocker is added to the procainamide and hypothermia. Generally, this combination successfully slows the rate sufficiently to allow hemodynamic stability until the rhythm self-terminates. Success with propafenone has been reported (Garson et al., 1987). Life-threatening cases of JET may necessitate surgical or catheter ablation of the bundle of His, with permanent pacing required thereafter (Hanisch & Perron, 1992). Long-term pharmacologic management is initiated with digoxin combined with propranolol. Treatment with procainamide, flecainide, or amiodarone may be considered (Ludomirsky & Garson, 1990).

AV Conduction Block

First degree heart block is the consequence of slowed conduction of an impulse through the AV node. It is characterized by a prolonged PR interval on the ECG with a P wave preceding each QRS complex. There is no significant hemodynamic impact, and this conduction disturbance does not necessitate intervention beyond the identification of its etiology. In pediatric patients digoxin administration is the most common cause of first degree heart block.

Second degree heart block occurs when an occasional or patterned block of AV conduction occurs. The ECG characteristics of Mobitz type I and Mobitz type II second degree heart block have been described. Mobitz type I second degree heart block may reflect AV node dysfunction in patients following intracardiac surgical procedures near the AV node or in those with digoxin, beta-blocker, calcium channel, or quinidine toxicity. It may be seen in patients without cardiovascular disease, especially during sleep. Most often, treatment is not required because this conduction delay does not compromise cardiac output and tissue perfusion unless the ventricular rate is excessively slow. In addition, it is unlikely to progress to complete heart block.

Mobitz type II second degree heart block is usually related to His bundle or bundle branch dysfunction, most often resulting from surgical injury. Progression to complete heart block is more common.

Complete heart block (CHB) is also called "third degree heart block" or "AV dissociation." It can be related to CHD, or it may occur congenitally in infants with normal cardiac structure, or it may be acquired. Regardless of etiology, the sinoatrial (SA) node paces the atria, whereas an independent junctional or ventricular pacemaker establishes the ventricular rhythm. Tissue perfusion is at risk for compromise, because CO may be inadequate.

Etiology and Clinical Presentation. Congenital complete heart block (CHB) occurs only about once in every 22,000 live births (Ross, 1990). Most infants with congenital CHB have normal cardiac structure, while about one third have associated CHDs. In infants with CHB and single ventricle, atrioventricular septal defect, tricuspid atresia, and coarctation of the aorta with endocardial fibroelastosis, the conduction block is thought to be the result of developmental abnormalities in the AV node. The most commonly associated CHD is L-transposition of the great arteries with ventricular inversion (Perry & Garson, 1989). It is possible that the abnormal twisting of the ventricles results in disruption of the AV node and His bundle. In infants without CHD there is a strong association between the incidence of congenital CHB and maternal connective tissue disease, typically systemic lupus erythematosus.

Low fetal heart rate usually leads to the diagnosis of congenital CHB. Fetal echocardiography detects asynchronous and independent contraction of the atria and ventricles. After birth, infants with congenital CHB may be severely symptomatic or may present without clinical findings suggestive of difficulty, save the slow heart rate. Severe CHF is manifested by hydrops fetalis, tachypnea, and lethargy. The presence of severe heart failure is associated with a neonatal mortality rate of 10% (Ross et al., 1990). Infants with CHD are more symptomatic, present sooner following birth, and are at increased risk of sudden death (Ross, 1990; Ross et al., 1990). After infancy, children with congenital CHB and a structurally normal heart may present with exercise intolerance, fatigue, or syncope. In these youngsters, the ventricular rate and the ability of the heart rate to increase with activity determine their symptomatology.

Acquired CHB is most often seen as a complication of intracardiac surgery near the AV junction, although it can also occur secondary to endocarditis, myocarditis, or Lyme disease. Surgical procedures with increased risk for complete heart block include repair of ventricular or atrioventricular septal defects, L-transposition of the great arteries, tetralogy of Fallot, aortic stenosis, mitral or tricuspid valve replacement, and a Fontan procedure requiring that the tricuspid valve be oversewn (Ross et al., 1990). Postoperative CHB may be transient or permanent, as is also the case with cardiac infection or inflammation. One quarter to one half of patients with AV block in the early postoperative period regain normal sinus rhythm within 2 weeks (Garson, 1984). However, CHB may occur late in these patients, and then is most often permanent (Ross et al., 1990). Implantation of a permanent pacemaker is recommended in patients with CHB that persists for 14 days.

ECG Characteristics. The P wave in patients with CHB originates in the SA node and is of normal morphology. However, transmission through the AV node is blocked and an escape rhythm, usually generated by a site high in the His bundle, ensues. The QRS complex is correspondingly wide. The P-P interval is regular, as is the R-R interval.

Critical Care Management. Acute management of congenital CHB is aimed at both treating heart failure and raising heart rate. Emergency cesarean section may be necessitated by evidence of fetal distress or hydrops. A continuous infusion of epinephrine (0.05–0.1 mcg/kg/minute) raises the heart rate to a safe level. Temporary pacing may be achieved via transthoracic or transvenous wires or by noninvasive transcutaneous electrodes; but often the infant remains on epinephrine until the clinical condition is stable enough to permit an operation and a permanent pacemaker is implanted.

Infants and children who are asymptomatic despite congenital CHB may undergo pacemaker implantation, although criteria for recommending the appropriate time, in the absence of symptoms, have not been established. There is general agreement that permanent pacing is recommended for asymptomatic infants with a ventricular rate less than 55 bpm and for infants or children with structural heart defects and congenital CHB. Exercise testing and Holter monitoring are used with older children to determine their exercise tolerance and the ability of the ventricular rate to increase, and to detect the presence of ventricular dysrhythmias. Ventricular ectopy, diminished capacity for exercise, and awake heart rate less than 50 bpm are usually considered indications for permanent pacing (Ross, 1990; Ross et al., 1990).

Ventricular Dysrhythmias

Infants and children have far fewer ventricular dysrhythmias than adults. Premature ventricular contractions and ventricular tachycardia are the ventricular rhythm disturbances most commonly encountered in pediatric patients.

Premature Ventricular Contractions

Premature ventricular contractions (PVCs) in children are recognized in the ECG as an early QRS complex with morphology different than that of the sinus QRS. Typically the duration of the QRS complex is prolonged in a PVC and the complex is bizarre in appearance, but nearly normal appearance and normal duration of the QRS complex for age are not uncommon, particularly in infants with PVCs.

PVCs can either be isolated or appear as bigeminy; but when PVC morphology is uniform and the PVCs decrease with exercise or increased heart rate in children without structural heart disease, hemodynamic consequence is exceptional. So-called benign PVCs are reported in as many as 33% of newborns and 10% to 20% of infants and children, based on Holter recordings (Garson, 1984). Conversely, children with structural heart defects or those with multiform PVCs, couplets, or PVCs that do not suppress with increased heart rate are at increased risk for hemodynamic compromise or deterioration of the PVCs into a lethal rhythm disturbance. Careful sur-

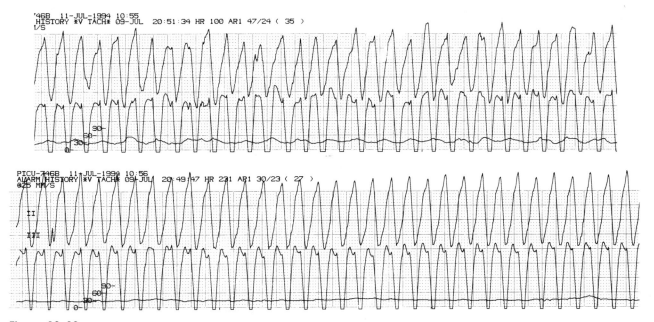

Figure 19–29 ● ● ● ● ● ●

Ventricular tachycardia in a 6-month-old with severe left ventricular outflow tract obstruction.

veillance is necessitated, although almost all PVCs require only observation without intervention.

Ventricular Tachycardia

Ventricular tachycardia (VT) is a serious ventricular rhythm disturbance with high potential for mortality. Because of its potential significance, *any wide complex tachycardia is treated as ventricular in origin until proved otherwise.*

Etiology and Clinical Presentation. Causes of VT in infants and children include profound electrolyte or metabolic disturbances including acidosis, hypoglycemia, hyperkalemia, hypokalemia, hypercalcemia, hypomagnesemia, and hypothermia. Other potential etiologies are drug toxicity (digoxin, quinidine, procainamide, sympathomimetics, anesthetic agents, cocaine, caffeine, nicotine) and cardiac pathology (cardiomyopathy, myocarditis, cardiac tumors, long QT interval syndrome). Cardiovascular collapse can develop rapidly with VT, with a typical presentation.

ECG Characteristics. VT occurs at a rate generally between 120 and 300 bpm. The complexes are wide and bizarre in appearance (Fig. 19–29). In patients with long QT interval syndrome, torsade de pointes, an unusual form of VT, may develop. Figure 19–30 illustrates the unique rotation of the ventricular complexes around the baseline.

Critical Care Management. Management of VT is initiated with assessment of the hemodynamic significance of the rhythm disturbance. Immediate synchronized cardioversion is necessary if the patient's condition is unstable. A lidocaine bolus (1 mg/kg) is followed by a continuous infusion (10–50 mcg/kg/minute). With the rhythm controlled, attention is directed toward correcting the initiating physiologic derangement, if possible.

If the patient's condition is stable, treatment proceeds with lidocaine, procainamide, propranolol, phenytoin, or amiodarone. Procainamide is contraindicated in patients with long QT interval syndrome or torsade de pointes VT. Overdrive pacing may also effectively terminate VT (Hanisch & Perron, 1992).

Long-term treatment of VT may include medical or surgical management. Surgical management is indicated in patients with cardiac tumors or severe left ventricular outflow obstruction. Long QT interval syndrome has been treated with left cardiac sympathectomy in a few patients (Case et al., 1990). An antitachycardia pacemaker or automatic implantable defibrillator may be necessary for patients with VT

Figure 19–30 ● ● ● ● ● ●

Ventricular tachycardia with torsade de pointes configuration. (From Holbrook, P.R. (1993). *Textbook of pediatric critical care*, p. 406. Philadelphia: W.B. Saunders.)

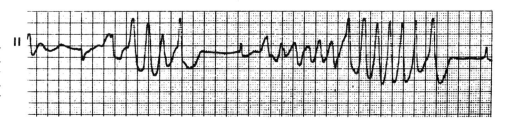

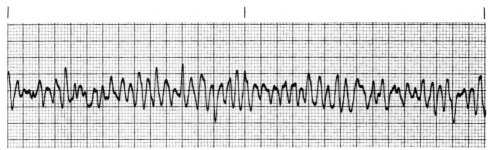

Figure 19–31 ● ● ● ● ● ●
Ventricular fibrillation. (From Curley, M.A.Q. (1985). *Pediatric cardiac dysrhythmias*, p. 125. Bowie, MD: Brady Communications Company, Inc. With permission of Appleton & Lange.)

refractory to medical management. Pharmacologic management includes beta-blockers, the medication of choice for patients with long QT interval syndrome, or phenytoin, mexiletine, tocainide, or amiodarone.

Ventricular Fibrillation

Ventricular fibrillation (VF) results from erratic firing of multiple ectopic foci in the ventricles, resulting in disorganized electrical activity and ineffective ventricular contraction.

Etiology and Clinical Presentation. VF is uncommon in infants and children. It may occur in patients with CHD or in those in whom resuscitation attempts are prolonged. The patient has obvious cardiovascular collapse, evidenced by pulselessness, apnea, and unresponsiveness. More often, severe bradycardia or idioventricular rhythm persists even in arrest situations.

ECG Characteristics. VF is documented by an ECG without measurable heart rate in which no P, QRS, or T waves can be identified. An erratic, wavy baseline is present (Fig. 19–31).

Critical Care Management. Cardiopulmonary resuscitation (CPR) is initiated to maintain circulation and oxygenation while the defibrillator is readied. Rapid asynchronous defibrillation is performed up to three times (2 watt-second/kg the first time and 4 watt-second/kg for subsequent attempts). If VF persists, IV epinephrine (0.01 mg/kg) and lidocaine (1 mg/kg) are administered while CPR continues. Defibrillation (4 watt-second/kg) is attempted 30 to 60 seconds after the medications are administered. Persistent VF is treated with second doses of epinephrine (0.1–0.2 mg/kg) and lidocaine (1 mg/kg). Epinephrine may be repeated every 3 to 5 minutes. Bretylium (5–10 mg/kg) is considered. Defibrillation (4 watt-second/kg) is repeated 30 to 60 seconds after medication is administered (Chameides, 1988) until VF is interrupted or the situation is deemed hopeless and resuscitation attempts are stopped.

SUMMARY

Cardiovascular dysfunction may be the consequence of congenital defects of cardiac structure, acquired heart diseases, or cardiac rhythm disturbances. Heart failure, cardiogenic shock, and hypoxemia are the potential final pathways.

This chapter provided an overview of cardiovascular dysfunction, which included assessment of patients with inadequate tissue perfusion and guidelines for providing baseline support. Congestive heart failure and hypoxemia were considered next from the perspective of the etiology, pathogenesis, clinical manifestations, and critical care management.

Congenital heart defects were discussed based on a classification system that examines the presence or absence of cyanosis and the volume of pulmonary blood flow. Intensive care of pediatric cardiac surgery patients was discussed in the next section. Critical care management was considered from the perspective of preventing potential complications.

The final sections of the chapter considered pediatric patients with acquired heart diseases and those with cardiac rhythm disturbances. Although these problems are less often the cause of critical illness in infants and children, their care is complex and requires expert and knowledgeable practitioners.

References

Abelman, W.H., & Lorell, B.H. (1989). The challenge of cardiomyopathy. *Journal of the American College of Cardiology*, 13:1219–1224.

Abramowitz, M. (1993). Drugs for chronic heart failure. *Medical Letter*, 8:40–42.

American Heart Association. Committee on Rheumatic Fever and Infectious Endocarditis of the Council on Cardiovascular Disease in the Young. (1984). Jones criteria (revised) for guidance in the diagnosis of rheumatic fever. *Circulation*, 60:204A.

Anand, K.J.S., & Hickey, P.R. (1992). Halothane-morphine compared with high dose sufentanyl for anesthesia and postoperative analgesia in neonatal cardiac surgery. *New England Journal of Medicine*, 326:1–11.

Artez, H.T. (1987). Myocarditis: The Dallas criteria. *Human Pathology*, 18:619–624.

Artman, M., & Graham, T.P. (1982). Congestive heart failure in infancy: Recognition and management. *American Heart Journal*, 103:1040–1055.

Artman, M., Parrish, M.D., & Graham, T.P. (1983). Congestive heart failure in childhood and adolescence: Recognition and management. *American Heart Journal*, 105:471–480.

Backer, C.L., & Mavroudis, C. (1993). Perioperative care. In C. Mavroudis & C.L. Backer (Eds.). *Pediatric cardiac surgery*. St Louis: C.V. Mosby.

Bailey, C.P., Cookson, B.A., Downing, D.F., et al. (1975). Cardiac surgery under hypothermia. *Journal of Thoracic and Cardiovascular Surgery*, 27:73–77.

Bailey, L.L., & Gundry, S.R. (1990). Hypoplastic left heart syndrome. *Pediatric Clinics of North America*, 37:137–150.

Bailey, L.L., Nehlsen-Cannarella, S.L., & Doroshow, R.W. (1986). Cardiac allotransplantation in newborns as therapy for hypoplastic left heart syndrome. *New England Journal of Medicine*, 315:949–951.

Baker, A. (1994). Acquired heart disease in infants and children. *Critical Care Nursing Clinics of North America*, 6:175–196.

Barratt-Boyes, B.G. (1990). Choreathetosis as a complication of cardiopulmonary bypass. *Annals of Thoracic Surgery*, 50:693–697.

Burch, G.E., Sun, S., Chu, K., et al. (1968). Interstitial and coxsackie B myocarditis in infants and children: Study of 50 autopsied hearts. *Journal of the American Medical Association*, 203:1–9.

Burtt, D.M., Pollack, P., Bianco, J.A. (1986). Intravenous streptokinase in an infant with Kawasaki disease complicated by myocardial infarction. *Pediatric Cardiology*, 6:307–311.

Cabinian, A.E., Kiel, R.J., Smith, F., et al. (1990). Modification of exercise-aggravated coxsackie B myocarditis by T lymphocyte suppression. *Journal of Laboratory and Clinical Medicine*, 115:454–459.

Case, C.L., Crawford, F.A., & Gillette, P.C. (1990). Surgical treatment of dysrhythmias in infants and children. *Pediatric Clinics of North America*, 37:79–92.

Castaneda, A.C., Jonas, R.A., Mayer, J.E., & Hanley, F.L. (1994). *Cardiac surgery of the neonate and infant*. Philadelphia: W.B. Saunders.

Chameides, L. (Ed.). (1988). *Textbook of pediatric advanced life support* (pp. 61–67). Dallas: American Heart Association.

Chang, A.D., Hanley, F.L., Weinding, S.N., et al. (1992). Left heart support with a ventricular assist device in an infant with acute myocarditis. *Critical Care Medicine*, 20:712–715.

Cohen, M.M., & Cameron, C.B. (1991). Should you cancel the operation when the child has an upper respiratory infection? *Anesthesia and Analgesia*, 72:282.

Combined Rheumatic Fever Study Group. (1960). A comparison of the effect of prednisone and aspirin therapy on the incidence of residual rheumatic heart disease. *New England Journal of Medicine*, 262:895–899.

Combined Rheumatic Fever Study Group. (1965). A comparison of short term intensive prednisone and aspirin therapy in the treatment of acute rheumatic fever. *New England Journal of Medicine*, 272:63–68.

Cooperative Rheumatic Fever Study Group. (1955). The treatment of acute rheumatic fever in children: A cooperative clinical trial of ACTH, cortisone and aspirin. *Circulation*, 11:343–348.

Craig, J. (1991). The postoperative cardiac infant: Physiologic basis for neonatal nursing. *Journal of Perinatal and Neonatal Nursing*, 5:60–70.

Crawford, F.A., Gillette, P.C., Zeigler, V., et al. (1990). Surgical management of Wolff-Parkinson-White syndrome in infants and small children. *Journal of Thoracic and Cardiovascular Surgery*, 99:234–240.

Dajani, A.S., Taubert, K.A., Gerber, M.A., et al. (1993). Diagnosis and therapy of Kawasaki disease in children. *Circulation*, 87:1776–1780.

Daniels, S.R., Specker, B., Capannari, T.E., et al. (1987). Correlates of coronary artery aneurysm formation in patients with Kawasaki disease. *American Journal of Diseases of Children*, 141:205–207.

Drucker, N.A., Colan, S.D., Lewis, A.B., et al. (1994). Gamma globulin treatment of acute myocarditis in the pediatric population. *Circulation*, 89:252–257.

Elixson, E.M. (1989). Hemodynamic monitoring modalities in pediatric cardiac surgical patients. *Critical Care Nursing Clinics of North America*, 1:263–273.

Fontan, F., & Baudet, E. (1971). Surgical repair of tricuspid atresia. *Thorax*, 26:240–248.

Friedman, R.A., Moak, J.P., Garson, A. (1991). Clinical course of idiopathic dilated cardiomyopathy in children. *Journal of the American College of Cardiology*, 18:152–156.

Fyler, D.C., Buckley, L.P., Hellenbrand, W.E., et al. (1980). Report of the NERICP. *Pediatrics*, 65([suppl]2):375–461.

Garson, A. (1984). Arrhythmias in pediatric patients. *Medical Clinics of North America*, 68:1171–1210.

Garson, A. (1990). Chronic postoperative arrhythmia. In P.C. Gillette & A. Garson (Eds.). *Pediatric arrhythmias: Electrophysiology and pacing* (pp. 667–678). Philadelphia: W.B. Saunders.

Garson, A., Moak, J., Smith, R.T., et al. (1987). Control of postoperative junctional ectopic tachycardia with propafenone. *American Journal of Cardiology*, 59:1422–1424.

Gillum, R.F. (1986). Idiopathic cardiomyopathy in the United States, 1970–1982. *American Heart Journal*, 111:752–760.

Gold, J., & Castaneda, A.R. (1987). Nonoperative removal of entrapped thoracic intracardiac monitoring catheters: A new bedside technique. *Annals of Thoracic Surgery*, 43:229–230.

Gordis, L. (1985). The virtual disappearance of rheumatic fever in the United States: Lessons in the rise and fall of a disease. *Circulation*, 72:1155–1159.

Greenwood, R.D., Nadas, A.S., Fyler, D.C. (1976). The clinical course of primary myocardial disease in infants and children. *American Heart Journal*, 92:549–555.

Griffin, M.L., Hernandez, A., Martin, T.C., et al. (1988). Dilated cardiomyopathy in infants and children. *Journal of the American College of Cardiology*, 11:139–144.

Hanisch, D.G., & Perron, L. (1992). Complex dysrhythmias in infants and children. *AACN Clinical Issues*, 3:255–267.

Iannettoni, M.D., & Bove, E.L. (1992). Myocardial preservation in the newborn. In M.L. Jacobs & W.I. Norwood (Eds.). *Pediatric cardiac surgery* (pp. 224–236). Boston: Butterworth-Heinemann.

Ichida, F., Fatica, N.S., Engle, M.A., et al. (1987). Coronary artery involvement in Kawasaki syndrome in Manhattan, New York: Risk factors and the role of aspirin. *Pediatrics*, 80:828–835.

Jatene, A.P., Fontas, V.F., Saoza, L.C., et al. (1976). Anatomic correction of transposition of the great arteries. *Journal of Thoracic and Cardiovascular Surgery*, 72:364–371.

Kato, H., Ichinose, E., Inoue, D., et al. (1987). Intracoronary thrombolytic therapy in Kawasaki disease: Treatment and prevention of acute myocardial infarction. *Prog Clin Biol Res*, 250:445–454.

Katz, A.M. (1990). Cardiomyopathy of overload. *New England Journal of Medicine*, 322:100–110.

Kay, E.B., & Cross, F.S. (1955). Surgical treatment of transposition of the great vessels. *Surgery*, 39:712.

Kirklin, J.W. (1986). Hypothermia, circulatory arrest, cardiopulmonary bypass. In J.W. Kirklin & B.G. Barrattt-Boyes (Eds.). *Cardiac surgery* (pp. 41–66). New York: John Wiley & Sons.

Klem, S.A. (1993). Cardiovascular support—mechanical. In P.R. Holbrook (Ed.). *Textbook of pediatric critical care* (pp. 279–287). Philadelphia: W.B. Saunders.

Koren, G., Lavi, S., Rose, V., et al. (1986). Kawasaki disease: Review of risk factors for coronary aneurysms. *Journal of Pediatrics*, 108:388–392.

Kreutzer, G., Galindez, E., Bono, H., et al. (1973). An operation for the correction of tricuspid atresia. *Journal of Thoracic and Cardiovascular Surgery*, 66:613–621.

Kugler, J.D. (1990). Sinus node dysfunction. In P.C. Gillette & A. Garson (Eds.). *Pediatric arrhythmias: Electrophysiology and pacing* (pp. 250–300). Philadelphia: W.B. Saunders.

Kulik, L.A. (1989). Caring for patients with lesions decreasing blood flow. *Critical Care Nursing Clinics of North America*, 1:215–229.

Lev, M. (1972). Pathogenesis of congenital atrioventricular block. *Progress in Cardiovascular Diseases*, 25:145–162.

Liu, P., McLaughlin, P.R., Sole, M.J. (1992). Treatment of myocarditis: Current recommendations and future approaches. *Heart Failure*, 8:33–40.

Ludomirsky, A., & Garson, A. (1990). Supraventricular tachycardia. In P.C. Gillette & A. Garson (Eds.). *Pediatric arrhythmias: Electrophysiology and pacing* (pp. 380–426). Philadelphia: W.B. Saunders.

Lux, K. (1991). New hope for children with Kawasaki disease. *Journal of Pediatric Nursing*, 6:159–164.

Maron, B.J., Nichols, P.F., Pickle, L.W., et al. (1984). Patterns of inheritance in hypertrophic cardiomyopathy: Assessment by M-mode two-dimensional echocardiography. *American Journal of Cardiology*, 53:1087–1091.

Matitiau, A., Colan, S.D., Perez, A., et al. (1991). Infantile congestive cardiomyopathy: Relation of outcome to LV function, hemodynamics, and histology. *Journal of the American College of Cardiology*, 17(suppl A):171A.

Mavroudis, C., & Greene, M.A. (1992). Cardiopulmonary bypass and hypothermic circulatory arrest in infants. In M.L. Jacobs & W.I. Norwood (Eds.). *Pediatric cardiac surgery: Current issues* (pp. 206–223). Boston: Butterworth–Heinemann.

Moak, J. (1990a). Pharmacology and electrophysiology of antiarrhythmic drugs. In P.C. Gillette & A. Garson (Eds.). *Pediatric arrhythmias: Electrophysiology and pacing* (pp. 37–115). Philadelphia: W.B. Saunders.

Moak, J. (1990b). Acute nonpharmacologic treatment of tachyarrhythmias and bradyarrhythmias. In P.C. Gillette & A. Garson (Eds.). *Pediatric arrhythmias: Electrophysiology and pacing* (pp. 516–527). Philadelphia: W.B. Saunders.

Monett, Z.J., & Moynihan, P.J. (1991). Cardiovascular assessment of the neonatal heart. *Journal of Perinatal and Neonatal Nursing,* 5:50–59.

Monrad, E.S., Matsumori, A., Murphy, J.C., et al. (1986). Therapy with cyclosporin in murine myocarditis with encephalomyocarditis virus. *Circulation,* 73:1058–1062.

Moore, P., & Soifer, S.J. (1993). Acquired heart disease. In P.R. Holbrook (Ed.). *Textbook of pediatric critical care* (pp. 370–383). Philadelphia: W.B. Saunders Co.

Moynihan, P.J., Wernovsky, G., Hickey, P.A., et al. (1992). Complication rates of transthoracic intracardiac lines removed by critical care nurses. *Circulation,* 86(suppl 1):4.

Mustard, W.T. (1964). Successful two-stage correction of transposition of the great arteries. *Surgery,* 55:469–474.

Newburger, J.W., & Burns, J.C. (1989). Kawasaki syndrome. *Cardiology Clinics of North America,* 7:453–465.

Newburger, J.W., Sanders, S.P., Burns, J.C., et al. (1989). Left ventricular contractility and function in Kawasaki syndrome. *Circulation,* 79:1237–1249.

Newburger, J.W., Takahashi, M., Beiser, A.S., et al. (1991). A single intravenous infusion of gamma globulin as compared with four infusions in the treatment of acute Kawasaki syndrome. *New England Journal of Medicine,* 324:1633–1639.

Norris, M.K., & Roland, J.A. (1994). Perioperative management of pulmonary circulation in children with congenital heart defects. *AACN Clinical Issues,* 5:255–262.

Norwood, W.I., Lang, P., & Hansen, D.D. (1983). Physiologic repair of hypoplastic left heart syndrome. *New England Journal of Medicine,* 308:23–26.

Norwood, W.I. (1989). Hypoplastic left heart syndrome. *Cardiology Clinics,* 7:377–385.

O'Connell, J.B., Reap, E.A., Robinson, J.A. (1986). The effects of cyclosporine on acute coxsackie B3 myocarditis. *Circulation,* 73:1058–1062.

Perry, J.C. & Garson, A. (1989). Diagnosis and treatment of arrhythmias. *Advances in Pediatrics,* 36:177–200.

Perry, J.C. (1990). Acute pharmacologic treatment of cardiac arrhythmias. In P.C. Gillette & A. Garson, (Eds.). *Pediatric arrhythmias: Electrophysiology and pacing* (pp. 234–240). Philadelphia: W.B. Saunders.

Pfeffer, M.A., Braunwald, E., Moye, L.A., et al. (1992). Effect of captopril on mortality and morbidity in patients with left ventricular dysfunction after myocardial infarction. *New England Journal of Medicine,* 327:669–677.

Pollack, M.M., Getson, P.R., Rurriman, U.E., et al. (1987). Efficiency of intensive care. *Journal of the American Medical Association,* 258:1481–1486.

Quigley, P.J., Richardson, P.J., Meany, B.T., et al. (1987). Long-term follow-up of acute myocarditis: Correlation of ventricular function and outcome. *European Heart Journal,* 8(suppl J):39.

Report of the Committee on Infectious Diseases. Georges P (ed). (1991). *Journal of Pediatrics,* 112:282–286.

Ross, B.A. (1990). Congenital complete atrioventricular block. *Pediatric Clinics of North America,* 37:69–78.

Ross, B.A., Pinsky, W.W., & Driscoll, D.J. (1990). Complete atrio-

ventricular block. In P.C. Gillette & A. Garson (Eds.). *Pediatric arrhythmias: Electrophysiology and pacing* (pp. 306–316). Philadelphia: W.B. Saunders.

Ruggerie, D. (1990). Cardiac arrhythmias. In J.L. Blumer (Ed.). *A practical guide to pediatric intensive care* (pp. 392–409). St Louis: Mosby–Year Book.

Sanders, S.P. (1992). Echocardiography. In D.C. Fyler (Ed.). *Nadas' pediatric cardiology* (pp. 159–186). Boston: Hanley & Belfus.

Senning, A. (1959). Surgical correction of transposition of the great vessels. *Surgery,* 45:966–972.

Smith, J.B., & Vernon-Levett, P. (1993). Care of infants with hypoplastic left heart syndrome. *AACN Clinical Issues,* 4:329–339.

Suzuki, A., Kamiya, T., Ono, Y., et al. (1990). Aortocoronary bypass surgery for coronary arterial lesions resulting from Kawasaki disease. *Journal of Pediatrics,* 116:567–573.

Talner, N.S. (1989). Heart failure. In F.H. Adams, G.C. Emmanouilides, & T.A. Riemenschneider (Eds.). *Moss' heart disease in infants, children and adolescents* (4th ed., pp. 890–910). Baltimore: Williams & Wilkins.

Terai, M., Ogata, M., Sugimoto, K., et al. (1985). Coronary artery thrombi in Kawasaki disease. *Journal of Pediatrics,* 106:76–78.

Tomioka, N., Kishimoto, C., Matsumori, A., et al. (1986). Effects of prednisone on acute viral myocarditis in mice. *Journal of the American College of Cardiology,* 73:1058.

Troug, R., Anand, K.J.S. (1989). Management of pain in the postoperative neonate. *Clinics in Perinatology,* 16:61–78.

Turina, M., Siehenmann, R., Nussbaumer, P., et al. (1988). Long-term outlook after atrial correction of transposition of the great arteries. *Journal of Thoracic and Cardiovascular Surgery,* 95:828–835.

Veasey, L.G., Blalock, R.C., Orth, J.L., et al. (1983). Intra-aortic balloon pumping in infants and children. *Circulation,* 68:1095–1100.

Veasey, L.G., Wiedmeier, S.E., Osmond, G.S., et al. (1987). Resurgence of acute rheumatic fever in the inter-mountain area of the United States. *New England Journal of Medicine,* 316:421–425.

Vincent, R.N., Lang, P., Elixson, E.M., et al. (1984). Measurement of extravascular lung water in infants and children after cardiac surgery. *American Journal of Cardiology,* 54:161–165.

Walsh, A.Z., Wernovsky, G., Wypij, D., et al. (1992). Postoperative course following the arterial switch operation. *Circulation* ([suppl] 1) 86:992–996.

Weindling, S.N., Wernovsky, G., Colan, S.H., et al. (1994). Myocardial perfusion, function, and exercise tolerance after the arterial switch operation. *Journal of the American College of Cardiology,* 23:424–433.

Woodruff, J. (1980) Viral myocarditis: A review. *American Journal of Pathology,* 101:425–435.

Wynne, J., & Braunwald, E. (1992). The cardiomyopathies and myocarditides: Toxic, chemical and physical damage to the heart. In E. Braunwald (Ed.). *Heart disease* (pp. 1394–1444). Philadelphia: W.B. Saunders.

Additional Reading

Lawrence, J.H., & Weixel, R.C. (1994). Pediatric arrhythmias. In Nichols, Cameron, Loppe, et al. (Eds.). *Critical heart disease in infants.* St. Louis: C.V. Mosby.

Medicus, L., & Thompson, L. (1995). Preventing pulmonary hypertensive crisis in the pediatric patient after cardiac surgery. *American Journal of Critical Care,* 4:49–55.

Zeigler, V.L. (1994). Postoperative rhythm disturbances. *Critical Care Nursing Clinics of North America,* 6:227–235.

CHAPTER 20

Pulmonary Critical Care Problems

BARBARA J. FEW

RESPIRATORY FAILURE
MECHANISMS OF ABNORMAL GAS
  EXCHANGE
INDICATIONS FOR VENTILATORY SUPPORT
MAINTAINING THE ARTIFICIAL AIRWAY

FINAL COMMON PATHWAYS
Mechanical Alterations
Circulatory Alterations
Alterations in the Control of Breathing
SUMMARY

Patients with pulmonary problems comprise 28% of pediatric critical care practice, more than any other clinical problem (AACN, 1991). Therefore, knowledge of respiratory anatomy and physiology as well as familiarity with the common pathologies leading to respiratory failure are essential. This chapter examines the physiology of the respiratory system and the means by which physiology is altered by disease. Respiratory failure is defined and the mechanisms of abnormal gas exchange are briefly reviewed. Next, the indications for ventilatory support are considered, as are the nursing implications when endotracheal intubation is required. A short review of the basic physiology of the developing respiratory system establishes the final common pathways of respiratory failure: mechanical, circulatory, and regulatory alterations. The remaining sections are devoted to specific disorders associated with these final common pathways in infants and children, exploring incidence, etiology, treatment, and nursing management. Whether resulting from chronic or acute processes, impending respiratory failure can be extremely frightening for infants, children, and their families. Consequently, sensitivity and attention to the impact of critical illness on children and their families is as important as knowledge of the causes and treatment of respiratory failure.

RESPIRATORY FAILURE

Respiratory failure is frequently defined simply in terms of blood gas abnormalities, for example, a Pa_{O_2} of less than 50 mmHg (in room air) and a Pa_{CO_2} greater than 50 mmHg. Quantifying respiratory failure in this fashion, however, lacks specificity and is ultimately inadequate. A child with a congenital heart defect, for example, may have a Pa_{O_2} less than 50 mmHg without respiratory failure. Similarly, a patient with a diuretic-induced metabolic alkalosis may have an increase in Pa_{CO_2} to greater than 50 mmHg, but this does not indicate respiratory failure. In addition, in clinical practice blood gas tensions are often maintained with supplemental oxygen. It follows that respiratory failure is more appropriately understood as an inability of the respiratory system to fulfill its role in transferring oxygen (O_2) and carbon dioxide (CO_2) to and from the venous blood in an amount commensurate with the needs of the patient.

The advantage of this definition is that it emphasizes the important link that exists between the function of the respiratory system and the metabolic requirements of the tissues. For example, the infant with bronchopulmonary dysplasia may be able to meet everyday metabolic demands, but when those demands are increased by an infectious process, the child's respiratory reserve may be inadequate and respiratory failure will ensue. In fact, fatigue from increased work of breathing, rather than hypoxia, usually precipitates respiratory failure in infants and children. Respiratory failure must also be differentiated from respiratory distress, which is manifested by retractions, tachypnea, nasal flaring, and so on. The latter is a judgment made by the clinician regarding the patient's work of breathing or the patient's own perception of dyspnea and does not necessarily imply respiratory failure. The child in status asthmaticus, for instance, may have respiratory distress yet be able to meet metabolic needs. Compensatory mechanisms, involving increased effort and use of additional respiratory muscles, can retard the development of respiratory failure, even if it is at an increased energy cost.

MECHANISMS OF ABNORMAL GAS EXCHANGE

Mechanisms of impaired gas exchange in the lungs may include hypoventilation, shunt, ventilation-per-fusion ($\dot{V}/\dot{Q}$) mismatch, and diffusion disorders. For reasons that are poorly understood, an impediment to oxygen diffusion does not represent a significant problem in children, therefore, we will concentrate on the remaining three.

Hypoventilation may be defined on the basis of reduced minute alveolar ventilation [(tidal volume − dead space) × respiratory rate] and inevitably results in an inability to eliminate carbon dioxide. Because the increased alveolar CO_2 occupies space, O_2 is displaced out of the alveolus and both alveolar and arterial PO_2 are decreased. Supplemental O_2, however, can overcome this displacement, and restore PaO_2 to normal (Fig. 20–1*B*).

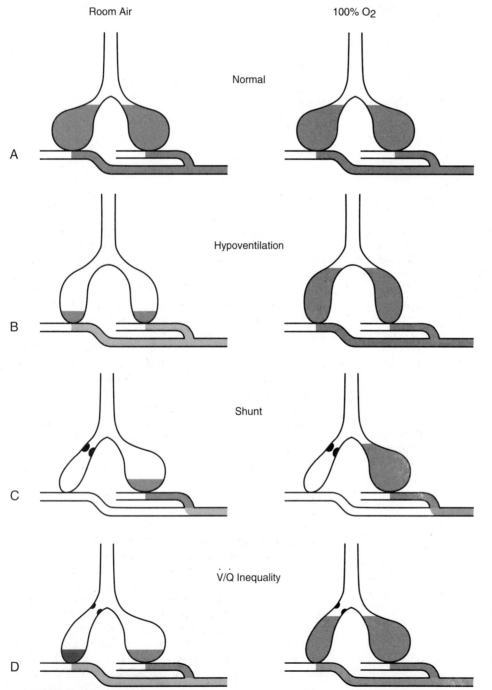

Room Air   100% O₂

Normal

A

Hypoventilation

B

Shunt

C

V/Q Inequality

D

Figure 20–1 ● ● ● ● ● ●

Mechanisms of hypoxemia and effect of increased FiO_2 in patients with lung disease. In this schematic representation, the normal lung is composed of two alveolar units with their respective capillaries. *A,* While breathing room air, on the left, the FiO_2 in the alveoli (shown by the level of filling of the alveolar units in the figure) is only 0.21. The alveolar PO_2 (PAO_2, indicated by the number of dots inside the alveoli), however, is sufficiently high to produce a normal O_2 hemoglobin saturation in the pulmonary capillaries (shown by the density of the dots inside the capillaries in the figure). Administration of an FiO_2 of 1.0 barely increased the O_2 content of the arterial blood. *B,* In the presence of hypoventilation, PAO_2 is reduced in room air, and the capillary blood is poorly saturated. Administration of an FiO_2 of 1.0 increases both the PAO_2 and O_2 content of the capillary blood. *C,* An intrapulmonary shunt allows mixed venous blood to pass through the lungs without being exposed to alveolar O_2. As a result, the arterial O_2 content is decreased. Supplemental O_2 raises only the O_2 content of the capillary blood that is not shunted; therefore, arterial O_2 content increased only to a limited extent. *D,* In $\dot{V}/\dot{Q}$ inequality, alveolar units that have a decreased PO_2 exist in combination with others that have a normal PO_2. Blood from these two types of units mixes, resulting in a lower than normal arterial O_2 content. Administration of O_2 increases the PAO_2 in both hypoventilated and normal units, and the O_2 content of the arterial blood increases as well. (The author wishes to acknowledge the assistance of J. Julio Perez Fontan, MD and George Lister, MD, of New Haven, Connecticut, in the development of this representation.)

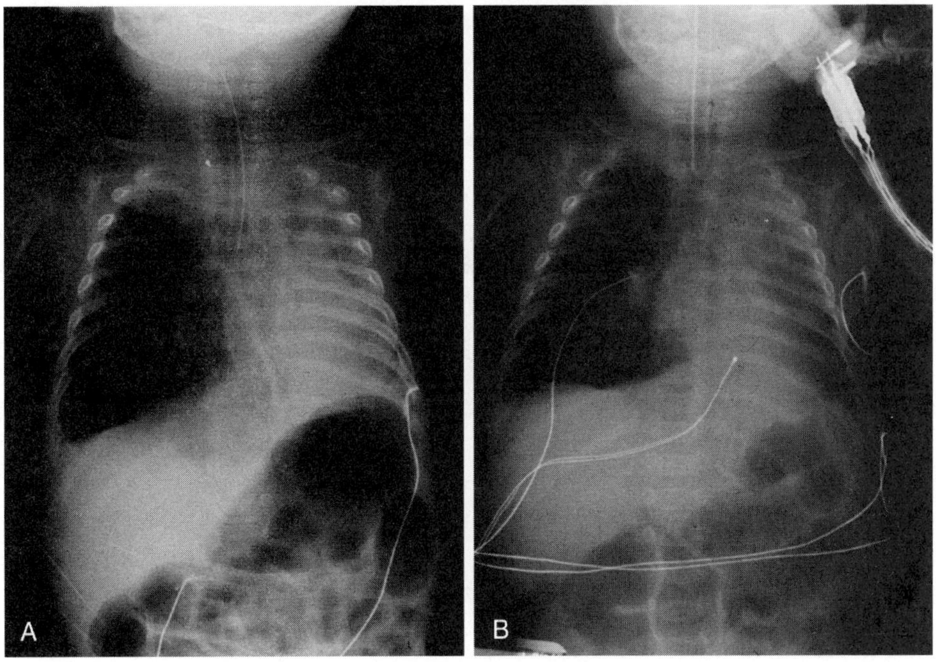

Figure 20–2 ● ● ● ● ● ●
Chest radiographs demonstrating the impact of small movements of an ETT. In the first radiograph *(A)*, the right mainstem bronchus is intubated and there is a collapse of the left lung. After withdrawing the ETT just 1 cm *(B)*, the left lung is partially re-inflated.

Normally a small percentage of right ventricular output is returned to the left atrium without passing through ventilated areas of the lung. This represents a physiologic right-to-left shunt. Additional shunting of blood occurs when collapsed alveoli continue to be perfused. Because these alveoli are no longer ventilated, the blood circulating through them is not oxygenated. This blood is mixed with oxygenated blood from other ventilated areas, thereby increasing pulmonary venous admixture, or causing an abnormal *right-to-left* shunt. PaO_2 decreases, but in this case, supplemental O_2 will not entirely abolish hypoxemia because the shunted blood is not exposed to inspired O_2 (see Fig. 20–1*C*). Intrapulmonary shunting does not usually result in an increase in $PaCO_2$ because the respiratory center responds to hypoxemia by increasing ventilation.

Ventilation-perfusion mismatching is the most common cause of abnormal gas exchange. If ventilation and blood flow are unequal in various regions of the lung, impairment of both O_2 and CO_2 transfer results. Supplemental O_2 will, however, increase the PaO_2 to normal (see Fig. 20–1*D*).

INDICATIONS FOR VENTILATORY SUPPORT

When respiratory failure occurs, whatever the cause, some sort of ventilatory support may be required to reestablish the adequacy of gas exchange. Established respiratory failure, however, is not the only circumstance in which ventilatory assistance is necessary. Examples of such circumstances are situations in which respiratory failure is anticipated because of the nature of the underlying disease process; providing support before respiratory failure de-

velops is essential to prevent secondary injury. For example, a child with Guillain-Barré syndrome (a condition characterized by progressive neuromuscular weakness) may need to be intubated at the first sign of dyspnea or airway obstruction. These signs suggest involvement in the disease of muscles essential for respiration. Muscle involvement poses an unacceptable risk of acute decompensation, and, in most cases, demands immediate intervention. Similarly, the child with extensive abdominal surgery who is likely to develop significant abdominal distension and impaired diaphragmatic function may require ventilatory support for a variable postoperative period, even if respiratory failure is not present. Ventilatory assistance may also be beneficial in a patient in moderate respiratory distress but with a limited ability to compensate, for example, in children with cardiogenic shock. With decreased cardiac output, respiratory muscle blood flow may be inadequate to meet increased needs, and muscle fatigue may occur, resulting in respiratory failure. It becomes apparent that, in a number of instances, providing ventilatory support before the development of respiratory failure may improve patient outcome.

MAINTAINING THE ARTIFICIAL AIRWAY

Regardless of the reason for airway intervention, when an infant or child has an endotracheal tube (ETT), maintaining the position and integrity of the artificial airway is a primary nursing responsibility.

Correct positioning of the ETT is usually confirmed radiographically at the time of intubation (Fig. 20–2, A and B). Once correct placement is established, continued assessment of ETT position can be accomplished by noting the depth of its insertion at regular

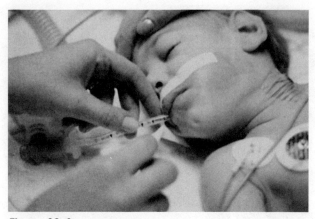

Figure 20–3 ● ● ● ● ● ●

ETT markings present at lip line are noted during ETT taping.

intervals; that is, documenting the mark on the tube that appears at the child's lip or nares and carefully monitoring bilateral breath sounds (Fig. 20–3).

The reported incidence of spontaneous or accidental extubation in PICUs ranges from 3% to 13% (Scott et al., 1985). Although it is unclear whether this variability is related to differences in patients or in patient care practices, several risk factors for accidental extubation have been identified. Infants may be at particular risk because their tracheas are shorter and head movement alone can dislocate the ETT (Franck, Vaughan, & Wallace, 1992) (Fig. 20–4). Scott and others (1985) found that spontaneous extubation was more likely to occur in a patient who is younger, has a large amount of secretions and ETT slippage, and a higher level of consciousness. In this particular study, 29% of those patients reintubated after an accidental extubation had at least one subsequent unplanned extubation, and 88% of the patients who had spontaneous extubation did so despite restraints. In another study (Little et al., 1990), level of sedation, lack of two-point or more restraints, and the performance of a patient procedure at the bedside were identified as critical factors contributing to accidental extubation. Various methods are employed to secure the ETT, but to avoid spontaneous extubation or inadvertent advancement of the tube, frequent assessment of the patient and the position and stability of the ETT are required. To rule out right mainstem bronchus intubation, auscultation compares bilateral air movement at the third intercostal space midaxillary line—a point at which referred breath sounds from the opposite lung are less likely to be heard. Restraints, which are necessary to prevent the child from removing the ETT, are not used in isolation. Measures to reduce anxiety should also be taken, including the use of anxiolytics and/or seda-

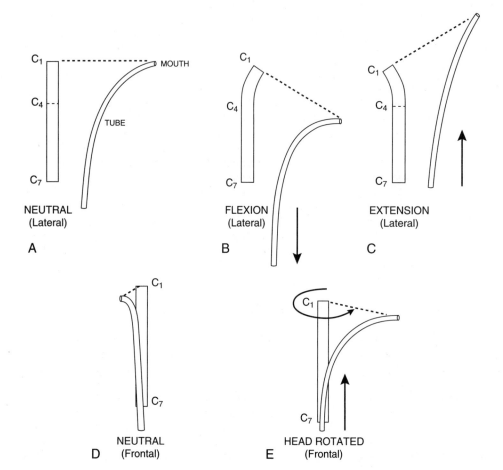

Figure 20–4 ● ● ● ● ● ●

A to *E*, The effect of head position on ETT position. (From Donn, S. M., Kuhns, L. R. 1980. Mechanism of endotracheal tube movement with change of head position in the neonate. *Pediatric Radiology*, 9, 37–40.)

tives, decreasing noxious or threatening stimuli, and encouraging family presence and participation in care.

Because endotracheal intubation prevents effective coughing and both bypasses and impairs normal mucociliary clearing mechanisms, endotracheal suctioning is an important nursing responsibility. ETT suctioning is not, however, a benign procedure. Suctioning has been associated with a host of negative side effects and complications including hypoxia, dysrhythmias, atelectasis, trauma to the trachea and bronchi, and increased intracranial pressure. It seems reasonable that one of the most frequently performed procedures in the PICU, which is associated with serious risks, should be guided by sound clinical research data. Unfortunately, much of what constitutes "routine suctioning technique" is guided more by ritual than scientific rationale (Capnell & Fergusson, 1995). A number of suctioning practices of concern to pediatric critical care nurses including hyperoxygenation, hyperinflation and/or hyperventilation, depth of suctioning, endotracheal instillation of normal saline, chest physiotherapy, and the frequency of endotracheal suctioning have been examined. Devices intended to minimize suction-induced hypoxemia have also been considered. Each will be discussed in the following section.

Hyperoxygenation is a maneuver designed to reduce hypoxemia associated with suctioning. This is accomplished in children by increasing the FiO_2 to 1.0 before, during, and after the suctioning procedure. Because hyperoxia should be avoided, the amount of supplemental O_2 administered during suctioning is determined by the infant's arterial oxygenation. Oxygen saturation, monitored continuously by pulse oximeter, can generally be maintained between 92% to 94% by increasing FiO_2 10% to 20% over baseline requirements, but the actual FiO_2 used is based on each individual infant's needs (Turner, 1990).

Hyperinflation and hyperventilation are additional techniques used during suctioning to lessen hypoxemia, presumably by reinflating collapsed lung segments. There is no uniform definition, however, for either maneuver. Generally, hyperinflation entails delivering several breaths before suctioning (and after each pass of the suction catheter) using either a manual resuscitation bag or the ventilator circuit. Each of these breaths is approximately 1.5 times the patient's usual tidal volume. Alternatively, peak inspiratory pressure (PIP) is increased approximately 10 cm H_2O above the patient's usual requirements. Using PIP to guide hyperinflation may be more appropriate in pediatrics because children are usually intubated with uncuffed ETTs and have a variably sized leak around the tube. In clinical practice, however, hyperinflation is often accomplished by a brief period of hand ventilation with the tidal volume and/or PIP determined by "feel," chest wall movement, and values shown on noninvasive monitors during the maneuver (for example, pulse oximetry and end tidal CO_2). Similarly, hyperventilation is frequently not standardized, but consists of some

increase in ventilatory frequency over the patient's respiratory rate.

Considerable research has focused on the efficacy of hyperoxygenation, hyperinflation, and/or hyperventilation in reducing suction-induced hypoxemia. Some combination of the three techniques probably provides the best protection from arterial oxygen desaturation (Turner, 1990). However, that combination has yet to be clearly defined, especially in infants and children. Until consensus is reached, guidelines should be flexible enough to encourage clinicians to design procedures tailored to the individual needs of the patient.

In contrast, research data already exist to direct the *depth of ETT suctioning*. Deep endotracheal suctioning has been routinely performed in PICUs. However, evidence associating that practice with bronchial perforation (Alpan et al., 1984; Anderson & Chandra, 1976) and acute histologic changes in the tracheobronchial tree should change that technique. Using an animal model, Kleiber and coworkers (1988) have demonstrated that merely inserting a suction catheter into the ETT until resistance is met (that is, to the carina or mainstem bronchus) causes as much tissue damage as insertion to resistance with the subsequent application of suction. Because of the alignment of the right middle lobe with the trachea, this type of chronic irritation of the bronchial mucosa can lead to persistent right middle lobe atelectasis (resulting from airway narrowing because of inflammation or stenosis), especially in infants. For these reasons, catheter insertion should stop short of the carina. An appropriate depth for endotracheal suctioning can be ensured by premeasuring and marking the suction catheter, or using a numerically calibrated catheter marked in centimeter increments and inserted 1 cm past the corresponding markings of the ETT (Kleiber et al., 1988).

The *endotracheal instillation of normal saline* is an example of a widely practiced nursing routine that is not supported by research. Normal saline has been used for the purpose of loosening or thinning tenacious secretions, but because mucus does not readily mix with saline, the effect is probably more that of a lavage (Shekleton & Nield, 1987). As such, it may enhance secretion clearance through cough stimulation (Gray et al., 1990) but may also cause mucosal irritation with little effect on mucus clearance (Ackerman, 1993). Bostick and Wendlegass (1987) found that the use of normal saline neither improved post-suctioning PaO_2 nor increased the amount of secretions retrieved. Other studies suggest that providing adequate systemic hydration (Chopra et al., 1977) and warming and humidifying inspired gases (Kahn, 1983) are more appropriate interventions for thinning secretions.

Chest physiotherapy (CPT) consists of a number of procedures including postural drainage, percussion, vibration, and coughing. The goals of these interventions are to improve mucociliary clearance, to increase the volume of sputum expectorated, and to improve airway function. Kirilloff and coworkers

(1985) reviewed the literature with regard to the efficacy of CPT in acute and chronic illness in adults. They concluded that CPT appeared beneficial in patients with large amounts of secretions and those with lobar atelectasis as well. Patients with chronic illnesses associated with increased mucus production (for example, cystic fibrosis) clearly benefitted from CPT. In contrast, CPT did not help patients in status asthmaticus and caused bronchospasm and hypoxemia in some acutely ill patients. The component activities of CPT were not uniformly associated with positive results. Postural drainage was usually effective, although directed coughing (teaching the patient cough techniques) may be as efficacious. There were no data showing a beneficial effect of percussion or vibration. Because these studies were of adult patients, caution should be used in generalizing the results to infants and children. The mixed findings suggest, however, that CPT is not uniformly effective in pediatric disorders and further research is certainly needed.

The *frequency of endotracheal suctioning* is determined by careful patient assessment. It should not be performed on a routine basis, but only when necessary to clear the airways of secretions. Assessments include respiratory rate and effort, auscultation of bilateral breath sounds for equality of air entry and the presence of adventitious sounds, amount and symmetry of chest expansion, peak airway pressures when on assisted ventilation, and data from noninvasive monitors. Evaluating a patient over time and documenting assessments permit early detection of clinical changes and recognition of individual patient responses that will guide subsequent interventions.

Several devices have been designed to ameliorate suction-induced hypoxemia. Two such devices, oxygen insufflation catheters and closed tracheal suction systems, may be especially useful when high levels of FiO_2 and positive end-expiratory pressure (PEEP) are required. *Oxygen insufflation catheters* can increase PaO_2 during suctioning by permitting simultaneous delivery of O_2 during the procedure (dual-lumen catheters) (Bodai et al., 1987; Friel et al., 1990), or alternate delivery of oxygen or suction (single-lumen catheters) (Taft et al., 1990). Unfortunately, their use is limited in infants and children because of the smaller ETT size.

One factor contributing to suction-induced hypoxemia is the necessity of interrupting the patient's regular ventilatory cycle during the procedure. A *closed tracheal suction system* (CTSS), however, permits mechanical ventilation (including PEEP) to continue during suctioning. One type of CTSS consists of a suction catheter in a plastic sheath that remains attached to the ventilator circuit with an adaptor, a suction control device, and an irrigation port for tracheal lavage and rinsing of the catheter (Fig. 20–5). While stabilizing the adaptor with one hand, the nurse uses the thumb and forefinger of the other hand to advance the catheter the desired depth into the ETT through the protective sheath; the procedure can easily be performed by one caregiver. Because the CTSS is left in place for 24 hours, suctioning can be accomplished quickly and immediately, without taking time to assemble supplies (Noll et al., 1990). This type of CTSS is as effective as conventional open suction technique in maintaining oxygenation (Carlon et al., 1987), and in clearing secretions (Witmer et al., 1990), and may have added benefits of preventing nosocomial lower respiratory tract infections (Baker et al., 1989) and avoiding aerosolization of contaminated secretions. Suction catheters as

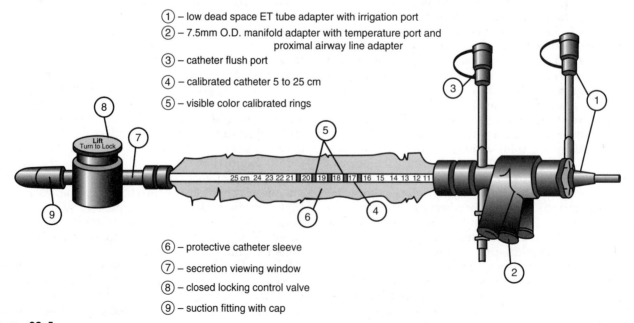

① – low dead space ET tube adapter with irrigation port
② – 7.5mm O.D. manifold adapter with temperature port and proximal airway line adapter
③ – catheter flush port
④ – calibrated catheter 5 to 25 cm
⑤ – visible color calibrated rings
⑥ – protective catheter sleeve
⑦ – secretion viewing window
⑧ – closed locking control valve
⑨ – suction fitting with cap

Figure 20–5 ● ● ● ● ● ●

Ballard's Trach Care closed-system suction catheter. (Courtesy of Ballard Medical Products, Draper, Utah.)

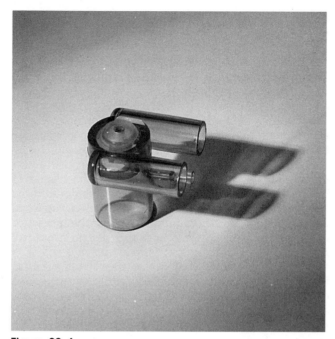

Figure 20–6 ● ● ● ● ● ●

The Bodai Neo$_2$-Safe Infant Suction Valve. (Courtesy of B&B Medical Technologies, Inc., Orangevale, California.)

small as 6 French are available; however, their use is currently limited and requires further investigation (Turner, 1990).

In contrast, the *Bodai* Neo$_2$-Safe valve is a closed suction system specifically designed for small infants (Fig. 20–6). Attached to the end of the ventilator circuit, this particular device permits a suction catheter to be passed through a valve that provides a seal to minimize the loss of PEEP during the procedure. The use of the valve does not totally eliminate the negative pressure induced by suctioning, but the ventilator continues to provide a flow of gas into the circuit, and may reduce suction-induced hypoxemia (Bodai et al., 1989).

FINAL COMMON PATHWAYS

The principal purpose of the respiratory system is to exchange gases, O$_2$ and CO$_2$, with the atmosphere. This process requires the combined function of heart, blood vessels, and lungs. It may be helpful to view the respiratory system as a mechanical pump controlled by a complex feedback system (Fig. 20–7). The pump includes the lung, the chest wall, and the respiratory muscles (primarily the diaphragm, but also the intercostal and abdominal muscles) which, when acting on the chest wall (rib cage and abdomen), expand and compress the lungs. Respiration is regulated by the respiratory center in the brainstem. This center is stimulated directly by CO$_2$ and hydrogen ions and indirectly via central and peripheral chemoreceptors. In addition, mechanoreceptors in the lung and chest wall convey information about

the status of the lungs. The central nervous system integrates all of the data and acts on the respiratory center where the respiratory pattern is established and conveyed through peripheral nerves like the phrenic nerve to the muscles of respiration. The pulmonary circulation completes the respiratory system by establishing a close interface between inspired gas and the blood, which permits delivery of O$_2$ to the blood and removal of CO$_2$.

This conceptual model of the respiratory system also delineates the three final common pathways of respiratory failure. These involve mechanical, circulatory, and regulatory alterations. Mechanical (or pump) alterations in pulmonary function can be classified into two major categories: illnesses that increase the work of breathing and diseases in which the respiratory muscles are unable to perform even the normal amount of work. The former include disorders that increase airway or pulmonary resistance (obstructive disease), those that decrease thoracic compliance (restrictive disease), and mixed disorders resulting in alterations in both resistance and compliance (for example, bronchopulmonary dysplasia). The diseases that affect the respiratory muscles, rendering them incapable of normal work, include disorders of the peripheral nerves (Guillain-Barré syndrome), the neuromuscular junction (infant botulism or myasthenia gravis), and the muscle itself (muscular dystrophy). Circulatory alterations involve disturbances in the normal contact between blood and gas within the lungs; pulmonary embolism and persistent pulmonary hypertension of the newborn are characteris-

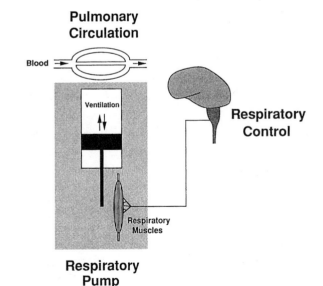

Figure 20–7 ● ● ● ● ●

Schematic drawing of the respiratory system. In this schematic representation, the respiratory system consists of a mechanical pump controlled by a complex feedback system. The respiratory pump includes the lung, chest wall, and respiratory muscles. Respiratory control is established by the respiratory center in the brainstem and conveyed (via peripheral nerves) to the muscles of respiration. Finally, the pulmonary circulation establishes an alveolar-capillary interface that permits gas exchange.

tic examples. In these conditions, pulmonary circulation is reduced, physiologic dead space increases and gas exchange may be impaired. Finally, alterations in the control of breathing include primary or secondary derangements in the breathing pattern such as apnea and alveolar hypoventilation syndromes.

Mechanical Alterations: Disorders That Increase the Work of Breathing

Obstructive Disease (Increased Resistance)

Mechanical alterations in pulmonary function in infants and children are frequently the result of illnesses that cause airway obstruction. Because the signs and symptoms of obstruction depend (in large part) upon location, it is helpful to delineate two categories of airway obstruction: extrathoracic (croup, epiglottitis, foreign body aspiration, and pharyngeal obstruction) and intrathoracic (asthma, bronchiolitis, and tracheobronchomalacia).

The diameter of an airway is determined by the compliance of the airway wall, coupled with the deforming force exerted upon it. The latter is the pressure difference between the gas inside the airway and the tissues surrounding the airway. This pressure difference, known as the transmural pressure, varies during inspiration and expiration and differs for extrathoracic and intrathoracic airways.

The signs and symptoms of obstruction depend upon location (extrathoracic or intrathoracic) and the direction of airflow (inspiration or expiration). During inspiration, airway pressure becomes progressively more negative as the alveoli are approached; a pressure gradient is necessary for airflow to occur inside the airways. On expiration, the pressure within the alveoli becomes positive and the gradient is reversed with pressures inside the airways being always positive, but diminishing toward the mouth. In contrast, the influence of inspiration and expiration on the pressure outside the airway is dependent upon whether the airways are extrathoracic or intrathoracic.

Extrathoracic airways (the pharynx, larynx, and a portion of the trachea) are included in the tissues of the neck, where the pressure can be considered to be zero or atmospheric. Because intrathoracic airways are embedded in the lung, however, the pressure affecting their airway caliber is the pleural pressure. During inspiration, extrathoracic airways have a transmural pressure that favors narrowing because intraluminal pressure decreases while the pressure exerted by tissues outside the airway remains constant. Intrathoracic airways dilate during inspiration as pleural pressure becomes more negative than intraluminal pressure (that is, transmural pressure decreases). During expiration the situation is reversed; extrathoracic airways dilate as intraluminal pressure becomes positive with respect to atmospheric pressure, and intrathoracic airways narrow as the pressure within those airways decreases with respect to pleural pressure. Airway obstruction causes an exaggeration of these normal changes in airway diameter (Fig. 20–8).

Typical clinical manifestations accompany airway

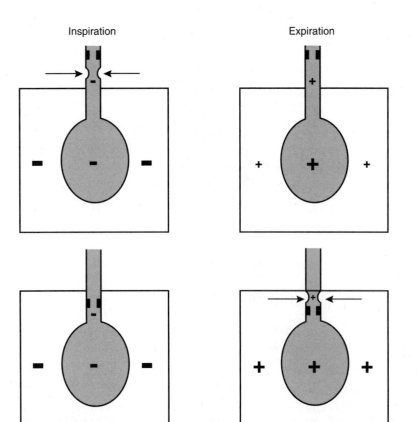

Inspiration   Expiration

Extrathoracic
Obstruction

Intrathoracic
Obstruction

Figure 20–8 ● ● ● ● ● ●

Effect of the respiratory cycle on extrathoracic and intrathoracic airway obstruction. Extrathoracic airway obstruction worsens during inspiration as intraluminal pressure decreases and the pressure outside the airways remains constant (atmospheric pressure). Intrathoracic obstruction worsens during expiration when positive pressures outside the airways (pleural pressure) exceed the pressure within the airways downstream from the obstruction. (Adapted from Fontan, J. P., Lister, G. 1990. Respiratory Failure, p. 53. In R. J. Touloukian (Ed.). *Pediatric trauma*. St. Louis: Mosby–Year Book.)

Table 20–1. DIFFERENCES BETWEEN EXTRATHORACIC AND INTRATHORACIC AIRWAY OBSTRUCTION ON PHYSICAL EXAMINATION

Sign	Extrathoracic	Intrathoracic
Respiratory rate	Slow	Slow
Duration of inspiration	↑	↔
Duration of expiration	↔	↑
Stridor	+	−
Wheezing	−	+
Gas trapping	−	+

↑, increased; ↔, unchanged; +, present; −, absent

obstruction. First, and perhaps foremost, a relatively slow respiratory rate helps to conserve energy. This can be readily appreciated by breathing through a straw; it is much more difficult to breathe rapidly than to breathe slowly. Additional signs of obstruction include intercostal and/or substernal retractions, which may be pronounced, and nasal flaring or the use of accessory muscles of respiration. Based on the previous discussion of airway dynamics, however, there are substantial differences between extrathoracic and intrathoracic obstruction—differences that can be detected by a careful clinical examination (Table 20–1). Inspiration is prolonged in extrathoracic obstruction, whereas the duration of expiration remains unchanged. The opposite is true in intrathoracic obstruction, in which expiration is prolonged and inspiratory time unchanged. The adventitious sounds heard on auscultation also differ in extrathoracic and intrathoracic obstruction. Inspiratory stridor occurs in extrathoracic obstruction; expiratory wheezing occurs in intrathoracic obstruction.

Gas trapping is not a predominant characteristic of extrathoracic obstruction, but occurs frequently in intrathoracic obstruction. Specific disorders that cause increased airway or pulmonary resistance and result in the clinical findings of obstruction include croup, epiglottis, foreign body aspiration, pharyngeal obstruction, asthma, bronchiolitis, and tracheobronchomalacia.

Extrathoracic Obstruction. The etiology of extrathoracic airway obstruction may vary considerably, but the dynamic consequences of the obstruction are the same: to overcome increased resistance during inspiration, the child must create greater negative pressure inside the airway segment downstream from the obstruction. This segment of the airway tends to collapse, worsening the obstruction and producing a characteristic inspiratory stridor. With extrathoracic obstruction the child's respiratory rate is relatively low, mainly because inspiration is prolonged. Suprasternal and subclavicular retractions occur. In addition, nasal flaring and head bobbing (neck extension during inspiration and flexion during expiration) may serve to keep the airway open during inspiration. In the PICU, frequent causes of extrathoracic obstruction are croup, epiglottitis, foreign body aspiration, and pharyngeal obstruction.

Croup. Croup (laryngotracheobronchitis), a viral

illness, is the most commonly occurring extrathoracic airway obstruction in pediatrics. It is characterized by airway obstruction that is primarily subglottic. It usually occurs in late autumn and winter, with parainfluenza and influenza viruses affecting the majority of patients with tracheobronchial inflammation. More prevalent in males, infants and toddlers 3 months to 3 years old are primarily affected, with incidence peaking at 9 to 18 months. Croup also affects other areas of the airway, but the subglottic area is the most narrow air passage at this age; therefore, the clinical manifestations are primarily related to this region. Older children, however, often have tracheitis and even bronchitis.

Inspiratory stridor and a harsh barky cough are usually preceded by a 2- to 3-day history of an upper respiratory tract infection. The child frequently has a low-grade fever, may complain of a sore throat, but does not appear very ill. Typically, croup is a mild disease and most children can be treated as outpatients. If increasing airway obstruction occurs, however, hospitalization may be required. Stridor and retractions even at rest, tachycardia, restlessness, and cyanosis indicate progressive airway obstruction necessitating close monitoring in a PICU and possibly airway intervention.

In most instances, treatment with cool mist oxygen is sufficient to ameliorate symptoms. In more severe cases, nebulized epinephrine is effective in reducing marked inspiratory stridor. Although racemic epinephrine is often used, there is no evidence that it is superior to natural epinephrine. The efficacy of steroids, however, is less clear. A prospective randomized double-blind study demonstrated a significant decrease in severity of symptoms in patients treated with 0.6 mg/kg of intravenous dexamethasone administered within 12 hours of hospital admission (Super et al., 1989). Endotracheal intubation is rarely required.

Nursing management of the child with croup includes limiting activity that may increase respiratory effort and exacerbate symptoms. The tachypnea that accompanies agitation, for example, may cause an increase in transmural pressure and airway turbulence, both of which lead to further narrowing of the airway. Therefore, it is essential to minimize the child's anxiety. Encouraging parental presence and participation in care may go a long way in reducing fears associated with hospitalization. Sedation should be used judiciously. Close observation and monitoring of the child's respiratory status includes respiratory rate and effort, heart rate, and pulse oximetry. Use of a croup scoring system (Table 20–2) may facilitate documentation of the progression or regression of symptoms, and provide a more objective evaluation of the efficacy of various interventions (Westley et al., 1978).

Epiglottitis. Epiglottitis is an acute inflammatory disease of the supraglottic structures of the airway that can result in rapidly progressive, life-threatening airway obstruction. Unlike croup, epiglottitis is a bacterial infection (usually caused by group A *Strep-*

Table 20–2. A CROUP SCORING SYSTEM BASED ON FOUR CLINICAL SIGNS

Level of consciousness	0 = Normal
	5 = Disoriented
Desaturation	0 = None
	4 = With agitation
	5 = At rest
Stridor	0 = Normal
	1 = With agitation
	2 = At rest
Air entry	0 = Normal
	1 = Decreased
	2 = Markedly decreased
Retractions	0 = None
	1 = Mild
	2 = Moderate
	3 = Severe

Zero represents the normal state or absence of the sign; the highest number represents the most severe distress. The range for each sign is weighted to reflect the clinical implications of the most severe form of that sign.

Adapted with permission from Westly, C.R., Cotton, E.K., & Brooks, J.G. (1978). Nebulized racemic epinephrine by IPPB for the treatment of croup. *American Journal of Diseases of Children, 132,* 486. Copyright 1978, American Medical Association.

tococcus or, occasionally, *Haemophilus influenzae* type B in the unimmunized patient) that characteristically occurs in older children, generally those 2 to 6 years of age.

There is an acute onset (usually less than a day) of sore throat, high fever, muffled voice, dysphagia, and lethargy. Dysphagia rapidly progresses to an inability to clear oropharyngeal secretions, and signs of obstruction develop including inspiratory stridor, tachypnea, cyanosis, and retractions. At this point, the child frequently appears pale and restless. Because ventilation can be maintained only in an upright position, the child sits upright with the chin extended and tongue held out, drooling.

The maintenance of a patent airway is the primary goal of therapy. Because agitation may precipitate laryngospasm and complete laryngeal obstruction, no detailed physical examination, blood drawing, or other invasive procedures are performed immediately on a child presenting with signs and symptoms suggestive of epiglottitis. It is especially important to avoid any attempt to examine the pharynx before the child can be taken to the operating room for direct visualization of the glottis under anesthesia. Oxygen is given as unobtrusively as possible. Before laryngoscopy, a lateral neck radiograph showing a very swollen epiglottic shadow is typical and may be helpful in cases if there is doubt about the diagnosis (Fig. 20–9). However, radiographic examination should not delay therapy in a child in severe distress. In those instances, the child is transported directly to the operating room in the parent's arms. Although respiratory arrest can occur from total airway obstruction, it is usually the result of a combination of partial obstruction and fatigue. Therefore, if the child's condition deteriorates, ventilation by bag and mask is frequently possible using sufficient positive

pressure to overcome the supraglottic obstruction, and is preferable to a clumsy attempt at intubation (Chameides & Hazinski, 1994). Once an appropriate level of inhalation anesthesia is reached, an intravenous line is placed, and visualization of the glottis and intubation are accomplished. Although epiglottitis can be treated without an artificial airway, most clinicians agree that the risk of sudden, total airway obstruction makes this practice unsafe (Griffith & Perkins, 1987). Laryngeal and blood cultures are obtained before initiating antibiotic therapy. Humidified gas is administered via a T-piece, ventilator circuit, or oxygen tent until swelling subsides and the child can be extubated; usually within 2 to 4 days. There is no evidence to suggest that corticosteroids are helpful in the treatment of epiglottitis.

Accidental extubation, particularly early in the course of epiglottitis, is potentially disastrous. Once the child has been intubated, therefore, a primary nursing goal is to maintain the position and patency of the artificial airway. The majority of patients with croup or epiglottitis are toddlers or preschoolers in whom egocentricity is prominent, freedom of movement is essential, and separation from parents is a major source of fear and stress. Elbow restraints are

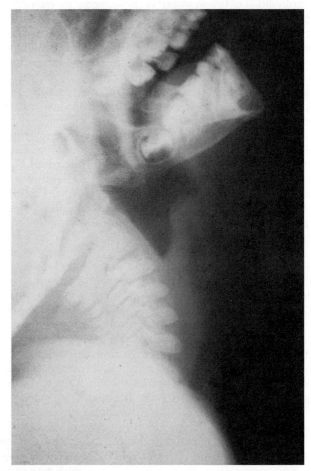

Figure 20–9 ● ● ● ● ● ●

Lateral neck radiograph in epiglottitis. Instead of its usual sharp appearance, the epiglottis is swollen. The supraglottic portion of the airway is dilated, while the air column below the laryngeal level is well preserved (i.e., there is no subglottic edema).

necessary to prevent the child from removing the endotracheal tube but are not used in isolation. Additional measures to keep the child calm and quiet should also be taken, including the administration of sedatives, decreasing noxious or threatening stimuli, and encouraging continued family presence and participation in care. If accidental extubation occurs, position the child in a sitting position and leaning forward to facilitate air entry. Bag and mask ventilation may be required if the child is unable to maintain spontaneous ventilation.

The child with epiglottitis secondary to *H. influenzae* will also require respiratory isolation until 24 hours after the start of effective antibiotic therapy.

Foreign Body Aspiration. A relatively common cause of airway obstruction in children is a foreign body lodged in the tracheobronchial tree, most commonly in the bronchi. The list of objects that can be aspirated is endless including crayons, coins, latex balloons and small toys, and frequently objects of vegetable matter (nuts and beans ranking high on the list) (Banerjee et al., 1988; Laks & Barzilay, 1988). Foreign body aspiration may affect any age, but occurs most frequently in young children ranging in age from 6 months to 3 years. Toddlers may be especially predisposed to aspiration because they lack molar teeth and, therefore, they may not be able to adequately chew their food. In addition, their swallowing coordination may not be fully developed and they have a well-known tendency to gain knowl-

edge of their environment by putting objects into their mouth (McGuirt et al., 1988). It is significant that, in one retrospective study, more than 25% of the 223 cases of aspiration reviewed did not have a history of a choking episode, and only 52% presented within 24 hours of inhalation (Banerjee et al., 1988). In many cases, the initial choking episode may be forgotten.

Signs and symptoms of foreign body aspiration vary, depending upon the location of the object in the airway. Children may present with acute asphyxia from tracheal obstruction, wheezing when a mainstem bronchus is occluded, or they may complain solely of a chronic cough or bloody sputum if a smaller or more peripheral airway is involved. Because foreign bodies are most often lodged in the bronchi, however, cough, respiratory distress, hemoptysis, and wheezing are the most common presenting complaints. Foreign bodies do not usually cause stridor unless the obstruction is at or near the larynx. When a foreign body is lodged in a lobar or segmental bronchus, unilateral physical findings become prominent. Asymmetric breath sounds, absent air entry, and unilateral prolongation of expiration may occur.

When foreign body aspiration is suspected, a careful history may reveal a choking episode days, weeks, or months before symptoms began. Although most aspirated objects are radiolucent, diagnosis may be aided by chest radiographs demonstrating unilateral hyperinflation, atelectasis, or infiltrate (Fig. 20–10).

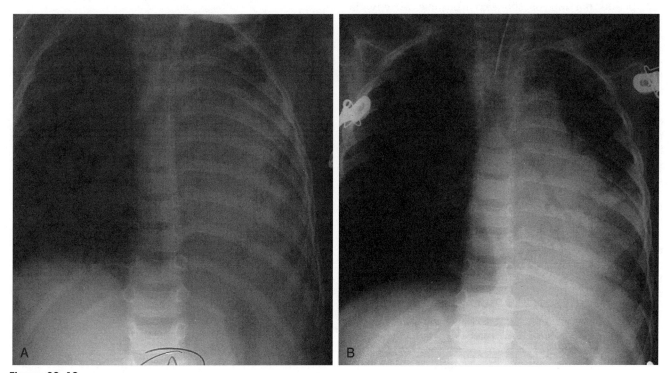

Figure 20–10 ● ● ● ● ● ●

Foreign body chest radiograph. *A,* This AP chest radiograph reveals complete collapse of the left lower lobe with partial aeration of the left upper lobe and lingula. The left main bronchus is well demonstrated containing air through its proximal course where there is an abrupt obstruction to the bronchial lumen. *B,* The AP view of the chest was obtained following the removal of bubble gum from the left mainstem bronchus. Air is now demonstrated throughout the central aspects of the left bronchus including into the periphery of the left lower lobe, which has undergone partial re-expansion compared with the view in *A.* There is partial re-expansion compared with of the upper lobe as well. (Courtesy of Robert Cleveland, MD, Radiology Department, Children's Hospital, Boston, MA.)

A forced expiration radiographic technique frequently reveals persistent air trapping in one location, a finding missed on a conventional chest films because there is increased and uniform expansion of the lung during inspiration. Fluoroscopy may also demonstrate persistent inflation during both phases of respiration, indicating airway obstruction and identifying the location of the foreign body. Even in the absence of a definitive diagnosis, bronchoscopy under general anesthesia is the diagnostic test and the treatment of choice when aspiration of a foreign body below the carina is suspected. The use of less direct methods, such as postural drainage, may lead to total airway obstruction by freeing an object that is too large to pass through the larynx. However, when an exact diagnosis cannot be made and a lobar or segmental obstruction is suspected, postural drainage and inhaled bronchodilators may be employed for several days. If there is no improvement, bronchoscopy is performed.

Residual irritation after removal of a foreign body by bronchoscopy or postural drainage may necessitate continued administration of supplemental oxygen, vigorous pulmonary toilet, and careful monitoring of the child's respiratory status in the PICU. Parent education is also important to help prevent future aspirations. This includes instructing parents that children under 3 years of age are prime candidates for aspiration accidents and aiding them in recognizing the importance of safeguarding their children from objects that are commonly aspirated.

Pharyngeal Obstruction. The pharynx, the most collapsible portion of the extrathoracic airway, is formed by constrictor muscles posteriorly and laterally and pharyngeal dilators located predominantly on the anterior and lateral walls of the pharynx. The constrictor muscles participate primarily in swallowing, whereas the pharyngeal dilators are believed to be important in airway maintenance (Mathew & Sant'Ambrogia, 1991). During states of decreased consciousness caused by sedatives, anesthesia, or primary central nervous system disease, the activity of these airway muscles and their responses to various stimuli may be depressed, leading to airway collapse during inspiration. In addition, muscle relaxation may cause airway obstruction by passive posterior displacement of the tongue. The largest group of patients at risk for pharyngeal obstruction in the PICU are patients who are comatose or are otherwise neurologically impaired. Other high-risk groups are patients who have been extubated after general anesthesia but are not yet fully awake, and those who are heavily sedated. These patients may have little difficulty maintaining a patent airway when awakened, but develop sonorous respirations and intermittent airway obstruction when permitted to rest in the supine position.

Pharyngeal obstruction can usually be overcome simply by side-lying or prone positioning. Placement of a nasopharyngeal airway may also be helpful if the child has an extremely flaccid pharynx or excessive oral secretions. If airway collapse is complete, endotracheal intubation is required.

Because level of consciousness may vary considerably, patients recovering from general anesthesia require close monitoring of both neurological function and respiratory status. Monitoring continuous pulse oximetry readings ensures adequate oxygenation; physical examination and arterial blood gases provide information about the adequacy of ventilation.

Intrathoracic Obstruction. As with extrathoracic obstruction, the respiratory rate of a child with an intrathoracic airway obstruction is relatively low. Other signs of respiratory distress may also be prominent including retractions, the use of accessory muscles of respiration (sternocleidomastoids, scaleni, and abdominals), and nasal flaring. However, additional clinical findings distinguish intrathoracic obstruction from its extrathoracic counterpart.

Normally, intrathoracic airways dilate during inspiration (as transmural pressure decreases), and narrow during expiration (see Fig. 20–8). These changes are exacerbated when there is obstruction, particularly during expiration, resulting in a prolonged expiratory phase and expiratory wheezes audible on auscultation. Variable regional air entry may also be present. The larger airways tend to collapse during forced expiration, and the combination of large and small airway obstruction leads to air trapping and hyperinflation of the lungs. This may be evidenced by downward displacement of the diaphragm on chest radiographs, and a tympanic chest on percussion. Three causes of intrathoracic airway obstruction that commonly lead to PICU admission are asthma, bronchiolitis, and tracheobronchomalacia.

Asthma. Asthma (reactive airways disease) is defined as recurrent, reversible episodes of wheezing or dyspnea caused by airway obstruction. It is classified as extrinsic (an immunologic, allergic response), intrinsic (nonallergic, often triggered by infection), exercise-induced, and/or aspirin induced (the last two types being rare during infancy or childhood). Although it may begin at any age, asthma most frequently begins within the first 5 years of life. It is one of the most prevalent childhood diseases and a major reason for emergency room visits and subsequent hospitalization. Asthma is an important cause of death, most often because its severity is underappreciated.

Asthma is characterized by a significant increase in intrathoracic airway resistance. This increased resistance to airflow results from the combined effect of spasm of bronchiolar smooth muscle, edema in the walls of small bronchioles, and obstruction of bronchial lumens by thick mucus. An extreme sensitivity of the airways to physical, chemical, and pharmacologic stimuli is a prominent feature of asthma and may implicate abnormalities in the autonomic regulation of airway smooth muscle in its pathogenesis.

Severe acute asthma, so-called *status asthmaticus*, does not respond to routine therapy and necessitates hospitalization. There is evidence to suggest that children whose asthma has caused even one episode of respiratory failure are more likely to have repeated episodes of respiratory failure and its catastrophic complications, including hypoxic brain injury and death (Newcomb & Akhter, 1988). These high-risk patients, as well as others judged on presentation to be at risk for respiratory failure, require PICU admission.

The child in status asthmaticus is usually pale and restless, has severe wheezing, and is sometimes cyanotic. Respiratory rate and heart rate are elevated, and a pulsus paradoxus of more than 15 mmHg may be detected. Vomiting and abdominal pain and distension are common, as is dehydration. As airway obstruction increases during an acute attack, arterial blood gases change through a characteristic series of stages. Arterial oxygen tension (PaO_2) is decreased because of reduced $\dot{V}/\dot{Q}$ ratios caused by the simultaneous occurrence of air trapping in some regions of the lung and atelectasis in others. Initially, hypoxemia stimulates respiratory drive, and the $PaCO_2$ decreases, with a normal or slightly elevated pH. Eventually, as muscle fatigue develops, and compensatory mechanisms fail, the $PaCO_2$ begins to rise, producing respiratory acidosis (Newcomb & Akhter, 1988). Respiratory rate and breath sounds decrease, and extreme restlessness is followed by stupor and unconsciousness. With progression, the $PaCO_2$ increases even more, pH falls with a superimposed metabolic acidosis, and PaO_2 becomes markedly reduced.

Treatment is directed at ensuring oxygenation and adequate alveolar ventilation while reversing the primary airway abnormalities: bronchospasm, mucosal edema, and overproduction of tenacious secretions.

Because patients in status asthmaticus are often hypoxic, it is essential to provide supplemental O_2 by oxyhood, mask, or nasal cannula. Preexisting $\dot{V}/\dot{Q}$ imbalances may be worsened by treatment with sympathomimetics (agents that ablate hypoxic vasoconstriction in the lungs, thereby increasing venous admixture [see later]); therefore, inspired O_2 is adjusted during treatment to maintain an O_2 saturation within normal limits.

Recently, sympathomimetics have replaced theophylline, with its narrow therapeutic margin, as the primary bronchodilators used in the treatment of status asthmaticus. To review, sympathomimetics are differentiated by the type of receptor they stimulate: alpha, beta$_1$, or beta$_2$. Alpha-adrenergic receptors are located in the smooth muscles of all vascular tissue. Stimulation of these receptors results in constriction of arterial and venous vasculature. Beta$_1$ receptors are found in the heart. Stimulating these receptors increases myocardial contractility, automaticity, and heart rate. Beta$_2$ receptors are primarily found in the smooth muscle of the lungs and skeletal muscle arterioles. Stimulation of these receptors results in smooth muscle relaxation, causing bronchodilation in the lungs and increased blood flow in skeletal muscle. The treatment of asthma calls for a beta$_2$ specific adrenergic agent. Sympathomimetics used in the treatment of asthma include noncatechol-amines (albuterol, metaproterenol, and terbutaline) and catecholamines (epinephrine, isoetharine, and isoproterenol). Aerosolized agents (albuterol, isoetharine, metaproterenol, or terbutaline) can be administered by continuous inhalation or as often as necessary to control symptoms (Moler et al., 1988; Schuh et al., 1990). Combining a nebulized beta$_2$ agonist with an anticholinergic (ipratropium bromide) may produce better bronchodilation (National Heart, Lung, and Blood Institute, 1991).

Parenteral corticosteroids are also started immediately. Steroids act not only as anti-inflammatory agents, but increase the number of beta-adrenergic receptors, enhancing the response of bronchial smooth muscle to both endogenous catecholamines and exogenous beta$_2$ agonists. Therefore, early steroid therapy combined with an adrenergic agent is significantly more effective than the adrenergic agent alone, even in infants and toddlers (Tal et al., 1990). An increase in PaO_2 in hypoxic patients may be seen as early as 3 hours after intravenous administration of corticosteroids (Piersen et al., 1974). Clinically, production of the thick tenacious sputum peculiar to asthma is also controlled, and mucosal edema appears to be decreased. Methylprednisolone (preferred over hydrocortisone because it has less effect on sodium and potassium metabolism at high doses) is given intravenously in a dose of 2 mg/kg/dose every 6 hours (maximum single dose 125 mg IV). Serious toxicity or adrenal suppression with short-term therapy (less than 2 weeks) is unlikely.

When continuous inhaled bronchodilators and steroids fail to correct hypoxemia and hypercarbia, intravenous terbutaline or isoproterenol may provide a dramatic reversal of bronchoconstriction and avert the need for endotracheal intubation and assisted ventilation. Terbutaline, a more selective beta$_2$ agonist, has few toxic effects. A loading dose of 10 mcg/kg of intravenous terbutaline is administered over 5 minutes followed by a continuous infusion of 3 to 6 mcg/kg/minute. This maintenance dose may be increased by 0.5 mcg/kg/minute as necessary keeping the heart rate under 200 beats per minute (bpm).

Alternatively, a continuous infusion of isoproterenol at 0.05 mcg/kg/minute may be increased by increments of 0.05 mcg/kg/minute until a clinical response is obtained. Stimulation of beta$_1$ receptors by isoproterenol, however, limits this therapy by causing an unacceptable increase in heart rate (greater than 20% from baseline or greater than 200 bpm) or dysrhythmias. More rarely in young children, isoproterenol may increase myocardial oxygen demands sufficiently to cause myocardial ischemia.

If deterioration continues despite therapeutic interventions, assisted ventilation may be necessary. Generally, severe acidosis despite aggressive management is reason enough for airway intervention and mechanical ventilation. The goal is to provide a pattern of ventilation that maintains adequate minute ventilation, while permitting a prolonged expiratory phase to reduce gas trapping. The use of PEEP may increase hyperinflation, but in some cases it improves oxygenation perhaps by stinting open airways that would ordinarily collapse during exhalation, and by facilitating alveolar emptying (Marini, 1989).

The importance of continuously monitoring the patient in status asthmaticus cannot be overemphasized. Frequent evaluations are necessary to assess the efficacy of sympathomimetics, and will direct the choice, and frequency of administration, of inhaled bronchodilators. Respiratory assessments include respiratory rate and effort, as well as the quality of air movement on auscultation. Oxygen saturation is monitored continuously by pulse oximetry; a fall in O_2 saturation below 90% is considered a sign of serious hypoxemia. Arterial blood gases also document progression in respiratory failure with an increase in $Paco_2$ and acidosis. The child's level of consciousness is frequently noted because a decrease in mental status may signal impending respiratory failure.

Fanta and coworkers (1986) noted that the severely bronchospastic patient with acute dyspnea was more likely to receive multiple pharmacologic agents to control symptoms. Skilled nursing assessment is necessary not only to monitor the effectiveness of interventions but also to detect negative effects of therapy (Table 20–3).

Caring for the child with asthma after endotracheal intubation presents additional nursing challenges. Routine maneuvers to maintain airway pat-

ency may irritate airway receptors and trigger bronchospasm and hypoxia. Even before airway intervention, chest physiotherapy may aggravate bronchospasm during status asthmaticus and is avoided until clinical improvement is assured. Heavy sedation and, in some patients, neuromuscular blockade may be required to achieve adequate ventilation and reduce the risks of barotrauma caused by positive pressure ventilation. In particular, the risk of developing a pneumothorax, already increased because of gas trapping, is great in mechanically ventilated patients with asthma. Pneumothorax should be suspected if there is sudden clinical deterioration with hypoxemia, acidosis, hypotension, or the unilateral absence of breath sounds. Equipment to needle aspirate extra-alveolar air (a large-bore intravenous catheter, stopcock, and large syringe) should be kept at the bedside, and equipment necessary for chest tube insertion readily available.

Patients in respiratory failure, especially those receiving steroids, routinely receive prophylactic treatment against stress-ulcer bleeding. One study, however, suggests that agents that elevate gastric pH may increase the risk of nosocomial pneumonia in endotracheally intubated patients by favoring gastric colonization with gram-negative bacilli (Driks et al., 1987). Retrograde colonization of the pharynx from the stomach may then occur. If this finding proves to be true in the pediatric population, agents such as sucralfate may be preferable to antacids or H_2 block-

Table 20–3. ACTIONS AND CLINICALLY SIGNIFICANT SIDE EFFECTS OF MEDICATIONS USED IN THE TREATMENT OF ASTHMA

Drug	Actions	Side Effects
Inhaled beta$_2$ agonist **Albuterol** (Ventolin) **Terbutaline** (Brethine) **Metaproterenol** (Alupent)	Bronchodilation (largely resulting from local drug effects in the lungs) Improve mucociliary clearance Metaproterenol is somewhat shorter acting and less selective for beta-adrenergic receptors	Tachycardia (less than with systemic drugs) Tremor and hyperactivity occur infrequently
Anticholingeric agent Ipratropium bromide	Enhance the magnitude of the response to beta$_2$ agonist.	
Corticosteroids: **Methylprednisolone**	Reduce inflammation ↑ Beta-adrenergic receptors (enhancing the response of bronchial smooth muscle to catecholamines)	Gastric ulcerations Adrenal insufficiency (with long-term therapy)
Systemic beta$_2$ agonist (Terbutaline is more selective for beta-adrenergic receptors)	Bronchodilation via: — Smooth muscle relaxation — Inhibition of antigen-induced release of histamine and other mediators of inflammation ↑ heart rate, contractility ↓ peripheral vascular resistance ↔ or ↑ systolic BP ↑ cardiac output	
Isoproterenol (Isuprel) **Terbutaline** (Brethine)		Tachycardia, dysrhythmias, myocardial ischemia Tachycardia, tremor, anxiety, restlessness, headache

ers. If gastric alkalinization is desired, gastric pH is periodically monitored.

Once the acute attack is controlled, parent and/or patient education becomes a nursing priority. This begins with a careful assessment of the family's understanding of the disease process and the measures necessary to help prevent future attacks.

Bronchiolitis. This is an acute viral infection of the small airways and a common cause of respiratory insufficiency in infancy. Although it may be associated with a number of other viruses, respiratory syncytial virus (RSV) is the etiologic agent in 75% of infants admitted to the hospital with bronchiolitis (Wohl & Chernick, 1978). Peak incidence is at 2 months of age, occurring most often in winter and spring. Mortality from RSV bronchiolitis is higher in infants with congenital heart disease (MacDonald et al., 1982), preexisting pulmonary disease (Hall et al., 1985), or acquired or congenital immunodeficiency. In infants without these underlying problems, smaller size, younger age (less than 2 months), and low gestational age at birth are more frequently associated with the need for mechanical ventilation (Lebel et al., 1989). In addition, Church and coworkers (1984) found that infants with bronchiolitis whose gestational age was 32 weeks or less at birth were at greater risk for developing apnea, both obstructive and central.

Respiratory distress in bronchiolitis is caused primarily by obstruction of small airways. This results from peribronchiolar cellular infiltration, interstitial edema, and the effects of plugging of small airways by sloughed epithelium and inflammatory exudates (Wohl & Chernick, 1978). The small size of the developing airways makes infants particularly vulnerable to obstruction owing to these mechanisms. Hypoxemia represents the major abnormality in gas exchange and is the result of underventilation of regions with relatively normal perfusion, that is, a low ventilation to perfusion ratio.

Bronchiolitis is also a disease of the lung parenchyma. Whether it is due to alveolar collapse from obstruction, or to primary involvement of the terminal airways and alveoli, many infants have a substantial restrictive component, which may predominate, usually causing a more severe form of the disease.

When a patient has obstructive lung disease, independent of its location, the respiratory rate tends to be low. This is because a low rate minimizes both energy expenditure and reduces the average pressure that the respiratory muscles must generate for a given minute alveolar ventilation (and CO_2 elimination). Infants with bronchiolitis, however, often breathe faster than predicted. This may represent the presence of a restrictive component (alveolitis, edema, or alveolar distension from hyperinflation); an overriding of the mechanism by the infant's cerebral cortex (because of agitation); and/or the work of a feedback mechanism initiated by stretch receptors of the lung and chest wall. Nevertheless, an infant with bronchiolitis still breathes slower and more

deeply than, for example, an infant with pulmonary edema from congestive heart failure. Crying, feeding, and agitation may exacerbate signs of respiratory distress, which include prolonged expiratory time, crackles and/or wheezing, and substernal and intercostal retractions. Respiratory insufficiency results when the infant, exhausted by the increased work of breathing, can no longer maintain adequate minute ventilation. At this point, air entry is greatly diminished, respiratory pauses and/or apnea may occur, and the infant may develop a respiratory or metabolic acidosis (Lebel et al., 1989). Rapidly progressing respiratory distress, increasing O_2 requirements, or an altered mental status are indications for PICU admission and, possibly, assisted ventilation. Smaller infants may also require PICU monitoring because a comparatively greater degree of obstruction is produced by exudate or edema in their small airways.

The management of infants with bronchiolitis has changed very little in the past 20 years. Therapy is still largely supportive consisting of O_2, mechanical ventilation, bronchodilators, and hydration. The use of the antiviral agent ribavirin is quite controversial and bears further discussion (see later) (Adams & McFadden, 1990).

Supplemental O_2 is generally required by all infants with bronchiolitis and generally reverses the hypoxemia caused by $\dot{V}/\dot{Q}$ abnormalities. Endotracheal intubation is indicated for signs of respiratory failure including worsening respiratory distress, severe tachycardia, listlessness or lethargy, and poor peripheral perfusion (Outwater & Crone, 1984). It may also be required for increasing hypoxemia (PaO_2 less than 60 mmHg or O_2 saturation less than 92% in an FiO_2 of 0.4), hypercarbia with respiratory acidosis, metabolic acidosis, apnea, or bradycardia (Lebel et al., 1989; Outwater & Crone, 1984). Apnea or hypercarbia with acidosis frequently necessitates positive pressure ventilation. Although continuous positive airway pressure (CPAP) or PEEP is generally contraindicated in cases of severe hyperinflation, either may help some infants by preventing airway closure and recruiting distal atelectatic regions (Outwater & Crone, 1984). A respiratory pattern with an increased expiratory time and lower respiratory rate also minimizes hyperinflation of the lungs. In two retrospective reviews of infants requiring assisted ventilation (Lebel et al., 1989; Outwater & Crone, 1984), the mean duration of ventilation was 5.4 and 4.3 days, respectively, and there were no serious complications.

Data regarding the use of bronchodilators in bronchiolitis are inconclusive (Stokes et al., 1983; Outwater & Crone, 1984). Inhaled agents may be beneficial; their use is determined by the individual infant's response.

Initially, fluid replacement may be necessary to correct fluid deficits resulting from increased insensible loss and poor intake. After replacing losses, fluids are restricted to maintenance requirements or somewhat less, to reduce the risk of developing pulmonary edema and further deterioration in respiratory function.

Ribavirin might provide an etiologic treatment for RSV infection. The Committee on Infectious Diseases of the American Academy of Pediatrics (1993), although not explicitly endorsing its use, recommends "consideration" of ribavirin for hospitalized infants at risk for severe or complicated RSV infections. Initial studies (Hall et al., 1983; Taber et al., 1983) indicated clinical improvement in respiratory status in RSV infected (but otherwise healthy) infants treated with aerosolized ribavirin. Subsequent research (Hall et al., 1985) purported therapeutic benefits for infants at increased risk of adverse outcomes from RSV infection, that is, those also suffering from underlying cardiac disease, pulmonary disease, or both. These conclusions, however, have been contradicted by some investigators (Barry et al., 1986), and severely criticized by others who suggest that "there is only marginal evidence for the clinical efficacy of ribavirin for the treatment of RSV infections" (Wald et al., 1988), and that more questions than answers exist concerning its use (Ray, 1988). In addition, ribavirin has been associated with increased respiratory difficulty in some infants, probably resulting from bronchospasm during its administration. The efficacy of ribavirin treatment, particularly in the intubated patient, remains unproven.

Because respiratory failure resulting from bronchiolitis may occur precipitously, it is important to identify high-risk patients upon hospital admission. Continuous monitoring includes heart rate, respiratory rate, and O_2 saturation. Frequent assessment of respiratory effort, breath sounds, and level of consciousness helps detect subtle changes in clinical status. The infant's response to interventions, for example, bronchodilators or chest physiotherapy directs future therapy and is closely evaluated and carefully documented. Any activity that increases the infant's work of breathing is avoided. The severely tachypneic infant may need to be fed by gavage. Before endotracheal intubation, placing an orogastric feeding tube is preferred because a nasogastric tube will occlude the infant's nare and may worsen respiratory distress by increasing airway resistance. Attempts are made to maximize ventilation, including elevating the head of the bed and positioning the infant prone to permit freer diaphragmatic movement. When mechanical ventilation is required, sedation may also be necessary to facilitate coordination of the infant's respiratory efforts with the ventilator and minimize coughing paroxysms.

If ribavirin is used, it is delivered via a face mask, oxyhood, or in the inspiratory limb of a ventilator circuit, by a small-particle aerosol generator (SPAG; Figure 20–11). The patient breathing spontaneously receives ribavirin, 6 g/100 mL, administered over 2 hours, three times daily for 3 to 5 days; the patient requiring mechanical ventilation receives ribavirin, 6 g per 300 mL, administered over 16 hours per day for 3 to 5 days. The drug may be deposited within the delivery system; therefore, careful observation is required, especially when ribavirin is delivered via a ventilator. Peak inspiratory pressures and end expir-

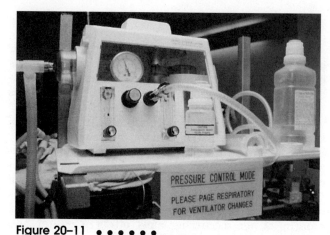

Figure 20–11 ● ● ● ● ● ●

The SPAG unit used for ribavirin administration.

atory pressures are monitored closely to detect obstruction of the expiratory circuit. Use of one-way valves on the inspiratory line and of a breathing circuit filter in the expiratory line have been helpful in preventing this problem (Outwater et al., 1988). To ensure tube patency, endotracheal suctioning is performed at least every 2 hours during the treatment period. Ribavirin is teratogenic and mutagenic in small animals; its long-term effect in humans is unknown. Therefore, additional precautions must be taken to limit others' exposure to the drug including patients, healthcare providers, and visitors. Ribavirin is administered in a private, negative-pressure room with the door kept closed. Because it may cause fetal harm, pregnant women should avoid contact with ribavirin (Adams, 1994).

The prevention of nosocomial RSV infections in high-risk patient populations requires meticulous handwashing. Moreover, because the virus can survive on surfaces for up to 6 hours (Hall et al., 1980), appropriate disinfection of surfaces and equipment contaminated by respiratory secretions is necessary to prevent the spread of infection by fomites.

Tracheobronchomalacia. This is a rare disease of infancy and childhood characterized by abnormally high compliance of the tracheal or bronchial wall. Severe congenital tracheobronchomalacia has been described in otherwise normal infants (Coghill et al., 1983), but is more often associated with other anomalies (tracheoesophageal fistula and esophageal atresia) or extrinsic compression of the airway by abnormal vascular structures (Sotomayor et al., 1986). Acquired tracheobronchomalacia may be the result of recurrent episodes of tracheitis and subsequent tracheal damage, local pressure, and irritation caused by an endotracheal tube (Sotomayor et al., 1986), or to barotrauma that may occur in very premature infants receiving positive pressure ventilation (Bhutani et al., 1986). Whatever its origin, expiratory collapse of the airway occurs because of inadequate cartilaginous and elastic supporting structures of the trachea and bronchi.

Clinical signs and symptoms depend on the location

and length of the malacic airway and the severity of the structural abnormality. If the affected segment encompasses both intrathoracic and extrathoracic portions of the trachea (as often occurs), the clinical presentation includes both stridor and wheezing. If the malacic area is only extrathoracic (larynx and trachea), there is only stridor. Airway obstruction may be episodic and is especially pronounced when intrathoracic pressure exceeds airway pressure, for example during forced expiration with Valsalva maneuvers, crying, or agitation. Increased respiratory rate (although slower than one would expect with the degree of respiratory distress), intercostal retractions, and grunting have been described in infants with severe tracheobronchomalacia. Wheezing and marked cyanotic spells requiring immediate intervention have also been reported (Sotomayor et al., 1986). During an acute obstructive episode, breath sounds may be markedly diminished and hypoxemia and hypercarbia may develop (Gordin, 1990). The diagnosis of tracheobronchomalacia is confirmed by examining the airways with bronchoscopy and/or fluoroscopy.

Many infants with minor degrees of tracheobronchomalacia and mild or moderate symptoms require no intervention and improve with growth. For infants with severe malacia, however, a tracheostomy is often required. The tracheostomy tube may stint open a semiflaccid trachea, as long as the cannula bypasses the affected area. However, a malacic segment very low in the trachea, or involving the bronchi, will not be supported by a tracheostomy tube alone. In this instance, positive airway pressure during expiration (PEEP or CPAP) may produce the same effect by increasing airway transmural pressure during the critical expiratory phase. Some patients may require a positive airway pressure as high as 25 cm H_2O to maintain airway patency (Kanter et al., 1982). Agitation and attempts by the infant to forcefully exhale cause airway collapse and complicate management; sedation and even muscle relaxation may be indicated in some patients undergoing mechanical ventilation.

In extreme cases of bronchomalacia, a pneumonectomy or lobectomy may be required because segmental bronchial resection and end-to-end anastomosis is not feasible. An alternative treatment for those patients is a surgically implanted splint that serves to support the collapsing bronchus (Filler et al., 1982).

Because tracheobronchomalacia is often a difficult problem to diagnose, it is important to carefully monitor and document episodes that may represent airway collapse. Unexplained periods of increased respiratory distress and arterial desaturation (with or without cyanosis) are noteworthy, especially in an infant on long-term ventilation. Documenting events immediately preceding hypoxic episodes is also important, because maneuvers that decrease transmural pressure, for example, crying or straining, may cause a malacic airway to collapse. When an infant with tracheobronchomalacia has acute respiratory

decompensation, slow hand ventilation with somewhat higher peak inspiratory pressures than the infant's baseline often relieve the obstruction (Gordin, 1990). For care of the patient with a tracheostomy, see Bronchopulmonary Dysplasia.

Restrictive Disease

Reduced pulmonary compliance is another mechanical alteration that can produce alterations in pulmonary function and respiratory pump failure. When pulmonary compliance is decreased, a greater airway pressure is needed to distend alveolar units to the same final lung volume; that is, it takes more pressure (and more work) to deliver normal lung volumes to a stiff lung. To reduce the work of breathing yet sustain minute alveolar ventilation, children with decreased thoracic compliance breathe rapidly and shallowly. Diminished compliance also results in intercostal and subcostal retractions, especially in the supple chest wall of the young infant.

In addition to increasing the work of breathing, decreased pulmonary compliance ultimately reduces functional residual capacity (FRC, the amount of air that remains in the lungs at the end of normal expiration). This reduction in FRC may lead to alveolar collapse and result in increased intrapulmonary shunting and hypoxemia.

Frequent causes of decreased lung compliance in PICU patients include adult respiratory distress syndrome (ARDS), pneumonia, pneumothorax, and congenital diaphragmatic hernia.

Adult Respiratory Distress Syndrome. Despite its name, adult respiratory distress syndrome (ARDS) is a condition well described in the pediatric patient population. ARDS is a symptom complex, not a specific disease entity, and represents the net result of various frequently unrelated but massive assaults to the lung. In 1967, Ashbaugh and others first described a group of patients who, after injuries such as trauma and sepsis, developed acute dyspnea and hypoxemia that failed to respond to conservative therapy. Today we recognize ARDS as a triad of clinical features, which include: (1) derangement in gas exchange sufficient to cause dyspnea and severe hypoxemia in room air; (2) decrease in pulmonary compliance, which results in a loss of FRC; and (3) bilateral, diffuse pulmonary infiltrates on chest radiographs consistent with pulmonary edema. The Pediatric Critical Care Study Group found the overall mortality from pediatric ARDS to be 43%. (Timmons, Havens, & Fackler, 1995).

A number of conditions are associated with the development of ARDS. Inhalation injuries are the most common cause of direct pulmonary injury, and include the aspiration of gastric contents, near drowning, and the inhalation of smoke or other toxic substances. ARDS also results from conditions that do not involve the lungs directly. Sepsis is most common of these conditions. In fact, in most studies, sepsis ranks highest of all conditions, direct or indirect, leading to ARDS.

The biochemical mediators and products of cellular damage that may contribute to the lung injury are not clearly delineated. Whatever the underlying mediator, the predominant physiologic disturbance is an alteration in the alveolar-capillary interface, which leads to increased capillary permeability and pulmonary edema. Under normal circumstances, the permeability of the alveolar epithelium is relatively constant. Fluid leaves the capillary bed via small clefts located at the junction of the endothelial cells lining the capillary walls, and the lymphatic system is capable of removing excesses. However, when the alveolar capillary membrane is disrupted, large amounts of fluid and protein leak first into the interstitial space, overwhelming the lymphatics, eventually entering the alveolus itself. This accumulation of abnormally large amounts of protein-rich interstitial and alveolar fluid is known as increased permeability, low pressure, or noncardiogenic pulmonary edema (Staub, 1980). As a result of this process, for any given pulmonary capillary pressure, lung water is greatly increased. Even at normal pulmonary capillary wedge pressures of 5 to 10 mmHg, there is fluid accumulation in ARDS. However, because measures of lung water and gas exchange correlate poorly, increased lung water is only partially responsible for the refractory hypoxemia seen in ARDS. Of greater consequence is the $\dot{V}/\dot{Q}$ mismatch associated with the multiple disturbances of pulmonary circulation and alveolar aeration seen in this disease.

The noncardiogenic pulmonary edema of ARDS results in decreased lung compliance (C_L); that is, it takes more pressure (and more work) to deliver normal tidal volumes because the lungs are stiffer. If the force required to inflate the lungs cannot be maintained, overall lung volume decreases, leading eventually to alveolar collapse and a net reduction in FRC. As alveoli collapse, intrapulmonary shunting occurs and hypoxemia develops. Ordinarily, the pulmonary vessels constrict in the face of alveolar hypoxia, a phenomenon called *reflex hypoxic vasoconstriction*. But in ARDS, reflex hypoxic vasoconstriction may not be intact and poorly ventilated areas continue to be perfused. Collapsed alveoli that remain perfused create a right-to-left shunt, increasing pulmonary venous admixture and causing hypoxemia. The opposite also occurs in the lungs with ARDS; some alveoli may remain ventilated but are not perfused. This may be the result of vasoconstriction, emboli, or destruction of the capillary structure by the disease process. Such areas behave as dead space, and may increase $PaCO_2$ (Fig. 20–12).

After the pulmonary insult, there may be a lag time of several hours to several days before respiratory distress develops. Then, dyspnea develops; the symptom is subjective and can be reported only by an older child. In an infant, increasing respiratory difficulty may be manifested as agitation, sometimes progressing to somnolence. Tachypnea, with intercostal and substernal retractions in smaller children and infants, may persist even after O_2 administration, reflecting the need for an increased minute ventilation. Central cyanosis is a late sign indicative of a marked decrease in PaO_2. Chest auscultation, which can be normal initially, eventually reveals course rales and bronchial breath sounds. The fine, basilar rales of congestive heart failure are often absent in ARDS. Wheezing may also occur because of narrowing of the terminal airways by peribronchial edema, decreased lung volume, or secretions. The majority of patients require intubation to ensure reliable ventilation and O_2 administration. PEEP increases FRC and lessens the work of breathing by improving lung compliance (Fig. 20–13).

The treatment for ARDS remains largely supportive. Supplemental O_2 is required by all patients. Although the extent to which the condition is made worse by O_2 is unknown, O_2 toxicity may occur after prolonged exposure to high concentration of inspired O_2. In addition, the nitrogen present in an FiO_2 less than 0.5 serves as an intra-alveolar splint. With higher concentrations of O_2, decreasing amounts of residual gas remain in the alveoli, and reabsorption atelectasis may occur. Therefore, it is prudent to reduce inspired O_2 concentrations as much and as rapidly as possible. Norwood and Civetta (1985) suggest a goal of maintaining a PaO_2 of 70 to 80 mmHg in an FiO_2 less than 0.5.

PEEP is considered the most effective treatment for ARDS. With positive pressure ventilation alone, high inspiratory pressures are required to open collapsed alveoli, pressures that to some extent hyperinflate normal alveoli. Perhaps more importantly, with-

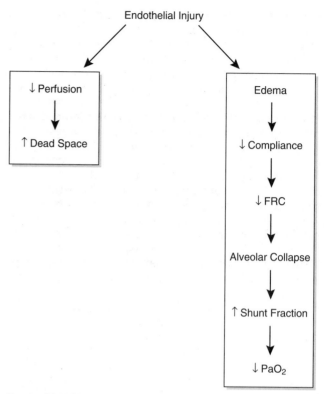

Figure 20–12 ● ● ● ● ● ●
Pathophysiology of ARDS.

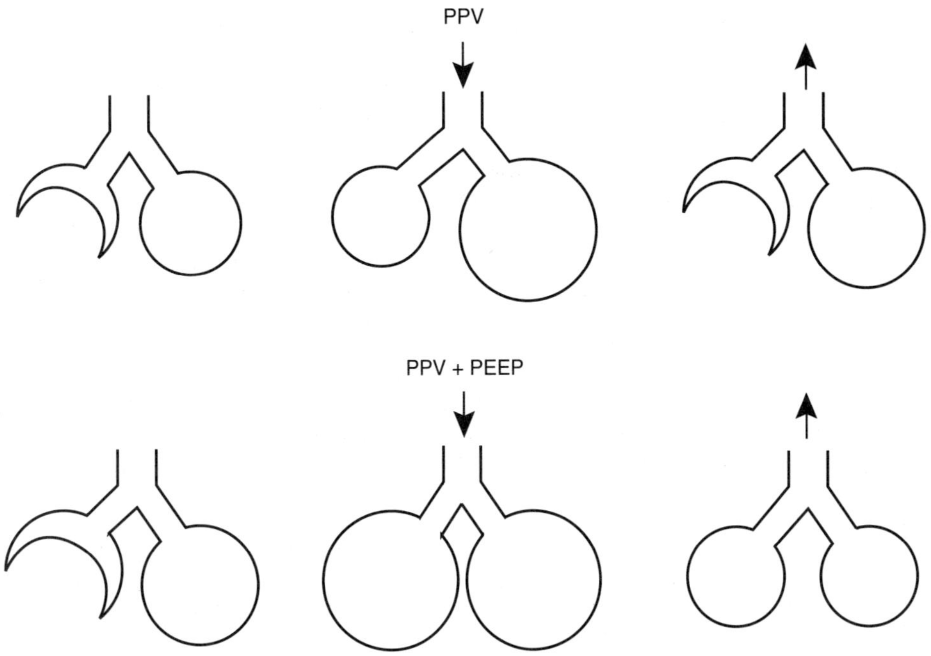

Figure 20–13 ● ● ● ● ● ●

Idealized schema of the effects of PEEP in restrictive lung disease. When lung compliance is decreased, functional residual capacity is reduced, alveolar structures become unstable and some alveoli collapse. Positive pressure ventilation (PPV) alone (top panel) will reduce the overall number of collapsed alveoli, but as the thorax is allowed to reach its relaxation volume at the end of expiration, some alveoli may still collapse. Reexpansion of the atelectasis following the application of PEEP, however, increases functional residual capacity (FRC) and provides more stable alveolar recruitment. Consequently, lung compliance and PaO_2 increase.

out PEEP, previously collapsed alveoli collapse again on exhalation (see Fig. 20–13). When PEEP is added to positive pressure ventilation, alveoli are opened by the PIP and remain open throughout all phases of the respiratory cycle to participate continually in gas exchange. PEEP increases FRC by augmenting the volume of expanded alveoli and by recruiting collapsed units. PEEP does not remove lung water but improves arterial oxygenation by increasing the number of ventilated alveoli. The implication for nursing is the need to be certain that prescribed levels of PEEP are maintained, including during endotracheal suctioning, after turning the child, and so on.

It should be noted that excessive PEEP can also have adverse effects. When PEEP is increased in an attempt to re-expand collapsed alveoli, more normal alveoli may become overdistended (Fig. 20–14). The proportion of nonoxygenated blood increases as the normal capillaries are compressed, increasing intrapulmonary shunting and hypoxemia. Dead space is increased in the overdistended units and $PaCO_2$ may climb. PEEP may also cause additional lung trauma. Frequent chest radiographs in patients with ARDS are necessary during the acute phase of the disease, not so much to follow the pulmonary edema, but to evaluate potential complications of therapy. Complications include pulmonary hyperinflation, interstitial gas, pneumomediastinum, and pneumothorax. Finally, PEEP may cause a decrease in cardiac output primarily by decreasing systemic venous return to the heart. Myocardial support may be necessary including both the judicious use of volume to increase preload, and the administration of inotropic agents.

Although controversies abound regarding fluid requirement and restriction in ARDS, it is generally advisable to keep patients relatively fluid restricted.

The ultimate goal of fluid therapy is to maintain an adequate cardiac output while keeping microvascular pressures as low as possible. Diuretics may be helpful in shifting extravascular water into the intravascular space if volume overload has occurred. Furo-

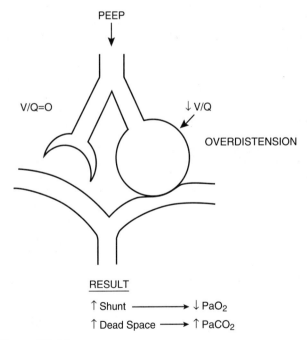

Figure 20–14 ● ● ● ● ● ●

Schema of effects of excessive PEEP in restrictive lung disease. When atelectatic alveoli have markedly decreased compliance, PEEP may go preferentially to more compliant alveoli. Intrapulmonary shunting and dead space ventilation occurs when the overdistended alveolus compresses the pulmonary capillary. This results in hypoxemia and hypercarbia, which are made worse by the collapsed alveolus that continues to be perfused.

semide is known to be effective in cardiogenic pulmonary edema by virtue of both its diuretic and nondiuretic vascular properties. By lowering central filling pressures through immediate vasodilation (independent of the later diuresis), furosemide can reduce pulmonary shunting and lung water in high permeability pulmonary edema as well.

Other treatment measures are attempts to maximize O_2 delivery. Because hypoxemia is a primary feature of ARDS, measures to reduce O_2 consumption ($\dot{V}O_2$) are critically important. In patients with very large intrapulmonary shunts, fever, anxiety, and physical activity can increase oxygen demand. This in turn decreases the PO_2 of mixed venous blood ($P\bar{v}O_2$), and ultimately lowers PaO_2. Therefore, treatment of fever, reduction of anxiety, and sedation are important. Muscle relaxants may be used, not so much to reduce O_2 consumption (neuromuscular blockade will not reduce $\dot{V}O_2$ beyond that achieved by adequate sedation [Palmisano et al., 1984]), but to overcome incoordination of the child's respiratory efforts with positive pressure ventilation and prevent the complications that may bring, for example, a pneumothorax or pneumomediastinum.

To maximize the availability of O_2 at the cellular level, attempts are made to correct factors that negatively influence oxyhemoglobin dissociation, that is, shift the oxyhemoglobin dissociation curve to the left and impair the release of O_2 to the tissues. Here normothermia is again important, as is the avoidance of metabolic or respiratory alkalosis.

The oxygen content of arterial blood (CaO_2) is maximized (see equation, later). Arterial O_2 saturations are maintained at 90% or more, and blood transfusions may be necessary to keep the hemoglobin between 12 and 15 g/dL.

Several experimental interventions have been suggested by research into the mechanisms of acute lung injury in ARDS. Steroids have long stimulated interest for their anti-inflammatory properties. In patients with ARDS, data regarding steroid use are contradictory. Several studies indicate no benefit in the use of pharmacologic doses of steroids even early in the course of the disease except in specific instances—radiation pneumonitis and fat embolism syndrome. As for treatment with high-dose steroids, no improvement in survival rates have been demonstrated and mortality may be higher because of an increase in the number of secondary infections (Bernard & Bradley, 1986). Nonsteroidal anti-inflammatory agents have been shown to decrease the degree of hypoxemia in animal ARDS models. In addition, agents that inhibit neutrophil activity, such as prostaglandin E_1, have been studied in adult patients with ARDS, but have had no effect on overall survival rates.

The child with ARDS has markedly impaired gas exchange related to intrapulmonary shunting, increased pulmonary dead space, and decreased FRC. In addition, an ineffective breathing pattern exists because of hypoxemia, hypercarbia, and pulmonary edema. Nursing interventions are directed at assessing, altering, or correcting these abnormalities.

Because the primary problem in ARDS is impaired gas exchange, the monitoring of that process is essential. Arterial blood gases provide information about oxygenation, ventilation, and acid-base balance. Arterial oxygenation, however, should be evaluated within the context of FiO_2 or alveolar PO_2 (PAO_2). Following PaO_2 alone is not enough to track the course of ARDS (Bernard & Bradley, 1986). Arterial oxygen content (CaO_2) is described by the following equation:

$$CaO_2 \text{ (mL/dL)} = [(\text{Hgb g/dL}) \times 1.36 \text{ (ml } O_2\text{/g hgb)}$$
$$\times \text{ hgb saturation (\%)}]$$
$$+ [PaO_2 \text{ (mmHg)}$$
$$\times 0.003 \text{ (mL/dL/mmHg)}]$$

The majority of oxygen is carried by hemoglobin; therefore, it becomes apparent that hemoglobin concentration and O_2 saturation are the important determinants of O_2 content. Maintaining the hemoglobin at normal levels optimizes O_2 carrying capacity without increasing viscosity and limiting tissue perfusion. Noninvasive pulse oximetry provides continuous data regarding O_2 saturation. This continuous information can prove invaluable in monitoring pulmonary perfusion changes that occur during various nursing interventions that may alter $\dot{V}/\dot{Q}$ matching, for example, when the patient is positioned prone. Hypercarbia is not a predominant feature of ARDS except in severe cases. Here, noninvasive end-tidal CO_2 monitoring may not be as useful except in providing trending information, because the difference between arterial CO_2 and end-tidal values widens with severe $\dot{V}/\dot{Q}$ mismatching. What is ultimately important, however, is not just the PaO_2 but the total amount of oxygen transported to the tissues. Therefore, monitoring gas exchange alone is insufficient.

Oxygen delivery (DO_2) is the product of the oxygen content of arterial blood (CaO_2) and the cardiac index (CI):

$$DO_2 = CaO_2 \times CI \times 10$$

Oxygen transport may be altered by various mechanisms in ARDS, by the primary disease process, by therapeutic interventions such as PEEP, or by anemia caused by blood sampling or hemorrhage. Monitoring the determinants or indices of O_2 transport, therefore, becomes as important as monitoring gas exchange. Blood pressure is a relatively poor index of cardiac output, which may be measured directly when a pulmonary artery catheter is in place. Noninvasive techniques for measuring cardiac output, such as those based on ultrasound results, may provide a valuable alternative in the future.

Those patients who require neuromuscular blockade present additional nursing challenges. Although the child may appear calm after neuromuscular blocking agents have been administered, sensory perception and level of consciousness are not altered. Neuromuscular blocking agents have no sedative or analgesic effects; therefore, sedatives and/or anxiolytics are *always* administered. Older children and adolescents require reassurance that the paralysis is

TOF Suppression and Degree of Neuromuscular Blockade

TOF Suppression					Approximate Percentage of Block
Four responses					0–75
Three responses					75–80
Two responses					80–90
One response					90
No response					100

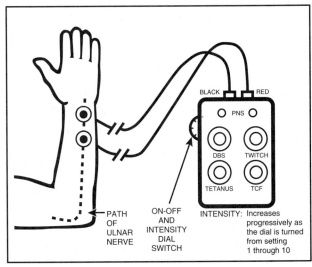

Figure 20–15 ● ● ● ● ● ●

Train-of-Four monitoring sites and procedures.

Clinically Relevant Levels of Neuromuscular Blockade

Percentage of Blockade	Clinical Interpretation
90–95	Conditions may be suitable for endotracheal intubation and long-term mechanical ventilation
80–90	Block may be adequate for short-term relaxation and long-term mechanical ventilation
75	Maintenance doses may be needed to extend duration of relaxation
≤75	Patient may be susceptible to rapid reversal with cholinesterase antagonists
<75	Patient's spontaneous recovery is probably satisfactory

drug-induced and reversible. If painful procedures are to be performed, or if the child's underlying condition or its treatment are inherently painful, analgesics are also administered. Every effort should be made to reduce noxious auditory stimuli around the child, scheduling care to permit quiet time for sleep. The child's response to these interventions can be assessed by monitoring the physiologic consequences of anxiety or pain, that is, tachycardia, hypertension, and pupillary dilatation.

Periodically, the neuromuscular blockade is permitted to wear off to perform at least a summary neurologic evaluation, as well as to determine the continued need for blockade. At times, it may be impossible to allow the neuromuscular blockade to wear off, for example, in the patient who requires high ventilator pressures who immediately has decompensation during dysynchronous breaths. Here, continuous infusion of intermediate-acting neuromuscular blocking agents may be beneficial.

Patients who require continuous or prolonged neuromuscular blockade benefit from monitoring of peripheral nerve stimulation. The most common of these techniques, the "train-of-four," was first described by Ali and coworkers in 1970. In a train-of-four, two electrodes placed in line along the distal ulnus are connected to a nerve stimulator that delivers four electrical stimuli at preset intervals (Davidson, 1991). Ordinarily, stimulation of the ulnar nerve produces four serial thumb adductions (Fig. 20–15). With neuromuscular blockade (induced by nondepolarization agents), this response fades; that is, each successive twitch becomes weaker. As blockade increases, the last twitch is obliterated, then the third, and so on. When only one twitch is elicited by a train-of-four stimulation, spontaneous respirations are suppressed. Continuous infusion rates are titrated or additional boluses of chemical muscle relaxants are administered to maintain a single twitch in the train-of-four response. Titrating these agents in this manner diminishes the likelihood of prolonged neuromuscular blockade.

Several researchers suggest that the consequences of prolonged muscle disuse brought about by neuromuscular blockade in young infants may be more severe than in adults. Reports of microscopic evidence of skeletal muscle growth failure with prolonged use of neuromuscular blockade in preterm infants (Rutledge et al., 1986) and residual muscle weakness in newborns after receiving pancuronium for several weeks (Torres et al., 1985) raise issues relating to the normal growth and development of muscle in the face of prolonged paralysis. It becomes obvious that neuromuscular blockade must be used judiciously, especially in infants.

When neuromuscular blockade is necessary, extreme vigilance is required to avoid tissue breakdown from immobility. Therapeutic surfaces that reduce pressure are indicated, as well as a routine turning schedule. Corneal abrasions are avoided by instilling artificial tears or other ophthalmic lubricant and ensuring that the child's eyes are closed. Chapter 17 provides a review of essential skin and eye care required of the chemically paralyzed patient.

ARDS is not a disorder of the respiratory system alone. Other organs may be adversely affected by the primary disease process (for example, sepsis), altered oxygen transport, or alteration in organ function directly. Monitoring of various organ function is, therefore, crucial. The brain may be negatively affected by inadequate O_2 delivery leading to altered levels of consciousness, for example, confusion, combativeness, or coma. Other organs may be involved because, in a more limited way, they undergo the same endothelial injury as the lungs. Therefore, disseminated intravascular coagulation (DIC), acute renal failure (ARF), and hepatic dysfunction are common in ARDS.

Oxygen is not the only nutrient important in ARDS; the overall nutritional status of the child cannot be ignored. Mechanical ventilation may be necessary for weeks or months, during which nutritional/caloric needs may greatly exceed maintenance requirement. Nutritional adequacy is established early in the development of ARDS because sustained malnutrition can result in abnormalities in pulmonary defense mechanisms and pulmonary structure and function (Rochester & Esau, 1984) and may limit the child's ability to wean from mechanical ventilation.

Because the child's prognosis is frequently uncertain and the intensive care course may be long and fraught with multiple setbacks, parents of the child with ARDS require a tremendous amount of nursing support. It is important to develop a therapeutic relationship with the family early on, to provide consistent and accurate information about their child, and to involve the family in nurturing behaviors.

Pneumonia. Pneumonia, whether an acute primary infection or a secondary process, is a common problem in PICU patients. Most pneumonias in infants and children are viral in origin. However, bacterial pneumonias are still an important cause of severe illness in childhood. In the immunocompetent pediatric patient, the major organisms causing bacterial pneumonia are pneumococcus, streptococcus, and staphylococcus. Certain infectious agents are more prevalent in certain age groups: Group B streptococci predominate in the newborn; pneumococcus in the

young child 1 month to 6 years of age; and pneumococcus in the older child. In the immunocompromised patient, *Pneumocystis carinii*, fungi, and opportunistic bacteria such as enteric and atypical mycobacteria are important causative agents.

Patients with endotracheal intubation are particularly vulnerable to nosocomially acquired pneumonia. Bacterial colonization of the upper respiratory tract frequently occurs in these patients and may promote pneumonia through aspiration of these pathogens. In addition, the child with an artificial airway may be at particularly high risk for pneumonia because of impaired mucociliary clearance, the frequency of airway invasion, and exposure to nosocomial pathogens.

Aspiration pneumonia is an important phenomenon in the PICU patient. When normal airway-protective mechanisms are impaired, gastric contents may be aspirated into the airways. This may occur because of a decreased level of consciousness or the presence of an endotracheal tube, which inhibits the child's ability to occlude the larynx.

A pneumonia can occur anywhere in the lung. As lobes or segments become filled with fluid and cellular debris, lung compliance and vital capacity decrease and the work of breathing increases. Increased venous admixture results from continued perfusion of consolidated, airless lung and may lead to hypoxemia. Signs and symptoms of respiratory distress may develop including tachypnea, dyspnea, cough, and intercostal retractions. Usually, there are localized findings over the affected lung segment with diminished breath sounds or adventitious noises.

When bacterial pneumonia is suspected, appropriate antibiotic therapy is started as soon as possible. Antibiotic coverage may be changed or extended when the causative organism is identified and antibiotic sensitivities established. Supplemental O_2 is administered to maintain normal O_2 saturation. If respiratory failure ensues, endotracheal intubation and mechanical ventilation are also required.

Nursing care of the patient with pneumonia is largely supportive. Impaired gas exchange is monitored by following arterial blood gases and pulse oximetry (SpO_2). When unilateral intrapulmonary shunting predominates, patient positioning becomes critically important. Pulmonary perfusion is gravity-dependent. The pattern of lung inflation depends upon how the patient is being ventilated; lungs inflate from bottom to top during spontaneous breaths and from top to bottom during positive pressure breaths. Optimal position to enhance matching of ventilation to perfusion is best determined at the bedside with the aid of continuous SpO_2 monitoring.

As in ARDS, O_2 delivery to the tissues can be maximized by avoiding factors that shift the oxyhemoglobin dissociation curve to the left including hypothermia and alkalosis.

Pneumothorax. A pneumothorax is a collection of air or gas in the pleural space that may occur spontaneously, but more frequently results from

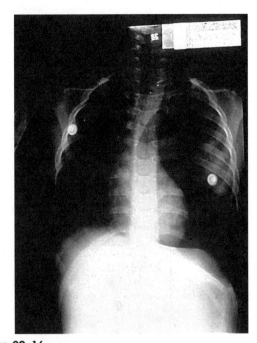

Figure 20-16 ● ● ● ● ● ●

Chest radiograph illustrating pneumothorax with mediastinal shift.

trauma to the lung parenchyma. A tension pneumothorax exists when air enters the pleural space at such a rate that pressure in the pleural space increases enough to produce circulatory and ventilatory impairment. As extra-alveolar air accumulates, it compresses and shifts the mediastinum toward the unaffected side. If a significant tension pneumothorax is not treated promptly, venous return to the heart falls, cardiac output decreases, and cardiopulmonary arrest ensues. Early detection and timely intervention, however, may prevent this catastrophic chain of events.

A small, stable pneumothorax may go completely undetected until a chest radiograph reveals its presence (Fig. 20-16). If the pneumothorax increases in size, the child may develop dyspnea, pleuritic chest pain, and tachypnea. However, a more dramatic presentation frequently occurs in the PICU setting. Commonly, the child undergoing positive pressure ventilation has a sudden deterioration in oxygenation and ventilation as reflected in noninvasive monitors and arterial blood gases. The child becomes tachycardic and hypotensive because of decreased venous return to the heart. A significant pulsus paradoxus (a decrease in blood pressure during inspiration) may also develop as left ventricular output is further compromised by increasing intrathoracic pressures. An infant who develops a large tension pneumothorax may rapidly become hypotensive and develop bradycardia from severe hypoxemia. On physical examination, there may be decreased breath sounds and hyperresonance to percussion on the affected side. However, in infants and small children, breath sounds may be readily transmitted from the

unaffected to the affected side, and a decrease in air entry may not be as apparent. Transillumination with a high-intensity light may be helpful in these patients; the side of the chest containing the free air will transmit light well. In older patients, there may also be a contralateral shift of the mediastinum with tracheal deviation toward the unaffected side and lateral displacement of the cardiac apical impulse. Occasionally, subcutaneous emphysema and crepitus may also occur.

A tension pneumothorax is a medical emergency that requires immediate intervention. Evacuation of pleural air is attempted whenever a patient has an acute deterioration that is likely to be the result of tension pneumothorax. Although a chest radiograph provides the definitive diagnosis, it should not delay treatment of a suspected pneumothorax in a patient with rapidly deteriorating circulatory function. In the absence of a chest radiograph, a pneumothorax can be localized by transillumination or physical examination. Initially, a large-bore needle or catheter, attached by a stopcock to a large syringe, may be used to rapidly evacuate the pneumothorax. Once the patient's condition has stabilized, a tube thoracostomy can be performed to permit full reexpansion of the lung and prevent reaccumulation of pleural air.

The primary nursing goals are to identify patients at risk, closely monitor for the signs and symptoms of a pneumothorax, and reduce or eliminate factors that may contribute to the development of extra-alveolar air.

To detect the development of a tension pneumothorax, it is necessary to identify and closely monitor those patients at higher risk for developing extra-alveolar air. First, alveolar rupture, resulting from overdistension, is not uncommon with the use of positive-pressure ventilation. Once the alveolus ruptures, the gas it contains moves into the interstitial space where it dissects into other fascial planes or compartments. This may result in interstitial emphysema, pneumopericardium, pneumothorax, pneumomediastinum, subcutaneous emphysema, pneumoretroperitoneum, and/or pneumoperitoneum. The incidence of these complications increases when it is necessary to use high peak inspiratory or end-expiratory pressures to achieve adequate oxygenation and ventilation.

Patients who have regional differences in lung compliance or airway resistance may also be predisposed to the development of extra-alveolar air. A pneumothorax may occur, for example, in a child with ARDS when less affected alveoli are overdistended by the pressure required to inflate noncompliant areas of the lung. In the child in status asthmaticus, a pneumothorax may result if airway obstruction during expiration leads to gas trapping and alveolar hyperinflation.

A pneumothorax may result from chest trauma. An open pneumothorax (or sucking chest wound) occurs when there is a penetrating injury that creates a communication between the pleural space and the environment. Pleural pressure and atmospheric pressure immediately equilibrate, the lung collapses, and the mediastinum shifts toward the unaffected lung. A small opening in the chest wall that permits air entry but blocks its exit (or a closed lung injury, caused by a broken rib, for example) may cause air to accumulate in the pleural space and result in a tension pneumothorax.

Patients receiving positive pressure ventilation are assessed frequently to determine the adequacy of their ventilation and detect untoward events, such as right mainstem intubation or asynchronous breathing, which may lead to a pneumothorax. Nursing vigilance in these patients can prevent what is sometimes an iatrogenic complication of treatment.

When a chest tube is required, assessment of the patient's respiratory status is followed by a thorough assessment of the chest tube and drainage system. The chest tube insertion site is covered with an occlusive dressing and kept dry to prevent maceration of the skin. Although usually sutured in at the time of insertion, the chest tube or drainage tubing is also taped to the child's chest wall to minimize the risk of dislodgement. The chest tube is usually connected to a drainage system by a length of latex rubber tubing. The tubing connections must be airtight and secured with ridged plastic straps. The tubing is kept free of kinks or dependent loops, which, if filled with fluid, may cause resistance to flow out of the chest. The tubing and drainage system should be positioned below the patient's chest to facilitate gravity drainage and prevent fluid backflow.

There are three interconnected chambers in all chest tube drainage systems: a chamber to collect drainage, a water-seal chamber to maintain a negative intrapleural pressure, and a suction control chamber that limits the amount of suction that can be applied to the pleural cavity. Bubbling in the water seal chamber indicates that there is a leak in the system. The source of the leak can be from the lung, from somewhere along the connecting tubing, or from the chest tube insertion site. If there is no bubbling, and the water level rises and falls as the child breathes, the system is reflecting normal pressure changes in the pleural cavity during respiration. Suction to the intrapleural space is regulated by the height of water in the suction chamber (usually 15 to 20 cm H_2O), not by the amount of suction applied to this chamber. Wall suction is regulated to produce gentle bubbling in the suction chamber. Water is replaced as it evaporates to maintain the prescribed water level. If suction is not applied, the suction chamber is left open to the atmosphere.

Congenital Diaphragmatic Hernia. Congenital diaphragmatic hernia occurs in approximately 1 in 2000 births when the fetal diaphragm fails to develop normally, leaving an opening between the thorax and the abdomen. This permits the abdominal contents to enter the thoracic cavity, interfering with normal development of the lungs.

The diaphragm forms during the eighth to tenth week of fetal life and separates the abdominal and thoracic cavities. Because the left posterior aspect of

the diaphragm is usually the last to close, the most common type of diaphragmatic hernia involves this area of the muscle (foramen of Bochdalek). While the diaphragm is forming, the midgut is developing within the umbilical pouch. If the diaphragm has not completely closed when the midgut returns to the abdominal cavity (about the tenth week of gestation), abdominal structures can enter the thoracic cavity—the stomach, large and small intestines in a left-sided defect, or part or all of the liver in the less common right-sided defect. The herniated gut then compresses the developing lung buds, arresting their growth on both the ipsilateral and, to a lesser degree, the contralateral side. As a result, the number of airways and alveoli is markedly reduced. The number of pulmonary arteries is also decreased and their distribution is abnormal. In addition, the amount of smooth muscle in pulmonary arterioles is greater than normal (Bohn et al., 1987). Therefore, infants with congenital diaphragmatic hernia have both lung hypoplasia and increased pulmonary vascular resistance.

At birth, the infant with a significant diaphragmatic hernia is tachypneic and has marked intercostal and substernal retractions. Breath sounds are decreased or absent on the affected side, and the PMI and heart sounds are shifted to the unaffected side. Typically, the infant's chest diameter is increased and the abdomen is scaphoid. Gas-filled loops of bowel may be evident within the chest on radiograph. Because the hypoplastic pulmonary vascular bed is unable to accommodate the normal increase in postnatal right ventricular output, pulmonary hypertension develops. Blood is shunted right to left across the foramen ovale and patent ductus resulting in refractory hypoxemia and cyanosis.

Treatment of infants with congenital diaphragmatic hernia involves the measures used in initial resuscitation of the newborn, ventilatory support, and surgical repair of the lesion. More aggressive support includes the use of extracorporeal membrane oxygenation (ECMO).

Not long ago, it was believed that immediate surgical repair of acutely symptomatic congenital diaphragmatic hernias would permit expansion of the lungs and improve ventilation. However, rather than improving pulmonary mechanics, Sakai and coworkers (1987) found that early repair frequently decreases lung compliance. They attribute this deterioration to postoperative distortion of the diaphragm and chest wall and abdominal distension. Additional clinical data now support a strategy of delaying surgical repair of the defect until the infant's cardiovascular status is more stable (Breaux et al., 1991; Langer et al., 1988; Shanbhogue et al., 1990). Cardiovascular stability is attained by correcting the acidosis, hypoxia, and hypotension that are often present in these critically ill infants. Preoperative stabilization may improve the infant's ability to tolerate surgery.

Often, infants with congenital diaphragmatic hernia are diagnosed prenatally by ultrasound technique, and maternal transport and delivery can be planned at a center equipped to manage the critically ill newborn. Because bag and mask ventilation may force air into the gastrointestinal tract and further compromise ventilation, endotracheal intubation is performed immediately after birth (Kent & Curley, 1992). Achieving adequate oxygenation (postductal PaO_2 greater than 100 mmHg) and purposefully producing a metabolic alkalosis may help reduce pulmonary vascular resistance. A metabolic alkalosis can be induced with an infusion of sodium bicarbonate or tromethamine (THAM). This approach may be preferable to aggressive hyperventilation, which poses the risk of barotrauma and pulmonary air leaks (Schreiber et al., 1986). Frequently, sedation and, as a last resort, neuromuscular blockade are necessary to achieve adequate ventilation. For a more thorough discussion of pulmonary hypertension see Persistent Pulmonary Hypertension of the Newborn (PPHN).

Umbilical arterial and venous access is immediately established to permit monitoring of arterial blood gases and pH and blood pressure and permit the administration of fluids and medications. Hemodynamic support may include crystalloids, transfusions, and/or inotropic agents as needed to maintain adequate peripheral perfusion.

Once the infant's condition has stabilized, the hernia is surgically reduced. A primary repair is attempted, but if this proves impossible, a prosthetic patch is used to close the defect.

In many centers, if maximal medical measures fail to support ventilation, the infant is placed on ECMO. ECMO serves as a modified heart-lung machine and consists of a servo-regulating blood pump, a membrane lung to exchange O_2 and CO_2, and a heat exchanger to maintain temperature (Ortiz et al., 1988). The defect is repaired after several days of stabilization. If necessary, surgery can be performed with the neonate on ECMO (Troug et al., 1990).

In large part, nursing care for the infant with a congenital diaphragmatic hernia focuses on avoiding conditions that increase pulmonary vascular resistance and is discussed within the context of PPHN.

Weaning mechanical ventilation in the infant with a congenital diaphragmatic hernia presents many of the challenges encountered in infants with bronchopulmonary dysplasia and is discussed more thoroughly later. Reductions in ventilatory support occur slowly, but steadily, while the infant's cardiopulmonary status is closely monitored (Kent & Curley, 1992).

Conditions that may increase pulmonary vascular resistance are prevented, including hypoxemia, hypothermia, and hypoglycemia. For the same reason, environmental stressors such as noise, excessive light, and invasive procedures are also minimized.

The infant's hydration and nutritional status are carefully monitored by evaluating the infant's intake and output, urine specific gravity, liver size, skin turgor, weight, and growth curve. A positive fluid balance may result in worsening respiratory status, which may improve with judicious use of diuretics.

Nutritional adequacy promotes healing and growth and decreases the risk of infection, which may prolong the need for ventilatory support (Kent & Curley, 1992).

The infant born with a diaphragmatic hernia typically has a lengthy hospital course that may include extremely intimidating, highly technical interventions. Parents, who may have begun anticipatory grieving at the time of an antenatal diagnosis, require considerable support and are encouraged to verbalize their questions and concerns. The nurse at the bedside can intervene to help parents cope with the sometimes frightening PICU environment and permit them to connect with their critically ill child.

Mixed Obstructive and Restrictive Disease

For the purpose of more clearly understanding mechanical alterations in pulmonary function, various illnesses are classified by their effect on airway resistance (obstructive disease) or pulmonary compliance (restrictive disease). However, characteristic abnormalities in bronchopulmonary dysplasia include both increased airway resistance (Kao et al., 1984; Kao et al., 1984; Loeber et al., 1980) and decreased compliance (Loeber et al., 1980; Wilkie & Bryan, 1987). Therefore, bronchopulmonary dysplasia is truly a "mixed" disorder, that is, both obstructive and restrictive in nature.

Bronchopulmonary Dysplasia. Bronchopulmonary dysplasia (BPD), a term originally coined by Northway and colleagues (1967), represents a form of unresolved lung injury of infancy. Clinically defined as oxygen dependency at 1 month postnatal age, BPD most commonly follows severe hyaline membrane disease, but may also occur after meconium aspiration, pulmonary hemorrhage, congestive heart failure, or severe neonatal pneumonia. Although disagreement exists regarding its primary cause, factors contributing to the development of BPD may include O_2 toxicity, positive pressure ventilation and resultant mechanical lung injury, chronic inflammation, and overhydration. Although not limited to the preterm infant, BPD is most frequently associated with prematurity and occurs in up to 40% of mechanically ventilated infants weighing less than 1500 g at birth (HiFi Study Group, 1990).

As stated earlier, infants with BPD have both increased airway resistance and decreased compliance. These changes in pulmonary mechanics are most likely the result of inflammation, atelectasis, overdistension, infiltration, increased mucus secretion, and fibrosis, all of which are known to occur in BPD (Bancalari & Gerhardt, 1986; Lee & O'Brodovich, 1988). Although minute ventilation can be increased by breathing rapidly, this respiratory pattern has the disadvantage of increasing dead space ventilation (Bancalari & Gerhardt, 1986). These disturbances in pulmonary function, along with an abnormal distribution of ventilation and perfusion ($\dot{V}/\dot{Q}$ mismatch), lead to characteristic hypoxemia and hypercarbia.

The mortality rate for infants who develop severe BPD is at least 25% in the first year of life (Bland & Tooley, 1987). Recovery in survivors is slow and hospital readmission common, usually because of recurrent respiratory tract infections or the development of significant reactive airway disease (Gibson et al., 1988).

As previously described, an infant with BPD typically breathes rapidly and shallowly. Increased work of breathing is evidenced by intercostal and substernal retractions. Eventually, respiratory muscle fatigue may lead to episodes of apnea and bradycardia. Crackles and bronchial sounds (sometimes associated with wheezing and decreased air entry when bronchospasm predominates) may be heard on auscultation. Both on physical examination and radiographically, the infant's chest is hyperinflated. Atelectasis also frequently occurs because of inadequate clearing of secretions and airway obstruction (Bancalari & Gerhardt, 1986). With prolonged respiratory failure, pulmonary hypertension develops, with signs of right-sided heart failure including cardiomegaly, hepatomegaly, and fluid retention (Bancalari & Gerhardt, 1986). Blood gas abnormalities include marked hypoxemia and hypercarbia.

Management of BPD includes ensuring adequate oxygenation, optimizing ventilation, and maximizing the infant's nutritional intake. Oxygen, although perhaps initially contributing to the development of BPD, is the most important medication for the infant with significant disease. Supplemental O_2 to maintain O_2 saturations of 92% to 97% ensures adequate tissue oxygenation and prevents the pulmonary hypertension and cor pulmonale that can result from chronic hypoxemia (Goodman et al., 1988). Improved growth has also been demonstrated in infants with BPD treated with oxygen during recovery (Groothuis & Rosenberg, 1987). However, because exposure to high concentrations of oxygen may contribute to lung microvascular and cellular injury, hyperoxia is avoided.

Oxygen therapy, however, is not enough; O_2 delivery to the tissues is also optimized. A hemoglobin of 12 to 15 g/dL maximizes O_2-carrying capacity, and blood transfusions may be necessary to maintain this level. In addition, factors that impair the release of O_2 to the tissues by negatively effecting oxyhemoglobin dissociation, that is, hypothermia and metabolic or respiratory alkalosis, are corrected or avoided. Persistent CO_2 retention results in a compensatory rise in serum bicarbonate concentration that may be further exaggerated by the use of diuretics; this requires close monitoring of serum electrolytes.

The infant with BPD has bronchiolar smooth muscle hypertrophy and hyperreactive airways (Smyth et al., 1981). Therefore, bronchospasm, a condition in which constriction of smooth muscle in the distal airway restricts airflow in and out of the alveoli, commonly occurs in these infants, especially during acute respiratory infections. Bronchodilators may be useful in these circumstances. Theophylline may also increase diaphragmatic strength and diuresis in in-

fants with BPD (Frank, 1987). Aerosolized beta-agonists (for example, metaproterenol, terbutaline, or albuteral) are also frequently used in the treatment of bronchospasm in BPD (Brudno et al., 1989; Gomez-Del-Rio et al., 1986; Kao et al., 1984; Motoyama et al., 1987). (See Asthma for more detailed information regarding the treatment of reactive airways.) In addition, diuretics may relieve airway obstruction and improve compliance, probably because of a reduction in interstitial pulmonary edema (Kao et al., 1984).

Because the infant with BPD is typically very slow to wean from ventilatory assistance, management of mechanical ventilation becomes a central issue. Attempts to rapidly reduce mechanical ventilation often meet with acute decompensation 24 to 48 hours later when the infant tires and $PaCO_2$ climbs. Therefore, it is important to move slowly and allow adequate time for the infant to adjust to decreased ventilator settings. In the infant with BPD, tachypnea and a $PaCO_2$ of 45 to 60 mmHg (or higher with a normal pH) may be "normal." Readiness for weaning from mechanical ventilation may best be demonstrated by a *persistent reduction in the infant's baseline spontaneous respiratory rate* and $PaCO_2$, accompanied by a sustained weight gain (Morray et al., 1981).

When the need for prolonged assisted ventilation is anticipated, a tracheostomy may be considered. A tracheostomy decreases anatomic dead space and permits care to be delivered outside of a critical care setting (at home in some instances), and may prevent the development of subglottic stenosis (Spitzer, 1995). However, decannulation may not be accomplished for 12 to 24 months even after assisted ventilation is no longer needed.

In the face of increased work of breathing, caloric intake as high as 170 to 200 Kcal/kg/day may be required for growth in BPD (Spitzer, 1995). Nutritional needs are difficult to meet in these infants, not only because of increased calorie demands, but also because of poor feeding tolerance and the need for fluid restriction. Therefore, nasogastric, nasojejunum, or gastrostomy tube feeding using concentrated formulas and diuretic therapy to prevent fluid overload are often necessary.

Nursing responsibilities in the care of infants with BPD include ensuring adequate oxygenation and ventilation, monitoring the efficacy of various interventions, and promoting growth and development. The infant with a tracheostomy presents additional challenges.

A thorough initial cardiopulmonary assessment and continued vigilant observation is essential to detect subtle clinical changes and permit early intervention when possible. Respiratory rate and effort (retractions, nasal flaring), heart rate, blood pressure, liver size, and fluid status (intake and output, urine specific gravity, and weight) are monitored carefully. The infant's baseline O_2 saturation (in room air and in supplemental O_2) is established and monitored continuously, preferably with a pulse oximeter.

To appropriately adjust FiO_2 and treatment regimens, it is especially important to follow SpO_2 during periods of stress (such as feeding), and while administering various treatments. Wheezing or bronchospastic episodes, so-called BPD spells, are treated promptly. Document the frequency and precipitating events when spells occur and assess the need for additional O_2, ventilatory support, and/or bronchodilators and the effect of each. That airway obstruction in BPD is, in part, reversible with bronchodilators, provides an opportunity for early intervention during the course of the disease and may possibly reduce its progression (Bancalari & Gerhardt, 1986).

Minimizing agitation, and the hypoxemia and bronchospasm that often accompany it, is a primary goal. The infant's individual temperament and sensitivities direct nursing measures to reduce stress. These measures may include controlling environmental noise and light, providing therapeutic touch, permitting non-nutritive sucking, and positioning for comfort. At times, sedation may also be required; however, sedation should be administered only after determining that agitation is not the result of inadequate ventilatory support or airway obstruction. Necessary procedures are spaced throughout the day to permit time for recovery, and unnecessary interventions are avoided. For example, clinical assessment and auscultation of breath sounds, not time alone, guide the frequency of chest physiotherapy and suctioning.

The nurse at the bedside may be in the best position to assess the infant's response to reductions in ventilatory support. Once readiness is established, weaning occurs slowly, but on a regular schedule; this is true during the infant's nursery course, and is also frequently necessary when mechanical ventilation is required for respiratory insufficiency later in life. Documenting the infant's respiratory rate and effort, response to activity, $ETCO_2$, and SpO_2 after ventilator changes permits objective evaluation of how well weaning is tolerated.

Infants with BPD are at high risk for growth failure into at least their second year (Meisels et al., 1986) and, ironically, growth is the key to recovery. Nutritional assessment includes trending weights, head circumference, and length (and plotting of the infant's growth against a normal curve). Complicating the task of providing sufficient caloric intake is the feeding intolerance frequently experienced in infants with BPD. Nasogastric feedings administered continuously or intermittently may be used, depending in part upon the infant's respiratory status. If gastric distension further compromises chest expansion, a continuous infusion is preferred. An intermittent feeding schedule and the use of a pacifier during feedings, however, may help stimulate gastric motility and reduce gastric residuals in some infants. Gastroesophageal reflux and aspiration may also occur and can be minimized by prone positioning with the head elevated to a 30- to 45-degree angle during and immediately after feedings. Infants with BPD are often described as disorganized feeders un-

able to coordinate suck, swallow, and breathing (Lund & Collier, 1990). In the chronically ill hospitalized infant, long-term use of tube feedings or parenteral nutrition can contribute to this behavior and may eventually lead to feeding resistance (Lund & Collier, 1990; Pridham et al., 1989). Helping parents assume the responsibility for feeding their infant and recognizing the social and emotional features of feeding, as well as the technical aspects, is an important part of discharge planning (Pridham et al., 1989).

Careful monitoring and early intervention are important in detecting and preventing developmental delay in the chronically ill infant. Parental involvement is important in establishing a routine for their infant and providing appropriate stimulation. Resources for ongoing care include child life, occupational, physical, and speech therapy.

Caring for the Infant With a Tracheostomy. These patients present additional nursing challenges including securing the artifical airway, maintaining airway patency and skin integrity, and supporting and educating the family.

Maintaining the position of the tracheostomy tube is especially important in the immediate postoperative period, because permanent cannulation does not occur for 4 to 5 days. Before that, a dislodged tube may not be easily reinserted. For this reason, the initial tracheostomy holder should be secure and not changed until the stoma is established. A protective barrier such as Duoderm (Convatec, Princeton, NJ) used beneath the ties on the infant's neck helps prevent skin breakdown.

Attention to skin integrity at and around the stoma is also important. Encrusted secretions or blood is removed with half-strength hydrogen peroxide solution. Applying a protective ointment, for example, Pericare (Sween Corp., North Mankato, MN) to the skin protects the area around the stoma from maceration. Alternatively, a protective skin barrier such as Comfeel (Coloplast, Inc; Denmark) or Duoderm can be cut in a U shape and applied beneath the tracheostomy tube to the edge of the stoma. These hydrocolloid dressings conform to the skin, absorb moisture, and provide both protection from skin maceration and padding to prevent pressure sores from the tracheostomy tube.

Maintaining the patency of a tracheostomy tube is similar to maintaining an endotracheal tube (see Maintaining the Artificial Airway). However, certain points should be emphasized. To avoid the development of granulomas or persistent right upper lobe atelectasis from trauma, measured suctioning technique is essential. Humidification of inspired gas is required in the dry hospital environment; adequate hydration is as important to keep secretions liquefied. Careful attention to handwashing and sterile technique helps prevent nosocomial infections that can cause significant morbidity in these small infants (Groothuis et al., 1988; Sawyer et al., 1987).

When an infant with BPD undergoes a tracheostomy, the chronicity of the illness can no longer be ignored. This may be a very difficult time for parents.

The nurse who has established a relationship with the family is in an ideal position to answer their questions and help parents cope with their feelings. Eventually, a tracheostomy may permit more parental participation in the care of their infant. When discharge to home is a possibility, parent education begins as soon as the infant's condition permits and the parents demonstrate a readiness to learn. Teaching should involve more than one caregiver in the family and be tailored to the learners' individual styles, abilities, and needs. It is important to teach not only specific procedures (for example, suctioning, skin care) and decision-making skills (for example, when to suction, when to call a healthcare provider), but also to respond to concerns about whether these responsibilities may upset family schedules and relationships (Kennelly, 1987). In addition, community resources are identified and mobilized to help meet the discharge needs of the infant/family.

Impairment of Respiratory Muscle Function

Another mechanical alteration affects the respiratory pump through impairment of respiratory muscle function. In this case, diminished respiratory muscle function results in respiratory failure despite normal lung mechanics. Guillain-Barré syndrome is one example of the numerous rare illnesses in which the chest wall and lungs are mechanically sound, but a failure of the respiratory muscles driving the pump leads to respiratory failure.

Guillain-Barré Syndrome. Guillain-Barré syndrome is an acute inflammatory disorder of the peripheral nerves and nerve roots characterized by progressive paresis, paralysis, paresthesia, and pain. Paralysis often involves the respiratory muscles. About 1 to 1.5 cases occur annually per 100,000 population. Although Guillain-Barré syndrome affects all ages (the youngest reported case is a 4-month-old infant [Carroll et al., 1977]), children appear to recover more quickly than adults.

The precise etiology of Guillain-Barré syndrome is unknown, but the demyelinative lesions seen throughout the peripheral nervous system are most likely the result of both cell-mediated and humoral factors (antibodies) (Koski et al., 1986; Prineas, 1981).

Criteria necessary to establish the diagnosis of Guillain-Barré are well established and are summarized in Table 20–4. Typically, symptoms occur within 4 weeks of some infectious process. The antecedent illness is often nonspecific, such as a mild respiratory infection or diarrhea. Symmetric weakness usually begins in the lower extremities, although it can rapidly ascend to the upper extremities, the trunk, and even the muscles innervated by the cranial nerves. Autonomic dysfunction also occurs frequently in children with Guillain-Barré syndrome, involving the sympathetic and parasympathetic systems. Signs and symptoms of autonomic neuropathy include orthostatic hypotension, hypertension, pupillary dis-

Table 20–4. CRITERIA FOR DIAGNOSIS OF GUILLAIN-BARRÉ SYNDROME

Features required for diagnosis	Progressive motor weakness of more than one limb
	Areflexia or marked hyporeflexia
Features strongly supportive of the diagnosis	Rapidly developing motor weakness, but no progression by 4 weeks into illness
	Mild sensory signs or symptoms
	Cranial nerve involvement
	Onset of recovery 2–4 weeks after halt of progression
	Autonomic dysfunction
	Initial absence of fever

Data from: Asbury, A.K., Arnason, B.G., Karp, H.R., & McFarlin, D.E. (1978). Criteria for diagnosis of Guillain-Barré syndrome. *Annals of Neurology, 3,* 565–567.

turbances, diaphoresis, cardiac dysrhythmias, constipation, and urinary retention.

Respiratory muscle involvement is seen in about half of the pediatric patients, and approximately 7% to 15% of those require mechanical ventilation (Ouvrier et al., 1990). When respiratory muscle weakness occurs, the child breathes shallowly and is unable to sigh. FRC is reduced, which leads to atelectasis, hypoxemia, and eventually CO_2 retention. Pooling of secretions with an absent or ineffective cough further contributes to alveolar collapse and respiratory compromise. Airway obstruction results from involvement of the pharyngeal muscles, leading to airway collapse during inspiration, passive posterior displacement of the tongue, or an inability to swallow oral secretions. Pharyngeal muscle function can be assessed by evaluating cranial nerves IX and X. When these nerves are involved, there is a decreased ability to swallow or cough, decreased voice volume, and a depressed gag reflex.

Supportive treatment is the mainstay of therapy. In the early stages of the illness, frequent careful assessments are necessary to detect impending respiratory failure, the most serious complication of muscle weakness. Respiratory function can be monitored in older children by measuring forced vital capacity (FVC). When FVC falls to 15mL/kg, intubation and mechanical ventilation are usually necessary. Although some children are not dyspneic at this level of ventilatory compromise, the risk of aspiration, atelectasis, and pneumonia is minimized by early intervention. Ventilatory support is also indicated whenever there is an increased risk of airway obstruction.

For older children with rapidly progressive disease, plasmapheresis is now the accepted therapy. Three controlled studies of patients over 12 years old have demonstrated that plasmapheresis decreases the severity and improves the outcome of patients with Guillain-Barré syndrome (French Cooperative Group, 1987; Guillain-Barré Study Group, 1985; Osterman et al., 1984). In addition, Epstein and Sladky (1989) retrospectively analyzed data from nine children treated with plasmapheresis, comparing them with

14 similarly affected historical controls. The time to achieve independent ambulation was significantly shorter in the treated patients and there were no significant complications from plasmapheresis. Therefore, plasmapheresis is generally recommended for children with severe and worsening disease (Shahar et al., 1990). The recommended protocol is an exchange of 200 to 250 mL of plasma per kg body weight over 7 to 14 days (Guillain-Barré Syndrome Study Group, 1985; McKann et al., 1988). Why plasmapheresis is helpful is not well known. It may be that antibodies, such as anti–peripheral-nerve antibody or other myelinotoxic or immunopathogenic factors are removed by pheresis.

The use of intravenous immunoglobulins is being explored as an alternative to plasmapheresis. Shahar and coworkers (1990) report rapid improvement in muscle strength in three children treated with intravenous immune serum globulin, but further studies are necessary to determine its efficacy.

When there is evidence of progressive disease and significant muscle weakness, the child is moved to the PICU, where frequent monitoring of respiratory status is possible. This is especially true for younger children in whom objective assessment of respiratory function is difficult (Ouvrier et al., 1990). Respiratory assessments include respiratory rate, pattern, and effort, as well as the quality of air entry on auscultation. Oxygen saturations are monitored continuously by pulse oximeter. In a cooperative child, serial measurements of FVC are obtained at least every 4 hours while muscle weakness is progressing. Arterial blood gases also document progression toward respiratory failure with an increase in $PaCO_2$ and acidosis. Swallowing ability is also evaluated, as well as the strength of the child's cough and voice. The child's gag reflex is tested periodically.

Estimates of peripheral muscle strength are valuable in tracking the course of the illness to determine whether muscle weakness is worsening, has reached a plateau, or strength is returning.

Because autonomic dysfunction is possible, cardiac monitoring is initiated and blood pressure carefully documented. Additional signs of excessive or inadequate activity of the parasympathetic or sympathetic systems are noted and treated as necessary (for example, placement of a drainage catheter in the case of urinary retention). Hypotension may be especially problematic during plasmapheresis, but is generally responsive to intravascular volume expansion.

Pain and paresthesias are also frequently present. A deep aching muscle pain is most often described, commonly in the back and lower extremities and correlating with the distribution of motor loss (Ouvrier et al., 1990). Lower back pain because of irritation of the nerve roots may be relieved with the careful application of heat, although more severe pain requires the use of analgesics. Successful pain control in adult patients with Guillain-Barré includes the use of epidural morphine (Connelly et al., 1990; Rosenfield et al., 1986).

Because both sensory and motor losses occur, it is important to turn and reposition the child at least every 2 hours. Therapeutic pressure-reducing devices may aid in maintaining skin integrity, but they do not eliminate the need for a routine turning schedule. Passive range of motion is also performed to prevent contractures.

Nutritional adequacy is established early in the course of the illness to avoid excessive muscle wasting. Weakness and dysphagia may necessitate the use of nasogastric feedings and parenteral nutrition.

Especially during the sometimes frightening progression of paralysis, it is important to reassure patients and their families that a near complete, if not full, recovery is expected.

Circulatory Alterations

The pulmonary circulation establishes the interface between inspired gas and the blood, thereby permitting delivery of O_2 to the blood and removal of CO_2. The second final common pathway of respiratory failure involves alterations in this circulation. Circulatory alterations disturb the normal contact between blood and gas within the lungs. Pulmonary embolism and PPHN are characteristic examples. In these conditions, pulmonary circulation is reduced, physiologic dead space increases, and gas exchange may be impaired.

Pulmonary Embolism

Pulmonary embolism occurs when materials traveling in the bloodstream become impacted in the pulmonary arterial bed. Although uncommon in childhood, pulmonary embolism may occur after trauma or surgery, and may complicate a number of illnesses and treatments. Thromboembolism is the most frequently occurring form of pulmonary embolism and appears when a blood clot travels from a peripheral vessel through the right side of the heart and lodges in the pulmonary arterial bed. Pulmonary thromboembolism may complicate sickle cell anemia, rheumatic fever, and bacterial endocarditis, or may occur with sepsis or severe dehydration. Thrombosis of the superior vena cava and right atrium resulting from a central venous catheter, or ventriculovenous shunt (Favara & Paul, 1967), may also serve as a source of thromboemboli in children. Fat and air emboli can occur after trauma or surgery. Air embolism may also be an iatrogenic complication in the care of critically ill children (Wetzel, 1987).

The child with a pulmonary embolism is dyspneic, tachypneic, and may complain of acute chest pain. Breath sounds may be clear or there may be scattered crackles. Radiographic findings are nonspecific and may include atelectasis, localized infiltrates, or a pleural effusion. Fever is also frequently present without other signs of infection.

Hypoxemia is common in acute pulmonary embolism. Regional bronchoconstriction and atelectasis result in $\dot{V}/\dot{Q}$ inequality and intrapulmonary shunting.

Because the right ventricle has poor tolerance for an increase in afterload, cardiac output may become inadequate, and mixed venous saturations fall. If pulmonary hypertension develops and there is a patent foramen ovale (or septal defect), right-to-left shunting within the heart also contributes to hypoxemia.

The child's increased respiratory rate usually compensates for the increase in physiologic dead space produced by the arterial occlusion. The $PaCO_2$ typically falls below 35 mmHg. However, $PaCO_2$ rises in children who cannot adequately increase their minute ventilation (for example, those with restrictive lung disease, neuromuscular disorders, or those receiving chemical paralyzing agents).

Treatment consists of O_2, hemodynamic support, anticoagulation, and thrombolytic therapy. Once the diagnosis is established, heparin therapy is initiated to prevent further thrombosis. A loading dose of 50 units/kg is followed by a continuous infusion of 10 to 25 units/kg/hour, and adjusted according to the child's activated partial thromboplastin time (aPTT). A clotting time of 1.5 to 2.0 times the normal mean aPTT value (usually 50 to 70 seconds) is therapeutic. Because heparin does not dissolve the clot, a thrombolytic agent such as streptokinase may also be used, although its efficacy in pulmonary embolism is questionable.

Nursing priorities in caring for the child with a pulmonary embolism include maintaining supplemental O_2 (and ventilatory support, if it becomes necessary), evaluating the child's cardiopulmonary status, and assessing the effects of therapy.

Continuous monitoring of O_2 saturation by pulse oximeter helps ensure adequate oxygenation. The adequacy of ventilation can be determined by evaluating the child's respiratory rate and effort and periodically measuring arterial blood gases. In addition, cardiovascular assessment including heart rate, blood pressure, strength of peripheral pulses, warmth of extremities, and adequacy of urine output helps determine the need for inotropic support or volume expansion.

Because hemorrhage is the major toxicity of heparin (an untoward effect that may be compounded by thrombolytics), it is especially important to carefully monitor coagulation studies. Initially, aPTT values are measured and the infusion rate adjusted frequently. Daily monitoring is sufficient when a steady dose is achieved. The child is also monitored for signs of bleeding including petechiae; bloody emesis, stools, or gastric aspirates; hemoptysis; and hematuria. Invasive procedures are avoided or minimized.

Persistent Pulmonary Hypertension of the Newborn

Persistent pulmonary hypertension of the newborn (PPHN) is a condition in which the high-resistance, low-flow pulmonary circulation of fetal life persists after birth. It is characterized by systemic or suprasystemic pulmonary artery pressures, with signifi-cant right-to-left shunting through the ductus arteriosus or foramen ovale. Desaturated venous blood is mixed with saturated arterial blood, resulting in arterial hypoxemia and tissue hypoxia. The etiology of PPHN is unknown. It has been suggested that PPHN results from an abnormal increase in the amount of smooth muscle in the wall of the peripheral pulmonary arteries (Murphy et al., 1981; Murphy et al., 1984). Alternatively, an accumulation of pulmonary vasoconstrictor substances in the blood perfusing the lung could be responsible (Hammerman et al., 1987). Whatever the underlying pathology, PPHN has been associated with a variety of pulmonary diseases (most commonly, meconium aspiration), congenital or acquired cardiovascular diseases, and a number of generalized disorders such as asphyxia, sepsis, and shock.

It is possible that PPHN is a process that starts well before birth, therefore birth history may be helpful in identifying those at greatest risk for developing PPHN. Typically, the infant born is born at term or postterm, is appropriate in size for gestational age, and had meconium staining or birth asphyxia at the time of delivery. In many cases, there are identifiable prenatal or perinatal risk factors such as increased maternal age, preeclampsia, abnormal presentation, cesarean section, or a precipitous delivery (Tiefenbrunn & Riemenschneider, 1986). Although the incidence of PPHN is fairly rare, approximately 1 in 1500 live births (Goetzman & Reimenschneider, 1980), it remains an important cause of neonatal death in term infants (Eden et al., 1987).

Typically, the infant with PPHN develops tachypnea and cyanosis soon after birth. Other signs of respiratory distress also appear including grunting, nasal flaring, and intercostal retractions. The quality of breath sounds depends upon the underlying clinical condition; adventitious sounds are prominent in meconium aspiration, for example, but may be absent in neonatal asphyxia. Neonates with PPHN also demonstrate a wide spectrum of myocardial abnormalities, ranging from mild dysfunction to severe biventricular congestive failure. On physical examination, the infant may have normal or diminished peripheral pulses and systemic blood pressure, a right ventricular heave, and often a single or narrowly split second heart sound (Tiefenbrunn & Riemenschneider, 1986). A systolic murmur may also be heard. Those with serious myocardial dysfunction show signs of congestive heart failure.

Right-to-left shunting through the ductus arteriosus and foramen ovale results in hypoxemia, which often proves refractory to supplemental O_2. Shunting can be demonstrated by simultaneous SpO_2 monitoring from probes placed on the infant's right hand and lower extremities. Preductal SpO_2 5% or more higher than postductal SpO_2 indicates clinically significant right-to-left shunting (Phillips et al., 1988). In severe PPHN, hypoxemia is followed rapidly by the development of hypercarbia and acidosis. Hypoxia and acidosis perpetuates the vicious cycle of pulmonary vasoconstriction, pulmonary artery hypertension,

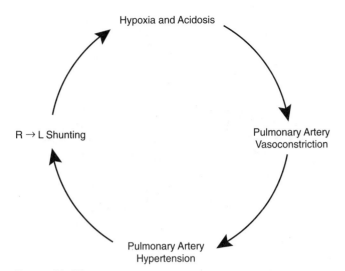

Figure 20–17 ● ● ● ● ● ●
PPHN. A vicious cycle.

and right-to-left intrapulmonary and intracardiac shunting (Fig. 20–17).

Treatment in PPHN is aimed at decreasing the ratio of pulmonary to systemic vascular resistance, thereby reducing or eliminating right-to-left shunting. Historically, this has been accomplished by hyperoxygenation, hyperventilation, and the use of nonspecific vasodilators such as tolazoline. However, mortality in infants with PPHN remained high, perhaps in part because of the complications of such aggressive therapy, that is, pneumothorax, pneumomediastinum, barotrauma, and chronic lung disease. Various therapies currently in use include oxygenation, alkalinization, high frequency ventilation, nitric oxide, and extracorporeal membrane oxygenation.

Hypoxemia causes reflex pulmonary vasoconstriction in fetal sheep and adult dogs, and may well contribute to the pathophysiology of PPHN. Therefore, in an attempt to reverse pulmonary hypertension, infants with PPHN usually receive high levels of supplemental O_2, the most potent pulmonary vasodilator available.

Through mechanisms that are unclear, an increase in pH also decreases pulmonary vascular resistance. By increasing arterial pH to a "critical level" at which there is a fall in pulmonary artery pressures, a reversal of right-to-left shunting and an increase in PaO_2 appear to be achieved in many cases. The degree of respiratory alkalosis necessary to reverse right-to-left shunting sometimes cannot be achieved with mechanical hyperventilation because of severe lung disease or the development of a metabolic acidosis. There is evidence to suggest, however, that respiratory alkalosis and metabolic alkalosis are equally effective in attenuating hypoxia-induced pulmonary vasoconstriction (Schreiber et al., 1986). Therefore, an infusion of sodium bicarbonate may produce the desired degree of alkalosis while avoiding the complications of aggressive mechanical hyperventilation. Generally, an infusion of sodium bicarbonate is begun

and adjusted to maintain a pH of 7.45 to 7.50. Alternatively, THAM may be used if CO_2 retention is a problem. A more conservative approach to mechanical ventilation can then be pursued. To prevent the complications of mechanical ventilation, the lowest PIP possible is used to achieve the therapeutic goals.

Wung et al (1985) first described a more conservative "kinder, gentler" approach to ventilation aimed at minimizing barotrauma while maintaining PaO_2 between 50 and 70 mmHg and permitting $PaCO_2$ to increase as high as 60 mmHg.

Because hypoxemia may put the infant with PPHN at risk for cerebral hypoxia, monitoring the infant's neurologic status is important. In a study of 19 infants with PPHN (the majority of whom had birth asphyxia), nine suffered cerebral infarctions (Klesh et al., 1987). Furthermore, eight of the nine infants with infarction had seizures detected by electroencephalogram (EEG) during periods of neuromuscular blockade. Routine EEGs may be warranted in these patients.

High-frequency ventilation is an alternative approach used in some centers, primarily as a rescue treatment when conventional therapy fails. In high-frequency ventilation, extremely small tidal volumes and high rates are used to provide gas exchange.

Nitric oxide (NO), a common environmental pollutant, has been identified as an important endothelial-derived relaxing factor (Frostell et al., 1991). Within 3 minutes of inhalation, NO selectively dilates the pulmonary vasculature, reversing hypoxia-induced pulmonary hypertension. Because NO is rapidly inactivated when combined with heme in hemoglobin, systemic effects are nonexistent. Researchers in a limited number of centers are investigating the affect of NO on pulmonary vascular resistance (Roberts, 1993; Pearl, 1993; Craig & Mullins, 1995).

Extracorporeal membrane oxygenation (ECMO) has been used to support patients with PPHN in whom conventional medical management has failed. In these cases, ECMO is a temporary rescue technique that permits correction of hypoxemia and acidosis, and a reduction of toxic levels of O_2 and high positive-pressure ventilation (McDermott & Curley, 1990).

The nursing care of the infant with PPHN is directed toward avoiding conditions that increase pulmonary vascular resistance, early detection of the complications of therapy, and whenever possible, minimizing those complications.

As stated earlier, hypoxemia results in increased pulmonary vascular resistance. In an infant in an unstable condition with PPHN, even small reductions in FiO_2 can lead to profound hypoxemia. Therefore, consistent delivery of O_2 must be assured. In the acutely ill infant during the first 24 hours, or in infants exhibiting wide fluctuations in oxygenation, attempts are made to maintain PaO_2 at approximately 100 mmHg. Furthermore, maneuvers that cause hypoxemia, for example, endotracheal suctioning, are avoided unless absolutely necessary. It is not uncommon for these infants to be exquisitely sensitive to any type of tactile stimulation, responding with precipitous drops in SpO$_2$ (Beachy & Powers, 1984). Prohibiting unnecessary handling will help limit episodes of hypoxemia, therefore routine care (for example, bathing or weighing the infant) is inappropriate. Finally, sedation is used to minimize agitation and its negative effect on pulmonary vascular resistance.

Cold stress, hypoglycemia, and hypoxemia may all result in acidosis that will increase pulmonary vascular resistance. These conditions are avoided by carefully controlling and monitoring the infant's environment and response to therapy. Because ready access to the critically ill infant is necessary, providing a neutral thermal environment is often not possible. Heat loss can be minimized, however, with a radiant warmer. Frequent bedside monitoring of blood glucose is also performed. Oxygen saturation or transcutaneous PaO$_2$ is monitored continuously and blood gases followed to monitor acid-base status, especially when alkalosis is being employed to reduce pulmonary vascular resistance.

Careful assessments of oxygenation and systemic perfusion accompany changes in ventilator settings. In the neonate, a tension pneumothorax may present as sudden hypotension, bradycardia, and hypoxemia, and requires immediate needle aspiration and eventual placement of a chest tube. In addition, excessive PEEP may cause an increase in pulmonary vascular resistance. This may increase right-to-left shunting and decrease pulmonary venous return and further reduce systemic flow of oxygenated blood.

Systemic blood pressure must be higher than pulmonary artery pressure to reverse right-to-left shunting; therefore, maintenance of adequate systemic blood pressure is essential to correct hypoxemia in PPHN. Intravascular volume is assessed frequently by monitoring heart rate, blood pressure, liver size, capillary refill time, and warmth of extremities. Hydration status can be further evaluated by assessing fluid intake and urine output, urine specific gravity, skin turgor, mucous membranes, and fontanelles. As stated earlier, infants with PPHN may have a variable degree of myocardial dysfunction, therefore myocardial depressants such as hypoglycemia, acidosis, and hypocalcemia are avoided. In addition, dopamine may be given to improve cardiac contractility.

The infant undergoing high-frequency jet ventilation presents additional nursing challenges. These are usually the most critically ill infants in whom conventional mechanical ventilation appears to be failing, or whose course has been complicated by pulmonary interstitial emphysema, pneumothorax, or pneumomediastinum. When high-frequency jet ventilation is begun, nursing vigilance becomes even more essential. The logistics of high-frequency jet ventilation will be briefly discussed with a focus on nursing implications.

To begin high-frequency jet ventilation, the endotracheal tube (ETT) must be replaced with a triple-lumen ETT (Fig. 20–18). The main port of the ETT

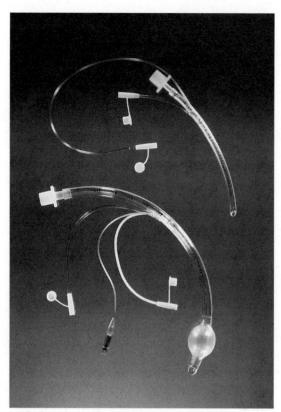

Figure 20–18 ● ● ● ● ● ●

Jet endotracheal tubes. The three lumens include (1) a main port that attaches to the conventional ventilator; (2) a jet port, which enters at the middle of the ETT; (3) a pressure sensing port, which opens at the tip of the ETT; and in larger ETTs (4) a balloon port. (Courtesy of Mallinckrodt Medical, Inc., St. Louis, MO.)

is usually connected to a conventional ventilator and is used to deliver PEEP. To prevent atelectasis because of the small tidal volumes used in high-frequency jet ventilation, low-rate (5 to 10 breaths per minute) positive pressure ventilation can also be delivered through this main port. The remaining two ports are the pressure-monitoring port, located near the tip of the ETT, and the jet-delivery port, located approximately 7 cm above the monitoring port.

The initial PIP used in high-frequency jet ventilation is based on the infant's requirements while on conventional mechanical ventilation. Ordinarily, PIP is set 20% to 33% below the pressure required during conventional treatment (White et al., 1990). Some infants with severe pulmonary hypertension, however, may have acute deterioration when high-frequency jet ventilation is initiated at lower inflating pressures. Therefore, some clinicians suggest that PIP not be lowered initially in infants with PPHN, but should be gradually decreased as determined by the infant's response to therapy (SpO$_2$ and arterial blood gases) (Spitzer et al., 1988). Ventilatory frequency can be adjusted to deliver 300 to 540 cycles per minute (6 to 9 Hz), and is usually started at a rate of 420 cycles per minute (7 Hz).

The infant receiving high-frequency jet ventilation requires continuous monitoring of heart rate, blood pressure, and transcutaneous O_2 and CO_2. Although vibration of the chest and body make monitoring of the infant's respiratory rate impractical, absence of vibration may signal tube obstruction or displacement, or a decrease in lung compliance, for example, with a tension pneumothorax (White et al., 1990). Breath sounds are also altered by the ventilator, but subtle changes can be detected with frequent, careful examination.

As with any artificial airway, maintaining airway patency is a primary nursing responsibility. It is possible to suction the endotracheal tube through its main port while maintaining high-frequency jet ventilation. However, some clinicians suggest that this practice may create shearing forces in the trachea (produced by the combination of negative pressure suction and high-frequency positive pressure breaths), which may contribute to the development of necrotizing tracheobronchitis (Spitzer et al., 1988). This particular complication, a severe airway injury that results in sloughing of the tracheal mucosa, is reported with varying frequency and may result from inadequate humidification of inspired gases, shearing forces in the airway, or other factors that have yet to be identified.

Alterations in the Control of Breathing

The last final common pathway of respiratory failure includes disorders resulting from abnormalities or deficiencies in the control of breathing, resulting in hypoventilation. This category includes alterations in the neuromuscular control of upper airway patency and abnormalities in respiratory drive that result in alveolar hypoventilation. Apnea, both central and obstructive, and alveolar hypoventilation syndromes are considered.

Apnea

Apnea is generally defined as the cessation of breathing for more than 20 seconds or for a shorter period when associated with hypoxemia or bradycardia. In recent years, the development of pulse oximetry has altered our perception of what is abnormal by greatly enhancing our ability to detect subtle changes in oxygenation associated with apnea. Central apnea is characterized by a respiratory pause. In contrast, respiratory efforts continue, sometimes quite vigorously, in obstructive apnea, but there is an absence of airway flow caused by airway obstruction. A mixed picture of central and obstructive apnea may also be observed.

Apnea of prematurity is most commonly central in origin, but obstructive apnea and mixed disorders also occur (Roberts et al., 1982). Although the cause is unknown, apnea of prematurity is thought to be related not only to an immaturity of the central nervous system, but also to an increase in chest wall compliance. More respiratory work is required to generate a constant tidal volume when the chest wall is highly compliant. Within this context, apnea may represent a strategy to avoid fatigue.

Although central apnea is the classic apnea of prematurity, it occurs in a number of other conditions in which the central nervous system is somehow altered. Sepsis, hypoglycemia, hypothermia, drug intoxication, trauma, and brain tumors may result in apnea. In addition, because their ventilatory response to hypoxia and sensitivity to CO_2 are already depressed, young infants may be especially vulnerable to periods of apnea when they receive narcotics and other respiratory depressants.

In obstructive apnea, upper airway collapse occurs because of poor coordination of the muscles responsible for airway maintenance. Obstructive apnea usually happens during sleep and, in children, it is most often caused by hypertrophy of the tonsils and adenoids. Although sleep is the most common functional condition predisposing to obstructive apnea, other factors that may depress airway-maintaining activity include narcotics, sedatives, alcohol, and some brainstem lesions, particularly those associated with Arnold-Chiari malformation.

Central apnea is evidenced by a cessation of respiratory activity and may be accompanied by a fall in O_2 saturation and heart rate. In the preterm infant, respiratory pauses occur more commonly in active sleep and often within the context of periodic breathing. Frequently, these infants also have an obstructive component to their apnea (Roberts et al., 1982).

Physical examination of the sleeping child with obstructive apnea reveals sonorous respirations, retractions, and breathing pauses that may be associated with hypoxemia and bradycardia. Often vigorous movement occurs during sleep in an attempt to overcome the airway obstruction. Brouillette and coworkers (1982) report serious sequelae including cor pulmonale, failure to thrive, permanent neurologic damage, and behavioral disturbances, hypersomnolence, or developmental delay in cases in which obstructive sleep apnea had gone untreated.

Although it is unclear what effect apneic periods may have on the preterm infant, frequent episodes accompanied by hypoxemia are usually treated because they may lead to additional neurologic complications. Nasal CPAP may help by preventing lung deflation and chest distortion. Pharmacologic approaches include the use of caffeine or theophylline to increase central respiratory drive and improve CO_2 sensitivity (Bairam et al., 1987). A loading dose of 20 mg/kg of caffeine citrate is administered orally or intravenously and followed by a maintenance dose of 5 mg/kg given once or twice a day. A serum caffeine level of 10 to 20 mg/L is considered therapeutic. Alternatively, a loading dose of 6 mg/kg of theophylline is followed by a dose of 2 mg/kg given two to three times a day to maintain a serum theophylline level of 8 to 12 mg/L.

Because adenotonsillar hypertrophy is the predominant anatomic cause of obstructive sleep apnea in childhood, tonsillectomy and adenoidectomy often provide the cure (Brouillette et al., 1982; Frank et al., 1983). Nasal CPAP may effectively relieve obstructive sleep apnea in preterm infants (Miller et al., 1985), but has rarely been used in children (Guilleminault, 1987). Tracheostomy is seldom required.

The primary nursing responsibilities in caring for the infant or child with apnea are early detection of the event and monitoring of the effects of treatment. All patients at risk for central or obstructive apnea have continuous cardiac and respiratory monitoring. Because thoracic impedance respiratory monitors may not detect obstructive apnea, O_2 saturation is monitored by pulse oximetry. Careful observation and documentation of apneic episodes is essential in establishing the etiology and guiding a treatment plan.

Alveolar Hypoventilation Syndromes

Alveolar hypoventilation syndromes are conditions in which there is no upper airway obstruction, but an insufficient respiratory drive results in hypoventilation. These respiratory control deficits, which originate within the central nervous system, may be congenital or acquired, and are characterized by progressive hypoxemia and hypercarbia during sleep, particularly quiet sleep.

The severity of hypopnea in congenital hypoventilation syndromes varies widely. The most severe form, central hypoventilation syndrome, is usually diagnosed soon after birth and may be associated with some degree of hypoventilation even during wakefulness.

Alveolar hypoventilation may also be acquired following a brainstem injury. Birth asphyxia can result in central hypoventilation syndrome (Brazy et al., 1987), as can encephalitis (Jensen et al., 1988), tumors, and brainstem trauma (Quera-Salva & Guilleminault, 1987).

The child with alveolar hypoventilation usually has a normal respiratory rate but breathes very shallowly (hypopnea). The respiratory rate is relatively fixed and does not increase in response to progressive hypoxemia or hypocarbia. This phenomenon occurs during quiet sleep when the child is totally dependent on automatic respiratory control systems.

Theophylline and caffeine may be helpful in milder forms of the disorder. A number of other respiratory stimulants have been evaluated in children with hypoventilation, but none has been uniformly effective. In severe cases, ventilatory assistance with positive pressure ventilation or phrenic pacing may be necessary.

SUMMARY

Caring for the patient with pulmonary dysfunction is inherent to the practice of pediatric critical care nursing. This chapter presents the pulmonary illnesses common to pediatric critical care. Within the final common pathway framework of mechanical, circulatory, and regulatory failure, emphasis is placed on nursing and collaborative interventions intended to both support the critically ill patient and prevent

iatrogenic injury. Much pediatric specific nursing research is needed to help guide practice related to the care of this vulnerable population and their families. Sensitivity and attention to the impact of critical illness on children and their families is as important as knowledge of the causes and treatment of respiratory failure.

References

AACN Certification Corporation (1991). Pediatric CCRN examination blueprint. *CCRN News*, Spring, 6.

Ackerman, M. H. (1985). The use of bolus normal saline instillations in artificial airways: Is it useful or necessary? *Heart & Lung*, 14, 505–506.

Ackerman, M. H. (1993). The effect of saline lavage prior to suctioning. *American Journal of Critical Care*, 2(4), 326–330.

Adams, D. A. (1993). Ribavirin administration via scavenger vacuum systems in the treatment of respiratory syncytial virus (RSV). *Journal of Pediatric Nursing*, 9(1), 51–53.

Adams, D. A. & McFadden, E. A. (1990). Respiratory syncytial viral infection in infants: Nursing implications. *Critical Care Nurse*, 10(2), 74–79.

Ali, H. H., Utting, J. E., and Grey, C. (1970). Stimulus frequency in the detection of neuromuscular block in humans. *British Journal of Anaesthesia*, 42, 967–977.

Alpan, G., Glick, B., Peleg, O., Amit, Y., & Eyal, F. (1984). Pneumothorax due to endotracheal tube suction. *American Journal of Perinatology*, 1, 345–348.

Anderson, K. D., & Chandra, R. (1976). Pneumothorax secondary to perforation of sequential bronchi by suction catheters. *Journal of Pediatric Surgery*, 11, 687–693.

Asbury, A. K., Arnason, B. G., Karp, H. R., & McFarlin, D. E. (1978). Criteria for diagnosis of Guillain-Barré syndrome. *Annals of Neurology*, 3, 565–567.

Ashbaugh, D. G., Bigelow, D. B., Petty, T. L., & Levine, B. E. (1967). Acute respiratory distress in adults. *Lancet*, 2, 319–323.

Bairam, A., Boutroy, M., Badonnel, Y., & Vert, P. (1987). Theophylline versus caffeine: Comparative effects in treatment of idiopathic apnea in the preterm infant. *Journal of Pediatrics*, 110, 636–639.

Baker, T., Taylor, M., Wilson, M., Rish, J., & Brazeal, S. (1989). Evaluation of a closed system endotracheal suction catheter. *American Journal of Infection Control*, 17, 97.

Bancalari, E., & Gerhardt, R. (1986). Bronchopulmonary dysplasia. *Pediatric Clinics of North America*, 33, 1–23.

Banerjee, A., Subba Rao, K. S. V. K., Khanna, S. K., Narayanan, P. S., Gupta, B. K., Sekar, J. C., Retnam, & Nachiappan, M. (1988). Laryngo-tracheo-bronchial foreign bodies in children. *Journal of Laryngology and Otology*, 102, 1029–1032.

Barry, W., Cockburn, R., Cornall, R., Price, J. F., Sutherland, G., & Vardag, A. (1986). Ribavirin aerosol for acute bronchiolitis. *Archives of Disease in Childhood*, 61, 593–597.

Beachy, P., & Powers, L. K. (1984). Nursing care of the infant with persistent pulmonary hypertension of the newborn. *Clinical Perinatology*, 11, 681–693.

Bell, C., Hughes, C. W., & Oh, T. H. (1991). *The Pediatric Anesthesia Handbook*. St. Louis: Mosby YearBook.

Bernard, G. R., & Bradley, R. B. (1986). Adult respiratory distress syndrome: diagnosis & management. *Heart & Lung*, 15, 250–255.

Bhutani, V. K., Ritchie, W. G., & Shaffer, T. H. (1986). Acquired tracheomegaly in very preterm neonates. *American Journal of Diseases of Children*, 140, 449–452.

Bland, R. D., & Tooley, W. H. (1987). Persistent respiratory distress syndromes. In A. M. Rudolph (Ed.). *Pediatrics* (pp. 1398–1401). Norwalk, CT: Appleton & Lange.

Bodai, B. I., Briggs, S. W., Goldstein, M., McLaughlin, G., & Haas, A. (1989). Evaluation of the ability of the Neo2Safe valve to minimize desaturation in neonates during suctioning. *Respiratory Care*, 34, 355–359.

Bodai, B. I., Walton, C. B., Briggs, S., & Goldstein, M. (1987). A clinical evaluation of an oxygen insufflation/suction catheter. *Heart & Lung*, 16, 39–46.

Bohn, D., Tamura, M., Perrin, D., Barker, G., & Rabinovitch, M. (1987). Ventilatory predictors of pulmonary hypoplasia in congenital diaphragmatic hernia, confirmed by morphologic assessment. *Journal of Pediatrics*, 111, 423–431.

Bostick, J., & Wendelgass, S. T. (1987). Normal saline instillation as part of the suction procedure: Effects on paO₂ and amount of secretions. *Heart & Lung*, 16, 532–537.

Brazy, J. E., Kinney, H. C., & Oakes, W. J. (1987). Central nervous system structural lesions causing apnea at birth. *Journal of Pediatrics*, 111, 163–175.

Breaux, C. W., Rouse, T. M., Cain, W. S., & Georgeson, K. E. (1991). Improvement in survival of patients with congenital diaphragmatic hernia utilizing a strategy of delayed repair after medical and/or extracorporeal membrane oxygenation stabilization. *Journal of Pediatric Surgery*, 26, 333–338.

Brouillette, R. T., Fernback, S. K., & Hunt, C. E. (1982). Obstructive sleep apnea in infants and children. *Journal of Pediatrics*, 100, 31–40.

Bruckheimer, E., & Eidelman, A. I. (1990). Persistent pulmonary hypertension and ECMO (letter). *Pediatrics*, 86, 809–810.

Brudno, D., Parder, D., & Slaton, G. (1989). Response of pulmonary mechanics to terbutaline in patients with bronchopulmonary dysplasia. *American Journal of Medical Science*, 297, 166–168.

Carlon, G. C., Fox, S. J., & Ackerman, N. J. (1987). Evaluation of a closed-tracheal suction system. *Critical Care Medicine*, 15, 522–525.

Carroll, J. E., Jedziniak, M., & Guggenheim, A. M. (1977). Guillain-Barré syndrome: Another cause of the "floppy infant." *American Journal of Diseases of Children*, 131, 699–700.

Chameides, L., & Hazinski, M. F. (Ed.) (1994). Chapter 4: Pediatric airway management. In *Pediatric Advanced Life Support* (pp. 4-1 to 4-22). Dallas, TX: American Heart Association.

Chopra, S. G., Taplin, V., Simmons, D. H., Robinson, G. D., Jr, Elam, D., & Coulson, A. (1977). Effects of hydration and physical therapy on tracheal transport velocity. *American Review of Respiratory Disease*, 115, 1009–1014.

Church, N. R., Anas, N. G., Hall, C. B., & Brooks, J. G. (1984). Respiratory syncytial virus-related apnea in infants. *American Journal of Diseases of Children*, 138, 247–250.

Coghill, T. H., Moore, F. A., Accurso, F. J., & Lilly, J. R. (1983). Primary tracheomalacia. *Annals of Thoracic Surgery*, 35, 538–541.

Committee on Infectious Diseases, American Academy of Pediatrics (1993). Use of ribavirin in the treatment of respiratory syncytial virus. *Pediatrics*, 92(3), 501–504.

Connelly, M., Shagrin, J., & Warfield, C. (1990). Epidural opioids for the management of pain in a patient with the Guillain-Barré syndrome. *Anesthesiology*, 72, 381–383.

Copnell, B., & Fergusson, D. (1995). Endotracheal suctioning: Time-worn ritual or timely intervention. *American Journal of Critical Care*, 4(2), 100–105.

Craig, J., & Mullins, D. (1995). Nitric oxide inhalation in infants and children: Physiologic and clinical implications. *American Journal of Critical Care*, 4(6), 443–450.

Davidson, J. E. (1991). Neuromuscular blockade. *Focus on Critical Care*, 18, 511–520.

Driks, M. R., Craven, D. E., Celli, B. R., Manning, M., Burke, R. A., Garvin, G., Kunches, L. M., Farber, H. W., Wedel, S. A., McCage, W. R. (1987). Nosocomial pneumonia in intubated patients given sucralfate as compared with antacids or histamine type 2 blockers: The role of gastric colonization. *New England Journal of Medicine*, 317, 1376–1382.

Dworetz, A. R., Moya, F. R., Sabo, B., Glandstone, I., & Gross, I. (1989). Survival of infants with persistent pulmonary hypertension without extracorporeal membrane oxygenation. *Pediatrics*, 84(1), 1–6.

Eden, R. D., Seifert, L. S., Winegar, A., Spellacy, W. N. (1987). Perinatal morbidity and mortality in a regional perinatal network. *Journal of Reproductive Medicine*, 32, 583–586.

Epstein, M. A., & Sladky, J. T. (1989). The role of plasmapheresis in childhood Guillain-Barré syndrome. *Annals of Neurology*, 26, 448.

Favara, B. E., & Paul, R. N. (1967). Thromboembolism and cor

pulmonale complicating ventriculo-venous shunts. *Journal of the American Medical Association*, 199, 668–671.

Filler, R. M., Buck, J. R., Bahoric, A., & Steward, D. J. (1982). Treatment of segmental tracheomalacia and bronchomalacia by implantation of an airway splint. *Journal of Pediatric Surgery*, 17, 597–603.

Frank, M. (1987). Theophylline: A closer look. *Neonatal Network*, 6(2), 7–13.

Frank, Y., Kravath, R. E., Pollak, C. P., & Weitzman, E. K. (1983). Obstructive sleep apnea and its therapy: clinical and polysomnographic manifestations. *Pediatrics*, 71, 737–742.

Franck, L. S., Vaughn, B., & Wallace, J. (1992). Extubation reintubation in the NICU: Identifying opportunities to improve care. *Pediatric Nursing* 18(3), 267–270.

French Cooperative Group of Plasma Exchange in Guillain-Barré Syndrome (1987). Efficiency of plasm exchange in Guillain-Barré syndrome: Role of replacement fluids. *Annals of Neurology*, 22, 753–761.

Friel, M. S., Quan, S. F., & Lohse, S. M. (1990). Comparison of the Jinotti oxygen-insufflation catheter to standard hyperoxygenation techniques in patients on high FiO₂ and high PEEP. *Respiratory Care*, 35, 1118.

Frostell, C., Fratacci, M. D., Wain, J. C., Jones, R., & Zapol, W. M. (1991). Inhaled nitric oxide. A selective pulmonary vasodilator reversing hypoxic pulmonary vasoconstriction. *Circulation*, 83(6), 2038–2047.

Gibson, R. L., Jackson, J. C., Twiggs, G. A., Redding, G. J., & Truog, W. E. (1988). Bronchopulmonary dysplasia. Survival after prolonged mechanical ventilation. *American Journal of Diseases of Children*, 142, 721–725.

Goetzman, B. W., & Reimenschneider, T. A. (1980). Persistence of the fetal circulation. *Pediatrics*, 2, 37–40.

Gomez-Del-Rio, M., Gehardt, T., Hehre, D., Feller, R., & Bancalari, E. (1986). Effect of a beta agonist nebulization on lung function in neonates with increased pulmonary resistance. *Pediatric Pulmonology*, 2, 289–291.

Goodman, G., Perkin, R. M., Anas, N. G., Sperling, D. R., Hicks, D. A., & Rowen, M. (1988). Pulmonary hypertension in infants with bronchopulmonary dysplasia. *Journal of Pediatrics*, 112, 67–72.

Gordin, P. C. (1990). Assessing and managing agitation in a critically ill infant. *Maternal and Child Nursing*, 15, 26–32.

Gray, J. E., MacIntyre, N. R., & Kronenberger, W. G. (1990). The effects of bolus normal-saline instillation in conjunction with endotracheal suctioning. *Respiratory Care*, 35, 785–790.

Griffith, J. A., & Perkin, R. M. (1987). Management of acute epiglottis in pediatric patients (letter). *Critical Care Medicine*, 15, 283.

Groothuis, J. R., Gutierrez, K. M., & Lauer, B. A. (1988). Respiratory syncytial virus infection in children with bronchopulmonary dysplasia. *Pediatrics*, 82(2), 199–203.

Groothuis, J. R., & Rosenberg, A. A. (1987). Home oxygen promotes weight gain in infants with bronchopulmonary dysplasia. *American Journal of Diseases of Children*, 141, 992–995.

Guilleminault, C. (1987). Obstructive sleep apnea syndrome and its treatment in children: areas of agreement and controversy. *Pediatric Pulmonology*, 3, 429–436.

Guillain-Barré Study Group (1985). Plasmapheresis and acute Guillain-Barré syndrome. *Neurology*, 35, 1096–1104.

Hall, C. B., Douglas, G., Jr., & Geiman, J. M. (1980). Possible transmission by fomites of respiratory syncytial virus. *Journal of Infectious Diseases*, 141, 98–102.

Hall, C. B., McBride, J. T., Gala, C. L., Hildreth, S. W., & Schnabel, K. C. (1985). Ribavirin treatment of respiratory syncytial viral infection in infants with underlying cardiopulmonary disease. *JAMA*, 254, 3047–3051.

Hall, C. B., McBride, J. R., Walsh, E. E., Bell, D. M., Gala, C. L., Hildreth, S., Ten Eyck, L. G., & Hall, W. J. (1983). Aerosolized ribavirin treatment of infants with respiratory syncytial viral infection. *New England Journal of Medicine*, 308, 1443–1447.

Hammerman, C., Lass, N., Strates, E., Komar, K., & Bui, K. I. (1987). Prostanoids in neonates with persistent pulmonary hypertension. *Journal of Pediatrics*, 110, 470–472.

Jensen, T. H., Hansen, P. B., & Brodersen, P. (1988). Ondines's curse in Listeria monocyto genes brain stem encephalitis. *Acta Neurologic Scandinavica*, 77, 505–506.

Johnston, P. W., Liberman, R., Gangitano, E., & Vogt, J. (1990). Ventilation parameters and arterial blood gases as a prediction of hypoplasia in congenital diaphragmatic hernia. *Journal of Pediatric Surgery*, 25, 496–499.

Kahn, R. C. (1983). Humidification of the airways: Adequate for function and integrity. *Chest*, 84, 510–511.

Kanter, R. K., Pollack, M. M., Wright, W. W., & Grundfast, K. M. (1982). Treatment of severe tracheobronchomalacia with continuous positive airway pressure (CPAP). *Anesthesiology*, 57, 54–56.

Kao, L. C., Warburton, D., Cheng, M. H., Cedeno, C., Platzker, A. C. G., & Keens, T. G. (1984). Effect of oral diuretics on pulmonary mechanics in infants with chronic bronchopulmonary dysplasia: Result of a double-blind crossover sequential trial. *Pediatrics*, 74(1), 37–44.

Kao, L. C., Warburton, D., Platzker, A. C. G., & Keens, R. G. (1984). Effects of isoproterenol inhalation on airway resistance in chronic bronchopulmonary dysplasia. *Pediatrics*, 74, 509–513.

Kennelly, C. (1987). Tracheostomy care: Parents as learners. *MCN*, 12, 264–267.

Kent, P. A., & Curley, M. A. Q. (1992). Challenges in nursing: Infants with congenital diaphragmatic hernia. *Heart & Lung*, 21(4), 381–389.

Kirilloff, L., Owens, G., Rogers, R., & Mazzocco, M. C. (1985). Does chest physical therapy work? *Chest*, 88, 436–444.

Kleiber, C., Krutzfield, N., & Rose, E. (1988). Acute histologic changes in the tracheobronchial tree associated with different suction catheter insertion techniques. *Heart & Lung*, 17, 10–14.

Klesh, K. W., Murphy, T. F., Scher, M. S., Buchanan, D. E., Maxwell, E. P., & Guthrie, R. D. (1987). Cerebral infarction in persistent pulmonary hypertension of the newborn. *American Journal of Diseases of Children*, 141, 852–857.

Koski, C. L., Gratz, E., Sutherland, J., & Mayer, R. F. (1986). Clinical correlation with anti-peripheral-nerve myelin antibodies in Guillain-Barré syndrome. *Annals of Neurology*, 19, 573–577.

Laks, Y., & Barzilay, Z. (1988). Foreign body aspiration in childhood. *Pediatric Emergency Care*, 4, 102–106.

Langer, J. C., Filler, R. M., Bohn, K. J., Shandling, B., Ein, S. H., Wesson, D. E., & Superina, R. A. (1988). Timing of surgery for congenital diaphragmatic hernia: Is emergency operation necessary? *Journal of Pediatric Surgery*, 23, 731–734.

Lebel, M. H., Gauthier, M., Lacroix, J., Rousseau, E., & Buithieu, M. (1989). Respiratory failure and mechanical ventilation in severe bronchiolitis. *Archives of Disease in Childhood*, 64, 1431–1437.

Lee, R., & O'Brodovich, H. (1988). Airway epithelial damage in premature infants with respiratory failure. *American Review of Respiratory Disease*, 137, 450–457.

Little, L. A., Koenig, J. C., Jr., & Newth, C. J. L. (1990). Factors affecting accidental extubations in neonatal and pediatric intensive care patients. *Critical Care Medicine*, 18, 163–165.

Loeber, N., Morray, J., Kettrick, R., & Downes, J. (1980). Pulmonary function in chronic respiratory failure of infancy. *Critical Care Medicine*, 8, 596–601.

Loisel, D. B., Smith, M. M., & MacDonald, M. G. (1987). Plasma theophylline levels as related to toxicity in infants with severe chronic lung disease. *Neonatal Network*, 6(2), 15–19.

Lund, C. H., & Collier, S. B. (1990). Nutrition and bronchopulmonary dysplasia. In C. H. Lund (Ed.). *Bronchopulmonary dysplasia*. Petaluma, CA: Neonatal Network.

McDermott, B. K., & Curley, M. A. Q. (1990). Extracorporeal membrane oxygenation: Current use and future directions. *AACN Clinical Issues in Critical Care Nursing*, 1, 348–364.

McGuirt, W. F., Holmes, K. D., Reehs, R., & Browne, J. D. (1988). Tracheobronchial foreign bodies. *Laryngoscope*, 98, 615–618.

McKann, G. M., Griffin, J. W., Cornblath, D. R., Mellits, E. D., Fisher, R. S., Quaskey, S. A., & The Guillaine-Barré Syndrome Study Group (1988). Plasmapheresis and Guillain-Barré syndrome: Analysis of prognostic factors and the effect of plasmapheresis. *Annals of Neurology*, 23, 347–353.

MacDonald, N. E., Hall, C. B., Suffin, S. C., Alexson, C., Harris, P. J., & Manning, J. A. (1982). Respiratory syncytial viral infection in infants with congenital heart disease. *New England Journal of Medicine*, 7, 397–400.

Marini, J. J. (1989). Should PEEP be used in airflow obstruction? *American Review of Respiratory Disease*, 140, 1–13.

Marx, G. (1988). Prediction of nonsurvival in critically ill infants with respiratory failure: Which patients are candidates for extracorporeal membrane oxygenation? *American Journal of Diseases of Children*, 142, 261–262.

Mathew, O. P., & Sant'Ambrogio, G. (1991). Development of upper airway reflexes. In V. Chernick & R. B. Mellins (Eds.). *Basic mechanisms of pediatric respiratory disease: Cellular and integrative* (pp. 55–71). Philadelphia: B. C. Decker.

Meisels, S. J., Plunkett, J. W., Roloff, D. W., Pasick, P. L., & Stiefel, G. S. (1986). Growth and development of preterm infants with respiratory distress syndrome and bronchopulmonary dysplasia. *Pediatrics*, 77, 345–352.

Miller, M. J., Carlo, W. A., & Martin, R. J. (1985). Continuous positive pressure selectively reduces obstructive apnea in preterm infants. *Journal of Pediatrics*, 106, 91–94.

Moler, R. W., Hurwitz, M. E., & Custer, J. R. (1988). Improvement in clinical asthma score and paCO$_2$ in children with severe asthma treated with continuously nebulized terbutaline. *Journal of Allergy and Clinical Immunology*, 81, 1101–1109.

Morray, J. P., Fox, W. W., Kettrick, R. G., & Downes, J. J. (1981). Clinical correlates of successful weaning from mechanical ventilation in severe bronchopulmonary dysplasia. *Critical Care Medicine*, 9, 815–818.

Motoyama, E., Fort, M., Klesh, K., Mutich, R., & Guthrie, R. (1987). Early onset of airway reactivity in premature infants with bronchopulmonary dysplasia. *American Review of Respiratory Disease*, 136, 50–57.

Murphy, J. D., Rabinovitch, M., Goldstein, J. D., & Reid, L. M. (1981). The structural basis of persistent pulmonary hypertension of the newborn infant. *Journal of Pediatrics*, 98, 962–967.

Murphy, J. D., Vawter, G. V., & Reid, L. M. (1984). Pulmonary vascular disease in fetal meconium aspiration. *Journal of Pediatrics*, 104, 758–762.

Nading, J. H. (1989). Historical controls for extracorporeal membrane oxygenation in neonates. *Critical Care Medicine*, 17, 423–425.

National Heart, Lung, and Blood Institute; National Institutes of Health (1991). *Executive summary: Guidelines for the diagnosis and management of asthma* (Publication No. 91–3042A). Washington, D.C.: U.S. Government Printing Office.

Newcomb, R. W., & Akhter, J. (1988). Respiratory failure from asthma. A marker for children with high morbidity and mortality. *American Journal of Diseases of Children*, 142, 1041–1044.

Noll, M. A., Hix, C. D., & Scott, G. (1990). Closed tracheal suction systems: Effectiveness and nursing implications. *AACN Clinical Issues*, 1, 318–326.

Northway, W. H., Rosan, R. C., & Porter, D. Y. (1967). Pulmonary disease following respirator therapy of hyaline membrane disease. Bronchopulmonary dysplasia. *New England Journal of Medicine*, 276, 357–368.

Norwood, S. H., & Civetta, J. M. (1985). Ventilatory support in patients with ARDS. *Surgical Clinics of North America*, 65, 895–916.

O'Rourke, P. P., Crone, R. K., Vacanti, J. P., Ware, J. H., Lillehei, C. W., Parad, R. B., & Epstein, M. F. (1989). Extracorporeal membrane oxygenation and conventional medical therapy in neonates with persistent pulmonary hypertension of the newborn: a prospective randomized study. *Pediatrics*, 84(6), 957–963.

Ortiz, R. M., Cilley, R. E., Bartlett, R. H. (1987). Extracorporeal membrane oxygenation in pediatric respiratory failure. *Pediatric Clinics of North America*, 34, 39–46.

Osterman, P. O., Lundmo, G., Pirskanen, R., Fagius, J., Pihlstedt, P., Siden, A., & Safwenberg, J. (1984). Beneficial effects of plasma exchange in acute inflammatory polyradiculoneuropathy. *Lancet*, 2, 1296–1299.

Outwater, K. M., & Crone, R. K. (1984). Management of respiratory failure in infants with acute viral bronchiolitis. *American Journal of Diseases of Children*, 138, 1071–1075.

Outwater, K. M., Meissner, C., & Peterson, M. B. (1988). Ribavirin administration to infants receiving mechanical ventilation. *American Journal of Diseases of Children*, 142, 512–515.

Ouvrier, R. A., McLeod, J. D., & Pollard, J. (Eds.) (1990). Acute inflammatory demyelinating polyradiculoneuropathy. In *Peripheral neuropathy in childhood* (pp. 39–49). New York: Raven Press.

Palmisano, B. W., Fisher, D. M., Willis, M., Gregory, G. A., & Ebert, P. A. (1984). The effect of paralysis on oxygen consumption in normoxic children after cardiac surgery. *Anesthesiology*, 61, 518–522.

Paneth, N., & Wallenstein, S. (1985). Extracorporeal membrane oxygenation and the play the winner rule. *Pediatrics*, 76(4), 622–623.

Pearl, R. G. (1993). Inhaled nitric oxide. *Anesthesiology*, 78(3), 413–416.

Perez Fontan, J. J., & Lister, G. (1990). Respiratory failure. In R. J. Touloukian (Ed.). *Pediatric trauma* (pp. 46–76). St. Louis: Mosby–YearBook.

Phillips, B. L., McQuitty, J., & Durand, D. J. (1988). Blood gases: Technical aspects and interpretation (p. 228). In J. P. Goldsmith & E. H. Karotkin. *Assisted Ventilation in the Neonate* (2nd ed.). Philadelphia: W. B. Saunders.

Piersen, W. E., Bierman, C. W., & Kelley, V. C. (1974). A double-blind trial of corticosteroid therapy in status asthmaticus. *Pediatrics*, 54, 782–788.

Pridham, K. F., Martin, R., Sondel, S., & Tluczek, A. (1989). Parental issues in feeding young children with bronchopulmonary dysplasia. *Journal of Pediatric Nursing*, 4, 177–185.

Prineas, J. W. (1981). Pathology of the Guillain-Barré syndrome. *Annals of Neurology*, 9[Suppl.], 6–19.

Quera-Salva, M. A. & Guilleminault, C. (1987). Post-traumatic central sleep apnea in a child. *Journal of Pediatrics*, 110, 906–909.

Rhine, W. D., Fischer, A. F., & Stevenson, D. K. (1990). The extracorporeal membrane oxygenation debate (letter). *Pediatrics*, 85(3), 381–382.

Roberts, J. D. (1993). Inhaled nitric oxide for treatment of pulmonary artery hypertension in the newborn and infant. *Critical Care Medicine*, 21(9[Suppl.]), 374–376.

Roberts, J. L., Mathew, O. P., & Thach, B. T. (1982). The efficacy of theophylline in premature infants with mixed and obstructive apnea and apnea associated with pulmonary and neurologic disease. *Journal of Pediatrics*, 100, 968–970.

Rochester, D. F., & Esau, S. A. (1984). Malnutrition and the respiratory system. *Chest*, 85, 411–415.

Rosenfield, B., Burel, C., & Hanley, D. (1986). Epidural morphine treatment of pain in Guillain-Barré syndrome. *Archives of Neurology*, 43, 1194–1196.

Rutledge, M. L., Hawkins, E. P., & Langston, C. (1986). Skeletal muscle growth failure induced in premature newborn infants by prolonged pancuronium treatment. *Journal of Pediatrics*, 109, 883–886.

Sakai, H., Tamura, M., Hosokawa, Y., Bryan, A. C., Barker, G. A., & Bohn, D. J. (1987). Effect of surgical repair on respiratory mechanics in congenital diaphragmatic hernia. *Journal of Pediatrics*, 111, 432–438.

Sawyer, M. H., Edwards, D. K., & Spector, S. A. (1987). Cytomegalovirus infection and bronchopulmonary dysplasia in premature infants. *American Journal of Diseases of Children*, 141, 303–305.

Schreiber, M. D., Heymann, M. A., & Soifer, S. J. (1986). Increased arterial pH, not decreased paCO$_2$, attenuates hypoxia-induced pulmonary vasoconstriction in newborn lambs. *Pediatric Research*, 20, 113–117.

Schuh, S., Reider, M. J., Canny, G., Pender, E., Forbes, T., Tan, Y. K., Bailey, D., & Levison, H. (1990). Nebulized albuterol in acute childhood asthma: Comparison of two doses. *Pediatrics*, 86, 509–513.

Scott, P. H., Eigen, H., Moye, L. A., Georgitis, J., & Laughlin, J. J. (1985). Predictability and consequences of spontaneous extubation in a pediatric ICU. *Critical Care Medicine*, 13, 228–232.

Shahar, E., Murphy, G., & Roifman, C. M. (1990). Benefit of intravenously administered immune serum globulin in patients with Guillain-Barré syndrome. *Journal of Pediatrics*, 116, 141–144.

Shanbhogue, L. K. R., Tam, P. K. H., Ninan, G., & Lloyd, D. A. (1990). Preoperative stabilization in congenital diaphragmatic hernia. *Archives of Disease in Childhood*, 65, 1043–1044.

Shekleton, M. E., & Nield, M. (1987). Ineffective airway clearance related to artificial airway. *Nursing Clinics of North America*, 22, 161–177.

Short, B. L. (1990). The extracorporeal membrane oxygenation debate (letter). *Pediatrics*, 85(3), 380–381.

Sladky, J. T. (1987). Neuropathy in childhood. *Seminars in Neurology*, 7, 67–75.

Smyth, J. A., Tabachnik, E., Duncan, W. J., Reilly, B. J., & Levison H. (1981). Pulmonary function and bronchial hyperreactivity in long-term survivors of bronchopulmonary dysplasia. *Pediatrics*, 68(3), 336–340.

Sotomayer, J. L., Godinez, R. I., Borden, S., & Wilmott, R. W. (1986). Large-airway collapse due to acquired tracheobronchomalacia in infancy. *American Journal of Diseases of Children*, 140, 367–371.

Spitzer, A. R. (1995). Neonatal respiratory care. In D. Dantzker, J. Marini, & E. Dakow (Eds.). *Comprehensive respiratory care*. Philadelphia: W. B. Saunders.

Spitzer, A. R., Davis, J., Clarke, W. T., Bernbaum, J., & Fox, W. W. (1988). Pulmonary hypertension and persistent fetal circulation in the newborn. *Clinics in Perinatology*, 15, 389–413.

Staub, N. C. (1980). The pathogenesis of pulmonary edema. *Progress in Cardiovascular Diseases*, 23, 53–80.

Stokes, G. M., Milner, A. D., Hodges, I. G. C., Henry, R. L., & Elphick, M. C. (1983). Nebulised therapy in acute severe bronchiolitis in infancy. *Archives of Disease in Childhood*, 58, 279–282.

Super, D. M., Cartelli, N. A., Brooks, L. J., Lembo, R. M., & Kumar, M. L. (1989). A prospective randomized double-blind study to evaluate the effect of dexamethasone in acute laryngotracheitis. *Journal of Pediatrics*, 115, 323–329.

Taber, L. H., Knight, V., Gilbert, B. E., McClung, H. W., Wilson, S. Z., Norton, H. J., Thurson, J. M., Gordon, W. H., Atmar, R. L., & Schlaudt, W. R. (1983). Ribavirin aerosol treatment of bronchiolitis associated with respiratory syncytial virus infection in infants. *Pediatrics*, 72, 613–618.

Taft, A. A., Mishoe, S. C., Dennison, F. H., Lain, D. C., & Chaudhary, B. A. (1990). A comparison of two methods of preoxygenation during endotracheal suction. *Respiratory Care*, 35, 1117.

Tal, A., Levy, N., & Bearman, J. E. (1990). Methylprednisolone therapy for acute asthma in infants and toddlers: A controlled clinical trial. *Pediatrics*, 86, 350–356.

Tiefenbrunn, L. J., & Riemenschneider, T. A. (1986). Persistent pulmonary hypertension of the newborn. *American Heart Journal*, 111, 564–572.

Timmons, O. D., Havens, P. L., & Fackler, J. C. (1995). Predicting death in pediatric patients with acute respiratory failure. *Chest*, 108(3), 789–797.

Troug, R. D., Schena, J. A., Hershenson, M. B., KoKa, B. V., & Lillihei, C. W. (1990). Repair of congenital diaphragmatic hernia during extracorporeal membrane oxygenation. *Anesthesiology*, 72, 750–753.

Turner, B. (1990). Maintaining the artificial airway: Current concepts. *Pediatric Nursing*, 16, 487–493.

Wald, E. R., Dashefsky, B., & Green, M. (1988). In re ribavirin: A case of premature adjudication? *Journal of Pediatrics*, 112, 154–158.

Westley, C. R., Cotton, E. K., & Brooks, J. G. (1978). Nebulized racemic epinephrine by IPPB treatment of croup. A double blind study. *American Journal of Diseases of Children*, 132, 484–487.

Wetzel, R. C. (1987). In M. C. Rogers (Ed.). *Textbook of pediatric intensive care* (p. 506). Baltimore: Williams & Wilkins.

White, C., Richardson, C., & Raibstein, L. (1990). High-frequency ventilation and extracorporeal membrane oxygenation. *AACN Clinical Issues in Critical Care Nursing*, 1, 427–444.

Wilkie, R., & Bryan, M. (1987). Effect of bronchodilators on airway resistance in ventilator dependent neonates with chronic lung disease. *Journal of Pediatrics*, 111, 278–282.

Witmer, M. T., Hess, D., & Simmons, M. (1990). An evaluation of the effectiveness of secretion removal with a closed-circuit suction catheter. *Respiratory Care*, 35, 1117.

Wohl, M. E. B., & Chernick, V. State of the art: Bronchiolitis. (1978). *American Review of Respiratory Disease*, 118, 759–781.

Wung, J., James, S., Kilchevsky, E., & James, E. (1985). Management of infants with severe respiratory failure and persistence of the fetal circulation, without hyperventilation. *Pediatrics*, 76(4), 488–494.

CHAPTER 21

Neurologic Critical Care Problems

PAULA VERNON-LEVETT

INTRACRANIAL HYPERTENSION
Brain Herniation Syndromes
Critical Care Management
Associated Pathologies
HYPOXIC ISCHEMIC ENCEPHALOPATHY
Terminology
Pathogenesis
Critical Care Management
Associated Pathologies

BRAIN DEATH
Controversies
Organ Donation
NEUROMUSCULAR DISORDERS
MUSCULOSKELETAL DISORDERS
Care of the Patient After Spinal Fusion
SUMMARY

Unique to pediatric critical care, a large percentage of intensive care admissions result from severe neurologic dysfunction. Numerous congenital and acquired neurologic disorders exist; however, most result in two final common pathways: intracranial hypertension and global hypoxic ischemia. This chapter focuses on these two major patient problems from a critical care nursing perspective.

Intracranial hypertension results from an uncompensated increase in one or more of the three intracranial volumes. Although the pathogenesis and medical management vary among these disorders, nursing care of patients with intracranial hypertension, regardless of the cause, is similar. The mechanisms and consequences of intracranial hypertension are presented, followed by a discussion of critical care management strategies intended to prevent secondary neuronal injury. After the general discussion, specific neurologic disorders that cause intracranial hypertension are presented, including the priorities in management.

The second final common pathway, global hypoxic ischemia, produces primary neuronal injury. Like intracranial hypertension, a number of pathophysiologic events and disorders can result in this final common pathway. A general discussion of the consequences of global hypoxic ischemia is presented, as well as common supportive strategies. Victims of near-drowning experience global hypoxic ischemia and are, unfortunately, common in the pediatric population (Quan et al., 1989); specific collaborative measures unique to this population are discussed.

Despite state-of-the-art critical care management, some patients develop irreversible brain damage. Specific guidelines and controversies in pediatric brain death, with a focus upon the care of the potential organ donor, are presented.

Because primary neuromuscular dysfunction is seldom the only reason for intensive care hospitalization, these disorders are briefly mentioned. Acquired disorders, for example, Guillain-Barré syndrome and spinal cord trauma, are presented in Chapters 20 and 30, respectively. To complement the discussion on care of the patient following craniotomy, care of the patient after spinal fusion is presented.

INTRACRANIAL HYPERTENSION

Intracranial hypertension is a term used to define a sustained elevation in intracranial pressure (ICP) above 15 mmHg (Hickey, 1986). Intracranial hypertension is not a disease itself, but is a final common pathway for a number of neuropathologies that elevate ICP. These diseases can be broadly classified into four groups: conditions that increase blood volume, increase brain volume, increase cerebrospinal fluid (CSF) volume, or increase a combination of the above three.

Uncontrolled intracranial hypertension eventually causes distortion and herniation of brain tissue, as well as a local or generalized reduction in cerebral perfusion pressure (CPP). Initially, an expanding intracranial mass occludes the subarachnoid spaces, preventing translocation of CSF into the spinal subarachnoid space. Eventually, the CSF cistern collapses and the arachnoid villi are compressed, preventing reabsorption of CSF. As intraparenchymal pressure increases, vascular collapse may occur with venous outflow obstruction (Shapiro, 1975). In an effort to maintain cerebral blood flow (CBF) with an elevated ICP, compensatory changes in the arterial vascular beds may occur with increased arterial resistance.

With an alteration in vascular resistance, capillary pressure may increase, promoting cerebral edema (Johnston & Rowan, 1974; Shapiro, 1975). At some critical point, autoregulation of CBF is lost and CBF becomes passively dependent on arterial pressure and CPP. Local or generalized brain ischemia, anoxia, and neuronal death results, as well as herniation and distortion of brain tissue. Figure 21–1 (A and B) shows drawings of normal intracranial contents and intracranial contents with intracranial hypertension.

Brain Herniation Syndromes

A pressure gradient between compartments may cause a shift in structures from one compartment to another. The cranial cavity is divided into compart-

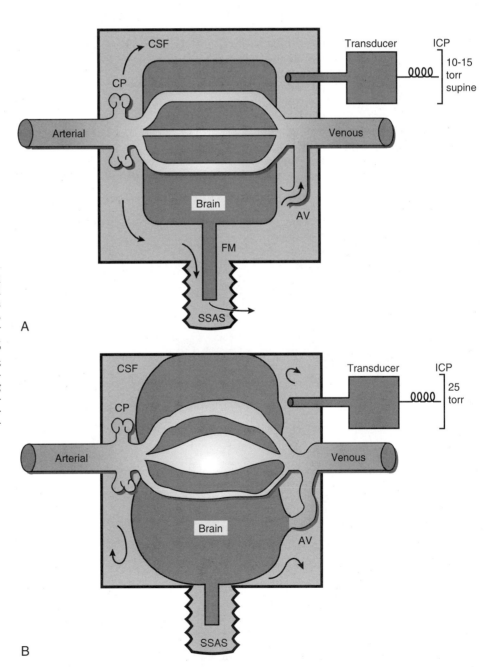

Figure 21–1 ● ● ● ● ● ●

A, Schematic representation of normal intracranial contents. SSAS—Spinal Subarachnoid Space, FM—Foramen magnum, CSF—Cerebrospinal fluid, ICP—Intracranial pressure, AV—Arachnoid villi, CP—Choroid plexus. Arrows indicate the direction of CSF flow and heavy dark lines represent the skull. B, Schematic representation of intracranial contents during intracranial hypertension. Abbreviations as in A. (A and B, From Shapiro, H.M. 1975. Intracranial hypertension. Anesthesiology, 43, 446.)

ments by the dura mater, which is fibrous and relatively rigid. The *falx cerebri* partially separates the supratentorial space as it drops into the longitudinal fissure. The *tentorium cerebelli* is a tent-like structure located in the posterior fossa. It separates the cerebellum and brainstem from the occipital lobe of the cerebral hemispheres. The tentorial notch refers to the central opening of the tentorium. The *foramen magnum* is a bony opening at the base of the skull that anatomically separates the intracranial contents from the spinal cord. Figure 21–2 illustrates the anatomic compartments of the brain.

Supratentorial Herniation

Brain herniation syndromes are usually classified into two broad categories: supratentorial and infratentorial. Supratentorial herniation syndromes are further classified into three types. First, *uncal herniation* refers to unilateral displacement of the uncus (medial aspect of the temporal lobe) from the middle fossa to the posterior fossa through the tentorium (Fig. 21–3). Second, *central herniation* refers to a symmetric downward displacement of both cerebral hemispheres through the tentorial notch. This syndrome occurs more frequently in infants and children, especially those with hydrocephalus (Milhorat, 1978). Last, *cingulate herniation* refers to displacement of the cingulate gyrus under the falx cerebri

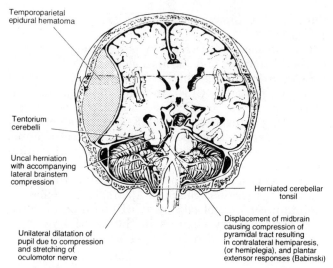

Figure 21–3 ● ● ● ● ● ●

Cross section showing herniation of part of the temporal lobe through the tentorium due to a temporoparietal epidural hematoma. (From Kintzel, K.C. 1977. *Advanced concepts on clinical nursing*, 2nd ed. Philadelphia: J.B. Lippincott.)

into the opposite hemisphere (Boss, 1990; Hickey, 1986; Morrison, 1987).

Infratentorial Herniation

Infratentorial herniation is less frequent than supratentorial herniation (Hickey, 1986). There are two types of infratentorial herniation syndromes. The most common type is downward displacement of one or both of the cerebellar tonsils through the foramen magnum (Fig. 21–4). The second type, which is rare,

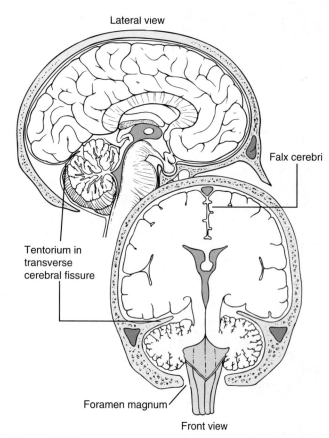

Figure 21–2 ● ● ● ● ● ●

Falx cerebri and tentorium. (From Snyder M., & Jackle, M. 1981. *Neurologic problems: A critical care nursing focus*, p. 21. Bowie, MD: Prentice-Hall.)

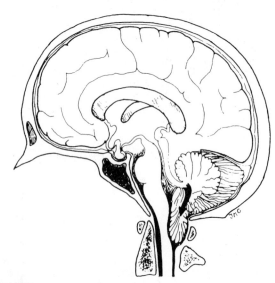

Figure 21–4 ● ● ● ● ● ●

Herniation of the cerebellar tonsils into the foramen magnum is the final outcome of increased intracranial pressure. Respiratory centers within the medulla oblongata are compressed and apnea in sleep frequently leads to cardiac arrest and death. (From Smith, R.R. 1980. *Essentials of neurosurgery*. Philadelphia: J.B. Lippincott.)

Table 21-1. PROGRESSIVE SIGNS AND SYMPTOMS OF CENTRAL AND UNCAL HERNIATION

	Uncal Herniation Syndrome	
	Early	Late
Level of consciousness	Restlessness, may progress quickly to coma	Coma
Motor function	May have contralateral hemiparesis, hemiplegia, decerebration	Flaccidity
Respirations	Normal	Progresses to Cheyne-Stokes (Diencephalon-Midbrain) → Central neurogenic hyperventilation (midbrain-upper pons) → Shallow (lower pons-upper medulla) → Ataxic, Apnea (medulla)
Pupil signs	Unilateral, sluggish, nonreactive/dilated ipsilateral pupil	Bilateral, fixed and dilated pupils
Extraocular signs	May have ipsilateral ptosis, slight weakness of oculomotor innervated muscles	Oculomotor paralysis

	Central Herniation Syndrome	
	Early	Late
Level of consciousness	Agitated, drowsy, then stuporous	Coma
Motor function	Contralateral hemiparesis to hemiplegia, progresses to decorticate posturing	Flaccidity with occasional decerebrate posturing
Respirations	Cheyne-Stokes, progresses as above	Ataxic, then apnea
Pupil signs	Bilateral small and reactive: may progress to unequal and nonreactive	Dilated and fixed
Extraocular signs	Normal or slightly roving, then difficulty with upward gaze	Dysconjugate gaze

Adapted with permission from Hickey, J. V. (1986). *The Clinical Practice of Neurologic and Neurosurgical Nursing* (2nd ed, pp. 259–260). Philadelphia: J. B. Lippincott.

is upward displacement of the cerebellum or lower brainstem through the tentorial notch into the supratentorial compartment (Boss, 1990; Hickey, 1986; Morrison, 1987).

Critical Care Management

Assessment

In the comatose patient, continuous ICP monitoring is the only accurate means of assessing early changes in intracranial pressure and compliance and determining the effectiveness of therapy. (See Chapter 12, Intracranial Dynamics, for a description of nursing care related to ICP monitoring). In the absence of intracranial pressure monitoring, serial assessments of the patient's neurologic status is the best means of identifying intracranial hypertension. Clinical signs and symptoms of increased intracranial pressure (IICP) are numerous and vary depending on a number of factors: the specific location or compartment of a mass or swelling, the acuteness of the rise in ICP, and the age of the patient.

With slowly expanding uncal or central herniation syndromes, neurologic signs are usually progressive in a rostral to caudal sequence with signs during the late stages being the same (Hickey, 1986; Shapiro, 1975.) In the infratentorial compartment, a clear-cut syndrome does not occur with IICP and herniation.

Clinical signs and symptoms of IICP also depend on how acutely ICP increases. Early signs and symptoms include an alteration in level of consciousness (restlessness or confusion), motor weakness or paresis, vomiting, headache, and pupillary changes. Late

signs and symptoms are more characteristic of brainstem dysfunction: depressed level of consciousness (coma), motor dysfunction (decorticate or decerebrate posturing), respiratory irregularities terminating with apnea, and impaired cranial nerve function (gag, corneal, oculocephalic, oculovestibular reflexes). Cushing's triad, a late sign indicative of brainstem compression, includes the classic signs of increased systolic pressure, which produces a wide pulse pressure, bradycardia, and bradypnea that is often irregular. Table 21–1 summarizes the progressive signs and symptoms of central and uncal herniation.

Neurologic signs of IICP can also be intermittent. Transient signs and symptoms usually last only a few minutes and are most often seen at the peak of plateau waves when CPP is compromised. Common clinical signs and symptoms include headache, blurred vision, change in level of consciousness, pallor, obtundation, paresis, and changes in pupillary reaction.

When chronic IICP exists (e.g., pseudotumor cerebri, slow-growing tumor, slowly increasing hydrocephalus), the patient clinically may be less symptomatic or may display more nonspecific symptoms. The absence of papilledema does not exclude the presence of IICP; however, when present it is almost always indicative of IICP. It can develop as early as 48 hours after IICP, but more often is seen as a chronic sign (Bell, 1978).

Many signs and symptoms of IICP are also age-dependent. In general, the younger the child, the more nonspecific the signs and symptoms. The older child typically complains of headache (especially upon awakening in the morning) and blurred vision. Infants and preverbal toddlers cannot report a headache. They usually express a headache by holding their head or exhibiting irritability and anorexia (Bell, 1978). Papilledema is less commonly seen in infants, presumably because of their expansible skull. Progressive signs and symptoms of IICP that are unique to the infant include a large full anterior fontanel, setting sun eyes, "cracked pot" sound upon skull percussion, and a progressive increase in head circumference. Separation of cranial sutures (diastasis) may be seen in both infants and young children with IICP because of unfused sutures. Late signs and symptoms of brainstem compression from IICP are more similar than different among the different age groups.

Collaborative Management

Intracranial hypertension results from loss of normal intracranial compensatory mechanisms. Management goals for patients with intracranial hypertension are directed toward improving the reduced intracranial compliance. In some patients with a localized mass, ICP is normalized following surgical excision. In other cases, the neuropathology is not amenable to surgical correction, and the complexity of the pathologic changes requires a combination of therapies to control intracranial hypertension. In general, specific interventions are introduced in a stepwise approach with the least invasive therapies used first and removed last.

Cerebral Blood Volume Reduction. Mechanisms that increase cerebral blood volume (CBV) and increase ICP include cerebrovascular vasodilation, hypercapnia, hypoxia, volatile anesthetics, and venous outflow obstruction (Mitchell, 1986; Reivich, 1964; Shapiro, 1975). Figure 21–5 illustrates the changes in CBF resulting from alterations in PaO_2, $PaCO_2$, and blood pressure.

Hyperventilation. Over the past 30 years, induced, controlled hyperventilation has been widely advocated during the first few days following a severe neurologic insult producing intracranial hypertension (Bruce, 1989a; Marshall & Marshall, 1987). Recently, hyperventilation is used as a rescue intervention when cerebral herniation and death are thought to be imminent or when all other means of reducing IICP have been exhausted (Marion, Firlik, & McLaughlin, 1995). Cerebral vascular changes are directly affected by the pH of surrounding interstitial fluid and indirectly by changes in $PaCO_2$. Low pH results in cerebral vasodilation, whereas high pH results in cerebral vasoconstriction (Muizelaar et al., 1988). Induced hypocarbia from hyperventilation may prevent or reverse brain and CSF acidosis, which, in turn, produces vasoconstriction of the precapillary cerebral arterioles and decreases CBF, cerebral blood volume (CBV), and ICP. Because CO_2 readily crosses the blood-brain barrier, there is an immediate reduction in cerebral interstitial CO_2 followed by a reduction in hydrogen ion concentration.

Controlled hyperventilation in the child is achieved with endotracheal intubation, muscle paralysis, and

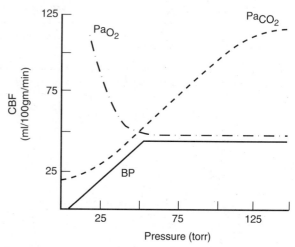

Figure 21–5 ● ● ● ● ● ●

Cerebral blood flow changes due to alterations in $PaCO_2$ (---), PaO_2 (.-.), and blood pressure (_). The other two variables remain stable at normal values when the remaining variable is altered. PaO_2—partial pressure of oxygen, $PaCO_2$—partial pressure of carbon dioxide, BP—blood pressure, CBF—cerebral blood flow. (From Shapiro, H.M. 1975. Intracranial hypertension. Anesthesiology, 43, 446.)

assisted ventilation. Arterial oxygen tension (PaO_2) is kept in a normal range; $PaCO_2$ is kept in a range of 25 to 30 mmHg and pH is kept slightly alkalotic (Marion, Firlik, & McLaughlin, 1995). Only rarely is $PaCO_2$ lowered significantly below this level because of the potential risk of cerebral ischemia. However, Bruce (1989a,b) reported a favorable decrease in ICP when $PaCO_2$ was lowered below 20 mmHg in children. When extreme hyperventilation is needed to decrease ICP, careful monitoring of CBF or cerebral arteriovenous difference of oxygen ($avDo_2$) is recommended (Bruce, 1989a,b; Walleck, 1989; Shapiro & Giller, 1991).

Despite the theoretical benefits of hyperventilation, it is no longer considered first-line therapy and prolonged use is controversial. It is thought that prophylactic hyperventilation may, in some patients, convert borderline cerebral ischemia to frank ischemia (Muizelaar et al., 1991). The beneficial effects of hyperventilation on CSF pH and thus arteriolar diameter are short-lived (less than 24 hours) (Muizelaar et al., 1988). This latter problem is believed to be the result of decreased buffer capacity associated with a low bicarbonate concentration. The cerebral vasculature may be more sensitive to changes in $PaCO_2$, and the patient may not tolerate transient increases in $PaCO_2$ that occur with nursing care, such as position changes or endotracheal suctioning. In short, how long hyperventilation should be maintained and how far $PaCO_2$ should be lowered and still have a beneficial effect are unknown.

Neuromuscular Blockade. Muscular paralysis with neuromuscular blocking agents is often used to facilitate ventilatory control and hyperventilation in the child with intracranial hypertension. Chemical paralyzing agents can also be used to prevent increases in arterial blood pressure associated with isometric muscle contraction (e.g., decerebrate or decorticate posturing) (Mitchell, 1988). Sedatives and analgesics are administered with neuromuscular agents to minimize anxiety and pain.

Anticonvulsants. In the patient with minimal intracranial buffering capacity, small increases in CBF can cause significant increases in ICP. Seizures increase CBF, CBV, and ICP, and therefore are prevented or controlled on an emergent basis. A variety of anticonvulsants are used depending on whether the therapy is to treat status epilepticus, prevent break-through seizures, or be used prophylactically. Electroencephalogram monitoring is necessary to detect seizures in the chemically paralyzed patient.

Barbiturates. Barbiturates have been used to treat intracranial hypertension since the early 1970s (Shapiro et al., 1973). Continuous intravenous infusion of barbiturates to induce coma is reserved for patients in whom conventional therapy has been unsuccessful in controlling intracranial hypertension. Barbiturates decrease ICP by reducing the cerebral metabolic rate, which is followed by a reduction in CBF and CBV (Donegan et al., 1985; Wilberger & Cantella, 1995). The most commonly used barbiturate is pentobarbital. Barbiturate coma is initiated with a loading dose of pentobarbital at 5 to 10 mg/kg followed by a continuous infusion at 1 to 5 mg/kg/hour (Dean, Rogers, & Traystman, 1992; Shapiro & Giller, 1991; Ward et al., 1985). The actual titration dose of a specific barbiturate varies among institutions. Some titrate the dose to a desired serum level, others titrate to obtain burst suppression on electroencephalogram (EEG), and still others titrate to a particular ICP level (Quandt & de los Reyes, 1984; Ward et al., 1985).

Barbiturate therapy is associated with significant cardiac effects: decreased cardiac output, decreased cardiac contractility, dysrhythmias, and subsequent hypotension. When continuous barbiturate therapy is administered, bedside EEG monitoring, as well as close monitoring of arterial blood pressure and thermodilution cardiac output measurements, are necessary. Vasopressors, specifically epinephrine, are often needed to counteract the hypotensive effects of barbiturate use.

Even when barbiturate therapy is successful in controlling ICP, long-term patient outcome has not been commensurately improved (Trauner, 1986; Ward et al., 1985). Few controlled studies exist to substantiate the efficacy of this therapy. As a result, barbiturate therapy is not routinely recommended for all cases of refractory intracranial hypertension.

Brain Volume Reduction. Brain tissue itself can also increase the total intracranial volume. The usual causes include tumors, infections, and edema. In the case of a tumor, definitive therapy is straightforward, at least theoretically, with surgical removal. Brain edema is not a disease entity but the consequence of other neuropathologies (e.g., infections, hypoxic-ischemic insult). Therapy is directed at preventing the development of edema or removing the excess fluid.

There are three types of cerebral edema that de-

velop in response to injury (Fishman, 1975). First, *cytotoxic edema* represents intracellular swelling resulting from hypoxia and ischemia. It reflects neuronal cell death and is not very amenable to therapy. *Vasogenic edema* is clinically the most common type of edema. It results from an alteration in permeability of brain capillary endothelial cells, allowing extravasation of protein-rich plasma into the brain. Vasogenic edema is commonly seen around abscesses, tumors, and hematomas. In contrast to cytotoxic edema, it is more easily treated. *Interstitial edema* results from increased CSF hydrostatic pressure commonly seen with obstructive hydrocephalus. There is transependymal movement of CSF from the ventricular system into adjacent tissue. It is easily treated with shunting procedures.

With many acute brain insults or neuropathologies, cerebral edema may result from a combination of the edema types described earlier. For example, an hypoxic ischemic insult may have components of both cytotoxic and vasogenic edema. Generalized cerebral swelling as a typical pattern of response to severe head injury has been reported (Zimmerman, 1979). However, computed tomography (CT) scan density measurements suggest that the increased brain bulk is not the result of edema but rather to increased blood volume (hyperemia).

Hyperosmolar Therapy. Several osmotic agents have been used to treat intracranial hypertension. It is theorized that they exert their effect by producing an osmotic gradient between the intravascular compartment and the surrounding brain tissue. There is a net influx of water into the bloodstream that is excreted by the kidneys. The end result is a reduction in brain bulk with a decrease in ICP.

Serum osmolality is routinely calculated to monitor hyperosmolar therapy, as well as detect inappropriate antidiuretic hormone (ADH) secretion or diabetes insipidus. Serum osmolality can be calculated by using the following formula:

$$2 \times [\text{Na}^+] + [\text{BUN}]/2.8 + [\text{glucose}]/18$$
(BUN, blood urea nitrogen; Na$^+$, sodium).

Normal serum osmolality is 270 to 290 mOsm/L. With hyperosmolar therapy, serum osmolality is maintained just above the high normal range (300–310 mOsm/L). When serum osmolality is above 320 to 330 mOsm/L there is an increased risk of cerebral infarction and renal tubular damage.

Currently, mannitol (Osmitrol) is the most commonly used osmotic agent to treat intracranial hypertension. In addition to its osmotic effects, there is evidence that mannitol reduces CBV and ICP by causing cerebral vasoconstriction (Muizelaar et al., 1983). It is hypothesized that in patients with intact autoregulation, low to moderate doses of mannitol (less than 1 g/kg) decrease blood viscosity, which causes autoregulatory vasoconstriction of cerebral arterioles. Because decreased blood viscosity reduces resistance to blood flow, CBF remains unchanged (Bullock, 1995; Muizelaar et al., 1984; Muizelaar et al., 1983).

A wide range of mannitol doses (0.25–2.0 g/kg) have been prescribed for either intermittent administration or as a continuous intravenous infusion. However, reports indicate that beneficial effects and fewer side effects are achieved with more frequently administered lower doses of mannitol (McGraw et al., 1978; McGraw & Howard, 1983). Mannitol, administered long-term or in high doses, may eventually move into the interstitial space, reducing or reversing the osmotic gradient between the intravascular and interstitial compartments. This "rebound" effect results in the movement of water into brain tissue.

Osmotic agents are contraindicated in patients with hyperemia associated with traumatic brain injury. In these patients, CBV is already increased and osmotic agents would further increase CBV and ICP. Osmotic agents are also contraindicated in patients with a suspected loss of an intact blood-brain barrier. In this situation, the osmotic agent readily crosses into brain interstitial fluid with a net influx of water into the surrounding brain tissue.

Oral glycerol (Osmoglyn) has been used to treat cerebral edema since the 1960s. However, the oral administration route has limited use in the patient with acute elevation in ICP because of delayed onset of action (30–60 minutes) and gastrointestinal side effects (Quandt & de los Reyes, 1984). Intravenous glycerol is available, but early studies reported severe side effects such as hemoglobinuria, hemolysis, and renal failure (Hagnevik et al., 1974; Gilsanz et al., 1975). More recent evidence shows fewer complications when 10% to 20% solutions are administered over several hours (MacDonald & Uden, 1982; Quandt & de los Reyes, 1984). The recommended intravenous dose of glycerol is 0.5 to 1.0 g/kg every 4 to 6 hours, not to exceed 1 g/kg/hour (Dean et al., 1992; Pitlick et al., 1982).

Clinical use of urea (Ureaphil) is rare today (Bullock, 1995). Urea is believed to cross the blood-brain barrier more readily than either mannitol and glycerol (Quandt & de los Reyes, 1984). Thus, there is a higher incidence of a "rebound" effect in intracranial pressure.

Diuretics. Furosemide (Lasix) is a potent loop diuretic that has been found to effectively lower ICP in some cases (Cottrell et al., 1977). Several mechanisms are thought to be responsible for the observed lowering of ICP: total reduction in body fluids, inhibition of CSF production, and a direct reduction in sodium transport into the brain (Cottrell et al., 1977; Wilkinson & Rosenfeld, 1983). Lasix has been successfully used alone and in combination with osmotic diuretics and oncotic agents (Wilkinson & Rosenfeld, 1983; Quandt & de los Reyes, 1984). It is used most successfully in patients with head injury and pulmonary edema or when used based upon pulmonary artery hemodynamic data (Bullock, 1995). The usual dose of Lasix in children is 0.5 to 1.0 mg/kg (Dean et al., 1992).

Corticosteroids. The utility of steroids in the treatment of intracranial hypertension is unclear. The theoretical basis for the use of steroids stems from its success in treating intracranial hypertension from neuropathologies (e.g., tumors, discrete hematomas) associated with vasogenic edema (French & Galicich, 1964). The exact mechanism of action is unknown. The use of high-dose steroids in the treatment of severe head injury has been found to have no beneficial effect (Braakman et al., 1983; Dearden et al., 1986). Furthermore, Dearden and coworkers (1986) reported a poorer outcome, assessed at 6 months with the Glasgow Outcome Scale, among head-injured patients with elevated ICP receiving steroids. Thus, steroid therapy is usually reserved for conditions associated with vasogenic edema.

Fluid and Electrolyte Monitoring. Fluid and electrolyte status is assessed in the patient with intracranial hypertension. In some patients, fluid intake is restricted to one-half to one-third maintenance to induce a mild dehydration state. It is thought that extracellular fluid will be reduced in all body tissue (including the brain) and thus intracranial pressure will decrease. The patient's hemodynamic status is closely monitored to prevent marked hypovolemia, which could compromise mean arterial pressure (MAP) and, subsequently, CPP.

Although hypotonic intravenous solutions are avoided, evidence supports the use of hypertonic intravenous solutions to reduce ICP (Gunnar et al., 1988; Prough et al., 1985). Fisher and coworkers (1992) compared the effects of 3% saline and 0.9% saline on IICP in children with traumatic brain injury. Three percent saline significantly reduced elevated ICP in patients compared with 0.9% solution. Intravascular dehydration did not occur during the study period, a more common risk with the use of diuretics and hyperosmotic agents.

Fluid and electrolyte imbalances may also occur in patients with neurologic dysfunction. Common etiologies include syndrome of inappropriate antidiuretic hormone (SIADH) secretion and diabetes insipidus. Serum and urine electrolytes and osmolalities are monitored.

Cerebrospinal Fluid Volume Reduction. Mechanisms that increase CSF volume may also cause elevated ICP. These mechanisms include increased CSF production, decreased CSF absorption, or obstruction of CSF circulation.

Cerebrospinal Fluid Drainage. Ventricular shunting is standard therapy for increased ICP related to hydrocephalus. In other situations, an intraventricular catheter may be placed in one of the lateral ventricles in patients with acute intracranial hypertension. The catheter is used to drain CSF to avoid significant increases in ICP (See Chapter 12). Ventricular drainage may be intermittent or continuous, depending on the size of the ventricles and the type of neuropathology.

Reduce Cerebrospinal Fluid Production. Cerebrospinal fluid formation can be reduced by a number of drugs. Medications that have been shown to transiently reduce ICP by slowing CSF production include acetazolamide (Diamox) and furosemide (Lasix). However, the efficacy of these agents for long-term control of ICP is unproven (Bruce, 1989a,b).

Nursing Care: Decreased Adaptive Capacity

Decreased adaptive capacity, intracranial, is a nursing diagnosis proposed by Mitchell (1986) to describe failure of normal intracranial compensatory mechanisms. It occurs in patients with intracranial hypertension, but is not synonymous with this pathophysiologic state. Rather, its use identifies patients at risk for disproportionate increases in ICP in response to a variety of nursing care activities. Nursing interventions are designed to reduce intracranial adaptive demands and increase adaptive capacity.

The goals for managing decreased intracranial adaptive capacity are to reduce intracranial volume and improve intracranial compliance. A number of nursing care activities have been shown to alter ICP (Farley, 1990; Hobdell et al., 1989). However, the patient's response to a specific nursing care measure is often variable and depends on the patient's intracranial compliance at a given point in time. Thus, all nursing interventions are specific to the patient. In addition to serial neurologic assessments, there are a number of independent nursing interventions that can be used to reduce adaptive demand (i.e., decrease CBV and CSF volume) and increase adaptive capacity (i.e., shift the intracranial volume/pressure [V/P] curve to the left).

Maintain Oxygenation and Ventilation. To avoid cerebral vasodilation, hypercarbia and hypoxemia are avoided or corrected expeditiously when they occur. Nursing measures to prevent hypercarbia and hypoxemia include maintaining a patent airway and judicious, careful airway suctioning. While considerable variation in patient response to suctioning does exist, routine suctioning of patients has been shown to increase ICP, presumably resulting from tracheal stimulation, hypercarbia, or hypoxemia (Fisher et al., 1982; Perlman & Volpe, 1983). Thus, suctioning is to be reserved for documented cases of accumulated airway secretions. The exact suctioning procedure is chosen according to patient response. However, usual steps in the procedure include preoxygenation with an FiO_2 of 1.0, limiting the suction time to less than 10 seconds per catheter insertion, and limiting the number of passes to two per procedure (Drummond, 1990; Hickey, 1986; Hobdell et al., 1989; Rudy et al., 1991).

Several investigators have found intravenous lidocaine (1.5 mg/kg) given 1 to 2 minutes before suctioning to be effective in blunting increases in ICP related to endotracheal suctioning (Donegan & Bedford, 1980; Yano et al., 1986). Yano and coworkers (1986) found that whereas both intravenous and endotracheal routes were effective, endotracheal tube (ETT) administration of lidocaine was significantly more effective in suppressing IICP associated with endotracheal suctioning. Few data are available comparing the relative effectiveness of other medications in preventing increases in ICP associated with endotracheal suctioning. White and coworkers (1982) found thiopental (Pentothal) 3 mg/kg and fentanyl 1 mcg/kg to be ineffective in altering an increase in ICP associated with endotracheal suctioning. However, this same study did find that succinylcholine (Anectine, Quelicin) 1 mg/kg was effective in blunting ICP associated with suctioning.

Serial monitoring of the patient's respiratory status allows for early detection of impaired oxygenation and ventilation. Respiratory rate, depth, and pattern should be regular. Breath sounds should be clear bilaterally without adventitious breath sounds. Further diagnostic monitoring includes the use of pulse oximetry, end-tidal CO_2 ($ETCO_2$) monitoring, and serial arterial blood gas (ABG) measurement.

Promote Venous Outflow. Patient position has a dramatic impact on CBV and ICP by altering venous outflow from the cranium. Nursing interventions that promote venous outflow from the cranium and may help to prevent increases in ICP include maintaining the head in the midline position, avoiding extreme flexion of the hips and neck, log rolling the patient while turning, and elevating the head of bed 15 to 30 degrees. Extreme elevation of the head of the bed is discouraged because of the possibility of compromising CPP and CBF. Rosner and Coley (1986) reported that the CPP declines as head elevation increases because of hydrostatic decreases in systemic arterial blood pressure as the head is positioned above the heart. These authors further state that as CPP reduction occurs, vasodilation follows, which increases CBV then ICP, further decreasing CPP and resulting in a vicious cycle. Thus, elevation of the head of the bed is individually determined in each patient while monitoring both ICP and CPP.

An increase in intra-abdominal or intrathoracic pressure can also impede cerebral venous outflow. Nursing measures to prevent or minimize increased abdominal and intrathoracic pressure include gastric decompression and prevention of coughing, gagging, vomiting, and a Valsalva maneuver. In addition, isometric muscle activity should be avoided and replaced with passive range of motion. Mechanical or manual ventilation with high tidal volume and positive end-expiratory pressure (PEEP) may also increase ICP and require close monitoring of the patient's response. Any procedure that normally requires the use of the Trendelenburg position (e.g., central line insertion, postural drainage) is avoided. In general, the need for any intervention that has the potential to obstruct venous outflow is assessed. Later, when the patient is able to tolerate enteral feedings, it is important to avoid gastric residuals, administer stool softeners, and maintain good hydration to prevent constipation and straining.

Minimize Noxious Stimuli. Many routine nursing interventions used to care for the child with IICP are unpleasant and painful and may cause elevations (spikes) in ICP (Boortz-Marx, 1985; Parsons et al., 1983). Painful procedures are minimized, physiologic pain controlled, and environmental stressors (e.g., loud noises, jarring of the bed, conversations about the patient) avoided. When noxious activities cannot be avoided, therapeutic touch may be used (Hickey,

1986; Walleck, 1989). Mitchell and coworkers (1985) studied the effect of touch on ICP in 13 children. They noted occasional, rather profound decreases in ICP with stabilization following parental stroking.

Data are conflicting when comparing the effects of rest between planned nursing care activities and clustering of care activities at one time (Bruya, 1981; Parsons et al., 1983). Because not all patients respond to noxious stimuli or to clustering of nursing care activities in the same way, specific nursing interventions and how and when they are performed are individually determined for each patient. Risks versus benefits need to be determined when identifying priorities in nursing care for a patient with intracranial hypertension. In patients who cannot tolerate multiple nursing care activities (i.e., respond with sustained elevations in ICP), nursing interventions are restricted to required care, eliminating less critical interventions.

Pain management in the patient with an alteration in consciousness is challenging. Pain assessment is often restricted to physiologic responses (e.g., increased heart rate, blood pressure, and ICP). Pain is especially detrimental in the patient with intracranial hypertension because pain can further increase ICP. Concern is often raised over pharmacologic management of pain because of blunting effects on neurologic assessment and potential decrease in mean arterial pressure and thus CPP. However, if the patient can perceive pain, appropriate analgesics are required to prevent further increases in ICP.

Control Cerebral Metabolism. Many patients with IICP cannot tolerate an increase in cerebral metabolism. Thus, any actual or potential situation that increases cerebral metabolism is monitored and aggressively treated. Core temperature is monitored frequently, and normothermia is maintained. If hyperthermia develops, the etiology is investigated and treated while the hyperthermic condition is reversed. Acetaminophen and a cooling blanket may be used to treat hyperthermia. Shivering is always prevented. Based upon recent clinical and laboratory work, there is renewed interest in the use of moderate systemic hypothermia (32°C) to protect the brain from secondary injury (Clifton, 1995; Prendergast, 1994).

Seizures may occur in patients with neurologic dysfunction. This complication significantly increases cerebral metabolism and may cause an uncoupling or imbalance of cerebral metabolic supply and demand. Further ischemic damage and elevated ICP may develop. Patients, especially if they are chemically paralyzed, are assessed closely for signs of seizure activity. If seizure activity does occur, oxygenation and ventilation requirements are met, and anticonvulsants are promptly administered.

Promote CSF Drainage. Most interventions to control CSF volume are collaboratively managed medical therapies. However, Mitchell (1988) demonstrates that patient position can transiently increase CSF obstruction. Body positions that obstruct venous outflow also obstruct CSF flow between the cranial and spinal subarachnoid spaces. A side-lying position with a neutral position of the head is recommended.

Even though the majority of nursing interventions are directed toward reducing adaptive demands, a few nursing interventions may improve intracranial compliance. Farley (1990) reviewed the literature and reported the stabilization of ICP with therapeutic touch. Preoxygenation and premedication with lidocaine prior to suctioning may also transiently improve intracranial compliance so that adaptive capacity is not reduced during a noxious stimulus (Mitchell, 1988).

Associated Pathologies

A number of neuropathologies can increase ICP by increasing one or more of the three volume components of the intracranial space. Common diseases or conditions among patients seen in the pediatric intensive care unit (PICU) that potentially increase ICP are status epilepticus and arteriovenous malformations (increased CBV); intracranial tumors, meningitis, and encephalitis (increased brain tissue); and hydrocephalus (increased CSF). There are also a large number of patients admitted to the PICU because of traumatic head injuries. Traumatic brain injury can potentially increase CBV, brain tissue, or CSF, resulting in IICP on a multidimensional basis.

Increased Cerebral Blood Volume

Status Epilepticus. A seizure is not a disease itself, but is a symptom of a number of diseases and conditions. Seizures represent a sudden abnormal electrical discharge from neurons within the cerebral cortex that produce a disturbance in behavior, sensation, or motor function. Status epilepticus is defined as "an epileptic seizure that is sufficiently prolonged or repeated at sufficiently brief intervals so as to produce an unvarying and enduring epileptic condition" (Gastaut, 1973). Minimum actual duration of a seizure necessary for definition as status epilepticus varies; however, most authorities use 30 minutes as the minimum duration.

The exact incidence of status epilepticus is unknown because it is not a reportable disease and it is not classified consistently among reported series. It is estimated that 60,000 to 160,000 persons in the United States have at least one episode of status epilepticus (Delgado-Escueta et al., 1982). The potential or actual causes of status epilepticus are numerous and include fever, CNS infection, inborn errors of metabolism, traumatic subarachnoid hemorrhage, metabolic derangements, CNS trauma, and anoxic-ischemic insult (Aicardi & Chevrie, 1970). The first four etiologies are unique to children (Lockman, 1990; Tasker & Dean, 1992). In many cases the etiology is unknown. Aicardi and Chevrie (1970) reviewed 239 cases of status epilepticus and found that approximately one-half of the cases were of idiopathic origin. In patients with known epilepsy, a frequent

Table 21-2. THE INTERNATIONAL CLASSIFICATION OF EPILEPTIC SEIZURES

I. **Partial (focal, local) seizures**
   A. Simple partial seizures (consciousness not impaired)
      1. With motor symptoms
      2. With somatosensory or special sensory symptoms
      3. With autonomic symptoms
      4. With psychic symptoms
   B. Complex partial seizures (with impairment of consciousness)
      1. Beginning as simple partial seizures and progressing to impairment of consciousness
      2. With impairment of consciousness at onset
   C. Partial seizures evolving to secondarily generalized seizures
      1. Simple partial seizures evolving to generalized seizures
      2. Complex partial seizures evolving into generalized seizures
      3. Simple partial seizures evolving to complex partial seizures to generalized seizures
II. **Generalized seizures (convulsive or nonconvulsive)**
   A. Absence seizures
      1. Absence seizures
      2. Atypical absence seizures
   B. Myoclonic seizures
   C. Clonic seizures
   D. Tonic seizures
   E. Tonic-clonic seizures
   F. Atonic seizures (astatic seizures)
III. **Unclassified epileptic seizures**
   Includes all seizures that cannot be classified because of inadequate or incomplete data and some that defy classification in hitherto described categories. This includes some neonatal seizures, e.g., rhythmic eye movements, chewing and swimming movements.

Adapted with permission from Dreifuss F. E. (1989). Classification of epileptic seizures and the epilepsies. *Pediatric Clinics of North America* 36, 265.

cause of status epilepticus is abrupt discontinuation of anticonvulsant drugs or a suboptimal drug level. Age is also related to the incidence of status epilepticus, with the average age in children being younger than three years (Dunn, 1990).

A number of classification systems have been used to categorize seizures according to clinical manifesta-tions, electrical activity, etiology, or response to therapy. The International Classification of Epileptic Seizures categorizes seizures according to the clinical nature of the onset of the seizure. Two major categories include generalized and partial seizures. Generalized tonic-clonic status epilepticus is the most common form in children. Table 21-2 provides a list of categories of epileptic seizures.

Pathogenesis. Injury to the CNS associated with status epilepticus can occur from one of three causes: acute insult precipitating the seizure, systemic effects from prolonged or repeated seizures, and injury from repeated electrical discharges within the CNS (Tasker & Dean, 1992). The specific effects of a prolonged seizure or repeated seizures on the developing human brain are unknown. Reports of systemic alterations and neurophysiologic changes associated with status epilepticus are for the most part based on adult studies and animal models. Table 21-3 summarizes the physiologic changes associated with seizures and status epilepticus.

If a seizure is allowed to progress beyond a critical point, cerebral blood flow may become inadequate to meet the increased metabolic demand of the brain. An uncoupling of cerebral oxygen supply and demand occurs with neuronal damage. In the patient with preexisting increased intracranial pressure, the increase in CBF associated with a seizure can cause further increases in ICP with herniation.

Clinical Manifestations. A significant number of patients in the PICU have the potential to develop seizures. Seizure activity associated with status epilepticus is most often described as generalized clonic (alternating rigidity and relaxation), tonic-clonic (muscle contraction with clonus), or unilateral clonic (Aicardi & Chevrie, 1970). During the tonic phase, signs and symptoms reflect autonomic overactivity: salivation, pupillary dilation, tachycardia, and increased blood pressure. Apneic episodes may occur, but are usually short in duration. In the postictal period, the patient is usually drowsy or sleeping, followed by lethargy and confusion.

In the patient with intracranial hypertension,

Table 21-3. PHYSIOLOGIC CHANGES ASSOCIATED WITH SEIZURES AND STATUS EPILEPTICUS

Parameter	Seizures		Status Epilepticus	Complications
Blood pressure	↑		↓	Shock
PaO_2		↓		Hypoxia
$PaCO_2$	↑		↓ →	↑ ICP
pH	↓		↓ →	Acidosis
Temperature		↑		Fever/hyperpyrexia
Autonomic activity		↑		Dysrhythmia
Pulmonary secretions		↑		Atelectasis shunt
K^+		↑		Dysrhythmias
CPK and myoglobin	Normal		↑	Renal failure
CBF	↑ (550%)		↑ (200%)	Intracranial hemorrhage
$CMRO_2$	↑ (300%)		↑ (300%)	Neuronal death
Blood glucose	↑		↓	Hypoglycemia, neuronal cell injury or death

CPK, creatinine phosphokinase; CBF, cerebral blood flow; $CMRO_2$, cerebral metabolic rate (O_2 consumption).
Modified with permission from Fuhrman, B. P., Zimmerman, J. J. *Pediatric Critical Care,* (p. 596). St. Louis: Mosby–YearBook, 1992.

signs and symptoms of cerebral herniation may be present. The chemically paralyzed patient experiencing a seizure may develop a sudden onset of tachycardia, systemic hypertension, elevated ICP and, occasionally, pupil dilatation.

The EEG is useful in evaluating some patients with seizures. Because generalized convulsive status epilepticus is easily diagnosed clinically, an ictal EEG is rarely helpful (Holmes, 1987). However, if there is any question regarding the seizure type, an EEG is done immediately. The sooner the EEG is obtained, the greater the likelihood a specific abnormality can be identified (Tauner, 1988). Continuous EEG monitoring is often used in patients considered to be at high risk for seizure activity.

Collaborative Management. Once the patient's airway is stabilized, oxygenation maintained, and perfusion is adequate, anticonvulsant therapy is initiated. The three most common classes of anticonvulsants used in children are benzodiazepines, phenytoin, and barbiturates. Table 21–4 lists the most commonly used anticonvulsants for status epilepticus.

When status epilepticus is refractory to conventional anticonvulsant therapy, a number of other therapies have been recommended. Refractory status epilepticus was controlled in one study with repeated bolus doses of 5 to 20 mg/kg of phenobarbital (Crawford et al., 1988). Other proposed methods of treating refractory status epilepticus include continuous intravenous infusion of diazepam or lorazepam, rectal paraldehyde or sodium valproate, and general anesthesia (Bell & Bertino, 1984; Lacey, 1988; Lowenstein et al., 1988). General anesthesia has included both intravenous (e.g., thiopental and pentobarbital) and inhalation agents (e.g., halothane). Methods, choice, and duration of anesthesia are variable.

Nursing Care. The goals in managing care of a child with status epilepticus are to ensure adequate cardiorespiratory function, reverse seizure activity, and assist in the identification and treatment of etiologic and precipitating factors. When observing a child during a seizure, specific assessments are noted (Fig. 21–6, pp. 668 and 669).

Initial management ensures adequate oxygenation and ventilation. The child's body is rolled to the side to facilitate drainage of secretions. If the airway is obstructed with secretions, the mouth is suctioned. Hard objects are not forced into the mouth. Oxygen is administered promptly. Frequently, patients in status epilepticus require intubation. For the patient who has recently eaten, intubation is performed using rapid-sequence induction.

The next step is directed toward protecting the patient from injury. The child is positioned to avoid injury, and the use of restraints is limited. Hard toys and other objects are removed from the child's bed and the siderails are padded.

Once intravenous access is secured, blood is obtained for study. Capillary blood is tested for glucose, and dextrose 25% in water is administered for hypoglycemia. A number of anticonvulsants may be required to stop the seizure.

Hyperthermia is commonly associated with status epilepticus. When present, antipyretics and sponging with tepid water is helpful.

Arteriovenous Malformations. Arteriovenous malformations (AVM) of the brain are anomalous connections between arteries and veins without an interposed capillary bed. Figure 21–7 (p. 669) is a drawing of an AVM over the cerebral cortex. AVMs vary in size from a few millimeters in diameter to more than 10 cm (Menkes, 1990). An AVM is characteristically cone-shaped with thin-walled vessels. Although the actual incidence of intracranial AVMs is unknown, there are approximately 2000 new cases identified each year (Williams, 1985).

Pathogenesis. Arteriovenous malformations occur early in fetal development from failure of capillaries to develop. Blood is shunted directly from the artery into the vein. As the child's brain grows, additional arterial contributions are acquired. The size of the vessels increases because they offer less resistance to blood flow than the surrounding vascular beds with capillaries (Dembo, 1982). As the AVM enlarges, blood is diverted from adjacent brain tissue (steal effect), resulting in tissue hypoxia (Vaiden & White, 1987). Gliosis (scarring) of the surrounding tissue from focal hemorrhage or ischemia is common. Neu-

Table 21–4. INITIAL ANTICONVULSANTS TO CONTROL STATUS EPILEPTICUS

Drug	Dose	Rate of Administration	Time to Effect	Side Effects
Rapid-Acting Agents				
Diazepam* (undiluted)	Begin 0.25 mg/kg IV and titrate to effect	<1 mg/min	1–2 min	Respiratory depression; thrombophlebitis
Lorazepam 2 mg/mL	0.1 mg/kg × 4, 20 min apart, max 4 mg	1 mg/min	2–3 min	Drowsiness, confusion, ataxia
Midazolam	0.075 mg/kg IV			Same as above; respiratory depression
Longer-Acting Agents				
Phenytoin 50 mg/mL; dilute in normal saline 1:10	15 mg/kg, up to 45 mg/kg	20–50 mg/min	~20 min	Heart block; hypotension
Phenobarbital 130 mg/mL	10 mg/kg, up to 30 mg/kg	30 mg/min	10–12 min	Respiratory depression; hypotension

Used with permission from Blumer, J. L. *A Practical Guide to Pediatric Intensive Care* (3rd ed.) (1990). Chicago, Mosby–YearBook, 1990.

rologic symptoms and dysfunction can occur as a result of direct compression of brain tissue. Hydrocephalus can develop from obstruction of CSF pathways or from extension of the AVM into the choroid plexus (Hickey, 1986). Intracranial hemorrhage is the most life-threatening complication.

Clinical Manifestations. Only half of patients with a known AVM are symptomatic, with the majority of manifestations presenting in adulthood (Menkes, 1990). The usual presentation of an AVM is from intracranial hemorrhage, a seizure, or symptoms associated with a space-occupying lesion. In children, spontaneous subarachnoid, intracerebral, or intraventricular hemorrhages are the most common initial manifestation (Golden, 1989; Humphreys, 1989; Menkes, 1990). With a hemorrhage, the child may present with a history of intermittent headaches or a sudden severe headache. Manifestations of meningeal irritation are common with a subarachnoid hemorrhage. Rapid deterioration in level of consciousness usually occurs with hemorrhage into the ventricular system (Humphreys, 1989). Focal neurologic deficits may also develop and are related to the location of the hemorrhage.

A seizure is the next most common initial manifestation of an AVM. The seizure may be simple or complex and focal or general. Seizures occur presumably from ischemic changes in tissue surrounding the AVM.

Less commonly, initial clinical manifestations of an AVM include headache, vomiting, developmental delay, visual disturbances, progressive hemiparesis, behavioral abnormalities, and hydrocephalus. Congestive heart failure is usually the presenting sign in the neonate because of the large runoff in the AVM producing increased blood return to the heart and high-output failure (Wiggins et al., 1991).

Bruits have been auscultated over the head in as many as 50% of children with an intracranial AVM. A cranial bruit in infants younger than 4 months of age almost always represents an AVM (Golden, 1989). In neonates, the bruit is loud, harsh, and best heard over the fontanels (Wiggins et al., 1991). A dural AVM is more likely to be auscultated than an intracranial AVM because of its close proximity to the skull. Bruits are less commonly audible in older children and adults.

The two studies most commonly used to diagnose an AVM are CT and arteriography. The CT scan can outline the blood clot and, on enhanced study, may detail feeding and draining vessels. Cerebral arteriography is the procedure of choice and most clearly identifies the numbers, size, and location of arterial feeders and draining vascular channels. Magnetic resonance imaging (MRI) can demonstrate flowing blood in AVMs and associated hematomas, but does not eliminate the need for angiography.

Collaborative Management. A number of treatment modalities are available to manage the child with an AVM. They include conservative medical management, surgical excision, radiation, embolization, and laser therapy. The specific strategy selected

depends on the size and location of the AVM, age of the patient, physician preference, cerebral dominance, technical support, condition of the patient, and characteristics of feeder vessels supplying the AVM.

Conservative management entails close observation without surgical intervention. The AVM is allowed to take its natural course. Investigators in one study reviewed 191 cases with cerebral AVM and found the average yearly risk for first hemorrhage between 2% and 3%. Risk of rebleeding increased with advancing age (Graf et al., 1983). The risk of death with each hemorrhage is 20% to 30% (Guertin, 1992).

Total surgical excision of an AVM is ideal, but is not always possible because of an inaccessible location. A rare but major complication of surgical excision is a phenomenon known as "normal perfusion pressure break-through" (McNair, 1988). It is characterized by massive dilation of vessels around the AVM and loss of autoregulation in these vessels. Without autoregulation, increased blood flow under high pressure occurs, resulting in cerebral edema or hemorrhage. This complication may be reduced with a staged surgical approach (i.e., removal of the AVM by surgical excision or embolization with more than one operation).

Proton-beam radiation is done as a stereotactic procedure and is noninvasive. Stereotactic neurosurgery employs a mechanical device to precisely position probes, electrodes, radiation, and other instruments in three-dimensional space. It is usually recommended for surgically inaccessible AVMs. Proton irradiation causes thickening of the vascular elements of the AVM with gradual shrinkage. There is minimal risk to the patient, and hospitalization time is short. The disadvantages are that it may take up to 2 years for optimal effects to occur, and the procedure may not completely eliminate the AVM.

Embolization of the AVM may also be recommended for surgically inaccessible lesions. This technique is usually done using a femoral artery approach. A catheter is advanced from the cervical area into one of the carotid vessels, depending on the feeder vessel of the AVM. The tip of the catheter is then positioned as close as is possible to the area requiring embolization. Embolization material is injected and carried by blood flow until it occludes a vessel. Total occlusion of an AVM may not be possible, but the lesion may be reduced to a more optimal size for surgical excision (Willis & Harbit, 1990).

Laser therapy is an alternative therapy for inaccessible lesions. Stereotactic technique is used to locate the target tissue so that the laser can be focused on a particular area. The light beam causes photocoagulation of vessels in the AVM with subsequent shrinkage of vessels (Hickey, 1986; McNair, 1988).

Nursing Care. In the patient with a suspected AVM without hemorrhage, nursing assessment and management is directed toward prevention of intracranial bleeding. An initial baseline neurologic assessment is performed, followed by serial assess-

DIRECTIONS:

1. Place date, time and duration of seizure in appropriate space.
2. Place (√) under all statements that apply. Only check statements that best describe the seizure.
3. The person witnessing the seizure should enter information on this record.
4. If you need to further explain the seizure, place (X) and describe on back of this sheet.
5. Place your initials in appropriate column.

ONSET							SEIZURE													POST ICTAL				SIGNATURE
Date	Time	Activity Before Seizure	Aura	Focal eyes, mouth, one area of body	Generalized	Focal Progressing to Generalized	Tonic Clonic	Tonic	Clonic	Brief Sudden Jerk	Less of Muscle Tone (drops)	Staring or Blinking	Chewing up Smacking	Unusual Behavior	Level of Consciousness	Eyes	Other: Incontinent vomit, tongue biting	Duration	Recovery Time	Sleep	Changes Behavior	Paralysis	

Figure 21–6 ● ● ● ● ● ●
See legend on opposite page

ments. If the child has a large AVM with a high risk for bleeding, special precautions are taken—maintenance of strict bedrest, control of hypertension, and provision of a quiet environment. If hemorrhage has occurred, signs and symptoms of intracranial hypertension are assessed and monitored. Management of intracranial hypertension has been discussed earlier. The principles of post-craniotomy nursing care are discussed in a later section on brain tumors.

If embolization therapy is performed using a femoral artery, post-procedure care is similar to post–cardiac catherization care. The leg is immobilized and the patient remains on bedrest for 24 hours. The catheter site dressing is assessed for bleeding. Distal

pulses and vital signs are monitored closely until stable.

Increased Brain Tissue

Brain Tumors. Primary intracranial tumors are the second most common form of childhood cancer and the most common solid tumor (Cohen & Duffner, 1989; Guertin, 1992). Various types of intracranial tumors have been identified in children, with astrocytomas having the highest incidence followed by medulloblastomas and ependymomas (Duffner et al., 1985). The majority of brain tumors in children are located in the posterior fossa.

GUIDELINES FOR SEIZURE RECORD DOCUMENTATION

Onset

1. Activity before seizure:	Describe what patient was doing, i.e., running, watching TV, sleeping, etc.
2. Aura:	Anything noticed at the start of the seizure activity. Example: bizarre behavior, chewing and lip smacking, yelling, sees lights, hears noises, etc.
3. Focal:	Only one area of the body involved. (Record area.)
4. Generalized:	Entire body involved.
5. Focal to generalized:	Begins in one area and progresses to involve the entire body (describe).

Seizure Activity

1. Tonic:	Becomes tense or stiff (arms and legs in extension).
2. Clonic:	Rapid rhythmic jerking/flexion of extremities.
3. Tonic/Clonic:	Tonic followed by clonic phase (may be repeated several times).
4. Brief sudden jerk:	Myoclonic jerks—may be focal or generalized.
5. Loss of muscle tone:	Example: falls to floor or slumps forward, remains limp.
6. Staring:	Does not respond to name. No blink response. Stares into space. May be seen alone or with eye blinking or other activity. (describe)
7. Chewing and lip smacking:	Check if present. (describe)
8. Unusual behavior:	Screaming, biting, pulling at clothing, non-purposeful behavior, etc. (describe)
9. Level of consciousness:	Unresponsive, confused, easily aroused, responds to commands.
10. Eyes:	Describe eye movements. Example: roll up, roll to side, nystagmus, etc. Status of pupils.
11. Other:	Incontinent, vomit, tongue biting.
12. Duration:	Time from onset of seizure activity to cessation of seizure activity.

Post-ictal State

1. Recovery time:	In seconds, minutes, etc.
2. Sleep:	Duration
3. Changes in behavior:	Becomes aggressive, fighting, combative, etc.
4. Paralysis:	Location, type (weakness or flaccidity) duration.
Staff Initials:	Initials of person witnessing seizure; complete name placed on back of sheet.
Right Margin:	Addressograph
If:	you do not see the onset of the seizure, write (unobserved) across the onset spaces.
If:	you are guessing at the duration of the seizure, write "approximately (time)" in duration column.

Figure 21–6 ● ● ● ● ● ● *Continued*

Seizure flow record. (Developed by Sarah M. Vaughn, RN, MSN; while a Pediatric Clinical Nurse Specialist at Baystate Medical Center, Springfield, Massachusetts.)

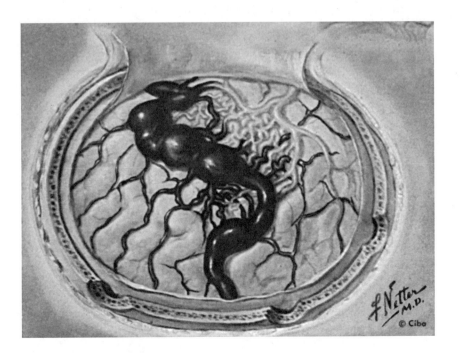

Figure 21–7 ● ● ● ● ● ●

AVM over the cerebral cortex. (© Copyright 1996. CIBA-GEIGY Corporation. Reprinted with permission from the Ciba Collection of Medical Illustrations, illustrated by Frank Netter, M.D. All rights reserved.)

Table 21–5. CLASSIFICATION OF BRAIN TUMORS IN CHILDREN

   I. Tumors of neuroepithelial tissue
      A. Glial tumors
      B. Neuronal tumors
      C. "Primitive" neuroepithelial tumors
      D. Pineal cell tumors
  II. Tumors of meningeal and related tissue
      A. Meningiomas
      B. Meningeal sarcomatous tumors
      C. Primary melanocytic tumors
 III. Tumors of nerve sheath cells
      A. Neurilemmoma
      B. Anaplastic neurilemmoma (schwannoma, neurinoma)
      C. Neurofibroma
      D. Anaplastic neurofibroma
  IV. Primary malignant lymphomas
   V. Tumors of blood vessel origin
  VI. Germ cell tumors
      A. Germinoma
      B. Embryonal carcinoma
      C. Choriocarcinoma
      D. Endodermal sinus tumor
      E. Teratomatous tumors
      F. Mixed
 VII. Malformative tumors
VIII. Tumors of neuroendocrine origin
  IX. Local extensions from regional tumors
   X. Metastatic tumors
  XI. Unclassified tumors

Adapted from Rorke L. B., et al. (1985). Revision of the WHO classification of brain tumors for childhood brain tumors. *Cancer* 56:1869.

A universally accepted histologic classification system for brain tumors does not exist. The most extensively used classification system was developed by the World Health Organization (WHO) and grades tumors based on site, histologic type, and degree of malignancy. In 1985, this classification system was modified to specifically address CNS tumors in children (Rorke et al., 1985). Table 21–5 is an abbreviated list of this revised classification of brain tumors.

Cerebellar astrocytomas represent approximately one-third of all posterior fossa tumors (Duffner et al., 1985; Sutton & Schut, 1989). They are derived from astrocytic neuroglial cells and typically consist of a single large cyst with a solid mural nodule.

Supratentorial astrocytomas are the most common form of supratentorial tumor (Duffner et al., 1985). Supratentorial astrocytomas are classified according to four grades that reflect their increasing tendency toward malignancy. Grades I and II are considered low-grade astrocytomas with a better outcome than grades III and IV.

Medulloblastoma is the most common tumor of the posterior fossa and accounts for 15% to 20% of intracranial tumors (Laurent & Cheek, 1986). Of all childhood tumors, it has shown the greatest improvement in survival. This rapidly growing tumor usually arises from midline cerebellar tissue in close contiguity to the fourth ventricle.

Ependymomas are derived from ependymal cells and may arise from any part of the ventricular system. Ependymomas occur more frequently in young children and most often are located in the fourth ventricle.

In contrast, ependymomas in older children and adolescents are more often located in the lateral ventricles (Hendrick & Raffel, 1989; Duffner et al., 1985).

Pathogenesis. The molecular and cellular origins of CNS tumors are not clear in all cases. There is evidence that genetic factors may play a role in the development of some tumors. Other tumors (e.g., craniopharyngiomas, some medulloblastomas) are congenital and may represent maldevelopment (Menkes & Till, 1990). The immune system may also play a role in the development of CNS tumors (Rudy, 1984). The effects of teratogens and other environmental factors in predisposing the brain to tumors is unclear.

The pathophysiology of intracranial tumors is based on an expanding mass that increases the intracranial volume. The expanding mass compresses and distorts adjacent tissue, compromises CBF, and obstructs CSF circulation. Left untreated, ischemic and herniation syndromes develop, resulting in death.

Clinical Manifestations. Clinical manifestations of CNS tumors can be classified into general and localized findings. General findings represent all of the potential signs and symptoms associated with increasing intracranial pressure. Classic signs and symptoms of increased ICP in a child with a posterior fossa tumor is one in which the child has flu-like gastrointestinal symptoms for several mornings. The symptoms resolve and are absent for several weeks followed by a return of symptoms that are more intense (Duffner et al., 1985). Localized symptoms vary and depend on the location and degree of involvement of the tumor. Table 21–6 highlights the clinical manifestations of brain tumors based on location.

The diagnostic evaluation of the child suspected of having a brain tumor is accomplished with CT scanning or MRI. Ancillary studies may be used to further evaluate the tumor. These studies include arteriogra-

Table 21–6. CLINICAL MANIFESTATIONS OF BRAIN TUMORS, ACCORDING TO LOCATION

Frontal lobe	Seizures
	Motor weakness
	Personality and behavioral changes
Parietal lobe	Perceptual problems
	Sensory disturbance
	Dyslexia
Occipital lobe	Visual disturbance
Temporal lobe	Auditory disturbance
	Impaired memory
	Visual field deficits
	Dysarthria
	Personality changes
Midline	Visual loss
	Endocrinopathies
	Nonlocalizing signs of IICP
	Personality changes
Cerebellum	Gait, balance, and coordination disturbance
Brain stem	Cranial neuropathies
	Hydrocephalus
	Hemiparesis/quadriparesis
	Late IICP
	Hyper/hypothermia

IICP, Increased intracranial pressure.

phy, EEG, plain skull films, ultrasound (infants), and position emission tomography (PET).

Collaborative Management. Standard medical management of childhood brain tumors involves one or more of the following therapies: surgery, radiation, and chemotherapy. Even though surgery has many limitations (e.g., accessibility, damage to adjacent tissues), it remains the procedure of choice for most brain tumors. Total removal of the tumor is usually not possible, but debulking surgery improves the effectiveness of radiation therapy and chemotherapy, as well as providing palliation of symptoms from mechanical obstruction or compression. In addition, tumor specimens can be obtained for histologic evaluation and more accurate chemotherapeutic treatment.

Radiation therapy can be delivered to the entire brain, a local area of the brain, or the craniospinal axis. The dosage, timing, and location of radiation is determined by the type of tumor and its potential to spread to other parts of the central nervous system (CNS) or seed in the CSF. Some patients with small, inoperable, benign tumors are treated with cobalt radiation using a stereotactic technique. This technique is able to deliver a single high dose of radiation to a precisely defined area, thus preserving surrounding normal tissue (Barker, 1990).

In general, chemotherapy has been less effective in treating CNS tumors compared with results for neoplasia in other parts of the body because of difficulty reaching the CNS. Several factors account for this. First, the blood-brain barrier provides a physiologic barrier that restricts choices for chemotherapeutic agents. Gliomas also have cellular characteristics that act as physiologic barriers. Astrocytomas have the ability to secrete a hormone that allows the tumor to increase its nutrient supply, thus reducing chemotherapeutic effectiveness. Last, many chemotherapeutic agents that successfully treat systemic tumors cannot be used in concentrations necessary to treat regionally confined tumors, for example, CNS tumors (Leahy, 1986). However, in recent years there has been an increase in clinical trials of chemotherapeutic agents for treating childhood tumors (Cohen & Duffner, 1989). Chemotherapy protocols continue to be developed and reexamined.

Nursing Care: Postoperative Craniotomy. Many children undergoing craniotomy require intensive care following surgery. Baseline postoperative cardiovascular and neurologic assessments are completed on admission to the PICU and compared with preoperative examination. Surgical dressings are assessed for blood and CSF drainage. Hemorrhage may occur postoperatively, especially in the posterior fossa, producing rapid neurologic deterioration. Signs include alternation in level of consciousness, ataxic respirations, quadriparesis, significant alterations in blood pressure associated with small pupils, and dysconjugate gaze (Marshall et al., 1990).

Routine care also involves proper positioning of the patient. For supratentorial craniotomy, the head of the bed is usually elevated 20 to 30 degrees with the patient positioned on either side or on the back. For infratentorial craniotomy, the head of the bed is usually flat with the patient positioned on either side. In both cases, the neck should not be flexed (Rudy, 1984).

The most common postoperative problems include elevated ICP, ineffective airway clearance, meningitis, hyperthermia, and seizures. Because of extensive manipulation and irritation of brain tissue, edema may develop and elevate ICP. Debulking surgery may also create a pressure gradient between intracranial compartments, causing shift and herniation of brain tissue. Intracranial pressure peaks at approximately 72 hours. ICP monitoring is not routine, but if a ventriculostomy is in place, monitoring is easily accomplished. Clinical manifestations and treatment of elevated ICP were described earlier.

Respiratory problems are a potential problem, especially in the unconscious child who cannot cough effectively and clear secretions. Pulmonary toilet, adequate hydration, and frequent position changes are required. Hypercarbia is avoided because of its adverse effects on CBV and ICP.

Inflammation of the meninges may occur from operative contaminants or from blood remaining in the subarachnoid space. Clinical signs are characteristic of meningeal irritation. Nursing care is similar to that provided to the child with bacterial meningitis. Aseptic technique is used with dressing changes and invasive procedures. Evidence of CSF drainage on the dressing (i.e., the halo sign, in which the center of the drainage is bloody or serosanguinous and the outer periphery is clear or yellow) is promptly reported. A dural tear may be present, placing the patient at risk for an intracranial infection.

Hyperthermia may result from infection or dehydration, as well as from alteration of the temperature-regulating centers in the hypothalamus and brainstem. Antibiotics are administered for infection and acetaminophen is administered for fever. Fluid and electrolyte status is assessed. Because diabetes insipidus (DI) and SIADH are potential postoperative complications, fluid and electrolyte status is vigilantly assessed. Urine output is closely monitored, as well as levels of serum and urine electrolytes and osmolalities. To prevent cerebral edema, fluids may be restricted or titrated to maintain a predetermined serum osmolality.

Seizures are a potential postoperative problem, especially after the child has recovered from anesthesia. It is at this time that the seizure threshold is lowered (Stewart-Amidei, 1991). However, seizures may occur at anytime before, during, or after surgery. Approximately one-third of all patients with a brain tumor have seizures (Barker, 1990). Many patients receive prophylactic anticonvulsants and seizure precautions are maintained.

Meningitis. A number of different types of pathogens (e.g., bacteria, viruses, fungi) can cause infection within the CNS. The most common types of CNS infections seen in children are bacterial and viral meningitis. The Pediatric Task Force on Diagnosis and Management of Meningitis (Klein et al., 1986) defines meningitis as an "inflammation of the meninges that is identified by an abnormal number of white blood cells (WBCs) in CSF." Aseptic meningitis is defined as meningitis without detectable bacterial pathogens in CSF by usual laboratory techniques (Klein et al., 1986). The overwhelming majority of cases of aseptic meningitis are caused by viruses (Rubenstein, 1992).

The incidence of bacterial meningitis is age-specific. Beyond the newborn period, the highest incidence is in infants between 3 and 8 months of age. After the second year of life, the incidence decreases with the lowest incidence in older children (Klein et al., 1986). Pathogens causing bacterial meningitis are also age-specific. In newborns the most common etiologic agents are Group B streptococcus and *Escherichia coli*. Between the ages of 2 months and 12 years, *Haemophilus influenzae, Neisseria meningitides,* and *Streptococcus pneumoniae* are responsible for the majority of cases (Klein et al., 1986; Kritchevsky, 1988; Vulcan, 1987).

Viral meningitis is less common than bacterial meningitis and occurs sporadically. It is present in all ages with the highest incidence in children. Enteroviruses are the most common cause of viral meningitis (Rubenstein, 1992).

Pathogenesis. In most cases of bacterial meningitis, pathogens enter the CNS indirectly from a distant site. Less commonly, pathogens may enter the CNS directly from penetrating trauma or from a ruptured intracranial abscess. Typically, colonization of a pathogen occurs in the upper respiratory tract and enters the bloodstream through small vessels (Rubenstein, 1992). The blood-borne organisms then seed in the meninges and colonize the CSF, producing inflammation of the brain and meninges. Throughout the progressive pathogenic stages, the inciting organism overcomes sequential host defenses resulting in invasion and replication in the CSF (Quagliarello & Scheld, 1992). The bacteria and subsequent inflammation produce a cascade of interrelated pathophysiologic events that, if left untreated, may result in cerebral edema, intracranial hypertension, and herniation.

The pathogenesis of viral meningitis remains unclear. Viral meningitis is spread from person to person with the mouth and nose as the usual port of entry. It is believed that viral pathogens disseminate through the bloodstream to the CNS. The clinical course is usually self-limiting, with improvement seen in 7 to 14 days.

Clinical Manifestations. Clinical manifestations of meningitis vary and result largely from the host response to pathogen invasion of the CSF. The most common clinical manifestations of bacterial meningitis in children are fever, vomiting, lethargy, headache, and alteration in level of consciousness. In progressive stages, signs and symptoms are characteristic of increased ICP, which, left untreated, can result in life-threatening cerebral herniation (e.g., oculomotor palsy, irregular respirations, and cardiovascular collapse). There is no one clinical sign that is pathognomic, but signs and symptoms of meningeal irritation include photophobia, back pain, nuchal rigidity, Brudzinski's sign (flexion of the hips and knees with passive flexion of the neck), and Kernig's sign (back pain and resistance after passive extension of the lower legs). Focal neurologic signs, (e.g., hemi- or quadriparesis, visual deficits), as well as hearing deficits and ataxia occur in some children. A petechial rash is commonly seen when *N. meningitides* is the etiologic agent and is most pronounced on the extremities. A diffuse maculopapular eruption with or without petechiae is commonly associated with viral illnesses. The clinical manifestations in infants are less specific and include fever, lethargy, poor feeding, vomiting, diarrhea, a bulging anterior fontanel, hypo- or hyperthermia, and hypo- or hyperglycemia. Seizures may occur in all age groups. Definitive diagnosis of bacterial meningitis is made by finding a bacterial pathogen in cultures of the CSF. Cerebrospinal fluid from a lumbar puncture is analyzed for color, glucose, protein, and white blood cell count. Usual abnormalities seen in the CSF of infants and children with bacterial and viral meningitis are contrasted in Table 21-7. Cerebrospinal fluid characteristics in the newborn with bacterial meningitis are less definitive and may not vary substantially from normal values (Klein et al., 1986).

Clinical manifestations of viral meningitis are those of meningeal irritation such as fever, photophobia, headache, and nuchal rigidity. Rarely, severe

Table 21–7. CHARACTERISTICS OF CEREBROSPINAL FLUID IN MENINGITIS*

CSF Analysis	Normal Values	Bacterial	Aseptic (Viral)
Pressure (mm H_2O)	60–100	Increased	Normal or increased
Color	Clear, odorless	Cloudy	Clear to slightly cloudy
WBC (mm³)	≤5	100–60,000	Usually <1000
Predominant WBC type	Mononuclear	Polymorphonuclear	Mononuclear†
Glucose (mg/dL)	>⅔ of blood glucose >60	Decreased, <½ to ⅔ of blood glucose	Normal to slightly decreased or increased
Protein (mg/dL)	15–45	>100	Normal to slightly increased 50–200
Gram stain	Negative	Positive	Negative

*Children beyond the neonatal period.
†An early polymorphonuclear reaction may be present.

Table 21–8. DOSE OF PARENTERAL ANTIMICROBIALS USED TO TREAT MENINGITIS IN CHILDREN

Children

Drug		Dose/kg/day	Interval
Ampicillin		400 mg IV	q4h
Gentamicin		7.5 mg IV*	q6–8h
Amikacin		22 mg IV*	q12h
Cefotaxime		200 mg IV	q8h
Ceftriaxone		100 mg IV	q12–24h
Chloramphenicol		100 mg IV*	q6h
		75 mg/kg PO*	
Nafcillin		200 mg IV*	q4h
Trimethoprim with		20 mg	q6 or 12h
sulfamethoxazole (1:5 ratio)		100 mg IV, PO	
Vancomycin		40–45 mg IV	q6h slow

Term Newborn

Drug	>2000 g (0–7 days)		>2000 g (>7 days)	
	Dose/kg/day	Interval	Dose/kg/day	Interval
Ampicillin	150 mg	q8h	200 mg	q6h
Penicillin	150,000 units	q8h	200,000 units	q6h
Gentamicin	5 mg	q12h	7.5 mg	q8h
Amikacin	15 mg	q12h	45 mg	q8h
Nafcillin	50 mg	q8h	75–150 mg	q6h
Vancomycin	30 mg	q12h	40–45 mg	q8h
Cefotaxime	100 mg	q12h	150–200 mg	q8h

*Drugs that require monitoring of serum concentrations and appropriate dosage requirements.
Adapted with permission from Blumer, J. L. *A Practical Guide to Pediatric Intensive Care,* 3rd ed. St. Louis: Mosby–Year Book.

systemic disease occurs in patients with viral meningitis. Cerebrospinal fluid characteristics of viral meningitis are increased white blood cells, normal or slightly increased protein, normal glucose, and no bacteria present on Gram stain or culture (Hickey, 1986; Rubenstein, 1992).

Collaborative Management. Antimicrobial therapy is the mainstay of treatment for bacterial meningitis. Before CSF results are known, broad-spectrum antibiotics are selected based on the most likely etiologic agent. Once CSF results are obtained, specific antibiotics are selected based on bacterial sensitivity and the age of patient. With the development of newer cephalosporins, a large selection of antimicrobials are now available. In the newborn, empiric therapy usually includes an aminoglycoside with ampicillin and sometimes cefotaxime or more recently, cefotaxime plus ampicillin. Recently, in the child over 6 weeks of age, empiric therapy includes cefotaxime or ceftriaxone with or without ampicillin (Goldfarb, 1990). Table 21–8 lists commonly used antibiotics and their dosages to treat bacterial meningitis. Beyond symptomatic treatment and supportive care, there is no specific therapy for viral meningitis.

Seizures have the potential to adversely effect the child with infectious meningitis. Whether prophylactic anticonvulsants are beneficial in all cases is unclear. However, when seizures do occur, prompt and aggressive treatment is recommended.

Several studies support the use of adjunctive dexamethasone (Decadron) for the treatment of bacterial meningitis in children, particularly in preventing deafness (Kennedy et al., 1991; Lebel et al., 1988). The Committee on Infectious Diseases, American Academy of Pediatrics (1990) also stated that dexamethasone probably reduces the likelihood of hearing loss after *H. influenzae* meningitis. However, they recommend individual consideration of dexamethasone use in the treatment of bacterial meningitis until placebo-controlled studies are complete. The benefits and possible risks (e.g., gastrointestinal bleeding) are weighed in each patient.

H. influenzae type b polysaccharide vaccine was first licensed in 1985 for administration for children 24 months or older. In October 1990, one of the currently licensed vaccines (HbOC) was approved for administration to infants beginning at 2 months of age (Committee of Infections Diseases, American Academy of Pediatrics, 1991). Although it is believed that the incidence of *H. influenzae* disease has decreased since the licensure of the vaccine, precise epidemiologic data do not exist.

The use of ICP monitoring for patients with clinical signs of intracranial hypertension is controversial. Controlled studies do not exist and decisions to monitor ICP are based on individual professional practice.

Nursing Care. Along with frequent measurements of vital signs and serial neurologic assessments, the neurologic examination includes assessment of meningeal irritation and increased intracranial pressure. Head circumference is measured daily in infants.

Nursing interventions include promoting patient comfort, preventing patient injury, and controlling elevated ICP. Patient comfort measures include maintaining normothermia, providing a quiet environment, shielding the patient from bright lights, and administering analgesics for headache. The patient is protected from injury by placing cribrails and bedrails up and maintaining seizure precautions. With bacterial meningitis, the infectious process should be halted and reversed as soon as possible. Intravenous antibiotics are administered promptly following blood and CSF culture collections. If intracranial hypertension is presumed, nursing measures to control ICP are instituted, as described earlier. Respiratory isolation is instituted in all patients with suspected meningitis until the specific pathogen is identified. If bacterial meningitis results from *N. meningitidis* or *H. influenzae,* an additional 24 hours of respiratory isolation after the start of antimicrobial therapy is required. Aseptic meningitis requires enteric precautions for seven days after the onset of disease (Centers for Disease Control [CDC], 1983).

Individuals who were in close contact (e.g., household, daycare, nursery school) to patients with known bacterial meningitis from *N. meningitidis* require chemoprophylaxis. The drug of choice is rifampin (Rifadin, Rimactane) 10 mg/kg (maximum dose, 600 mg/day) every 12 hours for a total of four doses during 2 days. Infants may require a lower dose. Household contacts (younger than 48 months of age) of patients with meningitis from *H. influenzae* also require chemoprophylaxis with rifampin. Prophylaxis is not recommended when household contacts are all 48 months or older. Rifampin 20 mg/kg (maximum dose, 600 mg/day) is administered once daily for 4 days. Again, infants younger than 1 month may require a lower dose. Definitive recommendations for chemoprophylaxis for daycare and nursery school contacts of *H. influenzae* meningitis have not been established (Committee on Infectious Diseases, American Academy of Pediatrics, 1991).

Viral Encephalitis. Viral encephalitis is an acute inflammation of the brain and meninges. The exact incidence is unknown. A large epidemiologic study conducted in Olmsted County, Minnesota, between 1950 and 1981 reported an incidence of 8.1 per 100,000 persons per year (Beghi et al., 1984). This same study reported the highest incidence in children 5 to 9 years of age. There are numerous viruses that are known to cause encephalitis; however, in the United States, the most common are the herpes simplex and arboviruses (California, Eastern equine, Western equine, St. Louis). With the advent of immunizations, encephalitis associated with measles, mumps, and rubella has disappeared almost entirely.

Pathogenesis. Viral growth begins in extraneural tissue and then spreads to the CNS via the bloodstream. It can enter the CSF by passing or growing through the choroid plexus. Passive transfer through the blood-brain barrier may also occur. Less commonly, spread can occur along the peripheral nerves or via the olfactory system (Weil, 1990). Injury to the CNS occurs from perivascular inflammation with neuronal destruction; demyelination; and subsequent necrosis, hemorrhage, and cavitation. Untreated herpes encephalitis may have associated cerebral edema and intracranial hypertension.

Clinical Manifestations. Many of the clinical features of viral encephalitis are similar to those of aseptic meningitis, as described earlier. However, changes in cortical function from parenchymal involvement differentiate the two. The patient may exhibit abnormal behavior, agitation, seizures, headache, fever, and severe alteration in consciousness. Meningeal signs may be present, depending on the age of the child and degree of meningeal involvement.

The extent of clinical features depend on the severity of the infection, specific focus of infection, and the specific viral pathogen. Patients may develop mild sensory loss or cranial nerve palsies characteristic of a specific area of brain involvement. Herpes simplex viruses are particularly virulent and devastating if untreated. Early manifestations include nausea and vomiting, headache, confusion, seizures, bizarre behavior, hallucinations, and focal neurologic deficits. Late manifestations represent increased ICP and herniation.

Presumptive evidence of encephalitis includes increased ICP, a rise in antibody titer to pathogen, and CSF alterations. Cerebrospinal fluid changes that are suggestive of encephalitis include elevated white blood cells with a predominance of lymphocytes, mildly elevated protein, and mildly reduced glucose. The CSF may also be completely normal. The EEG is abnormal in most cases. Computed tomography and MRI may demonstrate signs of cerebral edema, hyperemia, obstructive hydrocephalus, or disseminated lesions. Definitive diagnosis is made by isolating or culturing the viral pathogen from CSF or via a brain biopsy.

Collaborative Management. With few exceptions, treatment of viral encephalitis is primarily supportive and symptomatic. Anticonvulsants are used for seizures, analgesics for pain and headaches, and antipyretics for hyperthermia. Syndrome of inappropriate antidiuretic hormone secretion may occur. Thus, fluid and electrolyte status and signs of the development of cerebral edema are closely monitored. Antiviral therapy with intravenous acyclovir (Zovirax) (30 mg/kg/day) over 10 days is recommended for herpes encephalitis (Dyken, 1989). Acyclovir has been recommended in severe cases of varicella encephalitis (Krywanio, 1991).

Nursing Care. Nursing assessment of viral encephalitis is similar to that for meningitis. Management is largely supportive, and also similar to that for meningitis. Measures to ensure adequate respiratory and circulatory function, fluid and electrolyte balance, ICP control, and nutritional support are provided.

Increased CSF Volume

Hydrocephalus. Hydrocephalus is a condition characterized by a pathologic increase in CSF within the ventricular system that is, or has been, under

Table 21–9. ANATOMIC-ETIOLOGIC CLASSIFICATION OF HYDROCEPHALUS

Noncommunicating	Communicating
Congenital	*Congenital*
Aqueductal obstruction	Arnold-Chiari malformation
Atresia of foramen of Monro	Dandy-Walker malformation
Arnold-Chiari malformation	Leptomeningeal inflammation
Dandy-Walker malformation	Incompetent arachnoid villi
Neoplasms	Encephalocele
Benign intracranial cysts	Benign cysts
Skull base anomalies	
Neoplastic Inflammatory	*Neoplastic Inflammatory*
Infectious ventriculitis	Infectious meningitis
Intraventricular hemorrhage	Subarachnoid hemorrhage
Chemical ventriculitis	(spontaneous, traumatic, surgical)
	Chemical arachnoiditis

From Carey, C. M., Trillous, M. W., and Walker, M. L. (1994). In W. R. Check, et al. (eds). Pediatric neurosurgery, p. 189. Philadelphia: W. B. Saunders.

increased pressure. There is a discrepancy between the amount of CSF produced and absorbed, with a net increase causing dilation of the ventricles. The estimated incidence of hydrocephalus with spina bifida is approximately seven to nine cases per 10,000 births (McCullough, 1989). The estimated incidence of congenital hydrocephalus without spina bifida as reported by the Centers of Disease Control is 5.84 cases per 10,000 births (Edmonds & James, 1990).

Hydrocephalus is caused by obstruction, increased production, or reduced absorption of CSF. The majority of cases of hydrocephalus occur as a result of CSF obstruction.

Terms that more accurately describe the etiology of hydrocephalus are "communicating" and "noncommunicating" hydrocephalus. Communicating hydrocephalus indicates that CSF flows freely from the ventricular spaces into the spinal and cranial subarachnoid spaces. An accumulation of CSF occurs as a result of impaired absorption of CSF by the pacchionian granules or from a blockage within the subarachnoid space. Noncommunicating hydrocephalus indicates that there is a blockage somewhere

within the ventricular system. Communicating and noncommunicating hydrocephalus are often classified according to both etiology and anatomic site of obstruction or abnormality (see Table 21–9).

Pathogenesis. Regardless of etiology, the secondary effects of hydrocephalus on the CNS are potentially the same. The secondary effects result from transependymal flow of CSF and from increased ICP. With acute hydrocephalus, increased CSF pressure causes enlargement of the lateral ventricles, followed by enlargement of the third and fourth ventricles. Spontaneous rupture of the ventricles has been reported (Kapila & Naidich, 1981). Increased CSF pressure also splits the ependymal lining of the ventricles, enhancing its permeability. The net result is increased transependymal leak of CSF into the surrounding white matter. It is believed that interstitial edema is the likely cause of cerebral atrophy and may contribute to thinning of the cerebral mantle (gray matter covering the cerebral hemispheres). Cerebral mantle thinning also occurs from compression of the dilated ventricles and loss of extracellular water (Menkes et al., 1990). The increased mass effect and increased CSF pressure of hydrocephalus can also reduce cerebral blood flow to ischemic levels, and herniation of intracranial contents may occur.

Clinical Manifestations. The clinical manifestations of hydrocephalus depend on several factors: age of the patient, degree of obstruction, acuteness of progression, and etiology or associated neuropathology. In the infant, the most common clinical sign of hydrocephalus is enlargement of the head. In older children, focal neurologic signs are more common. Table 21–10 lists common clinical manifestations of hydrocephalus in infants and older children. Associated findings that may indicate infantile hydrocephalus include hypotonicity of the lower extremities, decreased active leg motion, and ankle clonus (McCullough, 1989).

Diagnostic studies used to confirm the clinical presentation of hydrocephalus include a number of neuroimaging procedures, as well as a variety of secondary procedures. The primary neuroimaging techniques used to diagnose hydrocephalus are CT scanning (Fig. 21–8), nuclear MRI, and cranial ultrasonogra-

Table 21–10. CLINICAL MANIFESTATIONS OF HYDROCEPHALUS

Infant	Increased head circumference	Child	Nausea
	"Setting sun" eyes		Vomiting
	Spread sutures		Headache
	Tense fontanel(s)		Alteration in consciousness
	Increased transillumination		Incontinence
	"Cracked pot" sound		Papilledema
	Dilated scalp veins		Diplopia
	Nonspecific signs		Seizures
	Irritability		Cranial nerve palsies
	Lethargy		
	Poor feeding		
	Vomiting		
	High-pitched cry		
	Seizures		
	Alteration in consciousness		

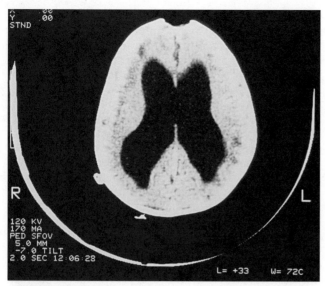

Figure 21–8 ● ● ● ● ● ●

Computed tomographic scan of infant with hydrocephalus, showing selection dilation of occipital horns. (From McLaurin R.L., et al., Eds., 1982. Pediatric neurosurgery: Surgery of the developing brain. Philadelphia: W.B. Saunders.)

phy. Secondary studies used to gather prognostic data include CSF analysis, radionuclide studies, ICP monitoring, perfusion and infusion studies, neuropsychologic tests, and cerebral blood flow studies.

Collaborative Management. Definitive treatment of hydrocephalus is to remove the obstruction. Although removal is the ideal, it is possible in only a small number of patients who have a resectable cyst or tumor. More commonly, the obstruction is bypassed with a shunt. The majority of children with hydrocephalus are treated with a valve-regulated shunt. There are a number of commercially available systems, but all have three major components: proximal catheter, distal catheter, and valve. The proximal catheter is most often placed in the lateral ventricle to drain CSF. The distal catheter can be placed in a number of receptacles, but the preferred site is the peritoneal cavity; the second is the right atrium. The last component of the shunt is a one-way valve that controls the flow of CSF from the proximal catheter into the distal catheter. A description of available shunt systems has been reviewed (Post, 1985).

Reservoirs or flush chambers can be added to most shunt systems. Flush devices are either single-chambered or double-chambered and can be used for withdrawing CSF, instilling medications or contrast material in the ventricles, and assessing shunt patency. Most reservoirs connect directly to the proximal ventricular catheter and provide access to the ventricles for instillation of medications and dye and for withdrawal of CSF. Unlike flush chambers, reservoirs cannot be flushed (Post, 1985).

For the most part, medical management of hydrocephalus has not been helpful. Intravenous mannitol (Osmitrol) and urea (Ureaphil) have been used to decrease brain extracellular fluid, but they are not practical agents for long-term management. One study reported a success rate of greater than 50% in avoiding a shunt with the use of acetazolamide (Diamox) and furosemide (Lasix) in infants (Shinnar et al., 1985).

Nursing Care. Nursing management of the infant or child with suspected hydrocephalus begins with obtaining a baseline neurologic assessment. Particular emphasis is placed on head circumference (in children younger than 2 years of age) and on progressive signs and symptoms of increased ICP. The nutritional status of the patient may be compromised because of anorexia and vomiting. Nutritional intake, fluid and electrolytes, and weight are closely monitored. Supportive nursing care includes frequent position changes and head support to prevent neck strain, discomfort, and pressure sores on the scalp.

Nursing care following a shunt insertion is similar to that for all patients following craniotomy. Ventricular shunting is not without complications. The most common complication is mechanical malfunction from obstruction or disconnection of the component parts of the shunt (McLaurin, 1989). Separation of the ventricular catheter from the rest of the shunt system has become less frequent as one-piece ventricular catheter reservoirs are used. Malfunction of a shunting device can produce signs and symptoms of increased ICP. If the obstruction is intermittent, the clinical manifestations may also be intermittent.

The second most common complication is infection. Infection may occur external to the shunt device, involving the subcutaneous tissue, or it may be internal (i.e., within the system). Signs and symptoms of external infection include the usual systemic signs of acute infection, as well as a detectable reddened streak along the subcutaneous tract of all or a portion of the shunt. Internal infection involves the CSF and is usually less virulent with less acute inflammation (McLaurin, 1989). Peritonitis and meningitis may develop. Managing shunt infections is variable and involves a combination of systemic and interventricular antibiotics with or without the removal of the shunt. Often the shunt is externalized, and antibiotics are administered into the shunt for a short period of time. Once the infection resolves, a new shunt is surgically placed.

Increased Intracranial Volume: Multidimensional

Traumatic Brain Injury (TBI). Traumatic brain injury is defined by the National Head Injury Foundation (1986) as:

an insult to the brain, not of a degenerative or congenital nature, but caused by an external physical force, that may produce a diminished or altered state of consciousness, which results in impairment of cognitive abilities or physical functioning. It can also result in the disturbance of behavioral or emotional functioning. These impairments may be either temporary or permanent and cause partial or total functional disability or psychosocial maladjustment.

Beyond the first year of life, head injury represents

the leading cause of death in children (Conroy & Kraus, 1988; Ward, 1995). Epidemiology, clinical manifestations, and description of specific head injuries are discussed in Chapter 30.

Pathogenesis. Central nervous system development is incomplete at birth and continues to mature over several years. As a consequence, the mechanisms of injury, specific types of injury, and the response to injury are age-specific. By far, the vast majority of acute intracranial injuries in children originate from a closed head injury. In contrast to adults, penetrating TBI with direct tissue disruption is less common in children. Although the most common cause of a TBI in adults is from motor vehicle and motorcycle accidents, infants most often sustain a TBI from a fall or abuse. The older child is commonly injured from a motor vehicle accident as a passenger, pedestrian, or cyclist.

Traumatic brain injuries are most commonly classified according to chronologic events. Primary injuries are those sustained at the time of impact or within milliseconds of the impact. Secondary injuries are conditions that develop in response to the initial impact injury. They develop in response to local or generalized ischemia, hypoxia, or increased ICP.

The CNS of the infant and young child is not only quantitatively different from that of adolescents and adults, but is qualitatively different as well. It is thought that the immature CNS responds to traumatic injury differently than the mature CNS. In general, diffuse cerebral swelling and increased ICP are more common in children. In contrast, brain contusions, focal parenchymal lesions, intracerebral hematomas, and diffuse brain injury (immediate impact type) are more common in adults (Shapiro, 1985). The primary conditions producing increased ICP in infants and children are cerebral hyperemia, hypoxia, and hypercarbia (increase CBV); cerebral edema, hematomas, and contusions (increase brain tissue); and subarachnoid hemorrhage obstructing CSF flow and absorption (increase CSF).

Skull radiographs have been used more frequently in the past to evaluate the child with a TBI. However, of more concern than skull disruption is intracranial damage. Thus, for those patients who require CT scanning, skull radiographs usually add very little to the neurodiagnostic evaluation, and vital therapy should not be delayed to obtain them. Skull radiographs can complement the CT scan with some pathologies (e.g., to evaluate those with depressed skull fractures and child abuse, or to localize foreign bodies). The CT scan is generally preferred over MRI because of its shorter examination time, ease of monitoring unstable patients, lower cost, and more accurate diagnosis of acute subarachnoid hemorrhage or acute parenchymal hemorrhage less than 72 hours old (Snow et al., 1986). MRI is useful in the subacute or chronic stages and to assess diffuse axonal injury and brainstem injury (Gean et al., 1995).

Collaborative Management. Principles of emergency management of the child with a TBI are similar to those for any resuscitation: respiratory and cardiovascular status are of primary concern. In a patient with an altered level of consciousness or suspected severe injury, intracranial hypertension is assumed and precautions are taken to avoid further increases in ICP. If the child's airway is patent, spontaneous hyperventilation usually occurs. Intubation may be necessary to control a compromised airway or to provide controlled hyperventilation. Sedation and paralysis are used to avoid increases in ICP induced by the intubation procedure. An $ETCO_2$ monitor is helpful to ensure adequate trending of CO_2. If intracranial hypertension is suspected, a fiberoptic ICP monitoring device is inserted in the emergency department. Mannitol is commonly used in the early treatment of head injuries in adults. In contrast, Bruce (1989) recommends that caution be used in children with early administration of osmotic agents because of the frequent occurrence of intracranial hypertension from hyperemia. A CT scan is obtained as soon as the patient's condition is stabilized.

Beyond the resuscitation phase, management is directed toward correcting the underlying pathology, when possible. When intracranial hypertension results from a hematoma, surgery is usually indicated. More frequently in children, TBI is diffusely distributed throughout the cerebral hemispheres and brainstem. A variety of therapies are available to treat intracranial hypertension, as discussed earlier. A specific regimen is selected based on the underlying pathology.

Early seizures (within 7 days of injury) are a frequent complication in children following TBI. However, they are thought to be an acute reaction to the injury rather than epilepsy (i.e., unprovoked seizures) (Temkin et al., 1995). Anticonvulsants are not usually given for an isolated, self-limited post-traumatic seizure, but are indicated for recurrent or late seizures, severe cortical contusions, cerebral lacerations, or a prior history of epilepsy. Phenytoin (Dilantin) is used more often than phenobarbital (Luminal) because it produces less CNS depression. In the patient with preexisting severe CNS depression (e.g., Glasgow Coma Score [GCS] less than 5) phenobarbital may be used because further CNS depression is irrelevant.

Other systemic complications observed in children following a TBI include neurogenic pulmonary edema, SIADH secretion, and infection. The exact mechanism for the development of neurogenic pulmonary edema is unclear. Treatment involves correcting the underlying neuropathology. Respiratory management may require ventilatory support with PEEP, diuretics, pulmonary toilet, and fluid restriction.

Signs and symptoms of SIADH include decreased urine output, hyponatremia, increased ICP, falling PaO_2, and decreased serum osmolality (sometimes difficult to recognize with mannitol administration). Serum and urine electrolytes and osmolality levels are monitored closely. Fluids are often restricted, and intake and output are accurately recorded.

All patients with traumatic stress are at risk for infection. Antibiotics are not routinely administered, but are reserved for patients with penetrating injuries or open fractures. Meticulous care of invasive lines, maximizing nutritional support, and close surveillance for signs of a local and systemic infection help prevent or reverse an infectious process.

Nursing Care. Key to preventing secondary brain injury in the child is control of hypoxia, hypercarbia, hypotension, and increased ICP. If the patient has inadequate oxygenation, ventilation, or perfusion, the neurologic assessment is delayed until they are restored.

The next step is to obtain a brief but pertinent history. Because the majority of TBIs are closed injuries, they are often anticipated based on history and mechanism of injury. Specific questions asked include how did the injury occur; where was the patient found; what (if any) type of restraint was used; was the patient unconscious when found, or was there a lucid interval; were drugs ingested; and did the patient require resuscitation. A brief, but thorough neurologic examination is performed followed by a complete systems review. Repeated assessments are performed during and after the initial management phase.

Beyond the initial stabilization phase, care is focused on correcting the primary TBI and preventing secondary injury from intracranial hypertension, hypoxia, and ischemia. Because operative lesions are less common in children, management is primarily directed toward controlling ICP.

As with all patients with intracranial hypertension, the guiding principles for management are to control the three components of the intracranial space: blood, brain tissue, and CSF. Nursing interventions to decrease CBV include promoting venous outflow from the cranium, reducing the caliber of the cerebral vasculature with controlled hyperventilation, maintaining normothermia, and controlling seizures. Nursing interventions to control increased brain bulk include administration and monitoring of hyperosmotic agents and diuretics, routine postoperative craniotomy care for operative lesions, and close monitoring of respiratory and cardiovascular status (to prevent hypoxia, ischemia, and cerebral edema). Nursing interventions directed toward controlling CSF include management and monitoring of CSF drainage (ventriculostomy) and administration and monitoring of medications to inhibit CSF production.

Complications of a TBI include gastric dysfunction, fluid and electrolyte imbalance, and malnutrition. Stress ulcers and paralytic ileus may occur in the head-injured patient. Gastric pH is monitored closely, and antacids are administered to correct low pH or maintain pH at a level above 4.0. Paralytic ileus is common in children following trauma and may compromise diaphragmatic movement. Gastric decompression with a orogastric tube may be required, but caution is used to prevent regurgitation and laryngospasm. An orogastric tube is used in place of a nasogastric tube when head and facial trauma is present and cribriform plate fracture may be a possibility.

Fluid and electrolyte imbalances may occur from volume resuscitation, diuretics, hyperosmotic agents, and SIADH. Fluid intake and output are closely monitored, as are serum and urine electrolyte levels, serum and urine osmolality, urine specific gravity, and blood component counts. With fluid overload, ICP is monitored for elevation, and the pulmonary system is assessed for the development of edema.

Patients with a severe TBI often develop a hypermetabolic response resulting in negative nitrogen balance and loss of lean body mass. Generally, nutritional support is instituted as soon as the patient's condition is stabilized with the primary goals of maintaining lean body mass and preventing complications. Enteral feedings are desired as the first choice of nutritional support (Roberts, 1995). If the patient is at risk for pulmonary aspiration related to ineffective airway protective reflexes, alternative therapies such as parenteral nutrition are considered.

Because accidental injuries are often thought to be preventable, families of victims with a TBI are at risk for family dysfunction. Whether or not feelings are justified, parents often feel guilty, ashamed, and defensive. The degree to which a family handles this situational crisis depends on many variables, such as age and developmental level of the child, severity of the injury, and preexisting family personalities and relationships. It is important that the family receive multidisciplinary support. Accurate explanations regarding the child's injuries and subsequent care are provided, directed toward dispelling irrational fears and guilt. Chapter 3 presents specific approaches in supporting the family.

HYPOXIC ISCHEMIC ENCEPHALOPATHY

Basic and advanced life support techniques have been increasingly successful in reversing cardiopulmonary arrest. However, irreversible brain damage continues to occur in a significant number of patients following the return of spontaneous circulation. As a result, cardiopulmonary-cerebral resuscitation (CPCR) and its science, reanimatology, have emerged to further elucidate the pathophysiology, reversibility, and treatment of patients suffering cardiopulmonary arrest.

Cardiopulmonary arrest is caused by a number of insults, which include asphyxiation, exsanguination, ventricular fibrillation, and electromechanical dissociation. In adults, primary cardiac arrest usually results from ventricular fibrillation associated with myocardial dysfunction because of coronary artery disease. In children, the usual event is a cardiopulmonary arrest from acute asphyxiation (e.g., airway obstruction or apnea). Asphyxial cardiac arrest is more injurious to the CNS than primary cardiac arrest, because of the period of hypoxic tissue acidosis that exists prior to cardiac standstill (Safar & Bircher, 1992).

Terminology

Ischemia and hypoxia are two mechanisms that can cause irreversible damage to the brain. Ischemia refers to a reduction in blood flow. The reduction may be global or focal and complete or incomplete. Global ischemia involves the entire brain and focal ischemia involves only a portion. With global or focal ischemia, perfusion can be completely absent, as with total circulatory arrest, or incomplete (i.e., on a continuum between perfusion and total absence, such as might occur with hypotension or bradycardia). Pathologic signs of decreased CBF can be detected when flow falls below 25 to 30 mL/minute per 100 g tissue; however, compensation usually occurs. When CBF falls below this level, a critical infarct threshold is reached and neuronal function will cease. The exact ischemic threshold varies among patients and depends on many factors (e.g., preexisting injury, age, medications) (Bouma & Muizelaar, 1995; Wauquier et al., 1987).

Hypoxia refers to a reduction in the delivery of oxygen. Oxygen delivery can be reduced from a number of causes such as anemia (anemic hypoxia), low cardiac output (ischemic hypoxia), severe pulmonary disease (hypoxic hypoxia), and carbon monoxide poisoning (anoxic hypoxia).

Clinically, hypoxia and ischemia are most often seen together. In the adult with a primary cardiac arrest, respirations stop shortly after cardiac standstill or electromechanical dissociation. In the child, asphyxia is the usual cause of a cardiopulmonary arrest. Typically, there is a prolonged period of anoxic or hypoxic perfusion of the brain before cardiac standstill. Global cerebral ischemia is the result of cardiopulmonary arrest, regardless of the events that precipitate the arrest.

The terms used to describe hypoxic brain insults and cerebral resuscitation are familiar. Primary and secondary cerebral injury, discussed in relation to traumatic brain injury, are also used when describing brain insults from hypoxia and ischemia. In both situations, the definition of the terms is the same. A primary brain injury describes the immediate damage to brain tissue, and secondary injury refers to the subsequent insults to brain tissue in response to the primary injury.

Treatment of brain injury because of hypoxic ischemia includes cerebral resuscitation, that is, application of therapeutic measures to prevent a secondary brain injury. Efforts in the PICU are aimed at preventing secondary brain injuries. In contrast, cerebral protection describes prophylactic measures to prevent a primary injury. An example is deep hypothermia used during circulatory arrest for congenital heart surgery.

Pathogenesis

Over the last decade, numerous studies have examined the pathophysiologic consequences of complete global ischemia (Wauquier et al., 1987; Kirsch et al., 1990; Rosenberg, 1986). However, research to date has been performed almost exclusively on animals of various species. In addition, different techniques to produce cardiac versus asphyxial insults have been used. In short, how precisely these experimental studies translate to the clinical situation especially in patients with a developing CNS remains unclear.

These laboratory studies identify numerous pathophysiologic processes following complete global ischemia to the brain (Michenfelder & Milde, 1990; Rosenberg, 1986). These biochemical changes begin with the initial ischemic anoxic period during total circulatory arrest and may continue with resumption of normal perfusion pressure.

Ischemic-anoxic Injury

The biochemical changes that occur in the brain during global cerebral ischemia result from the depletion of vital metabolic substrates and accumulation of toxic byproducts. The brain requirement for oxygen and glucose is very high compared with that for other organs. However, the storage capacity of these substrates is very limited. With the cessation of circulation, oxygen is depleted immediately, but glucose continues to be supplied briefly from the breakdown of brain glycogen stores. However, glycolysis in the brain is inefficient, and neuronal death occurs quickly. Lactic acidosis, which results from anaerobic metabolism, contributes to cellular damage. Hydrogen ion accumulation may cause disruption of adenosine triphosphate (ATP)-dependent ionic pumps and intracellular homeostasis (Kirsch et al., 1986). There is a loss of intracellular potassium with influxes of sodium, chloride, and calcium. Calcium influx causes uncoupling of oxidative phosphorylation and a reduction in ATP production. Lipid perioxidation also occurs with accumulation of free fatty acids. The combination of the above processes forms necrotizing cascades (Safar & Bircher, 1992). If complete circulatory arrest continues without reperfusion, uniform autolysis of the brain results after about 1 hour (Safar, 1986). Figure 21–9 is a schematic drawing of proposed mechanisms by which global cerebral ischemia may cause CNS injury.

Reperfusion Injury

In addition to injury that results from the ischemic phase, there is also evidence that additional injury occurs during reperfusion. Postischemic injury is believed to result from a number of interrelated pathophysiologic processes, including CBF alterations, calcium influx, increased oxygen free radial production, and microcirculatory obstruction.

A characteristic pattern of CBF following global cerebral ischemia has been supported by several studies using different animal models and different species (Kirsch et al., 1990; Michenfelder & Milde, 1990; Rosenberg, 1986). Safar (1986) describes the resumption of CBF progressing through four stages: (1) immediate multifocal absence of reperfusion ("no-flow phenomenon"); (2) transient increase in CBF (hyperemia) above the pre-ischemic level lasting 15 to 30 minutes; (3) delayed, prolonged global hypoper-

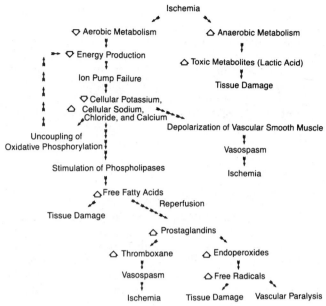

Figure 21–9 ● ● ● ● ● ●

Proposed mechanisms by which global ischemia may cause irreversible vascular and tissue injury. (From Kirsch, J.R., et al. 1986. Current concepts in brain resuscitation. *Archives of Internal Medicine*, 146, 1413–1419. Copyright 1986, American Medical Association.)

fusion lasting hours to days; and (4) resolution, continuance, or worsening. The ischemic threshold in adults as determined by CBF is reported to be below 10 mL/minute per 100 g of tissue (Kirsch et al., 1989). At this level, ionic pump failure occurs, which results in cell death. The ischemic threshold in infants and young children is unknown.

Calcium influx associated with cerebral ischemia also occurs in smooth muscle cells of the cerebral vasculature. This influx is believed to contribute, in part, to postischemic hypoperfusion by causing vasospasm in the smooth muscle of cerebral vessels (Kirsch et al., 1989). Other hypothetical detrimental effects of increased intracellular calcium in the brain include neurotransmitter release with neuronal excitability and postischemic hypermetabolism; energy depletion during reperfusion; and free fatty acid release, which may cause enzymatic dysfunction (Kochanek, 1988).

Oxygen-derived free radicals have also been implicated in reperfusion injury. Free radicals are molecules or molecular fragments that have an extra unpaired electron in the outer orbit, making them very reactive. Because of their reactivity they are also short-lived, making direct measurement difficult. During reperfusion following an episode of ischemia, it is thought that there is an increase in the production of oxygen free radicals from several pathways. In short, oxygen free radicals undergo a reaction enhanced by superoxide dismutase and form hydrogen peroxide. Hydroxyl radicals eventually form and cause a cascade of biochemical changes that produce widespread cellular injury (Rogers & Kirsch, 1989).

Safar (1986) also hypothesizes that blood sludges during the ischemic phase (stasis) and deteriorates. Once circulation is resumed, obstruction of the microcirculation occurs from red blood cell deformity, aggregates of thromocytes and granulocytes, calcium-induced vasopasm, and mediators of coagulopathy (Kirsch et al., 1989; Safar & Bircher, 1992). Thus, hypoperfusion or no perfusion exists locally or diffusely, producing more cellular damage.

Critical Care Management

Assessment

Following global cerebral ischemia, historical data are collected from the individuals witnessing the events leading to the cardiopulmonary arrest. In addition to routine questions concerning the patient's present and past medical history, it is also important to obtain details regarding the cardiopulmonary arrest and resuscitation. Specific questions include duration of apnea and circulatory arrest; precipitating event (e.g., aspiration, trauma, cardiac arrest); duration of basic and advanced life support; body temperature; and metabolic status (if hospitalized). The prehospital and in-hospital resuscitation records should also be reviewed for specific interventions and pharmacologic agents administered.

Clinical assessment of the patient begins with examination of the cardiopulmonary status. A good neurologic outcome is dependent on adequate oxygenation and cardiac output. Cardiopulmonary status is assessed in the usual fashion.

Once oxygenation, ventilation, and circulation are restored, the child's neurologic status can be assessed. Depending on specific variables of the global cerebral ischemia (e.g., duration of ischemia, type of arrest, metabolic status, etc.), the patient's neurologic status may range from complete orientation to coma. The comatose patient should be systematically assessed starting with level of consciousness, progressing to motor function, respiratory patterns, pupillary signs, and ocular movements. Because a number of resuscitative therapies and conditions can alter the child's neurologic response (e.g., catecholamines, atropine, hypothermia, chemical paralysis), special consideration is required when interpreting results. The Glasgow-Pittsburg coma scoring method is a useful tool used to assess the ongoing neurologic status of the child (beyond infancy) and adults (Table 21–11).

Routine ICP monitoring is not recommended following global cerebral ischemia; therefore, detection of intracranial hypertension is based on clinical manifestations. Increases in ICP occur transiently during the hyperemic phase of reperfusion, but quickly return to normal (Safar, 1986). Increased ICP may occur more often following asphyxial arrest (e.g., near-drowning); however, the threshold for poor outcome appears to be lower than the threshold for increased ICP development (Kochanek et al., 1992).

Table 21–11. GLASGOW-PITTSBURGH COMA SCORING METHOD

Glasgow Coma Score (GCS) (At Time of Examination)	Pittsburgh Brain Stem Score (PBSS) (At Time of Examination)
If patient is under the influence of anesthetics, sedatives or neuromuscular blockers, give best estimate of each item.	Add to GCS (A, B, C)
Write number in box to indicate status at time of this exam.	Lash reflex present (either side) yes = 2 / no = 1
(A) Eye opening	Corneal reflex present (either side) yes = 2 / no = 1
Spontaneous = 4	Doll's eye or iced water calorics reflex present (either side) yes = 5 / no = 1
To speech = 3	
To pain = 2	Right pupil: reacts to light yes = 2 / no = 1
None = 1	Left pupil: reacts to light yes = 2 / no = 1
(B) Best motor response (extremities of best side)	Gag or cough reflex present yes = 2 / no = 1
Obeys = 6	
Localizes = 5	Total PBSS (Best GCS = 15) (Worst GCS = 3)
Withdraws = 4	Patient condition at time of examination: Check (√) all that apply.
Abnormal flexion = 3	☐ Anesthesia/heavy sedation
Extends = 2	☐ Paralysis (partial or complete neuromuscular blockade)
None = 1	☐ Intubation
(C) Best verbal response (If patient intubated, give best estimate.)	☐ None of the above
Oriented = 5	
Confused conversation = 4	
Inappropriate words = 3	
Incomprehensible sounds = 2	
None = 1	
Total GCS (Best GCS = 15) (Worst GCS = 3)	

Note: The primary purpose of this scoring system is to identify a hierarchical *level* of function from brain stem to cerebrum, not to indicate laterality of disease.
Used with permission from Safar, P. & Bircher, N. G. (1988). *Cardiopulmonary cerebral resuscitation* (3rd ed). Philadelphia, W. B. Saunders.

That is, when increased ICP does develop, it most likely reflects the severity of the primary insult and not an opportunity to prevent secondary injury.

To prevent further uncoupling of supply (CBF) and demand (cerebral metabolic rate of oxygen [$CMRO_2$]), the presence of seizure activity is monitored closely. Body temperature is assessed for hyperthermia, and adequacy of pain control is optimized.

Airway patency and the ability to protect the airway are determined. Serial arterial blood gas (ABG) values quantify the adequacy of oxygenation and ventilation. Pulse oximetry and $ETCO_2$ monitoring are also helpful in assessing respiratory status.

Cardiovascular status is monitored closely for hypertension, hypotension, and dysrhythmias. Invasive hemodynamic monitoring is necessary if the cardiovascular system is unstable. Myocardial hypoxic damage is assessed with serial electrocardiograms (ECGs) and cardiac isoenzyme determinations. When induced hemodilution is used, the hematocrit level is monitored frequently.

Urine output is assessed and specific gravity monitored. Serum electrolytes are monitored at regular intervals. Syndrome of inappropriate secretion of ADH is detected by a drop in urine output, decreased serum osmolality, and hyponatremia. Infants may quickly become hypoglycemic following cardiopulmonary arrest; therefore, serum or capillary glucose is monitored.

Neurodiagnostic tests are often helpful in further assessing the child's neurologic status following a cardiopulmonary arrest. The EEG is extremely sensitive to cerebral cortical hypoxia or ischemia. Slight to moderate insults are demonstrated on the EEG as changes in peak frequency or asymmetric rhythms from homotopic regions in each hemisphere. With a severe hypoxic-ischemic insult, there is progressive flattening of the EEG tracing. Subcortical function can be assessed using evoked potential techniques (Wauquier et al., 1987). Cerebral blood flow can be assessed in the post-resuscitation phase using a variety of techniques. Limitations of each of these techniques needs to be considered when evaluating the patient and the response to therapy.

Collaborative Management

A multitude of inter-related biochemical changes have been identified during and following global cerebral ischemia. Consequently, the efficacy of traditional approaches to patient management during the postischemic phase is questioned, and novel approaches remain to be supported by clinical research.

Traditional. The single best therapy to treat global cerebral ischemia is prevention. Often, nothing can be done to prevent the initial cardiopulmonary arrest, but rapid response and effective intervention can reduce the cerebral ischemic time. Thus, basic and advanced pediatric life support are the first step in cerebral resuscitation.

The foundation for good neurointensive care following the ischemic phase is to ensure adequate oxygenation, ventilation, perfusion, and fluid and electrolyte homeostasis. In addition to post-arrest care, specific interventions to overcome the multifocal no-reflow phenomenon have been recommended. Safar (1986) suggests induced moderate arterial hypertension for 1 to 5 minutes with restoration of circulation. Beyond this period, normotension is maintained with plasma volume expansion and intravenous vasoactive medications. Induced arterial hypertension is contraindicated with cerebral trauma. Dextrose is combined with sodium chloride (0.25%–0.5%) to avoid cerebral edema. Seizures are always a threat with cerebral injury and are controlled immediately with anticonvulsants.

Hyperventilation. Although intracranial hypertension is rare after global cerebral ischemia, ICP-directed management continues to be used (Kochanek et al., 1992; Safar, 1986). In the past, induced hyperventilation was one of the most frequently recommended interventions in cerebral resuscitation protocols. However, the benefit of this intervention is unproven. Theoretically, hyperventilation may reduce CBV during the hyperemic phase; on the other hand, it may produce further ischemia during the hypoperfusion phase. To date, data do not exist comparing induced hyperventilation on CBF in humans during the reperfusion phase.

Barbiturates. Barbiturates have been shown to have a beneficial effect in controlling ICP and seizures. However, until recently, the effect of barbiturates in humans following global cerebral ischemia was unknown. In the early 1980s, a multi-institutional trial was devised to determine the risks and benefits of thiopental loading in 262 comatose cardiac arrest patients (Brain Resuscitation Clinical Trial I Study Group, 1986). Although barbiturates may be effective for focal cerebral ischemia or for cerebral protection in certain situations (e.g., coronary artery bypass), the results of this study do not support the routine use of thiopental after cardiac arrest (Haun et al., 1992; Kirsch et al., 1989).

Experimental. A number of novel therapeutic interventions have been proposed to treat global cerebral ischemia; the interventions remain in the experimental stage. These interventions stem from current understanding of the pathophysiologic processes described above.

Cerebral Blood Flow. A major emphasis in cerebral resuscitative therapies is to improve cerebral microcirculatory flow, especially during hypoperfusion. Therapies studied to enhance blood flow have

been directed toward decreasing coagulation and blood viscosity. Although heparin prophylaxis has not been widely supported, some protocols recommend moderate hemodilution (Safar, 1988; Wauquier et al., 1987).

Calcium Antagonists. Intracellular calcium influx has been hypothesized to cause neuronal injury by various mechanisms. As a result, numerous studies have investigated the potential beneficial effects of calcium antagonists. The most common experimental agents include flunarizine, lidoflazine, and nimodipine. Of the three, nimodipine has had the most encouraging results (Steen et al., 1985). Use of these drugs remains investigational.

Free Radical Scavengers. Because oxygen-derived free radicals have been hypothesized to be mediators of neuronal injury during reperfusion, the efficacy of free radical scavengers has been studied in animals. Some preliminary reports have been encouraging and have stimulated interest in the field (Imaizumi et al., 1990; Liu et al., 1989). Limitations of these agents include a short half-life, rapid rate of free radical reactions, and difficulty of some agents in crossing the blood-brain barrier (Brader & Jehle, 1989).

Numerous investigational therapies have been proposed to manage global cerebral ischemia (Table 21–12). However, the best therapeutic interventions have not yet been determined.

Nursing Care

Because cerebral resuscitation therapies remain experimental with less than enthusiastic results, the single best approach to preventing neuronal damage is to minimize the ischemic time. The significance of the prompt recognition of impending cardiopulmonary arrest and immediate intervention to restore circulation and breathing cannot be overstated.

Once circulation and breathing are restored, efforts to maintain hemodynamic stability may be required to ensure adequate CBF. Vasopressors and volume expanders are titrated to achieve optimal cardiac output. Dysrhythmias are treated promptly.

Secondary hypoxic hypoxia is prevented. Controlled ventilation with muscle paralysis may be re-

Table 21–12. INVESTIGATIONAL THERAPIES FOR CEREBRAL RESUSCITATION

Hemodilution	Opiate receptor antagonists
Barbiturates	Artificial blood substitutes
Calcium antagonists	Dimethylsulfoxide (DMSO)
Flunarizine	Indomethacin
Lidoflazine	Cardiopulmonary bypass
Nimodipine	Hypertension
Glutamate antagonists	Diazepam
Competitive	Hyperbaric oxygen
Noncompetitive	
Free radical scavengers	
Superoxide dismutase	
21-aminosteroids	

quired to ensure adequate oxygenation. Frequent turning and chest physiotherapy are used to avoid atelectasis and promote drainage of pulmonary secretions.

If intracranial hypertension develops, nursing care (as described earlier) to control ICP is instituted. Seizures are treated promptly with anticonvulsants, hyperthermia is reversed with antipyretics, and pain is controlled with analgesics.

Urine output is greater than 0.5 ml/kg/hour, serum electrolytes levels are in a normal range, and glucose is at a normal level. Stress ulcers are prevented with administration of antacids. Nutrition is supported with enteral and parenteral fluids as appropriate. Infection control is maintained with close surveillance of invasive lines, body temperature, and blood cell counts.

General supportive care is required. Skin integrity is maintained with frequent position changes and skin protective devices (e.g., sheepskin, heel pads, etc.) Passive range of motion and other physical therapy help to maintain muscle tone and joint mobility. Artificial tears are used to maintain eye moisture.

Associated Pathologies

Regardless of the etiology of cardiopulmonary arrest, the final common pathway is anoxia and ischemia. Drowning results in death from cerebral ischemic hypoxia in 2.8 per 100,000 children in the United States annually (Baker & Waller, 1989). This significant cause of global cerebral ischemia in pediatric patients is examined in the next section.

Near-drowning

Various terms are used to describe submersion injuries. *Drowning* refers to death by asphyxiation after submersion in water or some other type of liquid. *Near-drowning* is the term used to describe survival for at least 24 hours after a submersion episode. The term *secondary drowning* describes delayed death or complications from pulmonary insufficiency after a submersion episode (Sarnaik & Lieh-Lai, 1992; Spyker, 1985). *Dry drowning* describes an entity in which the drowning victim never aspirates water into the lungs or aspirates only a very small amount. It occurs in approximately 10% to 15% of all drownings.

Drowning is the second leading cause of accidental death in children and adolescents 0 to 14 years of age (Rivera, 1985). Within the pediatric population, the two age groups at greatest risk are toddlers and teenagers. As with most accidental injuries, males predominate. By far, the majority of drownings occur in fresh water, with the backyard swimming pool presenting the greatest risk. Domestic drownings (e.g., bathtub, hot tub, buckets of water, toilet) are greatest in infants and preschoolers. Drownings in lakes and rivers are greatest in teenagers (Quan et al., 1989).

Pathogenesis. Karpovich (1933), in his classic study with animals, described the sequence of events during drowning. Following submersion, there is an initial period of struggle and panic with a small amount of water entering the throat causing laryngospasm. Subsequently, large amounts of water are swallowed with vomiting and aspiration of water. In a small percentage of cases (10%–15%), laryngospasm persists without aspiration of water.

In the past, it was thought that the type of fluid (fresh versus salt) aspirated was important in terms of fluid and electrolyte balance. However, clinical information on near-drowning patients does not support this earlier animal research. The discrepancy between the laboratory and the clinical setting is attributed to the fact that humans do not aspirate as large a volume of fluid as was used to simulate drowning in animal studies.

Dramatic circulatory changes have been noted in some animals when submerged. These circulatory changes are commonly referred to as the "diving seal reflex." There is a redistribution of blood flow with selective shunting away from the cutaneous and splanchnic vascular beds to the coronary and cerebral circulations. Blood pressure is maintained, but heart rate drops significantly (Hochachka, 1981). Similar changes, to a lesser degree, were also noted in man with submersion of the face and were thought to be protective (Gooden, 1972). The diving reflex may be enhanced by cold water submersion and fear (Sarnaik & Vohra, 1986).

Hypothermia is commonly defined as a core temperature of less than 35 degrees C. Controlled hypothermia is known to have a protective effect against cerebral hypoxemia. Based on a recent review of prolonged (greater than or equal to 15 minutes) ice-water submersions, there are several reported cases of survival with good neurologic outcome (Orlowski, 1987). However, there are many more cases of death from ice-water submersion that go unreported. It is hypothesized that the accidental hypothermia that occurs in a few reported miraculous cases may simulate therapeutic hypothermia, which is routinely induced in a controlled setting and thus has a protective effect.

The initial pathologic event during submersion is anoxia. If the patient's airway is not resuscitated promptly, cardiac standstill occurs, causing ischemia. Potentially, every organ in the body can sustain injury from the combination of anoxia and ischemia. However, the CNS is most vulnerable and is primarily associated with outcome. The multiorgan effects of asphyxia are diagrammed in Figure 21–10.

Following submersion, anoxia occurs, but cardiac output usually continues for a brief period of time. During this period, blood continues to flow to the brain, delivering glucose and other nutrients in the absence of oxygen. Anaerobic metabolism develops, producing lactic acid and other toxic waste products. Once cardiac standstill occurs, all blood flow and substrate delivery ceases and cellular metabolism stops. The extent of neurologic injury depends on the

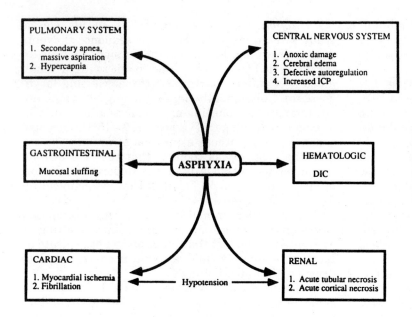

Figure 21-10 ● ● ● ● ● ●
Pathophysiology of anoxia and ischemia during submersion injury. DIC—disseminated intravascular coagulation, ICP—intracranial pressure. (From Rogers, M.C. 1992. *Textbook of pediatric intensive care*, 2nd ed., p. 887. © 1992, The Williams & Wilkins Co., Baltimore.)

duration of anoxia and ischemia. The pathobiologic processes that occur during ischemia and reperfusion are numerous, interrelated, and not well understood. In severe cases, diffuse neuronal death causes cytotoxic cerebral edema, which leads to a vicious cycle of increased ICP, decreased CBF, ischemia, and further CNS damage.

Regardless of the type of fluid aspirated, pulmonary surfactant is altered with submersion injuries. Fresh water causes dilution of surfactant, whereas salt water causes inactivation; both produce alveolar collapse (Christensen et al., 1992). Aspiration of stomach contents or contaminated water also produces pulmonary injury. Injury to the pulmonary capillaries and alveolar membranes results in abnormally increased permeability. Protein-rich fluid accumulates in the alveoli, causing pulmonary edema. The end result is intrapulmonary shunting and persistent hypoxia.

The heart, like all organs, can sustain injury from hypoxia and ischemia. Metabolic and electrolyte abnormalities may further compromise myocardial function. However, permanent damage is uncommon. Ventricular fibrillation may occur with severe hypothermia.

Other organs may also sustain damage and further complicate recovery. However, most extracerebral injuries and complications are responsive to therapy and rarely determine survival in a patient with intact neurologic function.

Clinical Manifestations. A large percentage of patients who have a submersion accident are rescued immediately and either do not require resuscitation or need only brief artificial ventilation. This group of patients usually recovers completely. On the other end of the spectrum, if cardiopulmonary resuscitation (CPR) is not begun promptly or the patient was submerged for a long period of time, significant anoxic-ischemic injury occurs. The primary clinical problems for these victims are related to the neurologic and pulmonary systems.

Following a mild to moderate submersion injury, neurologic findings most often include restlessness or lethargy and hyporeflexia, all of which are usually transient. Seizures may occur in the acute phase. In contrast, the patient with significant global cerebral ischemia presents to the hospital in a coma, is apneic and requires CPR, and has a low serum pH. The depth of coma varies, depending on the extent of neurologic injury. Hypothermia can depress neurologic function. Core temperatures below 30°C result in a clinical picture of brain death (i.e., unconscious, dilated pupils) (Sarnaik & Vohra, 1986). Signs and symptoms of intracranial hypertension may develop from cytotoxic cerebral edema.

Clinical features of respiratory dysfunction also vary considerably and depend on the degree of anoxic-ischemic injury and the amount and type of fluid aspirated. Common symptoms include cough, shallow rapid breathing, substernal burning, pleuritic chest pain, expectoration of pink frothy sputum, dyspnea, adventitious lung sounds, and shortness of breath (Hanke et al., 1992). Apnea may be present with severe submersion injuries but is due primarily to neurologic dysfunction. The chest radiographic findings vary and do not correlate well with other clinical findings. Arterial blood gas levels are usually abnormal, showing hypoxemia and metabolic acidosis (McKinley, 1989).

Atrial and ventricular fibrillation commonly occurs when the core temperature is lower than 28°C. Acute renal necrosis is the most common renal complication from anoxia and ischemia. Gastric dysfunction is often manifested by abdominal distension, vomiting, and bloody diarrhea.

Collaborative Management. The primary goal of managing near-drowning victims is prevention of secondary injury. Thus, intensive care management has focused efforts in four major areas: cardiopulmonary stabilization, hypothermia correction, ICP maintenance, and cerebral resuscitation.

Once the apneic and pulseless patient is rescued, CPR is begun immediately in hopes of limiting the anoxic-ischemic time. In the PICU, measures are taken to ensure adequate oxygenation, ventilation, and perfusion. Significant hypoxemia is corrected with supplemental oxygen, intubation, and ventilatory support. Positive end-expiratory pressure (PEEP) is used when pulmonary injury is present. Positive end-expiratory pressure restores functional residual capacity and improves gas exchange. When high levels of PEEP (10–15 cm H_2O) are used, pulmonary artery catherization is helpful to facilitate hemodynamic support. Diuretics may be required when pulmonary edema is present; however, caution is used in the presence of hypovolemia. Serial ABGs, PaO_2-FiO_2 ratio, and $ETCO_2$ are often used to assess effectiveness of therapy (Glankler, 1993).

Although fluid restriction is frequently used to manage cerebral edema, adequate cardiac output and CBF must be ensured. If shock is present, vasopressors and volume expanders may be required. Invasive monitoring is indicated for ongoing assessment, titration of drugs, and determination of therapeutic effectiveness. Cardiac dysrhythmias usually resolve spontaneously with correction of metabolic abnormalities and hypothermia.

Regardless of the air and water temperature, all patients with a submersion episode are at risk for *post-arrest* hypothermia. Children are particularly at risk because of their large body surface area. Hypothermic patients often require rewarming to stabilize their cardiopulmonary status. Hemodynamically stable patients with moderate hypothermia (32°C) can be safely rewarmed with active external rewarming, such as heating blankets, radiant warmer, and warm bath (Sarnaik & Vohra, 1986). Active core rewarming with warmed peritoneal or intravenous fluids and inhaled gas is recommended in patients with core temperatures below 32°C to avoid "afterdrop" of core temperature and rewarming shock (see Chapter 15).

In the past, authorities advocated the use of standard intracranial hypertension management (i.e., hyperventilation, mild hypothermia, osmotherapy, diuretics, ICP monitoring, and barbiturates). Despite effective control of ICP, patient outcome did not improve (Frewen et al., 1985; Nussbaum & Maggi, 1988; Sarnaik et al., 1985). Thus, most centers have abandoned routine ICP monitoring and aggressive ICP management. Increases in cerebral metabolism are avoided with aggressive treatment of seizures and maintenance of normothermia.

As described earlier, cerebral resuscitation therapies remain experimental without controlled human clinical trials. Thus, protocols for near-drowning victims continue to emphasize excellent cardiopulmonary care.

Nursing Care. Obtaining a clear history surrounding the submersion episode is very important in determining injuries and predicting outcome. Specific questions include location of submersion, type of water media, precipitating event (e.g., diving, seizure, etc.), duration of submersion, and water temperature. After the rescue, it is important to determine whether a pulse was present, how long apnea persisted, whether spontaneous breathing resumed, when resuscitation began, and what type of resuscitative efforts were performed.

Physical assessment begins with examining airway, breathing, and circulation. This rapid assessment is performed in the usual manner according to American Heart Association guidelines. Core temperature is an important parameter to assess early because of the neurologic depression that occurs with severe hypothermia. Even when the patient clinically appears to have severe irreversible neurologic damage, resuscitation continues until core body temperature is elevated above 32°C (Sarnaik & Vohra, 1986). Careful rewarming of the severely hypothermic patient is required to prevent ventricular fibrillation.

Once the patient's cardiopulmonary status is stabilized, a neurologic assessment is performed. Clinical signs and symptoms of intracranial hypertension may develop from cerebral cytotoxic edema. Emphasis is placed on excluding other potential causes of neurologic dysfunction, for example, drug or alcohol intoxication, spinal cord injury, head injury, or hypothermia.

Ongoing respiratory assessment includes monitoring physical assessment findings for significant changes; trending ABGs, $ETCO_2$, and pulse oximetry values; and determining effectiveness of ventilatory support. A baseline chest radiograph is obtained early to compare with follow-up radiographs.

Cardiovascular function is determined by assessing heart rate, blood pressure, peripheral pulses, and end-organ perfusion. When hemodynamically unstable, invasive monitoring of arterial, central, and pulmonary pressures is often required. Continuous infusions of vasopressors require close monitoring of patient response.

Hourly intake and output measurements are necessary to guide fluid therapy and assess renal function. Serum electrolytes, blood urea nitrogen (BUN), creatinine, glucose, and a complete blood count are followed for trends to assess for complications. Abdominal distension; gastric pH; and blood and stool Hematests are used to assess gastrointestinal function.

The goal of nursing management is to maintain or restore adequate oxygenation, ventilation, and perfusion so that secondary injury can be prevented or minimized. Hypoxia is the major threat for secondary injury to organs and is corrected promptly. Supplemental oxygen is the first-line management for respiratory support. If the patient cannot maintain a patent airway or has hypoxemia refractory to supplemental oxygen, manual ventilation followed by intubation is required. The early use of PEEP and generous tidal volumes (15–20 ml/kg) are often needed to overcome poor lung compliance (Beyda, 1991). Pulmonary toilet and chest physiotherapy is needed.

Cardiovascular management requires routine assessment of cardiac output. Determination of response to inotropic medications and titration of continuous vasopressor infusions are required in the hemodynamically unstable patient.

Effective management of neurologic damage is yet to be determined. Intracranial hypertension may develop in near-drowning victims. Noninvasive nursing interventions to control ICP are often used to increase adaptive capacity (e.g., head of bed elevated 30 degrees, alignment of head and neck, etc.). Patient complications that increase cerebral metabolic requirements (e.g., seizures, temperature alterations) are prevented or corrected promptly. There are a number of other nursing interventions that are commonly used in the care of near-drowning victims. They relate to complications that are observed in many pediatric patients with multisystem failure in the intensive care unit. These complications include infection, malnutrition, impaired physical mobility, and renal failure.

BRAIN DEATH

Despite state-of-the art technology and expert collaborative management, some pediatric critical care patients will sustain extensive and irreversible brain damage resulting in death. Prior to the 1960s, death was defined as the absence of breathing and circulation. However, with the advent of advanced life support techniques and artificial control and maintenance of breathing and circulation, an expanded definition of death was required. Currently in the United States, the diagnosis of death is determined by irreversible cessation of respiration and circulation or irreversible cessation of neurologic functions (brain death). Brain death is further defined as absence of cerebral and brainstem functions (i.e., whole brain death). Spinal reflexes may persist after death.

A diagnosis of brain death has never been required to withhold or withdraw life support when the patient's condition is terminal and life-sustaining procedures would only serve to prolong the inevitable. However, with the evolution of transplantation and organ procurement, it became critical both legally and ethically to establish criteria by which brain death can be determined. In 1968, the Ad Hoc Committee of the Harvard Medical School published the first set of guidelines for the determination of brain death in adults (A definition of irreversible coma, 1968). Since that time, numerous other reports have set forth specific guidelines for determining brain death, primarily in adults.

The legal and medical definition of death is the same for infants and children as it is for adults. However, there is concern about how brain death is accurately diagnosed in the infant and young child. In the past, caution was recommended when applying adult criteria to children younger than 5 years of age. This arbitrary "age of caution" was used because of the paucity of data describing pediatric

Table 21–13. GUIDELINES FOR THE DETERMINATION OF BRAIN DEATH IN CHILDREN

Physical examination*	1. Coma
	2. Absence of brainstem function
	  a. Midposition or fully dilated pupils, nonreactive to light
	  b. Absence of spontaneous eye movements, induced by oculocephalic and oculovestibular testing
	  c. Absence of bulbar musculature
	  d. Apnea
	3. Flaccid tone, absence of spontaneous or induced movements†

Observation period (for patient age)	1. Seven days to 2 months: two examinations separated by at least 48 hours 2. Two months to 1 year: two examinations separated by at least 24 hours 3. Over 1 year: observation period of at least 12 hours when irreversible cause known
Laboratory testing	1. Seven days to 2 months: two EEGs separated by at least 48 hours 2. Two months to 1 year: two EEGs separated by at least 24 hours 3. Over 1 year: laboratory testing not required when irreversible cause is known

*The physical examination should remain unchanged during the entire observation and laboratory testing periods. Severe hypothermia and hypotension must be excluded.
†Spinal cord reflexes may be present.
EEG, Electroencephalography.
Data from Task Force for the Determination of Brain Death in Children (1987). Guidelines for the determination of brain death in children. *Neurology*, 37:1007.

brain death, as well as a common, though unproven, belief that children are more resilient to neurologic damage (Ashwal & Schneider, 1987; President's Commission, 1981).

In 1987, the Ad Hoc Task Force for the Determination of Brain Death in Children published the first widely accepted guidelines for pediatric brain death. These guidelines apply to children and to term infants beyond the first 7 days of life. Specific issues addressed in these guidelines are critical historical information, physical examination criteria, age-related observation periods, and laboratory testing. Table 21–13 summarizes the guidelines developed by the Task Force for the Determination of Brain Death in Children (1987).

The most critical historical piece of information that must be determined is proximate cause of coma. By knowing exactly what caused the brain dysfunction, the possibility of a reversible condition can be more reliably eliminated. Reversible conditions that can invalidate the clinical examination include metabolic disorders, sedatives, paralytic agents, hypothermia, hypotension, and surgically treatable lesions.

To meet the medical and legal definition of brain death, the entire brain must be assessed as irreversibly damaged. The clinical determination of cortical death is difficult (Moshe, 1989; Vas, 1990). In general, the comatose patient with cortical dysfunction presents with flaccid tone, absence of spontaneous movement, and failure to respond to external stimuli. Cortical function is dependent on an intact reticular activating system, diffusely located in the brainstem, for maintenance of arousal.

Brainstem function is examined by eliciting various brainstem reflexes. Absence of a single brainstem reflex does not define brainstem death in all persons. Thus, it is the combination of absent brainstem reflexes that determines brainstem demise. The special Task Force of Determination of Brain Death in Children (1987) defines absence of brainstem function as fully dilated, midposition pupils that are nonreactive to light; no spontaneous or induced (i.e., oculocephalic or oculovestibular) eye movements; no movement of bulbar musculature including facial and oropharyngeal muscles; no corneal, gag, cough, sucking, and rooting reflexes; and no spontaneous respirations.

Apnea and coma must coexist for brain death to be diagnosed clinically. After all other physical examination criteria for brain death have been met, apnea testing is performed. Standard apnea testing for children has been described in the literature (Outwater & Rockoff, 1984).

For the apnea test to be valid, three conditions must be met while the patient is disconnected from the ventilator. First, the apneic period should be of sufficient duration for $PaCO_2$ to rise to a level normally sufficient to stimulate breathing. The exact apneic threshold in children is unknown. It is recommended that an apneic trial of 10 minutes be used initially. If the $PaCO_2$ does not reach 60 mmHg (corrected for altitude) after that period of time, a second apneic trial of 15 minutes is used (Ashwal & Schneider, 1991). The second condition that must be met during apnea testing is maintenance of adequate oxygenation. Thus, continuous flow of an FiO_2 of 1.0 is delivered by cannula in the airway. Oxygen saturations are monitored via pulse oximetry. The last condition that needs to be ensured during apnea testing is adequate perfusion. Hypotension must be corrected before apnea testing can be initiated. If cardiovascular deterioration occurs during the observation period, the test is discontinued and attempted at a later time.

The recommended observation period for infants and children suspected to be brain dead varies according to age and laboratory test used (Task Force Report, 1987). In general, the younger the age, the longer the observation period. Laboratory testing (i.e., EEG) is required for infants. However, when an irreversible cause is known in the child older than 1 year, laboratory testing is not required.

Although a number of tests exist to evaluate cerebral blood flow and brainstem evoked responses, the EEG remains that single most used laboratory test to confirm brain death. Electrocerebral silence must be demonstrated over a 30-minute period based on guidelines developed by the American Electroencephalographic Society (1986). Cerebral death may be confirmed with a cerebral radionuclide angiogram in infants older than 2 months of age. Figure 21–11 diagrams the decision-making process in determining brain death in children.

Controversies

Even though the Task Force Report (1987) on pediatric brain death is widely accepted and endorsed, it

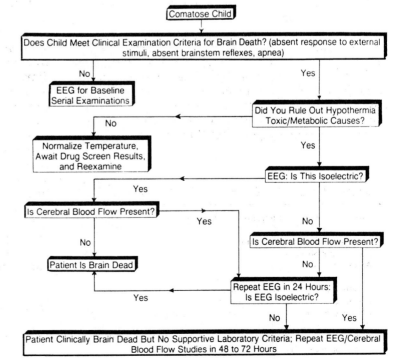

Figure 21-11 ● ● ● ● ● ●

Evaluation of the child suspected of brain death. Flow diagram indicates specific diagnostic studies and decision-making point for determination of brain death. (Reproduced by permission of *Pediatrics*, Vol. 78, p. 111, Copyright 1986.)

is not without controversy (Freeman & Ferry, 1988; Shewmon, 1988; Volpe, 1987). Uncertainty regarding the diagnosis of brain death persists in relation to newborns. The irreversibility of a condition is determined by knowing the etiology of absent brain functions. In newborns, most hypoxic-ischemic injuries occur in utero. Thus, the severity and possible reversibility of the injury is difficult to determine with certainty. There are also concerns regarding the accuracy of clinical criteria and EEG or angiographic studies during the neonatal period (Volpe, 1987). However, the Task Force (1988) maintains that there are no reported pediatric survivors that fulfilled the combination of criteria used to diagnose brain death. Until better scientific data are available, Freeman and Ferry (1988) recommend that brain death determination in children should remain a clinical decision by a qualified physician.

Organ Donation

The success of organ and tissue transplantation has created an increased demand for donor organs and tissue. Unfortunately, the demand outnumbers the supply. In an attempt to improve the supply of organs retrieved from potential donors, several laws have been adopted. The Uniform Anatomical Gift Act (UAGA), adopted by all 50 states in 1970, defines the process for the donation of organs and tissues once brain death has been determined. As a result, anatomical gifts can be specified by the Uniform Donor Card. More recently, the Omnibus Reconciliation Act of 1986 (PL-99-509) requires all hospitals participating in Medicare and Medicaid to develop protocols to identify potential organ donors. It is anticipated that these laws, as well as increased public awareness, will increase the donor supply of organs and tissues for transplantation.

Once a potential donor has been identified, specific criteria must be met to determine the acceptability of the donor (Table 21–14). However, individual transplant programs may have slightly different criteria based on a particular type of organ donor (Brink & Ballew, 1992). The selection of a donor recipient or recipients is processed through the local organ procurement agency (OPA) or tissue bank.

Table 21–14. GENERAL DONOR SELECTION CRITERIA*

Intact heart beat, adequate blood pressure and mechanical ventilator support
Etiology of brain death known
Age under 65 years
Absence of sepsis
Negative HIV titer
Absence of extra-cerebral malignancy
Absence of transmissible disease
Absence of end-organ dysfunction in the organ planned for procurement

*Organ-specific criteria may vary among transplant centers.

Nursing Care

The nurse's role in the organ donation process begins with identification of a potential donor. Once the patient is declared brain dead, determined to be a suitable donor, and the parents have consented to donation, the focus of care is directed toward donor stabilization and support of the family.

For the donor to remain acceptable for organ retrieval, adequate oxygenation and perfusion must be maintained. Respiratory function is stabilized with a ventilator. Ventilator settings are adjusted to maintain normocarbia, and supplemental oxygen is administered to maintain adequate tissue oxygenation. Avoiding excessive ventilatory pressures is recommended (Brink & Ballew, 1992). Positive end-expiratory pressure may be required to minimize atelectasis or pulmonary edema. Fluid administration is also closely monitored to avoid volume overload and pulmonary edema. Ongoing assessment of respiratory function is accomplished with ABGs, pulse oximetry, and chest radiographs.

Cardiovascular stability is critical for adequate tissue perfusion. Preload is supported with intravenous fluids. Hypotension is common, resulting from hypovolemia, dysfunction of the hypothalamic-pituitary-endocrine system, or myocardial ischemia. Intravascular volume is restored with isotonic crystalloid and colloids. Low-dose vasopressors are commonly used after restoration of intravascular volume. High-dose vasopressors are avoided to prevent decreased organ perfusion. Blood loss and coagulopathies are managed with appropriate blood components. When centrally mediated hypertension and tachycardia are present, adrenergic blocking agents are usually effective.

Maintenance of fluid and electrolyte balance may be a challenge. One study reported a 38% incidence of diabetes insipidus (DI) in children with brain death (Fisher et al., 1987). This same study reported diuresis in 76% of the same patient series. Several factors other than DI may contribute to diuresis in the child with brain death, including prior administration of diuretics, osmotic agents, and contrast media administered for radiographic studies. Hypovolemia and electrolyte alterations are corrected in the usual manner. Vasopressin (Pitressin) may be required when DI cannot be controlled.

Temperature instability is a potential problem in donors resulting from loss of hypothalmic control. As a result, there is a tendency for donor core temperature to be regulated by the external environment. This is especially true in the young child who has a large body surface area. Temperature is closely monitored and external heating devices (e.g., radiant warmers, thermal mattress) are used to provide thermal stability.

NEUROMUSCULAR DISORDERS

Although relatively rare, numerous diseases affect the motor unit in children, producing neuromuscular

Table 21-15. CLASSIFICATION OF NEUROMUSCULAR DISEASE

Anterior horn cell
  Inherited
    Werdnig-Hoffman disease
  Acquired
    Poliomyelitis

Peripheral nerves
  Axonal
    Lead poisoning
    Some organic compounds
  Trauma
    Phrenic nerve paralysis
    Brachial plexus injury
  Demyelination
    Guillain-Barré syndrome
    Diphtheria

Neuromuscular junction
  Autoimmune
    Myasthenia gravis
  Congenital
    Familial infantile myasthenia gravis
  Toxic
    Botulism
    Organophosphate poisoning

dysfunction. The motor unit is divided into four distinct parts: the anterior horn cell, the axon, the neuromuscular junction, and the muscle fibers innervated by the anterior horn cell. Descriptions of disorders are usually grouped together based on the primary level of motor unit involvement. The final common pathway of all disease entities affecting the motor unit is loss of motor output. Table 21–15 outlines the most commonly seen neuromuscular diseases in children based on the level of motor unit involvement.

Specific disease entities causing neuromuscular dysfunction are rarely the primary cause for PICU admission. When admission is required, it is usually from secondary respiratory failure or inability to protect the airway. The presentation of symptoms may be in the form of an acute illness or an exacerbation or progression of a chronic process. Many neuromuscular disorders are progressive and untreatable, and others are self-limiting. In both cases, the mainstay of therapy is supportive care. Chapter 20 presents a more detailed discussion of respiratory management of the pediatric patient with neuromuscular dysfunction.

MUSCULOSKELETAL DISORDERS

The only patients with musculoskeletal disorders that are frequently cared for in the PICU are those who require spinal fusion. Scoliosis is a lateral curvature of the spine that varies from minor alterations that are visually undetectable to severe curvatures with significant disfigurement. The curve is described according to the directed side of convexity and the location in the spinal column (e.g., right thoracolumbar). With severe cases, females predomi-

nate. Scoliosis is most often diagnosed in the preadolescent and adolescent years during routine physical examinations. In approximately 80% of the cases, the cause of scoliosis is idiopathic (unknown). Of the 20% known causes, they are most often congenital (e.g., congenital rib fusions, hemivertebrae, myelomeningocele) and neuromuscular (e.g., cerebral palsy, neurofibromatosis, and muscular dystrophy).

Scoliosis rarely presents as a life-threatening illness, but severe curvatures may compromise pulmonary function. There are no absolute indications, but surgery is usually recommended when the curvature progresses beyond a 45- to 50-degree range (Behrman, 1992). Surgical technique usually consists of spinal realignment and strengthening with bone grafts and internal fixation with metal rods or wires. The bone graft is taken from the iliac crests or tibia. The surgical approach traditionally has been posterior. However, an anterior approach with or without posterior spinal fusion has become more common in the treatment of spinal disorders. The anterior approach allows for a fewer number of vertebrae to be fused, but presents a greater degree of risk to the patient related to the thoracotomy (Ogilvie, 1988). The Harrington rod is the most frequently used apparatus for internal vertebral fixation. Table 21–16 describes additional surgical techniques for internal fixation.

Spinal fusion is an elective procedure that allows for adequate preparation of the acute- and long-term phases of care. Because of potential life-threatening complications and frequent monitoring, patients are usually admitted to the PICU for the first 24 hours following surgery. After 24 hours, the patient is transferred to a general care unit. The patient is usually discharged home with an external fixation device (e.g., splint, cast, jacket). The remaining section focuses on the postoperative nursing care in the intensive care unit.

Care of the Patient After Spinal Fusion

In addition to routine postoperative assessments, a baseline neurovascular assessment is performed on all extremities. Incisional pain and muscle spasms are common and are assessed immediately. The surgical procedure is long, and significant blood loss is common. The wound and graft sites are inspected for bleeding and hematoma formation. Surgical drains

Table 21-16. INTERNAL VERTEBRAL FIXATION DEVICES

Harrington rod instrumentation	Metal rod attached by hooks placed in vertebra at upper and lower portions of the curve
Dwyer instrumentation	Titanium cable attached to vertebra through cannulated screws
Luque rod instrumentation	Flexible L-shaped metal rod fixed by wires to the bases of the spinous processes

may be present. Suction is applied to these drains, and the admission output is recorded. If the chest was opened during surgery (as is the case for an anterior spinal fusion), the chest drainage system is evaluated for proper functioning. The patient is assessed for re-expansion of the lungs, as well as the presence of hemo- and pneumothoraces. A paralytic ileus is common postoperatively. The abdomen is assessed for distension and presence of bowel sounds. A nasogastric tube is assessed for patency. Baseline laboratory specimens are obtained including hemoglobin and hematocrit, serum electrolytes, and urine specific gravity levels. Continuing assessment focuses on three major objectives: early recognition of complications, promotion of comfort, and promotion of wound healing.

Thoracic excursion and subsequent tidal volume may be impeded from immobility, anesthesia, or pain. Ongoing respiratory assessment emphasizes adequacy of ventilation and oxygenation. The patient is positioned for comfort and optimal respiratory excursion. Careful log rolling is required. Ventilation and tidal volume may need to be supported with incentive spirometry or mechanical ventilation. Airway clearance is maintained with frequent turning, cough and deep-breathing, chest physiotherapy, and suctioning. Bronchodilators may be required in patients with reactive airways disease.

Because the surgical procedure is long and blood loss is significant, the adequacy of cardiac output and tissue perfusion is determined. It is normal for slight oozing of drainage to occur from the wound. The amount, consistency, and color of drainage is recorded. The spinal dressing may need to be reinforced. Clear, odorless drainage from the spinal dressing is reported immediately to rule out CSF leakage. Hemoglobin and hematocrit levels are followed for trends, and intravenous fluids and blood products are administered and adjusted as needed. Autotransfusion of blood is possible in some cases. Heart rate and rhythm, end-organ perfusion, and blood pressure are assessed frequently.

Significant postoperative pain may be present from the surgical incisions, immobility, surgical instrumentation, or muscle spasms. An age-appropriate assessment is performed at frequent intervals. Pain control management is specific to the patient. Frequently, a continuous morphine infusion is started in the immediate postoperative period and converted to a patient-controlled analgesia (PCA) device when appropriate. The patient is repositioned frequently, and uninterrupted rest periods are provided. Diversional activities and relaxation techniques are also helpful.

Spinal surgery can potentially damage or traumatize spinal nerves intraoperatively. Baseline and continuous neurovascular assessment of the lower extremities includes movement (dorsiflexion, plantar flexion, inversion, eversion, movement of toes); sensation (numbness, tingling, decreased sensation); and circulation (pedal and posterior tibial pulses, color, capillary refill, temperature). Significant alterations in assessment are reported immediately.

Fluid and electrolytes may be altered related to the lengthy anesthesia time and alteration in gastric function. Serum electrolytes, serum osmolarity, and urine specific gravity levels are monitored closely. Intake and output with close attention to nasogastric drainage is recorded at frequent intervals. Once bowel sounds are present, the nasogastric tube is discontinued and oral intake resumed.

SUMMARY

Pediatric critical care nurses are challenged to care for infants and children with a variety of neurologic insults. This chapter has discussed the most common neurologic disorders seen in the PICU in the context of two final common pathways: intracranial hypertension and global hypoxic ischemia. Each of these final common pathways included a general discussion of the pathophysiology and common elements of critical care management. Associated pathologies were described in terms of pathogenesis, clinical manifestations, and specific collaborative management approaches. Additional sections presented information on brain death and organ donation, neuromuscular disorders, and care of the child following spinal fusion.

As with all infants and children in the PICU, psychosocial support of the family is an essential component of critical care management. Parents of children with a CNS insult are at particular risk because of the unique threats of the CNS injury or illness and the potential chronicity of illness. In these situations, families benefit from multidisciplinary support. Parent-to-parent support groups and illness-specific organizations (e.g., the National Head Injury Foundation) are particularly helpful.

References

A definition of irreversible coma. Report of the Ad Hoc Committee of the Harvard medical school to examine the definition of brain death (1968). *Journal of the American Medical Association, 205*, 85–88.

Aicardi, J., & Chevrie, J. J. (1970). Convulsion status epilepticus in infants and children—a study of 239 cases. *Epilepsia, 11*, 187–197.

American Electroencephalographic Society (1986). Guidelines in EEG 1–7 (revised 1985). *Journal of Clinical Neurophysiology, 3*, 131–168.

Ashwal, S., & Schneider, S. (1987). Brain death in children: Part I. *Pediatric Neurology, 3*, 5–11.

Ashwal, S., & Schneider, S. (1991). Pediatric brain death: Current perspectives. *Advances in Pediatrics, 38*, 181–202.

Baker, S. P., & Waller, A. E. (1989). *Childhood injury state-by-state mortality facts.* Washington, D. C.: National Maternal and Child Health Clearinghouse.

Barker, E. (1990). Brain tumor. Frightening diagnosis, nursing challenge. *RN, 53*(9), 46–55.

Beckstead, J. E., Tweed, W. A., Lee, J., & Mackeen, W. L. (1978). Cerebral blood flow and metabolism in man following cardiac arrest. *Stroke, 9*, 569–573.

Beghi, E., Nicolosi, A., Kurland, L. T., Mulder, D. W., Hauser, W. A., & Shuster, L. (1984). Encephalitis and aseptic meningitis, Olmsted County, Minnesota, 1950–1981: I. Epidemiology. *Annals of Neurology, 16*, 283–294.

Behrman, R. E. (1992). *Nelson's textbook of pediatrics.* Philadelphia: W. B. Saunders.

Bell, W. E., & Bertino, J. S. (1984). Constant diazepam infusion in the treatment of continuous seizure activity. *Drug Intelligence and Clinical Pharmacy, 18,* 965–970.

Bell, H. E. (1978). Increased intracranial pressure-diagnosis and management. *Current Problems in Pediatrics, 8*(4), 1–62.

Beyda, D. H. (1991). Pathophysiology for near-drowning and treatment of the child with a submersion incident. *Critical Care Nursing Clinics of North America, 3,* 273–280.

Boortz-Marx, R. (1985). Factors affecting intracranial pressure: A descriptive study. *Journal of Neurosurgical Nursing, 17,* 89–94.

Boss, B. J. (1990). Concepts of neurologic dysfunction. In K. L. McCance & S. E. Huether (Eds.). *Pathophysiology: The biologic basis for disease in adults and children* (pp. 431–470). St. Louis: C. V. Mosby.

Bouma, G. J., & Muizelaar, J. P. (1995). Cerebral blood flow in severe clinical head injury. *New Horizons, 3,* 384–394.

Braakman, R., Schouten, H. J., Dishoeck, M. B., & Minderhoud, J. M. (1983). Megadose steroids in severe head injury: Results of a prospective double-blind clinical trial. *Journal of Neurosurgery, 58,* 326–330.

Brader, E., & Jehle, D. (1989). Cerebral resuscitation. *Topics in Emergency Medicine, 11*(2), 52–67.

Brain Resuscitation Clinical Trial I Study Group (1986). Randomized clinical study of thiopental loading in comatose survivors or cardiac arrest. *New England Journal of Medicine, 314,* 397–403.

Brink, L. W., & Ballew, A. (1992). Care of the pediatric donor. *American Journal of Diseases of Children, 146,* 1045–1050.

Bruce, D. (1983). Clinical care of the severely head injured child. In K. Shapiro (Ed.). *Pediatric head trauma* (pp. 31–40). Mt Kisco, NY: Futura.

Bruce, D. A. (1989a). Treatment of intracranial hypertension. In M. Wonsiewicz (Ed.). *Pediatric neurosurgery* (pp. 245–254). Philadelphia: W. B. Saunders.

Bruce, D. A. (1989b). Treatment of intracranial hypertension. In R. L. McLaurin, L. Schut, J. L. Venes, & F. Epstein (Eds.). *Pediatric neurosurgery: Surgery of the developing nervous system* (pp. 245–254). Philadelphia: W. B. Saunders.

Bruya, M. A. (1981). Planned periods of rest in the intensive care unit: Nursing care activities and intracranial pressure. *Journal of Neurosurgical Nursing, 13,* 184–194.

Bullock, R. (1995). Mannitol and other diuretics in severe neurotrauma. *New Horizons, 3,* 448–452.

Centers for Disease Control (1983). *Guidelines for prevention and control of nosocomial infections.* Atlanta: CDC.

Christensen, D. W., Dean, J. M., & Setzer, N. A. (1992). Near-drowning. In M. C. Rogers (Ed.). *Textbook of pediatric intensive care* (pp. 877–901). Baltimore: Williams & Wilkins.

Clifton, G. L. (1995). Hypothermia and hyperbaric oxygen as treatment modalities for severe head injury. *New Horizons, 3,* 474–478.

Cohan, S. L., Mun, S. K., Petite, J., Correia, J., DaSilva, A. T., & Waldhorn, R. E. (1989). Cerebral blood flow in humans following resuscitation from cardiac arrest. *Stroke, 20,* 761–765.

Cohen, M. E., & Duffner, P. K. (1989). Tumors of the brain and spinal cord including leukemic involvement. In K. F. Swaiman (Ed.). *Pediatric neurology: Principles and practice* (pp. 661–714). St. Louis: C. V. Mosby.

Committee on Infectious Disease, American Academy of Pediatrics (1990). Dexamethasone therapy for bacterial meningitis in infants and children. *Pediatrics, 86,* 130–133.

Committee on Infectious Disease, American Academy of Pediatrics (1991). *Report of the committee on infectious disease* (21st ed.). Elk Grove, IL: American Academy of Pediatrics.

Conroy, C., & Kraus, J. F. (1988). Survival after brain injury. Cause of death, length of survival, and prognostic variables in a cohort of brain injured people. *Neuroepidemiology, 7,* 13–22.

Cottrell, J. E., Robustelli, A., Post, K., & Turndorf, H. (1977). Furosemide-and mannitol-induced changes in intracranial pressure and serum osmolality and electrolytes. *Anesthesiology, 47*(1), 28–30.

Crawford, T. O., Mitchell, W. G., Fishman, L. S., & Snodgrass, S. R. (1988). Very-high-dose phenobarbital for refractory status epilepticus in children. *Neurology, 38,* 1035–1040.

Dean, J. M., Rogers, M. C., & Traystman, R. J. (1992). Pathophysiology and clinical management of the intracranial vault. In M. C. Rogers (Ed.). *Textbook of pediatric intensive care* (pp. 639–666). Baltimore: Williams & Wilkins.

Dearden, N. M., Gibson, J. S., McDowall, D. G., Gibson, R. M., & Cameron, M. M. (1986). Effect of high-dose dexamethasone on outcome from severe head injury. *Journal of Neurosurgery, 64,* 81–88.

Delgado-Escueta, R. V., Wasterlain, C., Treiman, D. M., et al. (1982). Management of status epilepticus. *New England Journal of Medicine, 306,* 1337–1340.

Dembo, M. (1982). Arteriovenous malformations of the brain: A review of the literature since 1960. *Archives of Physical Medicine and Rehabilitation, 63,* 565–568.

Donegan, J. H., Traystman, R. J., Koehler, R. C., Jones, M. D., & Rogers, M. C. (1985). Cerebrovascular hypoxic and autoregulatory responses during reduced brain metabolism. *American Journal of Physiology, 249,* H421–429.

Donegan, M. F., & Bedford, R. F. (1980). Intravenously administered lidocaine prevents intracranial hypertension during endotracheal suctioning. *Anesthesiology, 52,* 516–518.

Drummond, B. L. (1990). Preventing increased intracranial pressure. *Focus on Critical Care, 17*(2), 116–122.

Duffner, P. K., Cohen, M. E., & Freeman, A. I. (1985). Pediatric brain tumors: An overview. *CA, 35,* 287–301.

Dunn, D. W. (1990). Status epilepticus in infancy and childhood. *Neurologic Clinics, 8,* 647–658.

Dyken, P. R. (1989). Viral diseases of the nervous system. In K. F. Swaiman (Ed.). *Pediatric neurology: Principles and practice* (pp. 475–515). St. Louis: C. V. Mosby.

Edmonds, L. D., & James, L. M. (1990). Temporal trends in the prevalence of congenital malformations at birth based on the birth defects monitoring program, United States, 1979–1987. *Morbidity and Mortality Weekly Report, 39,* (SS-4), 19–23.

Farley, J. A. (1990). The comatose child: Analysis of factors affecting intracranial pressure. *Dimensions of Critical Care Nursing, 9,* 216–222.

Fisher, B., Thomas, D., & Peterson, B. (1992). Hypertonic saline lowers raised intracranial pressure in children after head trauma. *Journal of Neurosurgical Anesthesiology, 4,* 4–10.

Fisher, D. H., Jimenez, J. F., Wrape, V., & Woody, R. (1987). Diabetes insipidus in children with brain death. *Critical Care Medicine, 15,* 551–553.

Fisher, D. M., Swedlow, D., & Frewan, T. (1982). Increase in intracranial pressure during suctioning-stimulation vs rise in $PaCO_2$. *Anesthesiology, 57,* 416–417.

Fishmann, R. A. (1975). Brain edema. *New England Journal of Medicine, 293,* 706–711.

Frankowski, R. F., Annegars, J. F., & Whitman, S. (1985). The descriptive epidemiology of head trauma in the United States. In D. P. Becker & J. T. Povlischock (Eds.). *Central nervous system trauma: Status report.* National Institutes of Health.

Freeman, J. M., & Ferry, P. C. (1988). [Editorial]. New brain death guidelines in children: Further confusion. *Pediatrics, 81,* 301–303.

French, L. A., & Galicich, J. H. (1964). The use of steroids for control of cerebral edema. *Clinical Neurosurgery, 10,* 212–223.

Frewen, T. C., Sumabat, W. O., Han, V. K., Amacher, A. L., Del-Maestro, R. F., & Sibbald, W. J. (1985). Cerebral resuscitation therapy in pediatric near-drowning. *The Journal of Pediatrics, 106,* 615–617.

Gastaut, H. (1973). *Dictionary of epilepsies,* part 1: Definitions. Geneva: World Health Organization.

Gean, A. D., Kates, R. S., & Lee, S. (1995). Neuroimaging in head injury. *New Horizons, 3,* 549–561.

Gilsanz F., Rebollar, J. L., Buencuerpo, J., & Chantres, M. T. (1975). Controlled trial of glycerol vs. dexamethasone in the treatment of cerebral edema in acute cerebral infarction. *Lancet, 1,* 1049–1051.

Glankler, D. M. (1993). Caring for the victim of near drowning. *Critical Care Nurse, 13,* 25–32.

Golden, G. S. (1989). Cerebrovascular disease. In K. F. Swaiman (Ed.). *Pediatric neurology: Principles and practice* (pp. 603, 623). St. Louis: C. V. Mosby.

Goldfarb, J. (1990). Infections of the central nervous system. In J. L. Blumer (Ed.). *A pratical guide to pediatric intensive care* (pp. 464–474), St. Louis: Mosby–YearBook.

Gooden, B. A. (1972). Drowning and the diving reflex in man. *Medical Journal of Australia, 2,* 583–587.

Graf, C. J., Perret, G. E., & Torner, J. C. (1983). Bleeding from cerebral arteriovenous malformations as part of their natural history. *Journal of Neurosurgery, 58,* 331–337.

Grote, J., Zimmer, K., & Schubert, R. (1981). Effects of severe arterial hypocapnia on regional blood flow regulation, tissue PO_2 and metabolism in the brain cortex of cats. *Pflugers Archives, 391,* 195–199.

Guertin, S. R. (1992). Neurological intensive care: Selected aspects. In B. P. Fuhrman, & J. J. Zimmerman (Eds.). *Pediatric critical care* (pp. 621–635). St. Louis: Mosby–YearBook.

Gunnar, W. P., Jonasson, O., Merlotti, G. J., Stone, J., & Barrett, J. (1988). Head injury and hemorrhagic shock: Studies of the blood brain barrier and intracranial pressure after resuscitation with normal saline solution, 3% saline solution and dextran-40. *Surgery, 103,* 398–407.

Hagnevik, K., Gordon, E., Lins, L. E., Wilhelmsson S., & Forster, D. (1974). Glycerol-induced hemolysis with hemoglobinuria and acute renal failure. *Lancet, 1,* 75–77.

Hanke, B. K., Fields, A. I., Gerace, J. E., & Schwartz, G. R. (1992). Near-drowning. In G. R. Schwartz, C. G. Cayten, M. A. Mangelsen, T. A. Mayer, & B. K. Hanke (Eds.). *Principles and practice of emergency medicine* (pp. 2800–2806). Philadelphia: Lea & Febiger.

Haun, S. E., Dean, J. M., Kirsch, J. R., Ackerman, A. D., & Rogers, M. C. (1992). Theories of brain resuscitation. In M. C. Rogers (Ed.). *Textbook of pediatric intensive care.* (pp. 698–732). Baltimore: Williams & Wilkins.

Hayden, P. W., Foltz, E. L., & Shurtleff, D. B. (1968). Effect of an oral osmotic agent on ventricular fluid pressure of hydrocephalic children. *Pediatrics, 41,* 955–958.

Hendrick, E. B., & Raffel, C. (1989). Tumors of the fourth ventricle: Ependymomas, choroid plexus papillomas, and dermoid cysts. In M. Wonsiewicz (Ed.). *Pediatric neurosurgery.* (pp. 366–372). Philadelphia: W. B. Saunders.

Hickey, J. V. (1986). *The clinical practice of neurological and neurosurgical nursing* (2nd ed.). Philadelphia: J. B. Lippincott.

Hobdell, E. F., Adamo, F., Caruso, J., Dihoff, R., Neveling, E., & Roncoli, M. (1989). The effect of nursing activities on the intracranial pressure of children. *Critical Care Nurse, 9*(6), 75–79.

Hochachka, P. (1981). Brain, lung, and heart function during diving and recovery. *Science, 212,* 509–514.

Holmes, G. L. (1987). *Diagnosis and management of seizures in children.* Philadelphia: W. B. Saunders.

Humphreys, R. P. (1989). Arteriovenous malformations of the brain. In M. Wonsiewicz (Ed.). *Pediatric neurosurgery* (pp. 508–516), Philadelphia: W. B. Saunders.

Imaizumi, S., Woolworth, V., Fishman, R. A., & Cahn, P. H. (1990). Liposome-entrapped superoxide dismutase reduces cerebral infarction in cerebral ischemia in rats. *Stroke, 21,* 1312–1317.

Johnston, I. H., & Rowan, J. O. (1974). Raised intracranial pressure and cerebral blood flow. 3. Venous outflow tract pressure and vascular resistances in experimental intracranial hypertension. *Journal of Neurosurgery, Neurology, and Psychiatry, 37,* 392–402.

Kapila, A., & Naidick, T. P. (1981). Spontaneous lateral ventriculocisternostomy documented by metrizamide CT ventriculography. Case report. *Journal of Neurosurgery, 54,* 101–104.

Karpovich, P. V. (1933). Water in the lungs of drowned animals. *Archives of Pathology and Laboratory Medicine, 15,* 828–833.

Kennedy, W. A., Hoyt, M. J., & McCracken, G. H. (1991). The role of corticosteroid therapy in children with pneumococcal meningitis. *American Journal of Diseases of Children, 45,* 1374–1378.

Kirsch, J. R., Dean, M. J., & Rogers, M. C. (1986). Current concepts in brain resuscitation. *Archives in Internal Medicine, 146,* 1413–1419.

Kirsch, J. R., Diringer, M. N., Borel, C. O., Hart, G. K., & Hanley, D. F. (1989). Brain resuscitation: Medical management and innovations. *Critical Care Nursing Clinics of North America, 1,* 143–154.

Kirsch, J. R., Helfaer, M. A., Blizzard, K., Toung, T. J. K., & Traystman, R. J. (1990). Age-related cerebrovascular response to global ischemia in pigs. *American Journal of Physiology, 259,* H1551–H1556.

Klein, J. O., Feigin, B. D., & McCracken, G. H. (1986). Report of the task force on diagnosis and management of meningitis. *Pediatrics, 78*[suppl.], 959–982.

Kochanek, P. M. (1988). Novel pharmacologic approaches to brain resuscitation after cardiorespiratory arrest in the pediatric patient. *Critical Care Clinics, 4,* 661–677.

Kochanek, P. M., Uhl, M. W., & Schoettle, R. J. (1992). Hypoxic-ischemic encephalopathy: Pathobiology and therapy of the post-resuscitation syndrome in children. In B. P. Fuhrman & J. J. Zimmerman (Eds.). *Pediatric critical care* (pp. 637–658). St. Louis: Mosby–Year Book.

Kritchevsky, M. (1988). Infections of the nervous system. In W. C. Wiederholt (Ed.). *Neurology for the nonneurologist* (pp. 266–279). Philadelphia: Grune & Stratton.

Krywanio, M. L. (1991). Varicella encephalitis. *Journal of Neuroscience Nursing, 23,* 363–368.

Lacey, D. J. (1988). Status epilepticus in children and adults. *Journal of Clinical Psychiatry, 49*(12[suppl.]), 33–35.

Laurent, J. P., & Cheek, W. R. (1986). Brain tumors in children. In M. A. Fishman (Ed.). *Pediatric neurology* (pp. 325–340). New York: Grune & Stratton.

Leahy, N. M. (1986). Intraarterial cisplatin infusion: Nursing implications. *Journal of Neuroscience Nursing, 18,* 296–301.

Lebel, M. H., Freij, B. J., Syrogiannopoulos, G. A., Chrane, D. F., Hoyt, M. J., Stewart, S. M., Kennard, D. B., Olsen, K. D., & McCracken, G. H. (1988). Dexamethasone therapy for bacterial meningitis: Results of two double-blind, placebo-controlled trials. *New England Journal of Medicine, 3,* 964–971.

Liu, T. H., Beckman, J. S., Freeman, B. A., Hogan, E. L., & Hsu, C. Y. (1989). Polyethylene glycolconjugated superoxide dismutase and catalase reduce ischemic brain injury. *American Journal of Physiology, 256,* H589–H593.

Lockman, L. A. (1990). Treatment of status epilepticus in children. *Neurology, 40*(Suppl. 2), 43–46.

Lorber, J. (1973). Isosorbide in the medical treatment of infantile hydrocephalus. *Journal of Neurosurgery, 39,* 702–707.

Lowenstein, D. H., Aminoff, M. J., & Simon, R. P. (1988). Barbiturate anesthesia in the treatment of status epilepticus: Clinical experience with 14 patients. *Neurology, 38,* 395–400.

Marion, D. W., Firlik, A., & McLaughlin, M. R. (1995). Hyperventilation therapy for severe traumatic brain injury. *New Horizons, 3,* 439–447.

McCullough, D. C. (1989). Hydrocephalus: Etiology, pathologic effects, diagnosis, and natural history. In M. Wonsiewicz (Ed.). *Pediatric neurosurgery* (pp. 180–218). Philadelphia: W. B. Saunders.

McGraw, C. P., Alexander, E., & Howard, G. (1978). Effect of dose and dose schedule on the response of intracranial pressure to mannitol. *Surgical Neurology, 10,* 127–130.

McGraw, C. P., & Howard, G. (1983). Effect of mannitol on increased intracranial pressure. *Neurosurgery, 13,* 269–271.

McKinley, M. G. (1989). Near-drowning: A nursing challenge. *Critical Care Nurse, 9*(10), 52–60.

McLaurin, R. L. (1989). Ventricular shunts: Complications and results. In M. Wonsiewicz (Ed.). *Pediatric neurosurgery* (pp. 219–237). Philadelphia: W. B. Saunders.

McNair, N. (1988). Arteriovenous malformations. *Critical Care Nurse, 8*(4), 35–40.

MacDonald, J. T., & Uden, D. L. (1982). Intravenous glycerol and mannitol therapy in children with intracranial hypertension. *Neurology, 32,* 437–440.

Marshall, L. F., & Marshall, S. B. (1987). Medical management of intracranial pressure. In P. R. Cooper (Ed.). *Head injury* (pp. 177–196). Baltimore: Williams & Wilkins.

Marshall, S. B., Marshall, L. F., Vos, H. R., & Chestnut, R. M. (1990). *Neuroscience critical care: Pathophysiology and patient management.* Philadelphia: W. B. Saunders.

Menkes, J. H. (1990). Cerebrovascular disorders. In J. H. Menkes (Ed.). *Textbook of child neurology* (pp. 583–601). Philadelphia: Lea & Febiger.

Menkes, J. H. (1990). *Textbook of child neurology* (4th ed.). Philadelphia: Lea & Febiger.

Menkes, J. H., & Till, K. (1990). Tumors of the nervous system. In J. H. Menkes (Ed.). *Textbook of child neurology* (pp. 526–582). Philadelphia: Lea & Febiger.

Menkes, J. H., Till, K., & Gabriel, R. S. (1990). Malformations of the central nervous system. In J. H. Menkes (Ed.). *Textbook of child neurology* (pp. 209–283). Philadelphia: Lea & Febiger.

Michenfelder, J. D., & Milde, J. N. (1990). Postischemic canine cerebral blood flow appears to be determined by cerebral metabolic needs. *Journal of Cerebral Blood Flow Metabolism, 10,* 71–76.

Mitchell, P. H. (1986). Decreased adaptive capacity, intracranial: A proposal for a nursing diagnosis. *Journal of Neuroscience Nursing, 18,* 170–175.

Mitchell, P. H. (1988). Neurologic disorders. In M. G. Kinney, D. R. Packa, & S. B. Dunbar (Eds.). *AACN's clinical reference for critical-care nursing* (pp. 971–1028). New York: McGraw-Hill.

Mitchell, P. H., Habermann-Little, B., Johnson, F., VanInwegan-Scott, R., Tyler, D. (1985). Critically ill children: The importance of touch in a high-technology environment. *Nursing Administration Quarterly, 9*(4), 38–46.

Morrison, C. A. M. (1987). Brain herniation syndromes. *Critical Care Nurse, 7*(5), 34–38.

Moshe, S. L. (1989). Usefulness of EEG in the evaluation of brain death in children: The pros. *Electroencephalography and Clinical Neurophysiology, 73,* 272–275.

Muizelaar, J. P., Lutz, H. A., & Becker, D. P. (1984). Effect of mannitol in ICP and CBF and correlation with pressure autoregulation in severely head-injured patients. *Journal of Neurosurgery, 61,* 700–706.

Muizelaar, J. P., Marmarou, A., Ward, J. D., Kontos, H. A., Choi, S. C., Becker, D. P., Gruemer, N., & Young, H. F. (1991). Adverse effects of prolonged hyperventilation in patients with severe head injury: A randomized clinical trial. *Journal of Neurosurgery, 75,* 731–739.

Muizelaar, J. P., van der Poel, H. G., Li, Z., Kontos, N. A., & Levasseur, J. E., (1988). Pial arteriolar vessel diameter and CO_2 reactivity during prolonged hyperventilation in the rabbit. *Journal of Neurosurgery, 69,* 923–927.

Muizelaar, J. P., Wei, E. P., Kontos, H. A., & Becker, D. P. (1983). Mannitol causes compensatory cerebral vasoconstriction and vasodilation in response to blood viscosity changes. *Journal of Neurosurgery, 59,* 822–828.

National Head Injury Foundation (1986). *Definition of traumatic brain injury.* Southborough, MA: National Head Injury Foundation.

Nussbaum, E., & Maggie, J. C. (1988). Pentobarbital therapy does not improve neurologic outcome in nearly drowned, flaccid-comatose children. *Pediatrics, 81,* 630–634.

Ogilvie, J. W. (1988). Anterior spine fusion with Zielke instrumentation for idiopathic scoliosis in adolescents. *Orthopedic Clinics of North America, 19,* 313–317.

Orlowski, J. P. (1987). Drowning, near-drowning, and ice-water submersions. *Pediatric Clinics of North America, 34,* 75–92.

Outwater, K. K., & Rockoff, M. A. (1984). Apnea testing to confirm brain death in children. *Critical Care Medicine, 12,* 357–358.

Parsons, L. C., Peard, A. L., & Page, M. C. (1983). The effects of hygiene interventions on the cerebrovascular status of severe closed head injured persons. *Research in Nursing and Health, 8,* 173–181.

Perlman, J. M., & Volpe, J. J. (1983). Suctioning in the preterm infant: Effect on cerebral blood flow velocity, intracranial pressure, and arterial blood pressure. *Pediatrics, 72,* 329–334.

Pitlick, W. H., Pirikitakuhlr, P., Painter, M. J., & Wessel, H. B. (1982). Effects of glycerol and hyperosmolality on intracranial pressure. *Clinical Pharmacology and Therapy, 31,* 466–471.

Post, E. M. (1985). Currently available shunt systems: A review. *Neurosurgery, 16,* 257–260.

Prendergast, V. (1994). Current trends in research and treatment of intracranial hypertension. *Critical Care Nursing Quarterly, 17*(1), 1–8.

President's commission. Guidelines for the determination of death: Report of the medical consultants on the diagnosis of death to the President's Commission for the Study of Ethical Problems in Medicine and Biomedical and Behavioral Research (1981). *Journal of the American Medical Association, 246,* 2184–2186.

Prough, D. S., Johnson, J. C., Poole, G. V., Stullken, E. H., Johnston, W. E., & Royster, R. (1985). Effects on intracranial pressure of resuscitation from hemorrhagic shock with hypertonic saline versus lactated Ringer's solution. *Critical Care Medicine, 13,* 407–411.

Quagliarello, V., & Scheld, W. M. (1992). Bacterial meningitis: Pathogenesis, pathophysiology, and progress. *The New England Journal of Medicine, 327,* 864–872.

Quan, L., Gore, E. J., Wentz, K., Allen, J., & Novack, A. H. (1989). Ten year study of pediatric drownings and near-drownings in King County, Washington: Lessons in injury prevention. *Pediatrics, 83,* 1035–1040.

Quandt, C. M., & de los Reyes, R. A. (1984). Pharmacologic management of acute intracranial hypertension. *Drug Intelligence and Clinical Pharmacy, 18,* 105–112.

Reivich, M. (1964). Arterial PCO_2 and cerebral hemodynamics. *American Journal of Physiology, 206*(1), 25–35.

Rivara, F. P. (1985). Traumatic deaths of children in the United States: Currently available prevention strategies. *Pediatrics, 75,* 456–462.

Roberts, P. (1995). Nutrition in the head-injured patient. *New Horizons, 3,* 506–516.

Rogers, M. C., & Kirsch, J. R. (1989). Current concepts in brain resuscitation. *Journal of the American Medical Association, 261,* 3143–3147.

Rorke, L. B., Gilles, F. H., Davis, R. L., & Becker, L. E. (1985). Revision of the World Health Organization classification of brain tumors for childhood brain tumors. *Cancer, 56,* 1869–1886.

Rosenberg, A. A. (1986). Cerebral blood flow and O_2 metabolism after asphyxia in neonatal lambs. *Pediatric Research, 20,* 778–782.

Rosner, M. J., & Coley, I. B. (1986). Cerebral perfusion pressure, intracranial pressure, and head elevation. *The Journal of Neurosurgery, 65,* 636–641.

Rubenstein, J. S. (1992). Acute pediatric CNS infections. In B. P. Fuhrman & J. J. Zimmerman (Eds.). *Pediatric critical care* (pp. 613–620). St. Louis: Mosby–YearBook.

Rudy, E. B. (1984). *Advanced neurological and neurosurgical nursing.* St. Louis: C. V. Mosby.

Rudy, E. B., Turner, B. S., Baun, M., Stone, K. S., & Brucia, J. (1991). Endotracheal suctioning in adults with head injury. *Heart & Lung, 20,* 667–674.

Safar, P. (1986). Cerebral resuscitation after cardiac arrest: A review. *Circulation, 74*[Suppl IV], 138–153.

Safar, P. (1988). Resuscitation from clinical death: Pathophysiologic limits and therapeutic potentials. *Critical Care Medicine, 16,* 923–941.

Safar, P., & Bircher, N. G. (1992). The pathophysiology of dying and reanimation. In G. R. Schwartz, C. G. Cayten, M. A. Mangelsen, T. A. Mayer, & B. K. Hanke (Eds.). *Principles and practice of emergency medicine* (pp. 3–41). Philadelphia: Lea & Febiger.

Sarnaik, A. P., & Lieh-Lai, M. W. (1992). Near-drowning. In B. P. Fuhrman & J. J. Zimmerman (Eds.). *Pediatric Critical Care* (pp. 1201–1207). Philadelphia: Mosby–YearBook.

Sarnaik, A. P., Preston, G., Lich-Lai, M., & Eisenbrey, A. B. (1985). Intracranial pressure and cerebral perfusion pressure in near-drowning. *Critical Care Medicine, 13,* 224–227.

Sarnaik, A. P., & Vohra, M. P. (1986). Near-drowning: Fresh, salt, and cold water immersion. *Clinics in Sports Medicine, 5,* 33–46.

Shapiro, H. M. (1975). Intracranial hypertension: Therapeutic and anesthetic considerations. *Anesthesiology, 43,* 445–471.

Shapiro, H. M., Galindo, A., Wyte, S. R., & Harris, A. B. (1973). Rapid intraoperative reduction of intracranial pressure with thiopentone. *British Journal of Anesthesiology, 45,* 1057–1062.

Shapiro, K. (1985). Head injury in children. In D. Becker & J. Povlishock (Eds.). *CNS trauma status report* (pp. 243–253). Bethesda, MD: NINCDS, National Institue of Health.

Shapiro, K., & Giller, C. A. (1991). Increased intracranial pressure. In D. L. Levin & F. C. Morris (Eds.). *Essentials of pediatric intensive care* (pp. 49–53). St. Louis: Quality Medical Publishing.

Shewmon, A. (1988). Commentary on guidelines for the determination of brain death in children. *Issues in Clinical Neuroscience, 24,* 789–791.

Shinnar, S., Gammon, K., Bergman, E. W., Epstein, M., & Freeman, J. M. (1985). Management of hydrocephalus in infancy: Use of acetazolamide and furosemide to avoid cerebrospinal fluid shunts. *Journal of Pediatrics, 107,* 31–37.

Snow, R. B., Zimmerman, R. D., Gandy, S. E., & Derk, D. F. (1986). Comparison of magnetic resonance imaging and computed tomography in the evaluation of head injury. *Neurosurgery, 18,* 45–52.

Spyker, D. A. (1985). Submersion injury: Epidemiology, prevention, and management. *Pediatric Clinics of North America, 32,* 113–125.

Steen, P. A., Gisvold, S. E., Milde, J. H., Newberg, L. A., Scheithauer, B. W., Lanier, W. L, & Michenfelder, J. B. (1985). Nimodipine improves outcome when given after complete cerebral ischemia in primates. *Anesthesiology, 62,* 406–414.

Stewart-Amidei, C. (1991). Meningioma: Nursing care considerations. *Journal of Post Anesthesia Nursing, 6,* 269–278.

Sutton, L. N., & Schut, L. (1989). Cerebellar astrocytomas. In M. Wonsiewicz (Ed.). *Pediatric neurosurgery* (pp. 338–346). Philadelphia: W. B. Saunders.

Task Force for the Determination of Brain Death in Children (1987). Guidelines for the determination of brain death in children. *Neurology, 37,* 1077–1078.

Task Force on Brain Death in Children (1988). [Reply]. *Issues in Clinical Neuroscience, 24,* 791.

Tasker, R. C., & Dean, J. M. (1992). Status epilepticus. In M. C. Rogers (Ed.). *Textbook of pediatric intensive care* (pp. 751–777), Baltimore: Williams & Wilkins.

Trauner, D. (1986). Barbiturate therapy in acute brain injury. *The Journal of Pediatrics, 109,* 742–746.

Trauner, D. (1988). Seizure disorders. In W. C. Wiederholt (Ed.). *Neurology for the non-neurologist* (pp. 239–254). Philadelphia: Grune & Stratton.

Vaiden, R. E., & White, W. R. (1987). Arteriovenous malformations of the brain. *AORN Journal, 46(1),* 37–47.

Vas, C. J. (1990). Brain death in children. *Indian Journal of Pediatrics, 57,* 735–742.

Volpe, J. J. (1987). [Commentary]. Brain death determination in the newborn. *Pediatrics, 80,* 293–297.

Vulcan, B. M. (1987). Acute bacterial meningitis in infancy and childhood. *Critical Care Nurse, 7(5),* 53–65.

Walleck, C. A. (1989). Controversies in the management of the head-injured patient. *Critical Care Nursing Clinics of North America, 1,* 67–74.

Ward, J. D. (1995). Pediatric issues in head trauma. *New Horizons, 3,* 539–545.

Ward, J. D., Becker, D. P., Miller, J. D., Choi, S. C., Marmarou, A., Wood, C., Newlon, P. G., & Keenan, R. (1985). Failure of prophylactic barbiturate coma in the treatment of severe head injury. *Journal of Neurosurgery, 62,* 383–388.

Wauquier, A., Edmonds, H. L., & Clincke, G. H. C. (1987). Cerebral resuscitation: Pathophysiology and therapy. *Neuroscience & Biobehavioral Reviews, 11,* 287–306.

Weil, M. L. (1990). Infections of the nervous system. In J. H. Menkes (Ed.). *Textbook of child neurology* (pp. 327–423). Philadelphia: Lea & Febiger.

White, P. F., Schlobohm, R. M., Pitts, L. H., & Lindauer, J. M. (1982). A randomized study of drugs for preventing increases in intracranial pressure during endotracheal suctioning. *Anesthesiology, 57,* 242–244.

Wiggins, C. W., Loisel, D., & Budock, A. M. (1991). Intracranial arteriovenous malformation in a neonate: Aneurysm of the great vein of Galen. *Neonatal Network, 9(8),* 7–17.

Wilberger, J. E., & Cantella, D. (1995). High-dose barbiturates for intracranial pressure control. *New Horizons, 3,* 469–473.

Wilkinson, H. A., & Rosenfeld, S. (1983). Furosemide and mannitol in the treatment of acute experimental intracranial hypertension. *Neurosurgery, 12,* 405–410.

Williams, M. H. (1985). Arteriovenous malformations: Complications of surgical intervention and implications for nursing. *Journal of Neurosurgical Nursing, 17(1),* 14–21.

Willis, D., & Harbit, M. D. (1990). Transcatheter arterial embolization of cerebral arteriovenous malformations. *Journal of Neuroscience Nursing, 22,* 280–284.

Yano, M., Nishiyama, N., Yokota, N., Kato, K., Yamamoto, Y., & Otsuka, T. (1986). Effect of lidocaine on ICP response to endotracheal suctioning. *Anesthesiology, 64,* 651–653.

Young, J. L., & Miller, R. W. (1975). Incidence of malignant tumors in children. *Journal of Pediatrics, 86,* 254–258.

Zimmerman, R. A., Bilaniuk, L. T., Bruce, D., Dolinskas, C., Obrist, W., & Kuhl, D. (1978). Computed tomography of pediatric head trauma: Acute general cerebral swelling. *Radiology, 126,* 403–408.

CHAPTER 22

Renal Critical Care Problems

SUSAN MORGAN MADDER

PAMELA M. MILBERGER

Renal function affects all body systems through continuous adjustment of the internal environment. The vital nature of the renal system in maintaining homeostasis is typically appreciated when renal dysfunction occurs. The final common pathway of renal dysfunction is acute renal failure (ARF), defined as an abrupt discontinuation of kidney function.

ARF frequently occurs in critically ill infants and children and can significantly affect morbidity and mortality. Mortality rates ranging from 8% to 78% have been reported (Sweet et al., 1989). High mortality is associated with multisystem organ failure (MSOF); much lower rates occur when ARF is a primary disease. Several factors make the diagnosis of ARF in infants and children difficult. Urine output, commonly used to define ARF, is affected by multiple variables, and nonoliguric forms of ARF are often undetected.

The pathogenesis of ARF is multifactoral. Because renal function is dependent upon renal blood flow, any diminution in flow potentially alters kidney function. Over time, hypoperfusion results in altered renal function because of changes in the kidney itself. Intrinsic renal failure can occur as a result of ingestion or administration of nephrotoxic agents which impair renal cell function and cause an alteration in renal tubular reabsorption and/or secretion.

The clinical presentation and laboratory findings in ARF vary. Deteriorating renal function is best identified by following trends in a child's renal status over time. Early identification and management of ARF can prevent irreversible renal dysfunction. This chapter reviews the care required for the critically ill pediatric patient in ARF.

RENAL FUNCTION

The impact of an acute illness in infants and children may exceed the capacity of the kidneys to maintain normal renal function. The most commonly recognized role of the kidney is the formation of urine. The mechanisms of secretion, reabsorption, and active transport take place in the renal tubules (Fig. 22–1). Secretion clears the serum of unwanted substances. Reabsorption and active transport allow substances to be returned to the serum in appropriate proportions to maintain normal blood levels.

Renal function is not limited to the formation of urine, but is also responsible for a variety of other activities that maintain the internal stability of other body systems. Table 22–1 provides a summary of these functions.

Acid-base balance is regulated by the kidneys, lungs, and chemical buffering systems. The kidney selectively secretes or absorbs hydrogen and bicar-

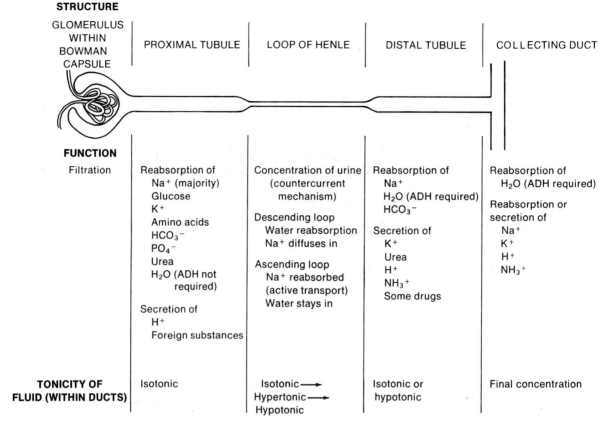

STRUCTURE

GLOMERULUS WITHIN BOWMAN CAPSULE	PROXIMAL TUBULE	LOOP OF HENLE	DISTAL TUBULE	COLLECTING DUCT
FUNCTION Filtration	Reabsorption of Na$^+$ (majority) Glucose K$^+$ Amino acids HCO$_3^-$ PO$_4^-$ Urea H$_2$O (ADH not required) Secretion of H$^+$ Foreign substances	Concentration of urine (countercurrent mechanism) Descending loop Water reabsorption Na$^+$ diffuses in Ascending loop Na$^+$ reabsorbed (active transport) Water stays in	Reabsorption of Na$^+$ H$_2$O (ADH required) HCO$_3^-$ Secretion of K$^+$ Urea H$^+$ NH$_3^+$ Some drugs	Reabsorption of H$_2$O (ADH required) Reabsorption or secretion of Na$^+$ K$^+$ H$^+$ NH$_3^+$
TONICITY OF FLUID (WITHIN DUCTS)	Isotonic	Isotonic → Hypertonic → Hypotonic	Isotonic or hypotonic	Final concentration

Figure 22–1 ● ● ● ● ● ●

Tubular components of the nephron. (From Whaley, L. F., & Wong, D. L. (1991). *Nursing Care of Infants and Children,* 4th ed. St. Louis: Mosby–YearBook.)

bonate ions to maintain the serum pH within normal range.

The kidneys maintain blood pressure by both direct and indirect means. This is accomplished by altering the circulating blood volume and activating the renin-angiotensin system. The outcome of renin-angiotensin system activation is contraction of vascular smooth muscle and aldosterone secretion, which results in renal tubular reabsorption of sodium and water (Fig. 22–2).

The kidney secretes erythropoietin, which stimu-

Table 22–1. RENAL FUNCTION

Function	Mechanism
Formation of urine	Secretion, reabsorption, and active transport
Acid-base balance	Hydrogen/bicarbonate ion secretion or absorption
Maintenance of blood pressure	Alteration in circulating blood volume, renin-angiotensin system
Erythrocyte production	Secretion of erythropoietin
Calcium and phosphorus balance	Activation of vitamin D
Vasodilation or vasoconstriction of the renal vasculature	Synthesis of prostaglandins

lates bone marrow to produce erythrocytes. Erythropoietin is released in response to decreased oxygen delivery to the kidneys resulting from low hematocrit and/or oxygen tension.

Several factors, including vitamin D$_3$ and parathyroid hormone (PTH), regulate calcium metabolism. Vitamin D$_3$ is an essential cofactor for PTH in both bone and kidney. After vitamin D$_3$ is absorbed by the jejunum and ileum, it must be metabolized into its active form first by the liver and then by the kidney. In its active form, vitamin D$_3$ promotes intestinal absorption of calcium and stimulates bone reabsorption of calcium. In the absence of vitamin D$_3$, hypocalcemia and disturbances in bone mineralization occur.

Serum calcium and phosphate levels share an inverse relationship (i.e., when serum calcium levels rise, serum phosphate levels decline and vice versa). The interrelationship of calcium-phosphate is progressively disrupted during ARF. When the glomerular filtration rate (GFR) decreases, phosphate is retained by the kidneys. Phosphate retention decreases serum calcium levels. The azotemic state also interferes with vitamin D activation by the kidneys, necessary for intestinal absorption of calcium. Both factors contribute to hypocalcemia.

The nephron also synthesizes prostaglandins, which are important in the maintenance of renal blood flow and glomerular perfusion during changes

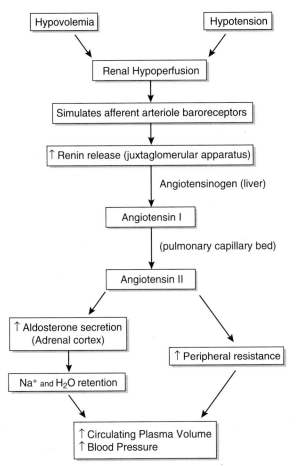

Figure 22-2 ● ● ● ● ● ●

The renin-angiotensin aldosterone cascade to maintain systemic perfusion pressure.

in renal vascular resistance. Vasodilation results in an increase in blood flow and GFR, whereas the opposite is true during vasoconstriction.

Maturational Factors

Maturation of renal function may require 2 years (Spitzer et al., 1985). During this time the immature kidney can ensure fluid and electrolyte balance, which is essential for growth in the developing infant; however, it is less capable of adjusting to the stress imposed by an acute illness. Table 22-2 summarizes the limitations of immature renal function.

In adults, renal blood flow normally constitutes 20% to 25% of the total cardiac output. Renal blood flow in infants may be 20 times lower because of lower mean arterial pressures and the high renal vascular resistance found in the immature kidney (Jose et al., 1987). The higher vascular resistance may be a response to the renin-angiotensin system and increased circulating catecholamines. The sympathetic nervous system may also play an important role in renal hemodynamics in infants. Sympathetic innervation may be incomplete, and most of the adrenergic receptor sites may be of alpha type, which

produce renal vasoconstriction when stimulated (Seikaly & Arant, 1992).

Increased vascular resistance causes vasoconstriction of the afferent arteriole, which decreases renal blood flow, ultrafiltration, and ultimately GFR. Because of the low GFR, the infant is unable to eliminate excessive water or solutes rapidly or efficiently. Renal blood flow increases with maturation mainly because of decreased vascular resistance within the afferent and efferent arterioles (Grupe, 1986). GFR and urine volume increase in direct relationship. GFR also increases as growth increases the surface area available for filtration. Thus, ultrafiltration pressure increases, and afferent arteriole resistance decreases (Seikaly & Avant, 1992).

Sodium balance is essential for tissue growth, and its conservation is important in the first year of life. However, immature tubular function results in less efficient maintenance of sodium and water balance. The decreased urinary excretion of sodium characteristic of the first year of life is directly related to the low GFR and high resorption rates at the level of the distal segment of the nephron (Robillard et al., 1992). A sodium load cannot be managed.

Functional limits also render the immature kidney less capable of excreting excessive water or concentrating urine to conserve water. The incomplete development of the concentration mechanisms is related to the short length of the loop of Henle and the abundance of interstitial tissue surrounding these anatomic structures. In the infant the shorter loop reduces the ability to either dilute or concentrate urine. During maturation the length and volume of the loop of Henle gradually increase and concentrating ability reaches adult levels by 2 years of age (Jose et al., 1987).

Associated with anatomic immaturity is an inability to build an adequate concentration gradient between solutes and water in the tubular structures (Spitzer et al., 1985). In the infant, this may be

Table 22-2. MATURATIONAL LIMITATIONS OF RENAL FUNCTION

Characteristics	Mechanism
Inability to excrete excessive sodium	Immature tubular function
Lower serum bicarbonate concentrations	Limited capacity to reabsorb bicarbonate and secrete hydrogen ions
Inability to concentrate urine	Cannot generate a sufficient concentration gradient in the inner medulla
Low GFR	Low perfusion pressures, decreased surface area available for filtration, glomerular permeability, and low glomerular plasma flow
Decreased percentage of cardiac output delivered to the kidney	High renal vascular resistance in afferent and efferent arterioles

related to the small amounts of urea excreted in the urine, reflecting the powerful anabolic state created by the demands of growth. As a result, the infant cannot excrete very dilute urine in states of overhydration and may be unable to excrete a very concentrated urine in response to dehydration. Maintenance of fluid balance is a challenge in an infant experiencing an acute illness.

Renal regulation of acid-base balance in the immature kidney has certain quantitative differences. Not reflecting acidosis, serum pH and bicarbonate levels are lower because of low renal threshold for bicarbonate (Grupe, 1986). The immature kidney has a limited ability to reabsorb bicarbonate and excretes it more freely from the renal tubules. Under normal conditions the immature kidney is able to maintain acid-base homeostasis but, when challenged with excess acid, the immature kidney is unable to clear it efficiently.

ACUTE RENAL FAILURE

Traditionally, ARF has been divided into three categories: prerenal, renal, and postrenal failure. These are not true divisions of "renal failure" but causes of

oliguria and azotemia (Fig. 22–3). True fixed renal failure occurs after a persistent state of prerenal or postrenal oliguria resulting in significant renal parenchymal damage. ARF can be prevented or attenuated with early recognition and appropriate intervention.

Prerenal Failure

Prerenal oliguria results from events that compromise renal perfusion prior to glomerular filtration (Table 22–3). Oliguria is a compensatory mechanism intended to restore intravascular volume when tissue perfusion is inadequate. Through conservation of sodium and water, venous return is increased and tissue perfusion to major organ systems may be improved.

The physiologic responses of the kidney to reduced blood flow depends upon the integrity of several intrarenal and extrarenal mechanisms. Intrarenal mechanisms control renal blood flow through autoregulation, defined as the intrinsic automatic adjustment of blood flow through an individual organ by modifications in the diameter of arterioles feeding the capillary bed (Maxwell et al., 1987). By varying

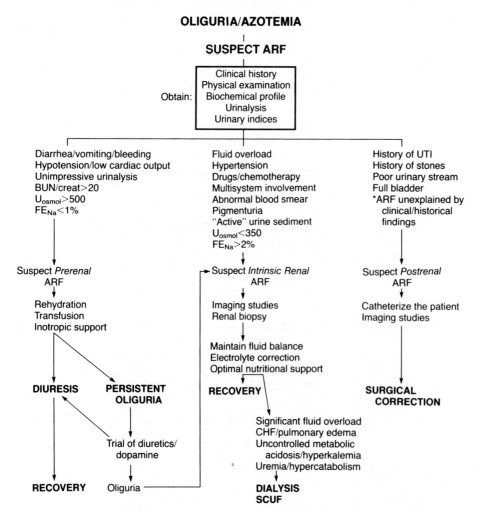

Figure 22-3 ● ● ● ● ● ●

Suggested approach to the basic diagnostic and therapeutic management of acute renal failure in infants and children. (From Ongkingco, J. R. C., & Block, G. H. (1933). Diagnosis and management of acute renal failure in the critical care unit. In Holbrook, P. R.: *Textbook of pediatric critical care,* p. 592. Philadelphia, W. B. Saunders.)

Table 22–3. CAUSES OF PRERENAL OLIGURIA

Altered Cardiac Performance	Vasodilation	Altered Vascular Volume	Altered Blood Supply to the Kidney
Cardiogenic shock	Septic shock	Intravascular volume loss	Surgical
Congestive heart failure	Anaphylaxis	Hemorrhage	Cardiac bypass
Congenital heart disease	Allergic	Third Space	Aortic cross-clamp
Postoperative myocardial dysfunction	Transfusion	Edema	Umbilical arterial catheter displacement
Dysrhythmias	Vasodilating agents	Peritonitis	Renal artery thrombosis
Cardiomyopathy		Burns	
Myocarditis		Gastrointestinal loss	
		Vomiting	
		Diarrhea	
		Renal Losses	
		Excessive diuresis	

arteriolar resistance, autoregulation allows organs to regulate blood flow in proportion to metabolic demand and maintain a constant blood flow over a wide range of perfusion pressures.

Autoregulation in the kidney is designed to maintain a relatively constant intraglomerular perfusion pressure despite a wide range of mean perfusion pressures (80–180 mmHg) (Maxwell et al., 1987). Because infants have lower systemic pressure, autoregulation is likely to have a much narrower range (30–60 mmHg). Autoregulation functions independent of extrarenal, humoral, or neurogenic factors. To maintain a relatively constant GFR, afferent arteriolar resistance varies in direct proportion to systemic pressure. Systemic hypotension is accompanied by afferent arteriolar vasodilation, which reduces renal vascular resistance and improves renal blood flow. The opposite is true during systemic hypertension. Because arterioles are present at either end of the glomerulus, constriction or dilation of these arterioles alters the perfusion pressure through the glomerular capillaries and regulates glomerular filtration. Changes in GFR ultimately affect the volume and content of the final urine product.

The extrarenal mechanisms that affect renal function include alterations in cardiac output, systemic vascular tone and corresponding distribution of systemic blood flow, and systemic blood pressure. The importance of the interplay of both intrarenal and extrarenal factors is evident during the physiologic response of the kidney to an acute episode of volume depletion or myocardial dysfunction. For example, a sudden reduction in renal perfusion activates the renin-angiotensin system to normalize renal perfusion and maintain GFR (see Fig. 22–2). The release of renin from the macula densa acts extrarenally to increase systemic vascular resistance and improve systemic blood pressure. In addition, renin stimulates the adrenal cortex to release aldosterone, which acts to increase tubular reabsorption of sodium followed by water. These responses also serve to normalize renal perfusion, thereby maintaining the GFR.

Primary or secondary renal vascular disease may cause a partial or complete obstruction to blood flow, resulting in renal ischemia. Renal artery thrombosis,

while rare in children, is an iatrogenic complication of umbilical artery cannulation and presents as acute hypertension. Acceleration of cortical ischemia contributes to acute hypertension activating the renin-angiotensin cascade, which results in a decrease in GFR. Renal vein thrombosis should be suspected in any infant who presents with hematuria, proteinuria, or an enlarging abdominal mass. Bilateral renal vein occlusion, a more common vascular lesion in infants, is associated with asphyxia, cyanotic congenital heart defects and maternal diabetes mellitus (Karlowicz & Adelman, 1992).

If compromised renal perfusion persists, the capacity of the intrarenal and extrarenal mechanisms to maintain homeostasis is jeopardized. Urine production decreases and azotemia may occur. If systemic pressure and volume are not restored after a finite period of time, true, fixed intrinsic renal failure ensues. Early detection of the subtle signs and symptoms of intrinsic renal failure is crucial to facilitate appropriate management to preserve renal function.

Clinical Presentation

Oliguria is no longer considered the cardinal sign of ARF, because ARF can be associated with any volume of urine excretion (Maxwell et al., 1987). *Nonoliguric ARF* describes renal dysfunction associated with a normal or excessive urine volume. The key to early recognition is to be alert for signs of decreased or increased urine volume in relation to overall fluid balance.

Acid-base disturbances may be detected early in patients with prerenal failure. An unexplained metabolic acidosis is a sign of decreased tissue perfusion, including renal perfusion.

The diagnosis of renal failure is based on the presence of azotemia. Serum blood urea nitrogen (BUN) and creatinine provide an index of glomerular filtration. Both of these substances are nitrogenous endproducts of protein metabolism normally excreted in urine. As GFR decreases, BUN and creatinine increase. In isolation, BUN is not a reliable indicator of renal function because the level may be affected by factors other than nitrogen excretion by the kidney. Extrarenal factors that affect BUN concentration are

Table 22–4. EXTRARENAL FACTORS THAT AFFECT BUN
AND CREATININE LEVELS

Blood Urea Nitrogen	
Increased by:	*Decreased by:*
Corticosteroid administration	Liver disease
Hypercatabolic states (e.g., fever, sepsis)	Hypometabolic state
GI hemorrhage	Hyperlipidemia
Dehydration	Low protein diet
High protein diet	High caloric diet
Starvation	

Creatinine	
Increased by:	*Decreased by:*
Dehydration	Loss of muscle mass
Rhabdomyolysis	Burns
Cephalosporins	Hyperlipidemia

listed in Table 22–4. Creatinine is an endproduct of
muscle metabolism, which is excreted and eliminated
at a constant rate. Serum creatinine is relatively
unaffected by extrarenal factors and, therefore, is a
more reliable indicator of glomerular function. Because the level of serum creatinine is a function of
muscle mass, plasma levels are affected by age, sex,
and body build (Ruley & Bock, 1989). In the face of
decreased tubular flow, a greater percentage of urea
is reabsorbed into the circulatory system, producing
a significant elevation in serum BUN. In the same
circumstance creatinine levels are usually only
slightly elevated. The serum BUN/creatinine ratio
may also help to differentiate prerenal from intrinsic
renal failure (Table 22–5).

Other laboratory values used to determine and
differentiate prerenal failure from intrinsic renal
failure include measuring tubular reabsorption of sodium and water. Unlike the kidney with parenchymal damage, the underperfused but functionally intact kidney has the capability to actively reabsorb
sodium as a compensatory response to hypovolemia.
A urinary sodium concentration less than 20 mEq/L

is more often present in prerenal failure, whereas
urinary sodium concentrations greater than 40 mEq/
L are consistent with parenchymal failure (Rudnick
et al., 1983). These levels may be altered by the
administration of diuretics. Loop diuretics inhibit the
reabsorption of sodium at the proximal tubule, which
improves solute excretion in the urine.

Reabsorption of water also requires a functionally
intact renal tubule. Measurement of urine specific
gravity is a simple and readily available procedure.
A urine specific gravity over 1.020 strongly suggests
prerenal failure. The increased concentration of
urine indicates decreased renal blood flow and functioning compensatory mechanisms intended to preserve circulating volume. However, falsely high values may occur in the presence of urine protein,
glucose, bilirubin, radiographic dyes, or other high-
molecular-weight substances (Rudnick et al., 1983).

Urine osmolality measurements are usually unaffected by protein, glucose, bilirubin, and radiographic
dyes (Ruley & Bock, 1989). Although there can be
considerable overlap among individuals, prerenal
failure is usually associated with a urine osmolality
greater than 500 mOsm/L, whereas parenchymal
failure is associated with a urine osmolality of less
than 350 mOsm/L.

Chemical testing of the urine has been simplified
by the introduction of multiple dipstick tests that
detect substances such as glucose, bilirubin, pH, protein, blood, and ketones on a single impregnated
paper strip. Dipstick tests can be done quickly and
accurately to gather information about the capacity
of the kidneys to maintain homeostasis during an
acute illness. Persistent proteinuria usually indicates
renal disease, evidencing an increase in glomerular
permeability to protein. Hematuria is a common
finding in a number of renal diseases and in processes involving the lower urinary tract, including
infection, trauma, and neoplasms. Hematuria is a
prominent feature in glomerulonephritis.

Numerous radiologic procedures are available to
evaluate the renal system. Imaging techniques are

Table 22–5. LABORATORY VALUES THAT DIFFERENTIATE CAUSES OF OLIGURIA

Laboratory Test	Normal	Prerenal Failure	Renal Failure
Urine specific gravity	1.015–1.022	>1.020	<1.010
Urine osmolality	50–1500 mOsm/L (infant: 50–650)	>500	<400
Urine sodium	40–80 mEq/L	<10 mEq/L	>30 mEq/L (infant >25)
Urine potassium	40–80 mEq/L	30–70 mEq/L	<20–40 mEq/L
Urine creatinine		>100 mg/dL	<70 mg/dL
Urine creatinine:plasma ratio		>30	<20 (infant <10)
Urine urea		>2000	<400
Urine urea:plasma ratio		>14	<6
Serum BUN/creatinine ratio	10:1–15:1	>20:1	<10:1
FE_{NA} (Fractional excretion of filtered sodium)	<1%	<1%	>2%

used to rule out obstruction when the etiology of ARF is unknown. Abdominal radiographs are used to determine kidney presence and size, or demonstrate calcification. Ultrasonography is also used to assess kidney size and identify urinary obstruction. Ultrasonography is particularly useful in differentiating solid tumors from fluid-filled cysts. Radionuclide studies evaluate both structure and function, and thus are helpful in differentiating parenchymal and obstructive renal failure. In addition to limitations of its use because of poor visualization in young infants, excretory urography is considered a high-risk procedure in the oliguric or anuric patient. Renal arteriogram allows for visualization of renal blood vessels and is helpful in assessing renal blood supply, renal artery stenosis, and neoplasm. Complications following arteriogram include thrombus or embolus formation and local inflammation or hematoma at the site of entry.

Renal biopsy is rarely helpful in differentiating prerenal from parenchymal failure (Ruley & Bock, 1989). However, in selected patients in whom there is inconclusive evidence of tubular necrosis, renal biopsy may be useful.

Emergent Management

Assessment and intervention to attenuate renal parenchymal damage is dependent upon recognizing high-risk situations that are associated with prerenal failure. Those conditions that alter fluid volume status and cardiac performance place patients at particular risk. Patient outcome depends on early diagnosis and management of inadequate renal perfusion and avoidance or careful monitoring of patient response to nephrotoxic agents listed in Table 22–6. Prompt discontinuation of both nephrotoxic agents and supplemental potassium may be warranted.

The first step in managing an oliguric patient is to assess and assure the adequacy of intravascular volume. On physical examination, dry mucous membranes, tachycardia, hypotension, a sunken fontanel, absence of tears, and decreased urine volume indicate hypovolemia. Ongoing assessment includes direct physical examination as well as monitoring hemodynamic variables that reflect volume status.

Table 22–6. NEPHROTOXIC AGENTS

Antibiotics	**Other**
Penicillins	Heavy metals:
Sulfonamides	lead, mercury, iron
Cephalosporins	copper, gold
Gentamicin	Organic solvents:
Amphotericin B	carbon tetrachloride
Diuretics	turpentine, ethylene glycol
Furosemide	
Mannitol	
Hyperuricemic agents	
Radiographic contrast agents	
Antineoplastic agents	
Salicylates	

Restoration of intravascular volume is the priority if hypovolemia is detected, to ensure adequate cardiac output regardless of whether renal damage has occurred. Except in the presence of hypervolemia, a 10- to 20-mL/kg fluid challenge, using any volume expander, is administered. The desired outcome is to restore circulating blood volume and increase urinary output. If the patient does not respond to the first fluid challenge, the same amount of volume may be repeated. Caution is taken to assess for signs of circulatory overload, which could jeopardize the patient if true renal parenchymal failure exists.

If the patient does not respond to the fluid bolus, diuretic therapy can be used to increase urine output. However, volume administration should always precede the administration of diuretics in the oliguric patient because diuretics may decrease renal perfusion by exacerbating preexisting dehydration (Maxwell et al., 1987). Diuretics can help distinguish prerenal from fixed renal failure and can convert an oliguric to a nonoliguric state. Diuretics may also be useful in restoring and maintaining normal water and electrolyte balance and preventing further renal damage.

Furosemide (Lasix) may be beneficial early in oliguria. The primary diuretic effect of furosemide is inhibition of chloride reabsorption in the ascending limb of the loop of Henle. Furosemide also increases renal blood flow and alters the intrarenal distribution of flow to augment filtration.

Mannitol administration should result in a urine output greater than 0.5 mL/kg/hour. Mannitol not only acts as an osmotic agent in the proximal tubule to inhibit the reabsorption of water, it also increases renal filtration pressure and causes a solute diuresis. Other theoretical benefits of mannitol include the maintenance of high urine flow, diminished renin secretion, and reduced endothelial cell swelling (Wells, 1990). Absence of a diuretic response suggests that tubular damage has occurred and that further mannitol therapy could be harmful. There is some concern that mannitol can cause hypervolemia and possibly pulmonary edema in patients who are unable to excrete the drug.

Diuretics can increase urine flow. However, increased urine flow is not necessarily the result of improved renal function, and diuretics appear to be limited in preventing, reversing or hastening recovery from renal failure (Maxwell et al., 1987). In addition, diuretics are not benign medications. Mannitol administration is associated with a dramatic increase in plasma volume and increased extracellular osmolality. The resultant fluid shifts may precipitate intraventricular hemorrhage in small infants or pulmonary edema in hypervolemic children with altered cardiac performance. Furosemide can cause interstitial nephritis, ototoxicity, and persistence of a patent ductus arteriosus (Ruley & Bock, 1989). The most common side effect of diuretic use is fluid and electrolyte imbalance. Major disturbances can occur rapidly in infants and small children, particularly when potent diuretics are administered. Fluid deficit impairs tissue perfusion to all organ systems. Electrolyte imbalance can occur rapidly, causing depletion of potassium, sodium, and chloride.

Dopamine may be effective at reversing oliguria in patients with early renal failure. Low-dose dopamine (1–5 μg/kg/min) results in renal vasodilation, increased renal blood flow, increased GFR, and sodium excretion. Infants may require higher doses of dopamine per kilogram of body weight because of immaturity of the sympathetic nervous system (Notterman, 1988). A synergistic effect of dopamine with diuretics has been proposed. Its vasodilator effects increase furosemide delivery to the renal tubular sites and subsequently increase urine output. The combination of low-dose dopamine and furosemide can result in conversion of oliguric to nonoliguric renal failure if adequate intravascular volume and cardiac output are present.

Recovery from prerenal failure depends upon astute nursing care focused to attenuate the progression of irreversible renal damage. Outcome is not only related to the underlying etiology of renal failure and extent of other organ system damage, but also to the ability of healthcare providers to recognize patients at risk and intervene effectively.

Intrinsic Renal Failure

Intrinsic renal failure refers to numerous conditions or primary physiologic events that produce renal parenchymal damage involving the glomerulus or tubular epithelium. Direct injury to the renal parenchyma also can be caused by episodes of acute hypoperfusion or adverse reactions to nephrotoxic agents.

Manifested by proteinuria and/or hematuria, intrinsic renal failure may occur after extensive injury to the glomerular capillary wall. Although the lesion is primarily glomerular, entire nephrons can be destroyed leading to chronic renal failure. The most common etiologies of intrinsic oliguria in the pediatric population are listed in Table 22–7. More than 50% of cases of intrinsic renal failure in children are the result of acute glomerulonephritis and hemolytic uremic syndrome.

Acute post-streptococcal glomerulonephritis occurs most frequently in children between the ages of 3 and 7 (Price & Wilson, 1986). The major physiologic disturbance is decreased GFR, despite normal renal blood flow, caused by fibrin deposition in the glomerular capillary. Consequently, excretion of water, sodium, and nitrogenous substances is compromised, resulting in oliguria and azotemia. Most children are not usually critically ill and recover completely following treatment. ARF can develop from renal microvascular disease.

The precise etiology of *hemolytic uremic syndrome* (HUS) is not known, but both infectious agents (viruses and bacteria) and endotoxin-mediated capillary endothelial injury have been suggested (Ruley & Bock, 1989). HUS occurs mainly in patients 2 months

Table 22–7. CAUSES OF INTRINSIC RENAL FAILURE

Immune-related
  Glomerulonephritis
  Systemic lupus erythematosus
Vascular
  Hemolytic-uremic syndrome
  Renal vein artery thrombosis
  Disseminated intravascular coagulation
  Thrombotic thrombocytopenia purpura
Interstitial nephritis
  Infectious
  Drug-related
  Malignant
Renal trauma
Nephrotoxins
  Endogenous
    Transfusion reaction
    Cytotoxic therapy
    Hyperalimentation
    Tumor lysis
  Exogenous
    Anesthetic agents
    Heavy metals
    Organic solvents
    Antibiotics
    Pesticides
    Radiographic contrast agents

to 8 years of age with no sex or racial predisposition (Price & Wilson, 1986). In HUS, damage occurs to the endothelial lining of blood vessels followed by fibrin and platelet aggregation. The occlusion of vessels leads to a microangiopathic hemolytic anemia, thrombocytopenia, and compromised renal function. As blood flows through the vessels that are lined with fibrin deposits, red blood cells (RBCs) become fragmented from mechanical stress. The damaged RBCs are quickly destroyed by the liver and spleen, resulting in a hemolytic anemia. Fibrin deposition in the renal blood vessels causes occlusion and damage to the glomeruli, resulting in ARF.

The term *acute tubular necrosis* (ATN) is commonly applied to nephrotoxic and ischemic renal injuries that damage the tubular epithelium. Two types of histologic changes are commonly observed in ATN: necrosis of the tubular epithelium leaving the basement membrane intact, commonly resulting from the ingestion of nephrotoxic agents, and necrosis of the tubular epithelium and basement membrane, commonly associated with renal ischemia. ATN is a common cause of eventual intrinsic renal failure in neonates following perinatal asphyxia, hypoxia, and sepsis.

Immature kidneys are uniquely sensitive to hypoxia. The reasons for this sensitivity include the high proportion of cardiac output normally delivered to the kidneys, the countercurrent concentrating mechanism in the renal medulla, and the relatively high oxygen requirement necessary for normal kidney function (Ruley & Bock, 1989). Nephrotoxic injury can also be produced by chemical agents that directly impair renal cell function, participate in immune or inflammatory reactions, and/or aggravate an underlying renal disorder (see Table 22–6) (Finn, 1990).

Ischemic injuries resulting in ATN occur during an acute period of renal hypoperfusion. If ischemia persists, irreversible renal damage occurs. The amount of renal cell damage depends upon the length of the ischemic episode. It has been reported that an ischemic time of 25 minutes or less causes reversible mild injury to renal cells; ischemia of 40 to 60 minutes results in severe damage that may resolve to some extent in 2 to 3 weeks; and ischemia lasting 60 to 90 minutes usually causes irreversible renal cell damage (Stahl, 1986). In low perfusion states, the autoregulatory properties of the afferent and efferent arterioles of the glomerulus become impaired. The pathologic change produced by renal ischemia is the destruction of tubular epithelium and basement membrane or *cortical necrosis*. When the basement membrane is destroyed, epithelial regeneration occurs in a random haphazard manner frequently leading to obstruction of the nephron at the site of necrosis. Prognosis is, therefore, dependent on the extent of necrosis.

The mechanisms that lead to a decrease in GFR and associated oliguria in patients with ATN have not been clearly defined. Tubular backleak and obstruction theories have been proposed to explain the oliguria associated with ATN. The tubular backleak hypothesis proposes that glomerular filtration continues normally but tubular fluid "leaks back" from the damaged tubular cells into the renal interstitium rather than being excreted as urine. Disruption and/or destruction of the basement membrane provides an anatomic basis for this mechanism (Baer & Lancaster, 1992). The tubular obstruction theory proposes that ATN leads to the desquamation of necrotic tubular cells and other protein materials, which then form casts that occlude the tubule lumina (Baer & Lancaster, 1992). Cellular swelling as a result of the initial ischemia may also contribute to obstruction and perpetuate the ischemia. Intratubular pressure increases, so that net glomerular filtration pressure is reduced. Tubular obstruction may be an important factor in ATN in situations where prolonged ischemia or ingestion of heavy metals or ethylene glycol occurs.

Clinical Presentation

Infants and children with ATN often present with abrupt-onset oliguria or anuria. It is important to recognize the onset of oliguria and differentiate the etiology leading to ATN from prerenal, intrinsic, and postrenal disorders that may cause oliguria. Three phases characterize the clinical course of ATN: oliguria, diuresis, and recovery.

After exposure to a nephrotoxic agent or following an ischemic event, oliguric ATN may develop immediately or several days after renal cell damage occurs. This phase is most often characterized by abrupt reduction in urine production that continues for 24 to 48 hours. However, severe oliguria may last from 1 day to 2 months with the average of 8 to 14 days (Maxwell et al., 1987). During the oliguric phase, serum BUN and creatinine rise. Other significant laboratory data resulting from tubular dysfunction and inability to concentrate urine include urine specific gravity less than 1.018, low urine osmolality, and urine sodium greater than 10 mEq/L. Potential complications during the oliguric phase include hypervolemia causing congestive heart failure and/or pulmonary edema and electrolyte imbalances, particularly hyponatremia and hyperkalemia; and acid-base disturbances.

The diuretic phase of ATN usually lasts 5 to 7 days. Early in the diuretic phase, urea clearance does not keep pace with endogenous urea production despite more than adequate urine output. BUN continues to rise. Later in the diuretic phase, BUN decreases and azotemia eventually disappears. Because glomerular filtration and subsequent production of urine is the first mechanism to recover, total body fluid and electrolytes may be depleted if replacement is inadequate. To achieve the goal of normovolemia with electrolyte and acid-base balance, astute monitoring is essential. Tubular reabsorption returns next and contributes significantly to the overall improvement in renal function.

The recovery phase from ATN in infants and children is usually longer than in adults: 2 to 4 months may elapse before normal renal function returns. BUN and urine laboratory values gradually return to normal, reflecting a progressive restoration of GFR and tubular function. The level of recovery is variable, especially if preexisting medical problems or renal insufficiency are present. Some patients may be left with some residual renal impairment, such as a permanent decrease in renal function or a urine concentrating defect. The primary cause of death during the recovery phase is infection and/or complications related to the primary illness that initially compromised renal function.

Nonoliguric ATN, increased urine output with elevated BUN and creatinine, is commonly associated with nephrotoxic agents. Compared with patients with oliguric ATN, morbidity and mortality rates are lower in patients with nonoliguric ATN (Gaudio & Siegel, 1987). Nonoliguria facilitates fluid and nutritional management of ARF.

Postrenal Failure

Postrenal oliguria results from an anatomic obstruction of the urinary tract and is uncommon in children. Table 22–8 outlines the causes of postrenal oliguria, which may result from obstruction of any portion of the urinary system. Most urinary obstruction is the result of a congenital problem. Obstruction increases intratubular pressure and leads to a reduction in renal blood flow and GFR that is manifested by a decrease in urinary output. Oliguria will not occur from unilateral obstruction unless the contralateral kidney is absent or nonfunctioning. In chil-

Table 22–8. POSTRENAL CAUSES OF OLIGURIA

Ureteral	
Intrinsic	*Extrinsic*
Stones	Tumor
Blood clot	Surgical ligation
Ureteropelvic stenosis	Radiation injury
Bladder	
Blood clots	
Neurogenic bladder	
Urethral	
Posterior urethral valves	
Urethral stricture	

dren, especially infants, who present with oliguria alone, the first consideration is to determine that the major anatomic components of the renal system: arteries, veins, ureters, and bladder outlet, are intact.

Anomalies in the urinary collecting system may restrict urinary flow from the bladder. Urinary reflux can ultimately increase hydrostatic pressure in the collecting ducts and renal tubules. When hydrostatic pressure in Bowman's capsule increases, GFR decreases, tubular reabsorption is enhanced, and oliguria or anuria develops. Eventually, renal insufficiency results from tissue atrophy.

Bilateral anatomic obstruction occurs more frequently in male infants than in females because of congenital posterior ureteral valves and/or urethral strictures. Postrenal oliguria may occur in older infants who have an undiagnosed solitary kidney that becomes acutely obstructed. This obstruction may be the result of an anatomic abnormality or an acquired intraluminal lesion such as renal calculi, blood clot, inflammation, and edema. Extrinsic compression of the urethral outflow tract by lesions such as periurethral abscess, trauma, Wilms' tumor or a neuroblastoma are rare but must be suspected in any patient with acute bilateral obstruction.

Clinical Presentation

The infrequent occurrence of obstructive uropathy in the critical care setting does not diminish its importance, because early diagnosis and correction can avert permanent parenchymal damage. Diagnostic imaging techniques are used to determine the etiology. Children with postrenal oliguria often present with abdominal or flank pain. A palpable mass may suggest an obstructed urinary system, although a mass may be associated with other causes of ARF such as renal vein thrombosis or polycystic kidney disease. A renal mass associated with a palpable bladder in a male suggests urinary tract obstruction from posterior ureteral valves. Young children may be completely asymptomatic except for failure to thrive. Analysis of urinary sediment associated with obstruction is usually normal unless there is a coexisting infection. Abdominal radiography and ultrasonography verify and reveal kidney size, demonstrate calcification, and help identify urinary obstruction.

Several invasive radiographic and urodynamic studies can be used to assess the function of the renal system through the detection of disturbances in voiding patterns and structural defects. These include intravenous pyelography (IVP), voiding cystourethrography (VCUG), renal angiography, and renal scan.

Emergent Management

The goal of treatment is decompression of the urinary collecting system by removal of the obstruction or by urinary diversion. Relief of the obstruction may result in a marked increase in urine formation because of increased renal blood flow and improved tubular function. However, hydrogen ion and potassium secretion may be impaired resulting in acidosis with hyperkalemia (Friedman, 1992). Management includes close surveillance of fluid and electrolyte balance to support kidney function during recovery.

Critical Care Management

As outlined in Table 22–9, altered renal function affects all body systems. Clinical presentation depends upon the length and acuity of the disease process.

Maintenance of Intravascular Volume

During ARF the regulatory factors that control *intravascular volume status* may be inadequate. Decreased or absent urine output deprives the body of a mechanism to eliminate fluid. Hypervolemia is a common manifestation of ARF. Hypertension may result from the increase in circulating volume and interplay of the renin-angiotensin system.

Deteriorating renal function may also result in excessive urinary output. Management strategies such as restricted fluid intake and diuretic therapy contribute to a fluid volume deficit. As a consequence, cardiac output and tissue perfusion may be impaired.

Maintenance fluid requirements are adjusted to the evolving needs of the patient. Daily total output determines intake. Daily output is the sum of urine output and insensible losses, which include gastroin-

Table 22–9. MANAGEMENT PRIORITIES DURING ARF

Alteration	Consequence
Intravascular volume status	Hyper- or hypovolemia manifested
Electrolyte balance	Abnormal K, Na, Ca, Mg, Phos levels
Uremia	Uremic syndrome
Acid-base balance	Metabolic acidosis
Nutritional status	Malnutrition
Immune function	Infection
Anemia, thrombocytopenia	Disruption in oxygen delivery, coagulation

testinal, respiratory, and evaporative losses. Other factors that influence precise calculation of fluid needs include the humidity and temperature of the environment, and the use of phototherapy, warming devices, and mechanical ventilation. Although fluid balance can be calculated, ongoing assessment of tissue perfusion is the best indicator of adequate intravascular volume.

Maintenance of Electrolyte Balance

Electrolyte disturbances commonly occur during the course of ARF. Alterations are related to changes in volume status and the inability of the kidneys to regulate electrolyte balance. Because the kidneys are responsible for 90% of potassium excretion, hyperkalemia is a major life-threatening complication of ARF. The catabolic state of the patient further elevates serum potassium.

Because of the potentially lethal nature of hyperkalemia, patients at risk require ongoing assessment of laboratory values along with cardiac rhythm assessment. Early ECG changes indicative of hyperkalemia are peaked or tented T waves. Later ECG changes include absent P waves, prolonged PR interval, and widened QRS complex. Physiologically significant hyperkalemia (>8.0 mEq/L) results in dysrhythmias. The most common dysrhythmias include second and third degree heart block, asystole, and ventricular fibrillation.

A primary goal in caring for the patient with ARF is the prevention of life-threatening hyperkalemia. Cautious attention to the administration of potassium containing intravenous fluid, medications (aqueous penicillin G) and cold stored blood is critical to attenuating the elevation of potassium levels.

Sodium imbalance is also prevalent in ARF. Hyponatremia is common. Important to consider is the variability in the amount of sodium excreted by the kidney. Induced diuresis or the diuretic phase of non-oliguric renal failure can significantly increase urine sodium loss. Hyponatremia also occurs because of dilutional effects related to retention of fluid in the oliguric patient or as a result of overestimation of intake needs.

Ongoing monitoring of serum sodium levels and urine sodium excretion determines the appropriate type and volume of fluid intake. Hyponatremia may deleteriously affect the clinical status and prognosis of the patient with acute renal failure. Cerebral edema, seizures, and coma result from adverse concentration gradients of sodium and osmolarity between the central nervous system and the systemic fluid compartment. Early clinical signs of neurologic dysfunction include decreased level of consciousness and changes in behavior. Serum sodium levels of 130 mEq/L indicate a need for further fluid restriction. Levels less than 120 mEq/L require aggressive therapy with intravenous administration of 3% sodium chloride (NaCl) solution or intravascular fluid removal.

Hypocalcemia and hyperphosphatemia are addi-

tional electrolyte disturbances that occur rapidly in ARF. Phosphate levels increase because of the limited ability of the kidney to excrete phosphate. This occurs simultaneously with catabolic increases in phosphate released from tissue. Hypocalcemia occurs along with hyperphosphatemia, although its exact etiology is not clearly defined. Decreased activation of vitamin D is another contributing factor resulting in decreased absorption of calcium (Feld et al, 1990).

Neurologic sequelae of hypocalcemia include seizures, muscle cramps, and tetany. Cardiovascular effects include diminished contractility and rhythm disturbance. Parenteral or enteral calcium replacement therapy is more efficient if hyperphosphatemia is managed first. Elevated plasma phosphate concentrations result in the precipitation of calcium phosphate in bone and soft tissues. Reduction of the serum phosphate level is accomplished by diminishing the absorption of phosphorus in the gastrointestinal tract. This usually results in an increase in the serum calcium level. Limiting the intake of parenteral and enteral sources of phosphate requires a thorough review of phosphorus content in all sources of intake.

Magnesium is another electrolyte that is affected by ARF. Generally, levels are normal or elevated. The manifestations of hypermagnesemia and depressed cardiac and neurologic functioning further compromise the patient with acute renal failure (Rice, 1983).

Maintenance of Acid-base Balance

The kidney maintains normal *acid-base balance* by the secretion and reabsorption of hydrogen and bicarbonate ions. Impairment of renal function results in the disturbance of acid-base homeostasis. Metabolic acidosis is the predominant finding. The causes of metabolic acidosis may be related to several etiologies. Renal tubular dysfunction results in the accumulation of acids and anion salts (Gaudio & Siegel, 1987). The mild acidosis that accompanies this isolated disturbance is compensated for by the respiratory system. Therefore, patients tolerate serum bicarbonate levels of 14 to 15 mEq/L (Gaudio & Siegel, 1987). Disturbances in normal cellular metabolism, resulting from hypoxemia and/or altered tissue perfusion, result in anaerobic metabolism and lactic acid production. Other conditions such as ethylene glycol intoxication, certain inborn errors of metabolism, diabetic ketoacidosis, or the administration of medications may overwhelm renal excretory capacity and worsen metabolic acidosis.

Symptoms of acid-base imbalance include hyperventilation, tachycardia, decreased level of consciousness, and decreased tissue perfusion. Patient assessment in combination with blood gas and serum potassium analysis facilitates patient care management. The inverse relationship of potassium and serum pH is considered when following trends of blood gases. Changes in pH are considered with respect to changes in both the arterial partial pressure of carbon dioxide ($PaCO_2$) and bicarbonate values. The bicarbonate level is the most reliable indicator of the ability of the kidneys to maintain acid-base balance.

Before initiating treatment for metabolic acidosis, the patient's ability to compensate for the imbalance is considered. Bicarbonate levels of 10 to 13 mEq/L may be managed with administration of intravenous sodium bicarbonate. Before administration, the extent to which the respiratory compensatory mechanisms are already in use and the potential effect the sodium and volume bolus will have, considering the clinical situation, are evaluated.

Maintenance of Adequate Nutrition

Many disease processes precipitating or occurring simultaneously with ARF place the child in a hypercatabolic state. The provision of appropriate caloric and protein intake and fluid and electrolytes minimize the accumulation of catabolic byproducts. Adequate nutrition also serves to maximize healing and promote growth (Finn, 1990). Protein intake should include essential and nonessential amino acids (Jones & Chesney, 1992), because a positive nitrogen balance provided through protein intake is desirable. The feasibility of doing this will be limited by the volumes of fluid and urea the child can tolerate (Compher et al., 1991). The metabolism of protein liberates nitrogenous residues that result in an increase in urea production, an increase in production of acid metabolites, and release of potassium (Baer & Lancaster, 1992). If the patient is not being treated with renal replacement therapy to remove these waste products, these disadvantages may preclude large protein intake. The nutritional support services department staff are best able to determine optimal protein and caloric intake. Patient age, weight, clinical status, previous nutritional status, and therapy all affect daily nutritional requirements.

Meeting a patient's nutritional requirements depends on the function of the gastrointestinal tract, vascular access, and severity of oliguria. Small and frequent enteral feedings are the method of choice. Advantages to the use of the enteral route include oral gratification and decreased risk for septicemia because vascular access is not required. Supplemental amino acid drinks are available. Although enteral feedings are the choice method of delivering nutrition, children may find it difficult to eat owing to the anorexia, nausea, and vomiting or impossible owing to critical illness.

When caloric needs cannot be met through the use of enteral feedings, parenteral nutrition is necessary. Essential amino acid infusions can decrease urea and nitrogen production and improve prognosis (Ruley & Bock, 1989). Attempts to aggressively meet nutritional needs may fail in the patient requiring fluid restriction. In this situation, some form of hemofiltration or dialysis may be required. One consideration for providing parenteral nutrition is the ability to administer maximal quantities of glucose and fat through the central access line.

Preventing Infection

The patient with ARF is at high risk for infection because of invasive monitoring and catheters, surgical procedures, and a highly catabolic metabolism. Difficulty in meeting the patient's nutritional needs compromises immune function. In addition, the patient's ability to fight infection is minimized owing to decreased neutrophil phagocytosis and chemotaxis caused by uremic toxins (Baer & Lancaster, 1992). In pediatric ARF, 33% to 67% of all deaths are due to *infection*. The most common site of infection is the urinary tract (Ruley & Bock, 1989). The need for indwelling bladder catheters to continuously monitor strict urine output and obtain sterile urine samples is reevaluated daily in light of this potential risk for infection.

Septicemia and lower respiratory tract infections also occur. Clearly, prevention of infection in an already sick patient is of concern. Sterility of intravascular catheters is maintained. Attention to the pulmonary system in the patient whose condition is compromised by immobility, nutritional depletion, and muscle weakness is required to prevent respiratory infections.

Because manifestations vary, infection during ARF is difficult to identify. Patient symptoms may include both hypothermia or hyperthermia. White blood cell count may be elevated or diminished. Other subtle signs include tachycardia, tachypnea, lethargy, flushing, and localized inflammatory response. Surveillance cultures are routinely indicated.

Prophylactic antibiotics are not recommended. Aggressive treatment with appropriate antibiotics is indicated in the case of proven infection. Dosage and frequency of antibiotics are based on renal function. Trending of serum drug peak and trough levels is used to determine appropriate dosage. Obtained in relation to the same dose of a given antibiotic, the trough level is drawn 30 minutes before the regularly scheduled dose, whereas the peak level is drawn 30 to 60 minutes after completion of the medication administration.

Maintenance of Hematologic Function

Because the kidney is responsible for the production of erythropoietin, the hematologic system is affected by ARF. *Anemia* often results from failure of the kidney to produce erythropoietin. Other causes of anemia include blood loss or hemodilution from volume expansion. The patient in ARF with altered cardiac output is further compromised by anemia as the delivery of oxygen and nutrients to the tissues is further diminished. *Thrombocytopenia* also occurs in ARF. The child in ARF may have multiple vascular access sites for blood sampling, intravenous intake, and hemodynamic monitoring. Surveillance of these sites for bleeding is important. Thrombocytopenia may also be associated with disseminated intravascular coagulation, hemolytic-uremic syndrome, cardiopulmonary bypass, and renal vein thrombosis.

RENAL REPLACEMENT THERAPY

The rationale for initiating renal replacement therapy includes the need to remove excessive intravascular volume and correct significant alterations in electrolyte and/or acid-base balance. Progressive hypervolemia may result in hypertension and, in the patient whose condition is previously compromised, congestive heart failure and pulmonary edema. Slow, steady increases in serum potassium levels (greater than 6.0 mEq/L) eventually produce lethal cardiac dysrhythmias. Persistent metabolic acidosis (arterial pH less than 7.2 or a serum bicarbonate less than 10 mEq/L) contributes to neurologic deterioration. Other electrolyte imbalances include hyponatremia (serum sodium less than 120 mEq/L), hypercalcemia (serum calcium greater than 12 mg/dL), and an imbalance in the calcium-to-phosphorus ratio. An elevation in BUN (greater than 150 mg/dL), with rapidly rising creatinine, influences the decision-making process to initiate more aggressive therapy.

Treatment options, intended to mimic renal function, include peritoneal dialysis (PD), continuous arteriovenous hemofiltration (CAVH), continuous venovenous hemofiltration (CVVH), and hemodialysis (HD). The benefits and limitations of each management option are compared in Table 22–10. Each is presented separately.

Peritoneal Dialysis

PD removes fluid and solutes slowly over a period of 2 to 3 days. Because of its time frame, the decision to initiate PD is usually made early, when progressive deterioration in patient status can be reasonably predicted. Earlier intervention is especially beneficial in some patients with multisystem organ failure, for example, in the patient with congenital heart disease and ARF following cardiovascular surgery. This population is at greater risk because the already compromised myocardium is especially sensitive to the deleterious effects of hypervolemia and hyperkalemia.

PD can be successfully initiated in patients with limited vascular access. In addition, because the removal of fluid and solutes is accomplished in a slow manner, patients who are especially sensitive to changes in vascular volume are ideal candidates. PD may be the treatment of choice for ARF in hemodynamically unstable patients or in patients with coagulopathy.

There are no absolute contraindications to PD. Patients better suited to another type of therapy include those with peritonitis, peritoneal adhesions, diaphragmatic defects, or those healing from recent abdominal surgery.

Principles of Therapy

With PD, the patient's peritoneum serves as a semipermeable membrane to allow movement of solutes by diffusion and water by osmosis (Fig. 22–4). As a semipermeable membrane, the peritoneum allows some but not all molecules to move across it. Diffusion is based upon the size of the molecules and the concentration gradient present on each side of

Table 22–10. ADVANTAGES AND DISADVANTAGES OF DIFFERENT FORMS OF RENAL REPLACEMENT THERAPY

Method	Advantages	Disadvantages
Peritoneal dialysis	Gradual process Can be used in hemodynamically unstable patients Vascular access beyond peripheral IV not required No complex equipment needed Inexpensive No heparinization required	Slow clearance of fluid and electrolytes—not helpful in hyperkalemic crises Risk for catheter-related sepsis, peritonitis Requires use of abdomen—not optimal status post laparotomy Large protein loss Failure of treatment results in worsened hypervolemia Fluid/electrolyte removal less controllable Diminished ventilation with decreased diaphragm compliance
CAVH/CVVH or hemofiltration	Very effective with hypervolemia Can be used in hemodynamically unstable patients Continuous treatment allows constant readjustment in therapy Relatively inexpensive Allows parenteral nutrition to be optimized without risk of hypervolemia	Access complications: infection, clotting, blood leaks, air emboli Requires vigilant monitoring Heparinization often required Not quickly effective with hyperkalemia Hemofilter clotting requires immediate intervention
Hemodialysis	Quickly effective in fluid and catabolic overload Intermittent therapy	Access complications: infection, clotting, bleeding Requires special equipment and specially trained personnel Heparinization required Fluid and electrolyte shift during therapy, hypotension Disequilibrium syndrome

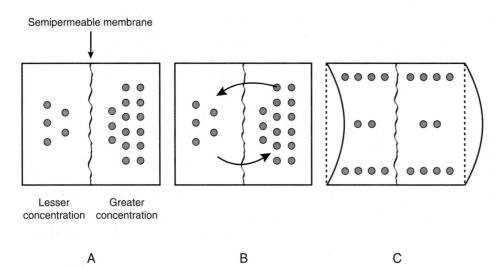

Semipermeable membrane

Lesser concentration   Greater concentration

A   B   C

Figure 22–4 ● ● ● ● ● ●
Osmosis and diffusion across a semipermeable membrane. *A,* the solute concentration is unequal on opposing sides of a semipermeable membrane. The volume on each side is equal. *B,* The process of osmosis and diffusion is occurring. *C,* The concentrations and fluid volumes have changed owing to the movement of both water and solutes in the direction of the arrows. (O, solute; →, direction of water movement; O →, direction of solute movement. (Adapted from Mitchell, P. H. (1977). *Concepts basic to nursing,* 2nd ed., p. 401. St. Louis: Mosby–Year Book.)

the peritoneum. Osmosis depends upon the osmolarity of the fluids separated by the peritoneum.

Dialysate fluid, containing a predetermined osmolality and concentration of ions, is infused into the peritoneal cavity. Exchange of solutes and water occurs over the peritoneal membrane. Osmotic pressure is determined by the glucose concentration in the dialysate. If the concentration of glucose in the dialysate is greater than that in the patient's serum, water will move from the intravascular space into the peritoneal fluid. Glucose may also move from the peritoneal space to the child's intravenous space, resulting in hyperglycemia. This occurrence is usually temporary until the pancreas is able to increase insulin production. Serum electrolytes diffuse across the peritoneum until equilibrium is reached with the dialysate. Urea and creatine diffuse against a zero concentration gradient because these two solutes are not present in dialysate. Therefore, they are readily cleared from the serum.

The smaller the patient the larger the ratio of peritoneal space to body mass. Therefore, in general, PD is more efficient in smaller pediatric patients.

Dialysate is commercially available as 1.5%, 2.5%, 4.25%, and 7.5% dextrose concentrations (Table 22–11). Except for the addition of glucose and the absence of potassium, dialysate is similar to normal serum. Dialysate contains either lactate or acetate as a buffering agent. Patients who are unable to metabolize lactate, such as those with liver disease, should receive dialysate containing acetate.

Additives to dialysate include potassium and heparin, xylocaine, or antibiotics. Initially, when significant hyperkalemia is present, potassium will not be added to the dialysate. Shortly thereafter, when the child's serum potassium begins to approach normal, 1 to 4 mEq of potassium chloride per liter of dialysate is added. Heparin, 100 to 1000 units per liter of dialysate, is sometimes added to prevent clot formation that can obstruct the PD catheter. Heparin does not cross the peritoneal membrane. Xylocaine 1%, 1 to 2 mL/L of dialysate (not to exceed 5 μg/kg),

is sometimes added to ease abdominal discomfort. Antibiotics may be added to diminish infection risk.

Procedure

PD can be initiated with relative ease in the ICU. Patient and parent preparation occurs prior to paracentesis. Accurate patient weight and abdominal girth are obtained and documented. Baseline laboratory results are reviewed. These include a complete blood count; serum chemistry levels including glucose, phosphorus, uric acid, BUN, creatinine; and coagulation studies. A blood sample is typed and crossmatched for blood to be made available.

There are several types of peritoneal catheters. The type of catheter selected depends upon the patient's risk of bleeding and potential for catheter obstruction. Pediatric catheters are usually the same size as adult catheters but the distal openings cluster over a shorter distance so that less catheter must be accommodated within the child's abdomen.

Before starting the procedure, the PD system, used both to deliver dialysate to the peritoneal cavity and

Table 22–11. COMPARISON OF DIALYSATE SOLUTIONS

	1.5%	2.5%	4.25%
Each 100 mL Contains:			
Dextrose (gm)	1.5	2.5	4.25
Sodium lactate (mEq)	448	448	448
NaCl (mg)	538	538	567
CaCl (mg)	25.7	25.7	25.7
MgCl (mg)	5.08	5.08	5.08
Electrolytes per 1000 mL:			
Na (mEq)	132	132	132
Ca (mEq)	3.5	3.5	3.5
Mg (mEq)	0.5	0.5	1.5
Cl (mEq)	96	96	102
Lactate	40	40	35
mOsmol/L	346	396	486
pH	5.2	5.2	5.2

collect peritoneal drainage, is prepared. Figure 22–5 illustrates an example of a pediatric system consisting of a Buretrol device, fluid warmer, tubing, roller clamps, and drainage bag. A closed system is required to limit the potential for peritonitis. The dialysate is warmed to 37°C to prevent heat loss, enhance solute clearance, and promote patient comfort (Elixson & Clancy, 1992).

The PD cycler (Fig. 22–6), a computerized system that automatically delivers the dialysate volume and weighs drainage accurately at programmed time intervals, is an alternative to manual PD. The PD cycler not only saves nursing time but allows fewer openings of the system and therefore decreases the patient's risk of peritonitis. PD cyclers are now available that accurately measure volumes as small as 50

mL, making it useful with infants weighing as little as 5 kg.

PD Catheter Insertion. Paracentesis is usually accomplished in the ICU. Patients younger than 2 years of age, those with poor abdominal tone, those that require chemical paralyzing agents for effective ventilation, or those with a history of abdominal surgery may warrant catheter placement in the operating room.

After adequate sedation is achieved, the PD catheter is inserted using aseptic technique under local anesthesia. A small incision is usually made below the umbilicus. After access to the peritoneal cavity is obtained, approximately 50 mL/kg of 1.5% dialysate solution is infused. This volume expands the peritoneal space to decrease the risk of bowel perforation

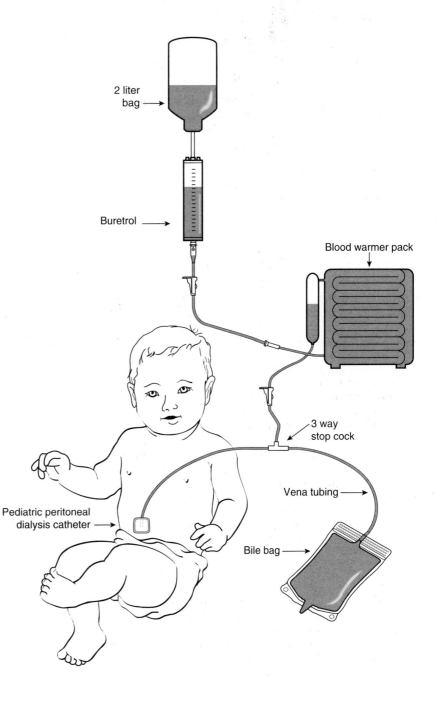

Figure 22–5 ● ● ● ● ● ●

Pediatric peritoneal dialysis setup. (Courtesy of GA Berzinsky.)

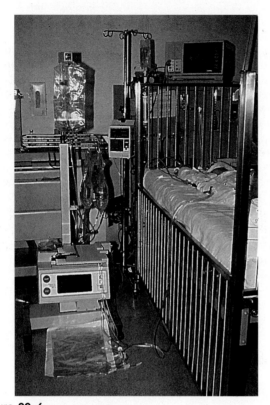

Figure 22–6 ● ● ● ● ● ●
Abbott Impersol Cycler 3000. (Courtesy of Abbott Laboratories, Renal Care, Abbott Park, Illinois.)

The drainage phase begins when the clamp on the outflow line leading to the drainage bag is opened. The time required for drainage varies for each patient. The average time required for drainage is 15 to 20 minutes. Drainage can be enhanced by repositioning the patient.

Critical Care Management. The goal of PD is established prior to instituting therapy and is reevaluated on a daily basis. For example, the daily goal may include removing a specified amount of fluid over a specific time, decreasing the serum potassium level to within normal limits, or decreasing the BUN to three times normal. Achievement of established multidisciplinary goals, ongoing monitoring of the patient's status, and prevention of complications requires vigilant assessment, intervention, and documentation.

Achievement of Established Goals. Modifications in PD therapy are made based on the patient's clinical status, renal function, and laboratory test results. The dialysate concentration is changed with relative simplicity. Variations in concentrations can be obtained by combining different osmolar solutions with each run. The 1.5% solution is used if fluid removal is not the primary and immediate goal. Generally, for fluid removal, 2.5% or 4.25% solutions are used. Use of 7.5% dialysate solution is associated with hyperglycemia, increased abdominal pain, and peritoneal irritation. Even though initial hyperglycemia may resolve with increased endogenous insulin production, other related side effects usually limit the use of highly osmolar solutions.

Monitoring. The volume of dialysate instilled depends upon patient tolerance during the dwell phase. Instillation of smaller, more frequent volumes may accomplish the desired goals in the patient who cannot tolerate runs of more than 20 mL/kg every hour.

Initial PD drainage is blood-tinged. This bloody drainage should clear after the first few runs. After this, PD drainage takes on a characteristic straw color. Changes in color or persistently bloody or cloudy drainage are significant observations and require further evaluation.

After the first few cycles a predictable drainage pattern should develop (Fig. 22–7). At times the catheter tip may migrate away from the dialysate in the peritoneal cavity or the catheter may become occluded by omentum. In these situations, dialysate freely flows into, but not out of, the peritoneal cavity. Interventions to increase fluid drainage include changing the child's position, elevating the head of the bed, or turning the child gently from side to side.

Catheter-related problems include obstruction and leakage at the insertion site. If the volume infused is greater than that drained, external obstruction in the drainage system may be present. This situation is evaluated by eliminating all potential external causes of obstruction such as kinked tubing or catheter. A clotted catheter requires replacement.

Catheter leakage at the insertion site may indicate catheter displacement. If all PD catheter infusion/drainage sites are contained within the abdomen, all

while the PD catheter is manipulated. Optimal catheter position is demonstrated by free flow of dialysate both in and out of the peritoneal cavity. During the initial cycle, patient assessment also includes evaluation of fluid infiltration around the insertion site, abdominal pain, grossly bloody drainage, fecal-contaminated drainage, and cardiovascular or respiratory compromise.

After optimal catheter position is established, a pursestring suture closes the incision around the PD catheter. An occlusive dry sterile dressing, which prevents kinking of the PD catheter, is applied.

Catheter Maintenance. Each PD cycle or run consists of three phases: installation, dwell, and drainage. During the instillation phase, dialysate runs into the peritoneum through the inflow line of the PD system. This occurs rapidly by gravitational flow over 5 to 15 minutes. The volume of dialysate instilled with each run is usually 10 to 20 mL/kg in infants and 35 to 40 mL/kg in children. Depending upon patient tolerance, initial volumes can be gradually increased.

The dwell phase follows. During this time both the inflow and outflow lines are clamped. The dialysate remains in the peritoneal cavity, allowing for water and solute movement across the peritoneum. This phase usually requires 30 to 60 minutes but is dependent upon many factors, such as surface area of the peritoneal membrane. Maximal solute transfer occurs at the beginning of the dwell phase.

PERITONEAL DIALYSIS WORKSHEET–CYCLER

PATIENT: _____ DATE: _____

NUMBER OF CYCLES: __24__   FILL/DWELL: __40__ MIN.   DRAIN: __20__ MIN.

MEDICATIONS ADDED: _____ KCl 3 mEq/L Heparin 200 units/L _____

Wt = 15 Kg

Cycle Number	Dialysis Fluid			Fill Volume	Drain Volume	Patient Balance		Remarks
	1.5%	2.5%	4.25%			Each Cycle	Cumulative	
1	2			300	295	+5	+5	Fluid pink in color
2	2			300	305	−5	0	
3	1	1		300	315	−15	−15	
4	1	1		300	300	0	−15	
5		2		300	330	−30	−45	Clearing
6		2		300	335	−35	−80	
7		2		300	330	−30	−110	Clear-straw in color

Figure 22–7 ● ● ● ● ● ●

Peritoneal dialysis cycler worksheet. (Courtesy of Children's Hospital of Philadelphia, Department of Nursing.)

that may be required is an extra external stitch to stop oozing of fluid from around the insertion site. Sometimes catheter leakage results from overfilling the abdomen. Assessment of abdominal tenseness with leakage during the dwell phase may indicate that smaller volumes of dialysate are warranted.

The need for accurate documentation of intake and output cannot be overstated. Twice-daily patient weights may be used to validate fluid assessments if the patient's condition permits. Weights are only useful if a consistent scale is used and the patient is weighed at the same time of day and during a specific phase in a PD cycle.

Laboratory studies are followed at a frequency determined by the acuity and lability of the patient's condition. Following trends of serum electrolytes, calcium, phosphorus, BUN, and creatinine levels is routine. Close monitoring of the patient's neurologic status is important because serum electrolyte and acid/base imbalance may manifest in neurologic changes. Sleep/wake cycle disturbances and parents' observations of behavior change affect nursing decision-making.

The impact of PD on the pharmacokinetics of all drugs the patient is receiving is evaluated. Medications that cross the peritoneal membrane require adjustment in dosage and scheduling. For example, aminoglycosides are removed by PD, and therefore increased doses of these antibiotics are necessary.

Monitoring of peak and trough antibiotic levels facilitates therapeutic dosing. Medications that may require adjustment are reviewed in Table 22–12.

The child's level of comfort is continuously monitored. Especially important is the patient's perception of comfort during the different phases of PD. Nonverbal signs of discomfort include tachycardia; tachypnea or shallow breathing; grimacing; splinting; and agitated, unsettled behaviors. In some instances, slowing the rate of dialysate infusion, decreasing the volume used per cycle, further warming of the dialysate, or repositioning the child may serve to alleviate some discomfort. Analgesics and sedatives are used in addition to comfort measures.

Monitoring for Complications. Distending the abdomen with large volumes of dialysate may compromise the patient's respiratory status. Increased abdominal volume and pressure prevent normal downward displacement of the diaphragm and limit functional residual capacity. This may predispose the patient to atelectasis with associated intrapulmonary shunting and increased work of breathing. Fatigue further compromises the patient's ability to compensate for existing alterations in oxygenation and ventilation.

Ongoing assessment of the patient's nutritional status includes an appreciation of the protein loss that occurs with PD. Losses of from 0.2 to 8.0 g of protein per liter of dialysate drained are anticipated.

Table 22-12. REMOVAL OF SELECTED MEDICATIONS BY HEMODIALYSIS, CAVH, AND PERITONEAL DIALYSIS

Drugs	Removal by Hemodialysis	Removal by Hemofiltration	Removal by Peritoneal Dialysis
Ampicillin	+	?	−
Cefazolin	+	+	+
Cefotaxime	+	+	+
Ceftazidime	+	+	+
Cefuroxime	+	+	−
Chloramphenicol	−	−	−
Clindamycin	−	−	−
Erythromycin	−	−	−
Gentamicin	+	+	+
Methicillin	−	−	−
Nafcillin	−	−	−
Netilmicin	+	+	+
Oxacillin	−	?	−
Penicillin	+	+**	+**
Ticarcillin	+	−	−
Tobramycin	+	+	+
Vancomycin	−	?	−
Amphotericin	−	−	−
Hydralazine	−	?	−
Sodium nitroprusside	−*	?	−
Digoxin	−	+	−
Furosemide	−	?	−
Cimetidine	−	?	−
Ranitidine	+	?	−
Theophylline	+	?	+
Phenobarbital	+	+	+
Dilantin	−	−	−
Cyclosporine	−	?	−

+ Removal of drug large enough to require a supplement to the dosage
  Removal of drug does not require supplement
? Information unknown
*Toxic metabolite, thiocyanate, is dialyzable
**For GFR <10

Data from: Bennett, W.M., Aronoff, G.R., Golper, T.A., Morrison, G., Singer, I., & Brater, D.C. (1991). *Drug prescribing in renal failure* (1st ed.). Philadelphia: American College of Physicians.

Bennett, W.M., Aronoff, G.R., Golper, T.A., Morrison, G., Singer, I., & Brater, D.C. (1991). *Drug prescribing in renal failure* (2nd ed.). Philadelphia: American College of Physicians.

Bernstein, J.M., & Erk, S.D. (1990). Choice antibiotics, pharmacokinetics and dose adjustment in acute and chronic renal failure. *Medical Clinics of North America*, 74(4), 1059–1076.

Without adequate replacement, protein loss further compromises the patient's respiratory status as it affects the diaphragm's ability to do work. Occasionally, supplemental glucose and amino acids are added to the dialysate to increase the patient's caloric intake while maintaining fluid restriction.

Instillation of large volumes of dialysate into the peritoneum may also compromise venous return and cardiac output. This is especially true when intravascular volume is limited. Close monitoring of cardiovascular status is necessary, especially during the instillation phase.

The greatest shift of water and solutes occurs within the first part of the dwell phase. Patient discomfort and respiratory and cardiovascular distress may force a time limit on the dwell phase. These adjustments eventually affect the number of cycles completed within the day, potentially influencing the effectiveness of therapy. As the patient's need for PD lessens, drainage time can be gradually increased, resulting in fewer runs per day.

Related probably to both the higher frequency of leakage around the catheter site and immaturity of immune function, there is an inverse relationship between age and the incidence of peritonitis. In general, the risk of peritonitis increases after day 3 of PD. Guidelines for practice regarding the frequency of system tubing change, catheter insertion site cleansing and dressing, and frequency of catheter change are policies determined within each institution. It is prudent to recommend care that is similar to guidelines for intravascular lines.

Signs of peritonitis include cloudy PD drainage, fever, abdominal pain and tenderness, and a change in the patient's level of consciousness. Daily culture, cell count with differential, and Gram stain of PD drainage are warranted. Maintaining a closed system, specimens should be aspirated from the PD outflow line and not the drainage bag. To prevent the possibility of contaminated fluid from flowing back into the peritoneum, the drainage bag is never elevated above the level of the abdomen.

Peritonitis does not preclude PD therapy. Treatment includes adding antibiotics to the dialysate and appropriate systemic antibiotic administration for positive blood cultures. Pancreatitis is also a frequent finding in patients on PD. Signs and symptoms include abdominal pain, nausea, vomiting, and low-grade fever.

Documentation. Documentation is crucial to patient management. Figure 22–8 illustrates a PD flow sheet that tracks patient information including patient weights, temperature, intake and output, and dialysate temperature. Included also are the volume and type of dialysate instilled, the volume drained from each cycle, and the number of cycles completed. If manually performed, documentation also includes the times at which: (1) instillation of dialysate begins; (2) instillation ends and dwell time begins; (3) dwell time ends and drainage time begins; (4) drainage time ends and a new run begins. If a PD cycler is used, the times are not important to record because they are automatically programmed.

Ongoing assessment of drainage volume, compared with instilled volume, is important in evaluating the patient's fluid balance. The patient's fluid status is considered to be "positive" when the volume instilled is greater than the volume drained. Positive fluid balance can be related to an increase in the patient's serum osmolarity or to an occlusion in the drainage system. A positive fluid balance for two or more runs requires a change in management strategy.

The patient is considered to be in "negative" fluid balance when the volume instilled is less than the volume drained. Negative balance, indicating removal of body fluid volume, is generally a goal of PD. However, rapid removal of volume may compromise the child's hemodynamic status. Continuous evaluation of the child's tolerance to fluid removal is necessary to determine the desired goal for hourly fluid balance.

PERITONEAL DIALYSIS WORKSHEET–MANUAL

DIALYSIS CYCLE

Fill/Dwell _____ minute   Amount of Dialysate Each Cycle _____

Drain _____ minute   Weight: _____

Medication Added: _____

Date	Cycle No.	Dialysis Fluid			Fill			Drainage			Patient			Remarks
		1.5%	2.5%	4.25%	Start Time	Finish Time	Volume In	Start Time	Finish Time	Volume Out	Balance	Cumulative Balance Shift	Cumulative Balance 24°	

Figure 22–8 ● ● ● ● ● ●

Manual peritoneal dialysis worksheet. (Courtesy of Children's Hospital of Philadelphia, Department of Nursing.)

The overall total of fluid instilled into the peritoneal cavity compared with the fluid volume drained in a 24-hour period yields the day's fluid balance. The volume, if positive, is added to the day's intake total and, if negative, to the day's output total.

Additional documentation specific to PD includes patient and parent education and assessment of their level of understanding and comfort with the information. It also describes the child's tolerance of PD. Appearance of the insertion site, the presence of any fluid leakage, and a description of the fluid drained out of the peritoneal cavity are documented each shift.

Continuous Arteriovenous/ Venovenous Hemofiltration

Continuous arteriovenous hemofiltration (CAVH) and continuous venovenous hemofiltration (CVVH) provide two conceptually similar methods for slow, continuous removal of fluid and solutes from the body, enabling continuous adjustment in the child's fluid status. Slow continuous hemofiltration is especially important in the critically ill patient in whom a predictable fluid and solute removal process allows a more liberal approach to intravenous intake of necessary nutrition and medications.

Hemofiltration can usually be successfully initiated in patients in whom PD and/or HD is contraindicated. Compared with HD, special equipment and the need for extra personnel are minimized with CAVH and CVVH.

Principles of Therapy

Uniquely different from PD and HD, CAVH/CVVH removes excessive fluid and solutes through ultrafiltration. The process requires continuous extracorporeal circulation of blood through a filter. The simplest system places a hemofilter and a collection bag between a patient's arterial and venous lines (CAVH; Fig. 22–9). Relying upon pressure gradients and the patient's cardiac output, blood flows from the arterial line through the hemofilter and returns to the patient by the venous line.

With CVVH a hemopump is used to pump blood through the hemofilter using two separate venous cannulas or two separate ports from a single multilumen cannula (CVVH, Fig. 22–10).

As blood moves through the highly permeable hemofilter, water and low-molecular-weight molecules are removed through ultrafiltration. Variations in hemofilter size and shape are commercially available. Cylindrical hollow filters or parallel plate filters are two commonly used types. Options in membrane type, surface area, clearance rate, and volume are commercially available.

Similar to that which occurs within the vascular space, ultrafiltration occurs as the net result of the opposing forces of hydrostatic and oncotic pressure. Hydrostatic pressure (determined by the patient's cardiac output or the hemopump's blood flow rate) provides the force necessary to filter blood on one side of the membrane, as oncotic pressure (determined by the concentration of plasma proteins) pulls fluid back into the system on the other side of the membrane (Fig. 22–11). Initially, hydrostatic pressure is greater than oncotic pressure, and thus water and small particles move out of the serum into the ultrafiltration collection area. At this point, depending upon the concentration of plasma protein that establishes the plasma oncotic pressure and the force of gravity exerted by the height of the collection bag, water is pulled back into the venous side of the circuit and ultrafiltrate (UF) is drained into the collection bag.

Ultrafiltrate has the same solute load as the patient's serum. Potassium, sodium, chloride, urea, and creatinine are all small molecules that freely move across the hemofilter. Glucose and other moderate size molecules move slowly across the hemofilter. Plasma proteins, which are large size molecules, do not cross the hemofilter. Therefore, all plasma proteins are returned to the patient and UF is protein free.

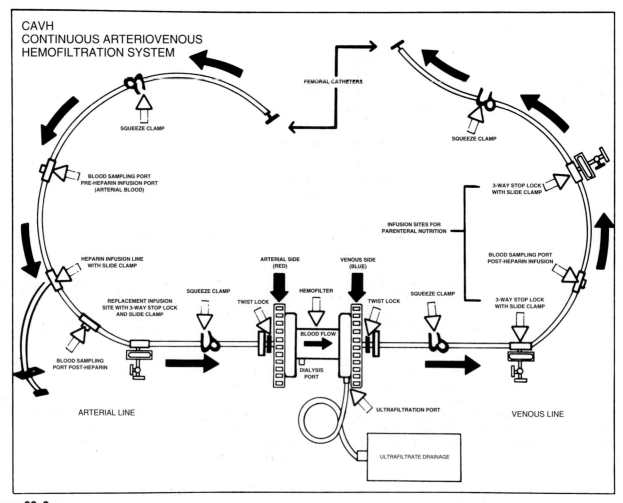

Figure 22–9 ● ● ● ● ● ●

CAVH—Continuous arteriovenous hemofiltration system. (From Coloski, D., Mastrianni, J., Dube, R., & Brown, L. H. (1990). *Dimensions of Critical Care Nursing,* 9(3), 130–141.)

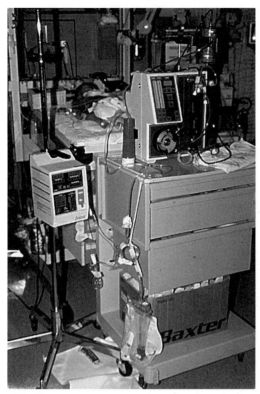

Figure 22–10 ● ● ● ● ● ●

Pump-assisted CVVH. Blood is pumped from the patient through the hemofilter, bubble trap, and air detector, then returned to the patient. An IV pump is used to control the amount of ultrafiltrate removed per hour. (Courtesy of Baxter Healthcare Corporation, Renal Division, Deerfield, IL.)

As water and small molecules are removed, plasma oncotic pressure increases. The net effect of oncotic and hydrostatic pressures becoming more equal is a decrease in the rate of ultrafiltration over time. At this point the patient's serum osmolarity is maintained as sodium, potassium, and chloride are removed and creatinine, urea, and glucose are filtered in concentrations equal to that of plasma.

The process of fluid and solute removal has distinct features that make hemofiltration the therapy of choice for many children with ARF. The slow process allows for relative hemodynamic stability during volume removal. In addition, it is a continuous therapy, allowing for constant readjustment in the treatment plan as the patient's needs change. Compared to HD, the extracorporeal circuit volume is small and there is a relatively low risk of bleeding. This is especially important in infants and in patients with existing coagulopathy. The major advantage over PD is that ventilation during hemofiltration is not affected by the abdominal distension that occurs during the dwell phase of each PD run.

A disadvantage to simple hemofiltration is that it does not remove solutes such as urea as efficiently as desired for some patients. Large solutes also are poorly cleared. Small ones, although cleared, are removed slowly. Therefore, hemofiltration may not be the therapy of choice for patients with azotemia.

The clearest indications for simple hemofiltration are fluid overload, which is resistant to diuretic therapy, and electrolyte imbalance. One common use of hemofiltration is to improve nutritional intake in patients who cannot tolerate a positive fluid balance. Increased amounts of parenteral nutrition can be administered because excessive fluid volume can be continuously removed. The controlled fluid management specifically benefits patients in multisystem organ failure. In addition, ultrafiltration may enhance the clearance of serum myocardial depressant factor and cytokines, mediators involved in the process of organ failure during shock (DiCarlo et al., 1990).

Procedure

Setup. Once the management plan includes hemofiltration, preparation for gaining large vessel access and priming of the extracorporeal circuit begins.

Arterial and/or venous cannulation sites must accommodate the largest size cannula as possible because system performance is directly related to the amount of blood flow through the hemofilter. Infants have adequate filter flow through 7 French (internal lumen) catheters, provided a blood pump is utilized within the system. In the pediatric population, femoral access is most common. To provide optimal filtration, drainage and return cannulas are generally the same size. When the gauge of the drainage cannula is less than optimal, improved circuit flow may be achieved when the return cannula is one to two gauge sizes larger than the drainage cannula. Return cannula size determines resistance of blood flow back to the patient and affects flow throughout the circuit. In CVVH, one venous cannula/line often pulls more effectively than the other. If this is the case, simply reversing the drainage and return lines may improve system performance. The procedure for gaining vascular access is the same as for any central line.

Preparation of the circuit is completed prior to gaining vascular access. If the arterial vessel is cannulated before the circuit is ready, a continuous heparin flush setup is used to maintain vessel patency. Venous cannulas are heparin flushed, then capped.

Assembly and priming of the circuit is institution-specific. General principles include the maintenance of aseptic technique during flushing of the circuit with 1 to 3 L of heparinized saline, the volume determined by the type of filter used. The concentration of heparin is 5000 units/L of saline. The system is flushed to remove air and all traces of glycerin, a byproduct of the sterilization process.

Most pediatric patients benefit from priming the hemofilter with packed red blood cells or 5% albumin. Depending upon the size of the hemofilter, the circuit volume is approximately 20 to 50 mL. Figure 22–12 illustrates the complete CAVH circuit during patient use.

Circuit pressures are monitored as a safety alarm to immediately identify inadvertent patient disconnection.

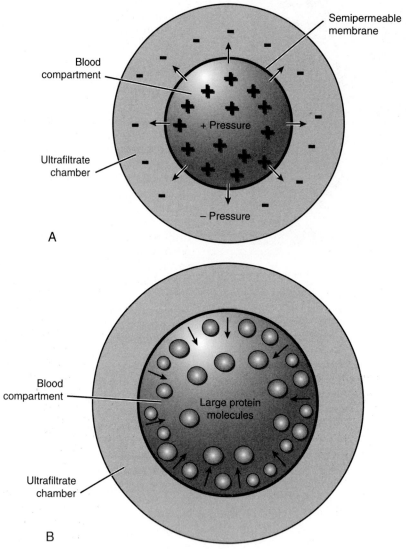

Figure 22–11 ● ● ● ● ● ●

Opposing mechanical forces in hemofiltration. *A,* Hydrostatic pressure is the positive force provided by the cardiac output or bleed pump that forces UF across the semipermeable membrane. *B,* Oncotic pressure, created by plasma protein concentration, attempts to keep fluid within the blood compartment. (Adapted from Coloski, D., Mastrianni, J., Dube, R., Brown, L. H. (1990). Continuous arteriovenous hemofiltration patient: nursing care plan. *Dimensions of Critical Care Nursing,* 9 (3), 130–141. Copyright 1990, Hall Johnson Communications, Inc. Reproduced with permission. For further use, contact the publisher at 9737 West Ohio Avenue, Lakewood, CO 80226.)

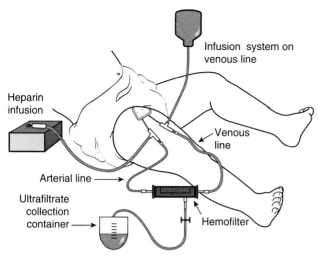

Figure 22-12 ● ● ● ● ●

CAVH setup. The patient's cardiac output propels blood from the arterial line through the hemofilter and returns it to the body via the venous line. (Courtesy of GA Berzinsky.)

An attached prefilter, a continuous heparin infusion, is necessary to keep the system from clotting. It is initially infused at a rate of 10 units/kg/hour then titrated to maintain an activating clotting time (ACT) within an individual therapeutic range (usually 180 sec or 10% over baseline). Patients with thrombocytopenia may not require anticoagulation. Some centers prefer regional heparinization of the hemofilter (Jones & Chesney, 1992). This is accomplished by the post-filter infusion of protamine sulfate in the dose of 1 mg protamine sulfate per 100 units heparin administered (Kaplan & Petrillo, 1987).

Insertion. Once vessel access has been achieved and the circuit has been assembled and primed, it is connected to the patient. The drainage side is connected to the patient first. Clamps are used to assist the team in establishing the extracorporeal circuit without air entry or unnecessary blood loss.

Maintenance. Because the patient's own cardiac output propels CAVH, decreasing arterial pressures automatically result in a decreased flow rate across the hemofilter and, therefore, decreased ultrafiltrate rate (UFR).

Similarly, any treatment that increases cardiac output, such as volume or vasoactive medication administration, increases UFR. Systolic blood pressures of at least 80 mmHg are required to maintain blood flow through the hemofilter.

Pump driven CVVH provides the hemofilter with constant blood flow, which results in a consistent ultrafiltration rate that can be precisely controlled. Ordered pump speed, adjusted in milliliters per minute, depends upon cannula size, intravascular volume, and desired UFR with solute clearance. Pump speeds greater than 15–30 mL/minute are required to prevent hemofilter clotting.

Use of a prefilter pump means that the child's cardiac output no longer affects the UFR. One advantage of this system is a decreased incidence of hemofilter clotting. Another is that the pump allows hemo-

filtration to be used in populations with low cardiac output or labile mean arterial pressures, such as infants or the hemodynamically unstable patient.

Disadvantages are associated with this same feature. Because the child's own cardiac output is no longer the driving force behind the UFR, changes in the child's hemodynamic status no longer automatically diminish blood flow through the filter. Therefore, vigilant monitoring of the patient's hemodynamic status is critical. Interventions to immediately stabilize a child's hemodynamic status are anticipated. This may simply include decreasing the speed of pump flow and resultant ultrafiltration.

Evaluation of Established Goals. Many interventions can alter UFR. For example, the level of the collection bag relative to the level of the circuit influences UFR. As gravity serves to draw the fluid away from the hemofilter, the difference between the hydrostatic and oncotic pressures increases, and increased drainage results. The length of tubing used also affects resistance in the circuit. The shorter the arteriovenous length of tubing, the better the extracorporeal flow.

Conversely, there are also interventions to decrease the UFR. Raising the collection bag, increasing the arteriovenous length of tubing, or partially clamping the venous return line all slow flow through the hemofilter, thereby decreasing the UFR.

During acute hypotensive episodes the collection bag is clamped. This maneuver prevents further drainage yet allows blood flow to continue through the hemofilter and prevent circuit occlusion. Clamping the circuit itself for more than a minute will lead to hemofilter occlusion.

One of the advantages of hemofiltration is that the UFR may exceed the vascular volume loss desired, and the child can receive replacement fluids in the form that best meets nutritional and electrolyte needs. Generally, a desired UF hourly volume is calculated and replacement fluid is ordered. At a regular frequency, over 1 to 4 hour blocks of time, the actual UF volume minus the desired UF volume is calculated and replaced over the next block of time. This recurring process provides the opportunity to replace UF with optimal fluids to meet the child's evolving needs. The more unstable the child's fluid and electrolyte status, the more frequently the volumes can be calculated and replaced. During the initial few hours of hemofiltration (or first block of time), careful attention to the UF volume is warranted because the patient is not receiving replacement fluid.

Except for albumin, replacement fluids are generally delivered before the filter. Fluid administration before the hemofilter serves to decrease the hematocrit, blood viscosity, and oncotic pressure. In combination, these factors improve blood flow through the hemofilter, decreasing the need for heparin therapy. Urea clearance also is improved through prefilter administration of replacement fluids (Paradiso, 1989).

Albumin is administered after the filter as it may

decrease the patency of the hemofilter. Medications are also administered post-filter to avoid hemofiltration of the medication.

The impact of hemofiltration on the pharmacokinetics of all drugs the patient is receiving is evaluated. Clearance of nonprotein-bound drugs is enhanced with hemofiltration. Anticipating enhanced clearance is critically important, especially in the child who is vasopressor-dependent. Enhanced clearance of insulin and some antibiotics, including the aminoglycosides and cefuroxime, also occurs. In general, because the extracorporeal circuit adds "body surface area" to the patient, the dosage of all nonprotein-bound drugs is increased (Table 22–12). Both dosage and timing of medication administration are best determined by evaluation of peak and trough drug levels. Sieving coefficients, which describe the concentration gradient of a molecule in the UF as compared with that of plasma, can be used to calculate therapeutic dosages during hemofiltration (Table 22–13).

Monitoring. Fluid balance assessment and calculations require vigilant monitoring and documentation. This activity may be time-consuming. Systems are available that assume the task of balancing UF flow rate and administration of replacement fluids. An infusion control device is used to draw off a predictable amount of UF every hour, thereby allowing a consistent amount of replacement to be infused. One such gravimetric controller is the Equaline system manufactured by Amicon (Amicon, Inc., Danvers, MA). The volume of UF removed and replacement volumes administered are separately and continuously weighed and stored in the computerized system. The system allows for intake and output assessment and documentation at a time that is optimal for the patient. When programmed, the system achieves a net fluid removal per unit of selected time. This saves nursing time by eliminating the need for routine calculations and pump manipulations. It benefits the child by providing immediate fluid replacement from continuously calculated data.

Hemofiltration requires ongoing monitoring of the patient and extracorporeal circuit. The child's volume status and cardiac output are affected over the time of fluid removal. Trends in laboratory results, intake and output totals, patient weights, and vital signs are critical assessment parameters. The cardiovascular examination is crucial. Hemodynamic pressure measurements obtained from the drainage side of the CAVH circuit are not accurate. Additional line monitoring or cuff blood pressures are necessary. Perfusion to the extremities distal to the cannulated vessels may diminish. Ongoing assessment of the presence and quality of pulses and sensation and movement of extremities is necessary.

Serum sodium, potassium, and chloride are removed in proportion to the fluid volume filtered, and shifts in these electrolytes occur as a result of the therapy. Changing acid-base status may also affect electrolyte levels. The volume and type of replacement fluid is readjusted, depending upon the needs

Table 22–13. SIEVING COEFFICIENTS IN CAVH

Drug	Sieving Coefficient	Drug	Sieving Coefficient
Amphotericin B	0.35 ± 0.06	Digoxin	0.96 ± 0.06
Ampicillin	0.69 ± 0.21	Phenobarbitone	0.86 ± 0.01
Cefotaxime	1.06 ± 0.34	Phenytoin	0.45 ± 0.06
Cefoxitin	0.32	Procainamide	0.86 ± 0.02
Ceftriaxone	0.52 ± 0.11	Theophylline	0.86 ± 0.01
Clindamycin	0.49 ± 0.25		
Erythromycin	0.37		
Gentamicin	0.81 ± 0.02		
Imipenem	0.76 ± 0.08		
Mezlocillin	0.71 ± 0.10		
Nafcillin	0.55 ± 0.12		
Oxacillin	0.02		
Penicillin	0.68		
Tobramycin	0.81 ± 0.06		
Vancomycin	0.76 ± 0.04		

The solute's ability to pass through the membrane is mathematically expressed.

Sieving coefficients closer to 1 indicate easier passage, whereas values closer to 0 indicate inability to cross.

Adapted with permission from Golper, T.A., & Bennett, W.M. (1988). Drug removal by continuous arteriovenous haemofiltration. *Medical toxicology, 3,* 341–349.

of the child. A reduction in the serum BUN and creatinine is gradually appreciated.

Nutritional management for the child receiving hemofiltration is usually welcomed in the previously fluid-restricted child with large metabolic needs. Provision of optimal fluid volume and calories are best determined by the renal team and nutrition support services. The replacement fluid, generally a modified solution of lactated Ringer's solution is a separate source of intake. The volume varies to assure that the desired volume of fluid removed matches the *net* volume of fluid removed.

The critical process of addressing the high risk of infection associated with this therapy begins with strict adherence to aseptic technique. Surveillance cultures from the circuit are routine. Cannula care is the same as for any central line. Meticulous attention to preventing contamination is necessary. Any need to enter the circuit warrants careful consideration. The need for conscientious preventative care cannot be overstated.

While on this therapy, the child's hematologic status may be compromised by anticoagulation. Initially, frequent ACTs are needed to evaluate the amount of heparin needed. After an appropriate rate for continuous infusion has been determined, the frequency of these tests may decrease to two to four times per day. Assessment of the child's ability to establish and maintain hemostasis is ongoing. This assessment includes checking for guaiac-positive nasogastric drainage or stool, hematuria, oral/nasal or mucosal bleeding, petechiae, and oozing from wounds or venipuncture sites. Neurologic assessment is critical in the coagulation evaluation, especially in infants.

The child's level of comfort is best evaluated with the patient and parents. Changes in the child's heart rate and blood pressure are integrated with assessments of behavior, facial expression, playfulness, and interaction with others. Hemofiltration should not cause pain. Use of analgesia is generally not indicated. Sedation, in a renal failure–adjusted dose, may be helpful in allowing the child to be less anxious and to rest. Provision of some environmental control, the presence of parents, and a routine of day-night activities may serve to minimize the child's fear and lessen discomfort from unfamiliar physical and emotional feelings.

Using a complex technology to provide ultrafiltration at the bedside has specific implications for the care of the child and parents. The appearance of the blood circulating outside the body can be frightening and worrisome to families. The need for continuous observation and hourly monitoring may minimize the parents' sense of control and may maximize their feelings of helplessness. Because of the presence of two large central cannulas, the child's mobility is usually restricted. It is a nursing challenge to help the child find a comfortable position and to include parents in the care of their child.

Parents can best identify how much information they would like about the care required of their child supported on CAVH/CVVH. Knowledge about the need for hourly collection of data and the frequency of blood draws from the line may be helpful for some parents. The security precautions inherent in the circuit and anticipatory information about the expected need for routine circuit changes are examples of other kinds of information some parents may find helpful.

Monitoring for Complications. Ongoing monitoring of the circuit requires skill and experience in troubleshooting complications. Unintentional decreases in ultrafiltration may be the result of changes within the child or circuit. As circuit flow diminishes, UFR decreases, and hemofilter patency is at risk. Any reduction in ultrafiltration in the CAVH circuit requires an initial assessment of the child to determine whether the etiology is reflective of decreased cardiac output. If this is the case, augmenting the child's cardiac output with intravascular volume or vasoactive medications may be the intervention of choice.

Inadequate blood flow through the circuit can also result from cannulas that are too small, vascular access thrombosis, kinks in the tubing, or clotting of the hemofilter or cannulas. Occlusion can occur anywhere in the circuit. Inspecting the entire circuit for kinks and clots is a first step. Prefilter hemodilution at 30 to 50 mL/kg/hour may be helpful in preventing clot formation. Prefilter volume is easily removed by the filter.

When the hemofilter begins to clot, dark red streaks appear. To assess hemofilter patency, a rapid prefilter flush, of normal saline solution or heparinized normal saline (1 unit/mL) through the hemofilter into the collection bag with both arterial and venous return lines clamped, is administered. If organized clot is present within the hemofilter, the dark streaks will not disappear with flushing.

Clotting within the hemofilter decreases the ultrafiltration rate and necessitates hemofilter change. If the hemofilter is totally occluded, the circuit must be replaced *immediately* to preserve patency of the cannulas. Once the new circuit is in place, fluid and heparin management is reevaluated. With the new circuit, one can anticipate improved ultrafiltration and fluid loss. An increase in the heparin infusion rate may be warranted to decrease the incidence of future clotting.

Location of the CAVH hemofilter above the level of the child's heart decreases the UFR and increases the incidence of clotting. The filter is generally placed at the level of the child's right atrium or fourth intercostal space midaxillary line. The location of the UF collection bag also affects blood flow through the filter. The higher the collection bag, the lower the UFR.

The potential for a lethal occurrence of cannula disconnection warrants the frequent inspection of the entire circuit for tight Luer-locked connections. Two major concerns include exsanguination and air emboli. If disconnection occurs, aseptic reconnection needs to rapidly occur. Immediate and temporary clamping of the circuit may prevent air entry. If air is present in a CAVH circuit, it is removed by syringe from the post-filter venous port before reconnecting and reestablishing flow through the circuit.

Hemofiltration systems require a post-filter bubble detection system. If air is detected, the pump is automatically turned off to stop the forward flow of blood. Air is then manually removed. An additional problem related to the actual circuit is spontaneous hemofilter capillary rupture. Rupture of hemofilter capillary fibers occurs if the transmembrane pressure exceeds the manufacturer's guidelines. Generally, these pressure limits are 100 to 200 mmHg. This is evidenced as a change in the UF color from a clear pale yellow color to pink or red. This requires immediate removal and replacement of the hemofilter.

Modifications

Ultrafiltration is dependent upon blood flow through the hemofilter (determined by the patient's cardiac output in CAVH or pump speed in CVVH), amount of free water available in the child's serum, and vertical distance between the heights of the hemofilter and the collection bag. In addition to interventions to optimize the role of each of these variables in enhancing UFR, some centers modify the CAVH circuit to better achieve patient outcomes.

SCUF, an acronym for slow continuous ultrafiltration, is one such modification of hemofiltration. Ultrafiltration occurs according to the same principles described for CAVH but at a slower rate. An IV pump is used to control the amount of UF removed per hour. Solute clearance is not as efficient because it is limited by the slow UFR. SCUF is used to prevent overhydration while maintaining intravenous fluids and nutritional balance. The desired hourly UFR rate is based on the patient's intake in order to maintain hemodynamic stability. Solute removal is ineffective.

Another variation to therapy, continuous arteriovenous hemodiafiltration (CAVHD) or continuous venovenous hemodiafiltration (CVVHD), differs from CAVH/CVVH because it enhances solute clearance. CAVHD/CVVHD is indicated for children with catabolic and uremic conditions complicating ARF.

The extracorporeal circuit is similar to that used in CAVH/CVVH. CAVHD/CVVHD involves a constant infusion of dialysate into the venous side of the hemofilter. The UF collection bag is positioned on the arterial side of the hemofilter. This system allows dialysate to flow over the outside surface of the filter countercurrent to blood flow on the inside surface of the filter. This provides for optimal diffusion and convective transport of solutes and urea from the patient's blood to the UF. CAVHD/CVVHD pulls larger molecules and proteins across the filter. Hourly measurements from the UF collection bag include the volumes of both dialysate infused and UF removed. Subtraction of the hourly dialysate volume infused from the volume collected in the UF collection bag results in the volume of actual UF removed.

The amount of UF produced can be altered through the interventions described under simple hemofiltration. A blood pump may be used to increase flow through the filter. A 1.5% dialysate solution with added KCl at very rapid rates to 900 mL/hour is frequently used (Bishof et al., 1990). Higher osmolar dialysate concentrations further increase UFR. Careful surveillance of the patient's hemodynamic status and routine monitoring of electrolyte levels are essential in evaluating the effectiveness of CAVHD/CVVHD for fluid and solute clearance.

Documentation. Accuracy in documentation during hemofiltration is critical to evaluate the effectiveness of the therapy. Depending on the specific features of the therapy used, equipment involved, and flexibility of the standard ICU flowsheet, the documentation of hemofiltration can take on many appearances.

Generally, sources of intake are recorded separately as IV fluid (including nutritional sources), replacement fluid, dialysate infusion and heparin infusions, and sources of gastrointestinal (GI) intake. Output includes drainage in the UF bag (which may include both dialysate and ultrafiltrate), urine, and GI losses. Total intake and output per hour are recorded, as well as the net UF volume per hour.

To calculate the amount of replacement fluid needed for infusion over an hour, the following equation can be used and is sometimes calculated on the documentation record:

Amount of replacement fluid to be given over the upcoming hour = total UF volume in bag − total amount dialysate infused over the previous hour − the total fluid intake for the previous hour (not including the last hour's replacement fluid) − the desired net UF volume per hour

Routine documentation also includes the child's ACT results, the blood pump speed, the appearance of the hemofilter, and the UF color. Observations of the system and the arming of bubble detector alarms for safety maintenance may be recorded in the form of a checklist.

Observations of the child's coagulation status, tolerance of the therapy, and the appearance of the catheter insertion sites are generally best documented in the narrative note. Education provided to the child and family and the identification of further learning needs is included in the record to assure continuity of care for the child and family.

Hemodialysis

Hemodialysis (HD) rapidly restores fluid, electrolyte, and acid-base balance and is more efficient in removing nitrogenous wastes than any other currently available form of therapy. HD may be the treatment of choice for several reasons. It is possible to calculate the amount of time necessary to remove a particular solute load for a given patient. This affords a sense of control and predictability in the management of life-threatening imbalances. In addition, depending upon the availability of an HD team and appropriate system, HD can be rapidly initiated in the intensive care unit. HD is also the only treatment available for certain toxic ingestions. The charcoal membrane used in HD removes some poisons, such as chloramphenicol and theophylline, that are not cleared by another type of membrane. Finally, HD may be the only available intervention when PD is contraindicated.

Principles of Therapy

PD and HD use the same principles that govern fluid and solute movement across a semipermeable membrane. Diffusion and osmosis occur relative to the concentrations and osmotic gradients present between the child's serum and the dialysate. Similar to PD, the goals of therapy determine which percentage of dialysate is used. Unlike PD, HD requires extracorporeal circulation. A dialyzer pumps blood and dialysate through the system in opposing directions. Similar to CAVHD, countercurrent flow provides an efficient exchange of solutes. The rate of flow through the dialyzer and the length of each exchange can be controlled.

Urea, creatinine, and potassium are usually present in greater concentration in the patient's serum than in dialysate; therefore, these solutes rapidly diffuse from the blood to the dialysate and are removed from the body. Bicarbonate, an alkalizing agent present in dialysate, moves from the dialysate to the blood and provides treatment for metabolic acidosis. Additional molecules can be removed through convective dialysis, where rapid fluid shifts from the blood to the dialysate tend to pull solutes along.

Significant protein loss during HD can be expected. Protein replacement as large as 2 g/kg/day may be necessary. The possibility of providing this level of nutrition is an essential consideration before beginning therapy.

Procedure, Setup, and Insertion. Before HD, intravenous access is evaluated and/or obtained. Although in rare situations native arteriovenous (AV) fistulas are available, femoral vein or superior vena cava cannulation is common. The use of peripheral veins in the pediatric population necessitates the use of smaller catheters. Difficult volume and hemodynamic management may be the consequence. The smaller catheters result in increased resistance to flow from the dialyzer returning to the patient. This increased resistance results in an increase in hydrostatic pressure in the dialyzer, thereby increasing UF and fluid removal. Despite the associated risk of infection with the use of femoral vessels, this location may be the best choice. Venous cannulation of two separate locations or one with double-lumen capacity may be used.

Several dialyzers are commercially available. The type of access and patient size are important considerations in the choice of an HD system. There are variations in the volume of dialyzer and the type and volume of tubing. The circuit volume is compared with the child's circulating blood volume (CBV). An acceptable circuit volume is calculated as 10% of the child's CBV or 8 mL/kg of body weight. The smallest circuit volume currently available is 45 mL. This system, primed with whole blood, can be used in infants.

Maintenance. Determined by the goals of therapy, the HD team prescribes the length of exchange time. Amounts of glucose, acetate, sodium, calcium, and potassium are variably added to the dialyzing fluid, depending upon the patient's situation. The length of one HD exchange usually extends over 2 to 6 hours. Some form of heparinization is required to prevent clot formation within the circuit. Baseline coagulation profiles are necessary before initiating HD. ACT levels are useful in evaluating the child's response to heparinization.

Solute clearance depends on several factors, including the rates of blood and dialysate flow and the surface area and permeability of the membrane. The rate of urea and water removal can be calculated. Information about the patient's serum level of solute is an important component of this calculation. The actual serum value, the rate of urea production, the patient's metabolic rate, and the child's protein intake all play a part in determining the rate of urea clearance.

The acceptable rate of solute clearance is affected by how the child tolerates HD. Because solutes are rapidly removed from the serum, but slowly removed from the brain, an osmolar gradient or disequilibrium between the intravascular and intracellular space may develop. This gradient results in fluid shifts and cerebral edema. The child with disequilibrium syndrome may exhibit confusion, irritability, headache, nausea, vomiting, and seizure activity.

Interventions for management of disequilibrium syndrome include changing to shorter exchanges, approximately 2 hours in length, on a daily basis during the initial stages of HD. Limiting the rate of blood flow through the dialyzer to 2 to 5 mL/kg/minute to decrease the solute exchange rate has also been recommended (Maxwell et al., 1992). Some centers use intravenous mannitol (0.5 g/kg) during the initial exchange to minimize disequilibrium effects.

Achievement of Established Goals. Bedside HD of critically ill pediatric patients requires the collaborative expertise of both PICU and HD nurses. Before beginning HD, the expectations of each nurse are clarified. Usually the PICU nurse continues to manage ongoing care, the HD nurse manages the therapy, and together they collaboratively manipulate vasopressors, volume, and fluid and solute removal within established guidelines to manage the patient through the procedure.

Monitoring. Assessment of the patient's intravascular volume status is an ongoing responsibility. When HD is initiated, a relative hypovolemia may develop owing to the external circulation of the child's blood in the amount of the circuit volume. Progressive hypovolemia and hypotension are not uncommon as therapy progresses. It is not uncommon to initiate or increase the dose of vasopressors during HD. The treatment objective is usually to establish and maintain intravascular normovolemia, but expedient and/or large volume removal challenges this objective.

The use of acetate as a buffer in dialysate may contribute to the development of relative hypovolemia because acetate decreases systemic vascular resistance. Therefore, despite the potential for calcium precipitation, sodium bicarbonate is frequently considered the dialysate buffer of choice (Maxwell et al., 1987).

Hypervolemia may occur if too much fluid is returned to the patient. A common time for this imbalance is at the end of an exchange when the child may be receiving additional blood products. Additional HD time for fluid removal may be required.

Dysrhythmias may occur from electrolyte or acid-base imbalance. Hypotension, which decreases coronary perfusion pressure, and hypokalemia are two of the most common causes of dysrhythmias during HD.

The goal of preventing clot formation can be approached in several ways. One method is through continuous heparinization. This entails increased risk for blood loss and requires meticulous attention to the patient's coagulation status. Another method is regional heparinization, which is accomplished by the administration of heparin in the blood line between the patient and the dialyzer and the administration of protamine sulfate in the venous line between the dialyzer and patient return blood line. The balance of heparin to protamine sulfate administration is crucial and requires close monitoring. The risks of too much heparin resulting in a coagulopathy or an oversupply or rapid administration of protamine sulfate resulting in hypotension are apparent. Some institutions have found the administration of small intermittent doses of heparin effective.

Part of the routine surveillance of the patient's coagulation status includes following trends in the platelet count. A relative thrombocytopenia may develop as platelets adhere to the dialyzer membrane over time.

Frequent monitoring of the dialysate and the child's temperature are important for several reasons. As for any patient with central vascular access, the risk of infection is increased. Daily surveillance cultures from dialysis tubing and dialysate are generally a part of institutional policy. Any elevation in temperature raises suspicion of infection, and a septic workup results. Urea may function as an antipyretic, and thus as the patient's serum urea begins to drop, an occult fever may appear, warranting further investigation.

A sudden rise of patient temperature, described as a "febrile reaction," may occur (Maxwell et al., 1987). One theory of the etiology of this hyperthermia is that the fever is a reaction to the dialyzer membrane materials. The patient care objective is to establish and maintain normothermia. Any deviation from this requires the collection of further patient data and laboratory testing.

Continuous monitoring of the child during HD includes observation of the blood in the circuit for color and clots, and inspection of the circuit for leaks, loose connection, and the characteristics of flow. It is necessary for nurses to assess the child's catheter insertion site or sites each shift for skin integrity, bleeding, and signs of infection. The HD circuit uses pumps, thereby increasing the risk of air embolism. An air bubble detector/alarm system is critical to safe care of the patient.

The impact of HD on the pharmacokinetics of all drugs the patient is receiving is evaluated (see Table 22–12). Additional doses may be needed at the end of each exchange. This is particularly true for drugs that are poorly bound to protein, such as the aminoglycosides.

Documentation. Documentation during HD is a shared responsibility between the HD and PICU nurse. The HD nurse usually documents procedural information, for example, fluid intake, laboratory results, medication administration, the amount of UF output. The PICU nurse usually documents the child's tolerance of the procedure and observations and assessments of the family, as well as identified needs and teaching. Documentation of information that is jointly monitored is institution-specific. Optimal use of the record by the entire healthcare team is considered.

SUMMARY

Various therapies are now available to support the patient in ARF. Despite these therapies, the mortality of ARF remains high. Currently, the frequency and mortality of pediatric ARF as a primary or sec-

ondary disease are unknown. Research in the identification of risk factors associated with ARF may allow earlier intervention, which may minimize the occurrence of ARF or limit mortality. Although ARF is associated with MSOF, low perfusion states, and the use of nephrotoxic drugs, concrete data to validate these perceptions are needed. Data linking supportive therapy to patient outcome are not available. Pediatric nursing research is needed to help guide practice related to the care of patients requiring renal replacement therapy.

Care of the patient in ARF is complex, requiring the combined expertise of an extensive multidisciplinary team. Collaboration within the team provides the best plan of care for each patient. The challenge for nursing is to help facilitate team communication and advocate for care that is in the best interest of the patient and family.

References

Baer, C.L., & Lancaster, L.E. (1992). Acute renal failure. *Critical Care Nursing Quarterly*, 14(4), 1–21.

Bishof, N.A., Welch, T.R., Strife, C.F., & Ryckman, F.C. (1990). Continuous hemofiltration in children. *Pediatrics*, 85(5), 819–823.

Compher, C., Mullen, J.L., & Barker, C.F. (1991). Nutritional support in renal failure. *Surgical Clinics of North America*, 71(3), 597–606.

DiCarlo, J.V., Dudley, T.E., Sherbotie, J.R., Kaplan, B.S., & Costarino, A.T. (1990). Continuous arteriovenous hemofiltration/dialysis improves pulmonary gas exchange in children with multiple organ system failure. *Critical Care Medicine*, 18(8), 822–826.

Elixson, E.M., & Clancy, G.T. (1992). Neonatal peritoneal dialysis in acute renal failure. *Critical Care Nursing Quarterly*, 14(4), 56–65.

Feld, L.G., Cachero, S., & Springate, J.E. (1990). Fluid needs in acute renal failure. *Pediatric Clinics of North America*, 37(2), 337–350.

Finn, W.I. (1990). Diagnosis and management of acute tubular necrosis. *Medical Clinics of North America*, 74(4), 873–891.

Friedman, A.L. (1992). Acute renal disease. In B.P. Fuhrman, & J.J. Zimmerman (Eds.). *Pediatric critical care* (pp. 723–740). St. Louis: C. V. Mosby.

Gaudio, K.M., & Siegel, N.J. (1987). Pathogenesis and treatment of acute renal failure. *Pediatric Clinics of North America*, 34(3), 771–786.

Grupe, W. E. (1986). The kidney. In M.H. Klaus, & A.A. Fanaroff (Eds.). *Care of the high-risk neonate*. (3rd ed., pp. 314–356). Philadelphia: W. B. Saunders.

Jochimsen, F., Schafer, J-H. Maurer, A., & Distler, A. (1990). Impairment of renal function in medical intensive care: Predictability of acute renal failure. *Critical Care Medicine*, 18(5), 480–485.

Jones, D.P., & Chesney, R.W. (1992). Glomerulotubular dysfunction and acute renal failure. In B.P. Fuhrman, & J.J. Zimmerman (Eds.). *Pediatric critical care* (pp. 697–706). St. Louis: C. V. Mosby.

Jose, P.A., Stewart, C.L., Tina, L.M., & Calcagno, P.L. (1987). In G.B. Avery (Ed.). *The third edition of neonatology: Pathophysiology and management of the newborn* (pp. 795–850). Philadelphia: J. B. Lippincott.

Kaplan, A., & Petrillo, R. (1987). Regional heparinization of continuous arterial-venous hemofiltration. *ASAIO Transplant*, 33, 312–315.

Karlowicz, M.G., & Adelman, R.D. (1992). Acute renal failure in the neonate. *Clinics in Perinatology*, 19(1), 139–157.

Maxwell, L.G., Colombani, P.M., & Fivush, B.A. (1992). Renal, metabolic and endocrine failure. In M.C. Rogers (Ed.). *Textbook* of *Pediatric Intensive Care* (Vol. 2, 2nd ed., pp 1182–1234). Baltimore: Williams & Wilkins.

Maxwell, L.G., Fivush, B.A., & McLean, R.H. (1987). Renal failure. In M.C. Rogers (Ed.). *Textbook of Pediatric Intensive Care.* (Vol. 2, pp. 1001–1055). Baltimore: Williams & Wilkins.

Notterman, D.A. (1988). Pediatric pharmacology. In B. Chernow (Ed.). *The pharmacologic approach to the critically ill patient* (2nd ed., pp. 131–198). Baltimore: Williams & Wilkins.

Paganini, E.P. (1987). Continuous renal prosthetic therapy in acute renal failure; An overview. *Pediatric Clinics of North America*, 34(1), 165–185.

Paradiso, C. (1989). Hemofiltration: An alternative to dialysis. *Heart and Lung*, 18(3), 282–290.

Price, S.A., Wilson, L.U. (1986). *Pathophysiology: Clinical concepts of disease process* (3rd ed.). New York: McGraw-Hill.

Rice, V. (1983). Magnesium, calcium, and phosphate imbalances; their clinical significance. *Critical Care Nurse*, 3(3), 90–112.

Robillard, J.E., Segar, J.L., Smith, F.G., & Jose, P.A. (1992). Regulation of sodium metabolism and extracellular fluid volume during development. *Clinics in Perinatology*, 19(1), 15–31.

Rudnick, M.R., Bastl, C.P., Elfinebein, I.B., & Narin, S.R. (1983). The differential diagnosis of acute renal failure. In B.M. Brenner, & J.M. Lazarus (Eds.). *Acute renal failure* (pp. 176–222). Philadelphia: W. B. Saunders.

Ruley, E.J., & Bock, G.H. (1989). Acute renal failure in infants and children. In W.C. Shoemaker (Ed.). *Textbook of critical care* (2nd ed., pp. 721–732). Philadelphia: W. B. Saunders.

Seikaly, M.G., & Arant, B.S. (1992). Development of renal hemodynamics: Glomerular filtration and renal blood flow. *Clinics in Perinatology*, 19(1), 1–13.

Spitzer, A., Bernstein, J., & Edelmann, C.M. (1985). Developmental morphology and physiology of the kidney: assessment of renal function and structure. In V.C. Kelley (Ed.). *Practice of pediatrics* (Vol. 8, pp. 1–25.) New York: Harper & Row.

Stahl, W. (1986). Kidney in shock. In J. Barrett, & L.M. Nyhus (Eds.). *Treatment of shock: Principles and practice* (2nd ed.). Philadelphia: Lea & Febiger.

Sweet, M., Kaher, K.K., & Makker, S.P. (1989). Acute renal failure in children: Etiology, diagnosis and management. *New York State Journal of Medicine*, June 89, 336–341.

Wells, T.G. (1990). The pharmacology and therapeutics of diuretics in the pediatric patient. *Pediatric Clinics of North America*, 37(2), 463–504.

CHAPTER 23

Gastrointestinal Critical Care Problems

DIANE S. JAKOBOWSKI
TWILA W. HARMON
SUSAN N. PECK
JUDITH J. STELLAR

A wide variety of gastrointestinal (GI) problems occur in infants and children that may require intensive nursing care. Problems of the GI tract range from intussusception, treated by simple reduction with barium enema, to fulminant liver disease with GI bleeding. GI disorders rarely occur in isolation but are often associated with other congenital defects or with multisystem dysfunction, placing infants and children with these disorders at high risk for morbidity and mortality.

GI problems result in the final common pathways of obstruction, GI and peritoneal inflammation, GI bleeding, and hepatic failure. The existence of one of these final common pathways often predisposes the child to the development of another. For example, the infant with an intestinal obstruction is at increased risk for developing perforation and/or necrosis of the bowel with peritoneal inflammation without prompt treatment. Critical care nurses play a vital role in the recognition and prevention of the progression of these final common pathways.

GASTROINTESTINAL ASSESSMENT

Abdominal Examination

Nursing assessment of the GI system is fundamental to the care of infants and children who are critically ill, particularly when GI dysfunction is suspected or confirmed. Assessment is initiated with serial abdominal examinations, employing the basic techniques of inspection, auscultation, percussion, and palpation. The abdomen is inspected for the presence of bruises, wounds, scars, erythema, or discolorations; peristaltic waves and/or pulsations; visible asymmetry, masses, bowel loops, or protuberances; a flat, full, or scaphoid contour; distension; and umbilical and muscular abnormalities.

Serial auscultation of the abdomen is performed in all four abdominal quadrants noting the presence, or absence, and character of bowel sounds with particular attention to changes in sounds over time. Intestinal obstruction produces high-pitched, tinkling sounds; nasogastric intubation causes decreased or absent sounds. A quiet abdomen is present during paralytic ileus, and an ominously silent abdomen may indicate perforation with peritonitis. Other sounds, such as bruits, hums, and rubs may also be heard with auscultation. A friction rub may indicate peritoneal inflammation.

Percussion is used to obtain information regarding abdominal contents, including air and fluid, as well as intra-abdominal organs and masses. Shifting dullness is elicited in the presence of intraperitoneal fluid. Absence of dullness over the liver may be found with pneumoperitoneum, or may be elicited when an air-filled loop of bowel is located over the liver. Percussion of the spleen or liver more than 2 cm below the costal margin indicates hepatosplenomegaly.

Palpation is used to obtain information regarding abdominal pain and tenderness and data regarding the size, shape, and location of organs and masses. Palpation also is used to detect free fluid. Superficial palpation is performed first, followed by deep palpation. It is important not to perform deep palpation on a patient with an "acute abdomen." In addition, deep palpation is not performed on any patient with a known or suspected abdominal mass.

The presence of rebound tenderness indicates peritoneal inflammation. The technique to elicit rebound tenderness consists of the examiner exerting firm pressure in an area away from the pain and then quickly releasing the pressure. A positive response is an unequivocally painful reaction. This technique is not used routinely with pediatric patients because it is unnecessarily painful for the child and does not reveal any new findings. Most children wince in response only to the change in pressure exerted, and children who have significant disease exhibit a painful reaction simply with light palpation.

Measurement of abdominal girth provides objective data regarding the degree of distension and is included in the assessment of the abdomen. If stooling and/or vomiting has occurred, nursing evaluation of this output is important. The color, character, and consistency of all GI output is noted; the amount is estimated or measured and included in output calculations. Gastric drainage is tested for pH and blood, and stool is tested for blood. The character and content of emesis and stool are helpful in understanding the underlying disorder. Bilious vomiting is a significant finding, indicative of a proximal mechanical obstruction. Hematemesis indicates an upper GI (UGI) bleeding site; hematochezia (bright red blood from the rectum) indicates brisk mid-GI or lower GI (LGI) tract bleeding. Melena is blood that has been digested during passage through the GI tract. Melanotic stools indicate slow upper or mid-GI tract bleeding (Harris, 1986).

Laboratory and Radiologic Assessment

Serial laboratory and radiologic studies are obtained on all patients with a GI disorder. If a peritoneal tap or laparotomy is performed, peritoneal fluid cultures are also obtained. Additional studies are warranted for specific disorders and are discussed specifically in the following sections.

Radiologic studies include plain films, contrast studies, nuclear medicine scans, computed tomography (CT), magnetic resonance imaging (MRI), ultrasound, and arteriography. Plain films are done in two views to identify air-fluid levels and provide an alternate view in addition to a flat plate. Small infants and older children who are critically ill cannot be put in the upright position for a second view and require either a cross-table lateral or left lateral decubitus film. Chest radiographs are also obtained to rule out abnormalities within the thorax, or concurrent disease processes such as right lower lobe pneumonia, or complications of severe GI dysfunction such as pleural effusion. Contrast studies help define GI anatomy, aid in diagnosis (of GE reflux, for example), or are treatment measures, such as in the reduction of an intussusception with a hydrostatic barium enema.

GENERAL PRINCIPLES OF MANAGEMENT

In addition to ongoing assessment and monitoring, gastric decompression, intravascular volume replacement and maintenance, and pharmacologic management are general interventions indicated in response to GI pathologic events.

Table 23–1. SOLUTION FOR REPLACING LOSSES OF GASTRIC SECRETIONS

	Gastric Secretion (mEq/L)	Replacement Fluid D5%, half NS + 30 mEq/KCl/L
Sodium	60–75	77
Chloride	105–130	107
Potassium	5–30	30
H+	0–65	0

From Filston, H.C. (1992). Fluid and electrolyte management in the pediatric surgical patient. *Surgical Clinics of North America, 72(6),* 1189–1205.

Gastric Decompression

Decompression of the GI tract is one of the primary interventions indicated in patients with a GI abnormality. The goal of gastric decompression is to actively remove air and secretions from an injured GI tract. In GI obstruction, which often precedes perforation, there is dilation of the proximal bowel as peristalsis continues against the distal obstruction. In addition, air and secretions collect in the bowel lumen proximal to the obstruction. Decompression is employed either continuously or intermittently to actively remove air and secretions from the upper GI tract.

The preferred position for intubation and gastric decompression in a child is semi-upright. A nasogastric (NG) or orogastric (OG) tube is inserted into the stomach via the esophagus. The oral route may be preferred for young infants who are obligate nose-breathers. For the purpose of decompression, the largest possible double-lumen vented tube is used, such as the Salem sump tube or a Replogle tube for neonates. Such tubes have a primary lumen to remove air and secretions; the other lumen serves as an air vent to keep the primary lumen from adhering to the stomach wall when suction is applied. It is important to note that the air vent lumen is not clamped off, and clogging with secretions is prevented. A slight hissing sound signals that the tube

is functioning properly. Patency may be maintained by instilling 5 to 30 mL of air (depending on the size of the child) into the air vent. The primary lumen can also be irrigated with saline. The child maintains a nothing by mouth (NPO) status, and excessive swallowing of air is discouraged.

Repositioning the tube, as well as irrigating as described earlier, may be indicated if there is doubt about the adequacy of gastric decompression. If inadequate, abdominal distension and diaphragmatic elevation can develop, which then compromise both respiratory and GI function. In addition to decompressing the GI tract, NG and OG tubes are used for gastric lavage, the administration of various medications, including antacids to prevent stress ulcer syndrome, and collection and analysis of gastric aspirate.

Intravascular Volume Replacement and Maintenance

Fluid administration takes into account insensible losses (supplied by maintenance fluids), estimated third-space losses, and measured losses, which include NG and OG tube secretions, ongoing GI bleeding, ostomy and fistula drainage, or losses from other tubes or drains and wounds (Filston, 1992). Measured losses are calculated and replaced at specified intervals. Table 23–1 outlines electrolyte content of GI secretions and comparable intravenous (IV) replacement fluids.

If hypovolemia is severe, fluid resuscitation may be required to correct hypovolemia and maintain a urine output of 1 to 2 mL/kg/hour. As fluid returns to the intravascular space, fluid retention or overload can occur and the administration of diuretics may be indicated to aid in the excretion of excess fluid. Meticulous monitoring of intake and output is mandatory for these patients, as is ongoing assessment for signs and symptoms of fluid volume deficit or excess.

Table 23–2. PHARMACOLOGIC AGENTS COMMONLY USED IN GI DISORDERS

I. Antimicrobials (Broad-spectrum) to Combat Infection	II. H2 Receptor Blockers and Topical Protectors to Combat Gastric Acid Secretion	III. Vasoconstrictive/Sclerosing Agents to Decrease Bleeding
Ampicillin	Cimetidine	Vasopressin
Gentamicin	Ranitidine	Somatostatin
Clindamycin	Antacids	Sodium morrhuate
Amiracin	Sucralfate	Tetradecylsulfate
Metronidazole		
Ticarcillin		
Clavulanate		
Erythromycin		
Cefoxitin		
Ceftazidime		
Cefotaxime		
Ceftriaxone		
Mezlocillin		

Table 23–3. CAUSES OF INTESTINAL OBSTRUCTION

| Mechanical Obstruction | | Paralytic Ileus | |
Intraluminal	Extrinsic	Abdominal Conditions	Systemic Conditions
Atresia or stenosis	Malrotation	Hirschsprung's disease	Trauma
Pyloric stenosis	Volvulus	Intestinal pseudoobstruction	Shock
Foreign body	Hernia	Severe gastroenteritis	Sepsis
Meconium	Annular pancreas	Perforation of viscus	Hypokalemia
Medications	Duplication cysts	Peritonitis	Drugs
• Cholestyramine	Adhesions/bands	Pancreatitis	Diabetic acidosis
• Antacid	Tumor	Necrotizing enterocolitis	General anesthesia
• Kaolin	Granulomatous process	Toxic megacolon	
Intussusception			
Parasitic infection			

From Quan, R. (1990). Bowel failure. In Levin, D.L., & Morriss, F.C. (Eds). *Essentials of pediatric intensive care* (pp. 147–150). St. Louis: Quality Medical Publishing.

Pharmacologic Management

In most cases of actual or potential GI dysfunction, a variety of pharmacologic agents are employed. These agents are used to treat infection, excessive gastric acid secretion, and GI bleeding. Pharmacologic agents include antimicrobials to combat infection; H2 receptor blockers and antacids to decrease and neutralize gastric acid secretion; and vasoconstrictive and sclerosing agents to decrease bleeding. Table 23–2 lists various medications within these categories.

GASTROINTESTINAL OBSTRUCTION

True GI obstructions occur most commonly in the newborn. Obstructions may be present in any portion of the gut from the esophagus to the anus and are related to a variety of causes (Table 23–3). The initial presentation, clinical findings, and patient management vary, depending upon the type and location of the obstruction. A maternal history of polyhydramnios may indicate a proximal obstruction because the fetus is unable to properly digest amnionic fluid. Bilious vomiting may be associated with malrotation with volvulus. Significant abdominal distension may signify a distal obstruction. Failure to pass meconium in the first 24 hours of life is suggestive of an obstruction related to Hirschsprung's disease. The pathophysiology of obstruction is depicted in Figure 23–1.

Esophageal Atresia

Esophageal atresia is a congenital anomaly in which the esophagus is segmented with a blind pouch separating the upper and lower portion. In most instances there is also a fistula connecting the distal

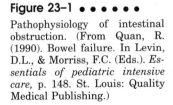

Figure 23–1 ● ● ● ● ● ●
Pathophysiology of intestinal obstruction. (From Quan, R. (1990). Bowel failure. In Levin, D.L., & Morriss, F.C. (Eds.). *Essentials of pediatric intensive care,* p. 148. St. Louis: Quality Medical Publishing.)

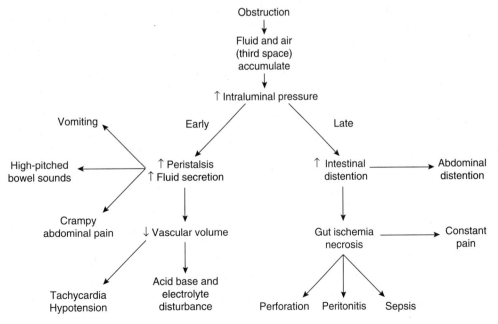

esophagus and trachea. However, the use of the term "tracheoesophageal fistula" (TEF) to describe all anomalies of the esophagus is incorrect. There are three main types of tracheoesophageal deformities (Fig. 23–2): esophageal atresia with distal TEF, isolated esophageal atresia, and TEF without esophageal atresia (H-type) (Holder et al., 1961).

Pathogenesis

The esophagus and trachea develop embryologically at the same time. These structures are first recognized as a ventral diverticulum of the foregut at 22 to 23 days after fertilization (Randolph, 1986). The development of the esophagus and trachea is felt to occur by the proliferation of endodermal cells on the lateral walls of the diverticulum. These cell masses becoming ridges of tissue that divide the foregut into the two separate channels of the esophagus and trachea (Rosenthal, 1931). This is completed by 34 to 36 days after fertilization. During the fourth week of fetal life, interruptions in development may result in abnormalities of the esophagus with and without fistula formation between the two structures.

Associated Anomalies

Deformities of the esophagus and trachea occur early in intrauterine development along with generalized organ differentiation and division. Mesodermal maldevelopment caused by some unknown intrauterine event is felt to be the cause for multisystem problems seen in many of these newborns. The majority of these defects are grouped under the name VACTERL (V—vertebral, A—anal, C—cardiac, TE—tracheoesophageal, R—renal, L—limb). Most series report the incidence of associated anomalies with esophageal atresia–TEF deformities to be between 30% and 55%. Cardiovascular disease is the most common associated anomaly, followed by limb and genitourinary defects (Ein et al., 1989).

Clinical Presentation

As with other causes of proximal obstruction, a maternal history of polyhydramnios is common. The infant typically presents with bubbly oral secretions and regurgitation of saliva, which cannot be swallowed because of the blind proximal esophageal pouch. Most babies with isolated esophageal atresia or esophageal atresia with TEF present with this problem soon after delivery. The diagnosis is made by careful placement of a nasogastric tube into the blind pouch. A simple chest radiograph subsequently reveals a curled tube in the proximal esophageal pouch. With esophageal atresia and distal TEF, an abdominal film typically reveals a distended stomach with gas patterns throughout the small bowel. However, in the infant with isolated esophageal atresia, the abdominal film shows a gasless bowel pattern.

An infant with an H-type TEF usually presents at 3 to 4 months of age with a history of respiratory distress, pneumonia, and some degree of cyanosis with feedings. Direct bronchoscopic visualization is the diagnostic study of choice. The tracheal end of the fistula can usually be visualized in the membranous portion of the trachea at the thoracic inlet (Martin & Alexander, 1985). Occasionally, a barium or water-soluble esophogram may be used for diagnosis, but often this does not demonstrate the fistula, and aspiration of the contrast material is a concern.

Critical Care Management

Once a diagnosis of esophageal atresia with or without TEF is made, preoperative stabilization of the newborn is essential. Decompression of the proximal pouch is of utmost importance in the preoperative phase. This is accomplished using the general principles of gastric decompression described earlier, except that the Replogle tube is placed in the proximal esophageal pouch, thereby removing oral secretions and preventing pulmonary aspiration.

Operative Management for Esophageal Atresia With Distal TEF. Primary repair is the best surgical option and may be performed even in the small preterm infant (Polson et al., 1988). The operative approach is through a right thoracotomy incision in which the fistula is first divided, and then the two segments of the esophagus are anastomosed.

Operative Management for Isolated Esophageal Atresia. In most cases of isolated EA there is a long gap between the proximal and distal segments of the esophagus, which precludes primary repair in the newborn period. For a full-term baby with no other abnormalities, usually only a feeding gastrostomy is placed. Over the next several months of life, it is felt that the esophageal segment will elongate spontaneously (Puri et al., 1981). During this waiting period, the surgeon may choose to manually stretch the upper and lower segments of the esophagus.

The second stage of surgical intervention typically occurs when the esophageal segments are separated by no more than one vertebral body, as seen on radiographic imaging. At this time a primary end-to-end anastomosis of the esophagus is attempted. If for some reason the segments do not come together easily, a circular or spiral myotomy of the upper esopha-

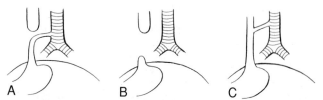

Figure 23–2 ● ● ● ● ● ●

Three forms of esophageal anomalies. A is the most common form of esophageal malformation; B is the next most common form; C is the classic "H" type fistula. (From Avery, M.E., et al. (1981). *The lung and its disorders in the newborn infant,* 4th edition, p. 151. Philadelphia: W.B. Saunders.)

gus is performed. This procedure usually provides 1 to 2 mm of extra length by dividing the outer layer of the esophagus.

Conversely, for the sick preterm infant this delayed type of primary closure may not be optimal. There also may be some infants in whom the gap between the esophageal segments is so wide that primary repair is impossible. In either of these cases, a cervical esophagostomy (exteriorizing the blind upper esophageal pouch in the neck region) and gastrostomy are performed in the newborn period. When the child reaches a weight of approximately 10 kg, an esophageal replacement procedure is performed using a piece of colon, small bowel, or stomach.

Operative Management of TEF. The operative approach to an isolated TEF is through a right thoracotomy or a right cervical incision. The fistula is divided primarily. Surgical complications are rare.

Postoperative Management. The respiratory system is managed with endotracheal intubation until it is absolutely no longer needed. Once the ET tube is removed, if the child again requires assisted ventilation, the operating surgeon must be present to make sure the intubation does not interrupt the anastomosis. Oro- or nasopharyngeal suctioning is performed with a suction catheter that is measured and marked at the time of surgery to avoid the anastomosis site during the suctioning procedure.

An extrapleural chest tube and drain are placed at the time of surgery; an assessment of the color and consistency of the drainage is important. The presence of saliva in the collecting chamber may indicate a leak at the site of anastomosis.

Gastric decompression remains essential in the postoperative period. This can be accomplished either with an NG tube or a gastrostomy tube. If the surgeon has placed an NG tube, it is important to remember that it passes through the esophageal anastomosis. It is critical not to accidentally remove or replace the tube in the immediate postoperative period. Passage of saliva through the tube indicates that the infant is able to swallow and that the esophagus is patent.

Enteral alimentation may begin on the third to fourth postoperative day via the NG or gastrostomy tube. Care is taken not to overdistend the stomach or allow the feeding to back up into the esophagus. This may be accomplished by using a Y-connector attached to the NG or gastrostomy tube allowing the stomach to be vented at the same time the feeding is delivered.

A water-soluble contrast swallow is performed at 7 to 10 postoperative days to evaluate the esophageal anastomosis. If a leak is present, it usually seals on its own. This is confirmed with a followup radiographic study. If no leak is encountered, the chest tube is removed and the baby may be allowed to attempt full nutrition by mouth. Successful transition to oral feedings usually takes several days to accomplish.

As the infant's condition stabilizes and transfer from the intensive care setting is considered, paren-

tal education becomes the nursing focus. The parents should be encouraged by this improvement in their child's health, but at the same time they need to be informed about possible future problems. There can be narrowing at the anastomosis requiring dilation, gastroesophageal reflux, and the characteristic "barking cough" related to tracheal irritation.

Duodenal Obstruction

Complete or partial duodenal obstruction may occur for a number of reasons. Atresia, stenosis, annular pancreas, and malrotation are the most common causes of duodenal obstruction. Each of these anomalies has unique characteristics that are important for appropriate management.

Pathogenesis

During the fifth to sixth week of intrauterine development there is a rapid growth of the epithelial lining of the duodenum. However, the cross-section of the gut cannot accommodate this growth, which obliterates the duodenal lumen. By the eighth to tenth week of gestation, recanalization of the duodenal lumen occurs. The absence of this recanalization process causes duodenal atresia, stenosis, or intrinsic web formation (Tandler, 1902).

Atresia results in complete obstruction of the duodenal lumen by an intrinsic duodenal membrane made up of mucosa or submucosa. Either two blind ends of the duodenum connected by a short fibrous cord with an intact mesentery; or two blind ends with no fibrous cord and a V-shaped defect in the mesentery separating the two pieces of the duodenum are found (Gray & Skandalakis, 1972) (Fig. 23-3A).

Duodenal stenosis is a partial obstruction of the lumen of the intestine. This narrowing may be caused by extrinsic indentation of the duodenal wall owing to mesenteric bands associated with malrotation, anterior preduodenal portal vein, or misplaced pancreatic tissue in the wall of the duodenum (Schnaufer, 1986). As with atresia, an intrinsic web or diaphragm can result in a partial obstruction. The child who has duodenal stenosis may not become symptomatic until later in life.

A congenital annular pancreas can create a situation of either atresia or stenosis, depending on the degree of pancreatic compression on the duodenum. The embryologic development of the pancreas occurs simultaneously with duodenal recanalization. The dorsal pancreas arises from the dorsal wall of the duodenum, and the ventral pancreas develops from the region between the duodenum and the hepatic diverticulum. As normal gut rotation occurs, the ventral pancreas grows around the right side of the duodenum until it meets with the dorsal pancreatic bud. An annular pancreas occurs when the tip of the ventral pancreas becomes fixed to the duodenal wall and during rotation wraps around the right side of

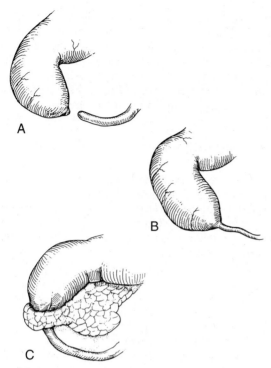

Figure 23–3 ● ● ● ● ● ●

Various types of duodenal atresia-stenosis. *A*, Complete duodenal atresia with discontinuity in the muscular wall of the bowel. *B*, Seromuscular layers may be in continuity with the atresia as represented by a complete membrane. *C*, An annular pancreas, which may create either atresia or stenosis depending on the degree of pancreatic compression on the duodenum. (From Ashcraft, K. W. (1994). *Atlas of pediatric surgery* (p. 92). Philadelphia: W.B. Saunders.)

the duodenum to fuse with the dorsal pancreas (Lecco, 1910). The intestinal compression from the pancreatic wrap causes the obstruction, as small segments of pancreatic tissue partially or completely encircle the second portion of the duodenum (Fig. 23–3*B*).

Another critical aspect of duodenal embryology is related to the positioning and fixation of the small bowel that may result in nonrotation. Obstruction can occur when rotation and fixation do not occur correctly during fetal development. During the fourth week of gestation the intestinal tract is elongating too rapidly for the abdominal cavity to accommodate its growth. The intestinal tract grows out of the abdomen into the umbilical cord. As the midgut begins to return to the abdomen at about 8 weeks' gestation, it rotates in a counterclockwise fashion around the superior mesentery artery. This rotation should be completed by the twelfth week. Fixation of the intestine inside the abdomen with the ligament of Treitz settling in the left upper quadrant and the cecum in the right lower quadrant should follow this rotation. When rotation and fixation do not occur, bowel obstruction as well as superior mesenteric artery occlusion may ensue with resultant ischemia and volvulus (Fig. 23–4*A*, *B*, *C*).

Associated Anomalies

Diaphragmatic hernia and abdominal wall defects are associated anomalies thought to occur because development of the diaphragm and abdominal wall is related to the return of the small bowel into the abdominal cavity. For example, if the pleuroperitoneal membranes have not closed completely before the gut reenters the abdominal cavity, the bowel is likely to pass through that opening and fill the space in the chest, resulting in a congenital diaphragmatic

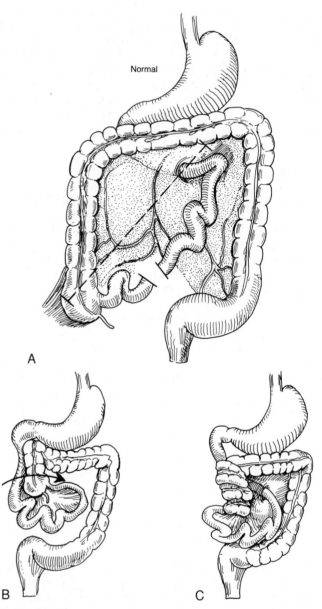

Figure 23–4 ● ● ● ● ● ●

Malrotation with volvulus. *A*, Normal small bowel mesenteric attachment (as demonstrated by line). This prevents twisting of the small bowel because of the broad fixation of the mesentery. *B*, Malrotation of the bowel with the cecum overlying the duodenum. *C*, Midgut volvulus around superior mesenteric artery due to narrow base of mesentery. (From Ross, A.J., III (1990). Malrotation of the intestine. In P.F. Nora (Ed.). *Operative surgery*, 3rd edition, p. 1048. Philadelphia: W.B. Saunders.)

hernia formation. Omphalocele occurs when the bowel does not completely return to the abdominal cavity. Nonrotation is present with these defects.

One genetic defect associated with duodenal obstruction is Down's syndrome. Down's syndrome is found in 30% of infants born with duodenal obstruction. The reason for this association is not known. There is also a recognizably higher incidence of congenital heart defects in children with duodenal obstruction (Schnaufer, 1986).

Clinical Presentation

A newborn with duodenal obstruction initially appears healthy, but quickly becomes symptomatic. An exception to this is the infant with an in-utero volvulus who presents with massive abdominal distension, respiratory distress, acidosis, and sepsis. A maternal history of polyhydramnios can alert the caregiver that an obstruction may be present. The child with simple duodenal atresia usually displays a normal-appearing abdomen but does not tolerate feedings, as demonstrated by bilious vomiting. When this occurs, management includes NG tube placement for decompression, IV fluids, and antibiotic administration. An abdominal radiograph is taken to aid in diagnosis and to rule out nonrotation. With pure duodenal atresia the abdominal film usually reveals the classic "double bubble" sign, in which the stomach and the first portion of the duodenum are dilated, and distal bowel gas is absent. This type of dilation can also be present with intestinal stenosis, but there is usually some air below the area of dilation.

Critical Care Management

Surgical correction of most duodenal obstructions is accomplished by a duodenoduodenostomy. Duodenoduodenostomy consists of excision of the atretic portion of the bowel and connects duodenum to duodenum. In rare situations, to avoid atretic bowel, duodenojejunostomy is performed connecting duodenum to jejunum, leaving a portion of the duodenum connected to the pancreas with the ability to drain bile. An intrinsic duodenal web is repaired with duodenoplasty, excision of the web, and closure of the lumen of the bowel.

Stabilization of infants with nonrotation and volvulus by gastric decompression, airway stabilization, and fluid resuscitation, must occur quickly with subsequent transport to the operating room. The Ladd's procedure is required for correction of nonrotation and volvulus. The intestines are untwisted, assessed for viability, and resected in areas of necrosis or perforation. Occasionally the entire small bowel is necrotic, making chances of the infant's survival grim. Once a full assessment of the bowel is made, the Ladd's bands are divided and the duodenum is mobilized and placed along the right side of the abdomen. An appendectomy is performed and the cecum and colon are placed on the left side. The appendix is removed to avoid a later misdiagnosis because the appendix is now located on the left rather than the right side. This type of abdominal placement allows for a broad base of mesentery, which prevents further volvulus (Ladd & Gross, 1941).

Adequate decompression of the GI tract is the first goal of postoperative management. Placement of a gastrostomy tube for long-term decompression until bowel patency is demonstrated is somewhat controversial. Some surgeons think this type of tube is essential, particularly in the preterm infant, whereas others favor decompression with a nasogastric tube (Schnaufer, 1986). Decompression is required until the upper GI tract drainage decreases, changes in color from green to clear, and the baby begins to stool.

Adequate nutritional support can be provided with operative placement of a transanastomotic feeding tube for early enteral feedings with an elemental infant formula. Peripheral or central total parenteral nutrition (TPN) is a temporary alternative to enteral nutrition with the initiation of feedings as soon as is possible.

Jejunoileal Obstruction

Atresia of the jejunum or ileum is defined as is duodenal atresia; that is, it is a complete congenital obstruction of the intestinal lumen at either of those locations. Stenosis of the jejunum or ileum is very rare and is not discussed.

Meconium ileus is one of the most common causes of obstruction in the small bowel. Meconium ileus occurs when inspissated meconium becomes lodged in the small bowel, usually in the ileum, and complete obstruction occurs owing to the tenacity of the meconium. The viscous nature of the meconium is usually caused by abnormal intestinal secretions and by pancreatic insufficiency related to cystic fibrosis (Thomaides & Arey, 1963). There are two types of meconium ileus. Simple ileus exists when there is an obstruction in the ileum with dilated proximal bowel and microcolon below the obstruction. Complicated ileus results in the same obstruction and intestinal findings, plus volvulus, necrosis, and perforation.

Pathogenesis

Defects in the arteriomesenteric arcade are thought to be primarily responsible for jejunoileal atresias. Atresia formation usually occurs early in gestation when a cord-like band separates the two ends of the bowel or when there is a total separation of the bowel due to a V-shaped deformity in the mesentery. This type of mesenteric vascular catastrophe, causing disruption of the bowel, can occur late in intrauterine life (Louw & Barnard, 1955). Meconium ileus is most often a newborn manifestation of cystic fibrosis.

Associated Anomalies

The relationship between meconium ileus and cystic fibrosis has been established. There are no other consistent abnormalities found in children with jejunoileal atresia. There are a few reported cases of trisomy 21 associated with these atresias (de Lorimier et al., 1969; Nixon & Tawes, 1971).

Clinical Presentation

An infant with jejunoileal atresia usually presents with subtle or delayed signs of obstruction, such as bilious vomiting and abdominal distension. A maternal history of polyhydramnios may also be present. Passage of meconium may or may not occur, depending on the level and extent of the obstruction (Grosfeld, 1986).

The diagnosis is made with an abdominal radiograph, which reveals significantly dilated loops of bowel, with multiple air fluid levels. This study alone may be all that is needed to make a definitive diagnosis. However, many surgeons also obtain a contrast enema to further define the exact area of the obstruction.

The clinical presentation of meconium ileus is similar to that of ileal atresia. An abdominal film demonstrates distended loops of bowel, and there may be a "soap bubble" appearance in the distal ileum as bubbles of gas mix with the tenacious meconium (Neuhauser, 1946).

Critical Care Management

Infants with simple meconium ileus may be treated nonoperatively with the use of a high hyperosmolar enema. Evidence of complicated meconium ileus is ruled out before performing the procedure. If complicated meconium ileus is suspected, fluid and electrolyte abnormalities are corrected, normal urine output is established, hypothermia corrected, and prophylactic antibiotics begun before operative correction.

In simple meconium ileus, the hyperosmolar enema used for treatment usually employs gastrographin, a water-soluble contrast solution. The infant is administered IV fluid, usually twice that which is established as maintenance, to counteract the hyperosmolality of the dye. The enema is administered with fluoroscopic guidance to prevent complications, especially perforation. With successful treatment, the infant passes a large amount of semisolid meconium for the next 24 to 48 hours. Failure to pass this meconium or progressive distension is an indication for operation (Noblett, 1969).

Surgical Management. Jejunal and ileal atresias are usually managed with end-to-end bowel anastomosis. The difficulty of the operative procedure is the result of the disparity in the size of the proximal dilated bowel and the small distal segment. The massively dilated segment is usually resected and the anastomosis is done in an oblique fashion to provide a wider opening.

Surgical repair of meconium ileus involves an enterostomy in the dilated segment of the ileum. The meconium is carefully expressed out of the proximal and distal segments, using saline or Mucomist as irrigants to help liquefy the meconium. In rare cases, when complete removal of the meconium plug is possible, primary anastomosis is done with bowel that appears healthy. Residual thick meconium usually remains, requiring an ileostomy to vent the bowel. The technique of ileostomy formation with meconium ileus is a Bishop-Koop anastomosis, in which the end of the proximal bowel is anastomosed to the side of the distal segment, leaving the end of the distal area as a stoma. This vents the bowel, but also allows for installation of Mucomist or other irrigants to flush out additional meconium or stool if needed. Because the normal fecal stream can continue with this operation, it is the procedure of choice for most surgeons (Lloyd, 1986).

Postoperative Management. The postoperative infant requires an NG tube for proximal decompression, respiratory support as needed, fluid and electrolyte replacement, and antibiotics. Close monitoring of temperature, other vital signs, and urine output is essential. The child is NPO and receives TPN for several weeks until normal GI function returns. Enteral alimentation usually begins with a predigested formula. The patient is observed closely for signs of malabsorption and diarrhea.

If an ileostomy is present, Mucomist may be instilled into the stoma to evacuate fecal contents from the distal bowel. Initially, most of the stool is expelled through the ileostomy, but with time, the infant has more output through the rectum. Once the meconium is cleared, an elemental enteral diet is started. Pancreatic enzymes are added when full-strength formula is begun, even if a firm diagnosis of cystic fibrosis has not yet been established. A complete cystic fibrosis workup is part of the postoperative management of any child with meconium ileus.

Intussusception

Intussusception is the telescoping or invagination of proximal bowel into distal bowel. It can be classified as idiopathic, associated with a specific lead point, postoperative, or chronic. The majority of cases are idiopathic, wherein the intussusception occurs at or near the ileocecal valve. Only about 5% of the cases have a specific lead point (Raffensperger, 1989). The most common lead point is a Meckel's diverticulum, followed by polyps, duplications, tumors, hemangiomas, and sutures lines or an appendiceal stump. Postoperative intussusception occurs within 2 weeks of a surgical procedure. It occurs most often in cases of intra-abdominal or retroperitoneal procedures, although it has also been reported following thoracic and other procedures (Kiesling & Tank, 1989). Intussusception is described as chronic when symptoms occur for 14 or more days and are less severe. This usually occurs in older children (Reijnan et al., 1989).

Etiology

The exact etiology of idiopathic intussusception is unknown. Possible causes include hypertrophied Peyer's patch, a localized area of hyperperistalsis, or viral gastroenteritis, with rotavirus and adenovirus being cited (Ravitch, 1986; Raffensperger, 1989). Older children with intussusception are usually found to have an anatomic abnormality, which is the associated lead point. Other types of lead points include the thick, inspissated fecal material seen in children with cystic fibrosis, or submucosal hemorrhage, exhibited in children with hemophilia and Henoch-Schönlein purpura (HSP).

Pathogenesis

When proximal bowel telescopes into distal bowel, it pulls the mesentery along with it (Fig. 23–5). The neck of the intussuscepted segment compresses the entrapped bowel. This compression, plus the traction on the mesentery, causes lymphatic and mesenteric venous obstruction, which eventually results in necrosis and gangrene of the entrapped bowel and subsequent perforation if treatment is delayed. Proximal to the intussusception, distension of the bowel increases.

Clinical Presentation

Typical presentation of intussusception is in an infant between 5 and 12 months of age, with a history of vomiting; intermittent crampy pain, where the legs are pulled up to the chest; and then bloody or "currant jelly" stools (blood mixed with mucus). Between episodes, the child appears pale and listless

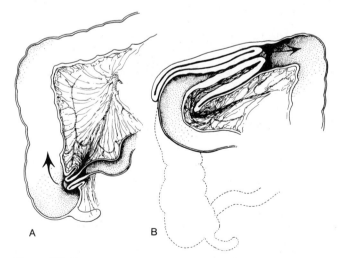

Figure 23–5 ● ● ● ● ● ●

Ileocolic intussusception. *A,* Beginning of an intussusception in which terminal ileum prolapses through the ileocecal valve. *B,* Ileocolic intussusception continuing through colon. This can be palpated as a mass in the right upper quadrant. (From Schnauffer, L.S., & Marboubi, S. (1988). Abdominal emergencies. In Fleischer, G.R., & Ludwig, S. (Eds.). *Pediatric emergency medicine,* p. 944. Baltimore: Williams & Wilkins.)

or lethargic. Altered level of consciousness maybe so severe that it is described as "intussusception encephalopathy" (Goetting et al., 1990). In some children altered level of consciousness is the initial symptom, prior to GI signs or symptoms. In such cases the differential diagnosis includes a postictal state and meningitis (Hickey et al., 1990). Later, the child develops abdominal distension, tenderness, and guarding. On rectal examination, there is bloody mucus and the tip of the intussusception may be felt. If symptoms persist longer than 6 to 12 hours, plain films reveal an obstruction, which includes distended bowel loops and air-fluid levels. Abdominal ultrasound may be helpful in the workup of intussusception before barium enema (BE). A positive or equivocal ultrasound indicates those patients that should undergo BE (Verscheldon et al., 1992).

In cases of postoperative intussusception the presentation is not as straightforward. The child may appear to be doing well in the first few days postoperatively, then develops vomiting or increased NG aspirate, which may be attributed to a paralytic ileus. Plain films, however, reveal an obstruction, with dilated loops of bowel and air-fluid levels.

Critical Care Management

Initially, management is with nasogastric decompression, IV fluid resuscitation, and IV antibiotics if symptoms have been present longer than 24 hours or if there is fever and leukocytosis. The child is then appropriately sedated before BE is performed, which serves as a diagnostic as well as treatment measure. One to three attempts at hydrostatic reduction of the intussusception by controlled BE are made, with the operating room team on standby for surgical reduction if necessary. In idiopathic intussusception, BE reduction is successful in 65% to 75% of patients. In cases in which there is a specific lead point, BE is less successful and surgical reduction is necessary. In children 6 years of age or older, where tumors (chiefly lymphosarcoma) and other abnormalities serve as a lead point, a BE may not be performed.

In patients who have had prolonged symptoms, bloody stools, severe distension and tenderness, and signs of shock, surgical intervention is warranted, after stabilization with IV fluid and blood products, intestinal decompression, and antibiotics. BE is not indicated in patients with postoperative intussusception because the site is high in the ileum or the jejunum. Most cases undergo successful manual reduction in the operating room.

A transverse right upper quadrant (RUQ) incision is performed and the intussusception is gently reduced with the surgeon's fingers "milking" the intussusception, without applying traction on the bowel. The bowel is then examined for areas of necrosis or gangrene, perforations, and any abnormalities that could have served as a lead point. Resection is indicated if the intussusception is not reducible; if there is nonviable bowel; if there are any perforations; or if there is a specific lead point. An end-to-end anastomosis is performed in most cases. Appendectomy may be done.

Postoperative complications are rare and are related to the underlying pathology. There is an average recurrence rate of 4%. Children are treated surgically if intussusception recurs (Raffensperger, 1989).

Toxic Megacolon

Toxic megacolon is dilation of the colon. It is the most serious complication of ulcerative colitis, occurring in up to 5% of all patients with ulcerative colitis. It is relatively rare in the pediatric population.

Clinical Presentation

Clinically, children present with abdominal distension, abdominal tenderness, and fever. Tachycardia, hypokalemia, hypoalbuminemia, and dehydration may also be present. High-dose steroid therapy may mask some of the signs of toxic megacolon, specifically fever and abdominal tenderness. The child with a toxic megacolon is at risk for colonic perforation, gram-negative sepsis, and massive hemorrhage. Diagnosis is made by clinical examination and confirming abdominal radiographs. There is also evidence of toxicity, as mentioned earlier (Caulfield & Michener, 1993).

Critical Care Management

Once the diagnosis of toxic megacolon is made, careful monitoring with serial radiographs of the abdomen and physical examinations are important. Gastric decompression is accomplished via a nasogastric tube or, if necessary, a small bowel tube. Enteral intake is restricted and parenteral nutrition initiated. If aggressive medical management fails and the toxic megacolon persists longer than 48 hours, or if perforation and hemorrhage develop, surgical intervention and colectomy are necessary (Jackson & Grand, 1991).

GASTROINTESTINAL INFLAMMATION

Inflammation can occur anywhere along the GI tract or on the surface of the peritoneum and occurs with varying levels of severity. For example, a child can exhibit mild esophagitis as a result of gastroesophageal reflux (GER) or present with septic shock due to an intestinal perforation and resultant peritonitis. GI inflammation, seen in critically ill infants and children, results from GER, inflammatory bowel disease, peritonitis, necrotizing enterocolitis, and pancreatitis.

Gastroesophageal Reflux

Gastroesophageal reflux (GER) is the return of stomach contents into the esophagus. It is the result of incompetence of the lower esophageal sphincter. It has been estimated that GER occurs in one in 500 live births.

Clinical Presentation

The major features of the syndrome are effortless vomiting, failure to gain weight, and aspiration pneumonia. GER may exist without obvious vomiting, and may produce such complications as protein-losing enteropathy, neuropsychiatric syndromes, and apnea.

Half of all infants vomit or spit up at some time during the first 2 years of life, with only 5% having a significant underlying cause. Most children with GER present by 6 weeks of age with symptoms of vomiting or failure to thrive, and outgrow the syndrome by approximately 18 months of age. The greatest improvement occurs at about 8 to 10 months of age when the child sits upright. Fifty percent of children with GER require medical evaluation and therapy of some degree.

Symptoms that lead to a differential diagnosis of GER are presented in Table 23–4.

Critical Care Management

In a child with uncomplicated GER, the self-limiting factor of the disease may preclude the need for medical therapy. Traditional noninvasive therapy consists of three elements: upright positioning, thickened feedings, and frequent feeding. Positioning at a 45- to 60-degree angle in an infant seat or car seat

Table 23–4. DIFFERENTIAL DIAGNOSIS OF REFLUX SYMPTOMS

Regurgitation, Vomiting
Pain, Esophagitis Symptoms
  Cardiac pain
  Pulmonary or mediastinal pain; chest wall pain (e.g., costrochondritis)
  Nonesophagitis upper gastrointestinal inflammation (e.g., peptic ulcer disease)
  Nonesophagitis dysphagia
  Many possible causes of nonspecific irritability in infants
  Functional; malingering
Respiratory Symptoms (wheeze, stridor, cough, etc.)
  Extrinsic compression (e.g., vascular ring)
  Intrinsic obstruction (e.g., malformation, foreign body, cyst, tumor)
  Airways reactive to other stimuli (e.g., allergens, infection)
  Infection; inflammation; cystic fibrosis; pertussis; asthma; other
  "Central" events (e.g., central apnea; "cough tic")
Neurobehavioral Symptoms (Sandifer's syndrome, seizure-like spells)
  Seizures
  Dystonic reaction to drugs
  Vestibular disorders
  Early pertussis

Adapted from Orenstein, S.R. (1991). Gastroesophageal reflux. In Stockman, J.A. II, Winter, R.J. (Eds.). *Current Problems in Pediatrics.* Chicago, YearBook Medical Publishers, May/June 1991; 21(5):223; reprinted from Wyllie, R., Hyams, J.S. (1993). *Pediatric gastrointestinal disease* (p. 358). Philadelphia: W.B. Saunders.

has been standard procedure for many years, but poor truncal tone makes the seated, upright position detrimental because of increased abdominal pressure. Placing a child supine with the head of the crib elevated 45 degrees is more beneficial than upright positioning. To prevent the baby from sliding, rolls of blankets or sandbags may be propped against the child's bottom, or a sling can be made from a diaper.

Thickened feedings are believed to be effective because of gravity: that is, it is more difficult to regurgitate a heavier mass. Small frequent feedings allow for adequate gastric emptying and decrease the chance of vomiting owing to gastric distension.

Many infants require medications to promote recovery. Bethanechol, a cholinergic agent, is used to treat GER because it elevates the lower esophageal sphincter pressure. Metaclopromide is also used to treat GER because it promotes gastric emptying. Cisapride is a newly released prokinetic agent that in early trials has proven effective in treating children with GER (Orenstein, 1993). Antacids, cimetidine, and ranitidine are used to neutralize the gastric contents, thus decreasing esophageal irritation.

Overnight continuous nasogastric feedings are also used to treat GER in selected infants. This has proved effective in infants with poor weight gain and delayed gastric emptying. It provides for optimal caloric intake, and has a soothing effect on an irritated esophagus.

Failure to respond to medical therapy or failure to promptly diagnose GER may require surgical intervention. Antireflux procedures are typically performed for children who have not responded to medical management and who continue to be unable to gain weight appropriately. The Nissen fundoplication is the most commonly performed antireflux procedure in children, followed by the Thal fundoplication and the uncut Collis-Nissen fundoplication.

The Nissen fundoplication involves a 360-degree wrap of the stomach around the distal esophagus, producing a tighter gastroesophageal (GE) junction, thereby decreasing the reflux of fluid back into the esophagus (Fig. 23–6). The Thal fundoplication only provides a 180-degree wrap of the stomach, which is thought to provide adequate pressure, producing antireflux (Ashcraft, 1978). The uncut Collis-Nissen uses a neoesophagus that is created out of stomach, around which the fundus is wrapped (Hoffman et al., 1990).

GI decompression using the gastrostomy tube that is typically placed during the operative procedure or an NG tube is of utmost importance. In some instances a transpyloric feeding tube is placed through the gastrostomy stoma to allow early introduction of enteral alimentation into the small bowel. Pain management and respiratory support are important aspects of postoperative care.

Inflammatory Bowel Disease

The term inflammatory bowel disease (IBD) is used to denote two disease processes, ulcerative colitis and

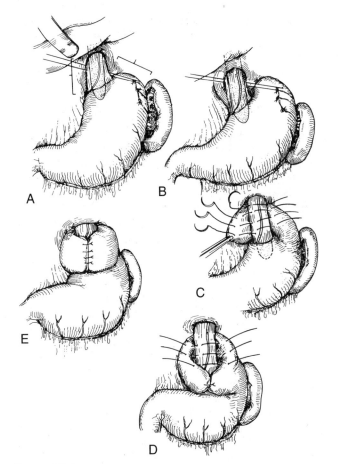

Figure 23–6 ● ● ● ● ● ●

A, A sizable bougie is placed in the patient's esophagus for the procedure to ensure that the wrap is not so tight that food passage is obstructed. *B,* The fundus is then drawn around behind the esophagus and *C,* interrupted sutures are used to construct the 360° wrap. *D,* When these sutures are tied, a cuff is formed around the lower esophagus. *E,* Distension of the stomach creates a valve that acts as a blood pressure cuff and can completely compress the lower esophagus. (From Ashcraft, K.W. (1994). *Atlas of pediatric surgery,* p. 73. Philadelphia: W.B. Saunders.)

Crohn's disease. IBD is inflammation of the GI tract and may extend from the mouth to the anus. It most commonly involves the small intestine (the ileum), large intestine, or both. It is a disease of school-age children, adolescents, and young adults. Most people are diagnosed when they are between ages 10 and 30 years. Complications of IBD (perforation, hemorrhage, abscess formation with sepsis, and toxic megacolon) and recovery from surgical interventions may require critical care attention.

Clinical Presentation

The symptoms of ulcerative colitis and Crohn's disease are similar. Diarrhea is the most common symptom for both diseases. In ulcerative colitis, diarrhea is accompanied by gross rectal bleeding, lower abdominal pain, mild anorexia, and weight loss. In Crohn's disease, gross rectal bleeding is rare; however, occult blood may be present. Other symptoms include anorexia, abdominal pain, weight loss, and growth failure. Complications of Crohn's disease include intestinal obstruction resulting from adhesions, strictures, and abscess formation.

The diagnosis of IBD is based on history, clinical presentation, biochemical parameters, radiographic findings, endoscopic findings, and biopsy information. The abdominal examination may reveal right lower quadrant tenderness or fullness along with diffuse tenderness in other quadrants. An important component of the physical examination is the rectal examination, in which evidence is sought for perianal disease, skin tags, fissures, or fistulas (commonly seen with Crohn's disease).

Initial biochemical parameters of complete blood count (CBC), chemistry panel, and erythrocyte sedimentation rate (ESR) provide important diagnostic information. The CBC documents anemic states and elevated platelet counts, often seen in inflammatory bowel disease. A chemistry panel is done to evaluate liver function (liver disease is associated with IBD). Albumin and total protein levels are also evaluated to determine the degree of mucosal damage and malnutrition. An elevated ESR is an indicator of inflammation. Stool cultures are also obtained to rule out an infectious process.

Colonoscopy is performed to document mucosal injury and extent of disease. Depending on symptoms, either an UGI with small bowel follow-through or a barium enema is also obtained. The UGI documents the presence or absence of small bowel disease. Barium enemas evaluate colonic disease and are not routinely obtained if a colonoscopy had been performed.

Critical Care Management

Medical management is aimed at quieting the acute event as quickly as possible and preventing the relapse of inflammation with maintenance therapy. Sulfasalazine, olsalazine or mesalamine (Asacol and Pentasa) are used initially. Sulfasalazine is a combination of a salicylate and sulfa antibiotic, whereas olsalazine, Asacal, and Pentasa are salicylate derivatives. The specific action remains unknown, but it is believed that the salicylate component acts locally within the intestinal lumen to reduce inflammation.

Corticosteroids may be necessary to induce a remission. Because the side effects of corticosteroids may be severe, children are given 2 mg/kg/day for a short period of time (4 to 6 weeks), and the dose is tapered to a maintenance level as quickly as possible. Other immunosuppressive medications such as azothriaprine, 6-mercaptopurine, and cyclosporine may be necessary in the treatment of IBD.

Nutritional therapy is often key to reversing the complications of Crohns's disease and ulcerative colitis. Bowel rest with parenteral and elemental enteral feedings may be necessary.

Surgical intervention may be necessary in selected situations. Surgery is curative in patients with ulcerative colitis. Removal of the colon eliminates the dis-

ease. However, in Crohn's disease the inflammation may recur at another site following resection.

Emotional and psychological factors have long been associated with IBD. However, a causal relationship has never been proved, nor is there evidence that stressful situations influence exacerbations of the disease (Hyams, 1993). Important nursing considerations are the emotional and psychological issues that a child with IBD faces. Even though these issues may not be the main priority in the critical care unit, awareness of them is important. It is essential that the effects of living with chronic illness are considered.

Peritoneal Inflammation

Peritoneal inflammation, or peritonitis, is associated with high morbidity and mortality. Peritoneal inflammation may occur with a rapid, abrupt onset or it may be the final outcome in a progression that begins with acute obstruction followed by necrosis and subsequent perforation. Peritonitis can be classified as either primary or secondary. Primary peritonitis is a condition wherein there is no obvious cause of contamination, but infection is indirectly introduced into the peritoneal cavity through the bloodstream or lymphatics. Common organisms include both gram-positive (*Streptococcus pneumoniae*, Pneumococcus) and gram-negative (*Escherichia coli*) bacteria. If more than one organism is found, perforation must be suspected (Mustata & Siegel, 1990).

Secondary peritonitis, also known as perforative peritonitis, occurs as a result of direct injury or contamination. This can develop after an injury to a main intra-abdominal blood vessel or solid organ, or after perforation of a hollow viscus.

Pathogenesis

Peritoneal inflammation occurs as a result of either direct or indirect injury or contamination. Contaminants include chemicals, blood, meconium, bacteria, or foreign bodies. A localized area of inflammation usually occurs first. This local inflammatory process causes exudation of fluid into the peritoneal cavity. The exudate, rich in antibodies, complement, neutrophils, and macrophages, plays an important role in the body's defense mechanism. The release of exudate into the peritoneal cavity can successfully resolve the inflammatory process. Otherwise, contamination of the peritoneum extends with subsequent abscess formation or generalized peritonitis. In the state of generalized peritonitis, bacteria and toxins are absorbed by the peritoneal surface into the bloodstream, causing bacteremia and endotoxemia. Hypovolemia occurs as fluid shifts into the peritoneal cavity. Concurrent sepsis from bacteremia can lead to the catastrophic result of septic shock and death.

Clinical Presentation

The clinical presentation of primary peritonitis consists of high fever, diffuse, generalized abdominal pain, vomiting, and an elevated white blood cell count. Onset of symptoms may be more abrupt in primary peritonitis than in perforative peritonitis. There may be a history of a minor preceding illness such as respiratory tract infection.

Abdominal pain is present in all children with peritoneal inflammation and increases with movement and with breathing, often leading to shallow, rapid respirations. Abdominal wall spasm is exhibited, and it progresses from voluntary guarding in the early stages to involuntary spasm as the inflammation worsens. Very young infants do not exhibit abdominal wall spasm, but rather abdominal wall erythema, discoloration, or cellulitis. Abdominal distension and rigidity are also manifested, and the child is febrile and tachycardic. Shifting dullness can be elicited on percussion because of the large amounts of free fluids in the peritoneal cavity. Anorexia, nausea, and vomiting are also exhibited, and bowel sounds may be decreased or absent. Occasionally diarrhea is present. As the inflammatory process progresses, signs of hypovolemia and sepsis become more apparent.

Critical Care Management

In addition to serial physical examinations done every 1 to 2 hours, serial abdominal girth measurements, laboratory monitoring, and chest and abdominal radiologic studies are needed. If a chronic condition exists such as cirrhosis, nephrosis, systemic lupus erythematosus or in a patient with a ventriculoperitoneal shunt, paracentesis is indicated and appropriate antibiotic therapy is initiated based on Gram stain results of the peritoneal fluid. Ongoing hemodynamic monitoring is indicated for these children in whom hypovolemic or septic shock may develop.

Supportive care of children with peritonitis includes ventilatory management, gastric decompression, IV fluids, colloids and blood products, early initiation of TPN, and broad-spectrum antibiotic coverage. Table 23–5 outlines recommendations for antibiotic coverage for intra-abdominal peritonitis and sepsis (Mustafa & Siegel, 1990).

If signs of perforation occur or if the child's clinical status deteriorates, surgery is warranted. Goals of surgery include closure of perforations, removal of necrotic tissue, drainage of abscesses, establishment of intestinal continuity, and preservation of intestinal length.

Necrotizing Enterocolitis

Necrotizing enterocolitis (NEC) is a condition of patchy or diffuse necrosis of the intestinal mucosa thought to result from a combination of decreased blood flow, hypoxia, and bacterial invasion (Rowe, 1986). The exact etiology of NEC remains unclear. It occurs most frequently in premature infants, but has been reported in full-term babies and in infants and children without recognized risk factors (Polin et al., 1975).

Pathogenesis

Neonatal asphyxia is most frequently associated with the development of NEC (Touloukian, 1976). The mucosal pathology may be caused by multiple factors or a microbiologic agent working alone (Kliegman & Fanaroff, 1984). Other predisposing factors include respiratory distress, hypothermia with asso-

Table 23–5. ANTIMICROBIAL AGENTS FREQUENTLY USED FOR TREATEMENT OF INTRA-ABDOMINAL SEPSIS

Drug	Dosage	Comments
Clindamycin*	30 divided q 8 hour	Resistant *Bacteroides* species in some areas of country
Metronidazole*	30 divided q 6 hour	Excellent activity against anaerobes; inactive against aerobes
Cefoxitin	160 divided q 6 hour	Poor activity against clostridial species
Chloramphenicol*	75 divided q 6 hour	Inactivated by anaerobic bacteria; bacteriostatic against aerobic gram-negative rods
Ceftazidime	150 divided q 8 hour	Variable activity against anaerobes; very active against aerobic gram-negative rods
Moxalactam	150 divided q 8 hour	Associated bleeding tendency makes this drug less desirable in surgical patients; variable activity against anaerobes; inactive against *Pseudomonas* species
Cefotaxime	150 divided q 6 hour	Variable activity against anaerobes; inactive against *Pseudomonas* species
Ceftriaxone	50–75 divided q 12 hour	Variable activity against anaerobes; inactive against *Pseudomonas* species
Ampicillin	100 divided q 6 hour	Active against *Enterococcus*
Ticarcillin	200–300 divided q 6 hour	Adequate activity against *Enterococcus* when combined with an aminoglycoside; variable activity against anaerobes
Mezlocillin	200–300 divided q 4 to 6 hour	Active against *Enterococcus*; variable activity against anaerobes
Gentamicin	5–7.5 divided q 8 hour	Reduced activity at acid pH and in anaerobic environment of abscesses and deep tissue infections
Tobramycin	5–7.5 divided q 8 hour	
Amikacin	22.5 divided q 8 hour	

*Oral route may be considered when gastrointestinal function is normal.
From Mustafa, M.M., & Siegel, J.D. (1990). Peritonitis. In Levin, D.L., & Morriss, F.C. (Eds.). *Essentials of pediatric intensive care* (p. 370). St. Louis: Quality Medical Publishing, Inc., 1990, 370.

ciated stress response, patent ductus arteriosus, umbilical artery catheters, and exchange transfusions.

In instances of asphyxia, blood is shunted to the brain and heart and away from less vital organs such as the bowel. Vasoconstriction of the intestinal vasculature occurs, followed by bowel ischemia and mucosal damage. Often, the baby is started on formula, and a combination of bacterial invasion from the formula and ischemia is thought to cause NEC.

Clinical Presentation

Any preterm infant in a neonatal nursery should be considered at risk for developing NEC. A high level of suspicion should be maintained even with subtle clinical changes such as an increased feeding residual, increased abdominal distension, temperature instability, lethargy, and apnea. Later indications of NEC include Hemoccult-positive stools, discoloration of the abdominal wall, and visibly dilated bowel loops. On physical examination the infant with NEC has abdominal tenderness, erythema, distension, and irritability along with respiratory compromise.

Critical Care Management

Radiographic studies are obtained when NEC is suspected to detect pneumatosis, persistent nonmobile loops of bowel, or pneumoperitoneum. Abdominal radiographs are routinely ordered every 6 hours. Blood work includes a CBC and differential with particular attention to platelets and white blood cell (WBC) shifts. Blood gases are also obtained to note changes in the pH. The child is kept NPO with active GI decompression. Nutrition is provided through the parenteral route. Intravenous antibiotic coverage is initiated immediately with the addition of anaerobic coverage if a pneumoperitoneum is observed on radiographic studies. This type of medical management may be maintained for 7 to 21 days or longer if the infant's condition remains stable.

If the child does not respond to medical management and exhibits an overall deterioration, surgical intervention may be necessary. Preparation for the operation includes stabilization with GI decompression, respiratory and cardiovascular support, thermoregulation, fluid resuscitation, and prevention of sepsis. The timing of surgical intervention for a child with NEC is critical but is a difficult management decision. Ideally the operation should take place when the bowel is truly necrotic but perforation has not occurred. If the operation occurs early, there may be a large gray, thin, edematous area of bowel that has no distinct boundaries, making surgical resection more difficult. On the other hand, if operation occurs too late the small bowel may be completely nonviable. Figure 23–7 provides an algorithm for treatment of the neonate with NEC.

Infants with fulminant NEC experience all the clinical signs and symptoms previously described within hours and exhibit rapid deterioration and multisystem failure. Immediate surgical intervention is required.

Postoperatively, fluid loss through the ileostomy is closely monitored, noting the presence of blood. Fluid management can be difficult in these patients because of the increased fluid output coupled with third-spacing of fluids. Nutritional support and antibiotic coverage are routine.

Long-term prognosis for infants with NEC is good if they survive the initial critical period. Stomal closure can occur between 6 weeks and 3 to 4 months of age, depending on the child's enteral feeding toler-

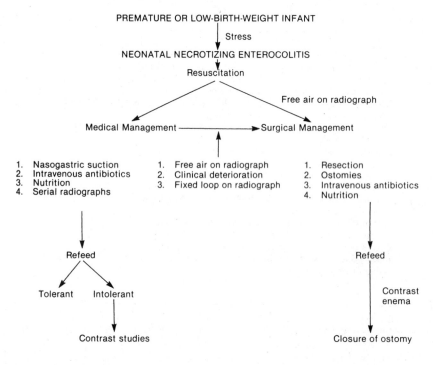

Figure 23–7 ● ● ● ● ● ●

Proposed algorithm for treatment of neonatal necrotizing enterocolitis. (From Ghoury, M.J., & Sheldon, C.A. (1985). Newborn surgical emergencies of the gastrointestinal tract. *Surgical Clinics of North America,* 65(5), 1083–1098.)

ance. In some children the increased water loss from the ileostomy can force earlier closure of the stoma. Before stomal closure, all children undergo a barium enema to assess the distal segment of bowel for stricture formation, a complication occurring after some episodes of NEC. Stricture formation and acquired short bowel syndrome are the two major complications that result from NEC.

Short Bowel Syndrome

Short bowel syndrome (SBS) is defined as the absence of more than 50% of the small bowel, which results in malabsorption of nutrients (Ziegler, 1986; Vanderhoff et al., 1992). Thirty years ago, children with this entity succumbed to the disease. Since that time major advances in venous access and parenteral-enteral nutrition, and understanding of bowel adaptation, have greatly improved the patients' quality of life and chances for survival.

Etiology

Massive bowel loss can occur owing to prenatal or postnatal causes. Before an infant is born, embryologic maldevelopment or vascular accidents necessitate emergent lifesaving surgery shortly after birth to correct the defect, but in many situations surgery leaves the child with a foreshortened small bowel. During infancy or childhood, disease processes, vascular thrombosis, or trauma can result in the same outcome. Intrauterine volvulus and necrotizing enterocolitis are the two leading causes of SBS (Wilmore, 1972; Cooper et al., 1984).

Pathogenesis

Following major small bowel resection, there is a loss of intestinal mucosal absorptive surface area, along with rapid transit time of intestinal contents, resulting in inadequate ability of the gut to digest and absorb nutrients (Ziegler, 1986). Depending on the severity of the symptoms, the child's nutritional rehabilitation course can be short and uncomplicated, or prolonged with multiple and severe complications, which ultimately lead to death.

With significant loss of small intestine, the bowel undergoes numerous changes. In many patients there is excessive secretion of gastric acid, which can lead to diarrhea, decreased function of pancreatic enzymes, bacteria overgrowth, ulceration, hemorrhage, and denuded perianal skin (Hennessey, 1989). Jejunal resection results in a loss of brush border enzymes, which impairs carbohydrate absorption. Stasis of carbohydrate substrate in the bowel further leads to bacteria overgrowth. Protein metabolism is hindered owing to malabsorption of peptides and amino acids. Loss of water-soluble vitamins including B_{12} is associated with a large jejunal resection. Ileal resection causes malabsorption of bile salts, which

leads to excessive fatty stools and malabsorption of fat-soluble vitamins (A, D, E, and K) (Ziegler, 1986).

Because of the ileum's potential for adaptation and ability to transport bile acids and B_{12}, the ileum, rather than the jejunum, is the more critical area to leave intact (Dowling & Booth, 1967). The presence of the ileocecal valve aids in both slowing small intestinal transit time, thus improving absorption of nutrients, and decreasing the risk of colonization by colonic bacteria (Cowen et al., 1984). But in many cases, especially in patients with NEC, preservation of the valve is impossible.

The exact length of the small bowel is difficult to ascertain but is thought to be approximately three times a person's linear length. For preterm infants it is important to note that the small bowel doubles in length from the 19th to the 35th week of gestation. Resection of the small bowel in a preterm infant may have more severe consequences than for full-term infants (Touloukian & Walker-Smith, 1983).

Intestinal "adaptation" is the normal physiologic response of the small intestine following major resection. During this process there is a gradual increase in surface area because of mucosal hyperplasia, villous lengthening, and increased depth of the intestinal crypts. Three mechanisms are involved in gut adaptation: luminal, hormonal, and cellular factors (Webster et al., 1991).

Critical Care Management

Following the initial resection of an extensive amount of bowel, nutrition is provided by TPN, to assure that nutrients, electrolytes, minerals, vitamins, and trace elements necessary for healing and growth are provided. It is important to remember that the central line is the "lifeline" for a child with SBS. It is critical that the integrity and sterility of the catheter be maintained to prevent iatrogenic catheter loss.

A complication of long-term TPN, especially in the preterm infant, is cholestatic liver disease. The cause for this is unknown but most likely is multifactoral. The responsible factors include toxicity of amino acids, bile acids, amino acid competition for transport across the canalicular membrane, toxins in the TPN solution, and lack of stimulation of biliary flow by the gut (Vanderhoff, 1992). To reduce the risk of TPN-induced jaundice, early enteral alimentation is provided and the concentration of amino acids in the TPN is limited to 2.5 g/kg/day.

Surgical intervention may increase the small bowel absorptive surface. A bowel-lengthening procedure, which involves longitudinal division of a dilated segment of the bowel, tubularization of the two segments and end-to-end anastomosis, has been successful. This procedure, in theory, doubles the segmental length of bowel (Bianchi, 1980). Other procedures included reversed small bowel segments, prejejunal isoperistaltic colonic interposition, and replacement of ileocecal value with a nipple valve intussusception (Garcia et al., 1981; Careskey et al., 1981). Unfortunately, none of these procedures has a high success rate. Small bowel transplantation is the procedure of choice to eliminate the problems associated with SBS.

Long-term survival of a child with SBS is dependent on transition from parenteral to enteral nutrition. When bowel function returns after surgery, slow continual enteral feeding of an isotonic, dilute, predigested formula is begun. Tolerance of the diet is determined by the number of stools per day, the absence of reducing substances in the stool, and consistent weight. Enteral nutrition is advanced usually in concentration first and then volume. As tolerance is observed the child can be advanced to small bolus feeds during the day with resumption of continual nasogastric or gastrostomy feeds at night. As the enteral product is increased, the TPN is tapered while maintaining optimal caloric intake. Cholestyramine and loperamide may be used to reduce GI motility, thereby increasing nutrient contact time with the mucosa. Supplementation of vitamin B_{12}, folic acid, electrolytes, and trace elements is essential if the levels are below normal. Cimetidine may be used to reduce gastric acid secretion. To prevent or treat bacteria overgrowth, oral antibiotics, usually metronidazole (Flagyl) and/or neomycin, are administered.

Pancreatitis

Pancreatitis is an acute inflammatory condition that results from an autodigestive process within the pancreas. It is relatively uncommon in children, but it can present at any age and ranges in severity from a mild to fulminant inflammatory process. It is associated with mortality as high as 30% (Stevenson, 1985).

Etiology

The most frequent cause of childhood pancreatitis is blunt abdominal trauma, with child abuse identified in as many as one third of these cases (Ziegler, 1987). In addition to traumatic pancreatitis, other causes include infection, drugs, heredity, and additional idiopathic and miscellaneous causes.

Pathogenesis

Regardless of the etiology of pancreatitis, the autodigestive process results from either the release and activation of proteolytic enzymes within the pancreas, or the reflux of activated enzymes into the pancreas from a distal obstruction. Both processes cause a localized inflammatory response. If autodigestion is severe and extensive, vascular damage may occur, causing hemorrhagic pancreatitis. In addition, release of lipase into surrounding tissues can cause fat necrosis and breakdown of calcium. Local inflammation in and around the pancreas causes third-spacing into the peritoneum and, if uncor-

rected, can lead to hypovolemia and cardiovascular collapse.

Clinical Presentation

Children with acute pancreatitis present with a variety of signs and symptoms. Abdominal pain is present in all cases and is described as constant, dull, epigastric, or periumbilical and may radiate to the back or be referred to the left shoulder. Diffuse peritoneal signs such as guarding, decreased bowel sounds, and distension are also present. In cases of hemorrhagic pancreatitis, a bluish discoloration may be seen in the flank area (Grey Turner's sign), indicating retroperitoneal bleeding. Periumbilical discoloration (Cullen's sign), indicating intra-abdominal bleeding, may also be seen in cases of hemorrhagic pancreatitis. Patients are febrile and exhibit nausea and vomiting. In patients with fulminant pancreatitis, signs of shock may be exhibited.

Initial laboratory analysis reveals markedly elevated amylase and amylase clearance levels, elevated liver function test (LFT) levels, elevated hematocrit (as a result of hemoconcentration due to intravascular fluid loss), and hypocalcemia. Radiologic workup may reveal a "sentinel loop," a dilated loop of bowel located near the pancreas, or a mass effect if a pseudocyst has developed, as demonstrated on plain films. A pseudocyst is a cyst-like mass filled with pancreatic fluids rising out of the pancreas. Although a pseudocyst may develop from any of the causes of pancreatitis, it is most frequently a complication of traumatic pancreatitis. Abdominal ultrasound examination is useful in identifying both the presence and extent of pancreatic damage and complications resulting from acute pancreatitis. In addition to pseudocyst formation, other complications include abscess formation, splenic vein thrombosis, diabetes (usually temporary), and pancreatic enzyme insufficiency (in cases of chronic, recurrent pancreatitis). Endoscopic retrograde cannulation of the pancreatic ducts (ERCP) is helpful in defining abnormalities of the pancreatic and biliary ducts that result in structural/obstructive pancreatitis.

Critical Care Management

Management of the patient with acute pancreatitis is multisystemic in approach, with the primary goal of suppressing or halting the autodigestive process. Strategies employed are aimed at decreasing the activity of the pancreas and include keeping the patient NPO, maintaining gastric decompression, and administering antacids and histamine 2 (H2) receptor blockers that act to decrease gastric acid secretion.

Other goals of management include prevention of hypovolemia and shock, provision of respiratory and nutritional support, and restoration of normal pancreatic functions. Patients presenting with or progressing to a fulminant form of acute pancreatitis require comprehensive hemodynamic monitoring.

Frequent serial abdominal examinations, including abdominal girth measurement, are an integral part of care. Meticulous monitoring of intake and output is mandatory, because renal failure and hypovolemia are complications of the disease process.

Laboratory studies to be monitored include amylase and amylase clearance, LFTs, serum glucose, electrolytes, albumin, total protein, CBC with differential, clotting studies, arterial blood gas (ABGs), BUN and creatinine, and serum calcium levels. Assessing for signs and symptoms of hypocalcemia, which include muscle twitching and irritability, is also indicated. If the patient has an ongoing or sudden temperature elevation, blood and urine cultures are obtained as well. Radiologic studies include serial abdominal plain films and ultrasound examination, as well as CT or MRI to assess the presence or progression of complications. For patients with suspected obstructive or structural etiology, endoscopic retrograde colangiopancreatography is also indicated. In addition, regular chest radiographs are obtained because patients are at risk for developing pleural effusions and adult respiratory distress syndrome (ARDS).

Because the child is kept NPO, administration of TPN is critical to provide nutritional support. Antibiotics are also given. These patients are at risk for respiratory complications, and thus respiratory support is another important focus of nursing care. Pain management is also important.

GASTROINTESTINAL BLEEDING

GI bleeding can vary in clinical presentation from acute life-threatening shock to asymptomatic bleeding with stools positive for occult blood. Bleeding can originate throughout the GI tract. Sudden onset of severe bleeding with hypovolemic shock is possible. Causes of GI bleeding are listed in Tables 23–6 and 23–7.

Acute Gastritis

A common cause of upper GI bleeding, regardless of age, is acute gastritis. Acute gastritis, also referred to as erosive or stress gastritis, is most commonly associated with severe stress in the acutely ill patient. Some patients develop isolated gastroduodenal erosions, and others develop mucosal ulcerations in multiple sites within the stomach and duodenum. Acute gastritis occurs in critically ill children suffering from burns, severe head trauma, major surgical procedures, sepsis, multiple trauma, and respiratory failure.

The etiology of acute gastritis secondary to stress is unknown but is, most likely, multifactoral. Potential causes include impaired blood flow, increased secretion of acid and pepsin, decreased production of mucus, decreased gastric somatostatin level, alterations in levels of adrenal steroids and catecholamines, and an impairment in the local production of prostaglandins.

Corticosteroids have been implicated in causing acute gastritis. There is an increased risk of ulcers and GI hemorrhage among patients who receive corticosteroids; however, the mechanism responsible is not known. Nonsteroidal anti-inflammatory drugs (NSAIDs) are known to cause both gastritis and mucosal ulceration.

Table 23–6. UPPER GASTROINTESTINAL BLEEDING

Age Group	Common	Less Common
Neonates (0–30 days)	Swallowed maternal blood Gastritis Duodenitis	Coagulopathy Vascular malformations Gastric/esophageal duplication Leiomyoma
Infants (30 days–1 year)	Gastritis and gastric ulcer Esophagitis Duodenitis	Esophageal varices Foreign body Aortoesophageal fistula
Children (1–12 years)	Esophagitis Esophageal varices Gastritis and gastric ulcer Duodenal ulcer Mallory-Weiss tear Nasopharyngeal bleeding	Leiomyoma Salicylates Vascular malformation Hematobilia
Adolescents (12 years–adult)	Duodenal ulcer Esophagitis Esophageal varices Gastritis Mallory-Weiss tear	Thrombocytopenia Dieulafoy's ulcer Hematobilia

From Olson, A.D., & Hillemeier, A.C. (1993). Gastrointestinal hemorrhage. In R. Wyllie & J.S. Hyams (Eds.). *Pediatric gastrointestinal disease: Pathophysiology, diagnosis, management* (p. 259). Philadelphia: W.B. Saunders.

Table 23–7. LOWER GASTROINTESTINAL BLEEDING

Age Group	Common	Less Common
Neonates (0–30 days)	Anorectal lesions Swallowed maternal blood Milk allergy Necrotizing enterocolitis Midgut volvulus	Vascular malformations Hirschsprung's enterocolitis Intestinal duplication Coagulopathy
Infants (30 days–1 year)	Anorectal lesions Midgut volvulus Intussusception (<3 yrs) Meckel's diverticulum Infectious diarrhea Milk allergy (<4 yrs)	Vascular malformations Intestinal duplication Acquired thrombocytopenia
Children (1–12 years)	Juvenile polyps Meckel's diverticulum Intussusception (<3 yrs) Infectious diarrhea Anal fissure Nodular lymphoid hyperplasia	Henoch-Schönlein purpura Hemolytic-uremic syndrome Vasculitis (SLE) Inflammatory bowel disease
Adolescents (12 years–adult)	Inflammatory bowel disease Polyps Hemorrhoids Anal fissure Infectious diarrhea	Arteriovascular malformation Adenocarcinomas Henoch-Schönlein purpura Pseudomembranous colitis

From Olson, A.D., & Hillemeier, A.C. (1993). Gastrointestinal hemorrhage. In R. Wyllie & J.S. Hyams (Eds.). *Pediatric gastrointestinal disease: Pathophysiology, diagnosis, management* (p. 262). Philadelphia: W.B. Saunders.

Lower GI Bleeding

Lower GI hemorrhage is rare in the pediatric population. Individuals at risk are those with known coagulopathies such as hemophilia A or B, chronic liver disease, and portal hypertension. Mucosal lesions, ulcers, polyps, arteriovenous malformations, and inflammatory bowel disease are also sources of lower tract bleeding.

Clinical Presentation

GI hemorrhage can present in several distinct ways (Table 23–8). Hematemesis describes bright red vomiting or coffee ground–like emesis. This suggests a bleeding source above the ligament of Treitz in the duodenum. Hematochezia is the passage of bright red blood or maroon-colored stool from the rectum. It is most commonly associated with a colonic source of bleeding. Melena is the passing of dark, black, tarry stools, which occurs in patients bleeding from a site located above the ileocecal valve. The black color is the result of the action of the bacteria on the hemoglobin that has been converted to hematin. Borborygmi is the deep rumbling abdominal sounds caused by the rapid transit of blood through the GI tract.

Critical Care Management

Acute GI bleeding can result in massive exsanguination and shock. An NG tube is inserted with UGI bleeding to prevent aspiration of blood. Hemodynamic assessment guides administration of fluid, red blood cells, and other blood products until the patient can be transported to the operating room for primary surgical intervention.

Esophageal Varices

Etiology

Esophageal varices are the result of portal hypertension, which can occur at any stage of liver disease. In hepatic disease, portal hypertension is caused by cirrhotic changes (intrahepatic scarring) that collapse and distort the hepatic vasculature.

Pathogenesis

When blood flow through the liver is obstructed, portal venous pressure increases. The development of collateral circulation redirects the portal venous blood flow through vessels of lower resistance and avoids the obstruction. Collateral vessels develop in the abdominal wall, rectum, lower esophagus, and stomach. These low pressure veins eventually become distended with blood, causing the veins to enlarge, developing into varices. The development of collateral portal circulation may reduce the portal pressure toward normal.

Clinical Presentation

The diagnosis of portal hypertension is based on clinical presentation, along with information ob-

Table 23–8. SIGNS AND SYMPTOMS IN GASTROINTESTINAL HEMORRHAGE

Sign	Indication	Site of Bleeding
Splenomegaly Caput medusa Jaundice	Portal hypertension	Esophageal varices Portal gastropathy
Hemangioma Telangiectasia	Multiple hemangioma syndrome	Vascular malformation of GI tract
Hematemesis	Bleeding from above the ligament of Treitz	Upper GI tract
Melena	Bleeding from above the ileocecal valve	Upper GI tract or small intestine
Hematochezia	Colonic bleeding, massive UGI bleeding	GI tract
Nasogastric aspirate: gross blood	Bleeding from above the ligament of Treitz	Upper GI tract
Palpable purpura	Henoch-Schönlein purpura	GI tract

From Olson, A.D., & Hillemeier, A.C. (1993). Gastrointestinal hemorrhage. In R. Wyllie & J.S. Hyams (Eds.). *Pediatric gastrointestinal disease: Pathophysiology, diagnosis, management* (p. 251). Philadelphia: W.B. Saunders.

tained from a variety of studies. Splenomegaly is generally the first sign of portal hypertension in children. Hematemesis, melena, nosebleeds, or an unexplained decrease in hemoglobin level may also indicate portal hypertension, although massive hematemesis is often the first clinical sign in children. A chest film may suggest the presence of esophageal varices by shadows in the esophagus. This is substantiated with a barium study. Ultrasound examination is useful in determining the presence and size of the portal vein and, with Doppler, can determine the direction of the blood flow through the portal system. An upper endoscopy determines the location of the varices and is able to document their size.

Critical Care Management

Hemorrhaging esophageal varices are a true medical emergency and require prompt action. The cause of a bleeding episode is usually unknown, but factors suggesting rupture include a sudden increase in abdominal venous pressure as a result of physical exertion, coughing, sneezing, vomiting, or stool straining. The first priorities are stabilization of airway, breathing, and circulation. The child is placed on the side in a semi-Fowler position with suction at the bedside to protect the airway against possible aspiration or occlusion. In addition to suction, accessibility of supplemental oxygen and equipment for intubation is assured.

Close monitoring of vital signs and determination of blood loss indicate the amount of fluid replacement necessary. During the resuscitation phase, it is vital that the blood pressure be maintained. Solutions of 5% albumin or normal saline are used until whole blood is available. As the child's condition stabilizes, the need for other blood products is determined by the CBC and coagulation indices.

Simultaneous with fluid resuscitation, an NG tube is inserted to determine the volume of bleeding. Suspicion of esophageal varices is not a contraindication for the insertion of an NG tube. A large-diameter tube (10–16 French) is passed to provide access for gastric lavage with room temperature normal saline. Room temperature solutions prevent hypothermia and its associated side effects, and are better tolerated by the patient.

Vasopressin, hypophysial antidiuretic hormone, is naturally excreted by the posterior pituitary. Administration of this hormone produces a pharmacologic effect that reduces bleeding in 35% to 50% of cases. It acts directly on GI smooth muscle and is able to contract vascular smooth muscle. Administration of vasopressin lowers portal venous pressure by vasoconstriction, which decreases arterial flow to the liver and subsequently reduces portal pressure.

Vasopressin is given through a central venous line. The drug is mixed in a solution of 5% dextrose and water to make a concentration of 1 unit/mL. Dosages of vasopressin are not weight-dependent. The universal dose is 0.2 to 0.4 units/minute, administered as a continuous infusion. Vasopressin infusion is continued for as long as 24 to 36 hours, and is slowly weaned if no evidence of rebleeding exists.

Because vasopressin vasoconstricts the coronary and renal arteries, it is important to closely monitor the heart rhythm and blood pressure. As a result of the vasoconstricting effects, hypertension is a complication with the induction of vasopressin. If bleeding does not cease or it reoccurs, further elevation of the vasopressin infusion creates increased intravascular pressure by further constricting the vessels. The increased pressure on the portal system can precipitate greater blood loss. Subsequent modes of therapy such as balloon tamponade and sclerotherapy are considered in this circumstance. In addition to hypertension, side effects such as dysrhythmias exist. Knowing the patient's normal electrocardiogram (ECG) pattern and following it closely are essential.

Renal complications that accompany the use of vasopressin include fluid retention. Fluid intake is limited to two-thirds maintenance requirements. Strict intake and output are measured. Urine output of less than 0.5 mL/kg/hour in a child is addressed.

Decreased urine output may be the result of fluid retention from the use of vasopressin.

Serum laboratory values are obtained every 6 hours simultaneous with collecting urine samples. Electrolyte and osmolality levels change significantly with fluid retention. Signs of fluid retention include decreased serum sodium and osmolality levels, whereas urine sodium and osmolality levels are increased. Liver dysfunction complicates the situation. The serum sodium may indicate hyponatremia due to vasopressin-induced free water retention. The total body sodium is actually increased due to hepatorenal disease. The interpretation of serum sodium and the administration of replacement sodium requires extreme caution.

Ascites and edema resulting from liver dysfunction are further complicated by vasopressin-induced water retention. Albumin is administered in an effort to draw fluids from the extracellular space into the vasculature. A preparation of 25% albumin is used for this purpose because it contains less fluid than 5% albumin. Following the infusion of albumin, a dose of furosemide (1 mg/kg) is administered to facilitate diuresis. It may be necessary to repeat this procedure until the serum albumin and total protein levels normalize and fluid retention resolves.

Somatostatin has been advocated for esophageal varices. Somatostatin reduces gastric blood flow and inhibits gastric acid and gastrin production. It has been found to be as effective as vasopressin with fewer complications in patients with cirrhosis and variceal bleeding (Reichlin, 1983; Basso et al., 1986).

If bleeding continues, the Sengstaken-Blakemore tube (SBT) may be used. With the availability of sclerotherapy, insertion of a tube is not as often performed as it was in the past, because sclerotherapy is less invasive. The SBT is available in two sizes, pediatric and adult. The pediatric tube consists of three lumens; one for gastric aspiration, one for inflating the esophageal balloon, and one for inflating the gastric balloon. The adult SBT has the addition of a fourth lumen for aspiration of esophageal secretions. The SBT provides a tamponade effect to the bleeding varices. Inflation of the gastric balloon applies pressure to the vessels feeding the varices and thus decreases the blood flow. Inflation of the esophageal balloon allows pressure to be placed directly on the varices. In children, the gastric balloon is inflated first and if the bleeding continues, inflation of the esophageal balloon is considered.

Once balloon tamponading is initiated, it is necessary to keep children immobile. Activity can increase abdominal and intravascular pressures, causing increased bleeding activity. Therefore, neuromuscular blockade may be necessary. Ventilatory support is necessary for as long as the SBT is in place.

Bleeding is monitored by the amount of blood aspirated with intermittent suction. The blood pressure and central venous pressure are continuously monitored and near-normal parameters are maintained by volume replacement. It is important that hypertension be avoided. CBC levels are monitored every

4 hours until the hematocrit is stable. A hematocrit of 30 to 36 is adequate for these patients because it has been noted that hematocrits higher than 36 may stimulate rebleeding, because increased intravascular pressure places stress on the varices. Packed RBCs are administered to raise the hematocrit. Coagulation indices and results of a platelet count determine the need for other blood products, such as platelets and fresh frozen plasma. Vitamin K may also be necessary.

Complications commonly seen with the SBT are atelectasis and aspiration pneumonia. Atelectasis is the result of increased intrathoracic pressure from the balloon, whereas aspiration pneumonia occurs because of aspiration of esophageal secretions. To

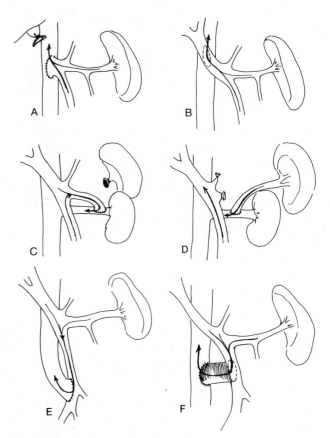

Figure 23–8 ● ● ● ● ● ●

Types of portosystemic shunts. *A,* End-to-side portocaval (all portal flow is diverted to systemic circulation). *B,* Side-to-side portocaval (the major direction of portal flow is to the systemic circulation, but the capacity for hepatic portal perfusion is retained, depending on the resistance within the liver. *C,* Proximal splenorenal (the principal direction of portal flow is to the systemic circulation; placing the shunt centrally minimizes the angulation of the splenic vein). *D,* Distal splenorenal (major direction of portal flow is to systemic circulation). *E,* Mesocaval (vena cava is transected and proximal cava is anastomosed to side of superior mesenteric vein. Major direction of visceral flow is toward vena cava). *F,* Interposition mesocaval (hemodynamically similar to mesocaval shunt. Autogenous vein graft is preferred for creation of this shunt in infants and children. (From Karrer, F., Lilly, J.R., & Hall, R.J. (1993). Biliary tract disorders and portal hypertension. In K.W. Ashcraft, & T.M. Holder (Eds.). *Pediatric surgery,* 2nd edition, p. 500. Philadelphia: W.B. Saunders.)

prevent respiratory complications, good pulmonary toilet is maintained. Balloon migration into the esophagus or airway can result in possible asphyxia and death. Esophageal perforation is a rare complication in children and is considered a surgical emergency.

Sclerotherapy is used to arrest active bleeding from esophageal varices and prevent rebleeding. The procedure is performed under general anesthesia, through a flexible fiberoptic endoscope. A fine needle attached to a catheter is passed through the biopsy channel of the endoscope. After identifying the varices, the endoscopist injects the sclerosing agent into the varix or the surrounding tissue. The most commonly used agents are sodium morrhuate and tetradecylsulfate. The sclerosing agent rapidly induces thrombosis and sclerosis of the vein, and does minimal damage to the esophageal mucosa and muscle (Conn & Grace, 1985).

Complications from sclerotherapy include hemorrhage. The bleeding is often self-limiting, but may be as severe as the original episode. Some oozing is to be expected after the procedure. Fever is a common complication, and alone is rarely considered serious. A persistent fever may indicate a bacteremia that is potentially lethal in the debilitated patient. Intense pain may indicate an erosion or perforation of the esophagus, which is rarely seen. The use of sucralfate following sclerotherapy has become common practice. Sucralfate has been demonstrated to be effective in the treatment of esophagitis, by binding tissues and promoting healing. No controlled studies have been done in children.

Surgical options are considered if medical therapy is ineffective. Shunting procedures divert the blood flow from the liver and allow for decompression of the portal system. Portacaval and splenorenal shunts are effective and control hemorrhage from esophageal varices (Fig. 23–8). In children, mesocaval and central splenorenal shunts have been successful even in very small infants. It was previously believed that the vessels needed for successful anastomosis and patent shunt were too small until a child was at least 7 years of age. It now seems that neither age nor size is a limitation to a successful shunt (Altman, 1986).

Liver transplantation is a consideration for children with portal hypertension resulting from liver diseases known to progress to liver failure and death. Liver transplantation is discussed in Chapter 27.

ABDOMINAL WALL DEFECTS

Omphalocele and Gastroschisis

Omphalocele is a midline, umbilical defect of the ventral abdominal wall in which the intestines herniate into a sac consisting of peritoneum and amnion. If the defect is larger than 4.0 cm it is said to be an omphalocele; but if it is smaller than 4.0 cm it is considered to be a hernia of the umbilical cord. The omphalocele can be extremely large, containing the entire midgut (distal duodenum, jejunum, ileum, ascending colon, and first portion of the transverse colon), liver, and spleen. The abdomen is, in this situation, small and scaphoid. If the sac remains intact, the appearance of the bowel may be fairly normal. Unfortunately in some cases the sac ruptures, leaving the organs exposed to the amniotic fluid or to the environment after birth.

Gastroschisis is an abdominal wall defect that usually occurs to the right and separate from the umbilical cord. There is no sac covering the defect and the bowel usually appears thick, foreshortened, hemorrhagic, and matted. The defect is usually small and contains only the bowel. The clinical differences between gastroschisis and omphalocele are shown in Table 23–9.

Etiology

The abdominal wall begins to develop by the fourth week of intrauterine life. It is formed by four separate embryonic layers; the cephalic layer, left and right lateral layers, and the caudal folds. Each of these are composed of sublayers known as the somatic and splanchnic layers. It is thought that if there is a failure of the normal embryonic folding and fusing of the somatic layers of the lateral folds,

Table 23–9. CLINICAL DIFFERENTIAL DIAGNOSIS

Factor	Gastroschisis	Omphalocele
Location	Lateral to cord	Umbilical ring
Size of defect	Less than 4 cm	2–10 cm
Umbilical cord	Normal insertion	Inserts in sac
Sac	None	Present
Contents	Bowel, stomach	Bowel, liver, spleen, bladder, uterus, ovaries
Bowel appearance	Matted, foreshortened	Normal
Malrotation	Present	Present
Small abdominal cavity	Present	Present
Associated anomalies	Unusual (15% atresia of the gut)	Common (37%–67%) GI, GU, CNS, cardiovascular, musculoskeletal
Coexisting syndromes	Not observed	Beckwith syndrome, cloaca, trisomy 13–15, trisomy 16–18, exstrophy of the bladder, pentalogy of Cantrell

Modified from Grosfeld, J.L., & Weber, T.R. (1982). Congenital abdominal wall defects: Gastroschisis and omphalocele. *Current Problems in Surgery.* 19(4), 165.

the anterior abdominal wall will not close completely (Schuster, 1986).

Omphalocele is thought to occur when the abdominal wall does not form completely as the midgut elongates out through the yolk sac, resulting in failure of the intestines to return to the abdominal cavity. There are many theories about the embryologic events resulting in gastroschisis, but one seems most likely. The developing embryo initially has both a left and right umbilical vein as well as two arteries (Brodel, 1916; Shaw, 1975). By the 11th week of gestation the right umbilical vein has been obliterated, leaving a weakness at this site in the abdominal wall (Cullen, 1916). It is theorized that this weakness of the abdominal wall allows a rupture of the lateral umbilical ring with bowel protruding through the defect, thus resulting in a gastroschisis.

Associated Abnormalities

Associated defects are more common with omphalocele than with gastroschisis. These can be divided into midline defects related to the failure of closure of the embryologic folds, chromosomal abnormalities, and other isolated abnormalities. Pentalogy of Cantrell occurs with the defective cephalic fold. This collection of defects includes intracardiac anomalies, ectopia cordis, sternal cleft, midline diaphragmatic hernia, and upper abdominal omphalocele. Lower midline abnormalities are related to defects in the caudal embryonic fold. These may include one or more of the following: cloacal exstrophy, imperforate anus, colonic atresia, sacral vertebral abnormalities, and meningomyelocele. Omphalocele has been identified as a component of the Bechwith-Wiedemann syndrome. Chromosomal abnormalities include trisomy 13 through 15, 16 through 18, and 21, many of which are incompatible with life. Associated cardiac disease is often significant. Omphalocele and congenital heart disease coexist 30 times more often than occurs by chance alone (Greenwood et al., 1974). Twenty percent of all children with omphalocele also have cardiac disease, and of those the most common defect is tetralogy of Fallot.

Clinical Presentation

Antenatal diagnosis of abdominal wall defects can usually be determined by ultrasound at approximately the 15th week of gestation. This prenatal determination assists the obstetrician to make a decision regarding transfer of the mother to a tertiary care setting. A cesarean section is usually indicated to prevent rupture of the sac or damage to the exposed viscera. If the defect has not been recognized before delivery, it is easily seen at birth, and thus treatment begins quickly.

Critical Care Management

If a sac is present, care must be taken to prevent rupture. The defect is usually covered with sterile gauze and wrapped in a figure-of-eight bandage to prevent pressure on the exposed viscera. There are two options for managing the exposed viscera. A saline-soaked gauze pad covered with occlusive plastic dressing or a bowel bag that covers the child's legs and abdomen, or dry gauze soaked with saline before removal may be used. These options prevent radiant heat loss that can occur with saline-soaked gauze alone.

Respiratory assessment and stabilization are critical, especially in the preterm infant in whom assisted ventilation may be necessary. This is accomplished with endotracheal intubation. Any mask or blow-by ventilation allows excess air to enter the GI track and is avoided.

Gastric decompression is essential to empty the stomach and prevent GI distension. Active decompression is accomplished with intermittent or continual suctioning, using a large-bore NG or OG tube. Comfortable positioning also calms the infant and prevents excessive crying and air swallowing. The head of the crib is elevated when possible to facilitate drainage.

Fluids are administered at twice maintenance requirement because of the fluid loss from the exposed bowel. Antibiotics are administered and the child is prepared for the operating room. As part of the preoperative workup, assessment of associated anomalies is completed. Part of this workup may be delayed until after surgery, but the cardiac examination is completed before surgery, as well as evaluation of any anomalies that may require emergency surgical care.

Operative Management. Omphalocele and gastroschisis are repaired using one of two surgical approaches—a primary repair or a staged repair. The primary repair involves removing the sac from an intact omphalocele, and opening the defect circumferentially. The bowel is examined for areas of atresia or perforation. The abdominal wall is stretched, and the viscera are carefully placed into the abdominal cavity. Attempts to correct the malrotation are not performed. The primary repair is successful if the defect is small and the infant does not have other major problems. With the primary repair, care is taken to avoid compromise of respiratory status resulting from marked elevation of the diaphragm; compression of the vena cava resulting in impaired venous return; and impaired intestinal blood supply. During the surgical procedure, when a primary repair is being attempted, careful communication with the anesthesiologist is essential to evaluate difficulty with ventilation or perfusion. If either is significant, the primary repair is aborted and a staged repair is done.

A staged repair is the procedure of choice for a large defect, especially one in which the liver is involved. With this technique, a single layer of Silastic material is sutured to the abdominal wall around the defect and the viscera that remains herniated. Over the next 7 to 10 days, the defect is slowly reduced, usually on a daily basis by squeezing down on the top of the Silastic silo, which pushes a small portion of the contents of the defect into the abdominal cavity. During this process, the infant is maintained on intravenous antibiotics and the silo is bathed in an antibiotic solution. When the defect is almost completely reduced, the infant returns to the operating room for final closure. This process of slowly reducing the defect needs to be completed within 1 to 2 weeks or there is significant risk of wound infection. With either surgical technique, there seems to be no difference in the length of hospitalization, adaptation of the GI system to enteral nutrition, or the development of complications.

Postoperative Management. The goal of postoperative management includes maintaining a normothermic environment; restoration of fluid and electrolyte balance; provision of nutrition; and prevention of respiratory, circulatory, GI, and infectious complications. On return from the OR, the infant is placed in an Isolette or warmer bed to maintain normal temperature. Vital signs are taken frequently. Respiratory assistance may be necessary regardless of whether a primary or staged repair is done. With the primary repair, there may be significant pressure on the diaphragm, warranting ventilatory support. Between reduction on a staged repair, the infant may have little need for respiratory support, but may require support immediately after the reduction. Therefore, the endotracheal tube usually remains in place until the defect is completely closed.

The possibility of vascular compromise requires that the lower extremities be assessed for color and capillary refill. Pedal pulses are checked frequently. Elevating the infant's legs may facilitate venous return. The infant will have third-space fluid loss, requiring twice-maintenance fluids and the administration of albumin to prevent intravascular hypovolemia.

Nutritional support is initially provided with TPN, but within 4 to 6 weeks, even those infants with a staged repair can begin elemental enteral feedings. The infant is observed frequently for signs of feeding intolerance, such as increased gastric residuals, vomiting, and water loss stools, which contain reducing substances.

Cloacal Exstrophy

Pathogenesis

Cloacal exstrophy, sometimes called *vesicointestinal fissure,* is the most severe abdominal wall defect. Cloacal exstrophy is a developmental abnormality that results from a perforation of the cloacal membrane during the descent of the urogenital sinus. This perforation is thought to occur before the cloaca is divided by the urogenital sinus at approximately the fifth week of embryonic life. Because the cloaca has not been divided into a bladder and rectum, the result is a midline defect exposing bladder, bowel and bifid external genitalia. It is thought that cloacal

exstrophy may be an early attempt at twinning (Ziegler et al., 1986).

Associated Anomalies

A number of anomalies are associated with cloacal exstrophy. Aside from the variety of genital anomalies with which these children present, renal problems such as hydronephrosis and small, absent, or multicystic kidneys are seen (Jeffs & Lepor, 1986). Nongenitourinary anomalies include the GI, musculoskeletal, cardiovascular, and central nervous systems. Because the spectrum of anomalies is so vast, it can be difficult to make generalizations about the care of children with cloacal exstrophy.

Clinical Presentation

The typical cloacal exstrophy consists of an omphalocele superiorly and two walls of hemibladder below. Children with cloacal exstrophy have a colon that is short accompanied by a blind rectal ending. In the male child the penis is bifid on widely separated pubic bones and is quite rudimentary. To date, most males with cloacal exstrophy are gender-converted to female because of the difficulty in reconstructing a functional male phenotype. The female typically has duplicate vaginas, a bifid clitoris, and uterine abnormalities (Ziegler et al., 1986).

Critical Care Management

Initial stabilization of the infant with cloacal exstrophy is necessary before the child is transferred to a tertiary center where surgical repair is initiated. The omphalocele is cared for as previously described. The hemibladders are loosely covered with plastic wrap to provide a covering that protects the bladder without adhering. Management of the child's airway and breathing, cardiovascular status, and fluid and electrolyte status is necessary.

Operative Management. Current surgical management of the infant with cloacal exstrophy may require a number of staged operations. The initial operation is the most critical and often the most complicated. The bowel and bladder are separated, an intestinal stoma created, the omphalocele closed, and the bladder closed or reapproximated, leaving the child with an exstrophied bladder if primary closure is impossible. The GI stoma of preference is an end or loop colostomy. When ileostomy is performed, absorption of nutrients and water may be inadequate (Ricketts et al., 1991). During the initial operation gender assignment to female is performed in almost all cases.

The issue of gender reassignment to female is a particularly delicate matter for the family and healthcare providers. This information is extremely upsetting to families, and gender issues are discussed in detail with the families, with careful attention given to confidentiality and informed consent.

At a subsequent operation, when the child is between 6 months and 2 years, formal bladder closure is achieved if primary closure was impossible at the initial operation. Bilateral ileac osteotomies are performed to realign the pelvis. At this time central nervous system anomalies like tethered cord may be repaired, and genital reconstruction, such as the creation of labial folds, is performed.

The remaining phases of reconstruction are based primarily on the individual child's growth and development. As the child matures and expresses desire for bowel and bladder control, surgical efforts may be made to achieve that control. Bowel control may be achieved through various pull-through procedures accompanied by some type of enema program. Urinary continence is also possible for these children through various modifications of the Mitrofanoff technique or bladder augmentation. Functional and cosmetic genital reconstruction can take place around the time of puberty (Ricketts et al., 1991).

Postoperative Management. Postoperative management after surgical repair of cloacal exstrophy is critical. Airway management, fluid and electrolyte regulation, and prevention of major system complications are provided. Nutritional support requires particular attention because of the congenital SBS that accompanies the anomaly. The infant is initially managed with TPN for a number of weeks before elemental enteral feedings are introduced slowly. Some may require long-term TPN with the introduction of enteral feedings taking months to accomplish. The GI stoma must be managed with an appliance to preserve skin integrity, because of the nature of GI output with SBS.

Management of the infant's pelvis requires special nursing attention if primary bladder closure has been achieved. The softness of the infant's bones and joints allows closure of the symphysis pubis without the need for osteotomy provided the pelvic bones remain approximated (Duckett & Caldemone, 1985). The infant returns from the operating room with the legs internally rotated and wrapped together at the knees and ankles. Known as a "mermaid wrap," the legs remain bound for approximately 6 weeks.

Maintenance of the mermaid wrap is dependent on optimal nursing care. The child is not diapered in the normal fashion but in a circular fashion around the abdomen so that the child's hips are never abducted. The straps or dressings around the knees and ankles are removed separately every 4 hours to assess skin integrity. The bony prominences of the knees and ankles are padded with sheepskin or some type of skin protector. Improper care of the legs and hips in this type of closure results in prolapse of the bladder, requiring repeat reconstruction.

HEPATIC FAILURE

Hepatic failure is the consequence of severe hepatocyte injury or dysfunction. It is characterized by hepatic encephalopathy; a severe and complex coagulopathy; alterations in intrahepatic metabolic pathways; and the complications of renal failure, cerebral

edema, susceptibility to infection, and hemodynamic instability (Treem, 1991). The injury to the liver may be acute, resulting in fulminant injury to the hepatocytes and rapid development of the clinical signs of hepatic failure, without previous history of liver disease. Known as fulminant hepatic failure, progression to a life-threatening condition is rapid. In other instances, hepatic failure is the result of chronic injury that has accumulated to cause serious compromise of hepatic function and results in end-stage disease. Regardless of the cause, the consequences and therapeutic modalities are the same. It is important that the clinical course of hepatic failure and the prognostic indicators be recognized early to facilitate medical therapies that promote hepatic regeneration and recovery. The alternative is to initiate the option of liver transplantation when necessary (Treem, 1991).

Etiology of Hepatic Dysfunction

Hepatic failure is rare in childhood. The causes of hepatic dysfunction and failure in infants and children are divided into two categories; fulminant failure and failure from chronic liver disease. The incidence of any one etiology of liver failure is difficult to assess. One pediatric center reported 81 children dying of hepatic failure between 1976 and 1983 (Lloyd-Still, 1985). Biliary atresia accounted for 20 cases, metabolic disorders (tyrosinemia, cystic fibrosis, alpha-1-antitrypsin deficiency, Wilson's disease, Zellweger syndrome) for 22, and infectious causes were responsible for 15 cases. Cholestatic liver disease (Alagille's syndrome, total parenteral nutrition–associated disease) accounted for 12. Miscellaneous causes were cited for the remaining 5 cases. One half to two thirds of all children receiving liver transplants have biliary atresia, whereas children with inborn errors of metabolism make up the second largest group requiring transplantation (Zitelli et al., 1986; Vacanti et al., 1987; Van Thiel, 1985).

Chronic Causes

Biliary Atresia

Biliary atresia occurs in approximately 1 in 25,000 live births. Biliary atresia is the absence of the extrahepatic biliary system between the hilus of the liver and the duodenum. The extent of involvement varies; however, there is complete obstruction of bile flow. Biliary cirrhosis is the result of unrelieved bile flow. The anatomic features of biliary atresia are atresia of the common bile duct and a patent proximal system; atresia involving the hepatic duct with patent proximal ducts; and atresia of the right and left hepatic ducts at the porta hepatis. Biliary atresia also occurs in infants with situs inversus and polysplenia syndrome.

Etiology. Biliary atresia is generally not a failure

of fetal development. It is an acquired lesion that probably begins late in fetal life. It is also associated with congenital malformations and anomalies, suggesting more than one etiology or cause that leads to a final common outcome. Many etiologic agents have been explored. The majority of viruses examined have proven negative. Reovirus causes a similar lesion in neonatal mice, but has been difficult to identify in human infants. Other causes are being explored. Environmental causes have been suggested because of the occurrence of biliary atresia in only one of HLA identical twins. However, biliary atresia has been reported to occur in siblings within a family (Piccoli et al., 1991).

Clinical Presentation. Infants with biliary atresia are generally full-term and appear healthy despite being jaundiced. The gestational history is unremarkable. Appetite and weight gain are initially normal, but stools progressively become pale and acholic during the first weeks of life. The infant may have physiologic unconjugated jaundice initially that merges into a conjugated hyperbilirubinemia. This is generally recognized between 2 and 6 weeks of age when the urine becomes dark and the stools acholic. The total serum bilirubin is between 6 and 12 mg/dL with a conjugated faction of 50% to 80% of the total (Piccoli et al., 1991). Serum aminotransferases (ALT, AST) are mildly elevated, whereas alkaline phosphatase and gamma glutamyl transpeptidase (GGT) are markedly elevated. Physical examination reveals hepatomegaly and often splenomegaly as well.

No single test confirms the diagnosis of biliary atresia. An abdominal ultrasound excludes other causes of obstructive jaundice such as choledochal cyst from the differential and is obtained for that purpose. The patency of the extrahepatic biliary system is demonstrated by a nuclear scintiscan (HIDA scan). Evidence of radioactivity in the duodenum confirms a patent biliary system, thus eliminating the possibility of biliary atresia. When there is no evidence of excretion with the HIDA scan, further diagnostic evaluation is necessary in the form of a percutaneous liver biopsy. The histologic finding of intrahepatic bile duct proliferation suggests a mechanical obstruction, indicating the need for laparotomy and operative cholangiogram. If the extrahepatic system cannot be demonstrated by cholangiogram, surgical intervention is necessary.

Critical Care Management. The most common surgical procedure performed to establish bile flow is the Kasai hepatoportoenterostomy (Fig. 23–9). The residual biliary system is removed. The surface of the liver is dissected and an area through which bile can drain is exposed. A limb of jejunum is made into a Roux-en-Y intestinal conduit to maintain the patency of the intestine. Success of the procedure varies, depending on the age of the infant at the time of surgery and the center performing the surgery, with one fourth to one half of patients having inadequate drainage despite the surgical intervention.

The two postoperative problems of consequence are

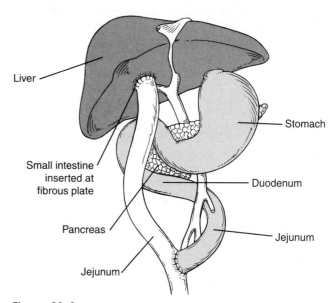

Figure 23–9 ● ● ● ● ● ●

Schematic representation of a hepatic portoenterostomy (Kasai procedure) providing bile drainage in a case of extrahepatic biliary atresia.

failure to establish bile flow and ascending cholangitis. Ascending cholangitis is a frequent and severe complication of a successful operation, occurring in 50% to 100% of patients with established bile flow following a Kasai procedure. Surgical and medical approaches have been attempted to decrease the incidence of ascending cholangitis. Surgical modifications of the Kasai procedure have not had great success. Medical approaches include choleretic agents to improve bile flow, postoperative antibiotics, and long-term prophylactic oral antibiotics, all with limited success.

Long-term prognosis is guarded in infants with biliary atresia. Establishment of bile flow and resolution of the jaundice appears to be correlated with the best outcome. Patients who remain jaundiced experience hepatic failure between the ages of 2 and 10 years of age and require a liver transplant. Those with established bile flow and resolution of jaundice have a 90% chance of surviving past age 10 years. Survival to the third decade with a high quality of life has been reported (Piccoli et al., 1991).

Arteriohepatic Dysplasia

Arteriohepatic dysplasia (Alagelle's syndrome, syndromic bile duct paucity) is characterized by a marked reduction of intrahepatic bile ducts and cholestasis. It occurs in association with cardiac, vertebral, ocular, facial, renal, and neurodevelopmental abnormalities. It is a familial disease that has a wide variation in clinical symptoms in affected individuals. The incidence of Alagille's syndrome is one in 100,000 births with an equal sex distribution (Mueller, 1987). It is believed that Alagille's syndrome is an inherited disorder; however, sporadic cases may occur. The exact genetic marker and autosomal penetration have not been decided.

It is now believed that infants with Alagille's syndrome may have a normal ratio of bile ducts, and in some cases a proliferation of bile ducts, resulting in confusion with biliary atresia at time of biopsy. Over a variable period of months to years, the intrahepatic ducts are lost and the condition becomes more definable. Progressive liver disease develops in 10% to 20% of patients with Alagille's disease (Perrault, 1981). There is no way of predicting the progression of significant pathology. The cause of the bile duct paucity is unknown. It has been suggested that an inability to secrete bile is related to the bile duct loss in Alagille's disease. The relationship of the liver disease to other systemic manifestations is unknown. Structural lesions involving the heart, eyes, kidneys, skeletal system, and genitalia are well described.

Clinical Presentation. Alagille's syndrome generally presents in the first 3 months of life in the symptomatic patient. It is among the more common causes for cholestasis and jaundice in the newborn period and must be distinguished from biliary atresia and choledochal cyst. Nonsymptomatic adults are frequently undiagnosed until a related child with symptoms is identified. Biochemically, infants with Alagille's syndrome have elevated bilirubin, alkaline phosphatase, GGT, and serum bile acids levels. There may also be elevations of the ALT and AST, up to 10 times normal. These elevations may persist through childhood. Hepatomegaly is present in nearly all patients, whereas splenomegaly is rare initially.

Jaundice is present in the majority of patients with symptomatic disease. Pruritus is severe, but rarely present before 3 to 5 months of age. Xanthomas resulting from cholestasis appear on the extensor surfaces of the fingers, the palmar creases, nape of the neck, buttocks, and inguinal area. The formation of xanthomas is related to the severity of the cholestasis and correlates with elevated serum cholesterol levels. Diminished bile salt excretion results in fat malabsorption and deficiency of fat-soluble vitamins, which has profound systemic effects. Growth failure is common with delayed pubertal development. Progression of the disease to cirrhosis and hepatic failure was initially believed to be an uncommon event that is now being recognized more frequently.

Alpha-1-Antitrypsin Deficiency

Alpha-1-antitrypsin deficiency is the most common metabolic disease in children requiring liver transplantation. It is an autosomal recessive disorder, specifically the PiZZ allele of the chromosome, that results in low serum concentrations of alpha-1-antitrypsin. The consequences include premature pulmonary emphysema and chronic liver disease in infants and children. In the United States, the prevalence has been described as one in 2000 individuals. It is more common among caucasians of Northern European ancestry (Perlmutter, 1991). The mecha-

nism by which alpha-1-antitrypsin deficiency causes liver disease is not understood.

Infants with alpha-1-antitrypsin deficiency generally present in the first 2 months of life with persistent jaundice. The ALT and AST are slightly elevated and the liver may be enlarged. The liver disease may also be discovered later in childhood or adolescence with hepatosplenomegaly, ascites, or hemorrhage from esophageal varices. Many of these children experience progressive liver dysfunction requiring transplantation. Diagnosis is confirmed by a serum alpha-1 concentration level and the determination of the alpha-1-antitrypsin phenotype (PiZZ).

Wilson's Disease

Wilson's disease is an autosomal recessive disorder of copper metabolism, in which biliary excretion of copper is inadequate and the excess accumulates in the liver, brain, kidneys, cornea, and skeletal system. The disease has been recognized for approximately 60 years; however, the biochemical defect has yet to be identified. Hepatic disease occurs when the copper overload leads to the destruction of liver tissue. It occurs in one in 30,000 individuals.

The clinical symptoms of Wilson's disease rarely present before the age of 5 years, more often in the second decade. Hepatic dysfunction is the most common presentation in children; however, the diagnosis must be considered in older children and adolescents with a neurologic abnormality. Symptoms may be subtle initially and include malaise, anorexia, and lethargy. Signs of progressive liver disease such as jaundice, petechiae, hematemesis, and ascites may also be present at diagnosis. Presentation with fulminant hepatitis with progression to liver failure requiring transplantation does occur. Neurologic symptoms include gradual onset of clumsiness, dysarthria, drooling, tremors, loss of fine motor skills, and psychological disturbances. Kayser-Fleischer rings, a greenish pigment encircling the cornea (the result of copper deposits) is considered diagnostic of Wilson's disease. Its absence, however, does not rule it out.

The diagnosis of Wilson's disease may be difficult. The majority of children with Wilson's disease have a low serum level of the copper-binding protein ceruloplasmin, implying a homozygosity (disease state) or heterozygosity (carrier state). Urinary copper excretion is usually elevated. An ophthalmologic examination for Kayser-Fleischer rings is necessary. A liver biopsy may be necessary to determine the amount of copper actually in the liver. Asymptomatic siblings should also be screened for Wilson's disease. Treatment of Wilson's disease is aimed at improving the excretion of copper and decreasing dietary intake of copper-containing foods.

Acute Causes

Infectious Causes

Fulminant hepatic failure in childhood is often idiopathic and a causative agent is not identified. The definition of fulminant hepatic failure is the development of hepatic encephalopathy within 8 weeks of the initial symptoms of the illness without a history of previous or underlying liver dysfunction (Trey & Davidson, 1970). Acute viral hepatitis may result in fulminant failure. The overall incidence of hepatitis A (HAV) in developed countries is relatively low, thus the incidence of HAV as a causative agent for fulminant hepatic failure is minimal (Treem, 1991). In the United States, fulminant hepatic failure resulting from hepatitis B (HBV) has been reported in infants vertically infected from their mothers and in older children from blood transfusions (Delaplane et al., 1983; Sinatra et al., 1982). Hepatitis C (HCV) non-A non-B hepatitis now accounts for a large percentage of fulminant hepatic failure.

Herpes simplex virus (HSV) and Epstein-Barr virus (EBV) have also been associated with fulminant hepatic failure in infancy and childhood. HSV infection is generally severe in the neonatal period, and is rare in immunocompetent children. EBV mononucleosis–associated fulminant hepatic failure has also been reported (Treem, 1991). Other congenital viral infections such as *Echovirus* and cytomegalovirus infections are known causes of fulminant hepatic failure in infancy.

Drug-Induced Hepatic Failure

Many drugs have been associated with fulminant hepatic failure owing to massive or centrilobular hepatic necrosis. Other drugs cause periportal necrosis and steatosis, also leading to liver failure. In children, the drugs most commonly linked with hepatic failure are acetaminophen, anticonvulsants (phenytoin, valproate), halothane anesthesia, and the antituberculous drug isoniazid (Treem, 1991). The relationship between a drug and fulminant hepatic failure is often ambiguous. Some medications such as acetaminophen are known to be hepatotoxic when taken in large doses. Levels of the drug can be measured, thus determining the diagnosis or cause of the liver failure. Other medications have known hepatotoxic effects that are monitored with serial liver function studies. If an elevation in these levels occurs, followed by evidence of hepatic failure, there is a high index of suspicion as to the causative agent. In the case of medications known to cause hypersensitivity reactions, extrahepatic manifestations such as rash, arthralgias, and peripheral eosinophilia may accompany the hepatic failure (Treem, 1991).

Consequences of Hepatic Failure

In children with hepatic disease, ongoing damage results in decreased function, which includes the metabolic and detoxification processes of the liver. The Kupffer cells' phagocytic process is diminished with hepatic failure, resulting in decreased filtration of blood. The child in hepatic failure is prone to infections, particularly bacteremias.

Decreased bile salt synthesis results in fat malabsorption. In children, fat accounts for a large percentage of calories consumed. Malnutrition and malabsorption of fat-soluble vitamins A, D, E, and K results. Vitamin A stores are long-lasting, approximately to 2 years; thus, a deficiency must be longstanding before ill effects are noted. Failure to absorb vitamin D results in demineralization of the bone leading to osteomalacia, rickets, and pathologic fractures. Vitamin E malabsorption has neurologic consequences, such as peripheral neuropathies and diminished deep tendon reflexes. Vitamin K deficiencies result in coagulopathies, which are discussed later in this section. Excessive accumulation of bile salts resulting from decreased extraction through the liver results in their deposition in the skin, causing intractable pruritus. Cholestasis (biliary obstruction) causes direct hyperbilirinemia and jaundice.

The liver is crucial in the process of carbohydrate metabolism. Initially, serum glucose levels are elevated, but glycogen stores are decreased. If the liver is unable to store glycogen or generate new glucose, the kidneys assume the process of gluconeogenesis. As the hepatic failure progresses, hypoglycemia becomes a problem.

Protein metabolism is altered in hepatic failure. Altered albumin synthesis results in low serum albumin levels. Without adequate levels, the body is unable to maintain oncotic pressure. Consequently, fluid leaks from the blood vessels into the abdominal cavity and tissues, resulting in ascites and edema.

The liver's ability to manufacture clotting factors is impaired. Vitamin K absorption is influenced by the decreased synthesis of bile salts resulting in a decreased production of vitamin K–dependent clotting factors II, VII, IX, and X. Alterations in hemostasis are evidenced by prolonged prothrombin time, easy bruising, and bleeding.

A failing liver is also unable to remove activated clotting factors from the circulating serum. Hepatic necrosis causes an inflammatory response, thus activating clotting factors. Once activated, clotting factors circulate in the plasma, form microthrombi, and consume platelets and fibrinogen. Disseminated intravascular coagulation (DIC) results when fibrinolysis occurs and the liver is unable to synthesize clotting factors.

The liver's inability to detoxify hormones, drugs, and other harmful compounds results in a variety of clinical manifestations. Continued circulation of aldosterone and antidiuretic hormone (ADH) contributes to the development of ascites and hepatorenal syndrome. Use of medications metabolized by the liver is avoided.

Complications of Hepatic Failure

Hepatic Encephalopathy

Hepatic encephalopathy is the change in mental status that accompanies hepatic failure. The encephalopathic agent responsible for these changes has not yet been identified. The appearance of hepatic encephalopathy is variable. It depends on the extent of the liver damage, speed of injury, degree of portal-systemic shunting, and contributing factors. The child with fulminant hepatic failure may progress to coma and unresponsiveness very rapidly, over several days, whereas the child with chronic liver disease may have intermittent alterations in mental status becoming more severe over time. Some with chronic liver disease do well until a major insult occurs, such as a variceal hemorrhage, or until an infection precipitates the onset of encephalopathic changes.

Hepatic encephalopathy is traditionally divided into 5 stages, which are outlined in Table 23–10. Passage through the stages may be rapid. It is important to monitor the progression so that therapeutic support can be escalated. In cases of chronic liver dysfunction, the deterioration may be subtle. Changes in behavior, school performance, and handwriting are the most commonly noticed.

Four hypotheses explain the pathophysiology of hepatic encephalopathy. No single hypothesis completely explains the process. The *ammonia* hypothesis suggests that ammonia accumulation in the brain results in encephalopathic changes. The *synergistic neurotoxins* hypothesis suggests that encephalopathy and coma are a result of accumulating toxins with synergistic effects augmented by other metabolic abnormalities. An excessive production of the brain inhibitory neurotransmitter, serotonin, and the false neurotransmitter, octopamine, accompanied by a deficient synthesis of excitatory neurotransmitters, nor-epinephrine and dopamine, result in encephalopathy and coma and are the basis of the *false neurotransmitter* hypothesis. The final hypothesis is the *GABA-ergic inhibitory* hypothesis. In this hypothesis, the brain amino acids are divided into excitatory and inhibitory neurotransmitters, concentrating on gamma-aminobutyric acid (GABA) and glycine as the main inhibitory neurotransmitters. Hepatic encephalopathy is the result of increased GABA-ergic and glycinergic neurotransmission (Treem, 1991).

Hepatic encephalopathy occurs as liver destruction progresses. The blood flow from the intestine is shunted around the liver completely, bypassing viable hepatocytes. Consequently, the filtration process of the liver does not occur. It is also believed that alterations in the function of the blood-brain barrier contribute to the development of hepatic encephalopathy. The blood-brain barrier is essential in preventing toxic substances in the systemic circulation from entering the brain. Animal studies have shown that accumulating toxins in hepatic encephalopathy may mediate their own entry into the brain (Treem, 1991).

Cerebral Edema

Cerebral edema is the major cause of mortality in patients with fulminant hepatic failure. The incidence of cerebral edema is much lower in people with encephalopathy and chronic liver disease. Thus, careful monitoring of intracranial pressure (ICP) by subdural or extradural pressure transducers is recommended for patients in stage III or IV encephalop-

Table 23–10. CLINICAL STAGING OF HEPATIC ENCEPHALOPATHY

Category of Physical Signs	Stage I	Stage II	Stage III	Stage IV	Stage V
Mental Status	Alert, oriented, slow mentation	Lethargic, confused, agitated	Stupor, arousal to voice	Unarousable	Unarousable
Behavior	Restless, irritable, short attention span, disordered sleep	Combative, sullen, euphoric	Sleeps most of time, marked confusion	None	None
Spontaneous motor activity	Incoordination, tremor, poor handwriting	Yawning, sucking, grimacing, intention tremor present, blinking	Decreased, marked intention tremor	Absent	None
Asterixis	Absent	Present	Present (if cooperates)	Absent	Absent
Muscle tone	Normal	Increased	Increased	Increased	Flaccid
Reflexes	Normal	Hyper-reflexic	Hyper-reflexic extensor plantars	Hyper-reflexic extensor plantars	Absent
Respirations	Regular or hyperventilation	Hyperventilation	Hyperventilation	Irregular	Apnea
Verbal response	Normal	Confused, dysarthric	Incoherent	None	None
Motor response	Obeys commands	Purposeful movements, may not respond to commands	Localized appropriately to pain	Abnormal flexor, abnormal extensor posturing	None
Pupils	Brisk	Brisk	Brisk	Sluggish	Fixed
Eye opening	Spontaneous	Verbal stimuli	Verbal stimuli	Noxious stimuli	None
Oculocephalic	Normal	Normal	Normal	Partial dysconjugate	Absent
Oculovestibular	Normal	Normal	Normal	Partial dysconjugate	Absent

From Treem, W.R. (1991). Hepatic failure. In W.A. Walker, et al. (Eds.). *Pediatric gastrointestinal diseases: Pathophysiology, diagnosis, management* (pp. 146–192). Toronto: B.C. Decker. By permission of C.V. Mosby.

athy to facilitate early recognition and treatment of increased ICP in these patients (Treem, 1991).

Impaired Coagulation

The liver is the site of synthesis of most of the coagulation factors, fibrinolytic agents, and inhibitors of coagulation. With the onset of hepatic failure, there are significant alterations in the coagulation process. Prothrombin time is often prolonged by more than 90 seconds and is unresponsive to vitamin K. Fibrinogen levels are reduced because of a decrease in synthesis and increase in consumption. Coagulation factor levels are decreased, most commonly factors II, V, VII, IX, and X. Platelet count is generally low, less than 100,000 per 10^9. Thrombocytopenia may be the result of platelet sequestration as a consequence of hypersplenism, or platelet-associated antibodies as seen in chronic active hepatitis, or DIC. With these coagulation abnormalities, patients with hepatic failure are at an increased risk for major hemorrhage, most commonly originating in the GI tract or the brain, resulting in death (Treem, 1991).

Hepatorenal Syndrome

Oliguria is common in both acute and chronic liver failure. Hepatorenal syndrome is defined as unexplained progressive renal dysfunction without obvious histologic lesions. It is characterized by significant sodium retention without urinary sodium. Urinary sediment is present but without protein, cells, or casts, and the oliguria is unresponsive to intravascular volume expansion. Hepatorenal syndrome accounts for the majority of renal impairment in fulminant hepatic failure and is often associated with a fatal outcome (Papper, 1983).

Management of Hepatic Failure

The management of fulminant hepatic failure is supportive therapy that requires a multisystem approach. General support measures are used to treat the complications of hepatic failure, which include hypokalemia, hypoglycemia, GI hemorrhage, and hypovolemia.

Electrolyte imbalances such as hypernatremia are treated by eliminating sodium chloride from IV solutions, including blood products and flushes. Hypokalemia is treated by adding KCl to IV solutions and discontinuing potassium-wasting diuretics. Hyperkalemia and azotemia warrant dialysis.

Metabolic disorders, such as hypoglycemia, are treated with IV dextrose. Acidosis is treated by ensuring adequate intravascular volume. Albumin may be administered to expand volume. Dialysis may be necessary to correct acidosis if hepatorenal syndrome is present. Hypoxemia is treated with administration of oxygen. If pulmonary edema develops, positive end expiratory pressure is employed.

Coagulopathies are treated when the platelet count drops to less than 50,000. Fresh frozen plasma is given for active bleeding. An H2 receptor antagonist is used to keep the gastric pH higher than 5.0 to prevent stress ulcers and GI bleeding. Vitamin K (up to 10 mg IM or IV) is administered for 3 days to correct a prolonged PT.

For the child with hepatic failure, sedatives and barbiturates, increased dietary protein, constipation, and infection may aggravate or precipitate hepatic encephalopathy. Sedatives and barbiturates are avoided; dietary protein is restricted. The child is intubated to protect the airway in stage III or IV coma. Increased ICP is treated. Lactulose is administered by NG tube at a dose of 30 mL every 6 hours. Enemas are given to clean the bowel of toxic proteins such as retained blood.

SUMMARY

Gastrointestinal problems in infants and children are extremely varied and can be complicated and severe. Although the pathology varies greatly, the nursing care and assessment follow common pathways. GI nursing assessment, gastric decompression, intravascular volume replacement and maintenance, and pharmacologic management are of critical importance to the survival of these infants and children.

References

Altman, R.P. (1986). Portal hypertension. In K.J. Welch, J.G. Randolph, M.M. Ravitch, J.A. O'Neill, & M.I. Rowe (Eds.). *Pediatric surgery* (pp. 1075–1085, 4th ed.). Chicago: YearBook Medical Publishers.

Ashcraft, K.M., & Holder, T.M. (Eds.) (1993). *Pediatric surgery.* Philadelphia: W.B. Saunders.

Ashcraft, K.W., Goodwin, C.G., & Amoury, R.W. (1978). Thal fundoplication: A simple and safe operative treatment for gastroesophageal reflux. *Journal of Pediatric Surgery, 13*, 643–647.

Basso, N., Bagarani, M. Bracci, F., et al. (1986). Ranititine and somatostin. Their effects on bleeding from the upper gastrointestinal tract. *Archives of Surgery, 121*, 833–835.

Bianchi, A. (1980). Intestinal loop lengthening: A technique for increasing small bowel length. *Journal of Pediatric Surgery, 15*, 145–151.

Careskey, J., Webster, T.R., & Grosfeld, J.L. (1981). Ileocecal valve replacement. *Archives of Surgery, 116*, 618–622.

Caulfield, M.E., & Michener, W. (1993). Ulcerative colitis. In R. Wyllie, & J.S. Hyams (Eds.). *Pediatric gastrointestinal disease: Pathophysiology, diagnosis, management* (pp. 765–787). Philadelphia: W.B. Saunders.

Conn, H.O., & Grace, N.D. (1985). Portal hypertension and sclerotherapy of esophageal varices: A point of view. *Endoscopy Review,* May/June, 39–55.

Cooper, H., Floyd, T.S., Ross, A.J., Bishop, H.C., Templeton, J.M., & Ziegler, M.M. (1984). Morbidity and mortality of short bowel syndrome acquired in infancy: An update. *Journal of Pediatric Surgery, 19*, 711–718.

Cullen, T.S. (1916). *The umbilicus and its diseases.* Philadelphia: W.B. Saunders.

Delaplane, D., Yogeu, R., Crussi, F., et al. (1983). Fatal hepatitis B in early infancy: The importance of identifying HBsAg-positive pregnant women and providing immunoprophylaxis to their newborns. *Pediatrics, 72*, 176–180.

de Lorimier, A.A., Fonhalsrud, E.W., & Hays, D.A. (1969). Congenital atresia and stenosis of the jejunum and ileum. *Surgery, 65*, 819.

Doughty, D.B., & Jackson, D.B. (1993). *Gastrointestinal disorders.* St. Louis: C.V. Mosby.

Duckett, J.W., & Caldemone, A.A. (1985). Bladder and urachus. In P.T. Kelalis, L.R. King, and A.B. Belman (Eds.). *Clinical pediatric urology* (2nd ed., pp. 726–751). Philadelphia: W.B. Saunders.

Ein, S.H., Shandling, B., Wesson, D., & Filler, R.M. (1989). Esophageal atresia with distal tracheoesophageal fistula: Associated anomalies and prognosis in the 1980's. *Journal of Pediatric Surgery,* 24(10), 1055–1059.

Fenter, S. (1987). *Neonatal Newborn,* Dec., 29–46.

Filston, H.C. (1992). Fluid and electrolyte management in the pediatric surgical patient. *Surgical Clinics of North America,* 72(6), 1189–1205.

Frenter, S. (1987). Abdominal wall defects: omphalocele and gastroschisis. *Neonatal Network.*

Garcia, V.G., Templeton, J.M., Eichelberger, M.R., Koop, C.E., & Vinograd, I. (1981). Colon interposition for the short bowel syndrome. *Journal of Pediatric Surgery,* 16, 994–995.

Goetting, M.G., Tiznado-Garcia, E., & Bakdash, T. (1990). Intussusception encephalopathy: an under-recognized cause of coma in children. *Pediatric Neurology,* 6(6), 419–421.

Greenwood, R.D., Rosenthal, A., & Nadas, A.S. (1974). Cardiovascular malformation associated with omphalocele. *Journal of Pediatrics,* 85, 818.

Grosfeld, J.L. (1986). Jejunoileal atresia and stenosis. In K.J. Welch, J.G. Randolph, M.M. Ravitch, et al. (Eds.). *Pediatric surgery* (pp. 839–857, 4th ed.). Chicago: YearBook Medical Publishers.

Harris, J.A. (1986). Pediatric abdominal assessment. *Pediatric Nursing,* 12(5), 355–361.

Harrison, M.W., Lindner, D.J., et al. (1984). Acute appendicitis in children: Factors affecting morbidity. *American Journal of Surgery,* 147, 605–610.

Hennessey, K. (1989). Nutritional support and gastrointenstestinal disease. *Nursing Clinics of North America,* 24(2), 373–384.

Hickey, R.W., Sodhi, S.K., & Johnson, W.R. (1990). Two children with lethargy and intussusception. *Annals of Emergency Medicine,* 19(4), 390–392.

Hillemeier, A.C. (1990). Reflux and esophagitis. In W.A. Walker (Ed.). *Pediatric gastrointestinal disease* (pp. 417–422). Philadelphia: B.C. Decker.

Hoffman, M.A., Stylianos, S., & Jacir, N.N. (1990). Technique of the transabdominal uncut Collis-Nissen fundoplication. *Pediatric Surgery International,* 5, 471–472.

Holder, T.M., Cloud, D.T., & Lewis, J.E. (1961). Esophageal atresia and tracheoesophageal fistula. A survey of its members by the Surgical Section of the American Academy of Pediatrics. *Pediatrics,* 34, 542.

Holman, R.C., Stehr-Green, J.K., & Zelasky, M.T. (1989). Necrotizing enterocolitis mortality in the United States, 1979–85. *American Journal of Public Health,* 79(8), 987–989.

Hornig, G.W., & Shillito, J., Jr. (1990). Intestinal perforation by peritoneal shunt tubing: Report of two cases. *Surgical Neurology,* 33(4), 288–290.

Hyams, J.S. (1993). Crohn's disease. In R. Wyllie, & J.S. Hyams (Eds.). *Pediatric gastrointestinal disease: Pathophysiology, diagnosis, management* (pp. 742–764). Philadelphia: W.B. Saunders.

Jackson, W.D., & Grand, R.J. (1991). Ulcerative colitis. In W.A. Walker, P.R. Durie, J.R. Hamilton, et al. (Eds.). *Pediatric gastrointestinal disease: Pathophysiology, diagnosis, management* (pp. 608–618). Toronto: B.C. Decker.

Jeffs, R.D., & Lepor, H. (1986). Management of exstrophy-epispadias complex. In P.C. Walsh, et al. (Eds.). *Campbell's urology* (5th ed., Vol. 2, pp. 1911–1921). Philadelphia: W.B. Saunders.

Kiesling, V.J. Jr., & Tank, E.S. (1989). Postoperative intussusception in children. *Urology,* 33(5), 387–389.

Kliegman, R.M., & Fanaroff, A.A. (1984). Necrotizing enterocolitis. *The New England Journal of Medicine,* 310(17), 1093–1103.

Ladd, W.E., & Gross, R.E. (1941). *Abdominal surgery of infancy and childhood.* Philadelphia: W.B. Saunders.

Lecco, T.M. (1910). Zur Morphologie des pankreas annulare. *Sitzungsb. Akad. Wissensch. Cl.* 119, 391.

Lloyd, D.A. (1986). Meconium ileus. In K.J. Welch, J.G. Randolph, M.M. Ravitch, J.A. O'Neill, & M.I. Rowe (Eds.). *Pediatric surgery* (pp. 849–858, 4th ed.). Chicago: YearBook Medical Publishers.

Lloyd-Still, J.D. (1985). Mortality from liver disease in children: Implications for hepatic transplantation programs. *American Journal of Diseases of Children,* 139, 381–384.

Louw, J.H., & Barnard, C.W. (1955). Congenital intestinal atresia: Observations on its origin. *Lancet,* 2, 1065.

Martin, L.W., & Alexander, F. (1985). Esophageal atresia. *Surgical Clinics of North America,* 65, 5.

Mueller, R.F. (1987). The Alagille's syndrome (arteriohepatic dysplasia). *Journal of Medical Genetics,* 24, 621–626.

Munn, J, et al. (1990). Ileal perforation due to arteriovenous malformation in a premature infant. *Journal of Pediatric Surgery,* 25(6), 701–703.

Mustafa, M.M., & Siegel, J.D. (1990). Peritonitis. In D.L. Levin, & F.C. Morriss (Eds.). *Essentials of pediatric intensive care* (pp. 366–371). St. Louis: Quality Medical Publishing.

Neuhauser, E.B.D. (1946). Roentgen changes associated with pancreatic insufficiency in early life. *Radiology,* 46, 319.

Noblett, H.R. (1969). Treatment of uncomplicated meconium ileus by gastrographin enema: A preliminary report. *Journal of Pediatric Surgery,* 4, 190.

Olson, A.D., & Hillemeier, A.C. (1993). Gastrointestinal hemorrhage. In R. Wyllie, & J.S. Hyams (Eds.). *Pediatric gastrointestinal disease: Pathophysiology, diagnosis and management* (pp. 251–270). Philadelphia: W.B. Saunders.

Orenstein, S.R. (1993). Gastroesophageal reflux. In R. Wyllie, & J.S. Hyams (Eds.). *Pediatric gastrointestinal disease: Pathophysiology, diagnosis and management* (pp. 337–369). Philadelphia: W.B. Saunders.

Orenstein, S.R., & Whittingham, P.F. (1983). Positioning for prevention of infant gastroesophageal reflux. *Journal of Pediatrics,* 103, 534–537.

Oshio, T., et al. (1991). Recurrent perforations of viscus due to ventriculoperitoneal shunt in a hydrocephalic child. *Journal of Pediatric Surgery,* 26(12), 1404–1405.

Papper, S. (1983). Renal failure in cirrhosis (the hepatorenal syndrome). In M. Epstein, (Ed.). *The kidney in liver disease* (pp. 84–94, 2nd ed.). New York: Elsevier Science.

Peck, S.N., & Griffith, D.J. (1988). Reducing portal hypertension and variceal bleeding. *Dimensions of Critical Care Nursing,* 7(5), 269–279.

Perlmutter, D.H. (1991). Alpha 1-antitrypsin deficiency. In W.A. Walker, et al. (Eds.) *Pediatric gastrointestinal disease* (pp. 976–991). Toronto: B.C. Decker.

Perrault, J. (1981). Paucity of interlobular bile ducts: Getting to know it better. *Digestive Disease Science,* 26, 41–44.

Piccoli, E.A., & Witzleben, C.L. (1991). Disorders of the extrahepatic bile ducts. In W.A. Walker, et al. (Eds.). *Pediatric gastrointestinal disease* (pp. 1140–1151). Toronto: B.C. Decker.

Polin, R.A., Pollack, P.F., Barlow, B., et al. (1975). Neonatal necrotizing enterocolitis in term infants. *Journal of Pediatrics,* 89, 460–462.

Polson, E.C., Schaller, R.T., & Tapper, D. (1988). Improved survival with primary anastomosis in the low birth weight neonate with esophageal atresia and tracheoesophageal fistula. *Journal of Pediatric Surgery,* 23, 418–421.

Puri, P., Blake, N., & O'Donnell, B. (1981). Delayed primary anastomosis following spontaneous growth of esophageal segments in esophageal atresia. *Journal of Pediatric Surgery,* 16, 180–183.

Quan, R. (1990). Bowel failure. In D.L. Levin, & F.C. Morriss (Eds.). *Essentials of pediatric intensive care* (pp. 147–150). St. Louis: Quality Medical Publishing.

Raffensperger, J.G. (Ed.). (1989). *Swenson's pediatric surgery* (5th ed.). Norwalk, CT: Appleton & Lange.

Randolph, J.G. (1986). Esophageal atresia and congenital stenosis. In K.J. Welch, J.C. Randolph, M.M. Ravitch, J.A. O'Neill, & M.I. Rowe (Eds.). *Pediatric Surgery* (pp. 682–693, 4th ed.). Chicago: YearBook Medical Publishers.

Ravitch, M.M. (1986). Intussusception. In K.J. Welch, et al. (Eds.). *Pediatric surgery* (pp. 868–882). Chicago: YearBook Medical Publishers.

Reichlin, S. (1983). Somatostatin (second of two parts). *The New England Journal of Medicine,* 309, 1556–1563.

Reijan, J.A., Festen, C., & Joosten, H.J. (1989). Chronic intussusception in children. *British Journal of Surgery,* 76(8), 815–816.

Ricketts, R.R., Woodard, J.R., Zwiren, G.T., Andrews, G., &

Broecker, B.H. (1991). Modern treatment of cloacal exstrophy. *Journal of Pediatric Surgery, 26,* 444–450.

Rosenthal, A.A. (1931). Congenital atresia of the esophagus with tracheoesophageal fistula. *Archives of Pathology, 12,* 756.

Rowe, M.L. (1986). Necrotizing enterocolitis. In K.J. Welch, J.C. Randolph, M.M. Ravitch, J.A. O'Neill, & M.I. Rowe (Eds.). *Pediatric surgery* (pp. 944–955, 4th ed.). Chicago: YearBook Medical Publishers.

Schnaufer, L. (1986). Duodenal atresia, stenosis and annular pancreas. In K.J. Welch, J.C. Randolph, M.M. Ravitch, J.A. O'Neill, & M.I. Rowe (Eds.). *Pediatric surgery* (pp. 829–836, 4th ed.). Chicago: YearBook Medical Publishers.

Schnauffer, L.S., & Mahboubi, S. (1988). Abdominal emergencies. In G.R. Fleischer, & S. Ludwig (Eds.). *Pediatric emergency medicine* (pp. 936–965). Baltimore: Williams & Wilkins.

Schuster, S.R. (1986). Omphalocele and gastroschesis. In K.J. Welch, J.C. Randolph, M.M. Ravitch, J.A. O'Neill, & M.I. Rowe (Eds.). *Pediatric surgery* (pp. 740–747. 4th ed.). Chicago: YearBook Medical Publishers.

Shaw, A. (1975). The myth of gastroscheses. *Journal of Pediatric Surgery, 10,* 973.

Sinatra, F.R., Shah, P., Weissman, J.Y., et al. (1982). Perinatal transmitted acute icteric hepatitis B in infants born to hepatitis B surface antigen-positive and antihepatitis B e-positive carrier mothers. *Pediatrics, 70,* 557–559.

Stevenson, R.J. (1985). Non-neonatal intestinal obstruction in children. *Surgical Clinics of North America, 65(5),* 1217–1235.

Stevenson, R.J. (1985). Abdominal pain unrelated to trauma. *Surgical Clinics of North America, 65(5),* 1181–1215.

Tandler, J. (1902). Entwich lungs geohicted es menschlich en duodenums. *Morphol. Jb, 29,* 187.

Thomaidis, T.S., & Arey, J.B. (1963). The intestinal lesions in cystic fibrosis of the pancreas. *Journal of Pediatric Surgery, 63,* 444.

Touloukian, R.J., & Walker-Smith, G.J. (1983). Normal intestinal length in preterm infants. *Journal of Pediatric Surgery, 18,* 720–723.

Touloukian, R.J. (1976). Neonatal necrotizing enterocolitis: An update. *Surgical Clinics of North America, 56(2),* 281–298.

Treem, W.R. (1991). Hepatic failure. In W.A. Walker, et al. (Eds.). *Pediatric gastrointestinal diseases: Pathophysiology, diagnosis, management* (pp. 146–192). Toronto: B.C. Decker.

Trey, C., & Davidson, C. (1970). The management of fulminant hepatic failure. *Progress in Liver Disease, 3,* 282–298.

Van Thiel, D.H. (1985). Liver transplantation. *Pediatric Annals, 14,* 474–480.

Vacanti, J.P., Lillehei, C.W., Jenkins, R.L., et al. (1987). Liver transplantation in children: The Boston Center experience in the first 30 months. *Transplant Proceedings, 29,* 3261–3266.

Vanderhoff, J.A., Langnas, A.N., Pinch, L.W., Thompson, J.S., & Kaugman, S.S. (1992). Short bowel syndrome. *Journal of Pediatric Gastroenterology and Nutrition, 14,* 359–370.

Verscheldon, P., et al. (1992). Intussusception in children: Reliability of ultrasound in diagnosis—a prospective study. *Radiology, 184(3),* 741–744.

Webster, T.R., Tracy, T., Jr., & Connors, R.H. (1991). Short-bowel syndrome in children. *Archives of Surgery, 126,* 841–846.

Wilmore, D.W. (1972). Factors correlating with a successful outcome following extensive intestinal resection in newborn infants. *Journal of Pediatrics, 80,* 88–95.

Ziegler, D.W., Long, J.A., et al. (1988). Pancreatitis in childhood. Experience with 49 Patients. *Annals of Surgery, 207(3),* 257–261.

Ziegler, M.M., Duckett, J.W., & Howell, C.G. (1986). Cloacal exstrophy. In K.J. Welch, J.C. Randolph, M.M. Ravitch, J.A. O'Neill, & M.I. Rowe (Eds). *Pediatric surgery* (pp. 764–771, 4th ed.). Chicago: YearBook Medical Publishers.

Ziegler, M.M. (1986). Short bowel syndrome in infancy: Etiology and management. *Clinics in Perinatology, 13(1),* 163–173.

Zitelli, B.J., Malatack, J.J., Gartner, J.C., et al. (1986). Evaluation of the pediatric patient for liver transplantation. *Pediatrics, 78,* 559–565.

CHAPTER 24

Oncologic Critical Care Problems

LORI J. KOZLOWSKI

Cancer has been perceived by many people, health professionals included, as a "terrible, hopeless disease that leads to certain death" (Fanslow, 1985, p. 43). But today pessimism is decreased and a degree of optimism prevails. The treatment of childhood cancers has made tremendous strides in recent years with 65% of children with cancer now surviving more than 5 years after diagnosis (Robison, 1993). Many childhood malignancies that were once universally fatal are now potentially curable. Examples include acute lymphocytic leukemia and Hodgkin's disease, which have significant chances of cure (Altman & Schwartz, 1983; Cohen, 1993; Liebhauser, 1993).

New drugs, combinations of existing drugs, and the use of drugs in combination with radiation therapy have led to more effective cancer therapy. Surgical techniques have also improved and have been combined with chemotherapy and radiation therapy to increase cure rates for many cancers. In addition, bone marrow transplantation offers new hope for many patients. Progress made in the research of biochemistry, genetics, and immunology may even lead to identification of causal agents in childhood cancer (Hockenberry et al., 1986).

Traditional conservative approaches to therapy for children with cancer, when the disease was considered fatal, have yielded to an aggressive philosophy in which cure is attempted. This change in focus has caused changes in implications for critical care nurses caring for these children. In the past, few of these children were admitted to critical care units, in most cases because it was felt that little benefit could be gained from intensive care. But with the use of more aggressive regimens and new immunologic and anti-infectious disease therapies, more of these children will be seen in critical care units (Gordon & Yeager, 1992).

Children with cancer may present to the critical care unit with dysfunction of several organ systems, leading to a variety of final common pathways. These

BONE MARROW TRANSPLANTATION

Bone marrow transplantation is being performed with increasing frequency in children with selected leukemias and solid neoplasms, as well as certain genetic, metabolic, and immune diseases (such as aplastic anemia, severe combined immunodeficiency syndrome, thalassemia major, and the leukodystrophies) (Frederick & Hanigan, 1993; Gordon & Yeager, 1992; Lie et al., 1988; Quinn, 1985). In past years, many of these diseases could not be successfully treated without very high doses of antineoplastic therapy. Unfortunately, the dose-limiting toxicity of these agents was bone marrow depression. Bone marrow transplantation was developed as a method of hematopoietic support for these patients. Successful bone marrow engraftment can mean long-term survival or cure (Cogliano-Shutta, Broda, & Gress, 1985; Dicke & Spitzer, 1986; Quinn, 1985).

Improvements in marrow-ablative therapies, supportive care, such as new treatments for infection and the use of hyperalimentation, and management of complications has dramatically increased the success rate for bone marrow transplants (Frederick & Hanigan, 1993; Quinn, 1985). This success continues to be limited, however, because of transplant-related toxicities. Many of these toxicities can be life-threatening and may require critical care resources. Acute complications described in this chapter include: acute respiratory failure, infections, veno-occlusive disease and graft-versus-host disease.

Bone marrow transplants are possible because stem cells, which are blood cell precursors, can be removed from one person and transplanted into another. By a process that is not yet understood, these stem cells move to the recipient's marrow, engraft, and produce a new hematopoietic and immune system (Frederick & Hanigan, 1993).

Three types of bone marrow transplants are available: autologous, syngeneic, and allogeneic. The difference between the types of transplants is the source of the bone marrow. Autologous transplantation uses the patient's own marrow. This type of transplant is an option for many children because the majority of those who could benefit from an allogeneic transplant do not have an acceptable donor. The marrow is collected during a period of disease remission. It is usually treated to destroy malignant cells that are present and then stored until a later date. Transplant protocols differ in the processing method of the bone marrow. The marrow is reinfused following patient treatment with marrow-ablative therapy such as high-dose chemotherapy and irradiation. Syngeneic transplantation uses bone marrow from an identical twin donor. The final type of bone marrow transplantation, allogeneic, uses a histocompatible transplant usually from a sibling or family member donor (Cogliano-Shutta et al., 1985; Quinn, 1985).

Pretransplant conditioning regimens usually involve high-dose chemotherapy alone or in combination with total body irradiation. These conditioning treatments are responsible for many of the complications that occur following transplantation. Protocols vary according to institutional practice and specific disease, with the most common regimen consisting of high-dose intravenous cyclophosphamide for 2 to 4 days and fractionated total body irradiation. These regimens serve to eradicate the recipient's malignant cells, suppress the body's immune system, and make room for the stem cells of the infused marrow. Bone marrow is infused intravenously, similar to the transfusion of a blood product, and stem cells repopulate the marrow cavities. Over the next several weeks the stem cells proliferate and differentiate. Immunosuppression is necessary to prevent rejection of the donor marrow (Meyers, 1986; Quinn, 1985, Rudder, 1990).

Extensive research is being conducted in bone marrow transplantation, which will allow even broader application of this treatment method. Currently under investigation are methods such as bone marrow T-cell depletion techniques that can decrease the risk of developing graft-versus-host disease and enable allogeneic transplants to be performed when donor and recipient are not histocompatible (i.e., donation by a carefully matched unrelated person). Biotherapy and immune technology are also being used to expand the application of bone marrow transplantation (Frederick & Hanigan, 1993). The use of peripheral blood stem cell transplantation has also emerged as an alternative method of transplantation, although the specific application of this technique in children is still being investigated (Demeocq et al., 1994; Kessinger & Armitage, 1991).

children may be admitted to the PICU at the time of diagnosis because of critical complications of the tumor itself. They may also require admission after a high-risk procedure such as an open lung biopsy, or because of life-threatening complications of antineoplastic therapy (Gordon & Yeager, 1992). Whatever the reason, the care of these children is often challenging. Critical care nurses must have an understanding of the child's underlying oncologic condition and the likely causes of life-threatening complications to appreciate the child's unique care needs.

Oncologic problems that may require critical care include acute respiratory failure, infection, renal failure, tumor mass effects, fluid accumulation, graft-versus-host disease, and veno-occlusive disease. This chapter will present these final common pathways as they relate to the critically ill child with an oncologic diagnosis. Management strategies particular to children with cancer will be discussed, whereas details regarding general therapies are outlined elsewhere in this book.

ACUTE RESPIRATORY FAILURE

The development of acute respiratory failure in the child with an oncologic disease frequently requires critical care resources. The inability to ventilate and adequately oxygenate can occur from a variety of infectious and noninfectious insults. These include pulmonary opportunistic infections and chemotherapy or radiation therapy–induced pulmonary disorders. Primary pulmonary malignancies are rare in children and do not account for many critical care unit admissions, with the exception of tracheal compression from a mediastinal mass (Gordon & Yeager, 1992; Freifeld, Hathorn & Pizzo, 1993).

A number of risk factors exist for the development of pulmonary problems in children with cancer. These include immunosuppression and resultant susceptibility to pulmonary infection, combination chemotherapy protocols, a history of radiation therapy to the lungs, and exposure to high oxygen concentrations after treatment with pulmonary-toxic chemotherapy (Sostman et al., 1977; Varricchio & Jassak, 1985).

Pathogenesis

In a non-neutropenic host, respiratory infections are attributed to the usual causes of community-acquired pneumonia. However, in the child with cancer who is neutropenic, intubated, or has a tumor mass that is obstructing the bronchus, bacterial pneumonias can be one of the most common causes of pulmonary infiltrates and can cause significant mortality. Gram-negative organisms are the most likely etiologic pathogens (Gordon & Yeager, 1992; White & Levine, 1991).

In the immunocompromised host, in particular those with extended periods of neutropenia (such as that which occurs with bone marrow transplantation) viral, fungal, or protozoal organisms may also be the cause of an infectious pneumonitis (Gordon & Yeager, 1992) (Table 24–1). These nonbacterial or interstitial pneumonias are among the most serious complications of bone marrow transplantation and can occur with varying severity in up to one half of all patients. Cytomegalovirus (CMV) is the most common causative organism in allogeneic bone marrow transplant recipients (Krowka et al., 1985; Quinn, 1985). The source of the virus may be from the donor in marrow transplants, from CMV-positive blood products administered to the child, or from reactivation of a latent infection (Gentry et al., 1987; Krowka et al.,

Table 24–1. DIFFERENTIAL DIAGNOSIS OF PULMONARY INFILTRATES IN THE CHILD WITH CANCER

Bacteria

Any gram-negative or gram-positive organism, including *Nocardia* and *Mycobacterium* species

Viruses

CMV
Herpes simplex
Varicella zoster
Measles

Parasites

Pneumocystis carinii
Toxoplasma gondii
Strongyloides stercoralis

Fungi

Aspergillus
Candida
Zygomycetes (mucor, absidia, rhizpus)
Cryptococcus

Miscellaneous

Chemotherapy
Radiation
Leukemic infiltrate

Data from Lode, H., et al. (1984). Diagnostic and therapeutic approach to nonbacterial pneumonias in immunosuppressed patients. In J. Klasterky (Ed.). *Infections in cancer patients* (p. 171). New York: Raven Press.

1985). Less commonly, cases can be attributed to herpes simplex and varicella zoster. Prophylactic therapy with acyclovir has reduced the morbidity of these infections. The incidence of protozoal *Pneumocystis carinii* pneumonitis, which was once quite common, has decreased greatly since the use of prophylactic trimethoprim-sulfamethoxazole, although it still does occur in immunocompromised hosts (Krowka et al., 1985; White & Levine, 1991). Fungal pneumonitis is most commonly diagnosed in a neutropenic host who has received prolonged antibacterial agents without evidence of clinical improvement. *Aspergillus* and *Candida* are the most common causative organisms (Freifeld et al., 1993; Krowka et al., 1985; Weiner et al., 1986).

In more than 50% of the cases of interstitial pneumonitis in bone marrow transplant patients, no pathogenic organism is identified. These cases are referred to as *idiopathic* and may represent unrecognized infections or the toxic effects of chemotherapy or radiation therapy that has been administered as part of the conditioning regimen. Mortality rates for idiopathic pneumonia can be as high as 60% (Quinn, 1985; Weiner et al., 1986).

As previously mentioned, pulmonary injury can be attributed to a variety of chemotherapeutic agents (Table 24–2). These can lead directly to respiratory dysfunction, or subclinical injury may be aggravated in the presence of additional respiratory complications (White & Levine, 1991). Lung damage from chemotherapeutic agents is often difficult to detect because such damage is usually insidious in onset and is caused by the presence of other sources of

Table 24–2. CHEMOTHERAPEUTIC AGENTS ASSOCIATED WITH PULMONARY INJURY

Adriamycin
Bleomycin
Busulfan
Cyclophosphamide
Cytosine arabinoside
Methotrexate

pulmonary injury such as infection, radiation, or metastatic lung disease, which can complicate diagnosis. Some chemotherapy agents may cause dose-dependent pulmonary changes, whereas others, such as methotrexate, may actually cause an inflammatory-type hypersensitivity reaction. Drug-associated lung injury appears histologically as diffuse alveolar damage. Pulmonary fibrosis may occur as interstitial and/or alveolar exudates worsen (Sostman et al., 1977; Varricchio & Jassak, 1985).

Radiation therapy can also cause toxic pulmonary changes (Fig. 24–1). Radiation to the lung fields can cause an acute inflammatory response of the lung tissue (Chernecky & Ramsey, 1984). In animal and human studies it appears that the initial injury in both chemotherapy and radiation therapy–induced injury occurs to the capillary endothelium soon after exposure. Subsequently, inflammation, alveolar involvement, and fibrosis develops (Gordon & Yeager, 1992). Radiation damage to the lungs is related to the total dose received, the dose rate, and the volume of lung tissue irradiated. The more radiation that is administered to the lung fields, the greater the damage (Meyers et al., 1982; Varricchio & Jassak, 1985).

All children undergoing bone marrow transplantation receive a conditioning regimen that is aimed at eradicating the recipient's malignancy while allowing engraftment of the donor marrow (Krowka et al., 1985). These regimens usually include combinations of chemotherapy and radiation therapy (Chessells, 1988). Chemotherapy-related damage to the lungs

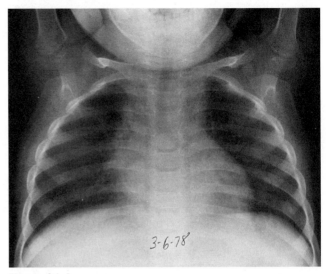

Figure 24–1 ● ● ● ● ● ●
Bilateral peritracheal and parahilar infiltrates resulting from radiation pneumonitis.

has been previously discussed. To minimize radiation damage to the lungs during total body irradiation, the radiation is fractionated. This process causes less damage to normal tissue. Shielding of the lungs during certain portions of the therapy can also minimize lung risks (Brochstein et al., 1987; Quinn, 1985).

Pulmonary complications occurring from bone marrow transplantation are often described according to the time that they occur in the transplant process (Fig. 24–2). The period from conditioning therapy to 1 month following transplant is the time when severe neutropenia makes the child more susceptible to gram-negative and fungal pneumonia. Fluid management is also a problem at this time. During the 1- to 6-month post-transplant period, the neutrophil count is recovering but the immune system is not yet reconstituted and interstitial pneumonias are common. Causative organisms during this time include CMV

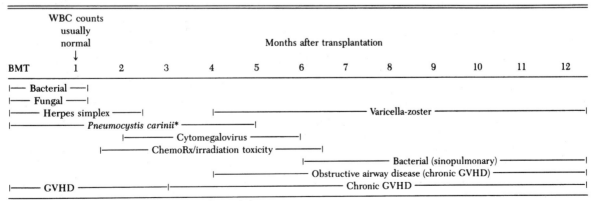

Figure 24–2 ● ● ● ● ● ●
Usual approximate time of onset of major complications after bone marrow transplantation (BMT). (From Krowka, M.J., Rosenow, E.C., & Hoagland, H.C. (1985). Pulmonary complications of bone marrow transplantation. *Chest*, 87(2), 239.)

as well as idiopathic lung problems. After 6 months, pulmonary dysfunction can be related to chronic graft-versus-host disease or continued immunologic deficiencies. Bacterial pneumonias continue to occur during this time (Krowka et al., 1985; White & Levine, 1991).

Pulmonary edema is another respiratory complication that can occur in the second and third week following bone marrow transplantation. The mechanism for this problem appears to be pulmonary endothelial cell damage caused by chemotherapy and radiation, compounded by iatrogenic fluid overloading. This leads to a capillary leak syndrome (Dickout et al., 1987). Some children are more susceptible to fluid management problems resulting from anthracycline administration and subsequent cardiotoxicity. Even without this history, the multiple antibiotics, hyperalimentation, blood products, and pre-chemotherapy hydration that most of these children receive complicate fluid management (White & Levine, 1991).

There are also reports in the literature of severe obstructive lung disease following bone marrow transplantation, which appears to be related to chronic graft-versus-host disease or a complex interaction of transplant, chemotherapy, radiation therapy, and infection (Krowka et al., 1985). Lung function tests may show obstructive ventilatory impairment that does not respond to bronchodilator administration. The onset usually occurs more than 3 months following transplant in patients with chronic graft-versus-host disease. The onset can be insidious or sudden and is manifested by cough, wheezing, and dyspnea. The chest radiograph may be normal or may show hyperventilation and air trapping. The condition is often progressive, with significant morbidity and mortality (Johnson et al., 1984).

Clinical Presentation

Clinical manifestations of acute respiratory failure in the child with an oncologic disorder include fever, cough (usually dry and hacking), rales, dyspnea, hypoxia, cyanosis, and tachypnea. The chest radiograph typically demonstrates a diffuse infiltrative pattern (Krowka et al., 1985; Sostman et al., 1977; Weiner et al., 1986) (Fig. 24–3).

Differential diagnosis of respiratory dysfunction in the child with cancer can be difficult and often requires invasive techniques. Diagnostic testing includes cultures, serology, radiologic studies including x-ray and chest computerized tomography (CT) scans, arterial blood gas analysis, and ventilatory function tests. Bronchoalveolar lavage (BAL) may be used to obtain samples for testing and isolate the causative organism. If this is unsuccessful, an open lung biopsy may be necessary to differentiate infectious and noninfectious causes (Freifeld et al., 1993; Krowka et al., 1985).

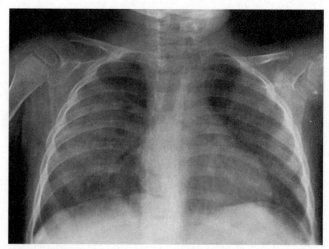

Figure 24–3 ● ● ● ● ● ●
Bilateral diffuse peripheral infiltrates in a 2-year-old boy with lymphoma proven to be *Pneumocystis carinii* pneumonia, which is sparing the central portions of the lung that are involved with radiation fibrosis.

Critical Care Management

Impaired Gas Exchange. Management of the child with cancer in acute respiratory failure focuses on the support of respiratory and circulatory function, minimizing the risk of pulmonary edema, aggressively identifying and treating infectious processes, and avoiding iatrogenic complications such as fluid overload.

Broad-spectrum antibiotics are started immediately in the child who develops fever and pulmonary symptoms. These are instituted even before receiving results of diagnostic testing because rapid progression to an overwhelming pneumonia and sepsis can occur (White & Levine, 1991). If the child is not already receiving trimethoprim-sulfamethoxazole, the preparation is usually initiated because of the risk of *P. carinii* infection (Gordon & Yeager, 1992). Antiviral agents, such as ganciclovir (DHPG), are currently being investigated for the treatment of CMV pneumonia and require confirmatory evidence of infection before use (Winston et al., 1987; White & Levine, 1991).

Supplemental oxygen is an essential aspect of therapy. The amount of oxygen that is required can be determined by usual methods of arterial blood gas monitoring and pulse oximetry. The child with cancer has the potential for enhanced oxygen toxicity as a consequence of previous chemotherapy or radiation therapy, and thus should be maintained on the lowest amount of oxygen that results in sufficient oxygenation.

The indications for mechanical ventilation in the child with cancer are similar to those for any child suffering from a diffuse interstitial-alveolar process. There are, however, some unique problems to consider in the population with cancer if intubation is required. The child may suffer upper airway bleeding from the trauma of intubation because of thrombocytopenia, coagulation abnormalities, or mucositis that already exists. Platelets, fresh frozen plasma, or vitamin K may be necessary before intubation to minimize the risk of bleeding. If intubation needs to be performed as an emergency, the oral route is preferred to the nasal route to diminish the risk of serious bleeding. Intubation can also increase the risk of infection in the immunosuppressed patient population (Carlon, 1985; Gordon & Yeager, 1992; White & Levine, 1991). Once the child has an airway in place, positive end-expiratory pressure (PEEP) is used at a level high enough to maintain the oxygen concentration at 40% to 50% or less to minimize the risk of toxicity. High airway pressures and rapid ventilatory rates may be necessary to maintain adequate gas exchange. It is imperative that the child be adequately sedated (Gordon & Yeager, 1992; Stokes, 1990).

General principles of nursing management of the critically ill child with respiratory compromise should be applied while caring for this patient population. Deterioration in respiratory function, however, may be sudden and dramatic warranting frequent respiratory assessments. In addition, an increased awareness of the need for strict aseptic technique when performing an invasive procedure, such as suctioning, is necessary for the immunocompromised child. Tracheal aspirate cultures should be obtained at least twice weekly and with any changes in the color, odor, or amount of secretions.

The child with cancer in a critical care unit is at increased risk for barotrauma because of the high levels of positive pressure ventilation that are often used. The respiratory assessment must therefore include observing for signs and symptoms of pneumothorax or pneumomediastinum.

If the child with acute respiratory failure is still receiving potentially toxic chemotherapy or radiation therapy, these treatments may need to be discontinued or modified to prevent further lung damage. Prevention of lung injury is important because there is no specific effective therapy for these causes of pulmonary dysfunction (Sostman et al., 1977; Varricchio & Jassak, 1985). High-dose corticosteroids may also be added to the treatment regimen to decrease lung inflammation (Gale & Quinn, 1989).

Decreased Cardiac Output. Inotropic support with agents such as dopamine and dobutamine may be necessary to maintain cardiac output, which is often compromised by high levels of PEEP. Swan-Ganz catheters are frequently inserted to assist in management (Gordon & Yeager, 1992; White & Levine, 1991). Frequent clinical assessment of cardiac output is imperative, including monitoring of all hemodynamic parameters.

Fluid Volume Excess. Diuretics are often used because of the oncology patient's increased susceptibility to fluid management problems (Carlon, 1985). The challenge of treatment of the child with cancer is to avoid fluid overload of the lungs while maintaining cardiac output, oxygen delivery, and urine output. Renal doses of dopamine may assist in maintaining effective diuresis in the face of poor cardiac function. Blood products and antibiotic infusions should be concentrated to reduce volume.

The frequent use of diuretic therapy requires close monitoring of intake and output records and twice-daily patient weights. Careful attention must also be made to hemodynamic data and serum electrolyte levels.

INFECTION

Despite progress made in the treatment of children with cancer, complications related to infection remain a leading cause of morbidity and mortality. (Altman & Schwartz, 1983; Griffin, 1986, Freifeld et al., 1993). As more intensive and aggressive treatments are used in the treatment of childhood cancer, more children become immunocompromised for a longer period of time and subsequently become more susceptible to infection. In addition to treatment intensity, the type of tumor and the state of the disease also contribute to the frequency and types of infection that occur (Freifeld et al., 1993). The critical care nurse must have an understanding of the risk factors for infection in the immunocompromised child, assess for the clinical syndromes that may occur, and initiate appropriate interventions.

Pathogenesis

The development of infection in children with cancer can be related to compromise in a variety of host defenses. The nature of the disease and the myelosuppressive action of chemotherapy and radiation therapy result in immune alterations that compromise the child's ability to combat infection. Specifically, there can be neutropenia caused by malignancy of the bone marrow or resulting from chemotherapy; cellular or humoral immunity defects; loss of the body's protective barriers to infection; direct access to the bloodstream by a variety of foreign bodies; malnutrition; and urinary, cerebrospinal fluid (CSF), or gastrointestinal obstructions (Gold, 1985; Weintraub, 1993) (Fig. 24–4).

The tumor itself can predispose the child to infection. Primary or metastatic tumors can cause obstruction that promotes infection by the colonizing of organisms at the site of the obstruction. For example, children with Wilms' tumor may experience an increased incidence of urinary tract infections as a result of urinary obstruction caused by the tumor (Altman & Schwartz, 1983; Freifeld et al., 1993; Weintraub, 1993). The tumor may erode through the body's protective barriers, such as the skin and mucosal surfaces, and permit the entrance of pathogens into the bloodstream. These protective barriers can

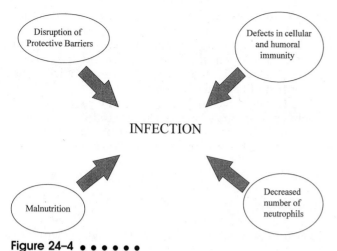

Figure 24–4 ● ● ● ● ● ●
Alterations in host defenses that result in infection.

also be broken by the numerous invasive diagnostic and therapeutic procedures performed on the critically ill child with cancer. Venous access devices, biopsies, pressure monitoring devices, respiratory care equipment and indwelling catheters all provide direct access to the bloodstream for a variety of pathogens.

Defects in cellular or humoral immunity further increase the susceptibility to infection in children with certain malignancies. Children with Hodgkin's disease and non-Hodgkin's lymphoma are known to have impaired T cell and monocyte function as well as diminished B cell function. Patients with leukemia may have defective cell-mediated immunity. Children who have undergone splenectomies, for example those undergoing staging procedures for Hodgkin's disease or cytoreductive therapy for chronic myelogenous leukemia (CML), are found to experience diminished antibody responses, the loss of specific phagocytosis factors, and loss of the spleen's filtering functions. These factors make these children more susceptible to infection with encapsulated organisms. Chemotherapy and radiation therapy regimens before bone marrow transplantation contribute to impairment of cellular and humoral immunity. Corticosteroids that are often used in therapy can alter leukocyte mobilization, diminish cell-mediated immunity, and impair phagocytosis (Allegretta et al., 1985a; Freifeld et al., 1993; Gold, 1985; Pizzo, 1981; Weintraub, 1993). In addition, any critically ill child will be at an increased risk for infection secondary to being in a debilitated state and being in a critical care environment (Gold, 1985; Gordon & Yeager, 1992; White & Levine, 1991).

Neutropenia, which is defined as an absolute neutrophil count (ANC) of 500/mm³ or less, is the most common immunologic defect in children with cancer and the single most important factor predisposing them to infection (Allegretta et al., 1985a; Freifeld et al., 1993). The ANC can be calculated by multiplying the total white blood cell count by the percentage of

band cells plus polymorphonuclear neutrophils (Altman & Schwartz, 1983).

The risk of serious infection has been shown to increase when the number of circulating neutrophils is less than 1000/mm³ (Gold, 1985). Pizzo (1981) adds that this infection risk is directly related to the extent and duration of neutropenia. The decreased number of neutrophils can be the result of the bone marrow–producing inadequate neutrophils, as seen in acute leukemias. Neutropenia also results because the bone marrow produces abnormal granulocytes that are not capable of participating in phagocytosis. In addition, antineoplastic chemotherapy or radiation therapy can also contribute to neutropenia (Freifeld et al., 1993; Gold, 1985).

Cancer treatment may contribute to new sources of infection. Stomatitis is a frequent side effect of certain chemotherapeutic agents, such as methotrexate, actinomycin-D, adriamycin, and transplant chemotherapy. Under certain conditions, septicemia can develop from stomatitis. Damage that occurs to the gastrointestinal (GI) mucosa from antineoplastic therapy may be the reason that enteric organisms are often isolated in the cancer patient with infection. Rectal fissures can occur and can be a source of fulminant infection, usually by gram-negative bacteria (Gold, 1985).

Malnutrition that often occurs in children with malignancies can increase susceptibility to infection. Nutritional alterations can have a direct impact on immune functioning, leading to impaired phagocytosis, decreased macrophage mobilization, and depressed lymphocyte function. Broad-spectrum antibiotic therapy, which is frequently used, can lead to alterations in microbial colonization and overgrowth of resistant organisms present in the critical care environment (Pizzo, 1981).

All of these factors put children with cancer at a significant risk for bacterial, fungal, viral, and protozoal infections. Bacterial infections are often the most serious acute infections occurring in children with cancer. As previously mentioned, neutropenia is the most common cause leading to bacterial infection. The organisms most often responsible for these infections include the gram-negative enteric bacilli, specifically *Escherichia coli, Klebsiella pneumoniae,* and *Pseudomonas aeruginosa.* The GI tract is the major portal for infection because of the multitude of organisms present there. *Staphylococcus aureus, S. epidermis,* and streptococci are the most common gram-positive organisms isolated in serious infections. Their source is most likely from venous access devices (Ellerhorst-Ryan, 1985; Freifeld et al., 1993).

Children with cancer are at risk for fungal infections because of the intensive use of broad-spectrum antibiotics (Weintraub, 1993). The most frequently encountered fungal infections in affected children include those from *Candida* and *Aspergillus.* The most common sites of infection include the oral cavity, sinuses, lungs, blood, and liver (Gordon & Yeager, 1992).

Candida infections can range from local infections

such as thrush to widespread dissemination. Mucosal lesions, which often occur as a result of cancer therapy, can provide a portal for *Candida* septicemia. *Candida* urinary tract infections can also occur in catheterized patients (Ellerhorst-Ryan, 1985). *Aspergillus* infection is usually characterized by a necrotizing pneumonia in children with cancer. The respiratory tract, GI tract, and brain are most often affected. Diagnosis of *Aspergillus* infection is often problematic because of difficulties in culturing the organism (Ellerhorst-Ryan, 1985; Gordon & Yeager, 1992).

Viral infections may cause significant morbidity and mortality in children with cancer, because they have the potential for rapid dissemination in these immunocompromised hosts. The most common viruses encountered in this population include herpes simplex, varicella zoster, and cytomegalovirus (Weintraub, 1993).

The herpesvirus group can be responsible for a variety of infections. Herpes simplex infections are usually more severe and prolonged in children with malignancies. Dissemination can occur with mucosal lesions, cellulitis, or pneumonia. Abnormalities in T cell function and diminished cell-mediated response to varicella zoster can cause fulminant varicella, which may disseminate to the liver, lung, and central nervous system. Every attempt is made to avoid exposure of immunocompromised patients to this virus. In children who have had varicella zoster infection, herpes zoster infection (shingles) can occur as a reactivation of this virus. Children with lymphomas appear to have the greatest risk for development of herpes zoster infection (Freifeld et al., 1993).

The most common cause of viral pneumonia in the immunocompromised host is CMV, especially in those who have undergone bone marrow transplantation. Pneumonitis is the most common clinical consequence of CMV infection in these children. The parainfluenza virus may also cause significant respiratory failure (Altman & Schwartz, 1983; Freifeld et al., 1993; Weintraub, 1993).

Protozoal infections in children with cancer are most commonly attributed to *P. carinii*. This organism is responsible for serious pneumonitis in this population. If untreated it is fatal in these patients. Prophylactic use of trimethoprim-sulfamethoxazole has proved to be very effective in decreasing the incidence of this infection (Pursell & Telzak, 1991). The prophylactic dose used by the Johns Hopkins Hospital Division of Pediatric Oncology is 150 mg/m^2/day by mouth in divided doses twice daily for 3 consecutive days each week.

Infection is the leading cause of morbidity and mortality in patients who have undergone a bone marrow transplant (Fig. 24–5). As the transplanted marrow engrafts, the immune system recovers (Pursell & Telzak, 1991). Mature blood cells are usually produced in 3 to 4 weeks (Quinn, 1985). The initial phase of severe neutropenia is characterized by bacterial and candidal infections as well as reactivation of latent herpes simplex virus, which can cause significant oropharyngeal infections. In the 1-

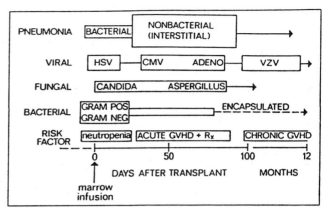

Figure 24–5 ● ● ● ● ● ●

Predisposing risk factors and common infections by time after marrow transplant. (Reproduced from Meyers, J.D. Infections in marrow recipients. In G.L. Mandell, et al., Eds. (1984). *Principles and practice of infectious diseases*, p. 1674. New York: Churchill Livingstone.)

to 3-month period following transplantation, infections from viruses, fungi, and protozoans develop, especially in patients with graft-versus-host disease. Serious viral infections, in particular those caused by CMV, are a major concern (Meyers, 1986). After this time, the possible development of chronic graft-versus-host disease and persistent immune defects lead to additional infections. Reactivation of varicella zoster is also responsible for infection during this period (Meyers, 1986; Pursell & Telzak, 1991).

Clinical Presentation

Because shock can ensue rapidly in these children, and host responses may be subtle, early recognition and prompt treatment of infections are imperative (Freifeld et al., 1993). If infection is undetected and left untreated in a patient with cancer, especially one who is neutropenic, it can prove to be fatal in a very short course. Detection of infection requires strong clinical judgment and a careful search for signs and symptoms, which are often covert (Gordon & Yeager, 1992). Fever is the single most consistent indicator of infection in the granulocytopenic patient because the lack of an inflammatory response prevents many of the classic signs and symptoms of infection from appearing. Common sites of infection in granulocytopenic patients include the skin, lungs, perioral region, GI tract, perirectal areas, and insertion sites of intravenous devices (Allegretta et al., 1985a; Griffin, 1986; Freifeld et al., 1993).

Diagnosis requires careful physical examination, with particular attention to the ears, nose, throat, abdomen, perirectal and perineal area, radiologic and laboratory evaluation (blood counts, electrolyte levels, and coagulation studies), and cultures of any potential infection source. Surveillance bacterial and fungal culture results of throat, urine, stool, and blood are often monitored twice weekly to allow for

early detection of infection. Even so, causes for fever
in children with cancer may be demonstrated in less
than one half of children with granulocytopenia during the initial evaluation. If invasive lines are in
place when the child becomes febrile, they must be
considered as potential infective sources (Freifeld et
al., 1993).

Critical Care Management

Potential for Infection. Any organism that
grows in cultures should be regarded as significant
and the child should be treated with an antibiotic
specific for that organism. However, as previously
mentioned, broad-spectrum antibiotic coverage is instituted promptly, once adequate cultures are obtained, at any time infection is suspected in a neutropenic patient until the etiologic agent is identified
(Freifeld et al., 1993; Gold, 1985; Gordon & Yeager,
1992). Subsequent management of the infection depends on the identification or lack of identification of
the causative organism and the duration of neutropenia. Children with a documented infection whose
fever is resolving and show an increase in the ANC
typically receive antibiotic therapy for 10 to 14 days.
If no infection is documented and fever and neutropenia resolve, antibiotic therapy is discontinued. For
children who are afebrile, without a documented infection, but are still neutropenic, Freifeld and coworkers (1993) recommend continuation of therapy
for 14 days and monitoring for further signs and
symptoms of infection.

Individual centers have varying protocols for specific antibiotics, but most give a combination of a
cephalosporin and/or a semisynthetic penicillin and
an aminoglycoside (Gold, 1985). When the child has
a venous access device, vancomycin is usually added
(Weintraub, 1993). Alternative regimens are available including agents such as imipenum and ceftazi-
dine as single-agent therapy (Freifeld et al., 1993).

In children with persistent fever and neutropenia,
antifungal treatment should be added. Amphotericin
B has been found to be the most reliable agent for
treatment of fungal infections (Allegretta et al.,
1985a; Freifeld et al., 1993; Gordon & Yeager, 1992).
A test dose of 0.1 mg/kg (up to a maximum of 1 mg)
is usually administered intravenously over 1 hour to
assess for anaphylaxis and other side effects. The
maintenance dose of 0.5 to 1.0 mg/kg/day is given
over 4 to 6 hours. Although it is very useful in the
treatment of fungal infections, amphotericin B is often accompanied by side effects that can complicate
care of the patient receiving this drug. Fever, chills,
and rigors can be minimized by the administration
of diphenhydramine (1 mg/kg intravenous) and acetaminophen (10–15 mg/kg) with meperidine (1 mg/
kg intravenously) as needed. When side effects are
severe, hydrocortisone (25–50 mg) may be added to
the infusion. Hypokalemia, hypomagnesemia, and
nephrotoxicity, including elevations in plasma urea
and creatinine and renal tubular acidosis, have also

been noted with amphotericin B. If renal function is
impaired, lowering the dose of amphotericin B or
administering the drug on alternate days may be
necessary. Documented fungal infections should be
treated for 4 to 6 weeks (Allegretta et al., 1985a;
Pursell & Telzak, 1991; Weintraub, 1993).

Protozoal and viral organisms must also be suspected, especially in the event of pulmonary infection. Acyclovir (250–500 mg/m^2 every 8 hours) is often used for the treatment of varicella zoster, herpes
simplex, and herpes zoster infections. It is also administered prophylactically to bone marrow transplant patients who are seropositive for herpes simplex to prevent stomatitis (125 mg/m^2). Studies are
in progress to examine prophylactic infusion of ganciclovir and intravenous immunoglobulin for CMV
prevention (Freifeld et al., 1993; Gale & Quinn,
1989).

The use of granulocyte transfusions to replace
these elements in the neutropenic patients remains
controversial. Freifeld and coworkers (1993) report
that data do not support their use for neutropenic
patients. Granulocyte-macrophage colony stimulating factor (GM-CSF) and granulocyte colony-stimulating factor (G-CSF) have been used as an alternative therapy to accelerate granulocyte recovery.
These cytokines, which accelerate hematopoiesis
when given following chemotherapy-induced neutropenia, have been shown to reduce the severity and
duration of neutropenia for some children (Freifeld
et al., 1993).

Varying degrees of protective isolation for the immunocompromised child are used by different institutions. Studies have demonstrated that reverse isolation has not been shown to reduce the acquisition
of new organisms in areas in which strict handwashing is followed. For most children with cancer, a
total protected environment is usually not necessary
(Freifeld et al., 1993; Griffin, 1986). When available,
however, the child with cancer should be placed in a
private room in the critical care unit. In all cases,
the benefits of invasive procedures must always be
weighed against the risks in this vulnerable population. Strict attention to handwashing technique is
crucial.

Because infection is a major cause of morbidity
and mortality for children with cancer, its prevention
and detection are the major goals of nursing management. Nursing measures to prevent and detect infection and specific management of sepsis and septic
shock are outlined elsewhere in this book, but monitoring vital signs, especially temperature, and obtaining cultures of suspicious sites with prompt physician notification are imperative for early detection.
The skin, oral, and rectal areas are assessed at least
every 4 hours to observe for irritation or breakdown.
Scrupulous mouth care should be performed several
times daily while assessing the oral cavity for leuko-
plakia or vesicles in the mouth. All breaks in the
skin integrity require ongoing evaluation as potential
sources of infection. Rectal procedures, such as temperatures, suppositories, or enemas are avoided to

minimize the risks of bacteremia and local infection. The child is also monitored for nonspecific signs of infection such as lethargy and irritability (Ellerhorst-Ryan, 1985).

Antibiotic therapy is administered as soon as it is ordered and is given promptly as scheduled. Infusion of antibiotics is usually given priority over other intravenous therapies.

The child who is receiving amphotericin B is monitored for nephrotoxicity (including blood urea nitrogen and creatinine levels and strict intake and output records), fever, chills, rigors, and electrolyte imbalances (in particular, serum potassium and magnesium levels). Potassium and magnesium supplements may be necessary. Premedication with antihistamines and antipyretics, as previously described, diminishes the fevers and chills associated with amphotericin B. Intravenous meperidine for severe rigors is usually most effective if given during chilling rather than as a premedication (Varricchio & Jassak, 1985; Weintraub, 1993).

RENAL FAILURE

Acute Tumor Lysis Syndrome

Renal failure in the child with cancer is often related to acute tumor lysis syndrome (ATLS). ATLS refers to a metabolic imbalance that occurs from the rapid release of intracellular components as a result of the degradation or lysis of tumor cells. The intracellular components uric acid, potassium, and phosphate may be released in amounts that the kidneys may not be able to clear adequately. These products can accumulate in the collecting ducts and cause renal failure (Allegretta et al., 1985b; Patterson & Klopovich, 1987).

Manifestations of ATLS are most often seen 1 to 5 days following cytotoxic therapy in tumors with rapid tumor cell proliferation, which are especially sensitive to chemotherapy. ATLS may also occur prior to cytoreductive therapy because spontaneous cytolysis can occur (Cohen et al., 1980; Lange et al., 1993).

ATLS occurs most frequently in cancers that have a rapidly dividing cell population. It is seen in lymphomas, especially Burkitt's lymphoma, as well as T cell leukemia/lymphoma, acute myeloid and lymphocytic leukemia, and chronic myeloid leukemia (Allegretta, Weisman, & Altman, 1985b; Lange et al., 1993; Patterson & Klopovich, 1987).

Pathogenesis

This syndrome consists of three metabolic imbalances that can occur individually or in combination. These include hyperuricemia, hyperkalemia, and hyperphosphatemia. Renal failure and hypocalcemia, which occurs from the interaction of calcium and phosphorus, are often resultant complications (Allegretta et al., 1985b; Lange et al., 1993).

Hyperuricemia can develop because uric acid is produced by the breakdown of purines that are released by fragmented tumor nuclei (Allegretta et al., 1985b). In an alkaline renal environment uric acid exists in a solution, however, in an acidic environment it is insoluble and tends to precipitate in the collecting ducts as crystals. The deposition of these crystals throughout the renal system can lead to renal failure (Lange et al., 1993; Patterson & Klopovich, 1987).

Hyperkalemia can occur because of potassium release during tumor cell lysis. It is usually the most immediate threat to life in children experiencing ATLS. Hyperkalemia can develop not only as a result of ATLS, but also from oliguric renal failure caused by hyperuricemia or hyperphosphatemia (Allegretta et al., 1985b; Lange et al., 1993).

Hyperphosphatemia occurs when phosphate is released with tumor cell lysis. In addition, the interaction of hyperphosphatemia with extracellular calcium causes calcium-phosphorus precipitation in the renal tubules, which can lead to hypocalcemia and possibly renal failure. If renal failure ensues, it also results in an increase in serum phosphorus because the body clears phosphorus only by glomerular filtration (Altman & Schwartz, 1983; Lange et al., 1993; Patterson & Klopovich, 1987).

Clinical Presentation

When caring for a child whose cancer has a large cell burden of tumor, the critical care nurse becomes alert for signs and symptoms of ATLS. Renal, cardiac, and neuromuscular complications can occur and are listed in Table 24–3. Laboratory analysis reveals elevated uric acid, phosphate, and potassium levels. Decreased serum calcium levels can also occur.

Various diagnostic measures are employed if the child is at risk for ATLS. Most importantly, renal function should be assessed prior to the institution of chemotherapy (Allegretta et al., 1985b). Studies have shown that children with pre-existing renal insufficiency are more likely to experience the metabolic imbalances of ATLS (Cohen et al., 1980; Lange et al., 1993).

Critical Care Management

Altered Urinary Elimination Patterns. The key to management of patients at risk for ATLS is prevention and identification of those who are most at risk for its development. To prevent progression to renal failure, management involves hydration, alkalinization, and allopurinol administration (Patterson & Klopovich, 1987). Admission to the critical care unit may be necessary before hydration of any child with preexisting respiratory compromise or of children with renal impairment, infiltration, or obstruction. Fluid balance is monitored to maintain renal perfusion without causing volume overload and pulmonary edema (Stokes, 1990).

The most important aspects of management in the prevention of renal failure are hydration and alkalin-

Table 24–3. CLINICAL MANIFESTATIONS OF ACUTE TUMOR LYSIS SYNDROME

Hyperuricemia
    Lethargy
    Nausea/vomiting
    Renal colic
    Flank pain
    Hematuria
    Oliguria
    Azotemia

Hyperphosphatemia
    Pruritic tissue changes
    Inflammation of the eyes and joints

Hypocalcemia (resultant)
    Anorexia
    Vomiting
    Cramps
    Tetany
    Altered level of consciousness
    Neuromuscular irritability
    Seizures
    Lethargy
    Numbness
    Tingling of the extremities
    Prolonged QT intervals

Hyperkalemia
    Muscles weakness
    Paresthesia
    Nausea
    Diarrhea
    Abdominal cramps
    Acidosis
    Asystole
    Elevated T waves
    Prolonged PR intervals
    Depressed ST segments
    Widened QRS

ization. The goal for the child is to reduce urate deposition in the kidneys and enhance the clearance of phosphate and urate. To accomplish this, intravenous fluids are infused at two to four times maintenance to keep a high rate of urine flow. Sodium bicarbonate is added to the fluid so that the urine pH is maintained at 7.0 to 7.5 with a specific gravity no greater than 1.010. Because uric acid is more soluble in alkaline urine, alkalinizing the urine during tumor lysis prevents the development of uric acid crystals. Diuretics may be administered to maintain a urine output of at least 1 ml/kg/hour. Vigorous urine alkalinization must be used with caution when hyperphosphatemia and hypocalcemia are present because crystals are less soluble at a urine pH above 6.0. Alkalinization is discontinued when uric acid levels are normalized, usually within 24 hours of starting therapy (Allegretta et al., 1985b; Lange et al., 1993; Panzarella & Duncan, 1993; Stokes, 1990).

Allopurinol should be administered to decrease uric acid production. It accomplishes this by inhibiting the enzyme xanthine oxidase, which is responsible for the formation of uric acid from the purine breakdown products hypoxanthine and xanthine (Lange et al., 1993; Patterson & Klopovich, 1987) (Fig. 24–6). The dose is usually 100 mg/m^2 orally every 8 hours (maximum dose is 600 mg/day). Allopurinol is also available in intravenous form as an investigational agent.

Hyperphosphatemia may be prevented by the use of binding resins such as aluminum hydroxide (100–150 mg/kg/day by mouth) which enhances phosphate excretion in the stool. Calcium supplements are used with caution because an increase in serum calcium while the patient is hyperphosphatemic may accelerate calcium-phosphorus precipitation (Allegretta et al., 1985b).

If hyperkalemia or renal failure develop, immediate intervention is necessary when the serum potassium is greater than 6.5 mEq/L or there are characteristic electrocardiogram (ECG) changes indicative of hyperkalemia (QRS widening and peaked T waves) (Allegretta et al., 1985b). Intravenous calcium gluconate (100–200 mg/kg) can be administered to induce intracellular shift of potassium and stabilize myocardial conduction. Intravenous insulin (0.1 unit/kg) with 25% glucose (2ml/kg) also induces an intracellular influx of potassium. Potassium intake is eliminated and Kayexalate (1 g/kg) with 50% sorbitol is administered orally. Intravenous sodium bicarbonate (1–2 mEq/kg) may also be administered to facilitate an intracellular shift of potassium (Allegretta et al., 1985b; Lange et al., 1993).

Emergent dialysis may be necessary in situations where hyperkalemia and renal failure cannot be managed with the measures described. It may also be used in cases when neurologic symptoms develop. Hemodialysis is preferred to peritoneal dialysis for its ability to remove uric acid more efficiently (Allegretta et al., 1985b; Lange et al., 1993; Patterson & Klopovich, 1987). Continuous venovenous hemofiltration (CVVH) has been used in children with renal failure from ATLS.

The critical care nurse ensures that hydration, alkalinization, and allopurinol administration are instituted at least 24 hours before starting chemotherapy (Patterson & Klopovich, 1987). Additional nursing interventions are similar to those for critically ill children who are experiencing acute renal failure from any cause. Monitoring, including hourly urine outputs, urine pH and urine specific gravity with each void, and frequent electrolyte levels (at least every 6–8 hours) is imperative.

TUMOR MASS EFFECTS

Specific complications may occur in the child with cancer that are related to the effect of the tumor itself. These include leukostasis, superior vena cava syndrome, and spinal cord compression.

Leukostasis

Leukostasis is the clinical symptom of hyperleukocytosis, which is defined as a peripheral white blood cell count exceeding 100,000/mm^3 (Lange et al.,

Figure 24–6 ● ● ● ● ● ●

Mechanism of uric acid formation from purine break-down. (Adapted from Altman, A.J., Schwartz, A.D. (1983). *Malignant diseases of infancy, childhood, and adolescence*, 2nd ed, p. 138. Philadelphia: W.B. Saunders.)

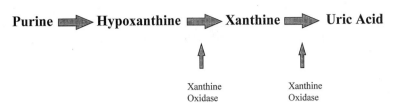

1993). The high numbers of circulating blasts cause capillary obstruction, microinfarction, and organ dysfunction. The lungs and brain are usually involved as target organs for this damage (Allegretta et al., 1985b). Leukostasis is most often associated with the myeloid leukemias, as compared with the lymphoid leukemias (Allegretta et al., 1985b; White & Levine, 1991). Lange and coworkers (1993) describe leukostasis as occurring in 9% to 13% of children with acute lymphocytic leukemia (ALL), in 5% to 22% of children with acute non-lymphocytic leukemia (ANLL), and in most children with chronic myelogenous leukemia (CML) in chronic phase. Rowe and Lichtman (1984) found in their group of 10 children with CML that hyperleukocytosis and leukostasis were much more common in children than in adults with CML, and that it required immediate cytoreduction. The increased prevalence in ANLL and CML occurs because of the large cell myeloblast, rather than smaller cell lymphoblasts, which do not move as freely through the microcirculation (Bunin & Pui, 1985; Lange et al., 1993).

Pathogenesis

The many blasts impair blood flow by causing sludging and thrombi formation in the small vessels of the lung and brain. Accumulation and vessel wall invasion by these blasts can also lead to rupture and bleeding. Often, lactic acidosis develops from the diminished tissue perfusion and anaerobic metabolism of the blast cells (Lange et al., 1993; Lichtman & Rowe, 1982).

Leukostasis in the capillary beds of the brain or lung can cause life-threatening complications. In the cerebral vasculature, local cell proliferation occurs with resultant vessel damage and secondary hemorrhage. In the lungs, alveolar damage occurs as blast cells degenerate in the pulmonary vessels and interstitium, releasing their intracellular contents. Leukostasis can cause death by intracerebral hemorrhage or thrombosis, pulmonary leukostasis, or metabolic imbalances that can occur with acute tumor lysis syndrome (Lange et al., 1993; Sheridan, 1990).

Clinical Presentation

The clinical presentation is most often related to the pulmonary and central nervous systems, although many children experiencing leukostasis do not exhibit specific signs and symptoms. Pulmonary leukostasis can lead to a variety of clinical manifestations, from infiltrates and dyspnea to hypoxia requiring intubation. Additional signs and symptoms include acidosis, blurred vision, agitation and confusion, ataxia, delirium or stupor. Plethora, cyanosis and papilledema are noted on physical examination (Lange et al., 1993; Sheridan, 1990).

Diagnostic workup of children suspected of experiencing leukostasis includes a complete blood count with clotting times, arterial blood gas analysis, chest radiograph, and CT scan. In addition, a venogram or arteriogram may be performed.

Critical Care Management

Potential for Injury Related to Leukostatic-Induced Complications. Treatment for leukostasis is aimed at reducing the number of circulating leukocytes. Management includes the immediate institution of hydration, alkalinization, and allopurinol administration, as discussed in ATLS management, as well as the prompt initiation of specific cytoreductive therapy (Lange et al., 1993).

As with any child with an oncologic disorder, these children may require platelet and red blood cell transfusions. Platelet transfusions are administered when the platelet count falls below 20,000/mm³ to minimize the risk of cerebral hemorrhage. Red blood cell transfusions are used cautiously because their use causes a further increase in blood viscosity. It is often recommended that the hemoglobin level not be higher than 10 g/dL or the whole blood viscosity maintained at or below a hematocrit equivalent to 45% (Allegretta et al., 1985b; Lange et al., 1993).

To reduce a large tumor cell burden and the metabolic load on the kidneys, children presenting with high white blood cell counts (usually higher than 300,000/mm³) may undergo exchange transfusions or leukapheresis (Allegretta et al., 1985b; Lange et al., 1993). In small children, exchange transfusion is often less difficult than leukapheresis (Lichtman & Rowe, 1982). Some centers also recommend the use of cranial irradiation to prevent central nervous system hemorrhage. All of these procedures are controversial; therefore, institutions differ on their approaches to the management of children with hyperleukocytosis (Lange et al., 1993).

Children with leukostasis require careful pulmonary and neurologic assessment for the development of complications such as respiratory failure and cerebrovascular accident. In addition, hematologic laboratory data must be monitored frequently. The nurse prepares the child and family for immediate chemotherapy as well as for the possibility of cranial irradiation or exchange transfusions. Ventilatory management may be needed in situations of severe neurologic or respiratory deterioration.

Superior Vena Cava Syndrome

Superior vena cava syndrome (SVCS) occurs when the superior vena cava (SVC) is compressed by external pressure, such as that produced by enlarged lymph nodes or tumor, invasion by tumor, or obstruction internally (Chernecky & Ramsey, 1984). The SVC is very susceptible to obstruction and does not resist extrinsic mechanical compression. It is a thin-walled, potentially collapsible vessel with a relatively low intravascular pressure that is located within a tight compartment formed by the mediastinum and sternum. In addition, the location of the lymph nodes, which surround the SVC, and the thymus may also cause compression of the vena cava when involved with tumor (Ahmann, 1984; Faro, 1987; Lange et al., 1993; Morse et al., 1985).

Although this is a relatively rare condition in children, it can occur in about 12% of children with malignant anterior mediastinal tumors at presentation (Faro, 1987; Issa et al., 1983; Lange et al., 1993) (Fig. 24-7). SVCS occurs most frequently in children with metastatic diseases such as Hodgkin's disease and non-Hodgkin's lymphomas (Allegretta et al., 1985b). Other related malignancies include mediastinal granulomas, neuroblastoma, rhabdomyosarcoma,

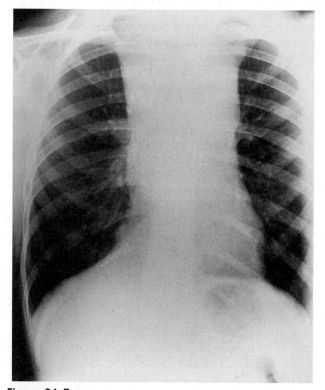

Figure 24–7 • • • • • •

Superior mediastinal mass with superior vena cava syndrome in a child with lymphosarcoma.

and Ewing's sarcoma. Non-neoplastic etiologies include thrombotic complications of venous access devices, which are used frequently in children with cancer (Faro, 1987; Issa et al., 1983; Lange et al., 1993).

Pathogenesis

Blood and air flow can both be decreased as a result of compression, clotting, and edema of the SVC. Venous drainage from the head, upper thorax, and upper extremities is decreased or completely blocked, resulting in venous hypertension (Faro, 1987; Lange et al., 1993).

In children, tracheal compression and respiratory distress can occur in addition to the SVC obstruction that occurs in adults. This variation is termed *superior mediastinal syndrome* (Ingram et al., 1990; Lange et al., 1993). Despite the relative rigidity of the trachea and right mainstem bronchus as compared with the SVC, these structures can become compressed with certain types of tumors, such as Hodgkin's or T cell lymphomas. In infants, very little edema is needed in the trachea and bronchi before obstruction occurs (Issa et al., 1983; Lange et al., 1993).

Clinical Presentation

Diagnosis of SVCS is often determined by evaluation of the child's clinical condition. Symptoms may not be as severe with the development of adequate collateral circulation, which allows blood to be circulated around the obstruction (Sculier & Feld, 1985; Morse et al., 1985). Tachypnea, wheezing, cough, and stridor may be among the presenting symptoms in a child who has compression of the trachea or bronchus. The child may avoid lying supine to minimize respiratory distress (Faro, 1987).

Other signs and symptoms include hoarseness, dyspnea, and chest pain. Dilation of the collateral veins of the head and neck may be evident along with facial swelling and neck and upper torso edema. Fullness may be noted in the brachial veins if the right arm is raised above the chest. Conjunctival edema is an additional manifestation. Signs and symptoms of increased intracranial pressure may be observed, which results from venous obstruction. Signs and symptoms include drowsiness, lethargy, confusion, headache, and distorted vision (Ahmann, 1984; Faro, 1987; Lange et al., 1993; Sculier & Feld, 1985).

Severe airway obstruction and cerebral anoxia can occur if SVCS is not detected promptly. The extent of the diagnostic workup and initial management is dictated by the respiratory status of the child. Invasive procedures are done only if severe respiratory compromise does not exist. Diagnosis should be attempted by the least invasive means possible, because many measures can carry a high risk and may lead to respiratory distress. Blood counts and bone marrow studies may demonstrate a malignant process. Biopsy of an accessible peripheral node may be performed under local anesthesia, because general anesthesia can be a risk due to the cardiovascular and respiratory alterations that occur and may aggravate SVCS by increasing the effects of extrinsic compression (Allegretta et al., 1985b). A chest radiograph may demonstrate a mass in the anterior mediastinum as well as tracheal compression. Chest computed tomography (CT) or magnetic resonance imaging (MRI) are necessary to determine the location and extent of the tumor and to quantitate the degree of obstruction. If there is a suspected thrombus within a central catheter believed to be the etiology for SVCS, MRI or venograms may be used as a diagnostic tool (Faro, 1987; Lange et al., 1993; Issa et al., 1983; Sculier & Feld, 1985).

Critical Care Management

Potential for Injury Related to Compression. Radiation therapy and chemotherapy are the initial and primary modes of treatment (Allegretta et al., 1985b; Altman & Schwartz, 1983). The goal of therapy is to relieve symptoms and decrease growth of the mass. The aggressiveness of initial management is dependent upon the child's clinical condition on presentation. Empiric prebiopsy radiation therapy and/or chemotherapy is instituted if respiratory compromise is evident. Otherwise, there is time for biopsy and diagnosis (Faro, 1987; Morse et al., Flynn, 1985).

Diuretics are administered to reduce edema but should be used with care to prevent dehydration and further decrease in blood flow. Steroids may be given for cytoreduction of the tumor and to reduce inflammation caused by tumor invasion or compression, providing symptomatic relief (Faro, 1987; Morse et al., 1985; Sculier & Feld, 1985).

Most children demonstrate subjective relief of symptoms within 72 hours and objective improvement within 1 week (Allegretta et al., 1985b; Morse et al., 1985). Thrombolytic therapy is instituted in those situations when SVCS is associated with intracaval thrombosis (Faro, 1987). Lange and coworkers (1993) describe success with infusion of urokinase at 200 mg/kg/hour.

Mechanical ventilation may be required, if airway obstruction exists, until the tumor bulk decreases. Children experiencing SVCS are at a much higher risk for complications, including death, during intubation. They may suffer cardiac arrest when placed in a supine position for sedation and/or anesthesia, which may cause further impedance of venous return and airflow. These children are at risk to develop complete airway obstruction if they are given neuromuscular blockades or general anesthesia (Gordon & Yeager, 1992; Lange et al., 1993; White & Levine, 1991). Halothane induction of anesthesia and fiberoptic tracheal intubation are recommended by Gordon and Yeager (1992) in cases of severe airway obstruction.

SVCS is an emergency that requires prompt inter-

vention to maintain airway patency and to monitor and maintain oxygenation and ventilation. The critical care nurse observes for changes in status and prevents further side effects of therapy. The nurse frequently assesses for the development of respiratory distress. The child is positioned in a semi-Fowler position to improve gas exchange with supplemental oxygen administered as needed (Faro, 1987).

The child is assessed for neck distension, facial and periorbital edema, or trunk edema. If swelling of the upper extremities does exist, the lower extremities should be used for venous access and blood pressure measurements. The upper extremities may be elevated to promote venous return (Altman & Schwartz, 1983).

Because SVCS may produce cerebral anoxia, frequent neurologic assessments including pupillary changes, level of consciousness, sensory/motor function, and vision changes are important. Siderails are kept up at all times with restraints used as necessary for patient safety.

Spinal Cord Compression

Although primary spinal cord tumors are rare in children, when they do occur the effects can lead to severe neurologic morbidity (Lange et al., 1993; Pack & Maria, 1987). Lange and associates (1993) report that 4% of children with cancer develop spinal cord dysfunction, usually related to tumor compression. These children require critical care if they have acute decompensation with increased intracranial pressure, seizures, or a rapidly developing paraplegia.

Pathogenesis

Spinal cord compression can result from a primary tumor of the spine or from spinal metastases (Fig. 24–8). Epidural compression occurs most frequently (Altman & Schwartz, 1983; Lange et al., 1993). The cord can be damaged as a result of tumor infiltration or edema and ischemia, which cause significant neurologic sequela.

The majority of cases of spinal cord disease in children are caused by metastatic sarcomas (Lewis et al., 1986). Others include metastatic neuroblastoma, lymphomas and leukemias, Wilms' tumor or primary tumors of the central nervous system (Lange et al., 1993; Pack & Maria, 1987). Spinal cord compression is most often seen in the late stages of a metastatic malignancy, but it may also be the presenting symptom in neuroblastomas or lymphomas (Lange et al., 1993).

Clinical Presentation

Signs and symptoms of spinal cord compression (SCC) are dependent upon tumor location and age of the child. In infants and toddlers, it may be especially difficult to detect SCC because many of the

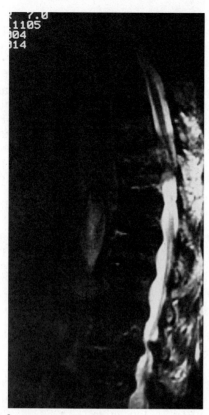

Figure 24–8 ● ● ● ● ● ●

Metastatic tumor at T9 with epidural disease and spinal cord compression.

clinical manifestations may be subtle, and children may find it difficult to describe their symptoms (Allegretta et al., 1985b; Pack & Maria, 1987).

Back pain is seen in up to 80% of children with SCC (Lange et al., 1993). This pain may be exaggerated by activities such as coughing and sneezing, straining, flexion of the back, and leg raising. Any pain must be assessed for location, intensity, radiation, duration, character, and aggravating and alleviating factors (Altman & Schwartz, 1983; Lange et al., 1993; Pack & Maria, 1987; Rodriguez & Dinapoli, 1980).

Motor weakness is another common manifestation of SCC (Allegretta et al., 1985b; Pack & Maria, 1987). Muscles must be assessed for strength and tone. Sensory deficits are often noted but may be difficult to assess in children. Numbness, tingling, and sensation loss may occur. Their location can help determine the extent of spinal cord involvement. Changes in bowel or bladder habits can also indicate spinal cord involvement. Respiratory dysfunction may occur from paresis of diaphragmatic and intercostal muscles (Allegretta et al., 1985b; Pack & Maria, 1987; Panzarella & Duncan, 1993; Rodriguez & Dinapoli, 1980).

Attempts must be made to diagnose promptly and begin therapy for SCC. Any child with neoplastic disease and complaints of back pain must be presumed to have SCC until proved otherwise. Prognosis

for the child's recovery is usually determined by the extent and duration of spinal cord involvement when treatment is instituted (Klein, 1985; Lange et al., 1993).

Lumbar myelography is the most useful diagnostic tool for SCC (Allegretta et al., 1985b; Altman & Schwartz, 1983). Results demonstrate tumor location and the degree of cord block. During myelography, CSF can be obtained for cytologic and chemical studies (Allegretta et al., 1985b; Lewis et al., 1986; Pack & Maria, 1987).

MRI may be a beneficial tool for diagnostic workup, although its use in the detection of certain lesions has not been yet determined (Packer et al., 1986). In addition, spine radiographs may be obtained because they may aid in localization. A normal-appearing bone scan or spine films, however, does not rule out the possibility of epidural disease (Lange et al., 1993).

Critical Care Management

The current method of treatment for children with SCC depends on tumor type and status of disease and may include surgical decompression of the spine (laminectomy), radiotherapy, and/or chemotherapy. Surgery is indicated when tumor identification has not been made because this can be accomplished during the procedure (Altman & Schwartz, 1983; Klein, 1985; Lange et al., 1993).

In children whose disease is widely metastatic, palliation can be achieved with radiotherapy. Children who have tumors sensitive to chemotherapy may require the use of these agents as an alternative treatment, in particular those children with lymphoma or neuroblastoma (Hayes et al., 1984). If compression signs occur or are severe or progressive, dexamethasone is given at a dose of 1 to 2 mg/kg intravenously, followed by immediate myelogram or MRI (Lange et al., 1993; Lewis et al., 1986).

Potential for Ineffective Breathing Patterns Related to Ventilatory Dysfunction. The child is frequently monitored for signs of ventilatory dysfunction, which may be caused by thoracic or cervical tumors (Pack & Maria, 1987). Chest wall movements must be monitored as well as the presence of cough, gag, and swallow reflexes. Supplemental oxygen and ventilatory support may be needed, as arterial blood gas results and pulmonary function data indicate. Pulmonary toilet measures are important to minimize the risk of pneumonia and atelectasis (Couillard-Getreuer, 1985).

Decreased Cardiac Output Related to Diminished Vasomotor Tone. Vital signs are assessed to monitor for hypotension related to decreased vasomotor tone, hypothermia from central nervous system (CNS) alterations, and bradycardia, which may be indicative of sympathetic or parasympathetic nervous system involvement (Couillard-Getreuer, 1985; Pack & Maria, 1987). Additional interventions are those used for any critically ill child with decreased cardiac output.

Alteration in Bowel and Urinary Elimination Related to Cord Compression. Assessment for urinary retention and constipation are critical. The presence of urinary retention may require the use of an indwelling urinary catheter to monitor renal function and fluid status. An intermittent catheterization program is instituted as soon as possible to promote reflex bladder emptying.

Maintenance of a nasogastric tube to low intermittent suction may be necessary for the child with impaired bowel function. Assessment of the abdomen, including abdominal girth measurements, should take place at least every 8 hours. A bowel program, including the use of stool softeners, may be indicated. Because of their increased susceptibility to infection, children with cancer require meticulous perianal skin care.

Impaired Physical Mobility Related to Neuron Damage. Children with impaired mobility require frequent assessments of muscle strength, tone, reflexes, and upper and lower extremity movement (Couillard-Getreuer, 1985). Lower extremity denervation may result in loss of tone and sensation. This can lead to pressure sores, contractures, loss of skin integrity and muscle atrophy. Careful attention is directed toward maintaining proper body alignment and passive range of motion exercises.

Alteration in Comfort and Pain Related to Spinal Cord and Spinal Root Compression. The child may experience a wide variety of pain symptoms related to cord compression. Interventions include the administration of analgesics while providing ongoing pain assessment and evaluation of effectiveness.

FLUID ACCUMULATION

Pleural Effusion

Pathogenesis

Pleural effusions in the child with cancer may occur for a variety of reasons. These include irritation of the pleural membrane by cancer cells, an extension of the tumor itself, lymphatic or venous obstruction of the pleura by a mediastinal mass, or infection. In addition, chylous effusions may occur from obstruction of the lymphatics (Lange et al., 1993). Children at risk for this complication include those with leukemia, Hodgkin's disease and non-Hodgkin's lymphoma, sarcomas, neuroblastoma, and Wilms' tumor (Altman & Schwartz, 1983; Chernecky & Ramsey, 1984; Lange et al., 1993).

Clinical Presentation

Signs and symptoms of pleural effusion include dyspnea, cough, pleuritic chest pain, tachypnea, and tachycardia. Physical examination may reveal dullness on percussion over the infected area (Altman & Schwartz, 1983).

Diagnosis of pleural effusion involves techniques similar to those used with pleural effusion from other disease processes. Chest radiographs help confirm the presence of fluid in the pleural space. Pleural fluid can also be examined for the presence of malignant cells or to rule out infection (Altman & Schwartz, 1983).

Critical Care Management

Ineffective Breathing Patterns Related to Fluid Accumulation and Decreased Pulmonary Function. Thoracentesis and possibly chest tube placement are indicated to drain the fluid when it is causing respiratory distress, or to make a diagnosis. In addition, sclerotherapy may be necessary to prevent or delay formation of a new effusion (Lange et al., 1993). Sclerotherapy employs agents such as tetracycline, talc, or bleomycin to cause adhesions and irritation in the pleural or pericardial spaces. The procedure consists of the injection of these agents into the respective spaces, which may be repeated for several days as needed. Ultrasound examination may be helpful to guide the physician to the effusion area, especially when the effusion is loculated. Therapy specific to the disease process should be instituted (Chernecky & Ramsey, 1984).

Careful respiratory assessment and monitoring are necessary for the child with a pleural effusion. In addition, the nurse needs to be aware of the procedure and possible side effects of various sclerotherapy techniques. These side effects are dependent upon agents used but can include pain, nausea and vomiting, infection, inflammation, hypoxia, pneumothorax, and hemothorax.

Pericardial Effusion and Cardiac Tamponade

In children with cancer, the etiology of pericardial effusion can be much different than that in other children who present to the critical care unit with this clinical syndrome. Pericardial effusion in this population can be caused by compression of the heart by pericardial fluid from tumor invasion or infection, a resultant constrictive fibrosis from radiation therapy, metastatic spread of tumor, or actual tumors of the cardiac muscle or pericardium. Pericardial effusions may be seen in children with Wilms' tumor in whom a thrombus can extend into the heart, in those children who have received radiation therapy to the chest, and in children with lymphomas and other primary mediastinal tumors (Altman & Schwartz, 1983; Lange et al., 1993).

Pericardial effusions are a rare presentation for children with malignancies. Chronic accumulation of fluid permits the pericardium to stretch gradually over time and allow it to accommodate large fluid volumes before cardiac tamponade occurs. However, if the fluid accumulates rapidly, circulatory effects are more profound (Concilus & Bohachick, 1984; Lange et al., 1993).

Clinical Presentation

The signs and symptoms of cardiac tamponade and diagnostic techniques have been discussed earlier in Chapter 19. As always, prompt recognition and treatment are imperative.

Critical Care Management

Decreased Cardiac Output Related to Impaired Ventricular Filling. The management of pericardial effusions is dictated by the degree of existing circulatory compromise. Supportive care includes hydration, oxygen, and positioning to achieve maximum patient comfort. Definitive therapy involves removal of the accumulated fluid, usually under echocardiography (Lange et al., 1993). Pericardiocentesis in children with cancer is not only therapeutic but also allows collection of a specimen for malignancy diagnosis. For those children who are thrombocytopenic or have evidence of other coagulopathies, platelets and fresh frozen plasma may be needed before pericardiocentesis. In situations where prolonged palliation is warranted, a pericardial window may be placed. Sclerotherapy may be indicated for those children with recurrent pericardial effusions (Altman & Schwartz, 1983).

GRAFT-VERSUS-HOST DISEASE

Graft-versus-host disease (GvHD) remains a significant cause of morbidity and mortality following bone marrow transplantation (Nimer et al., 1994). It is most commonly seen following allogeneic bone marrow transplantation but can also occur after autologous transplants. In addition, GvHD may develop from the administration of non-irradiated blood products to an immunoincompetent patient because of the presence of donor lymphocytes in the blood products (Altman & Schwartz, 1983; Quinn, 1985).

Pathogenesis

Unlike typical rejection that occurs in organ transplantation, graft-versus-host disease is caused by an immunologic reaction of the donor's graft to the bone marrow transplant recipient (host). It results from immunocompetent donor T cells recognizing the immunocompromised host as foreign and trying to reject the host. Specific tissues affected include the skin, liver, and GI tract (Cogliano-Shutta et al., 1985; Deeg & Storb, 1986).

GvHD is distinguished as acute or chronic. Acute GvHD occurs during the first 100 days following transplant and affects the previously mentioned organ systems. Chronic GvHD typically develops more than 100 days after transplant and has distinct clinical and pathologic changes that resemble those of an autoimmune disease (Quinn, 1985). There is an increased severity of acute GvHD in adults and a decreased incidence of chronic GvHD in children as compared with adults (Locatelli et al., 1993).

Clinical Presentation

Manifestations of acute GvHD may occur as early as 1 to 3 weeks following transplantation. Skin manifestations usually begin with a maculopapular rash involving the palms and soles, which is often intensely pruritic. This rash may resolve spontaneously or progress to severe sloughing and desquamation of the skin (Deeg & Storb, 1986; Parker & Cohen, 1983; Quinn, 1985).

Liver involvement can range from minimal jaundice and mild elevations in liver function test values to complete liver dysfunction (Quinn, 1985). Intestinal manifestations include secretory diarrhea, crampy abdominal pain, nausea, and anorexia that can progress to severe bloody diarrhea and sloughing of the intestinal mucosa. Immunologic deficiencies can also occur with GvHD and may lead to increased susceptibility to certain infections (Deeg & Storb, 1986; Parker & Cohen, 1983).

Chronic GvHD typically affects the lungs, joints, oral mucosa, and eyes. It is characterized by scleroderma-like skin lesions. Additional symptoms include ocular and oropharyngeal dryness, chronic hepatitis, esophagitis, and malabsorption. Bone marrow failure can occur with all types of GvHD (Quinn, 1985).

A histologic diagnosis is usually necessary to rule out other causative factors for the clinical signs and symptoms, including chemotherapy, radiation, or infection. Diagnosis is accomplished by biopsy of the involved organ. The severity of GvHD is then graded on a scale of I to IV based on the extent of damage to the organ (Table 24–4). This "stage" is then used to judge the severity of illness and to determine therapy and response to therapy (Parker & Cohen, 1983).

Critical Care Management

The ideal treatment for GvHD is to prevent its occurence. Selection of histocompatible (i.e., when human leukocyte antigens are closely matched) bone marrow donors is the first step in GvHD prophylaxis (Parker & Cohen, 1983; Quinn, 1985). The use of agents to suppress, remove, or inactivate T lymphocytes is also important in prevention. Methotrexate, cyclosporin, and prednisone have all been used (Cassano, et al., 1990; Deeg & Storb, 1986; Tollemar, et al., 1988). The donor marrow may be depleted of T cells to reduce the risk and severity of GvHD; however, this technique is associated with a greater risk of graft failure and relapse owing to an immune-mediated antileukemic effect of GvHD (Nimer et al., 1994; Vowels et al., 1988). Research is currently fo-

Table 24–4. STAGING AND GRADING OF SEVERITY OF GRAFT-VERSUS-HOST DISEASE

Proposed Clinical Stage of Graft-versus-Host Disease According to Organ System

Stage	Skin	Liver	Intestinal Tract
+	Maculopapular rash <25% of body surface	Bilirubin 2–3 mg/100 ml	>500 ml diarrhea/day
+ +	Maculopapular rash <25–50% of body surface	Bilirubin 3–6 mg/100 ml	>1000 ml diarrhea/day
+ + +	Generalized erythroderma	Bilirubin 6–15 mg/100 ml	>1500 ml diarrhea/day
+ + + +	Generalized erythroderma with bullous formation & desquamation	Bilirubin >15 mg/100 ml	Severe abdominal pain, with or without ileus

Overall Clinical Grading of Severity of Graft-versus-Host Disease

Grade	Degree of Organ Involvement
I	+ to + + skin rash; no gut involvement; no liver involvement; no decrease in clinical performance
II	+ to + + + skin rash; + gut involvement or + liver involvement (or both); mild decrease in clinical performance
III	+ + to + + + skin rash; + + to + + + gut involvement or + + to + + + + liver involvement (or both); marked decrease in clinical performance
IV	Similar to grade III with + + to + + + + organ involvement & extreme decrease in clinical performance

Reprinted, by permission of the New England Journal of Medicine, 292, 896, 1975.

cusing on alternate methods to prevent GvHD without increasing the relapse rate. Prevention of GvHD also includes the irradiation of all blood products administered to transplant patients to prevent the transfusion of active T lymphocytes from product donors. This process does not affect the function of the transfused blood product (Chernecky & Ramsey, 1984; Parker & Cohen, 1983; Quinn, 1985).

When GvHD does occur, treatment is based upon immunosuppression and supportive care. Mild (Grade I) cases may not always require intervention, but more extensive disease requires therapy with cyclosporin and corticosteroids. Thalidomide and monoclonal antibodies to T cells may also be used. Intestinal manifestations are often treated with hyperalimentation and bowel rest (Cogliano-Shutta et al., 1985; Deeg & Storb, 1986; Gale & Quinn, 1989).

Impaired Skin Integrity Related to T Cell Reaction to Host Cells. The skin should be assessed at least every 8 hours. In cases of Grade I and II GvHD of the skin, minor maculopapular rashes, dry skin, and itching can be treated with meticulous skin care and lubrication with lotions and creams. In addition, mild nonirritating soaps are used. Antihistamines may be administered for pruritus. More severe cases may require actual debridement of the skin.

The skin must be kept clean and dry, and adhesive tape is avoided. Skin lesions should be cultured as indicated.

Awareness of high infection risk to these children because of the loss of skin integrity is critical. Care to open areas of denuded skin may involve sulfadiazine (Silvadene) and Xeroform dressings similar to those used for burn patients (Parker & Cohen, 1983).

Alteration in Bowel Elimination Related to Diarrhea From GI Tract Effects. GvHD of the GI tract requires strict intake and output records, frequent (usually twice daily) weights, monitoring of electrolytes because stool output may be excessive, control of nausea and vomiting with antiemetics, meticulous rectal care after each stool, and nutritional support with hyperalimentation. The perianal area is assessed at least every 8 hours for redness, fissures, or signs of abscess formation. The stool is assessed for amount, color, and consistency. Frequent monitoring of hematocrit and platelet values may be necessary due to the potential blood loss through the GI tract. All stools should be tested for blood. These children are also at an increased risk for infection because of GI mucosal breakdown. Universal precautions and isolation procedures are followed carefully (Parker & Cohen, 1983).

Alteration in Comfort and Pain Related to Manifestations of GvHD. For children experiencing pain from the manifestations of GvHD, continuous infusions of narcotics are often required. The nurse constantly assesses the effectiveness of pain relief mechanisms and monitors the child's hemodynamic and respiratory parameters for changes associated with pain relief measures.

VENO-OCCLUSIVE DISEASE

In the early days of bone marrow transplantation, veno-occlusive disease (VOD) went essentially unrecognized as a separate disease process because liver problems were common in the post-transplant period. Patients often suffered from viral hepatitis, bacterial and fungal infections, GvHD, and liver complications from hyperalimentation. Recently, however, the role of VOD in liver dysfunction following transplant has been appreciated (Ford et al., 1983; Shulman et al., 1980). VOD is now recognized as a major complication of bone marrow transplantation (Baglin, 1994).

In the oncology population, several risk factors exist for the development of VOD. The most important risk factor is an elevated alanine aminotransferase (ALT) before transplantation. This has obvious implications for those responsible for choosing potential BMT candidates (Baglin, 1994; McDonald et al., 1984). Other risk factors include a diagnosis of acute myelogenous leukemia or chronic myelogenous leukemia, increased age, pretransplant conditioning regimens (in particular those that use busulfan), and having a second BMT (owing to previous exposure to intensive chemotherapy and radiation therapy, which injures the tissues of the hepatic cells and venous epithelium) (Frederick & Hanigan, 1993; Ford et al., 1983; Jones et al., 1987; McDonald et al., 1984).

Pathogenesis

VOD is characterized by deposits of fibrous materials that block small venules of the liver, causing an obstruction to blood flow leaving the liver. Sinusoidal outflow obstruction causes the fluid content of the blood to be drained through the lymphatic system and into the peritoneal cavity, leading to ascites. Over time, the disruption of normal blood flow through the liver also affects the pericentral hepatocytes, which may embolize into the central vein (Ford et al., 1983; Jones et al., 1987).

Clinical Presentation

Symptoms typically develop 1 to 3 weeks following BMT and are initially the result of intrahepatic portal hypertension. Not all symptoms may occur in all children. Clinical characteristics depend on the degree of obstruction of hepatic blood flow. They include sudden weight gain, right upper quadrant pain, hepatomegaly, ascites, jaundice, encephalopathy, increased total bilirubin with normal or mildly elevated liver function tests, and coagulopathy. Some cases of VOD are self-limited with spontaneous resolution, whereas others are progressive and lethal (Baglin, 1994; Ford et al., 1983; Jones et al., 1987).

Other liver diseases that may have more specific treatments, such as hepatitis or GvHD, must be ruled out. Typically, jaundice appears later in GvHD, and ascites is not common in liver dysfunction caused by GvHD, hepatitis, and viral or fungal infections (Baglin, 1994). Diagnostic testing includes ultrasound and CT scanning, which may reveal a congested liver, ascites, or an enlarged portal vein (Ford et al., 1983). Doppler detection of reduced portal vein blood flow in VOD has also been described (Zieger & Koscielniak, 1993). Liver biopsies may also be performed, although they can be associated with a significant risk in the oncology population, because of thrombocytopenia (Baglin, 1994).

Critical Care Management

Potential for Injury Related to Liver Dysfunction. There is no known way to open the occluded liver vessels (Ford et al., 1983). Therefore, management is supportive to allow the liver to recover. This is achieved by treating the side effects of liver failure, which are fluid overload, third-spacing, electrolyte imbalances, and coagulation abnormalities. Other strategies specific to the child experiencing liver dysfunction from VOD include dose adjustment of transplant chemotherapy (busulfan) and use of low-dose heparin. Orthotopic liver transplantation and thrombolytic therapy with agents such as tissue plasmino-

gen activator have been suggested as treatment options (Baglin, 1994; Nimer et al., 1990). Prophylactic use of prostaglandin E_1 has also been described (Gluckman et al., 1990).

SUMMARY

New cancer treatment modalities are increasingly complex and aggressive. With the refinement of these treatment regimens, the use of high-dose intensive therapy, including BMT, will find broader application in cancer patients. Children receiving these regimens will more likely need critical care resources at various points during their initial diagnosis and therapy. Only by careful observation and frequent clinical updates will the care of these patients be managed successfully.

The transition to the critical care unit can often be a difficult one. Most children have been hospitalized often. Families are familiar with the oncology unit staff and routines. This transition can be facilitated by the primary nurse who can disseminate information regarding the child's previous history and response to procedures to the entire critical care team before the child's arrival, when time allows. Multidisciplinary patient care conferences can be useful to discuss treatment plans and allow expression of concerns regarding therapy. Parents should be empowered to remain involved in their child's care to the fullest extent possible.

It is essential that critical care nurses strive to incorporate knowledge of the complexities of care of the child with cancer into their practice. The nursing contribution to the team approach is a crucial and central one that will lead to improvement in outcomes for these children.

ACKNOWLEDGMENT

The author wishes to acknowledge Joseph M. Wiley, M.D. for his review of this chapter.

References

Ahmann, F.R. (1984). A reassessment of the clinical implications of the superior vena caval syndrome. *Journal of Clinical Oncology*, 2(8), 961–969.

Allegretta, G.J., Weisman, S.J., & Altman, A.J. (1985a). Oncologic emergencies: Hematologic and infectious complications of cancer and cancer treatment. *Pediatric Clinics of North America*, 32(3), 613–623.

Allegretta, G.J., Weisman, S.J., & Altman, A.J. (1985b). Oncologic emergencies: Metabolic and space-occupying consequences of cancer and cancer treatment. *Pediatric Clinics of North America*, 32(3), 601–611.

Altman, A.J., & Schwartz, A.D. (1983). *Malignant diseases of infancy, childhood and adolescence*. Philadelphia: W.B. Saunders.

Baglin, T.P. (1994). Veno-occlusive disease of the liver complicating bone marrow transplantation. *Bone Marrow Transplantation*, 13, 1–4.

Brochstein, J.A., Kernan, N.A., Groshen, S., Cirrincione, C.,

Shank, B., Emanuel, D., Laver, J., & O'Reilly, R.J. (1987). Allogeneic bone marrow transplantation after hyperfractionated total-body irradiation and cyclophosphamide in children with acute leukemia. *The New England Journal of Medicine*, 317(26), 1618–1624.

Bunin, N.J., & Pui, C-H. (1985). Differing complications of hyperleukocytosis in children with acute lymphoblastic or acute non-lymphoblastic leukemia. *Journal of Clinical Oncology*, 3(12), 1590–1595.

Carlon, G.C. (1985). Acute respiratory failure in the cancer patient. In W.S. Howland & G.C. Carlon (Eds.). *Critical care of the cancer patient* (pp. 39–60). Chicago: YearBook Medical Publishers.

Cassano, W.F., Gross, S., Graham-Pole, J., & Rudder, S. (1990). Graft versus host disease. In J.L. Blumer (Ed.). *A practical guide to pediatric intensive care* (pp. 509–514). St. Louis: Mosby–YearBook.

Chernecky, C.C., & Ramsey, P.W. (1984). *Critical nursing care of the client with cancer*. Norwalk, CT: Appleton-Century-Crofts.

Chessells, J.M. (1988). Bone marrow transplantation for leukaemia. *Archives of Diseases in Childhood*, 63(8), 879–882.

Cogliano-Shutta, N.A., Broda, E.J., & Gress, J.S. (1985). Bone marrow transplantation. An overview and comparison of autologous, syngeneic, and allogeneic treatment modalities. *Nursing Clinics of North America*, 20(1), 49–66.

Cohen, D.G. (1993). Acute lymphocytic leukemia. In G.V. Foley, D. Fochtman, & K.H. Mooney (Eds.). *Nursing care of the child with cancer* (pp. 208–225). Philadelphia: W.B. Saunders.

Cohen, L.F., Balow, J.E., Magrath, I.T., Poplack, D.G., & Ziegler, J.L. (1980). Acute tumor lysis syndrome. A review of 37 patients with Burkitt's lymphoma. *The American Journal of Medicine*, 68(4), 486–491.

Concilus, E.M., & Bohachick, P.A. (1984). Cancer: Pericardial effusion and tamponade. *Cancer Nursing*, 7, 391–398.

Couillard-Getreuer, D.L. (1985). Spinal cord compression. In B.L. Johnson, & J. Gross (Eds.). *Handbook of oncology nursing* (pp. 412–429). New York: Wiley Medical.

Deeg, H.J., & Storb, R. (1986). Acute and chronic graft-versus-host disease: Clinical manifestations, prophylaxis, and treatment. *Journal of the National Cancer Institute*, 76(6), 1325–1328.

Demeocq, F., Kanold, J., Chassagne, J., Bezou, M.J., Lutz, P., deLumley, L., Philip, I., Vannier, J.P., Margueritte, G., Lamagnere, J.P., Baranzelli, M.C., Lenat, A., Carla, H., & Malpuech, G. (1994). Successful blood stem cell collection and transplant in children weighing less than 25 kg. *Bone Marrow Transplantation*, 13, 43–50.

Dicke, K.A., & Spitzer, G. (1986). Evaluation of the use of high-dose cytoreduction with autologous marrow rescue in various malignancies. *Transplantation*, 41(1), 4–20.

Ellerhorst-Ryan, J.M. (1985). Complications of the myeloproliferative system: Infection and sepsis. *Seminars in Oncology Nursing*, 1(4), 244–250.

Fanslow, J. (1985). Attitudes of nurses toward cancer and cancer therapies. *Oncology Nursing Forum*, 12(1), 43–47.

Faro, V. (1987). Superior vena cava syndrome in pediatric oncology. *Journal of the Association of Pediatric Oncology Nurses*, 4(3&4), 32–35.

Ford, R., McClain, K., & Cunningham, B.A. (1983). Veno-occlusive disease following marrow transplantation. *Nursing Clinics of North America*, 18(3), 563–568.

Frederick, B., & Hanigan, M.J. (1993). Bone marrow transplantation. In G.V. Foley, D. Fochtman, & K.H. Mooney (Eds.). *Nursing care of the child with cancer* (pp. 130–178). Philadelphia: W.B. Saunders.

Freifeld, A.G., Hathorn, J.W., & Pizzo, P.A. (1993). Infectious complications in the pediatric cancer patient. In P.A. Pizzo & D.G. Poplack (Eds.). *Principles and practice of pediatric oncology* (pp. 987–1014). Philadelphia: J.B. Lippincott.

Gale, R.P., & Quinn, S.J. (1989). The management of acute leukemias. *Clinical Advances in Oncology Nursing*, 1(2), 1–7.

Gentry, L.O., Price, M.F., & Zeluff, B. (1987). Cytomegalovirus infection in the post-transplant patient. *Mediguide to Infectious Diseases*, 8(4), 1–3.

Gluckman, E., Jolivet, I., Scrobohaci, M.L., Devergie, A., Traineau, R., Bordeau-Esperou, H., Lehn, P., Faure, P., & Drouet, L. (1990). Use of prostaglandin E1 for prevention of liver veno-occlusive disease in leukaemic patients treated by allogeneic bone marrow transplantation. *British Journal of Haematology*, 74, 277–281.

Gold, J.W.M. (1985). Infectious complications of neoplastic diseases in the critical care unit. In W.S. Howland & G.C. Carlon (Eds.). *Critical care of the cancer patient* (pp. 261–274). Chicago: YearBook Medical Publishers.

Gordon, J.B., & Yeager, A.M. (1992). Management of the child with malignant disease in the pediatric intensive care unit. In M.C. Rogers (Ed.). *Textbook of pediatric intensive care* (pp. 1403–1440). Baltimore: Williams & Wilkins.

Griffin, J.P. (1986). Nursing care of the critically ill immunocompromised patient. *Critical Care Quarterly*, 9(1), 25–34.

Hayes, F.A., Thompson, E.I., Hvizdala, E., O'Connor, D., & Green, A.A. (1984). Chemotherapy as an alternative to laminectomy and radiation in the management of epidural tumor. *The Journal of Pediatrics*, 104(2), 221–224.

Hockenberry, M.J., Coody, D.K., & Falletta, J.M. (1986). Introduction to childhood cancer. In M.J. Hockenberry & D.K. Coody (Eds.). *Pediatric oncology and hematology. Perspectives on care* (pp. 3–13). St. Louis: C.V. Mosby.

Ingram, L., Rivera, G.K., & Shapiro, D.N. (1990). Superior vena cava syndrome associated with childhood malignancy: Analysis of 24 cases. *Medical and Pediatric Oncology*, 18, 476–481.

Issa, P.Y., Brihi, E.R., Janin, Y., & Slim, M.S. (1983). Superior vena cava syndrome in childhood: Report of ten cases and review of the literature. *Pediatrics*, 71(3), 337–341.

Johnson, F.L., Stokes, D.C., Ruggiero, M., Dalla-Pozza, L., & Callihan, T.R. (1984). Chronic obstructive airways disease after bone marrow transplantation. *The Journal of Pediatrics*, 105(3), 370–376.

Jones, R.J., Lee, K.S.K., Beschorner, W.E., Vogel, V.G., Grochow, L.B., Braine, H.G., Vogelsang, G.B., Sensenbrenner, L.L., Santos, G.W., & Saral, R. (1987). Venoocclusive disease of the liver following bone marrow transplantation. *Transplantation*, 44(6), 778–783.

Kessinger, A., & Armitage, J.O. (1991). The evolving role of autologous peripheral stem cell transplantation following high-dose therapy for malignancies. *The Journal of the American Society of Hematology*, 77, 211–212.

Klein, P.W. (1985). Neurologic emergencies in oncology. *Seminars in Oncology Nursing*, 1(4), 278–284.

Krowka, M.J., Rosenow, E.C., & Hoagland, H.C. (1985). Pulmonary complications of bone marrow transplantation. *Chest*, 87(2), 237–246.

Lange, B., D'Angio, G., Ross, A.J., O'Neill, Jr., J.A., & Packer, R.J. (1993). Oncologic emergencies. In P.A. Pizzo & D.G. Poplack (Eds.). *Principles and practice of pediatric oncology* (pp. 951–972). Philadelphia: J.B. Lippincott.

Lewis, D.W., Packer, R.J., Raney, B., Rak, I.W., Belasco, J., & Lange, B. (1986). Incidence, presentation, and outcome of spinal cord disease in children with systemic cancer. *Pediatrics*, 78(3), 438–443.

Lichtman, M.A., & Rowe, J.M. (1982). Hyperleukocytic leukemias: Rheological, clinical and therapeutic considerations. *Blood*, 60(2), 279–283.

Lie, S.O., Glomstein, A., Slordahl, S.H., Storm-Mathisen, I., Albrechtsen, D., Young, E.P., & Patrick, A. (1988). Bone marrow transplantation in metabolic diseases. *Transplantation Proceedings*, 20(3), 499–500.

Liebhauser, P. (1993). Hodgkin's disease. In G.V. Foley, D. Fochtman, & K.H. Mooney (Eds.). *Nursing care of the child with cancer*, (pp. 254–263). Philadelphia: W.B. Saunders.

Locatelli, F., Uderzo, C., Dini, G., Zecca, M., Arcese, W., Messina, C., Andolina, M., Miniero, R., Porta, F., Rovelli, A., Pession, A., Rondelli, R., Paolucci, P. (1993). Graft-versus-host disease in children: The AIEOP-BMT Group experience with cyclosporin A. *Bone Marrow Transplantation*, 12, 627–633.

McDonald, G.B., Sharma, P., Matthews, D.E., Shulman, H.M., & Thomas, E.D. (1984). Venocclusive disease of the liver after bone marrow transplantation: Diagnosis, incidence, and predisposing factors. *Hepatology*, 4(1), 116–122.

Meyers, J.D. (1986). Infection in bone marrow transplant recipients. *The American Journal of Medicine*, 81 [Suppl. 1A], 27–38.

Meyers, J.D., Flournoy, N., & Thomas, E.D. (1982). Nonbacterial pneumonia after allogeneic marrow transplantation: A review of ten years' experience. *Reviews of Infectious Diseases*, 4(6), 1119–1132.

Morse, L.K., Heery, M.L., & Flynn, K.T. (1985). Early detection to avert the crisis of superior vena cava syndrome. *Cancer Nursing*, 8(4), 228–232.

Nimer, S.D., Giorgi, J., Gajewski, J.L., Ku, N., Schiller, G.J., Lee, K., Territo, M., Ho, W., Feig, S., Selch, M., Isacescu, V., Reichert, T.A., & Champlin, R.E. (1994). Selective depletion of CD8 + cells for prevention of graft-versus-host disease after bone marrow transplantation. *Transplantation*, 57(1), 82–87.

Nimer, S.D., Milewicz, A.L., Champlin, R.E., & Busuttil, R.W. (1990). Successful treatment of hepatic venoocclusive disease in a bone marrow transplant patient with orthotopic liver transplantation. *Transplantation*, 49(4), 819–821.

Pack, B., & Maria, B.L. (1987). Neurological emergencies in pediatric oncology. *Journal of the Association of Pediatric Oncology Nurses*, 4(3&4), 8–18.

Packer, R.J., Zimmerman, R.A., Sutton, L.N., Bilaniuk, L.T., Bruce, D.A., & Schut, L. (1986). Magnetic resonance imaging of spinal cord disease of childhood. *Pediatrics*, 78(2), 251–256.

Panzarella, C., & Duncan, J. (1993). Nursing management of physical care needs. In G.V. Foley, D. Fochtman, & K.H. Mooney (Eds.). *Nursing care of the child with cancer* (pp. 335–352). Philadelphia: W.B. Saunders.

Parker, N., & Cohen, T. (1983). Acute graft-versus-host disease in allogeneic marrow transplantation. *Nursing Clinics of North America*, 18(3), 569–577.

Patterson, K.L., & Klopovich, P. (1987). Metabolic emergencies in pediatric oncology: The acute tumor lysis syndrome. *Journal of the Association of Pediatric Oncology Nurses*, 4(3&4), 19–24.

Pizzo, P.A. (1981). Infectious complications in the child with cancer. I. Pathophysiology of the compromised host and the initial evaluation and management of the febrile cancer patient. *The Journal of Pediatrics*, 98(3), 341–354.

Pursell, K.J. & Telzak, E.E. (1991). Infectious complications of neoplastic diseases in the intensive care unit. In J.S. Groeger (Ed.). *Critical care of the cancer patient* (pp. 40–63). St. Louis: Mosby–YearBook.

Quinn, J.J. (1985). Bone marrow transplantation in the management of childhood cancer. *Pediatric Clinics of North America*, 32(3), 811–828.

Robison, L.L. (1993). General principles of the epidemiology of childhood cancer. In P.A. Pizzo & D.G. Poplack (Eds.). *Principles and practice of pediatric oncology* (pp. 3–10). Philadelphia: J.B. Lippincott.

Rodriguez, M., & Dinapoli, R.P. (1980). Spinal cord compression: With special reference to metastatic epidural tumors. *Mayo Clinic Proceedings*, 55, 442–448.

Rowe, J.M., & Lichtman, M.A. (1984). Hyperleukocytosis and leukostasis: Common features of childhood chronic myelogenous leukemia. *Blood*, 63(5), 1230–1234.

Rudder, S. (1990). Bone marrow transplant. In J.L. Blumer (Ed.). *A practical guide to pediatric intensive care* (pp. 505–508). St. Louis: Mosby–YearBook.

Sculier, J.P., & Feld, R. (1985). Superior vena cava obstruction syndrome: Recommendations for management. *Cancer Treatment Reviews*, 12, 209–218.

Sheridan, C.A. (1990). Uncommon leukemias: Implications for clinical practice. *Seminars in Oncology Nursing*, 6(1), 44–49.

Shulman, H.M., McDonald, G.B., Matthews, D., Doney, K.C., Kopecky, K.J., Gauvreau, J.M., & Thomas, E.D. (1980). An analysis of hepatic venocclusive disease and centrilobular hepatic degeneration following bone marrow transplantation. *Gastroenterology*, 79(6), 1178–1191.

Solodky, M., Mikos, K., Bordieri, J., & Modesitt, R. (1986). Nurses' prognosis for oncology and coronary heart disease patients. *Cancer Nursing*, 9, 243–247.

Sostman, H.D., Matthay, R.A., & Putman, C.E. (1977). Cytotoxic drug-induced lung disease. *The American Journal of Medicine*, 62(4), 608–615.

Stokes, D.N. (1990). Tumour lysis syndrome and the anesthesiologist: Intensive care aspects of pediatric oncology. *Seminars in Surgical Oncology*, 6, 156–161.

Tollemar, J., Ringden, O., Heimdahl, A., Lonnqvist, & Sundberg, B. (1988). Decreased incidence and severity of graft-versus-host disease in HLA matched and mismatched marrow recipients of cyclosporine and methotrexate. *Transplantation Proceedings*, 20 [Suppl. 3], 470–479.

Varricchio, C.G., & Jassak, P.F. (1985). Acute pulmonary disorders associated with cancer. *Seminars in Oncology Nursing*, 1(4), 269–277.

Vowels, M.R., Lam-Po-Tang, R., Ziegler, J., Ford, D., Trickett, A., White, L., & Mameghan, H. (1988). T cell depletion for matched marrow transplants. *Transplantation Proceedings*, 20(1), 38–39.

Weiner, R.S., Bortin, M.M., Gale, R.P., Gluckman, E. Kay, H.E.M., Kolb, H-J., Hartz, A.J., & Rimm, A.A. (1986). Interstitial pneumonitis after bone marrow transplantation: Assessment of risk factors. *Annals of Internal Medicine*, 104(2), 168–175.

Weintraub, M.H. (1993). Nursing management of the child or adolescent with infection. In G.V. Foley, D. Fochtman, & K.H. Mooney (Eds.). *Nursing care of the child with cancer* (pp. 372–384). Philadelphia: W.B. Saunders.

White, D.A., & Levine, S.J. (1991). Respiratory failure. In J.S. Groeger (Ed.). *Critical care of the cancer patient* (pp. 13–39). St. Louis: Mosby–YearBook.

Winston, D.J., Ho, W.G., Lin, C.-H., Bartoni, K., Budinger, M.D., Gale, R.P., & Champlin, R.E. (1987). Intravenous immune globulin for prevention of cytomegalovirus infection and interstitial pneumonia after bone marrow transplantation. *Annals of Internal Medicine*, 106(1), 12–18.

Zieger, M.H., & Koscielniak, E. (1993). Diagnosis and follow-up of veno-occlusive disease of the liver by use of doppler ultrasound. *Pediatric Radiology*, 23(2), 137–139.

CHAPTER *25*

Endocrine Critical Care Problems

KATHRYN M. MURPHY
CRAIG ALTER

**ENDOCRINE REGULATION OF WATER
  BALANCE**
Antidiuretic Hormone
Mineralocorticoids (Aldosterone)
Glucocorticoids
**DISTURBANCES OF WATER BALANCE:
  FLUID VOLUME DEFICIT**
ADH Deficit (Diabetes Insipidus)
**DISTURBANCES OF WATER BALANCE:
  FLUID VOLUME EXCESS**
ADH Excess (Syndrome of
  Inappropriate ADH Secretion)
**ADRENOCORTICAL INSUFFICIENCY:
FLUID VOLUME DEFICIT**

**ENDOCRINE REGULATION OF GLUCOSE
  HOMEOSTASIS**
Hormonal Regulation of Glucose Balance
Glucose, Protein, and Fat Metabolism
**DISTURBANCES OF GLUCOSE
  HOMEOSTASIS: HYPOGLYCEMIA**
Insulin Excess
Deficits of Counterregulatory Hormones
Disorders of Fasting Adaptation
**DISTURBANCES OF GLUCOSE
  HOMEOSTASIS: HYPERGLYCEMIA**
Excess of Counterregulatory Enzymes
Insulin Resistance and Deficit (Diabetic
  Ketoacidosis)

The endocrine system is a complex communication network that allows the body to regulate growth, development, metabolism, and sexual differentiation. This integrated system of feedback loops is dependent on glands that facilitate or inhibit the secretion of hormones into the bloodstream. Figure 25–1 provides an overview of the endocrine system and the glands involved in this regulatory process.

The most frequently encountered endocrine emergencies in children can be grouped into two final common pathways: (1) alterations in fluid and electrolyte balance, and (2) alterations in glucose homeostasis. This chapter will review basic pathophysiology, diagnosis, and treatment of selected endocrine conditions. Recommendations for nursing management of the infant or child with a serious endocrine disturbance will be discussed within the context of fluid deficit or excess and hypoglycemia or hyperglycemia.

ENDOCRINE REGULATION OF WATER BALANCE

Water is distributed in the human body in two compartments: (1) intracellular fluids (70% of total body water), and (2) extracellular fluids, which includes plasma and interstitial fluids (30% of total body water). Osmolality is an important factor regulating fluid balance between the intracellular fluid (ICF) and the extracellular fluid (ECF) compartments. Normal plasma osmolality ranges between 270 and 285 mOsm/L. Sodium is the major cation of the ECF and usually accounts for 90% of the plasma osmolality. Hormonal action on the kidney influences the reabsorption and excretion of sodium and water and thereby permits the concentration, composition, and volume of body fluids to be maintained within this narrow osmotic range.

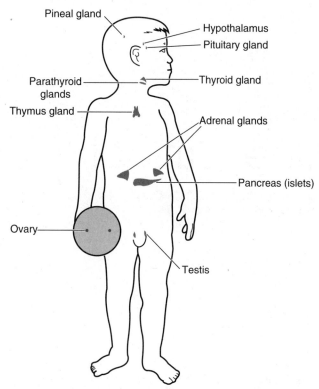

Figure 25–1 ● ● ● ● ● ●

The anatomic loci of the principal endocrine glands of the body. (Modified from Thompson, E.D., Ed. (1995). *Introduction to maternity and pediatric nursing,* 2nd ed., p. 835. Philadelphia: W.B. Saunders.)

Antidiuretic Hormone

Antidiuretic hormone (ADH) is formed in the supraoptic and paraventricular nuclei of the hypothalamus and is stored in the posterior pituitary. The effect of ADH is to increase the reabsorption of water in the collecting ducts of the kidneys. Through the action of ADH, water is returned to the vascular space and water loss in the urine is minimized. ADH secretion is governed by (1) plasma osmolality (receptors located in the third ventricle of the brain), and (2) blood pressure and plasma volume (stretch receptors located in the ascending aorta and left atrium). When the plasma osmolality is higher than 285 mOsm/L, the osmoreceptors in the hypothalamus are stimulated, resulting in a thirst sensation and ADH secretion. Hypovolemia is a potent stimulus for ADH secretion and thirst. Figure 25–2 illustrates the role of thirst and ADH in the process of osmotic regulation.

Mineralocorticoids (Aldosterone)

Aldosterone is secreted by the adrenal cortex. It acts on the renal tubules, resulting in the conservation of sodium and the excretion of potassium in the urine. Under the influence of aldosterone, water and sodium are returned to the vascular space and urine output is decreased. Aldosterone secretion is stimulated by hyperkalemia and the renin-angiotensin system. The renin-angiotensin system is stimulated by (1) decreased renal perfusion, (2) decreased blood volume, or (3) decreased blood pressure. In states of decreased circulatory volume, the kidney releases renin, which eventually leads to the formation of angiotensin II. The effect of the renin-angiotensin system on aldosterone and ADH is outlined in Figure 25–3.

Glucocorticoids

Glucocorticoids (cortisol) are produced and secreted by the adrenal cortex. Glucocorticoid production is regulated by the anterior pituitary. As circulating cortisol levels decrease, adrenocorticotropic hormone (ACTH) is secreted by the anterior pituitary. ACTH signals the adrenals to secrete cortisol. Glucocorticoids have a weak mineralocorticoid effect. As such,

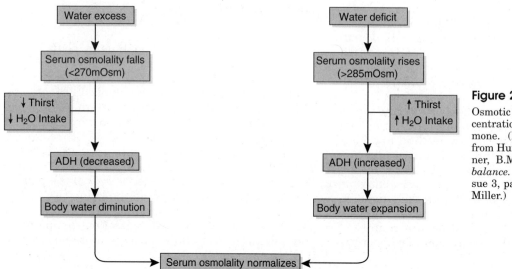

Figure 25–2 ● ● ● ● ● ●

Osmotic regulation of body fluids concentration. ADH, antidiuretic hormone. (Reproduced with permission from Humes, D., Narins, R.G., & Brenner, B.M. (1979). *Disorders of water balance.* Hospital Practice, Vol. 14, issue 3, page 136. Illustration by Albert Miller.)

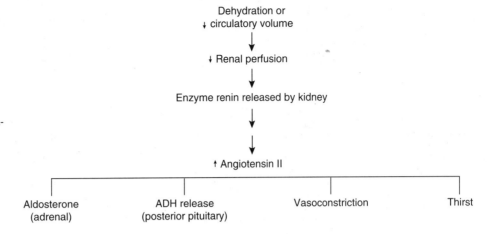

Figure 25-3 ● ● ● ● ● ●

Stimulation and effects of the renin-angiotensin system.

they enhance the reabsorption of water and sodium in the kidney, resulting in the return of water to the vascular space.

During illness, surgery, and trauma, increased production of glucocorticoid hormones is essential to support the body's stress response. Inadequate cortisol production may result in profound hypotension because of myocardial depression, poor arterial tone, and decreased responsiveness and synthesis of catecholamines. The hypothalamic-pituitary-adrenal axis is depicted in Figure 25-4.

DISTURBANCES OF WATER BALANCE: FLUID VOLUME DEFICIT

ADH Deficit (Diabetes Insipidus)

Central diabetes insipidus (DI) is a condition in which there is a deficit of ADH, resulting in decreased permeability of the renal distal tubules and loss of free water in the urine. Diabetes insipidus is usually associated with a central nervous system disorder that produces damage or pressure in the area of the hypothalamus, pituitary stalk, or posterior pituitary. The most common causes of central DI in children are outlined in Table 25-1.

Diabetes insipidus may also be the result of a primary renal defect. Primary renal DI is seen when the kidney's inherent ability to respond to ADH fails. Secondary renal DI is associated with intrinsic renal disease or other factors that interfere with the kidney's ability to concentrate water, such as protein deficiency, limited sodium intake, hypokalemia, hypercalcemia, and some drugs (lithium, demeclocycline).

The signs and symptoms of central DI and underlying pathology are outlined in Table 25-2. Urinary water losses result in an ECF deficit that may be significant enough to precipitate hypovolemic shock and cardiovascular collapse. Serum sodium may be extremely high because of the ECF volume depletion. The child with an intact thirst mechanism who is allowed to drink at will may be able to keep up with

urinary fluid losses and thereby maintain a normal serum sodium and serum osmolality. However, interference with usual access to water may rapidly precipitate volume depletion. Critical illness interferes with normal thirst, as well.

Diagnostic Presentation

Diagnostic findings are outlined in Table 25-3. The diagnosis of central DI hinges on the demonstration that urinary osmolality is inappropriately low (generally <100-200 mOsm/L) when serum osmolality is high (>285 mOsm/L) and serum sodium is high.

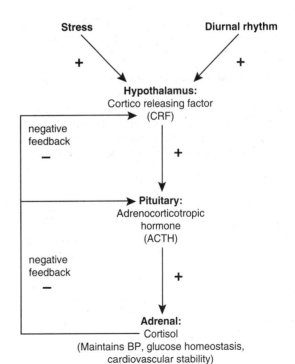

Figure 25-4 ● ● ● ● ● ●

Elements of the hypothalamic-pituitary-adrenal axis. Production of cortisol by the adrenals is not the result of local stimuli, but rather to signals from the pituitary (ACTH). Similarly, high cortisol or exogenous steroid suppresses the hypothalamus and pituitary and, therefore, the adrenal gland.

Table 25–1. ENDOCRINE CAUSES OF FLUID AND ELECTROLYTE IMBALANCE

Examples	Etiology
Diabetes insipidus	Central nervous system lesions: suprasellar tumor, trauma, ischemia, infection, granulomatous disease Congenital anomaly
Syndrome of inappropriate antidiuretic hormone (SIADH)	Central nervous system lesions: brain tumor, trauma, hemorrhage, seizures, hydrocephalus Pneumonia or other pulmonary disorders Mechanical ventilation with positive end-expiratory pressure Endocrine (hypopituitarism, adrenal insufficiency)
Adrenal insufficiency	Primary disease: Congenital adrenal hyperplasia Addison's disease Adrenoleukodystrophy Secondary disease: Hypothalamic pituitary disorder CNS trauma, tumor Iatrogenic: Abrupt withdrawal of high-dose steroids

These values demonstrate that water is inappropriately lost in the urine in the face of an ECF deficit and plasma hyperosmolality. Stimulation tests such as the water deprivation test and vasopressin test may be used to confirm the diagnosis. The water deprivation test involves the restriction of all fluids until 3% to 5% of body weight has been lost. Because of the risk of hypovolemic shock, vital signs are monitored closely along with hourly serum sodium, serum osmolality, urine osmolality, and body weight. At the completion of the test, vasopressin is administered subcutaneously or intranasally. A rise in urinary concentration and decreased output following the administration of vasopressin supports the diagnosis of

Table 25–2. ANTIDIURETIC HORMONE (ADH) DEFICIENCY (DIABETES INSIPIDUS)

Signs/Symptoms	Underlying Mechanism
Polyuria	ADH effect (decreased permeability of renal collecting tubules secondary to ADH deficit)
Urine hypoosmolar for plasma osmolarity	
Hypernatremia	ECF volume depletion
Plasma hyperosmolar	
Thirst, polydipsia, fatigue, anorexia	Dehydration
Shock Tachycardia, hypotension, decreased perfusion, weak thready pulse, cold clammy skin	Hypovolemia secondary to ECF volume depletion

ECF, extracellular fluid.

central DI. No detectable response in urine-concentrating ability is seen with nephrogenic DI.

Critical Care Management

Care of the child with central DI is outlined in Table 25–3. Nursing care is directed at the prevention of complications associated with hypovolemic shock and hyperosmolar encephalopathy. Urinary losses in these children may be significant, and failure to replace losses may result in hypovolemic shock and cardiovascular collapse. Urine losses may require replacement on a half-hourly or hourly basis. Careful monitoring of the child's neurologic status is essential so as to detect early signs of encephalopathy (headache, mental status changes, seizures, and cerebral edema). Encephalopathy is associated with over-rapid correction of hypernatremia. Children who are unconscious, who do not have an intact thirst mechanism, or who have an intact thirst mechanism but who are receiving fluids intravenously are at high risk both for the development of hypovolemia and water intoxication. These children require close monitoring of fluid intake, urine output, and body weight.

Vasopressin replacement is one approach to the treatment of central DI. The intravenous, subcutaneous, or intranasal routes are all viable options for vasopressin replacement. Children with DI who are receiving ADH replacement are at risk for problems with both underhydration (because of inadequate replacement of both ADH and fluids) and water intoxication (because of over-replacement of water in relation to renal losses). The unconscious child or infant presents a special challenge because of the risk of water intoxication. Therefore, shorter acting preparations such as vasopressin (Pitressin) or lypressin (Diapid) are preferred in this population. Desmopressin acetate (DDAVP), given intranasally, is a commonly used intermediate-acting preparation for home management. However, because of variability in absorption, it is not the preparation of choice in the critically ill patient.

A rise in urine specific gravity within 1 hour following the administration signals that the vasopressin has taken effect. Intravenous fluid rates must be readjusted once antidiuresis has been achieved to prevent volume overload and water intoxication. Serum sodium and osmolality are useful indices of water balance and are usually obtained hourly until intravenous infusion rates have been determined. Hourly monitoring of urine volume and specific gravity are necessary to provide data essential in determining vasopressin dosing.

A second approach to treatment may be selected to avoid the risk of water intoxication associated with vasopressin administration in the unconscious child. This approach involves withholding vasopressin and replacing urinary water losses on a half-hourly or hourly basis. Careful monitoring of fluid intake and output is essential, and laboratory studies (serum

Table 25–3. MANAGING ADH DEFICIENCY (DIABETES INSIPIDUS)

1. Participate in diagnostic workup
   History: Polyuria, enuresis, thirst, weight loss, fatigue, anorexia, poor growth

   Risk factors: Recent head trauma or surgery, CNS infection or ischemia, midline defects

   Physical examination: Dehydration
                           Hypovolemia/shock/cardiovascular collapse:
                              Tachycardia, weak, thready pulse
                              Skin cold, clammy; delayed capillary refill
                              Hypotension

   Laboratory tests: Serum osmolality increased (>290) / urine osmolality decreased (<200)
                           Hypernatremia
                           Urine specific gravity decreased
                           BUN increased

   Stimulation tests: Water deprivation test
                           Vasopressin test

2. Prevent complications associated with hypovolemia/shock/cardiovascular collapse
   Evaluate fluid balance: Compare urine output to fluid intake
                             Measure urine specific gravity
                             Monitor weight trends every 8 hours
                             Assess orthostatic blood pressure

   Observe for dehydration hypovolemia/shock/cardiovascular collapse (listed above)

   Replace deficit and ongoing losses: Bolus with 10–20 mL/kg of normal saline if hypotensive
                           Then 0.45% normal saline until perfusion improves
                           Replace urine losses until vasopressin effects are seen (urine specific gravity >1.010, and urine
                             output decreased)

   Replace ADH   Aqueous Pitressin (subcutaneous, IV infusion): 4–6 hour duration
                     DDAVP (intranasally): 8–24 hour duration
                     Diapid (intranasally): 4–6 hour duration
                     Desired effect: urine volume decreased to <2 mL/kg/hr
                                 urine specific gravity increased to >1.010
                                 urine osmolality increased
                                 normalization of serum sodium/osmolality

   Observe for signs of water intoxication secondary to overtreatment. (Correction of hypernatremia should be no greater than a decrease of 2 mEq/L/hr):   Mental status changes, headache
                             Nausea, vomiting
                             Lethargy, weakness
                             Seizures, coma

ADH, antidiuretic hormone; DDAVP, desmopressin acetate.

sodium, osmolality) are used to determine water and electrolyte replacement regimens.

The child who presents with significant hypernatremia (>155 mEq/L) is at risk for hyperosmolar encephalopathy and requires slow correction, usually over a 36- to 48-hour period to prevent hyperosmolar encephalopathy.

DISTURBANCES OF WATER BALANCE: FLUID VOLUME EXCESS

ADH Excess (Syndrome of Inappropriate ADH Secretion)

The syndrome of inappropriate secretion of antidiuretic hormone (SIADH) is a condition in which ADH is secreted in the face of serum hypoosmolality, hyponatremia, and euvolemia. Inappropriate ADH secretion results in increased permeability of the renal distal tubules and collecting ducts, increased water reabsorption, and a resultant decrease in urine volume.

As with DI, the underlying problem may stem from the hypothalamus, pituitary stalk, or posterior pituitary. However, various other factors are associated with the development of this disorder. The most common underlying causes of SIADH in children are outlined in Table 25–1.

The classic signs and symptoms of SIADH and the underlying mechanisms are outlined in Table 25–4. Hyponatremia and hypoosmolality both result from the dilutional effect of the ECF volume expansion. Worsening of the hypoosmolar state may precipitate a fluid shift of free water from the ECF to the ICF, which may result in cerebral edema.

Diagnostic Presentation

Diagnostic findings are outlined in Table 25–5. The diagnosis of SIADH hinges on the demonstration that urinary osmolality is inappropriately high for the low serum osmolality, in the face of euvolemia.

Critical Care Management

Treatment of the child with SIADH is outlined in Table 25–5. Nursing care is focused on the prevention

Table 25–4. ADH EXCESS (SIADH)

Signs/Symptoms	Underlying Mechanisms
Serum hypoosmolality	Dilutional effect
Serum hyponatremia	
Concentrated urine	ADH concentrates urine by
High urine sodium (>10–20 mEq/L)	increasing permeability of renal collection tubule
High fractional excretion of sodium	Decreased renin-angiotensin II and aldosterone result in sodium excretion
Nausea, vomiting, weakness	Hyponatremia
Mental status changes: Lethargy, irritability, headache (early) Pupillary changes, seizures, coma, death (late)	Cerebral edema resulting from fluid shift

SIADH, syndrome of inappropriate antidiuretic hormone.

of complications associated with water intoxication and hyponatremia. As with the child with DI, meticulous attention to fluid balance is essential. Fluid restriction is the mainstay of treatment. Early detection of neurologic changes associated with water intoxication is critical. Children with SIADH are at risk for cerebral edema because the hyponatremic state allows free water to move from the ECF space to the ICF space, from plasma to the intracellular space, including brain cells. The unconscious child who is receiving fluids intravenously and is thereby unable to regulate fluid intake is at increased risk for fluid overload. Emergency treatment of hyponatremia may be necessary if the hyponatremia is accompanied by neurologic symptoms. A standard approach involves the administration of a loop diuretic such as furosemide (Lasix) followed by infusion of a 3% sodium chloride solution to correct the hyponatremia.

ADRENOCORTICAL INSUFFICIENCY: FLUID VOLUME DEFICIT

Adrenocortical insufficiency is associated with a variety of conditions in which there is a deficiency of glucocorticoids (primarily cortisol), mineralocorticoids (aldosterone), or both. These conditions will be considered as a group because problems associated with an isolated mineralocorticoid deficiency are rare in children.

The adrenal glands also produce androgens. However, because these hormones have no direct effect on fluid balance, conditions associated with androgen excess or deficit will not be considered in this discussion.

Aldosterone deficiency causes decreased sodium and water reabsorption and increased potassium reabsorption in the renal distal tubules. Glucocorticoid deficits result in myocardial depression, poor arterial tone and decreased responsiveness, and synthesis of catecholamines, all of which contribute to the profound hypotension seen in these children. An isolated glucocorticoid deficit in the face of a significant stressor is sufficient to produce hypovolemia and shock.

Primary adrenocortical disease is associated with

Table 25–5. MANAGING ADH EXCESS (SIADH)

1. Participate in diagnostic workup	
History:	Nausea, vomiting, headache, weakness
Risk factors:	CNS infection, trauma, surgery Pneumonia, mechanical ventilation with positive end-expiratory pressure Adrenocortical hypofunction
Physical examination:	Nausea, vomiting, weakness Urine output decreased, normal skin turgor Mental status changes (lethargy, irritability, headache, seizures, coma, pupillary changes) Hypertension, tachycardia (late)
Laboratory tests:	Hyponatremia Serum osmolality decreased in the face of a high urine osmolality BUN normal or decreased Increased fractional excretion of urine sodium Urine sodium increased Urine osmolality increased
2. Prevent complications associated with water intoxication/hyponatremia	
Evaluate fluid balance:	Compare urine output to fluid intake Measure urine specific gravity Monitor weight trends every 8 hours
Evaluate for signs of water intoxication:	Headache, nausea, vomiting Lethargy, weakness, irritability Mental status changes, pupillary changes, seizures, coma
Restrict fluids:	Usually equal to amount of insensible losses or ½ to ¾ maintenance *After sodium correction* intake equivalent to output plus insensible losses
Treat acute hyponatremia:	Loop diuretic (furosemide) Followed by infusion of 3% NaCl solution

SIADH, syndrome of inappropriate ADH.

conditions that impair the ability of the adrenals to produce cortisol and/or aldosterone. Secondary adrenocortical disease reflects intrinsic hypothalamic or anterior pituitary dysfunction in which there is a problem with the production or excretion of ACTH. Although adrenal function is intact, cortisol is not produced because the adrenal glands do not receive an ACTH signal from the pituitary. Conditions such as congenital hypopituitarism, central nervous system trauma, or tumor are causes of secondary disease. Adrenal crisis may be precipitated in the child with known adrenal insufficiency who is not covered with higher doses of steroids during illness, surgery, or other significant stress. Figure 25–4 illustrates the hypothalamic-pituitary-adrenal axis.

Adrenocortical insufficiency may also be iatrogenic, as is seen with the administration of high-dose steroids over an extended period, resulting in the suppression of the hypothalamic-pituitary-adrenal axis. A fixed dose of exogenous cortisol is sufficient to meet normal daily needs. However, if exogenous steroids are abruptly withdrawn, or if additional coverage is not provided during stress or illness, the adrenals are unable to respond to the demands for increased cortisol production because the hypothalamic-pituitary axis has been suppressed. Regardless of the underlying dysfunction (whether primary, secondary, or iatrogenic), adrenal crisis may be precipitated when the body is unable to respond to the demand for increased glucocorticoid production.

The most common underlying causes of adrenocortical insufficiency in children are outlined in Table 25–1. Signs and symptoms of adrenocortical insufficiency and the underlying mechanisms are outlined in Table 25–6.

Diagnosis

Diagnostic findings are outlined in Table 25–7. The overall picture at the time of presentation is often that of profound hypovolemic shock. In primary adrenal insufficiency, the skin may appear tanned as a result of high levels of pituitary ACTH precursors. Associated electrolyte imbalances include hyponatremia, hyperkalemia, and hypoglycemia.

Critical Care Management

The treatment of the child with adrenal insufficiency is outlined in Table 25–7. Nursing care is focused on the prevention of complications associated with hypovolemic shock and the correction of electrolyte imbalances. Emergency resuscitation usually includes the use of a solution of normal saline to expand the vascular volume. Vasopressors (e.g., dopamine, epinephrine) may be used to exert a vasoconstrictive effect. Plasma expanders (e.g., 5% albumin) may be necessary if these interventions are not successful in reversing hypovolemic shock. If the serum potassium exceeds 5.5 mEq/L, strategies outlined in Table 25–7 may be used to manage acute hyperkalemia.

Emergency replacement of glucocorticoids is achieved intravenously using a soluble cortisol preparation such as hemisuccinate or 21-phosphate. Cortisol replacement may be given by continuous infusion or intravenous (IV) bolus every 4 to 6 hours. When the child can take medications orally, mineralocorticoid replacement is accomplished by giving fludrocortisone acetate (Florinef) daily. As with the previous disorders discussed in this section, meticulous attention to fluid and electrolyte balance is an important aspect of the nursing care of the child with acute adrenocortical hypofunction.

ENDOCRINE REGULATION OF GLUCOSE HOMEOSTASIS

Glucose is a primary fuel source for all body cells. Plasma glucose is normally maintained between 80 and 120 mg/dL. Five hormones are key contributors to the regulation of blood glucose. Insulin is the only one of the five that acts to lower blood glucose. The four counterregulatory hormones—glucagon, epinephrine, cortisol, and growth hormone—all oppose the effects of insulin and act to elevate the blood glucose during periods of hypoglycemia and stress.

Hormonal Regulation of Glucose Balance

Insulin is produced by the beta cells of the pancreas and has widespread effects on glucose, protein, and fat metabolism. Insulin lowers blood glucose, enhances protein synthesis, and inhibits lipolysis. Insulin release is regulated by blood glucose levels.

Glucagon is produced by the alpha cells of the pancreas. The action of glucagon is opposite to that of insulin. Glucagon raises blood glucose, facilitates the breakdown of proteins (thereby making amino

Table 25–6. ADRENOCORTICAL INSUFFICIENCY

Signs/Symptoms	Underlying Mechanisms
Serum hyponatremia Serum hyperkalemia	Mineralocorticoid effect (decreased sodium and increased potassium reabsorption in distal tubule)
	Glucocorticoid effect (decreased free water clearance)
Shock	Volume depletion
Tachycardia, hypotension, weak rapid pulse, cold clammy skin, decreased perfusion, fever	Vasodilation, myocardial depression, poor arterial tone, decreased responsiveness and synthesis of catecholamines
Nausea, vomiting, diarrhea, poor feeding, weakness, fatigue	Electrolyte imbalance and other less well understood mechanisms
Mental status changes, irritability	CNS changes resulting from fluid deficit or hypoglycemia
Hypoglycemia	Decreased gluconeogenesis

Table 25–7. TREATING WATER DEFICIT RELATED TO ADRENOCORTICAL HYPOFUNCTION

1. Participate in diagnostic workup

History:	Nausea, vomiting, diarrhea, fatigue, weakness, headache
Risk factors:	Hypopituitarism, congenital adrenal hyperplasia, abrupt discontinuation of high-dose steroids, known adrenally insufficient child who was ill and failed to receive stress coverage, CNS lesions (trauma, tumor, hemorrhage, seizures, hydrocephalus)
Physical examination:	Dehydration, fever Mental status changes, headache, irritability Shock (tachycardia, weak thready pulse, cold clammy skin, decreased perfusion, hypotension)
Laboratory tests:	Hyperkalemia Hyponatremia Hypoglycemia Serum cortisol level decreased
Stimulation tests:	Cortrosyn (adrenal function) Metyrapone (pituitary function)

2. Prevent complications related to hypovolemic shock, hyperkalemia, hypoglycemia

Evaluate fluid balance:	Compare urine output and fluid intake Monitor weight trends Measure urine specific gravity Assess orthostatic blood pressure
Monitor electrocardiogram for changes related to serum potassium level	
Treat acute hypovolemia, hyponatremia, and/or hypoglycemia:	Normal saline bolus then 5% glucose in normal saline Vasopressors Plasma expanders
Treat acute hyperkalemia:	Administer bicarbonate Calcium Lasix Glucose and insulin infusion Kayexalate enema
Replace mineralocorticoids:	Florinef orally daily (0.05–0.2 mg)

Replace glucocorticoids:	Emergency management:
	  Soluble cortisol (hydrocortisone: hemisuccinate or 21-phosphate)
	  Give 0.5–1 mg/kg/dose every 4–6 hours intravenously until showing signs of improvement

Observe for undertreatment:	Dehydration, shock

acids available for gluconeogenesis), and stimulates lipolysis. Glucagon release is stimulated by hypoglycemia and neural impulses associated with the stress response.

Epinephrine is produced in the adrenal medulla and is released in response to sympathetic nervous system stimulation during stress. Epinephrine raises blood glucose and stimulates lipolysis.

Glucocorticoids (primarily cortisol) are produced by the adrenal cortex and increase blood glucose. Cortisol release is under the control of ACTH and, for the purpose of this discussion, is stimulated by a stress response. Glucocorticoids increase blood glucose and stimulate lipolysis.

Growth hormone, produced by the anterior lobe of the pituitary, stimulates protein synthesis and lipolysis. Growth hormone also raises blood glucose. As with cortisol and epinephrine, growth hormone increases with stress.

Glucose, Protein, and Fat Metabolism

Insulin is the dominant hormone in the postprandial state. As nutrients are absorbed by the gut, blood glucose rises. The release of insulin is stimulated by a rise in blood glucose. High insulin levels have an inhibitory effect on the counterregulatory hormones. Insulin places the body in an anabolic state. Glucose is taken up in the liver and skeletal muscles. Amino acids are converted into protein; excess glucose, amino acids, and fatty acids are stored in adipose tissue. The effects of insulin on glucose, fat, and protein metabolism in the fed state are outlined in Table 25–8.

The counterregulatory hormones are the dominant hormones in the fasting state and in times of stress. These hormones work collectively to maintain blood glucose and meet the body's energy requirements. As blood glucose falls, insulin production is suppressed, and the inhibitory effects of insulin on the counterregulatory hormones are lost. Catabolic processes including gluconeogenesis, glycogenolysis, and lipolysis are called upon to meet energy requirements. Table 25–9 outlines the effects of insulin and the counterregulatory hormones on glucose, fat, and protein metabolism in the fasting state.

Hepatic glycogen stores are the initial glucose source in the fasting state. Healthy children may have sufficient glycogen stores to last up to 8 hours.

Table 25–8. GLUCOSE, FAT, AND PROTEIN METABOLISM FED STATE

Glucose

Glucose stored as glycogen in liver and skeletal muscles
  (↑ insulin)
Glycogenolysis inhibited (↑ insulin)
Gluconeogenesis inhibited (↑ insulin)

Fat

Excess glucose converted into fatty acids and stored in fat cells
  as triglycerides (↑ insulin)
Fatty acids and triglycerides stored in adipose tissue (↑ insulin)
Lipolysis inhibited (↑ insulin)

Protein

Excess amino acids converted to fatty acids and stored in adipose
  tissue (↑ insulin)
Amino acids converted into protein (↑ insulin)
Protein breakdown inhibited (↑ insulin)

The stores of the infant are limited and may be sufficient to maintain blood glucose for only approximately 4 to 6 hours. Following the depletion of glycogen stores, gluconeogenesis (the synthesis of glucose from noncarbohydrate substrates) accounts for the primary glucose source. The healthy young child can maintain blood glucose in the normal range for approximately 12 to 18 hours by switching to fatty acid oxygenation as a primary fuel source. Fasts extending longer than 12 hours necessitate the use of fatty acids as an alternative fuel source to spare body protein. Fatty acids can be used by muscle, heart, and kidney cells to meet energy requirements. Fatty acids are also oxidized in the liver to produce ketone bodies (beta-hydroxybutyrate and acetoacetate), which can be used as a fuel source by muscle and brain cells. Triglycerides become the primary fuel source by 18 hours of fasting.

Table 25–9. GLUCOSE, FAT, AND PROTEIN METABOLISM FASTING STATE

Glucose

Gluconeogenesis: synthesis of new glucose from noncarbohydrate
  sources (↑ growth hormone; ↑ cortisol; ↑ glucagon)
Glycogenolysis: breakdown of stored glycogen in liver and
  skeletal muscles (↑ epinephrine; ↑ glucagon)
Glucose uptake by body cells decreased (↑ glucagon; ↑ cortisol
  ↑ growth hormone)
Insulin release from beta cells inhibited (↑ epinephrine)

Fat

Triglycerides broken down into fatty acids and glycerol
  (↑ epinephrine; ↑ growth hormone; ↑ glucagon; ↑ insulin)
Fatty acids used by liver cells as an energy source
  (↑ epinephrine; ↑ growth hormone; ↑ glucagon)
Fatty acids converted to ketone bodies and used as an energy
  source (↑ epinephrine; ↑ growth hormone; ↑ glucagon)

Protein

Amino acids an important substrate for gluconeogenesis
  (↑ growth hormone; ↑ cortisol; ↑ glucagon)

DISTURBANCES OF GLUCOSE HOMEOSTASIS: HYPOGLYCEMIA

Hypoglycemia has been previously defined by various authors to be blood glucose less than 60 mg/dL in a child to under 20 mg/dL in the premature neonate. Although blood glucose in premature infants tends to run lower than in a full-term baby, it is difficult to prove that serum glucose levels in the 20 to 60 mg/dL range are safe. Therefore, in light of the profound effects of hypoglycemia on the developing brain, a blood glucose level less than 60 mg/dL should be considered hypoglycemic, even in the neonate. The therapeutic goal should be to maintain blood glucose above 65 to 70 mg/dL.

The most frequent underlying causes of hypoglycemia in the pediatric age group are outlined in Table 25–10.

Insulin Excess

Transient hypoglycemia may be seen in infants of diabetic mothers, infants with erythroblastosis fetalis, and when concentrations of glucose infused intravenously are abruptly discontinued. A period of transient hypoglycemia may follow this hyperglycemic state while the beta cells reregulate insulin production. All of these conditions result from a temporary hyperglycemic environment, which stimulates insulin production by the pancreas.

Table 25–10. ENDOCRINE CAUSES OF HYPOGLYCEMIA

Causes	Examples
Insulin overproduction	
Transient	Infants of diabetic mothers
	Rapid discontinuation of high-concentration dextrose infusion
	Erythroblastosis fetalis
	Exogenous insulin
Persistent	Hyperinsulinism
	Beckwith-Wiedemann syndrome
	Islet cell adenoma
Counterregulatory hormone deficits	Primary: adrenocortical dysfunction
	Secondary: pituitary/hypothalamic dysfunction
	Iatrogenic (adrenal suppression by high-dose steroids)
Problems with fasting adaptation	
Inadequate/inaccessible glycogen stores	Preterm, SGA, hypoxic, cold stressed, or septic infants;
Transient	congenital heart disease; starvation/malabsorption
	Hepatic failure (Reye's syndrome) toxins; cirrhosis
Persistent	Glycogen storage disease (types 1, 3)
Disorders of fatty acid metabolism	Medium chain acyl-dehydrogenase deficiency (MCAD)
	Carnitine deficiency

SGA, small for gestational age.

Persistent hypoglycemia is seen with beta cell hyperplasia (nesidioblastosis) and beta cell adenomas. These conditions are associated with an overproduction of insulin and a dramatic increase in the demand for glucose. Normal hepatic glucose production rates in the fasting state during infancy are in the 5 to 8 mg/kg/minute range. This decreases to 1.7 mg/kg/minute in the adult. The infant with one of these conditions often requires up to 20 mg/kg/min of glucose to maintain a normal blood glucose. Children with hyperinsulinism are particularly vulnerable because high insulin levels inhibit the safety net afforded by the counterregulatory response, including not only glycogenolysis and gluconeogenesis but also ketone production. (The brain can use ketone bodies for a significant portion of its energy demands.)

Deficits of Counterregulatory Hormones

Hypopituitarism and adrenal insufficiency are associated with a deficiency of either cortisol, growth hormone, or both. Hypoglycemia in both cases is the result of impaired gluconeogenesis and lipolysis.

Disorders of Fasting Adaptation

Hypoglycemia may stem from failure of one of the body's fasting adaptation systems. Problems with inadequate or inaccessible glycogen stores are seen with glycogen storage disease, in hepatic failure, and with infants with inadequate glycogen stores (such as infants who are preterm, small for gestational age, stressed, septic, or have congenital heart disease). Problems with gluconeogenesis are seen with glycogen storage disease (type I), fructose 1,6-diphosphatase deficiency, or hepatic failure. Disorders of fatty acid metabolism precipitate hypoglycemia with prolonged fasting. Drugs that may precipitate hypoglycemia include alcohol, sulfonamides, beta-adrenergic antagonists, salicylates, and insulin.

Clinical signs and symptoms of hypoglycemia are summarized in Table 25–11. Adrenergic and cholinergic stimulation responses are responsible for the early signs and symptoms of hypoglycemia. Because the brain has an obligatory glucose requirement, central nervous system symptoms are precipitated by neuroglycopenia.

Diagnostic Evaluation

Bedside blood glucose monitoring instruments are useful screening devices for the detection of hypoglycemia. However, they should not be used to diagnose hypoglycemia because they lack the degree of precision required to document the degree of hypoglycemia. All hypoglycemic events documented by a bedside glucose monitoring require confirmation by a laboratory sample. Such samples should be immediately transported to the laboratory because red blood cells metabolize glucose. Therefore, a delay in processing the sample results in falsely low readings.

Accurate documentation of a blood glucose value less than 60 mg/dL may be all that is needed to diagnose transient hypoglycemia in the infant with a history of prenatal stress, sepsis, maternal diabetes, prematurity, or congenital heart disease or in the infant or child who becomes hypoglycemic following rapid discontinuation of high-concentration glucose infusions.

Persistent hypoglycemia suspected to be associated with glycogen storage disease, hyperinsulinism, adrenocortical hypofunction (hypopituitarism, or primary adrenal insufficiency) and disorders of fatty acid metabolism often require confirmation during a controlled fasting study. The intent of the fasting study is to determine the child's ability to use alternative fuel sources and, if abnormal, to diagnose the underlying problem. Fasting is begun following a feeding or meal and is continued until the blood glucose drops to 40 or 50 mg/dL, or for a maximum of 24 to 36 hours. The child needs intravenous access and a 10% dextrose solution at the bedside to be used at the end of the fast, if the child is symptomatic and unable to take glucose-containing fluids orally. The child should be observed closely throughout the fast. All urine output is checked for ketones, and vital signs are monitored frequently. Blood glucose is measured every 1 to 2 hours while the glucose level is higher than 80 mg/dL, every 1 hour while the glucose level is between 60 and 80 mg/dL, and every 30 minutes when the glucose level is less than 60 mg/dL. When the blood glucose level is less than 45 to 50 mg/dL or if the child is symptomatic (pallor, diaphoresis, tremors, tachycardia, drowsiness), the critical blood sample is drawn. The critical sample is sent for glucose, insulin, cortisol, growth hormone, fatty acid, and ketone levels. The fast may end with a glucagon challenge, which provides information about the availability of unused glycogen stores.

In the face of hypoglycemia, the infant or child with hyperinsulinism demonstrates inappropriately high insulin levels and normal to high cortisol and growth hormone levels. Unlike other fasting children who cannot respond to glucagon because their glyco-

Table 25–11. HYPOGLYCEMIA

Signs/Symptoms	Underlying Mechanisms
Weakness Tachycardia Pallor Anxiety Tremors Rebound hyperglycemia	Adrenergic response
Diaphoresis Sudden hunger	Cholinergic response
Drowsiness Headache Dizziness Decreased mental capacity	Neuroglycopenia

gen stores are depleted, these patients typically respond to the glucagon challenge with a glucose level rise of more than 30 mg/dL within 30 minutes. High insulin levels inhibit the release of glucagon; therefore, glycogen stores are present in the liver in the face of hypoglycemia.

During hypoglycemia, the infant or child with glucocorticoid deficiency demonstrates abnormally low cortisol levels. An appropriate insulin level for the measured blood glucose is documented. These children may be able to mobilize fatty acids and show a modest response in the way of ketone body production. Cortrosyn (ACTH) and metyrapone stimulation tests may be used to distinguish primary from secondary (ACTH) deficiency.

In the face of hypoglycemia, the child with glycogen storage disease (GSD) (type I) demonstrates high lactate levels. High levels of free fatty acids document the child's ability to mobilize free fatty acids. Response to glucagon in the fed state is abnormal in that stored glycogen is not released in response to the glucagon stimulus, and lactate levels increase.

In the face of hypoglycemia, the child with GSD (type III) has a normal serum lactate and can mobilize fatty acids. A normal response to glucagon is seen in the fed state, and a lower than normal glucose response is seen after a relatively brief period of fasting.

The child with a disorder of fatty acid metabolism usually is seen when acutely ill with lethargy, coma, or seizures. A high ammonia level and an absence of urinary ketones are usually found in the face of hypoglycemia. Diagnosis of any of the disorders of fatty acid oxygenation is confirmed by the presence of specific organic acids in the urine during hypoglycemia.

Critical Care Management

The care of the child with hypoglycemia is outlined in Table 25–12. Goals for care are to minimize the short- and long-term effects of hypoglycemia on the central nervous system. If the child is able to take fluids orally, treatment may simply involve the provision of calorie-containing fluids such as glucose water, formula, or juice. Simple carbohydrates are absorbed most quickly and are therefore more desirable than more complex ones such as chocolate or cookies. If the child is unconscious or unable to take fluids orally, glucose is administered intravenously. Glucose

Table 25–12. MANAGING HYPOGLYCEMIA

1. Participate in diagnostic workup	
History:	Child's age, length of fast
Risk factors:	Infants: (large or small for gestational age; history of maternal diabetes; preterm; hypoxic, stressed, septic, congenital heart disease) Rapid discontinuation of high-concentration dextrose infusion Adrenocortical hypofunction (primary, secondary, iatrogenic)
Physical examination:	Adrenergic response Signs of neuroglycopenia
Laboratory tests:	Glucose (decreased)
Fasting study laboratory tests:	Insulin, growth hormone, cortisol Serum ketones Lactates Free fatty acids Carnitine Urine ketones, organic acids
2. Prevent central nervous system complications associated with hypoglycemia	

Measure blood glucose:	STAT if symptomatic (pallor, irritability, difficult to arouse, diaphoretic)
	q 15 min if blood glucose <50 mg/dL
	q 30 min–1 hour:
	    Until blood glucose is consistently in 80–120 mg/dL range *or* if making changes in glucose infusion
	      rate/concentration
	q 2–4 hours if blood glucose is consistently in 80–120 mg/dL range and child is on glucose infusion
	Before meals/feeds if blood glucose in 80–120 range and child is no longer on glucose infusion doses

Manage acute hypoglycemia (blood glucose <60 mg/dL):	1. if no IV access and able to take PO/NG, give 4–6 oz formula, glucose water, juice 2. if IV access, increase IV glucose rate/concentration (5–20 mL/kg 10% DW IV or 2 mL/kg 25% DW) 3. if no IV access, symptomatic and unable to take PO, give 1 mg glucagon intramuscularly, subcutaneously. (Will not work with GSD and children who are glycogen depleted.)
Limit fasting demands:	High-risk infant: Provide glucose supplements orally or via IV infusion to maintain glucose levels GSD: Limit fasting to 3–4 hours (type 1) or 6–8 hours (type 3) Supplement with uncooked cornstarch and/or overnight nasogastric feedings Fatty acid oxygenation defects: Limit fasting to 10–12 hours
Treat underlying problem:	Hyperinsulinism: Diazoxide, somatostatin, subtotal pancreatectomy Hypopituitarism: Cortisol, growth hormone replacement

GSD, glycogen storage disease.

Table 25–13. HYPERGLYCEMIA

Signs and Symptoms	Underlying Mechanisms
Glucosuria	Glucose is spilled in urine when blood glucose exceeds renal threshold (approximately 180 mg/dL). Glucosuria creates an osmotic drag of fluid in renal tubules
Calorie wasting/weight loss	Glucosuria Tissue starvation from inability to uptake glucose without insulin
Polyuria, polydipsia, dehydration	Osmotic diuresis secondary to urinary excretion of glucose Insensible water loss (secondary to intercurrent illness; tachypnea, hyperpnea)
Tachycardia, hypotension, shock, cardiovascular collapse	Hyperosmolality (hyperglycemia results in creation of osmotic gradient of free water between ICF and ECF). ECF volume remains expanded at the expense of ICF and hemodynamic consequences are minimized. Severity of dehydration is often masked.

Electrolyte imbalance
   Hyponatremia
   Hypokalemia
	Passive loss of electrolytes in urine due to osmotic diuresis

Hyperosmolality	Hyperglycemia Decreased glomerular filtration rate when approximately 6–10% dehydrated. Therefore, kidney is less able to excrete glucose resulting in worsening of the hyperglycemia and further increase in osmolality of ECF. Hypernatremia secondary to hemoconcentration BUN rises from decreased renal clearance secondary to dehydration

ECF, extracellular fluid; ICF, intracellular fluid.

0.5 to 2 g/kg given as a 10% to 25% glucose solution can be administered via intravenous drip or bolus. Blood glucose is remeasured immediately to determine the effectiveness of treatment. This process is repeated until the blood glucose reaches the 80 to 120 mg/dL range. Blood glucose measurements are obtained at least hourly until the blood glucose level has stabilized in this range. Guidelines for the frequency of measuring blood glucose for the child at risk are outlined in Table 25–12.

Long-term treatment of the child with persistent hypoglycemia is determined by the underlying cause. Mild hyperinsulinism may be managed initially with oral diazoxide (Proglycem) and frequent feedings. If this regimen fails, a trial of a somatostatin analogue octreotide (Sandostatin) given subcutaneously three to four times daily may be initiated. Children who do not improve on either of these regimens usually require a subtotal pancreatectomy. Children with GSD and fatty acid oxygenation disorders are generally treated by limiting fasting periods by providing the child with small, frequent feedings or continuous nasogastric feedings. Hypoglycemia related to cortisol or growth hormone deficiency is treated by replacing the deficient hormones.

DISTURBANCES OF GLUCOSE HOMEOSTASIS: HYPERGLYCEMIA

Hyperglycemia is defined as a serum glucose level higher than 120 mg/dL. Blood glucose values that exceed the renal threshold (approximately 180 mg/dL) result in glucosuria. The excretion of glucose in the urine may result in (1) osmotic diuresis leading to dehydration and cardiovascular collapse, (2) calorie wasting, and (3) electrolyte imbalance. The effects of hyperglycemia and resultant osmotic diuresis are outlined in Table 25–13. As the blood glucose exceeds the renal threshold, glucose is spilled into the urine, creating an osmotic diuresis that may be profound enough to precipitate shock and cardiovascular collapse. Passive loss of sodium and potassium in the urine accompanies the osmotic diuresis. Although there is likely to be a total body deficit of both potassium and sodium, the serum sodium may be elevated, reflecting hemoconcentration. Serum is hyperosmolar because of hyperglycemia, hypernatremia, and azotemia. Weight loss is the result of both calorie wasting and fluid losses.

Underlying causes of hyperglycemia are outlined in Table 25–14. Drugs that are associated with hyperglycemia include epinephrine, glucocorticosteroids, diuretics, beta-adrenergic agonists, and phenytoin.

Table 25–14. ENDOCRINE CAUSES OF HYPERGLYCEMIA

Causes	Examples
Excess of counterregulatory hormone	
Cortisol	Primary: adrenocortical dysfunction Secondary: pituitary/hypothalamic dysfunction Iatrogenic: High-dose steroids
Epinephrine	Pheochromocytoma Stress Exogenous epinephrine
Glucagon	Glucagonoma
Insulin deficiency	Type I diabetes Pancreatitis Cystic fibrosis

Excess of Counterregulatory Hormones

Adrenocortical hyperfunction (Cushing's syndrome) is associated with an overproduction of glucocorticoids resulting in hyperglycemia. As with adrenocortical hypofunction, the underlying problem may be at one of three levels: (1) the pituitary (resulting in an overproduction of ACTH), (2) the adrenals (resulting in overproduction of cortisol), or (3) iatrogenic (stemming from administration of high doses of steroids). Ectopic ACTH production by a tumor is seen in the adult population.

High catecholamine levels may be a result of stimulation of the sympathetic nervous system (stress response), adrenal overproduction (pheochromocytoma), or exogenous sources (infusion or subcutaneous injection). All have the potential to increase blood glucose.

Transient hyperglycemia may be seen in the acutely ill child and is associated with an increased production of cortisol and epinephrine, which accompany a stress response. Any child receiving exogenous epinephrine is at risk. Children undergoing chemotherapy with high-dose steroids and L-asparaginase frequently experience a transient period of hyperglycemia. Hyperglycemia accompanying a glucagonoma, pheochromocytoma, and Cushing's disease are more persistent in nature and are accompanied by their own unique configuration of diagnostic cues.

Hyperglucagonemia may be the result of a glucagonoma (tumor of the alpha cells of the pancreas). This very rare source of hyperglycemia in children is caused by the stimulation of gluconeogenesis and glycogenolysis by high glucagon levels.

Diagnosis

Diagnostic findings in hyperglycemia are outlined in Table 25–15. Urinary glucose measurements provide a useful initial screening device for identifying the patient at risk. When the urine test is positive for glucose, a blood sample is obtained to estimate the blood glucose (using Dextrostix, Chemstrips, etc.). This bedside estimate is confirmed by a simultaneous laboratory measure.

Critical Care Management

Care of the child with hyperglycemia is outlined in Table 25–15. Definitive therapy involves the identification and treatment of the underlying cause of hyperglycemia. Nursing care is directed at the prevention of complications associated with weight loss and dehydration. A systematic process for screening patients at risk for hyperglycemia is also outlined in Table 25–15.

Mild dehydration (<5%) may be managed with oral fluid replacement of calorie-free liquids. More severe dehydration (>5%), or the child who is unconscious

or refusing to drink requires intravenous fluid replacement.

Dietary management may be all that is required in some cases of transient and mild hyperglycemia. Placing the child on a low concentrated carbohydrate diet may be sufficient to prevent significant hyperglycemia. Otherwise, insulin may be given as four short-acting doses (before each meal and again at the time of a bedtime snack). A second option is a split-mixed dose of short- and long-acting insulin before breakfast and again before dinner. Frequent monitoring of blood glucose and monitoring for signs of hypoglycemia (see Table 25–11) is essential with insulin administration. Children receiving most or all of their calories intravenously are most easily managed using an intravenous insulin infusion titrated to maintain blood glucose values between 100 and 200 mg/dL.

Insulin Resistance and Deficit (Diabetic Ketoacidosis)

Underproduction of insulin is associated with beta cell injury or destruction. Beta cell destruction is

Table 25–15. TREATING HYPERGLYCEMIA

1. Participate in diagnostic workup
   History: Polyuria, polydipsia, weight loss, fatigue
   Risk factors: Diabetes, significant stress, exogenous epinephrine, steroid or L-asparaginase administration, Cushing's syndrome, pheochromocytoma, glucagonoma
   Physical examination: Dehydration, mental status changes
   Laboratory tests: Hyperglycemia, hypernatremia, Cortisol increased, glucagon increased Glucosuria

2. Detect hyperglycemia in patients at risk:
   Measure urine for glucose q 12 hours and
   If urine positive for glucose, measure blood glucose
   If blood glucose is >180 mg/dL, measure blood glucose qid until blood glucose consistently <180 mg/dL
   When blood glucose is consistently <180 mg/dL, resume measuring urine for glucose q 12 hours
   If on subcutaneous insulin, measure blood glucose 5 times per day (pre-breakfast, pre-lunch, pre-dinner, pre-bedtime snack and 2 A.M.)
   Additional measurements should be obtained as needed when clinical symptoms of hypoglycemia or hyperglycemia are detected

3. Prevent complications of hyperglycemia (dehydration, cerebral edema, weight loss)
   Correct fluid/electrolyte imbalance:
   Replace fluids lost as a result of osmotic diuresis orally or intravenously
   Low concentrated carbohydrate diet
   Administer insulin subcutaneously as ordered
   Evaluate fluid balance:
   Compare urine output to fluid intake
   Assess for orthostatic blood pressure
   Weigh daily while spilling glucose in urine
   Correct underlying cause:
   Surgery: Pheochromocytoma, glucagonoma, Cushing's syndrome
   Supportive: L-asparaginase, high-dose steroids, stress

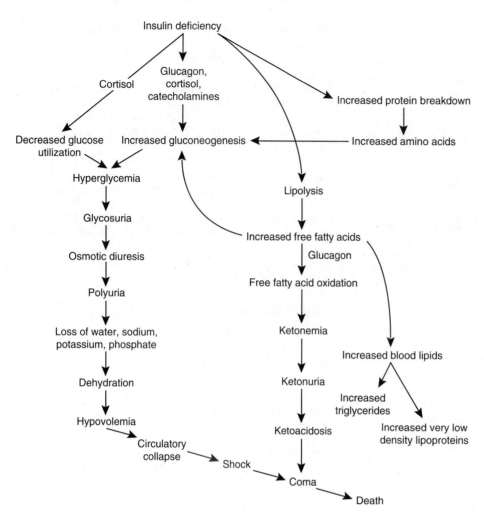

Insulin deficiency

Figure 25–5 ● ● ● ● ● ●
Diabetic ketoacidosis. (Modified from Mosby's Manual of Clinical Nursing, 2nd ed., p. 931. St. Louis: C.V. Mosby.)

the pathophysiologic mechanism underlying type 1 diabetes. Acute pancreatitis may result in temporary interference with beta cell function and hyperglycemia until the inflammatory process subsides. Cystic fibrosis produces sclerotic changes in the pancreas, which may interfere with insulin production and may result in permanent destruction of the beta cells and functional diabetes.

Hormonal regulation in diabetic ketoacidosis (DKA) is outlined in Figure 25–5. Insulin deficiency results in hyperglycemia and mobilization of fatty acids. Hyperglycemia is a function of the inability of

Table 25–16. DIABETIC KETOACIDOSIS

Signs and Symptoms	Underlying Mechanisms
Hyperglycemia, dehydration, cardiovascular collapse	Osmotic diuresis secondary to hyperglycemia
Acidosis	Buildup of ketoacids and lactic acid in serum from lipolysis resulting in increased H^+ ion concentration in serum
Electrolyte imbalance Sodium	Total body hyponatremia because of passive loss of electrolytes as a result of osmotic diuresis. However, serum sodium may be high as a result of hemoconcentration
Potassium	In acidosis, potassium shifts from ICF to ECF. Therefore, initially serum potassium may increase, then decrease as a result of osmotic diuresis
Cardiac arrhythmia	Hypokalemia Hyperkalemia
Ketonuria	Serum ketone levels rise above the renal threshold and are spilled in the urine
Hyperpnea	A compensatory mechanism. An effort to blow off excess carbonic acid as water and CO_2 and thereby correct the degree of acidosis
Mental status changes/cerebral edema	Possibly related to rate of correction, level of acidosis, fluid shifts

ICF, intracellular fluid; ECF, extracellular fluid; H^+, hydrogen.

glucose to enter body cells and decreased utilization of glucose. The relative excess of counterregulatory hormones signals gluconeogenesis. Body proteins are broken down, thereby making amino acid substrates available for gluconeogenesis. A relative lack of insulin in relation to epinephrine, growth hormone, and, to lesser extent, cortisol stimulates the mobilization of fatty acids, the production of ketone bodies, and resultant ketoacidosis.

As depicted in Figure 25–5, significant hyperglycemia results in a profound osmotic diuresis and urinary electrolyte loss. Dehydration may be severe enough to precipitate cardiovascular collapse. The accumulation of ketone bodies produces a severe acidosis, with pH levels occasionally falling below 7.0. As perfusion status worsens, lactic acidosis contributes to the falling pH.

As previously noted, DKA is accompanied by total body sodium and potassium deficits resulting from osmotic diuresis. However, fluid shifts between the intracellular fluid (ICF) and extracellular fluid (ECF) and significant hemoconcentration result in variable measured serum electrolyte values. Serum potassium and sodium levels may be high, normal, or low depending on the degree of dehydration and/or the stage of fluid correction. Acidosis complicates the interpretation of the electrolyte picture because of the shifts of potassium (from the ICF to the ECF) in the acidotic state and the return of potassium from the ECF to the ICF during correction of acidosis. As a result, serum hyperkalemia or hypokalemia may precipitate life-threatening cardiac arrhythmias.

Cerebral edema is a complication of treatment of DKA, the cause of which is unknown. It may occur at any time during the 24-hour period following the initiation of therapy. Risk factors believed to be associated with cerebral edema include a pH less than 7.0; glucose level higher than 800 mg/dL; hyperosmolality and hypernatremia; use of bicarbonate to correct acidosis; too rapid correction of blood glucose, creating an osmotic gradient; and an infant younger than 1 year of age.

Diagnosis

Diagnostic findings are outlined in Table 25–16. A history of polyuria, polydipsia, and weight loss with documented hyperglycemia is usually a sufficient history to diagnose diabetes mellitus, particularly if accompanied by a metabolic acidosis. Blood urea nitrogen (BUN) and creatinine levels provide some index of the degree of dehydration. Arterial pH provides an index of the degree of acidosis and the $Paco_2$ (partial pressure of carbon dioxide in arterial blood) value provides an index of the body's ability to compensate.

Critical Care Management

The prevention of complications related to dehydration, cardiovascular collapse, acidosis, electrolyte imbalance, and cerebral edema are the primary goals of the treatment of the child in DKA (Table 25–17).

Table 25–17. TREATING DIABETIC KETOACIDOSIS

1. Participate in diagnostic workup
   History:
   Polyuria, polydipsia, weight loss, fatigue, nausea, vomiting

   Physical examination:
   Dehydration, Kussmaul's respirations, facial flushing, abdominal tenderness, mental status changes

   Laboratory tests: Blood glucose, blood gas, electrolytes, BUN, creatinine, urine ketones/sugar

2. Prevent complications related to dehydration/cardiovascular collapse, acidosis, hypokalemia, hyperkalemia, cerebral edema

   Replace fluid/electrolytes lost as a result of osmotic diuresis:
   Resuscitate with 20 mL/kg of normal saline over a 1-hour period
   Repeat bolus if heart rate elevated and/or hypotensive following first bolus
   Replace remaining deficit over the next 24–48 hours with 0.45 normal saline
   While on insulin infusion:
   Add 5% glucose to infusion when blood glucose reaches 300 mg/dL to prevent hypoglycemia
   Add 10% glucose to infusion when blood glucose reaches 200 mg/dL (and patient is on 5% dextrose) to prevent hypoglycemia
   Replace potassium losses in IV fluids
   Monitor ECG for signs of hyperkalemia and hypokalemia

   Correct acidosis:
   Insulin infusion (0.1 μ/kg/hr)
   Sodium bicarbonate for severe acidosis (pH < 7.0) infused over 1–2 hour period, *not* IV push

   Measure blood glucose:
   Every hour until insulin infusion is discontinued
   Every 2 hours until taking fluids orally and IV fluids are discontinued
   Five times per day after discontinuing IV fluids (pre-breakfast, pre-lunch, pre-dinner, pre-bedtime snack and 2 A.M.)
   Additional measurements should be obtained as needed when clinical symptoms of hypoglycemia are detected

   Monitor response to therapy:
   Vital signs (pulse, respirations, blood pressure)
   q 30–60 min while on insulin infusion
   q shift until ketones cleared
   Weigh daily
   Compare fluid intake to output
   Measure urine ketones/sugar whenever blood glucose >240 mg/dL

   Detect and treat cerebral edema in a timely fashion:
   Neurosigns hourly for 24 hours (mental status changes, pupillary response)
   Treat signs of cerebral edema immediately (hyperventilation, mannitol, fluid restriction, intracranial pressure monitoring, high-dose steroids)

The first priority of care is to manage the dehydration. An initial fluid bolus (approximately 20 mL/kg of normal saline) is given over a 1-hour period. If the child continues to appear poorly perfused after the initial bolus, a second fluid bolus may be necessary. Remaining fluid deficits are usually replaced over a 24-hour period, often as 0.45% normal saline with potassium supplements (once voiding has been established). Ongoing urine losses in excess of 2 to 3 mL/kg/hour may be replaced with 0.45% normal saline.

The second priority of care is to correct the acidosis

and to prevent further lipolysis. Insulin has an inhibitory effect on ketone production; therefore, the administration of insulin is the key to correcting metabolic acidosis. An intravenous infusion is the preferred method of administering insulin in the poorly perfused patient. Initial rates that exceed normal physiologic requirements (approximately 0.1 unit/kg/hour) are used to achieve the desired inhibitory affect on further lipolysis. A 5% solution of glucose is added to the intravenous fluid as the blood glucose drifts down to the 200 to 300 mg/dL range. Blood glucose is measured at least hourly while insulin infusion is maintained and within 30 minutes following a change in either the rate of the insulin infusion or the concentration of the glucose being infused. When the child's blood glucose again drifts down into the 200 range, the concentration of glucose is increased to 10%. The rate of the insulin infusion is usually held constant at supraphysiologic levels to achieve serum insulin levels high enough to inhibit further lipolysis and resultant ketone production.

Infusion of sodium bicarbonate to correct severe acidosis may be considered if the pH is less than 7.0 or if there is evidence of inadequate respiratory compensation (HCO_3 <5). Bicarbonate is given slowly by infusion over a 2-hour period. The aim is to correct the pH to the 7.15 range. Infusing sodium bicarbonate too rapidly is associated with a worsening of the intracellular acidosis and may be a factor associated with the development of cerebral edema.

Life-threatening cardiac arrhythmias precipitated by either hypokalemia or hyperkalemia may be detected during the period of the initial correction. It is essential that the child in severe DKA be monitored closely for ECG changes associated with hyperkalemia and hypokalemia.

Signs of cerebral edema include mental status changes and pupillary changes. Treatment must proceed rapidly because mortality is high. Treatment involves efforts to decrease intracranial volume including hyperventilation, administration of mannitol, fluid restriction, intracerebral pressure monitoring, and possibly steroid administration. Neurologic signs and intracranial pressure monitoring provide important data for emergency management of the child with cerebral edema.

Bibliography

Baxter, J.D., & Tyrrell, J.B. (1987). Adrenal disease. In P. Felig, J.D. Baxter, A.E. Broadus, & L.A. Frohman (Eds.). *Endocrinology and metabolism* (2nd ed., pp. 511–650). New York: McGraw-Hill.

Chin, R. (1991). Adrenal crisis. *Critical Care Clinics, 1,* 23–42.

Constant, R.B., & Barth, R.J. (1988). Adrenal disease. In J.M. Civetta, R.W. Taylor, & R.R. Kirby (Eds.). *Critical care* (pp. 1405–1413). Philadelphia: J.B. Lippincott.

Egger, M., Gschwend, S., Smith, G., Zuppinger, K. (1991). Increasing incidence of hypoglycemic coma in children with IDDM. *Diabetes Care,* 11, 1001–1005.

Felicetta, J.V. (1987). Endocrine changes with critical illness. *Critical Care Clinics,* 5, 855–869.

Finegold, D. (1984). Hypoglycemia. *Topics in Emergency Medicine,* 5, 57–63.

Ganong, W.F. (1991). Neuroendocrinology. In F.S. Greenspan, (Ed.). *Basic and clinical endocrinology* (2nd ed., pp. 66–78). Norwalk, CT: Appleton & Lang.

Germon, K. (1987). Fluid and electrolyte problems associated with diabetes insipidus and syndrome of inappropriate anti-diuretic hormone. *Nursing Clinics of North America,* 22, 785–796.

Guthrie, D., & Guthrie, R. (1991). *Nursing management of diabetes mellitus.* New York: Springer.

Guyton, H. (1991). *Textbook of medical physiology* (8th ed). Philadelphia: W.B. Saunders.

Halloran, T.H. (1990). Nursing responsibilities in endocrine emergencies. *Critical Care Nursing Quarterly,* 13, 74–81.

Hartshorn, J., & Hartshorn, E. (1988). Vasopressin in the treatment of diabetes insipidus. *J Neuroscience Nursing,* 20, 58–59.

Humes, D., Narins, R., & Brenner, B. (1979). Disorders of water balance. *Hospital Practice,* 133–145.

Johndrow, P.D. & Thornton, S. (1985). Syndrome of inappropriate anti-diuretic hormone. *Focus on Critical Care,* 12, 29–34.

Kessler, C.A. (1992). Disorders of glucose metabolism. In G. Alspach (Ed.). *Instructor's manual for AACN's core curriculum* (pp. 250–259). Philadelphia: W.B. Saunders.

Kessler, C.A. (1992). Endocrine emergencies. In G. Alspach (Ed.). *Instructor's manual for AACN's core curriculum* (pp. 250–259). Philadelphia: W.B. Saunders.

Kitabachi, A., & Rumback, M. (1989). The management of diabetic emergencies. *Hospital Practice,* 129–133.

LaFranchi, S. (1987). Hypoglycemia of infancy and childhood. *Pediatric Clinics of North America,* 34(4), 961–983.

Munch, A., Guyre, P.M., & Holbrook, N.J. (1984). Physiologic functions of glucocorticoids in stress and their relation to pharmacological actions. *Endocrine Review,* 5, 25.

Ober, K.P. (1991). Diabetes insipidus. *Critical Care Clinics,* 7, 109–125.

Patterson, L.M., & Noroinan, E.L. (1989). Diabetes insipidus versus syndrome of inappropriate antidiuretic hormone. *Dimensions of Critical Care Nursing,* 20, 226–234.

Ramsay, D.J. (1991). Posterior pituitary gland. In F.S. Greenspan (Ed.). *Basic and clinical endocrinology* (2nd ed., pp. 177–187). Norwalk, CT: Appleton & Lange.

Reasner, C.A. (1990). Adrenal disorder. *Critical Care Nursing Quarterly,* 13, 67–73.

Sabo, C., & Michael, S.R. (1989). Diabetic ketoacidosis: pathophysiology, nursing diagnosis, and nursing interventions. *Focus on Critical Care,* 16, 21–28.

Sanford, S.J. (1990). Endocrine anatomy and physiology. In L.A. Thelan, J.K. Davie, & L.D. Urden (Eds.). *Textbook of critical care nursing.* Philadelphia: C.V. Mosby.

Schira, M.G. (1987). Steroid-dependent states and adrenal insufficiency fluid and electrolyte disturbances. *Nursing Clinics of North America,* 22, 837–841.

Stanley, C.A., & Baker, L. (1976). Hyperinsulinism in infants and children: Diagnosis and therapy. *Advances in Pediatrics,* 23, 315–354.

Stanley, C.A., & Baker, L. (1976). Hyperinsulinism in infancy: Diagnosis by demonstration of abnormal response to fasting hypoglycemia. *Pediatrics,* 57, 702–711.

Thompson, J., McFarland, G., Hirsch, J., Tucker, S., & Bauers, A. (1989). *Mosby's manual of clinical nursing* (2nd ed.). Philadelphia: C.V. Mosby.

Tyrell, J.B., Aron, D.C., & Forsham, P.H. (1991). Glucocorticoids and adrenal androgens. In F.S. Greenspan (Ed.). *Basic and clinical endocrinology* (2nd ed., pp. 323–362). Norwalk, CT: Appleton & Lange.

Zucher, A., & Chernow, B. (1986). Diabetes insipidus and the syndrome of inappropriate anti-diuretic release. *Critical Care Quarterly,* 3, 63–74.

CHAPTER 26

Hematologic Critical Care Problems

CHERYL CAHILL-ALSIP
BETH McDERMOTT

Children in the pediatric intensive care unit experience a variety of hematologic problems with wide ranges of etiology, severity, interventions, and prognoses. This is partially because of the complex structure and function of blood and the multiple functions of blood components, which affect every cell in the body. In addition, organs of the hematopoietic system such as bone marrow are prone to the adverse effects of sepsis, trauma, shock, and drugs used for critically ill children. The majority of hematologic problems seen in critically ill children are acquired and often present as an acute episode (Baker & Finklestein, 1989). The more common causes are disseminated intravascular coagulation (DIC), anemias, liver and/or renal disease, hemolytic uremic syndrome (HUS), and blood dyscrasias.

The final common pathways of altered hematologic function include disorders of coagulation and disorders of oxygen-carrying capacity. This chapter focuses on these final common pathways with an emphasis on DIC, sickle cell anemia, and HUS. Because hematologic intervention is one of the most frequently used therapeutic modalities in the PICU, this chapter will discuss the administration of blood

products and apheresis, with an emphasis on nursing implications.

ESSENTIAL EMBRYOLOGY

During embryologic development blood formation can be recognized as early as 3 weeks after conception. By the sixth week of gestation, hematopoiesis (the production of red cells, white cells, and platelets) moves from the yolk sac to the liver, which is the main site of blood formation during the middle portion of fetal life. Following the 20th week of gestation, hematopoiesis then moves to the bone marrow, and following birth, it takes place almost entirely in the bone marrow.

ESSENTIAL ANATOMY AND PHYSIOLOGY

Hematopoietic Organs

Bone marrow is the chief site for hematopoiesis. There are two types of bone marrow: yellow marrow, which contains a large percentage of fat cells; and red marrow, which contains mostly blood cells. The infant and young child have a larger proportion of red marrow because of the high requirements for red cell production. Early in life the red marrow is contained in the medullary cavities of the long bones. These cavities gradually fill with fat as the demands for red cell production decrease until the adult distribution of hematopoiesis (sternum, pelvis, vertebrae, cranium, ribs, and epiphyses of long bones) is reached at puberty. In disease states associated with anemias, hematopoiesis can return to its former sites including the long bones, liver, spleen, and lymph nodes. It may also take place in the adrenal glands, cartilage, adipose tissues, and kidneys.

The production of red blood cells (RBCs) also takes place in the lymphoid tissue and the thymus glands, as well as in the bone marrow. Therefore, these organs are also important components of hematopoiesis. Figure 26–1 illustrates the formation and maturation of blood cells.

Blood Stem Cell

Human bone marrow contains a pluripotent hematopoietic stem cell precursor that is capable of differentiating into erythroid, granulocytic, monocytic, megakaryocytic, and certain lymphoid cell lines. This cell gives rise to the marrow stem cell, which produces the precursor for erythrocytes, granulocytes, monocytes, and platelets. Stem cells are present in small numbers in blood and bone marrow. Their turnover depends upon the needs of the body. It has been suggested that the structure of the stem cell is similar to that of the lymphocyte.

Composition of Blood

Blood is composed of plasma in which are suspended certain proteins (such as albumin, globulin), clotting factors, and the blood cells. These include erythrocytes (red blood cells [RBCs]), leukocytes (white blood cells [WBCs]), and thrombocytes (platelets). The main function of the leukocytes are to fight infection; defend the body against foreign organisms through phagocytosis; and produce, transport, and distribute antibodies in the immune system. Leukocytes are discussed in detail in Chapter 16.

Erythrocytes

Erythrocytes (RBCs) are the most abundant component in the blood. They have biconcave discs without nuclei and are extremely flexible. This allows them to travel extremely fast and bend and twist as they pass through tiny capillaries. Their elongated shape in the capillaries allows for more surface area for the exchange of oxygen and carbon dioxide.

After birth, the rate of hemoglobin synthesis and production of RBCs decreases dramatically during the first few days of life. The rate of production of RBCs and hemoglobin reaches a minimum during the second week of life, increases during the following month, and reaches its maximum at about 3 months of age, when production is at about 2 mL of packed RBCs per day (Oski, 1987).

The main function of erythrocytes is the transport of oxygen and carbon dioxide, which is accomplished through hemoglobin (hgb), the major component of RBCs. Oxygen binds with hgb and then is released at tissue sites where gas exchange takes place.

Fetal hemoglobin (hgb F) is present at birth and allows for more efficient binding of oxygen at lower surface tensions. Hgb F constitutes 70% of the total hgb at birth but declines rapidly. By 6 to 12 months of age, hgb F has been mostly replaced by adult hemoglobin, although levels of 1% to 2% of hgb F remain throughout life. Hgb F shifts the oxyhemoglobin dissociation curve to the left so that oxygen bound to hemoglobin is not readily released to the tissues. This may compromise tissue oxygenation in newborns with diminished cardiovascular reserves.

RBCs are formed in the red bone marrow and progress through the stages of development outlined in Table 26–1. The mature erythrocyte is released into the circulation where the average lifespan is about 120 days. This span of time represents the interval between the cell's release into the circulation from the bone marrow and its destruction. When the RBC ages, it is removed from the circulation by the spleen, liver, and red bone marrow. When the hematopoietic system is faced with a heavy demand for the production of RBCs, such as with hemorrhage, immature RBCs are released into the circulation. The number of immature cells and their degree of immaturity reflect the severity of stress placed on this body system. When the demand is great, the number of reticulocytes may increase by 30% to 50%. With an increased demand, the number of normoblasts may appear in large numbers. In severe anemias, the percentage of normoblasts may be as high as 5% to 20% of the circulating RBCs. Prorubricytes may also appear at this time. This informa-

Table 26–1. DEVELOPMENT OF RED BLOOD CELLS

HEMOCYTOBLAST
(Precursor of all blood cells)
↓
PRORUBRICYTE OR BASOPHIL ERYTHROBLAST
(Synthesis of hgb begins)
↓
RUBRICYTE
(Nucleus begins to shrink, more synthesis of hgb)
↓
NORMOBLAST
(Nucleus begins to disintegrate, more synthesis of hgb)
↓
RETICULOCYTE
(Nucleus absorbed, strands of endoplasmic reticulum seen)
↓
ERYTHROCYTE
(Mature RBC without nucleus or reticulum)

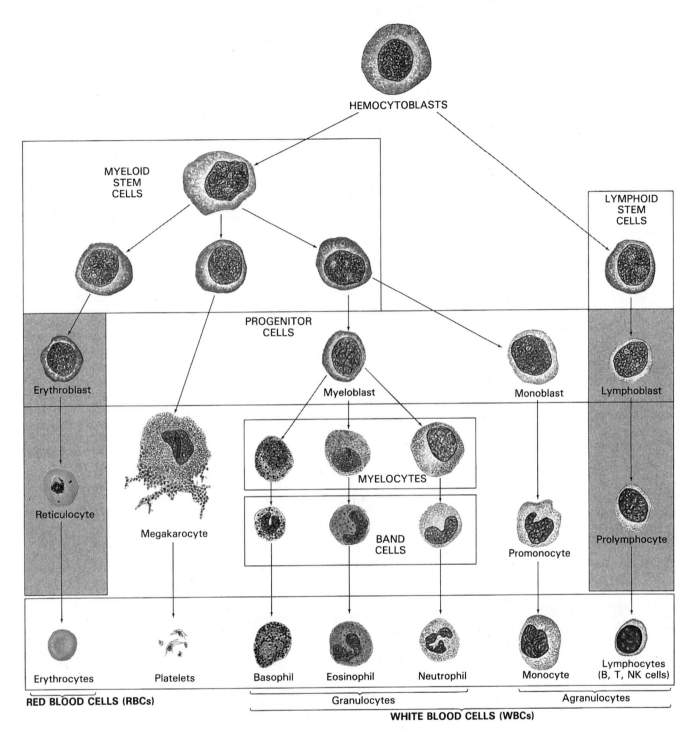

Figure 26–1 ● ● ● ● ● ●

The origins and differentiation of blood cells. (From Martini, Frederic, FUNDAMENTALS OF ANATOMY AND PHYSIOLOGY, 3/E © 1995, p. 669. Adapted by permission of Prentice-Hall, Upper Saddle River, New Jersey.)

tion is also important in differentiating various types of anemias.

RBC production is also stimulated by decreased tissue oxygenation, because RBC production depends not only upon the actual number present in the circulation but also upon their ability to carry oxygen and carbon dioxide. When tissue oxygenation is decreased, erythropoietin stimulates the stem cells in the bone marrow to produce mature RBCs. Erythropoietin is produced in the kidney and is released in response to hypoxia and anemia. Table 26–2 lists the normal RBC values at various ages.

Thrombocytes (Platelets)

Platelet development takes place primarily in the bone marrow. Platelets are the smallest of the blood

Table 26–2. RED BLOOD CELL STUDIES

Test	Normal Values		Purpose	Clinical Signficance
Red blood count (RBC)	*Millions of cells/mm³*		Measures total number of circulating red blood cells	Increased in polycythemia, severe diarrhea, dehydration, acute poisoning, during and immediately following hemorrhage
	1 wk	3.9–6.3		
	2 wk	3.6–6.2		
	1 mo	3.0–5.4		
	2 mo	2.7–4.9		Decreased in anemias, diseases of bone marrow function, hemolytic and pernicious anemia, subacute endocarditis
	3–6 mo	3.1–4.5		
	0.5–2 yr	3.7–5.3		
	2–6 yr	3.9–5.3		
	6–12 yr	4.0–5.2		
	12–18 yr			
	M	4.5–5.3		
	F	4.1–5.1		
Hematocrit (Hct)	*% of Packed Cells*		Measures percentage of red blood cells in a volume of blood	Increased in erythrocytosis, polycythemia, severe dehydration, shock—when hemoconcentration rises considerably
	3 d	44–72		
	2 mo	28–42		
	6–12 yr	35–45		Decreased in anemia, leukemia, acute massive blood loss, hemolytic reactions
	12–18 yr			
	M	37–49		Unreliable immediately after transfusions, hemorrhage
	F	36–46		
Hemoglobin (Hgb)	*g/dL*		Measures oxygen-carrying capacity of the blood	Increased in hemoconcentration of the blood, CHF
	1–3 d	14.5–22.5		
	2 mo	9.0–14.0		Decreased in anemias; severe hemorrhage, hemolytic reactions
	6–12 yr	11.5–15.5		
	12–18 yr			Unreliable immediately after transfusions, hemorrhage
	M	13.0–16.0		
	F	12.0–16.0		
Erythrocyte sedimentation rate (ESR)	0–10 mm/hr		Measures the rate at which RBCs settle out of unclotted blood in one hour	Increased values found in infections, inflammatory diseases, carcinomas, cell or tissue destruction, toxemia, nephritis, pneumonia, severe anemia
			Based on the fact that inflammatory and necrotic processes result in aggregation of RBCs, which makes them heavier and more likely to settle	Decreased values found in polycythemia vera, sickle cell anemia, congestive heart failure
Reticulocyte count	Infants:	2–5% of total RBCs	Measures the number of immature RBCs (reticulocytes) compared with total RBCs	Increased in hemolytic anemia, sickle cell disease, leukemia, 3–4 days following hemorrhage, after splenectomy, following treatment of anemias
	Children:	0.5–4.0% of total RBCs	Indicates an increase in RBC production and/or a decrease in RBC destruction	Decreased levels indicate that the bone marrow is not producing enough erythrocytes and is seen in iron-deficiency anemia, aplastic anemia, chronic infection, radiation therapy
Mean corpuscular volume (MCV)	*um³*		Measures the volume occupied by a single red blood cell and indicates size of the cell: Normocytic—of normal size Microcytic—smaller than normal Macrocytic—larger than normal	Decreased in anemias, thalassemia
	1–3 d	95–121		Increased in liver diseases, deficiency of folate or vitamin B_{12}
	0.5–2 yr	70–86		
	6–12 yr	77–95		
	12–18 yr			
	M	78–98		
	F	78–102		

Table 26–2. RED BLOOD CELL STUDIES *Continued*

Test	Normal Values		Purpose	Clinical Signficance
Mean corpuscular hemoglobin concentration (MCHC)	*% hgb/cell or g hgb/dL RBC*		Measure of the concentration of hemoglobin in an average cell	Most valuable in evaluating therapy for anemia because the two most accurate hematologic determinations (Hgb & Hct) are used in this test
	1–3 d	30–36		
	1–2 wk	29–37		
	1–2 mo	29–37		Increased MCHC usually indicates spherocytosis
	3 mo–2 yr	30–36		
	2–18 yr	31–37		Decreased MCHC indicates that a unit volume of packed RBCs contains less hemoglobin than normal
				May be seen in iron-deficiency anemia, thalassemia
Mean corpuscular hemoglobin (MCH)	*%/cell*		Measure of the average weight of hemoglobin in the red blood cell	Increased MCH associated with macrocytic anemia
	1 d–3 d	31–37		
	1 wk–1 mo	28–40	Less accurate than MCHC because uses RBC count in the calculation and that count may be inaccurate	Decreased value associated with iron-deficiency anemia
	2 mo	26–34		
	3–6 mo	25–35		
	0.5–2 yr	23–31		
	2–6 yr	24–30		
	6–12 yr	25–33		
	12–18 yr	25–35		

Data from Fischbach, F. (1980). *A manual of laboratory diagnostic tests.* Philadelphia: J. B. Lippincott; Foster, R. L., Hunsberger, M. M., Anderson, J. J. (1989). *Family-centered nursing care of children.* Philadelphia: W. B. Saunders.

cell components. They are fragments of megakaryocytes. Megakaryocytes mature in the bone marrow and fragment, where each one releases approximately 5000 platelets into the blood. The lifespan of platelets is approximately 7 to 14 days. Approximately 10% to 15% of the circulating platelets is consumed in the daily repair of small vascular injuries.

The rate of platelet production and the level of circulating platelets are thought to be controlled by thrombopoietin or thrombopoiesis-stimulating factor. The level of circulating catecholamines also has an effect on platelet levels. The administration of epinephrine can immediately produce a 20% to 50% increase in the platelet count. This response is likely to be the result of mobilization from the splenic pool. Hypoxia also increases the number of circulating platelets.

Platelets play a primary role in the process of hemostasis. Hemostasis is achieved by vascular spasm, formation of a platelet plug, formation of a blood clot, and formation of connective tissue, which permanently repairs the damaged vessel. Vascular spasm reduces blood flow through a damaged blood vessel to prevent further blood loss. When platelets come in contact with the damaged blood vessel, they adhere to the walls of the vessel at the site of damage. Other platelets in the area are activated, and aggregation occurs when these cells adhere to the first. Thus, platelets group together to repair the damaged vessel.

Coagulation is a complex process involving an intricate series of reactions that include a number of different factors present in the blood or the tissues.

These substances influence the mechanisms of clotting by promoting clotting with procoagulants (clotting factors) or inhibiting clotting with anticoagulants. Some are also involved in the removal of a clot once it is formed. Each clotting factor acts as an enzyme, which, when activated, proceeds in a stepwise fashion to the next reaction. This is referred to as the *clotting cascade*, and each step must be completed for the next step to occur (Fig. 26–2).

The first step of coagulation is the formation of prothrombin activator. This step is the most complex because it involves a group of clotting factors involved in the extrinsic and intrinsic pathways. The extrinsic pathway is activated by trauma to the vascular walls and surrounding tissues. Factor III must be released from the endothelial cells and other tissues before activation can begin. When chemicals released into the tissues at time of injury (tissue factor) contacts factor VII, sequential activation of factors X, V, II, and I takes place. These factors then convert factor X to activated factor X.

When factor XII and platelets come in contact with collagen in the damaged wall of a vessel, the intrinsic pathway is activated. Factors XI, IX, VIII, X, II, and I are then activated, followed by the activation of factor X.

With the help of factor V, activated factor X forms prothrombin activator. Once this is formed, with the assistance of calcium ions, prothrombin is activated. Prothrombin is converted to thrombin with assistance of factor V. In the presence of thrombin and calcium ions, fibrinogen is converted into fibrin. The fibrin threads form a network over the damaged area of the vessel, which traps blood cells, platelets, and

Intrinsic system

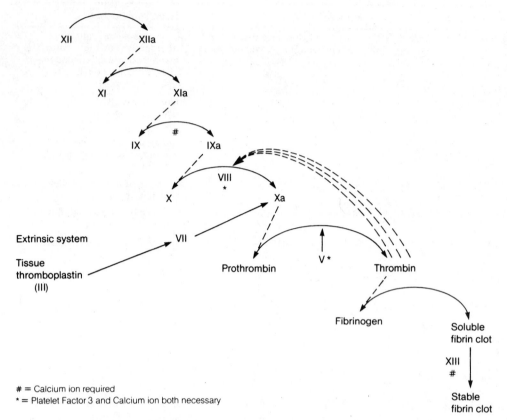

Figure 26–2 ● ● ● ● ● ●

The coagulation sequence. (From Hudak, C., Gallo, B., Lohr, T. (Eds.) (1973). *Critical care nursing*. Philadelphia: J.B. Lippincott.)

\# = Calcium ion required
* = Platelet Factor 3 and Calcium ion both necessary

plasma. A blood clot is formed and prevents further leakage through the damaged vessel. Within minutes of formation, clot retraction pulls together the sides of the damaged vessel.

Once formed, the clot may be the basis for new connective tissue or undergoes the processes of lysis and dissolution. After a few hours, fibroblasts invades the clot, and within 7 to 10 days, fibrous connective tissue is formed. Plasminogen and plasminogen activator, which are trapped within the clot with platelets and RBCs, ultimately produce plasmin, which lyses the clot.

The extrinsic pathway is activated when factor III gains access to the bloodstream; the intrinsic pathway is activated when blood comes in contact with an abnormal surface. Regardless of the initiating mechanism, the end is the same. Large amounts of thrombin are produced, which is then followed by the transformation of fibrinogen to fibrin. Table 26–3 lists the various factors involved in the clotting mechanism.

Various laboratory tests are used to assess coagulation function. These tests with normal values are reviewed in Table 26–4.

TRANSFUSION THERAPY

Pediatric critically ill patients may require blood product administration for a variety of reasons.

Nurses must be familiar with modifications of the blood products or unusual transfusion procedures required by individual patients, and with the potential risks of transfusions. Table 26–5 presents blood products commonly used in the PICU, indications for these blood products, dosage, and nursing implications.

Modifications of Blood Products

Various methods are available to modify blood products before administration to minimize the risks

Table 26–3. CLOTTING FACTORS

Factor	Synonym
I	Fibrinogen
II	Prothrombin
III	Tissue thromboplastin
IV	Calcium
V	Proaccelerin
VI	Proconvertin
VII:C	Antihemophilic factor A
IX	Christmas factor
X	Stuart-Prower factor
XI	Plasma thromboplastin antecedent
XII	Hageman factor
XIII	Fibrin stabilizing factor

From Gordon, J. B., Bernstein, M. L., Rogers, M. C. (1992). Hematologic disorders in the pediatric intensive care unit. In M. C. Rogers (Ed.). *Textbook of pediatric intensive care* (2nd ed.) (pp. 1380). Baltimore: Williams & Wilkins.

of transfusions for patients with special needs. One such modification is the irradiation of blood products. Leukocytes present in the transfused blood component can react against an immunosuppressed patient, causing graft-vs-host disease (GVHD). Irradiation destroys the leukocytes' ability to engraft in the patient. Patients susceptible to transfusion-associated GVHD (TA-GVHD) include transplant recipients and those with lymphoma or acute leukemia. The incidence of TA-GVHD is not known, but many oncology units and some neonatal centers routinely use irradiated blood (Luban & DePalma, 1993). It is generally recommended that patients at risk for TA-GVHD in the PICU receive irradiated blood products. Irradiated blood products pose no danger to health-care personnel (Committee on Transfusion Practices, 1986; National Blood Resource Education Program [NBREP], 1991).

To reduce the risk of nonhemolytic febrile reactions, leukocyte-depleted blood products may be transfused, especially to patients receiving frequent transfusions. They are ordered primarily when it has been demonstrated or suspected that the patient has previously experienced a febrile transfusion reaction. Other indications for leukocyte-depleted blood products are to prevent alloimmunization in recipients of frequent platelet transfusions, to prevent cytomega-

lovirus (CMV) infection when CMV-negative blood products are not available, and in prospective renal allograft recipients. Leukocyte depletion is usually achieved by filtration—a process that removes 70% to 99% of WBCs. Leukocytes can also be removed by washing RBCs or by freezing and deglycerolyzing RBCs (Folkes, 1990; NBREP, 1991).

Most transfusions can be administered without the use of a blood warmer. However, transfusions of more than one unit of blood every 10 minutes, and exchange transfusions in neonates, mandate the use of a blood warmer to prevent severe hypothermia, dysrhythmias, and cardiac arrest. Patients who are hypothermic prior to the transfusion, and those who have cold agglutinin disease, also require warmed blood products. When blood must be warmed, it is heated via an inline system. Because RBCs heated above 37°C may hemolyze, only temperature-controlled devices designed specifically to warm blood should be used (Committee on Transfusion Practices, 1986; NBREP, 1991).

Potential Complications

The most important potential complication associated with blood product administration is transfusion

Table 26–4. COAGULATION STUDIES

Test	Normal Values	Purpose	Clinical Significance
Platelet count	150,000–400,000/mm³	Measures total number of circulating platelets	Abnormally decreased in idiopathic thrombocytopenic purpura; pernicious, aplastic, and hemolytic anemias; drugs, especially chemotherapeutic agents; bone marrow malignancies. Abnormally increased after splenectomy and in certain cancers; may predispose to thrombotic episodes
Prothrombin time (PT)	11–15 sec	Indirectly measures the ability of the blood to clot and directly measures a defect in phase II clotting mechanisms (prothrombin, fibrinogen, factors V, VII, X)	Prolonged in prothrombin deficiency; vitamin K deficiency; deficiencies of fibrinogen; factors V, VII, X; anticoagulant therapy; severe liver disease; DIC
Partial thromboplastin time (PTT)	30–45 sec	Measures time required for clotting of plasma, fibrin clot formation; assesses phase I of clotting mechanism (adequacy of factors XII, XI, IX, VIII)	Prolonged in deficiencies of factors VIII, IX, XI, XII, fibrinogen; antocoagulant therapy; severe liver disease; DIC
Activated partial thromboplastin time (APTT)	16–25 sec	Same as for PTT but more sensitive and faster to perform	Same as PTT
Thrombin time (TT); thrombin clotting time	9–13 sec	Measures fibrinogen to fibrin formation; detects stage III of fibrinogen abnormalities	Prolonged with low fibrinogen levels; anticoagulaant therapy; liver disease; DIC
Thromboplastin generation time (TGT)	12 sec or less	Measures ability to form thromboplastin	Prolonged with thrombocytopenia; deficiencies of factors VIII to XII; anticoagulant therapy

Data from Fischbach, F. (1980). *A manual of laboratory diagnostic tests.* Philadelphia: J. B. Lippincott.
Foster, R. L., Hunsberger, M. M., Anderson, J. J. (1989). *Family-centered nursing care of children.* Philadelphia: W. B. Saunders.
Jackson, B. S. & Jones, M. B. (1988). Hematologic anatomy & physiology. In M. R. Kinney, D. R. Packa, S. B. Dunbar (Eds.). *AACN's clinical reference for critical-care nursing* (2nd ed.). New York: McGraw-Hill.

Table 26–5. BLOOD PRODUCTS COMMONLY USED IN THE PICU

Blood Product	Indication	Dosage	Must Be ABO Compatible	Requires Compatibility Testing	Rate of Administration	Available Modifications	Special Considerations
Whole blood	Symptomatic deficit of oxygen-carrying capacity plus hypovolemic shock Massive blood loss Exchange transfusions	20 mL/kg initially, followed by volume necessary to stabilize child's condition	Yes (must be ABO identical)	Yes	As fast as tolerated	Warmed Irradiated Leukocyte-depleted CMV neg, frozen, deglycerolyzed	Rarely used, usually for massive acute blood loss Platelets, WBCs, and clotting factors within stored whole blood are not functional
Packed red blood cells (PRBC)	Anemia/symptomatic deficit of oxygen-carrying capacity ± hypovolemia	10–20 mL/kg	Yes	Yes	2–4 hours (not greater than 6 hours)	Washed Warmed Irradiated Leukocyte-depleted CMV neg, frozen, deglycerolyzed	Multiple transfusions may result in dilution of coagulation factors Wait 4–6 hours after transfusion to check hematocrit
Platelets	Thrombocytopenia (usually platelet count <20,000 or <50,000 with active bleeding) Abnormal platelet function	1–2 units/10 kg	Yes (preferred)	No	As fast as tolerated, but usually not faster than 1 mL/kg/min	Irradiated Leukocyte-depleted CMV neg Volume-reduced Single donor HLA matched	Do not use microaggregate filters High risk of alloimmunization with repeated transfusions Transfusion not indicated in platelet-destruction conditions, except with hemorrhage
Fresh frozen plasma	Deficit of plasma coagulation factors (prolonged PT, PTT)	Clotting deficiency: 10–15 mL/kg Acute hemorrhage: 15–30 mL/kg	Yes	No	Depends on patient tolerance. Not faster than 1 mL/kg/min, not slower than 4 hours	Irradiated	Should not be used for hypovolemia/hypoproteinemia unless coagulation values are prolonged Must be used within 6 hours of thawing
Cryoprecipitate	Hemophilia A Hypofibrinogenemia Factor XIII deficiency Von Willebrand disease	1 unit per 5 kg	Yes	No	As fast as tolerated, usually not faster than 1 mL/kg/min	Irradiated	Must be used within 6 hours of thawing
Albumin	Hypovolemia	5%: 10–20 mL/kg 25%: 2–4 mL/kg	No	No	5%: As fast as tolerated 25%: 20–60 minutes	NA	No infectious risk Risk of circulatory overload secondary to increased oncotic pressure, especially with 25% albumin. Use within 6 hours of entering container

reaction. Transfusion reactions are generally classified as hemolytic or nonhemolytic reactions. Each reaction has some characteristic signs and symptoms, but the type of reaction may be difficult to ascertain initially.

Acute Hemolytic Reactions

Acute hemolytic reactions are potentially the most serious of transfusion reactions. A hemolytic reaction occurs when the blood product recipient has antibodies to some antigen on the transfused RBCs. The most common etiology of this antibody-antigen reaction is ABO incompatibility. The most frequent source of hemolytic reactions is mismatched blood, usually as a result of clerical error. Other possible causes of hemolysis of transfused blood are heating or freezing blood improperly, combining blood with

incompatible solutions (e.g., dextrose), and rapid infusion of blood through a small needle (Folkes, 1990; NBREP, 1991).

The signs and symptoms associated with a hemolytic reaction are fever, chills, flushing, low back pain, chest pain, tachycardia, tachypnea, and hypotension, which may progress to shock and cardiac arrest. Laboratory examination of blood and urine samples shows hemoglobinemia and hemoglobinuria, respectively. Acute renal failure may develop as a result of mechanical renal tubule obstruction from lysed cells (Bonato, 1989; Committee on Transfusion Practices, 1986; Folkes, 1990; NBREP, 1991).

If a hemolytic reaction is suspected, the transfusion is stopped immediately and the intravenous line kept patent with a normal saline solution. After notification of the physician, the patient is physiologically supported depending on the symptomatology (e.g., shock or respiratory distress are treated appropriately). Osmotic diuresis may be attempted to "flush out" the kidneys to prevent renal failure. The blood bank should be notified, and blood and urine samples should be sent for analysis (Bonato, 1989; Committee on Transfusion Practices, 1986; Folkes, 1990; NBREP, 1991). Bleeding that occurs as the result of DIC should be treated with fresh frozen plasma and platelet infusions.

Nonhemolytic Reactions

Nonhemolytic reactions are generally classified into febrile and allergic reactions. Febrile reactions, which are characterized by fever and possibly shaking chills, are the result of an immune response to infused WBCs or plasma proteins. Febrile reactions usually occur in frequently transfused patients, and are rarely serious. However, because fever can be the initial manifestation of a life-threatening hemolytic reaction, the transfusion should be discontinued if the patient's temperature rises 1°C or more above baseline. Antipyretics may be administered to control the fever. Febrile reactions can be prevented by providing frequently transfused patients with leukocyte-depleted blood products (Bonato, 1989; Committee on Transfusion Practices, 1986; Folkes, 1990; NBREP, 1991).

The other common type of nonhemolytic reaction is an allergic reaction. Most allergic reactions are mild, characterized by local erythema, pruritus, and urticaria. The transfusion should be stopped temporarily, and an antihistamine preparation should be administered. If the symptoms are mild and resolving, the transfusion may be restarted slowly. Patients who have had an allergic reaction to a transfusion may be pretreated with an antihistamine drug before subsequent transfusions.

Rarely, an anaphylactic reaction may occur. Features that distinguish an anaphylactic reaction are bronchospasm, hypotension, and absence of fever. These reactions, which are typically apparent after administration of only a few milliliters of the transfused blood product, occur almost exclusively in IgA-deficient recipients. Collaborative interventions include the administration of epinephrine, fluids, and corticosteroids (Bonato, 1989; Committee on Transfusion Practices, 1986; Folkes, 1990; NBREP, 1991).

Alloimmunization

Alloimmunization is another potential risk of receiving blood products, especially in patients who receive multiple transfusions. Such patients develop antibodies against antigens that they intrinsically lack, but that are present on the surface of the cells that have been transfused. Subsequent transfusions are affected; these newly formed antibodies may destroy future transfused cells that possess the targeted antigens. When platelets are transfused to a patient alloimmunized against platelets, there is no therapeutic effect; the patient is considered refractory to platelet therapy. Single-donor or HLA-matched platelets may offset the effects of alloimmunization. When RBCs are transfused to a patient alloimmunized against red cell antigens, hemolysis of the donor's cells may result. Appropriate cross-matching should prevent a serious hemolytic reaction. Using leukocyte-depleted blood components reduces the risk of alloimmunization (Folkes, 1989; NBREP, 1991).

Circulatory Overload

Circulatory overload is a potential complication of blood product administration, which occurs when the transfusion volume exceeds circulatory system capacity. Critically ill pediatric patients are at increased risk of circulatory overload because of their relatively small baseline blood volume and potentially compromised cardiovascular, pulmonary, and/or renal systems.

Symptoms of circulatory overload include dyspnea, tachycardia, tachypnea, hypertension, and even frank pulmonary edema. This complication can usually be prevented by adjusting the transfusion volume and flow rate based on the patient's size and clinical status. The blood bank can divide packed cells into smaller aliquots and can provide "volume-reduced" platelets to fluid-sensitive patients. Increased respiratory support and diuretics may be necessary to treat circulatory overload (Bonato, 1989; Folkes, 1990; NBREP, 1991).

Citrate Toxicity

Citrate is a substance that is present in the anticoagulant preservative solution added to most blood products. In the body, citrate binds with serum calcium, potentially causing hypocalcemia. The patients most at risk for symptomatic citrate toxicity are those who receive very rapid transfusions, those who receive multiple transfusions over a relatively short period of time, and patients with existing hepatic or renal dysfunction, because citrate is metabolized in the liver and excreted by the kidneys (Bonato, 1989).

The serum calcium level of patients at risk for citrate toxicity is checked before and during transfusions. When toxicity in the presence of hypocalcemia is anticipated, intravenous calcium chloride or calcium gluconate may be administered prophylactically.

Transmission of Infectious Diseases

Transmission of infectious diseases is a potential risk of blood product administration. Although fear of acquiring the human immunodeficiency virus (HIV) causing acquired immunodeficiency syndrome (AIDS) is generally the dominant concern of transfusion recipients and their families, the chances of contracting other infectious diseases, such as hepatitis or CMV poses a more significant health risk.

Approximately 2.5% of adult AIDS cases reported

to the Centers of Disease Control (CDC) have been related to transfusions. However, pediatric AIDS cases have a much higher proportion of post-transfusion etiology. As of August 1990, CDC statistics indicate that 15% of children with AIDS were infected by blood transfusions. The vast majority of patients with transfusion-acquired AIDS were infected before 1985. Since 1985, all blood-collecting facilities have used the HIV antibody test to screen donated blood, which has significantly decreased the risk of HIV transmission. The current risk of acquiring HIV from a blood transfusion is unknown, but it is estimated to be 1 in 88,000 to 1 in 300,000. There is evidence that the risk is declining by 30% per year (Bonato, 1989; DePalma & Luban, 1991).

The exact incidence of post-transfusion hepatitis is unknown. Hepatitis A virus (HAV) is usually transmitted by fecal-oral contact. At one time it was believed that post-transfusion HAV infection was virtually nonexistent. More recently, there have been reports in the literature that document HAV transmission by transfusion. For example, several nursery-wide outbreaks of post-transfusion HAV infection among newborns have been reported. Fortunately, none of these studies has demonstrated significant morbidity from HAV (DePalma & Luban, 1991).

In contrast, hepatitis B virus (HBV) has long been known to produce post-transfusion infection, which can cause significant morbidity and mortality. Despite the fact that all blood is screened for hepatitis B surface antigen (HBsAg), several prospective studies have documented that up to 1.7% of transfusion recipients develop HBV infection. Possible explanations for this phenomenon include the presence of infectious donors who are in the incubation phase, before HBsAg testing would be positive, and infectious donors with a serum level below the limits of detectability with current assays (DePalma & Luban, 1991).

Non-A non-B hepatitis (NANBH) is the most common post-transfusion hepatitis, accounting for about 60% of all cases. Hepatitis C virus (HCV) has been confirmed to be the cause of most, if not all, cases of NANBH. In adults, the sequelae of NANBH are chronic active hepatitis in 40% to 50% of cases, and cirrhosis in 20%. No data are available on long-term morbidity of post-transfusion NANBH in infants and children (Bonato, 1989).

Since May 1990, all units of blood and blood products have been tested for HCV antibody. Before routine testing, the risk of transfusion-associated HCV infection was estimated to be as high as 1 in 100. The current risk of transmission is not known (DePalma & Luban, 1991).

CMV transmission is another potential infectious risk of blood transfusions. Approximately 50% of the population are potential transmitters of CMV. Fortunately, in the majority of patients, CMV infection does not cause a clinical illness.

However, two populations at risk for serious complications from CMV infection are neonates and immunocompromised patients. In infants born to mothers without detectable CMV antibodies, acquired CMV infections can lead to atypical lymphocytosis, hepatosplenomegaly, pneumonia, or death. In immunosuppressed children, such as patients with oncologic disease and transplant recipients, CMV infection can cause life-threatening pneumonitis or hepatitis. Patients at risk for clinical CMV disease should receive blood that has been screened for antibodies to CMV (Bonato, 1989).

Coagulopathy

Coagulopathy can occur during massive transfusion, which is defined as the replacement of more than one blood volume (Fosburg & Kevy, 1987). During a rapid blood loss, the body cannot replace more than a small fraction of coagulation factors and platelets. Stored blood also has lost platelets and coagulation factors, such as factor VIII, which have become less active. When multiple transfusions are given over a short period of time, it is generally recommended that for every three units of packed RBCs administered, the child also receives one unit of fresh frozen plasma and one unit of platelets (Mehta et al., 1990). Coagulation studies may be done to determine specific component replacement.

APHERESIS

The term *apheresis* is derived from the Greek word for removal. Apheresis is a therapeutic process used to selectively extract abnormal blood components from the circulation. All apheresis procedures have certain basic principles in common. Blood is withdrawn from the patient, pumped through a cell separator that removes the desired component by centrifugal force, then the blood is returned to the patient. Each procedure is labeled according to the major component removed. Thus, removal of leukocytes is termed *leukapheresis*, red cell removal is *erythropheresis*, and so forth. *Plasmapheresis*, which is also called *intensive plasma exchange*, refers to the removal of plasma (Cohen, 1983; Kevy & Fosburg, 1990).

As with many advanced technologies, apheresis has been used more extensively in adults than in children. However, pediatric apheresis use has increased substantially since the early 1980s, with documented safety and efficacy for a variety of conditions. Apheresis has been successfully performed on very young and critically ill patients, but the smaller and sicker the patient, the greater the risks involved (Fosburg et al., 1983; Kasprisin, 1984a & b, 1989; Kevy & Fosburg, 1990).

Indications

Most of the accepted uses of apheresis in adults are for diseases that rarely occur in children, such as multiple myeloma and myasthenia gravis (Cohen,

1983). There are a number of pediatric conditions that are treated with apheresis on an outpatient basis, such as hyperviscosity in cyanotic congenital heart disease, familial hypercholesterolemia, and hyperproteinemia syndromes (Fosburg et al., 1983). This discussion will be limited to the indications for pediatric apheresis in the PICU patient.

HUS is a pediatric condition for which plasmapheresis has been used, with variable success rates. HUS is clinically similar to a primarily adult syndrome called thrombotic thrombocytopenia purpura (TTP), for which plasmapheresis has documented efficacy. The hypothesized mechanism of action of plasmapheresis in HUS and TTP is the removal of circulating endotoxin and/or the replacement of normal platelet aggregating factors (Cohen, 1983; Fosburg et al., 1983; Kasprisin, 1989; Kevy & Fosburg, 1990).

An acute condition that can be helped transiently by plasmapheresis is the severe coagulopathy associated with end-stage liver failure. In children, the massive amount of plasma volume necessary to correct this condition can result in severe circulatory overload, if the plasma is provided in the form of ongoing transfusions. Plasmapheresis allows the patient to remain relatively euvolemic, as the intrinsic coagulant-poor plasma is replaced with fresh coagulant-rich plasma and cryoprecipitate. This technique is a temporary supportive measure, generally used in life-threatening situations immediately before and after liver transplant (Kevy & Fosburg, 1990).

Other indications for pediatric plasmapheresis include autoimmune hemolytic disorders, hyperacute graft rejection after renal transplant, Guillain-Barré syndrome, and acute transfusion reactions. The rationale for plasmapheresis in these situations is to deplete the circulation of deleterious antibodies and immune complexes. Plasmapheresis is frequently successful in these cases (Cohen, 1983; Fosburg et al., 1983; Kevy & Fosburg, 1990).

There are two pediatric conditions that are commonly treated with cytopheresis (the removal of a specific cellular component from the blood). Erythropheresis is used for RBC exchange in some acute situations associated with sickle cell disease, such as stroke, acute chest syndrome, and priapism. Erythropheresis has a fairly high success rate for clinical improvement in these conditions, especially acute chest syndrome (Kevy & Fosburg, 1990).

Leukapheresis is a form of cytopheresis used to remove excessive leukocytes from the pediatric leukemic patient who presents with massive leukocytosis (leukocyte blast counts in excess of 150,000/mm³). Hyperleukocytosis causes hyperviscosity, which puts these patients at risk for acutely diminished organ perfusion, especially of the lungs and central nervous system. Two or more sessions of leukapheresis will generally reduce the WBC count to less than 100,000/mm³ (Cohen, 1983; Fosburg et al., 1983; Kasprisin, 1989; Kevy & Fosburg, 1990). Leukapheresis can enhance the efficacy of chemotherapeutic agents, whose action against a smaller tumor burden is enhanced (Cohen, 1983).

Procedure

The preparation and implementation of the apheresis procedure is typically the responsibility of the apheresis team (usually a hematologist and a specially trained apheresis nurse), but PICU nurses must be knowledgeable about the technical aspects of the process that affect the physiologic status of the patient in the PICU.

Vascular Access

The first, and often the most challenging, technical aspect to be considered in pediatric apheresis is the establishment of vascular access. This is especially problematic in small children and infants because peripheral vessels can rarely accommodate catheters of sufficient caliber to sustain the minimum flow rates (20–40 mL/minute) required for apheresis. Antecubital sites have occasionally been successfully used in children as young as 3 years old, but more commonly, jugular, femoral, or subclavian veins are cannulated for the procedure (Fosburg et al., 1983; Kasprisin, 1984, 1989; Kevy & Fosburg, 1990).

Catheters are generally inserted percutaneously at the bedside for acute short-term therapy. Two ports are required to simultaneously remove and return blood, necessary in the pediatric patient to prevent hypovolemia. Frequently, double-lumen catheters that are designed for short-term hemodialysis are used (Kevy & Fosburg, 1990). If the patient already has a double-lumen catheter in place, it may be adequate if it is large enough to accommodate high flow rates, and if the patient has other access available for the infusion of maintenance fluids and medications during apheresis procedures.

Priming

The procedures followed to prime the apheresis circuit are quite different in adult than pediatric apheresis. In children, the amount of extracorporeal blood necessary to fill the apheresis equipment may represent a significant proportion of the patient's blood volume (i.e., greater than 10%). As a result, pediatric patients can become hypovolemic if the tubing is not primed with a solution to replace the blood being drawn off at the onset of the procedure (Fosburg et al., 1983; Kaprisin, 1984a & b, 1989; Kevy & Fosburg, 1990).

The composition of the priming solution must also be given careful consideration in the pediatric patient. If the machine is primed with saline, the child's hematocrit level is diluted by the percentage of blood volume that the priming solution represents. The smaller and more seriously ill the child, the less able to tolerate abrupt fluctuations in RBC concentration. The technique most commonly used to offset this phenomenon involves preparing a priming solution consisting of packed RBCs diluted with saline to a hematocrit level equal to the patient's hematocrit level (or greater if the child is anemic). Alternatively, the child may be transfused with packed RBCs immediately before the procedure (Fosburg et al., 1983; Kasprisin, 1984a & b, 1989; Kevy & Fosburg, 1990).

Anticoagulation

Anticoagulation is another technical issue that must be considered for the apheresis procedure. The blood circulating through the apheresis equipment must be anticoagulated to avoid thrombus formation in the tubing. The amount and type of anticoagulating agent used is based upon the patient's age and intrinsic coagulation status, and on the type of apheresis machine used. Young children and those with coagulopathies receive smaller doses of anticoagulants (Kevy & Fosburg, 1990).

The two agents most commonly used are acid-citrate-dextrose (referred to as ACD or citrate) and heparin. It is crucial to monitor the patient for side effects of the anticoagulants used (Fosburg et al., 1983; Kasprisin, 1984a & b; Kevy & Fosburg, 1990). The side effect of heparin is bleeding; the side effect of citrate toxicity is symptomatic hypocalcemia.

Nursing Implications

There are a number of potential physiologic derangements associated with apheresis procedures in the PICU. Patients are monitored carefully for changes in condition to permit timely and appropriate intervention. The apheresis team is responsible to manage the apheresis procedure itself, whereas the critical care team is responsible for continuing patient assessment and monitoring.

Fluid Volume Deficit

Apheresis can cause fluid depletion in the critically ill child if an excessive amount of the child's circulating blood volume is in the extracorporeal circulation at one time. Apheresis can also cause hypoproteinemia resulting from the depletion of albumin from the bloodstream. Hypovolemia may result from fluid shifts from the intravascular space (Kasprisin, 1989).

To minimize intravascular depletion, it is standard to prevent more than 15% of the child's blood volume from being in the extracorporeal circulation at any time (Fosburg et al., 1983; Kasprisin, 1984a & b, 1989). The patient's heart rate, blood pressure, and tissue perfusion status are continuously monitored. In addition, serum albumin and total protein are measured to ensure stable oncotic pressure. The team coordinating the apheresis procedure should be alert for signs of hypovolemia. The rate of blood removed may be slowed and/or albumin or another fluid infused to correct hypovolemia.

Fluid Volume Excess

The pediatric apheresis patient is also at risk for circulatory overload. If the patient receives a large amount of albumin to correct hypoproteinemia or requires a substantially greater volume of fluid than is removed, fluid volume excess may occur.

The patient is monitored for signs of hypervolemia, such as an increased central venous pressure (CVP), pulmonary edema, a "gallop" rhythm heard upon cardiac auscultation, peripheral edema, and increased weight after the procedure. The net fluid balance during and after apheresis is calculated and the physician notified of signs of hypervolemia. The fluid calculations may be adjusted, or a diuretic may be administered after the procedure, in the event of symptomatic circulatory overload.

Potential for Injury Related to Alteration in Calcium Metabolism

Calcium is lost from plasma that is removed during plasmapheresis, putting the patient at risk for hypocalcemia. In addition, during apheresis the use of citrate as an anticoagulant poses significant risks for hypocalcemia because citrate inactivates calcium. Patients at greatest risk for citrate toxicity are those who are prone to hypocalcemia for other reasons, such as shock, renal failure, or the infusion of large amounts of citrated blood products (Cohen, 1983; Fosburg et al., 1983; Kasprisin, 1984a & b; Kevy & Fosburg, 1990).

If citrate is administered during apheresis, the patient is assessed for clinical signs of hypocalcemia. In critically ill children, the first apparent sign of hypocalcemia is usually hypotension. Hypotension in patients receiving citrate is assumed to be caused by hypocalcemia until proved otherwise (Fosburg et al., 1983; Kevy & Fosburg, 1990).

Ionized calcium is monitored during the procedure, especially if citrate is administered (total calcium values are inaccurate because of fluctuating albumin levels). The frequency of monitoring depends upon the size of the child and the amount of blood being administered. Calcium gluconate is administered for clinical and/or laboratory evidence of hypocalcemia. Calcium is administered slowly because rapid infusion can cause bradycardia and cardiac arrest. If a patient who has developed citrate toxicity requires repeated apheresis procedures, using heparin alone as an anticoagulant is considered (Fosburg et al., 1983).

Ineffective Thermoregulation

Infants and young children are at increased risk for heat loss. In addition, when critically ill, disruptions in thermoregulation related to sepsis or neurologic compromise may result in temperature instability. When blood is circulated outside the body, as in the apheresis procedure, and exposed to room temperature, hypothermia may result.

The child should be monitored for signs of hypothermia, such as shivering, bradycardia, diminished perfusion, and decreased level of consciousness. The patient's temperature should be monitored every 15 to 30 minutes, by the axillary or rectal route in infants, young children, and unconscious patients. Increasing the room temperature and applying blanket layers and heating pads (cautiously) can prevent or correct hypothermia in these patients.

In addition, depending on the apheresis machine used, and the judgment of the apheresis physician, blood may be warmed before it is returned to the patient (Fosburg et al., 1983; Kasprisin, 1984a & b). In patients whose reinfusion line terminates in or near the right atrium, the rapid infusion of relatively "cold" blood can cause severe ventricular dysrhythmias (Kasprisin, 1984a & b). These patients require electrocardiogram (ECG) monitoring for dysrhythmias, and warming the reinfused blood may be warranted.

Potential for Injury Related to Bleeding

A number of factors put the pediatric apheresis patient at risk for bleeding complications, including preexisting coagulopathy, systemic anticoagulation, depletion of fibrinogen and platelets owing to the apheresis process, and the presence of a large intravascular line.

Prothrombin time (PT), partial thromboplastin time (PTT), fibrinogen level, platelet count, hematocrit, and activated clotting time (ACT) are measured before and after apheresis. These values help to determine the type and amount of anticoagulant used during the procedure. The ACT is generally measured at the bedside at regular intervals by the apheresis nurse, and the citrate and/or heparin doses are titrated accordingly. Normal ACT is 90 seconds; the desired ACT during apheresis is usually 150 to 180 seconds (Fosburg et al., 1983; Kasprisin, 1984a & b; Kevy & Fosburg, 1990).

The child is monitored for clinical signs of bleeding during and after the procedure. Platelets or other clotting factor transfusions may be necessary to replace those depleted during apheresis. In rare instances, protamine sulfate may be administered to reverse the anticoagulant effects of heparin. All hematologic values should be rechecked 24 hours after the apheresis procedure.

DISORDERS OF COAGULATION

Disseminated Intravascular Coagulation

DIC is not a distinct disease, but rather an abnormal coagulation syndrome which occurs secondary to another disease process (Young, 1990). It is characterized by excessive use of coagulation factors that exceeds the ability to replenish these factors and results in the rapid production of thrombin and activated factor X or excessive bleeding as a result of failure of clot formation. Critically ill children may develop this syndrome as a final common pathway

complicating their underlying illness. The onset of DIC is usually preceded by massive activation of the hemostatic processes. The leading cause is infection. Many bacterial processes invoke activating factors that initiate the intrinsic coagulation system. Endothelial damage and tissue damage also enhance intrinsic stimulation as well as activate the extrinsic coagulation pathway.

DIC may also occur secondary to shock, burns, malignancies, fat emboli, hemolytic transfusion reactions or immune disease. Other precipitating factors are hypoxia, acidosis, and hypotension. DIC has actually been reported to complicate more than 100 clinical disorders (Esparaz & Green, 1990).

Pathogenesis

In DIC there is acceleration of normal coagulation, but the end result is bleeding. Excessive production of thrombin and plasmin degrades fibrinogen to fibrin, leading to further activation of the coagulation system, deposition of fibrin in the microvasculature, activation of the fibrinolytic system, and platelet activation. Consumption of clotting factors and platelets occurs and, as the process continues, fibrin split products (FSP) are produced. If FSP are not cleared from the circulation by the reticuloendothelial system (RES), anticoagulation will be enhanced. Normally the RES removes fibrin, activated clotting factors, endotoxins, and FSP from the circulation. Dysfunction of the RES owing to shock or liver disease impairs removal of these substances, leading to hypercoagulability and DIC. With an increase in circulating FSP, there is decreased platelet function and adherence, inhibition of thrombin, activation of complement, and further endothelial damage. The development of microvascular thrombi and bleeding leads to cellular ischemia (Fig. 26–3).

Clinical Presentation

The clinical presentation of DIC varies dramatically from one patient to another. Onset may be sud-

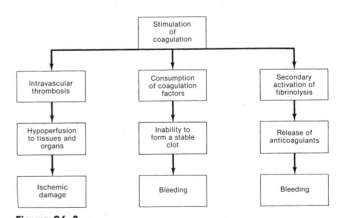

Figure 26–3 ● ● ● ● ● ●

The pathophysiology of DIC. (From Dressler, D.K. (1992). Patients with coagulopathies. In J.M. Clochesy, et al. (Eds.). *Critical care nursing*, p. 1056. Philadelphia: W.B. Saunders.)

den or gradual. It may be difficult to differentiate clinical signs from those of the underlying disease state. DIC may be suspected only because of its known association with certain pathologic states. Bleeding is the most obvious clinical sign of DIC. In the child, abnormal bleeding is often identified from ecchymoses or petechiae or in oozing from intravenous and venipuncture sites (Flug & Karpatkin, 1985).

In its most extreme case, the child with DIC shows pallor and circulatory failure, which is manifested by tachycardia and hypotension. Purpura and overt bleeding that may involve the pulmonary, cerebral, and intraventricular systems may be seen. In addition, thrombosis of the central and peripheral veins may lead to gangrene and tissue necrosis.

Abnormal serum coagulation values are an early indication of DIC. Typical findings include anemia with RBC fragmentation, and prolonged PT, PTT, and thrombin time. An increase in FSP is the cardinal sign of DIC. The greatest degree of diagnostic specificity is the measurement of the D-dimer FSP fragment, which is a breakdown product of cross-linked fibrin in either plasma or serum (Kruskal et al., 1987). Fibrinogen levels are usually decreased but may be normal in some cases. Factors V and VIII are normal or may be extremely elevated. The presence of fragmented blood cells or shistocytes may be seen and indicates fibrin deposition in small vessels and a thrombolytic occurrence.

Critical Care Management

Many patients in the PICU are at risk to develop DIC. Thorough nursing assessment is essential in the prompt recognition and subsequent management of patients with DIC. The skin, mucous membranes, and all drainage or secretions should be observed for obvious or occult bleeding.

Vital sign changes that may be indicative of bleeding and hypovolemia are tachycardia, tachypnea, and hypotension. It is important to remember that hypotension is a late sign in the child. Changes in mental status such as irritability, restlessness, and lethargy are signs of decreased cerebral perfusion related to hypovolemia and may present in the child with bleeding related to DIC.

Critical care management of patients with DIC is supportive, aimed at stabilization of cardiac status and restoration of fluid and electrolyte balance. Specific treatment of the underlying disorder includes correction of shock, acidosis, and electrolyte imbalance, and antibiotic therapy for bacterial infections. Replacement of coagulation factors is often necessary. Packed red blood cells (PRBCs) may be administered for active bleeding. In addition, if the child is actively bleeding and has a low platelet count (<20,000/μL), platelets are administered to increase the platelet count to 60,000/μL. If the platelet count is higher than 50,000/μL and the child is still bleeding, fresh frozen plasma (FFP) 10 to 15 mL/kg body weight is administered to replace consumed clotting compo-

nents. Cryoprecipitate is administered for fibrinogen levels below 75 g/dL to elevate fibrinogen levels. Table 26–5 presents specific implications associated with the use of these blood products.

Nursing care for the child receiving these blood products consists of monitoring for reactions to blood products, signs of fluid imbalance, and vital signs, including central venous pressure. Intake and output volumes are also strictly measured.

Controlling and preventing further bleeding is of paramount importance in caring for the critically ill child with DIC. Vital signs and laboratory studies must be monitored frequently for changes that indicate bleeding. All output, including urine, stool, and nasogastric drainage, should be tested for the presence of blood. All invasive sites should be closely observed for oozing or active bleeding. Intramuscular injections and rectal procedures must be avoided because of the increased risk for bleeding.

Heparin Therapy. Heparin therapy for DIC is controversial because its efficacy has not been proven (Bray, 1993). The rationale for administering heparin is the enhancement of antithrombin (AT) III activity, a major inhibitor of thrombin. With thrombin activity inhibited, degradation of fibrinogen to fibrin is impeded and further development of microvascular thrombi is slowed or halted. The concern about heparin therapy is the potential risk of further bleeding. When heparin is administered, the child receives an initial intravenous loading dose of 50 units/kg, followed by a continuous intravenous infusion of 10 to 20 units/kg/hour. Supportive therapy with platelet, FFP, and cryoprecipitate transfusions is continued.

The most valuable test for evaluating the effectiveness of heparin is the fibrinogen level. Even with a severe decrease in fibrinogen, the level should rise to a normal or near-normal level within 24 hours of effective heparin therapy (Lusher, 1987). The PT and PTT are not particularly useful in evaluating heparin therapy in DIC because test results in both are prolonged with heparin. The platelet count is also of little value as an early guide to the efficacy of heparin therapy because it may take several days for the count to return to normal even though the platelet count is not affected by heparin.

Assessing the child closely for the exacerbation of bleeding related to heparin is critical because this is the indication for discontinuation of heparin therapy. The child is also reevaluated regarding the need for further replacement of platelets and coagulation factors. Protamine sulfate may be administered to counteract the effects of heparin (1 mg for every 100 units of heparin). However, this is only rarely necessary owing to the short half-life of heparin.

The duration of heparin therapy for DIC may vary from 12 to 24 hours in conditions when the underlying disease may be treated effectively. Other conditions, such as leukemia, may require therapy for as long as 2 to 3 weeks.

Apheresis. Partial exchange transfusions with heparinized fresh blood or reconstituted FFP and packed RBCs may be necessary if fluid overload becomes a persistent problem and the child continues to require large volumes of blood or clotting factors. Removal of selected mediators also may break the vicious, self-perpetuating cycle of DIC. Nursing responsibilities related to apheresis have been discussed previously.

ALTERATIONS IN OXYGEN-CARRYING CAPACITY

Anemias

Anemia is defined as an inadequate amount of hemoglobin or RBCs necessary to meet the patient's oxygen transport needs (Pascucci, 1989). Anemia results from an excessive loss or destruction of blood, an inadequate production of hemoglobin and RBCs resulting from bone marrow failure or a deficiency state, or a combination of both (Platt & Nathan, 1989).

Patients with anemia may present to the PICU as an emergency or with an acute exacerbation of a chronic anemia. Overall, the main problems seen in children with anemia of any etiology are impaired gas exchange, altered tissue perfusion, and altered fluid volume. Nursing care is directed toward assessment and management of these problems.

Impaired Gas Exchange

Children with anemia may show signs of respiratory distress related to the decreased oxygen-carrying capacity of the RBCs. A thorough assessment of their respiratory status is essential. Monitoring oxygen saturation and arterial blood gases on a regular basis is included in this assessment. The need for supplemental oxygen and/or mechanical ventilation is based on the results of this assessment and other problems produced by the severity of the anemia.

Alteration in Tissue Perfusion

Children who present with anemia from excessive blood loss have the potential for altered tissue perfusion related to hypovolemia. Cold extremities, pallor, mottled skin, decreased or absent peripheral pulses, and blood pressure changes all are seen as the result of altered tissue perfusion.

Treatment is aimed at restoring circulating blood volume. Initially this may be done with a crystalloid solution, followed by blood products, if necessary. Nursing implications associated with blood transfusions are presented in Table 26–5.

Alteration in Fluid Volume

Children with hypovolemia from excessive blood loss or dehydration (which is often seen with sickle cell anemia) may present with inadequate fluid volume. Children should be monitored for signs of hypo-

volemia and dehydration and therapy implemented when appropriate.

Children with anemia and hypovolemia may require the administration of large amounts of fluids and blood products, placing them at risk for fluid overload. Edema, weight gain, intake greater than output, abnormal breath sounds including rales and crackles, and an increase in CVP and blood pressure are seen. It is critical for the nurse caring for children requiring administration of large volumes of fluid or blood product to closely monitor for the development of these symptoms.

The anemias seen in children are reviewed in Table 26–6 and discussed briefly later. Sickle cell anemia is discussed in more detail because children with this disease present to the PICU more frequently than do children with other types of chronic anemia.

Anemia Related to Blood Loss

Acute or chronic blood loss may produce anemia. With acute blood loss, the anemia is present after the loss of blood volume is replaced with ECF. Chronic blood loss produces anemia when the body has expended its iron reserve.

Table 26–6. CLASSIFICATION OF ANEMIAS OF CHILDHOOD

A. Abnormal red blood cell production
  1. Disorder of proliferation/differentiation
    a. Aplastic anemia
    b. Pure red cell aplasia
    c. Erythropoietin deficiency
  2. Disorder of DNA synthesis
    a. Vitamin B_{12} deficiency
    b. Folate deficiency
  3. Disorder of hemoglobin synthesis
    a. Iron deficiency
    b. Thalassemia
B. Increased RBC destruction
  1. Intrinsic RBC abnormalities
    a. Membrane defects
      Hereditary spherocytosis
      Liver disease
    b. Abnormal red cell metabolism
      Glucose-6-phosphate dehydrogenase deficiency
      Pyruvate kinase deficiency
  2. Extrinsic abnormalties
    a. Mechanical destruction
      Microangiopathic hemolytic anemia
      Traumatic hemolysis (cardiac valve prosthesis)
    b. Infection
      Bacterial
      Viral
      Parasitic
    c. Antibody-mediated
      Alloimmune hemolytic disease of the newborn
      Drug reaction
      Autoantibody-mediated destruction of erythrocytes
    d. Hypersplenism
C. Blood loss
  1. Traumatic/gastrointestinal hemorrhage
  2. Surgical

From Nugent, D. J., & Tarantino, M. D. (1992). Hematology-oncology problems in the intensive care unit. In B. P. Fuhrman, & J. J. Zimmerman (Eds.). *Pediatric critical care* (pp. 816). St. Louis: Mosby–Year Book.

Critical Care Management. The clinical presentation of a child with anemia related to blood loss varies greatly. Those with chronic anemia often adapt to a low hematocrit and hemoglobin without compromise. On the other hand, a previously healthy child who has a sudden and dramatic reduction in hematocrit and hemoglobin may present as an acutely ill child in shock and requires aggressive intervention.

Laboratory tests to evaluate this type of anemia include a complete blood count (CBC) with RBC indices, platelet count, PT, PTT, serum fibrinogen level, and FSP. During and shortly after an episode of bleeding, the platelet count and serum fibrinogen level may transiently decrease. The hematocrit and hemoglobin remain unchanged in the acutely bleeding child because 24 to 72 hours are necessary for the hematocrit and hemoglobin levels to equilibrate and accurately reflect the total amount of blood loss.

Treatment for acute blood loss is aimed at restoring intravascular volume. Chronic anemia is generally well tolerated, and transfusion is not usually necessary unless the hemoglobin falls below 6 to 7 g/dL.

Hemolytic Anemia

The average lifespan of a RBC is 100 to 120 days. About 1% of RBCs are removed from the circulation each day and the same percentage is replaced by new red cells (reticulocytes) released from the bone marrow. Hemolytic anemia results when RBC destruction is abnormally high and the bone marrow compensatory mechanism cannot keep pace with the loss of RBCs. Hemolysis of RBCs may be caused by a variety of etiologies. These include DIC, HUS, hemolytic transfusion reactions, Rh hemolytic disease of the newborn, and thalassemia syndromes.

Critical Care Management. Because hemolysis of RBCs is the cause of this anemia, diagnosis is based on the fact that RBCs are undergoing premature disruption. An elevated reticulocyte count and elevated serum levels of unconjugated bilirubin are seen. Erythroid hyperplasia and a decrease in the granulocyte to erythrocyte level are revealed in examination of the bone marrow.

If the child is experiencing signs of diminished oxygenation and/or tissue perfusion, packed RBCs are administered. If the child is experiencing an immune hemolytic reaction owing to an underlying disorder such as lupus or lymphoma, a cross-match may be difficult to obtain. However, if the anemia is causing hemodynamic instability, the child should be transfused with type-specific blood in a sufficient amount to stabilize the cardiovascular system, in spite of incompatibility.

Aplastic Anemia

Aplastic anemia refers to a pronounced reduction in the number of RBCs, WBCs, and platelets resulting from hypoplasia or aplasia of the bone marrow in the absence of malignant disease. This type of anemia may be congenital or acquired, resulting from medications, infections, chemical exposure, or radiation.

Critical Care Management. Children show the classic signs of a low blood count. Anemia, pallor, and fatigue may be present because of a decreased RBC count; increased susceptibility to infections from a low WBC count; and ecchymosis, petechiae, and epistaxis resulting from a low platelet count. Bone marrow biopsy reveals a marked reduction in all cells. Children with severe aplastic anemia may present to the PICU with signs of decreased oxygenation resulting from a reduction in the oxygen-carrying capacity of the blood, cardiac failure, overwhelming infection, or massive bleeding.

The treatment priority for the child with life-threatening complications of aplastic anemia is cardiopulmonary stabilization. RBC transfusions are administered and platelet transfusions are indicated for the child with signs of severe bleeding (e.g., gastrointestinal bleeding). All blood products are irradiated and filtered before transfusion because of the risk of post-transfusion GVHD related to sensitization of the recipient to HLA antigens in the donated blood. Infections are treated with broad-spectrum antibiotics or antifungal agents, if a fungal infection is present.

Treatment specific to aplastic anemia includes androgen therapy, immunosuppressive therapy, and bone marrow transplantation. Bone marrow transplantation is the treatment of choice if a compatible donor is available. Chapter 24 provides information on the care of the child receiving a bone marrow transplant.

Iron Deficiency Anemia

Iron deficiency anemia is the result of a disturbance of heme synthesis. The most common causes are inadequate intake of daily iron requirements or malabsorption.

Critical Care Management. Signs and symptoms of iron deficiency anemia tend to be vague and nonspecific. Irritability, anorexia, and pallor may be present. Some degree of growth retardation may be seen in the child with long-term iron deficiency.

Laboratory studies demonstrate a hemoglobin of less than 10 g/dL. The RBC count is normal or only slightly decreased, but because the cells are lacking hemoglobin, they are microcytic and hypochromic. Red cell indices reveal mean corpuscular volume (MCV) less than 80 μm, mean corpuscular hemoglobin (MCH) less than 27 picograms, and MCH concentration (MCHC) less than 30%.

PICU admission is not warranted solely for iron deficiency anemia, but anemia may be concurrent with another disease process. Iron deficiency anemia is easily treated with iron therapy.

Sickle Cell Disease

Sickle cell disease (SCD) refers to a group of hemoglobinopathies distinguished by the development of sickled cells in response to deoxygenation. Sickle cell anemia (SCA) is the most common cause of SCD. SCA is an autosomal recessive disorder in which the child produces sickle hemoglobin (hgb S) rather than hgb A. The child with sickle cell trait has inherited a sickle gene (Hb S) from one parent and a normal hemoglobin gene (Hb A) from the other parent. This child is always a carrier of SCA, although the trait does not progress to anemia.

When the child inherits two Hb S genes, SCA results. The red cells of SCA contain up to 80% to 100% of Hb S. This is a potentially fatal disease that occurs predominantly in the black race.

Pathogenesis. Sickling of the RBC describes the change of a normal round RBC to a sickle-shaped one. The sickling process begins with the substitution of valine for glutamic acid on the beta chain of the hemoglobin molecule. This process produces Hb S, which is less soluble than the normal cell when deoxygenated. The decreased solubility causes Hb S to become more viscous and change to the sickle shape.

Once RBCs sickle, they are more fragile and easily destroyed. They cannot flow easily through the capillary beds and tend to become clumped, causing obstruction and impediment to blood flow. Tissue hypoxia develops, which promotes further sickling. As the hypoxia worsens, infarctions and necrosis can develop (Fig. 26–4).

There are several factors that cause Hb S to sickle (Table 26–7). Hypoxia is a major determinant. Characteristics of blood flow can also increase the tendency toward sickling. Under normal circumstances, the cardiac output of the child with SCD is elevated. This compensatory mechanism ensures that the transit time of blood between the capillary and the lung is rapid so that sickling cannot occur. However, any pathophysiologic process that affects pressure (such as hypotension or pulmonary hypertension), or increases resistance (such as vasoconstriction or increased hematocrit) promotes sickling.

Critical Care Management. The clinical presentation of children with SCD varies greatly. The symptoms seen are usually the result of (1) hemolysis of the cells and the compensatory mechanisms invoked

Table 26–7. FACTORS THAT MAY PROMOTE SICKLING

1. Pressure-related
a. Hypotension
b. Pulmonary hypertension
2. Resistance-related
a. Vasoconstriction
b. Increased hematocrit (>35%)
3. Desaturation-related
a. Hypoxemia
b. Acidosis

From Gordon, J. B., Bernstein, M. L., Rogers, M. C. (1992). Hematologic disorders in the pediatric intensive care unit. In M. C. Rogers (Ed.). *Textbook of Pediatric Intensive Care* (2nd ed., pp. 1359). Baltimore: Williams & Wilkins.

by the subsequent anemia; and (2) thrombi in the small vessels of various organs resulting from the sickling. General symptoms seen in the child with SCA include weakness, pallor, fatigue, tissue hypoxia, and jaundice, as the result of RBC hemolysis. The heart may become enlarged because of the higher cardiac output demanded by the chronic anemia. Thrombi from the sickle cells may cause progressive damage to multiple organs, including the eyes, liver, and lungs.

Diagnosis of SCA and sickle cell trait are made through a variety of tests. The most commonly used is a hemoglobin electrophoresis. This assay separates the various types of hemoglobin and quantifies the percentages of various hemoglobins present. There are less sensitive tests that determine the presence or absence of Hb S; however, positive results require further screening with hemoglobin electrophoresis. Diagnosis may be made prenatally by using fetal blood obtained in placental aspiration or photoscope.

A PICU admission often signals a life-threatening episode with a high risk of morbidity and mortality for children with SCA. Outcome is often dependent upon which organs are affected, the type of virus and/or bacteria causing the infection, if one is present, and the degree of progressive damage that has already occurred because of the disease. Nursing care is critical in managing the effects of the SCD crises.

Impaired Gas Exchange. The child with sickle cell anemia may have signs of respiratory distress for a number of reasons. Pneumonia and pulmonary infarctions occur more frequently in this patient population. Splenic sequestration may also cause respiratory distress as the engorged spleen pushes up on the diaphragm (Morrison & Vedro, 1989). Hypoxemia causes increased sickling and, in turn, a vicious cycle of deoxygenation related to anemia and vasoocclusive crisis.

Assessment of breath sounds on a regular basis is imperative. The patient is observed for signs of respiratory distress, and the lungs are auscultated to detect decreased breath sounds along with abnormal sounds. Monitoring arterial blood gases on a regular schedule and continuous monitoring of oxygen saturation is essential. Oxygen by face mask or nasal cannula may be the only respiratory support that is needed. However, if the blood gases do not demon-

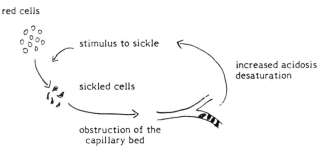

Figure 26–4 ● ● ● ● ● ●

The "vicious cycle" of progressive sickling causing intravascular occlusion. (From Gordon, J.B., Bernstein, M.L., Rogers, M.C. (1992). Hematologic disorders in the intensive care unit. In M.C. Rogers (Ed.). *Textbook of pediatric intensive care*, 2nd ed., p. 1360. Baltimore: Williams & Wilkins.)

strate improved oxygenation and the child's respiratory status continues to deteriorate, intubation and ventilatory support are necessary. Daily chest films are routinely done to monitor progression or resolution of pulmonary complications.

Alteration in Comfort, Pain. Vasoocclusive crises can vary in location, duration, and intensity. The pain associated with the crises may be mild, moderate, or severe. Nursing assessment of the child in pain should include physiologic and behavioral indicators (see Chapter 18). On admission to the PICU, the child's pain and level of analgesia should be assessed, and opioid bolus given if necessary. Pain assessment and treatment should continue every 30 minutes to 1 hour, until the pain is tolerable.

A recommended regimen for initial pain management is 0.10 to 0.15 mg/kg/dose of morphine sulfate given every 2.5 hours around the clock (Shapiro, 1989). Another alternative is to administer a continuous narcotic infusion, since bolus injections may not provide satisfactory analgesia because of the short plasma half-life of the narcotic (Morrison & Vedro, 1989). An infusion of 0.05 to 0.10 mg/kg/hour of morphine is recommended, with close assessment of level of sedation and respiratory depression (Shapiro, 1989). Patient-controlled analgesia (PCA) provides yet another method of pain management for children who are able to and want to manage their own pain relief.

Regional anesthetic techniques, such as epidural infusions and nerve blocks, may be necessary for pain control. These techniques are used when the pain is persistent despite large doses of narcotics to avoid narcotics' life-threatening side effects.

A parenteral anti-inflammatory drug (ketorolac) is being used for crisis pain and has dramatically decreased the amount of narcotic these patients previously required.

Fluid Volume Deficit. Hypovolemia is often seen in children with SCA in the PICU. Fluid replacement depends upon the clinical condition and the results of the serum electrolytes, hematocrit, and coagulation studies. Children with splenic sequestration require crystalloid and RBCs immediately to restore circulating blood volume. Children in aplastic crisis require packed RBCs because of their decreased hematocrit level. Crystalloids may be the only fluid replacement in vasoocclusive crisis, depending on the degree of sickling and whether or not there is ischemia or infarction of the affected organ.

Patients with SCA tolerate a low hematocrit level extremely well, and transfusions should only be initiated when absolutely necessary. The potential for significant complications related to multiple transfusions include infection, iron overload, and alloimmunization.

The nurse monitors for reactions to blood products and for signs of fluid imbalance. Children with SCA may require frequent transfusions during an acute episode, which increases the risk of volume overload. It is critical to closely monitor the patient for signs of fluid overload. The use of short-acting diuretics before or after the transfusion may help to prevent this complication. Other nursing responsibilities include monitoring vital signs and laboratory values, and maintaining an accurate intake and output.

Exchange or partial exchange transfusions are often used for acute complications of sickle cell anemia. The advantage of an exchange or partial exchange transfusion over a simple transfusion is that there is less risk for volume overload and a more rapid reduction in the percentage of cells containing Hb S. Preoperative exchange transfusions may be done for children with SCA requiring surgery to reduce the risk of postoperative vasoocclusive complications. Apheresis may also be used in the treatment of acute complications of SCA. Nursing responsibilities related to these procedures have been discussed in the previous section.

Alteration in Tissue Perfusion. SCA is considered a multiorgan disease because of the risk of ischemia or infarction of many organs caused by sickling of RBCs and vasoocclusion. The organs most frequently affected are the spleen, kidneys, and bone marrow; however, involvement of the lungs and the brain can also occur. Children with frequent episodes of intravascular sickling are at risk for progressive organ dysfunction because of decreased tissue perfusion, ischemia, and necrosis. All organs can be affected during an acute episode, as well as chronically. A complete and ongoing assessment of all organ systems during an intensive care admission is imperative.

Complications of SCD

The most frequent clinical manifestations of SCD are (1) vasoocclusive crises; (2) sequestration crises; and (3) aplastic crises. These may lead to life-threatening complications such as acute chest syndrome, stroke, acute anemia, and sepsis, which require admission to the PICU.

Vasoocclusive Crises. The most common reason for admission to the PICU is vasoocclusive crisis with ischemia or infarction of the occluded organ. Vasoocclusive crisis is an acute, painful episode that is the result of intravascular sickling, occlusion of small vessels, and tissue ischemia and infarction. The onset is acute and may be precipitated by infection, hypoxia, fever, acidosis, dehydration, change in climate, and psychological factors. However, many times a predetermining factor cannot be identified. The joints and the extremities are most often affected.

CRITICAL CARE MANAGEMENT. Therapy for the child with vasoocclusive crisis is aimed at removing the precipitating cause, treating complications, and preventing further crises. Treatment is supportive and includes hydration, antibiotics, and pain management. Moderate pain may be treated with oral narcotics. Severe pain requires intravenous analgesia, usually morphine sulfate at 0.1 to 0.2 mg/kg IV every 4 hour, or by constant infusion. Oxygen should be provided if the child is hypoxemic in order to prevent further sickling and possibly promote conversion of sickled RBCs to normal shape.

Acute Chest Syndrome. Acute chest syndrome often requires admission to the PICU. Acute chest syndrome is the result of sickling of RBCs in the pulmonary vasculature, which may cause intrapulmonary shunting and abnormalities in gas exchange. These patients are also at high risk for pulmonary infarctions from recurrent sickling and pneumonia.

Signs and symptoms include pleuritic chest pain, hypoxia, tachypnea, retractions, and nasal flaring. The radiographic picture is consistent with pulmonary infiltrates. This may progress to a complete "whiteout" of lung fields and respiratory failure. Fever and an increased WBC count may be seen with both infection and infarction.

CRITICAL CARE MANAGEMENT. Therapy for acute chest syndrome follows the general principles of therapy for vasoocclusive crises. Pain relief is critical to allow effective pulmonary toilet and coughing. Antibiotics are recommended in any febrile child with acute chest syndrome because untreated bacterial infections can be devastating for children with SCD. Oxygen is necessary for the hypoxemic child to promote normal oxygenation and prevent further sickling. Partial exchange transfusion may be necessary even in the child with mild symptoms to halt progression of the disorder (Table 26–8).

Cerebrovascular Accident (CVA). CVA is another vasoocclusive crisis that results in admission to the PICU. CVA is most often the result of thrombosis in the major cerebral arteries in younger children and to hemorrhage in older children. CVA affects 6% to 12% of children with SCA (Charache et al., 1989).

The diagnosis of CVA is made on the basis of clinical signs. Unfortunately, warning signs of an impending CVA are rare. Some children may complain of headache or dizziness, but often the first signs are apparent only with the CVA itself. These signs may be hemiplegia, aphasia, speech difficulties, visual disturbances, seizures, or coma.

Upon admission of a child with neurologic signs suggesting CVA, assessment includes a history and a detailed neurologic examination. A CT or MRI must be done to rule out a lesion such as subdural hematoma if the history (such as recent head trauma) suggests this. The CT should be done without contrast materials because they may precipitate sickling by drying out the RBCs. If there are no signs of increased intracranial pressure, a lumbar puncture may be done to rule out an infectious process. Angiography should be postponed until the child's condition is stable and the Hb S has been decreased to below 10% by exchange transfusion.

CRITICAL CARE MANAGEMENT. The most critical intervention for the child presenting with a CVA is a partial exchange transfusion to prevent progression of the CVA. Other therapy is supportive. If the child has experienced a large infarction, close monitoring for intracranial hypertension is necessary. Anticoagulant therapy is contraindicated.

Other Crises. The child with SCD admitted to the PICU may experience a variety of other crises. As with acute chest syndrome and CVA, any crisis may be precipitated by infection, dehydration, fatigue, and hypoxia.

Bony crises may involve the marrow or the cortex of the bone itself. The small bones of the hands and feet are frequently affected in infants and toddlers, giving rise to dactylitis or hand-foot syndrome. In all bone crises, pain, fever, and leukocytosis are present. With bone cortex involvement, pain, redness, and swelling over the affected area are seen.

Abdominal crises are often the result of occlusion of the mesenteric vessels or vessels of some of the viscera, such as the spleen or the kidney. These crises are characterized by acute abdominal pain, fever, malaise, anorexia, nausea, and an increased WBC count. These symptoms are often indistinguishable from an acute "surgical abdomen," and a thorough history and surgical evaluation are required. Patients with "crisis pain" usually remain in stable condition or improve slightly with supportive measures such as hydration and analgesics. Those patients with an acute surgical abdomen do not improve with these measures, and instead become more acutely ill.

CRITICAL CARE MANAGEMENT. Therapy for other crises is supportive. Adequate hydration must be maintained. Antibiotic therapy is indicated if there is redness and swelling over a bone. Pain management is crucial with all crises. For the child with an abdomi-

Table 26–8. PARTIAL EXCHANGE TRANSFUSION IN THE PICU

1. Preparation
   a. Decision to transfuse
   b. Insertion of venous and arterial catheters (or two large-bore venous catheters, if possible)
   c. Blood sent to laboratory for:
      i. Complete blood count
      ii. Quantitative sickle cell preparation (this appears to correlate well with the quantity of hgb S noted at electrophoresis)
      iii. Electrolytes and calcium determination
      iv. Cross-match with PRBC (sickle negative)
2. Procedure
   a. Volume of packed cells: (2 × hematocrit × 0.7 × wt [kg])
   b. Rate
      i. Adjust intravenous line so transfusion occurs over 4–6 hours (more difficult if over 1000 mL are to be exchanged)
      ii. Withdraw blood at 10- to 15-min intervals from arterial line or large-bore venous catheter
      iii. Balance maintained within 5% of blood volume (blood volume, 80 mL/kg)
   c. Monitoring
      i. Heart rate and blood pressure (continuously)
      ii. Hematocrit (every 2 hr, and at last hour)
      iii. Electrolytes, calcium (at last hour)
   d. Endpoint
      i. Hematocrit 33% to 37% (add FFP to remainder of PRBC if hematocrit is >35%)
      ii. % Hgb S is <40% (initial screening by quantitative sickle cell preparation, followed by chromatography or electrophoresis)

From Gordon, J. B., Bernstein, M. L., Rogers, M. C. (1992). Hematologic disorders in the pediatric intensive care unit. In M. C. Rogers (Ed.). *Textbook of pediatric intensive care* (2nd ed, pp. 1363). Baltimore: Williams & Wilkins.

nal crisis, pain management prevents atelectasis that occurs because of splinting of the abdomen.

Splenic Sequestration Crises. Splenic sequestration is a life-threatening complication of SCA and one of the leading causes of death in children with this disease. There is massive engorgement of the splenic sinuses with blood and a significant amount of the RBC mass becomes trapped in the spleen. The result is an abrupt fall in hemoglobin levels, which may result in death from circulatory failure. The etiology of this complication is unknown and the severity of the crisis ranges from mild splenic enlargement with minimal decrease in hemoglobin level to substantial splenomegaly, life-threatening anemia, and shock.

Splenic sequestration is normally seen in infants and children younger than 6 years of age because these children have not yet undergone autosplenectomy. Autosplenectomy is a process by which repeated episodes of infarction reduce the spleen to fibrotic tissue with deposits of iron. By age 7 most patients with SCA have become permanently asplenic because of this process (Platt & Nathan, 1987).

Children with splenic sequestration have acute, severe left upper quadrant pain, vomiting, acute onset of anemia, a rapidly distending abdomen, and signs of hypovolemia. On physical examination, there is severe hypotension, cardiac enlargement, and splenomegaly. The hematocrit is often half the patient's normal value, and there is usually a rapid reticulocytosis with increased immature RBCs and moderate to severe thrombocytopenia.

CRITICAL CARE MANAGEMENT. Therapy for this crisis is the immediate transfusion of packed RBCs to restore intravascular volume and oxygen-carrying capacity. Once the cardiovascular status stabilizes, the child usually improves rapidly. The spleen shrinks within a few days, and the thrombocytopenia resolves. Splenic sequestration may recur, usually within 4 months of the initial episode. Emergency splenectomy for an acute crises is not indicated; however, some recommend splenectomy after one episode to prevent further crises (Edmond et al., 1984).

Aplastic Crisis. Aplastic crisis is a condition that results from a primary erythropoietic failure often associated with a parvovirus infection. The cessation of bone marrow function causes the hematocrit to decrease dramatically (Pascucci, 1989). If the anemia is severe and the child is symptomatic or general condition compromised, an intensive care admission may be necessary.

The child with aplastic crisis usually appears listless and pale. Hemoglobin values are decreased and the reticulocyte count is less than 1%.

CRITICAL CARE MANAGEMENT. Most aplastic episodes are mild and require no treatment. Recovery is usually spontaneous with an elevated nucleated RBC count, followed by reticulocytosis in 1 or 2 days. Packed RBCs may be administered if the anemia is severe to maintain a hemoglobin of 8 g/dL or more.

Sepsis. Infection is the most common cause of death in children with SCA. These children are immunocompromised because of decreased splenic function with the loss of its filtering capabilities and diminished antibody function. Infections in children with altered splenic function are usually caused by organisms such as *Streptococcus pneumoniae, Haemophilus influenzae,* and *Neisseria meningitidis* (Pearson et al., 1985). Other gram-negative organisms, such as *Salmonella* species, may also cause infection because of impaired neutrophil function that appears to exist in these children (Humbert et al., 1990). Children with SCA seem to be at particular risk for septic shock caused by *S. pneumoniae.*

CRITICAL CARE MANAGEMENT. In children with SCA, a temperature higher than 38.5°C, band count greater than 1000/mm^3, or a high ESR are treated with antibiotic therapy regardless of whether they appear septic. Children who appear septic are treated with antibiotics regardless of their temperature.

MIXED DISORDERS

Hemolytic Uremic Syndrome

Hemolytic uremic syndrome (HUS) is a clinical syndrome characterized by the triad of microangiopathic hemolytic anemia, thrombocytopenia, and acute renal failure. HUS is the most common cause of acquired renal failure in children. Although the primary systemic effects are hematologic and renal, there is potential for multisystem involvement, primarily of the gastrointestinal and neurologic systems.

HUS does not appear to have a single etiology, but is a syndrome of diverse causes. Numerous agents and predisposing factors have been associated with HUS, including infectious organisms, medications, and hereditary traits, but causality has not been definitively established.

Etiologic investigations of HUS have focused on infectious agents, specifically verotoxin-producing organisms such as *Escherichia coli.* One particular strain of *E. coli* (*E. coli* 0157:H7) has been identified as the most common pathogen associated with HUS; 40% to 50% of stools cultured from children with HUS are positive for *E. coli* 0157:H7 (Coad et al., 1991; Kaplan et al., 1990; Martin et al., 1990; Robson & Leung, 1990; Rowe et al., 1991).

Other infectious organisms that have been less frequently associated with HUS are *Shigella dysenteriae, Salmonella typhi, Camphylobacter jejuni, S. pneumoniae, Yersinia* pseudotuberculosis, and coxsackie virus (Beattie, 1990; Drummond, 1985; Kaplan et al., 1990; Robson & Leung, 1990). HUS patients who have positive cultures for one of these enteropathogens at the onset of their illness are "postinfectious" or "typical" HUS patients. The postenteropathic form of HUS differs from other forms in etiology, clinical manifestations, and prognosis.

There is a familial form of HUS that appears to be

hereditary, which is inherited by either autosomal recessive or dominant patterns. There is evidence that a genetic deficiency of prostacycline-stimulating hormone underlies this less common recurrent form of HUS (Beattie, 1990; Drummond, 1985; Kaplan et al., 1990). Other potential precipitating agents or factors associated with HUS are medications (e.g., cyclosporin A, mitomycin, chemotherapeutic agents, oral contraceptives), pregnancy, malignancy, lupus erythematosus, and malignant hypertension (Beattie, 1990; Drummond, 1985; Kaplan et al., 1990). It is unclear which of these may cause HUS, which are chance simultaneous occurrences, or which are related to some third unidentified causal factor.

HUS most commonly affects children between the ages of 6 months and 4 years. Approximately 80% of the cases of HUS occur in children under the age of 5 years (Coad et al., 1991; Graham, 1988; Grodinsky et al., 1990; Martin et al., 1990; Robson & Leung, 1990; Rowe et al., 1991). The majority of reported cases of HUS (75%–80%) occur between the months of April and September (Coad et al., 1991; Grodinsky et al., 1990; Martin et al., 1990; Rowe et al., 1991). No explanation for the age distribution or seasonal variation of HUS has been established.

The incidence of HUS in North America has been reported as three to five cases per 100,000 children under the age of 5 years (Robson & Leung, 1990; Rowe et al., 1991). Some studies have documented an increasing incidence of HUS since the early 1980s. The increased occurrence of HUS has coincided with an increased appearance of verotoxin-producing strains of *E. coli* as pathogens in humans (Coad et al., 1991; Martin et al., 1990). The most likely route of transmission of *E. coli* to humans is through the ingestion of undercooked beef (Coad et al., 1991; Robson & Leung, 1990).

Pathogenesis

The major underlying mechanism of injury in HUS is vascular endothelial damage. In the postenteropathic form of HUS, the verotoxin released by *E. coli* or other organisms initiates the endothelial damage (Kaplan et al., 1990; Robson & Leung, 1990). There is some evidence that the endothelial injury in other forms of HUS is immune complex–mediated (Beattie, 1990). The kidneys are the primary site of endothelial disruption, but extrarenal sites may experience similar microangiopathic changes.

Typically, damaged endothelial cells within the vasculature of the renal glomerulus swell and become separated from the basement membrane, creating a widened subendothelial space. Fibrin, platelets, and lipids are deposited in the subendothelial space, which, combined with the swollen endothelial cells, produce thickened glomerular capillary walls and thus reduced capillary lumen size. Small arterioles become thrombosed as a result of local intravascular coagulation activation. Thus, the renal vasculature becomes obstructed by endothelial swelling and/or thrombi, resulting in a reduced filtering surface and

renal ischemia. Consequently, the glomerular filtration rate is significantly diminished, and acute renal failure develops (Argyle et al., 1990; Drummond, 1985; Kaplan et al., 1990). Histopathologic studies of renal tissue in children with HUS have demonstrated glomerular thrombotic microangiopathy and cortical necrosis (Argyle et al., 1990).

Thrombocytopenia in HUS is the result of both aggregation and destruction of platelets within the damaged microvasculature. Normally, an anticlumping substance released from the endothelium (prostacycline) keeps platelet aggregation in check. However, there is evidence that in HUS, inappropriate platelet aggregation is facilitated by diminished prostacycline activity. "Familial" HUS may be seen in patients who have a hereditary prostacycline deficiency. The mechanism of prostacycline inhibition in other forms of HUS is unknown. The result is that significant numbers of platelets are "trapped" in multiple microvascular thrombi or are injured and removed from the circulation by the spleen (Beattie, 1990; Drummond, 1985; Robson & Leung, 1990).

The pathogenesis of the hemolytic anemia of HUS is also related to renal endothelial disruption. Erythrocytes are mechanically damaged as they pass through the swollen and occluded arterioles. The spleen and liver remove these fragmented RBCs from the circulation, causing a progressive and severe anemia. The body attempts to compensate by accelerating RBC production, as evidenced by reticulocyte counts as high as 10% (Robson & Leung, 1990).

Although the kidneys are the primary location of pathologic changes in HUS, extrarenal involvement occurs in a significant proportion of patients. The gastrointestinal system is actually the first site of physiologic derangement in most cases of "typical" HUS. Hemorrhagic colitis, frequently caused by *E. coli*, precedes the onset of HUS in up to 70% of patients. The mechanism of bowel injury is similar to the renal pathophysiologic process: endothelial disruption and thrombosis of the microvasculature, leading to ischemic/necrotic tissue damage. Gastrointestinal complications of HUS are perforation, obstruction, stricture, or intussusception of the bowel (Argyle et al., 1990; Grodinsky et al., 1990; Robson & Leung, 1990).

It has recently been recognized that in up to 20% of HUS patients, the pancreas suffers comparable hemorrhagic and necrotic damage. These microangiopathic changes are hypothesized to be endotoxin-mediated. Similar hemorrhagic, thrombotic, and necrotic lesions have been documented in the central nervous system, lungs, adrenal glands, and hearts of some patients with HUS (Argyle et al., 1990; Grodinsky et al., 1990; Robson & Leung, 1990).

HUS is not limited to renal, hematologic, and gastrointestinal involvement. Approximately 30% of patients with HUS experience neurologic dysfunction owing to involvement of the microvasculature of the brain and the direct neurologic effects of the toxins. Approximately 40% of patients with neurologic involvement develops further neurologic impairment from HUS, including hemiparesis, cortical blindness, and a persistent state of altered consciousness.

Critical Care Management

In the majority of HUS patients, the syndrome is preceded by a prodromal illness. Approximately 80% of children diagnosed with HUS have experienced gastroenteritis with some combination of diarrhea (usually bloody), vomiting, and/or abdominal pain at the onset of their illness. Less commonly, the diagnosis of HUS may be preceded by an upper respiratory infection, or by no specific signs of illness at all. The average interval between onset of diarrhea and diagnosis of HUS is 4 days. Patients with "atypical" HUS are less likely to present with diarrhea. Approximately one-third of HUS patients are febrile in the prodromal period (Argyle et al., 1990; Coad et al., 1991; Grodinsky et al., 1990; Martin et al., 1990; Robson & Leung, 1990; Rowe et al., 1991).

Initial physical assessment of the child with HUS generally reveals a pale, lethargic, and/or irritable child, with evidence of abdominal pain or tenderness. Inspection of the skin may reveal hemorrhagic manifestations, such as bruising, petechiae, or purpura. Admission vital signs are usually within normal limits for age, although some children may have tachycardia and/or tachypnea if anemia is severe at presentation. Tachypnea may also reflect an attempt to compensate for metabolic acidosis resulting from renal failure. Hypertension may be present, but usually it develops later in the course of the disease.

Up to 20% of children with HUS present with seizure activity. The etiology of seizures at presentation is usually hyponatremia, but seizures may be the result of early central nervous system microangiopathy (Argyle et al., 1990; Coad et al., 1991; Grodinsky et al., 1990; Hahn, 1989; Martin et al., 1990; Robson & Leung, 1990; Rowe et al., 1991).

Oliguria or anuria is present in more than 89% of children who develop HUS (Argyle et al., 1990; Robson & Leung, 1990; Rowe et al., 1991). Urine is usually grossly hematuric. Laboratory analysis confirms acute renal failure, with rapidly increasing blood urea nitrogen (BUN) and creatinine levels. It is not unusual for a child with HUS to have a BUN level higher than 100 mg/dL and a creatinine level higher than 4 mg/dL within the first 2 days of diagnosis with HUS. Urinalysis reveals proteinuria and the presence of urinary casts. Serum electrolyte values may be initially normal, or consistent with acute renal failure (decreased sodium and calcium, increased potassium and phosphorus) (Graham, 1988).

Hematologic analysis confirms the diagnosis of HUS. Microangiopathic anemia is present, with a hematocrit typically less than 25%. Microscopic smear reveals burr-shaped, fragmented erythrocytes. Thrombocytopenia (platelet count less than 100,000/mm^3) is present, but other coagulation values (PT, PTT) are typically within normal limits, differentiating this disorder from DIC. Frequently, the CBC also reveals leukocytosis upon presentation (Robson & Leung, 1990).

If stool cultures are sent, the most common organism identified is *E. coli* 0157:H7. Other potential enteropathogens are listed within the discussion of HUS etiologies. Cultures from other sites are generally negative at presentation.

Diagnostic workup of the patient with HUS is generally limited to laboratory analysis. Occasionally, abdominal pain and colitis lead to an exploratory laparotomy before the diagnosis of HUS is made, especially if the rest of the clinical picture is not consistent with "typical" HUS (Grodinsky et al., 1990). In addition, a brain computerized tomography (CT) scan may be performed to rule out an intracerebral lesion as the source of seizures (Hahn, 1989).

Planning care for the child with HUS admitted to the PICU begins with the identification of appropriate nursing diagnoses, which are based upon the child's clinical status and knowledge of the potential complications of HUS.

Fluid Volume Imbalance. Initially, the child with HUS may present with dehydration resulting from gastrointestinal (GI) losses (diarrhea, vomiting) and decreased oral intake. As the disease progresses, GI losses generally diminish, and the child is at risk for fluid overload from acute renal failure.

Initial fluid replacement with intravenous solutions is administered cautiously, with careful monitoring of serum electrolytes and an ongoing assessment for fluid overload. Subsequently, the patient with HUS must be monitored closely for signs of hypervolemia, including peripheral edema, tachycardia, hypertension, pulmonary edema, and increased weight. In the oliguric or anuric patient, fluid intake should be restricted to insensible losses (approximately 30% maintenance) plus urine output replacement.

Nursing responsibilities include assessing for signs of pulmonary edema, such as crackly breath sounds, hypoxemia, frothy sputum, tachypnea, and increased heart size and infiltrates, which are seen on chest radiographs. Serum electrolyte values must be monitored closely (every 6–8 hours), along with assessment for complications of electrolyte imbalances (e.g., hyperkalemia, hyponatremia).

Management of hypertension in the HUS patient is a collaborative responsibility. In addition to fluid overload, hypertension is exacerbated by excessive renin release by the kidneys caused by decreased renal perfusion. Antihypertensives are required to control blood pressure in up to 40% of critically ill HUS patients (Argyle et al., 1990; Coad et al., 1991).

The majority of patients admitted to the PICU with HUS require dialysis during the acute phase of their illness. The decision to dialyze a patient is not based on absolute criteria, but on an overall assessment of the individual patient's status. Indications for dialysis include one or more of the following: anuria for longer than 24 hours, hypertension, pulmonary edema, hyperkalemia, and severe azotemia (Graham, 1988; Robson & Leung, 1990).

Patients with HUS may receive peritoneal dialysis (PD) or hemodialysis (HD). The advantages of PD are that fluid is removed gradually, so that hemodynamic stability is assured, and that PD does not require vascular access. However, there are a number of disadvantages to PD as compared with HD for the HUS patient. The high glucose solutions used in PD may cause hyperglycemia, especially if the patient has pancreatic insufficiency caused by HUS. Probably the biggest disadvantage to PD in this population is the risk of precipitating or exacerbating the abdominal complications associated with HUS.

The main advantage of HD, aside from avoiding involvement of the GI tract, is that it provides more precise correction of fluid imbalance, electrolyte values, and acidosis. One disadvantage is that patients who are hemodialyzed must be systemically heparinized for each procedure, which may transiently increase their risk of bleeding.

Potential for Bleeding. The primary risk factor for bleeding in HUS patients is thrombocytopenia. However, in addition to a decrease in the absolute number of platelets, there is evidence that the HUS patient's circulating platelets are hyporesponsive to aggregating agents (Beattie, 1990; Drummond, 1985). It has been established that the platelets of uremic patients in general do not function properly; it is unclear whether there is an additional mechanism compounding this "malfunctioning" in HUS patients.

The nurse closely monitors the HUS patient for signs of bleeding, such as bruising, petechiae, oozing from invasive line sites, epistaxis, or upper and/or lower GI bleeding. Procedures that may promote bleeding, such as intramuscular injections and rectal instrumentation, are avoided. In addition, the child is assessed for signs of occult bleeding, such as increased abdominal girth, increased pulse and respiratory rate, diminished peripheral perfusion, a change in neurologic status, or hypotension (a late sign of hypovolemia) (Geller, 1990).

Blood component replacement is generally not aggressive in patients with HUS, because there is evidence that transfused platelets and RBCs suffer the same damage in the microvasculature as the child's intrinsic blood components, and may exacerbate the risk of thrombus formation. Consequently, RBCs are generally transfused only when the hematocrit falls below 20%. Most HUS patients receive at least one blood transfusion during the acute phase of their illness. Platelets are usually not administered until the platelet count is below 10,000 to 20,000/mm^3, or if there is active bleeding.

All blood products should be administered slowly and timed to coincide with dialysis when possible, to minimize the risks of circulatory overload. All patients should be monitored for signs of a transfusion reaction.

Potential for Altered Cerebral Perfusion. There are a number of potential risk factors for an alteration in cerebral perfusion in the HUS patient. There is evidence that the microangiopathic process that obstructs perfusion in the renal vasculature can develop in the cerebral vasculature. Thus, there is a risk of microthrombi or even large thrombus formation in the cerebral arterioles, potentially leading to infarction. In addition, thrombocytopenia coupled with hypertension puts the patient with HUS at significant risk for an intracranial hemorrhage.

It is the responsibility of the critical care nurse to carefully monitor the patient with HUS for changes that may indicate neurologic damage. This can be challenging, because patients are typically lethargic and/or irritable upon admission, because of uremia, anemia, and/or a postictal state. Signs of focal infarction or hemorrhage include hemiparesis, seizures, change in motor strength, cranial nerve deficits, and a change in level of consciousness. Signs of increased intracranial pressure include decreased responsiveness to stimuli, pupillary changes, change in respiratory pattern, (late) decreased pulse, and increased blood pressure with widened pulse pressure. A CT scan of the brain may be required to identify infarctions, edema, or hemorrhage, so that neurologic recovery can be optimized.

If there is clinical or radiologic evidence of neurologic deterioration, therapeutic modalities aimed at the removal of circulating endotoxin and the normalization of platelet-aggregating factors may be instituted. Fresh plasma infusion and plasmapheresis are the two most commonly employed therapies. There is some evidence that these interventions may improve neurologic outcomes, but their efficacy has not been definitively demonstrated in clinical studies (Coad et al., 1991; Robson & Leung, 1990). Other therapies studied at various times include heparin, thrombolytic agents, prostacyclin infusion, gamma globulin, and vitamin E. None of these therapies has consistently proved effective for HUS, but some are still used in cases of severe disease, especially with cerebrovascular involvement (Coad et al., 1991; Robson & Leung, 1990).

Collaborative interventions to optimize neurologic functioning include control of seizures with anticonvulsants and electrolyte balance. Standard interventions to reduce or prevent rises in intracranial pressure are instituted if the patient with HUS demonstrates cerebral edema on CT (e.g., hyperventilation, midline and elevated head positioning, and fluid restriction). The only modification for the anuric patient is that osmotic diuretics are not used, because they draw fluid into the intravascular space, which can not be excreted, thereby exacerbating hypervolemia.

Potential for Altered Gastrointestinal Perfusion. The patient with HUS is at risk for GI complications resulting from vascular endothelial damage, thrombi, and necrosis of bowel tissue. Careful monitoring of the patient is the cornerstone of managing GI complications. The child is assessed for abdominal tenderness, cramping, and distension, especially as compared with baseline status upon admission. Abdominal girth is measured and recorded each shift, and all gastric output is tested for the presence of blood. Gastric pH is maintained above 5 with hydrogen ion blockers or antacids to prevent gastric ulceration.

If a paralytic ileus or an acute abdominal process develops, the patient with HUS should be kept NPO and a nasogastric tube should be inserted to decompress the stomach. Approximately half the children with HUS require parenteral nutrition during the acute phase of their illness. The GI tract may require serial evaluation with kidney, ureter, and bladder (KUB) x-ray and/or abdominal ultrasound examination. Signs of an acute bowel infarction, perforation, obstruction, or necrosis include tachycardia, hypotension, acidosis, vomiting, and abdominal distension. Surgical intervention may be necessary (Grodinsky et al., 1990).

Potential for Altered Pancreatic Perfusion. Pancreatitis, with both endocrine and exocrine involvement, has recently been recognized as a potential complication of HUS, presumably resulting from the same mechanisms that injure renal, GI, and cerebral tissue (Argyle et al., 1990; Grodinsky et al., 1990).

It may be difficult to evaluate the patient with HUS for pancreatitis because the clinical signs, abdominal pain and vomiting, may be present because of another etiology. Patients with these signs should be made NPO regardless of whether a definitive diagnosis is made. Serum amylase and lipase levels are followed, but because these enzymes are partially excreted by the renal route, levels greater than four times normal are necessary to diagnose pancreatitis in patients with renal failure (Grodinsky et al., 1990). Abdominal ultrasound examinations may be performed; enlargement and sonolucence of the pancreas is consistent with pancreatitis.

The nurse assesses the patient with HUS for hyperglycemia resulting from pancreatic insufficiency, which may necessitate exogenous insulin administration. The anuric patient cannot be monitored for glycosuria; therefore, serum glucose is measured every 4 to 8 hours. Serum glucose should be maintained at 100 to 200 mg/dL with insulin administration carefully titrated by the nurse.

Outcome

The average length of hospitalization for a patient with HUS is 10 to 14 days, but there is a wide range depending on the occurrence of complications and rate of recovery of renal function. Fully 60% to 80% of children with a one-time occurrence of HUS recover completely. Another 10% to 30% are left with long-term sequelae, which include hypertension, chronic renal failure, and neurologic complications such as hemiparesis, seizures, blindness, and cognitive deficits. Currently, less than 5% of all patients studied progressed to end-stage renal disease and renal transplantation, but recent long-term studies show evidence that in some post-HUS patients, renal function declines after apparent recovery (Siegler et al., 1991). Overall, the mortality rate for HUS in North America is 3% to 10%, but it may be higher for the proportion of patients with disease severe enough to warrant admission to the ICU (Coad et al., 1991; Drummond, 1985; Martin et al., 1990; Robson & Leung, 1990; Rowe et al., 1991; Siegler et al., 1991).

Extensive analysis has been done to identify patients at high risk for a poor outcome from HUS. Poor outcome is generally defined as chronic renal failure, neurologic sequelae, or death. Some investigators differentiate between typical (or classic) and atypical HUS when discussing prognosis. The typical form, which has a better prognosis, affects young children (usually younger than 3 years old), has a prodrome of bloody diarrhea, occurs during the summer, and is nonrecurrent. Hereditary and other atypical forms of HUS have a poorer prognosis (Drummond, 1985).

Other factors that have been statistically correlated with a poor outcome are high neutrophil count upon admission (which may reflect the degree of endotoxin exposure), short diarrhea prodrome before admission (which may reflect a higher infectious dose of circulating toxin), higher hemoglobin count upon admission (more invasive disease may prompt admission before hemolysis has occurred), seizures upon admission, bowel necrosis during the acute phase, and longer duration of anuria during the acute phase (Coad et al., 1991; Havens et al., 1988; Martin et al., 1990; Siegler et al., 1991). Though it is still difficult to predict the long-term outcome for an individual patient, even limited prognostic information may be useful in guiding therapies and in counseling parents of patients with HUS in the ICU.

SUMMARY

Critically ill children may experience a wide range of hematologic problems during their hospital stay related to a variety of causes. Anemia and thrombocytopenia also may be part of the pathologic process that brings children to the PICU. Children's response to medical and nursing interventions depends on their preexisting state, the severity of their illness, and length of time before treatment is initiated.

Caring for these children requires a collaborative approach. It is imperative that the nurse caring for these children be vigilant for subtle but significant signs that occur because of the complexity of the patient's needs and the potential for rapid changes in the patient's condition. Expert nursing management is essential to maximize the potential for a positive outcome.

References

Argyle, J.C., et al. (1990). A clinicopathological study of 24 children with hemolytic uremic syndrome. *Pediatric Nephrology*, 4(1), 52–58.
Baker, J.A., & Finklestein, J.Z. (1989). Bleeding and clotting disorders. In E. Nussbaum (Ed.). *Pediatric intensive care* (pp. 653–671). New York: Future Publishing.

Beattie, T.J. (1990). Recent developments in the pathogenesis of hemolytic uremic syndrome. *Renal Failure*, 12(1), 3–7.

Bonato, J. (1989). Blood transfusions: Are they safe? *Critical Care Nurse*, 9, 40–44.

Bray, G.L. (1993). Inherited and acquired disorders of homeostasis. In P.R. Holbrook (Ed.). *Textbook of pediatric intensive care* (pp. 783–801). Philadelphia: W.B. Saunders.

Charache, S., Lubin, B., & Reid, C.D. (1989). Management and therapy of sickle cell disease (NIH Publication No. 89-2117). Washington, DC: National Institutes of Health.

Coad, N.A.G., et al. (1991). Changes in the postenteropathic form of the hemolytic uremic syndrome in children. *Clinical Nephrology*, 35(1), 10–16.

Cohen, R.J. (1983). Apheresis in hematologic and oncologic disease. *Hospital Practice*, 18(10), 199–205.

Committee on Transfusion Practices (1986). The latest protocols for blood transfusions. *Nursing 86*, 16, 34–41.

DePalma, L., & Luban, N.L.C. (1991). Transfusion-transmitted diseases: AIDS and hepatitis. *Contemporary Pediatrics*, 8, 22–39.

Drummond, K.N. (1985). Hemolytic uremic syndrome—then and now. *New England Journal of Medicine*, 312, 116–118.

Edmond, A.M., et al. (1984). Role of splenectomy in homozygous sickle cell disease in childhood. *Lancet*, 1, 88–90.

Esparaz, B., & Green, D. (1990). Disseminated intravascular coagulation. *Critical Care Nurse Quarterly*, 13(2), 7–13.

Folkes, M.E. (1990). Transfusion therapy in critical care nursing. *Critical Care Nursing Quarterly*, 13, 15–28.

Fosburg, M., et al. (1983). Intensive plasma exchange in small and critically ill pediatric patients: Techniques and clinical outcomes. *Journal of Clinical Apheresis*, 1, 215–224.

Fosburg, M., & Kevy, S.V. (1987). Red cell transfusion. In D.G. Nathan & F.A. Oski (Eds.). *Hematology of infancy and childhood* (Vol. 2, pp. 1580–1587). Philadelphia: W.B. Saunders.

Flug, F., & Karpatkin, M. (1985). Acquired disorders of hemostasis. In S. Zimmerman, & J.H. Gildea (Eds.). *Critical care pediatrics* (pp. 426–436). Philadelphia: W.B. Saunders.

Geller, M. (1990). Multisystem failure in a child with HUS. *Critical Care Nurse*, 10(4), 56–64.

Graham, M. (1988). Classic hemolytic uremic syndrome and current treatment modalities. *Canadian Critical Care Nursing Journal*, 5(4), 7–14.

Grodinsky, S., et al. (1990). Gastrointestinal manifestations of hemolytic uremic syndrome: Recognition of pancreatitis. *Journal of Pediatric Gastroenterology and Nutrition*, 11(4), 518–524.

Hahn, J. (1989). Neurological complications of hemolytic uremic syndrome. *Journal of Child Neurology*, 4(2), 108–113.

Havens, P.L., et al. (1988). Laboratory and clinical variables to predict outcome in hemolytic uremic syndrome. *American Journal of Diseases of Children*, 142, 961–964.

Humbert, J.R. (1990). Neutrophil dysfunction in sickle cell disease. *Biomed Pharmacotherapeutics*, 44, 153–158.

Kaplan, B.S., et al. (1990). Recent advances in understanding the pathogenesis of the hemolytic uremic syndromes. *Pediatric Nephrology*, 4(1), 276–283.

Kasprisin, D. (1984a). Clinical considerations in pediatric apheresis. *Plasma Therapy Transfusion Technology*, 5, 207–212.

Kasprisin, D. (1984b). Guidelines for performing therapeutic apheresis in children. *Plasma Therapy Transfusion Technology*, 5, 213–218.

Kasprisin, D. (1989). Techniques, indications, and toxicity of therapeutic hemapheresis in children. *Journal of Therapeutic Apheresis*, 5, 21–24.

Kevy, S., & Fosburg, M. (1990). Therapeutic apheresis in childhood. *Journal of Clinical Apheresis*, 5, 87–90.

Kruskal, J.B., et al. (1987). Fibrin and fibrinogen-related antigens in patients with stable and unstable coronary artery disease. *New England Journal of Medicine* 317, 1361.

Luban, N.L.C., & DePalma, L. (1993). Transfusion therapy in the pediatric intensive care unit. In P.R. Holbrook (Ed.). *Textbook of pediatric intensive care* (pp. 773–782). Philadelphia: W.B. Saunders.

Lusher, J.M. (1987). Diseases of coagulation: The fluid phase. In D.G. Nathan, & F.A. Oski (Eds.). Hematology of infancy and childhood (3rd ed., Vol. 2, pp. 1248–1270). Philadelphia: W.B. Saunders.

Martin, D.L., et al. (1990). The epidemiology and clinical aspects of the hemolytic uremic syndrome in Minnesota. *New England Journal of Medicine*, 323, 1161–1167.

Mehta, P., Gross, S., & Kao, K. (1990). Transfusion with packed red blood cells. In J.L. Blumer (Ed.). *A practical guide to pediatric intensive care* (pp. 1001–1007). St. Louis: Mosby–YearBook.

Morrison, R.A., & Vedro, D.A. (1989). Pain management in the child with sickle cell disease. *Pediatric Nursing*, 15(6), 595–599.

National Blood Resource Education Program's Nursing Education Working Group (1991). Choosing blood components and equipment. *American Journal of Nursing*, 91, 42–50.

Oski, F.A. (1987). The erythrocyte and its disorders. In D.G. Nathan & F.A. Oski (Eds.). *Hematology of infancy and childhood* (3rd ed., Vol. 1, pp. 16–43). Philadelphia: W.B. Saunders.

Pascucci, R.C. (1989). Pediatric intensive care. In G. Gregory (Ed.). *Pediatric Anesthesia* (Vol. 2, pp. 1289–1388). New York: Churchill Livingstone.

Pearson, H.A. (1985). Developmental pattern of splenic dysfunction in sickle cell disorders. *Pediatrics*, 76, 392–397.

Platt, O.S., & Nathan, D.G. (1987). Sickle cell disease. In D.G. Nathan & F.A. Oski (Eds.). *Hematology of infancy and childhood* (3rd ed., Vol. 1, pp. 655–698). Philadelphia: W.B. Saunders.

Platt, O.S., & Nathan, D.G. (1989). Hematology. In M.E. Avery & L. First (Eds.). *Pediatric medicine* (pp. 495–545). Baltimore: Williams & Wilkins.

Robson, W.L.M., & Leung, A.K.C. (1990). Hemolytic uremic syndrome in children. *Postgraduate Medicine*, 88(5), 135–136, 139–142.

Rowe, P.C., et al. (1991). Epidemiology of hemolytic uremic syndrome in Canadian children from 1986 to 1988. *Journal of Pediatrics*, 119(2), 218–224.

Shapiro, B. (1989). The management of pain in sickle cell disease. *Pediatric Clinics of North America*, 36(4), 1029–1045.

Siegler, R.L., et al. (1991). Long-term outcome and prognostic indicators in the hemolytic uremic syndrome. *Journal of Pediatrics*, 118(2), 195–200.

Young, L. (1990). DIC: The insidious killer. *Critical Care Nurse*, 10(9), 26–33.

Multisystem Problems

This section addresses the needs of patients experiencing multiple system dysfunction and their complicated demands and unique needs. Because these patients' illnesses involve more than a single body system, they present a distinctive challenge to the care team.

CHAPTER 27

Organ Transplantation

BARBARA GILL
PATRICIA O'BRIEN
KAREN ZAMBERLAN*
SARAH MARTIN
MICHELE TOPOR

INTRODUCTION

Solid organ transplantation, the replacement of a diseased organ with a healthy one, has become accepted therapy for end-stage failure of the heart, liver, and kidney and is now being extended to the lung, intestine, and pancreas. Generally, successful transplantation in adult patients precedes widespread application of these new procedures in the pediatric population. Transplantation has been performed in children in increasing numbers, extended to newborns and infants, and appears to parallel the successful outcomes reported in adults (Table 27–1). There are many concerns of nurses caring for infants and children that are of no consequence in adult

programs. These include differences in technical detail owing to the small size of children; the urgency of transplantation to maximize neurologic, psychological, and physical growth; and the need for awareness of the psychological changes maturing patients undergo when making transitions from infancy to childhood, adolescence, and young adulthood.

History

The history of solid organ transplantation spans less than 40 years. The first successful solid organ transplant performed in humans was a kidney transplant between twin brothers in 1954 by Merrill and Murray in Boston. In 1963, the first patient to undergo liver transplantation was a 3-year-old with

*Deceased.

Table 27–1. TRANSPLANTS BY ORGAN AND AGE

Recipient Age Group	Cadaveric Kidney		Live-Donor Kidney		Liver		Pancreas		Heart		Heart and Lung		Lung	
	N	%	N	%	N	%	N	%	N	%	N	%	N	%
0–5	341	0	419	3	1918	12	8	0	786	6	20	6	23	1
6–17	1608	4	1418	11	973	6	7	0	480	4	38	11	97	5
18–49	30399	66	9581	71	7339	46	2930	96	4325	36	264	75	1043	53
50–64	11551	25	1811	13	5185	32	108	4	6094	50	30	8	743	38
65+	1758	4	170	2	645	4			399	3			25	1
Not reported	40		50		5				9				1	
Total	45697		13449		16065		3053		12093		352		1932	

Data from donor registration entered at UNOS from 1988 to 1993; subject to change based upon future data submission or correction. Percentages are based upon totals excluding "not reported" category.

extrahepatic biliary atresia who died of hemorrhage on the day of transplantation. Subsequent attempts in Denver, Boston, and Paris were unsuccessful until 1967, when the first extended human liver recipient success was achieved by Starzl. This 18-month-old child with hepatocellular carcinoma survived for 13 months before dying of metastatic disease despite good graft function (Starzl et al., 1982). After extensive experimental work by Shumway and Lower at Stanford University, the first successful clinical cardiac transplant was preempted by Barnard in South Africa in 1967. Demekov performed the first recorded orthotopic experimental pulmonary transplant in 1947 without immunosuppression. However, the longest survival period achieved was 10 days. Generally, experience with single lung transplants was unsuccessful before the introduction of cyclosporine. As early as 1959, Lillehei of Minnesota developed the surgical techniques for small bowel transplantation. Intestinal allografts were found not only to be subject to rejection but also to be able to mount a graft-versus-host (GVH) reaction. The first pancreas transplant in a human was performed in 1966; however, few have been performed in children.

In the early 1960s, three events occurred that changed the course of clinical transplantation. First, the development of tissue typing established methods to enhance histocompatibility. Second, methods for regular dialysis treatment were developed that could be integrated with transplantation. Third, and most importantly, new, potent immunosuppressant drugs were developed.

Pioneering work during this time vastly increased knowledge of the immune system. From a greater understanding of the immune system came a description of the process of rejection and then attempts to alter the immune response to prevent rejection. John Lutit used total body irradiation in the 1950s in experiments in rodents undergoing skin grafting; this method was extended to humans by Murray and others in attempts to prevent rejection of transplanted organs. In 1959, Schwartz and Dameshek found that 6-mercaptopurine could suppress the immune response of the rabbit to human serum albumin and to rabbit skin allografts (Schwartz, 1959). Hitchings and Elion (1963) of the Burroughs Well-come Research Laboratories, working to synthesize purine and pyrimidine derivatives to act as antimetabolites, developed azathioprine (Imuran), which quickly replaced 6-mercaptopurine and continues in clinical use today. Calne, working in John Merrill's laboratory in Boston, successfully used this drug in kidney transplantation in dogs. The addition of steroids to azathioprine was reported by Starzl (1963) to have a synergistic immunosuppressive effect.

Over the years, other immunosuppressive treatments were introduced. One of the more popular agents was the antilymphocyte or antithymocyte globulin preparation raised in other species against lymphocytes of the species to be grafted. It was shown in 1960 that antilymphocyte serum prolonged rat skin allografts; in 1963, this agent was used clinically.

In the mid-1970s, Jean Borel discovered the fungal peptide cyclosporin A, which is a powerful immunosuppressant that has been found to be particularly effective when combined with azathioprine and steroids. Following the availability of cyclosporine in 1982, improved survival led to a rapid increase in the number of transplants. The use of this drug ushered in the present era of transplantation.

The monoclonal antibody OKT3 was introduced to treat rejection episodes in 1983. A new immunosuppressive agent, FK-506 (Prograf), was approved by the Food and Drug Administration (FDA) in April 1994. Research efforts continue to identify and develop improved immunosuppressive agents with fewer side effects.

Current Challenges

While organ transplantation has generated great excitement and been life-saving for many children, it has also raised many questions and concerns. The shortage of donor organs is the primary limiting factor in treating patients who could benefit from the procedure. Future ethical issues will arise as controversial solutions to the shortage of pediatric donor organs are proposed. There are currently approximately 1600 children between 0 and 18 years awaiting organ transplants (UNOS, 1995). Many of these children will die due to the shortage of organs; thus, solutions that have been proposed include payment for donor organs, use of living-related donors, use of xenografts (cross-species transplantation), and segmental organ-sharing between recipients. Anencephalic infants have been proposed as potential organ donors for infants, and this possibility has raised many ethical questions. The balance of risks and benefits for donors and recipients, ability to obtain informed consent for these innovative procedures, considerations of human and animal rights, and equitable access and distribution of needed organs are challenging issues.

The imbalance between donor supply and patient demand necessitates a procedure for selecting patients for transplantation considered most likely to benefit from the operation. Selection criteria vary between organs and between transplant programs and include both medical and psychosocial considerations.

Transplantation is the embodiment of high technology and, therefore, high-cost medical care. The average hospital charge for a kidney transplant is $87,700; a heart transplant is $210,000; a liver transplant is $303,000 (UNOS, 1993). Legitimate questions are raised about who pays for the cost of organ transplants and about the fairness of spending large sums of money to benefit a few children when many preventive health programs, which would potentially benefit many children, are underfunded.

The financial requirements for transplantation can be prohibitive if adequate funding or insurance coverage is not available. The financial requirements must be met by each candidate in order to maintain financial stability of the institution's transplant program. Private insurance companies, Medicare, or individual fundraising may serve as sources of financial support for patients. In the future, it is uncertain whether children who receive transplants will maintain their eligibility for health insurance coverage. Additionally, it is unclear whether these children will face employment discrimination issues as adults.

This chapter discusses cardiac, lung, liver, intestine, renal, and pancreas transplantation in the pediatric patient population. Pathophysiologic final common pathways in the care of all organ transplants are rejection and infection. The different organ transplant procedures will be described, as well as the critical care nursing of the patient in the immediate postoperative period. The chapter concludes with a discussion of the long-term issues in pediatric solid organ transplantation, including growth and development, psychosocial adjustment, and physiologic concerns of chronic rejection and chronic immunosuppression.

EVALUATION PROCESS

A multidisciplinary approach is taken in evaluating infants and children for transplantation. The evaluation process has several goals: (1) to determine that transplantation is the only treatment option, that conventional therapies are not applicable, nor better treatment options; (2) to rule out other major systemic diseases or permanent damage in other organ systems that would increase the risk or preclude transplantation; (3) to assess the ability of the child and family to cope with the stresses of transplantation and comply with the complex medical regimen; (4) to educate the child and family about transplantation so they can make an informed decision about this treatment option; and (5) to establish rapport between the child and family and the transplant team.

A thorough evaluation of the clinical status of the patient and of the failing organ is undertaken to establish severity of disease and prognosis. The principal indications for organ transplantation in children are outlined in Table 27–2. Generally, contraindications to organ transplantation include active infection, malignancy, active substance abuse, and severe, permanent damage in another major organ system that would result in the patient's demise.

An adequate social support system is crucial in considering transplantation in children, since they are dependent on others to provide care and nurturance. A dedicated caregiver who will take responsibility for the child's care following transplant must be identified; ideally, two or more caregivers share responsibility. Generally, every effort is made to support the family unit to enable their coping with the stress of transplantation and the provision of adequate care for the child. Psychosocial assessment and ongoing support and intervention by social service and child psychiatry are important.

Nurses play an active role in educating the child (at the appropriate developmental level) and the family about transplantation so they are able to make an informed choice. The development of a trusting relationship with the transplant team and incorporating the family as members of the child's caregiving team during and following transplantation are important goals of the initial evaluation period.

Maintaining an optimal level of physical and emotional wellness in the transplant candidate facilitates the necessary strength to tolerate the evaluation and waiting phase of transplantation and contributes to a successful outcome. Ongoing physical assessment, educating the patient and family about signs and symptoms of illness or progressive failure, and promotion of health-related activities are nursing interventions.

An important part of a transplant evaluation, particularly in renal transplantation, involves tissue typing in an attempt to match a recipient with the most compatible donor. The body identifies the transplanted organ as foreign and sets in motion a number of physiologic mechanisms to destroy the new organ. In addition to immunosuppressive medications, another method to reduce the incidence of rejection is to minimize the differences between the donor and recipient. Histocompatibility testing is performed to match donor and recipient as closely as possible in

Table 27–2. PRINCIPAL INDICATIONS FOR PEDIATRIC SOLID ORGAN TRANSPLANT

Cardiac	Acquired heart disease
	  Cardiomyopathy
	  Acute myocarditis
	  Cardiac tumor
	  Anthracycline myocardial toxicity
		Congenital heart disease
		  Ventricular failure following surgical correction
		  Complex defects not amenable to surgery

Heart/lung & lung	Primary pulmonary hypertension Pulmonary vascular obstructive disease (Eisenmenger's syndrome) Cystic fibrosis Pulmonary fibrosis Emphysema	
Liver	Primary disease: biliary atresia, arteriohepatic dysplasia (Alagille's syndrome), familial cholestasis, choledochal cyst, Byler's disease Secondary disease: primary hepatic tumor, histiocytosis, cystic fibrosis Metabolic disease: alpha$_1$-antitrypsin deficiency, tyrosinemia, glycogen storage disease, Wilson's disease Infectious: neonatal hepatitis, hepatitis A, B, C, hepatitis non-A, non-B, fulminant hepatic failure	

Liver/intestine	*Short gut syndrome*
	Prenatal: intestinal atresia
	  type I-IV, gastroschisis,
	  mid-gut volvulus
		Postnatal: Necrotizing enterocolitis, trauma,
		  microvillus atrophy, pseudo-obstruction

Renal	End-stage renal disease	
Pancreas	Diabetes mellitus with uremia or severe sequela	
All organs	End-stage organ failure refractory to maximum medical or surgical therapy Limited lifespan	

order to reduce the immune system response to foreign antigens.

Histocompatibility testing varies with each organ. Some organs, like the heart, exist singly and the entire organ must be used, so donations must come from cadaveric donors. The kidney and segments of the liver may be removed from living-related donors, where tissue typing can be more exact. Organs vary in their immunogenicity (likelihood of inducing rejection). The heart is most immunogenic, followed by the kidney and then the liver (Roitt, 1989). Most organs can now be preserved for many hours outside the body. This allows for tissue typing to be performed. Other organs, the heart and lung in particular, have shorter preservation times, which may preclude many tissue typing procedures.

The less antigenic the graft, the less the host will react against it. In human transplantation when the donor and recipient are identical twins and there is no antigenic difference, the tissue is accepted without immunosuppressive agents. When the donor and recipient are siblings or when a parent donor is used for an offspring, there is greater statistical likelihood for antigen sharing between the donor and the recipient than when a cadaveric or unrelated donor is used. Patient outcomes are better when either a sibling graft or a parent-child graft is used as compared with a cadaveric transplant.

The ABO and HLA systems are the main antigen systems in the body. Both tissue typing and tissue matching procedures may be performed prior to transplantation. Some of these procedures are described.

ABO typing: The ABO system identifies the presence or absence of antibodies on most body tissues and on red blood cells. The major blood groups are O (universal donor), A, B, and AB (universal recipient). Transplants are performed within blood groups but may be done with donors from a compatible blood group; for example, B recipient receives an O heart. Because O-type organs can be used by any blood type and type O patients can only receive O organs, public policy dictates that O-type organs be used in O patients first. There is some evidence that liver transplants may cross ABO-compatible groups (Gordon, 1986).

RHO antigens: RHO antigens, positive or negative, appear to have no role in graft rejection. Therefore, an O− recipient may receive an O+ donor organ.

HLA typing: The human lymphocyte antigen (HLA) molecules are present on most cells and allow the body to distinguish self from non-self (foreign antibodies). The presence of these antigens plays an important role in graft rejection. The major histocompatibility complex is the HLA genetic complex for each individual. HLA molecules are divided into class I antigens (HLA, A, B, and C antigens) and class II antigens (HLA-DR, DQ, and DP antigens).

Matching procedures are performed to identify preformed circulating patient antibodies to donor antigens. Crossmatching can be done between a specific donor and recipient prior to transplant to identify compatibility. Crossmatching is also performed between a recipient and a randomly selected panel of donor lymphocytes to measure recipient level of antibody reactivity. This is known as a percentage panel reactive antibody (PRA) and is established as part of the evaluation process. A positive crossmatch denotes the presence of antibodies in the recipient serum against donor lymphocytes and is a predictor of hyperacute rejection. A high PRA means the recipient has been sensitized to many possible donor antigens and makes finding a suitable donor much more difficult. Patients with preformed antibodies indicated by a high PRA are crossmatched with specific donor serum prior to transplant. The transplant can occur if the crossmatch is negative.

The *United Network for Organ Sharing (UNOS)* is a nonprofit organization under contract with the U.S. Department of Health and Human Services to operate the Organ Procurement and Transplantation Network (OPTN). In accordance with government guidelines administered by the Health Care Finance Administration (HCFA) in 1988, regional organ procurement organizations (OPOs) were designated to coordinate identification of potential donors and organ recovery with transplant centers and participate in public and professional educational activities to increase organ donation. OPOs are involved in the procurement of all solid organs in the United States. All organ transplant candidates are listed on the UNOS computer. In collaboration with UNOS, each solid organ group has agreed upon a national organ distribution scheme to match organs with recipients based on criteria such as ABO compatibility, patient weight, recipient medical status, HLA compatibility, presensitization, waiting time, and distance between donor and recipient.

The major factor that limits organ transplantation for all who could benefit is the lack of donors. Patients with end-stage renal disease can be managed with dialysis until a donor becomes available, but patients needing a heart or liver often have little time to wait and may die before a donor organ is found. The shortage of donor organs has prompted some innovative changes in practice in recent years. The age and weight range for pediatric transplants has been broadened. Improvements in organ preservation have increased the length of time the organ remains viable outside the body and therefore allows organs to be transported greater distances. A preservation solution containing hydroxyethyl starch was developed at the University of Wisconsin (Viaspan) and has lengthened kidney and liver preservation times. Segmental liver transplants increase the donor pool for young infants.

All cadaveric organ donors are declared brain dead prior to removal of any vascular organ. Most states have enacted brain death legislation in accordance with the Uniform Determination of Death Act (see Chap. 21 for brain death criteria). Critical care nurses play a vital role in identifying potential donors and participating with the healthcare team and OPO in approaching family members about organ donation. Federal Required Request legislation requires that all family members be given the option to donate, or refuse to donate, the organs of their loved one. Additionally, the OPO in the region must be notified by every hospital if there is a potential donor.

The period spent waiting for an appropriate donor and for the transplant to occur is one of great stress and anxiety for patients and their families. The fear that the patient will die before an organ can be found

is ever-present. Children normally regress in the face of serious illness and return to their previous developmental level following recovery. Older children and adolescents may grieve the loss of their good health and former lifestyle, especially if their illness has had a sudden onset. The forced dependence and lack of control are very difficult during the waiting period. All feel a sense of being interminably "on hold," unable to make future plans. Children and families need much emotional support and reassurance during the waiting period.

While many organ transplant candidates are stable and can wait at home, some are critically ill and require hospitalization. The fear that an organ will not be found in time is heightened for these patients and families. The need for invasive procedures, intravascular lines, ventilators, and other mechanical support increases the risk of infection, which would temporarily place a patient's candidacy on hold until the infection is treated. Critically ill patients may develop multisystem organ failure that would preclude organ transplantation.

Critically ill patients waiting for organ transplant present a challenge and a frustration to critical care nurses. They require constant monitoring and frequent adjustment of treatment to maintain their tenuous hold on life, as well as meticulous care to prevent complications. The critical care team's efforts are temporizing, at best, because the therapeutic answer to the patient's problem is organ transplantation.

FINAL COMMON PATHWAYS

After organ transplantation, all patients are at risk for two pathophysiologic final common pathways: organ rejection and infection. General principles are presented, followed by a discussion of organ-specific issues.

Rejection

Since all the physiologic properties of the human immune system have not been fully explained, the phenomenon of rejection is not completely understood. Rejection is the result of a series of complex immunologic responses in which the recipient recognizes the donor organ as being different from itself. Foreign antigens on the donor organ are recognized by the host organism, and then, through a number of pathways, destruction of the donor graft occurs. This process involves lymphocyte infiltration, cellular edema, eventual cellular necrosis leading to organ dysfunction, and later, if untreated, graft loss. A more complete discussion of the immune system is found in Chapter 16. Three types of rejection have been described.

Hyperacute rejection is a humoral immune response, which occurs within minutes or hours of transplantation as the result of preformed circulating antibodies to the donor. The organ sustains intense endothelial damage with interstitial edema and clotting of the microvasculature. The kidney appears most prone to hyperacute rejection, while the liver appears most tolerant of ABO incompatibility and transplant antigen incompatibility (Najarian, 1969; Gordon, 1986). Hyperacute rejection is rare in heart transplantation (Weil, 1981). Using ABO-compatible donors and avoiding implants in crossmatch-positive recipients are standard practices to prevent hyperacute rejection in renal and cardiac transplantation.

Acute rejection is a cellular mediated immune response, which may occur 1 to 2 weeks following transplantation and any time thereafter. The T lymphocytes of the recipient are activated by the surface antigens of the donor organ, causing cellular infiltration of the transplanted organ with resultant interstitial edema and cellular necrosis. Because of cellular damage, acute rejection may interfere with normal organ function. Immunosuppressive therapy following transplantation is designed to prevent and treat acute rejection episodes.

Chronic rejection is a combination of both humoral and cellular immune responses, which may occur 3 months after transplantation but is more common after the first year. It has an insidious onset, appears to be progressive, and results in vascular damage to the organ eventually leading to organ failure. There is no known treatment except retransplantation.

The diagnosis of acute rejection is different for each solid organ transplant. The following discussion describes the clinical signs of rejection and use of procedures to diagnose rejection.

Organ-Specific Rejection

Cardiac Rejection. Clinical signs of acute rejection of the heart in infants and children are often subtle and nonspecific and may be absent until rejection is severe. This is especially true in patients treated with cyclosporine, which appears to lessen the clinical severity of rejection episodes. Signs and symptoms of rejection in infants include irritability, lethargy, poor feeding, tachypnea, and tachycardia. Children may demonstrate decreased exercise tolerance, marked fatigue, elevated temperature, and signs of congestive heart failure. On auscultation, a gallop or pericardial friction rub may be appreciated and dysrhythmias may be detected.

Additional diagnostic tests may be helpful. Cardiomegaly may be seen on chest x-ray. EKG may show atrial or ventricular dysrhythmias, and summation of EKG voltages may be decreased from the patient's baseline. Because cyclosporine blunts the rejection response, changes in EKG voltages are less common with rejection in these patients. Echocardiograms may show pericardial effusion, increasing posterior wall thickness, decreased LV volumes, and decreased ventricular function demonstrated by decreased shortening fraction. Hemodynamic data obtained via intracardiac lines or during cardiac biopsy procedures may show increased filling pressures, increased right ventricular end-diastolic pressure (RVEDP), and decreased cardiac output during rejection episodes.

Despite a number of possible noninvasive parameters, endomyocardial biopsy remains the "gold standard" in the diagnosis of cardiac rejection. Pathologists have agreed on a rating system to interpret cardiac biopsies (Billingham, 1990). Mild rejection is characterized by perivascular and interstitial infiltrates. Moderate rejection involves increased infiltrates and focal myocyte necrosis. Severe rejection is manifested by increased inflammatory infiltrates, multiple sites of myocyte necrosis, and interstitial edema. While endomyocardial biopsy is the most reliable method currently available to diagnose cardiac rejection, it is not infallible. There are many anecdotal reports of patients with clinical signs of severe rejection who had a negative cardiac biopsy and, conversely, patients who appeared well but had a biopsy demonstrating rejection. The importance of experience and clinical judgment in weighing all available data to reach a diagnosis and prescribe appropriate treatment cannot be overemphasized in the field of transplantation, especially when dealing with infants and children.

Biopsies are performed most frequently in the first few months following transplantation because risk of rejection is highest. The length of time between biopsies is gradually increased over the first year. Many programs biopsy patients several times a year for an indefinite period.

The endomyocardial biopsy involves advancing a bioptome catheter into the right ventricle under fluoroscopy and obtaining four to five tissue samples for microscopic analysis. Vascular access is through a neck vein, usually the right internal jugular, in older children and adults. Infants and young children are usually approached via femoral veins. Sedation with chloral hydrate or diazepam (Valium) is usually adequate, with a local anesthetic being given at the puncture site. The procedure is usually performed on an outpatient basis in the cardiac catheterization laboratory and takes approximately one half hour. Pneumothorax and bleeding at the puncture site are possible complications; perforation of the heart muscle is rare.

The endomyocardial biopsy technique and the size of the bioptomes used have been modified so that endomyocardial biopsies can be performed in neonates as well as in older children. However, endomyocardial biopsy has some disadvantages in children: (1) a sampling error is inherent in the technique; (2) it is an invasive technique, which is more difficult to repeat in young children; and (3) anesthesia is an added risk that is sometimes required.

In the Stanford experience, Billingham (1991) reported that 521 endomyocardial biopsies were performed in 30 children ranging in age from 1 month to 15 years (mean, 8.1 years). Only 1.5% (8/521) of the biopsy specimens were inadequate for diagnosis, and 23.2% (121/521) were positive for acute rejection. One biopsy-related death occurred in this series. The patient, a 2-month-old infant, died as a result of right ventricular perforation, highlighting the danger of endomyocardial biopsy in infants. Thus, the recommendation of these investigators is that cardiac biopsy should be performed in infants only when clinically indicated, and that it may not be justified for routine surveillance.

Acute rejection, along with infection, remains the leading cause of death in the first year following cardiac transplantation (Kriett, 1990). Most patients will have at least one rejection episode, usually within the first 3 months following transplantation. There is some evidence that children have a higher rate of rejection than adults (Addonizio, 1990; Fricker, 1987). The critical care nurse plays a vital role in monitoring infants and children for signs of rejection in the early postoperative period. Prompt recognition of rejection and the institution of immunosuppressive therapy increase the likelihood of successful treatment.

Lung Rejection. Three distinct patterns of lung allograft rejection have been defined (Veith, 1972). The first of these is the classic form, in which there is decreased transplant ventilation and perfusion occurring concomitantly. This form of rejection is always observed in nonimmunosuppressed recipients. The second form of rejection, termed atypical or alveolar rejection, is observed in some patients receiving standard immunosuppressive agents. This form of rejection is characterized by the presence of fibrinous alveolar exudates. Radiographically and functionally, alveolar rejection is associated with transplant opacification and decreased ventilation without a corresponding reduction in blood flow. The third form, vascular rejection, involving primarily the small and medium-sized blood vessels, is manifested by an increase in vascular resistance and a decrease in blood flow to the allografted lung. Results of plain chest x-ray and ventilation scans may be completely normal, although in the later stages, some abnormalities caused by alveolar involvement may appear.

Lung rejection can be diagnosed with reasonable accuracy on the basis of the chest x-ray, presence of fever and hypoxemia, and examination of the sputum. Alveolar lavage provides a direct sample of cellular and noncellular material from the transplanted lung. Routine bronchoscopy (approximately every 3 months) or open lung biopsy for troublesome diagnoses may be utilized to monitor the transplanted lung(s). Patients can also be provided with a handheld peak flow meter, which measures peak expiratory flow (PEF) in a very reproducible manner. Even small decreases in PEF have proven to be reliable predictors of a problem in most patients and provide a sensitive indicator of early rejection (Augustine, 1991).

Liver Rejection. Hyperacute, acute, and chronic rejection can occur after hepatic transplantation. Hyperacute rejection is rarely seen with liver transplantation except if donor and recipient blood groups are crossed. Acute, or cellular, rejection most commonly occurs 7 to 10 days after transplant and is characterized by the invasion of mononuclear cells in the portal triads (Tzakis & Starzl, 1992).

Symptoms of rejection are variable and often vague. Symptoms include fever, flush, tachypnea, distended abdomen, irritability, loss of appetite, myalgia, right upper quadrant tenderness, and septic appearance. Changes in liver function laboratory studies may provide the first indication that rejection is occurring (Table 27–3). An early but nonspecific indicator of rejection may be a rapid increase in gamma-glutamyl transpeptidase (GGTP) levels. A subsequent increase in serum bilirubin, alkaline phosphatase, and variable changes with alanine aminotransferase (ALT) and aspartate aminotransferase (AST) levels may be observed (Shaw, 1989). A liver biopsy may be performed if rejection is suspected from liver function tests and the patient is unresponsive to medical therapy. With acute rejection, some degree of mononuclear cellular infiltrate in the portal tracts is found on biopsy (Shaw, 1988b). With chronic rejection, there is disappearance of the intrahepatic bile ducts with varying degrees of bridging fibrosis.

Intestinal Rejection. Rejection of the transplanted intestine is assessed by clinical, radiologic, and histologic evaluation (Todo, Tzakis, Abu-Elmagd, 1992). There are no biochemical indices that reflect rejection of the transplanted intestine. Clinical signs of acute rejection include fever, abdominal distension, abdominal pain, increased or decreased enteric output, and watery diarrhea. Dusky stomal mucosa, mucosal edema, and decreased peristalsis may be associated endoscopic findings. Severe, acute rejection is characterized by severe diarrhea, abdominal pain, abdominal distension, and metabolic acidosis. Endo-

Table 27–3. LIVER FUNCTION TESTS

Biochemical Indices	Newborn/Infant Values	Child Values
Alanine aminotransferase (ALT)/(SGPT)	<48 U/L	<37 U/L
Asparate aminotransferase (AST)/(SGOT)	<50 U/L	<34 U/L
Alkaline phosphatase (ALP)	Newborn	<310 U/L
	1 month–1 year	<360 U/L
	1–10 years	<290 U/L
	10–15 years	<400 U/L
	>15 years	<110 U/L
Gamma-glutamyltransferase (GGT)	<120 U/L	<44 U/L
Ammonia	50–84 µmol/L	12–38 µmol/L
Direct bilirubin		0.1–0.4 mg/dL
Total bilirubin	1–12 mg/dL	0.2–1.3 mg/dL
Prothrombin time (PT)		10.5–13.5 seconds
Partial thromboplastin time (PTT)		18–30 seconds
Total protein	4–7 g/dL	6.5–8.6 g/dL
Albumin	3.9–4.6 g/dL	

Data from Children's Hospital of Pittsburgh, Department of Pathology, Manual of Laboratory Information, 1988.

scopic findings with severe acute rejection include ulceration, mucosal sloughing, bleeding, and loss of peristalsis. Chronic rejection is characterized by chronic diarrhea, malabsorption, and weight loss. Gastric emptying times may be evaluated radiologically, with prolonged emptying times indicative of rejection.

Endoscopic examinations are performed on a periodic basis and if intestinal rejection is suspected from clinical observations. The endoscopic examination yields valuable information about the appearance of the graft's mucosa and intestinal motility.

Renal Rejection. Acute rejection most commonly occurs during the first 6 months following transplantation but may occur at any time. Renal biopsy is important in the diagnosis and management of acute rejection, as the histologic severity of rejection can be used to determine the optimal therapy for the patient. The parameters for diagnosing acute rejection in renal transplantation include fever, decreased urinary output, graft pain and tenderness, increased blood urea nitrogen (BUN) and creatinine levels, weight gain, and hypertension. Small children who receive an adult kidney may not have early significant changes in the BUN and creatinine because of the abundance of renal parenchyma compared with their small size. The introduction of cyclosporine has made the diagnosis of acute rejection more difficult due to potential nephrotoxicity. Urinary obstruction, acute tubular necrosis (ATN), and urinary extravasation can usually be ruled out by ultrasound and radionuclide scan. A biopsy may be required to differentiate between cyclosporine nephrotoxicity and early recurrence of the original disease.

Chronic rejection may occur following an episode of severe acute rejection as early as the first few weeks post transplantation, but, often, it is a disorder characterized by progressive ischemic loss of nephron mass secondary to vascular lesions. Chronic rejection is characterized by a gradual decline in glomerular filtration and an increase in permeability of the glomerulus to protein. The most common signs of chronic rejection are hypertension, proteinuria, edema, gradual rise in BUN and creatinine levels, and decreased creatinine clearance.

Pancreas Rejection. Monitoring for rejection is based on functional parameters specific to the pancreas. The most important parameter to monitor in a pancreas transplant recipient is plasma glucose levels. A functioning graft will maintain plasma glucose levels less than 200 mg/dL in the absence of exogenous insulin, and usually plasma glucose levels are entirely within the normal range (Sutherland, 1988).

Serum amylase levels are usually elevated in the immediate post-transplant period but eventually return to normal. A precipitous decline may indicate deterioration of graft function. On the other hand, a precipitous rise followed by an immediate drop may also be an indication of rejection. If such is the case, a rise in plasma glucose would soon follow.

In recipients of a kidney and pancreas transplant from the same donor, serum creatinine levels are important to monitor for possible isolated renal allograft rejection. A rise in serum creatinine level as a manifestation of renal rejection will, in general, occur before a rise in plasma glucose as a manifestation of pancreas rejection. Thus, in recipients of both a kidney and a pancreas graft from the same donor, rejection of the pancreas can be treated earlier in its course than in recipients of pancreas grafts alone.

In patients in whom the pancreas graft exocrine secretions have been drained into the urinary system, the exocrine function of the graft can be monitored by measurement of urine amylase levels. A decrease in urine amylase activity will precede a rise in plasma glucose levels during a rejection episode (Prieto, 1987). A decline of urine amylase activity of more than 255 U/L is suggestive of rejection, and a decline of 50% is virtually diagnostic. A decline in urine amylase activity associated with a moderate rise in plasma glucose levels is considered rejection and leads to treatment. Severe or advancing rejection will produce significant hyperglycemia; the management objective is to treat rejection before this stage occurs.

Immunosuppression

The rationale for immunosuppressive therapy is to suppress the natural immune response of the host and prevent or limit rejection of the transplanted organ. Some drugs, used on a long-term basis to prevent rejection, are referred to as maintenance immunosuppressants. Other drugs are used on a short-term basis to treat rejection episodes. Because the host does not appear to develop immunologic tolerance to the transplanted organ over time, immunosuppressant medications must be continued for a lifetime to prevent rejection.

Immunosuppressant regimens vary between transplant centers and organ groups, but combination therapy using double- or triple-drug protocols is most common. The advantages of combination therapy are enhanced immunosuppression and a reduction in drug toxicities because of the lower dosages of each individual drug. As Figure 27–1 depicts, the immunosuppressive drugs act on different sites in the immune system, therefore having varying effects on the process of rejection and the extent of systemic side effects experienced by the patient. Azathioprine and prednisone affect many immune system functions, while the monoclonal antibodies act at specific receptor sites for T cell antigens. Cyclosporine and corticosteroids have been the primary maintenance drugs in solid organ transplantation since the early 1980s. Cyclosporine is also T lymphocyte–specific in its action. Improved patient outcomes with triple-drug therapy have prompted many centers to add azathioprine to the prescribed immunosupressive regimen. The long-term side effects of chronic corticosteroids, in particular the negative effects on growth in children, have led clinicians to substantially reduce ste-

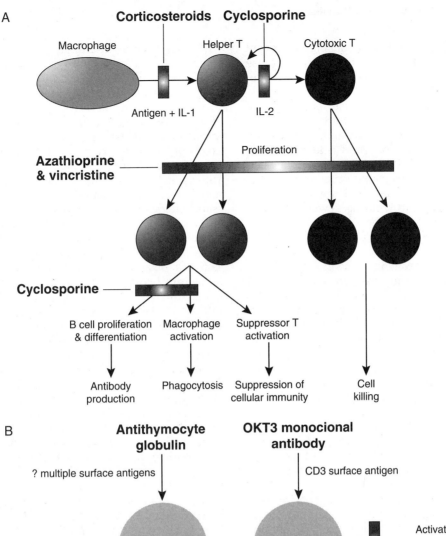

Figure 27-1 • • • • • •

A, Outline of putative activation sequence of cell-mediated immunity. Macrophages present antigen to helper T lymphocytes and secrete interleukin-1 (IL-1), leading to activation of helper T lymphocyte and its production of interleukin-2 (IL-2). IL-2 stimulates proliferation of other helper T cells and cytotoxic T lymphocytes. Activated helper T cells also secrete several other lymphokines, including B cell growth differentiation factors, gamma interferon, and a factor that stimulates suppressor T lymphocytes. Activated cytotoxic T lymphocytes lyse cells that are recognized as non-self. After activation by B cell growth and differentiation factors, B lymphocytes proliferate and produce antibody. Gamma interferon stimulates macrophage phagocytosis and augments T and B cell responses. Activated suppressor T lymphocytes inhibit B cells and other T cells. Sites of action of immunosuppressive agents are indicated by open rectangles. Corticosteroids inhibit release of IL-1, which indirectly inhibits IL-1–dependent release of IL-2. Cyclosporine inhibits release of IL-2, B cell growth and differentiation factors, and gamma interferon. Suppressor T lymphocyte activation is not inhibited. Azathioprine blocks deoxyribonucleic acid replication, and vincristine inhibits microtubular formation necessary for cell divisions. Agents thus inhibit proliferation of effector lymphocytes. *B,* Outline of sites of action for antithymocyte globulin and OKT3 monoclonal antibody. Antithymocyte globulin binds to multiple surface antigens present on T lymphocytes. OKT3 monoclonal antibody binds specifically to CD3 surface antigen. Both agents result in opsonization of T lymphocytes and their clearance from circulation by reticuloendothelial system. In addition, administration of OKT3 monoclonal antibody results in antigenic modulation of remaining T lymphocytes with loss of functional properties caused by loss of antigen recognition receptor. (Adapted from Bristow, M. R., Gilbert, E. M., Renlund, D. G., DeWit, C. W., Burton, W. A., & O'Connell, J. (1988). Use of OKT-3 monoclonal antibody in heart transplantation: Review of the initial experience. *Journal of Heart Transplantation, 7* (1) Jan/Feb 1988.)

roid doses, provide alternate-day dosing, or avoid maintenance steroids altogether, reserving their use for rejection episodes. Unfortunately, eliminating steroids has met with variable results.

The search continues for a more perfect immunosuppressive agent, one that is more specific in blocking the process of rejection without suppressing other immune system functions and that has fewer toxicities. A new drug, FK-506 (Prograf), has been FDA approved. This antirejection medication, derived from a soil fungus, has had success at the University of Pittsburgh in treating severe rejection and possibly has fewer side effects than cyclosporine in long-term use (Tzakis, Fung, Todo, Reyes, Green, & Starzl, 1991).

As with any pharmacologic therapy, knowledge about the immunosuppressant medications including the action, dosage and administration, adverse effects, drug interactions, assessment parameters, and nursing implications is required. Because of the many medical problems of transplant patients, complex immunosuppressant protocols, and the large number of medications each patient receives, correctly administering medications and assessing patients for side effects become a challenging and vital nursing and family responsibility.

The following discussion briefly describes the most commonly used immunosuppressant medications. Other treatments for severe rejection are briefly described. Drug side effects and nursing implications are outlined in Table 27–4.

Cyclosporine (Sandimmune). Cyclosporine is a potent immunosuppressive medication that is a metabolite of a soil fungus. Introduced in 1978, it has substantially improved survival in patients following transplantation. The drug's main mechanism of action is blocking the responsiveness of T lymphocytes to interleukin-2 (IL-2). This prevents the development of mature cytotoxic T cells, also known as killer T cells, which mediate rejection. Cyclosporine appears to have minimal effects on B lymphocytes and does not directly inhibit macrophage activity such as phagocytosis (though it may have indirect effects). Cyclosporine does not cause bone marrow suppression or effect neutrophil response; therefore, some infection-fighting mechanisms remain intact. There is a correspondingly lower incidence of severe infections in cyclosporine-treated patients. Cyclosporine is metabolized by the liver and excreted via bile into the feces.

Cyclosporine is available in an oral form (a liquid in an olive oil base and capsules) and in an intravenous solution. Absorption of the drug following oral administration varies widely, and it is usually given on an empty stomach to reduce the interference of food with absorption. Cyclosporine is fat-soluble, so its bioavailability in patients with severe liver dysfunction is reduced. Children metabolize cyclosporine more rapidly than adults and thus require higher doses per kilogram of body weight and often a more frequent dosing schedule to maintain adequate levels of immunosuppression. Many medications interfere

with cyclosporine metabolism. Table 27–5 outlines some of the more common drugs and their effects on cyclosporine blood levels.

Cyclosporine is often administered intravenously in the immediate post-transplant period. It is given as an infusion over 2 to 6 hours or as a continuous infusion. IV cyclosporine may be given until adequate levels of the drug are reached with the oral preparation. Cyclosporine dosages are adjusted based on trough levels, evidence of nephrotoxicity or other major side effects, and during rejection. Generally, trough levels are maintained at a higher level in the early transplant period and then doses are gradually tapered to a lower long-term maintenance level.

Seizures associated with cyclosporine administration are more prevalent in children than in adults following transplantation (Addonizio, 1990). Post-transplant patients are at risk for seizures due to infection, metabolic derangements, fluid overload, use of steroids, or hypertension. Cyclosporine use, especially at high blood levels, may also predispose patients to seizures (Walker, 1988). A decrease in cyclosporine dose or temporary discontinuation of the drug will stop seizure activity. Valproic acid is the preferable anticonvulsant because both phenytoin (Dilantin) and phenobarbital interfere with the action of cyclosporine. Long-term morbidity from cyclosporine-related seizures is unusual.

Azathioprine (Imuran). Azathioprine, an antimetabolite to DNA synthesis, is closely related to 6-mercaptopurine (6-MP). It was first used as an immunosuppressant with renal transplant patients in 1963. The combination of corticosteroids and azathioprine was found to be more effective than either drug alone and became the basic therapy for those patients receiving other grafts as well. Subsequently, many other drugs were added to this combination, but they generally failed to improve the therapeutic index until the development of cyclosporine. Azathioprine prevents the rapid cell division that occurs in the immune response, thus limiting the ability of the body to generate cytotoxic T cells. Azathioprine is toxic primarily to the bone marrow, and its use may result in leukopenia. This results in an increased risk of infection when azathioprine is used in higher doses.

Azathioprine is metabolized by the liver and excreted by the kidney. It is available in oral and intravenous forms. The oral form is readily absorbed from the GI tract.

Corticosteroids. Corticosteroids are potent anti-inflammatory agents that exert systemic effects in humans. Included in this group of agents are the endogenous glucocorticoids, cortisol, and the exogenous agents prednisone and methylprednisolone (Solu-Medrol). Steroids have several immunosuppressive properties and are used both to prevent rejection and treat rejection episodes. Steroids interfere with macrophage function, impairing antigen recognition. They inhibit both interleukin-1 (IL-1) and interleukin-2 (IL-2), causing a decrease in the production of cytotoxic T cells. At high doses, cortico-

Table 27–4. IMMUNOSUPPRESSION AGENTS

Drug	Side Effects	Nursing Implications
Cyclosporine (Sandimmune) 　Inhibits T cell proliferation 　Metabolized by liver 　Excreted through bile in feces	CNS toxicity: tremors, seizures, headaches, paresthesia, flushing, confusion Nephrotoxicity: >BUN, Cr, Cr clearance, >K, >uric acid Hypomagnesemia Hypertension Hepatotoxicity Infection GI: anorexia, N, V, D, Dermatology: gum hyperplasia and hirsutism Lymphoma	Observe for CNS symptoms Seizures managed with antiseizure medication, usually valproic acid (Depakene) Tremors more pronounced at higher doses Headache—symptomatic treatment Monitor renal function closely; monitor I&O Monitor CyA levels—drawn at trough = just before next dose given Monitor BP, may need antihypertensive medications Monitor LFTs Observe for S&S of infection GI—symptomatic treatment, adjust dose if possible Good oral hygiene: routine dental care May use depilatory cautiously to remove hair Monitor CXR; frequent PE
Azathioprine (Imuran) 　Antimetabolite—depresses AB production 　Metabolized by the liver 　Excreted in the urine	Bone marrow suppression 　Leukopenia 　Thrombocytopenia 　Anemia Hepatotoxicity Infection GI: N, V, D, mouth sores Pancreatitis Muscle wasting	Monitor CBC & platelet counts May hold dose if WBC <3000 Monitor for signs of bleeding Monitor for signs of infection Administer blood products as indicated Monitor LFTs Observe for signs of liver dysfunction Administer with food Good oral hygiene Monitor serum amylase levels
Corticosteroids 　Prednisone 　Solu-Medrol 　　Anti-inflammatory 　　Suppresses T and B lymphocytes 　　Metabolized by liver 　　Excreted in the urine	Infection Fluid retention: >Wt, >Na reabsorption >BP, >uric acid Osteoporosis: <calcium absorption, leaches calcium from bone Increased appetite Mood swings, depression, psychosis Cushingoid appearance GI distress: ulcers and GI bleeding Fragile skin and sun sensitivity, slow wound healing, stomatitis Steroid-induced diabetes: >glucose in blood and urine Cataracts Acne, hirsutism Muscle weakness—proximal more pronounced Aseptic necrosis of large joints Insomnia Headaches Neutrophilia/lymphocytopenia	Observe for S&S of infection Monitor weight, low-sodium diet Monitor BP, administer antihypertensives Monitor serum calcium, give supplements as needed Diet to maintain ideal body weight Adequate exercise Emotional support, treatment as indicated Cushingoid appearance may decrease with decreased dose, emotional support Give with food, antacid therapy, guaiac stools Good oral hygeine Avoid trauma to skin Limit intake of concentrated sugars Monitor lab values, dipstick urine Insulin therapy if needed Routine ophthalmology exams Symptomatic treatment of acne and hirsutism Physical therapy Evaluate C/O joint pain—ortho referral Avoid sudden withdrawal of drug—dose must be tapered
Antithymocyte globulin (ATG) Antilymphocyte sera (ALS) 　Suppresses T lymphocytes	Leukopenia Infection (especially opportunistic infections) Anaphylactic reaction Fever, chills, decreased BP, respiratory distress Thrombocytopenia Very caustic to blood vessels Serum sickness—usually 1–2 weeks after beginning therapy Skin rashes	Follow CBC and differential Monitor for S&S of infection Perform skin test prior to administration Premedicate with Tylenol and Benadryl Have epinephrine, corticosteroids, and intubation equipment readily available Follow platelet counts—observe for bleeding Fever and chills—symptomatic treatment Give in large vein, preferable central line Slow infusion over 6–8 hours, use inline filter Monitor for serum sickness—symptomatic treatment
OKT3 (orthoclone OKT3) Monoclonal antibody (Muromonab-CD3) 　Blocks T cell function	Fever and chills Pulmonary edema (renal transplant patients) Aseptic meningitis (temperature, headache, stiff neck; increased and WBC protein in CSF) Infection—especially herpes and CMV Acute joint pain Diarrhea Lymphopenia (decreased CD-3 cells)	Premedicate with Tylenol and Benadryl Most often occurs in the first 48 hours Assess respiratory function and fluid balance Observe for seizures—supportive therapy Observe for S&S of infection Joint pain is self-limiting Symptomatic treatment of diarrhea Follow WBC differential Monitor T cell subsets CD-3
FK-506 (Prograf) 　Inhibits T cell proliferation 　Inhibits interleukin-2 production 　Suppresses lymphokine production 　Metabolized and excreted in bile	Headaches Irritability, insomnia Nausea, vomiting Tremors Hyperkalemia Nephrotoxic effects	Side effects increased with intravenous administration Follow BUN & creatinine With IV, do not mix with NaHCO$_3$ Administer as a constant infusion With PO, give 4 hours apart from alkalizing drugs (NaHCO$_3$)

Table 27–5. DRUG INTERACTIONS THAT AFFECT CYCLOSPORINE METABOLISM

Increase Cyclosporine Levels	Decrease Cyclosporine Levels
Erythromycin	Phenobarbital
Ketoconazole	Phenytoin
	Rifampin
	Calcium channel blockers

steroids have a profound negative effect on the function of lymphocytes. The ability to recognize their target antigens is impaired, and circulating lymphocytes are redistributed into lymphoid compartments where they avoid contact with the transplanted organ.

Steroids are predominantly metabolized by the liver and excreted by the kidney. Steroids are most commonly given intravenously (as Solu-Medrol) and then orally (as prednisone) following transplantation. The oral preparation is readily absorbed from the GI tract. High doses of corticosteroids are given immediately post transplant to prevent rejection and then weaned to lower maintenance levels over several weeks or months. Because of the many toxic side effects of steroids, especially their negative effect on linear growth in prepubertal children, low maintenance doses are advantageous. The goal is to reach a very low maintenance dose, or ideally, an every-other-day dose schedule to improve growth in prepubertal children. Prednisone inhibits normal adrenocorticoid production of cortisol, so the drug dosage is weaned prior to discontinuation to avoid symptoms of adrenal corticoid insufficiency that occur if the drug is abruptly stopped.

High-dose steroid therapy is usually the initial treatment for rejection episodes. A 3 to 8 day "pulse" of high-dose Solu-Medrol given IV or oral therapy with high doses of prednisone for 3 days and then tapered to maintenance levels over 7 to 10 days is a common treatment option. Many rejection episodes are successfully treated with steroid treatment alone.

Antithymocyte Globulin (ATG)/(ATGAM). ATG is an immune globulin preparation produced by injecting an animal with human thymocytes. The animal produces antibodies to the human thymocytes, which are then separated and purified into an immune globulin preparation. The antilymphocyte sera is then infused into the patient, and the immunosuppressive effect is achieved through the depletion of circulating lymphocytes in the lymph nodes and spleen.

This therapy has been used primarily to treat rejection episodes that are resistant to corticosteroid treatment. In addition, ATGAM is used to prevent cyclosporine nephrotoxicity and rejection in the newly transplanted kidney and is also used as an adjunct to other immunosuppressive therapy to delay the onset of the first rejection episode.

ATGAM comes as an IV preparation given daily for 14 days as treatment for allograft rejection and usually used in combination with other immunosuppressants, in particular steroids and azathioprine. It may also be used to delay the onset of allograft rejection. Before administration, prior sensitization to the heterologous globulin is assessed by giving a subcutaneous test dose diluted with normal saline. During administration, premedication with an antihistamine will decrease the incidence of toxic reactions such as flushing, chills, fever, occasional anaphylactic reactions, and serum sickness (Flye, 1989). Dose is regulated by monitoring T cell subsets.

Monoclonal Antibodies (Orthoclone OKT3, Muromonab-CD3). Monoclonal antibodies are produced by a hybridization technique that joins sensitized B cell lymphocytes with murine myeloma cells and produces monoclonal antibodies. The antibodies are targeted to react with a specific subset of lymphocytes defined by surface cell antigens (Goldstein, 1986). Monoclonal antibodies are derived from a single clone, so each molecule is an identical, highly specific antibody to a specific antigen. In the case of OKT3, the antigen is the CD3 cell surface antigen of the T lymphocytes.

OKT3 administration has two actions on the immune system. It causes an immediate decline in circulating T cells, and it interferes with the antigen recognition complex on the surface of the T lymphocytes. This prevents the lymphocytes from reacting with foreign antigens and inhibiting T cell function. The advantages of OKT3 as an immunosuppressant are its specificity for interfering with antigen recognition on the T lymphocytes and its different toxic effects from the other immunosuppressants. Experience in renal, liver, and cardiac transplantation has demonstrated its efficacy in treating rejection.

OKT3 has also been used prophylactically in the immediate transplant period by some heart and renal transplant programs (Bristow, 1988; Carpenter, 1989). The goal was to induce early graft tolerance by reducing the circulating transplant antigens and therefore decrease later rejection episodes. The efficacy of prophylactic use of OKT3 in decreasing rejection has not been established. There is now some evidence that prophylactic use of OKT3 may be associated with an increased risk of lymphoma following heart transplantation in adults (Swinnen, 1990).

OKT3 comes as an IV preparation and is given once daily as an IV bolus infusion over 1 minute. Treatment for rejection is usually a 10- to 14-day course. Premedication is given to decrease adverse reactions, especially common with the first dose. OKT3 administration has been associated with an increased incidence of cytomegalovirus (CMV) infection. Therefore, many patients receive CMV prophylaxis concomitant with a course of OKT3. Because OKT3 is a foreign protein, patients may develop antibodies to the drug, which could limit the potency of the drug in the future treatment of the patient. The manufacturer (Ortho Pharmaceutical Co.) offers an immunoassay service to measure antibody titers to OKT3.

FK-506 (Prograf). FK-506 is a potent, selective anti-T cell immunosuppressant drug whose mode of action is similar to that of cyclosporine (Macleod & Thomson, 1991). FK-506 is a novel macrolide antibiotic derived from the soil fungus *Streptomyces tsukubaensis,* found in the Tsukuba region of northern Japan. Compared with cyclosporine, FK-506 is 100 times more potent and has the same ability to inhibit T cell function (Bierer, 1990). Like cyclosporine, FK-506 is believed to act by inhibiting T cell receptor–mediated activation of CD4 T (helper) lymphocytes and selectively inhibiting various cell growth prompting cytokines (interleukin-2, 3, 4 and interferon-alpha). There is no evidence that FK-506 directly affects B cell or macrophage function (Thomson, 1988).

FK-506 holds promise for transplant recipients because of associated potency and relatively low toxicity. The first human trials of FK-506 were conducted as rescue therapy for liver graft rejection, despite administration of conventional immunosuppressive therapy (Starzl, 1989). FK-506's efficacy has been demonstrated with pediatric cardiac, liver, intestinal, renal, and pancreas transplant recipients. Improved graft and patient survival, enhanced steroid-free growth, and successful treatment of autoimmune disorders indicate that FK-506 is an effective immunosuppressant agent (Tzakis, Fung, Todo, Reyes, Green, & Starzl, 1991).

Clinical studies completed to this date indicate that FK-506 has fewer side effects than cyclosporine (Starzl, Abu-Elmagd, Tzakis, Fung, & Todo, 1991). Reported toxicities in children are dose related and include impaired renal function, headaches, nausea and vomiting, paresthesias, and insomnia (Shapiro, Fung, Jain, Parks, Todo, & Starzl, 1990). Since the introduction of FK-506 as primary immunosuppression in October 1989, hypertension has been infrequently observed (Tzakis & Starzl, 1992).

Absorption of FK-506 appears to occur more rapidly than cyclosporine, with peak plasma concentrations of FK-506 achieved in 0.5 to 4 hours. FK-506 is metabolized and excreted in the bile with an associated half-life of 4 to 14 hours (Venkataramanan, Jain, Warty, Abu-Elmagd, Furakawa, Imventarza, Fung, Todo, & Starzl, 1991). Current FK-506 pediatric intravenous dosing is 0.15 mg/kg/day via a 24-hour continuous infusion. The drug is administered through central or peripheral intravenous access. Once blood levels of 0.5 to 2.5 ng/mL by ELISA are achieved with the child tolerating oral intake, oral doses are prescribed. As increased side effects of FK-506 have been reported with intravenous use, the child is switched to oral dosing as soon as tolerated. The initial oral dose is 0.15 mg/kg twice per day (Tzakis, Fung, Todo, Reyes, Green, & Starzl, 1991). The current maintenance oral dose is 0.075 mg/kg/day. Drug interactions reported with FK-506 are listed in Table 27–6. Monotherapy with FK-506 in the majority of patients is achieved in 1 to 3 months (Tzakis & Starzl, 1992).

Other Agents. Several other treatments have been tried to prevent or treat rejection following transplantation. Some centers have used the anticancer agents cyclophosphamide (Cytoxan) and vincristine in patients with severe rejection. Total lymphoid irradiation (TLI) has been used in small groups of patients. With renal transplant patients, it was used prior to transplantation in an attempt to induce immune tolerance to the donor organ and decrease later rejection (Levin, 1985). It has also been used after heart transplantation to treat intractable rejection (Hunt, 1989). New monoclonal antibodies are being sought. Ideally, scientists hope to find a method for inducing a state of true tolerance to the transplanted organ.

Table 27–6. DRUG INTERACTIONS WITH FK-506

Increase FK-506 Levels	Decrease FK-506 Levels
Erythromycin	Carbamazepine
Clotrimazole	Rifampin
Ketoconazole	Phenobarbital
Diltiazem	Phenytoin
Verapamil	

Infection

Infection in the immunocompromised child following organ transplantation is a significant problem and, along with rejection, a leading cause of death. The risk of infection is highest in the first few months following transplantation, when immunosuppression is greatest. The incidence of infection has declined in the past decade for several reasons. Cyclosporine is more specific in altering the immune response that causes rejection, sparing other immunologic functions that defend against infection. With combination therapy, lower doses of prednisone and azathioprine are used, reducing the infection risk. Increased knowledge about post-transplant infections allows for improved detection and treatment. The development of antiviral agents, acyclovir and the newer ganciclovir, has aided in the treatment of viral infections. Improvements in the diagnosis and management of rejection have decreased the time interval of intense immunosuppression, which was often associated with infections. The following section reviews the risk factors for infection in the child following transplantation; types of infections, their presentation and treatment; and outlines the vital role of the nurse in prevention and surveillance.

Risk factors for infection include the use of intense immunosuppression, host characteristics, and the PICU environment. Immunosuppression is at its highest level in the immediate post-transplant period in order to hope to induce immune tolerance of the new organ and prevent rejection. At the present time, all pharmacologic therapies disturb normal immune defenses to some extent; none is specific enough to block only the processes that cause rejection. In the field of transplantation, it is recognized that the greater the amount and duration of immunosuppression, the greater the likelihood of infection (Rubin, 1981).

Many patients, prior to transplantation, are immunocompromised secondary to their debilitating chronic illness, poor nutrition, or end-stage organ failure. A weakened host then undergoes a major operation and requires complex postoperative care involving the use of invasive equipment and procedures that further compromise the body's defenses. The presence of an endotracheal tube, multiple invasive lines, catheters, and drainage tubes breach the normal external defense mechanism of the body and carry a risk of infection. The PICU environment also predisposes transplant patients to an infectious risk with exposure to multiple organisms common in the hospital environment and numerous caregivers. Immunosuppression, a compromised host, and environmental concerns combine to make infection a significant risk for the child following transplantation (see Chapter 16, Host Defenses).

A pattern of infections following transplantation has been identified (Rubin, 1988). Most infections in the first month are nosocomial infections primarily involving bacteria and occur as a result of multiple lines and invasive procedures or are related to pre-existing disease conditions and surgical manipulation. From 1 month to 6 months, opportunistic infections are most common and may cause significant morbidity and mortality. It has been reported that approximately one third of renal allograft recipients will require hospitalization for infection over a 4-year period (Peterson, 1982).

Opportunistic infections are caused by organisms common in the environment that rarely cause disease in an immunocompetent host. In the immunosuppressed patient, however, these organisms are capable of causing illness. Infection can also result from exposure to an exogenous source of a virulent pathogen, such as meningococcal meningitis; reactivation of an organism such as herpes or cytomegalovirus (CMV); or from endogenous invasion of a normally present organism, such as overgrowth of GI flora. Sites of infection following transplant include the lungs, central nervous system, wounds, skin, mucous membranes, gastrointestinal tract, and urinary tract.

Bacterial Infections

Bacterial infections are most common in the first month following transplantation and are similar to the organisms found in the postoperative surgical patient. Gram-negative bacilli including *Pseudomonas aeruginosa, Proteus* species, *Klebsiella* species, and *E. coli* are common infecting organisms, and both *Staphylococcus epidermidis* and *aureus* are seen. Bacterial infections usually arise from organisms already colonizing the patient. Because of a disruption of anatomic and mechanical defense systems such as the skin, mucous membranes, cilia, and mucosa of the gastrointestinal tract, bacteria are able to enter the body and cause infection. Common types of bacterial infections are pneumonias, wound infections, line sepsis, and urinary tract infections.

Unusual bacterial infections include *Legionella,* an aquatic organism that causes pneumonia; and *Nocardia,* commonly present in soil and decaying matter that enters the body by inhalation and can cause pneumonia and infections of the central nervous system. Both are often associated with environmental hazards such as construction or contamination in air filtration systems.

Most surgical patients receive prophylactic antibiotics at the time of surgery and for a short period following surgery to prevent bacterial infection. The antibiotic chosen is a broad-spectrum agent effective against the common organisms causing wound infections in a particular healthcare setting. Prolonged use of prophylactic antibiotics raises concerns about the growth of antibiotic-resistant bacteria and fungi. Equally important in the prevention of bacterial infections is removal of all invasive monitoring lines, tubes, and catheters as soon as possible.

Viral Infections

Viruses comprise an important group of infecting organisms following transplantation and include herpes simplex viruses, varicella zoster, CMV, Epstein-Barr virus, hepatitis virus, and the human immunodeficiency virus (HIV). Viral infections can be primary or secondary. Primary infections are caused the first time the individual is exposed to the organism, including those that can be transmitted from donor to recipient. A secondary infection is a reactivation of the virus. Infants and young children are more likely to have primary infections, while adolescents and adults are more likely to have been exposed to most common viruses and have a reactivation of a previous infection. Prospective recipients and donors are carefully screened for pre-existing titers to the more common viral agents in order to assist with the prevention of infection.

Herpes simplex viruses are divided into two types: HSV-1 is responsible for most herpes infections above the waist, most commonly of the lips, face, and mouth; HSV-2 is responsible for herpes genitalis. HSV-1 infections are usually acquired during childhood and establish a permanent residence in most hosts. Herpes genitalis is acquired through sexual activity.

HSV-1 is usually a localized infection of recurrent vesicles and low ulcerations on the lips and oral mucosa. It can be diagnosed by its classic appearance, but viral cultures provide the definitive diagnosis. HSV-1 infection is common in the first month following transplantation. Treatment of both HSV-1 and HSV-2 infections is with acyclovir. Some programs use acyclovir prophylactically in the first few months following transplant to prevent herpes infections (Dresdale & Diehl, 1990).

Varicella zoster can be a dangerous infection for children following transplantation. Outbreaks of chickenpox are common in childhood, and transplant patients may be exposed many times. The disease is likely to be more virulent in the immunocompromised host and can cause pneumonitis and significant respiratory compromise. Children may be given V-ZIG, varicella immune globulin, upon exposure to provide them with antibodies to fight the disease. Treatment of active infection is with intravenous acyclovir and reduction of immunosuppressant drug dosages.

CMV is a significant viral infection following transplantation and is associated with the greatest morbidity and mortality (Smith, S., 1990). Infection with CMV can be a primary infection in which a seronegative recipient receives a CMV-positive blood transfusion, a CMV-positive donor organ, or is exposed to infected individuals. Reactivated, or secondary, infection occurs when a seropositive patient then becomes immunosuppressed. Primary infections appear to be associated with more serious and symptomatic morbidity.

The symptoms and severity of CMV infection are variable. Some patients may have a mild, subclinical infection; others a self-limiting syndrome of fever, arthralgias, and fatigue. Disseminated disease can affect many organ systems, including the lung, liver, pancreas, kidneys, stomach, intestine, and brain, and is associated with significant mortality (Schumann, 1987). CMV infection is most commonly seen from 1 to 4 months following transplantation. Definitive diagnosis is by tissue biopsy, but a fourfold increase in antibody titers, conversion from IgM to IgG antibodies, positive buffy coat cell cultures, and presence of the clinical syndrome are strongly suggestive of infection.

In addition to infection with CMV, transplant patients may develop superinfections, most often in the lung. CMV infection has been shown to suppress cell-mediated immunity, further impairing the body's ability to fight infection (Pollard, 1978). Superinfections with opportunistic organisms such as *Pneumocystis carinii* may occur simultaneously.

The only treatment for CMV is ganciclovir (DHPG), a derivative acyclovir that prevents replication of CMV. Ganciclovir has led to improved outcomes for CMV-infected patients, with a clinical response evident 5 to 7 days after initiation of therapy (Green & Michaels, 1991). Because of the high morbidity and mortality associated with CMV infection following transplant and, until recently, a lack of treatment for the disease, there is much interest in preventing the infection. The use of acyclovir for CMV prophylaxis with high-dose oral therapy (650 mg/M^2/dose) is supported in some protocols. The efficacy of prophylactic use of CMV immune globulin in patients who are seronegative and receive a seropositive organ has been demonstrated in renal transplant patients and extrapolated for use in other organ groups (Snydman, 1987).

Epstein-Barr virus (EBV) is known to cause mild infections similar to mononucleosis in patients following transplant, but its most important association is with lymphoproliferative malignancies seen months or years following organ transplantation. EBV is implicated in the development of these lymphomas. There is some evidence that sharp reduction in cyclosporine dosage will cause regression of the tumor (Starzl, 1984).

Fungal Infections

The most common fungal infections following transplantation are those caused by the *Candida* species of organisms and are seen in the mouth, gastrointestinal tract, and vagina. Oral candidiasis, known as thrush, is a common infection in infants and also prevalent in immunocompromised patients and those receiving broad-spectrum antibiotics. Thrush appears as wet, white lesions on the tongue and mucous membranes of the mouth, which are painful and can impair oral nutritional intake. The infection can spread through the gastrointestinal tract, causing esophagitis, and can cause a *Candida* diaper rash. Transplant patients often receive the topical antifungal drug nystatin prophylactically to prevent *Candida* infections. Vaginal infections caused by *Candida* present with itching, irritation, and a malodorous white discharge. The offending organism must be identified through appropriate diagnostic tests because *Trichomonas* has a similar presentation. The treatment of choice is clotrimazole suppositories.

Candida can become disseminated throughout the body, usually through the gastrointestinal mucosa, and cause serious infection. The diagnosis can be difficult, and signs and symptoms include a disseminated rash and swollen tender muscles, persistent fever, eye pain, and eventual signs of central nervous system disease. Treatment involves administration of intravenous amphotericin B.

Several unusual fungal infections can present later in the post-transplant period and are generally community acquired. All have an insidious onset and are difficult to diagnose. *Aspergillus* can cause pneumonia, pulmonary infarction, gastrointestinal bleeding, and brain abscesses. *Cryptococcus* enters the body through the lungs and disseminates to the central nervous system. Coccidioidomycosis disseminates to the lungs, central nervous system, joints, and liver. Histoplasmosis causes disease in lungs and central nervous system, liver, spleen, and lymph nodes. All these fungal infections are treated with systemic amphotericin B.

Parasitic Infections

The most common parasitic infections seen following transplantation are pneumonia caused by *Pneumocystis carinii* (PCP) and infections with toxoplasmosis. *Pneumocystis* presents with an abrupt onset of dyspnea, cough, hypoxemia, and fever. Bilateral alveolar infiltrates are seen on chest x-ray, and definitive diagnosis is made with bronchoalveolar lavage or transbronchial biopsy. Treatment is with IV trimethoprim-sulfamethoxazole (Bactrim) or IV pentamidine. Many programs use Bactrim prophylactically for a period of time following transplantation to prevent *Pneumocystis* infection. Toxoplasmosis is caused by a protozoan parasite present in the environment, and infection is usually acquired through ingestion of undercooked or raw meat, inhalation of dust containing the spores, or contaminated food. It can be transmitted through blood transfusions and through the donor organ. Transplant patients at greatest risk include those who are seronegative for toxoplasmosis and receive a seropositive organ. Toxoplasmosis can affect multiple organs, including the central nervous system, lungs, and heart, and has a wide range of clinical signs. Treatment is with pyrimethamine and sulfadiazine. Folic acid deficiency may occur as a side effect of pharmacologic treatment and must be supplemented.

The critical care nurse plays a vital role in the assessment of transplant patients for infection. All caregivers must have a very high index of suspicion for infection in this patient population. Signs of infection may be subtle; may be masked by the use of immunosuppressive agents, especially steroids; or may be confused with rejection or other problems. An aggressive approach to diagnosis is warranted because the consequences of untreated infection can be life-threatening.

A complete head-to-toe physical assessment specifically focused on possible signs or symptoms of infection should be performed daily. All fevers should be taken seriously, though many serious infections may present with little or no fever. Complaints of headache, subtle mental status changes, and fever are important signs of potential CNS infection. Assessment of responsiveness, alertness, mental status, evidence of impairment of cranial nerves or sensory or motor function, and the presence of meningeal signs are all critical elements of a neurologic assessment. The mouth, tongue, and oral mucosa should be carefully examined for evidence of thrush or herpetic lesions. The lymph node chains of the head and neck should be examined for signs of infection and inflammation. Alterations in respiratory function can be key signs of an infectious process, especially since pneumonia is a common type of infection following transplantation. Tachypnea, dyspnea, cough, labored respirations, retractions, hypoxia, and rales and rhonchi on auscultation are all important observations. Tachycardia, pulsus paradoxus, a new murmur, and signs of pericardial effusion can sometimes be associated with an infectious process. Abdominal distension, cramping and pain, nausea, vomiting, diarrhea, and changes in the stool may be a result of infection. Cloudy urine, burning on urination, or a change in the frequency of urination may suggest a urinary tract infection. Pain or inflammation of the joints should be noted. All skin surfaces and mucous membranes should be examined closely for any signs of infection.

Preventing infection is a critical nursing responsibility. Isolation techniques following transplantation vary between institutions and organ types, but the mainstay of all is the simple measure of good handwashing. Surveillance of visitors and caregivers to prevent contact with anyone actively infected is important. All invasive lines are cared for with aseptic technique. All lines and equipment are discontinued as soon as possible. Patients are extubated as early as possible and aggressive pulmonary toilet carried out. Early ambulation is an important goal. Meticulous skin care and mouth care are crucial to prevent further breaks in the body's defensive barrier. The physical environment is kept clean and infection-free. The importance of good nutrition in preventing infection is recognized.

CARDIAC TRANSPLANTATION

The treatment of end-stage heart disease in infants and children with heart transplantation has become available only in the last decade following improved outcomes in adults and the advent of cyclosporine. Data from the Registry of the International Society for Heart Transplantation show that between 1980 and 1988, 206 patients under 10 years of age had heart transplant operations compared with approximately 9000 patients over age 10 years (Heck, 1989). Although the annual number of adult heart transplants has leveled off during the last 3 years, the number of pediatric heart transplants has continued to rise. Transplants in children (ages 0–18 years) currently account for 9% of all heart transplants annually. The actuarial survival associated with pediatric heart transplantation since 1984 is a 1-year survival rate of 73.5% and a 5-year survival rate of slightly more than 60%. More than half of the early deaths have resulted from cardiac complications, which include donor preservation failure, right heart failure caused by elevated pulmonary vascular resistance, cardiac arrest, hemorrhage, and other nonspecified technical problems. An additional 15% of early deaths have been attributed to infection and 13% to acute rejection. As in the adult population, rejection has continued to be the major cause of late deaths in children following heart transplantation. An additional 25% of late deaths occur secondary to infection (Kaye, 1991). The long-term results of pediatric heart transplantation are not fully known.

Cardiac transplantation in children presents some unique concerns. The optimal timing of transplantation in children is unknown. There is less information on the course of illness in end-stage heart disease in children than in adults. Unlike adults, children with severe cardiac disease may have few symptoms until they acutely decompensate. The small numbers of children with dilated cardiomyopathy make it difficult to prognosticate for this group; however, age greater than 2 years at onset appears to correlate with poor outcome (Griffin, 1988). There are little data on the time course of illness in patients with surgically palliated congenital heart disease (CHD) who develop ventricular failure; some may remain well compensated for years, others may die suddenly of dysrhythmias.

Powerful arguments have been made on both sides of the "palliate or transplant" controversy in care of children with complex CHD. Those who argue in favor of palliation cite the relative scarcity of donors and the sometimes dismal results with transplantation at inexperienced centers. They propose that using pieces of an infant's own heart to fashion some form of circulation capable of sustaining life is preferable to using someone else's tissue (i.e., a transplanted organ), with its attendant need for immunosuppression. It is further argued that because the long-term results of transplantation are not known, this procedure is best reserved for conditions that cannot be palliated any longer or could never be palliated, as in the case with dilated cardiomyopathy. Proponents of transplantation believe it is a better alternative for severe cardiac defects such as hypoplastic left heart syndrome (HLHS), which require several high-risk palliative procedures without achieving normal cardiac function. They argue that having a normal heart offsets the risks of chronic immunosuppression.

Donor selection and organ recovery require some adjustments for infants and younger children. Hearts can come from donors larger than the recipient, sometimes more than double the recipient's body weight (Johnston, 1991). The recipient's failing heart is often markedly hypertrophied, so the mediastinum can accommodate a larger heart. This may be especially advantageous if increased pulmonary vascular resistance (PVR) is present. Surgeons usually remove extra donor aorta and pulmonary artery to use in reconstruction of these vessels in patients with congenital heart disease. Surgical techniques for cardiac transplantation in patients with many congenital cardiac anomalies have been described (Bailey, 1986; Baumgartner, 1990; Mayer, 1990).

There is evidence that the neonatal myocardium is more vulnerable to ischemic injury and that long ischemic times are less well tolerated. Thus, the time between identifying a suitable donor and the transplant operation is short. Coordination and cooperation between all transplant personnel are critical to a successful outcome.

Transplant Procedure

The operative technique for cardiac transplantation in infants and children is similar to that in adults except for modifications in those with congenital cardiac anomalies. The operation is performed through a median sternotomy and cardiopulmonary bypass. *Orthotopic* heart transplantation involves the removal of the recipient's diseased heart, retaining the great arteries and back wall of the atrium, and replacing it with a donor organ. *Heterotopic* heart transplantation leaves the recipient's own heart in place and attaches the donor heart, via conduits to the great arteries as a "piggyback" heart.

Rarely performed, heterotopic transplantation might have a role in patients with increased PVR as an alternative to heart-lung transplantation (Griffin, 1987).

Postoperative Care

Many aspects of postoperative nursing care following heart transplantation are similar to the care of infants and children following cardiac surgery (see Chap. 19). Therapy is based on the clinical course of the pediatric recipient. The unique aspects of rejection, immunosuppression, and infection are similar to other solid organ transplants and have been discussed earlier. The hemodynamic alterations seen in the early postoperative period following heart transplantation result from ventricular dysfunction and denervation of the allograft heart.

Decreased Cardiac Output Related to Ventricular Dysfunction

Ventricular dysfunction leading to low cardiac output following transplantation can be caused by several factors. An ischemic injury to the donor heart causing poor contractility can occur during retrieval, during the cold ischemic time while the heart is being transported, or during the implantation. Inadequate preservation and prolonged ischemia times (longer than 4–5 hours) can contribute to global ventricular dysfunction (Rosado, 1990). Clinical signs of decreased cardiac output and elevated filling pressures are seen.

Increased PVR in the recipient resulting from long-standing congestive heart failure prior to transplantation can cause acute right ventricular failure in the immediate postoperative period. The donor heart, already stressed by a period of cold arrest and cardiopulmonary bypass, must attempt to pump against elevated PVR and may not be able to meet the challenge. Right ventricular dilation and signs of right-sided heart failure ensue with elevated right atrial pressures, tachycardia, dilated neck veins, hepatomegaly, pericardial and pleural effusions, a gallop rhythm or tricuspid regurgitation murmur, and marked right ventricular dysfunction seen on echocardiography.

Rejection is unusual in the first postoperative week but possible in the second and subsequent weeks. Rejection can also impair contractility and result in low cardiac output.

Postoperative mediastinal bleeding and the risk of cardiac tamponade are of particular concern following heart transplantation. The native pericardium is often stretched by severe cardiac hypertrophy and dilatation. The donor heart may be smaller than the patient's native heart, resulting in a large potential space in the pericardial sac. Blood can easily accumulate and may contribute to hypovolemia, decreased cardiac output, and possible tamponade. Chest tube drainage is closely monitored, and measures to ensure adequate drainage of the mediastinum are followed. Coagulopathies are monitored and corrected. The patient is closely observed for signs of tamponade and prompt treatment instituted if tamponade is suspected. Reoperation for bleeding is sometimes necessary.

Hypovolemia and hypothermia are commonly seen following cardiopulmonary bypass and may contribute to decreased contractility in the newly transplanted heart. Careful assessment of fluid balance and temperature is followed by appropriate fluid replacement and rewarming.

Severe ventricular dysfunction, due to an increased PVR or acute ventricular failure, is a life-threatening event and has led to death following transplantation (Smith, C.R., 1990; Trento, 1989). Assist devices such as the intra-aortic balloon pump, extracorporeal membrane oxygenation (ECMO), or ventricular assist devices have been tried when conventional measures have failed.

Decreased Cardiac Output Related to Heart Rate and Rhythm

Change in heart rate because of denervation of the donor heart and rhythm disturbances may also lead to alterations in cardiac output following transplantation. Because nervous system connections to the heart are permanently severed during transplantation, there is no autonomic control of heart rate. In the absence of parasympathetic control, the resting heart rate is elevated. The Valsalva maneuver and carotid massage are no longer effective following transplantation. The sympathetic nervous system normally acts to increase heart rate. Loss of sympathetic control impairs the ability to respond quickly to the need for increased cardiac output. Slower mechanisms that increase cardiac output include the Starling response, which increases venous return and therefore stroke volume, and the release of endogenous catecholamines with both inotropic and chronotropic properties. Changes in heart rate in response to increased metabolic demands such as fever or exercise occur more slowly and are dependent on an appropriate circulating blood volume to provide adequate preload and normal contractility. The absence of a normal compensatory reflex tachycardia may cause orthostatic hypotension because of venous pooling. Vasodilation (especially resulting from vasodilating drugs or rewarming early postoperatively) may lead to hypotension and a rapid decrease in cardiac output because of reduced preload.

Medications that act on the autonomic nervous system will be ineffective (Horak, 1984). Digoxin loses its influence on heart rate and rhythm but may be a useful inotropic agent. Atropine has no effect on heart rate in the transplanted heart. Calcium channel blockers such as verapamil, which have negative inotropic effects, are used cautiously. Because beta-blockers inhibit circulating catecholamines, which are important in increasing heart rate in the trans-

planted heart, they may blunt the heart rate response and are used with caution (Funk, 1986).

The electrocardiogram (EKG) following transplantation demonstrates two P waves representing both the donor sinoatrial (SA) node and the recipient SA node, which was left as part of the wall of the right atrium (Fig. 27–2). Because the impulse from the recipient SA node cannot cross the suture line, there is no further stimulation of the conduction system or cardiac contraction. The donor SA node initiates the electrical stimulation through the conduction system, which results in contraction.

Dysrhythmias are often seen in the early postoperative period. Because children following cardiac transplantation are dependent on an adequate heart rate to maintain cardiac output, any dysrhythmia can have a negative consequence on cardiac output. Bradydysrhythmias may be due to temporary swelling near the SA node following surgery or ischemic injury during preservation. These difficulties often resolve with time. Use of a temporary external pacemaker or continuous intravenous isoproterenol will provide a faster heart rate and enhance cardiac output. Tachydysrhythmias, both ventricular and supraventricular, may be seen and are more difficult to manage. Pharmacologic therapy is limited because the heart is denervated. Tachycardia limits the use of many inotropic agents, and the negative inotropic effects of most antidysrhythmics can have a deleterious effect on contractility in the early postoperative period. Drug therapy is used cautiously. Overdrive pacing or cardioversion may be utilized as alternatives.

Interventions to maintain adequate cardiac output are directed at providing inotropic support, decreasing pulmonary vascular resistance, preventing increased cardiac work, and maintaining an adequate heart rate and rhythm. Inotropic agents such as dopamine, dobutamine, and isoproterenol are used to enhance contractility. Isoproterenol is favored because of its positive chronotropic effects and its vasodilator effects on the pulmonary vascular bed. Afterload reducers such as nitroprusside or amrinone are used to lower PVR. Prostaglandin E_1 (PGE$_1$) has also been used to lower PVR (Smith, C.R., 1990). Other measures to reduce PVR include sedation, careful suctioning, good pulmonary toilet to prevent atelectasis, and adequate diuresis. Nursing interventions to decrease cardiac workload include maintaining normal temperature, ensuring adequate pain control, reducing environmental stressors, providing emotional support to decrease anxiety, proper nutrition, careful ambulation, and adequate rest.

Experience at Loma Linda and elsewhere has suggested that the clinical course of the newborn heart recipient can be divided into three consecutive stages (Assaad, 1991). The first stage, the first 24 to 48 hours after transplantation, is characterized by generalized edema including pulmonary edema and possibly brain edema. During this stage, urine output may be decreased. Chest x-ray shows mild diffuse pulmonary edema, and blood gas values reflect a

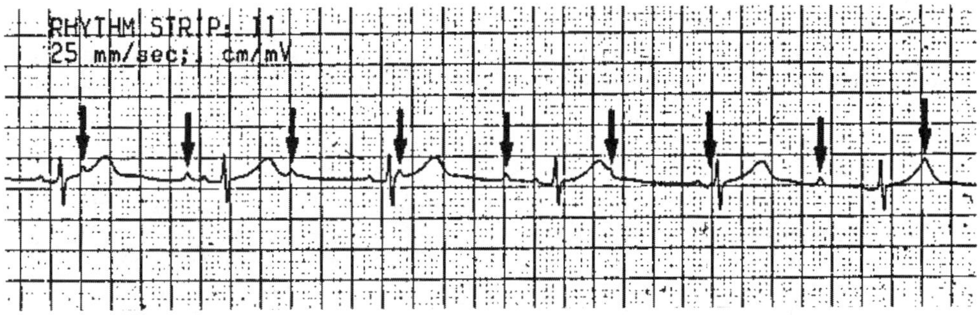

Figure 27–2 ● ● ● ● ● ●
Rhythm strip after cardiac transplant. *Arrows* indicate the recipient's native (but unconducted) P waves.

mixed metabolic and respiratory alkalosis resulting from induced hyperventilation and diuresis. Therapy during this stage is directed toward fluid restriction (to about 80–100 mL/kg/day), induced diuresis, and mechanical-assisted ventilation. Patients are maintained on low-dose inotropic support therapy consisting of dopamine and isoproterenol. Pulmonary vasodilators, such as tolazoline and PGE_1, are not routinely used unless pulmonary hypertension is a significant problem. An antibiotic, usually cefazolin, is used while central lines are in place. Cyclosporine, started before transplantation, is continued; and azathioprine (3 mg/kg) is added on the first post-transplant day, and intravenous methylprednisolone (25 mg/kg/dose) is given every 12 hours for a total of four doses. In selected cases, immunoglobulin, 400 mg/kg, is started on the third day and given every other day for a total of three doses.

The second stage, between the second and the fourth postoperative days, is characterized by increased diuresis, decreased edema, and increased activity including spontaneous respirations. The chest x-ray shows clearing of lung fluid. Atelectasis, especially of the right upper lobe, may be encountered and is managed with aggressive chest physiotherapy. Fluid restriction continues, and diuretics are used to maintain the patient's weight at or around the preoperative "dry weight." Inotropic drugs are gradually withdrawn. Ventilatory support is progressively decreased, and the infant is extubated. Enteral feedings are introduced and individualized according to each patient's clinical condition. Intolerance to feedings may be present during the early post-transplantation stages, but this improves with time. Total parenteral nutrition is not routinely used but may be specifically indicated for the occasional infant.

The third stage begins on about the fifth day after transplantation. By this time, most of the patients have been extubated and require little or no oxygen supplementation; however, diuretics may still be necessary. Feedings are advanced as tolerated; breastfeeding is encouraged.

HEART-LUNG AND LUNG TRANSPLANTATION

The Registry of the International Society for Heart and Lung Transplantation (1991) has received data on more than 1500 lung transplants from a total of 83 centers worldwide, including 1025 combined heart-lung procedures from 67 centers, 447 single lung procedures from 54 centers, and 120 double lung procedures from 25 centers. More than 90% of all lung transplant procedures have occurred since 1985. The number of heart-lung procedures has declined, most likely related to both the limitations in donor availability and the rapid expansion in both single and double lung transplantation during the past 2 years. A bilateral lung transplant is preferred over heart-lung transplant for persons with adequate cardiac function who require removal of all diseased lung tissue (Cooper, 1984). Single lung transplantation offers a therapeutic option for patients with pulmonary hypertension and adequate cardiac reserve.

Of the combined heart-lung procedures, the major indications have been primary pulmonary hypertension, pulmonary vascular obstructive disease (Eisenmenger's syndrome), or other congenital heart diseases. Of the double lung procedures, cystic fibrosis has been the major indication; whereas in the single lung procedures, primary pulmonary hypertension, pulmonary fibrosis, and emphysema each account for one third of recipients.

The operative mortality (<30 days) associated with lung transplantation is approximately 18%. In contrast with heart transplantation, early mortality in lung transplantation has not been higher in the pediatric age group, but fewer children under 2 years of age have had lung transplantation.

Causes of death in lung recipients are similar for all forms of lung transplantation. As in heart transplantation, intraoperative technical complications (including primary graft failure and hemorrhage) and cardiac complications account for about one third of all deaths. Infections have been reported in an additional one third of deaths, higher than in heart recipients. Rejection has been reported in 19% of deaths in lung recipients.

Survival in lung recipients has been lower than that in heart recipients. Currently, little difference in survival rate is apparent between the specific types of lung transplant procedures. One-year actuarial survival is 59% for heart-lung, 67% for single lung, and 57% for double lung transplantation. The 5-year actuarial survival for heart-lung transplantation has been 41%.

The increased success of lung transplantation and

the donor shortage (only 1 in 20 donors has suitable lungs for transplantation) have prompted some surgeons to look to living-related segmental lung donors. Regarding the donor shortage, it is important to recognize that procurement of the cadaveric lung allograft does not preclude the use of the heart for standard orthotopic heart transplantation. Removal of the heart-lung bloc is performed first, and removal of the heart at the midatrial level can be accomplished with adequate atrial and pulmonary venous cuffs (Baldwin, 1988). Donors deemed unsuitable for heart-lung transplantation on the basis of unilateral lung pathology, including trauma, atelectasis, and even pneumonia, may be suitable for single lung and orthotopic heart graft procurement. Furthermore, selected donors with excessive pressor requirements, cardiac contusions, or arrhythmias must be viewed as potential double lung or single lung donors.

Transplant Procedure

Transplant techniques have been refined over the past 20 years. In the past, bronchial anastomosis disruption was an early cause of death. Use of steroids impeded vascular supply to the transplanted donor bronchus, leading to bronchial air leaks, bleeding, stenosis, mucosal necrosis with aspiration pneumonia, and infection (Veith, 1983). Consequently, steroid has been reduced and cyclosporine was added to the immunosuppressive regimen, as it was found not to inhibit healing by altering the blood supply. A surgical omental wrap has been found to provide bronchial anastomosis increased vascularization and stability (Cooper, 1984). Currently, any available tissue in the chest (for example, thymus) is used to separate the pulmonary artery and bronchial anastomoses.

Briefly, the operative procedure entails removing the heart and lungs, or isolated lung(s), preserving both the phrenic and recurrent laryngeal nerves. The trachea is divided one ring above the carina. The donor heart and lungs are prepared and removed en bloc after core cooling and administration of cardioplegia to the heart. Reimplantation of the heart-lung graft is accomplished by sequential anastomoses of the trachea, followed by the aorta and then the right atrium.

In a single lung transplant, the recipient undergoes a thoracotomy on the side of implantation with usually at least one rib resection, often the sixth rib. Choice of which lung to transplant will be affected by previous surgery, such as lobectomy (the opposite lung is then chosen for transplant because no scar tissue is present), the size of the donor (if a relatively large lung is to be transplanted, the left side is preferred because the left hemidiaphragm is easier to mobilize downwards to accommodate the lung tissue), and lung condition (if one side is damaged more than another, the worse lung is replaced).

Clamping the recipient's pulmonary artery is initially attempted to determine if the patient can toler-

ate the implantation without the use of extracorporeal membrane oxygenation (ECMO) or lung bypass. This avoids the potential complication of platelet destruction and risks of infection through cannulation sites. Once oxygenation methods have been established, the recipient's organ is removed in sections to cauterize any bleeding and to preserve essential nerves (vagus and phrenic). The donor organ is placed through the thoracotomy, and three major anastomoses are completed. First, the bronchial anastomosis is completed. Second, the two major pulmonary veins from the one lung of the donor are attached to the recipient's left atrium. Lastly, the pulmonary artery is anastomosed. This anastomosis must be able to accommodate changes in right ventricular output, although it will be a low-flow artery. The recipient and donor pulmonary arteries are spread, and an anastomosis is performed with very small "bites" through all the layers of the vessel. An extra piece of pericardium may also be wrapped on this vessel for support (Veith, 1983).

In a bilateral lung transplant a clamshell incision is used to provide full exposure of the operative field (Fig. 27–3). Patients over 20 kg are intubated with a double-lumen endotracheal tube (a blocker is used in patients under 20 kg) to allow for unilateral lung ventilation. A pulmonary artery (PA) catheter is placed to provide continuous assessment of pulmonary artery pressures and cardiac output. After cannulation of the PA, right ventricular tolerance of both left and right PA clamping is assessed, as well identification of the "best lung" by sequential ventilation and assessment of ABGs. If there is any question of right ventricular dysfunction, cardiopulmonary bypass is used to support the patient through the transplant. If the patient is able to tolerate unilateral lung ventilation and pulmonary artery clamping, then similar to single lung transplant, each lung is sequentially implanted.

Postoperative Care

Table 27–7 outlines critical care management of the lung transplant patient in the immediate postop-

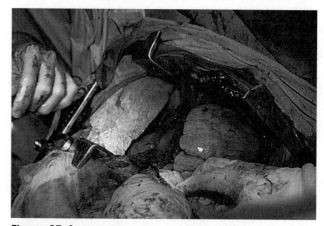

Figure 27–3 ● ● ● ● ● ●

The clamshell incision for bilateral lung transplantation.

Table 27–7. MANAGEMENT PLAN: POSTOPERATIVE LUNG TRANSPLANT

Actual Problems

#1 Problem: Impaired Gas Exchange RT "reimplantation response" as evidenced by pulmonary edema occurring secondary to lymphatic interruption, cold injury, and ischemia
Need: To reduce or eliminate hypoxemia and hypercapnia
Outcome Criteria: Normal ABGs
Process Criteria:
1. Maintain hemodynamic stability while minimizing fluid overload and pulmonary edema
2. Strict I&O
3. Maintain negative fluid balance: consider diuretics & ultrafiltration
Individualized:
Parameters: PaO_2 _____ mmHg (100–150) PvO_2 _____ mmHg
SaO_2 _____ % SvO_2 _____ %
$PaCO_2$ _____ mmHg (35–40)   _____ Maintenance fluids (3/4)
MAP _____ mmHg
UO _____ mL/hr

#2 Problem: V/Q Mismatch
Need: To optimize V/Q matching
Outcome Criteria: Normal ABGs
Process Criteria:
1. Correlate A/VBGs to "best" position
2. Assess pulmonary perfusion by monitoring $ETCO_2$
3. *Isolated transplant:* (Usually preferential V/Q to denervated transplanted lung.) Position patient so that perfusion to transplanted lung is enhanced—operative side down; position patient so that ventilation to transplanted lung is enhanced (position variable—compliance dependent)—operative side _____
3. *Bilateral transplant:* Place on rotating bed: begin with 30° turns every hour. Progress to 90° turns every hour as tolerated
4. *Preferential Ventilation:* If unilateral pulmonary edema present, position affected side down to optimize ABGs. After stabilization, gradually start to turn on a more equal basis
Double-lumen Roche ETT: _____ ; _____ at lip line
Individualized:
PEEP: _____ cm/H_2O
Turning schedule:
Currently on _____° turns per hour

#3 Problem: Ineffective Airway Clearance & Breathing Pattern RT denervated transplanted lung, loss of cough reflex, and slowing of mucociliary clearance & sedation
Need: Maintain adequate pulmonary clearance to prevent atelectasis and pneumonia
Outcome Criteria: Clear airways & improved breathing pattern
Process Criteria:
1. After assessing for an adequate level of analgesia, aggressive pulmonary care every 2 hours except during planned periods of rest. *Aggressive* pulmonary care to include CPT & vibration to *all* involved lobes. Instill NS, provide an inspiratory hold, and suction (ABOVE ANASTOMOSIS SITE) after each position change
2. Consider bronchodilator treatments
3. Coach patient to cough
4. Use BP, HR, SaO_2 to assess tolerance to pulmonary care
5. Use CXR, breath sounds, and sputum characteristics to guide pulmonary care (expect clear sputum)
6. May increase FiO_2 to accomplish pulmonary care regimen
7. Assist with flexible bronchoscopy
8. Use incentive spirometer after extubation (both inspiration & expiration)
9. Daily CXR and sputum culture/Gram stain
10. Observe for high fevers, hypoxemia, increased WBCs, and increased neutrophils in sputum/positive sputum cultures. Assess CXR findings that are consistent with pneumonia
Individualized:
Inspiratory hold at ___ cm/H_2O
Depth of suctioning not to exceed ___ cm
May increase FiO_2 ___ % over baseline
Modify care as indicated by MAP _____ , HR _____ , SaO_2 >90%

#4 Problem: RV Dysfunction related to pulmonary hypertension
Need: To optimize oxygen delivery
Outcome Criteria: Adequate cardiac output
Process Criteria:
1. Monitor RV ejection fraction
2. Monitor hemodynamic profile
3. Monitor oxygenation profile
Individualized;
Parameters: PA mean _____ mmHg (20–25)

Table continued on following page

Table 27-7. MANAGEMENT PLAN: POSTOPERATIVE LUNG TRANSPLANT *Continued*

#5 Problem: Alterations in Hemostasis RT perioperative blood product replacement &/or cardiopulmonary bypass
Need: Prevent hemorrhage
Outcome Criteria: No hemorrhage
Process Criteria:
1. Insitute care precautions
2. Monitor hematologic status
3. Keep Hct 35–40
4. Administer blood components or assist with phlebotomy as indicated
Individualized:
    Maximal total blood loss per hour: _____ mL/kg

#6 Problem: Alteration in Nutrition
Need: Provide adequate nutrition for physiologic stability
Outcome Criteria: Need is _____ kcal/day; CHO intake = _____ /day
Process Criteria:
1. Until paralytic gastric ileus resolved, NGT
2. Consult with nutritional support service
3. Maintain TPN and IL; consider CHO to decrease CO_2 production
4. Consider early NGT feeds
5. In CF patients consider Peptamen (cut pancrease in ½), Reabilan, & Colace
Individualized:

#7 Problem: Alteration in Comfort
Need: Maintain comfort
Outcome Criteria: patient says s/he is comfortable
Process Criteria:
1. Maintain epidural anesthesia until chest tubes DCed
2. Supplement with fentanyl or Ativan, midazepam, and chloral hydrate as needed
3. Consider PCA
4. Support parents' ability to comfort child
Individualized:

#8 Problem: Sleep Pattern Disturbance
Need: Provide adequate rest to promote physiologic stability
Outcome Criteria: Patient says s/he is not tired
Process Criteria:
1. Provide a protective environment with day/night cycling
Individualized:
    Daily scheduled rest periods are: _____

Potential Problems

#9 Problem: Potential for airway necrosis, dehiscence, and/or stenosis
Need: Maintain an intact tracheal anastomosis site
Outcome Criteria: Intact tracheal anastomosis site
Process Criteria:
1. Rapidly manage postoperative hypotension and hypoxemia
2. Observe for mediastinal abscess, mediastinitis, and air leaks
3. Assist with flexible bronchoscopy, BAL, & biopsy
4. Consider the possibility of associated infection &/or rejection
Individualized:

#10 Problem: Potential for Infection RT immunosuppression
Need: Prevent infection
Outcome Criteria: No infection
Process Criteria:
1. Isolation room, keeping doors closed, & positive room pressure
2. Strictly enforce infection control standards
3. Screen for opportunistic infections
4. Assist ORL in clearing sinuses
5. Wound care every shift after dressing discontinued
Individualized:

#11 Problem: Potential for Nephro/Hepatotoxicity RT cyclosporine
Need: Rapidly detect and manage side effects
Outcome Criteria: To minimize the side effects of cyclosporine
Process Criteria:
1. Monitor liver enzymes, BUN, and creatinine
2. Monitor blood pressure
3. Assess cyclosporine blood levels (nl 200–300 ng/dL).
Individualized:

Table 27–7. MANAGEMENT PLAN: POSTOPERATIVE LUNG TRANSPLANT *Continued*

#12 Problem: Potential for Organ Rejection
Need: Prevent organ rejection (peaks at 5–9 days then after 11 days)
Outcome Criteria: To rapidly detect and manage early signs of rejection
Process Criteria:
1. Observe for persistent low-grade fever and hypoxemia
2. Assess CXR and breath sounds for pleural effusion
3. Assess for an increase in chest tube or pleural drainage
4. Monitor sputum for increased lymphocytes
5. Monitor exercise tolerance; observe for earlier desaturations with exercise
6. Monitor for increased platelet counts within 72 hours
Individualized: Isolated lung Tx: Position operative side down to improve pulmonary perfusion

#13 Problem: Potential for Injury RT Immobilization
Need: Prevent iatrogenic injury
Outcome Criteria: No problems RT immobilization will occur
Process Criteria:
1. Consider TEDs and/or compression boots
2. Consider low-dose heparin therapy
3. Ambulate after extubation
Individualized:

See also Practice Guideline:
  #14 Problem: Impaired coping: Individual
  #15 Problem: Impaired coping: Parent/Family

Lab Schedule:
Q2°: ABGs, chem strip
Q6°: Lytes, BUN, BS, ICal, Spun Hct
Q12°: CBC with Diff (Imuran), Cr, platelets, PT, PTT, D-dimer
Q24°: Cyclosporine level, CXR, sputum culture/Gram stain
Q48°: Clot to blood bank

From the Multidisciplinary ICU, Children's Hospital, Boston, Boston, MA.

erative period. Nursing responsibilities include a complete physical assessment, including hemodynamic assessment. A pulmonary artery catheter is routinely used to monitor right ventricular performance and pulmonary artery pressures. Cardiac output is assessed noninvasively by the quality of peripheral pulses, capillary refill, skin temperature and color, and urinary output. Serum electrolyte levels, ABGs and chest tube drainage are documented. Careful evaluation of heart and respiratory sounds is necessary. A negative fluid balance is maintained for the first 2 weeks to decrease interstitial edema (Jamieson, 1986). Renal function is monitored carefully, with adjustments of cyclosporine or infusion of low-dose dopamine to augment renal perfusion.

Of particular interest in the postoperative lung transplant patient is the reimplantation response. This is defined as the morphologic, radiologic, and functional changes that occur in a transplanted lung in the early postoperative period as the result of surgical trauma, ischemia, denervation, lymphatic interruption, and other injurious processes (exclusive of rejection) that are unavoidable aspects of the transplant operation (Montefusco, 1989). Functionally, the reimplantation response produces a temporary impairment of the ventilation-perfusion ratio in the transplanted lung. There may also be some transient impairment of blood flow. The patient may present with symptoms of adult respiratory distress syndrome (ARDS), manifested as defects in pulmonary gas exchange, compliance, and vascular resistance, as well as an inability of the disrupted lym-

phatic system to clear interstitial fluid. Subjectively, the patient becomes very anxious and complains of shortness of breath. Examination of the patient reveals diffuse rales, and chest x-ray demonstrates pulmonary edema. Treatment includes vigorous diuresis, chest physiotherapy, and reintubation if necessary. Differential diagnoses include rejection, infection, and reimplantation response. Distinguishing among these diagnoses, though often difficult, is essential to formulating a treatment and nursing care plan. The incidence and severity of the reimplantation response seem to be decreasing, possibly due to better preservation techniques (Borkon, 1988).

Assessing for clinical signs of infection is a primary nursing function. A small increase in temperature can indicate infection. Fevers greater than 38°C require prompt and aggressive workup. Persistent or productive cough with or without fever, or decrease in forced expiratory volume in 1 second (FEV_1), requires further investigation by chest x-ray and, frequently, bronchoscopy.

CMV and *Pneumocystis carinii* are common opportunistic infections in heart-lung or lung transplant recipients. The risks of infection by any organism are directly related to potency and duration of immunosuppression, donor selection, operating room technique, and postoperative exposure to pathogens.

Monitoring for rejection includes physical assessment, chest x-ray, simple pulmonary function testing, and bronchoscopy with biopsy and, in some centers, bronchoalveolar lavage. Once infection has been ruled out, the presence of fever, respiratory insufficiency, and a diffuse pulmonary infiltrate after the first postoperative week should be regarded as lung rejection.

LIVER TRANSPLANTATION

Liver transplantation for children with end-stage liver disease is currently available in over 76 centers worldwide. Approximately 350 children each year undergo liver transplantation (Whitington, 1990). Since 1983, liver transplantation has been recognized as a nonexperimental treatment option for children with end-stage liver disease. In the pre-cyclosporine era, 5-year survival statistics for children treated with azathioprine were a dismal 30% (Starzl et al., 1987). With advances in preservation methods, refined surgical techniques, and improved immunosuppression protocols, centers are reporting 85% to 90% 1-year survival rates (Gordon, 1991; Whitington, 1990).

Indications for pediatric liver transplantation include biliary atresia, intrahepatic cholestasis, hepatitis, metabolic diseases, and hepatic tumors (see Table 27–2). Biliary atresia is the most common indication for liver transplantation in the child (over 50% of the cases per center). Liver and cluster transplantation are being increasingly utilized for children with primary liver tumors (hepatoma and hepatoblastoma).

A current medical debate exists over the use of the portoenterostomy (Kasai procedure) prior to transplantation for children with biliary atresia (Shaw et al., 1988a; Tzakis & Starzl, 1992; Wood et al., 1990). Tzakis and Starzl contend that even with the relief of jaundice in the postoperative period following the Kasai procedure, cirrhosis occurs in most patients. The Kasai procedure with associated surgical scarring complicates the transplant procedure.

In January 1991, the UNOS system for classifying liver transplant candidates was revised (UNOS, 1991). Within the present system, patients are grouped within a four-tier system. Status one patients are at home with stable liver function. Status two patients require continuous medical care and are at home or near a transplant center. Status three patients are continuously hospitalized because of their medical condition. Status four patients are ICU-bound and are expected to live less than 7 days. In addition, the patient must be experiencing at least one of the following: mechanical ventilation, vasopressors for blood pressure support, prothrombin time >25 seconds, primary nonfunction post transplant, grade III or IV encephalopathy, dialysis, or experiencing uncontrollable variceal bleeding. Status four patients are allowed to remain at this status for 14 days. After 14 days, these patients revert to a status three listing or an extension can be requested.

Due to the shortage of pediatric organs, deviations from the standard orthotopic liver transplantation procedure have been developed and are currently being refined. These procedures include reduced-sized liver transplantation (RSLT), split-liver transplantation (SLT), and living-related liver trans-

plantation (LRLT). The use of University of Wisconsin (UW) solution (Viaspan) has lengthened acceptable ischemic times up to 16 to 18 hours, providing recovering surgical teams additional time required to prepare recovered organs for RSLT and SLT procedures (Furukawa et al., 1991). All of these procedures are orthotopic procedures, which means replacement of the native liver with the allograft. Back table preparation of the newly recovered liver includes identifying vessels, reducing graft size, and sending tissue for pathology examination of graft quality prior to the recipient operation.

Transplant Procedure

The standard orthotopic liver transplant procedure involves three phases: preanhepatic, anhepatic, and postanhepatic. After the child has been anesthetized and positioned, a bilateral subcostal incision with xiphoid extension and removal of the xiphoid process is performed. The suprahepatic inferior vena cava (IVC), the infrahepatic IVC, the portal vein, and the hepatic artery are dissected and then clamped, after which the native liver is removed. This begins the anhepatic phase which ends when the donor liver is reperfused. For children over 15 kg, venovenous bypass is utilized during the anhepatic phase (Tzakis & Starzl, 1992). Venovenous bypass consists of extracorporeal circulation whereby blood from the IVC and portal vein is returned to the superior vena cava via the left axillary vein. Heparin-bonded shunts inserted into the left common femoral vein and the left common axillary vein allow pump-assisted return of systemic blood from the lower part of the body back to the heart. An additional shunt is placed in the portal vein to allow for decompression of the portal system. In addition to the patient's preexisting coagulopathies, appropriate tubing size and regulation of pump flow provide protection from shunt clotting (Tzakis & Starzl, 1992).

During the anhepatic phase, four vascular anastomoses are completed using polypropylene suture in a running technique: (1) suprahepatic IVC anastomoses, (2) infrahepatic IVC anastomoses, (3) portal vein, and (4) hepatic artery. After completion of the infrahepatic IVC anastomosis, the donor liver is flushed with cold lactated Ringer's solution to remove air and University of Wisconsin (UW) solution. Once the portal vein anastomosis is completed, portal venous blood flow is reestablished to the graft. At this time, venovenous bypass is discontinued. A color change in the allograft can be observed. Patchy areas of poorly perfused parenchyma may persist until the hepatic artery anastomosis is completed. Hemostasis is achieved during this operative phase by suture ligation and cautery.

Biliary reconstruction in pediatric recipients is typically performed with a Roux-en-Y limb of intestine (choledochojejunostomy), as the patient's native bile duct is absent in the most common pediatric indication for surgery, biliary atresia. In more than 90%

of pediatric cases, the Roux technique is required (Tzakis & Starzl, 1992). The bile duct may be reconstructed by anastomosing the native bile duct to the donor bile duct over a T tube (choledochocholedochostomy). Vascular anomalies may require complex arterial reconstructions or interposition grafts to the aorta. Jackson-Pratt drains are placed under the diaphragm, and the incision is then closed.

Reduced-size liver transplants are performed in the pediatric patient, as there is a limited supply of appropriate size organs. Organs that are 0.8 to 10 times the size of the recipient's liver can be utilized (Woodle et al., 1990). Whitington (1990) recommends the following donor to recipient ratios: right lobe grafts 1.5–3:1, the left lobe graft 2–4:1, and the left lateral lobe graft 3–10:1. The procedure requires two surgical teams—one to perform the graft reduction, and one to perform the recipient hepatectomy. Preparation of the graft involves dissection of the bile duct system, followed by the hepatic artery, portal vein, and hepatic veins. The recipient procedure parallels standard orthotopic liver transplantation, except in situations where there is significant disproportion in donor organ size, in which case the recipient IVC is preserved and the donor liver is placed in a "piggyback" position with only one caval anastomosis to the recipient hepatic veins (Tzakis & Starzl, 1992).

The split-liver technique utilizes one donor organ for two recipients. The smaller recipient receives the left lateral or left lobe, and the larger recipient the right lobe. The donor liver graft is prepared in the recipient operating room, where hepatic resection is performed through the principal fissure between the right and left lobes. The right lobe graft is identical to that prepared for a reduced-sized graft, retaining the portal vein and hepatic artery. The left lobe graft usually requires vascular interposition grafts (Whitington, 1990).

Living-related transplantation has evolved from the split-liver transplant procedure. The donor (usually a parent) undergoes a left hepatectomy, which is prepared as in split-liver transplantation. Implantation of the graft is similar to the split-liver procedure. Current experience with the procedure has required hepatic artery and portal vein grafts (Broelsch et al., 1990).

Postoperative Care

A preliminary nursing assessment is completed prior to admitting the patient to the PICU. This assessment includes an evaluation of preexisting disease factors and significant psychosocial information. Tzakis and Starzl (1992) reported improved transplant outcomes with better patient condition at the time of transplant. According to Williams and Rzucidlo (1985), transplant candidates fall into one of two disease categories. These categories are (1) those in whom the disease is lethal with a clearly defined downhill course; and (2) those in whom the disease has a less well-defined history, with signs of progressive liver deterioration. At the time of transplant, the child may have numerous physical signs and symptoms. These include bleeding, severe ascites, pruritus, hepatorenal syndrome, malnutrition, and hepatic encephalopathy. Knowledge of the child's developmental status and family dynamics at the time of transplant will assist with meeting identified psychosocial needs.

Admitting the postoperative liver transplant patient to the PICU employs the same principles as admitting a patient after a major abdominal surgical procedure. As with any patient, universal precautions for body fluids are maintained. Isolation procedures are not required. Standard PICU monitoring is used. A central line is used to continuously monitor central venous pressure (CVP); pulmonary artery catheters are infrequently inserted.

"Liver ABCs" are completed first. "A" is for aeration. As with any patient, airway management is the first priority. All patients will return to the PICU intubated and on a ventilator. "B" is for blood pressure. A cuff blood pressure check is a priority; hypertension or hypotension is a common postoperative assessment finding. "C" is for coagulopathies. All drains and incision sites are carefully assessed for bleeding. The patient's prothrombin time (PT), partial thromboplastin time (PTT), and platelet counts are assessed at admission.

Coagulopathies and technical aspects of liver transplantation can precipitate the need for massive intraoperative transfusions. The lengthy 12- to 14-hour operation, and/or the use of massive volume exchange, and prolonged bowel exposure can predispose the patient to hypothermia. Normothermia can be achieved with heating lamps or a warming blanket.

After the "liver ABCs," a quick system check is performed. The incision and Jackson-Pratt drainage are assessed. The incision is often covered with an occlusive dressing. The dressing should be dry and intact. At this time, Jackson-Pratt drainage will appear bloody. Laboratory tests are drawn expediently. Routine lab tests include hematology studies, a coagulation profile, electrolytes, liver function tests, and an ABG. A chest x-ray is obtained.

The nurse receives a complete report from anesthesia. The report includes organ ischemic time, the length of surgery, current laboratory values, and a summary of the operative course including complications. The intraoperative use of venovenous bypass is included in the operative report. If a reduction hepatectomy was performed, assessment for signs of increased bleeding, biliary fistulas, and infection from the raw surface is appropriate, as the incidence of these complications is greater with reduced-sized grafts (Tzakis & Starzl, 1992). If a living-related transplant is performed, the nurse should receive information about the donor's condition.

Report on the visible condition of the liver is useful information. The allograft should change from a pale tan color to a reddish-brown after anastomoses are complete. After the arterial grafts are anastomosed, bile production should occur. If hyperbilirubinemia exists preoperatively, the urine appears dark orange in the early postoperative period. The presence of these signs are excellent early prognostic indicators of graft function.

The patient's fluid status is reviewed. Because of third-space loss, the need for intraoperative fluid resuscitation is common. Several blood volume replacements may be administered. Within 48 hours after admission to the PICU, the patient should diurese.

Intraoperative medications are reviewed. The transplant operation is lengthy (8–24 hours), and often there are changes in anesthesia personnel. During report, immunosuppressive medications and doses are double-checked by the nurse and operating room personnel.

Related medical problems and associated nursing interventions are dependent on allograft function. With a well-functioning graft, the patient may be normotensive or hypertensive. Laboratory values may reveal normoglycemia and resolving hypokalemia, hypocalcemia, and coagulopathies. The child should wake up 4 to 6 hours after admission to the PICU.

Signs of poor graft function may include hypotension, hyperkalemia, hypoglycemia, coagulopathies, and decreased level of consciousness. Poor initial function may be associated with a phenomenon called primary graft dysfunction from ischemia-reperfusion injury in the donor organ during the preservation period. Fishbein and Whitington (1990) reported that in 10% of these cases, there is an urgent need for retransplantation.

Ineffective Airway Clearance and Breathing Patterns, Impaired Gas Exchange

The liver-lung relationship has been described (Krowka & Cortese, 1985, 1989). Patients with fulminant and chronic hepatic failure may manifest signs of the failing liver in the lungs. The pulmonary effects of chronic liver disease are more prevalent in the adult population; however, such complications have been reported in children (Mews et al., 1990). Pleural effusions and arteriovenous collateral vessels with resultant intrapulmonary shunting and ventilation-perfusion mismatches are reported complications.

Ineffective airway clearance is related to a long abdominal procedure, large transverse abdominal incision, and postoperative pain. Fifty percent of the patients are extubated by the end of the second postoperative day (Thompson, 1987). However, 40% of the children will experience collapse of the right upper and right middle lobes of the lung. Phrenic nerve paresis due to clamping of the upper vena cava and right mainstem bronchus intubation contribute to lobar collapse (Shaw et al., 1988b).

Pulmonary assessment includes frequent auscultation of breath sounds, interpretation of arterial blood gases, and monitoring of chest x-rays. The child's

coagulopathy status determines the appropriateness of chest physiotherapy. Gentle chest physiotherapy is performed if coagulopathies persist. Once hemostasis is achieved, aggressive chest physiotherapy is initiated.

Ineffective breathing patterns may be related to diaphragm paralysis and abdominal distension secondary to ascites, large donor liver, and/or bleeding. The potential for diaphragmatic paralysis exists if the right phrenic nerve is injured during surgery. An elevated diaphragm on chest x-ray and decreased expansion of the right lower lobe with spontaneous respiration may indicate phrenic nerve damage. Generally, if the child is unable to tolerate extubation twice, an ultrasound examination is used to confirm the suspected diagnosis.

Persistent ascites may also limit tidal volume and impair ventilation. As well, a large donor liver may reduce intrathoracic space and tidal volume. The optimal liver size is within 20% of the patient's weight (Shaw et al., 1988b). Emergent indications for liver transplantation may necessitate widening the candidate's weight range with an increased mismatch in donor to recipient size. Inability to close the abdominal incision may further impair the patient's respiratory effort, as supportive musculature and associated resistance will not assist the patient's ventilatory efforts.

Impaired gas exchange may be related to right pleural effusion and intrapulmonary shunting. Right-sided pleural effusion is a common postoperative finding. Shaw (1989) reported that preoperative ascites promoted rapid fluid accumulation postoperatively. The sympathetic response observed with acute rejection may increase ascites accumulation (Whitington, 1990). Treatment measures include the use of diuretics, albumin administration with diuretics, and drainage of the accumulated pleural fluid by thoracentesis or insertion of a pigtail catheter in the pleural space.

Pulmonary infection is common. Viral organisms include CMV, respiratory syncytial virus, adenovirus, herpes simplex, and herpes zoster. Pulmonary *Aspergillus* and systemic candidiasis may contribute to pulmonary dysfunction (Thompson, 1987).

Alterations in Tissue Perfusion

Park et al. (1985) described the hemodynamic profile of 73 children with chronic liver disease. Eighty-two percent of the children had high cardiac output with a cardiac index greater than 4 L/min/M². In four of the children, there was evidence of intrapulmonary and arteriovenous shunting. After transplant, cardiac index decreased by a mean of 35% ($P < .001$). The authors concluded that transplantation improved chronic hemodynamic abnormalities (hyperdynamic state) in children with chronic liver disease.

Greater than 70% of liver transplant recipients experience hypertension, with approximately 10% of these patients requiring long-term antihypertensive medications (Whitington, 1990). Mean arterial blood pressure in excess of 90 mmHg or systolic blood pressure greater than 140 mmHg requires treatment. Severe hypertension is most problematic within the first postoperative week (Thompson, 1987).

There are several hypotheses regarding the etiology of hypertension in liver transplant patients. These include alterations in renin levels and steroid and cyclosporine administration. Whitington (1990) contends the etiology is unknown; however, cyclosporine and sodium overload are contributing factors. Hypertension may be associated with good graft function. Vigilant nursing assessment of blood pressure will ensure prompt treatment and minimize associated side effects, which include seizures, subarachnoid hemorrhage, intraparenchymal hemorrhage, and coma (Thompson, 1987).

Pharmacologic treatment of hypertension is institution-specific. Initially, the use of a nitroprusside infusion may be necessary. Intravenous and oral drug therapy may include use of renin-angiotensin inhibitors, peripheral vasodilators, beta-blockers, and alpha-adrenergic blockers. Commonly prescribed antihypertensives include nifedipine (Procardia), hydralazine (Apresoline), captopril (Capoten), and labetalol (Normodyne). Combination therapy is frequently prescribed.

Hypotension is infrequently seen and is usually associated with complications, for example, hemorrhage, graft failure, or sepsis. With graft dysfunction, coagulopathies will persist despite ongoing administration of fresh-frozen plasma, platelets, and crystalloids. Hypotension in the presence of primary graft dysfunction is associated with alterations in blood chemistries. Hypotension after the first 72 hours may be an indication of intra-abdominal sepsis (Thompson, 1987). Several factors are evaluated if hypotension persists. Every 4 hours, hematology laboratory tests, coagulation profile, and serum pH are monitored.

Treatment measures are initiated in the immediate postoperative period to prevent hepatic artery thrombosis (HAT). The patient may be maintained on intravenous dextran 40 (Gentran 40), subcutaneous heparin, oral aspirin, and dipyridamole (Persantine). Dextran 40 draws water from the extravascular space, decreasing blood viscosity and platelet adhesiveness. Rapid corrections of coagulopathies are avoided. The patient's hematocrit is maintained at 30% to minimize the incidence of HAT. Within 12 hours after transplantation, daily ultrasound examinations are initiated to evaluate vessel patency.

Abdominal drainage and incisional oozing are carefully assessed. The abdominal girth is assessed as frequently as every hour. If drainage from the Jackson-Pratt is excessive, a hematocrit of the drainage is obtained. Drainage of greater than 80 mL/kg/hour usually indicates surgical bleeding (Thompson, 1987).

Intra-abdominal bleeding and increased abdominal girth impede venous return and may impair effective ventilation and oxygenation. If the patient is extubated, mechanical ventilation is reestablished. Fluid replacement is ongoing. Often vasopressor therapy is prescribed to maintain an acceptable blood pressure. If surgical bleeding is suspected, the child should return to the operating room for an exploratory laparotomy. When graft failure is suspected, the patient is relisted for a replacement graft. Fluid resuscitation may be ongoing until retransplantation occurs.

Metabolic/Nutritional Deficits

Common electrolyte derangements seen after transplant include hypocalcemia, hypokalemia, hypo/hyperglycemia, and hypomagnesemia. Electrolytes, calcium, and serum glucose are obtained every 6 hours. Hourly Dextrostix per the glucometer are obtained until normoglycemia is achieved.

Hypocalcemia occurs in approximately one half of patients. Causes of hypocalcemia include citrate intoxification from the large quantities of blood products administered, hypoproteinemia, liver membrane damage with subsequent shift of calcium from the extracellular to the intracellular space, and decreased ionized calcium due to metabolic or respiratory alkalosis (Thompson, 1987).

Shaw et al. (1988b) describe a "syndrome" of hypertension, metabolic alkalosis, hypernatremia, hypokalemia, and relative oliguria. Proposed causes include large citrate load, multiple doses of diuretics, and nasogastric suction. However, none of these adequately explains the "syndrome," as it is short lived. Preoperative respiratory alkalosis may be replaced by postoperative metabolic alkalosis due to the citrate load in the blood products, nasogastric drainage, fluid restriction, and diuretic therapy.

Hypokalemia or hyperkalemia may be present after surgery. Potassium is usually not added to intravenous fluids, due to the risks of renal failure and possible graft necrosis with a resultant increase in serum potassium.

Hypomagnesemia is common with end-stage renal disease and can be exacerbated in the early postoperative period. Magnesium-containing antacids, oral magnesium gluconate, and intravenous magnesium sulfate may be prescribed. Effects of magnesium on blood pressure may be direct or through the influences on the internal balance of potassium, sodium, and calcium (Dyckner & Wester, 1983). Hypophosphatemia may be observed. Increased phosphate needs of the allograft for the repletion of adenosine triphosphate may be the contributing factor.

Hypoglycemia or hyperglycemia may be present in the immediate postoperative period. Normal amounts of glucose with maintenance infusions of 5 to 7 mg/kg/min should achieve normoglycemia (Thompson, 1987).

A related problem is alteration in nutrition: less than body requirements. Total parenteral nutrition is usually administered within 24 hours postoperatively. Feedings are initiated as soon as postoperative ileus resolves. Malabsorption and diarrhea are common problems experienced postoperatively. Causes of infectious diarrhea include CMV, *Clostridium diffi-*

cile, and other enteric organisms. The malabsorption syndrome may be transient, with an unclear etiology. Hypothesized causes include manipulation of the bowel during surgery and immunosuppressive drugs.

Altered Skin Integrity

The patient is returned from the operating room with Jackson-Pratt drains in place (see Fig. 27–4). These drains are strategically placed to prevent and allow for early recognition of complications. The lateral drain on the right side of the patient is placed posteriorly in the right subdiaphragmatic space. This drain allows the dome of the right lobe to seal against the diaphragm. The second drain on the right is placed under the right hepatic lobe, leading up to the area of the bile duct anastomoses. This drain allows for the assessment of a bile leak. The third drain, on the patient's left side, is positioned in the posterior aspect of the left subdiaphragmatic space. Unusual bloody drainage could be observed in any of the Jackson-Pratt drains. Drainage is initially bloody. Drains are emptied every 2 hours. The hematocrit of the drain contents is checked if drainage is excessive.

The skin and visceral layers are generally closed. Normally, the abdominal dressing is removed after 24 hours and the incision left open to air to promote healing. If liver size or bowel edema precludes surgical closure, complex wound care is required. An enterostomal therapy consult can assist the bedside nurse and surgeons in providing optimal wound care. Dressing changes over draining wounds are required frequently and are accomplished with the use of Montgomery straps to limit patient discomfort associated with tape removal (see Chapter 17, Skin Integrity).

For the majority of pediatric patients, a Roux-en-Y biliary reconstruction is indicated; therefore, a T tube is not usually inserted. If present, T tube drainage is carefully assessed, with normal drainage appearing bilious. Absence of a color change in the drainage may be indicative of graft dysfunction. T tube drainage is emptied every 8 hours.

Altered Renal Function

Impairment in renal function is common postoperatively due to fluid shifts, persistent hypoproteinemia, diuretics, tense abdominal pressure affecting renal filtration pressure, and cyclosporine nephrotoxicity (Thompson, 1987). In the immediate postoperative period, fluids are restricted to 3/4 of maintenance.

Oliguria is reported in over 50% of liver transplant recipients on postoperative day 1 or 2 (Whitington, 1990). Management of the patient includes fluid restriction, diuretics, and low-dose dopamine. Shaw et al. (1988b) reported that oliguria may coincide with the second dose of cyclosporine and is usually associated with hypovolemia. Crystalloid replacement may be useful for ensuring adequate intravascular volume; however, rarely is urine output increased. Additional fluids are administered with caution, as fluid overload may precipitate edema and ascites and worsen hypertension.

Polyuria rarely occurs but may be seen in patients recovering from hepatorenal failure or acute tubular necrosis (Shaw, 1989). Hepatorenal syndrome is associated with liver failure and is usually irreversible (Munoz, 1989).

Drug and fluid management is adjusted for the liver transplant recipient with presumed renal dysfunction. Immunosuppressant drug levels are carefully monitored, with dosage adjusted accordingly. All potentially nephrotoxic pharmacologic agents are administered with caution.

Alterations in Comfort

After liver transplantation, the goal of pain management is to achieve a balance between comfort and ability to assess the patient's level of consciousness, as hepatic metabolism of pain medication may be impaired. The importance of evaluating mental status is crucial, as graft function is imperative for metabolizing narcotics. Small intravenous narcotic doses are preferable to the use of benzodiazopines or phenothiazines because, in an emergency, narcotic antagonists can be used to reverse the narcotics and permit evaluation of hepatic encephalopathy (Shaw, 1988b).

There are transplant center variations in narcotic dosing for pain management. In some centers, there is a general avoidance of the administration of narcotics and when they are used, they are prescribed in reduced doses. Shaw (1989) contends that once the liver demonstrates adequate functioning, with the patient awake and complaining of pain, narcotics can be administered safely. Sommerauer et al. (1988)

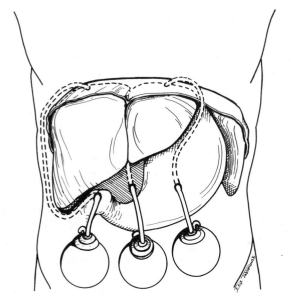

Figure 27–4 ● ● ● ● ● ●
Placement of Jackson-Pratt drains post orthotopic liver transplantation.

reported that associated hypertension was not related to pain. Patients treated with appropriate analgesia dosing (morphine infusions and narcotic boluses) were sedated without resolution of hypertension.

Potential Complications

Complications after liver transplantation are common. One complication often leads to a cascade of additional complications. Common complications in the early postoperative course include bleeding, infection, rejection, primary graft dysfunction, bile leaks, and hepatic artery thrombosis (HAT). Post-transplant lymphoproliferative disorder (PTLD) may be experienced early or late (weeks to months) following transplant.

Infection is the leading cause of death in the liver transplant recipient (Shaw, 1989). For the liver patient, infections frequently originate in the abdomen and are due to local ischemia, associated bleeding, and/or bowel contamination. Children with a failed Kasai procedure are prone to recurrent episodes of cholangitis (Green, 1991). As most children undergo Roux-en-Y choledochojejunostomy, intraoperative infectious complications include contamination of the bile ducts with yeast and bacteria (Green, 1991).

Infectious complications associated with HAT generally occur within the first 30 days after transplant (Green, 1991). HAT can precipitate areas of necrosed liver, abscesses, and bacteremia. Bile duct strictures with resultant cholangitis can occur following HAT. Technical difficulties may necessitate reexploration of the abdomen with associated increased incidence of fungal infection.

Bacterial and fungal sources are the most common infectious agents in the liver transplant recipient maintained on cyclosporine and prednisone; the rate of bacterial infection is 40% to 50%, whereas the rate of fungal infection is 63% (Green, 1991). CMV is the most important viral infection (Whitington, 1990). *Candida albicans* is the most common fungal infection in the pediatric liver transplant recipient (Green, 1991; Whitington, 1990). Adenovirus is the third most important infection.

According to Tzakis and Starzl (1992), the rate of biliary tract complication is 10% to 15%. Two percent to ten percent of the global mortality in reported series is related to biliary tract complications. The rate has decreased due to improved surgical techniques, the avoidance of gallbladder conduits, and cholecystenterostomy. Many children with biliary obstructions do not develop dilated ducts because of the relationship between biliary secretory pressure and the radius of the bile duct (Whitington, 1990). Characteristic laboratory values and histologic findings may preclude percutaneous cholangiogram. Depending on findings, an exploratory laparotomy may be performed to correct strictures on the visceral surface of the liver.

Further biliary complications include cholangitis and bile leaks. Hepatic abscesses can occur if biliary obstruction is not detected. Bile leaks are more prevalent with reduced-size grafts. HAT should be suspected in patients with biliary complications, as arterial blood is the principal blood supply to the bile duct graft.

In the patient with a T tube, the nurse may observe biliary sludge in the drainage. Sludge is a chalk-like substance composed of organic fibrous matrix from the sloughing of the bile duct lining (Traiger & Bohachick, 1983). Cholangitis and biliary tract obstruction can occur with severe biliary sloughing.

HAT occurs in 5% to 30% of pediatric patients. HAT can lead to graft failure if adequate collateral circulation is not established. HAT is suspected if liver function studies do not begin to decrease within the first 48 hours after transplantation. In one third of the cases, the patient may be asymptomatic (Tzakis & Starzl, 1992). Symptoms occur in three forms: fulminant hepatic failure with liver gangrene, biliary complications such as a bile leak or biliary stricture, or chronic bacteremia with visible intrahepatic abscesses.

Several causes of HAT are documented. Tzakis and Starzl (1992) report that HAT is usually caused by technical problems, with contributing nontechnical factors. A lower incidence of HAT is associated with transplantation of liver fragments due to the larger size hepatic artery.

Patients at risk due to technical difficulties or other factors are placed on a protocol to maintain and enhance blood flow through anastomoses. Subclinical anticoagulation is achieved with intravenous dextran, subcutaneous low-dose heparin, oral aspirin, and/or Persantine.

Post-transplant lymphoproliferative disorder (PTLD) occurs in 7% of liver transplant recipients. This complication is generally seen weeks to months postoperatively. The lymphomas are generally Epstein-Barr virus associated with B cell tumors. Patients may present with fever, atypical lymphocytosis, lymphadenopathy, and diarrhea. If the disease is organ-specific, local symptoms may provide the first signs of the disease. Definitive diagnosis may require an open biopsy of enlarged lymph nodes. Conventional cancer treatments for PTLD have not been successful in patients following transplantation. Successful treatment has included reducing or discontinuing immunosuppression. Mortality-associated PTLD for children greater than 7 years post transplant maintained on cyclosporine has risen to nearly 20% (Malatack et al., 1991). Children receiving FK-506 immunosuppression have developed PTLD as early as 3 months after transplant; no data are available for patients maintained on FK-506. Current treatment by lowering or discontinuing immunosuppression has been successful, with resultant tumor resolution and good graft function. Knowledge of PTLD is important, as patients may be diagnosed early in the postoperative course or return to the ICU if there is significant cerebral or pulmonary involvement.

LIVER/SMALL INTESTINE TRANSPLANTATION

Liver/small intestine transplants offer new hope for children with short gut syndrome. Promising outcomes have been achieved with replacement of the liver and small intestine in 23 children, isolated intestinal transplants in 7 children, and 7 multivisceral procedures at the University of Pittsburgh/Children's Hospital of Pittsburgh. Twenty-two children have survived, representing the world's most successful series of intestinal transplants.

The indications for small intestine transplantation are varied; however, for the majority of pediatric patients, the operation is indicated for short gut syndrome. Short gut syndrome is a disorder characterized by the loss of a significant portion of the intestine with resultant rapid intestinal transit, inadequate digestion, and malabsorption of nutrients (Schwartz & Maeda, 1985). Thus far, the majority of candidates have required liver/small intestine transplants due to the resultant cholestasis from long-term hyperalimentation use.

Each candidate is unique, and evaluation is tailored by the transplant team depending on the child's diagnosis. Evaluative testing includes D-xylose determination and an upper GI with a small bowel follow-through. Contraindications for small bowel transplant include metastatic disease or cardiac, pulmonary, renal, or neurologic impairment that may contribute to a poor surgical outcome and quality of life. Sepsis is a relative contraindication for any transplant candidate at the time of operation. Sepsis with multisystem organ failure is a relative contraindication for surgery. All of the small bowel/liver recipients in Pittsburgh have experienced complications of total parenteral nutrition, including line sepsis, associated cholestasis, and other related complications (Todo et al., 1992).

These candidates are listed according to current UNOS intestine criteria. Status 1 patients have liver dysfunction and line access problems as evidenced by no access through the subclavian, jugular, or femoral veins. Status 2 patients have no liver dysfunction and have line access available in standard sites. The candidate may be listed for an isolated intestinal graft, if cholestatic liver disease is not present. If the child needs a liver graft, the child is also listed with UNOS as a liver candidate. The ideal donor is of the same blood type and of the same size to 25% less in body weight of the recipient. HLA matching is random and not considered in recipient selection.

Tzakis et al. (1991) and Funovits et al. (1993) have detailed the intraoperative course. Prior to recovery of the donor's intestine, bowel decontamination is initiated. Bowel decontamination consists of Go-LYTELY and an antibiotic combination of polymyxin B (colistin), gentamicin/tobramycin, and Mycostatin (nystatin)/amphotericin B. Preoperatively, bowel decontamination is also initiated in the recipient and is continued for 4 postoperative weeks.

Additional vascular anastomoses in the liver/small intestine transplant include the anastomosis of the donor's superior mesenteric vein (SMV) to the recipient's SMV. The donor's proximal jejunum is anastomosed to the recipient's jejunum or duodenum. Distally, the donor ileum is connected to the recipient's colon (if present). An ileostomy is performed for drainage and early assessment of the transplanted graft. A jejunostomy feeding tube is placed at the time of the operation for venting and initiation of enteral feedings.

The critical care management in the postoperative period is difficult and complicated. Stormy postoperative courses are anticipated for the liver/small intestine recipient. Lengthy recovery periods are anticipated, as time is needed for the intestine to become functional.

Care of children post intestine transplant is similar to the care required of a liver transplant patient. Additional concerns include care of the large abdominal incision and an ileostomy. Consultation with an enterostomal therapist in the immediate postoperative period is necessary to prevent impairment of skin integrity.

Careful measurement of enteric output is essential. The surgeon is notified of extremes of output. Excessive output may indicate rejection and reflects poor absorption. Enteral feedings are introduced to stimulate absorption as soon as tolerated in the postoperative period. Total caloric intake is maintained with parenteral nutrition, which is decreased once enteral feedings are tolerated.

Initiation of enteral feedings is a gradual process, as the achievement of the alimentation process has taken from 6 weeks to 9 months (Todo et al., 1992). Enteral feedings are initiated with Peptamen, with Modified Compleat B started later. Peptamen is a low-osmolality, dipeptide, lactose-free formula. Modified Compleat B is a lactose- and gluten-free formula that contains dietary fiber to promote normal intestinal motility.

Graft function is evaluated for motility and absorption. Motility is evaluated by barium gastrointestinal series with determination of duration of gastric emptying and intestinal transit time. Fifty percent of the recipients experienced delayed gastric emptying that improved in 4 to 6 months (Todo et al., 1992). Intestinal motility was increased in 7 recipients and prolonged in 3 recipients, with these same abnormalities improving with time (Todo et al., 1992). D-Xylose testing and fecal fat content are performed to evaluate intestinal absorption abilities, assessing carbohydrate absorption and fat metabolism.

Pharmacologic measures including the administration of camphorated opium tincture (Paregoric), Lomotil, loperamide (Imodium), and propantheline (Pro-Banthine) are administered to decrease gastrointestinal motility. Pectin is administered to decrease stool fluid content. Many children requiring intestinal transplant have never eaten prior to surgery, and an occupational therapist or feeding specialist is utilized during the postoperative period to assist these children with mastery of this task.

FK-506 (Prograf) is the primary immunosuppressive agent for the liver/small intestine recipient. Initially, the intravenous form of the drug is prescribed, with the patient switched to the oral preparation when tolerating enteral feedings. Compared with other immunosuppressants, FK-506 is less influenced by the presence or absence of bile, bile acids, and intestinal motility (Furukawa et al., 1992). Daily measurement of FK-506 levels is performed due to the potential erratic absorption of the drug in the intestinal recipient. In addition, in the immediate postoperative period patients are usually prescribed methylprednisolone (Solu-Medrol). Intravenous steroids are tapered to oral prednisone, with the doses decreased as tolerated.

Infection is a common complication. Translocation of bacteria from the intestine to the bloodstream can occur, if bacteria seeps through damaged intestinal mucosa into the bloodstream. Causes of translocation include intestinal overgrowth, sloughing of the mucosa, and rejection. Thus, bowel decontamination is continued for the first 4 postoperative weeks to minimize translocation due to bowel overgrowth.

Quantitative stool cultures are obtained daily in the immediate postoperative period. Stool organisms present in quantities of greater than 10^9 are treated with antibiotics, and surveillance for systemic infection is initiated.

Graft-versus-host disease (GVHD) is another potential complication due to the large quantities of lymphoid tissue present in the intestine. Recipients of liver/intestine and intestine have been treated with increased immunosuppression for GVHD, which is diagnosed by the presence of a fine intermittent pink skin rash and histologic diagnoses per intestinal and skin biopsy.

RENAL TRANSPLANTATION

During the last 20 years, substantial experience has been gained in providing care and treatment to children with end-stage renal disease (ESRD). These developments have allowed this patient population the opportunity to live far longer than would ordinarily be expected. Experience has also assured us that infants and very small children, although a high-risk group, are not only acceptable candidates for treatment but also favored candidates when outcome and quality of life are measured.

The Report of the North American Pediatric Transplant Cooperative Study (Alexander, 1990) has summarized data contributed by 57 participating centers on 754 children who received 761 transplants from January 1, 1987 to February 16, 1989. The results indicated the following:

1. One-year graft survival was 88% for living-related donor (LRD) grafts and 71% for cadaver grafts. Live donor sources accounted for 42% of the transplants. The median times to first rejection were 36 days for cadaver transplants and 156 days for living donor transplants. Overall, 57% of treated rejections were completely reversible, although the complete reversal rate decreased to 37% for four or more rejections.
2. One-year patient survival was 96% for LRD grafts and 92% for cadaver grafts. The main cause of death was infection (16/35).
3. Rehospitalization during months 1 to 5 occurred in 62% of the patients, with treatment of rejection and infection being the main causes.

The incidence of ESRD in children differs markedly from that in adults. ESRD is an unusual disorder in children, with an estimated incidence of one to three new cases in children under 16 years of age per million total population per year (Potter, 1980; Donckerwolcke, 1983).

The etiology of ESRD in children is also in striking contrast to the adult ESRD population, in which more than 80% of patients have acquired renal disease. Approximately half of the children needing treatment have a congenital or hereditary renal disorder and half an acquired renal lesion. The congenital anomalies, vascular nephropathies, and embryonal tumors are characteristically seen in children under 5 years of age. Hereditary nephropathies and cystic diseases are found in children and adolescents, often not reaching terminal stage until the mid to late teens. Glomerular disease continues to be the most prevalent cause of ESRD in the older pediatric age group. On the average, there seems to be an interval of about 4 to 5 years between the onset of glomerular disease and the onset of ESRD. The etiology of renal failure is important information for the healthcare team, patients, and their families. The identification of a hereditary renal disease has implications for family members who may wish to be considered as kidney donors. Since certain renal diseases tend to recur in the transplanted kidney, this information can influence the timing of the transplant as well as the choice of LRD versus cadaveric donor.

The principles of conservative treatment of ESRD in children are based on maintaining metabolic balance and growth and development by diet and drug therapy. With the availability of dialysis and transplantation, conservative treatment should exclude the need for drastic limitations on diet and activity. When conservative management can no longer relieve the symptoms of uremia and permit the child to function in peer, school, or family life, it is necessary to institute alternate forms of treatment. Treatment options include chronic hemodialysis, chronic continuous ambulatory peritoneal dialysis (CAPD) or continuous cycling peritoneal dialysis (CCPD), and transplantation. Although most patients are brought to an optimal metabolic state with dialysis prior to transplantation, it is not unusual to undergo transplantation without dialysis.

Once dialysis is begun and thereafter, the child's surgical and urologic abnormalities are corrected. A voiding cystourethrogram is used to evaluate the bladder. Many children whose bladders were thought to be unusable may in fact be surgically augmented so that these children may void normally. Children with neurogenic bladders may require intermittent clean catheterization after transplantation. Every effort is made to use the bladder; however, when it absolutely cannot be used, diversion to an ileal or colonic conduit may be performed.

Bilateral nephrectomy is indicated to manage malignant hypertension that has failed to respond to maximal antihypertensive therapy and ultrafiltration by dialysis and for persistent infections and structural upper tract uropathies. There has also been some discussion that very young children might be more prone to graft thrombosis when the native kidneys have not been previously removed (Harmon, 1991). It is possible that the cardiac output of young recipients may not be sufficient to adequately perfuse the native kidneys and the larger graft.

The recurrence of the primary renal disease in the allograft is of great concern in the pediatric recipient. Focal segmental glomerulosclerosis, hemolytic-uremic syndrome, oxalosis, and membranoproliferative glomerulonephritis have all been reported to recur. Cystinosis, another inherited metabolic disorder, results in the reappearance of cystine crystals in the allograft, but graft dysfunction due to cystinosis does not occur. Unfortunately, the extrarenal manifestations of cystinosis, such as deposition of cystine crystals in other major organs, continue to persist after successful transplantation.

Some centers question the acceptability of a mentally retarded child for treatment of ESRD. Others hold that the child who is educable, functioning in society, and does not need custodial care is an acceptable candidate.

Recipient age is a highly controversial consideration to transplantation. Results of transplantation in infants less than 2 years of age historically have been poor. The 12-month graft survival for these infants is reported to be only 39% for cadaver (CAD) and 80% for living-related donor (LRD) grafts, compared with 72% and 98%, respectively, for older pediatric graft recipients. Infants also have increased mortality risks following renal transplantation, even when compared with only slightly older children. One-year patient survival rates among infants less than 12 months of age at transplant were only 80% (LRD) and 78% (CAD), compared with 100% (LRD) and 94% (CAD) among 3-year-olds. The 1-year mortality risk for infants who received a CAD graft between 12 and 24 months of age was nearly 35% (Alexander, 1990). Since outcome appears to be dramatically improved when LRDs are used in this age group, it would seem that these infants should undergo transplantation only in the most experienced centers accustomed to technical problems inherent in the transplantation of an adult kidney into an infant. These centers have reported transplantation into infants weighing as little as 5 kg and as small as 62 cm in length. Most centers prefer to maintain infants on dialysis until the infant weighs at least 8 kg or is

more than 2 years of age. It is also important to recognize that renal transplantation is not the only treatment option for children with ESRD. A study in long-term mortality has shown no significant difference in the 5-year patient survival of those treated with hemodialysis (95%), LRD renal transplant (88%), and CAD renal transplant (85%) (Kim, 1991). This is particularly important in caring for the newborn/infant where increased linear growth is preferred prior to transplantation. Dialysis can also provide optimal recovery in the medically unstable child and should a transplant fail, dialysis is an acceptable alternative until another transplant can be performed.

The decision to use a living-related or cadaver kidney donor is dependent on the philosophy of the particular program, as well as the availability of a living-related kidney and the preference of the particular family. However, living-related donors should be used whenever possible, considering the improved graft survival. An LRD must be at least 18 years of age; highly motivated; and meet the individual program's immunologic, medical, and psychosocial parameters. Since graft loss is most frequently due to rejection, it follows that an important goal in transplantation is to identify those dissimilarities that provoke an immunologic response. In addition to absolute ABO compatibility, it is also preferable to select that donor who shares at least one haplotype for the serologically detectible antigens, against whom the recipient has no specific lymphocytotoxic antibody (negative crossmatch), and who is least stimulatory in mixed lymphocyte culture. The medical evaluation will determine that the donor is in excellent health, that the operation carries only a small risk, and that the renal function in the donor is normal. So as not to be influenced by the patient's medical condition, by family pressures, or by the urgency of the transplant, this evaluation is usually conducted by a physician independent from the transplantation team.

When an LRD cannot be identified, the child is placed on the waiting list for a cadaveric kidney. Monthly determinations of sensitivity against a representative panel of lymphocytes are made. The kidney is selected on the basis of a negative crossmatch between the recipient's serum and lymphocytes from the donor. Other criteria include current sensitization, length of time waiting, and recipient's age. The donor should be greater than 6 and less than 65 years old, normotensive, and otherwise healthy and free of transmissible disease. Moreover, these donors have been declared brain dead and are maintained on life support systems until the kidneys can be recovered. While awaiting the final determination of brain death, histocompatibility typing and crossmatching with potential recipients can be performed.

At present, UNOS is considering modification in the point system for renal allocation to provide pediatric recipients an enhanced opportunity to receive a transplant in a shorter period of time than the present system allows. The rationale for early transplantation is that these children suffer potentially irreversible impediments to growth and neuropsychological development as the result of their disease.

Random third-party blood transfusions as well as deliberate donor-specific blood transfusions prior to living-related renal transplantation were thought to improve graft survival. More recent studies, however, have suggested that current immunosuppressive techniques lead to graft survival rates that are not improved by deliberate transfusions. Therefore, possible sensitization by transfusions is no longer warranted (Ahmed & Terasaki, 1991).

Transplant Procedure

The surgical placement of the transplanted kidney in the older child is generally similar to that in adults. The donor kidney is placed retroperitoneally in the right or left iliac fossa, anastomosing the donor vessels to the recipient's iliac vessels. Transplantation in the very small child poses several problems because the donor kidney is usually relatively large. Therefore, in the infant it is usually necessary to use a transabdominal approach with intraperitoneal placement of the kidney, anastomosing the renal vessels to the abdominal aorta and the lower inferior vena cava. Transfusions of blood and colloid may be necessary to provide a circulating blood volume that is adequate to perfuse the new kidney. The donor's ureter is tunneled into the bladder through a ureteroneocystostomy.

Large adult kidneys that are transplanted into children will decrease in size with time but will function adequately. Conversely, cadaveric kidneys from small children that are transplanted into adolescents undergo hypertrophy and increase in function.

Postoperative Care

The patient usually goes directly from the operating room to the PICU, where monitoring continues. A chest x-ray confirms central line placement. A renal ultrasound is obtained to serve as a baseline for future comparison, as is a radionuclide scan, which confirms perfusion to the newly grafted kidney.

It is not unusual to keep the small infant who has received a large adult kidney placed intraperitoneally, intubated, and on a ventilator for several days. A central line is usually inserted to monitor the effects of fluid loss on circulating blood volume and to determine replacement therapy. An additional peripheral IV line is used to replace insensible losses. Intraoperative bowel manipulation usually results in an ileus. The patient will require a nasogastric tube and parenteral nutrition until bowel function returns. A bladder catheter is placed for bladder decompression and urine output measurement.

Fluid and Electrolyte Imbalance

Following surgery, the kidney may produce a massive diuresis, may remain totally anuric, or may produce urine volumes between these extremes. Serum and urine electrolytes are determined frequently to monitor the patient's chemical balance. Intravenous fluids are administered based on the serum electrolyte levels and urine volumes. Inadequate fluid and electrolyte replacement may precipitate hyponatremia, hypokalemia, and hypotension. This is especially important in the very small child, in whom fluid shifts occur very rapidly. Hypotension heralding hypovolemia must be prevented in order to maintain adequate perfusion to the new graft and prevent possible graft thrombosis.

Most patients with good allograft function will have normal BUN and serum creatinine levels by the third or fourth postoperative day. At this time, they are managed on routine fluid volumes. Often these patients have been maintained on hemodialysis prior to transplantation with concomitant fluid intake restriction. An unlimited or 2-L requirement may be met with resistance.

Hypocalcemia, except in the patient with severe hyperparathyroidism, usually ceases to be a problem in the presence of good renal function. Phosphorus regulation, however, may continue to be problematic for the patient, now in the form of hypophosphatemia. It is not unusual for the newly grafted kidney to develop a "phosphate leak," requiring oral phosphate supplementation for an indefinite period of time.

Decreased Urine Output

Post-transplant oliguria or anuria is commonly caused by acute tubular necrosis (ATN) or rejection. If the transplanted kidney is undergoing ATN, it may produce a diuresis for a day and then become anuric and may not secrete urine for days or weeks. This is more commonly found as the result of prolonged ischemia during cadaveric organ retrieval. The reversibility of this ischemic disease is difficult to predict, and anuria may persist for several weeks before adequate renal function begins. The patient is then maintained on dialysis until the ATN has resolved. If hemodialysis is used, it is important not to aggressively ultrafiltrate, as excessive fluid loss could result in thrombosis of the allograft. Careful regulation of immunosuppressive agents and other drugs excreted by the kidney is especially important during this period.

Rejection must be ruled out whenever the volume of urine decreases. Acute rejection most commonly occurs during the first few weeks but can occur at any time during the life of the graft. It is usually reversible when identified and treated early. Serial creatinine, ultrasound, radionuclide scans, and percutaneous renal biopsy are often needed to confirm the diagnosis of rejection.

Other causes for oliguria and anuria cannot be overlooked and are equally investigated. Hypovolemia may be due to surgical blood loss or third spacing of fluids, particularly common in patients who have been previously maintained on peritoneal dialysis. Occasionally a very small child will return from the operating room in congestive heart failure after having received a substantial amount of fluids and colloids within a few hours. Careful fluid replacement, diuretics, and/or dialysis will be necessary until the intravascular volume status has become near normal.

Diminished urinary flow may also be caused by obstruction of the bladder catheter by a simple kink or a clot. Very gentle irrigation may be necessary to ensure drainage.

Occasionally the distal ureter, which is minimally vascularized, becomes necrotic from ischemia, causing obstruction and subsequent extravasation of urine into the lower abdomen. If the leak is very small, a bladder catheter may be able to provide adequate drainage until the leak has healed. Placement of a nephrostomy tube or ureteral stent, or reimplantation of the ureter may be necessary. Although rare, obstruction of the ureter may also be caused by a clot or a kidney stone.

Also unusual and potentially preventable is graft thrombosis. Preliminary data suggest that graft thrombosis may be an increased risk for recipients less than 6 years of age who have not had prior dialysis, as well as children who receive cadaveric grafts from young donors.

Potential Complications

Hypertension is commonly seen in children who have received a renal transplant. The multiple potential factors include acute and/or chronic rejection, side effects of prednisone and/or cyclosporine, recurrence of primary renal disease, transplant artery stenosis, ischemia of native kidneys, and excessive sodium and fluid retention. Effective treatment for hypertension is essential, since poor control can cause seizures and intracerebral bleeding as well as accelerated deterioration of the graft.

The postoperative management of the renal transplant patient can be complicated by a variety of problems largely related to the toxic effects of immunosuppression. Infection is the most frequent and most often fatal complication. Prominent among these infections are those with a large number of pathogens, mainly gram-negative bacteria and opportunistic organisms such as *Pneumocystis carinii* and CMV.

Patients who lack the antibody to CMV and are going to receive a kidney from a donor who is positive for the CMV antibody may be treated with prophylactic IV CMV immunoglobulin. The first dose must be administered within 72 hours of the transplant, then subsequent doses are given up to 16 weeks following the transplant. Reports of using ganciclovir to treat tissue-invasive CMV infections are also encouraging (Dunn, 1991). The patient who tolerates the graft poorly and requires large amounts of immunosuppressive drugs is the one most likely to develop serious infections. For this reason, vigorous immunosuppressive therapy is not pursued. Instead, rejection is

allowed to proceed, and the kidney is then removed and later replaced with a second transplant.

PANCREAS TRANSPLANTATION

The number of pancreas transplantations performed for the treatment of diabetes mellitus has increased dramatically in the last few years. More than one half of the transplants reported to the International Pancreas Transplant Registry have been performed since 1991 (UNOS, 1995). In 1995, there were a total of 3900 pancreas transplants performed. However, only 11 transplants were reported in the age group 0 to 5 years and 9 transplants in the age group 6 to 18 years. The survival data from October 1987 to December 1993 are reported as 62% graft survival and 83% patient survival (UNOS, 1995).

Diabetes is a chronic disease that affects more than 12 million Americans and is associated with permanent and irreversible functional and structural changes in body cells (Guyton, 1977). The financial impact of this disease is staggering both to the patient and to society. The goals of pancreas transplantation are to restore glucose control, permit independence from insulin, and halt the progression of complications.

Pancreatic transplantation procedures are being performed in rigorously selected diabetic patients at this time, and in very few children. Because generalized immunosuppression is needed to prevent rejection, pancreas transplantation has been limited to patients whose secondary complications of diabetes are, or predictably will be, more serious than the potential side effects of antirejection therapy. Patients who require or who have had a kidney transplant, and who are obligated to immunosuppressive therapy, meet this criterion. However, many nonuremic, non–kidney transplant patients are also in this category, for example, those with preproliferative retinopathy who are at great risk for loss of vision, or those with albuminuria who thus have early, but progressive, diabetic nephropathy. When it becomes possible to abrogate a specific immune response in humans, and when the risks of immunosuppression and transplantation are minimal, the limiting factor will be the availability of donor pancreases.

Currently, most pancreas transplants are performed in uremic patients either simultaneously with or 6 months to 1 year following renal transplantation. The rationale is that a functioning endocrine pancreas will protect the renal graft and stabilize diabetic complications. It also assists in monitoring pancreatic rejection. Renal biopsies can be performed to monitor rejection, but pancreatic biopsies are not indicated because the pancreas is highly vascular.

Patient selection is often based on age, stage of renal failure, ophthalmic examination to assess for diabetic retinopathy, electromyography, cardiac workup, ability to withstand surgery, noninvasive vascular studies, and emotional and psychological stability. The primary age of this population ranges from 22 to 44 years.

Cadaveric pancreas transplantation is indicated for two subpopulations. One is the patient who has had a previous renal transplant and is currently immunosuppressed. The other is the patient who exhibits renal failure and is a candidate for renal transplantation. Pancreas transplantation in nonuremic diabetics who have not had a renal transplant and would be subjected to the side effects of immunosuppressants has been tried. It is being debated whether the risks outweigh the benefits (Sutherland, 1988).

Clinical attempts at islet cell allotransplantation have not yet reached a high level of success. The manipulations that can lead to a relatively high success rate in experimental animal models are difficult to apply in the human clinical situation. Islet cell transplantation is not a simple procedure for the transplant team. It is very difficult to procure a sufficient quantity of viable islet cell tissue from one donor pancreas, and techniques to alter graft immunogenicity need to be made practical.

Transplant Procedure

Surgical technique and transplantation of whole or segmental pancreas vary between centers. The type of surgical technique is based solely on how exocrine secretion is to be directed. Although the pancreas has a dual function, exocrine and endocrine, in which the exocrine portion excretes enzymes that aid digestion, and the endocrine portion secretes insulin, only the endocrine function is needed. Exocrine function in the native pancreas remains intact despite diabetes mellitus.

The three most common techniques to occlude duct drainage of exocrine secretions are (1) polymer injection into the pancreatic duct, (2) intestinal drainage, and (3) bladder drainage. The pancreatic graft is placed intraperitoneally and anastomosed to the common iliac vessels with the tail of the graft lying downward with the omentum. A renal graft can be placed using the opposite common iliac vessels in all techniques. In the intestinal drainage technique, anastomosis of the graft to either duodenum or jejunum with a temporary pancreatic duct tube draining to the exterior is known as pancreaticoenterostomy (Corry, 1986). Wound sepsis is a potential disadvantage for this technique if the bowel anastomosis should leak.

In the bladder drainage technique, which is the most usual approach, the pancreatic vessels are anastomosed to iliac vessels as in the previous techniques. Both pancreas and a portion of duodenum containing the pancreatic duct are anastomosed to the bladder. Pancreatic enzymes are secreted in an inactive form and do not cause any damage to the bladder or ureter. The advantage of this technique is that the nurse can monitor the amylase in urine as an aid in diagnosing rejection of the pancreatic graft

if simultaneous pancreas and renal grafts are not used.

The International Pancreas Transplant Registry reports that no major differences have been shown with 1-year graft survival between whole organ versus segmental transplantation. There is also no difference in graft survival related to selected exocrine drainage technique. Differences do occur in graft survival statistics between centers. The treatment of rejection based upon renal dysfunction in simultaneous pancreas and renal grafts has allowed for the successful treatment of pancreatic rejection. Graft survival statistics for simultaneous transplants are much higher than those for a pancreas transplanted alone.

Postoperative Care

Careful monitoring for rapid changes in the recipient's status and potential complications are the primary intensive care nursing responsibility during the post-transplant period. Fluid balance, respiratory care, and potential for bleeding are focal points. The patient's abdominal girth is monitored to assess for graft edema. A central line is utilized to facilitate blood sampling, as an access for medication administration, and to monitor central venous pressure.

Assessment of anastomosis leakage is important. A Foley catheter is placed during surgery and remains in place for approximately 10 to 14 days. This provides constant decompression of the bladder to minimize pressure on the anastomosis site. Before the catheter is removed, a cystogram is obtained to ensure that the anastomosis of the pancreas and duodenal segment is well healed to the bladder without leakage. The catheter will remain in place for several weeks if a leak is noted. Frequent cultures are obtained with aggressive treatment of pathogens. The patency of the catheter is vital to avoid urine retention. Urine is often bloody due to the anastomosis and vascularity of the bladder and clears within a week postoperatively. Hematuria after clearing may indicate a complication.

Vital signs, daily weights, and serial central venous pressure readings help to assess hydration and avoid volume depletion, which can cause decreased perfusion to transplanted organs. Metabolic acidosis can occur in pancreas transplants with bicarbonate levels well below normal. Loss of bicarbonate in the urine from the duodenal transplanted segment may be excessive, necessitating replacement. Hypokalemia may occur secondary to fluid replacement, diuresis, or diuretic therapy. Potassium supplements are administered when necessary. Hyponatremia may occur with osmotic diuresis and is usually treated by changing the intravenous solution.

Daily serum laboratory values are assessed to monitor for signs of rejection, infection, bleeding, and electrolyte imbalance. Blood glucose, serum amylase, and urinary amylase levels are obtained frequently for the first 48 hours. Frequency is then tapered with the patient's progress.

Monitoring for pancreatitis is a primary nursing function. Elevation of serum amylase occurred frequently postoperatively prior to the use of University of Wisconsin (UW) preservation solution. This rise was self-limited and did not require treatment. The use of this solution has eliminated the initial pancreatitis seen postoperatively at some centers. Reflux pancreatitis can occur later in the postoperative course from bladder overdistension and reflux into the pancreatic duct. Bladder distension is assessed regularly. Voiding patterns, including frequency and volume, are noted. A persistent pancreatitis may indicate infected ascites, necessitating surgical intervention. Elevation of serum amylase is a marker to predict pancreas rejection but has not consistently been a reliable indicator (Stratta, 1988).

Serum glucose levels are monitored every 2 hours postoperatively. Euglycemia usually occurs within 6 hours after transplant without the administration of insulin (Groshek, 1991). Glucose intolerance is not manifested in the face of rejection until most of the pancreas is destroyed. Only 10% of islet cells are needed for glycemia control. Therefore, reversal of rejection after the onset of hyperglycemia has a low success rate. Early manifestations of a rejection episode can be assessed by noting slight changes in normal patterns of glucose levels for that patient at comparable times of the day. An elevation of 30 to 40 mg/dL is reported.

ISSUES IN PEDIATRIC TRANSPLANTATION

The commitment to transplant children with end-stage organ failure can be one of the most challenging yet rewarding programs undertaken by a transplant center. It provides many avenues for highly skilled and sensitive nursing care. Cardiac, liver, and kidney transplantations are viable therapeutic options for critically ill children who will either be limited in their lifestyle or their lifespan. Lung, small bowel, and pancreatic transplantations have been shown to be feasible but are still in the developmental stages.

Children and families facing the process of transplantation deal with multiple issues. The developmental level of the child, the family dynamics, and the fact that many of the children are very young and have little or no participation in or control over their own care require the attention of the families as well as the nurses providing care.

End-stage organ failure differs from other life-threatening childhood diseases in that transplantation offers the chance of long-term survival and rehabilitation. However, children with organ failure are at risk of experiencing physical and emotional problems similar to those of children with other chronic or life-threatening illnesses (Williams, 1991). Prior to transplantation, children often incur repeated hospitalizations, which may involve separation from family members, school, friends, and familiar environments. Throughout the process of transplantation, the child is influenced by previous experiences with hospitals and healthcare professionals. As well, perceptions are affected by the child's developmental age.

Severe stress for patients, family, and staff occurs during the post-transplant period with rejection, delay in or interruption in the progress of the clinical course, and infections. Constant efforts at reassurance, support, and promotion of normal life patterns for child and family must be provided. The PICU staff must be aware of the individual family's coping patterns, as well as their need to participate in the patient's care. Not to be forgotten is the living-related donor, who is usually a parent. The donor who needs to mourn the loss of a body part can easily feel unappreciated and ignored while the recipient is the focus of care.

Alterations in parenting is a key nursing diagnosis in the immediate postoperative period. Weichler (1990) reported on an exploratory study determining information needs of mothers of liver transplant recipients. A 13-item, open-ended interview guide was completed by eight mothers. The most prominent maternal emotions were fear of the child's death and fear of organ rejection. In the PICU phase, mothers reported feelings of guilt over seeing their child with numerous invasive tubes in place. The mothers perceived that the most important way for parents to cope with these fears was to be as prepared as possible for the transplant process.

In the PICU, mothers reported five consistent information needs. These were: (1) the purpose of the tubes, (2) liver enzyme laboratory values, (3) child's blood pressure, (4) medications, and (5) child's overall well-being. Three of the eight mothers reported they were too stressed to seek information during the PICU phase.

Supervised viewing of the native organ with pathology personnel may provide support to the parents. Parents have reported that seeing their child's liver relieved the lingering question of the necessity of the transplant at this time. If the diagnosis or etiology of liver failure (or other organ failure) is unknown, meeting with the pathologist allows for parental questions to be asked. However, answers may not be known.

Returning the transplant patient to his home and community may prove to be a very stressful occasion. The very small child will tend to be overactive for a few months until the excitement of being well becomes exhausting and normal childhood activity resumes. The adolescent, who is already in a period of structural ego alteration, may have conflicts about body image, identity, and dependency. A cushingoid appearance and struggles with weight gain may make returning to school a nightmare.

Quality of life issues in children following liver transplantation have been reported (Kosmach, 1990; Zamberlan, 1989; Zitelli, 1988). Zitelli and associates

(1988) noted that objective lifestyle changes in 65 children had improved from their pretransplant status and that the children overall attended school, took fewer medications, and experienced fewer days of hospitalization. Zamberlan (1989) interviewed 20 school-age children, 3 to 6 years after liver transplantation, who perceived their quality of life to be good; however, many negative feelings about physical appearance were expressed. The 20 children expressed feelings of insecurity and loneliness, had difficulties in peer relations, and had higher anxiety scale scores as compared with a normal group on the Piers-Harris Self-Concept Scale. Kosmach (1990) interviewed 7 adolescents, 1 to 4 years following liver transplantation, and reported disruptions in their life related to rejection and concerns about physical appearance.

The family, having previously cared for the ill patient, may find it difficult to let go and permit independent activity. Previously submerged intrafamilial tensions may become overt with the stresses of chronic illness, and the family structure may disintegrate.

Consideration must also be given to the financial stresses that burden families of transplant patients. Fortunately for patients undergoing renal transplantation, the financial burden is eased through federal legislation. This program entitles every citizen and his or her dependents who are either currently or fully insured by the Social Security program to Medicare reimbursement for dialysis and transplantation. Coverage extends for 3 years after the transplant and is reinstituted if the graft fails and the patient returns to dialysis. The current extent of coverage is constantly changing. The recipient insurance would also cover the costs of care for actual or potential kidney donors, including all reasonable preparatory, surgical, and postoperative recovery expenses associated with the donation. However, not covered are lost wages due to time from work lost while undergoing the donor evaluation, followed by recuperation post nephrectomy. The costs for other transplants must largely be covered by each individual family's resources and/or private insurance.

The future of transplantation includes issues such as organ donation, management with improved immunosuppression, and the facilitation of a return to a more normal lifestyle by the patient and family. Segmental organs, xenografts, anencephalic donors, and living-related donors are possibilities to increase the supply of available organs. Extensive examination of the long-term effects on growth and development, school performance, and emotional status of children must occur now that there is a larger population of pediatric transplant patients. Future patient issues of sexual maturation, fertility, and long-term drug effects during the first and second generations will become important. Creative approaches to facilitate treatment compliance must be developed and tested.

Transplantation provides nurses the unique opportunity to combine aspects of planning and providing care that meets each child's developmental level in the setting of highly technical and challenging science.

References

Addonizio, L. (1990). Cardiac transplantation in the pediatric patient. *Progress in Cardiovascular Disease, 33* (1), 19–34.

Ahmed, K., & Terasaki, P. (1991). Effect of transfusions. In P. Terasaki. (Ed.). *Clinical transplants 1991.* Los Angeles: UCLA Tissue Typing Laboratory.

Alexander, S. R., Arbus, C. S., Butt, K. M., Conley, S., Fine, R. N., et al. (1990). *The 1989 report of the North American Pediatric Renal Transplant Cooperative Study, 4,* 542–553.

Assaad, A. (1991). Management of the newborn after cardiac transplantation. *Journal of Heart Transplantation, 10* (5), 823–824.

Augustine, S. M. (1991). Heart-lung and single lung transplantation. In Norris & House (Eds.), *Organ and tissue transplantation: Nursing care from procurement through rehabilitation* (pp. 89–111). Philadelphia: F. A. Davis.

Bailey, L. L., Nehlsen-Cannarella, S., Concepcion, W., et al. (1985). Baboon to human cardiac xenotransplantation in a neonate. *Journal of the American Medical Association, 254,* 3321.

Bailey, L. L., Nehlsen-Cannarella, S., Doroshow, R. W., et al. (1986). Cardiac allotransplant in newborns as therapy for hypoplastic left heart syndrome. *New England Journal of Medicine, 315,* 949–951.

Baumgartner, W. A., Reitz, B. A., & Achuff, S. C. (Eds.) (1990). *Heart and heart-lung transplantation.* Philadelphia: W. B. Saunders.

Bierer, B. E., Schreiber, S. L., & Burakoff, S. J. (1990). Mechanisms of immunosuppression by FK-506. *Transplantation, 49* (6), 1168–1169.

Billingham, M. E. (1982). Diagnosis of cardiac rejection by endomyocardial biopsy. *Journal of Heart Transplantation, 164,* 25–30.

Billingham, M. E. (1991). Endomyocardial biopsy in pediatric heart recipients: The gold standard. *Journal of Heart Transplantation, 10* (5), 841–842.

Billingham, M. E., Cary, N. R. B., Hammond, M. E., Kemnitz, J., Marboe, C., McCallister, H. A., Snovar, D. C., Winters, G. L., & Zerbe, A. (1990). A working formulation for the standardization of nomenclature in the diagnosis of heart and lung rejection: Heart rejection study group. *Journal of Heart Transplantation, 9* (6), 587–593.

Borkon, A. M., & Reitz, B. A. (1988). Heart-lung transplantation. In M. A. Konstam & I. M. Isner (Eds.). *The right ventricle* (p. 321). Boston: Martinus Nijhoff Publishing.

Bristow, M. R., Gilbert, E. M., Renlund, D. G., et al. (1988). Use of OKT3 monoclonal antibody in heart transplantation: Review of the initial experience. *Journal of Heart Transplantation, 7,* 1–11.

Broelsch, C. E., Emond, J. C., Whitington, P. F., Thistlethwaite, J. R., Baker, A. L., & Lichtor, J. L. (1990). Application of reduced-size liver transplants as split grafts, auxiliary orthotopic grafts, and living related segmental transplants. *Annals of Surgery, 212* (3), 368–375.

Carpenter, C. B., & Suthanthiran, M. (1989). The prophylactic use of monoclonal antibodies in renal transplantation: A consensus conference sponsored by the American Society of Transplant Physicians. *American Journal of Kidney Disease, 14* (Suppl. 2), 1–77.

Cate, F. H., & Laudicina, S. S. (1991). *Transplantation white paper* (p. 16). Annenberg Washington Program; Communications Policy Studies; Northwestern University and UNOS.

Chiu, R. C., & Bindon, W. (1987). Why are newborn hearts vulnerable to global ischemia? The lactate hypothesis. *Circulation, 76,* V-146.

Cooper, J. D. (1984). Experience with lung transplant at the Toronto General Hospital. *Transplant Today, 1* (1), 26–27.

Corry, R., & Nghiem, D. (1986). *Transplantation and Immunology Letter, 3.*1. New York: Immunology Information Network.

Deodher, S. D. (1986). Review of xenografts in organ transplantation. *Transplantation Proceedings, 18,* 83.

Donckerwolcke, R., Broyer, M., & Brunner, F. (1983). Combined report on regular dialysis and transplantation in Europe. *Proceedings of the European Dialysis Transplant Association, 19,* 61.

Dresdale, A., & Diehl, J. (1990). Early postoperative care: Infectious disease considerations. *Progress in Cardiovascular Disease, 33*(1), 1–9.

Dunn, D. L., Mayoral, J. L., Gillingham, K. J., et al. (1991). Treatment of invasive cytomegalovirus disease in solid organ transplant patients with ganciclovir. *Transplantation, 51,* 98–106.

Dyckner, T., & Wester, P. O. (1983). Effect of magnesium on blood pressure. *British Medical Journal, 286,* 1847–1849.

Emond, J. C., Whitington, P. F., Thistlethwaite, J. R., et al. (1989). Reduced size liver transplantation: Use in the management of children with chronic liver disease. *Hepatology, 10,* 867–872.

Firth, B. (1987). Southwestern Internal Medicine Conference: Replacement of the failing heart. *American Journal of Medical Sciences, 293* (1), 50–65.

Fishbein, M. H., & Whitington, P. F. (1990). Update on pediatric liver transplantation in the treatment of end-stage liver disease. *International Pediatrics, 5* (1), 9–17.

Flye, M. W. (1989). Immunosuppressive therapy. In M. W. Flye, (Ed.). *Principles of organ transplantation* (p. 166). Philadelphia: W. B. Saunders.

Francione, G. L. (1990). Xenografts and animal rights. *Transplantation Proceedings, 22* (3), 1044–1046.

Fricker, F., Trento, A., Griffith, B., et al. (1987). Cardiac allograft rejection is more frequent in children than in adults. *American Journal of Cardiology, 60,* 642.

Funk, M. (1986). Heart transplantation: Postoperative care during the acute period. *Critical Care Nurse, 6* (2), 27–45.

Funovits, M., Altieri, K., Kovalak, J., & Staschak, S. (1993). Small intestine transplantation: A nursing perspective. *Critical Care Nursing Clinics of North America, 5* (1), 203–213.

Furukawa, H., Imventarza, O., Venkataramanan, R., Suzuki, M., Zhu, Y., Warty, V. S., Fung, J., Todo, S., & Starzl, T. E. (1992). The effect of bile duct ligation and bile diversion on FK-506 pharmacokinetics in dogs. *Transplantation, 53,* 722–725.

Furukawa, H., Todo, S., Inventarza, O., Casavilla, A., Wu, Y. M., Fogloeni, C., Broznick, B. M., Bryant, J., Dau, R., & Starzl, T. E. (1991). Effect of cold ischemic time on the early outcome of human hepatic allografts preserved with UW solution. *Transplantation, 51,* 1000–1004.

Goldstein, G. (1986). An overview of orthoclone OKT-3. *Transplant Proceedings, 18,* 927.

Gordon, R. D., Iwatsuki, S., Esquivel, C. O., et al. (1986). Liver transplantation across ABO groups. *Surgery, 100,* 342–348.

Gordon, R. D., Todo, S., Tzakis, A. G., Fung, J. J., Stieber, A., Staschak, S., Iwatsuki, S., & Starzl, T. E. (1991). Liver transplantation under cyclosporine: A decade of experience. *Transplantation Proceedings, 23*(1), 1393–1396.

Green, M., & Michaels, M. G. (1991). Infectious complications of solid-organ transplantation in children. *Advances in Pediatric Infectious Diseases, 7,* 181–203.

Griffin, B., Kormos, R. L., & Hardesty, R. (1987). Heterotopic cardiac transplantation: Current status. *Journal of Cardiac Surgery, 2* (2), 283–289.

Griffin, M. L., Hernandez, A., Martin, T. C., et al. (1988). Dilated cardiomyopathy in infants and children. *Journal of the American College of Cardiology, 11* (1), 139–144.

Groshek, M., & Smith, V. L. (1991). Pancreas transplant. In Norris & House (Eds.). *Organ and tissue transplantation* (p. 163). Philadelphia: F. A. Davis.

Groth, C. (1988). *Pancreatic transplantation* (p. 181). Philadelphia: W. B. Saunders.

Guyton, A. (1977). *Basic human physiology: Normal function and mechanisms of disease.* Philadelphia: W. B. Saunders.

Harmon, W. E., Stablein, D., Alexander, S. R., & Tejani, A. (1991). Graft thrombosis in pediatric renal transplant recipients. *Transplantation, 51,* 406–412.

Heck, C. F., Shumway, S. J., & Kaye, M. P. (1989). The Registry of the International Society for Heart Transplantation. *Journal of Heart Transplantation, 8,* 271–276.

Hitchings, G. H., & Elion, G. B. (1963). Chemical suppression of the immune response. *Pharmacol Review, 15,* 365.

Horak, A. R. (1984). Physiology and pharmacology of the transplanted heart. In D. K. Cooper & R. P. Lanza (Eds.). *Transplantation* (pp. 147–146). Boston: MTP Press Limited.

Hunt, S., Strober, S., Hoppe, R., et al. (1989). Use of total lymphoid irradiation for therapy of intractable cardiac allograft rejection. *Journal of Heart Transplantation, 8,* 104.

Jamieson, S. W., & Oguannaike, H. O. (1986). Cardiopulmonary transplantation. *Surgical Clinics of North America, 66,* 491.

Johnston, J. (1991). A new beginning: Current trends in pediatric heart transplantation. *Focus on Critical Care, 18* (1).

Johnston, J., & Mathis, C. (1988). Determination of rejection using noninvasive parameters after cardiac transplantation in very early infancy. *Progress in Cardiovascular Nursing, 3* (2), 13–18.

Jordan, R. D., Iwatsuki, S., Esqvivel, C. O. Tsakis, A., Todo, S., & Starzl, T. E. (1986). Liver transplantation across ABO blood groups. *Surgery, 100,* 342–348.

Kaye, M. P., & Kriett, J. M. (1991). Pediatric heart transplantations: The world experience. *Journal of Heart Transplantation, 10* (5), 823–824.

Kim, M. S., Jabs, K., & Harmon, W. E. (1991). Long-term patient survival in a pediatric renal transplantation program. *Transplantation, 51,* 413–417.

Kosmach, B. (1990). *Adolescents' responses to quality of life issues following liver transplantation.* Master's thesis, University of Pittsburgh.

Kriett, J. M., & Kaye, M. K. (1990). The Registry of the International Society for Heart Transplantation: Seventh Official Report. *Journal of Heart Transplantation, 9* (4), 323–330.

Krowka, M. J., & Cortese, D. A. (1985). Pulmonary aspects of chronic liver disease and liver transplantation. *Mayo Clinic Proceedings, 60,* 407–418.

Krowka, J. J., & Cortese, D. A. (1989). Pulmonary aspects of liver disease and liver transplantation. *Clinics in Chest Medicine, 10* (4), 593–616.

Kusne, S., Dummer, J. S., Singh, N., Iwatsuki, S., Makowka, L., Esquivel, C., Tzakis, H., Starzl, T., & Ho, M. (1988). Infection after liver transplantation. An analysis of 101 consecutive cases. *Medicine, 67,* 132–143.

Landwirth, J. (1986). Should anencephalic infants be used as organ donors? *Pediatrics 82,* 257–259.

Levin, B., Hoppe, R. T., Collins, G., et al. (1985). Treatment of cadaveric renal transplantation recipients with total lymphoid irradiation, antithymocyte globulin, and low dose prednisone. *Lancet, 2,* 1321.

Lillehei, R. C., Goott, B., & Miller, F. A. (1959). The physiological response of the small bowel of dog to ischemia including prolonged in vitro preservation of the bowel with successful replacement and survival. *Annals of Surgery, 150,* 543.

Macleod, A. M., & Thomson, A. W. (1991). FK-506: An immunosuppressant for the 1990s? *Lancet, 337,* 25–27.

Malatack, J. J., Gartner, J. C., Urbach, A. H., & Zitelli, B. J. (1991). Orthotopic liver transplantation, Epstein-Barr virus, cyclosporine, and lymphoproliferative disease: A growing concern. *The Journal of Pediatrics, 118* (5), 667–675.

Mayer, J. E., Perry, S., O'Brien, P., et al. (1990). Orthotopic heart transplantation for complex congenital heart disease. *Journal of Thoracic and Cardiovascular Surgery, 99,* 484–492.

Mews, C. F., Dorney, S. F., Sheil, A. G., Forbes, D. A., & Hill, R. E. (1990). Failure of liver transplantation in Wilson's disease with pulmonary arteriovenous shunting. *Journal of Pediatric Gastroenterology and Nutrition, 10,* 230–233.

Montefusco, C. M., & Veith, F. J. (1989). Lung transplantation. In M. W. Flye (Ed.). *Principles of organ transplantation* (pp. 413–435). Philadelphia: W. B. Saunders Co.

Moskop, J. (1987). Organ transplantation in children: Ethical issues. *Journal of Pediatrics, 110* (2), 175–179.

Munoz, S. J., & Friedman, L. S. (1989). Liver transplantation. *Medical Clinics of North America, 73* (4), 1011–1038.

Najarian, J. S., & Forker, J. E. (1969). Mechanisms of kidney allograft rejection. *Transplantation Proceedings, 1,* 184–193.

Omery, A., & Caswell, D. (1988). A nursing perspective of the ethical issues surrounding liver transplantation. *Heart & Lung, 17* (2), 626–638.

Park, S. C., Beerman, L. B., Gartner, J. C., Zitelli, B. J., Malatack,

J. J., Fricker, F. J., Fisher, D. R., Mathews, R. A., Neches, W. H., & Zuberbuhler, J. R. (1985). Echocardiographic findings before and after liver transplantation. *The American Journal of Cardiology, 55,* 1373–1378.

Parness, I. P., & Nadas, A. S. (1988). Cardiac transplantation in children. *Pediatrics in Review, 10* (4), 111–117.

Peabody, J., Emery, J., & Ashwal, S. (1988). Experience with anencephalic infants as prospective organ donors. *New England Journal of Medicine 321,* 334–350.

Peterson, P. K., Ferguson, R., Fryd, D. S., et al. (1982). Infectious diseases in hospitalized renal transplant recipients: A prospective study of a complex and evolving problem. *Medicine, 61,* 360–372.

Pollard, R. B., Rand, K. H., Arvin, A. M., et al. (1978). Cell mediated immunity in CMV infection in normal subjects and cardiac transplant patients. *Journal of Infectious Diseases, 137,* 541.

Potter, D. E., Holliday, M. A., Peil, C. F., Feduska, N. J., & Salvatierra, O. (1980). Treatment of end-stage renal disease in children: A 15-year experience. *Kidney International, 18,* 103–109.

Prieto, M., Sutherland, D. E. R., Fernandez-Cruz, L. et al. (1987). Diagnosis of rejection in pancreas transplantation. *Transplantation Proceedings, 19,* 2348–2349.

Roitt, I. M. (Ed.). (1989). *Immunology* (2nd ed). St. Louis: C. V. Mosby.

Rosado, L. J., & Copeland, J. G. (1990). Orthotopic heart transplantation: Recent advances. *Primary Cardiology, 16* (4), 33–47.

Rubin, R. H., & Young, L. S. (1988). *Clinical approach to infection in the compromised host* (2nd ed., pp. 557–621). New York: Plenum.

Rubin, R. H., Wolfson, J. S., Losini, A. S., et al. (1981). Infection in the renal transplant recipient. *American Journal of Medicine, 70,* 405.

Schumann, D. (1987). CMV infection in renal allograft recipients: Indications for intervention in the surgical intensive care unit. *Focus on Critical Care, 14* (3), 40–47.

Schwartz, M. Z., & Maeda, K. (1985). Short bowel syndrome in infants and children. *Pediatric Clinics of North America, 32* (5), 1265–1279.

Schwartz, R., Dameshek, W., & Donovan, J. (1959). The effects of 6-mercaptopurine on primary and secondary immune responses. *Journal of Clinical Investigation, 38,* 1394.

Shapiro, R., Fung, J. J., Jain, A. B., Parks, P., Todo, S., & Starzl, T. E. (1990). The side effects of FK-506 in humans. *Transplantation Proceedings, 22* (1), 35–36.

Shaw, B. W., Stratta, R., Donovan, J. P., Langnas, A. N., Wood, R. P., & Markin, R. J. (1989). Postoperative care after liver transplantation. *Seminars in Liver Disease, 9* (3), 202–230.

Shaw, B. W., Wood, R. P., Kauffman, S. S., Williams, L., Antonson, D. L., & Vanderhoof, V. (1988a). Liver transplantation therapy for children: Part I. *Journal of Pediatric Gastroenterology, 7,* 157–166.

Shaw, B. W., Wood, R. P., Kauffman, S. S., Williams, L., Antonson, D. L., Kelly, D. A., & Vanderhoof, J. A. (1988b). Liver transplantation therapy for children: Part II. *Journal of Pediatric Gastroenterology, 7,* 797–815.

Singer, P. A., Siegler, M., Whitington, P., Lantos, J. D., Emond, J. C., Thistlethwaite, J. R., & Broelsch, C. E. (1989). Ethics of liver transplantation with living related donors. *New England Journal of Medicine, 321* (9), 620–621.

Smith, C. R. (1990). Techniques in cardiac transplantation. *Progress in Cardiovascular Diseases, 32* (6), 383–404.

Smith, S. L. (Ed.). (1990). *Tissue and Organ Transplantation: Implications for Professional Nursing Practice.* St. Louis: Mosby–Year Book.

Snydman, D. R., Werner, B. G., Heinze-Lacey, B., et al. (1987). Use of CMV immune globin to prevent CMV disease in renal transplant recipients. *New England Journal of Medicine, 317,* 1049.

Sommerauer, J., Gayle, M., Frewen, T., Wall, W., Grant, D., Girvan, D., Ghent, C., Jenner, M., & Stiller, C. (1988). Intensive care course following liver transplantation in children. *Journal of Pediatric Surgery, 23* (8), 705–708.

Starzl, T. E., Abu-Elmagd, K., Tzakis, A., Fung, J. J., & Todo, S. (1991). Selected topics on FK-506, with special references to rescue of extrahepatic whole organ grafts, transplantation of

"forbidden organs," side effects, mechanisms, and practical pharmacokinetics. *Transplantation Proceedings, 23* (1), 914–919.

Starzl, T. E., Esquivel, C., Gordon, R., & Todo, S. (1987). Pediatric liver transplantation. *Transplantation Proceedings, 19* (4), 3230–3235.

Starzl, T. E., Iwatsuki, S., Van Thiel, D. H., Gartner, J. C., Zitelli, B. J., Malatack, J. H., Schade, R. R., Shaw, B. W., Hakala, T. R., Rosenthal, J. T., & Porter, K. A. (1982). Evolution of liver transplantation. *Hepatology, 2* (5), 614–636.

Starzl, T. E., Marchioro, G. L., & Waddell, W. R. (1963). The reversal of rejection in human renal homografts with subsequent development of homograft tolerance. *Surgery, Gynecology and Obstetrics, 117,* 385.

Starzl, T. E., Nalesnik, M. A., Porter, K. A., et al. (1984). Reversibility of lymphomas and lymphoproliferative lesions developing under cyclosporine-steroid therapy. *Lancet, 1,* 583–587.

Starzl, T. E., Todo, S., Fung, J., Demetris, A. J., Venkataramanan, R., & Jain, A. (1989). FK-506 for liver, kidney, and pancreas transplantation. *Lancet, 2,* 1002–1004.

Stratta, R. (1988). Early diagnosis and treatment of pancreas allograft rejection. *Transplant International, 1,* 6.

Sutherland, D. E. R., & Moudry-Munns, K. C. (1988). International Pancreas Transplant Registry report. In D. I. Terasaki (Ed.). *Clinical transplants* (pp. 53–63). Los Angeles: UCLA Tissue Typing Laboratory.

Sutherland, D. E. R., Moudry, K. C., & Najarian, J. S. (1988). Pancreas transplantation. In Cerilli (Ed.), *Organ transplantation and replacement* (pp. 535–574). Philadelphia: J.B. Lippincott.

Swinnen, L. J., Costanzo-Norton, M., Fisher, S. G., et al. (1990). Increased incidence of lymphoproliferative disorder after immunosuppression with the monoclonal antibody OKT3 in cardiac transplant recipients. *New England Journal of Medicine, 324* (20), 1437–1439.

Thompson, A. E. (1987). Aspects of pediatric intensive care for after liver transplantation. *Transplantation Proceedings, 19* (4), Suppl. 4, 34–39.

Thomson, A. W. (1988). FK 506: How much potential? *Immunology Today, 10,* 6–9.

Todo, S., Tzakis, A. G., Abu-Elmagd, K., Reyes, J., Fung, J. J., Casavilla, A., Nakamura, K., Yagihashi, A., Jain, A., Murase, N., Iwaki, Y., Demetris, A. J., Van Theil, D. H., & Starzl, T. (1992). Cadaveric small bowel and small bowel-liver transplantation in humans. *Transplantation, 53* (2), 365–369.

Todo, S., Tzakis, A., Abu-Elmagd, K., Reyes, J., Nakamura, K., Casavilla, A., Selby, R., Nour, B., Wright, H., Fung, J. J., Demetris, A. J., Van Thiel, D. H., & Starzl, T. E. (1992). Intestinal transplantation in composite visceral grafts or alone. *Annals of Surgery,* (3), 223–234.

Traiger, G., & Bohachick, P. (1983). Liver transplantation: Care of the patient in the acute postoperative period. *Critical Care Nurse, 3* (5), 96–103.

Trento, A., Griffith, B. P., Fricker, F. J., et al. (1989). Lessons learned in pediatric heart transplantation. *Annals of Thoracic Surgery, 48* (5), 617–623.

Tzakis, A., Fung, J. J., Todo, S., Reyes, J., Green, M., & Starzl, T. (1991). Use of FK-506 in pediatric patients. *Transplantation Proceedings, 23* (1), 924–927.

Tzakis, A., & Starzl, T. E. (1992). Pediatric liver transplantation. In K. W. Ashcraft & T. M. Holder (Eds.). *Pediatric surgery* (2nd ed., pp. 505–524). Philadelphia: W. B. Saunders.

Tzakis, A. G., Todo, S., Reyes, J., & Starzl, T. E. (1991). Liver and small bowel transplantation for short gut syndrome in a child. *Transplantation Science, 1* (1), 27–33.

Uniform Determination of Death Act: President's Commission for the Study of Ethical Problems in Medicine and Biomedical and Behavioral Research (1981). *Defining death: Medical, legal and ethical issues in the determination of death.* Washington, DC: US Government Printing Office.

UNOS Update (1991). 7 (1).

UNOS Update (1992). 8 (9), 39.

UNOS Update (1995). 11 (12), 26.

Veith, F., Kamholz, S., Mollenkopf, F., et al. (1983). Lung transplantation. *Transplantation 35* (4), 271–278.

Veith, F. J., Sinha, S. B. P., Dougherty, J. C., et al. (1972). Nature and evolution of lung allograft rejection with and without immunosuppression. *Journal of Thoracic and Cardiovascular Surgery,* 63, 509.

Venkataramanan, R., Jain, A., Warty, V. W., Abu-Elmagd, K., Furakawa, H., Imventarza, O., Fung, J., Todo, S., & Starzl, T. E. (1991). Pharmacokinetics of FK-506 following oral administration: A comparison of FK-506 and cyclosporine. *Transplantation Proceedings,* 23 (1), 931–933.

Vernon, W. B., & Sollinger, H. W. (1989). Management of combined pancreatico-renal allograft recipients. *Transplant Management,* 1, 565.

Walker, R. W., & Brochstein, J. A. (1988). Neurologic complications of immunosuppressive agents. *Neurologic Clinics,* 6 (2), 261–278.

Weichler, N. K. (1990). Information needs of mothers of children who have had liver transplants. *Journal of Pediatric Nursing,* 6 (2), 88–96.

Weil, R. (1981). Hyperacute rejection of a transplanted human heart. *Transplantation,* 32, 71.

Whitington, P. (1990). Advances in pediatric liver transplantation. In L. A. Barnes (Ed.). *Advances in pediatrics* (pp. 357–389). St. Louis: C.V. Mosby.

Williams, L., & Rzucidlo, S. E. (1985). Care of the pediatric liver transplant patient in the ICU. *Critical Care Quarterly,* 8 (1), 13–25.

Williams, L., House, M. A., & Hill, C. (1991). The pediatric transplant patient: Donor and recipient. In Norris & House (Eds.). *Organ and tissue transplantation* (p. 175). Philadelphia: F. A. Davis.

Wood, R. P., Langnas, A. N., Stratta, R. J., Pillen, T. J., Williams, L., Lindsay, S., Meiergerd, D., & Shaw, B. W. (1990). Optimal therapy for patients with biliary atresia: Portoenterostomy ("Kasai" procedures) versus primary transplantation. *Journal of Pediatric Surgery,* 25 (1), 153–162.

Woodle, E. S., Budzinski, J., Pitman, M., Flanagan, L., Boone, P., Smith, C., Whitington, P. F., Emond, J. C., & Broelsh, C. E. (1990). Reduced-size liver transplantation. *AORN Journal,* 52 (2), 252–260.

Zamberlan, K. (1989). Quality of life in school-age children following liver transplantation. *Dissertation Abstracts International,* SO: 150-Osb.

Zitelli, B., Miller, J., Gartner, J., Malatack, I., Urbach, A., Belle, S., Williams, L., Kirkpatrick, B., & Starzl, T. (1988). Changes in lifestyle after liver transplantation. *Pediatrics,* 82 (2), 173–180.

Zuberbuhler, J. R., Fricker, F. J., & Griffith, B. P. (1989). Cardiac transplantation in children. *Cardiology Clinics,* 7 (2), 411–418.

CHAPTER *28*

HIV in the Critically Ill Child

KIMMITH M. JONES
MARY BERRY LeBOEUF
PATRICIA DILLMAN

EPIDEMIOLOGY
Viral Transmission
Incubation Period
PATHOPHYSIOLOGY
Immune System
Immune Response
Viral Replication
CLASSIFICATION
**LABORATORY DIAGNOSIS OF HIV
    INFECTION**
Antibody Testing
Tests Utilized in Research
AIDS-DEFINING ILLNESSES
ACUTE RESPIRATORY FAILURE (ARF)
Pneumocystis carinii Pneumonia (PCP)

Lymphoid Interstitial Pneumonitis (LIP)
Tuberculosis
DECREASED CARDIAC OUTPUT
Septic Shock
Cardiomyopathy
**CENTRAL NERVOUS SYSTEM
    DYSFUNCTION**
HEMATOLOGIC DYSFUNCTION
OTHER ORGAN DYSFUNCTION
ANTIRETROVIRAL THERAPY
PSYCHOSOCIAL ISSUES
EFFECTS ON PICU RESOURCES
EFFECTS ON THE PICU NURSING STAFF
SUMMARY

The first reported case of acquired immunodeficiency syndrome (AIDS) was made in 1981 by a physician in New York who noticed the rare cancer Kaposi's sarcoma in a group of gay men (Friedman-Kien, 1981). At the same time, a physician in Los Angeles identified a rare pneumonia, *Pneumocystis carinii* pneumonia (PCP), in another group of gay men (Farthing, 1991; Gottlieb, Schroff, Schanker, Weisman, Fan, Woolf, & Saxon, 1981). In 1981, 16 cases of AIDS were reported among children below the age of 13 (CDC, 1993). The number of pediatric cases of AIDS that has been reported to the Centers for Disease Control and Prevention (CDC) has progressively increased from 1981.

Human immunodeficiency virus (HIV) disease is defined as the spectrum from exposure to the virus until death. AIDS is that part of the HIV disease spectrum where opportunistic illnesses have begun to develop until death. Pediatric AIDS refers to those cases that have been reported in children under 13 years of age.

Critical care nurses are being challenged by children with HIV disease and AIDS. Because of multisystem organ involvement and eventual failure, more children affected by this disease are being admitted to pediatric intensive care units for intense medical and nursing management. The final common pathway of this immune deficit affects all organ systems, and critical care nurses need to understand the disease process and causes of life-threatening complications. This chapter presents an overview of the disease process and discusses collaborative interventions specific to the critically ill child with HIV disease and AIDS.

EPIDEMIOLOGY

From 1981 through June 1995, 6611 pediatric cases of AIDS have been diagnosed (CDC, 1995a). Children may acquire HIV by one of several routes of transmission. The most common is perinatal transmission, which accounts for 6124, or 90% of the cases (CDC, 1995a). Five thousand nine hundred twenty-five pediatric cases of AIDS were acquired from women who had HIV disease, or were at risk for HIV disease. In the majority of these cases, the primary risk behavior of the mother was IV drug use (CDC, 1994). The remainder of the pediatric cases have been attributed to hemophilia/coagulation disorders or blood product transfusion. One hundred one cases of AIDS in children under 13 years of age could not be associated with a risk behavior (CDC, 1993).

Adolescents tend to become infected by routes of transmission that are associated with adult risk behavior. These include unprotected sex with an infected partner, IV drug use, and contamination with infected blood (Gayle & D'Angelo, 1990).

Viral Transmission

A great deal of information has been learned about the transmission of HIV since it was first isolated in 1983. It is known that HIV is a very fragile virus. HIV cannot survive for long periods of time once it is outside the body. The length of time it does survive depends upon the size of the droplet that the virus is in, and the concentration of HIV within that droplet (CDC, 1987). The larger the droplet, the longer the survival time of the virus. HIV is killed as the droplet dries.

HIV has been isolated from all body fluids, including blood, semen, vaginal fluid, tears, saliva, sweat, sputum, urine, breast milk, and cerebrospinal fluid. It has also been isolated from some body tissues, including bone marrow, lymph nodes, and brain tissue (Levy, 1990; McMahon, 1988; Newman & Quinn, 1988). Blood, semen, vaginal fluid, and breast milk are the only fluids that have been implicated in the transmission of HIV (Wofsy, 1990).

The infectiousness of a body fluid is dependent upon two variables: the amount of viral particles present within the fluid, and the ability of that fluid to reach the target T4 lymphocytes. In order for HIV to produce an infection, it must be able to enter the recipient's bloodstream and attach itself to the T4 lymphocyte.

There are three modes of transmission for HIV (Barrick, 1990; Bartlett, 1994; Michael & Burke, 1991; Newman & Quinn, 1988; Flaskerud, 1995). The first is unsafe vaginal or anal sexual contact with an infected individual.

Direct inoculation with infected blood or blood products is the second mode of transmission. Mechanisms that allow this transmission to occur include inoculation through transfusions, needles not cleansed properly following IV drug use, inoculation with infected blood through small cuts, and inoculation through needle sticks.

The risk of transmission through blood transfusions has significantly decreased since 1985, when the enzyme-linked immunosorbent assay (ELISA) was implemented into the process of blood screening. Since 1985, all donated blood has been screened for the presence of HIV (Boland & Czarniecki, 1995).

The third mode of transmission is from mother to fetus or during birth. Seven thousand infants are born to HIV-positive women each year, with approximately 1000 to 2000 infants actually becoming HIV-positive (CDC, 1994). Being an HIV-positive mother does not guarantee that her baby will develop HIV disease. However, babies born to infected women will test positive because of maternal antibody transmission to the fetus during development (Bastin, Tamaya, Tinkle, Amaya, Trejo, & Herrera, 1992; Tinkle, Amaya, & Tomayo, 1992). Maternal antibodies remain in the baby's system for up to 15 months (Boland & Czarniecki, 1995). Therefore, it is not currently possible to determine the true HIV status of a baby until the effects of maternal antibodies have resolved. Current statistics indicate that 25% to 35% of the babies born to HIV-positive women will develop HIV disease (Ellerbrock, Bush, Chamberland, & Oxtoby, 1991; Tinkle, Amaya, & Tomayo, 1992). Unfortunately, researchers are unsure why 100% of the babies do not become HIV-positive. If a woman has given birth to an HIV-positive baby in the past, there is a 65% chance that the woman will give birth to another HIV-positive baby (Smeltzer & Whipple, 1991).

Zidovudine (AZT) is proving to be effective in the prevention of perinatal transmission of HIV (CDC, 1994a). In a study of 364 HIV-positive women, AZT therapy was associated with a 67.5% decrease in perinatal transmission. As a result of this study, The Public Health Service recommends that HIV-positive women be informed that AZT substantially reduces the risk of HIV transmission to their unborn baby but does not eliminate it. Also, because this study did not examine teratogenicity, it is recommended that AZT not be started before the fourteenth week of gestation if it is being given for the sole purpose of reducing perinatal transmission (CDC, 1994a).

Incubation Period

When HIV was first identified, it was thought that individuals were diagnosed as being HIV-positive, developed AIDS, and then died within a very short period of time. Adults are now being diagnosed as HIV-positive and are living healthy, productive lives for 10 to 15 years before they develop AIDS, and then living 3 to 4 years with AIDS before they die (Michael & Burke, 1991). However, the length of time from asymptomatic HIV disease to the development of AIDS is shorter in children than in adults (Falloon, Eddy, Wiener, & Pizzo, 1989). The mean age of AIDS diagnosis is 12 months for children with disease acquired through perinatal transmission and 24.4 months for children with transfusion-acquired disease (Mendez, 1992). The progression to AIDS has been as long as 7 years in some children (Falloon, Eddy, Wiener, & Pizzo, 1989).

PATHOPHYSIOLOGY

Immune System

There are two types of immunity: humoral and cellular. Humoral immunity is responsible for the production of antibodies, also called immunoglobulin. The primary cell of humoral immunity is the B cell, which accounts for 10% to 20% of the total lymphocyte count and has a lifespan of about 16 days. The B cell is produced in the bone marrow and is programmed for only one antigen. After a B cell has been exposed to an antigen, it differentiates into a plasma cell. The plasma cell then produces the antibodies that will attach to the antigen, or invading organism, and kill it (Robins, 1989; Tribett, 1989). The humoral system has the ability to produce millions of different antibodies and is used to protect the host against bacteria and viruses (Tribett, 1989).

Cellular immunity is the second type of immunity and protects the host against viruses, fungi, and parasites. The cells involved with this type of immunity are the T cells, which account for about 80% of the total circulating lymphocytes. T cells are produced in the bone marrow and then migrate to the thymus gland, where they mature. There are two subsets of T cells: the T4 and T8 cells. T4 cells are also called inducer, or helper, cells and are sometimes referred to as the conductor of the immune system because of their function (Grady, 1989). The T4 cells release lymphokines, which stimulate or activate the other cells of the immune system (Grady, 1989). The other cells would not know an invader was present without lymphokines being released.

The second set of cells are the T8 cells, which are referred to as cytotoxic or suppressor cells. The T8 cells stop the production of antibodies or lymphokines when an acceptable level has been reached (Grady, 1989). Normally, there are twice as many T4 cells than T8 cells.

A third subset of cells are the natural killer cells. They are nonspecific and attack and kill any cell that has mutated or is infected with a virus. Chapter 16 presents a detailed discussion about the immune system.

Immune Response

There is a normal sequence of events that occurs when an organism enters the body. When a microorganism enters the body, it attaches to a macrophage and is phagocytized and digested. A piece of the invader is then made available on the surface of the macrophage. The T4 cells recognize that piece of mi-croorganism as an antigen and become activated. Once activated, these cells differentiate into lymphokine-producing cells and memory cells. Lymphokines are then released to stimulate the type of immunity that would be most appropriate to cleanse the body of the invader. The T4 cell decides which type of immunity would work best and may stimulate B cells, natural killer cells, T4 cells, T8 cells, phagocytes, or any combination of these to achieve a pure system (Grady, 1989). See Chapter 16 for a further discussion about immune response.

Viral Replication

HIV is classified as a retrovirus. A retrovirus is a virus that must translate, or convert, its RNA into DNA in order for it to replicate. Once this translation has taken place, the virus can then insert itself into the host DNA, which then allows the host cell to produce more retroviral particles (Tramont, 1991).

The translation from RNA to DNA must occur in the presence of reverse transcriptase, which is an enzyme that is present in HIV and other retroviruses but is not present in normal host cells (Levy, 1990). Reverse transcriptase is important because current therapies to slow the progression of HIV disease are reverse transcriptase inhibitors that prevent this translation from taking place.

Once translation is complete, the process of HIV replication continues. Initially, HIV enters the bloodstream of the host and attaches itself to the CD4 receptor, a receptor site located on the T4 lymphocyte. Once this attachment has taken place, an uncoating process occurs in which the virus sheds the outer envelope. The HIV RNA is transcribed into DNA via reverse transcriptase after the virus is uncoated and inside the host cell. Next, the viral DNA is incorporated into the host DNA. At this point, the virus can either remain dormant for months to years or begin to replicate. At the end of the latent stage, the cell in which the virus is located becomes activated by an antigen. Unfortunately, it is uncertain what the antigen is that causes the cell to become activated. New virons are formed and released into the general bloodstream through a process called budding. These new viral cells then attach to other uninfected cells. It appears that the host cell ruptures, releasing many viral particles at once and causing death to that cell. All the particles released into the bloodstream can now continue the cycle. It is by this mechanism that the immune system is gradually depleted of the T4 cells, leaving the host open to massive infections and malignancies, which eventually lead to the individual's death (Grady, 1989; Levy, 1990; Michael & Burke, 1991; Tramont, 1991). Figure 28–1 illustrates the process of viral replication.

CLASSIFICATION

The Centers for Disease Control and Prevention (CDC) has developed a classification system to assist

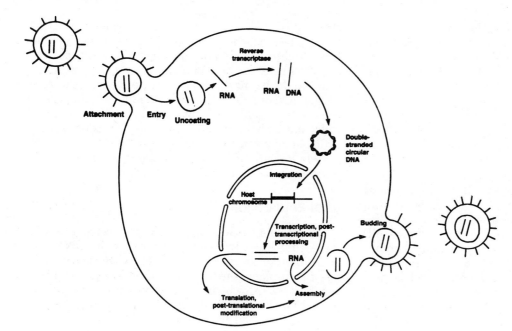

Figure 28–1 ● ● ● ● ● ●
Replication cycle of the human immunodeficiency virus. (From Fallon, J., Eddy, J., Weiner, L., & Pizzo, P.A. (1989). *Journal of Pediatrics,* 114 (1), 1–30.)

the healthcare provider in staging the progression of HIV disease because of the huge spectrum that exists. Children over the age of 13 are classified according to the adult system that has been developed. However, this system has proved insufficient for classification of pediatric HIV infection. In 1987, the CDC proposed a classification system specific to children under 13 years of age. This system defined symptomatic pediatric HIV infection based on pediatric symptoms and categorized infants under 15 months of age born to anti-HIV-antibody seropositive mothers (Berkowitz, Berkowitz, and Johnson, 1992). In 1994, a revised classification system for HIV replaced the system developed in 1987. The new system classifies infected children into mutually exclusive categories according to infection status, clinical status, and immunologic status (CDC, 1994b). This system is outlined in Table 28–1. The adult classification system was revised in 1993 along with the case definition of AIDS (CDC, 1992).

LABORATORY DIAGNOSIS OF HIV INFECTION

Antibody Testing

Once a person is exposed to HIV, that individual's blood can be tested to determine the presence of antibodies. The most common test used is the enzyme-linked immunosorbent assay (ELISA), which was developed in 1983. The ELISA detects the presence of antibodies to the whole virus (Grady & Vogel, 1993). The ELISA is very sensitive, with a sensitivity index of 99%. It also is very specific, with an index of 99% (Grady & Vogel, 1993). Unfortunately, other antibodies within the patient's body can react with the material used in the ELISA to produce a false-

positive result (CDC, 1987). A positive ELISA is always repeated.

If the second ELISA is positive, an even more specific test is performed, called the Western blot analysis (McMahon, 1988). The Western blot confirms the presence of antibodies reacting to individual viral components, which makes it more specific than the ELISA (Grady & Vogel, 1993). The Western blot is more expensive than the ELISA, due to the advanced technology and skill needed to perform it. The Western blot also has pitfalls. The criteria used for interpretation of this test are not standardized, which means that a degree of subjectivity is used in the final analysis. Western blot tests that are indeterminate need to be repeated (McMahon, 1988).

The ELISA and the Western blot tests are not necessarily definitive for the diagnosis of perinatally acquired HIV infection in infants. This is because of the placental transfer of immunoglobulin G to the fetal circulation and the fact that the routine tests cannot differentiate between maternal antibodies and those antibodies synthesized by the infant in response to the infection. The presence of anti-HIV IgG only verifies that the mother had HIV, and up to 15 months may be required for the maternal antibodies to dissipate from the infant's circulation. Beyond 15 months, a positive ELISA or Western blot is indicative of HIV infection.

Since the routine tests are limited in infants, an alternative approach is the repeated (longitudinal) collection of serum samples and batch assay to establish a rising anti-HIV antibody titer. The increasing titer is evidence of HIV infection. Johnson et al. demonstrated that up to 85% to 90% of infected infants will be detected by 6 months of age (Johnson, Nair, O'Neil, Alger, & Hines, 1989).

Another method to establish IgG synthesis against HIV is the demonstration of new antibody specifici-

Table 28-1. PEDIATRIC HUMAN IMMUNODEFICIENCY VIRUS (HIV) CLASSIFICATION*

	Clinical Categories			
Immunologic Categories	*N: No Signs/Symptoms*	*A: Mild Signs/Symptoms*	*B:† Moderate Signs/Symptoms*	*C:† Severe Signs/Symptoms*
1: No evidence of suppression	N1	A1	B1	C1
2: Evidence of moderate suppression	N2	A2	B2	C2
3: Severe suppression	N3	A3	B3	C3

*Children whose HIV infection status is not confirmed are classified by using the above grid with a letter E (for perinatally exposed) placed before the appropriate classification code (e.g., EN2).

†All clinical conditions in Category C and lymphoid interstitial pneumonitis are reportable to state and local health departments as acquired immunodeficiency syndrome (AIDS).

From Centers for Disease Control and Prevention (1994). 1994 revised classification system for human immunodeficiency virus infection in children less than 13 years of age. *Morbidity and Mortality Weekly Report, 43* (RR-12), 1–10.

ties against antigens of HIV by Western blot. Synthesis of new antigen-specific antibodies may be seen even with declining total anti-HIV antibody titer during the same period (Johnson, Nair, & Alexander, 1987).

The disadvantage of all tests that require assessment of the onset of IgG antibody synthesis is the length of time that longitudinal study requires. This delay diminishes the usefulness of such tests in the PICU, where rapid diagnosis is necessary. Another major disadvantage is that not all children synthesize IgG against HIV in the first 15 months of life. Therefore, lack of synthesis against HIV during the first 15 months cannot be the sole basis for diagnosis.

Detection of neonatal IgM against HIV is another possible test. Assessing for IgM against other infectious agents has been used to diagnose other congenital infections. Current tests for IgM against HIV are about 50% sensitive (Johnson et al., 1989). Even though detection of IgM will not mark all infected infants, it may be the only serologic marker in some. The specificity of tests using IgM response has been questioned because of the tendency to high false-positive results (Johnson & Vink, 1992). A reason for this is the high quantity of maternal IgG against HIV in infant serum that may block IgM binding. Also, IgM may bind nonspecifically. Techniques have been applied to remove IgG from serum, which enhances other isotype detection.

There are some indications that salivary IgA synthesis against HIV infection can be highly specific and diagnostic within the first few months of life (Pyun, Ochs, Dufford, Wedgewood, 1987). In addition, promising results have been obtained with study of the measurement of anti-HIV synthesis by B cells drawn from infant or cord blood, though further modification will be necessary before there can be widespread application (Pahwa, Chirmule, Leombruno, et al., 1989).

Tests Utilized in Research

There are tests utilized in HIV research that are not used in clinical practice. The first is the p24 antigen test. The p24 antigen is the core protein found inside HIV (Grady & Vogel, 1993). Initially, when a person becomes infected, p24 can be detected in the blood. The p24 antigen becomes nondetectable as the person develops antibodies and HIV enters its latent phase. When the virus becomes active again, the amount of p24 antigen in the blood becomes detectable (Farthing, 1991; Michael & Burke, 1991; Tindall, Imrie, Donovan, Penny, & Cooper, 1990). The p24 antigen test is not used routinely as a clinical marker of disease progression; however, it is sometimes performed to determine if HIV is active or latent. The sensitivity of p24 is only about 50% in children; and children with measurable p24 appear to have a poorer prognosis (Berkowitz, Berkowitz, & Johnson, 1992).

Polymerase chain reaction (PCR) is a procedure that examines the individual's genes within the DNA strand to detect the presence of HIV. PCR is extremely expensive. It may be used to detect HIV in HIV-negative individuals before they develop antibodies, to confirm a positive ELISA when an indeterminate Western blot is present, to isolate the exact strain of HIV, to screen newborns for HIV, or to follow viral burden over time (Grady & Vogel, 1993).

Viral cultures are another way to detect HIV. However, this is also very expensive and not performed in the clinical setting.

It is not uncommon for HIV antibody tests to be ordered and performed in the PICU. Anxiety can develop in the patient and/or parent due to a lack of understanding concerning the meaning of the test or the possibility that the test will be positive. Pretest and posttest counseling, therefore, is very important. It is essential for PICU nurses to understand these tests, be able to explain their meaning and purpose, and clarify the misconception that a positive HIV test equals AIDS.

AIDS-DEFINING ILLNESSES

A wide range of manifestations of HIV infection are present in children. There are generally two patterns of disease presentation: one that is associated with a rapidly progressive disease with a poorer prognosis, and the other associated with a slower process.

Table 28–2. CLINICAL MANIFESTATIONS OF PEDIATRIC HIV INFECTION

Nonspecific	Infectious Complications
Recurrent fever	Pyogenic infections
Failure to thrive*	Mycobacterial
Parotiditis	Tuberculosis
Diffuse lymphadenopathy	Atypical*
Hepatosplenomegaly	Candidal infections
Anorexia*	Tineal infections
Hyperviscosity	Viral infections
	Measles*
Organ System–Related Diseases	Cytomegalovirus*
	Hepatitis A, B, C
Progressive encephalopathy*	Herpes zoster virus
Peripheral neuropathy	Herpes simplex virus
Lymphoid interstitial	Epstein-Barr virus
pneumonia	*Pneumocystis carinii**
Cardiomyopathy*	*Toxoplasma gondii**
Arteriopathy*	Cryptosporidiosis
Hepatitis	Cryptococcal infections*
Chronic diarrhea/malabsorption	Malignancies*
Neuropathy/nephritis	Lymphomas, particularly non-
Hypertension	Hodgkin's type
Anemia/leukopenia/	
thrombocytopenia	
Endocrinopathies	
Dermatitis	

*Associated with a graver prognosis.
From Hoyt, L.G., & Oleske, J.M. (1992). The clinical spectrum of HIV infection in infants and children: An overview. In R. Yogev & E. Connor (Eds.). *Management of HIV infection in infants and children* (pp. 227–246). St. Louis: Mosby–Year Book.

However, regardless of the manifestation, once a child develops an AIDS-defining illness, the prognosis is poor.

AIDS-defining illness can be caused by viruses, fungi, parasites, bacteria, or cancers (CDC, 1992). One of these opportunists must be present for the diagnosis of AIDS to be used. All of the organisms that cause these illnesses are ubiquitous in nature. The person who is HIV-negative has the ability, through the normal immune system, to fight these opportunists. Unfortunately, the HIV-positive person's immune system loses the ability to keep these opportunists under control, through depletion of the T4 cells, leading to overwhelming infection.

The most common clinical manifestations of HIV infection in infants and children are listed in Table 28–2. The presenting signs and symptoms are often nonspecific and may include recurrent fevers, failure to thrive, diffuse lymphadenopathy, hepatosplenomegaly, and anorexia. These may be caused by chronic viral infection, malnutrition, and immunodeficiency.

The most common clinical manifestation early in the disease process is lymphadenopathy. This is often associated with hypergammaglobulinemia and splenomegaly. In addition, skin disorders, candidal dermatitis in particular, are common clinical manifestations.

There are several organ system–related diseases, including those related to the central and peripheral nervous system, lungs, heart, blood vessels, gastroin-

testinal tract, kidneys, immune system, hematologic system, endocrine system, and skin. Many of these are described in detail throughout the rest of this chapter.

ACUTE RESPIRATORY FAILURE (ARF)

Pulmonary complications leading to acute respiratory failure are the most common reason for admission of pediatric AIDS patients to the PICU. In fact, ARF is the leading cause of morbidity and mortality in these children. Notterman et al. report a mortality rate of 81% (Notterman, Greenwald, Di Maio-Hunter et al., 1990). Table 28–3 outlines the infectious and noninfectious pulmonary diseases that can occur in HIV-infected children.

Pneumonias caused by *Pneumocystis carinii* pneumonia (PCP), respiratory syncytial virus (RSV), cytomegalovirus (CMV), *Mycobacterium avium–intracellulare, Pseudomonas aeruginosa, Candida albicans, Haemophilus influenzae, Streptococcus aureus, Klebsiella,* and lymphoid interstitial pneumonitis (LIP) have all been reported as reasons for ARF. Of these, PCP and LIP are by far the most common. Respiratory failure secondary to overwhelming bacterial sepsis has also been identified (Vernon et al., 1988).

Table 28–3. PULMONARY DISEASES IN CHILDREN WITH AIDS

Infectious	
1. Parasitic	*Pneumocystis carinii, Toxoplasma gondii, Strongyloides stercoralis*
2. Viral	Respiratory viruses: respiratory syncytial virus, influenza virus, parainfluenza virus, adenovirus
	Measles
	Opportunists: cytomegalovirus, herpes simplex, varicella zoster virus
3. Bacterial	*Streptococcus pneumoniae, Haemophilus influenzae, Staphylococcus aureus*
	Nosocomial: enteric bacilli, *Pseudomonas aeruginosa*
	Actinomycetes: *Nocardia* species
	Mycobacterial: *M. tuberculosis, M. avium–intracellulare*
4. Fungal	*Cryptococcus neoformans, Histoplasma capsulatum, Coccidioides immitis, Candida* sp., *Aspergillus* sp.
Noninfectious	
1. Lymphoid diseases	Pulmonary lymphoid hyperplasia Lymphocytic interstitial pneumonia Polyclonal polymorphic B cell lymphoproliferative disorder
2. Bronchiectasis	
3. Kaposi's sarcoma	

From Berkowitz, I. D., Berkowitz, F. E., & Johnson, J. P. (1992). The critically ill child and human immunodeficiency virus. In M. C. Rogers (Ed.). *Textbook of pediatric intensive care* (pp. 953–975). Baltimore: Williams & Wilkins.

Pneumocystis carinii Pneumonia (PCP)

PCP is the most common opportunistic infection in children with HIV infection and has affected approximately 39% of children with AIDS (Scott & Mastrucci, 1992). The incidence of PCP varies with age at diagnosis: in a national survey, it was reported that 54% of children less than 1 year of age had PCP; 18% between the ages of 1 and 4 years had PCP; and that in the 5- to 12-year age group, 16% were diagnosed as having PCP. In addition to this, a correlation between age at diagnosis and prognosis may be suggested: children less than 1 year of age diagnosed with PCP have a poorer prognosis for survival (Falloon, Eddy, Wiener, & Pizzo, 1989).

Etiology and Pathogenesis

P. carinii is considered either a protozoan parasite or a fungus, which exists as a cyst that contains eight intracystic bodies (Berkowitz, Berkowitz, Johnson, 1992). These bodies are released from the cysts and form new cysts, which then attach to type I alveolar cells. As a result, alveolitis and interstitial edema develop. The consequence of this is ventilation-perfusion mismatch, decreased pulmonary compliance, hypoxia, and an increased A-a gradient (Berkowitz, Berkowitz, Johnson, 1992).

Clinical Manifestations

The clinical course of PCP is highly variable, ranging from the acute onset of fever and marked respiratory distress to a more insidious onset with a subacute course. The presenting signs are often nonspecific and include fever, cough, tachypnea, and hypoxemia. Chest auscultation may be normal even with the presence of tachypnea and clinical evidence of respiratory distress. Early in the course, the chest radiograph may also be normal. As roentgenographic findings develop, a diffuse bilateral interstitial pattern is most often seen.

Guidelines for prophylaxis against PCP for children infected with or perinatally exposed to HIV exist (CDC, 1995b). Prophylaxis is determined by the child's CD4+ count, CD4+ percent, and age. Trimethoprim-sulfamethoxazole remains the drug of choice for prophylaxis. Alternative regimens include the use of Dapsone or aerosolized pentamidine (CDC, 1995b).

Diagnosis

PCP may be diagnosed with noninvasive or invasive techniques. Analysis of sputum, endotracheal secretions, and gastric washings may show evidence of the organism and is attempted first. Other methods may include bronchoalveolar lavage, transbronchial biopsy, or open lung biopsy (Broaddus et al., 1985). Open lung biopsy is reserved for children in whom other methods have not provided a diagnosis.

The latter three are the most reliable methods for diagnosis (Tribett, 1993).

Critical Care Management

Management of the child with PCP includes oxygen therapy, mechanical ventilation, positive end-expiratory pressure (PEEP), antibiotic therapy, and steroids.

The standard antibiotic therapy for PCP is the administration of trimethoprim/sulfamethoxazole (TMP-SMX) or pentamidine isethionate. TMP-SMX is given orally or intravenously at 20 mg/kg/day, with the initial administration being intravenous. Oral administration can begin once improvement has taken place. Because many patients become neutropenic when treated daily with TMP/SMX, administration three times a week may be used; this appears equally effective and causes less neutropenia (Wasserman, 1990). Therapy is recommended to continue for 21 days.

Intravenous pentamidine is instituted when no response to TMP/SMX is seen. Aerosol pentamidine, although effective in adults with less severe cases of PCP, is of limited use in children because of uneven delivery of the drug to the smaller airways (Hauger & Powell, 1990). The recommended dose is 4 mg/kg/day given in a single dose for 14 to 21 days. The drug is administered by slow intravenous infusion, since hypotension may result if administered rapidly. Side effects that may result with use of pentamidine are hypoglycemia, hyperglycemia, neutropenia, thrombocytopenia, and azotemia. Table 28–4 lists the dosage and side effects of these drugs.

Lymphoid Interstitial Pneumonitis (LIP)

Lymphoid interstitial pneumonitis is a common symptom of pulmonary involvement in children with HIV infection. The incidence of LIP, like PCP, varies with age. In children less than 1 year of age, approximately 18% were diagnosed with LIP. Children 1 to 4 years showed an incidence of approximately 36%, while children 5 to 12 years of age showed an incidence of about 29% (Caldwell & Rogers, 1991).

Etiology and Pathogenesis

Most children who develop lymphoid disease of the lung acquired HIV infection through perinatal transmission (Berkowitz, Berkowitz, Johnson, 1992). LIP is identified by diffuse interstitial infiltration of the alveolar septa with lymphocytes and plasma cells (Joshi, 1991). This results in restrictive lung disease with hypoxia and hypercapnia.

Clinical Manifestations

Most children who present with LIP exhibit their symptoms after the first year of life with an insidious onset of tachypnea, coughing, and wheezing. Other

Table 28–4. ANTIBIOTIC THERAPY FOR *PNEUMOCYSTIS CARINII* PNEUMONIA (PCP)

Drug	Dosage	Side Effects/Precautions
TMP/SMX	Severe infections and PCP: 20 mg/kg/ 24 hours divided every 6–8 hours	May cause kernicterus in newborns, blood dyscrasias, crystalluria, glossitis, renal or hepatic injury, GI irritation, allergy, or hemolysis in G-6-PD Reduce dose in renal impairment
Pentamidine	4 mg/kg/day	Risks of therapy >12–14 days is not well defined May cause hypoglycemia, transient hypotension, tachycardia, nausea, vomiting, mild hepatotoxicity, megaloblastic anemia and granulocytopenia, hypocalcemia, renal toxicity Infuse over minimum of 1 hour to reduce risk of hypotension

From Johnson, K.B. (Ed.). (1993). *Harriet Lane handbook* (p. 363). St. Louis: Mosby–Year Book.

symptoms include progressive bilateral diffuse infiltrates resulting in symptomatic hypoxemia, generalized lymphadenopathy, hepatosplenomegaly, salivary gland enlargement, and digital clubbing (Stewart, 1989).

Diagnosis

Clinical and x-ray findings may lead to a presumptive diagnosis. However, the definitive diagnosis is made by lung biopsy, in which the specimen shows the typical lymphocytic infiltrates.

Critical Care Management

Management of the child with LIP is mostly supportive because there is no specific therapy. Oxygen and bronchodilators may be helpful. As the disease progresses and the child chronically has a PaO_2 of less than 65 mmHg on room air, corticosteroids may be considered (Scott & Mastrucci, 1992). Prednisone may be started at 2 mg/kg/day and is given orally for 2 to 4 weeks until oxygen saturation improves. The dose is then tapered over the next several weeks to 0.5 mg/kg/day (Scott & Mastrucci, 1992).

Upon arrival of the child with HIV infection to the PICU, nursing assessment would be consistent for any child with impending ARF.

Although ventilatory management is similar to that for any child in ARF, it should be noted that many HIV children in ARF require higher levels of PEEP to maintain acceptable oxygenation. Suctioning should be performed carefully and only when necessary through a swivel-type connector, with hyperoxygenation being accomplished by increasing the FIO_2 on the ventilator.

Tuberculosis

Tuberculosis is common in adult patients with AIDS. It is less common in the child with AIDS, with little information on the incidence and clinical characteristics. Nonimmunocompromised children who develop primary tuberculosis demonstrate lymph node enlargement in the hilar, mediastinal, and cervical areas; along with pulmonary infiltrates with consolidation, atelectasis, pleural effusion, and tuberculous meningitis (Stamos & Rowley, 1995). The clinical manifestations in HIV-infected children are usually nonspecific and include fever, weight loss, and cough. On chest x-ray, localized patchy infiltrates and hilar lymphadenopathy are seen. Due to the immunosuppression that accompanies the disease, skin testing alone is not conclusive for diagnosis of tuberculosis. Cerebrospinal fluid and blood cultures, in addition to gastric and bronchial washings, need to be obtained.

The initial treatment includes four drugs. Isoniazid, rifampin, pyrazinamide and ethambutol or streptomycin are recommended while awaiting susceptibility results. In the case of disseminated disease, a bactericidal agent may be used. The duration of therapy ranges from 6 to 9 months, decided by infection site, response to therapy, and the sensitivity of the organism. A 12 month duration of therapy is recommended for those children with miliary tuberculosis, bone and joint tuberculosis, or tuberculosis meningitis (CDC, 1994c).

Infection control is a critical nursing concern in caring for children with HIV infection and tuberculosis. Children with cavitary lesions, endobronchial tuberculosis, or positive gastric washing or sputum cultures are placed on respiratory isolation (Burroughs & Edelson, 1991). Family members should wear a mask during visits, and careful monitoring of the infection status of these children is necessary.

DECREASED CARDIAC OUTPUT

It is now known that cardiac disease in children with HIV infection may be common, extensive, and clinically significant. It has been suggested that approximately 20% of HIV-infected children will have some type of cardiac complication, the two most common being cardiovascular failure secondary to septic shock and cardiomyopathy (Stewart, 1989).

Septic Shock

Septic shock is the primary cardiovascular etiology for PICU admission of HIV-infected children. Serious bacterial infections frequently occur in children with AIDS. *Streptococcus pneumoniae; Salmonella, Pseu-*

domonas, and *Enterobacter* species; *Haemophilus influenzae*; *Enterococcus*; *Staphylococcus aureus* and *S. epidermidis*; and *Escherichia coli* have all been identified as causative pathogens.

Cardiomyopathy

Cardiomyopathy is the second most frequent cardiac PICU presentation of children with AIDS. Although the degree of cardiac dysfunction may be difficult to determine because of multi-organ involvement, autopsy findings of these children have shown biventricular dilatation, myocardial hypertrophy, interstitial fibrosis, myocardial necrosis, and endocardial thickening (Joshi, Gadol, Connor et al., 1988). Conduction disturbances secondary to vasculitis, myocarditis, or fibrosis have also been described (Bharati, Joshi, Connor et al., 1989).

Etiology and Pathogenesis

The etiology of HIV-associated cardiomyopathy is unknown. It is suggested the cause has many factors, including HIV infection, infection with other agents, an abnormal host response, and drug toxicity (Kavanaugh-McHugh, Ruff, Rowes, Herskowitz, & Modlin, 1991). Despite the autopsy findings, the pathogenesis of this dilated cardiomyopathy has yet to be fully explained. The virus itself may cause myocardial damage by releasing mediator-infected monocytes, or the host immune system may play a role by producing an autoimmune response (Vogel, 1992).

Clinical Manifestations

Congestive heart failure is the predominant clinical manifestation of later stage cardiac involvement, though it may be difficult to diagnose in the HIV-infected child. Tachypnea and rales may be secondary to pulmonary disease/insufficiency, tachycardia may be due to fever and/or anemia, and hepatosplenomegaly is typically present in many children with HIV infection. Therefore, these symptoms cannot be relied upon as specific of congestive heart failure. From the experience gained at several institutions, the most reliable clinical indicators of congestive heart failure in these children are the presence of a gallop rhythm associated with tachypnea and tachycardia, and cardiomegaly on chest x-ray (Castello & Pena, 1990; Stewart et al., 1989).

Cardiac dysrhythmias have been reported in HIV-infected children, although the occurrence is uncommon and nonspecific. Isolated incidences of ventricular and atrial ectopy have been reported (Lipschultz, Chanock, Sanders, Colan, Perez-Atayde, & McIntosh, 1989).

Although there are not echocardiographic findings specific for HIV infection, this procedure does reveal information about cardiac anatomy, pump function, valvular dysfunction, and the presence of pericardial effusions. These findings, however, have not been shown to be predictive of the severity of the cardiac manifestations of HIV infection.

Critical Care Management

Nursing care for the HIV-infected child is the same as for any child exhibiting low cardiac output secondary to septic shock or cardiomyopathy and would include inotropic support, afterload reduction, and appropriate antimicrobial therapy. Treatment of congestive heart failure secondary to cardiomyopathy is directed at preload reduction and the administration of digoxin for diminished pump function.

CENTRAL NERVOUS SYSTEM DYSFUNCTION

Central nervous system dysfunction in the HIV-positive child may be caused by secondary infection by usual or opportunistic pathogens as well as by primary HIV infection of the brain. The primary neurologic manifestation of HIV infection of the brain is HIV encephalopathy and is present in more than 50% of HIV-infected children (Berkowitz, Berkowitz, & Johnson, 1992). This can present as a rapid course of deterioration or may be static.

Children can present with static encephalopathy, demonstrated by an inability to achieve developmental milestones in some or all areas (Belman, 1992). Also, progressive encephalopathy has been reported in children. It has been described as either a loss of developmental milestones or intellectual deficits, associated with impaired brain growth; weakness with bilateral pyramidal tract signs, ataxia, and, less commonly, seizures; and coma (Belman, 1992; Caldwell & Rogers, 1991). In a study performed by Epstein et al., the most common CT scan finding was cerebral atrophy, with secondary enlargement of the subarachnoid spaces and ventricles (Epstein, Sharer, Oleske et al., 1986). The damage to the central nervous system is believed to be caused by the direct effect of the virus in the brain tissue. Progressive encephalopathy develops and worsens proportionally to the increasing immunodeficiency (Mintz, Rapaport, Oleske et al., 1989).

Although these children are rarely admitted to the critical care unit for a neurologic problem, an awareness of the developmental level of the child by the nurse is critical to keep explanations at an age-appropriate level, to provide for the psychosocial needs of the child, and to ensure that proper referrals are made for rehabilitation. Developmental delay is a common factor in children with HIV infection. The predominant features are a pattern of developmental delay in infancy with progressive impairment in the older child. The most pronounced areas of delay are in fine and gross motor skills and in speech.

The most common neurologic diagnoses that necessitate admission of the HIV-infected child to the PICU are central nervous system infection, lymphoma, and strokes.

Children may develop bacterial meningitis associated with usual pathogens such as *H. influenzae, S. pneumoniae,* and *Neisseria meningitidis* as well as various gram-negative bacilli. Meningitis and encephalitis may also result from infection by numerous viral pathogens. Other CNS infections include mycobacterial and fungal meningitis (Wilkinson & Greenwald, 1988).

Primary central nervous system lymphomas are the most common intracranial mass lesions that develop in children with HIV, though they are relatively rare. The symptoms usually seen are seizure activity, mental status changes, and neurologic deficits.

Strokes are an infrequent complication of AIDS but very devastating when they do occur. They may result from the inflammation of the cerebral blood vessels, causing an ischemic infarction, or they may result from cerebral hemorrhage. Bleeding is usually the consequence of autoimmune thrombocytopenia (Mintz, 1992).

HEMATOLOGIC DYSFUNCTION

Hematologic manifestations related to HIV infection include autoimmune thrombocytopenia, anemia, leukopenia, granulocytopenia, and lymphomas (Wasserman, 1990). Primary bone marrow failure also occurs in some children (Wilkinson & Greenwald, 1988).

Thrombocytopenia may be an early manifestation of HIV infection. B cell dysfunction is postulated to lead to the production of autoantibodies and immune complexes, resulting in peripheral platelet destruction (Warrier & Lusher, 1992). Therapies to treat thrombocytopenia in the HIV-infected child include corticosteroids, splenectomy, danazol, vincristine, and intravenous IgG (Warrier & Lusher, 1992).

Anemia is a prominent diagnosis of HIV disease. Although the anemia is generally mild and nonprogressive, in a child with multiple opportunistic infections this may be significant. There may be many factors that cause anemia, one being that the virus may infect erythroid precursors in the bone marrow, inhibit the production of red cells, and cause sequestration of the red cells in the spleen and liver (Warrier & Lusher, 1992). Zidovudine (AZT) may also cause anemia.

HIV-infected patients with anemia who are symptomatic are recommended to receive transfusion of irradiated packed RBCs. Also, granulocyte colony-stimulating factor (G-CSF) with erythropoietin for children with zidovudine toxicity has been found to be effective in correcting anemia (Warrier & Lusher, 1992). Further information regarding red blood cell and platelet disorders is found in Chapter 26.

Leukopenia occurs frequently in children with HIV infection, often in combination with anemia. Granulocytopenia can also occur and is usually accompanied by a left shift. Causes are probably multifactorial, including immune dysfunction that results in hypogammaglobulinemia, and production of auto-

antibodies and immune complexes. Antibodies against granulocytes have also been observed. The primary method of treatment of HIV-associated leukopenia and granulocytopenia is the use of granulocyte growth factors. Both recombinant granulocyte-macrophage colony-stimulating factor (GM-CSF) and G-CSF have been found to be effective.

Malignancies, such as non-Hodgkin's lymphoma, have been reported in HIV-infected children. These tumors are almost always of B cell origin. Also, primary CNS lymphoma has been reported in children with perinatally acquired infection. Short-term chemotherapy is usually the treatment of choice, since most of these children will not tolerate the immunosuppressive effects of long-term chemotherapy (Warrier & Lusher, 1992).

OTHER ORGAN DYSFUNCTION

Abnormalities of all organ systems can be seen in HIV-infected children, whether induced by the HIV infection itself or by opportunistic infections. Hepatitis is commonly seen without an easily documented infectious cause. Pancreatitis with elevated serum amylase and lipase levels has also been seen in HIV-infected children. An HIV-associated renal disease with azotemia and proteinuria has also been described in children (Falloon, Eddy, Wiener, & Pizzo, 1989). As many as 30% of HIV-infected children may develop one of several forms of renal disease (Berkowitz, Berkowitz, Johnson, 1992).

ANTIRETROVIRAL THERAPY

Drug therapy begins when an individual's T4 cell count drops below 500/mm^3 and remains at that level (Bartlett, 1994). The first-line drug for HIV disease is zidovudine (AZT, Retrovir). AZT is a reverse transcriptase inhibitor. Reverse transcriptase is needed to convert viral RNA into DNA before it can become incorporated into the host DNA. Some individuals who take AZT continue to progress along the HIV continuum with the development of opportunistic illnesses despite AZT therapy. This may be due, in part, to drug resistance (Lifson, Hessol, & Rutherford, 1992). However, current data support that early AZT therapy slows down the progression to AIDS and prolongs survival in those individuals who have already been diagnosed with AIDS (Kozal & Merigan, 1994).

AZT has both short- and long-term side effects. Short-term side effects include nausea, headache, insomnia, myalgia, and vomiting. All of these usually resolve if the individual continues with therapy. The major long-term side effect is bone marrow suppression with anemia. If this occurs, the dose of AZT is decreased (Bartlett, 1994). Transfusions may be necessary if the individual's hematocrit continues to decline. Monitoring of patients on AZT includes a complete blood count (CBC) at the initiation of therapy, every 2 weeks for 1 month, every month for 3 months, then every 3 months if values are normal.

Didanosine (ddI) (trade name, Videx) is the second drug used to slow the progression of HIV disease. This drug was approved by the Federal Drug Administration (FDA) in 1991. Didanosine is indicated in those individuals who do not tolerate AZT, who have significant clinical or immunologic deterioration on AZT, or who have decreased bone marrow reserve (Volberding, 1994; Kahn, Lagakos, Richman et al., 1992). Like AZT, ddI is a reverse transcriptase inhibitor; however, it does not appear to possess the bone marrow suppression that AZT may stimulate (Anastasi & Rivera, 1991). It does have side effects, which include peripheral neuropathy, pancreatitis (which is the most frequent reason for discontinuation), hyperuricemia, confusion, and hepatotoxicity (Anastasi & Rivera, 1991; Bartlett, 1994).

Dideoxycytidine (ddC) (trade name, Zalcitabine) is a newer antiviral that may promise greater efficacy with less toxic effects than AZT. Currently, multicenter trials are underway to evaluate the use of ddC for children who do not respond to or cannot tolerate zidovudine. Initial studies have shown evidence of antiretroviral activity without hematologic toxicity (Pizzo, Butler, Balis et al., 1990). The most common side effect is peripheral neuropathy, which is usually dose related and reversible. Other "less frequent" side effects include arthralgia, myalgia, ulcers, headache, abdominal pain, allergic reactions, diarrhea, and nausea (Unguarski, 1993). Alternating treatment with zidovudine and ddC may augment antiretroviral activity of both drugs while decreasing toxic effects. ddC has been approved for combination therapy with zidovudine, but not for monotherapy use (Kozal & Merigan, 1994; Unguarski, 1993).

PSYCHOSOCIAL ISSUES

As previously stated, developmental delays are a common occurrence in the child with HIV infection. Nursing care involves assessment of the child's developmental level and gearing communication at that level. In addition, some children may present with depressive symptoms such as apathy, social withdrawal, or anorexia (Spiegel & Mayers, 1991). These symptoms are often an indication of other issues, and a psychotherapist should be consulted. Nurses caring for the child may also need to consider that the child may have lost a parent to the same disease. Excellent communication skills and support will be necessary.

A diagnosis of HIV infection also has a major impact on the family. Frequently, the child may be diagnosed before the parent. The psychosocial stress that the diagnosis of HIV places on the family is unique in that, in most cases, the child and parent are both ill (Spiegel & Mayers, 1991). Problems that must be faced include (1) coping with the diagnosis of a potentially fatal illness; (2) dealing with the healthcare of the child; (3) approaching the emotional, financial, and time-demanding aspects of a sick child;

and (4) facing potential ostracism from family members and the community (Falloon, Eddy, Wiener, & Pizzo, 1989).

Working with these families often poses a major challenge for the PICU nurse. The sight of the ICU to a parent who is also infected may be overwhelming, since it may represent to the parent his or her future (Czarniecki & Dillman, 1992). Parents may blame themselves and have difficulty even visiting their child.

Many parents are also dealing with the problem of substance abuse. Working with these families may be especially difficult for the nursing staff. Open communication, establishment of a relationship, and referral to appropriate resources are critical to family-centered care of the child.

EFFECTS ON PICU RESOURCES

It is difficult to estimate the amount of resources spent on caring for the pediatric HIV-infected patient in the critical care unit. Results from an ongoing study at the New York Hospital–Cornell Medical Center showed that infants and children with AIDS composed 4 per cent of all PICU admissions for the period July 1986 through October 1987, but accounted for 6.7% of PICU patient days and used nearly 12% of available PICU resources for the same period (Wilkinson & Greenwald, 1988). Studies have shown that pediatric HIV-infected patients have longer durations of hospitalization than do other HIV-positive subgroups, with the exception of intravenous drug users. Some of the proposed reasons include loss of home care secondary to parents who are also incapacitated or who have died of AIDS and the difficulty in obtaining alternative care settings (Wilkinson & Greenwald, 1988). At present, data collection continues in an attempt to determine the dollar value attached to the PICU care of pediatric AIDS patients.

EFFECTS ON THE PICU NURSING STAFF

Previously, ICUs were reserved for patients who had some hope for improvement or cure. Caring for children in critical care units with a disease that is incurable is stressful on staff. The clinical conditions associated with admission to PICUs demand the utmost in staff efforts and sophisticated technology. The staff's awareness that these efforts are on behalf of a child with a futile illness can cause feelings of failure, low professional self-esteem, and depression, and can lead to the development of burnout (Wilkinson & Greenwald, 1988). The staff members need to be supported through times of frustration and need to be allowed to vent their feelings in private.

Lastly, the PICU staff members face the natural fear of acquiring HIV infection in the course of caring for infected children. Educational updates regarding HIV disease and consistent enforcement of universal precautions with all patients is the rational response to these fears. Due to the nature of procedures performed in the PICU, a thorough understanding of and compliance with universal precautions are mandatory.

SUMMARY

HIV disease attacks and destroys an individual's immune system through depletion of the T4 lymphocytes. The decreased number of T4 cells allows ubiquitous organisms to cause massive and life-threatening infections in the compromised host. There is a list of organisms that, when present, allow the diagnosis of AIDS to be made in the HIV-positive individual. Pediatric critical care nurses can deliver care more effectively when the pathophysiologic process of their patient is understood. With a clearer understanding of the chronicity of HIV disease, pediatric critical care nurses can provide hope and support to HIV-infected children and their parents, thus assisting them in achieving and maintaining quality of life.

References

Anastasi, J. K., & Rivera, J. L. (1991). Nursing considerations in administering ddI and ddC. *AIDS Patient Care,* 5 (1), 9–12.

Barrick, B. (1990). Light at the end of a decade. *American Journal of Nursing,* 90 (11), 37–40.

Bartlett, J. (1994). Medical Management of HIV Infection. Coleview, IL: Physicians & Scientists Publishing Co.

Bastin, N., Tamayo, O. W., Tinkle, M. B., Amaya, M. A., Trejo, L. R., & Herrera, C. (1992). HIV disease and pregnancy. Part 3. Postpartum care of the HIV-positive woman and her newborn. *Journal of Obstetric, Gynecologic, and Neonatal Nursing,* 21 (2), 105–111.

Belman, A. L. (1992). Acquired immunodeficiency syndrome and the child's central nervous system. Pediatric Neurology, 39 (4), 691–714.

Berkowitz, I. D., Berkowitz, F. E., and Johnson, J. P. (1992). The critically ill child and human immunodeficiency virus. In M. C. Rogers (Ed.). *Textbook of pediatric intensive care* (pp. 953–975). Baltimore: Williams & Wilkins.

Bharati, S., Joshi, V. V., Connor, E. M., et al. (1989). Conduction system in children with acquired immunodeficiency syndrome. *Chest,* 96 (2), 406–413.

Boland, M., & Czarniecki, L. (1995). Nursing care of the child. In J. H. Flaskerud & P. J. Unguarski (Eds.). HIV/AIDS: A Guide to Nursing Care, 3rd ed. (pp. 185–219). Philadelphia: W.B. Saunders.

Broaddus, C., et al. (1985). Bronchoalveolar lavage and transbronchial biopsy for the diagnosis of pulmonary infections in the acquired immunodeficiency syndrome. *Annals of Internal Medicine,* 102, 747–752.

Burroughs, M. H., & Edelson, P. J. (1991). Medical care of the HIV-infected child. *Pediatric Clinics of North America,* 38 (1), 45–67.

Caldwell, M. B., & Rogers, M. F. (1991). Epidemiology of pediatric HIV infection. *Pediatric Clinics of North America,* 38 (1), 1–16.

Castello, F. V., & Pena, R. M. (1990). Adult respiratory distress syndrome (ARDS) in children with AIDS. *Critical Care Medicine,* 18 (4), s232.

Centers for Disease Control and Prevention (1995a). HIV-AIDS Surveillance Report. US HIV and AIDS Cases Reported through June, 1995. Mid-Year Edition, 7 (1), 1–34.

Centers for Disease Control and Prevention (1995b). 1995 revised guidelines for prophylaxis against *Pneumocystis carinii* pneumonia for children infected with or perinatally exposed to human immunodeficiency virus. *Morbidity & Mortality Weekly Report,* 44 (RR-4), 1–11.

Centers for Disease Control and Prevention (1994a). Zidovudine for the prevention of HIV transmission from mother to infant. *Morbidity and Mortality Weekly Report,* 43 (16), 285–287.

Centers for Disease Control and Prevention (1994b). 1994 revised classification system for human immunodeficiency virus infection in children less than 13 years of age. *Morbidity & Mortality Weekly Report,* 43 (RR-12), 1–10.

Centers for Disease Control and Prevention (1994c). Core Curriculum on Tuberculosis: What the Clinician Should Know, 3rd ed. Atlanta: CDC.

Centers for Disease Control (1993). HIV/AIDS surveillance report. First quarter edition. 5 (1), 1–19.

Centers for Disease Control (1992). 1993 revised classification system for HIV infection and expanded surveillance case definition for AIDS among adolescents and adults. *Morbidity and Mortality Weekly Report,* 41 (RR-17), 1–10.

Centers for Disease Control (1987). Recommendations for prevention of HIV transmission in health-care settings. *Morbidity and Mortality Weekly Report,* 36 (2S), 3S–18S.

Czarniecki, L., & Dillman, P. (1992). Pediatric HIV/AIDS. *Critical Care Nursing Clinics of North America,* 4 (3), 447–456.

Ellerbrook, T. V., Bush, T. J., Chamberland, M. E., & Oxtoby, M. T. (1991). Epidemiology of women with AIDS in the United States, 1981 through 1990. *Journal of the American Medical Association,* 265 (22), 2971–2975.

Epstein, L. G., Sharer, L. R., Oleske, J. M., et al. (1986). Neurologic manifestations of human immunodeficiency virus in children. *Pediatrics,* 78 (4), 678–687.

Falloon, J., Eddy, J., Wiener, L., & Pizzo, P. A. (1989). Human immunodeficiency virus infection in children. *Journal of Pediatrics,* 114 (1), 1–30.

Farthing, C. (1991). AIDS: A historical overview. *Dermatologic Clinics of North America,* 9 (3), 391–396.

Flaskerud, J. H. (1995). Health promotion and disease prevention. In J. H. Flaskerud & P. J. Unguarski (Eds.). HIV/AIDS: A Guide to Nursing Care, 3rd ed. (pp. 30–63). Philadelphia: W.B. Saunders.

Friedman-Kien, A. E. (1981). Disseminated Kaposi's sarcoma syndrome in young homosexual men. *Journal of the American Academy of Dermatology,* 5, 468–471.

Gayle, H. B., & D'Angelo, J. (1990). The epidemiology of AIDS and HIV infection in adolescents. In P. A. Pizzo & C. M. Wilfert (Eds). *Pediatric AIDS. The challenge of HIV infection in infants, children and adolescents* (pp. 38–52). Baltimore: Williams & Wilkins.

Gottlieb, M. S., Schroff, R., Schanker, H. M., Weisman, J. D., Fan, P. T., Woolf, R. A., & Saxon, A. (1981). *Pneumocystis carinii* pneumonia and mucosal candidiasis in previously healthy homosexual men: Evidence of a new acquired cellular immunodeficiency. *New England Journal of Medicine,* 305 (24), 1425–1431.

Grady, C. (1989). The immune system and AIDS/HIV infection. In J. H. Flaskerud (Ed.). *AIDS/HIV infection: A reference guide for nursing professionals* (pp. 37–57). Philadelphia: W.B. Saunders.

Grady, C., & Vogel, S. (1993). Laboratory methods for diagnosing and monitoring HIV infection. *Journal of the Association of Nurses in AIDS Care,* 4 (2), 11–21.

Hauger, S. B., & Powell, K. R. (1990). Infectious complications in children with HIV infection. *Pediatric Annals,* 19 (71), 422–433.

Johnson, J. P., Nair, P., O'Neil, K. M., Alger, L., & Hines, S. E. (1989). HIV infection in infants: Natural history and serologic diagnosis of children. *American Journal of the Diseases of Children,* 143, 1147–1153.

Johnson, J. P., & Vink, P. E. (1992). Diagnosis and classification of HIV infection in children. In R. Yogev & E. Connor (Eds.), *Management of HIV Infection in Infants and Children* (pp. 117–128). St. Louis: Mosby–Year Book.

Johnson, J. P., Nair, P., & Alexander, S. (1987). Early diagnosis of HIV infection in the neonate. *New England Journal of Medicine,* 316, 273–274.

Joshi, V. (1991). Pathology of children with AIDS. *Pediatric Clinics of North America,* 38 (1), 97–120.

Joshi, V. V., Gadol, C., Connor, E., et al. (1988). Dilated cardiomyopathy in children with acquired immunodeficiency syndrome. *Human Pathology, 19,* 69–73.

Kahn, J. O., Lagakos, S. W., Richman, D. D., et al. (1992). The NIAID AIDS Clinical Trials Group. A controlled trial comparing continued zidovudine with didanosine in human immunodeficiency virus infection. *New England Journal of Medicine, 327* (9), 581–587.

Kavanaugh-McHugh, A., Ruff, A. J., Rowes, A., Herskowitz, A., & Modlin, J. F. (1991). The challenge of HIV infection in infants, children, and adolescents. In P. A. Pizzo & C. M. Wilfert (Eds.), *Pediatric AIDS* (pp. 355–372). Baltimore: Williams & Wilkins.

Kozal, M. J., & Merigan, T. C. (1994). Therapy of HIV-1 infection. *Current Opinion in Infectious Diseases, 7* (1), 72–81.

Levy, J. A. (1990). Features of HIV and the host response that influence progression of disease. In M. A. Sande & P. A. Volberding (Eds.). *The medical management of AIDS* (2nd ed., pp. 23–37). Philadelphia: W.B. Saunders.

Lifson, A. R., Hessol, N. A., & Rutherford, G. W. (1992). Progression and clinical outcome of infection due to human immunodeficiency virus. *Clinical Infectious Disease, 4,* 966–972.

Lipschultz, S. E., Chanock, S., Sanders, S. P., Colan, S. D., Perez-Atayde, A., & McIntosh, K. (1989). Cardiovascular manifestations of human immunodeficiency virus infection in infants and children. *The American Journal of Cardiology, 63,* 1489–1497.

McMahon, K. M. (1988). The integration of HIV testing and counseling into nursing practice. *Nursing Clinics of North America, 23* (4), 803–821.

Mendez, H. (1992). Natural history and prognostic factors. In R. Yogev & E. Connor (Eds.). *Management of HIV infection in infants, children and adolescents* (pp. 89–106). St. Louis: Mosby–Year Book.

Michael, N. L., & Burke, D. S. (1991). Natural history of human immunodeficiency virus infection. *Dermatologic Clinics of North America, 9* (3), 429–441.

Mintz, M. (1992). Neurologic abnormalities. In R. Yogev & E. Connor (Eds.). *Management of HIV infection in infants and children* (pp. 247–285). St. Louis: Mosby–Year Book.

Mintz, M., Rapaport, R., Oleske, J. M., et al. (1989). Elevated serum levels of tumor necrosis factor are associated with progressive encephalopathy in children with acquired immunodeficiency syndrome. *American Journal of the Diseases of Children, 143,* 771.

Newman, C. L., & Quinn, T. C. (1988). Acquired immunodeficiency syndrome. In A. M. Harvey, R. J. Johns, V. A. McKusick, A. H. Owens, & R. S. Ross (Eds.). *The principles and practice of medicine* (22nd ed.). Norwalk, CT: Appleton & Lange.

Notterman, D. A., Greenwald, B. M., Di Maio-Hunter, A., Wilkinson, J. D., Krasinski, K., & Borkowsky, W. (1990). Outcome after assisted ventilation in children with acquired immunodeficiency syndrome. *Critical Care Medicine, 18* (1), 18–20.

Pahwa, S., Chirmule, N., Leombruno, C., et al. (1989). In vitro synthesis of human immunodeficiency virus–specific antibodies in peripheral blood lymphocytes of infants. *Proceedings of the National Academy of Sciences, 86,* 7532–7536.

Pizzo, P. A., Butler, K., Balis, F., et al. (1990). Dideoxycytidine alone and in an alternating schedule with zidovudine in children with symptomatic human immunodeficiency virus infection. *Journal of Pediatrics, 117,* 799–808.

Pyun, K. H., Ochs, H., Dufford, M. T. W., & Wedgewood, R. J. (1987). Perinatal infection with human immunodeficiency virus: Specific antibody response by the neonate. *New England Journal of Medicine, 317,* 611–614.

Robins, E. V. (1989). Immunosuppression of the burned patient. *Critical Care Nursing Clinics of North America, 1* (4), 767–774.

Scott, G. B., & Mastrucci, M. T. (1992). Pulmonary complications of HIV-1 infection in children. In R. Yogev & E. Connor (Eds.). *Management of HIV Infection in Infants and Children* (pp. 323–356). St. Louis: Mosby–Year Book.

Smeltzer, S. C., & Whipple, B. (1991). Women and HIV infection. *Image: Journal of Nursing Scholarship, 23* (4), 249–256.

Spiegel, L., & Mayers, A. (1991). Psychosocial aspects of AIDS in children and adolescents. *Pediatric Clinics of North America, 38* (1), 153–167.

Stamos, J. K., & Rowley, A. H. (1995). Pediatric Tuberculosis: An Update. Current Problems in Pediatrics, 25, 131–136.

Stewart, J. M., et al. (1989). Symptomatic cardiac dysfunction in children with human immunodeficiency virus infection. *American Heart Journal, 117,* 140–144.

Tindall, B., Imrie, A., Donovan, B., Penny, R., & Cooper, D. A. (1990). Primary HIV infection: Clinical immunologic and serologic aspects. In M. A. Sande & P. A. Volberding (Eds.). *The medical management of AIDS* (2nd ed., pp. 68–84). Philadelphia: W.B. Saunders.

Tinkle, M. B., Amaya, M. A., & Tamayo, O. W. (1992). HIV disease and pregnancy. Part 1. Epidemiology, pathogenesis, and natural history. *Journal of Obstetric, Gynecologic, and Neonatal Nursing, 21* (2), 86–93.

Tramont, E. C. (1991). The human immunodeficiency virus. *Dermatologic Clinics of North America, 9* (3), 397–401.

Tribett, D. (1989). Immune system function: Implications for critical care nursing practice. *Critical Care Nursing Clinics of North America, 1* (4), 725–740.

Tribett, D. (1993). The patient with human immunodeficiency virus (HIV). In M. R. Kinney, D. R. Packa, & S. B. Dunbar (Eds.). *AACN's clinical reference for critical care nursing* (pp. 1059–1067). St. Louis: Mosby–Year Book.

Unguarski, P. (1993). Zalcitabine. *Journal of the Association of Nurses in AIDS Care, 4* (3), 53–54.

Vernon, D. D., et al. (1988). Respiratory failure in children with acquired immunodeficiency syndrome and immunodeficiency syndrome–related complex. *Pediatrics, 82* (2), 223–228.

Vogel, R. L. (1992). Cardiac manifestations of pediatric acquired immunodeficiency syndrome. In R. Yogev & E. Connor (Eds.), *Management of HIV infection in infants and children* (pp. 357–369). St. Louis: Mosby–Year Book.

Volberding, P. A. (1994). Strategies for antiretroviral therapy in adult HIV disease: The San Francisco perspective. In S. Broder, T. C. Merigan, & D. Bolognesi (Eds.). *Textbook of AIDS medicine* (pp. 773–787). Baltimore: Williams & Wilkins.

Warrier, I., and Lusher, J. M. (1992). Hematologic manifestations of HIV infection. In R. Yogev & E. Connor (Eds.). *Management of HIV infection in infants and children* (pp. 447–460). St. Louis: Mosby–Year Book.

Wasserman, R. (1990). AIDS. In D. L. Levin & F. C. Morriss (Eds.). *Essentials of pediatric intensive care* (pp. 378–382). St. Louis: Quality Medical Publishing.

Wilkinson, J. D., & Greenwald, B. M. (1988). The acquired immunodeficiency syndrome: Impact on the pediatric intensive care unit. *Critical Care Clinics, 4* (4), 831–843.

Wofsy, C. B. (1990). Prevention of HIV transmission. In M. A. Sande & P. A. Volberding (Eds.). *The Management of AIDS* (2nd ed., pp. 38–56). Philadelphia: W.B. Saunders.

CHAPTER *29*

Shock

MARTHA A. Q. CURLEY

One of the most challenging clinical problems in pediatric critical care is caring for the patient in shock. Shock is a progressive syndrome characterized by circulatory dysfunction and *insufficient* tissue perfusion. Shock results from the loss of integrity of one or more of the four essential components of circulation: blood volume, cardiac pump, vascular tone, and cell function (Table 29–1). Regardless of the etiology, the final common pathway of shock is **cell destruction** caused by either inadequate tissue delivery or impaired utilization of essential cellular substrates.

The extent to which shock contributes to morbidity and mortality among critically ill infants and children is directly related to the ability of caregivers to (1) rapidly recognize the cluster of symptoms characteristic of shock; (2) vigilantly attend to the administration and titration of collaborative management strategies intended to interrupt the numerous pathophysiologic cascades associated with shock; and (3) provide intensive nursing care.

CATEGORIES OF SHOCK

Although classified in a variety of ways, shock can be divided into two major categories. Based on char-

acteristic blood flow, the categories are *low-flow shock* and *maldistributive shock*. Low-flow shock states are characterized by decreased cardiac output (CO). The low-flow state may be due to hypovolemia, cardiac

Table 29–1. SHOCK STATES

Altered Component of Circulation	Shock
Blood volume: Insufficient circulating blood volume in relation to the vascular space	**Low-flow: hypovolemic**
Cardiac pump: Insufficient cardiac output despite adequate ventricular preload	**Low-flow: cardiogenic**
Vascular tone: Inappropriate systemic and/or pulmonary vascular tone	**Maldistributive: distributive**
Cellular function: Ineffective tissue utilization of oxygen and nutrients	**Maldistributive: septic**

failure, and/or critical obstruction of blood flow from the heart. Maldistributive shock states are characterized by normal or increased cardiac output but an abnormal distribution of blood flow. This category of shock includes neurogenic shock, anaphylaxis, and, most commonly, septic shock. Clustering all shock states into these two major categories provides clinically relevant information. Not only do these two categories of shock present differently from one another, but also the primary interventions in each are different. However, it is crucial to acknowledge that clinically, there is much overlap among shock states. For example, septic shock presents as maldistributive shock but may progress to low-flow shock secondary to myocardial failure.

Low-Flow Shock

The most common shock syndrome in infants and children is low-flow shock due to acute hypovolemia. Any illness or injury that results in an acute reduction in circulating blood volume—that is, severe blood, plasma, or body fluid loss—can cause hypovolemia and shock. The decrease in intravascular volume can be absolute, as in hemorrhage after trauma; or relative, as in nephrotic syndrome when plasma moves out of the vascular space into the interstitial space. Other common causes of hypovolemia and low-flow shock in infants and children are listed in Table 29–2.

The progressive pathophysiologic effects of intravascular volume loss include decreased venous return, decreased ventricular filling, decreased stroke volume, and decreased cardiac output, then inade-

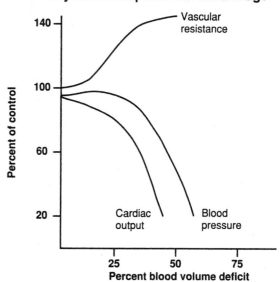

Hemodynamic Response to Hemorrhage

Figure 29–1 ● ● ● ● ● ●

Model for cardiovascular response to hypovolemia from hemorrhage. (Reproduced with permission. © *Textbook of pediatric advanced life support*, 1990. Copyright American Heart Association.)

quate tissue perfusion. Following the loss of volume, a series of cardiac and peripheral hemostatic adjustments are stimulated in an attempt to support myocardial and cerebral perfusion pressures. In previously healthy hypovolemic patients, systolic and mean arterial blood pressures are often maintained until the blood volume deficit reaches 25% (Fig. 29–1). The degree to which compensatory mechanisms succeed in maintaining blood pressure is determined by the infant's or child's preexisting health status as well as the volume and rate of blood or fluid loss and resuscitation.

Insufficient CO despite adequate ventricular preload is the second cause of low-flow shock. In addition to congenital or acquired heart disease, other important causes of cardiogenic low-flow shock in the pediatric population include hypoxemia, acidosis, post–hypoxic-ischemic arrest, hypoglycemia, severe electrolyte imbalance, dysrhythmias, drug intoxication, chest trauma (myocardial contusion), and outflow obstructions. The term obstructive shock is sometimes used to describe the low-flow state that results from mechanical obstruction to ventricular outflow from tension pneumothorax, tension pneumopericardium, pericardial effusion, cardiac tamponade, or massive pulmonary embolus. Compensatory mechanisms designed to support perfusion pressures often contribute to the progression of cardiogenic shock.

Maldistributive Shock

Maldistributive shock results from an abnormal distribution of blood volume. Vasomotor paralysis,

Table 29–2. CAUSES OF SHOCK

Low-Flow Shock (Hypovolemia)	
Blood loss	**Water loss**
Inadequate replacement	Vomiting and diarrhea
Trauma—splenic rupture	Diabetes mellitus
Gastrointestinal bleeding	Diabetes insipidus
Plasma loss	
Capillary leak syndrome	
Hypoproteinemia	
Nephrotic syndrome	
Burns	
Peritonitis	
Bowel obstruction	

Low-Flow Shock (Cardiogenic)
Metabolic: hypoxemia, acidosis, hypoglycemia, severe electrolyte imbalance
Dysrhythmias: drug toxicity
Cardiac tamponade
Coexisting disorders: cardiac failure secondary to congenital or acquired heart disease

Maldistributive Shock
Neurogenic: anesthesia, spinal cord injury
Anaphylactic
Septic shock: any infectious organism

increased venous capacity, or abnormal shunting of blood past capillary beds results in the abnormal apportionment of circulating blood volume that is characteristic of maldistributive shock. In infants and children, maldistributive shock may be neurogenic, or precipitated by anaphylaxis or sepsis.

Neurogenic maldistributive shock is characterized by massive vasodilation from loss of sympathetic vasomotor tone. Alterations in the regulation of vasomotor tone may be due to either pharmacologic blockade (anesthetic agents, morphine, barbiturates, antihypertensives) or traumatic damage to the sympathetic nervous system (spinal cord transection above T-1). The resulting vasodilation leads to increased vascular capacity in affected body parts, usually the extremities, depriving vital organs of oxygen and nutrients.

Anaphylactic maldistributive shock is a severe antigen-antibody reaction occurring after sensitized individuals are exposed to drugs, foods, or insect venoms. The antigen-antibody reaction triggers a massive release of vasoactive mediators (such as histamine from mast cells), producing vasodilation, capillary leak, severe bronchoconstriction, and an urticarial rash. Unlike in the emergency department, anaphylactic shock is a rare phenomenon in the intensive care unit.

The most common etiology of maldistributive shock in pediatrics is sepsis. Zimmerman and Dietrich (1987) describe septic shock as a disease of interme-

diary metabolism induced by an infectious agent, which results in fuel energy deficits and corresponding physiologic and destructive host responses resulting in multiple organ dysfunction syndrome (MODS). Septic shock results from an amplified activation of the normal immune response. Once activated, these systems trigger the release of multiple endogenously produced mediators that produce the deleterious effects associated with septic shock. Not only is vascular resistance inappropriately diminished, altering normal hemodynamics, but also cellular function is impaired as utilization of oxygen and nutrients is disrupted.

Consensus on the use of terminology is important so that clinicians can compare the results of clinical research studies related to sepsis. Bone (1991a) proposed the initial framework that was later adopted by the American College of Chest Physicians and the Society of Critical Care Medicine (1992). See Table 29–3.

The hallmark of septic shock is a maldistribution of blood flow. The pathophysiologic events (see Fig. 29–2), produced by chemical mediators and dysfunctional cascades, include endothelial cell destruction; massive vasodilation; increased capillary permeability; microemboli formation; vasoconstriction of the pulmonary, renal, and splanchnic vasculature; and depressed myocardial contractility.

Risk factors that increase the individual's risk of sepsis diminish either the effectiveness of the im-

Table 29–3. DEFINITIONS OF SEPSIS

Infection:
Microbial phenomenon characterized by an inflammatory response to the presence of microorganisms or the invasion of normally sterile host tissue by those organisms

Bacteremia:
The presence of viable bacteria in the blood

Systemic inflammatory response syndrome (SIRS):
The systemic inflammatory response to a variety of severe clinical insults. The response is manifested by two or more of the following conditions:
  Temperature >38°C or <36°C
  Tachycardia
  Tachypnea
  WBC >12,000 cells/mm³, <4000 cells/mm³, or 10% immature (band) forms

Sepsis:
The systemic response to infection. This systemic response is manifested by two or more of the following conditions as a result of infection:
  Temperature >38°C or <36°C
  Tachycardia
  Tachypnea
  WBC >12,000 cells/mm³, <4,000 cells/mm³, or 10% immature (band) forms

Severe sepsis:
Sepsis associated with organ dysfunction, hypoperfusion, or hypotension (for example, lactic acidosis, oliguria, an acute change in mental status)

Septic shock:
Sepsis with hypotension, despite adequate fluid resuscitation, along with the presence of perfusion abnormalities that may include, but are not limited to, lactic acidosis, oliguria, or an acute alteration in mental status. Patients who are on inotropic or vasopressor agents may not be hypotensive at the time that perfusion abnormalities are measured

Multiple organ dysfunction syndrome (MODS):
Presence of altered organ function in an acutely ill patient such that homeostasis cannot be maintained without interventions

From the American College of Chest Physicians/Society of Critical Care Medicine Consensus Conference (1992). Definitions for sepsis and organ failure and guidelines for the use of innovative therapies in sepsis. *Critical Care Medicine,* 20(6), 864–874. ©1992.

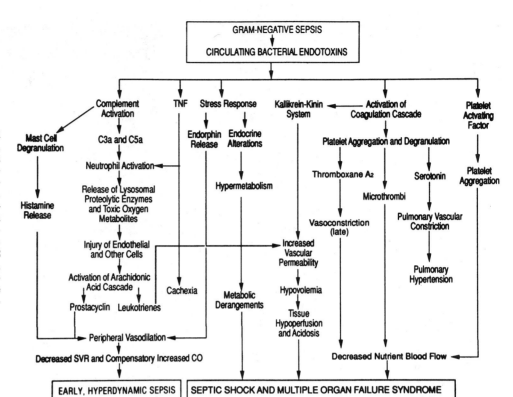

Figure 29–2 ● ● ● ● ● ●
Biochemical mediators involved in the pathophysiology of sepsis, septic shock, and multiple organ failure. TNF, tumor necrosis factor; SVR, systemic vascular resistance; CO, cardiac output. (From Klein, D.M., & Witek-Janusek, L. (1992). Advances in immunotherapy of sepsis. *Dimensions of Critical Care Nursing*, 11 (2), 77. Copyright 1992 Hall Johnson Communications, Inc. Reproduced with permission. For further use contact the publisher at 9737 West Ohio Avenue, Lakewood, CO 80226.)

mune system or the body's protective barriers against infection (Klein & Witek-Janusek, 1992). Host-related factors include functional immaturity (infancy), malnutrition, and either primary or secondary immunodeficiency related to disease or drug therapy. Treatment-related risk factors include surgical or invasive procedures, invasive devices, antibiotics, steroids, immunosuppression, hypothermia, and the presence of virulent antibiotic-resistant organisms within the hospital environment. Translocation of normal gut flora into the lymphatic or portal system may occur secondary to mesenteric hypoperfusion (Fink, 1993). Considering the patient population and therapies provided in the intensive care unit, sepsis in this high-risk population continues to rise (Bone, 1991b).

All organisms (gram-negative bacteria, gram-positive bacteria, viruses, fungi, rickettsiae, spirochetes, protozoa, and parasites) can initiate the multisystem, subcellular metabolic derangements associated with septic shock (Table 29–4). In pediatrics, gram-negative and gram-positive nosocomial infections occur in almost equal proportions; the foci primarily include skin and lungs (Jarvis, 1987). Endotoxin release from gram-negative bacteria (Fig. 29–3) or exotoxins and cell wall component release from gram-positive bacteria are two of probably several bacterial products that trigger the body's immune response (NIH, 1990).

Meningococcemia, caused by the gram-negative diplococcus *Neisseria meningitidis*, is a particularly virulent infection in children. Clinical presentation is often dramatic, with death ensuing in a matter of hours. Classic presentation includes purpura fulmi-

nans, initially described as petechiae coalescing to diffuse purpuric ecchymotic lesions (Fig. 29–4). Poor prognostic indicators include purpura fulminans along with hypothermia, seizures, or hypotension on presentation; WBC <5000 mm³; and platelet count <100,000 mm³ (Wong, Hitchcock, & Mason, 1989). Fulminant disease is often associated with bilateral adrenal hemorrhage referred to as Waterhouse-Friderichsen syndrome. The severe, rapidly progressive cardiovascular collapse associated with meningococcemia is thought to be a result of endotoxin-induced myocardial depression.

Table 29–4. COMMON ETIOLOGIC AGENTS OF SEPTIC SHOCK

Neonate
β-Hemolytic streptococci
Escherichia coli
Herpes simplex virus

Older Infant and Child
Haemophilus influenzae
Neisseria meningitidis
Streptococcus pneumoniae
β-Hemolytic streptococci

Nosocomial
Staphylococcus aureus
Staphylococcus epidermidis
Pseudomonas
Candida

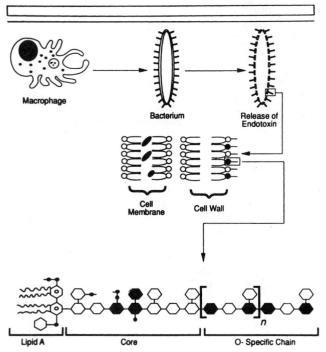

Figure 29–3 ● ● ● ● ● ●

Phagocytosis of gram-negative bacteria releases endotoxin, which is a component of the bacterial cell wall. Endotoxin is a lipopolysaccharide molecule with three components: lipid A, a polysaccharide core, and an O-specific chain. The lipid A contains most of the biologic effects of endotoxin, and the O-specific chain is a major antigen recognized by the body. (From Klein, D.M., & Witek-Janusek, L. (1992). Advances in immunotherapy of sepsis. *Dimensions of Critical Care Nursing*, 11 (2), 79. Copyright 1992 Hall Johnson Communications, Inc. Reproduced with permission. For further use contact the publisher at 9737 West Ohio Avenue, Lakewood, CO 80226.)

Toxic shock syndrome (TSS), septic shock resulting from toxin-producing strains of *Staphylococcus aureus,* can occur in non-menstruating women and in males. Diagnostic criteria are included in Table 29–5. Individualized treatment includes antistaphylococcal antibiotics and control of the focus of infection.

TRAJECTORY OF ILLNESS

Shock is a syndrome that reflects the body's attempt to adapt to an insult and preserve vital organ function. The trajectory of adaptation in shock can be divided into three phases: a compensated stage during which vital organ function is maintained, an uncompensated stage that reflects the inadequacy of compensatory mechanisms in the maintenance of adequate tissue perfusion, and a refractory stage. Response to therapy varies during these stages.

In the *first phase,* the body's intrinsic supportive mechanisms can generally maintain normal vital organ function. Systemic blood flow is usually normal or increased. Hemodynamic values and vital signs may be normal or actually enhanced, reflecting the physiologic attempt to maintain vital organ perfusion. The success of the body's intrinsic supportive mecha-

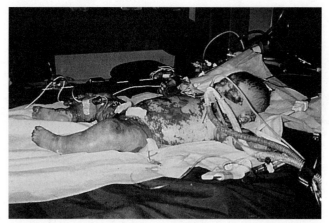

Figure 29–4 ● ● ● ● ● ●

Infant with purpura fulminans associated with meningococcemia.

nisms is determined by the patient's preexisting state (for example, volume status and myocardial function), illness, time elapsed, and treatment provided.

In the *second phase,* compensatory mechanisms are insufficient to maintain adequate oxygen and nutrient delivery to the tissues. Delayed or inadequate maintenance of intravascular volume or other iatrogenic causes may play some role in the patient's

Table 29–5. DIAGNOSTIC CRITERIA OF TOXIC SHOCK SYNDROME

Fever	>38.9°C
Rash	Diffuse macular erythroderma Desquamation (palms and soles) 1–2 weeks after onset of illness
Hypotension	Systolic pressure less than the 5th percentile for children <16 yr
Three or more organ system involvement:	
Gastrointestinal	Vomiting or diarrhea or both
Muscular	Severe muscle pain or creatine phosphokinase over twice upper normal
Mucous membrane	Hyperemia (conjunctival, oral, vaginal)
Renal	BUN over twice upper normal and increased WBC in urine (without UTI)
Hepatic	Total bilirubin, AST (SGOT), or ALT (SGPT) over twice upper normal
Hematologic	Platelets <100,000/mm³
Central nervous system	Change in consciousness when fever and hypotension absent
Negative laboratory results	Blood, throat, CSF cultures (except for *Staphylococcus aureus),* serologic test for Rocky Mountain spotted fever, leptospirosis, or measles

Modified from Yogev, R. (1990). Toxic shock syndrome. In J. L. Blummer (Ed.). *A practical guide to pediatric intensive care* (3rd ed., p. 461). Philadelphia: Mosby–Year Book. Adapted from the Centers for Disease Control: MMWR 31:201, 1982.

deterioration. More often, though, the body simply lacks sufficient substrate for metabolic processes, or the cellular damage sustained is such that available substrate cannot be utilized. During this uncompensated period, associated problems such as adult respiratory distress syndrome (ARDS) or disseminated intravascular coagulation (DIC) may develop and hasten the onset of the final stage and preclude recovery.

In the *third phase,* shock becomes irreversible. Damage to vital organs such as the heart and brain cannot be reversed with either time or therapeutic maneuvers.

Refractory or unresponsive septic shock has been described as progressing through three phases: a hyperdynamic-compensated phase, a hyperdynamic-uncompensated phase, followed by a hypodynamic or cardiogenic shock phase (Perkin & Levin, 1982). Bone (1991a) advises against using the terms "warm" and "cold" shock when referring to septic shock. In the past, warm shock referred to the early phase of septic shock characterized by decreased systemic vascular resistance (SVR) and increased CO. We now know that progression to what had been traditionally referred to as cold shock, characterized by increased SVR and decreased CO, is a rare phenomenon. In refractory septic shock, decreased SVR persists but CO falls because of unresponsive myocardial depression.

PHYSIOLOGIC RESPONSES TO SHOCK

Although physiologic responses to the different types of shock vary, patterns do exist within each category. The common physiologic characteristic of all early shock states is either reduced or inadequate oxygen *supply* relative to tissue *demand.* Physiologic mechanisms such as increased oxygen extraction in low-flow shock and increased cardiac output in maldistributive shock attempt to compensate for the uncoupling of oxygen supply and demand. Autoregulation maintains perfusion to the brain and heart by diverting blood flow from the nonessential areas of the skin, gut, and kidneys. With time, ongoing redistribution of blood flow can lead to progressive destruction of major organ systems.

Sympathetic Stimulation

The stress response, activated by stimulation of the cardiac centers in the brainstem, increases cardiac output. The adrenal medulla releases massive amounts of catecholamines; epinephrine levels increase 50-fold. Epinephrine increases both heart rate and myocardial contractility (unless limited by reduced or impaired myocardial function) and increases tissue perfusion pressure by direct vasoconstriction of all vascular beds except those in skeletal muscle and the liver. Norepinephrine levels also increase 10-fold to produce vasoconstriction in all vascular beds.

Reduction in mean arterial pressure and/or pulse pressure results in baroreceptor stimulation. Baroreceptor stimulation leads to diminished parasympathetic stimulation and enhanced sympathetic stimulation of the heart producing positive cardiac inotropy and chronotropy (β effects) and arterial and venous vasoconstriction (α effects). Low capillary hydrostatic pressure relative to plasma oncotic pressure shifts interstitial fluid into the intravascular compartment. The benefits of this "autotransfusion" are self-limiting, since dilution of the hematocrit and plasma oncotic pressure eventually results. Because extracellular fluid volume is higher in children than in adults, this mechanism may play a greater role in pediatric shock than in adult shock.

When cerebral perfusion pressures reach very low levels (below cerebral autoregulation—about 40 mmHg in older children) there is a sympathetic surge that produces massive vasoconstriction and a *temporary* arrest in the decline of the blood pressure (BP) and cardiac output. The CNS ischemic reflex maintains blood pressure by doubling SVR and producing a fivefold increase in pulmonary vascular resistance (PVR).

Anaerobic Metabolism

By definition, shock is inadequate tissue perfusion leading to anaerobic metabolism, an accumulation of lactic acids, and metabolic acidosis. At a time when oxygen demands are greatest for tissue repair, adequate oxygen delivery is unavailable. Cellular processes therefore occur without oxygen (anaerobic metabolism), and lactic acid accumulates. Decreased oxygen consumption (VO_2) occurs secondary to reduced blood flow and/or maldistribution of flow. Arterial pH and base deficit determination serve as readily available markers of adequate tissue perfusion and oxygenation.

In the future, gastric intramucosal pH monitoring may provide a noninvasive method for the indirect measurement of tissue oxygenation (Clark & Gutierrez, 1992). Gastrointestinal tonometry uses a standard vented nasogastric tube combined with a silicone balloon system that is permeable to CO_2. When the saline-filled balloon is placed in close proximity to the gastric mucosa, CO_2 gas diffuses from the gastrointestinal mucosa into the balloon tonometer. The CO_2 measurement, used in conjunction with the arterial blood bicarbonate, serves as an indirect estimate of the intramucosal pH of the gut. Mucosal acidosis correlates well with the onset of anaerobic metabolism in response to sepsis or hypoxia (Gutierrez et al., 1992). Current limitations in infants and children include the size of the adapted nasogastric tube.

Lactate levels help to determine the degree of tissue perfusion. Lactate levels greater than 2.0 mmol/L are generally considered to be indicative of shock (Tuchschmidt, Oblitas, & Fried, 1991). However, lactate levels reflect total body homeostasis and normal levels do not ensure that any particular organ is adequately perfused. More importantly, increased lactate levels lag behind alterations in tissue oxygenation.

An increase in alveolar ventilation attempts to compensate for the evolving metabolic acidosis associated with shock. Decreased central nervous system pH is a potent stimulus to chemoreceptors located in the medulla to increase minute ventilation. The rise in minute ventilation results in respiratory alkalosis in the early stages of shock. When respiratory alkalosis is present, the seriousness of a patient's condition may be underestimated.

Fluid Shifts

In addition, there are some category-specific hemodynamic changes and responses. Hypovolemic shock is characterized by low circulating blood volume and decreased preload. Compensatory, generalized vasoconstriction takes place, decreasing venous capacity and translocating venous blood to the central circulation, thereby increasing preload. A rise in blood pressure and cardiac output may follow.

The renin-angiotensin-aldosterone system (RAAS) and antidiuretic hormone (ADH) also help restore intravascular volume within minutes after hemorrhage or trauma. Renal vasoconstriction and hypoperfusion activate the RAAS with increased production and secretion of renin. Increased plasma renin activity stimulates the release of angiotensin I. Angiotensin I is converted to angiotensin II by the angiotensin-converting enzyme (ACE) in the vascular epithelium of the lungs as well as other tissues, including the heart, adrenals, kidneys, and brain. Angiotensin II is a potent vasoconstrictor that also stimulates the production of aldosterone by the adrenal gland, increasing sodium and water reabsorption in the renal tubules. Stimulated by an increase in serum osmolality, vasopressin (ADH) secretion from the posterior pituitary gland results in peripheral vasoconstriction and increased reabsorption of water from the renal tubules and collecting ducts. Stress precipitates the release of adrenocorticotropic hormone (ACTH) from the anterior pituitary, which then stimulates the adrenal glands to release cortisol. Cortisol sensitizes arteriolar smooth muscle to the effects of catecholamines.

In contrast to the low ventricular filling pressures seen in patients with hypovolemic shock, the ventricular filling pressures in those with cardiogenic shock are high. This is a consequence of both myocardial dysfunction and loss of ventricular diastolic compliance and the additional venous return brought about by the compensatory venous constriction.

Metabolic Changes

A number of metabolic and endocrine changes are characteristic of hypovolemic shock and may also occur in other types of shock. Alterations in metabolic rate, carbohydrate metabolism, and temperature are common. Initially, due to epinephrine secretion, hyperglycemia is present. Later, hypoglycemia develops as hepatic glycogen stores are depleted and gluconeogenesis fails. Anaerobic glycolysis results in increased blood lactate and pyruvate, and protein is catabolized for energy. Plasma levels of catecholamine, 17-hydroxyketosteroids, and potassium also increase.

Chemical Mediators

A number of chemical mediators are released into the bloodstream during septic shock. Tumor necrosis factor (TNF, cachectin), a cytokine released from leukocytes, modulates the inflammatory response including fever, the hyperdynamic state, and stress hormone response. TNF is thought to be *the major* endogenous mediator of the septic cascade (NIH, 1990). TNF stimulates the release of interleukin-1 (IL-1), stimulates arachidonic acid metabolism, activates the complement system and clotting cascade, and stimulates the production of platelet-activating factor (Hazinski et al., 1993). The net result is sequestration of platelets, vasodilation, increased capillary permeability, and microvascular constriction.

IL-1 is a cytokine that is released by phagocytosis that works in synergy with TNF to perpetuate the inflammatory response and release of platelet-activating factor (PAF). PAF produces vasodilation, activates platelet aggregation, and increases tissue permeability.

Arachidonic acid, a normal constituent of cell membranes, is released after cell injury. Arachidonic acid is metabolized through two major pathways: the cyclooxygenase and lipoxygenase pathways. Metabolism of arachidonic acid through the cyclooxygenase pathway results in the formation of the cytokines thromboxane A_2, prostacyclin, and prostaglandins E_2 and D_2. Thromboxane produces pulmonary and systemic vasoconstriction and enhances platelet aggregation. Prostacyclin decreases SVR and PVR, increases vascular permeability, and inhibits platelet aggregation. Prostaglandins decrease SVR, inhibit platelet aggregation, increase vascular permeability, activate production of cAMP, and increase gastrointestinal smooth muscle contraction. The metabolism of arachidonic acid through the lipoxygenase pathway results in the formation of leukotrienes that stimulate neutrophil and eosinophil chemotaxis and lysosomal release. The leukotrienes also increase SVR, produce smooth muscle contraction, and increase vascular permeability. In total, arachidonic acid metabolism increases capillary permeability, platelet dysfunction, maldistribution of blood flow, and organ ischemia; causes pulmonary edema and intrapulmonary shunting; and thus contributes significantly to MODS associated with septic shock. The kidney, gastrointestinal tract, liver, lungs, and brain are at particular risk. Dysfunction of any of these organs may preclude successful treatment of shock.

Unremitting activation of the complement cascade with associated histamine activation also contributes to the clinical findings and the eventual outcomes of septic shock. Continued activation of the complement cascade results in increased capillary permeability, vasodilation, and lysosome release. Histamine, derived from mast cells in damaged tissues and from basophils in the blood, decreases SVR, increases vascular permeability, and augments gastrointestinal motility. As part of the complement system, the clotting system also becomes dysfunctional.

The Hageman factor (factor XII) may also become activated, which in turn activates the coagulation and fibrinolytic systems contributing to the development of DIC. The Hageman factor also stimulates the production of bradykinin, a potent vasoactive peptide found in plasma or tissue fluid. Bradykinin causes venodilation, increased vascular permeability, bronchoconstriction, and constriction of gastrointestinal smooth muscle.

Endorphins, the brain's natural opiate, are released from the autonomic and central nervous systems. Similar to systemic narcotic administration, endorphin release may decrease SVR, reduce CO and BP, diminish gastrointestinal motility, relieve pain and alter mood, and enhance parasympathetic activity while inhibiting the sympathetic nervous system.

Patients in septic shock typically exhibit reduced left ventricular ejection fraction and LV dilation (Natanson, Hoffman, & Parrillo, 1989). In addition to adrenergenic receptor dysfunction and impaired myocardial intracellular calcium flux, myocardial dysfunction occurs secondary to the negative inotropic effects of numerous chemical mediators, including myocardial depressant factors, endotoxin, TNF, complement products, and leukotrienes. Myocardial depressant factors are hemodynamic inhibitory peptides released secondary to ischemia to the splanchnic region. As occurs in other organs, eventually myocardial perfusion and oxygen consumption are disrupted in septic shock.

CLINICAL ASSESSMENT: RED FLAGS OF CARDIOVASCULAR COLLAPSE

Shock is a dynamic process that requires vigilant assessment and continuous patient reevaluation. Physical findings and hemodynamic indices reflect the consequences of impaired tissue perfusion. Progressive circulatory dysfunction and cellular oxygen and nutrient deprivation must be detected early if interventions are to be successful.

Unexplained and persistent tachycardia—that is, tachycardia not related to fever, anemia, pain, and/ or agitation—is often the first indicator of circulatory impairment and physiologic distress. Increased heart rate may compensate for inadequate stroke volume. In addition, dysrhythmias, which impair cardiac function, are not uncommon in pediatric patients

with electrolyte imbalance, metabolic acidosis, and hypoxemia. All of these can occur in shock.

Early in shock states, minute ventilation increases in an attempt to compensate for the evolving metabolic acidosis reflective of inadequate tissue perfusion. Unexplained persistent tachypnea is a valuable early sign of shock.

Low-Flow Shock

The red flags of low-flow shock are the signs of increased SVR and decreased CO. In order to maintain blood pressure in low-flow states, SVR increases, as blood pressure is the product of CO and SVR (BP = CO × SVR). Symptoms of increased SVR can be assessed in three major organ systems: the skin, kidneys, and brain.

Impairment of peripheral circulation is assessed by examination of skin temperature, color, and capillary refill. Normally, a child's extremities are warm and pink with brisk capillary refill (<2 seconds). The child in low-flow shock, however, presents with cool skin, mottled or gray extremities, and sluggish capillary refill. (Note: to assess capillary refill from the arterial side of the circulation, the extremity should be slightly elevated above heart level.) Skin color changes may progress from pink, to pale, to mottled, then to marbleized in appearance. A core-to-skin temperature gradient greater than 2°C is considered significant. The temperature gradient widens with progressive decreases in peripheral perfusion (Fagan, 1988). Proximal-to-distal skin temperature gradients—that is, changes in the position of the demarcation line between warmth and coolness—can be trended as well. Pale skin color may be noted when the hemoglobin and hematocrit are decreased.

In low-flow shock, peripheral pulses are difficult to palpate. Weak pulses result from the narrow pulse pressure characteristic of a diminished stroke volume (SV) and increased SVR. The narrow pulse pressure occurs before systolic pressures fall. Diastolic blood pressure reflects SVR, while systolic blood pressure is determined by stroke volume and SVR. When cardiac output falls, SVR increases to maintain the blood pressure. The increased SVR increases the diastolic component of the blood pressure and maintains the systolic component. Because pulse pressure is a sensitive indicator of stroke volume, it is an important parameter to monitor.

Urine output is an extremely important measurement when assessing infants and children in shock. Particularly in hypovolemic patients, urine output may decrease long before other signs of impaired tissue perfusion are evident. Renal blood flow is dependent on cardiac output. Sudden decreases in renal blood flow or pressure decrease the glomerular filtration rate and result in decreased urine output and increased urine specific gravity. Low urine output is defined as less than 0.5 to 1.0 mL/kg/hour in infants and children, and less than 1.0 to 2.0 mL/kg/hour during the newborn period.

Signs and symptoms of inadequate cerebral perfusion are often subtle in the early stages of shock. The child's sensorium may be clouded; response to stimuli may be limited; and anxious, irritable, or lethargic behavior may be present. Infants frequently exhibit a weak cry and/or poor suck. As shock progresses, somnolence advances to obtundation. Level of consciousness is assessed developmentally. Infants normally do not tolerate missed feedings or wet/soiled diapers, especially if they have a diaper rash. Toddlers normally do not tolerate their parents' absence in a foreign environment for any period of time.

Unique to *hypovolemic* low-flow shock, signs of dehydration may also be present. Skin turgor may be poor, and, in extreme situations, the skin may remain "tented" when gently pinched. Mucous membranes are often dry, the patient will cry without producing tears, the fontanelle may be sunken, and weight may decrease. Skin tone will be pale in low-flow shock secondary to hemorrhage.

The patient in *cardiogenic* low-flow shock is in sharp contrast to the patient with hypovolemic low-flow shock. In cardiogenic shock secondary to congestive heart failure, the patient may have a gallop rhythm and often appears "wet." For example, diaphoresis, periorbital/sacral or dependent edema, hepatomegaly, jugular venous distension, and rales with increased work of breathing are often present. In cardiogenic shock secondary to an outflow obstruction, the patient may exhibit a low-voltage EKG and electromechanical dissociation (EMD). If a cardiac tamponade is present, a significant pulsus paradoxus greater than 10 mmHg may be present.

Late signs and symptoms of low-flow shock include progressive neurologic deterioration, hypotension, and bradycardia. Table 29–6 reviews the lower limits of normal systolic blood pressure (Chameides, 1990).

Maldistributive Shock

The red flags of maldistributive shock are the signs of decreased SVR and increased CO. In order to maintain blood pressure in low SVR states, CO must increase. Associated with normal or increased CO, septic shock patients have warm and dry skin. They are often febrile (>38°C), but may be hypothermic (<36°C). They often appear flushed and well perfused, with normal or brisk capillary refill, despite the ominous nature of their illness. Because neutrophil activation produces many of the early signs of infection and the inflammatory response, septic patients who are neutropenic may not present in the typical fashion.

In patients with high cardiac output, pulses are easily palpated. Bounding pulses, a rare finding in a pediatric physical examination, reflect widened pulse pressure that occurs secondary to an increased stroke volume and decreased SVR. Urine output may initially be normal or increased, despite a relative hypovolemia. Subtle changes in mental status (for example, confusion) may be present.

Tissue injury may progress secondary to both compromised tissue perfusion and impaired cellular metabolism, evidenced by lactic acidemia. Other signs and symptoms of tissue ischemia include hypoglycemia, increased bilirubin, decreased albumin, and increased BUN and creatinine.

Disseminated intravascular coagulation (DIC) may become evident, as demonstrated by thrombocytopenia, prolonged prothrombin and partial thromboplastin times, reduced activity of clotting factors V and VII, hypofibrinogenemia, and increased fibrin split products. Other assessment parameters include prolonged bleeding from old puncture sites and the presence of petechiae.

The quiet tachypnic respiratory pattern may become shallow and labored, reflecting respiratory muscle fatigue and failure to compensate for acidosis. Microthrombi formation contributes to pulmonary vascular plugging and increased PVR. ARDS symptomatology, including decreased pulmonary compliance, intrapulmonary shunting (contributing to hypoxemia), then increased PVR, becomes evident.

Late symptoms include those present in low-flow shock states and MODS. The patient manifests signs and symptoms of low cardiac output. A narrowed pulse pressure is present and correlates with reduced stroke volume; progressive hypotension accompanies decreased CO. Clot and interstitial edema obstruct blood flow through the periphery. Tissue acidosis causes arterioles to dilate and venules to constrict, causing further pooling and stasis of blood. There is marked capillary leak and interstitial and pulmonary edema.

Hemodynamic and Oxygenation Profiles

Table 29–7 provides a summary of the numerous hemodynamic and oxygenation profile changes associated with low-flow and maldistributive shock states. Currently, there is a lack of pediatric research to help guide collaborative practice. Normal values are not necessarily optimal values in shock (Pollack, Fields, Ruttimann, 1985).

Heart rate increases in all shock states. Mean arterial pressure remains normal when compensatory mechanisms are effective but falls when compensatory mechanisms fail. Right atrial pressure (RAP) and pulmonary artery wedge pressure (PAWP) reflect right and left ventricular preload, respectively. Both

Table 29–6. LOWER LIMITS OF SYSTOLIC BLOOD PRESSURE

Greater than 1 year of age	70 mmHg + 2 × age in years
1–12 months of age	>70 mmHg
0–1 month of age	>60 mmHg

Fifth percentile systolic blood pressure for age. Data from Chameides, L. (1990). *Textbook of pediatric advanced life support.* Chapter 1: Recognition of respiratory failure and shock: Anticipating cardiopulmonary arrest, p. 5. American Heart Association.

Table 29–7. HEMODYNAMIC AND OXYGENATON PROFILE CHANGES IN SHOCK

Parameter	Norms	Hypovolemic	Cardiogenic	Septic Early	Septic Late
HR	NB–3 mo: 85–205; 3 mo–2 yr: 100–190; 2–10 yr: 60–140; >10 yr: 60–100	Increased			
MAP	>60 mmHg	Normal$_{Compensated}$ → Decreased$_{Decompensated}$			
CI	2.5–5.5 L/min/M²	↓	↓	↑ then ↓	
RAP/PAW	2–6 mmHg/6–12 mmHg		↑	↓ then ↓	
PVRI	PVRI = mean PA − PCWP/CI × 80 Norm: 80–240 dyne-sec/cm⁵/M²		Normal Increased		
SVRI	SVRI = MAP − RAP/CI × 80 Norm: 800–1600 dyne-sec/cm⁵/M²	↑		↓	
Do$_2$	Do$_2$ = CaO$_2$ × CI × 10 Norm: 620 ± 50 mL/min/M²	↓		↑ then ↓	
Vo$_2$	Vo$_2$ = arterial Do$_2$ − venous Do$_2$ Norm: 120–200 mL/min/M²	↑ then ↓			
OER	CaO$_2$ − Cvo$_2$/CaO$_2$ × 100 Norm: 25 ± 2%	↑ then ↓		Nl/↑ then ↓	
SvO$_2$	Norm: 75% (60–80%)	↓ then ↑		Nl/↓ then ↑	

MAP, mean arterial blood pressure; PAW, pulmonary artery wedge; PVRI, pulmonary vascular resistance index; SVRI, systemic vascular resistance index; Do$_2$, oxygen delivery; Vo$_2$, oxygen consumption; OER, O$_2$ extraction ratio.

are decreased in hypovolemic shock, as circulating blood volume is inadequate. As ventricular function deteriorates in cardiogenic shock, RAP and PAWP increase. RAP and PAWP are initially decreased in early septic shock as vasodilation leads to venous pooling and decreased venous return. Both RAP and PAWP pressures increase in late septic shock, reflecting myocardial failure.

Pulmonary vascular resistance index (PVRI), reflecting right ventricular afterload, is high in all shock states. In septic shock, many factors, including pulmonary vasoconstriction, microembolic occlusion, and lung injury, necessitate the use of high positive end-expiratory pressure (PEEP). All these factors increase PVRI and may contribute to right ventricular dysfunction, placing the requisite hyperdynamic state at risk. Systemic vascular resistance index (SVRI), reflecting left ventricular afterload, increases to maintain blood pressure in low-flow shock. SVRI remains low in septic shock.

The cardiac index (CI) is decreased in low-flow states, is high in early septic shock, but falls in late septic shock. Skin temperature is directly proportional to CO and inversely proportional to SVRI. Even though CO is increased in septic shock, the left ventricular ejection fraction (LVEF) is significantly decreased. The increased CO in septic shock occurs secondary to an increase in heart rate and ventricular dilation, not an increase in contractility. Overall myocardial performance is frequently compromised by diffuse myocardial edema, circulating myocardial depressant factor from splenic hypoperfusion, adrenergic receptor dysfunction, and impaired sarcolemma calcium flux (NIH, 1990).

Considering that shock represents an imbalance of oxygen supply and demand, oxygenation profile monitoring provides data necessary for informed individualized titration of therapy. Oxygen delivery (Do$_2$) and extraction ratio (OER) balance to maintain

tissue oxygen consumption (Vo$_2$) over a very wide range (Fig. 29–5). When Do$_2$ decreases in low-flow states, OER increases to maintain Vo$_2$. This continues until a critical Do$_2$ range is reached, after which Vo$_2$ depends upon Do$_2$. This is referred to as supply-dependent Vo$_2$. Patients in septic shock require higher Do$_2$ to maintain adequate tissue perfusion and to avoid anaerobic metabolism (Tuchschmidt, Oblitas, & Fried, 1991). Associated with poor outcome, a pathologic supply-dependent Vo$_2$ may exist

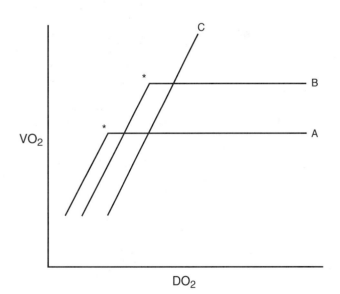

Figure 29–5 ● ● ● ● ● ●

Abnormal Vo$_2$ in sepsis. Sepsis may result in a hyperutilization state (b) with increased Vo$_2$ and intact OER or in (c) a pathologic supply-dependence state in which OER is nonexistent. *Critical Do$_2$ range; A = normal Vo$_2$/Do$_2$ curve; B = elevated critical Do$_2$ range; C = supply-dependent Vo$_2$. (Adapted from Carcillo, J.A. (1993). Management of pediatric septic shock. In P.R. Holbrook (Ed.). *Textbook of pediatric critical care* (p. 130). Philadelphia: W.B. Saunders.)

in patients with septic shock. In this state, Vo_2 is abnormally supply-dependent at normal or supernormal Do_2 rates (Schumacker & Cain, 1987). Late in septic shock, there may be an uncoupling of the Do_2-Vo_2 relationship. Supply-independent Vo_2 occurs secondary to an endotoxin-induced impairment of oxidative metabolism, a redistribution of blood flow away from the microcirculation, and a severe impairment of mitochondrial oxygen utilization.

Continuous mixed venous oxygen saturation monitoring (Svo_2) provides valuable on-line information about tissue perfusion. In low-flow shock, the Svo_2 is low, reflecting decreased CO and an increased OER. In septic shock, the Svo_2 reflects the adequacy of the cardiac output to maintain the hyperdynamic state and tissue extraction of oxygen.

Like Svo_2, the arteriovenous difference in oxygen (a-vDo_2) gradient is inversely related to cardiac output. The a-vDo_2 gradient increases in low-flow states because tissues extract more oxygen. In late septic shock, decreased Do_2 and a narrow a-vDo_2 are ominous signs.

Pollack and others (1984) identified several pediatric predictors of outcome from septic shock. Survivors of septic shock were able to maintain a normal or hyperdynamic state—that is, increased CI (3.3–6.0 L/min/M^2), higher Vo_2 (>200 mL/min/M^2) and, higher OER (>28%)—and did not experience significant pulmonary disease. On the other hand, nonsurvivors demonstrated low CI (<3.3 L/min/M^2) and low and poor O_2 utilization (<Vo_2, <a-vDo_2, and OER), had lower temperatures (<37°C), and experienced pulmonary disease. In adult survivors of septic shock, the characteristic hyperdynamic state (increased HR and CO with decreased SVR) begins to resolve within 24 hours. Nonsurvivors develop unresponsive hypotension and progressive MODS (Parrillo, 1990). Implications for management of septic shock patients include supporting factors associated with positive outcomes and eliminating factors associated with negative outcomes.

Interpreting and predicting hemodynamic and oxygenation profile changes in any shock state is done cautiously. Changes may be due to the disease process, interventional strategy (for example, inadequate fluid resuscitation, catecholamine selection), or the impact of the two on system maturation. More clinical research is definitely needed in this area.

COLLABORATIVE MANAGEMENT

Patient management is directed toward resolution of the primary problem while titrating therapy to achieve an *optimal* physiologic, oxygenation, and hemodynamic state. Optimal states may not reflect "normal" values but values that meet the dynamic individual needs of the patient. The primary focus of therapy is on improving tissue perfusion and oxygenation. Objective criteria may include supporting supply *in*dependent Vo_2 and a normal OER while preventing metabolic acidosis.

"ABCs"

When prioritizing the care of the critically ill patient in shock, the "ABCs" of resuscitation are helpful. Immediate therapy includes establishing a patent airway, maintaining oxygenation and ventilation, and improving perfusion while the underlying problem is assessed. Endotracheal intubation and assisted ventilation with adequate Fio_2 and PEEP may be indicated.

Establishing and maintaining vascular access is a priority in shock. Two central lines provide optimal intravenous access. Small-gauge percutaneous multilumen central lines have improved the ability to continuously monitor venous pressure and maintain direct access to the central circulation. Supradiaphragmatic central lines are preferred because catecholamine infusions are administered closer to myocardial receptor sites and because they limit iatrogenic injury associated with the administration of numerous caustic medications. In an emergency, intraosseous lines are considered in children less than 6 years of age for short-term volume expansion and/or catecholamine infusion.

Stop the Process

Identification and treatment of the patient's primary problem is of critical importance. For example, controlling hemorrhage, cardioverting the tachydysrhythmia, or providing appropriate broad-spectrum antibiotic coverage as soon as possible if sepsis is documented or suspected is a priority. Other interventions in sepsis include locating, excising, draining, and removing the focus of the infection, i.e., draining an abscess or replacing the central line.

Monitoring

Continuous noninvasive and invasive monitoring is essential to adequately manage patients in shock. Changes in the patient's physiologic status occur rapidly, and mechanisms to quickly evaluate the effectiveness of therapy are invaluable. Alterations in tissue perfusion may affect the accuracy of several of the standard noninvasive monitoring modalities available in the PICU, that is, end-tidal CO_2 ($ETco_2$) and pulse oximetry monitors. While this may be considered a limitation, considering the lack of available methods to quantify tissue perfusion, these limitations can be considered benefits. For example, the $ETco_2$ reading may not correlate with the $Paco_2$. However, $ETco_2$ reflects pulmonary capillary blood flow. Alterations in pulmonary perfusion associated with shock and the effectiveness of therapy can be evaluated by assessment and trending of the $ETco_2$-$Paco_2$ gradient. Pulse oximetry depends upon a reliable pulse, which may not be present in low-flow shock states.

The RAP normally quantifies right ventricular preload, the equivalent of circulating blood volume. Because ventricular compliance affects atrial pressure, an abnormal relationship between ventricular preload and work is seen. In order to provide and titrate optimal therapy in maldistributive shock states, hemodynamic and oxygenation variables require quantification. Pulmonary artery catheters are necessary to evaluate left ventricular filling pressures and CO, and provide a route to obtain true mixed venous blood samples or provide continuous SvO_2 monitoring. Strategies to enhance successful pulmonary artery (PA) catheter insertion during low cardiac output states include stiffening the 5F PA catheter with iced saline through the PA port and planning PA catheter insertion after a fluid bolus.

Sequential echocardiograms are also helpful in monitoring cardiac function. Echocardiography quantifies ventricular ejection fraction (normal 65%), quantifies the disparity between right and left ventricular function, and will determine whether pericardial effusions are present.

Enhance Substrate Delivery

The therapeutic goal in any shock state is to enhance substrate delivery (DO_2) to the tissues. This is accomplished by maximizing cardiovascular performance and optimizing arterial oxygen content (CaO_2). The major emphasis is to improve tissue perfusion.

Maximize Cardiovascular Performance

Optimize Preload. Rapid intravascular volume expansion guided by clinical examination, RAP monitoring, and urine output is the most important immediate therapeutic intervention for patients in shock. Early correction of intravascular volume deficit is necessary to increase CO and to reestablish microcirculatory flow. Maintenance of the hyperdynamic septic state and improvement of oxygen consumption are critically dependent on fluid administration (Carcillo, Davis, & Zaritsky, 1991). Improvement in perfusion pressure, oxygen delivery, and consumption indicates successful fluid therapy.

Colloids or crystalloids may be used for acute volume expansion in patients in shock. Colloids—for example, albumin, synthetic plasma substitutes (hetastarch, dextran), whole blood, packed cells, and fresh-frozen plasma (FFP)—stay within the vascular space. Isotonic crystalloid (electrolyte) solutions—for example, normal saline and lactated Ringer's solution—will equilibrate between the intravascular and interstitial spaces.

Colloid infusion may be more effective than crystalloid in achieving optimum hemodynamic and oxygen transport goals. Colloids are important for maintaining plasma osmotic pressure and minimizing interstitial edema. In shock, the ideal solution would expand the intravascular space but limit interstitial accumulation. Prevention of interstitial pulmonary edema is critically important to prevent alterations in gas exchange. In patients with capillary leak syndrome, colloid therapy may actually increase the risk of pulmonary edema. In addition, colloids are expensive and difficult to titrate, making the possibility of fluid overload much greater than when crystalloid is used.

Albumin is commonly used if the hematocrit is adequate. FFP and platelets are administered if clotting abnormalities or thrombocytopenia exists. Synthetic plasma substitutes (dextran and hetastarch) are relatively inexpensive but cause diminished platelet function.

In an emergency, crystalloids are immediately available and can be rapidly infused to restore and maintain effective extracellular fluid volume. However, more than twice the amount of crystalloid as colloid is usually necessary to achieve the same degree of hemodynamic stability. Under-replacement is more likely to occur with crystalloid therapy, as about one third of infused crystalloids remain in the vascular space after 20 minutes. Use of lactated solutions in patients with impaired liver function may alter acid-base balance by increasing blood lactate concentrations and renal loss of sodium and potassium (Perkin & Levin, 1982).

Clinically, a variety of volume expanders in a 4:1 crystalloid to colloid ratio are usually employed, depending upon the type of volume loss suffered by the child and the availability of various colloids. The amount and rate of infusion will depend upon the child's condition; 20 mL/kg of an isotonic crystalloid infused over several minutes is a reasonable starting point. A second bolus of the same amount is infused if there is no improvement in the child's condition, e.g., increased mean arterial pressure, improved perfusion, increased urine output, and decreased acidosis.

Carcillo, Davis, and Zaritsky (1991) reported that aggressive fluid administration in excess of 40 mL/kg in the first hour after presentation to the emergency department is associated with improved survival, decreased occurrence of persistent hypovolemia, and no increase in the risk of cardiogenic pulmonary edema or ARDS in pediatric patients in septic shock. The researchers did not control for type of fluid used, crystalloids were used preferentially, and colloids were used if the blood pressure was unresponsive to crystalloids. Blood products were also used if coagulation was a problem.

If the patient with nonhemorrhagic hypovolemic shock fails to respond to 40 mL/kg of crystalloid infusions, complicating factors are suspected. Common causes of **unresponsive shock** include pneumothorax, pericardial effusion, ongoing intra-abdominal fluid loss (for example, due to volvulus, intussusception), gastrointestinal ischemia, brainstem dysfunction, adrenocortical insufficiency, and pulmonary hypertensive crisis.

Blood is administered as soon as possible to replace whole blood loss and/or correct anemia. Autotransfusion devices, for example, cell saving devices, scavenge then return blood lost during spinal fusion and intrathoracic surgical cases (when no enteric contamination has occurred). If there is evidence of continued bleeding or consumption of clotting factors, FFP may be given as well.

When managing children with cardiogenic or septic shock, efforts to improve cardiac output and tissue perfusion by volume augmentation are carefully monitored. The volume of fluid that can be safely administered is contingent on ventricular compliance. Continuous measurement of ventricular end-diastolic pressure (that is, RAP, LAP, or PAWP) permits early detection of cardiac decompensation and provides an important guide for fluid replacement. The vascular congestion associated with cardiogenic shock may be improved by concurrent administration of albumin with diuretics (furosemide [Lasix]).

Perkin and Levin (1990) described a helpful method of evaluating the effectiveness of volume replacement. Fluid is administered until the patient's hemodynamic status is corrected or the RAP exceeds the preinfusion value by 2 mmHg or the PCWP within 3 mmHg. A RAP greater than 7 to 10 indicates myocardial dysfunction, excessive right ventricular afterload, or volume overload. The authors note that the absolute limitation to fluid administration is persistent increase in ventricular filling pressure without improvement in CO.

Emergency autotransfusion to maintain an adequate perfusion pressure is enhanced by elevating the patient's limbs or by gentle compression on the liver. The Trendelenburg position is used cautiously, especially when cerebral perfusion pressures are questionable.

Optimize Contractility. Prior to, or concurrent with, the administration of positive inotropic medications, negative inotropic states—for example, hypoxia, acidosis, hypoglycemia, hypokalemia, and hypocalcemia—must be rectified (Fig. 29–6). Acidosis depresses myocardial function and renders sympathomimetic drugs ineffective. Poor outcomes have been associated with a base deficit greater than 10 mEq/L in patients with cardiogenic or septic shock. Base deficits greater than a negative 6 require correction. The *primary correction* for metabolic acidosis secondary to cardiovascular collapse is restoration of *tissue perfusion*. With adequate tissue perfusion and oxygenation, metabolic acidosis will self-correct. When the arterial pH is less than 7.20 and adequate ventilation has been established (that is, the $Paco_2$ is normal), correction with $NaHCO_3$ is indicated. The dose is calculated from the base deficit (mEq $NaHCO_3$ = 0.3 [weight in kg] × base deficit). The calculated dose usually approximates 1 to 2 mEq/kg. If the serum sodium is greater than 150, tris-hydroxymethyl-amino-methane (THAM), a non-CO_2 generating buffer, can be used with cautious evaluation of hypoglycemia and hyperkalemia.

Electrolyte shifts will occur when correcting metabolic acidosis. As the pH increases, ionized calcium levels fall and potassium shifts into the intracellular space, decreasing the serum potassium level. Cal-

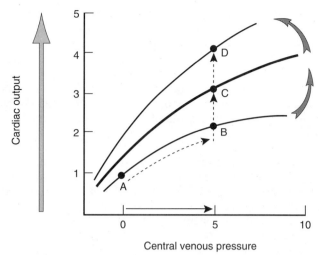

Figure 29–6 ● ● ● ● ● ●

Starling's law. Stroke volume and cardiac output are increased in the hypovolemic, acidotic child (point A) by increasing preload through volume infusion (point B), and by restoring the ventricular function curve to a more normal one (point C) by correcting acidosis and metabolic abnormalities. The myocardial function curve (and cardiac output) can potentially be shifted to a supranormal value (point D) with the infusion of a positive inotropic agent. (Modified from Crone, R.K. (1980). Acute circulatory failure in children. *Pediatric Clinics of North America*, 27 (3), 525–537.)

cium replacement may be necessary to correct hypocalcemia (ionized calcium level less than 1.3 mg/dL), occurring frequently in circulatory failure, especially after administration of large amounts of albumin, whole blood, or FFP.

After fluid resuscitation, pharmacologic therapy is then used to enhance cardiovascular performance (Table 29–8). Sympathomimetics stimulate alpha, beta, and dopaminergic receptors throughout the body, causing a variety of effects. It is difficult to predict the dose response of any catecholamine in patients in shock. Also, stress may deplete endogenous catecholamine stores and down-regulate alpha-adrenergic receptor sites (Zaritsky & Chernow, 1984). Pharmacologic management requires individual titration at the bedside. Frequently, more than one catecholamine is administered at a time; finding the best combination and dosage requires continuous patient assessment and invasive hemodynamic monitoring.

The rapid onset, controllable dosage, and ultra-short half-life of catecholamines make them effective for treating shock. Dopamine, epinephrine, norepinephrine, and dobutamine are the most frequently used exogenous catecholamines.

Dopamine is an endogenous catecholamine whose effects depend upon the patient's own endogenous catecholamine response (related to maturation) and releasable norepinephrine stores (related to chronic illness). Dopamine activates the dopamine and adrenergic receptors in a dose-dependent manner. Low doses (1–5 µg/kg/min) produce splanchnic and renal vasodilation and a decrease in SVR. The dopaminergic effect on renal blood flow results in increased

Table 29–8. PHARMACOLOGIC THERAPY USED IN SHOCK

Drug	Site of Action	Dose (μg/kg/min)	Primary Effect*	Secondary Effect
Dopamine	Dopam Dopam β_1 α	2–5 2–10 10–20	Increase renal perfusion Inotropy Chronotropy Increased renal perfusion Vasoconstriction	Dysrhythmias
Norepinephrine	$\alpha > \beta$	2–10	Vasoconstriction Inotropy	>MVo$_2$ Dysrhythmias <Renal BF
Epinephrine	α & β	0.05–1.5	Vasoconstriction Inotropy Chronotropy	>MVo$_2$ Dysrhythmias <Renal BF
Dobutamine	β_1	5–20	Inotropy	Tachycardia Dysrhythmias Vasodilation Hypotension
Sodium nitroprusside	NA	1–10 (light-sensitive)	Vasodilation (balanced)	<PVR >V/Q mismatch Cyanide toxicity
Nitroglycerin	NA	0.2–20	Vasodilation (venous)	<PVR >ICP
Amrinone	NA	5–10 (load with up to 3 mg/kg over 20 minutes)	Inotropy Vasodilation	Dysrhythmias <PVR Thrombocytopenia

*Difficult to predict the dose → response effect. Management requires individual titration at the bedside.
MVo$_2$, myocardial oxygen consumption; BF, blood flow; PVR, pulmonary vascular resistance; V/Q, ventilation/perfusion; ICP, intracranial pressure.

urine output. Dopamine stimulates beta$_1$-adrenergic receptors at moderate doses (5–10 μg/kg/min), resulting in a moderate positive inotropic effect in patients with normal myocardial function. At high doses (>10 μg/kg/min), dopamine is primarily an alpha-adrenergic agonist that causes tachycardia, renal vasoconstriction, and increased SVR. The increased afterload may decrease cardiac output. When dosages greater than 20 μg/kg/min are required to maintain blood pressure, an epinephrine drip should be considered as an alternative (Chameides, 1990). Dopamine is used either in less severely ill patients who do not require doses greater than 10 μg/kg/min or at low doses for its selective effect on renal and splanchnic perfusion in sicker patients who require other inotropes.

Epinephrine, also an endogenous catecholamine, mimics sympathetic nervous system stimulation by providing a perfect balance of both alpha and beta stimulation. Epinephrine increases myocardial and cerebral perfusion pressures. Its most pronounced action is on the beta receptors of the heart, vascular, and other smooth muscle. Epinephrine may be particularly helpful in septic shock and anaphylaxis when SVR is significantly low. Hypotensive septic patients may not respond to alpha agents in a normal manner, so higher doses (1.0 to 1.5 μg/kg/min) may be needed (Chameides, 1990). Renal blood flow will improve if perfusion pressure improves. Because catecholamines increase myocardial oxygen consumption, signs of myocardial hypoxia or ischemia such as

ST segment and T wave changes on the EKG may occur during administration.

Norepinephrine (Levophed) has been repopularized in septic shock. Also an endogenous catecholamine, norepinephrine's potent vasoconstrictor effects overshadow its positive inotropic effects. Starting dosage is 0.05 to 0.1 μg/kg/min. Beta effects are pronounced at the lower dosage, while alpha effects predominate at the higher dosage. Norepinephrine, administered with low-dose dopamine, is useful in early septic shock.

Dobutamine, a synthetic catecholamine, is a beta$_1$ stimulant that increases cardiac contractility but causes only a slight increase in heart rate. Since the alpha- and beta$_2$-adrenergic receptors are not stimulated by dobutamine, SVR is usually decreased and only minimal vasoconstriction is occasionally observed. Effects do not depend upon releasable norepinephrine stores. Dobutamine is very effective as a selective inotropic agent in a patient with poor perfusion but normal blood pressure. The starting dose is 5 to 10 μg/kg/min; if greater than 20 μg/kg/min is required to maintain blood pressure, epinephrine should be used instead (Chameides, 1990). Dobutamine is not as effective as dopamine in infants less than 1 year of age and in patients with septic shock. In cardiogenic shock, dobutamine will increase CO and decrease PAW and SVR. In a volume-depleted patient, dobutamine may cause systemic and pulmonary vasodilation and increased R-L intrapulmonary shunting, and thus decrease cardiac output and oxygen delivery despite improved contractility.

Optimize Afterload. In low-flow states, blood pressure is usually supported by an increase in SVR. However, in cardiogenic low-flow shock, the increased SVR may further compromise myocardial function and further limit CO (Fig. 29–7). When heart failure coexists with increased resistance to ventricular outflow (as evidenced by increased SVRI or PVRI), the use of vasodilators, often in combination with a positive inotropic agent, is indicated. Factors that increase afterload—for example, hypothermia, acidosis, hypoxia, pain, and anxiety—should be managed prior to considering vasodilator therapy.

By reducing the resistance to left ventricular outflow, arterial vasodilators increase the cardiac ejection fraction and increase stroke volume. In contrast, venous vasodilators shift blood into the periphery and reduce right and left ventricular end-diastolic volume. Decreased end-diastolic volume reduces myocardial wall stress and improves myocardial perfusion. Most vasodilators are classified as "balanced" and exert both arterial and venous effects.

Afterload reduction may be accomplished with a direct vasodilator, a beta-agonist, or alpha-antagonist. Note that *hypotension will result if a vasodilator is administered in the hypovolemic patient.* Fluids should be readily available at the bedside.

Amrinone and milrinone are nonglycoside, nonadrenergic, phosphodiesterase inhibitors that produce positive inotropic and vasodilator effects. An initial bolus of amrinone 0.75 to 3.0 mg/kg is required, followed by a continuous infusion of 5 to 10 μg/kg/min. In this dose range, amrinone reduces afterload and preload by its direct effect on vascular smooth muscle. In children with depressed myocardial function, amrinone produces a prompt increase in CO. Because amrinone is a nonsympathomimetic inotropic agent, it may be of particular value in patients with clinical problems that down-regulate adrenergic receptor sites, e.g., septic shock.

Sodium nitroprusside is a direct-acting vasodilator that relaxes both arteriolar and venous smooth muscle. The subsequent fall in afterload and preload improves CO only when the reduction of outflow resistance predominates over the effects of the reduced venous return. The dose range for nitroprusside is 0.5 to 8 μg/kg/min. Manifestations of toxicity (headache, nausea, palpitations, hyperventilation, metabolic acidosis, and unexplained elevation of venous oxygen tension) have occurred at relatively low doses, leading some to suggest a maximum infusion rate of 4 to 8 μg/kg/min for adults and less for infants and young children. Some precautions are necessary when the drug is administered: monitor serum levels of thiocyanate and cyanide, the toxic metabolites of nitroprusside; protect the 5% dextrose infusion containing the drug from light.

Other vasodilator drugs include nitroglycerin, a potent venodilator and pulmonary vasodilator; and captopril, an angiotensin-converting enzyme inhibitor that generally causes a decrease in both peripheral arterial pressure and resistance. Hydralazine exerts a peripheral vasodilating effect through direct relaxation of vascular smooth muscle, primarily arterial muscle, with little effect on venous beds. SVR decreases, but the change in filling pressure is minimal.

Tolazoline is a direct peripheral vasodilator with moderate alpha-adrenergic blocking activity. It decreases peripheral resistance, increases venous capacitance, and causes cardiac stimulation. In addition, tolazoline usually reduces pulmonary artery pressure and vascular resistance, which decreases right ventricular afterload and improves left ventricular preload. The use of epinephrine with large doses of tolazoline may cause epinephrine reversal, a further reduction of blood pressure that is followed by an exaggerated rebound.

Nitric oxide (NO) has been identified as the endothelial-derived relaxing factor (EDRF). Inhaled in a dose range less than 80 ppm, NO acts as a selective local pulmonary vasodilator within 3 minutes without causing systemic effects (Roberts, Polaner, Lang, Zapol, 1992). NO is selective to the pulmonary vascular bed because it is rapidly inactivated when combined with hemoglobin. NO stimulates the release of cyclic guanosine monophosphate (GMP); and, unlike arginine, a precursor for NO synthesis, NO works on sick pulmonary endothelium. NO affects only ventilated areas and thus may improve oxygenation when V/Q mismatch is present.

Optimizing Heart Rate and Rhythm. Changes in heart rate directly impact cardiac output. However, increasing the heart rate to optimize cardiac output is usually not an option among pediatric patients. When tissue perfusion is inadequate, heart rate is usually at or near peak capacity. Excessively rapid heart rates associated with fever, volume depletion, and endogenous catecholamine release secondary to the stress response may limit ventricular diastolic filling and compromise stroke volume and cardiac output. Aggressive management of dysrhythmias that occur secondary to electrolyte imbalance and metabolic acidosis is warranted.

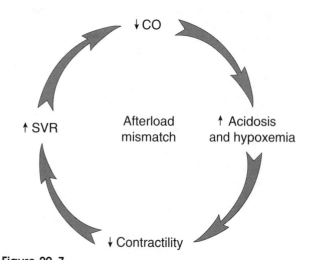

Figure 29–7 ● ● ● ● ● ●

"Afterload mismatch" present in low-flow cardiogenic shock.

Maximize Substrate Transport

Arterial Oxygen Content. While much clinical attention is appropriately focused on optimizing cardiovascular performance in patients with shock, an equal amount of attention must also be placed on the oxygen content of blood perfusing the cardiovascular bed. Oxygen content is optimized by maintaining adequate hemoglobin levels, that is, a hematocrit that optimizes DO_2. Blood administration is required to correct both whole blood loss and severe anemia.

Lucking and others (1990), studying children in hyperdynamic septic shock post volume loading and pharmacologic support, found that despite an initial low OER, VO_2 could be increased by augmenting DO_2 through packed RBC tranfusion. The researchers noted that since VO_2 correlates with survival, one should consider enhancing VO_2 despite an initial low OER and high DO_2. Mink and Pollack (1990) reported a similar study but found that although DO_2 significantly increased after a similar RBC transfusion, VO_2 did not change.

Not only are adequate levels of hemoglobin important, but also hemoglobin saturation with oxygen is ensured by providing adequate oxygenation and ventilation. Extreme shifts in the oxyhemoglobin dissociation curve are avoided by maintaining normal pH and body temperature.

Minimize Energy Expenditure

In addition to enhancing substrate delivery to the tissues, an adjunctive strategy is to limit the patient's metabolic demands. Early identification of clinical states that increase demand and initiation of interventions to decrease physiologic work benefit patients with little or no metabolic reserve. Interventions include providing adequate support of ventilation to decrease the work of breathing, early identification of both heat and cold stress (for each degree Celsius, the metabolic demands change 13%), prevention of shivering, and providing periods of rest and adequate sedation/analgesia. Nurses play an invaluable role in reducing the anxiety and fear that patients and families experience during critical illness and intensive care. The unfamiliar environment, painful procedures, and the potential for death that accompany advanced shock are issues that nurses are in a unique position to address.

Optimize Nutrition

Critically ill infants and children are at risk for malnutrition because their metabolic needs far exceed their nutritional stores and also because of the nature and duration of their illnesses. Previously well-nourished infants and children may develop nutritional deficiencies after 3 to 5 days of serious illness and intensive care; infants and children who have been hospitalized for some time before the de-velopment of shock may already be malnourished. In septic shock, there is a sequential alteration in the utilization of glucose, then fat, and finally protein as sources of energy. Parenteral support of nutrition is initiated as soon as possible (see Chapter 14). Continuous venovenous hemofiltration (CVVH) can be used to facilitate caloric delivery in patients who are fluid restricted and/or in acute renal failure (see Chapter 22).

PROACTIVE CARE: VIGILANCE

Preventing the often lethal complications of shock through anticipatory monitoring of evolving problems is an important nursing activity. All organ systems are at risk from hypoxia and acidosis, and irreparable MODS may preclude successful management of shock.

Newborns

The newborn in shock presents with additional challenges to the critical care nurse. The newborn in stress is often hypothermic due to immature thermoregulation and has low serum glucose and calcium levels due to limited intracellular stores. Because of their large surface area/volume ratio, infants will lose heat rapidly to the environment. Alterations in carbohydrate metabolism occur secondary to endogenous epinephrine release. Epinephrine produces an initial increase in serum glucose levels that decrease rapidly with depletion of hepatic glycogen stores and failure of gluconeogenesis. Anaerobic glycolysis elevates blood lactate and pyruvate levels, contributing to acidosis. Stressed neonates are at high risk for apnea, necrotizing enterocolitis as blood is shunted away from the gut, and seizures due to hypoglycemia and hypocalcemia.

Multiple Organ Dysfunction Syndrome

ARDS, DIC, acute tubular necrosis (ATN), hepatic dysfunction, pancreatic ischemia, and gastrointestinal hemorrhage are not uncommon in critically ill children with shock. Even with normal or increased cardiac output, the child in shock may suffer myocardial injury as evidenced by ST segment changes on the EKG and abnormal cardiac enzyme values.

Ongoing assessment of pulmonary function is important so that early detection and management of respiratory failure can be assured. Oxygen reserve is limited and compensatory mechanisms are maximized in shock states, sharply decreasing the patient's tolerance of even brief periods of hypoxia and respiratory acidosis. In patients who develop ARDS, the mechanism of injury may involve activation of complement proteins that promote aggregation of granulocytes in the lung. Granulocytes release proteolytic enzymes and toxic oxygen radicals that cause direct lung injury. Decreased pulmonary compliance and altered V/Q relationship result in increased intrapulmonary shunting and venous admixture. In cardiogenic shock, left ventricular end-diastolic pressure of approximately 20 to 25 mmHg directly results in the development of pulmonary edema. In septic shock, damage to the alveolar pulmonary capillary epithelium produces a protein fluid leak into the interstitium and alveoli. Early and appropriate intervention in either case includes oxygen administration and colloid-diuretic therapy. Endotracheal intubation, mechanical ventilation, and PEEP are used to support an adequate functional residual capacity and limit intrapulmonary shunting.

Since DIC frequently accompanies shock states, blood coagulation studies are assessed early in the patient's course and component therapy is provided as indicated. What is accepted as a minimum platelet count varies from one institution to another. FFP and cryoprecipitate are used to correct prolonged prothrombin time, activated partial thromboplastin time, and abnormal fibrinogen levels when necessary.

Renal hypoperfusion reduces glomerular filtration and stimulates aldosterone and antidiuretic hormone secretion, which contribute to progressive azotemia with or without oliguria. In shock, acute renal failure occurs on a continuum from acute tubular necrosis to cortical necrosis. Albumin with diuretics and low-dose dopamine augment renal perfusion and urine output. Progressive hyperkalemia, refractory acidosis, and hypervolemia may require dialysis.

Gastrointestinal hypoperfusion may lead to ulceration of the stomach and intestines. Ulceration not only increases the risk of bleeding but also disrupts the patient's natural barrier to infection. Stress ulcer prevention with antacid and histamine (H_2)–receptor antagonist administration may control gastric acidity and prevent gastric bleeding.

The liver may also fail to perform many functions, for example, metabolism of drugs and hormones and conjugation of bilirubin. Medications that require hepatic metabolism are limited or administered with caution.

Purpura fulminans describes the extensive, patchy, purpuric, and ischemic areas of the extremities and buttocks noted in patients with fever, septic shock, and DIC (Irazuzta, McManus, 1990). The massive tissue destruction is commonly associated with meningococcal or *Haemophilus influenzae* infection. The pathophysiology involves endotoxemia, vasculitis, DIC, and a low blood flow state resulting in widespread thrombosis of the venules and capillaries, particularly of the superficial vascular plexus (Wong, Hitchcock, Mason, 1989). Numerous therapies intended to limit tissue loss and prevent gangrene are under investigation. Current therapies include heparinization, dextran infusion, sympathetic blockade (Chiafery, Stephany, & Holliday, 1993), and nitroglycerin. Irazuzta and McManus (1990) reported an increase in skin perfusion with the use of topical nitropaste 2% (15 mg/2.5 cm; total 15 cm; every 6 hours). In the patient with meningococcemia, household contacts receive prophylaxis with rifampin.

ALTERNATIVE THERAPIES

Clinical management of the septic shock patient is in transition from helping the patient defend against invading microorganisms to helping the patient defend against them him/herself. Numerous agents for the treatment of shock (particularly septic shock) are under investigation (Table 29–9). It is likely that a number of individual therapies used in combination will prove beneficial for patients in septic shock (Giroir, 1993).

Ziegler et al. (1991) reported a multicenter, randomized, double-blind, placebo-controlled clinical trial of the HA-1A human antiendotoxin IgM monoclonal antibody specific for the lipid A portion of bacterial endotoxin. Either HA-1A or placebo was given in a single infusion over 15 to 20 minutes to severely ill septic adult patients along with conventional therapy. The experimental group had reduced mortality (49%–30%), but there were several methodologic flaws. More patients in the control group had received inappropriate antibiotics and had more system dysfunction than the experimental group. Warren, Danner, and Munford (1992) noted that the results were suggestive but not conclusive. They rec-

Table 29–9. EXPERIMENTAL THERAPIES FOR SEPSIS

Monoclonal antibodies to:
  Endotoxin
  Exotoxin
  TNF
  Interleukin-1
  Complement fragment C5a
Receptor antagonists to:
  TNF
  Interleukin-1
  Platelet-activating factor
  Thromboxane
  Bradykinin
Prostaglandin
Other inhibitors of inflammation
  C1 inhibitor
  Arachidonic acid inhibitors
    Cyclooxygenase pathway (ibuprofen)
    Thromboxane synthetase (imidazole)
    Lipoxygenase pathway (diethylcarbamazine)
    Leukotriene inhibitors
  Neutrophil inhibitors
    Pentoxifylline
    Adenosine
    Antioxidants
    Heavy metal chelators
    Oxygen radical scavengers
    Protease inhibitors
Modulators of coagulation
  Antithrombin III
  Protein C
  Plasminogen activators
Other
  Gut decontamination
  Antihistamines
  Naloxone
  Calcium channel blockers

Adapted from Bone, R.C. (1991). A critical evaluation of new agents for the treatment of sepsis. *JAMA*, 266 (12), 1686–1691. © 1989, American Medical Association.

ommend that HA-1A remain experimental until a second randomized placebo-controlled trial is conducted. Limitations also include cost ($4000 per patient per course) and timing. Successful use of immunotherapy requires early intervention, before the mediator cascade is initiated. Monoclonal antibodies to TNF are also under development.

Endogenous endorphins play an important role in modulating sympathetic nervous system responses in all types of shock. Peripheral endorphin effects may involve vascular and myocardial depression, calcium transport, and modulation of macrophage responses. The opioid antagonist naloxone has been found to rapidly reverse hypotension secondary to endotoxin and blood loss in animals. Naloxone has been used successfully in some children with septic shock who failed to respond to conventional therapy. The response to naloxone therapy has been inconsistent, and severe reactions may occur.

Similar variable results have been obtained with the use of corticosteroid in shock. In certain subgroups of septic shock patients, corticosteroid administration may improve short-term survival and permit reversal of shock. In contrast, adverse effects include superinfection, electrolyte imbalance, hyperglycemia, and gastrointestinal bleeding (Bone, Fisher, Clemmer et al., 1987). In septic shock, Zimmerman (1990) postulated that steroid administration *before* antibiotic administration may help attenuate the inflammatory response that occurs secondary to endotoxin release. Steroid administration may be efficacious in patients with sepsis from specific organisms, for example, gram-negative bacteremia (Veterans Administration, 1987).

Steroid administration is considered when adrenocortical insufficiency is suspected, for example, in patients whose adrenal tissue is destroyed as in Waterhouse-Friderichsen syndrome associated with meningococcemia. Also at risk are chronically ill patients who may not be able to increase their cortisol output in response to stress.

Plasmapheresis (removal of the child's blood, separation of the plasma and blood cells, and reinfusion of the packed cells in fresh plasma) and continuous arteriovenous/venovenous hemofiltration (CAVH/CVVH) have also been used to remove septic shock mediators, endotoxin, and/or bacterial byproducts. McManus and Churchwell (1991) identified coagulopathy (defined as PTT >50 seconds and fibrinogen <150 mg/dL) as a poor prognostic indicator in meningococcemia and purpura fulminans. The authors used plasmapheresis in severely coagulopathic patients as a means of restoring normal clotting factors without fluid overload. Although the sample size was small, plasmapheresis was found to be safe and effective in correcting coagulopathy and stabilizing hemodynamics.

CONCLUSIONS

In summary, care of the pediatric patient in shock requires multidisciplinary collaboration. Recognizing the child's condition early, diligently tending to the administration and evaluation of treatment, and preventing the onset of common complications compose a challenging nursing role.

References

Bone, R.C. (1991a). Let's agree on terminology: Definition of sepsis. *Critical Care Medicine*, 19 (7), 973–976.

Bone R.C. (1991b). Gram-negative sepsis: Background, clinical features, and intervention. *Chest*, 100 (3), 802–808.

Bone, R.C., Fisher, C.J., Clemmer, T.P., Slotman, G.J., Metz, C.A., & Balk, R.A. (1987). A controlled clinical trial of high-dose methylprednisolone in the treatment of severe sepsis and septic shock. *New England Journal of Medicine*, 317 (11), 653–658.

Carcillo, J.A., Davis, A.L., & Zaritsky, A. (1991). Role of early fluid resuscitation in pediatric septic shock. *JAMA*, 266 (9), 1242–1245.

Chiafery, M.C., Stephany, R.A., & Holliday, K.J. (1993). Epidural sympathetic blockade to relieve vascular insufficiency in an infant with purpura fulminans. *Critical Care Nurse*, 13 (3) 71–76.

Clark, C.H., & Gutierrez, G. (1992). Gastric intramucosal pH: A noninvasive method for the indirect measurement of tissue oxygenation. *American Journal of Critical Care*, 1 (2), 53–60.

Curley, M.A.Q. (1989). *Red flags in the critically unstable pediatric patient* (videotape). New York: American Journal of Nursing.

Fagan, M.J. (1988). Relationship between nurses' assessments of perfusion and toe temperature in pediatric patients with cardiovascular disease. *Heart & Lung*, 17 (2), 157–165.

Fink, M.P. (1993). Adequacy of gut oxygenation in endotoxemia and sepsis (review). *Critical Care Medicine*, 21 (2 Suppl.), S4–8.

Giroir, B.P. (1993). Mediators of septic shock: New approaches for interrupting the endogenous inflammatory cascade. *Critical Care Medicine*, 21 (5), 780–789.

Gutierrez, G., Palizas, F., Doglio, G., Wainsztein, N., Gallesio, A., Pacin, J., Dubin, A., Schiavi, E., Jorge, M., Pasajo, J., Klein, F., San Roman, E., Dorfman, B., Shottlender, J., & Giniger, R. (1992). Gastric intramucosal pH as a therapeutic index of tissue oxygenation in critically ill patients. *Lancet*, 339 (8787), 195–199.

Hazinski, M.F., Iberti, T.J., MacIntyre, N.R., Parker, M.M., Tribett, D., Prion, S., & Chmel, H. (1993). Epidemiology, pathophysiology and clinical presentation of gram negative sepsis. *American Journal of Critical Care*, 2 (3), 224–237.

Irazuzta, J., & McManus, M.L. (1990). Use of topically applied nitroglycerin in the treatment of purpura fulminans. *The Journal of Pediatrics*, 117 (6), 993–995.

Jarvis, W.R. (1987). Epidemiology of nosocomial infections in pediatric patients. *Journal of Pediatric Infectious Disease*, 6, 344–351.

Klein, D.M., & Witek-Janusek, L. (1992). Advances in immunotherapy of sepsis. *Dimensions of Critical Care Nursing*, 11 (2), 75–89.

Lister, G. (1991). Oxygen supply/demand in the critically ill. In R. Taylor (Ed.). *Critical care: State of the art* (Vol. 12, pp. 311–350). Fullerton, CA: Society of Critical Care Medicine.

Lucking, S.E., Williams, T.M., Chaten, F.C., Metz, R.I., & Mickell, J.J. (1990). Dependence of oxygen consumption on oxygen delivery in children with hyperdynamic septic shock. *Critical Care Medicine*, 18 (12), 1316–1319.

McManus, M.L., & Churchwell, K.B. (1991). Consumptive coagulopathy as predictor of outcome in purpura fulminans. *Anesthesiology*, 75, A286.

Mink, R.B., & Pollack, M.M. (1990). Effect of blood transfusion on oxygen consumption in pediatric septic shock. *Critical Care Medicine*, 18 (10), 1087–1091.

Natanson, C., Hoffman, W.D., & Parrillo, J.E. (1989). Septic shock: The cardiovascular abnormality and therapy. *Journal of Cardiothoracic Anesthesia*, 3 (2), 215–227.

NIH Conference: Parrillo, J.E. (Moderator) (1990). Septic shock in humans, advances in the understanding of pathogenesis, cardiovascular dysfunction, and therapy. *Annals of Internal Medicine*, 113 (3), 227–242.

Parrillo, J.E. (1990). Septic shock in humans: Advances in the understanding of pathogenesis, cardiovascular dysfunction, and therapy. *Annals of Internal Medicine, 111,* 227–242.

Perkin, R.M., & Levin, D.L. (1982). Shock in the pediatric patient. Part I. *The Journal of Pediatrics, 101* (2), 163–169; Shock in the pediatric patient. Part II. Therapy. *The Journal of Pediatrics,* 101 (3), 319–332.

Perkin R.M., & Levin D.L. (1990). Shock. In D.L. Levin & F.C. Morriss (Eds.). *Essentials of pediatric intensive care* (pp. 78–97). St. Louis: Quality Medical Publishing.

Pollack, M.M., Fields, A.I., & Ruttimann, U.E. (1984). Sequential cardiopulmonary variables of infants and children in septic shock. *Critical Care Medicine, 12* (7), 554–559.

Pollack, M.M., Fields, A.I., & Ruttimann, U.E. (1985). Distributions of cardiopulmonary variables in pediatric survivors and nonsurvivors of septic shock. *Critical Care Medicine, 13* (6), 454–459.

Roberts, J.D., Polaner, D.M., Lang, P., & Zapol, W.M. (1992). Inhaled nitric oxide in persistent pulmonary hypertension of the newborn. *Lancet, 340* (8823), 818–819.

Schumacker, P.T., & Cain, S.M. (1987). The concept of a critical oxygen delivery. *Intensive Care Medicine, 13,* 223–229.

Tuchschmidt, J., Oblitas, D., & Fried, J.C. (1991). Oxygen consumption in sepsis and septic shock. *Critical Care Medicine, 19* (5), 664–671.

Veterans Administration Systemic Sepsis Cooperative Group (1987). Effect of high-dose glucocorticoid therapy on mortality in patients with clinical signs of systemic sepsis. *New England Journal of Medicine, 317* (11), 659–665.

Warren, H.S., Danner, R.L., & Munford, R.S. (1992). Sounding board: Anti-endotoxin monoclonal antibodies. *New England Journal of Medicine, 326* (17), 1153–1156.

Wong, V.K., Hitchcock, W., & Mason, W. (1989). Meningococcal infection in children: A review of 100 cases. *Journal of Pediatric Infectious Disease, 8,* 224–227.

Zaritsky, A., & Chernow, B. (1984). Use of catecholamines in pediatrics. *The Journal of Pediatrics, 105* (3), 341–350.

Ziegler, E.J., Fisher, C.J., Sprung, C.L., Straube, R.C., Sadoff, J.C., Foulke, G.E., Wortel, C.H., Fink, M.P., Dellinger, R.P., Teng, N.N.H., Allen, I.E., Berger, H.J., Knatterud, G.L., LoBuglio, A.F., & Smith, C.R. (1991). Treatment of gram-negative bacteremia and septic shock with HA-1A human monoclonal antibody against endotoxin. *New England Journal of Medicine, 324,* 429–436.

Zimmerman, J.J., & Dietrich, K.A. (1987). Current perspectives on septic shock. *Pediatric Clinics of North America, 34* (1), 131–163.

CHAPTER 30

Trauma

PATRICIA A. MOLONEY-HARMON
PATRICIA SRNEC
REGINA MUIR

Trauma remains the leading cause of death in children. In children between the ages of 1 and 19 years, injuries cause more deaths than all diseases combined and are a leading cause of disability (Division of Injury Control, 1990). The single largest cause of trauma-related death is motor vehicle accidents. Other causes of death include homicides, suicides, drownings, burns, and falls.

It is estimated that in the United States, more than 30,000 children suffer permanent disabilities from injury every year (Division of Injury Control, 1990). An estimated 600,000 children annually are hospitalized for their injuries, and almost 16 million injured children are seen in hospital emergency departments. The cost of injuries to children is estimated to be over $7.5 billion a year and is higher when the cost of lost future productivity is taken into account (Division of Injury Control, 1990).

Two out of three childhood accidents occur in males, with the peak accidental age range between 4 and 12 years (Widner-Kolberg & Moloney-Harmon, 1994). Blunt trauma accounts for 80% of all accidental injuries. Blunt injuries are associated with rapid deceleration, which may occur with motor vehicle accidents; or from direct blows, the result of contact sports or child abuse. Penetrating trauma accounts for the other 20% of injuries.

Head injury is the most common injury seen in children and accounts for 80% of all pediatric trauma deaths. This is because the head of a child accounts for a larger proportion of body weight. Skeletal injuries usually involve the long bones, especially of the lower limbs. Other common injuries include abdominal and thoracic. The kidneys, spleen, and liver are not well protected in the child and thus are more susceptible to trauma.

Regardless of the type of injury, the final common pathways of trauma are tissue hypoxia secondary to inadequate oxygenation and ventilation, fluid volume deficit, and cerebral hypertension. The goal of pediatric trauma care is to stabilize the effects of traumatic injury before irreversible damage occurs. Frequently, children will survive the initial insult only to die later because of complications such as malignant intracranial hypertension, sepsis, respiratory failure, or multiple organ dysfunction syndrome (MODS).

The purpose of this chapter is to provide information about caring for the critically injured child. Initial resuscitation is presented, followed by a discussion of specific system injuries with collaborative management. Prevention strategies are also reviewed.

INITIAL RESUSCITATION

The initial resuscitation of the pediatric trauma victim is guided by the principles of the primary and secondary survey. The primary survey allows for the rapid identification of any life-threatening injuries.

Primary Survey

Airway

The first assessment priority for the pediatric trauma patient is airway patency. The child is observed for signs of respiratory distress, such as tachypnea, nasal flaring, retractions, stridor, the use of accessory muscles, and decreased level of consciousness. These symptoms require immediate intervention.

Stabilization of the airway is based on observed symptoms and progresses for simple to complex interventions. The child is assumed to have a cervical spine injury until proven otherwise, so that manual in-line immobilization is a critical aspect of airway management. An appropriately sized rigid cervical collar can be applied, but immobilization must be maintained manually if a collar is not available. To determine the correct size, the collar is measured in width from the top of the shoulder to the chin with the head in neutral position.

While in-line manual cervical immobilization is maintained, the airway is opened using the jaw-thrust method. The jaw-thrust maneuver alone may relieve airway obstruction. If the child does not respond, vomit, blood, or broken teeth may be obstructing the airway. Severe maxillofacial injuries or injuries to the larynx may also produce airway obstruction.

If the child does not respond to positioning and suctioning, artificial ventilation with 100% oxygen and intubation is indicated. Following intubation, an nasogastric tube is inserted for gastric decompression. An oral gastric tube is inserted if there is any question of a basilar skull fracture.

A rapid-sequence intubation is appropriate for the child with a full stomach or in the child with the potential for increased intracranial pressure. All pediatric trauma victims are assumed to have a full stomach, and a rapid-sequence intubation will minimize the possibility of regurgitation (Fackler & Yaster, 1992). This technique will also blunt the response of increased intracranial pressure that can be stimulated by intubation. Prior to the administration of the intubation medications, the child is preoxygenated with 100% oxygen. The sedatives and muscle relaxants are given in a rapid sequence intravenously while cricoid pressure is applied (Table 30–1).

The technique of cricoid pressure (Sellick's maneuver) is used during a rapid-sequence intubation to prevent passive regurgitation of stomach contents into the pharynx. In this technique, the upper esophagus is compressed against the cervical vertebral column by applying anteroposterior pressure on the cricoid cartilage (Rice & Britton, 1993). Cricoid pressure is maintained until correct placement of the endotracheal tube has been confirmed.

In some uncommon instances, the child will require a needle cricothyroidotomy. This technique is indicated in the child with an obstruction below the larynx or with a significant maxillofacial or airway injury. A 14- or 16-gauge needle is inserted through the cricothyroid membrane to establish the airway. If this is not possible, a surgical tracheostomy is performed.

Breathing

Assessment of the child's breathing status includes observation for signs of respiratory distress, especially once the airway is established. In addition to signs described under airway assessment, the child may exhibit "see-saw" breathing (paradoxic movement of the chest and abdomen). Although this is normal in children, it will become greatly exaggerated in respiratory distress. Assessment also includes an examination of the chest for contusions, lacerations, unequal chest movement, and deformities in rib structure. Breath sounds are auscultated in both the apices and the bases bilaterally, with careful attention to the quality of the breath sounds. Significant thoracic injury may be present even with minimal outward signs of trauma. Stabilization of the child's respiratory status is accomplished by 100% oxygen and artificial ventilation at a rate that is age- and condition-specific.

Table 30–1. SUGGESTED DRUGS FOR RAPID-SEQUENCE INTUBATION IN CHILDREN

Atropine
   0.02 mg/kg (1 mg maximum, 0.15 mg minimum)
Muscle relaxant (vecuronium or succinylcholine)
   Vecuronium 0.1 mg/kg
   Succinylcholine 2.0 mg/kg (infants), 1.5 mg/kg (children)
Sedation agent: problem-specific
   No hypotension/hypovolemia (excluding status asthmaticus)
      Thiopental 4–5 mg/kg
   Mild hypotension/hypovolemia with suspected head injury
      Thiopental 2–4 mg/kg
   Mild hypotension/hypovolemia without head injury
      Ketamine 1–2 mg/kg
   Severe hypotension/hypovolemia
      No sedative or ketamine 0.35–0.7 mg/kg
   Status asthmaticus
      Ketamine 1–2 mg/kg

Adapted from Yamamoto, L. G., Yim, G. K., & Britten, A. G. (1990). Rapid sequence induction for emergency intubation. *Pediatric Emergency Care, 6* (3), 205.

If respiratory distress, unequal breath sounds, and unstable vital signs are present, a pneumothorax or hemothorax is suspected and warrants immediate intervention. For a pneumothorax, needle decompression of the chest is performed without waiting for confirmation of the diagnosis by chest roentgenogram. A 14- to 20-gauge needle is inserted into the fourth or fifth intercostal space at the midaxillary line. After the initial rush of air occurs, a chest tube is inserted into the same space.

If a hemothorax is suspected, a large-bore needle is inserted at the same site used for evacuation of a pneumothorax. Fluid resuscitation is started before evacuation of the hemothorax to prevent exsanguination. Excessive bleeding through the chest tube may require clamping of the tube to tamponade bleeding. If bleeding persists at a rate of equal to or greater than 2 mL/kg/hour, an emergency thoracotomy is indicated (Eichelberger & Anderson, 1987).

Circulation

A small amount of blood loss can quickly produce hypovolemic shock in the child. Assessment of the child for hypovolemic shock consists of close observation and measurement of heart rate, systemic perfusion, and blood pressure. Symptoms of shock include tachycardia, capillary refill greater than 2 seconds, cool and mottled extremities, pallor, narrowed pulse pressure, decreased urine output, and decreased level of consciousness. A decrease in systolic blood pressure is a late sign of shock; the child who is hypotensive can be assumed to have lost between 25% and 50% of the total blood volume (King, 1985). Bleeding in excess of one half of the circulating blood volume is associated with profound hypotension and is often fatal (King, 1985). Table 30–2 presents the four classes of hemorrhage, with clinical signs and initial treatment for each stage.

The most crucial aspect of treatment for the hypotensive pediatric trauma victim is restoration of the circulating blood volume. An intravenous line is inserted, although this may be difficult in the hypovolemic child. If venous access cannot be obtained quickly, intraosseous access may be attempted.

Once venous or intraosseous access has been obtained, Ringer's lactate is administered at 20 mL/kg by IV push. The child's response to the fluid bolus is evaluated by looking for a decrease in heart rate; increased capillary refill time, pulse pressure, urine output, and warmth of the extremities; a return of color; and an improvement in the level of consciousness. If the response to fluid administration is inadequate, a second fluid bolus of Ringer's lactate is given at 20 mL/kg. If shock still persists, packed cells are administered at 10 mL/kg (Waisman & Eichelberger, 1993). All fluids are warmed by a fluid warmer prior to administration to prevent hypothermia. Once shock has been controlled, fluids can be delivered at the maintenance rate.

Use of pneumatic antishock garments (PASG) is not indicated in children for several reasons. The inflation of the abdominal compartment may cause respiratory arrest by interfering with diaphragmatic excursion. In addition, pulmonary edema may result when fluid infusion is accompanied by a sudden increase in afterload, which is produced by the application of PASG. Finally, there is evidence that suggests outcome is worsened by application of PASG (Maddox, Bichell, Pete et al., 1987). Generally, PASG are

Table 30–2. CLASSES OF HEMORRHAGE FOR CHILDREN

Class	Blood Loss	Signs	Treatment
Class I	15% or less 40-kg child = 500 mL blood	Pulse: slight increase BP: normal Respiration: normal Capillary refill: normal Tilt test:* normal	Crystalloids Rule 3:1 (3 mL of RL:1 mL blood loss), e.g., 500 mL blood loss = 1200–1500 mL RL
Class II	20–30% 40-kg child = 800 mL blood	Tachycardia > 150 BP: systolic decreased, decreased pulse pressure Tachypnea > 35–40 Delayed capillary refill Positive tilt test Urine output normal (1 mL/kg/h)	Crystalloids Rule 3:1 as above, e.g., 800 mL blood loss = 2100–2400 mL RL
Class III	30–35% 40-kg child = 1200 mL blood	Blood pressure drop Narrow pulse pressure Urine output affected	Crystalloids 20 mL/kg Packed red cells 10 mL/kg
Class IV	40–50% 40-kg child = 1600 mL blood	Nonpalpable blood pressure and pulse No response to verbal or painful stimuli	Crystalloids 20 mL/kg Packed red cells 10 mL/kg

*A tilt test is performed by sitting the child upright. The test is normal if the child can stay up more than 90 seconds and maintain blood pressure.
BP, blood pressure; RL, Ringer's lactate.
From Widner-Kolberg, M. R., & Moloney-Harmon, P. A. (1994). Pediatric trauma. In V. D. Cardona, P. D. Hurn, P. J. B. Mason, et al. (Eds.): *Trauma nursing: From resuscitation through rehabilitation* (2nd ed., p. 703). Philadelphia: W. B. Saunders.

indicated for ongoing hemorrhage resulting from a pelvic fracture (Waisman & Eichelberger, 1993).

If shock continues despite all interventions, other causes of shock are considered. The child may have developed a tension pneumothorax, which requires immediate intervention. If muffled heart sounds and pulsus paradoxus are present, the child may have developed pericardial tamponade, which requires an immediate pericardiocentesis. If these are not present and shock persists, immediate surgical intervention, such as an exploratory laparotomy, is warranted.

Disability

Once airway, breathing, and circulation have been stabilized, a rapid assessment for neurologic injury takes place. Head injuries are common in children, with a high incidence of mortality and morbidity.

Neurologic assessment during the primary survey consists of observation of the level of consciousness, pupil size and reaction, and motor response. The Glasgow Coma Scale (GCS) or the AVPU scale can be used to determine initial level of consciousness. The AVPU scale is defined in Table 30–3.

Control of intracranial hypertension, maintenance of adequate cerebral perfusion, and prevention of hypoxia are the goals of stabilization for the child with a neurologic injury. A secure airway is critical, since hypoxia and hypercapnia must be avoided. If the child is hypotensive, fluids are given at the resuscitation dose, even if neurologic injury is present. One must keep in mind, however, that an isolated head injury rarely causes shock. If shock is present, a high index of suspicion for another source of bleeding should exist.

Once the cervical spine has been cleared by roentgenography, the head of the bed may be elevated. This will help to decrease cerebral venous pressure and control intracranial hypertension.

Exposure

Exposure is an important component of the primary survey. The child is completely exposed, to examine for life-threatening injuries. This does, however, place the child at risk for hypothermia. Hypothermia produces various physiologic consequences, such as metabolic acidosis and dysrhythmias, and can interfere with resuscitation efforts.

Radiant warmers and warmed IV fluids and blood are used with pediatric trauma patients during resuscitation. The child's core temperature is maintained between 36° and 38°C. If the child is hypother-

mic on arrival to the unit, a warming blanket on the bed and warm, humidified oxygen are used. Refer to Chapter 15 for more information on the management of hypothermia in the child.

Secondary Survey

The secondary survey follows the primary survey and the initial stabilization of the cardiorespiratory system. The secondary survey is the systematic evaluation of each body system for injury. The order of the examination may vary but normally proceeds in descending order of urgency (Fackler & Yaster, 1992). The examination of the abdomen and perineum occurs last unless otherwise indicated, because this assessment produces pain and the child's response may obscure other findings. As the secondary survey is initiated, it is important to remember that any child with one injury is assumed to have another until proven otherwise. The examination is as gentle as possible, and reassessment is continuous. In-depth assessment of each system is covered under system-specific injuries.

TRAUMA SCORES

Reliable means of measuring injury severity and resulting disability are necessary to scientifically assess care provided to injured children (Sacco, Copes, & Gotschall, 1993). Numerous scoring systems that use measures of anatomic or physiologic derangements to quantify severity of injury have been developed. These scores include the Glasgow Coma Score (GCS); Trauma Score (TS); Circulation, Respiration, Abdomen, Motor, Speech (CRAMS) Scale; Revised Trauma Score (RTS); Abbreviated Injury Scale (AIS); and Injury Severity Score (ISS). These scores may be used for field triage, quality assessment, scientific comparison of trauma patients, and epidemiologic research (Sacco, Copes, & Gotschall, 1993).

A pediatric trauma score was developed in the 1980s because the existing scores did not take into account normal pediatric physiologic parameters. The Pediatric Trauma Score (PTS) considers the unique anatomic and physiologic characteristics of the child and uses these measures to predict childhood injury severity (Tepas, Ramenofsky, Mollitt, et al., 1988). Table 30–4 illustrates the PTS. A score of 8 or less warrants transport to a pediatric trauma center (Eichelberger, Gotschall, Sacco et al., 1989).

The current focus on the variety of scores available is further refinement and validation. Scores are often revised and modified as use demonstrates limitations.

Table 30–3 AVPU SCALE

A = patient is alert
V = patient responds to verbal commands
P = patient responds to pain
U = patient is unresponsive

Table 30–4. PEDIATRIC TRAUMA SCORE

Component	Category		
	+2	+1	-1
Size	>20 kg	10–20 kg	<10 kg
Airway	Normal	Maintainable	Unmaintainable
Systolic BP	>90 mmHg	50–90 mmHg	<50 mmHg
CNS	Awake	Obtunded/LOC	Comatose
Skeletal	None	Closed fracture	Open/multiple fractures
Cutaneous	None	Minor	Major
			Sum _____

From Tepas, J. J., Ramenofsky, M. L., Mollitt, D. L., et al. (1988). The pediatric trauma score as a predictor of injury severity: An objective assessment. *The Journal of Trauma, 28* (4), 427.

SYSTEM-SPECIFIC INJURIES

Alteration in Cerebral Tissue Perfusion Related to Head Injury

Etiology

Head injury is a common pediatric injury and the most common cause of traumatic death in children (Ghajar & Hariri, 1992). The cranial bones are thinner in children and offer less protection to the growing brain. In addition, the size of the infant head is large in proportion to body size. These anatomic considerations predispose children to head injury. Children's response to head injury differs in that they have a lower incidence of mass lesions but a higher one of intracranial hypertension (Walker, Storrs, & Mayer, 1985). Children also more commonly suffer from "malignant brain edema," which is actually significant cerebral hyperemia. As many as 50% of head-injured children may develop this (Bruce, Alavi, Bilaniuk et al., 1981). Because children experience intracranial hypertension and cerebral hyperemia more frequently, they are more susceptible to a secondary head injury rather than a primary head injury.

Pathogenesis

Traumatic brain injury is characterized by primary and secondary injury. Primary injury is produced by the trauma itself. It occurs immediately in the CNS following impact and may cause damage and/or death of the neuronal cells. Axonal injuries, laceration of brain tissue, contusions, skull fractures, and scalp injuries are examples of a primary head injury. Hypoxic injury may also cause a primary head injury if any of the neurons or astrocytes are injured by hypoxia or ischemia. This can be seen following a cardiac arrest. Secondary injury is produced by the brain's response to trauma. Secondary injury is a dynamic process that evolves over a period of hours to days and generally peaks at 3 to 5 days after injury (Walker, Storrs, & Mayer, 1985). Secondary injury involves the loss of cerebral autoregulation, development of extracellular and intracellular edema, and a breakdown of the blood-brain barrier. Secondary injury is compounded by systemic hyper- and hypotension, hypoxia, and hypercapnia. Secondary injury can often be prevented.

Specific Head Injuries. There are a number of specific head injuries that may be seen in children. Even though these are discussed separately, each one may be an element of a more serious brain injury.

Scalp lacerations are common in infants and young children and usually do not require a hospital stay for treatment. Because of the vascularity of the scalp, a large amount of bleeding may result from a laceration. Once underlying pathology has been ruled out, treatment is minimal and consists of stopping bleeding, inspection, irrigation, and suturing. An underlying skull fracture may be ruled out by palpation and possibly a skull film.

Many children with head trauma will have a concomitant *skull fracture*. Most of these children will have linear fractures. The majority of linear fractures are uncomplicated and heal spontaneously in 2 to 3 months. However, there are some linear fractures that are considered serious, based on their location. A fracture that crosses a major vascular structure, such as the middle meningeal artery or the dural venous sinus, has the potential of bleeding into the subdural or epidural space. A complication of a linear fracture seen in children is the growing fracture. With this complication, a portion of the arachnoid membrane becomes trapped between two edges of the fractured bone, producing a leptomeningeal cyst. The child may present with a soft and pulsating skull defect, seizures, and other neurologic defects (Vernon-Levett, 1991). This defect may resolve with age, or surgical intervention may be necessary.

A depressed skull fracture is a fracture where the inner table of the skull is displaced by more than the thickness of the entire bone. This represents a more severe injury, since a great deal of force is required to produce this situation. The treatment of a depressed skull fracture is debridement and elevation of the fragment within 4 hours (Davis, Tait, Dean et al., 1992).

A basilar skull fracture is a common type of skull fracture in children and represents a significant blow to the head. A basilar skull fracture usually involves a break in the base of the frontal, ethmoid, sphenoid, temporal, or occipital bone. The diagnosis is generally made on clinical presentation. A history of impact at the back of the head raises the index of suspicion. There may also be a loss of consciousness, seizures, or other signs of neurologic deficit. On physical examination, the child may show certain findings that are indicative of a basilar skull fracture. Rhinorrhea, raccoon eyes (periorbital ecchymosis), anosmia, and ocular motor palsies may occur with anterior fossa fractures. Hematotympanum, otorrhea, vertigo, Battle's sign (mastoid ecchymosis), or unilateral hearing loss may occur with middle fossa fractures. Hypotension, tachycardia, and changes in the respiratory pattern may be indicative of brainstem compression that can occur with posterior fossa fractures (Vernon-Levett, 1991). CSF leakage from the ear indicates disruption of the leptomeninges, and CSF leakage from the nose indicates leakage through the perinasal sinuses. Clear drainage from the ears or nose is tested for the presence of glucose, since glucose is present in CSF. However, since CSF is often mixed with blood and blood contains glucose, the presence of glucose does not always confirm that the fluid is CSF. If CSF is mixed with blood, as the blood dries, an xanthochromic (yellow) halo will appear on a dressing. The presence of a halo confirms the presence of CSF. A serious potential complication of CSF leakage is the development of meningitis. This is unusual, however, and the use of prophylactic antibiotics is controversial. The trend has been to treat only documented cases of meningitis (Davis, Tait, Dean et al., 1992).

In general, most basilar skull fractures are uncomplicated. Skull films identify basilar skull fractures in only 10% of cases. CT scans are indicated to identify the area of the fracture and any underlying brain injury. Because the cribriform plate is disrupted, insertion of nasotracheal and nasogastric tubes is avoided. Most children with basilar skull fractures require only 24 to 48 hours of observation with frequent neurologic checks and can expect a full recovery.

Concussion is the mildest form of traumatic injury to the brain. With a concussion, the child momentarily loses consciousness at the time of injury. The loss of consciousness is the result of the stretching and shearing forces in the brainstem (Davis, Tait, Dean et al., 1992). Diagnosis is usually made on a historical basis based on a temporary loss of consciousness.

The nature of concussion is varied based on the age group. Infants tend to have a less specific clinical presentation. They usually exhibit benign posttraumatic seizures, vomiting, diaphoresis, pallor, and lethargy (Davis, Tait, Dean et al., 1992) and do not usually experience a loss of consciousness. In the older child, posttraumatic amnesia becomes an important finding. The child may also complain of headaches, dizziness, and fatigue and may show some behavioral changes. The child's neurologic function usually normalizes in about 1 week, though some symptoms may persist for months or even to 1 year. This postconcussive syndrome is expected to resolve completely.

Cerebral contusion is defined as an actual bruising or microscopic bleeding of the brain, associated with temporary or permanent structural damage. A contusion is similar to a concussion in that a transient or actual loss of consciousness may occur; however, a contusion causes an actual disruption of cerebral tissue to varying degrees, often accompanied by parenchymal hemorrhage and focal edema. The contusion may occur at the site of impact (coup injury) or at a site opposite the impact (contrecoup injury). The degree of injury is reflected by alterations in the child's mental status. In a mild contusion, the return of consciousness is not as rapid as with a concussion and there is retrograde amnesia. With mild retrograde amnesia, the loss is only that of exact details of events occurring immediately before impact. More severe amnesia manifests itself by extending for a period of hours before the impact occurred. Children with more severe amnesia often have some disorientation, slowed reaction, headache, vomiting, and other mild neurologic abnormalities. Diagnosis of contusion is made based on focal neurologic signs and CT scan. The most common pattern seen on CT is that of multiple small hemorrhages surrounded by varying degrees of edema.

Return to consciousness following rapid neurologic deterioration may be seen in children with a cerebral contusion. The cause in children is usually due to diffuse generalized cerebral swelling. The most common CT scan finding among all children with an acceleration/deceleration injury is diffuse cerebral swelling. This is produced by cerebral hyperemia rather than by an increase in cerebral water content.

The incidence of cerebral contusion in infants is rare compared with older children. This is attributed to several factors. The skull of the infant is more pliable, and there are less convolutional markers on the inner table. Because the surface between bone and brain tissue is smoother, there is less resistance to movement and surface injury is minimized. Also, the infant's brain is less myelinized; and demyelinized brain tissue has a softer consistency, which may reduce injury (Walker, Storrs, & Mayer, 1985).

Treatment of a cerebral contusion depends upon the severity of the contusion. Treatment may be supportive medical therapy, involving treatment of increased intracranial pressure if it exists. Surgical treatment, removal of the contused tissue, may be necessary if medical management does not control increased intracranial pressure or if significant shifts are seen on CT scan.

An *epidural hematoma* refers to a collection of blood above the dura. Epidural hematomas are less common in children, especially infants, due to several reasons. The dura is tightly adherent to the inner table of the skull, especially at suture lines in infants and young children. Also, the fixation of the middle meningeal artery does not occur until approximately 2 years of age. Since the artery is not embedded into the temporal bone until fixation occurs, it can rotate and possibly avoid injury.

An epidural hematoma is a readily correctable lesion if identified and removed before secondary injury to the brainstem occurs. The classic lucid interval between the initial loss of consciousness and subsequent rapid neurologic deterioration is much less common in children (Davis, Tait, Dean et al., 1992). More often, the symptoms tend to be vague depending on the age of the child and the location of the bleeding. Infants may experience bulging fontanelles, separation of the sutures, decreased hematocrit, and shock with significant bleeding. In older children, an enlarging hematoma may cause herniation into other areas of the brain, producing corresponding signs. The child may exhibit hemiparesis, hemiplegia, ipsilateral pupil dilatation, posturing, or contralateral limb weakness (Vernon-Levett, 1991). Symptoms may be delayed for hours or days, if the source of bleeding is venous rather than arterial. If the hematoma continues to enlarge and the compensatory mechanisms of the brain become exhausted, temporal lobe herniation and brainstem compression will occur. A progressive decrease in the level of consciousness is the most significant diagnostic sign for all age groups. If time permits, a CT scan can be performed which will show a localized, high-density lesion with mass effect. If the child demonstrates rapid clinical deterioration, immediate surgical intervention without the benefit of a CT scan is necessary.

Treatment of choice is surgical evacuation of the hematoma. This is done as quickly as possible to avoid increasing morbidity or mortality. Evacuation of the hematoma is by craniotomy with removal of the clot and control of bleeding. Burr holes are technically difficult but may be useful as a diagnostic procedure in the absence of CT scan evaluation (Davis, Tait, Dean et al., 1992). With prompt surgical intervention, the prognosis for the child with an epidural hematoma is good.

A *subdural hematoma* is a collection of blood in the subdural space, often with associated cortical damage from lacerated vessels or direct contusion. Acute subdural hematomas are almost always caused by a traumatic incident. They are usually associated with a high mortality and morbidity due to the fact that the lesion is often caused by disruption of a cortical artery or a large bridging vein. The impact required to produce this type of injury is significant and is associated with severe contusion of the underlying vein. Common causes of a subdural hematoma are high-speed motor vehicle accidents, falls, assaults, and violent shaking.

The clinical presentation of a child with a subdural hematoma is routinely that of a youngster who has sustained a major head injury. The lucid interval seen with epidural hematoma is not seen here because the brain is so severely injured. The child will present with profound neurologic deterioration, and because of the force of impact, the mental status will almost always be affected.

Confirmation of the diagnosis of subdural hema-toma can be made with CT scan. The most effective treatment is evacuation of the clot with control of bleeding and possible resection of damaged brain tissue (Teasdale, Murray, Anderson et al., 1990). Even with aggressive treatment, the prognosis for the child with a subdural hematoma is less favorable than for the child with an epidural hematoma. This is due to the associated damage to the underlying brain tissue.

Chapter 21 provides in-depth information regarding collaborative management of the child with a head injury.

Impaired Mobility Related to Spinal Cord Injury

Etiology

Spinal cord injury occurs in over 1000 children per year in the United States, and an even higher number experience injury to the vertebral column (Kewalramani, Kraus, & Sterling, 1980; Dickman, Rekate, Sonntag et al., 1989). Motor vehicle accidents are the leading cause of spinal cord injury in children. In addition to occupant motor vehicle accidents, pedestrian and bicycle motor vehicle accidents are common causes of spinal injury in children (Ruge, Sinson, McLone et al., 1988). Sports-related and recreational injuries, child abuse, falls, and birth-related injuries also account for a large proportion of pediatric spinal cord injuries (Kling, 1986). Adolescents and young adults in the 16- to 24-year age range have the highest incidence of spinal cord injury (Kewalramani, Kraus, & Sterling, 1980). Children and adolescents in the 9- to 16-year age range experience spinal cord injury 10 times the incidence in younger children (Kewalramani, Kraus, & Sterling, 1980).

The type and severity of injuries seen in children differ than from those seen in adults (Dickman & Rekate, 1993). Children experience a higher incidence of cervical injuries and spinal cord injury without radiographic abnormality (SCIWORA). There are a number of factors related to this, but the most significant factor is the inherent differences between the pediatric and adult spine. The development of the pediatric spine is a continuous, dynamic process. Development is characterized by changes in the geometric configuration of the vertebrae; development of the ossification centers; closure of the epiphyseal plates; changes in the characteristics of the ligaments and soft tissues; and changes in osseous shape, size, strength, and integrity (Dickman, Rekate, Sonntag et al., 1989). Even though the epiphyses fuse at different ages, most epiphyseal plates are fused by 8 years of age. Multiple ossification centers are present at birth but continue to develop throughout childhood. The vertebral bodies are wedge shaped, and the vertebrae are mostly cartilaginous. The vertebral facets tend to have a horizontal orientation, and they become more vertical and ossify between 7 and 10 years of age. Before this time, they provide minimum stability to the vertebral column. The head of the infant and young child is large in relation to the neck, and the paraspinous muscles are not well developed. The vertebral ligaments and soft tissue are more elastic than in adults. These features all contribute to creating hypermobility of the neck and a tendency toward SCIWORA, severe ligamentous injury, and upper cervical spine injuries (Dickman, Rekate, Sonntag et al., 1989).

These differences make the children susceptible to different patterns of injury compared with adults. The types of injuries change as the biomechanical and anatomic features of the spine become more adult-like; however, the adult spinal characteristics and patterns of injury are not fully seen until after the age of 15 years (Dickman, Rekate, Sonntag et al., 1989).

Pathogenesis

Younger children between the ages of 0 and 8 years often sustain soft tissue injury without fractures. This is related to hypermobility and osseous immaturity. Manifestations of soft tissue injuries include SCIWORA, ligamentous dislocations, subluxation without fracture, growth plate injuries, and epiphyseal separations. In contrast, adolescents experience more "true" fractures than ligamentous or growth plate injuries.

Hypermobility of the child's spine is the most critical determinant of injury (Dickman, Rekate, Sonntag et al., 1989). Hypermobility protects the spinal cord from injury because force is dispersed over multiple vertebral levels. Hypermobility also accounts for the low incidence of spinal injury in the child and the patterns of injury. When spinal injury does occur, it is usually severe and accounts more often for complete loss of function in the child than in any other age group (Dickman & Rekate, 1993).

Most spinal cord injuries in the first 10 years of life involve the cervical region, especially the upper portion (occiput through C-3). Sixty percent to eighty percent of vertebral injuries in children affect the cervical spine (Hill, Miller, Kosnik et al., 1984). Significant ligamentous injuries have a propensity for the upper cervical spine. Atlanto-occipital dislocation (separation of the occipital condyles from the atlas) results in severe craniovertebral junction instability and can cause fatal neurologic injury. Immediate internal fixation is necessary to preserve neurologic function, since halo immobilization may not maintain alignment and traction with tongs may cause distraction of the craniovertebral junction, even with a small amount of weight.

Atlantoaxial dislocations (subluxations) are usually not fatal. Subluxation at the C1-C2 level is better tolerated than subluxation at the lower levels because the spinal canal is larger at C-1. Rotatory subluxation occurs with injury to the capsular ligaments. Anterior subluxations often occur in conjunction with rupture of the transverse ligament of the atlas and with relaxation of other atlantoaxial ligaments. Posterior subluxations occur with injury to the dens.

Anterior or posterior instability is seen best on flexion and extension radiographs. Rotatory subluxa-

tions are apparent with a CT scan. Rotatory subluxations greater than 40 degrees cause facet interlock and require external reduction and internal fixation (Godersky & Menezes, 1989).

Young children are susceptible to dislocations without fractures at all levels of the vertebrae, though this tends to occur mostly in the cervical region. Fracture characteristics change with vertebral maturation. Younger children tend to experience epiphyseal separations and growth plate fractures, while adolescents usually sustain more adult-like fracture patterns. Most cervical spine injuries in adolescents, like adults, occur at the C5-C6 level.

Occipital condyle fractures are extremely rare in children. These fractures are usually stable, though they can cause cranial nerve dysfunction. Fractures of the atlas or axis are also uncommon in young children; these fractures tend to occur more often in adolescence.

Fractures of the thoracic or lumbar spine in children often occur in the T11-L2 region where the rigid thoracic segments join the more mobile lumbar segments. Again, these injuries tend to involve the soft tissues and the ligaments, which result in cartilaginous or growth plate injuries. Children restrained by lap belts involved in motor vehicle accidents may sustain fractures in the midlumbar region.

As previously mentioned, a group of children experience SCIWORA. The hallmark of this entity is the presence of a spinal cord injury even though radiographic studies are normal. Flexion-extension views and CT scans are also normal. The injury occurs due to the immature pediatric spine where momentary intersegmental damage causes disruption of the cord without disrupting bones or ligaments.

Hyperextension is proposed as a mechanism of injury in SCIWORA (Osenbach & Menezes, 1989). Hyperextension of the cervical spine causes inward bulging of the ligamentum flavum and increased thickness in the spinal cord. This can reduce the diameter of the spinal canal by as much as 50% and allow for direct damage to the spinal cord. In addition, the anatomy and biomechanics of the occipitoatlantal junction cause the vertebral arteries to be susceptible to compression during hyperextension. This can result in temporary occlusion leading to ischemia and infarction.

Injuries experienced by children with SCIWORA tend to be devastating. Children with SCIWORA often present with delayed onset of neurologic deficit, though the reasons for this are not known. The delayed onset follows what appears to be a insignificant injury but once onset ensues, it progresses rapidly to a severe, permanent neurologic deficit. This may occur several hours to days after injury; however, in retrospect a history of subtle neurologic symptoms is often elicited (Pang & Pollack, 1989).

Patient Management

Assessment. Any child who has experienced head or facial trauma or who complains of neck pain is suspected of having a spinal cord injury. Clearance of the cervical spine requires anteroposterior, lateral, and open-mouth views of the cervical spine (Kling, 1986). It is critical that the cervical spine films include C7 and T1. These films may be obtained by gently pulling the shoulders downward to visualize the seven cervical vertebrae.

Due to the possibility of SCIWORA, occult fractures and vertebral malalignment are ruled out by CT scan. In addition, children with head and neck injuries are questioned for the presence of transient neurologic symptoms that may indicate SCIWORA.

There are some considerations when evaluating cervical spine films in the child. The vertebral bodies of the child are less rectangular than those of the adult. These bodies have a bioconcave appearance, which can give the impression of a compression fracture. This can be ruled out by comparing all the vertebral bodies, as the normal vertebral bodies will all appear the same. In addition, angulation in the infant spine is more extreme than in the adult. This is due to the fact that the infant spine is very cartilaginous and, especially at the C2-C3 level, vertebral offsets may appear. These may give the impression of subluxation.

Critical Care Management. Initial management of spinal cord injury begins with appropriate resuscitation and stabilization of the spine. Data indicate that a high proportion of children under 15 years of age die immediately or within the first hour after injury (Kling, 1986). As many as 50% of children with spinal cord injuries may die in the field, and among the children who survive the initial injury, another 25% will die during the initial period of hospitalization (Kewalramani, Kraus, & Sterling, 1980). Children who do survive the initial 3 months have a better chance of survival after 5 years compared with other age groups with spinal cord injury (Kewalramani, Kraus, & Sterling, 1980). The high initial mortality suggests that critically injured children do not tolerate severe neurologic injury or multisystem trauma.

Initial immobilization of the child with suspected spinal cord trauma is standard. However, using a standard backboard to achieve immobilization may be problematic. Young children have a disproportionately large head, and when positioned on a flat surface, the head may be forced forward, causing it to flex. Therefore, when immobilizing the young child, the occiput needs to be lower than the body. There are also commercially available spinal immobilization devices made especially for children.

Initial management includes attention to airway, breathing, and circulation. Hypotension is assumed to result from bleeding until proven otherwise. Spinal neurogenic shock, often resulting from complete upper spinal cord injury, may occur at the time of injury. The triad of symptoms are hypotension, bradycardia, and hypothermia. These symptoms are the result of sudden loss of sympathetic outflow from the cervicothoracic region. The loss of vasomotor tone that results can be treated with phenylephrine hy-

drochloride (Neo-Synephrine) (50 mg in 250 mL of 5% dextrose in water titrated at 50 to 100 µg/hour) (Dickman & Rekate, 1993). Volume expansion is also appropriate. In addition, with spinal shock, there is a temporary but complete loss of segmental reflex activity (Dickman & Rekate, 1993). These children have flaccid, areflexic limbs with no sensory or sphincter function. Priapism may also be present. Gradually, after 7 to 21 days, segmental reflex function returns and spasticity occurs (Dickman & Rekate, 1993).

The administration of methylprednisolone may have significant benefit if administered within the first 8 hours after injury. An intravenous bolus of 30 mg/kg followed by a continuous infusion of 5.4 mg/kg/hr for 23 hours has been recommended (Bracken, Shepard, Collins et al., 1990).

The use of external orthotic devices depends on the nature of the injury and the age of the child. A stiff molded collar may be useful to restrict cervical movement and is suitable for muscular injuries, atlantoaxial rotatory subluxation, and nondisplaced atlas fractures. However, these collars are not truly effective in immobilizing the cervical spine but serve more as a reminder not to move the neck.

Complete reduction and immobilization of the cervical spine may be accomplished by the use of traction. However, the halo jacket is considered the preferred immobilization device because it completely stabilizes the head, yet allows for patient mobility (Fig. 30–1). Nursing care focuses on prevention of dislodgment, loosening, and pin protrusion, especially in young children. Other potential complications are decubitus ulcers, brain abscesses, and pin site infection.

Treatment of thoracic and lumbar spine injuries is based on the characteristic of the fracture and the presence of pain, spinal deformity, or neurologic deficits. Children with more than 50% compression of the height of the vertebral body, spinal instability, kyphotic deformity, or severe intractable pain are treated with open reduction and internal fixation. Children with less than 50% compression are treated with surgical decompression of the spinal cord and/or nerve roots (Dickman & Rekate, 1993).

Unstable fractures and dislocations, progressive neurologic deficits with an incomplete cord injury, or compound wounds are treated surgically. Persistent instability despite the use of external orthotic devices requires internal fixation.

Ongoing nursing care of the child with a spinal cord injury revolves around supporting the child's physiologic and psychosocial needs. In addition to managing the initial resuscitation and care of the stabilization device, attention is focused on supporting the child's oxygenation and ventilation status, if necessary. The child with a spinal cord injury will suffer neuromuscular failure if the lesion is at C4 or above. Injuries above the T1 level result in paralysis of the intercostal muscles, and injuries above T10–12 result in paralysis of the abdominal muscles. This may have implications for younger children who are

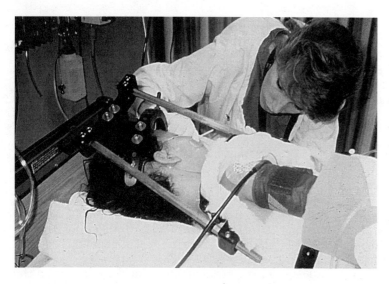

Figure 30-1 • • • • • •
Halo traction.

abdominal breathers. Also, abdominal muscle involvement will limit effective coughing.

Assessment of ventilatory parameters is important, especially vital capacity. Once baseline vital capacity has been obtained, values are obtained at least every 4 hours. If vital capacity decreases over time, diaphragmatic failure is occurring and ventilatory support is necessary. Ventilatory support may be permanent or temporary, depending on the level of the injury. If the injury is at C3-4 or above, lifelong ventilatory support will be necessary.

The psychosocial needs of the child with a spinal cord injury and the family of the child are tremendous. Especially with a high cord injury, the child no longer has control over the most basic bodily functions. For the adolescent, a time of developing complete independence has now become a time of complete dependence. Nursing interventions revolve around a sensitivity to the needs of children or adolescents as they experience changes in their ability to interact and be independent.

Family needs are also enormous as they face the prospects of a permanent change in their lives as well as the life of the child. The family is assisted with coping with the change and with regaining their pre-injury level of functioning or attaining a higher level of functioning.

Early involvement in a rehabilitation program is critical. If the child is in a center that has a rehabilitation program, involvement may begin on the day of injury. Concentration on a bladder and bowel program, prevention of contractures and decubitus ulcers, and relief of spasticity are three major areas focused on by the rehabilitation program.

Impaired Gas Exchange Related to Thoracic Injury

Etiology

Thoracic trauma accounts for one of the highest mortality rates in children, second only to head injury (Eichelberger, 1987). Morbidity associated with thoracic injury is also an issue. Peclet, Newman, Eichelberger et al. (1990) found that children who suffered thoracic injury were more severely injured than those who did not. Seventy percent of the children in this study required admission to the intensive care unit, and twenty percent required surgical intervention. Thoracic injury, when combined with injuries to other systems, increases the severity of injury and requires extensive resource use.

Thoracic injury is most commonly the result of blunt trauma. Motor vehicle–related injuries account for the majority of thoracic injury. Falls and child abuse are also frequent causes of thoracic injury in children.

Pathogenesis

The pathogenesis of thoracic injury is related to the specific injury. Regardless of the injury, the pathogenesis may include ineffective airway, impaired breathing pattern, impaired gas exchange, and/or alteration in cardiac output.

Rib Fractures. The incidence of rib fractures in children is less than in the adult. The decreased incidence can be attributed to the incomplete ossification of the pediatric skeleton, which results in more flexibility in the bones. The presence of rib fractures in a child suggests severe traumatic force. Fractures of multiple ribs have been directly correlated with an increase in mortality (Garcia, Gotschall, Eichelberger, 1990).

Injuries associated with rib fractures vary according to the fracture site. The four upper ribs are protected by the shoulder girdle and are less likely to fracture. Fractures of ribs one through four suggests injury to the bronchial, tracheal, or great vessels.

The most commonly fractured ribs are the middle ones (4 through 9). Often, these ribs penetrate lung tissue, causing serious damage. Pneumothorax and hemothorax often accompany middle rib fractures.

The lowest three ribs are not attached to the sternum and can withstand a great deal of force without breaking. Fractures of these free-floating ribs are often accompanied by liver, spleen, or kidney laceration.

Signs of rib fractures are localized pain on movement or deep breathing and crepitus on palpation. The child may breathe shallowly to decrease pain, leading to hypoventilation. Treatment of rib fractures is aimed at rest and pain relief.

Flail Chest. Flail chest occurs when there are multiple fractures of the same rib, or when there are fractures of the rib and sternum. The configuration of the fractures results in a floating rib segment. The chest wall becomes unstable as the flail segment moves paradoxically to the rest of the chest wall (Fig. 30–2).

As the diaphragm descends with inspiration, subatmospheric pressure allows the flail segment to move inward toward the negative pressure. The flail segment moves outward as the diaphragm rises with expiration. The paradoxic movement causes a decrease in tidal volume by preventing the lung from fully expanding and causing atelectasis. Ventilation-perfusion mismatch results. Children with a flail chest often have an accompanying pulmonary contusion. Hypoventilation, combined with the contusion and shunting, accounts for the morbidity associated with a flail chest.

Treatment of an uncomplicated flail chest is similar to that of rib fractures. Rest, analgesia, and meticulous pulmonary toilet are the primary treatments. Children with significant impairment of gas exchange may require pneumatic stabilization, which consists of intubation and positive-pressure ventilation. Judicious use of intravenous fluid and good pulmonary toilet are also recommended.

Traumatic Asphyxia. Traumatic asphyxia occurs almost exclusively in children because of their complaint chest wall and absence of valves in the superior and inferior vena cava. Direct compression against a closed glottis causes an acute increase in intrathoracic pressure with accompanying obstruc-

tion of vena caval drainage. A marked increase in venous pressure occurs, causing extravasation from the capillary bed and hemorrhage from the brain and other organs. Traumatic asphyxia may occur as the result of automobile wheels passing over the chest of the child or when the child is trampled. Often the child is lying on soft ground, which allows for compression without sternal or rib fractures.

Signs and symptoms of traumatic asphyxia include cyanosis of the face and neck; petechiae of the head, neck, and chest; and retinal and subconjunctival hemorrhages. Signs of disorientation and respiratory distress may be present. Traumatic asphyxia is often accompanied by pulmonary contusion and pneumothorax.

Treatment for traumatic asphyxia and associated injuries is symptomatic. Increased intracranial pressure may result in prolonged asphyxia and is treated accordingly.

Pneumothorax. Pneumothorax is the most common manifestation of thoracic injury, caused by blunt or penetrating trauma. Pneumothorax can range from a small, single pneumothorax to a life-threatening tension pneumothorax or open pneumothorax.

Simple pneumothorax occurs when air enters the pleural space, secondary to tears in the tracheobronchial tree, the esophagus, or the chest wall itself. Since the thorax is flexible, a pneumothorax may be present without rib fractures. Symptoms of a pneumothorax range from none to severe respiratory distress. Physical examination may reveal decreased breath sounds and hyperresonance to percussion over the injured area (Eichelberger, 1987). If the child is stable, a chest roentgenogram may be obtained to confirm the diagnosis.

Treatment of a pneumothorax varies. The child in severe respiratory distress will require needle thoracostomy first, followed by tube thoracostomy. The child who is stable will require only a tube thoracostomy. A very small pneumothorax (<15%) in the asymptomatic child may only require observation.

Tension pneumothorax results when air enters the pleural space but is unable to exit. The trapped air accumulates, increasing intrapleural pressure, which causes the affected lung to collapse. The air continues to accumulate, causing the mediastinum to shift and compress the contralateral lung. Excessive shift in the mediastinum results in vena cava compression, a decrease in venous return to the right side of the heart, and, ultimately, a decrease in cardiac output. If tension pneumothorax is not corrected immediately, cardiovascular collapse and death will occur.

Signs of tension pneumothorax include severe respiratory distress, absence of breath sounds and hyperresonance over the affected lung, cardiovascular instability, and tracheal shift to the unaffected side. A needle thoracentesis is the immediate treatment of choice. This relieves the tension, allowing the mediastinum to shift back. Once the air is evacuated, a chest tube insertion is performed.

The third type of pneumothorax is an open pneu-

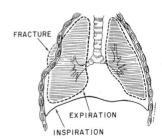

INJURY

ACTIVE BREATHING

FRACTURE

EXPIRATION

INSPIRATION

Figure 30–2 ● ● ● ● ● ●
Flail chest. There is a paradoxic segment of the chest wall and loss of the normal bellows mechanism. (From Jones, K.W. (1985). Thoracic trauma. In T.A. Mayer (Ed.). *Emergency management of pediatric trauma* (p. 258). Philadelphia: W.B. Saunders.)

mothorax. An open pneumothorax occurs when there is an opening in the chest wall, usually due to penetrating trauma. The opening allows air to move freely in and out of the pleural space. With a large wound, the mediastinum moves to one side or the other, depending on the phase of respiration. During inspiration, air moves through the wound. The lung collapses, and the mediastinum moves toward the functioning lung. During expiration, air exits through the wound, the lung partially reexpands, and the mediastinum shifts back (Fig. 30–3).

The child with an open pneumothorax often shows signs of restlessness, cyanosis, subcutaneous emphysema, and mediastinal shift. In addition, a sucking sound may be heard as air moves through the open wound. The open wound is covered immediately with an airtight seal. Sterile towels or a gloved hand can be used until a dressing is applied. Once the patient has stabilized, a petroleum jelly–gauze is applied.

Hemothorax. Hemothorax occurs when blood accumulates in the pleural space causing collapse of the affected lung. Hemothorax can occur secondary to blunt or penetrating injury. Blood collects in the pleural space, causing the affected lung to collapse. Injury to the heart, great vessels, or other thoracic structures may lead to the development of a hemothorax.

Signs and symptoms of hemothorax include respiratory distress, decreased or absent breath sounds, and dullness to percussion over the affected area. Shock may develop, as children can lose up to 40% of their total blood volume into a hemothorax (Eichelberger, 1987).

Treatment of a hemothorax varies slightly from that of a pneumothorax. Blood is immediately evacuated from the pleural space with a chest tube; however, intravenous access is established before evacuation to allow for fluid resuscitation. The chest tube is placed in the seventh or eighth intercostal space, which drains the hemothorax, reexpands the lung, and allows for monitoring of ongoing bleeding. Blood volume is rapidly replaced. Any child who exhibits blood loss of more than 1 to 2 mL/kg/hr is prepared for a thoracotomy.

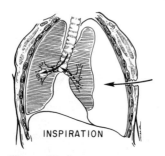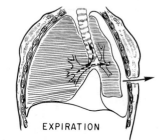

Figure 30–3 ● ● ● ● ● ●

Open pneumothorax results in ipsilateral lung collapse, mediastinal shift, and impaired ventilation of the opposite lung. (From Jones, K.W. (1985). Thoracic trauma. In T.A. Mayer (Ed.). *Emergency management of pediatric trauma* (p. 259). Philadelphia: W.B. Saunders.)

Pulmonary Contusion. Pulmonary contusion is one of the most frequent thoracic injuries seen in the child and is the most common cause of potentially fatal chest injury. It is often seen in the absence of bony injury. Pulmonary contusion is suspected whenever the child has a thoracic injury, especially if there is bruising noted on the chest.

Pulmonary contusion occurs when the lung is traumatized, causing bleeding from the capillary endothelium. Resultant increased capillary permeability allows for the development of both alveolar and interstitial edema. Impaired gas exchange results, causing ventilation-perfusion mismatch and decreased compliance (Luchtefield, 1990).

Signs and symptoms of pulmonary contusion may not initially be evident. Signs of respiratory distress may develop within several hours after injury and may include wheezing, hemoptysis, fever, rales, and signs of hypoxemia. Chest roentgenograms will demonstrate patchy densities, but this may not occur for 24 to 48 hours after the initial injury.

Treatment of pulmonary contusion is dependent upon the severity. Mild contusions may be managed with oxygen, analgesia, pulmonary toilet, and judicious fluid management to prevent large increases in interstitial pulmonary edema. Severe pulmonary contusions, which significantly alter respiratory function, may require intubation and mechanical ventilation. A pulmonary artery catheter is often placed to monitor pulmonary capillary wedge pressure to closely monitor fluid status. Albumin may be used for osmotic purposes; serum osmolarity is maintained at 300 mOsm. Diuretics may also be used to decrease the amount of pulmonary interstitial fluid.

Ventilatory interventions include the use of high-flow oxygen and positive end-expiratory pressure (PEEP). The pulmonary status is continuously evaluated with serial monitoring of arterial blood gases and continuous monitoring of SaO_2 and end-tidal CO_2. Since the child may be on a high amount of PEEP, close monitoring for the development of barotrauma is critical.

Some children with a large pulmonary contusion may not respond well to conventional mechanical ventilation. Volume delivered by the conventional ventilator will tend to go to the more compliant lung; therefore, the "good" lung will be at risk for hyperinflation and barotrauma while the affected lung receives insufficient volume. The use of independent lung ventilation using an double-lumen endobronchial tube may be useful for these children. Its effectiveness has been reported in the adult population (Simon & Borg, 1990), and anecdotal cases of use in children have been reported (Frame, Marshall, & Clifford, 1989). The tubes may be connected to various circuits. These include two separate, synchronized ventilators and a modified circuit that allows independent, synchronized ventilation.

Other nursing interventions for the child with a pulmonary contusion include positioning, observation for signs of infection, and meticulous pulmonary toilet. Positioning the child who is receiving positive-pressure ventilation with the injured lung up will optimize oxygenation and ventilation in the patient with a unilateral contusion. The child who is spontaneously breathing is positioned with the injured lung down. The child with bilateral contusions is placed in the right lateral decubitus position (Luchtefeld, 1990).

The child with pulmonary contusion may be at risk for the development of adult respiratory distress syndrome (ARDS), although one study demonstrated a low incidence of ARDS following pulmonary contusion or multiple trauma (Davis, Furman, & Costarino, 1993). It is critical to monitor for the development of ARDS, since failure of the respiratory system is strongly correlated with multiple organ dysfunction syndrome (MODS) (Philichi, 1994).

Cardiac Tamponade. Cardiac tamponade occurs when blood accumulates in the pericardial sac, increasing pericardial pressure. The increase in pressure alters the pumping mechanism of the heart, resulting in a decrease in cardiac output. Signs and symptoms of acute tamponade are the classic triad of jugular venous distension, hypotension, and muffled heart sounds, though these may be difficult to detect in the child. The short, fat neck of the child makes assessment of venous distention difficult. Also, the thin chest wall allows for increased transmission of sound. Another classic sign is the presence of a pulsus paradoxus of greater than 10 mmHg. Tamponade is suspected in children with persistent hypotension despite fluid resuscitation. In the absence of hypovolemia, an increased central venous pressure may be noted. Initial treatment of pericardial tamponade is pericardiocentesis. If pericardiocentesis is not successful, or if tamponade reoccurs, operative intervention is warranted.

Myocardial Contusion. Myocardial contusion occurs when traumatic forces cause local injury to the myocardium. Dysrhythmias may occur secondary to injury. Children suffering from myocardial contusion are less likely than adults to have dysrhythmias or alterations in cardiac function (Mueller-Dickinson, 1991).

Signs of myocardial contusion are chest pain and alteration in cardiac function. Chest wall bruising and tenderness may not be present, making a high suspicion of injury an important diagnostic factor. A 12-lead echocardiogram is obtained on all patients with a suspected contusion. One third of children with nonpenetrating myocardial trauma will develop S-T segment and T wave changes during the first 24 to 48 hours after injury like those seen with myocardial ischemia and infarction (Othersen, 1990). Using serial cardiac isozyme studies may be helpful in making the diagnosis of contusion, but the more recent literature has questioned the value of enzyme use (Fabian, Cicala, Croce et al., 1991). For example, the myocardial band of creatinine kinase (CK-MB) may be elevated, but false-positive results are often seen in trauma patients (Tellelz, Harden, Takehashi, et al., 1987). In addition, significant elevations in serum glutamic-oxaloacetic transaminase (SGOT) and lactate dehydrogenase (LDH) occur with hemorrhagic shock, so these alterations are not significant for myocardial contusion (Othersen, 1990). Two-dimensional echocardiography may also be used to detect ventricular wall motion abnormalities and determine ventricular ejection fraction.

Treatment of myocardial contusion involves treatment of symptoms. Long-term sequelae of myocardial contusion in children are unknown. Aneurysm, myocardial rupture, and postcontusion pericarditis have been reported in adults (Reynolds, 1987).

Aortic Rupture. Aortic rupture, although rare in the pediatric population, can occur secondary to blunt trauma. Common sites of injury are the descending aorta distal to the level of the ligamentum arteriosum, which is associated with horizontal deceleration injuries; and disruption of the ascending aorta, secondary to vertical deceleration injuries (Stiles, Cohlemia, & Smith, 1985).

Injuries may vary from a small tear in the intimal lining to complete transection. Signs and symptoms of injury will range from cardiopulmonary arrest to no external sign of injury. Discrepancies between pulse in the upper and lower extremities and between blood pressure in the limbs is suggestive of aortic trauma.

Nursing interventions for the patient with aortic injury is to assist with diagnostic procedures such as a aortogram. Fluid resuscitation is started immediately, and the patient is prepared for immediate thoracotomy.

Diaphragmatic Rupture. Rupture of the diaphragm occurs most commonly following blunt trauma in which there is a sudden increase in intraabdominal or intrathoracic pressure against a fixed diaphragm. The left hemidiaphragm is most commonly injured. The diagnosis is often missed when the child is asymptomatic.

The most common presenting symptoms are chest pain and shortness of breath. Unilateral diaphragm dysfunction accompanied by herniation of intra-abdominal contents into the chest cavity causes these symptoms. Physical examination may reveal decreased breath sounds or auscultation of bowel sounds over the affected lung. The mediastinum may shift to the contralateral side and the abdomen will appear scaphoid in the infant and young child. Chest roentgenogram may reveal diaphragmatic displacement, loops of bowel in the thorax, or the presence of a nasogastric tube in the thoracic cavity (Fig. 30–4). Surgical repair of the diaphragmatic tear is required.

Tracheobronchial Injury. Tracheobronchial tree injury is rare in the child because of the elasticity of the thorax and the mobility of the mediastinum. Blunt tracheobronchial injury can result from a variety of forces, including shearing, compression, and vertical stretch. Injuries most frequently occur at the take-off point of a mainstem or upper lobe bronchus (Eichelberger, 1987).

Signs of a tracheobronchial disruption include mediastinal or subcutaneous emphysema, hemoptysis,

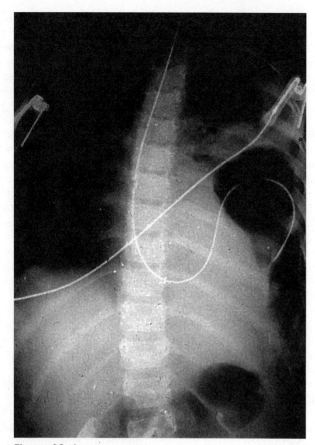

Figure 30–4 ● ● ● ● ● ●

X-ray positive for diaphragmatic hernia.

airway obstruction, pneumothorax with persistent airleak, and massive atelectasis refractory to treatment. Bronchoscopy is the most reliable means of diagnosing the site and extent of injury. Treatment involves symptom relief (for example, relief of airway obstruction) and surgical repair of the lesion.

Patient Management

The final common pathways in the pediatric thoracic trauma victim are impaired gas exchange and low cardiac output (see Chapters 9, 10, 19, and 20).

Fluid Volume Deficit Related to Abdominal Injury

Etiology

Abdominal injuries in children are not common; however, the failure to diagnose these injuries promptly and manage them successfully accounts for increased mortality and morbidity. Usually, serious injury to the head or limbs is obvious, whereas serious abdominal injury tends to be subtle.

Features of a child's physical maturity may place the youngster at greater risk for injury. The child's abdominal contents are more vulnerable to injury due to poorly developed abdominal musculature and a relatively smaller anteroposterior diameter. The rib cage, although very resilient in children and less prone to fractures, provides only partial protection for intraperitoneal contents (McAnena, Moore, & Marx, 1990). The abdominal organs in children also have unique characteristics. Compared with other abdominal organs, the liver is more vascular and larger in size. The right lobe, which comprises greater than 50% of the total liver volume, is the section most commonly injured (Lebet, 1991). The child's spleen has a thicker capsule, which allows for increased protection, and the spleen's higher proportion of epithelial cells tends to promote tamponade of bleeding (Lebet, 1991).

Blunt injury continues to be the most common form of abdominal trauma in children, accounting for approximately 90% of all injuries (Ramenofsky, 1987). Automobile-related injuries account for approximately 40% of childhood abdominal trauma; this includes children injured as passengers or pedestrians and when riding on bicycles and motorcycles. Falls from heights comprise the second largest category of injury, accountable for 39% of all injuries (Ramenofsky, 1987).

Penetrating injury is rare in children and accounts for approximately 10% of injuries (Ramenofsky, 1987). Penetrating injuries may result from gunshot or stab wounds, or impalement on an object (Haller & Beaver, 1990).

Pathogenesis

Blunt trauma produces injury by compression against the spine or by rapid deceleration with subsequent tearing of structures (Matlak, 1985). Such forces may result in the crushing of solid organs such as the liver or spleen, or rupture of the hollow viscera such as the bladder or stomach. Solid organs are injured more frequently than the hollow viscera, with laceration of the spleen being the most common injury. Other sites of potential injury include the liver, pancreas, small bowel mesentery, duodenum, and proximal jejunum. Associated injury to the urinary tract is also suspected and evaluated in the child with abdominal trauma (Matlak, 1985).

Hollow viscus injury is very common with penetrating trauma; as a result, peritonitis may be quickly evident if a segment of intestine full of food or stool evacuates into the peritoneal cavity. Life-threatening hemorrhage due to major vascular injury is also more likely with penetrating injury. The majority of penetrating abdominal injuries require operative surgical management (Haller & Beaver, 1990).

Specific Injuries. Spleen. The spleen is the most commonly injured abdominal organ in childhood. Splenic injury usually follows blunt trauma to the upper abdomen or lower thorax. Approximately 50% of these injuries occur during recreational or athletic activities; the remainder occur as the result of vehicular trauma. Abuse may also be a cause and should be considered in the child with a splenic injury under 4 years of age when an unreliable history is provided (Touloukian, 1990).

The spleen is located in the left hypochondrium, where in older children and adolescents, the lower rib cage covers the spleen entirely. In infants and small children, the rib cage does not extend down far enough and is also more pliable than the ossified adult rib cage. Therefore, the pediatric spleen is not adequately protected by the rib cage.

The child with a splenic injury has usually received a blow to the left upper quadrant with or without an associated rib fracture. The child will often experience pain in the left shoulder, in the left upper quadrant, or in the left part of the chest with breathing. Bruising, abrasions, nausea, and vomiting may be present. Heart rate and blood pressure may be normal, or mild tachycardia and hypotension may occur. A mass may be palpable in the left upper quadrant. The child may have a positive Kehr sign (pain in the left shoulder), Turner sign (ecchymosis in the left flank), and/or Cullen sign (ecchymosis around the umbilicus). Ecchymosis in the left upper quadrant or left flank is a strong indication of injury (Scorpio & Wesson, 1993).

Laboratory analysis is often normal in a child with splenic injury, but if abnormalities are seen, they are usually a decreased hematocrit and leukocytosis in the 20,000 to 30,000 mm^3 range. Both chest and abdominal x-rays may be suggestive of splenic trauma; Table 30–5 presents these findings. An abdominal x-ray alone will not confirm the diagnosis of splenic trauma. It will, however, provide evidence to confirm the clinical findings. The CT scan is the method of choice for diagnosis of splenic trauma in the hemodynamically stable child. Diagnostic peritoneal lavage (DPL) is usually not indicated for the child who will be managed nonoperatively, since a positive DPL does not mandate surgery. DPL is most useful for the child who is hypotensive and who is not responding to fluid resuscitation or who requires emergency surgery for abdominal injuries (Scorpio & Wesson, 1993).

Treatment is aimed toward splenic preservation. Appreciation of the increased risk of overwhelming

Table 30–5. X-RAY FINDINGS SUGGESTIVE OF SPLENIC INJURY

Chest X-ray Findings
Lower left rib fractures
Elevation of the left hemidiaphragm
Pleural effusion

Abdominal X-ray Findings
Raised left hemidiaphragm
Stomach dilatation or medial displacement
Opacification of the left hypochondrium
Downward displacement of the transverse colon
Fluid between coils of intestines

From Scorpio, R.J., & Wesson, D.E. (1993). Splenic trauma. In M.R. Eichelberger (Ed.). *Pediatric trauma: Prevention, acute care, rehabilitation* (p. 458). St. Louis: Mosby–Year Book.

postsplenectomy sepsis in children has led to a heightened awareness of the importance of splenic preservation, especially in the pediatric age group. For many years, the spleen was thought to be expendable; however, in the 1950s, a number of infants who had undergone splenectomy developed overwhelming bacterial sepsis or meningitis (Schiffman, 1989). Currently, postsplenectomy sepsis is a well-recognized syndrome that can occur days to years following removal of the spleen. The syndrome of overwhelming postsplenectomy infection (OPSI) occurs in 1.5% of children who have undergone splenectomy after trauma, with a 50% mortality rate. The incidence of OPSI is higher in younger children (Schiffman, 1989).

Because the spleen is recognized as a source of antibodies against *Haemophilus influenzae*, pneumococcus and Meningococcus, the goal in the management of injury to the spleen is preservation. The presence of even a portion of the spleen provides some protection against postsplenectomy infection. As a result, strategies for splenic conservation have been developed and splenorrhaphy, which is debridement of the injury and surgical repair, is preferred to splenectomy (Schiffman, 1989).

The spleen may be preserved by nonoperative means as well; in fact, most children with splenic trauma can be treated this way. Nonoperative management is recommended for the child who maintains stable vital signs, requires less than one-half blood volume replacement, and is free of other abdominal injuries that would require surgery. If the child is monitored nonoperatively, close monitoring in the ICU is required for at least 48 hours. Vital signs are monitored frequently, and hematocrit and hemoglobin are measured at least daily. Strict bedrest is maintained until there have been no requirements for blood for 48 hours. At this point, ambulation may occur and the child may be discharged home after 5 to 7 days after ambulation. After discharge, the child may return to school but should refrain from vigorous activities for at least 8 weeks.

Complications of nonoperative management are associated mainly with rebleeding. This would be indicated by unstable vital signs, decreasing hematocrit and hemoglobin, and worsening findings on abdominal examination.

If the child requires operative management and splenic preservation is not possible, a splenectomy will be required. Indications for splenectomy are (1) a spleen that is completely separated from its blood supply; (2) children with a positive DPL, unstable hemodynamics, and associated injuries; (3) children with severe head injury who cannot tolerate massive volume resuscitation necessary for blood loss; (4) children with continuous blood loss of unknown causes; and (5) children who have experienced fecal contamination of the peritoneal cavity (Touloukian, 1990). Standard principles of postoperative care will apply; however, since these children are at risk for OPSI, protection from infection is critical. This is accomplished through vaccination and prophylactic antibiotics. Vaccines available are those against pneumococcus, *H. influenzae* type B (HIB), and *Neisseria meningitidis*. The use of the pneumococcal and HIB vaccines is strongly recommended. These vaccines are administered in the postoperative period.

Even with vaccines, antibiotic prophylaxis is suggested, especially in infants and young children. Penicillin prophylaxis is recommended to continue until adolescence. Amoxicillin is advocated by some instead of penicillin because it is effective against HIB. Erythromycin may be used as an alternative to penicillin for those children with a penicillin allergy (Scorpio & Wesson, 1993).

Not surprisingly, patient compliance with antibiotic regimen prophylaxis is poor. In addition, infections can still occur. Therefore, it is critical that parent teaching include recognition of signs of infection and prompt medical attention for initiation of antibiotics.

Liver. Injury to the liver is the second most common injury in blunt abdominal trauma and the most common fatal abdominal injury (Buntain, Lynch, & Ramenofsky, 1987). Because most liver injuries are the result of blunt trauma, additional organs are often involved, such as the head, chest, and musculoskeletal system.

Injuries are classified as contusions, parenchymal lacerations, or injuries to the hepatic veins or vena cava (Haller & Beaver, 1990). The most severe injuries are usually fatal early on due to massive bleeding. Severe bleeding can result from the intrahepatic vessels, the vena cava, or the hepatic veins. The majority of liver injuries are to the right lobe, and the majority of these tend to be simple (Torres & Garcia, 1993). Left-sided injuries tend to be more complex.

Children with liver injuries experience pain in the right upper shoulder or right upper quadrant tenderness. They may also have bruising, seatbelt markings, and abrasions. Hypotension may be present if major bleeding is occurring. Fractured ribs are a common concomitant finding.

Initial laboratory tests include a CBC, urinalysis, serum glutamic-oxaloacetic transaminase (SGOT), serum glutamic-pyruvic transaminase (SGPT), and amylase. Elevations in SGOT and SGPT appear to correlate with hepatic injury (Torres & Garcia, 1993). As with splenic injury, DPL is of limited use; the preferred method of diagnosis in the hemodynamically stable child is CT scan.

Management of children with hepatic injuries is similar to the treatment for splenic injuries. Nonoperative management for the hemodynamically stable child is the treatment of choice. Potential complications of nonoperative management include continued bleeding or bile accumulation, which may lead to delayed healing, hepatic necrosis, or abscess formation. Such complications may not be noted until weeks after the injury (Cooney & Bellmire, 1990). Nonoperative management does mandate that the child be followed closely in the ICU with frequent monitoring of blood work. Hematocrit levels may

need to be assessed every 4 hours or more often, if indicated by clinical condition. Once the liver transaminase normalizes, the child can ambulate; however, activity is restricted until complete healing has occurred as documented by CT scan. Delayed bleeding has been reported to occur as late as 1 month after injury (Torres & Garcia, 1993).

Operative management is indicated if the child exhibits hemodynamic instability, transfusion requirements of greater than 33% to 50% of the circulating blood volume in 24 hours, signs of peritoneal irritation, or a pneumoperitoneum or other abdominal injuries that require surgical repair (Lebet, 1991; Torres & Garcia, 1993). In the case of a severely injured liver, such as a lobar fracture, the initial management is to control the massive bleeding. If liver resection is required, it does carry a high mortality rate (Torres & Garcia, 1993).

Pancreas. Pancreatic injury is relatively infrequent in children. When it does occur, recognition is often delayed due to the retroperitoneal location of the pancreas. Traumatic pancreatitis commonly results from blunt trauma compressing the pancreas over the body of the vertebral column, causing contusion and/or parenchymal disruption with or without ductal disruption. Because of the retroperitoneal location of the pancreas, associated injuries involving the duodenum, stomach, extrahepatic biliary system, and the spleen are common. Injury resulting from pancreatic trauma is usually devastating because of extensive bleeding and tissue damage from pancreatic and biliary secretions.

Children who have experienced pancreatic trauma usually have diffuse abdominal tenderness, abdominal pain, vomiting, and findings of associated injuries. Hemodynamic instability may be present, resulting from massive retroperitoneal bleeding or massive sequestration of third space fluid losses.

Laboratory studies to confirm the diagnosis of pancreatic injury include serum amylase levels. However, this elevation may not occur for 3 to 5 days after injury and may be missed completely. Also, an elevated serum amylase level is a nonspecific finding that may occur with bowel perforation, appendicitis, intestinal obstruction, and mesenteric thrombosis (Moosa, 1984). X-rays and contrast-enhanced CT scans will assist in confirming the diagnosis.

The preferred treatment of traumatic pancreatitis is nonoperative, if there is no evidence of ductal disruption. The use of nasogastric suction to rest the GI system is a major treatment modality. Also, total parenteral nutrition is important and is continued for at least 3 weeks to allow for bowel rest. In addition, serial physical examinations are important and the child is monitored for signs of infection. Complications include the development of pancreatic fistulas and pseudocyst formation.

Operative management is indicated for patients who have pain, fever, ileus, or elevated serum amylase levels that persist or develop. Also, for children who have findings of traumatic pancreatitis at the time of operative exploration for other intra-abdominal injuries, external drainage or partial or total pancreatectomy may be performed.

Stomach and Small and Large Intestines. Hollow viscus disruption in the child is frequently subtle in its presentation, especially that which results from blunt trauma (Ramenofsky, 1987). Injuries to the stomach and small and large bowel are significant even though they constitute only a small number of abdominal injuries. However, the incidence of gastric and intestinal injuries has been increasing. This is due to improved ability to recognize these injuries and to societal factors, such as the increase in urban violence and child abuse (Newman, 1993).

Hollow viscus injuries are difficult to diagnose, yet a missed diagnosis can result in sepsis due to a slow but continuous peritoneal contamination (Ramenofsky, 1987; Schiffman, 1989). The only early sign of this type of injury may be a subtle degree of abdominal tenderness. Abrasions or contusions in the upper abdomen should raise the index of suspicion for stomach injury. Bloody gastric drainage, tympanic sounds when percussion is performed over the liver, detection of free air, and a NG tube in abnormal position on x-ray are all indicative of stomach injury. If the stomach perforates, the child will develop a board-like abdomen with intense pain. Peritonitis will develop within hours, and surgery is always required.

The small intestine can be ruptured by even mild abdominal trauma. Perforation of the small intestine may result from compression, such as that which occurs with lap belts. The child with ruptured intestines may have minimal symptoms, yet frank peritonitis is inevitable. Surgical repair is always required.

Colon and Rectum. The colon and rectum are rarely injured, and when they are, injury is usually due to penetrating trauma (Rouse, 1993). The child will present with signs of free air or peritonitis on x-ray. Surgical repair is necessary.

Patient Management

Assessment. The initial assessment of pediatric patients with abdominal trauma is often challenging due to age-related difficulties in communication, fear, anxiety, uncooperative behavior, or concomitant head injury (McAnena, Moore, & Marx, 1990). However, initial evaluation is not geared at identifying a specific abdominal organ injury; instead, the recognition and treatment of difficulties with airway, breathing, or circulation are first addressed. After initial stabilization, specific organ injury assessment is begun.

Once secondary survey of the abdomen commences, the mechanism of injury can be used to guide the physical examination. Knowing the mechanism should produce a high index of suspicion for certain injuries; for example, a fall over bicycle handlebars with a subsequent blow to the left upper quadrant should lead to a suspicion of splenic injury.

The child is assessed for contusions, lacerations, abdominal distension, patterns of bruising, pulsations, and peristaltic waves. Upper gastric distension usually suggests gastric dilatation, while lower quadrant distension suggests bleeding. Certain manifestations indicate the presence of injury. Kehr sign is pain in the left shoulder that occurs when free blood in the abdomen irritates the diaphragm and phrenic nerve. Pain is referred along the nerve to the left shoulder and indicates splenic injury. Cullen sign, periumbilical ecchymosis, is a rare indication of a ruptured spleen that is caused by intra-abdominal bleeding. Turner sign, ecchymosis in the left flank, also indicates splenic injury. Another manifestation is the seat belt sign, which is ecchymosis over the lower abdomen. This results from compression of the abdomen by a lap belt against the iliac crest and the lower abdomen. It indicates that a severe force has been applied against the abdominal viscera.

Bowel sounds are auscultated. Decreased bowel sounds are often caused by irritants outside the bowel. Irritants decrease or cause cessation of peristalsis, resulting in diminished or absent bowel sounds. Increased bowel sounds are caused by irritants within the bowel. Absent bowel sounds are more indicative of pathology than increased bowel sounds (Peckham & Kitchen, 1989).

Abdominal pain will be present with most injuries; the location, duration, and character of the pain are assessed and documented. All four quadrants of the abdomen are palpated to elicit tenderness or rigidity. The fingers are pressed firmly over an area and released quickly. Pain felt on release is rebound tenderness and is a sign of peritoneal irritation.

As mentioned previously for specific injuries, the CT scan is considered the most appropriate and accurate method of assessing solid organ injuries (Kane, Cronan, Dorfman et al., 1988). It is noninvasive, safe, reliable, injury-specific, and available in most institutions that care for trauma patients. Since many patients with abdominal injuries have sustained multisystem trauma, it is convenient to obtain an abdominal CT along with a head CT.

Some children will require a DPL. Indications for DPL include ambiguous abdominal findings, hemodynamic instability while ruling out an abdominal examination, an altered level of consciousness affecting pain response, and a stab injury without peritonitis. Before the actual technique is performed, the bladder is emptied and the stomach decompressed with a nasogastric tube. The site below the umbilicus is prepared and the incision made. A long 18-gauge needle is advanced into the peritoneal cavity, followed by a guidewire and Silastic catheter. The contents of the peritoneal cavity are aspirated, and if no blood is present, 10 to 20 mL/kg of balanced saline solution is instilled into the abdomen (warmed, if possible). Dependent drainage is used to evacuate the lavage fluid after a short dwell time, usually less than 10 minutes. The fluid is evaluated for the presence of RBCs, WBCs, amylase, bile, bacteria, and intestinal contents (Table 30–6).

DPL is sensitive for the diagnosis of hemoperitoneum; however, in the stable child, hemoperitoneum is not an indication for surgery. Since most children are managed nonoperatively, it is more important to

Table 30–6. PERITONEAL LAVAGE RESULTS

	Result	Indication
Aspirate	Gross blood > 20 mL	Positive
	Pink fluid	Intermediate*
	Clean	Negative
Lavage fluid	Bloody	Positive
	Clear	Negative
RBC	>100,000 cells/mm³	Positive
	50,000–100,000 cells/mm³	Intermediate*
WBC	>500 cells/mm³	Positive
	100–500 cells/mm³	Intermediate*
Amylase	>175 U/dL	Positive
	75–175 U/dL	Intermediate*
	<75 U/dL	Negative
Bacteria	Present	Positive
Fecal material	Present	Positive
Bile	Present	Positive
Food particles	Present	Positive

*Intermediate lavage results require further observation of the patient, possible repeat lavage, and interventions based on clinical presentation.

From Mason, P. J. B. (1994). Abdominal injuries. In V. D. Cardona, P. D. Hurn, P. J. B. Mason, et al. (Eds.). *Trauma nursing: From resuscitation through rehabilitation* (2nd ed., p. 524). Philadelphia: W. B. Saunders.

define the source of injury rather than determine the presence of a hemoperitoneum. Therefore, for most abdominal injuries in children, DPL is not indicated or useful.

The child's breathing pattern may be a strong indicator of abdominal injury. Peritoneal irritation from blood or intestinal contents may dramatically change a child's breathing pattern; such a change is demonstrated when the child breathes with the chest rather than the abdomen, and avoids deep inspiration and expiration because it causes severe pain. A conscious child may also be still and avoid crying loudly to prevent pain. Such signs may be indicative of peritonitis (Matlak, 1985).

Critical Care Management. The management of blunt abdominal trauma in children has changed significantly in the past decade as a result of both advances in diagnostic imaging and an improved understanding of the healing processes in the spleen and liver. In the past, mandatory laparotomy was the accepted mode of treatment for proven or suspected hemoperitoneum. Such treatment modalities have been replaced with intensive observation of patients able to be stabilized with supportive therapy. The result since this change in treatment method has been a reduction in morbidity because of anesthetic complications, postsplenectomy sepsis, and peritoneal adhesions (Schiffman, 1989).

Although nonoperative management of abdominal injuries is both the most frequent and preferred treatment of choice, it is essential to clarify that "nonoperative" is not synonymous with "nonsurgical." Expert surgical consultation is required in all but the most trivial of abdominal injuries. If nonoperative management is to be successful, meticulous observation in an intensive care setting with expert nursing care is essential.

Immediate treatment focuses on stabilization of

the cardiopulmonary status, if appropriate. If the child is hemodynamically unstable, an intravenous line is placed, ideally above the diaphragm in case of rupture of the hepatic vein and the inferior vena cava. Resuscitation fluids are administered. If the child is managed nonoperatively, close monitoring of vital signs (especially trends) and appropriate serum levels is mandatory. Indications for laparotomy include massive bleeding, unstable vital signs in spite of aggressive fluid resuscitation, requirements for more than one half of the child's circulating blood volume for replacement, severe abdominal distension associated with hypotension, penetrating injuries, and some blunt injuries.

Altered Patterns of Urinary Elimination Related to Genitourinary Injuries

Etiology

Genitourinary injuries occur frequently in children, with 90% the result of blunt abdominal trauma. Trauma to the genitourinary tract is strongly suspected in the patient with multiple injuries, as signs and symptoms may be obscured by concomitant injuries.

Anatomic features of the child's genitourinary system allow for an increased risk of renal and bladder injury. A child's bladder lies higher in the abdomen, as compared with an adult's bladder, resting in the pelvic region; poorly developed abdominal muscles in the child are thus less protective of the bladder. In addition, underdeveloped abdominal musculature along with a lack of extensive perirenal fat offers less protection to the kidney. The kidney is proportionately larger, and the child's total body mass is small (Kass, 1988). Also, the kidney may retain fetal lobulations, which allows for easier parenchymal disruption because these lobulations are less resistant to blunt forces (Kuzmarov, Morehouse, & Gibson, 1981).

As many as 10% of children who experience renal trauma have a preexisting renal anomaly. Anomalous kidneys are injured more easily; the extent of trauma required to damage anomalous kidneys is minimal and unimpressive (Brower, Paul, & Brosman, 1978; Livine & Gonzales, 1985). Often, renal abnormalities are first recognized after a child presents with minor, blunt abdominal trauma.

Pathogenesis

The kidney is the most commonly injured organ in the genitourinary tract in children; over 90% of renal injuries are the result of blunt abdominal trauma. Though rare, penetrating stab wounds are potentially serious, with the possibility of severed renal vessels and lacerations to the collecting system.

The mechanism of renal injury due to blunt abdominal trauma may be direct or indirect. With a direct injury, the kidney is crushed between the 12th rib and the lumbar spine; examples include sporting injuries, seat belt injuries, and those instances when a child is run over by a car or another vehicle (Terry, 1990). An indirect injury, which is less common, results from a rapid deceleration, such as when a child falls from a tree or ladder. In this scenario, the body's momentum is abruptly halted as it strikes the ground yet the kidney continues to move. This results in shearing forces that may tear the major renal vessels or rupture the ureter at the pelvic-ureteric junction. Renal injuries as a result of indirect mechanisms are difficult to detect, and only an accurate description of the injury will lead to the correct diagnosis.

A variety of classifications of renal injuries are described in the literature—some in terms of minor and major; others in terms of degree of contusions, lacerations, and tears. A classification of renal injuries is presented in Figure 30–5.

Any child with abdominal or flank pain, pelvic fractures, lower rib fractures, or perineal swelling is suspected of having renal injury. Manifestations of renal trauma include hematuria (a hallmark of renal

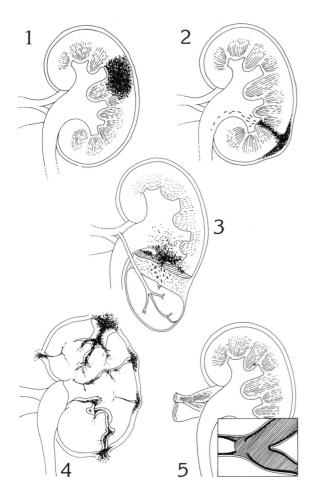

Figure 30–5 ● ● ● ● ● ●
Composite of the five classes of blunt renal injury: 1, contusion; 2, laceration; 3, transection; 4, fragmentation; 5, pedicle injury. (From Hensle, T.W., & Dillon, P. (1990). Renal injuries. In R.J. Touloukian (Ed.). *Pediatric Trauma* (2nd ed., p. 359). St. Louis: Mosby–Year Book.)

trauma), flank and/or abdominal pain, an inability to void, superficial abrasions, contusions, and ecchymoses. An intravenous pyelography (excretory urogram) (IVP) may be useful to assess asymptomatic hematuria with minimal trauma. A CT scan, however, is superior with more accurate diagnostic capabilities. Ultrasound is also valuable as a rapid initial screening tool, as it provides an overall assessment of liver, spleen, kidneys, and retroperitoneum. In addition, it can determine the presence of a hemoperitoneum (Hensle & Dillon, 1990).

Appropriate diagnostic evaluation will allow for identification of the type, location, and extent of injury, and the status of the contralateral kidney. Status of the contralateral kidney may significantly impact treatment decisions; for example, congenital absence of a kidney mandates an attempt to salvage a severely injured kidney (Middleton, Matlak, Nixon et al., 1985).

Although significant controversy exists with regard to the management of renal trauma, the ultimate goals are to prevent mortality, reduce immediate and long-term morbidity, and preserve as much functioning renal parenchyma as possible (Quinlan & Gearhart, 1990). Considering that patients with renal trauma frequently have associated injuries, the immediate management of the patient is determined more by the patient's general clinical state than by the renal injuries. Renal injuries, in and of themselves, are rarely life-threatening; hypovolemic shock in patients with renal injury is nearly always due to associated trauma.

Approximately 85% to 95% of renal injuries are best managed nonoperatively (Terry, 1990; Lebet, 1991). Injuries in this category include contusions and simple lacerations. Successful results can be anticipated with nonoperative management if the child is maintained on bedrest with monitoring of laboratory studies, vital signs, and urinary status.

The remaining 5% to 15% of clinically stable patients with major renal trauma elicit controversial opinions with regard to operative versus nonoperative treatment. Some centers advocate routine exploration and repair of such injuries, while others advocate conservative management. Proponents of early surgical intervention believe that it results in less morbidity, such as blood loss, sepsis, hypertension, abscess formation, and a decreased hospital stay. They also believe it allows for a better salvage rate of functional tissue. Finally, they believe that the majority of serious complications arise from conservative treatment (Middleton, Matlak, Nixon et al., 1985; Kass, 1988).

In contrast, others favor an initial period of conservative management for all clinically stable patients. They believe early surgery results in a significantly higher nephrectomy rate and does not necessarily reduce long-term complications of hypertension, hydronephrosis, or loss of renal function (Middleton, Matlak, Nixon et al., 1985; Kass, 1988; Terry, 1990).

The incidence of ureteral trauma in children is low but is suspected after severe blunt trauma or penetrating injury to the abdomen. When ureteral injury does occur, the most common is the separation of the ureter at its junction with the renal pelvis. This may occur as a result of a sudden extreme flexion of the trunk that stretches the ureter. This injury is more likely in children because of increased mobility of a child's spine (Livine & Gonzales, 1985).

Attention to the description of injury is essential for a correct diagnosis; intravenous urography will also demonstrate extravasation of contrast media at the level of disruption. Operative repair is required for such injuries, and recovery is usually without sequelae if the injury is recognized early and treated appropriately (Middleton, Matlak, Nixon et al., 1985).

Bladder injuries may occur as a result of penetrating or blunt trauma. Approximately 10% to 15% of children with a fractured pelvis also exhibit an associated bladder injury (Middleton, Matlak, Nixon et al., 1985; Kass, 1988). Bladder injury is most often defined as extraperitoneal rupture, which is the most common injury, and intraperitoneal rupture. Extraperitoneal rupture is usually associated with pelvic fracture, where the bladder has been penetrated by a bony structure. Management includes surgical debridement and urethral or suprapubic urinary drainage until healing occurs, usually 7 to 14 days (Livine & Gonzales, 1985; Middleton, Matlak, Nixon et al., 1985).

Intraperitoneal rupture occurs when urine, and possibly blood, extravasates into the peritoneal cavity. These injuries usually occur in the posterior bladder wall; the patient has usually suffered a compression injury with a full bladder (Guerriero, 1982). The symptoms of a bladder rupture include an inability to void, abdominal tenderness, and anuria. Failure to diagnose this condition may lead to azotemia, acidosis, and death. Thus, it becomes essential to consider the diagnosis with children who have experienced major abdominal trauma. Treatment of intraperitoneal rupture requires surgical repair.

The majority of urethral injuries result from pelvic fractures, straddle injuries, or urethral manipulation. Complications may include strictures, incontinence, impotence, and fistulas (Livine & Gonzales, 1985). Urethral injuries are most often seen in males, as the male's urethra is longer and less well protected. Signs of urethral injury include blood in the external urethral meatus, perineal hematoma or edema, a distended bladder with the inability to void, and a high-riding prostate in male children (Kass, 1988; Lebet, 1991).

If there is any suspicion of urethral injury, a retrograde urethrogram is performed before any attempt at urethral instrumentation. Difficulty encountered in placing an indwelling catheter also dictates that a urethrogram be performed, as repeated unsuccessful attempts at catheterization may lead to urethral injury and stricture formation that may last a lifetime (Kass, 1988).

Surgical repair is usually required, but there is controversy about whether the repair should be early or delayed. Neither approach has demonstrated a lower complication rate or potential for success. With delayed repair, a suprapubic tube is placed to allow for urinary drainage.

Injuries to the male genitalia may be the result of blunt trauma or penetrating injury. Examples of blunt trauma include falls or kicks, while penetrating injuries may be due to falls onto sharp objects such as glass, fences, sticks, etc. Injury to the penis may be caused by a falling toilet seat in a child being toilet trained; zipper injuries are also common, particularly in uncircumcised males who catch the redundant foreskin in the zipper of their pants. Testicular trauma in males can also occur during sporting events when the child is hit or kicked in the scrotum. Management of such injuries depends upon the type and severity of the injury.

Perineal injuries of young females may occur as a result of falls on sharp or blunt objects or straddle injuries. It is important to pay careful attention to the history; if it is not consistent with the type and degree of injury, sexual abuse is suspected. In any injury to the female vulva or vagina, urethral or rectal injuries must also be considered. Management of the injury will depend on the extent and severity of the injury.

Patient Management

Assessment. The abdomen and flank are examined carefully during the assessment process to detect the presence of pain, masses, abrasions, contusions, or flank ecchymosis (Grey Turner sign), all of which may suggest retroperitoneal bleeding. Considering that genitourinary injuries are rarely life-threatening, knowledge about the location, type, and extent of injury is necessary as a guide to determine appropriate treatment. A detailed history and physical examination are critical. Details of the method of injury are elicited from the patient, family, or others who may have been present. Signs and symptoms of genitourinary trauma will vary depending upon severity, location, presence of associated injuries, and the child's general condition. Urinalysis is performed early in the evaluation of every child who suffers significant trauma. Hematuria is the hallmark of renal trauma and occurs in 80% to 90% of patients with renal injury. The degree of hematuria, however, does not necessarily correlate with the severity of injury (Kass, 1988). In children, it may be particularly difficult to quickly obtain a urine sample; thus, a small feeding tube or catheter can be passed into the bladder (if there are no signs of urethral injury) to facilitate a rapid evaluation. The absence of hematuria, however, does not exclude the possibility of renal injury if there are other findings that strongly suggest it.

Some form of radiographic investigation is necessary to exclude injury to the urinary tract if a child presents with hematuria, a history of a deceleration injury, or abdominal trauma. The specific imaging method may vary depending upon the clinical status of the patient, the capability of the institution, and practitioner preference. Radiographic imaging may include IVP, renal scan, ultrasonography, CT scan, and renal angiography. The type and role of radiographic evaluation is a controversial subject. In the past, IVP was recommended for all patients with hematuria; today, many practitioners are reluctant to expose all children to a potentially serious reaction to contrast medium, and unnecessary radiation and expense. Instead, they recommend that IVP be used in children with physical findings of renal injury, evidence of significant blood loss or hematuria, or when renal artery injury is suspected. CT scans have become more widely used and are often the procedure of choice for many practitioners. The major benefit of CT is that all organs in the upper abdominal and retroperitoneal areas can be simultaneously evaluated (Middleton, Matlak, Nixon et al., 1985).

Critical Care Management. The management of the child with genitourinary trauma will depend on the specific injury as described above. Nursing management involves close monitoring for signs of complications and progress of healing.

Immobility Related to Orthopedic Trauma

Etiology

Musculoskeletal trauma is common in children; it occurs in approximately 20% of all trauma sustained by children (Thomas, 1993). Skull and clavicle fractures are most common at birth; however, during the first year of life, fractures are rare. Fractures that occur during the first 2 years of life may be an indication of skeletal problems, bone disease, or child abuse. In children 2 years of age through adolescence, fractures of the upper extremity occur more often than fractures of the lower extremity (Thomas, 1993).

Motor vehicle accidents are a common cause of fractures and are associated with the more serious injuries. For example, the unrestrained child in a car can be tossed around the inside in a crash and actually ricochet off the interior structures multiple times. A child pedestrian can be thrown a long way with significant force upon impact.

Falls are another common cause of fractures. Children may fall from great heights, resulting in numerous fractures along with other injuries. Additional causes of fractures include sports-related trauma, penetrating injuries, and child abuse. With child abuse, fractures are a common manifestation, second only to skin injuries.

Children are susceptible to fractures because of the types of activities they engage in and because their immature skeleton. Many fractures, such as hairline or greenstick fractures, are not serious, but intra-articular or epiphyseal plate fractures have serious potential for growth plate disruption.

Children have different complications from fractures than adults. Growth disturbances will follow epiphyseal plate fractures. Osteomyelitis resulting from an open fracture or an open reduction from a closed fracture tends to be more extensive in a child. This infection has the potential to damage the epiphyseal plate, resulting in growth disturbance. Volkman ischemia (resulting from vascular compromise) of the nerves and muscles, posttraumatic myositis ossificans, and refracture are more common in children (Salter, 1985).

Torn ligaments and dislocation are less common in children. The ligaments are strong and resilient; in fact, the ligaments are stronger than the associated epiphyseal plates. A sudden extension on a ligament at the time of injury results in the separation of the epiphyseal plate rather than a torn ligament.

This is also true of the fibrous joint capsule. The type of injury that would produce a traumatic dislocation of the shoulder in an adult will produce a separation fracture of the proximal humeral epiphysis in a child.

Children's fractures heal more rapidly because of the osteogenic activity of the periosteum and endosteum. The osteogenic activity is very active at birth, decreases progressively throughout childhood, and remains constant from adulthood to old age.

Pathogenesis

The mechanism of bone injury involves external forces acting on the body and the bony structures (direct impact) or internal forces caused by muscle contraction or ligament stress (bending force). Bone breakage is produced by loading forces where the ability of the bone to store and dissipate energy by temporary deformation has been exceeded (Joy, 1989). Loading forces include bending, tension, compression, torsion, and combined loading. These forces can be applied along the bone's long axis or along the traverse axis. The magnitude and rate of loading will determine the extent of bone deformation.

Epiphyseal fractures are of particular concern in children. As mentioned earlier, these have the potential to produce growth disturbances in children by causing progressive angular deformity and limb length discrepancies (Campbell & Campbell, 1991). Epiphyseal fractures have been classified according to the Salter-Harris classification (Table 30–7).

Types of fractures seen in children are presented in Figure 30–6. Greenstick fractures are common in small children and are characterized by an incomplete fracture of the bone with a portion of the cortex and periosteum still intact. Transverse fractures are seen in infants and small children with the fracture line across the bone at a right angle to the longitudinal axis of the bone. Spiral fractures are caused by torsional forces such as when the extremity rotates while in a fixed position. This is commonly associated with child abuse. Comminuted fractures are seen more in older children and adolescents and are the result of a high-impact force such as a fall from a long height or a high-speed motor vehicle accident.

Table 30–7. SALTER AND HARRIS'S CLASSIFICATION OF EPIPHYSEAL PLATE FRACTURES

Type	Description	Management	Prognosis
I	Complete epiphyseal separation without fracture. Most common in younger children with thick epiphyseal plates	Closed reduction and cast immobilization	Excellent unless the blood supply to the epiphysis is compromised
II	Most common epiphyseal fracture. Separation of epiphyseal plate with a fracture through the metaphysis, producing a triangular fragment	Closed reduction and cast immobilization	Excellent unless the blood supply to the epiphysis is compromised
III	Fracture through part of the epiphyseal plate and extending into the joint	Open reduction and internal fixation usually required	Good, with restoration of normal joint surface and vascularity
IV	Fracture completely through the epiphyseal plate and extending through a portion of the metaphysis	Open reduction and internal fixation	At risk for interrupted longitudinal growth unless there is perfect anatomic alignment, which must be maintained until complete healing
V	Crush injury to an area of the epiphyseal plate that is nondisplaced with no fracture line visible on roentgenography	Immobilization and non–weight bearing for a minimum of 3 weeks to prevent further compression	Poor. Injury is frequently identified only in retrospect after growth disturbance has occurred

Pelvic fractures may occur as the result of a severe injury, such as that associated with a motor vehicle accident. The most important aspect of the fractures is not the fracture itself but associated complications such as internal bleeding from torn vessels and extravasation of urine from bladder rupture or urethral injury. Pelvic fractures are classified as stable or unstable, depending on whether the fracture interferes with the stability and integrity of the pelvic ring. Stable fractures do not transgress the pelvic ring; therefore, they do not interfere with the stability of the pelvis in relation to weight bearing and do not require reduction. Unstable fractures include separation of the symphysis pubis; an opening in the pelvic ring; movement of one half of the pelvis; or a bucket handle fracture, in which the fractured half of the pelvis rolls forward and inward (Salter, 1985). Usually these fractures result from a crush injury that occurs when the child is run over.

A serious musculoskeletal injury that may be seen is an amputation. Amputations may occur as the result of power tools, farm machinery, railroad accidents, or sharp objects. Amputations are classified as partial or complete with varying degrees of tissue and bone injury. A guillotine type of amputation involves a wound that has clean, well-defined edges, and has the best prognosis for reimplantation. A crush amputation is the separation of the body part with extensive damage to the soft tissue, bone, nerve, and blood vessels. This wound has a poor prognosis for limb salvage.

Patient Management

Assessment. As with any trauma patient, the first focus is on the ABCs. A detailed musculoskeletal assessment takes place during the secondary survey. Observation along with palpation of each bone and joint will help to identify abnormalities. These abnor-

Table 30–8. ABNORMALITIES ASSOCIATED WITH MUSCULOSKELETAL TRAUMA

Blood loss associated with a specific injury
Neurologic or vascular deficit distal to the injury
Visible deformity, shortening, or angulation of a limb
Partial or complete loss of a digit or limb
Increase in limb circumference that worsens
Manifestations of pelvic fracture
Crush injury
Any injury suspected of resulting in compartment syndrome
Abnormal muscle or tendon function
Point tenderness or muscle spasms
Bruising
Swelling
Crepitus
Abnormal movement between joints or a joint

Table 30–9. COMPONENTS OF A NEUROVASCULAR ASSESSMENT

Circulation

Color
Temperature
Capillary refill
Edema
Pulses above and below the injury

Sensation

Numbness
Tingling
Level of pain

Motion of Extremities

Coordinated
Symmetric
Strength

Transverse – Results from angulation force or direct trauma.

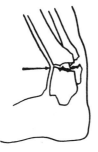

Impacted – Results from severe trauma causing fracture ends to jam together.

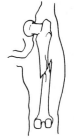

Oblique – Results from twisting force.

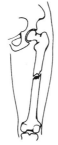

Compressed – Results from severe force to top of head or os calcis or acceleration/deceleration injury.

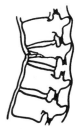

Spiral – Results from twisting force with firmly planted foot.

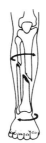

Greenstick – Results from compression force; usually occurs in children under 10 years of age.

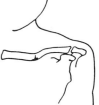

Comminuted – Results from severe direct trauma; has more than two fragments.

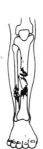

Avulsion – Results from muscle mass contracting forcefully, causing bone fragment to tear off at insertion.

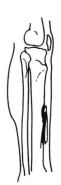

Figure 30–6 • • • • • •
Types of fractures. (From Budassi-Sheehy, S. (Ed.) (1990). *Manual of emergency care*. St. Louis: Mosby–Year Book.)

malities are listed in Table 30–8 and are documented once identified. Observation for spontaneous movement always takes place before manipulation of the extremity. Manipulation of the injured extremity may inflict pain and interfere with further examination.

Once the injuries are recognized, the first priority is to estimate blood loss and then follow with a neurovascular assessment. Components of the neurovascular assessment are included in Table 30–9. It is critical to compare extremities bilaterally. Neurovascular status is monitored frequently for the first 24 hours after injury; after application of a cast or traction; after surgery; and after any treatment, including temporary splinting.

Assessment following an amputation injury also

first focuses on the ABCs. Blood loss is estimated, but with a complete amputation, the severed blood vessels retract and clamp down, resulting in effective clotting and minimal bleeding.

It is critical for the nurse caring for the child with an orthopedic injury to monitor for the develop of compartment syndrome. Compartment syndrome is progressive vascular compromise caused by an increase in pressure within an anatomic space that causes circulatory impairment and compromised tissue function within that space. Direct bleeding and inflammation may cause increased pressure within a compartment. In addition, a decrease in the size of the compartment caused by the constriction of a splint or cast may produce compartment syndrome. This syndrome can occur anywhere where fascia binds muscle groups, but it tends to occur most frequently in the four components of the lower leg (Fig. 30–7).

The manifestations of compartment syndrome are seen with the "5 Ps." Pain, which is described as extreme, occurs out of proportion to the apparent injury. Pain may also occur with passive movement of the affected extremity. Parethesia, specifically numbness or tingling, may occur. The child may also exhibit a decreased ability to discriminate between two points on the affected extremity. Pallor is a late sign, and delayed capillary refill may be present. Another late sign is paralysis or a progressively weakening muscle. Pulselessness will occur only after compartment pressures are extremely high because the larger arteries will remain open until then. Therefore, an injured extremity with a strong pulse does not rule out compartment syndrome.

Diagnosis of compartment syndrome is based on the presence of these symptoms and on increased interstitial pressure. This pressure can be directly measured using a variety of systems that use a needle or a catheter connected to a pressure transducer and monitor. Interstitial pressures exceeding 30 to 35 mmHg are indicative of compartment syndrome.

Critical Care Management. The initial treatment of fractures involves controlling bleeding, assessing neurovascular status, and then applying splints or traction. A closed fracture will require anatomic alignment and splinting. An open fracture requires wound irrigation, debridement, fracture alignment, and stabilization in the OR. Continuous monitoring for signs of complications, such as infections or compartment syndrome, is critical.

Amputations require special attention. Initially, if severe bleeding is occurring, direct pressure with a soft dressing is applied and the extremity is elevated.

If there is minimal bleeding, a sterile dressing is applied to the stump, which is then splinted and elevated. Tourniquets and clamps are contraindicated, since they may cause tissue ischemia and vessel damage. Intravenous access is obtained for fluid resuscitation and antibiotics.

The goal of care for the amputated body part is to reduce ischemia time. The body part is gently rinsed with normal saline to remove visible dirt. It is then wrapped in moist, sterile gauze, placed in a sealable plastic bag, and then put on ice for transport to the OR or to another center. The body part is never placed directly in saline or ice, as moisture absorbed by the tissue will result in swelling and necrosis.

Postoperatively, the child's neurovascular status is frequently assessed. Anticoagulants may be given to prevent hemostasis in the reimplanted vessels, so measures to prevent bleeding are initiated. Antibiotics are administered to prevent or treat infection. Psychosocial support is crucial, especially if the child loses the body part, to help the child and family cope with a changed body image.

Compartment syndrome requires immediate treatment if pressures exceed normal limits. The limb is placed in a neutral position, since elevation results in further compromise of arterial flow. Cast or constricting bandages are opened and removed. If the symptoms and excessive pressures continue, a fasciotomy may be performed to release pressure and maintain extremity circulation. The incision will be left open for a period of time with the limb splinted in a functional position. A dressing is applied to the open wound, and, if after 24 hours the muscle is considered viable, saline dressings are applied and changed daily until the wound is closed (Willis & Rorabeck, 1990).

Pain management is an important issue for those caring for the child with a musculoskeletal injury. Results of a study examining pain in children suggest that children hospitalized with orthopedic conditions experience a higher number of painful occurrences and symptoms than children hospitalized with other conditions (Wong & Baker, 1988). Occurrences such as postoperative pain, pain with moving, and pain associated with traction and pins were rated as causing more pain than injections, venipuncture, and IV insertion. Recommended methods for pain control include oral or intravenous medication, patient-controlled analgesia, and nonpharmacologic methods. Chapter 18 provides in-depth information regarding pain management.

CHILD MALTREATMENT

History

Varying forms of child abuse have been accepted by society for many centuries. In earlier times, children who were considered undesirable due to religious or economic reasons or because they were defective or female were often destroyed; such actions

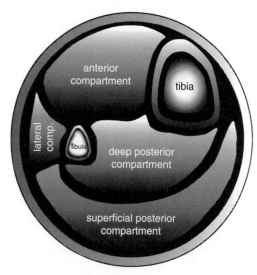

Figure 30–7 ● ● ● ● ● ●

The four compartments of the lower leg. (From Robertson, W.W. (1993). Crush injury and compartment syndrome. In M.R. Eichelberger (Ed.). *Pediatric trauma: Prevention, acute care, rehabilitation.* St. Louis: Mosby–Year Book.)

were culturally sanctioned. During the 14th century, unwanted children were thrown into the Thames; during the Industrial Revolution, young children were forced to work long hours in hazardous settings with unhealthy conditions. Throughout history, there are many examples of young boys or girls being sold or kept for the purposes of sexual pleasure.

The first legal intervention on behalf of a child occurred in 1874 in the United States. Ironically, the case was brought to court by the American Society for the Prevention of Cruelty to Animals (SPCA). The SPCA was able to demand legal protection for a child who was regularly beaten by her adoptive parents on the basis that she belonged to the Animal Kingdom. Most states did not adopt laws requiring reporting of abuse until the 1960s and 1970s. Today, all 50 of the United States have laws requiring the reporting of child abuse. The public became more acutely aware of this concern when Dr. Henry Kempe coined the phrase "battered-child syndrome" in 1962. Despite the progress that has been made in the arena of child maltreatment, it continues to be a serious social problem.

The Changing Spectrum of Abuse

Children of any race, age, religion, sex, and socio-economic group can be victims of child maltreatment. It is believed that many more children fall prey to abuse than are ever reported to the authorities. A few decades ago, children who were treated for abuse fit the pattern of the "battered child"—one who was malnourished or presented with multiple fractures sustained at different times. Today's abused child is likely to have severe injuries resulting from a sudden, impulsive act of violence. The perpetrator has also changed, from almost exclusively in the past being a parent, to now frequently being a live-in babysitting boyfriend (Kessler & New, 1989).

Incidence of Abuse

Reports of child maltreatment continue to increase; it is estimated that tens of thousands of children suffer major inflicted physical injuries and are at risk for fatality and permanent disability in the United States each year (Kerns, 1985). The true incidence of child abuse is unknown. It is believed to be underestimated and under-reported because of undiagnosed cases, the lack of a uniformly accepted definition, varying diagnostic methods and documentation standards, and identified cases that are never reported.

Defining Child Maltreatment

Child abuse can take on many forms and is difficult to define and standardize. Physical abuse is a form that is often easy to identify and recognize; other forms such as emotional and psychological abuse are

just beginning to be acknowledged. Still other forms of abuse such as child pornography and prostitution remain difficult to identify and manage.

Unfortunately, the term *child maltreatment* is subject to a variety of interpretations and definitions. In addition to a lack of clear definitions, inadequate professional experience, and training and motivation to report, disagreement exists about how responsible parents should be for the safety of their children. A general definition of child maltreatment may be described as an act that endangers a child such that substantial risk to his or her health, safety, development, or mental well-being is created. Various forms of child maltreatment exist, including physical abuse and neglect, sexual abuse, and emotional abuse and neglect.

Physical Abuse

Physical abuse may be difficult to define in a society such as the United States that condones corporal punishment as a method of discipline. A definition of physical abuse used by Children's Hospital, Columbus, Ohio, is an injury caused by a child's caretaker for any reason, including a caretaker's reaction to an unwanted behavior. "Injury" includes tissue damage beyond erythema such as bruises, burns, tears, punctures, fractures, organ rupture, and disruption of functions (Johnson, 1990). When investigating a physical injury, it is important to question whether the injury is in keeping with the developmental capability of the child. Physical injuries labeled by the parents as self-inflicted accidents require certain motor skills on the part of the child; thus, knowledge of child development is essential.

Physical Neglect

Identifying the scope of the problem of neglect is nearly impossible because of the inability to give clear and consistent answers to the question of what constitutes neglect of a child. In general, child neglect is believed to occur when those responsible for meeting the basic needs of children fail to do so (Helfer, 1990). It also includes the failure to provide the basic necessities of life such as medical care, food, clothing, shelter, and supervision. A note of caution, however, is not to define as willful neglect a case in which an impoverished or uneducated family is providing, in truth, the best care possible within their means.

Sexual Abuse

Sexual abuse refers to contacts or interactions between a child and an adult when the child is being used for sexual stimulation of the perpetrator or another person. Sexual abuse may also be committed by a person under the age of 18 if that person is significantly older than the victim or when the perpetrator is in a position of power or control over the victim. Key elements of this broad definition emphasize developmental inappropriateness and coercion

(Paradise, 1990). Such sexual activity violates the norm of informed consent, as the child has neither an appreciation of the deviance of the act nor the autonomy necessary to consent freely (Garbarino, 1989).

Sexual abuse can be assaultive or nonassaultive. Assaultive abuse produces physical injury and often severe emotional trauma. Nonassaultive abuse often results in little or no physical injury, yet the child who is chronically sexually misused often suffers a severe disruption in the development of his or her sexuality. Sexual abuse is the least reported form of child abuse, particularly nonassaultive, chronic abuse. Often, the abuser is a parent of the child and family members are reluctant to acknowledge and reveal such abuse (McNeese & Hebeler, 1977; Cheek, 1985; Paradise, 1990).

Emotional Abuse and Neglect

Emotional and psychological maltreatment is very difficult to define and manage. In general, such abuse occurs when caretakers fail to provide an environment in which a child can thrive, learn, and develop (McNeese & Hebeler, 1977). Garbarino (1989) discusses psychological maltreatment in terms of five categories: rejecting, isolating, terrorizing, ignoring, and corrupting. Rejecting behavior is the refusal to acknowledge a child's worth and the legitimacy of his or her needs. Isolating a child implies cutting the youngster off from normal social experiences, preventing friendship formation, and making the child believe that he or she is alone in the world. One terrorizes a child by verbally assaulting, creating a climate of fear, and making the child believe that the world is a dangerous and hostile place. Ignoring behavior is demonstrated when the caretaker is psychologically unavailable to the child and deprives the child of essential stimulation, responsiveness, and a sense of protection. Corrupting is the "missocializing" of the child, encouraging the child to engage in antisocial behavior, reinforcing deviant behavior, and thus setting the child up for rejection by peers and adults (Garbarino, 1989).

Collaborative Interventions

Evaluation of the child with traumatic injuries serves to validate plausible justification for suspicion of abuse and neglect. Gathering initial information is critical, as is a thorough examination of physical injuries. Regardless of suspicion, the family is questioned in a nonjudgmental, nonthreatening manner.

Histories Suggestive of Child Maltreatment

Obtaining an accurate history in cases of pediatric injury is usually challenging but even more so in the case of suspected child maltreatment. Parents or caretakers may be anxious, angry, guilt-ridden, or intimidating (Kerns, 1985). Physicians and nurses are often dependent on family members for an explanation of an injured child's condition, as many children may be too frightened, too young, or too ill to give an explanation. Even when they are able to do so, many children are unwilling to accuse the adult who cares for them of abuse. It is rare for an adult to spontaneously admit to inflicting injuries; however, an admission of partial or possible responsibility may be indicative of child abuse and should be pursued (Schmitt, 1987).

Other clues or presentations suggestive of child abuse include denial of the existence of injuries or how they occurred, an explanation inconsistent with the physical findings, and a marked delay in seeking medical attention. Delays in presentation result in the near moribund state seen in many seriously abused children when they eventually are brought to the hospital (Kerns, 1985; Ledbetter & Tapper, 1989). A history of prior trauma is important to note, and review of the medical record may reveal a pattern indicative of prior abuse. It may also be helpful to review the records of siblings if they are available. All details of the elected history should be carefully reviewed and evaluated in the context of their consistency or discrepancy with the physical findings.

Physical Examination

The physical examination of the battered, sexually abused, or neglected child is critical. Sometimes, physical injuries not revealed in the history may be discovered. The absence of external injury, however, does not rule out abuse. Children with significant head or abdominal trauma may not have any outward visible signs of trauma. Documentation of physical findings is an important component of the examination. Physical signs of possible abuse are listed in Table 30–10.

Radiographic Examination

Radiographic studies are invaluable in the diagnosis of intentional injuries. Skeletal surveys, CT scans, bone scans, and MRIs are all useful. Radiographic evidence of intentional injuries is presented in Table 30–11.

Psychosocial Interventions

The child victim of abuse and the family need comprehensive psychosocial intervention. This intervention is best provided by a trained mental health professional such as a clinical nurse specialist, social worker, or psychologist who specializes in the care of victims of child maltreatment. The status of the child and the parent-child relationship are assessed and treatment based on that assessment. The approach is one of nonjudgmental support and probing for relevant information. Even though the nurse caring for the child will probably not do the in-depth psychosocial intervention, it is still essential that the parent or caretaker be treated in a nonjudgmental manner.

Table 30–10. PHYSICAL SIGNS OF POSSIBLE ABUSE IN THE CHILD

Skin and Subcutaneous Tissue

Cradle cap, diaper rash, uncleanliness, and other evidence of unconcern or unawareness of infant needs

Cigarette burns, bite marks (human, insect, etc.; infected or not), grab marks, belt lashes (also the characteristic loop lamp cord welts)

Ecchymosis, hematomas, abrasions, and lacerations unusual for the child's developmental age

Injury to the external genitalia, anus, and rectum

Marks on the neck from strangling by hand or rope

External ears traumatized by pinching, twisting, or pulling

Unusual skin rashes that defy dermatologic diagnosis

Burns, particularly of the soles of the feet, hands, or buttocks

Skeletal System

Tenderness, swelling, and limitation of motion of an extremity

Periosteal swelling

Deformities of the long bones

Head

Cephalhematomas

Irregularities of contour resulting from skull fractures

Signs of intracranial trauma

Eyes

Subconjunctival hemorrhages

Traumatic cataracts

Retinal hemorrhages

Papilledema

Ears

Ruptured eardrums from blows to the head

Face

Periorbital ecchymosis

Displaced nasal cartilages

Bleeding from the nasal septum

Fracture of the mandible

Mouth

Lacerated frenulum of the upper lip

Loosened or missing teeth

Burns of the lips or tongues

Chest

Deformity of the chest and limitation of motion due to fracture of the ribs

Subcutaneous edema

Hemothorax

Abdomen

Signs of peritoneal irritation from ruptured organs

Abdominal masses from hematomas

Central Nervous System

Lower motor neuron paralysis from spinal cord injury

Upper motor neuron paralysis from intracranial injury

Neurologic signs varying with location and extent of the injury

From Widner-Kolberg, M.R. (1991). Recognizing child abuse and neglect and what to do about it. Presented at Pediatric Issues in Multisystem Trauma Conference (pp. 105–107). Walnut Creek, CA: Symposia Medicus.

Considerations for the Practitioner in Suspected Child Maltreatment Cases

Protection for the Child

Abused and neglected children are often too young and too frightened to seek help themselves. Because of their physical and psychological immaturity, they are helpless against the cruelty of their caretakers. In the instance of suspected abuse, a decision must be made whether it is safe to return the child to his or her home. If hospitalization is required due to a medical condition, the matter is temporarily solved; if hospitalization is not medically warranted, the practitioner, in concert with a social worker or protective services worker, must make the decision. Such a decision must not be made lightly, as it could result in additional harm to the child, even a potentially fatal injury. Essential factors to consider are the age of the child, nature of the injury, past treatment of injuries, and family characteristics. If the circumstances are marginal, it is best to err on the side of protecting the child (Kerns, 1985).

Documentation

Because the patient's medical record will become a critical piece of evidence, it is imperative that all assessments and findings be meticulously and legibly documented. Interactions with and actions by the caretakers will be of great importance and should also be carefully recorded.

Reporting to Protective Services

All 50 states have laws requiring that practitioners report cases of suspected child abuse to the local protection services agency. Anyone reporting a case

Table 30–11. RADIOGRAPHIC EVIDENCE OF INTENTION INJURIES

Multiple Fractures

In different stages of healing, including:
  Single blow fractures in infant
  Epiphyseal separation
  Spiral fracture in the young
  Fractured ribs
  Fractured spine†

Cortical Metaphyseal Fragmentation

"Chip" fractures or "corner spurs" partially separated from the metaphysis

Traumatic Involucrum‡

Exuberant calcifying new bone formation secondary to subperiosteal forces and hematoma (grasping, shaking, and torsion forces); may produce "bucket-handle" images (extension of hematoma beyond the end of the shaft)

Skull Fracture*

With† or without subdural hematoma

Suture Separation‡

Hemorrhage† without fracture

Increasing head circumference in infant—whiplash forces from shaking alone can cause

*Evident immediately after trauma.

†Cerebrospinal injury, subdural, intraventricular, and/or intracerebral hemorrhage are most serious complications and principle causes of death and permanent crippling.

‡Not visible radiographically until 7–18 days after trauma.

From Widner-Kolberg, M.R. (1991). Recognizing child abuse and what to do about it. Presented at Pediatric Issues in Multisystem Trauma Conference (p. 108). Walnut Creek, CA: Symposia Medicus.

of suspected abuse, who does so in good faith, is immune from civil and criminal liability for having done so. If a practitioner fails to report, penalties varying from nominal fines to imprisonment may be imposed. Failure to report has led to medical malpractice claims in a number of cases (Kerns, 1985).

Testifying in Court

Although many persons are reluctant to testify in court, the practitioner's knowledge may be essential in allowing for the future protection of the child. When testifying in a case, the following guidelines may be helpful:

1. Arrange for a pretrial interview with the attorney—this will allow for review of both the process and the content of the testimony. Expectations can be clarified and any questions answered at this time.
2. Request to go to court "on call"—delays and rescheduling are frequent, and requesting "on call" status will eliminate many wasted hours waiting in anterooms prior to testimony.
3. Review the facts—review the medical records in detail; a prepared practitioner allows for a more helpful witness and a smoother testimony.
4. Take the time to prepare responses—it is helpful to take a few moments to formulate a verbal response. Testimony should be presented in a logical and orderly way and articulated calmly and slowly.
5. Maintain a neutral position—the practitioner testifies on behalf of the truth, not one side or the other.
6. Refuse to answer complex questions with simple answers—should a yes or no response be requested for a complex or subtle question, simply state that the question cannot be answered in such a fashion. Usually, the judge will then allow the witness to give a more comprehensive answer.
7. Do not be intimidated—if an attorney attempts to confuse or embarrass, keep in mind that the attorney's goal is to "win" the case for the client. Various tactics may be used to do so; therefore, remember not to take it personally. Rarely will a judge allow any significant harassment of a professional witness (Kern, 1985).

PREVENTION OF PEDIATRIC TRAUMA

Traumatic injury continues to be a serious threat to a child's well-being and life. Attention to injury prevention is lacking, as many injuries are viewed as acts of chance or random occurrences that cannot be predicted or prevented (Srnec, 1991). The reality is that injuries are no more likely to occur by chance than are diseases (Brent, Perper, Allman, 1987). Accidental injury and death cannot be regarded as an inescapable part of life.

Children must live in an environment that is cre-ated and regulated by adults; thus, adults must accept the responsibility to consider the needs of children. However, all too often, the needs of children and their right to a safe environment are misunderstood, ignored, neglected, or made subservient to economic considerations (Wheatley & Cass, 1989).

Premature mortality as a result of pediatric trauma results in years of potential life lost. There is also a significant amount of hidden morbidity associated with pediatric trauma that may not become obvious until long after the injury occurs. Such morbidity is defined as psychosocial disabilities and is evidenced by events such as changes in family structure (marital difficulties, divorce, sibling effects), economic difficulties, and cognitive and behavioral symptoms (Harris, Schwaitzberg, Seman, et al., 1989).

It is generally believed that the majority of childhood injuries are preventable once the causative factors have been identified. It is also known that many preventative strategies are currently available; however, they are frequently not applied or are used incorrectly. Rivara calculated a possible further 29% reduction in accidental deaths in the United States if the existing preventative strategies (air bags, seat restraints, cycle helmets, pool barriers, window bars, smoke detectors, handgun legislation, and appropriate packaging of poisonings) were applied consistently and conscientiously (Rivara, 1985).

The likelihood that prevention methods will be used is often dependent upon the ease with which they can be used. The most effective and successful measures are passive, those that require no action on the part of the user. Such measures include flame retardant sleepwear for children and air bags in automobiles. The next most effective measures are those that require a simple, one-time action, such as installing window locks or window guards to prevent children from opening or falling out of windows. Least effective measures are those that require frequent and consistent actions by the user, such as replacing smoke detector batteries and putting guns, matches, and medicines in safe places (Widner-Kolberg, 1991).

The majority of pediatric injuries and deaths are due to car passenger injuries, pedestrian injuries, drownings, and bicycle injuries (Wheatley and Cass, 1989). Programs that are designed to decrease childhood trauma must concentrate on these four areas.

With regard to car passenger injuries, safety measures such as seat belts and safety seats are available, yet many times restraint measures are not used, particularly for infants. Because children are smaller and lighter than adults, they are thrown about the interior of a vehicle much more easily than an adult. Thus, accidents that may result in only minor trauma to an adult may result in serious or even fatal injury to a child. Other factors that put children and infants who are unrestrained at greater risk include their proportionately larger head size, which makes them more susceptible to deceleration forces and neck muscles less able to support the head.

It is clear that the safety of infants and children in motor vehicles is dependent on the behavior of adults. Strategies to influence adult behavior must be developed and enforced if childhood injuries related to motor vehicle accidents are to be prevented. Such strategies include education related to safe driving habits, laws created and enforced to maintain safe driving, and harsh penalties for those violating safety laws. The use of passive protection is another measure that can help to prevent pediatric injuries; such measures include better engineering of roads and highways and the development of safer automobiles (Widner-Kolberg, 1991).

Pedestrian-auto injuries continue to be a serious threat to children. The majority of pedestrian-auto injuries occur in children under 12 years of age, with children in the 5- to 9-year age group being at greatest risk (Zuckerman & Duby, 1983). The normal impulsiveness of children at this young age combined with their inability to assess distances and speed and localize sounds adequately often results in unsafe traffic behavior. Although behavior modification through safety education may lead to a small reduction in traumatic injuries, many believe that children should be taught avoidance of the roadway unless they are in the company of an adult (Wheatley & Cass, 1989; Widner-Kolberg, 1991).

Bicycles and cycle injuries are a cause of serious head injuries in children. Once again, it seems that children have been neglected when one considers the legislation, or lack of it, with regard to bicycle helmet laws. While adults who are riding motorcycles are required by law in many states to wear a helmet, pedal-cyclists are not. Requiring children to wear bicycle helmets is probably the single most effective way of making riding safer. Although many argue that such legislation would be too difficult to enforce, one would expect a higher rate of compliance following legislation.

Although appropriate postinjury care is essential in the management of pediatric trauma, attention to the area of prevention has the greatest potential for reducing morbidity and mortality. Nurses can and must play a major role in injury prevention. Through education, role modeling, lobbying for legislation, and research, nurses can play a part in the development and initiation of prevention strategies that will decrease the problem of traumatic injuries in children.

SUMMARY

Pediatric trauma is a national epidemic. It is the leading killer of children between the ages of 1 and 14 years and is a major cause of disabling injuries. This is a major concern to society when one considers not only the tragedy to the family, but also the implications of the loss of work potential, the length and cost of rehabilitation, and the effects on growth and development.

Children have been shown to have a better potential for recovery, especially after head injury (Pfen-ninger, Kaiser, Lutschg, et al., 1983; Alberico, Ward, Choi, et al., 1987). This potential can be maximized by expert nursing care. Nursing care includes precise assessment, formulation of nursing diagnoses based on assessment, and collaborative interventions guided by appropriate nursing diagnoses. Research has demonstrated the positive impact nursing care has on the trauma patient; however, more study is needed, especially in the pediatric population. Research priorities for trauma nursing have been identified (Bayley, Richmond, Noroian, et al., 1994).

Nurses are in a key position to provide leadership in the area of pediatric injury prevention. They can educate legislators and the public about how to manage this public health epidemic. Children can be protected by further research in all areas of pediatric trauma, including trauma prevention, resuscitation, and nursing interventions to further maximize outcome.

References

Alberico, A.M., Ward, J.O., Choi, S.C., et al. (1987). Outcome after severe head injury: Relationship to mass lesions, diffuse injury and ICP course in pediatric and adult patients. *Journal of Neurosurgery, 67,* 648.

Bayley, E.W., Richmond, T., Noroian, E.L., et al. (1994). A Delphi study on research priorities for trauma nursing. *American Journal of Critical Care, 3* (3), 208–216.

Bracken, M.B., Shepard, M.J., Collins, W.F., et al. (1990). A randomized, controlled trial of methylprednisolone or naloxone in the treatment of acute spinal-cord injury. *New England Journal of Medicine, 322,* 1405–1411.

Brent, D.A., Perper, J.A., & Allman, C.J. (1987). Alcohol, firearms, and suicide among youth. *JAMA, 257,* 3369–3372.

Brower, P., Paul, J., & Brosman, S.A. (1978). Urinary tract abnormalities presenting as a result of blunt abdominal trauma. *Journal of Trauma, 18,* 719.

Bruce, D.A., Alavi, A., Bilaniuk, L., et al. (1981). Diffuse cerebral swelling following head injuries in children: The syndrome of "malignant brain edema." *Journal of Neurosurgery, 54,* 170.

Buntain, W.L., Lynch, F.P., & Ramenofsky, M.L. (1987). Management of the acutely injured child. *Advances in Trauma, 2,* 43–86.

Campbell, L.S., & Campbell, J.D. (1991). Musculoskeletal trauma in children. *Critical Care Nursing Clinics of North America, 3* (3), 445–456.

Cheek, J.G. (1985). Sexual abuse of children. In T.A. Mayer (Ed.). *Emergency management of pediatric trauma* (pp. 435–443). Philadelphia: W.B. Saunders.

Cooney, D.R., & Bellmire, D.F. (1990). Hepatic, biliary tree and pancreatic injury. In R.J. Touloukian (Ed.). *Pediatric trauma* (2nd ed., pp. 312–331). St. Louis: Mosby–Year Book.

Davis, R.J., Tait, V.F., Dean, J.M., Goldberg, A.L., & Rogers, M.C. (1992). Head and spinal cord injury. In M.C. Rogers (Ed.). *Textbook of pediatric intensive care* (2nd ed., Vol. 1, pp. 805–857). Baltimore: Williams & Wilkins.

Davis, S.L., Furman, D.F., & Costarino, A.T. (1993). Adult respiratory distress syndrome in children: Associated disease, clinical course, and predictors of death. *The Journal of Pediatrics, 123* (1), 35–45.

Dickman, C.A., & Rekate, H.L. (1993). In M.E. Eichelberger (Ed.). *Pediatric trauma: Prevention, acute care, rehabilitation* (pp. 362–377). St. Louis: Mosby–Year Book.

Dickman, C.A., Rekate, H.L., Sonntag, V.K.H., et al. (1989). Pediatric spinal trauma: Vertebral column and spinal cord injuries in children. *Pediatric Neuroscience, 15,* 237–256.

Division of Injury Control, Center for Environmental Health and Injury Control, Centers for Disease Control (1990). Childhood injuries in the United States. *American Journal of the Diseases of Children, 144,* 627–646.

Eichelberger, M.R. (1987). Trauma of the airway and thorax. *Pediatric Annals*, 16 (4), 307–316.

Eichelberger, M.R., & Anderson, K.D. (1987). Sequelae of thoracic injury in children. In W.R. Hix & B.L. Aaron (Eds.). *Residual of thoracic trauma* (p. 252). Mt Kisco, NY: Futura.

Eichelberger, M.R., Gotschall, C.S., Sacco, W.J., et al. (1989). A comparison of the Trauma Score, the Revised Trauma Score, and the Pediatric Trauma Score. *Annals of Emergency Medicine*, 18, 1053–1058.

Fabian, T., Cicala, R., Croce, M., et al. (1991). A prospective evaluation of myocardial contusion: Correlation of significant arrhythmias and cardiac output with CPK-MB measurements. *Journal of Trauma*, 31 (5), 653–659.

Fackler, J.C., & Yaster, M. (1992). Multiple trauma in the pediatric patient. In M.C. Rogers (Ed.). *Textbook of pediatric intensive care* (2nd ed., Vol. 2, pp. 1443–1475). Baltimore: Williams & Wilkins.

Frame, S.B., Marshall, W.T., & Clifford, T.G. (1989). Synchronized independent lung ventilation in the management of pediatric unilateral pulmonary contusion: Case report. *Journal of Trauma*, 29 (3), 395–397.

Garbarino, J. (1989). The psychologically battered child: Toward a definition. *Pediatric Annals*, 18, 8.

Garcia, V.F., Gotschall, C.S., & Eichelberger, M.R. (1990). Rib fractures in trauma: A marker of severe trauma. *Journal of Trauma*, 30, 697–698.

Ghajar, J., & Hariri, R.J. (1992). Management of pediatric head injury. *Pediatric Clinics of North America*, 39 (5), 1093–1125.

Godersky, J.C., & Menezes, A.H. (1989). Optimal management for children with spinal cord injury. *Contemporary Neurosurgery*, 11, 1–6.

Guerriero, W.G. (1982). Trauma to the kidneys, ureters, bladder, and urethra. *Surgical Clinics of North America*, 62 (6), 1047–1074.

Haller, J.A., & Beaver, B.L. (1990). Overview of pediatric trauma. In R.J. Touloukian (Ed.). *Pediatric trauma* (2nd ed., pp. 3–13). St. Louis: Mosby–Year Book.

Harris, B.H., Schwaitzberg, S.D., Seman, T.M., et al. (1989). The hidden mortality of pediatric trauma. *Journal of Pediatric Surgery*, 24 (1), 103–106.

Helfer, R.E. (1990). The neglect of our children. *Pediatric Clinics of North America*, 37 (4), 923–941.

Hensle, T.W., & Dillon, P. (1990). Renal injuries. In R.J. Touloukian (Ed.). *Pediatric trauma* (2nd ed., pp. 358–370). St. Louis: Mosby–Year Book.

Hill, S.A., Miller, C.A., Kosnik, E.J., et al. (1984). Pediatric neck injuries: A clinical study. *Journal of Neurosurgery*, 60, 700–706.

Johnson, C.F. (1990). Inflicted injury versus accidental injury. *Pediatric Clinics of North America*, 37 (4), 791–813.

Joy, C. (1989). Musculoskeletal trauma. In C. Joy (Ed.). *Pediatric trauma nursing* (pp. 119–142). Rockville, MD: Aspen.

Kane, N.M., Cronan, J.J., Dorfman, G.S., & DeLuca, F. (1988). Pediatric abdominal trauma: Evaluation by computed tomography. *Pediatrics*, 82 (1), 4–15.

Kass, E.J. (1988). Genitourinary trauma. In M.R. Eichelberger, G.L. Pratsch (Eds.). *Pediatric trauma care* (pp. 105–112). Rockville, MD: Aspen.

Kerns, D.L. Child abuse. (1985). In T.A. Mayer (Ed.). *Emergency management of pediatric trauma* (pp. 421–434). Philadelphia: W.B. Saunders.

Kessler, D.B., & New, M.I. (1989). Emerging trends in child abuse and neglect. *Pediatric Annals*, 18 (8), 472–475.

Kewalramani, L.S., Kraus, J.F., & Sterling, H.M. (1980). Acute spinal cord lesions in a pediatric population: Epidemiological and clinical features. *Paraplegia*, 18, 206–219.

King, D.R. (1985). Trauma in infancy and childhood: Initial evaluation and management. *Pediatric Clinics of North America*, 32 (5), 1299–1310.

Kling, T.F. (1986). Spine injury in the multiply injured child. In R.E. Marcus (Ed.). *Trauma in children* (pp. 175–197). Rockville, MD: Aspen.

Kuzmarov, I.N., Morehouse, D.D., & Gibson, S. (1981). Blunt renal trauma in the pediatric population: A retrospective study. *Journal of Urology*, 126, 648.

Lebet, R.M. (1991). Abdominal and genitourinary trauma in children. *Critical Care Nursing Clinics of North America*, 3 (3), 433–444.

Ledbetter, D.J., & Tapper, D. (1989). Injuries caused by child abuse. *Pediatrics*, 15 (10), 9–13.

Livine, P.M., & Gonzales, E.T. (1985). Genitourinary trauma in children. *Urology Clinics of North America*, 12 (1), 53–65.

Luchtefield, W.B. (1990). Pulmonary contusion. *Focus on Critical Care*, 17, 482–485.

Maddox, K.L., Bichell, W.H., Pete, P.E., et al. (1987). Prospective MAST study in 911 patients. *Journal of Trauma*, 29, 1104–1107.

Matlak, M.E. (1985). Abdominal injuries. In T.A. Mayer (Ed.). *Emergency management of pediatric trauma* (pp. 328–340). Philadelphia: W.B. Saunders.

McAnena, O.J., Moore, E.E., & Marx, J.A. (1990). Initial evaluation of the patient with blunt abdominal trauma. *Surgical Clinics of North America*, 70 (3), 495.

McNeese, M.C., & Hebeler, J.R. (1977). The abused child: A clinical approach to identification and management. *Clinical Symposia*, 29 (2).

Middleton, R.G., Matlak, M.E., Nixon, G.W., et al. (1985). Genitourinary injuries in children. In T.A. Mayer (Ed.). *Emergency management of pediatric trauma* (pp. 341–352). Philadelphia: W.B. Saunders.

Moosa, A.R. (1984). Diagnostic tests and procedures in acute pancreatitis. *New England Journal of Medicine*, 311, 639–643.

Mueller-Dickinson, C. (1991). Thoracic trauma in children. *Critical Care Nursing Clinics of North America*, 3 (3), 423.

Newman, K.D. (1993). Gastric and intestinal injury. In M.R. Eichelberger (Ed.). *Pediatric trauma: Prevention, acute care, rehabilitation* (pp. 475–481). St. Louis: Mosby–Year Book.

Newman, K.D., Eichelberger, M.R., & Randolph, J.G. (1988). Abdominal injury. In M.R. Eichelberger & G.L. Pratsch (Eds.). *Pediatric trauma care* (pp. 101–104). Rockville, MD: Aspen.

Osenbach, R.K., & Menezes, A.H. (1989). Spinal cord injury without radiographic abnormality in children. *Pediatric Neurosurgery*, 15, 168–175.

Othersen, H.B. (1990). Cardiothoracic injuries. In R.J. Touloukian (Ed.). *Pediatric trauma* (2nd ed., pp. 266–311). St. Louis: Mosby–Year Book.

Pang, D., & Pollack, I.F. (1989). Spinal cord injury without radiographic abnormality in children—the SCIWORA syndrome. *The Journal of Trauma*, 29 (5), 654–664.

Paradise, J.E. (1990). The medical evaluation of the sexually abused child. *Pediatric Clinics of North America*, 37 (4), 839–863.

Peckham, L.M., & Kitchen, L.A. (1989). Abdominal and genitourinary trauma. In C. Joy (Ed.). *Pediatric trauma nursing* (pp. 102–118). Rockville, MD: Aspen.

Peclet, M., Newman, K., Eichelberger, M., et al. (1990). Patterns of injury in children. *Journal of Pediatric Surgery*, 25 (1), 85–91.

Pfenninger, J., Kaiser, G., Lutschg, J., et al. (1983). Treatment and outcome of the severely head-injured child. *Intensive Care Medicine*, 9, 13.

Philichi, L.M. (1994). Multiple organ system in the pediatric population. *Critical Care Nursing Quarterly*, 16 (4), 96–105.

Quinlan, D.M., & Gearhart, J.P. (1990). Blunt renal trauma in childhood: Features indicating severe injury. *British Journal of Urology*, 66, 526–531.

Ramenofsky, M.L. (1987). Pediatric abdominal trauma. *Pediatric Annals*, 16 (4), 318–326.

Reynolds, S.F. (1987). Cardiac trauma and tamponade. *Critical Care Quarterly*, 12, 30–31.

Rice, L.J., & Britton, J.T. (1993). Airway management. In M.R. Eichelberger (Ed.). *Pediatric trauma: Prevention, acute care, rehabilitation* (pp. 162–168). St. Louis: Mosby–Year Book.

Rivara, F.P. (1985). Traumatic deaths of children in the United States: Currently available prevention strategies. *Pediatrics*, 75, 456–462.

Rouse, T.M. (1993). Colonic, rectal, and perineal injury. In M.R. Eichelberger (Ed.). *Pediatric trauma: Prevention, acute care, rehabilitation* (pp. 482–489). St. Louis: Mosby–Year Book.

Ruge, J.R., Sinson, G.P., McLone, D.G., et al. (1988). Pediatric spinal injury: The very young. *Journal of Neurosurgery*, 68, 25–30.

Sacco, W.J., Copes, W.S., & Gotschall, C.S. (1993). Measurement and assessment of outcomes. In M.R. Eichelberger (Ed.). *Pediatric trauma: Prevention, acute care, rehabilitation* (pp. 641–649). St. Louis: Mosby–Year Book.

Salter, R.B. (1985). Musculoskeletal injuries. In T.A. Mayer (Ed.). *Emergency management of pediatric trauma* (pp. 353–389). Philadelphia: W.B. Saunders.

Schiffman, M.A. (1989). Nonoperative management of blunt abdominal trauma in pediatrics. *Emergency Medicine Clinics of North America*, 7 (3), 519–535.

Schmitt, B.D. (1987). The child with nonaccidental trauma. In R.E. Helfer & R.S. Kempe (Eds.). *The battered child* (pp. 178–196). Chicago: University of Chicago Press.

Scorpio, R.J., & Wesson, D.E. (1993). Splenic trauma. In M.R. Eichelberger (Ed.). *Pediatric trauma: Prevention, acute care, rehabilitation* (pp. 456–463). St. Louis: Mosby–Year Book.

Simon, B., & Borg, U. (1990). Independent lung ventilation. *Critical Care Report*, 1 (3), 398–407.

Srnec, P. (1991). Children, violence, and intentional injuries. *Critical Care Nursing Clinics of North America*, 3 (3), 471–478.

Stiles, Q.R., Cohlemia, G.S., & Smith, J.H. (1985). Management of injuries to the thoracic and abdominal aorta. *American Journal of Surgery*, 150, 133.

Teasdale, G.M., Murray, G., Anderson, E., Mendelow, A.D., MacMillan, R., Jennett, B., & Brookes, M. (1990). Risks of acute traumatic intracranial hematoma in children and adults: Implications for managing head injuries. *British Medical Journal*, 300, 363–367.

Tellelz, D.W., Harden, W.D., Takehaski, M., et al. (1987). Blunt cardiac injury in children. *Journal of Pediatric Surgery*, 22, 1123–1128.

Tepas, J.J., Ramenofsky, M.L., Mollitt, D.L., et al. (1988). The pediatric trauma score as a predictor of injury severity: An objective assessment. *Journal of Trauma*, 28 (4), 425–429.

Terry, T. (1990). ABC of major trauma: Trauma of the upper urinary tract. *British Medical Journal*, 301 (6750), 485–488.

Thomas, M.D. (1993). Musculoskeletal injury. In M.R. Eichelberger (Ed.). *Pediatric trauma: Prevention, acute care, rehabilitation* (pp. 533–554). St. Louis: Mosby–Year Book.

Torres, A.M., & Garcia, V.F. (1993). Hepatobiliary trauma. In M.R. Eichelberger (Ed.). *Pediatric trauma: Prevention, acute care, rehabilitation* (pp. 464–474). St. Louis: Mosby–Year Book.

Touloukian, R.J. (1990). Splenic injury. In R.J. Touloukian (Ed.). *Pediatric trauma* (2nd ed., pp. 332–348). St. Louis: Mosby–Year Book.

Vernon-Levett, P. (1991). Head injuries in children. *Critical Care Nursing Clinics of North America*, 3 (3), 411–421.

Waisman, Y., & Eichelberger, M.R. (1993). Hypovolemic shock. In M.R. Eichelberger (Ed.). *Pediatric trauma: Prevention, acute care, rehabilitation* (pp. 178–185). St. Louis: Mosby–Year Book.

Walker, M.L., Storrs, B.B., & Mayer, T.A. (1985). Head injuries. In T.A. Mayer (Ed.). *Emergency management of pediatric trauma* (pp. 272–286). Philadelphia: W.B. Saunders.

Wheatley, J., & Cass, D.T. (1989). Traumatic deaths in children: The importance of prevention. *The Medical Journal of Australia*, 150, 72–78.

Widner-Kolberg, M.R. (1991). The nurse's role in pediatric injury prevention. *Critical Care Nursing Clinics of North America*, 3 (3), 391–398.

Widner-Kolberg, M.R., & Moloney-Harmon, P.A. (1994). Pediatric trauma. In V.D. Cardona, P.D. Hurn, P.J.B. Mason, et al. (Eds.). *Trauma nursing: From resuscitation through rehabilitation* (2nd ed., pp. 693–720). Philadelphia: W.B. Saunders.

Willis, R.B., & Rorabeck, C. (1990). Treatment of compartment syndrome in children. *Orthopedic Clinics of North America*, 21, 401–412.

Wong, D., & Baker, C. (1988). Pain in children: Comparison of assessment scales. *Pediatric Nursing*, 14, 9–17.

Zuckerman, B.S., & Duby, J.C. (1983). Developmental approach to injury prevention. *Pediatric Clinics of North America*, 32, 17–29.

CHAPTER *31*

Thermal Injury

PATRICIA M. LYBARGER
WENDY ROBERTS

Fire and/or burn injuries are second only to motor vehicle accidents as the leading cause of death in children aged 1 to 4 years in the United States. They are among the leading causes of injury and death in children aged 1 to 19 years. Severe burns are considered the most catastrophic injury a person can survive, resulting in disfigurement, pain, emotional distress, and tremendous economic costs. Costs for caring for burned children are extremely high.

Burn care has progressed dramatically in the last 10 years, in large part as result of the establishment of specialized burn centers. Advances in medical knowledge, surgical techniques, and nursing care in this area have increased the probability of surviving massive burns.

Every organ system is affected by an injury to the skin that involves more than 25% total body surface area (TBSA) or more. Burns affecting more than 50% TBSA have a prolonged critical care phase that may last weeks or months.

ETIOLOGY OF PEDIATRIC BURN INJURIES

Most childhood burn deaths occur in house fires, in which children are unable to escape the heat and smoke. Many causes, including careless handling of smoking materials, unsafe cooking and heating practices, faulty wiring, and match play have been associated with these fatal fires.

Burn injuries in children tend to follow patterns related to both developmental level and the socioeconomic environment of the child. The causes of injury are varied, and most are unintentional injuries. It is important to be alert to the possibility of intentional injury, because it has been reported that between 4% and 39% of admissions to burn units are related to child abuse by burning (Showers & Garrison, 1988). A physical presentation that is incongruent with the history of injury should be clarified, with appropriate followup initiated (Tofrino, 1991).

Scalds are the leading cause of burn injury for young children. Most scald injuries are related to the handling and consumption of hot food and liquids. Food prepared in microwave ovens, as well as hot coffee and soup, are often involved. The pattern of splash and dripping is a common finding across the upper body and lap. These wounds are painful and may be very deep, depending on the nature of the scalding liquid and the time that the skin was exposed to it. Grease scalds from kitchen fryers can produce serious injury because the hot grease cools slowly and is difficult to remove.

Hot household tapwater is an important cause of lower body scald injuries, especially in the bath. Because children's skin is thinner than that of a young adult, even short exposure to water at 130°F can cause full-thickness damage. Children may unintentionally turn on the hot water faucet and be unable to get away from it. Water heaters should be set between 120 and 130°F and the bath water temperature checked before placing a child in the tub. Adult supervision and protection are key to preventing these injuries.

As children become more mobile and curious, their exposure to household burn hazards expands. Electrical burns to the oral cavity are seen in infants chewing on wires. Contact burns from hot irons, ovens, and radiators occur in all ages. Ingestion of household chemicals can lead to devastating gastrointestinal damage. Even when diluted, these chemicals can cause full-thickness injury.

Match and fire play are a problem for the schoolage population, but have been recognized in children as young as 2 years of age. Flame burns associated with clothing ignition can cause serious injury from both heat and melting fabrics. Ignition of flammable liquids is seen in children old enough to work on their bikes or mow the lawn. Flash burns involving flammable liquids and explosives add a chemical component to the burn. Cigarette smoking and other risk-taking behaviors contribute to the burn problem for adolescents.

There are seasonal and regional differences that affect the pattern of burn injury. Summer brings fireworks, outdoor cooking, and sunburn. Winter brings alternative heating sources, such as kerosene heaters and woodstoves. Traditional birthday celebrations may involve lighted candles. Cultural and socioeconomic factors, such as housing, heating, and cooking traditions, may also influence the patterns of burn injury in any community.

Inhalation injury can occur with or without associated burns. Most who die in housefires are overcome by the smoke and are unable to escape. Anyone who is burned in an enclosed space or has burned facial areas should be evaluated for inhalation injury. Inhalation injury may not always be evident initially, but carbon monoxide (CO) poisoning, thermal damage, and toxic damage all affect survival.

Children at greatest risk are those who cannot protect themselves. An infant relies totally on others for protection, whereas a preschooler can be taught to stay away from matches and to "stop-drop-and-roll." Every home should have smoke detectors and an escape plan. Children with neurologic disorders, disabilities, and developmental delays must be protected appropriately, because they are at risk for burn injuries of all types.

PATHOGENESIS

Burn severity is dependent both on the intensity of the heat and the duration of its contact with the skin. The magnitude of the physiologic response depends on the type, size, location, and depth of the burn. All body systems are potentially affected as the body adapts to compensate for the alterations in normal function.

Zones of Injury

Thermal damage to tissue is described as having three zones (Fig. 31–1). The area of superficial damage is the *zone of hyperemia*, appearing warm and red. The middle area of damage is the *zone of stasis*, where the microcirculation is damaged and changes in capillary permeability allow fluids to leak from the vascular system into the interstitial space. This leads to local edema and shock when extensive wounds are present. The deepest area is the *zone of coagulation*, wherein blood vessels are occluded by heat-damaged cells. The obstructed microcirculation prevents the humoral components of the immune response from reaching the burned tissue.

Cardiovascular Response

In large body surface area (BSA) burns, there are profound vascular changes that lead to fluid shifts in burned and nonburned tissue. There is a loss of intravascular volume into the interstitium. Local increases in vascular permeability are the result of direct heat damage that causes large fluid and protein losses through the wound itself. Mediator-induced cell damage appears to contribute to changes in cellular function in nonburned tissue, contributing to the overall edema that occurs following a large burn injury. The fluid and protein shifts are most pronounced in the first several hours, because of the combined effect of increased permeability and an imbalance in osmotic pressures. If not treated, these changes lead to burn shock, characterized by hypovolemia, hypoproteinemia, decreased oxygen tension and increased tissue pressure.

Cardiac compromise is a factor in burn injury. Initially, cardiac output falls abruptly but returns to 30% of the preburn level within 30 minutes of injury. If resuscitation is adequate, cardiac output returns to preburn levels within 36 hours (Aikawa et al., 1978). Thereafter, cardiac output increases to supernormal levels and may remain elevated for a period of time, which is typical of the hypermetabolic response to thermal injury. Both metabolic and immune factors play a role in myocardial dysfunction following burn injury, but the exact mechanism has not been identified (Rieg & Jenkins, 1991).

Metabolic Response

Immediately following thermal injury, the shock phase ensues. This phase, lasting for 24 to 48 hours, is characterized by decreases in cardiac output, oxygen consumption, and body temperature. Following the shock phase is the flow phase, wherein the metabolic rate increases and persistent tachycardia,

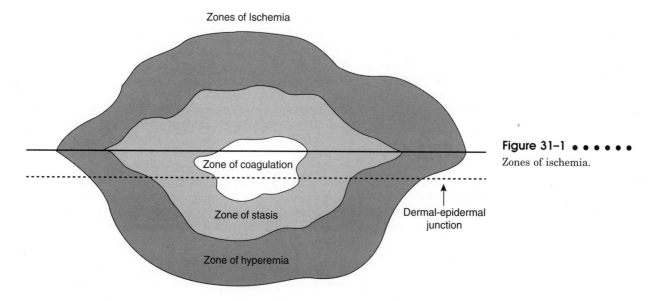

Figure 31-1 ● ● ● ● ● ●
Zones of ischemia.

tachypnea, hyperpyrexia, and body wasting are seen (Wilmore & Aulick, 1978). The metabolic rate increases in proportion to burn size in a linear relationship to a maximum of two and one-half times basal levels (Wilmore et al., 1977). Maximal levels are attained between the fifth and twelfth postburn day; however, increased metabolic output remains until wound closure occurs (Rieg & Jenkins, 1991).

Hypermetabolism mandates increased cardiac output and oxygen utilization, which produces an increase in blood flow to the visceral organs and burn wound. The visceral organs do not increase oxygen consumption; however, the burn wound requires increased blood flow to provide nutrients for wound healing to occur.

Immune Response

Infection is the leading cause of morbidity for burn patients. Persistently open wounds, increased meta-

bolic needs, decreased nutritional intake, loss of plasma protein, and suppression of the host defense mechanism all contribute to the burned patient's susceptibility to infection. There is an altered immune response following thermal injury, with defects related to both the altered host environment and the injury-triggered host deficiency state. The skin barrier is lost, providing an open portal of entry for microorganisms. Neutrophil function is diminished and opsonization is decreased, leaving the child increasingly susceptible to local and systemic infections.

CLASSIFICATION OF BURN WOUNDS

Classification of burn depth involves skilled clinical judgment. Surface appearance provides only a clue to the actual tissue damage below. Burns are rarely of uniform depth throughout. Appearance,

Table 31-1. BURN DEPTH CATEGORIES

	First Degree	Second Degree Partial Thickness	Third Degree Full Thickness
Cause	Scald, flash, flame, contact, chemical, ultraviolet light	Scald, flash, flame, contact, chemical, ultraviolet light	Scald, flash, flame, contact, chemical, electrical
Surface Appearance	Dry, no blisters	Moist blebs, blisters	Dry, leathery eschar
	Minimal or no edema	Underlying tissue mottled pink and white	Mixed white, waxy, pearly
	Erythematous	Good capillary refill	Khaki, mahogany, soot-stained
Pain and Temperature	Very painful	Very painful	Insensate
	Rapid heat loss	Rapid heat loss	Less rapid heat loss
Histologic Depth	Epidermal layers only	Epidermis, papillary and reticular layers of dermis	Down to and may include subcutaneous tissue
		May include fat domes of subcutaneous layer	May include fascia, muscle, and bone
Healing Time	2 to 5 days with NO scarring	Superficial, 5–21 days with no grafting	Large areas require grafting, which may require months
	May have some discoloration	Deep partial, 21–35 days with no infection	Small areas may heal from the edges after weeks
		If infected, converts to full thickness	

pain, and tissue pliability are used to assess wound depth. The type of burning agent and the extent of skin exposure combine to form challenging clinical presentations.

Burn depth is classified as partial thickness or full thickness (Table 31–1). Superficial partial thickness burns involve only the epidermis. Deep partial-thickness burns involve the epidermis and the dermis, but spare epidermal appendages necessary for epidermal regeneration. Full-thickness burns involve the epidermis, dermis, epidermal appendages, and sometimes subcutaneous tissues such as fat, muscle, and bone. Any burn wound can be converted to a deeper thickness if there is infection, hypoxia, or further mechanical tissue damage.

Burns are also described by measuring the size of the BSA that is burned. For children this size is determined using a Lund and Browder or Berkow chart, which takes into account the proportional body changes that occur during growth (Fig. 31–2). Deep partial- and full-thickness burns on body parts are charted as a percent of the whole. Affected areas are measured and combined to determine total body surface area (TBSA) burned. This percent BSA becomes important in calculating fluid resuscitation and nutritional needs after burns.

A number of other methods are used for determining TBSA burned in children. The Palmar method may be used in smaller or more scattered burns. This method equates the palm of the child's hand with 1%

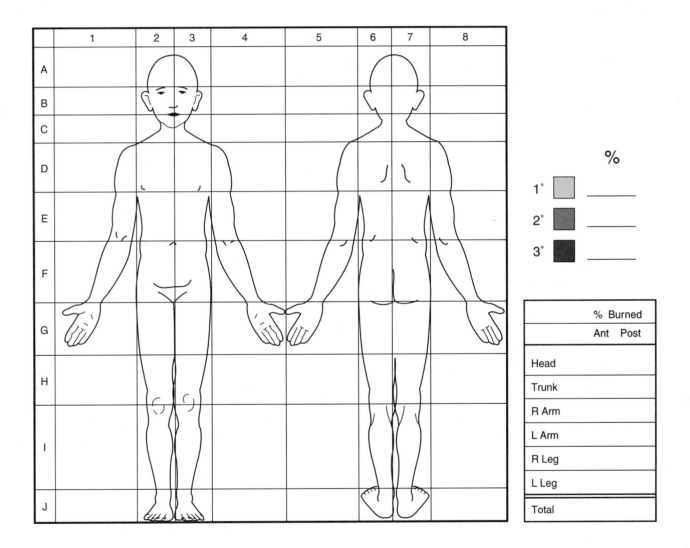

	Newborn	3 Years	6 Years	12+ Years
Head	18%	15%	12%	6%
Trunk	40%	40%	40%	38%
Arms	16%	16%	16%	18%
Legs	26%	29%	32%	38%

Figure 31–2 ● ● ● ● ● ●
Lund and Browder chart.

of the body surface area. Another method is the Baby Rule of Nines (Fig. 31–3). This method is used primarily in children younger than 3 years of age and allows for the relative difference in head size and lower extremity size in children compared with adults. The head is 18% of TBSA in children versus 9% of TBSA in adults. The lower extremity is 14% TBSA in children versus 18% of TBSA in adults. Of all the methods, the Lund and Browder chart is preferred for children because it takes into account the variation in distribution of BSA in different aged children (Rieg & Jenkins, 1991).

SPECIFIC INJURIES

Electrical Injuries

Electrical injuries are caused by the conversion of electrical energy into heat energy, which coagulates body tissues. Electrical injuries in children occur most often in the infant and adolescent age groups.

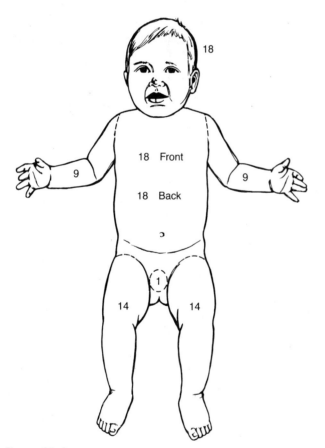

Figure 31–3 ● ● ● ● ●

The Baby Rule of Nines allows for the proportionate difference in head size related to lower extremity size in children younger than 3 years of age compared with adults. Note that the head is 18% of the TBSA in children versus 9% TBSA in adults. The lower extremity is then 14% rather than the 18% in adults. (From Kravitz, M. (1994). Thermal injuries. In V. Cardona, et al. (Eds.). *Trauma nursing: Resuscitation through rehabilitation*, p. 710. Philadelphia: W.B. Saunders.)

Infants, while exploring their environment, often put everything they find into their mouth. Saliva, which is an excellent conductor, creates a current pathway from the cord or plug to and through the child's tissues.

The adolescent usually comes in contact with electricity as an unintentional sequela of risk-taking behavior, such as climbing power poles or going into electrical substations on a dare.

When electrical current comes in contact with skin, the skin acts as an insulator to protect the internal organs from the electrical charge. The degree of protection provided depends on the voltage of the current and the degree of resistance the skin presents to current flow. Voltage refers to the intensity of current flow. It can range from house current (115–120 volts) to high voltage lines (up to 250,000 volts). Current higher than 1000 volts is referred to as *high voltage*. The resistance of the skin can be overcome by wetting, immersing in water, or actually grounding the body.

The damage created by the electrical current that enters the body is both direct and indirect. Direct effects include those that cause inappropriate depolarization of cardiac and neuromuscular cells, changes in the medial layer of blood vessels, and damage to the lens of the eye. Ventricular fibrillation more likely results from contact with alternating current than direct current. Current flow at 10 to 15 mA can produce tetanic muscle contractions that prevent the victim from letting go of the current source, thus prolonging exposure and subsequent damage.

Indirect effects refer to the soft tissue destruction that occurs from the heat produced by the passage of current through these tissues. Once the skin has been breached, the electrical current travels through the interior of the body as a single mass. Therefore, the greatest heat is generated in areas where current must pass through small cross-sectional areas. Distal extremities are excellent examples of this principle. Hands and feet are often the location of the greatest tissue destruction, because the greatest amount of heat has been generated in these tissues.

The child may not have to actually touch the current source to sustain injury. Electrical current has been known to jump or "arc" from the source to electrically conductive substances in its search for a path in which to "ground." Current also arcs from one area of the body to another (e.g., across flexed joints).

Electrical contact with the child's clothing can cause ignition with consequent surface burns from burning fabrics. If not extinguished promptly, the smoke and toxic chemicals produced by the burning clothing can produce an inhalation injury.

The physiologic impact of current upon the body is very unpredictable. Where the current enters the body, there is a small entrance wound. The current usually explodes out of the body, at one or more points, where the body is in contact with a ground. Cardiac dysrhythmias and myocardial ischemia and infarction may occur as the current passes through the body. The child may sustain traumatic injuries as a result of falls from high places following contact. Because the extent of tissue destruction is often hidden under normal-appearing skin, fluid loss into the interstitial spaces may go undetected. This can lead to inadequate restoration of the circulating blood volume during fluid resuscitation. Massive tissue edema can result in compartment syndrome with further tissue destruction. Destruction of muscle and red blood cells by the current can produce myoglobinuria and hemoglobinuria. These large molecules occlude renal tubules, resulting in renal failure. Extensive cellular destruction can also result in massive infusion of intracellular potassium into the circulation. The resulting hyperkalemia can rapidly reach lethal levels, resulting in lethal dysrhythmias. Local tissue destruction and intravascular coagulation can often be so severe that amputation of the necrotic tissue becomes essential.

Chemical Injuries

Chemical injuries result from the thermal energy produced when strong acids or alkalis come in contact with body tissue. Strong acids and alkalis are the most common causes of chemical burns in children. In infants, injury is common from household cleaning chemicals, such as lye, ammonia, sulfuric acid, and laundry detergent. Older children are injured in school laboratory accidents, or when "experimenting" at home. They may be injured by gasoline-soaked clothing or by exposures related to their first jobs or helping around the house.

Chemicals destroy skin by coagulation necrosis, which may progress over time. The severity of the injury is dependent on the chemical properties, the concentration of the chemical, and the duration of contact with skin or mucous membranes. Collagen, a primary component of the skin, is denatured by the chemical and precipitates to form eschar.

Inhalation Injury

Inhalation injury, often called smoke inhalation, is a condition associated with exposure to the heat and toxic fumes produced by fire conditions in a closed space. Complete and incomplete combustion of materials commonly found in the everyday environment produces extreme heat, toxic fumes, and a reduction in the environmental oxygen concentration, often reducing it to 16% or less (Heimbach, 1983).

The identification of a person who has sustained an inhalation injury is often difficult. Clinically, a person who is at risk has the following characteristics:

- Burned in a closed space or standing upright as their clothing burned
- Burns of the face or neck
- Singed eyebrows, nasal hairs, and hairline or facial hair

- Carbon particles in the mouth or nose or carbonaceous sputum
- Brassy cough, hoarseness, or stridor
- Significant serum carboxyhemoglobin level

These children warrant close observation and immediate intervention if respiratory distress develops. Early or prophylactic intervention, particularly in young children, is essential for survival.

The inhalation injury that is produced by fire conditions has four components. First, thermal injury occurs in the upper airways because of exposure to high environmental temperatures and superheated gases. Direct heat damage is usually limited to the upper airway, because the moist mucous membranes act as a heat exchanger, lowering the temperature of the inhaled gases before they cross the vocal cords. In fire conditions, the upper airway extracts excess heat from inhaled gases. This protects the lower airway (below the vocal cords) from thermal damage. The sole exception to this is the inhalation of steam. Steam has a heat-carrying capacity that is approximately 400 times the capacity of ambient air. This allows the steam to pass through the vocal cords with little heat loss in the upper airway, thus creating thermal burns below the vocal cords.

Exposure to hot gases produces diffuse edema throughout the upper airway, resulting in airway obstruction. The edema rapidly advances and peaks at about 6 to 12 hours after injury. Extensive scald burns of the head and neck can produce such massive edema in local tissues that the airway is compromised. Although not a true inhalation injury, this type of scald burn is treated by protecting the airway with an endotracheal tube until the edema resolves. Because of the small comparative size of children's airways, intervention in the form of endotracheal intubation is often required.

The second aspect of inhalation injury is when CO combines with the hemoglobin molecule to reduce the oxygen-carrying capacity of blood. CO is a clear, colorless, odorless gas produced by the incomplete combustion of organic materials, such as wood, paper, cotton, gasoline, and others. Incomplete combustion occurs because there is insufficient oxygen available in fire conditions. Depending on the carboxyhemoglobin levels, the child may experience anything from mild intellectual dysfunction to apnea and cardiac arrest (Table 31–2). The CO binding to hemoglobin can be reversed by the administration of 100% oxygen. It takes approximately 40 minutes to clear CO in normally breathing or mechanically ventilated patients at this concentration.

A third aspect of inhalation injury is hypoxia caused by exposure to fire conditions wherein environmental oxygen is rapidly consumed by combustion. This results in environmental oxygen concentrations that reduce the inspired oxygen concentrations, so that PaO_2 levels of 50 to 60 mmHg are commonplace. Combined with CO exposure, the reduced FiO_2 worsens the tissue hypoxia and its consequences.

As a fourth aspect of injury, the inhalation of toxic

Table 31–2. PHYSIOLOGIC EFFECTS OF CARBON MONOXIDE EXPOSURE

Carboxyhemoglobin Level (%)	Physiologic Effects
<20	Headache, dyspnea, confusion, lapse of attention, loss of peripheral vision
20–40	Irritability, faulty judgment, dim vision, nausea, vomiting, easily fatigued
40–60	Tachycardia, tachypnea, confusion, hallucinations, ataxia, syncope, convulsions, coma
>60	Often fatal

Adapted from Cohen, M.A., & Guzzardi, W. (1983). Inhalation of products of combustion. *Annals of Emergency Medicine, 12,* 628–632.

gases from the fire may produce a chemical pneumonia. The combustion of commonly found materials results in the liberation of toxic gases, which can include hydrogen sulfide, hydrogen cyanide, hydrogen chloride, acrolein, mustard gas, nerve gas, and many others. When these gases come in contact with the epithelium lining the tracheobronchial tree, they form corrosive acids that destroy the cilia and underlying tissue. Toxic materials also adhere to soot particles that are inhaled, providing an additional source of toxic exposure and debris that must be cleared. Toxins are also absorbed into the general circulation where they can have systemic effects (for example, hydrogen cyanide). This toxin produces respiratory dysfunction that is seen immediately. The initial response of the lung is bronchorrhea followed by a sloughing of necrotic tissues. The increased debris formation plus the loss of the cilia results in atelectasis. The effects may not be evident immediately; instead, the clinical symptomatology may present itself only hours to days later.

There are three time periods following injury when the damage caused by these toxic agents occurs. Immediately after the exposure to fire conditions, hypoxia associated with decreased environmental oxygen concentrations, CO poisoning, and airway edema from exposure to hot gases develops. During the 24 to 48 hours following injury, pulmonary edema is associated with the toxicity of inhaled gases and fluid resuscitation. After 48 hours, the effects of atelectasis and pneumonia become evident as a clinical picture similar to adult respiratory distress syndrome (ARDS) develops.

Inhalation injury may occur without surface burns. The presence of skin involvement further complicates the management of inhalation injury. Skin damage that involves more than 25% TBSA results in diffuse capillary leak throughout the body, including the lung. The increase in interstitial water surrounding the alveoli reduces effective gas exchange and increases the patient's volume requirements. Inhalation injury can increase the body's fluid requirement up to 37% over calculated fluid resuscitation needs. The assessment of fluid balance becomes increasingly complicated, and pulmonary edema is a common complication. The treatment of the pulmonary edema is usually reduction of the infused fluid volume in increments until the rales disappear (Demling & LaLonde, 1989).

Full-thickness, circumferential surface burns of the neck and chest wall can compromise pulmonary function even further. When inelastic eschar surrounds the chest, a corset-like effect is created. Edema continues to occur in the burn wound, compressing the tissues of the chest wall inward and compromising the vital capacity. The patient is unable to take a deep breath and cannot be provided with manual ventilation. Relief is provided by escharotomies, incisions through the eschar, that allow the chest wall to expand. This problem must usually be dealt with within the first 24 hours following injury.

Surviving the initial inhalation injury is not the end of the child's pulmonary problems. The child may develop ARDS following hypoxic or hypovolemic insult or as a component of septic shock associated with bacteremia from wound debridement, intravascular lines, urinary tract infections, or pneumonia.

The long-term sequelae of inhalation injury include bronchiolitis obliterans, cylindrical bronchiectasis, and tracheal stenosis, associated with prolonged intubation or tracheostomy. The destruction of respiratory units at a young age has a better prognosis for long-term respiratory function than do injuries that occur in schoolage or adolescent children. As the young child grows following the injury, the remaining respiratory units can increase in surface area more than would normally be expected to compensate for the units that were destroyed.

The spectrum of disease that is inhalation injury varies from very mild symptoms to acute respiratory failure. Inhalation injury is the second leading cause of death for individuals who sustain burn injuries.

Toxic Epidermal Necrolysis

Toxic epidermal necrolysis (TEN) is a rare, severe form of epidermal sloughing occurring in patients with more than 20% TBSA. In addition to epidermal sloughing, the epithelial linings of the gastrointestinal tract and respiratory tract, and the mucous membranes of the eye and oropharynx may also slough. The epidermis separates at the dermoepidermal junction. The mortality rate associated with TEN ranges from 25% to 70% (Taylor, 1989).

The syndrome is manifested by sore throat, fever, malaise, rash with a positive Nikolsky sign (sloughing of sheets of epidermis in response to light touch), and exposure to known trigger agents. These agents include sulfonamides, anticonvulsants, penicillins, and allopurinol. Milder forms of the same disease process include erythema multiforme and Stevens-Johnson syndrome. These forms are localized to less than 20% of the TBSA, with mild to no systemic manifestations.

TEN must be differentiated from staphylococcal

scalded skin syndrome (SSSS), a clinically similar syndrome that is caused by a staphylococcal skin infection usually occurring in children younger than 5 years of age. Some strains of staphylococci produce an epidermolytic toxin that causes the epidermis to cleave at the upper malpighian and granular layers. The mortality rate from SSSS is about 3% (Roujeau, 1990).

The clinical problems that TEN patients present are identical to those presented by large surface area, partial-thickness burns. Over the past 10 years, these patients have been successfully treated in burn units.

Circumferential Burns

Full-thickness circumferential burns of the torso or an extremity present a special problem for the child. Areas of full-thickness burns are nonelastic and produce a tourniquet effect that diminishes blood flow to the affected area. As mentioned earlier, circumferential burns of the chest can compromise pulmonary function.

As edema occurs in the affected area and the tissue cannot stretch, the child experiences numbness and tingling distal to the injured area, loss of motor function and sensation, and severe pain. Release of the pressure must occur and requires surgical intervention by escharotomy or fasciotomy (Fig. 31–4). An escharotomy involves an incision through the burned tissue down to the subcutaneous fat layers to restore

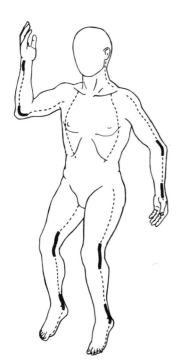

Figure 31–4 ● ● ● ● ● ●
Diagram shows preferred site of escharotomy incisions. (From Finkelstein, J.L., et al. (1992). Pediatric burns: An overview. *Pediatric Clinics of North America*, 39 (5), 1145–1163.)

blood supply. A fasciotomy is necessary when the escharotomy has not restored adequate perfusion. This procedure involves a deeper incision into the muscle compartments.

The best time to perform an escharotomy varies and is based on frequent assessment of the affected area, pulses, and respiratory effort (with torso burns). If the escharotomy is performed too early, blood loss may be a problem. If it is too late, necrosis and gangrene can develop.

CRITICAL CARE MANAGEMENT

Resuscitative Phase

As with any other trauma, the initial management priorities focus on support of the airway, breathing, and circulation. For the burned patient, the first priority is to stop the burning process, then proceed with the ABCs.

Thorough and ongoing assessment of the airway is key in the initial nursing care. Immediate intubation should be considered if there is a facial burn, upper airway edema, or an inhalation injury. It is important to ensure an adequate airway, because delay may make intubation difficult or impossible owing to massive swelling. It is important to select the largest appropriate-size endotracheal tube and place it nasally, if possible, to improve comfort and nursing management of the airway. Maintenance of a stable airway may require creativity, including the use of tracheal ties or other nonadhesive stabilization techniques, because adhesives do not stick to slippery, wet, edematous skin. Loss of the artificial airway has serious consequences, because reintubation may be impossible. Ventilatory support is provided as needed. Oxygen at 100% is continued for any child with CO poisoning until carboxyhemoglobin levels are below 15%.

Maintenance of fluid balance is an important component of the emergent phase. Establishment of intravenous access with a large-caliber catheter is essential, because fluid resuscitation is a vital part of the initial management of a major burn. Insertion of monitoring lines is considered early when site access is less obscured by edema.

Peripheral circulation is monitored in the extremities with large or circumferential burns. Escharotomies may be necessary to restore circulation to the extremity. Patients with large chest or back burns may require escharotomies to allow sufficient chest wall excursion for adequate ventilation.

A bladder catheter is inserted, so that the character and amount of urine output can be used to evaluate the patient's response to the burn and fluid resuscitation efforts. Patients are initially kept NPO. A nasogastric tube is considered for gastric decompression in patients with major injuries. Children with major burns are at risk for postinjury paralytic ileus. Thus, the nasogastric tube is critical to prevent vomiting and aspiration (Finkelstein et al., 1992).

Pertinent information about the circumstances of injury is obtained and a secondary survey for other injuries performed. Other important data include weight; known allergies; medical history; chronic medication, drug, or alcohol use; and immunization status.

Burn Shock Resuscitation

The fluid requirements for the first 24 hours vary between 2 and 4 mL/kg of body weight multiplied by the percent BSA burn. Various formulas are used for determining the volume of fluid resuscitation (Table 31–3). These calculations are only guidelines. Rate and fluid choices vary depending on the type of fluid used, patient age, size of burn, and the presence of associated injury. The rate of infusion is systematically decreased over the first 24 to 48 hours to adjust

for expected fluid shifts. Insensible losses and maintenance needs are added to these formulas to accurately meet patient requirements.

Fluid overload has serious consequences for children, resulting in pulmonary, cerebral, and local tissue edema. Tissue oxygenation is compromised because of extracellular edema. Individual patient response is monitored closely and fluid replacement optimized. Cardiac filling pressures and cardiac index can be used to titrate vasopressors, such as dopamine, during the resuscitative phase. Cardiac filling pressures are often low in the initial phase. Fluid replacement and circulatory support should be planned to adjust for anticipated fluid shifts. Changes in electrolyte balance, hematocrit level, or osmolality are treated in the context of known burn pathophysiology. Colloid solutions may be included in the resuscitation therapy, in an attempt to maintain

Table 31–3. FLUID RESUSCITATION FORMULAS

Formula	Type and Volume of Fluid		Special Monitoring Recommendations
	First 24 Hours	Second 24 Hours	
Evans	Colloid: 1 mL/kg/% burn Crystalloid: Lactated Ringer's 1 mL/kg/% burn 5% D/W: 2000 mL/m² Urine: 30–50 mL/hr (adult) Rate: ½ in first 8 hrs ¼ in next 8 hrs ¼ in last 8 hrs Calculation of volume: Use burn area up to 50% TBSA, >50% TBSA calculate at 50% TBSA	0.5 mL/kg/% burn Lactated Ringer's 0.5 mL/kg/% burn 1500–2000 mL/m² ½ of first 24 hours	Urine output Vital signs
Brooke	Colloid: 0.5 mL/kg/% burn Crystalloid: Lactated Ringer's 1.5 mL/kg/% burn 5% D/W: 2000 mL/m² Urine: 30–50 mL/hr (adult) Rate: ½ in first 8 hrs ¼ in next 8 hrs ¼ in last 8 hrs Calculations of volume: same as Evans	0.25 mL/kg/% Lactated Ringer's 0.75 mL/kg/% burn 1500–2000 mL Same ½ of first 24 hour's colloids + crystalloids	Urine output 30–50 mL/hr
Parkland	Colloid: None Crystalloid: Lactated Ringer's 4 mL/kg/% burn 5% D/W: None Urine: 50–70 mL/hr (adult) Rate: ½ in first 8 hrs ¼ in next 8 hrs ¼ in last 8 hrs Calculation of volume: Use total burn area for ALL size burns	700–2000 mL (adult) as needed to maintain urine output None Sufficient to maintain urine output Same ½ first day's lactated Ringer's	Urine output: 50–70 mL/hr (adults) 1 mL/kg/hr (children <3 years) 15–25 mL/hr (children >3 years)
Hypertonic saline	Colloid: None Crystalloid: Na⁺ 250 mEq/L Cl⁻ 150 mEq/L lactate 100 mEq/L 5% D/W: "liberal" free water by mouth Urine: 30–40 mL/hr (adult) Rate: average 30 mL/hr Calculation of volume: Titrate to urine output not burn size	None 5% D/W	Adjust formula to urine output to 30–40 mL/hr (adult), mental state, peripheral capillary filling, vital signs

fluids in the intravascular space or provide necessary plasma elements.

Evaluation of Fluid Resuscitation

The adequacy of fluid resuscitation for the burned child can be monitored by assessment of urine output, cardiovascular status, acid-base changes, mental status, and body temperature.

Hourly urine output is a critical criterion for the evaluation of fluid resuscitation. A gauge for the resolution of burn shock is the point at which the child is able to maintain adequate urine output for 2 hours while receiving fluids at the calculated maintenance rate (Kravitz, 1994). The goal for urine output is 1.0 mL/kg/hour in the child and 0.5 mL/kg/hour in the adolescent.

Heart rate is a useful assessment of the degree of shock. Following successful resuscitation, the heart rate should move toward normal limits for age. The blood pressure also returns to normal as shock is resolved. In addition to monitoring these parameters, central venous pressure monitoring is helpful during resuscitation.

A mild metabolic acidosis occurs with burn shock but usually resolves within 18 to 24 hours of injury. Children younger than 2 years of age, because of their inadequately developed buffer system, are especially prone to the development of metabolic acidosis (Helvig, 1993). Serum pH is monitored closely and bicarbonate given if the acidosis becomes severe or if circulating blood volume is restored without resolution of the acidosis.

Mental status is a critical guide to evaluate the adequacy of fluid resuscitation. A child in an obtunded state requires a thorough assessment because the burn injury itself does not directly affect mental status. If obtunded due to shock, fluid resuscitation should restore the child's normal sensorium. If this is not the case, other causes of altered level of consciousness are considered.

Pediatric burn patients are particularly affected by alteration in temperature. Patients with large burns are at risk for hypothermia until skin coverage is achieved. Exposure during procedures and dressing changes may produce rapid hypothermia. Efforts by patients to maintain temperature increase oxygen consumption and energy expenditure, and add to the stress of the burn injury.

The environment is kept draft-free and warmer than normal to allow for maintenance of normal temperature (37–37.5°C). Use of warm blankets, head covering, reflective blankets, and warming shields are nursing measures that effectively raise the body temperature. Increasing environmental humidity can decrease evaporative losses from wet dressings and exposed body surfaces. Continuous monitoring with a rectal probe may be appropriate initially. Warmed intravenous (IV) and irrigation solutions and a warming blanket may be considered if there is profound hypothermia.

Pain Management

Most extensive burn injuries have components of superficial and partial- and full-thickness injuries. Superficial and partial-thickness injuries are very painful. Full-thickness injuries initially are anesthetic, but as the wounds are debrided, the nerve endings in the deeper layers of tissue become exposed, resulting in very painful lesions. In addition, wound contraction inhibits joint mobility, so that range-of-motion exercises, activities of daily living, and dressing changes are painful and anxiety-producing.

Intravenous narcotics are indicated for the pain associated with burns. The drugs of choice are morphine sulfate and fentanyl (see Chapter 18). Anxiolytic drugs may also be needed. Medications are given in small doses and titrated to relieve distress without complicating ventilation. It is recommended that all medications be given intravenously during the critical phase because of unreliable uptake from edematous tissues.

In addition to pharmacologic management of pain, interventions such as relaxation techniques and distraction may be appropriate. These approaches also provide a means for family members to be involved in the care of the child. Every effort is made to meet the patient's need for comfort and psychological support. Consideration is given to associated injuries, past medical history, and the developmental needs of the child.

Psychological Support

During the resuscitative phase of care, patients may be awake and alert. Survival, loss of control, and adaptation to an unfamiliar environment are the focus of psychosocial support systems. The ability to communicate needs is impaired as a result of the treatment of pain, anxiety, and respiratory function.

The child and family should be informed of the procedures taking place and included in the overall plan of care. Efforts to reassure and calm the family are important components. Social services, psychiatry, chaplaincy, and other hospital resources can be involved as needed.

Wound Care

As the child's respiratory and cardiovascular status is stabilized, attention can be directed toward the management of the burn wounds. All clothing is removed and a total survey of the body performed in a clean, warm environment. It may be necessary in children with large burns to assess only a portion of the body at a time to maintain the child's temperature. This becomes increasingly important in the infant and young child because heat loss is rapid and physiologic consequences are significant. Classification of depth and determination of TBSA involvement are verified. Less obvious areas of injury, such as scalp and oropharynx, are examined for evidence of thermal injury. Regular assessment of peripheral pulses is performed on involved extremities.

Surgical escharotomies may be required during the resuscitation phase to restore effective circulation to extremities and digits. After the escharotomy has been performed, the neurologic status of the affected limb is assessed frequently because peak edema formation does not occur until 24 hours after the burn (Kravitz, 1993).

Wounds are cleansed with antibacterial soap and sterile water or normal saline. Loose tissue is mechanically debrided, and the prescribed topical agent applied. Topical agents are not applied if the child is to be transferred to a burn center. The initial dressings are wrapped loosely to allow for anticipated swelling. The head and extremities are elevated for comfort and to minimize fluid accumulation. Access to peripheral pulses is anticipated and dressings wrapped to allow periodic assessment of circulation. Wound management varies with physician preference, but current therapy generally involves total removal of all devitalized tissue as soon as feasible.

Hyperbaric Oxygen Therapy

Hyperbaric oxygen therapy (HBO) may be used for the child with CO poisoning. The child is put into a hyperbaric chamber and breathes 100% oxygen at a pressure higher than atmospheric pressure. HBO reverses the toxic effects of CO by rapidly displacing CO from the hemoglobin molecule and providing increased amounts of available oxygen (Thorp, 1993). The half-life of carboxyhemoglobin (HbCO) is 5 hours when breathing room air; the half-life decreases to 23 minutes when breathing 100% oxygen in a hyperbaric chamber at three atmospheres (Grimes & Baker, 1990).

Recommended indications for HBO are a HbCO level greater than 40%, shock, severe acidosis, electrocardiogram (ECG) changes, or focal neurologic abnormalities (Thorp, 1993). Complications of HBO include barotrauma, especially of the ears, and oxygen toxicity. Barotrauma of the ears may be prevented by performing myringotomies before the child is placed in the chamber. The use of hyberbaric oxygen therapy continues to be controversial in the management of inhalation injury.

Transfer and Referral Priorities

The American Burn Association has identified the type of injuries that require referral to a specialized burn center (Table 31–4). Initial assessment and treatment should be performed at the nearest appropriate hospital (Nebraska Burn Institute, 1990). The very young patient, or one with associated trauma, is at increased risk for complications and is considered for transfer to a specialized burn center as soon as feasible.

Table 31–4. AMERICAN BURN ASSOCIATION CRITERIA FOR PATIENT TRANSFER TO A BURN CENTER

1. Deep partial- and full-thickness burns greater than 10% BSA in patients under 10 years and over 50 years of age.
2. Deep partial- and full-thickness burns greater than 20% BSA in all other age groups.
3. Deep partial- and full-thickness burns with serious threat of functional or cosmetic impairment that involve face, hands, feet, genitalia, perineum, and major joints.
4. Full-thickness burns greater than 5% BSA in any age group.
5. Electrical burns, including lightning injury.
6. Chemical burns with serious threat of functional or cosmetic impairment.
7. Inhalation injury.
8. Pediatric burn patients of any kind, when the local hospital does not have appropriate pediatric care capabilities.
9. Burn injury in patients with preexisting medical disorders that could complicate management.
10. Burn patient with concomitant trauma.

Acute Phase

Wound Care and Coverage

After stabilization has been achieved in the resuscitative phase, attention is directed toward closing the burn wound. The first step in this process is the assessment of wound depth and the surface area involved. The depth and extent are variable, depending on the intensity of the source and the duration of contact with the source of injury. Over the first 3 to 5 days following injury, the wounds continue to evolve. The ultimate depth of the injury, especially in scald and chemical injuries, may not be evident until this evolution is complete.

The goals of wound care become the preservation of as much viable tissue as possible, removal of all necrotic tissue, control of the growth of microorganisms on the wound, and creation of an environment that is conducive to wound healing. Where extensive full-thickness skin loss has occurred, the deficit must be replaced by some form of autograft or permanent skin substitute. These goals are achieved in a myriad of ways, but the ultimate outcome is the same—wound closure with intact, durable skin.

The first step in the preservation of viable tissue is the recognition of that which is viable. Viable tissue is pink, moist, warm, and sensate (depending on the depth of the wound). Viability is a reflection of the degree of perfusion of the tissue, the availability of adequate substrates for tissue repair, and the degree of exposure to such noxious agents as bacteria and fungus, some topical agents, and cleansing solutions. Debriding dressings, mechanical trauma, shearing forces caused by movement, and desiccation (drying) of the wound bed also contribute to loss of viable tissue. Episodes of hypotension, hypoxia, and poor perfusion of the wound bed can reduce tissue viability.

The activities of the burn care team are directed toward the preservation of viable tissue. Specifically, the focus of care is to maintain adequate tissue perfusion, provide adequate nutritional resources, prevent desiccation, reduce shear and mechanical trauma, critically evaluate dressing materials that are being used on a particular wound, keep the wound free of debris and necrotic tissue, reduce the exposure of the wound to toxic topical agents and cleansing solutions, and provide permanent wound closure as soon as possible.

It is not possible to control all of the variables that influence tissue viability, but care should be taken to reduce known risks to tissue survival while considering the requirements of the whole child. When it is not possible to tell whether a specific tissue is viable, it is often best to allow the body to demarcate the line between viable and nonviable. This dilemma often occurs when the viability of fingers or toes is in question.

Debridement of necrotic tissue is the second component in wound care. It can be achieved in a number of ways including dressings, blunt and sharp debridement, with hydrotherapy or showers, and primary excision under anesthesia. Regardless of the methods selected by the burn team for the individual patient, it is essential that adequate pain and anxiety relief be provided. Intravenous or oral narcotics and anxiolytic agents must be provided in adequate doses during these procedures. Assessment of the child's pain and anxiety is performed throughout the procedure and additional medication administered, as needed (Tompkins, 1988).

Many dressing materials are on the market, with new ones being introduced frequently. It is imperative that the specific properties and recommended uses for a product be understood by caregivers. Inappropriate use of a product can actually be detrimental to the wound.

If debridement of the wound is the goal, one of the least expensive and most commonly available materials is wide mesh gauze (WMG). WMG is laid in a single layer over the wound. It may be impregnated with a cream topical agent before application or soaked with a liquid topical agent after a bulky outer dressing has been applied.

An environment that is conducive to wound healing is one that is warm and moist and has sufficient substrates for cell maturation and division (David, 1986). Unfortunately, this is also the environment that is conducive to the growth of microorganisms. These organisms compete with the body's cells for available substrate and produce toxins that inhibit the repair of the damaged tissue. The wound, therefore, is kept warm, moist, and as clean as possible, if wound healing is to be facilitated (David, 1986).

A number of biologic dressings are available. These materials include human cadaver allografts, porcine xenografts, and several biosynthetic materials (manmade materials impregnated with collagen).

It is necessary that biologic dressings be applied to clean wound beds, because they decrease evaporative water loss from the wound and create a warm moist environment. Biologic dressings placed over contaminated wounds facilitate the growth of microorgan-

isms and result in deepening the wound. At the first sign of purulent drainage, increasing local inflammation, or systemic signs of sepsis, the biologic dressing that is not adherent to the wound bed is removed and the wound inspected and cultured.

The ideal coverage of the debrided full-thickness burn wound is skin grafts from the child's own body. Autologous skin grafts, the patient's own skin, remains the only permanent, durable closure for the burn wound.

Autografts may be harvested from unburned areas of the body. Split-thickness autografts include both epidermal and dermal elements and vary in thickness from 0.015 cm to 0.04 cm. Epidermal appendages are spared so that the donor site will heal in 10 to 14 days. The donor site is then available for reharvesting.

Full-thickness grafts include epidermis, dermis, and sometimes fat and muscle tissue. Because no epidermal appendages remain, the donor site must be either primarily closed or grafted with a split-thickness skin graft. Full-thickness grafts in large surface area burns are a very limited resource. They are therefore reserved for hand and facial reconstructions and for coverage of open joints.

Several artificial skin replacement products are in the research and development phases or newly available on the market. These products, in whole or part, remain integrated with the patient's body or are gradually replaced by the body's own tissue (Gordon, 1988).

The artificial skin Integra, developed by Burke and Yannis, provides a replacement dermis with a temporary "epidermal" membrane. The artificial skin consists of a collagen mat with a Silastic membrane (temporary epidermis) on one side. The full-thickness burn wound is excised and the artificial skin sutured in place with the collagen side down. Over a period of about 3 weeks the collagen mat becomes vascularized. The Silastic membrane, which until this time has reduced evaporative water losses from the wound, is removed. A very thin split-thickness skin graft is then applied to the vascularized collagen mat. The neodermis (vascularized collagen mat) and split-thickness graft form a durable skin replacement with a cosmetically acceptable appearance.

Epithelial cell cultures (e.g., BioSurface Technology) are other commercially available products that can be used as part of the coverage plan for the extensively burned child. A postage stamp–sized skin biopsy of normal skin is obtained and sent to specific tissue culture laboratories. In the laboratory, the epidermis is mechanically separated from the dermis. Enzymes are then added to the epidermal tissue to produce a single-cell suspension. The single-cell suspension is then inoculated into special tissue culture media. In about 10 days, the epidermal cells have grown into confluent sheets. These sheets are treated with Dispase, an enzyme, to release them from their attachments to the plastic flasks. At this time they can be transferred to the patient's tissue; however, in most instances, the surface that they would cover would be insufficient to meet the patient's needs. These primary cultures are then treated with enzymes to produce a single-cell suspension that is again inoculated into tissue culture media and incubated for another 10 days. The cultured epithelial sheets are then Dispase-released from the flasks, clipped to Vaseline gauze carriers with surgical clips, and transported to the operating room for application to the patient.

This process requires approximately 21 days. At this time, the equivalent of 2 square meters of epithelial cell cultures become available to the patient. During this waiting period, it is necessary to excise the wounds and cover them with some form of biologic dressing.

The epithelial cell cultures are applied to the excised wound beds and are secured in place with either sutures or surgical staples. Care must be taken to handle the cultures as little as possible, because even minor mechanical trauma results in the death of the epithelial cells involved. Postoperatively, the wounds are dressed with dry dressings and the areas immobilized. In approximately 7 days, the Vaseline gauze backings are gently removed. Thin glistening sheets of epithelial cells can be seen as the backings are very gently removed from the tissue. The coverage remains very fragile for several weeks, requiring nonadherent dressings and great care in handling.

The durability of epithelial cell cultures is never the same as normal skin but rather is like that of thin split-thickness grafts. They can, however, provide lifesaving coverage for the child with extensive full-thickness burns. Whatever the method of wound coverage selected by the burn team, coverage must be pursued aggressively if the child is to survive and avoid systemic sepsis and shock.

Regardless of the type of wound covering, it is critical that the child's wound be assessed at least daily for signs of deterioration. Signs of wound infection must be identified early before systemic infection develops. Clinical manifestations include discoloration of eschar (dark red, brown, or black), conversion of a split-thickness injury to a full-thickness one, rapid acceleration of the eschar, reddened necrotic lesions in unburned skin, discoloration of unburned skin at the wound edge, and accelerated circular subcutaneous edema with central necrosis (Finkelstein et al., 1992). Once a burn wound is identified, surgical excision of the burn eschar is necessary. Antibiotics are administered systemically to treat proven bacteremias, not wound infections.

Infection Control

The goals for the burned child related to infection control include the following:

- Prevent the transmission of microorganisms from the child to the environment and other patients.
- Prevent the transmission of microorganisms from the environment and other patients to the child.

- Control or eradicate microorganisms that are not part of the child's normal flora.

Creating physical barriers between the burned child and the environment helps to prevent the transmission of microorganisms from the child to the environment and other patients, and from the environment and other patients to the child (Lee, 1990). These barriers can be created in a number of ways, depending on the architecture and resources of the individual unit. The child can be cared for in a single room or in a laminar flow unit on an open ward. Barriers can include plastic aprons, gauntlets, gloves, hats and masks or isolation gowns, gloves, hats and masks. Universal precautions require the addition of goggles or face shields if there is a reasonable risk of splash and splatter of body fluids or tissues.

Topical agents are applied to the wounds to control the growth of microorganisms on the wound until permanent coverage is achieved. The appropriateness of a specific agent for a specific wound is dependent on the characteristics of the topical agent, the wound, and the clinical experience or preference of the burn team. Table 31–5 lists the properties of the various agents and their limitations.

Respiratory Care

The increased tissue oxygen requirements and the load of carbon dioxide (CO_2) from the hypermetabolic state following burn injury place heavy demands on the respiratory system. The work of breathing is increased following injury. It is important to recognize the early signs of deterioration before a hypoxic emergency occurs, because any impairment of tissue oxygenation has multisystem consequences. After recovering from the initial inhalation injury, children remain at risk for the development of ARDS.

Nutritional Management

The burned child has increased nutritional requirements related to the hypermetabolic state and the energy needed to heal wounds. Calculated nutritional needs are based on basal metabolic rate, physical activity, and stress-induced energy needs (Table 31–6). Caloric requirements are estimated based on the body surface area involved in a burn injury, as well as the child's daily requirements based on growth needs. A nutritional consult is planned on admission to determine caloric, carbohydrate, and protein goals. A systematic plan is established to meet these goals. Formulas vary for determining the exact nutritional needs, and some may calculate as much as twice the normal caloric and protein requirements. Adequacy of nutritional support can be evaluated from calorie counts, laboratory values, metabolic cart measurements, weekly weights, and the status of wound healing.

Although patients are often kept NPO with a nasogastric tube initially, enteral feeding is begun as

Table 31–5. TOPICAL AGENTS

Topical Agent	Effectiveness	Side Effects	Ease of Use	Available	Pain	Cost
Silver sulfadiazene Silvadene Flamazene 1% in water-miscible cream base	Broad-spectrum Deeper penetration than AgNO₃	Dose-related neutropenia Sulfa allergies *Do not use* in pts. with TEN Development of pseudoeschar	Semi-closed dressings Changed BID–QID Residue *must* be washed off with each dressing change	Yes	Cooling	$15.64 (400 g) Retail $25.00 (400 g)
Silver nitrate solution 0.5% in water	Broad-spectrum Only penetrates 2–4 mm into burn wound	Hypoallergenic Leaches electrolytes from wound, especially sodium and potassium Can precipitate methemaglobinemia	Bulky (½″ thick), wet dressings Changed BID–QID Must be soaked q2h to maintain wetness Stains the skin and environment black Surrounding normal skin must be protected from staining with petrolatum-based gauze	Yes	Stings briefly on application or soaking	$ 6.00 (Liter)
Mafenide acetate Sulfamylon 10% in water-miscible cream base	Broad-spectrum including *pseudomonas* Rapid and deep wound penetration	Inhibits spontaneous epithelial regeneration Carbonic anhydrase inhibitor causing metabolic acidosis due to HCO₃ wasting Sensitivity rash	Semi-closed dressings Changed BID–QID Residue *must* be washed off with each dressing change	Yes	Burning feeling for 15–20 minutes	$49.39 (400 g) Retail $64.50 (400 g)
Povidone iodine Betadine 1%	Broad-spectrum, including some fungi	Iodine absorption through wound increasing serum iodine levels Iodine allergies	Semi-closed or wet dressings Changed BID–QID Line care Foley care	Yes	Stinging pain	$17.46 (gal.) Retail $25.00 (gal.)
Hypochlorite Dakin's Eusol	Broad-spectrum Safe for use as a wet dressing over tendons and open joints (used rarely in U.S.)	Can macerate normal tissue Unstable-use fresh Keep in a dark place Drying to tissue	Wet–wet dressings Wet–dry dressings (debriding) Changed BID-QID Soak q2h	Yes	Stings	<$1.00 (gal.)
Normal saline 0.45% or 0.9%	No antimicrobial properties Keeps wound moist	Can macerate tissue	Wet–wet dressings Wet–dry dressings (debriding) Changed BID–QID Soak q2h	Yes	Stings	¢

Data from Gilman, A. G., et al. (1990). *Goodman & Gilman's the pharmacological basis of therapeutics* (8th ed.). New York: Pergamon Press.

Table 31–6. NUTRITIONAL SUPPORT FOR PEDIATRIC BURNS*

Age (yr)	Ideal Body Weight IBW Kilograms	Surface BSA m²	Energy kcal/day	Protein g/day	Ratio** kcal/gN
0.25–1.5	5–10	0.27–0.47	100 × kg	3 × kg	200
1.5–3	11–15	0.48–0.65	90 × kg	3 × kg	185
3–6	15–20	0.65–0.80	80 × kg	3 × kg	165
6–10	21–30	0.80–1.00	70 × kg	2.5 × kg	175
10–12	31–40	1.0–1.3	1000 +(40 × kg)	2.5 × kg	170
12–14	41–50	1.3–1.5	1000 +(35 × kg)	2.5 × kg	140
15–18	50–70	1.5–1.7	45 × kg	2.5 × kg	110
adults	50–75	1.5–2.0	40 × kg	2.5 × kg	100

*Approximations of goals for energy and protein (amino acids) for infants, children, adolescents, and adults during acute recovery from moderate to severe burns.

**Subtract 25 to obtain *nonprotein kcal:N ratio*, if desired.

Note: the *individual* calorie goal is more precisely calculated by the Nutritional Support staff from the IBW (or BSA).

From Cunningham, J. (1995). Nutritional support for pediatric burns. In Payne-James et al. (Eds.). *Artificial nutritional support*, (p. 461). London: Edward Arnold.

soon as practical. Oral nutrition is the preferred method of feeding. However, oral intake is often insufficient because of anorexia and an inability to voluntarily take in all the calories required. Supplemental enteral feedings via flexible feeding tubes are helpful in achieving calorie and protein goals. In some cases holding the feedings before meals, or increasing the night time feedings can encourage oral intake, even when supplemental tube feedings are used. Some burn centers continue enteral feedings during surgical procedures to make it possible to achieve nutritional goals (Trofino, 1991).

Intravenous hyperalimentation may be required in patients with prolonged paralytic ileus, an inability to meet caloric needs by other routes, or other gastrointestinal abnormalities making the enteral route impractical. Consideration must be given to providing necessary proteins, vitamins, trace elements, and lipids necessary for wound healing and growth (Young, 1988).

Comfort Management

Comfort management is an important issue in the acute phase as it was in the resuscitative phase. Comfort management for the acutely ill child with a large surface area burn is complicated by many factors. The hypermetabolic state of the patient accelerates their utilization of narcotic and anxiolytic medications (Osgood & Szyfelbein, 1989). It is often difficult to assess the severity of the child's pain and fear because of the child's growth and developmental level, level of consciousness, and ability to communicate. All of these factors influence the nurse's ability to assess the level of discomfort and the child's responses to interventions. Pain assessment tools are useful in helping the alert child to express his pain (Osgood & Szyfelbein, 1989).

Often the child is too ill to express discomfort and the only parameters the nurse has to rely on are physiologic. This is particularly true if the child has been chemically paralyzed to facilitate mechanical ventilation. Such children should always be provided with liberal amounts of analgesics and anxiolytic drugs.

Intravenous narcotics, particularly morphine sulfate and fentanyl, have become the standards for pain management. Continuous pain requires continuous infusions of IV narcotics. For very painful procedures, such as dressing changes, bolus doses of narcotics and anxiolytic drugs are used before and during the procedure. For the alert schoolage child and adolescent, patient-controlled analgesia has been effective (Atchison, 1991).

Psychological pain management strategies, such as distraction, guided imagery, hypnosis, music, and providing the child with opportunities to exercise control can be effective in the acute phase as well as in the resuscitative phase. They are very successful adjuncts to the pharmacologic management of pain and anxiety (Osgood & Szyfelbein, 1989). Their application for a specific child is dependent on the child's growth and developmental level, level of consciousness, and willingness to participate in these strategies, as well as the skill of the nurse. Further information regarding pain management strategies in the critically ill child is found in Chapter 18.

Mobility

Patients with burns are often immobilized for periods of time, placing them at risk for associated complications. Movement is restricted initially by pain, bulky dressings, and splints. Bedrest and sedation also place the burned child at risk for the hazards of immobility. Later, scar contractures, discomfort of healed wounds, and loss of stamina affect the ability to move about comfortably. To maintain optimal physical functioning, the patient's mobility should be considered from admission. Active and passive range of motion (ROM) exercises are done with every dressing change and throughout rehabilitation and recreational therapy activities. Nursing care involves routine position changes for the patient on bedrest, comfort and protection from nerve damage, and maintenance of joints in extended functional positions.

Physical and occupational therapy consultation and participation in their own daily care can maximize burned children's functioning through the hospital stay and beyond. Involvement in exercise and self-care activities has important short- and long-term benefits for the child. Patients benefit from being out of bed as soon as feasible. Pressure wraps or garments need to be applied to grafted legs to help compensate for vascular instability in the newly grafted skin when the child is out of bed or ambulating. Many problems of wound contracture, hypertrophic scarring, and impaired mobility can be limited when these issues are addressed early.

Psychosocial Issues

Emotional support for the family and patient are critical throughout this prolonged critical illness. Nurses are instrumental in providing this support and in coordinating support from others. The early involvement of social service and mental health professionals is essential in supporting the child and family. Maintaining contact with the child's peers, school teachers, and other members of the community ultimately eases the child's return to a normal life (Bernstein, 1976).

As the child begins to recover and passes through critical illness toward rehabilitation, the concerns of the child and family shift toward the child's ability to physically function and the child's ultimate appearance. Children with facial and hand scars have the most difficult time dealing with their changed appearance. The child's body image changes with growth and development, producing new challenges to coping through the different developmental stages. Parents and siblings share these struggles.

For the child who is unable to survive the injury,

support for the family becomes the focus of resources. The team's goals are to help them grieve for their lost child and begin to rebuild their lives as they heal their own emotional scars (Arnold & Gemma, 1983).

Nursing staff and other caregivers need to support themselves and each other through this emotionally draining experience. Support groups, workshops, and individual discussions help professionals to support the family and care for themselves. Open discussions surrounding the ethical issues that often surround the care of these children are an invaluable resource to the staff who participate.

SUMMARY

The child who sustains a major burn injury faces and overcomes multisystem assault with the help of a multidisciplinary team. A vast array of professionals participate in the effort to restore the child's physiologic and emotional integrity. An integral part of this team is the child's parents, who must help the child with integration into the community and development into a productive member of society. Today, physical survival from devastating burn injury can almost be assured. The challenge for professionals in the future is to ensure that survival is meaningful for the child, family, and the community.

References

Aikawa, N., Martyn, J.A.J., & Burke, J.F. (1978). Pulmonary artery catheterization and thermodilution cardiac output determination in the management of critically burned patients. *American Journal of Surgery*, 135, 811–817.

Arnold, J.H., & Gemma, P.B. (1983). *A child dies: A portrait of family grief*. Rockville, MD: Aspen Publications.

Atchison, N.E., et al. (1991). Pain during burn dressing change in children: Relationship to burn area, depth and analgesic regimens. *Pain*, 47, 41–45.

Bernstein, N.R. (1976). *Emotional care of the facially burned and disfigured*. Boston: Little, Brown.

David, J.A. (1986). *Wound management: A comprehensive guide to dressing and healing*. Springhouse, PA: Springhouse Corporation.

Demling, R.H., & LaLonde, C. (1989). *Burn trauma*. New York: Thieme Medical Publishers.

Finkelstein, J.L., Schwartz, S.B., Madden, M.R., Marano, M.A., & Goodwin, C.W. (1992). Pediatric burns: An overview. *Pediatric Clinics of North America*, 39(5), 1145–1163.

Goodman-Gilman, A. (1990). *The pharmacological basis of therapeutics*. New York: Pergamon Press.

Gordon, M.D. (1988). Synthetic and biosynthetic skin substitutes. *Journal of Burn Care and Rehabilitation*, 9(2), 209–217.

Grimes, B., & Baker, T. (1990). Smoke inhalation. In R.H. Welton & K.A. Shane (Eds.). *Case studies in trauma nursing* (pp. 63–67). Baltimore: Williams & Wilkins.

Heimbach, D. (1983). *Smoke inhalation: Current concepts in current topics in burn care*. Rockville, MD: Aspen Publishers.

Helvig, E. (1993). Pediatric burn injuries. *AACN Clinical Issues in Critical Care Nursing*, 4(2), 433–442.

Kravitz, M. (1994). Thermal injuries. In V. Cardona, P. Hurn, P. Bastnagel-Mason, A. Scanlon-Schilpp, & S. Veise-Berry (Eds.). *Trauma nursing: From resuscitation through rehabilitation* (Ed. 2). Philadelphia: W.B. Saunders.

Lee, J.J., et al. (1990). Infection control in a burn center. *Journal of Burn Care and Rehabilitation*, 11(8), 575–580.

Nebraska Burn Institute. (1990). *Advanced burn life support course manual*. Nebraska Burn Institute, Lincoln, NE.

Osgood, P.F., & Szyfelbein, S.K. (1989). Management of burn pain in children. *Pediatric Clinics of North America*, 36(4), 1001–1013.

Rieg, L.S., & Jenkins, M. (1991). Burn injuries in children. *Critical Care Nursing Clinics of North America*, 3(3), 457–470.

Roujeau, J.C., et al. (1990). Toxic epidermal necrolysis (Lyell Syndrome). *Archives of Dermatology*, 126(1), 37–47.

Showers, J., & Garrison, K.M. (1988). Burn abuse: A four-year study. *Journal of Trauma*, 28, 1581–1583.

Taylor, J.A., et al. (1989). Toxic epidermal necrolysis: A comprehensive approach. *Clinical Pediatrics*, 28(9), 404–407.

Thorp, J.W. (1993). Hyperbaric oxygen therapy. In P.R. Holbrook (Ed.). *Textbook of pediatric critical care* (pp. 493–500). Philadelphia: W.B. Saunders.

Tofrino, R.B. (1991). *Nursing care of the burn injured patient*. Philadelphia: F.A. Davis.

Tompkins, R.G., et al. (1988). Significant reductions in mortality for children with burn injuries through the use of prompt eschar excision. *Annals of Surgery*, 208(5), 577–585.

Wilmore, D.W., & Aulick, L.H. (1978). Metabolic changes in the burned patient. *Surgical Clinics of North America*, 58, 1173–1187.

Wilmore, D.W., Aulick, L.H., Mason, A.D., & Pruitt, B.A. (1977). Influence of the burn wound on local and systemic responses to injury. *Annals of Surgery*, 186, 44–458.

Young, M.E. (1988). Malnutrition and wound healing. *Heart and Lung*, 17(1), 60–67.

CHAPTER 32

Toxic Ingestions

CATHLEEN B. LONGO
CHRISTINE M. DICKENSON

INTRODUCTION

Accidental poisoning continues to occur in the pediatric population despite the efforts and publicity of regional poison control centers. Methods of exposure to toxic agents vary but occur by a number of different routes. Exposures occur in order of frequency, by ingestion, dermal, inhalation, ocular, bites and stings, parenteral, and aspiration routes.

Developmental characteristics typical of the toddler period increase the likelihood of ingestions in this age group. These children are newly mobile, curious, and anxious to explore their environment through reaching, climbing, and tasting. Other factors that put children at risk are a family illness, pregnancy, recent move, an unemployed or single parent household, accessibility to toxic agents, and lack of proper supervision. These risk factors combined explain why 5% of all accidental childhood deaths are related to poisoning.

Most adolescent ingestions that occur in the home are suicide attempts and involve the use of household products. They are commonly associated with academic difficulty, the termination of a romance, family difficulties, or the death of a loved one.

Incidence of Poisoning

According to data from the 1994 Annual Report of the American Association of Poison Control Centers, 1,926,438 human exposures to toxins were reported that year. Children under the age of 6 were involved in 54% of all cases, while 40% of all cases occurred in children 0 to 3 years of age. Most of the 766 fatalities were caused by the ingestion and inhalation routes. Children younger than 6 accounted for 3.4% (26) of the fatalities. Males predominated in the ingestions under age 13, while teenage cases involved more females (Litovitz et al., 1995). The difference in percentage of deaths between young children and adolescents may occur because most ingestions under the age of 6 involve one agent, happen by accident, and are discovered shortly after they occur. Adolescent ingestions, however, frequently involve multiple substances, occur as suicidal attempts, and have a delay between the time the ingestion occurs and when medical attention is sought. One study indicated that acute poisoning accounted for 1% of all hospitalizations and 4.5% of all pediatric intensive care unit admissions (Fazen et al., 1986).

Ingestion Frequency Versus Severity

The substances involved most frequently in human exposure do not produce toxic effects. Some of the more common agents involved are cleaning fluids, analgesics, cosmetics, plants, cough and cold preparations, and bites and stings. Toxic effects do not often occur with these substances, predominantly because most children usually do not ingest amounts sufficient to produce harm.

Other agents ingested less frequently but that do not require large exposures to produce toxic effects are alcohols, tricyclic antidepressants, theophylline, barbiturates, cocaine, iron, clonidine, and caustics. Acetaminophen is considered toxic when consumed in amounts greater than 140 mg/kg. The ingestion of these substances causes the greatest percentage of hospitalizations, ICU admissions, and fatalities in pediatric poisonings. Table 32–1 compares the most common with the most toxic substances ingested.

Table 32–1. MOST COMMON VERSUS MOST TOXIC AGENTS INGESTED*

Most Common	Most Toxic
Cleaning substances	Analgesics
Analgesics	Antidepressants
Cosmetics	Sedatives/hypnotics
Plants	Stimulants/street drugs
Cough/cold preparations	Cardiovascular drugs
Bites/envenomations	Alcohols
Pesticides	Gases and fumes
Topicals	Asthma therapies
Foreign bodies	Automotive products
Food products	Chemicals
Hydrocarbons	Hydrocarbons
Antimicrobials	Antihistamines
Sedatives/hypnotics	Cleaning substances
Alcohols	
Antidepressants	
Chemicals	
Vitamins	

*Listed in order of frequency of ingestion.

From Litovitz, T.L., Felberg, L., Soloway, R.A., Ford, M., & Geller, R. (1995). 1994 Annual Report of the American Association of Poison Control Centers National Data Collection System. *American Journal of Emergency Medicine,* 13 (5), 551–597.

Poison Prevention

The concept of regional poison control centers evolved because of the need for a central source of information on ingredients, toxicology, symptoms, and treatment of ingestions. Poison control centers have streamlined the most efficient methods of accessing current diagnostic and therapeutic modalities for the management of poisonings. At the present time, 65 centers serve a population of 215.9 million of the estimated 260.3 million in the United States (Litovitz et al., 1995). Other significant contributions made by the centers include education, prevention, legislation, and research. The Poison Prevention Packaging Act of 1970, issued by the Consumer Product Safety Commission, was designed to make access to hazardous substances more difficult for children under the age of 5 years. Over a 5-year period in which poison prevention packaging was mandated, emergency department visits for treatment of accidental ingestion of prescribed drugs or household substances were reduced 45%. Child-resistant containers have reduced accidental ingestion of children's aspirin by 45% to 55% and regular aspirin by 40% to 45% (Gill, 1989). Death related to poisoning has declined over the last two decades as well, reflecting the positive results of the legislative and preventive efforts of poison control centers.

EMERGENCY MANAGEMENT

Initial evaluation of the patient in whom a toxic ingestion is suspected includes establishing stable cardiorespiratory status evidenced by a patent airway, effective ventilatory pattern, and adequate perfusion (Table 32–2). Primary measures to stabilize the patient's condition are based on the priorities of resuscitation (i.e., the ABCs) in the event of respiratory or hemodynamic compromise. Regardless of the substance ingested by a child or adolescent, serum, gastric, and urine toxicology screens are necessary to rule out the possibility of multiple ingestants. Further management in the emergency department is guided by the principles of (1) identifying the poison; (2) decreasing its absorption; and (3) increasing its elimination.

Identification of the Ingestant

History-taking is the first vital step in the identification of the ingestant when a child presents with a suspected toxic exposure. Obtaining information about the time the ingestion occurred, the substance and amount involved, who was present, and what interventions were employed are all necessary for a thorough evaluation.

Decreasing Absorption

Reducing the life-threatening potential of an ingested substance depends on the effectiveness of sev-

Table 32–2. MANAGEMENT OF THE PATIENT WITH A SUSPECTED TOXIC INGESTION

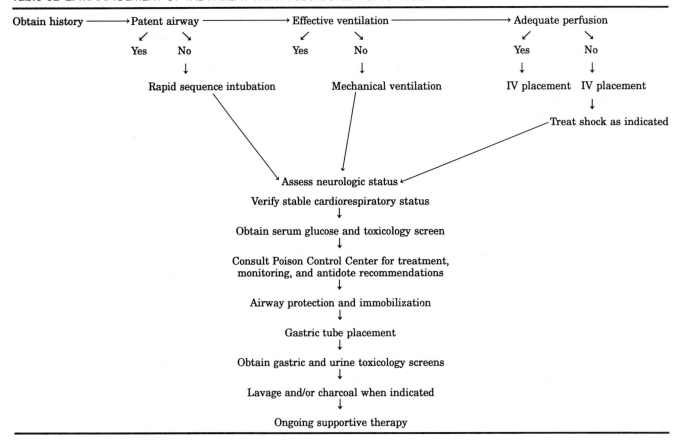

eral different treatment modalities. Gastric emesis and gastric lavage are used to limit toxic absorption.

Gastric Emesis

Ipecac, when recommended, is the agent of choice for forced emesis. Ipecac is very useful in the home for accidental ingestions discovered immediately after they occur, but it is no longer favored in the clinical setting because it causes significant delay in the administration of activated charcoal due to prolonged vomiting. Ipecac acts as both a local gastric irritant and a central stimulant, triggering the chemoreceptors in the fourth ventricle to activate the vomiting center in the reticular formation. The result is coordinated muscular activity of the stomach and small intestine and emesis. Dosages of 10 mL for infants older than 6 months, 15 mL for children 1 to 5 years, and 30 mL for children over 5 years usually produce emesis in 20 minutes.

Ipecac is contraindicated with the ingestion of strong acids, alkali, or hydrocarbons; in infants younger than 6 months of age; and in the presence of neurologic impairment. Other contraindications are loss of the gag reflex and ingestion of agents likely to cause a rapid onset of central nervous system (CNS) depression or seizures (i.e., clonidine, tricyclic antidepressants, lindave, and camphor). When indicated, forced emesis with ipecac is considered more likely to be effective than gastric lavage at removing gastric contents. The use of ipecac in cases when the substance is readily absorbed (e.g., alcohols) and was ingested more than an hour before ipecac administration remains controversial.

Gastric Lavage

Gastric lavage evacuates the stomach and augments decontamination in the presence of residual toxin. The substance is flushed through a large-bore naso- or orogastric tube (28 to 38 French) with room temperature normal saline until the yield is clear. This method has limited utility in the clinical setting when the ingestion has occurred more than 30 minutes before its institution. In addition, the large tube size required for effective lavage may not be possible in pediatric patients. Pill fragments can rarely be removed with pediatric-sized gastric tubes. The largest bore tube, known as an Ewald, can only be placed in the adolescent patient. Consequently, the utility of gastric lavage in the management of pediatric patients who have ingested pill fragments is controversial. Tracheal intubation must precede lavage in patients in whom the gag reflex is diminished and ability to protect the airway is compromised to avoid the hazards of vomiting and subsequent aspiration.

Increasing Elimination

Promotion of Excretion

Activated charcoal reduces absorption and enhances excretion of a toxin by binding with it in the gastrointestinal tract. It is best administered by nasal or orogastric tube to patients such as small children who may refuse to drink it because of its poor palatability and gritty texture. A dose of 1 g/kg (to a maximum of 50 g) is administered. To prevent tube obstruction and ensure complete administration, the consistency of charcoal is made less viscous by mixing it with water.

Ideally, charcoal is administered within 2 hours of the ingestion, after emesis has subsided and lavage is complete. Repeated doses of activated charcoal (0.5 g/kg every 4 hours) enhance elimination by interrupting hepatic recirculation, adsorbing the drug secreted across the gastric membrane into the bowel lumen, and continued adsorption throughout the gastrointestinal tract.

The first dose of activated charcoal is most effective in children when combined with a cathartic such as sorbitol. Once bound to the charcoal, sorbitol propels the toxin rapidly through the intestinal tract, decreasing intestinal transit time. Subsequent doses of activated charcoal are administered without sorbitol to avoid severe diarrhea and subsequent electrolyte abnormalities that may result in additional problems such as hypernatremia and seizures.

The patient's ability to tolerate charcoal varies. Charcoal administration is usually followed by periods of vomiting, especially when its administration has been preceded by a dose of ipecac. It is difficult to detect that nausea has subsided in young children who are unable to completely describe physical symptoms. This further complicates the decision about when charcoal therapy should begin. No effective treatment exists to limit vomiting episodes and enhance the tolerance of charcoal. In patients with diminished ability to protect the airway, the potential hazards of vomiting and aspiration are significant and airway intubation is indicated.

Priorities for the nursing care of patients who are administered charcoal include positioning on the right side with the head of the bed elevated, ensuring that suction is readily available to protect the airway if vomiting occurs, and immobilization of the child to maintain intravenous patency and the position of the gastric tube. Protecting both the child's and parents' clothing is also necessary because of the mess that charcoal creates.

Other Methods of Toxin Elimination

Extracorporeal drug removal can be used to cleanse the blood of harmful toxins by forced diuresis, peritoneal dialysis, hemodialysis, hemoperfusion, and plasmapheresis (Berkowitz et al., 1992). Forced diuresis with alteration of urine pH reduces the concentration of the drug in the distal segment of the nephron by filtration and secretion via "ion trapping." Altering the pH of the urine by alkalinization traps the compound in the tubular lumen, reducing reabsorption and enhancing excretion. Drugs that are not highly lipid-soluble or protein-bound and have a primarily renal route of excretion are removed most effectively by this method.

Dialysis eliminates toxic substances by movement of solutes through a semipermeable membrane across a concentration gradient. The effectiveness of hemodialysis and peritoneal dialysis depends on the molecular weight, lipid-water solubility, protein-binding properties, and plasma concentration of the drug.

Hemoperfusion involves the passage of blood over an adsorbent matrix material of charcoal or resin. Plasmapheresis separates harmful substances from the plasma by continuous centrifugation. Substances that are eliminated best by this method have small volumes of distribution and tight plasma protein-binding properties. Hypotension and thrombocytopenia are possible complications of hemoperfusion.

The Unknown Toxin

When the name or the amount of a poison ingested is unknown, the incident unwitnessed, or the history at all vague; the child is treated as though a harmful substance was consumed. If elements of the history provided are contradictory or questionable, it is especially important to rule out the possibility of trauma as a cause of the child's physical injuries. Physical assessment focuses on the potential for unreported traumatic injuries, as well as on significant details related to the ingestion, such as altered mental status or unusual odors on the skin or clothing.

Cardiorespiratory status is monitored and intravenous access is achieved immediately upon the patient's arrival in the emergency department. Gastric, serum, and urine specimens are obtained for toxic analysis. A patent airway is maintained and supportive care is rendered until definitive care can be prescribed. The availability of antidotes such as naloxone (Narcan), glucose, oxygen, diphenhydramine (Benadryl), physostigmine, flumazenil (Mazicon), digoxin immune Fab (Digibind), methylene blue, deferoxamine, acetylcysteine (Mucomyst), calcium gluconate, and glucagon is assured when the ingestion of a toxic substance is suspected (Gill, 1989). The local poison control center can provide details regarding the indications and guidelines for use of these antidotes.

The sections that follow detail the care of children who have ingested potentially harmful toxic substances. Pharmaceutical agents include acetaminophen, barbiturates, carbamazepine, clonidine, cocaine, iron, theophylline, and tricyclic antidepressants. Nonpharmaceutical agents discussed are the alcohols (methanol, ethanol, isopropanol, and ethylene glycol), caustics, and hydrocarbons. Tables 32–3 and 32–4 list these substances and also indicate the body system(s) most often affected.

PHARMACEUTICAL TOXINS

Acetaminophen

Acetaminophen is used commonly as an antipyretic and analgesic in the pediatric population. This is the result of studies that imply a relationship between the use of salicylates and the incidence of Reye's syndrome. Its availability in the home makes it more accessible to children than other household products. Acetaminophen ingestions are potentially more harmful in adolescents than in young children because the quantity consumed is usually greater. Therefore, adolescents are two times more likely to manifest toxic blood levels (>140 mg/kg), and six more times more likely to develop hepatotoxicity than are young children (Rumack, 1986).

Pathogenesis

Acetaminophen reaches peak serum levels 30 to 60 minutes after administration (Selbst & Henretig, 1985). However, peak plasma levels (>140 mg/kg) may not occur with an overdose until 4 hours after ingestion (Rumack, 1986).

There are three primary pathways by which acetaminophen is metabolized in the liver and ultimately excreted in the urine (Fig. 32–1). It can be detoxified by:

1. Sulfation (the reaction between benzene and sulfuric acid), the primary metabolic pathway in children.
2. Glucaronidation (glucose is conjugated to become water-soluble), the primary metabolic pathway in adults.
3. Cytochrome P-450 chain (molecules conjugate with glutathione to form the nontoxic mercapturic acid) (Rumack, 1986).

When toxic amounts of acetominophen are ingested metabolism by the P-450 chain increases, ultimately causing rapid depletion of glutathione stores.

The depletion of glutathione inhibits normal formation of the nontoxic mercapturic acid that would otherwise be excreted. Instead of mercapturic acid, a toxic intermediate agent accumulates and combines with hepatic macromolecules to cause cellular necrosis.

Final Common Pathways

Hepatic Failure. Altered hepatic function becomes evident when aspartate transaminase (AST), alanine aminotransferase (ALT), bilirubin, and prothrombin times are elevated. Four stages best characterize the progression of hepatotoxicity in acetaminophen overdoses.

Table 32–3. SYSTEMS MOST COMMONLY AFFECTED BY PHARMACEUTICAL TOXINS

Agent	Systems Involved
Acetaminophen	Hepatic
Barbiturates	Neurologic Cardiovascular Renal
Carbamazepine	Neurologic Cardiovascular Hepatic Renal
Clonidine	Neurologic Cardiovascular
Cocaine	Cardiovascular Neurologic
Iron	Cardiovascular Neurologic Metabolic Hepatic Renal Gastrointestinal
Theophylline	Cardiovascular Neurologic Gastrointestinal Metabolic
Tricyclic antidepressants	Neurologic Cardiovascular

Stage 1 occurs within 12 to 24 hours following ingestion. The patient is assessed for symptoms of generalized malaise, nausea, vomiting, and diaphoresis. Young children often vomit earlier than those who are older and rarely exhibit diaphoresis. AST and bilirubin level and prothrombin time are normal. The severity of the overdose is predicted most accurately from the serum level of acetaminophen 4 hours

Table 32–4. SYSTEMS MOST COMMONLY AFFECTED BY NONPHARMACEUTICAL TOXINS

Agent	Systems Involved
Alcohols	
Methanol	Neurologic
Ethanol	Neurologic
Isopropyl alcohol	Neurologic Cardiovascular Gastrointestinal Renal
Ethylene glycol	Neurologic Cardiovascular Respiratory Renal
Caustics	Gastrointestinal
Hydrocarbons	Respiratory Neurologic Cardiovascular Gastrointestinal Hepatic Renal

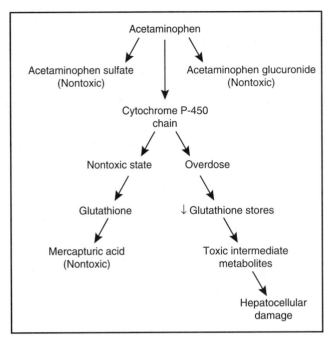

Acetaminophen

Acetaminophen sulfate
(Nontoxic)

Acetaminophen glucuronide
(Nontoxic)

Cytochrome P-450
chain

Nontoxic state   Overdose

Glutathione   ↓ Glutathione stores

Mercapturic acid
(Nontoxic)

Toxic intermediate
metabolites

Hepatocellular
damage

Figure 32–1 ● ● ● ● ● ●

Metabolism of acetaminophen. (From Agran, P.F., Zenk, K.E., & Romansky, S.G.: Acute liver failure and encephalopathy in a 15 month old infant. *American Journal of Diseases of Children*, 137:1107–1114. © 1983, American Medical Association.)

after ingestion. Figure 32–2 shows the relationship between the peak serum level of acetaminophen and probable hepatotoxicity.

Stage 2 occurs 24 to 48 hours after ingestion. The patient appears to feel better. However, AST, bilirubin level, and prothrombin time increase if treatment has been delayed.

Stage 3 develops 72 to 96 hours after ingestion. Jaundice and right upper quadrant tenderness are present. Hepatotoxicity is indicated by elevated AST (>1000 IU/L). Peak elevation of AST occurs during this stage. It is not unusual to care for patients with levels higher than 20,000 IU/L. In this period, centrilobular necrosis takes place in the hepatocytes.

Stage 4 is characterized by AST levels returning to normal 7 to 8 days after the ingestion. However, 2% to 4% of patients with toxic serum levels develop hepatic failure or die (Selbst & Henretig, 1985).

Initial Management

A reliable history is obtained to determine the time of the poisoning and to rule out the possibility of coingestants. Activated charcoal with sorbitol is recommended to prevent development of a toxic serum level. A peak plasma level is drawn 4 hours after ingestion.

Critical Care Management

If the peak serum level of acetaminophen exceeds 140 mcg/mL, N-acetylcysteine (NAC or Mucomyst) is

administered. NAC acts as a chemical substitute for glutathione, detoxifying the toxic intermediate so that it does not accumulate and normal P-450 metabolism can occur. NAC is available in both 10% and 20% solutions but is diluted to a 5% concentration before administration. If vomiting occurs within 1 hour, the dose is repeated. It can be mixed with a citrus or carbonated beverage to decrease its pungent smell and is administered orally or by lavage tube.

NAC may be administered within 16 hours of toxic acetaminophen ingestion. An intravenous form is available in Canada and Europe, but is available only as an investigational drug in the United States. Intravenous administration may be more effective because of better patient tolerance, because it is not affected by vomiting, and the administration protocol is shorter (Tenenbein, 1986). However, enteral administration produces higher concentrations of NAC in the portal circulation. The initial enteral dose of NAC is 140 mg/kg, administered within 16 hours of the ingestion and followed by 70 mg/kg every 4 hours for a total of 17 doses (Rumack, 1986).

Nursing interventions focus on monitoring liver function studies and neurologic status to assess for signs of hepatic encephalopathy. Altered mental status in the presence of elevated liver enzymes can progress to hepatic coma and death in severe acetaminophen ingestions.

Barbiturates

Barbiturates are a class of sedative-hypnotic agents. Indications for prescribed use include induc-

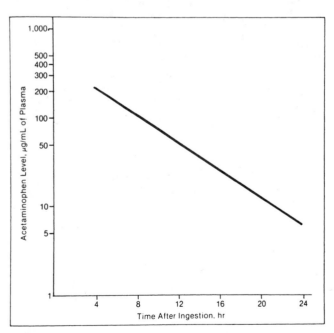

Figure 32–2 ● ● ● ● ● ●

Acetaminophen toxicity nomogram. Area above line indicates probable hepatotoxic reaction. Area below line indicates no hepatotoxic reaction. (From Rumack, B.H., Peterson, R.C., Koch, C.G., et al. Acetaminophen overdose. *Archives of Internal Medicine*, 141:380, © 1981, American Medical Association.)

tion of sleep and sedation. Known as "downers," barbiturates may be illegally obtained on the street. Barbiturates are classified according to their duration of action: ultrashort, short, intermediate, or long-acting (Table 32–5). In this drug class, those barbiturates that are highly lipid-soluble have a more rapid onset and a shorter duration of action, as well as a greater degree of hypnotic activity, than those that are less lipophilic (Bertino & Reed, 1986). Duration of action, however, does not correlate with the serum half-life of these medications.

Central nervous system effects are related to the brain tissue concentration of barbiturate. The effect of barbiturates is primarily on the CNS through depression of the response of synapses, delaying their recovery time. Therapeutic doses of barbiturates do not produce side effects likely to bring a patient to a tertiary care setting, unless used in combination with other medications or alcohol. Approximately three times the therapeutic dose of a barbiturate is necessary to produce the side effects of overdose.

Pathogenesis

Barbiturates have a very narrow therapeutic index (i.e., the difference between an effective dose and a lethal dose is small). Barbiturates are usually taken orally, and when taken with liquids, absorption is hastened; when taken with food, absorption is slowed. Serum levels are only somewhat indicative of toxicity, because of the discrepancy between plasma and brain tissue concentration. In general, those patients most at risk for death as a result of barbiturate overdose are those who are not treated despite the following serum levels: greater than or equal to 3 mg/dL for short-acting barbiturates, greater than or equal to 7 mg/dL for intermediate-acting barbiturates, and greater than or equal to 10 mg/dL for long-acting barbiturates (Bertino & Reed, 1986). Short-acting barbiturates, particularly those with high lipid solubility, are considered more toxic than the longer-acting forms (Winchester, 1990). These short-acting agents are absorbed in the small intestine and transformed in the liver to inactive metabolites, which are excreted predominantly in urine.

The effects of barbiturate intoxication include depression of the central nervous, respiratory, and cardiovascular systems, and renal dysfunction. Smooth muscle activity is also depressed in barbiturate overdose.

Final Common Pathways

CNS Dysfunction. Nervous system dysfunction is evidenced by a spectrum of presentations from mild sedation to coma with loss of deep tendon reflexes. The medication, dose, and route of the ingestion all play a part in the effect of the overdose on the child. Early in barbiturate overdose, the child may demonstrate miosis, although a common late presentation in serious overdose is dilated pupils that are unresponsive to light. Hypothermia may result from hypothalamic depression.

Respiratory dysfunction results from depression of the respiratory control centers in the brainstem. The neurogenic drive to breathe may be obliterated and the mechanisms that affect respiratory rhythm may be altered. Breathing patterns may range from slow to rapid and shallow, and may progress to Cheyne-Stokes respiration. As respiratory depression continues, the respiratory rate and volume of gas exchanged decrease, causing hypoxemia and hypercarbia. The cough reflex may be suppressed, and the child may experience laryngospasm resulting from inhibition of smooth muscle activity.

Cardiovascular Dysfunction. Cardiovascular dysfunction is caused by the direct effect of barbiturates on the heart, i.e., depressed myocardial contractility, as well as by central effects on the brain. Depression of the midbrain's regulation of cardiovascular function is evidenced by hypotension and bradycardia. Dilation of vascular smooth muscle causes venous pooling, which, in turn, decreases intravascular volume.

Vascular smooth muscle dilation results from loss of blood pressure control mechanisms. The loss of these mechanisms causes decreased motility through the gastrointestinal tract and depressed muscular activity of the ureters and urinary bladder.

Renal Dysfunction. Renal dysfunction may be present for two reasons. First, barbiturates stimulate the release of antidiuretic hormone, producing a decrease in urine output. In addition, renal function may be compromised by hypotension that can lead to acute tubular necrosis.

Initial Management

If barbiturate overdose is suspected in the unconscious patient, the airway is protected with endotracheal intubation. The child may undergo gastric aspiration to remove remaining pill fragments, followed

Table 32–5. CLASSIFICATION OF BARBITURATES BY DURATION OF ACTION

Long-acting	Short to Intermediate	Ultrashort
Phenobarbital	Amobarbital	Hexobarbital
Mephobarbital	Butabarbital sodium	Methohexital sodium
Metharbital	Pentobarbital sodium	Thiopental sodium
	Secobarbital	

From Bertino, J.S., & Reed, M.D. (1986). Barbiturate and nonbarbiturate sedative hypnotic intoxication in children. *Pediatric Clinics of North America,* 33(3), 705.

by gastric lavage. Activated charcoal and a cathartic are subsequently administered.

If warranted by inadequate gas exchange, the unconscious patient is placed on mechanical ventilation. For the patient who presents in shock, aggressive intravascular volume replacement is begun with crystalloid fluid (20 mL/kg). Assessment for adequate renal function is essential.

Critical Care Management

Nervous system dysfunction is treated with supportive care. Temperature is assessed regularly to prevent hypothermia-induced ventricular fibrillation. If the child is hypothermic, the first line of treatment is to prevent further heat loss. Warming with external devices may be considered, but is not universally recommended (Harvey, 1975).

Respiratory dysfunction is managed by ensuring a patent airway and adequate gas exchange. Assessment of arterial blood gases and serum pH guides intervention. The presence of aspiration pneumonitis requires treatment with antibiotic therapy.

Cardiovascular dysfunction treatment includes volume replacement as needed. If volume replacement does not resolve hypotension, continuous infusion of dopamine (1–20 mcg/kg/minute) or dobutamine (2–12 mcg/kg/minute) may be required.

Renal dysfunction may be treated with forced diuresis. Forced diuresis is achieved by administration of one or more fluid boluses followed by intravenous administration of furosemide (1–2 mg/kg), with the goal of achieving urine flow at 0.1 mL/kg/minute (Mann & Sandberg, 1970). In the case of overdose with phenobarbital, urinary alkalinization (maintaining urine pH >7.5) is the therapy of choice. This is best accomplished by intravenous administration of 1 to 2 mEq/kg of sodium bicarbonate and followed by 2 to 4 mEq/kg for the next 6 to 12 hours. Long-acting barbiturate overdose may respond well to hemodialysis or hemoperfusion as the lower protein-binding capability of the long-acting preparations allows them to be removed through hemodialysis or hemoperfusion. Patients who are considered for these therapies are those in profound coma with high barbiturate levels who are not responding to conventional intensive care therapies (Winchester, 1990).

Carbamazepine

Carbamazepine (Tegretol) is used for treatment of partial complex and tonic-clonic seizures and trigeminal neuralgia in children and adults. It is structurally related to tricyclic antidepressants, sharing some of the cardiac and CNS effects of these medications. The mechanism of action is unknown, although it is known to elevate the seizure threshold. Carbamazepine is available for oral administration in 100-mg and 200-mg tablets.

Pathogenesis

Plasma drug concentration in carbamazepine ingestion is influenced by the length of therapy (single dose versus long-term therapy), the patient's age, and interactions with other medications. The half-life of carbamazepine is 18 to 54 hours following a single dose and 10 to 20 hours in long-term therapy (Seger, 1990). After several weeks of carbamazepine therapy, hepatic microsomal enzymes are autoinduced and begin to metabolize carbamazepine more quickly. Peak serum levels occur in a range between 4 and 24 hours after ingestion (Seger, 1990). Children metabolize carbamazepine more rapidly than adults. The metabolism of carbamazepine is increased when administered with phenobarbital and phenytoin, and decreased when administered with erythromycin. Carbamazepine is highly bound to tissue and plasma proteins. Therapeutic serum concentrations differ, depending on whether carbamazepine is used alone or in conjunction with other medications. For single drug therapy, a therapeutic level of carbamazepine is 8 to 12 mcg/mL. When used with other antiepileptic medications, a serum concentration of 4 to 8 mcg/mL is in the therapeutic range (Goldfrank, 1990). Because of the varying nature of serum concentration, treatment of overdose is directed by the patient's clinical course rather than the serum level. Table 32–6 correlates the stages of intoxication with serum levels and signs and symptoms.

Carbamazepine is absorbed slowly because of its low water solubility. It is metabolized by the liver via oxidation and conjugation into a compound that is as active as carbamazepine, and other inactive products, and excreted in the urine. It exerts some anticholinergic effects, delaying gastric emptying time. The system most affected by carbamazepine overdose is the CNS, although the cardiovascular, hepatic, and renal systems may also be involved.

Final Common Pathways

CNS Dysfunction. Neurologic system dysfunction is evidenced following a toxic ingestion of carbamazepine by a spectrum of symptoms from irritability to coma with seizure activity, depending on the

Table 32–6. STAGES OF CARBAMAZEPINE OVERDOSE WITH SERUM LEVEL AND CLINICAL SIGNS

Stage	Serum Level	Clinical Signs
I	>25 mcg/mL	Stupor or coma, abnormal pupillary reaction to light, respiratory depression
II	15–25 mcg/mL	Irritability, combativeness, choreiform movements, hallucinations
III	11–15 mcg/mL	Nystagmus, drowsiness, ataxia
IV	<11 mcg/mL	Normal mental examination, mild ataxia, may relapse to earlier stages

From Weaver, D.F., Camfield, P., & Fraser, A. (1988). Massive carbamazepine overdose: Clinical and pharmacologic observations in five episodes. *Neurology, 38,* 756–757.

amount of drug ingested. The neurologic presentation following overdose is similar to that found with tricyclic antidepressant overdose because of the chemical similarity between tricyclic antidepressants and carbamazepine. The patient's neurologic status may wax and wane with the stage of absorption following carbamazepine overdose, with increased absorption of this medication in stage 4, when normal peristalsis resumes.

Cardiovascular Dysfunction. Cardiovascular system dysfunction is manifested by cardiac conduction delays, dysrhythmias, and hypotension. These effects are most likely the result of the tricyclic antidepressant–like chemical structure of carbamazepine.

Other Effects. Acute hepatic dysfunction occasionally occurs following carbamazepine overdose. Alteration in renal function may include hyponatremia and syndrome of inappropriate antidiuretic hormone (SIADH). These side effects can be present with long-term administration of carbamazepine and aggravated by overdose.

Initial Management

Gastric lavage is initiated upon the patient's arrival to the emergency department. Undigested tablets can form a concretion in the stomach, which is detectable by an abdominal radiograph using contrast medium. If a concretion is present, surgical gastrotomy is considered.

Repeated doses (two or three) of activated charcoal are recommended because the serum half-life of carbamazepine may be reduced by as much as 50% with this therapy (Neuvonen & Elonen, 1980; Wason et al., 1992). Activated charcoal binds with carbamazepine, decreasing its half-life and increasing its elimination. If the patient's condition worsens, charcoal hemoperfusion may be considered. Catharsis is not recommended because of the potential for increased systemic absorption as a result of increased drug distribution throughout the gastrointestinal tract (Weaver et al., 1988).

Critical Care Management

The treatment of carbamazepine overdose is supportive and symptom-based. Children are monitored in the intensive care unit until their condition has remained stable for 24 hours. Because of the risks of relapse from stage 4 to the previous stages, lavage followed by activated charcoal administration is continued until the patient is no longer comatose (Weaver et al., 1988).

Neurologic dysfunction resulting in respiratory depression may require tracheal intubation and mechanical ventilation. The combative patient must be protected from injury. Seizures, if they occur, are treated with diazepam or phenytoin in conventional doses (Weaver et al., 1988). Seizures from hyponatremia are treated with intravenous sodium replace-

ment. Patients in status epilepticus are considered candidates for charcoal hemoperfusion.

Cardiovascular dysfunction is assessed with EKG monitoring for conduction delays and dysrhythmias, and hemodynamic monitoring for hypotension. Charcoal hemoperfusion is used when dysrhythmias resulting from carbamazepine overdose are evident.

Alteration in hepatic function is assessed with liver function studies. Conventional therapy, including monitoring serum glucose levels and administration of clotting factors for prolonged clotting time, is recommended for hepatic dysfunction.

Alteration in renal function requires monitoring of serum electrolyte levels, particularly that of sodium. Serum sodium and urine output are assessed for evidence of SIADH. Treatment with water restriction and sodium supplementation is initiated promptly.

Clonidine

Clonidine is used primarily in the treatment of hypertension in adults, but may also be used in children for treatment of Tourette syndrome and attention deficit disorder with hyperactivity (Cohen et al., 1979; Hunt et al., 1985). Its exact mechanism of action is unknown, but it is hypothesized that clonidine centrally stimulates presynaptic alpha-adrenergic receptors, which inhibits sympathetic discharge and produces a decrease in peripheral vascular resistance and decreased heart rate, stroke volume, and cardiac output (Mack, 1988; Artman & Boerth, 1983). Clonidine also inhibits uptake of norepinephrine by neuronal tissues, producing CNS depression. Clonidine is available in 0.1-, 0.2-, and 0.3-mg tablets and in transdermal patches. The transdermal patches contain 2.5, 5.0, or 7.5 mg of clonidine, and are designed to release 0.1, 0.2, or 0.3 mg of clonidine per day over a period of one week's time (Roberts & Zink, 1990).

Pathogenesis

Clonidine is absorbed in the gastrointestinal tract, metabolized by the liver, and excreted primarily in urine. Its effects are evident 30 minutes after ingestion, with peak effects occurring approximately 2 hours following oral administration. Antihypertensive effects are present for as long as 24 hours following an oral dose. Overdose in children has been documented with as little as a 0.1-mg dose, or by application or ingestion of a transdermal patch. A discarded transdermal patch contains enough clonidine to produce overdose symptoms in a child. Clonidine is not part of a routine toxicology screen, but serum levels can be obtained if a clonidine ingestion is suspected.

Clonidine overdose affects the CNS and the cardiovascular and respiratory systems. The majority of children present within 1 hour of a clonidine overdose, and symptoms may persist for up to 24 hours following overdose. However, progression of symptoms or new clonidine-related toxic effects do not develop more than 4 hours after presentation to the hospital (Wiley et al., 1990). No pediatric deaths have been reported following clonidine overdose (Artman & Boerth, 1983; Roberts & Zink, 1990).

Final Common Pathways

CNS Dysfunction. CNS dysfunction mimics narcotic overdose, where miosis, coma, and respiratory depression are the hallmarks. Respiratory depression may progress to apnea as a result of clonidine's presumed involvement in endogenous opiate receptor pathways.

Symptoms vary from a depressed level of consciousness to coma, and are postulated to be from inhibition of the uptake of norepinephrine by the neurons, which then decreases noradrenergic activity (Mack, 1988). Other CNS symptoms include hypothermia, which is attributed to alpha-adrenergic receptor stimulation of the serotonin-acetylcholine pathways, causing decreased metabolic heat production and increased heat loss (Roberts & Zink, 1990). Cool, pale skin is presumed to be the result of vasoconstriction. Hypotonia may also be seen.

Cardiovascular Dysfunction. Cardiovascular system dysfunction depends on the plasma level of clonidine. Serum levels higher than 10 to 15 mg/mL cause the peripheral alpha receptors to vasoconstrict, resulting in transient hypertension. The hypertensive period is followed by a hypotensive phase. Patients with a serum level lower than 10 mg/mL present with normotension or hypotension. Bradycardia, a known side effect of clonidine in normal doses, is commonly noted in children with clonidine overdose (Wiley et al., 1990). Other dysrhythmias, including first degree atrioventricular block and premature atrial contractions, may be noted. Bradycardia and hypotension are seen in clonidine ingestions of 0.01 mg/kg or more (Fiser et al., 1990).

Initial Management

If clonidine ingestion is suspected, emesis is contraindicated because CNS and respiratory depression occur rapidly. Gastric lavage is initiated in an attempt to recover remaining pills or pill fragments. Activated charcoal is then administered, although no studies have proven its efficacy (Roberts & Zink, 1990).

If hypotension and shock are present, the child is treated with infusion of 20 mL/kg of intravenous fluid and placed in Trendelenburg position. If signs of shock do not resolve with those measures, an infusion of dopamine (5–10 mcg/kg/minute) is begun.

Critical Care Management

Patients usually require supportive and symptomatic treatment in the critical care setting for less than 24 hours following clonidine overdose. Careful monitoring of vital signs, including temperature, is

necessary. Hypothermia is treated with passive warming to maintain a normal body temperature. Tracheal intubation and mechanical ventilation are instituted if respiratory effort is absent or inadequate to maintain normal serum oxygen (O_2) and carbon dioxide (CO_2) levels. Control of the airway protects the child from aspiration and subsequent respiratory compromise.

Cardiovascular system dysfunction treatment is based on the child's symptoms. Bradycardia associated with cardiovascular compromise is responsive to IV atropine (10 mcg/kg), although repeated doses may be necessary because of the long half-life of clonidine (Wiley et al., 1990). Hypotension is treated first with volume infusion, and then with dopamine infusion, as described in the initial management section. If a hypertensive phase occurs, treatment with a nitroprusside infusion (0.5–8 mcg/kg/minute) is instituted only if end-organ compromise is noted. The ensuing hypotensive period must be anticipated (Lewin & Howland, 1990). Dysrhythmias resolve with decreasing serum clonidine levels and usually do not require treatment.

Naloxone (Narcan) is recommended for treatment of all patients with clonidine overdoses in which CNS, cardiovascular, or respiratory depression is present (Lewin & Howland, 1990; Mack, 1988). The exact mechanism of action of naloxone in these patients is unknown, and identification of those patients who will benefit from naloxone has not been determined, but improvement in symptoms has been noted in some. The initial naloxone dose is 0.01 mg/kg, and if no response is noted, a repeat dose of 0.1 mg/kg is administered.

Cocaine

Grown in Peru and Bolivia, cocaine is an alkaloid that is extracted from the leaves of the *Erythroxylum coca* plant. It is crystallized as hydrochloride salt, prescribed as a local anesthetic and mucous membrane vasoconstrictor, and used illicitly as a CNS stimulant. Its anesthetic properties are regarded as highly efficient and relatively toxic (Gay, 1982). The adulterants with which cocaine is diluted for illicit use, including local anesthetics, sugars, stimulants, toxins, and inert compounds, may also exert toxic effects (Shannon, 1988).

Cocaine may be injected intravenously, sniffed intranasally, ingested, or applied to the mucous membranes. Cocaine can also be smoked in its free-base form known as "crack." Children may be exposed to cocaine by passive transmission via the placenta in utero, or in breast milk, or by inhalation of crack vapors (Bateman & Heagerty, 1989). Cocaine is well absorbed by all mucous membranes, metabolized in the blood and in the liver, and excreted in the urine as its primary metabolite, benzoylecgonine (Gay, 1982). Cocaine levels in blood may be detected within several minutes of ingestion. They peak in 15 to 30 minutes and persist for up to 8 hours (Kulberg, 1986;

Shannon et al., 1989). Cocaine may be detected in urine within 1 hour of ingestion or administration and persists for up to 3 days in children and 5 days in neonates following exposure (Shannon et al., 1989).

Pathogenesis

Three systems primarily affected by cocaine's toxic effects are the neurologic system, the cardiovascular system, and the respiratory system. Cocaine stimulates the sympathetic nervous system, and an overdose is especially toxic to the brain and heart. Cocaine alters normal intraneural communication by augmenting the effects of the catecholamines norepinephrine and dopamine. Cocaine stimulates the "fight or flight" mechanism, demonstrated by an increase in heart rate, stimulation of norepinephrine secretion, vasoconstriction, rise in blood glucose, dilation of pupils, and an increase in body temperature (Gay, 1982). As cocaine continues to stimulate norepinephrine and dopamine release, the cardiovascular and neurologic systems demonstrate progressive stimulation that may progress to exhaustion, producing coma and cardiac and respiratory arrest. Signs and symptoms become more severe with larger cocaine doses.

Final Common Pathways

Cardiovascular Dysfunction. Cardiovascular dysfunction is first manifested by sinus tachycardia, hypertension, ventricular ectopy (premature ventricular contractions—PVCs) and peripheral vasoconstriction. These signs may occur as a result of the toxic action cocaine exerts on the tissues of the myocardium directly, and/or because of its effect of sensitizing the heart to the actions of norepinephrine and dopamine (Howard et al., 1985). As a patient shows evidence of a toxic dose, heart rate and blood pressure peak and begin to fall, ventricular dysrhythmias become more frequent, and the patient begins to show signs of shock with decreased peripheral perfusion and cyanosis. Progression of signs includes ventricular fibrillation, circulatory collapse, and an ashen appearance before cardiac arrest. Cocaine-induced coronary artery vasoconstriction may also cause myocardial ischemia or infarction (Minor et al., 1991).

CNS Dysfunction. Neurologic dysfunction begins as the cerebral cortex is stimulated. Dysfunction is demonstrated by talkativeness, evidence of euphoria and emotional lability, overalertness, mydriasis, and nausea and/or vomiting. As stimulation continues and cocaine affects the functions of the medulla, the child becomes hyperthermic and develops hyperreflexia and may have seizures. As the CNS becomes exhausted, the child becomes comatose with flaccid paralysis.

Respiratory dysfunction in cocaine overdose is caused by the effects of cocaine on the respiratory centers within the medulla. The early stimulation phase is evidenced by tachypnea and increased depth of respirations. The child becomes more dyspneic as CNS stimulation continues, and the condition may progress to respiratory failure. Seizures, or the side effects of the medications used to control seizures, may also contribute to respiratory failure in cocaine toxicity.

Initial Management

Because cocaine is absorbed within minutes, no treatment can decrease its absorption or enhance its excretion. Initial management of cocaine exposure depends on the phase at which the patient presents for care. Adequate cardiovascular and respiratory function must be ensured. Assessment of cardiovascular function includes heart rate and rhythm, blood pressure, and peripheral perfusion. Respiratory evaluation includes assessment of both respiratory rate and depth, with pulse oximetry or arterial blood gas analysis as needed. Intravenous access is obtained promptly and vital signs are monitored frequently. Continuous core temperature monitoring is initiated to assess for hyperthermia.

Critical Care Management

Cardiovascular dysfunction is initially treated with fluid resuscitation. Labetalol (100 mcg/kg/dose) may be given to treat tachycardia and ventricular dysrhythmias (Haddad & Winchester, 1990). A lidocaine bolus (1 mg/kg) and continuous infusion (10–50 mcg/kg/minute) may be required to suppress ventricular arrhythmias. Severe hypertension resulting from vasoconstriction is best treated with sedatives such as diazepam (40–200 mcg/kg IV) or lorazepam (30 mcg/kg/day in three or four doses IV) in an effort to control hypertension, calm the patient, prevent seizures, and decrease hypertonicity. If these measures fail, the use of a continuous infusion of nitroprusside (0.2–10 mcg/kg/minute) may be necessary. Pulmonary artery pressure monitoring may be indicated to estimate the left heart filling pressures and to guide management.

Assessment of neurologic function begins on the patient's arrival to the healthcare setting. Use of a tool such as the Glasgow Coma Scale or the Pediatric Coma Scale guides assessment. Seizures may be treated with diazepam (100–250 mcg/kg) or lorazepam (50 mcg/kg) given intravenously over 3 minutes. Hyperpyrexia should be aggressively treated with cooling blankets or tepid baths, avoiding shivering, which increases body temperature.

Respiratory dysfunction management includes maintenance of a patent airway as the first priority. Oxygen may be administered to prevent complications of hypoxemia. Tracheal intubation is considered if the child is unable to maintain a patent airway and adequate cough and gag reflexes, if seizures compromise respiratory function, or if arterial blood gas analysis demonstrates hypercarbia. Mechanical ventilation may be required to treat respiratory insufficiency or respiratory failure.

Iron

Iron ingestion is one of the more common childhood ingestions because of the availability of iron and iron-containing compounds in the household and the appearance of these compounds. The similarity of colors, shapes, and flavorings between multivitamins and other iron-containing products and candy makes them especially enticing to children. Iron supplementation is prescribed for pregnant women, and iron is a common component in both pediatric and adult multivitamins. Elemental iron is available in combination with gluconate, sulfate, or fumarate salts, each having differing amounts of elemental iron. Although only rare cases of iron ingestion require intensive care management, the number of fatalities from accidental iron overdose has doubled in the past decade. In 1990 it was considered the most toxic substance ingested by children, having caused 11 fatalities (Litovitz et al., 1990).

After ingestion in normal doses, 10 to 15 mg of iron is absorbed daily through the gastrointestinal tract (Berkowitz et al., 1992). Iron is absorbed in the duodenum and jejunum and is transported to the hepatocytes and the reticuloendothelial system, where it is stored, and to the bone marrow, where it is used for hemoglobin synthesis.

With an acute iron overdosage, the total serum concentration of iron exceeds the total iron binding capacity, and free iron circulates in the blood, causing vasodilation and increased capillary permeability (Steinhart et al., 1988). Fluid moves out of the intravascular space, causing relative hypovolemia and hypotension. The free iron is distributed into cells, particularly the hepatocytes, causing pathophysiologic changes in the mitochondria that lead to widespread cellular dysfunction. Serum iron levels peak 2 to 4 hours following ingestion, and begin to fall 6 hours after ingestion (Henretig & Temple, 1984). Table 32–7 shows the correlation between serum iron levels and toxicity. An iron concentration higher than 350 mcg/dL is indicative of moderate to severe toxicity (Mann et al., 1989).

Pathogenesis

The effects of acute iron overdose have been described in four phases (Covey, 1964). The first phase of iron toxicity occurs within 6 hours of the ingestion and is the result of the corrosive effects of iron on the gastrointestinal mucosa. The child complains of nausea and moderate to severe abdominal pain, and presents with vomiting, diarrhea, and/or gastrointestinal hemorrhage. Vomitus and stools may be dark gray or black because of the presence of iron. In cases of severe poisoning, the child may present in coma with hypotension or shock.

The second phase of iron toxicity is described as one of symptom abatement, with the child demonstrating only mild lethargy. It generally occurs 6 to 24 hours following the ingestion, but this phase may be absent in children with severe poisoning.

The third phase, 12 to 48 hours following the ingestion, is one of critical illness. Metabolic acidosis, renal tubular and hepatic necrosis, and severe lethargy progressing to coma with cardiovascular collapse may be seen.

The fourth and final phase of iron toxicity occurs 4 to 6 weeks following an ingestion that involved severe gastrointestinal effects. This phase involves the development of gastric and pyloric strictures that may require surgical correction.

Final Common Pathways

Cardiovascular Dysfunction. Hypotension is one of the known side effects of iron toxicity. This finding may be a result of blood loss through the gastrointestinal tract or from vasodilation and increased capillary permeability. Intravenous deferoxamine can also cause hypotension, particularly if infused at a rate higher than 15 mg/kg/hour.

Neurologic Dysfunction. Neurologic dysfunction varies from slightly depressed sensorium to coma as a result of the toxic effects of free iron on the CNS. If a child presents in coma shortly following an iron ingestion, the prognosis for neurologic recovery is poor (Henretig & Temple, 1984).

Other Effects. Metabolic acidosis develops as a result of poisoning of the mitochondria by iron. Cellular respiration is compromised as a consequence, producing lactic acidosis.

Hepatic failure can result from iron poisoning of the mitochondria within hepatocytes, causing cell death. Alterations in glucose metabolism, coagulopathy, and hepatic encephalopathy accompany liver failure.

Renal failure may occur following iron intoxication. Treatment of this problem is especially important as the iron-deferoxamine compound, feroxamine (the end-product of chelation treatment), is excreted by the kidney.

Gastrointestinal dysfunction occurs from the corrosive effects of iron on the mucosa. Signs and symptoms may be mild (nausea and vomiting) or indicative of necrosis with perforation and peritonitis. Children with severe iron overdoses are at risk for intestinal obstruction from fibrosis, which may develop as a late effect of gastrointestinal tract scarring.

Table 32–7. SERUM IRON LEVEL AND POTENTIAL SEVERITY OF INTOXICATION

Serum Iron Level	Potential Toxicity
<100	None
100–350	Minimal toxicity
350–500	Moderate toxicity; chelation usually not necessary
500–1000	Severe toxicity; start chelation immediately
>1000	Potentially lethal; start maximum chelation immediately

From Henretig, F.M., & Temple, A.R. (1984). Acute iron poisoning in children. *Clinics in Laboratory Medicine, 4,* 579.

Initial Management

When iron ingestion is suspected in an unconscious child, lavage is initiated with a large-bore nasogastric tube with the goal of blocking absorption and decreasing mucosal injury. Sodium bicarbonate may be added to lavage solutions to form ferrous sulfate, which is less absorbable. A 1% to 1.5% sodium bicarbonate solution is the solution of choice for lavage, because it avoids the complications of hyperphosphatemia and subsequent hypocalcemia reported with sodium phosphate solutions (Henretig & Temple, 1984). In severe toxicity, deferoxamine, a heavy-metal antagonist (2 g/L in 1.5% sodium bicarbonate) may also be administered as a lavage solution, although the clear benefit of deferoxamine in lavage has not been documented by improved patient outcomes (Mann et al., 1970). Charcoal administration is ineffective because it binds poorly with iron (Tenenbein et al., 1991) and is contraindicated because it may decrease the visibility of iron tablets on abdominal radiographs.

Following lavage, an abdominal radiograph is obtained to document the presence of retained iron tablets in the stomach and pylorus. If present, whole bowel irrigation with polyethylene glycol electrolyte lavage solution (GoLYTELY) enhances stooling while quickly emptying iron from the gastrointestinal tract (Durbin, 1989; Everson et al., 1991). This solution is instilled at room temperature into the stomach via nasogastric tube at 300 to 500 mL/hour for children younger than 5 years and up to 2 L/hour for adolescents. Whole bowel irrigation continues until diarrhea is produced and the effluent resembles the infusate. This process can require 6 to 12 hours of treatment (Tenenbein, 1987). If lavage and whole bowel irrigation are unsuccessful in removing intact iron tablets, emergency gastrotomy may be considered (Mann et al., 1989).

Chelation therapy, which binds iron into a soluble complex, is initiated in the emergency department with IV deferoxamine at a maximum dose of 15 mg/kg/hour for children in whom severe intoxication is suspected. The daily maximum recommended dose is 360 mg/kg/day, with a limit of 6 g. Deferoxamine combines with iron to form feroxamine, which is excreted by the renal system; although the mechanism of action is unclear (Berkowitz et al., 1992). The urine becomes pink shortly after chelation begins. Serum iron levels are followed during chelation therapy. Chelation is discontinued when the serum iron level falls below 100 mcg/dL, or when the urine color returns to pale yellow (Henretig & Temple, 1984). The child's blood pressure should be assessed frequently during chelation therapy owing to the peripheral vasodilation caused by deferoxamine.

Initial management also includes close monitoring for the known side effects of iron toxicity. Intravenous access is obtained in any child with suspected moderate to severe toxicity so that hypotension, metabolic acidosis, hypoglycemia, and blood dyscrasias can be treated promptly. Continuous monitoring of the adequacy of the child's airway, breathing, and circulation is necessary.

Critical Care Management

Cardiovascular assessment includes central venous pressure monitoring to provide a guide to the patient's volume status and fluid management. Periodic assessment of serum hemoglobin and hematocrit levels is necessary to track blood loss via the gastrointestinal tract. Volume replacement with blood components or other fluids is initiated early in the treatment of hypotension. Intravenous infusion of catecholamines, such as epinephrine (0.2–2.0 mcg/kg/minute) or dopamine (1–20 mcg/kg/minute), may be required to treat hypotension that is refractory to volume replacement.

Neurologic dysfunction management is primarily supportive. If the child has inadequate cough and/or gag reflexes, tracheal intubation is performed and mechanical ventilation instituted as needed. Acid-base balance is assessed by serial measurement of serum pH and bicarbonate ions. Intravenous sodium bicarbonate is administered as necessary to treat metabolic acidosis.

Hepatic failure requires assessment and treatment of hypoglycemia and coagulopathy. Hypoglycemia is treated with intravenous infusion of dextrose-containing solutions, the concentrations of which are titrated to maintain the serum glucose level above 80 to 100 mg/dL. Increased prothrombin time (PT) or partial thromboplastin time (PTT) or clinical signs of bleeding are treated with infusion of the appropriate clotting factors. Plasmapheresis may be instituted to temporarily remove toxins if hepatic encephalopathy becomes evident. Liver transplantation may be the therapy of last resort if liver biopsy demonstrates significant hepatic cell death.

Renal function is assessed by hourly measurement of urine output and periodic monitoring of specific gravity, blood urea nitrogen (BUN), and serum creatinine. If acute renal failure occurs, continuous hemofiltration, hemodialysis, or peritoneal dialysis can be utilized to remove feroxamine, as well as other metabolic end-products (Banner et al., 1989). Exchange transfusion is another alternative for removal of the iron-deferoxamine complex in the setting of acute renal failure. Renal transplantation may be necessary if the renal system does not recover following iron toxicity.

Gastrointestinal dysfunction is monitored by serial assessment of abdominal girth and tenseness and for the presence of blood in gastric contents and stool, and by abdominal radiographs. Blood loss in vomitus or stools is treated. If gastrointestinal perforation is suspected, the child is taken for an exploratory laparotomy to identify and manage areas of necrosis. Peritonitis is treated with appropriate antibiotic therapy. Gastrointestinal scarring causing strictures within the stomach or pylorus may cause obstruction within those areas, requiring surgical intervention.

Theophylline

Theophylline is most commonly used as a bronchodilator in children to relieve the bronchospasm associated with asthma. The therapeutic serum level ranges from 10 to 20 mg/L. Dosages to achieve a therapeutic level via bolus administration are 6 mg/kg orally and 7 mg/kg intravenously. Each 1 mg/kg of theophylline raises the serum level by 2 mg/L. Maintenance dosages vary with each child based on weight, concentration of the preparation, and extent of illness. Theophylline toxicity is characterized by serum levels higher than 20 mg/L. Precipitating factors associated with theophylline overdoses include dosage errors, accidental ingestions, suicide attempts, respiratory tract infections, or erythromycin administration (Baker, 1986).

Pathogenesis

The normal pharmacologic properties of theophylline include CNS stimulation, stimulation of the respiratory and vomiting centers in the medulla, positive chronotropic and inotropic effects, reduction of peripheral arteriolar resistance, relaxation of bronchial smooth muscle, inhibition of mast cell degranulation, increase in renal blood flow and glomerular filtration rate, and increases in gastric acid and pepsin secretion. These processes are accelerated in situations when theophylline toxicity occurs. Three systems primarily affected by toxic effects of theophylline are the cardiovascular system, CNS, and gastrointestinal system (Gaudreault & Guay, 1986).

Final Common Pathways

Cardiovascular Dysfunction. Patients with theophylline toxicity are at risk for dysrhythmias because theophylline decreases the ventricular fibrillation threshold, increases conduction velocity (predisposing the heart to reentry phenomenon), increases catecholamine release, and reduces myocardial oxygen supply (Gaudreault & Guay, 1986).

Altered cardiac output results from supraventricular dysrhythmias such as sinus tachycardia, atrial tachycardia, atrial flutter, and atrial fibrillation. Ventricular dysrhythmias may develop and include PVCs and ventricular tachycardia and fibrillation. Serious dysrhythmias occur most often in young patients with acute theophylline overdoses when serum levels exceed 50 mcg/mL (Gaudreault et al., 1983).

Other toxic effects associated with the development of dysrhythmias include hypokalemia, hypophosphatemia, and acidemia. Theophylline's beta-2 effects, which reduce peripheral vascular resistance, are responsible for severe hypotension and reduced myocardial perfusion associated with toxicity.

Neurologic Dysfunction. CNS disturbances include agitation, hyperreflexia from cerebral excitation, and seizures. Theophylline causes cerebral vasoconstriction and an increase in the cerebral concentration of cyclic adenosine monophosphate (cAMP).

Gastrointestinal Dysfunction. The gastrointestinal system is affected by increased secretion of gastric acid, which irritates the mucosa and causes vomiting. Vomiting is also the result of the local emetic effect of decreased esophageal tone and central stimulation of the vomiting center.

Other Effects. Other metabolic disorders that may result from theophylline overdose are hyperglycemia from increased gluconeogenesis, and glycogenolysis caused by catecholamine release. Hyperglycemia, in turn, causes an intracellular potassium shift resulting in hypokalemia.

Initial Management

Ipecac is contraindicated in the treatment of theophylline toxicity because the patient often continues to vomit as a result of the theophylline overdose. Treatment of seizures includes intubation and gastric lavage followed by repeated doses of activated charcoal with cathartic every 2 to 4 hours. This is performed until serum levels are within normal limits.

Critical Care Management

Nursing priorities include monitoring for cardiac dysrhythmias. Dysrhythmias are best treated with low doses of propranolol (0.02 mg/kg IV) repeated every 5 to 10 minutes with a maximum of 0.1 mg/kg IV (Gaudreault & Guay, 1986). Propranolol is also effective at reversing hypotension and is preferred over administration of fluid boluses because of its beta blocking effect (Gaudreault & Guay, 1986). The absence of dysrhythmias allows the nurse to evaluate the effectiveness of propranolol. The desired response to propranolol when treating hypotension, sinus tachycardia, atrial fibrillation, and rapid ventricular rates is a return to the patient's baseline parameters for blood pressure and cardiac rhythm. One case study reports effective treatment of tachycardia and hypotension with administration of intravenous esmolol, an ultra–short-acting beta-blocker, in a 500 mcg/kg bolus over 1 minute, followed by a 50 mcg/kg/minute continuous infusion (Seneff et al., 1990).

Repeated doses of activated charcoal are effective at increasing the clearance of theophylline in an overdose. Because of the persistant vomiting associated with theophylline toxicity, smaller doses of activated charcoal (0.25 g/kg) every 2 hours orally or by nasogastric tube and metoclopramide hydrochloride (Reglan) administration may be indicated.

Hemoperfusion is effective at enhancing the elimination of theophylline. Indications for hemoperfusion are unstable hemodynamics, seizures, or theophylline serum levels between 40 and 60 mcg/mL in chronic overdoses or 90 and 100 mcg/mL in acute overdoses (Gaudreault & Guay, 1986). The patient is assessed for signs of thrombocytopenia, hypocalcemia, and infection at the catheter insertion site when hemoperfusion is in progress.

Maintaining seizure precautions and ongoing assessment of level of consciousness is necessary to limit the degree of cerebral anoxia caused by seizure activity. Because a correlation exists between the length of seizure activity and morbidity and mortality, seizures are controlled as soon as possible. Lorazepam (0.05 mg/kg IV) is indicated for immediate cessation of seizure activity and is administered with phenobarbital (10 mg/kg) for continued seizure control.

Other nursing interventions include administration of potassium, phosphate, and sodium bicarbonate with subsequent monitoring of laboratory values to evaluate the resolution of toxic effects.

The effectiveness of antiemetics in theophylline toxicity is variable. Recommendations include the use of metoclopramide (2 mg/kg IV) or ranitidine (1–2 mg/kg/day IV) to control vomiting and increase the tolerance of charcoal.

Tricyclic Antidepressants

Tricyclic antidepressant medications are widely prescribed in the United States for both adult and pediatric patients. Indications in children include treatment of depression, hyperkinesis, sleep disorders, school phobias, and enuresis (Byck, 1975; Pettit & Biggs, 1977; Herson et al., 1979). Most adults are prescribed tricyclic antidepressants for depression, chronic pain, and sleep disorders.

Pathogenesis

Most patients with tricyclic antidepressant overdose present within several hours of ingestion (Frommer et al., 1987). When ingested, tricyclic antidepressants may be absorbed erratically because they exert an anticholinergic effect, delaying gastric emptying. Tricyclics are highly lipid-soluble, and a large portion binds to plasma proteins shortly after ingestion. Serum levels are of little use in the clinical setting, because they vary with the extent of protein-binding and distribution. A prolonged QRS duration on EKG or Glasgow Coma Scale score less than 8 is most predictive of toxicity (Emerman et al., 1987). Tricyclic antidepressant overdose affects the parasympathetic nervous system, CNS, and cardiovascular system.

Final Common Pathways

Neurologic Dysfunction. Neurologic dysfunction may cause life-threatening complications. CNS effects of tricyclic antidepressant overdose include a period of agitation and restlessness followed by sedation that may progress to coma or seizures. More than 50% of patients with tricyclic antidepressant overdose demonstrate pseudoseizures seen as myoclonus, tremors, chorea, or choreoathetosis (Goldfrank et al., 1990). Seizures occur in 10% to 20% of patients with tricyclic antidepressant overdose and are most likely to occur in comatose patients (Braden et al., 1986).

Neurologic dysfunction may cause respiratory compromise through several pathways. The child is at risk for both impaired gas exchange following aspiration and for ineffective airway clearance with upper airway obstruction (Braden et al., 1986). Respiratory failure can also occur as a result of seizure-related apnea.

Cardiovascular Dysfunction. Cardiovascular dysfunction frequently accompanies tricyclic antidepressant overdose. Decreased cardiac output evidenced by hypotension may occur as a result of myocardial depression or dysrhythmias.

Tricyclic antidepressants exert quinidine-like effects on the conduction system of the heart. These effects can include a decreased rate of conduction, increased repolarization period, and decreased inotropy (Marshal & Forker, 1982). A QRS complex longer than 100 to 160 milliseconds is indicative of decreased conduction rate through the His-Purkinje system, and identifies patients at high risk for the development of seizures or ventricular dysrhythmias (Boehnert & Lovejoy, 1985). The standard lead for pediatric QRS measurement is the precordial lead V_5 (Braden et al., 1986). Increased repolarization time is seen on EKG as increased PR and QTc intervals and ST segment and T wave changes (Fig. 32–3) facilitating ventricular tachycardia, ventricular fibrillation, or asystole (Braden et al., 1986). Decreased ionotropy is demonstrated by general signs of decreased cardiac output. Metabolic acidosis may potentiate dysrhythmias and aggravate the poor inotropic performance of the myocardium.

Parasympathetic Overstimulation. Parasympathetic nervous system dysfunction may be evident following tricyclic antidepressant overdose. Characteristic signs of parasympathetic overstimulation include dry skin, axilla, and mouth; mydriasis, flushed skin; agitation; and hyperpyrexia. Alterations in both gastrointestinal and urinary elimination may also be present.

Initial Management

Diagnosis of tricyclic antidepressant overdose is considered if a child presents in coma or with hypotension, seizures, sinus tachycardia, a widened QRS interval, or other ventricular dysrhythmias on EKG. Ipecac is contraindicated because of the potential for rapid onset of CNS depression or seizures. Lavage is recommended for patients with altered level of consciousness. Following lavage, activated charcoal and a cathartic are recommended.

Critical Care Management

Primary treatment of respiratory dysfunction is directed toward achieving and maintaining the patency of the airway. Endotracheal intubation and mechanical ventilation are initiated promptly for patients whose oxygenation and ventilation are at risk.

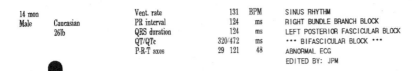

14 mon		Vent. rate	131	BPM	SINUS RHYTHM
Male	Caucasian	PR interval	124	ms	RIGHT BUNDLE BRANCH BLOCK
	26lb	QRS duration	124	ms	LEFT POSTERIOR FASCICULAR BLOCK
		QT/QTc	320/472	ms	*** BIFASCICULAR BLOCK ***
		P-R-T axes	29 121	48	ABNORMAL ECG
					EDITED BY: JPM

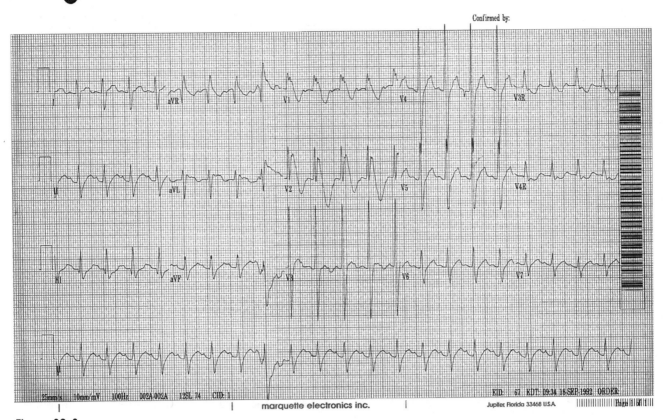

Figure 32–3 ● ● ● ● ● ●

Electrocardiogram in a patient with a prolonged QT interval following tricyclic antidepressant overdose.

Arterial blood gases are assessed for both hypoxia and acidosis, because these problems are known to increase the frequency and recurrence of dysrhythmias.

Cardiovascular dysfunction may result in hypotension. Treatment begins with Trendelenburg positioning and a 20 mL/kg fluid bolus of normal saline or lactated Ringer's solution. If these measures are ineffective in returning the blood pressure to normal range, a continuous infusion of phenylephrine (0.1–0.5 mcg/kg/minute), norepinephrine (0.05–1.0 mcg/kg/minute) or dopamine (5–30 mcg/kg/minute) may be required (Vernon et al., 1991). These medications exert predominantly alpha-agonistic effects and counteract the alpha-adrenergic blockade of the tricyclic antidepressants.

Treatment of dysrhythmias begins with ensuring adequate ventilation, followed by sodium bicarbonate infusion. Mild metabolic alkalosis (pH >7.45–7.55) has proven to be effective in narrowing widened QRS complexes, correcting hypotension, and in decreasing the incidence of dysrhythmias in tricyclic antidepressant overdoses (Berkowitz et al., 1992; Pentel & Be-

nowitz, 1986). Hyperventilation to induce respiratory alkalosis is thought to be less effective for controlling dysrhythmias. Serum sodium levels are monitored during and following administration of sodium bicarbonate. If sodium bicarbonate therapy is ineffective for controlling dysrhythmias, lidocaine (1 mg/kg IV) is given as a bolus and followed with a continuous infusion (10–50 mcg/kg/minute).

Neurologic dysfunction may be evidenced by seizures or coma. Diazepam (100–250 mcg/kg IV over 3 minutes) is the drug of choice for immediate use in tricyclic-related seizures. Phenytoin 3 to 8 mg/kg/day is the choice for long-term seizure management. Coma usually resolves within 24 hours of ingestion.

Parasympathetic nervous system dysfunction requires intervention as necessary. Urinary retention, evidenced by bladder distension, may require placement of an indwelling catheter. Constipation may result from slowed peristalsis, although the use of activated charcoal and cathartics may promote elimination and relieve this symptom. It is important to assess the patient for the presence of active bowel sounds before the administration of charcoal, because paralytic ileus is common and is a contraindication to its use.

NONPHARMACEUTICAL TOXINS: THE ALCOHOLS

Methanol

Methanol, also known as wood alcohol, is a common household item found in substances like windshield washer fluid, antifreeze, carburetor fluid, and paint stripper or remover. Methanol ingestions most often occur as epidemics among socially vulnerable people. Unsuspecting drinkers, particularly adolescents, may consume beverages to which methanol has been added.

Pathogenesis

Methanol is rapidly absorbed into the blood 30 to 90 minutes after ingestion. Methanol is excreted unchanged, in part. The lungs excrete 30% of methanol and 5% is excreted by the kidneys. However, the majority is metabolized in the liver to toxic substances including formaldehyde and formic acid (Berkowitz et al., 1992). The effects of methanol produce signs of CNS depression. Formic acid and formaldehyde also cause visual disturbances. Metabolic acidosis is the result of methanol metabolism.

Final Common Pathways

Neurologic Dysfunction. Methanol affects the CNS causing restlessness, headache, vertigo, and depression. These signs normally occur 6 to 24 hours following ingestion and are accompanied by abdominal pain and vomiting, metabolic acidosis, Kussmaul respirations, and formaldehyde odor on the breath.

Ophthalmic disturbances that result include photophobia, blurred vision, the appearance of "snowflakes" in the visual field, hyperemia of the optic disks, retinal edema, and fixed dilated pupils. The accumulation of formaldehyde in the retina causes optic papillitis, retinal disease, and optic atrophy, all of which can result in blindness.

In patients who develop coma, convulsions, and apnea, the prognosis is poor. Death usually results from circulatory collapse or respiratory arrest.

Initial Management

Methanol ingestion results in an elevation in the osmolal gap because it alters the volume of water in serum. Osmolal gap is defined as the difference between measured and calculated osmolality. Early in a patient's clinical course (under 12–24 hours), before methanol has been completely metabolized, rapid diagnosis of methanol toxicity can be made on the basis of the presence of an osmolal gap (Table 32–8). Calculated osmolality is subtracted from measured osmolality and normally does not exceed 10

Table 32–8. CALCULATION OF ANION AND OSMOLAL GAPS

Anion gap = (Na + K) − (Cl + HCO_3)
  (Normal anion gap = 12–16 mmol/L)
Example: (135 + 4) − (102 + 22)
  = 139 − 124
  = 15
Elevated anion gap: (148 + 4) − (100 + 18)
  = 152 − 118
  = 34
Osmolal gap = Measured osmolality − calculated osmolality
  (Normal osmolal gap ≤ 10 mOsm/kg)
  Normal measured osmolality = 285–290 mOsm/kg
  Calculated osmolality = (2Na) + (glu/18) + (BUN/2.8)
Example: (2 × 138) + (108/18) + (14/2.8)
  = 276 + 6 + 5
  = 287
Elevated osmolal gap: >10 mOsm/kg
  = measured − calculated osm
  = 299 − 287
  = 12

mOsm/kg. Elevated osmolal gap gradually resolves as methanol is metabolized, toxic metabolites form, and an anion gap metabolic acidosis develops (Litovitz, 1986).

Under normal circumstances, the anion gap is 12 to 16 mmol/L. An elevated anion gap occurs later in the clinical course of patients with methanol ingestion because of retention of nonvolatile organic acids. Calculation of the osmolal and anion gap is useful in the initial management of patients in whom methanol ingestion is suspected because it identifies the presence of harmful substances, eliminating delay in treatment while specific laboratory levels are awaited.

Patients who appear in an obtunded or neurologically impaired condition are intubated to ensure an adequate airway and effective ventilation. Although the benefits of charcoal administration are unknown in methanol ingestions, charcoal is usually recommended.

Critical Care Management

Treatment of metabolic acidosis includes correction of pH and base deficit by administration of sodium bicarbonate. Although acidosis may be reversed, ocular damage associated with the toxic effects of methanol metabolism often persists.

Ethanol administration slows the production of formaldehyde and formic acid by blocking methanol metabolism, which promotes its excretion unchanged by the lungs and kidneys. Ethanol is administered in a 5% to 10% solution intravenously or orally in a 20% to 30% solution. A loading dose (0.8 g/kg) is administered intravenously in 10% dextrose solution over 30 minutes. Maintenance dosage is 130 mg/kg/hour of ethanol until a serum level of 100 mg/dL is achieved.

Dialysis enhances the elimination of methanol and its toxic byproducts and is indicated in patients with a serum level of 50 mg/dL and severe metabolic acidosis, or in the presence of neurologic or visual disturbances (Berkowitz et al., 1992). Higher doses of ethanol are required during hemodialysis because ethanol is easily dialyzed (Jacobson & McMartin, 1986). Maintenance doses of 250 to 350 mg/kg/hour are required to achieve and maintain the necessary serum level.

Patient monitoring during critical care includes evaluating arterial blood gases, blood alcohol level, and serum glucose level to assess the effectiveness of ethanol administration. Glucose is monitored closely because glycogen stores are depleted rapidly after methanol ingestion. Complications of dialysis such as infection and hypoglycemia must be recognized and treated early.

Ethanol

Ethanol is found in perfume, cologne, aftershave, mouthwash, and antiseptics. As little as 3 mg/kg (i.e., 5–10 oz mouthwash or 1–2 oz cologne) may be lethal in children (Litovitz, 1986). Ethanol is more likely to be ingested than some other substances because these products are used daily and are usually within reach of young children.

Pathogenesis

Ethanol is rapidly absorbed from the gastric tract, peaking in the serum 30 to 60 minutes after ingestion. A total of 90% is metabolized by the liver via oxidation. The other 2% to 10% is excreted by the kidney. Ethanol directly affects the reticular activating system, causing CNS depression.

Final Common Pathways

Neurologic Dysfunction. Ethanol overdose produces alteration in CNS function including dyskinesia, slurred speech, blurred or double vision, hypothermia, and depression. Significant intoxications are characterized by the presence of an osmolal gap (see Table 32–8). Ethanol metabolism causes impaired gluconeogenesis during the Krebs cycle. Profound hypoglycemia can ultimately lead to convulsions and coma in the pediatric patient, but the prognosis for children who ingest ethanol is generally good.

Initial Management

Gastric lavage may be recommended when CNS depression is present. Charcoal and forced diuresis are ineffective because the liver is the primary metabolic pathway. Cardiac and respiratory support are necessary in addition to the initiation of an intravenous infusion of 10% dextrose if hypoglycemia exists.

Critical Care Management

Supportive therapy with ongoing monitoring of vital functions until toxic effects subside is the primary focus of intensive care. Children who ingest ethanol require frequent serum glucose and ethanol determination and assessment for changes in mental status. Reassuring parents by noting signs of improvement in clinical status is helpful as the child progresses through the recovery period. Maintaining seizure precautions is necessary until symptoms of neurologic toxicity abate.

Isopropanol

Isopropyl alcohol is a clear, colorless solution, most commonly found in the form of rubbing alcohol. Parents may use isopropanol for sponging a child to reduce fever, and isolated cases have resulted in stupor or coma. Consequently, this practice is strongly discouraged.

Pathogenesis

The absorption of alcohol occurs after 30 minutes, usually from the ingestion or inhalation of rubbing alcohol or other household substance. The liver is responsible for about 80% of isopropanol metabolism. Hepatic detoxification of isopropanol results in acetone formation, which is primarily excreted by the kidney, and, to a lesser degree, by the lungs. As a myocardial depressant, acetone causes altered cardiac function with profound hypotension. Acetone acts as a CNS depressant and produces prolonged alteration in cerebral functioning. Impaired gastrointestinal system function results from the effects of isopropanol as a local irritant.

Final Common Pathways

Neurologic Dysfunction. Isopropanol toxicity produces CNS effects including depression, ataxia, confusion, stupor, and coma. The depression has been described to be 2 to 2 1/2 times more profound than in ethanol ingestions (Litovitz, 1986). Hyperglycemia, inconsistent pupil size, miosis, and depressed or absent deep tendon reflexes are other CNS manifestations characteristic of isopropanol toxicity.

Other Effects. Direct cardiac depression causing hypotension has been noted to be a poor prognostic sign. Gastrointestinal symptoms such as gastritis, abdominal pain, vomiting, and hematemesis usually occur as a result of isopropanol ingestion. Renal tubular necrosis, myopathy, and hemolytic anemia have also developed as a result of ingestion of isopropanol.

Initial Management

Airway protection is crucial to prevent aspiration should vomiting occur. Continuous gastric lavage is recommended because isopropanol is resecreted into the stomach and saliva. Lavage limits absorption and helps to decrease the local irritation in the lining of the stomach.

Critical Care Management

Therapy for isopropanol ingestion is fairly nonspecific, focusing mostly on general supportive care. Maintaining adequate ventilation and normotension is the primary goal. Care of children with isopropanol toxicity necessitates close monitoring for and correction of fluid and electrolyte imbalances.

Ethylene Glycol

Ethylene glycol is a colorless, odorless liquid found in permanent types of antifreezes and coolants. In the past, before its toxicity was known, it was used as a glycerine substitute in pharmaceuticals and as a preservative in juices. Ethylene glycol ingestions have been attributed to its bittersweet taste. Ethylene glycol poisonings usually occur as isolated instances.

Pathogenesis

Metabolism of ethylene glycol occurs predominantly in the liver and kidneys. It is rapidly absorbed, peaking in the bloodstream within 1 to 4 hours of ingestion. A small percentage is excreted unchanged in the urine (25%). Ingestion of an amount as small as 1.4 to 1.6 mL/kg can be lethal. The toxic byproduct of ethylene glycol metabolism, oxalic acid, chelates serum calcium and, as calcium oxalate crystals, is deposited in many tissues. Widespread injury to metabolic, cardiorespiratory, renal, and central nervous systems results.

Final Common Pathways

Multisystem organ dysfunction results from ingestion of ethylene glycol. Hyperemia of the CNS produces symptoms of inebriation such as ataxia, stupor, and coma. Other manifestations of neurologic dysfunction are nystagmus, depressed deep tendon reflexes, myoclonic jerks, and seizures. A result of calcium oxalate crystal deposition in the leptomeninges, vessel walls, and perivascular spaces is meningoencephalitis. Symptoms of neurologic injury during the first phase (30 minutes–12 hours) are slurred speech, ataxia, confusion, nausea, and vomiting in the absence of an ethanol odor on the breath. An elevated anion gap and oxalate crystalluria develop during this phase.

After the first 12 to 18 hours, the second stage is characterized by tachycardia, tachypnea, cyanosis, and pulmonary edema leading to cardiorespiratory failure. Myocardial and pulmonary dysfunction occur as a result of accumulation of the toxic intermediate and deposition of calcium oxalate crystals in the heart and lungs.

The third stage occurs 1 to 3 days after ingestion and is marked by flank pain, hematuria, and proteinuria as a result of oliguric renal failure. Damage to the renal tubules is thought to be caused by the byproducts glycolaldehyde, glycolic and glyoxylic acid, during ethylene glycol metabolism (Berkowitz et al., 1992).

Initial Management

Gastric lavage is indicated only in patients presenting within several hours of ingestion. Ventilatory support, if needed, is initiated immediately. Ethanol administration blocks ethylene glycol metabolism, thus allowing more time for the renal excretion of unchanged ethylene glycol. In cases when ethylene glycol concentration is higher than 50 mg/dL or renal failure exists, hemodialysis is recommended. Thiamine (0.25–0.5 mg/kg) and pyridoxine (1–2 mg/kg) administration are thought to decrease oxalate production. The prevention of oxalate crystal formation and subsequent deposition in the kidney are benefits of forced diuresis in the treatment of ethylene glycol intoxication.

Critical Care Management

Priorities for critical care management include meticulous assessment of intake and output to ensure adequate hydration despite forced diuresis. Care is aimed toward enhancing clearance of ethylene glycol and its metabolites. If hemodialysis is required, critical care is focused on the maintenance of normal hemodynamics and fluid and electrolyte balance during therapy. Ethanol administration is continued until the ethylene glycol level reaches zero.

Close monitoring of blood gas and calcium determinations are necessary for early detection and treatment of metabolic acidosis and hypocalcemia. Intravenous sodium bicarbonate (1–2 mEq/kg) is indicated because ethylene glycol is metabolized faster than methanol, resulting in a more profound metabolic acidosis. Calcium chloride (10–20 mg/kg/dose) is required to reverse the hypocalcemic effects of calcium oxalate precipitation in the serum.

NONPHARMACEUTICAL TOXINS: CAUSTICS

The incidence of caustic injuries to the esophagus has increased significantly since the 1960s when the use of concentrated liquid alkaline cleansers became popular. Substances that cause direct chemical burns to the esophageal mucosa are oxidizing and reducing agents, corrosives, and desiccants. They are usually strong acids or alkalis and can be found in most homes.

The majority of caustic burns to the esophagus are a result of sodium hydroxide or lye ingestions and most often occur in children younger than 5 years (Rothstein, 1986). Commercial ammonia is an alkali that causes ulcers or full-thickness burns to the esophagus after ingestion and irritation to the lungs or pulmonary edema after inhalation. Toilet bowl cleaners that contain sulfuric, hydrochloric, or phosphoric acid burn the oropharyngeal mucosa and are usually spit out on contact. Detergents and bleach are commonly ingested by children and produce local irritation without causing necrosis.

Pathogenesis

Esophageal burns produced by the ingestion of caustic agents are classified as first degree burns, which produce hyperemia and superficial desquamation; second degree burns, resulting in blisters and shallow mucosal ulcers; and third degree burns, producing deeper ulceration into the esophageal muscle. Caustics can affect a variety of regions along the gastrointestinal tract in addition to the esophagus because of the agents' low surface tension and ability to spread to a large surface area.

The location of the injury varies but can involve the cricopharyngeal area, impression of the aortic arch and left bronchus, lower esophageal sphincter, and stomach. Greater damage occurs in these locations because the ingested agent may become stagnated. Granular agents may imbed in the tissues of the oropharynx or proximal esophagus, whereas liquid agents produce damage along the entire esophagus to the stomach lining. When the lower esophageal sphincter is involved, the resting pressure decreases, causing reflux of the agent back and forth between the esophagus and stomach. This is usually followed by violent regurgitation.

Acids produce a coagulating necrosis in the stomach and esophagus, resulting in eschar formation. This limits deep penetration into the tissue, but leads to metabolic acidosis and pooling of acids in the stomach.

Final Common Pathways

Gastrointestinal Dysfunction. Alkaline agents usually affect the mouth, esophagus, and stomach. However, it is possible to have esophageal burns without oral involvement if the agent was swallowed rapidly. The alkali acts as a solvent on the lipoprotein lining, causing a liquefaction necrosis with inflammation and deep penetration into the mucosal, submucosal, and muscular layers of the esophagus and stomach. This is followed several days later by saponification of mucosal fats and proteins, thrombosis of adjacent blood vessels, cell necrosis, and tissue degeneration. Sloughing occurs 4 to 7 days after ingestion when bacteria invade the injured areas. The development of strictures can occur anytime between 21 and 42 days after exposure (Rothstein, 1986).

Initial Management

If the gag reflex is intact, the child can be given a small amount of milk or water to dilute the substance. An esophagoscopy may be indicated for the ingestion of a strong alkali or acid because the extent of injury cannot be determined by external examination. Activated charcoal should not be given because it can impede the view of the endoscopist.

Critical Care Management

Airway protection and general supportive care are the first priorities of critical care. Initiating IV therapy, not allowing the child to drink anything by mouth (NPO) for 12 to 24 hours, and observing closely to assess for drooling or the presence of lesions in the oral mucosa are also necessary in the early stages of hospitalization. The child who has sustained first degree burns must be assessed for the ability to tolerate liquids and slowly advanced to a regular diet. For children with second and third degree burns, the administration of antibiotics and antacids may be indicated. These children may also need parenteral nutrition and an endoscopy 2 to 3 weeks after the ingestion to evaluate the extent of esophageal dysmotility or stricture formation. Repeated esophageal dilations may be required if strictures develop (Rothstein, 1986). Long-term sequelae may require surgical replacement of the severely damaged esophagus.

NONPHARMACEUTICAL TOXINS: HYDROCARBONS

Fully 80% to 90% of hydrocarbon ingestions occur in children younger than 5 years largely because of the agents' pleasant scent and color (Litovitz, 1986). Hydrocarbons can be divided into four different categories: aliphatics, aromatics, alicyclics, and halogenated products. Aliphatic hydrocarbons are found in the form of petroleum distillates such as furniture polish, lamp oil, and lighter fluid. Aromatic hydrocarbons such as benzene, toluene, and xylene are found in glues, nail polish, paints, and paint removers. Alicyclic hydrocarbons are otherwise known as turpentine, cyclopropane, and cyclohexane. Halogenated hydrocarbons such as carbon tetrachloride, chloroform, methylene chloride, freon, and trichloromethane are particularly harmful because they produce various forms of systemic toxicity.

Pathogenesis

Aliphatic hydrocarbons produce minimal systemic toxicity but may cause pulmonary injury, depending on their viscosity and ease of aspiration. Alicyclics can produce pulmonary aspiration and direct CNS depression. Aromatic and halogenated hydrocarbons can cause cardiac arrhythmias in addition to aspiration and CNS depression (Table 32–9).

The risk of aspiration depends on the viscosity, surface tension, and volatility of the substance. The lower the viscosity and surface tension and the

Table 32–9. CLINICAL MANIFESTATIONS OF HYDROCARBON INGESTION

1. Pulmonary dysfunction
   Tachypnea, dyspnea, adventitious breath sounds, oxygen desaturation, cyanosis
2. CNS dysfunction
   Euphoria, agitation, restlessness, confusion, seizures, coma
3. Cardiovascular dysfunction
   Ventricular dysrhythmias (tachycardia, fibrillation)
4. Gastrointestinal dysfunction
   Oropharyngeal irritation, gastric irritation, vomiting, hematemesis
5. Hepatic dysfunction
   Elevated liver enzymes, hepatomegaly
6. Renal dysfunction
   Urine positive for albumin, cells, casts

higher the volatility, the greater the risk of aspiration (Henretig & Shannon, 1993). The ingestion of 0.2 mL of a low-viscosity hydrocarbon may produce chemical pneumonitis (Litovitz, 1986). Agents that are not aspirated easily but that cause systemic toxicity (i.e., the halogenated hydrocarbons) induce neurotoxicity. Benzene, in addition, is associated with aplastic and acute myeloblastic anemia because of its ability to injure bone marrow.

Final Common Pathways

Respiratory Dysfunction. The ingestion of a hydrocarbon causes irritation of the mouth, pharynx, and gastric mucosa and is usually followed by vomiting. Aspiration of these substances, which are lipid solvents, causes loss of surfactant leading to hydrocarbon pneumonitis within 12 to 24 hours after exposure (Henretig & Shannon, 1993). Alveolar instability and collapse produce atelectasis and pulmonary edema exhibited by tachypnea, dyspnea, cyanosis, and severe hypoxia. Physical examination is characterized by rales on auscultation, rhonchi, wheezing, or decreased breath sounds. Positive radiographic findings such as perihilar densities, basilar pneumonitis, atelectasis, and consolidation have been noted as early as 2 hours after ingestion (Litovitz, 1986). Other pulmonary complications include pneumatoceles, emphysema, pleural effusion, pneumothorax, pneumomediastinum, and pneumopericardium.

Neurologic Dysfunction. Halogenated and aromatic hydrocarbons are well absorbed by the gastrointestinal tract and pulmonary system. This enables them to cause direct CNS depression resulting in symptoms of changes in mental status. Patients can exhibit signs of narcosis, inebriation, or coma (Henretig & Shannon, 1993).

Cardiovascular Dysfunction. Inhalation of halogenated hydrocarbons has been known to cause fatal ventricular dysrhythmias resulting from myocardial sensitization to catecholamines. The pathophysiologic effect of inhalation of these substances causes increased ventricular irritability, predisposing the heart to ventricular fibrillation.

Gastrointestinal Dysfunction. All hydrocarbons produce symptoms of gastrointestinal distress including nausea, hematemesis, and diarrhea. Absorption varies, depending on the type of hydrocarbon. Aliphatic hydrocarbons have minimal absorption, whereas alicyclic, aromatic, and halogenated hydrocarbons can have significant gastrointestinal absorption.

Hepatic Dysfunction. Halogenated hydrocarbons have been known to produce centrilobular necrosis. Specific types include carbon tetrachloride and chloroform, which induce fatty degeneration of the liver, resulting in necrosis (Keaton, 1990).

Renal Dysfunction. Many halogenated hydrocarbons that produce hepatic dysfunction also cause renal tubular acidosis. Damage occurs directly to the proximal tubule and the loop of Henle from carbon tetrachloride. This leads to acute renal failure between 1 and 7 days after exposure (Keaton, 1990).

Initial Management

Because aliphatic hydrocarbons do not produce systemic toxicity, but are harmful when aspirated, ipecac administration and gastric lavage are usually contraindicated to reduce the risk of aspiration. Ipecac, when recommended, is preferable to lavage for hydrocarbons that must be removed because of their systemic toxicity (halogenated and aromatic).

Children with a history of hydrocarbon ingestion are monitored for signs of pulmonary aspiration, including coughing, choking, or gagging and oxygen desaturation on pulse oximetry. If these signs are present, a chest radiograph is necessary to evaluate potential parenchymal injury. Clothes are removed, copious bathing is done, and eye irrigation performed if necessary to reduce absorption by other routes.

Critical Care Management

Admission to the PICU is warranted in children with severe parenchymal injury and pneumonia. Care of these patients includes mechanical ventilation and close attention to maintenance of a patent airway, effective pulmonary toilet, and routine monitoring of arterial blood gases until symptoms of respiratory compromise subside. Pulmonary dysfunction and radiographic changes determine the degree of mechanical support required in the acute phase of parenchymal injury. Severe injuries may require the use of extracorporal membrane oxygenation.

SUMMARY

Children who have ingested pharmaceutical or nonpharmaceutical toxins are a critical care nursing challenge in the emergency department and the intensive care unit. The effects of a toxic ingestion may be systemic, involving many organ systems. Finely tuned collaboration between nurses, physicians, and poison experts is necessary for a positive outcome for these patients.

ACKNOWLEDGMENTS

The authors wish to acknowledge the assistance of Frances Gill, R.N., M.S.N., C.E.N., C.P.N., Advanced Practice Nurse, Department of Pediatric Surgery, A.I. DuPont Institute of the Nemours Foundation, Wilmington, Delaware; Maria Picciotti, Managing Director, The Poison Control Center serving Philadelphia, Pennsylvania; and Steven Selbst, M.D., Director, Emergency Department, The Children's Hospital of Philadelphia, and Associate Professor of Pediatrics, University of Pennsylvania School of Medicine, Philadelphia, Pennsylvania, for their assistance in the preparation of this chapter.

References

Anderson, K.D., et al. (1990). A controlled trial of corticosteroids in children with corrosive injury of the esophagus. *New England Journal of Medicine, 323*(10), 637–640.

Artman, M. & Boerth, M.D. (1983). Clonidine poisoning: A complex problem. *The American Journal Diseases of Childhood, 137,* 171–174.

Baker, M.D. (1986). Theophylline toxicity in children. *Journal of Pediatrics, 109,* 538–542.

Banner, W., Vernon, D.D., Ward, R.M., Sweeley, J.C., & Dean, J.M. (1989). Continuous arteriovenous hemofiltration in experimental iron intoxication. *Critical Care Medicine, 17*(11), 1187–1190.

Bateman, D.A., & Heagerty, M.C. (1989). Passive freebase cocaine ("crack") inhalation by infants and toddlers. *The American Journal of Diseases of Childhood, 143,* 25–27.

Berkowitz, I.D., Banner Jr. W., & Rogers, M.C. (1992). Poisoning and the critically ill child. In M. Rogers (Ed.). *Textbook of pediatric intensive care* (pp. 1290–1354). Baltimore: Williams & Wilkins.

Bertino, J.S., & Reed, M.D. (1986). Barbiturate and nonbarbiturate sedative intoxication in children. *Pediatric Clinics of North America, 33,* 703–722.

Boehnert, N.T., & Lovejoy, F.H. (1985). Value of the QRS duration vs. the serum drug level in predicting seizures and ventricular arrhythmias after an acute overdose of tricyclic antidepressants. *New England Journal of Medicine, 313,* 474–479.

Braden, N.J., Jackson, J.E., & Walson, P.D. (1986). Tricyclic antidepressant overdose. *Pediatric Clinics of North America, 33*(2), 287–297.

Brown, T.C.K., Barker, G.A., & Dunlop, M.E. (1973). The use of sodium bicarbonate therapy in the treatment of tricyclic antidepressant-induced arrhythmias. *Anaesthesia & Intensive Care, 1,* 203–210.

Burckart, G.J., & Ternullo, S.R. (1980). Management of anticonvulsant overdosages. *Clinical Toxicology Consultant, 2*(3), 88–99.

Byck, R. (1975). Drugs and the treatment of psychiatric disorders. In L.S. Goodman & A. Gilman (Eds.). *The pharmacologic basis of therapeutics* (5th ed., pp. 152–200). New York: McMillan Publishing Corp.

Cohen, D.J., Young, J.G., Nathanson, J.A., & Shaywitz, B.A. (1979). Clonidine in Tourette's syndrome. *Lancet, 2,* 551–553.

Covey, T.J. (1964). Ferrous sulfate poisoning: A review, case summaries and therapeutic regimen. *Journal of Pediatrics, 64,* 218–266.

Durbin, D. (1989). Whole bowel irrigation for iron ingestion. *Toxtalk, 2*(2), 2.

Emerman, C.L., et al. (1990). Risk of toxicity in patients with elevated theophylline levels. *Annals of Emergency Medicine, 19*(6), 643–648.

Emerman, C.L., Connors, A.F., & Burma, G.M. (1987). Level of consciousness as a predictor of complications following tricyclic overdose. *Annals of Emergency Medicine, 16*(3), 326–330.

Everson, G.W., Bertoccini, E.J., & O'Leary, J. (1991). Use of whole bowel irrigation in an infant following iron overdose. *American Journal of Emergency Medicine, 9,* 366–369.

Fazen, L.E., Lovejoy, F.H., & Crone, R.K. (1986). Acute poisoning in a children's hospital: A 2-year experience. *Pediatrics, 77*(2), 144–151.

Fiser, D.H., Moss, M., & Walker, W. (1990). Critical care for clonidine poisoning in toddlers. *Critical Care Medicine, 18*(10), 1124–1128.

Fleisher, G., & Ludwig, S. (Eds.). (1993). *Textbook of pediatric emergency medicine* (3rd ed.). Baltimore: Williams & Wilkins.

Frommer, D.A., Kulig, K.W., Marx, J.A., & Rumack, B. (1987). Tricyclic antidepressant overdose: A review. *Journal of the American Medical Association, 257*(4), 521–526.

Gaudreault, P., Wason, S., & Lovejoy, Jr., F.H. (1983). Acute pediatric theophylline overdose: A summary of 28 cases. *Journal of Pediatrics, 102,* 474–476.

Gaudreault, P., & Guay, J. (1986). Theophylline poisoning: Pharmacologic considerations and clinical management. *Medical Toxicology and Adverse Drug Exposures, 1,* 169–191.

Gay, G.R. (1982). Clinical management of acute and chronic cocaine poisoning. *Annals of Emergency Medicine, 11*(10), 562–572.

Gershman, H., & Steeper, J. (1991). Rate of clearance of ethanol from the blood of intoxicated patients in the emergency department. *Journal of Emergency Medicine, 9,* 307–311.

Gill, F. (1989). Pediatric poisonings. In C. Joy (Ed.). *Pediatric trauma nursing* (pp. 173–192). Rockville, MD: Aspen Publishers.

Goldfrank, L.R., Lewin, N.A., & Flomenbaum, N.E. (1990). Tricyclic antidepressants. In L.R. Goldfrank, N.E. Flomenbaum, N.A. Lewin, R.S. Weismanm, & M.A. Howland (Eds.). *Goldfrank's toxicologic emergencies* (4th ed., pp. 401–412). Norwalk, CT: Appleton & Lange.

Goldfrank, L.R., Osborn, H., & Bresnitz, E.A. (1990). Phenytoin and other anticonvulsants. In L.R. Goldfrank, N.E. Flomenbaum, N.A. Lewin, R.S. Weisman, & M.A. Howland (Eds.). *Goldfrank's toxicologic emergencies* (4th ed., pp. 327–335). Norwalk, CT: Appleton & Lange.

Gorman, R.L., et al. (1992). Initial symptoms as predictors of esophageal injury in alkaline corrosive ingestions. *American Journal of Emergency Medicine, 10*(3), 189–194.

Haddad, L.M., & Winchester, J.F. (Eds.). (1990). *Clinical management of poisoning and drug overdose* (2nd ed.). Philadelphia: W.B. Saunders.

Harvey, S.C. (1975). Hypnotics and sedatives. In L.S. Goodman, & A. Gilman (Eds.). *The pharmacologic basis of therapeutics* (5th ed., pp. 102–123). New York: Macmillan.

Henretig, F.M., & Shannon, M. (1993). Toxicologic emergencies. In G. Fleisher, S. Ludwig (Eds.). *Textbook of pediatric emergency medicine* (3rd ed., pp. 745–801). Baltimore: Williams & Wilkins.

Henretig, F.M., Karl, S.R., & Weintraub, W.H. (1983). Severe iron poisoning treated with enteral and intravenous deferoxamine. *Annals of Emergency Medicine, 12*(5), 306–309.

Henretig, F.M., & Temple, A.R. (1984). Acute iron poisoning in children. *Clinics in Laboratory Medicine, 4,* 575–586.

Herson, V.C., Schmitt, B.D., & Rumack, B.H. (1979). Magical thinking and imipramine poisoning in two school-aged children. *Journal of the American Medical Association, 1926–1927.*

Howard, R.E., Heuter, D.C., & Davis, G.J. (1985). Acute myocardial infarction following cocaine abuse in a young woman with normal coronary arteries. *Journal of the American Medical Association, 254,* 95–96.

Hunt, R.D., Minderaa, R.B., & Cohen, D.J. (1985). Clonidine benefits children with attention deficit disorder and hyperactivity: Report of a double-blind placebo–crossover therapeutic trial. *Journal of the American Academy of Child Psychiatry, 24,* 617–629.

Jacobsen, D., & McMartin, K.E.(1986). Methanol and ethylene glycol poisonings. Mechanism of toxicity, clinical course, diagnosis and treatment. *Medical Toxicology, 1,* 309–334.

Janes, J., & Routledge, P.A. (1992). Recent developments in the management of paracetamol (acetaminophen) poisoning. *Drug Safety, 7*(3), 170–177.

Keaton, B.F. (1990). Chlorinated hydrocarbons. In L.M. Haddad, &

J.F. Winchester (Eds.). *Clinical management of poisoning and drug overdose* (2nd ed., pp. 1216–1222). Philadelphia: W.B. Saunders.

Jay, M.S., Graham, C.J., & Flowers, C. (1989). Adolescent suicide attempters presenting to a pediatric facility. *Adolescence, 24*(94), 467–472.

Kogan, M.J., Verebey, K. G., DePace, A.C., Resnick, R.B., & Mule, S.J. (1977). Quantitative determination of benzoylecgonine and cocaine in human biofluids by gas-liquid chromatography. *Annals of Chemistry, 49*(13), 1965–1969.

Kulberg, A. (1986). Substance abuse: Clinical identification and management. *Pediatric Clinics of North America, 33*(2), 325–361.

Laussen, P., et al. (1991). Use of plasmapheresis in acute theophylline toxicity. *Critical Care Medicine, 19*(2), 288–290.

Lewin, N.A., & Howland, M.A. (1990). Antihypertensive agents: Including beta blockers and calcium channel blockers. In L.R. Goldfrank, N.E. Flomenbaum, N.A. Lewin, R.S. Weisman, & M.A. Howland (Eds.). *Goldfrank's toxicologic emergencies* (4th ed., pp. 369–377). Norwalk, CT: Appleton & Lange.

Lewis, R.K., & Paloucek, F.P. (1991). Assessment and treatment of acetaminophen overdose. *Clinical Pharmacy, 10*, 765–774.

Litovitz, T.L., Felberg, L., Soloway, R.A., Ford, M., & Geller, R. (1995). 1994 Annual Report of the American Association of Poison Control Centers National Data Collection System. *American Journal of Emergency Medicine, 13* (5), 551–597.

Litovitz, T.L., Schmitz, B.F., & Bailey, K.M. (1991). 1989 Annual Report of the American Association of Poison Control Centers National Data Collection System. *American Journal of Emergency Medicine, 8*, 394–442.

Litovitz, T.L. (1986). The alcohols: Ethanol, methanol, isopropanol, ethylene glycol. *Pediatric Clinics of North America, 33*(2), 311–323.

Lovejoy, F.H. (1990). Corrosive injury of the esophagus in children. *New England Journal of Medicine, 323* (10), 668–669.

Mack, R.B. (1988). Clonidine overdose—kingdom of the temporarily infirm. *Contemporary Pediatrics, 5*(10), 149–154.

Mann, J.B., & Sandberg, D.H. (1970). Therapy of sedative overdosage. *Pediatric Clinics of North America, 17*(3), 617–629.

Mann, K.V., Picciotti, M.A., Spevack, T.A., & Durbin, D.R. (1989). Management of acute iron overdose. *Clinical Pharmacy, 8*, 428–440.

Marshal, J.B., & Forker, A.D. (1982). Cardiovascular effects of tricyclic antidepressant drugs: Therapeutic usage, overdose, and management of complications. *American Heart Journal, 103*, 401–414.

Minor, R.L., Scott, B.D., Brown, D.D., & Winniford, M.D. (1991). Cocaine-induced myocardial infarction in patients with normal coronary arteries. *Annals of Internal Medicine, 115*, 797–806.

Neuvonen, P.J., & Elonen, E. (1980). Effect of activated charcoal on absorption and elimination of phenobarbitone, carbamazepine, and phenylbutazone in man. *European Journal of Clinical Pharmacology, 17*, 51–57.

Osborn, H., Goldfrank, L.R., Howland, M.A., Bresnitz, E.A., & Kirstien, R.H. (1990). Barbiturates and other sedative-hypnotics. In L.R. Goldfrank, et al. (Eds.). *Goldfrank's toxicologic emergencies,* (4th ed., pp. 449–463). Norwalk, CT: Appleton & Lange.

Pentel, P.R., & Benowitz, N.L. (1986). Tricyclic antidepressant poisoning: Management of arrhythmias. *Medical Toxicology, 1*, 101–121.

Pettit, J.M., & Biggs, J.T. (1977). Tricyclic antidepressant overdoses in adolescent patients. *Pediatrics, 59*, 283–287.

Roberts, J.R., & Zink, B. J. (1990). Clonidine. In L.M. Haddad, & J.F. Winchester (Eds.). *Clinical management of poisoning and drug overdose* (2nd ed., pp. 1351–1359). Philadelphia: W.B. Saunders.

Rothstein, F.C. (1986). Caustic injuries to the esophagus in children. *Pediatric Clinics of North America, 33*(3), 665–689.

Rumack, B.H. (1986). Acetaminophen overdose in children and adolescents. *Pediatric Clinics of North America, 33*(3), 691–701.

Seger, D. (1990). Phenytoin and other anticonvulsants. In L.M. Haddad, & J.F. Winchester (Eds.). *Clinical management of poisoning and drug overdose* (2nd ed., pp. 887–891). Philadelphia: W.B. Saunders.

Selbst, S., & Henretig, F.M. (1985). Acute treatment of toxicologic emergencies. *Clinics in Emergency Medicine, 7*, 199–248.

Seneff, M., et al. (1990). Acute theophylline toxicity and the use of esmolol to reverse cardiovascular instability. *Annals of Emergency Medicine, 19*(6), 671–673.

Shannon, M. (1988). Clinical toxicity of cocaine adulterants. *Annals of Emergency Medicine, 7*(11), 1243–1247.

Shannon, M., Lacouture, P.G., Roa, J., & Woolf, A. (1989). Cocaine exposure among children seen at a pediatric hospital. *Pediatrics, 83*(3), 337–342.

Steinhart, C.M., & Pearson-Shaver, A.L. (1988). Poisoning. *Critical Care Clinics, 4*(4), 845–872.

Tenenbein, M. (1986). Pediatric toxicology: Current controversies and recent advances. *Current Problems in Pediatrics, 16*(4), 185–233.

Tenenbein, M. (1987). Whole bowel irrigation in iron poisoning. *Journal of Pediatrics, 111*, 142–145.

Tenenbein, M., Wiseman, N., & Yatscoff, R.W. (1991). Gastrotomy and whole bowel irrigation in iron poisoning. *Pediatric Emergency Care, 7* (5), 286–288.

Thorstrand, C. (1976). Clinical features in poisoning by tricyclic antidepressants with special reference to the ECG. *Acta Medica Scandinavica, 199*, 337–344.

Vernon, D.D., Banner, W., Garrett, J.S., & Dean, J.M. (1991). Efficacy of dopamine and norepinephrine for treatment of hemodynamic compromise in amitriptyline intoxication. *Critical Care Medicine, 19* (4), 544–549.

Wason, S., Baker, R.C., Carolan, P., Seigel, R., & Druckenbrod, R.W. (1992). Carbamazepine overdose—the effects of multiple dose activated charcoal. *Clinical Toxicology, 30*, (1), 39–48.

Weaver, D.F., Camfield, P., & Fraser, A. (1988). Massive carbamazepine overdose: Clinical and pharmacologic observations in five episodes. *Neurology, 38*, 755–759.

Wiley, J.F. II, Wiley, C.C., Torrey, S.B., & Henretig, F.M. (1990). Clonidine poisoning in young children. *Journal of Pediatrics, 116*(4), 654–658.

Winchester, J.F. (1990). Barbiturates, methaqualone, and primidone. In L.M. Haddad, & J.F. Winchester (Eds.). *Clinical management of poisoning and drug overdose* (pp. 718–729). Philadelphia: W.B. Saunders Co.

Woodbury, D.M., & Fingl, E. (1975). Drugs effective in the therapy of the epilepsies. In L.S. Goodman, & A. Gilman (Eds.). *The pharmacologic basis of therapeutics,* (5th ed., pp. 201–226). New York: Macmillan.

CHAPTER *33*

Resuscitation of Infants and Children

MARTHA A. Q. CURLEY
NEIL EAD

In 1986 the American Heart Association (AHA) celebrated the silver anniversary of contemporary cardiopulmonary resuscitation (CPR) by publishing the third edition of the *Standards and Guidelines for Cardiopulmonary Resuscitation and Emergency Cardiac Care.* Within this publication, for the first time ever, advanced pediatric life support received its own section. Not only did this publication present the needs of the pediatric patient requiring resuscitation as different from those of the adult, it also created the framework for the pediatric advanced life support (PALS) programs, which are now available throughout the country. The focus of PALS is on prevention of pediatric arrest, early recognition of the distressed pediatric patient, and a maturational approach to patient care management.

Pediatric resuscitation offers a challenge to the pediatric critical care nurse. Participating in resuscitation attempts requires specialized knowledge and skill. Consideration of the potential impact of the child's developmental maturity integrated with nursing's humanistic approach to supporting families in crises are vital aspects of care.

This chapter will begin with a discussion of the final common pathways that lead to cardiopulmonary arrest in infants and children. Resuscitation research that influenced the PALS standards will be discussed. The standards for pediatric advanced life support will be reviewed, emphasizing nursing care issues.

FINAL COMMON PATHWAYS

Cardiac arrest resulting from primary cardiac dysfunction is a rare occurrence in the pediatric population (O'Rourke, 1986). Primary cardiac arrest, the most frequent type of arrest in the adult population, produces an acute loss of perfusion at a time of relative homeostasis. Thus, most organs are well perfused and functioning normally immediately before the event. In contrast, most pediatric cardiac arrests occur after a prolonged disruption in homeostasis produced by the final common pathways of *respiratory failure* and/or *cardiovascular collapse.*

In a secondary cardiac arrest, widespread organ dysfunction occurs not only during the arrest but also during the period preceding the arrest. Pediatric resuscitation attempts are often very difficult and prolonged because the precipitating events such as a prolonged period of hypoxemia, acidosis, and organ

963

hypoperfusion must be corrected, and ongoing secondary organ dysfunction must be reversed. Secondary cardiac arrest also predisposes patients to severe or irreversible organ damage, for example, poor neurologic outcome and/or multisystem organ failure (MSOF).

Respiratory failure is imminent when the respiratory system is unable to fulfill its role in gas exchange. The etiologies of respiratory failure are varied and result from both intrinsic and/or extrinsic factors. Any shock state can contribute to insufficient tissue perfusion and cardiovascular collapse. In contrast, there is a small segment of the pediatric population who suffers from significant cardiac disease such as complex congenital heart disease (CHD), post–cardiac surgery myocardial/conduction system dysfunction, myocarditis, and cardiomyopathy. These children may present with a primary cardiac arrest or "sudden cardiac death" (Silka, 1991).

DIVERSE ETIOLOGIES

One of the major features that distinguishes pediatric patients suffering cardiac arrest from adults is that the etiologies in children are diverse. An extensive data base from which to draw conclusions about the distribution of etiologies in pediatric secondary cardiac arrest does not exist.

Zaritsky and coworkers (1987) studied 113 arrests in 93 children in a large regional referral center. Most patients were younger than 1 year of age and had at least one underlying chronic disease. Fifty-three patients experienced cardiac arrest and 40 patients experienced respiratory arrest. Eighteen percent of the sample suffered primary cardiac arrest resulting from congenital heart disease. Seventeen percent suffered secondary cardiac arrest due to respiratory disease. Table 33–1 contains the overall distribution of etiology of cardiac arrest in this study. It should be noted that because data were collected in a pediatric cardiac referral center, high numbers of children with CHD were included and thus the population may not truly reflect the distribution of cardiac arrest in the general pediatric population.

Eisenberg and coworkers (1983) compiled data on 119 cardiac arrests in children younger than 18 years who presented to the emergency department. All pediatric nontrauma patients with asystole (77%), idioventricular rhythm (11%), and/or ventricular fibrillation (9%) were included. As illustrated in Table 33–1, the primary etiologies of cardiac arrest in this population were different from those occurring in the inpatient setting. Another interesting finding in this study was that during the same time period, only 7% of pediatric cardiac arrests patients were discharged alive compared with 20% of adult cardiac arrests patients. The vast majority of adult survivors (95%) presented in ventricular fibrillation (VF), a primary cardiac dysrhythmia amenable to therapy.

O'Rourke's data (1986) reporting the etiology of cardiac arrest in children presenting to the emer-

Table 33–1. COMPARISON OF IN-HOSPITAL AND OUT-OF-HOSPITAL ARRESTS

Etiology	In-hospital		Out-of-hospital			
	Zaritsky (n = 69)		Eisenberg (n = 119)		O'Rourke (n = 34)	
Respiratory	14	20%	11	9%	3	9%
Primary cardiac	26	38%	9	7%		
Issues RT prematurity	1	2%				
Hematologic	6	9%				
Oncologic	1	2%	4	3%		
Neurologic	5	7%	5	4%		
Trauma	5	7%			10	29%
SIDS			38	32%	10	29%
Near drowning			26	22%	5	15%
Sepsis	9	13%			4	12%
Overdose			4	3%		
Burns/smoke inhalation			2	2%	2	6%
Anaphylaxis			2	2%		
Endocrine			1	1%		
Other—unknown	2	3%	17	14%		

Data from Zaritsky, A., Nadkarni, V., Getson, P., & Kuehl, K. (1987). CPR in children. *Annals of Emergency Medicine*, 16(10), 1107–1111. Eisenberg, M., Bergner, L., & Hallstrom, A. (1983). Epidemiology of cardiac arrest and resuscitation in children. *Annals of Emergency Medicine*, 12(11), 672–674. O'Rourke, P. (1986). Outcome of children who are apneic and pulseless in the emergency room. *Critical Care Medicine*, 14(5), 466–468.

gency department in a pulseless apneic state is somewhat different than that of Eisenberg and coworkers' (1983) study. Trauma was the most frequent underlying cause of cardiac arrest in her sample (see Table 33–3). Second only to trauma was sudden infant death syndrome (SIDS). SIDS accounts for 8,000 infant deaths per year in the United States. Some hypothesize that SIDS is the result of a primary cardiac arrest (Valdez-Dapena, 1985); however, this has not been substantiated by research.

Unlike most pediatric arrests, arrests that occur in the pediatric intensive care unit (PICU) are seldom unanticipated, are commonly nonrespiratory in origin, and occur in spite of aggressive support (Von Seggern et al., 1986). Von Seggern and coworkers (1986) described patients requiring a great deal of nursing support before the arrest; nurse-patient staffing ratio was greater than 1:1. The number of medical versus surgical patients was approximately the same. The largest single group requiring resuscitation were patients with cardiovascular disease. Level of consciousness was identified as an important factor in predicting 24-hour outcome; 76% of patients alert before CPR survived at least 24 hours compared with only 30% of patients comatose before CPR.

Respiratory Arrest Versus Cardiopulmonary Arrest

Regardless of the setting, one dramatic finding in pediatric resuscitation research is that the type of arrest significantly influences outcome. Although the etiologies of pediatric cardiac arrest vary across settings, the outcomes are equally dismal. The survival rate and long-term neurologic outcome for children who suffer pure respiratory arrest with timely intervention are dramatically better than those of secondary cardiac arrest, even when intervention is rapidly initiated.

Lewis and coworkers (1983) conducted a 1-year prospective study of 105 resuscitation attempts in 74 children in all inpatient areas of a large midwestern children's hospital. Outcome was correlated with the location of the arrest, level of monitoring at the time of the arrest, and type of arrest. The type of arrest was the only variable that significantly influenced outcome. They reported a 25% mortality rate for children who experienced a respiratory arrest and an 87% mortality rate when cardiac arrest occurred.

Zaritsky and coworkers (1987) reported similar findings: a 33% mortality rate in patients who experienced a respiratory arrest compared with a 91% mortality rate in those who experienced a secondary cardiac arrest. The poor outcomes were not influenced by the well-coordinated resuscitation team available in the large tertiary center. In addition, no significant relationship was found between outcome and the location of the inpatient arrest, laboratory values, or demographics variables.

The etiology of cardiac arrest also influences outcome. Friesen and coworkers (1982) reported that respiratory failure accounted for most of the cardiac arrests occurring in both the inpatient and outpatient setting. Cardiac arrest resulting from respiratory failure carried a 79% mortality rate, whereas none of their patients survived cardiac arrest resulting from trauma or sepsis.

Factors That May Improve Outcome

Although the outcome for pediatric patients who suffer cardiac arrest is grim, existing research has identified a number of factors that may improve outcome. These factors include prevention, early recognition, and monitoring of children in distress (Friesen et al., 1982).

Prevention of a pulseless state *is* critical. Earlier application of both basic and advanced life support to prevent a pulseless state has been related to improved outcome (Torphy et al., 1984). In addition, selected subgroups in the pediatric population such as submersion victims have experienced improved survival when prompt intervention is available (Quan et al., 1990).

One major factor influencing outcome in the pediatric population that has probably received the least amount of empiric review is the role nurses play in the recognition of the pre-arrest state. Nurses play a critical role by recognizing the *red flags* of respiratory distress and cardiovascular compromise that are present in the clinically unstable pediatric patient. The mark of a true nursing expert is skill in assessing these *red flags*, anticipating deterioration in patient status, and advocating for changes in collabo-

rative management when early signs of distress are evident (Curley, 1989).

RED FLAGS OF COMPENSATION

Nurses, by early recognition of the pre-arrest state, can significantly affect patient outcome. This requires expertise in recognizing the *red flags* of *compensation* to respiratory distress and cardiovascular collapse that are present in the clinically unstable pediatric patient. Many believe that "children deteriorate rapidly" but, in reality, they are exquisitely capable of compensating until they can no longer support vital organ function.

Even if vital signs are within the normal range for the patient's age, if they are incongruent with the child's clinical need they are considered red flags. Faster heart rates can be expected when, for example, the patient is active, anxious, anemic, dehydrated, febrile, or in pain. Faster respiratory rates can be expected, for example, in the active, febrile child or when there is significant past medical history of chronic pulmonary disease. Faster heart and respiratory rates indicate that there is a need for increased cardiac output or minute ventilation. Rates incongruent with need are considered red flags.

Red flags of respiratory distress are listed in Table 33–2. Tachypnea, a salient symptom, occurs as the patient attempts to maintain minute ventilation when tidal volume is compromised. Retractions become more pronounced when lung compliance continues to decrease within the highly compliant chest wall of the pediatric patient.

Airway problems frequently precipitate pediatric arrests because pathologic processes that cause airway narrowing exponentially compromise gas flow within the airway. Patients position themselves to maximize their airway; they sit up, lean forward, and extend their neck. Inspiratory stridor is present with upper airway disease, whereas wheezing may be heard on auscultation in lower airway disease. Inspiratory times are prolonged in upper airway disease; the opposite is true in lower airway disease.

Table 33–2. RESPIRATORY DISTRESS—RED FLAGS

Tachypnea
Mechanics of breathing
  Retractions
  Nasal flaring
  Head bobbing
  Grunting on exhalation
  Air entry: Stridor/wheezing
Change in breath sounds
  Prolonged inspiratory time—stridor
  Prolonged expiratory time—wheezing
Late signs
  Skin color changes—dusky/cyanotic
  Apnea/irregular respirations
  Change in level of consciousness/activity
  Bradycardia

Grunting on expiration occurs as an infant attempts to maintain functional residual capacity (FRC).

Changes in the patient's level of consciousness and/or activity depend upon the patient's primary alteration in gas exchange. With hypoxia the patient usually becomes restless, agitated, and irritable. Hypercapnea usually produces opposite symptoms; the patient usually becomes somnolent and lethargic, has decreased muscle tone, loses interest in the environment, or even more ominous in a toddler, is less reactive to a parent's departure.

Late signs of respiratory distress often include apnea, decreasing level of consciousness and/or activity, followed by bradycardia. Skin color changes also occur and include a pale, dusky, or cyanotic appearance. Much energy is expended trying to maintain oxygenation and ventilation. Infants, especially, tire and exhibit periods of apnea.

Arterial blood gases (ABGs) that are incongruent with the patient's clinical presentation serve to quantify the patient's ominous status. When a patient begins to tire, $Paco_2$ levels climb despite tachypnea and Pao_2 falls despite increasing Fio_2. Pulse oximeters have facilitated rapid detection and intervention during transient periods of arterial desaturation. The $ETco_2$ increases with the $Paco_2$, then precipitously falls as pulmonary perfusion becomes compromised (Curley & Thompson, 1990).

Red flags of cardiovascular compromise include tachycardia and alterations in perfusion to the skin, brain, and kidneys (Table 33–3). Tachycardia, the first sign of a stressed cardiac state, serves to maintain cardiac output when stroke volume is compromised by inadequate preload, increased afterload, or myocardial dysfunction. The smaller the child, the more reliant upon heart rate to maintain cardiac output. Blood pressure is usually not helpful as an early sign of deterioration because increased systemic vascular resistance (SVR) maintains blood pressure when the cardiac output is decreased.

Hypotension is not evident until approximately 25% of the intravascular volume is lost. The estimated circulating blood volume in children represents approximately 8% of the body weight or 80 mL/kg. For example, a 5-kg infant may be expected to have a circulating blood volume of 400 mL; 8% of 5 kg is equal to 400 g or mLs (1 g = 1 mL). A 25% blood loss in a 5 kg infant is 100 mL.

Early symptoms of low cardiac output are the signs of increased SVR and are best assessed in end-organ perfusion of the skin, brain, and kidney. Signs include capillary refill longer than 2 seconds; a mottled or marblized skin appearance; an increased core-to-skin temperature gradient; an altered level of consciousness; a worried appearance; and decreased urine output, less than 1 mL/kg in an infant or 0.5 mL/kg in a child older than 2 years.

Infants' temperatures drop, and serum glucose and calcium levels fall when infants are stressed. Late symptoms of cardiovascular collapse include decreased response to pain, flaccid muscle tone, hypotension, and bradycardia. These symptoms are directly related to progressive intracellular acidosis and hypoxia.

COLLABORATIVE MANAGEMENT

The alphabetical approach to resuscitation is the same for all age groups, but pediatric resuscitation requires an emphasis on support of ventilation as well as an awareness of the influence of maturation on respiratory and cardiovascular system performance. The goal is to restore stability as soon as possible by reestablishing vital organ perfusion and oxygenation, especially to the brain. Neurologic outcome appears to be directly related to the child's response to initial resuscitation efforts rather than post-resuscitation brain resuscitation. Postischemic reperfusion injuries, a progressive state of cerebral hypoperfusion after a global or incomplete ischemic insult, is a poorly defined phenomenon in infants and children (Rogers & Kirsch, 1989).

It is essential to note that very little clinical research on resuscitation of pediatric patients exists. This is largely because the overall incidence of cardiopulmonary arrest in infants and children is low. Much of the data that guides pediatric practice has been extrapolated from resuscitation studies with adult patients or is derived from animal models. Many studies are flawed by poor controls and/or small sample size. As a result, the current standards in pediatric resuscitation are derived from the best information available. As new research becomes available, revisions to the existing standards can be anticipated. Standards create controversy; controversy provides the foundation for clinical research.

Airway Management and Breathing

Positioning is the first step in airway management. Infants should be placed in the "sniffing position" by a head tilt–chin lift or jaw thrust maneuver that brings the angle of the chin up 90 degrees from the

Table 33–3. CARDIOVASCULAR COLLAPSE—RED FLAGS

Tachycardia
Altered perfusion
  Skin
    Prolonged capillary refill
    Increased core to skin temperature gradient
  Brain
    Altered level of consciousness/activity
    Decreased response to parents
    "Worried" appearance
  Kidneys
    Decreased urine output
Decrease in pulse quality
Late signs
  Decreased response to pain
  Flaccid tone
  Hypotension
  Bradycardia

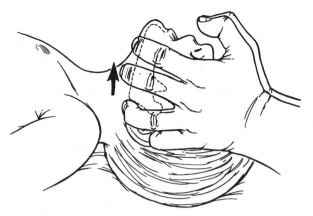

Figure 33–1 ● ● ● ● ● ●

Opening the airway with the jaw-thrust maneuver. The airway is opened by lifting the angle of the mandible. The rescuer uses two or three fingers of each hand to lift the jaw while other fingers guide the jaw upward and outward. (Reproduced with permission. © *Textbook of Pediatric Advanced Life Support*, 1994. Copyright American Heart Association.)

bed (Figs. 33–1 and 33–2). This prevents hyperextension of the airway and allows for maximal ventilation. In contrast to the neutral head position in the infant, a child's head is positioned slightly further back.

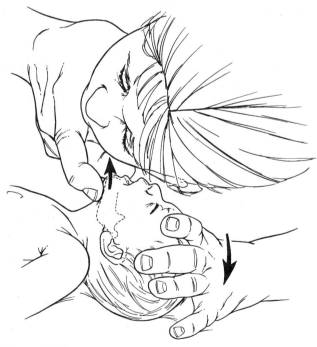

Figure 33–2 ● ● ● ● ● ●

Opening the airway with the head tilt—chin lift maneuver. One hand is used to tilt the head, extending the neck. The index finger of the rescuer's other hand lifts the mandible outward by lifting on the chin. Note that the angle of the chin is 90 degrees from the bed. Head tilt should not be performed if cervical spine injury is suspect. (Reproduced with permission. © *Textbook of Pediatric Advanced Life Support*, 1994. Copyright American Heart Association.)

After the airway is opened, two slow breaths with a pause in between are recommended (Melker, 1986). Two slow breaths provide long inspiratory times and low flow rates, keeping the peak inspiratory pressures (PIPs) less than the opening pressure of the lower esophageal sphincter, which is 15 cmH_2O in the anesthetized child (Moynihan et al., 1993). This technique promotes lung inflation while decreasing the risk of gastric distention. When pressures greater than 15 cmH_2O are necessary to adequately ventilate the patient, the Sellick maneuver, pressure over the larynx on the anterolateral surface of the cricoid cartilage, can be used to collapse the esophagus against the cervical vertebrae (Fig. 33–3). This maneuver may prevent aspiration in the unintubated patient.

Healthy lungs of infants and children are normally very compliant and accept large tidal volumes (V_T) at low pressures. The delivered V_T is the amount needed to provide normal chest excursion; usually 7 to 10 mL/kg. Care is taken because most pediaric resuscitation bags are capable of delivering volumes in excess of the individual needs of the patient. Self-inflating bags deliver volume until the pressure exceeds that of the pop-off valve, which is usually 30 to 35 cmH_2O. Self-inflating bags only deliver an FiO_2 of 0.5 to 0.6 unless a gas reservoir is present. In contrast, anesthesia bags refill with fresh gas, thus delivering an FiO_2 of 1.0. Anesthesia bags are also capable of a wider range of PIPs and positive end-expiratory pressure (PEEP) and thus are useful in patients with poor lung compliance. Use of excessive pressures places the patient at risk for barotrauma. Therefore, anesthesia bags should be operated by experienced personnel with pressures monitored and

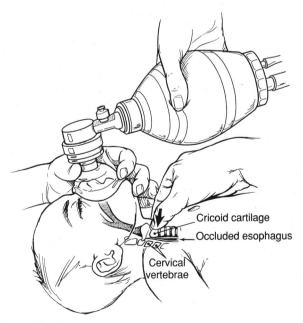

Figure 33–3 ● ● ● ● ● ●

Cricoid pressure (Sellick maneuver). (Reproduced with permission. © *Textbook of Pediatric Advanced Life Support*, 1994. Copyright American Heart Association.)

controlled using an attached pressure gauge and gas escape valve.

Children have a greater propensity for air swallowing when distressed. This, along with increased tracheal-esophageal proximity, places the child at risk for gastric distension during positive pressure bag-valve-mask ventilation. In addition to the risk of pulmonary aspiration, gastric distension elevates the diaphragm, compromising lung expansion and tidal volume. Gastric decompression, using the largest nasogastric tube that the nares can accommodate comfortably, should be accomplished early in the resuscitation effort.

Early endotracheal intubation is recommended because it secures the airway, facilitates the use of PEEP, and provides a route for the administration of select resuscitation drugs when venous access is delayed. Anatomic differences make endotracheal tube (ETT) intubation difficult (see Chapter 10). Until experienced personnel are available, adequate ventilation can usually be provided by using an appropriate-size resuscitation bag and mask; a correct size mask provides an airtight seal and minimizes rebreathing. Because of the close proximity of the cricoid cartilage to the vocal cords, a cricothyrotomy is always considered as a last resort especially in children younger than 12.

Various methods for determining correct ETT size have been proposed. Appropriate ETT size often approximates the diameter of the patient's little or fifth finger, but this method is somewhat inaccurate and does not offer an opportunity to anticipate equipment needs before a patient's arrival in the emergency department or critical care unit. The formula *age in years plus 16 divided by four* also accurately predicts correct ETT size.

Clearly, the ETT size chosen should be the largest that adequately ventilates the lungs while fitting comfortably through the glottis and the cricoid cartilage. Smaller sizes increase airway resistance, result in excessive air leaks, plug easily with secretions, and by themselves may ultimately cause respiratory failure. The nurse may anticipate anatomic variation by choosing three ETT sizes (one larger and one smaller than the calculated size).

Stylets are used to provide rigidity and direct the tip of the ETT up through the glottic opening. To avoid airway trauma, caution is taken to ensure that the stylet does not extend beyond the tip of the ETT during intubation.

Confirmation of ETT placement is achieved by auscultating breath sounds high along the midaxillary line. Because of the thin chest wall and subsequent prevalence of referred breath sounds, slight change in the pitch of the patient's breath sounds may be the only indication of right mainstem intubation in infants and children. Right mainstem intubation is a frequent problem in the pediatric population because of the standard length of ETTs and the variation in sizes of children. Additional clinical indicators of correct ETT placement include the presence of condensation in the ETT on expiration and symmetric chest excursion with manual ventilation. On chest radiographs, the ETT should be 1 to 2 cm above the carina or halfway between the carina and clavicles; the carina approximates the level of the fourth rib; therefore, the tube should approximate the level of the third.

Once intubated, the ETT is held firmly in place, and markings on the ETT in relation to the nares or lip line are noted while the tube is taped. The head should be positioned at midline or maintained in a neutral position, particularly during radiographic determination of placement. Excessive flexion of the patient's neck may force uncuffed ETTs down onto the carina, and extension of the neck or rotation of the head may dislodge the ETT completely.

Continuous assessment of the adequacy of ventilation is always a priority. The magnitude and duration of hypoxia sustained during a period of respiratory distress or arrest adversely affect the myocardium, ultimately influencing myocardial response to resuscitation if cardiac arrest develops. Spontaneous breaths are supported with humidified oxygen at an FiO_2 of 1.0.

Short-term hyperventilation may be advantageous in the initial management of hypercapnea, and it provides a compensatory alkalosis in the patient with metabolic acidosis. However, sustained hyperventilation should be avoided because it may compromise cerebral blood flow and promote cerebral anoxia.

Circulation

In the event of cardiac arrest, the primary goal in resuscitation is restoration of hemodynamic stability. Following stabilization of the airway and delivery of the initial breaths, pulses are immediately assessed to determine the need for cardiac compressions. This section expands upon the traditional concept of circulation to include measures focused to improve tissue perfusion: vascular access and the administration of intravenous fluids, then resuscitation medications.

Cardiac Compressions

Initial recommendations for hand placement during cardiac compressions came from postmortem anatomic studies that located the heart at midsternum in infants and at the lower sternum in older children (Fetterolf & Gittings, 1911; Thaler, 1963). It was not until much later that these data were questioned. Because the data were derived from cadaver models, the lungs were deflated. Positive pressure ventilation during resuscitation locates both the heart and the diaphragm lower in the chest.

Orlowski (1984), Finholt and coworkers (1986), and Phillips & Zideman (1986) studied anteroposterior chest radiographs and right-sided cardiac angiography in patients of all age groups. These studies demonstrated that the geometric center of the heart lies under the lower third of the sternum in patients of all ages. In addition Orlowski (1984) studied children

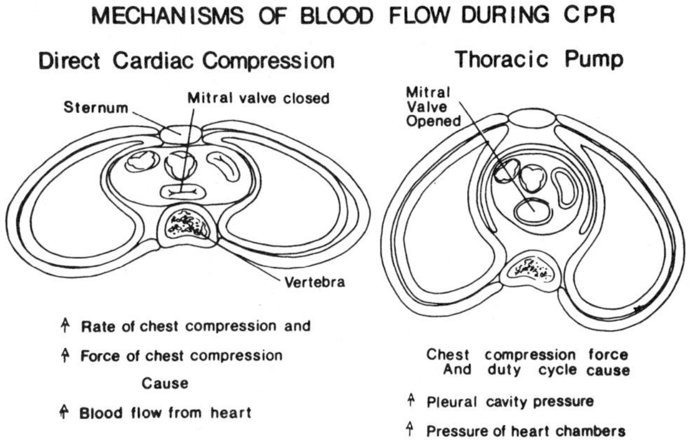

MECHANISMS OF BLOOD FLOW DURING CPR

Direct Cardiac Compression   **Thoracic Pump**

↑ Rate of chest compression and

↑ Force of chest compression

Cause

↑ Blood flow from heart

Chest   compression force
And duty cycle cause

↑ Pleural cavity pressure

↑ Pressure of heart chambers

Figure 33–4 ● ● ● ● ● ●

Mechanism of blood flow during CPR; direct cardiac compression versus thoracic pump. (From Schleien, O.L., Berkowitz, I.D., Traysman, R., & Rogers, M.C. (1989). Controversial issues in cardiopulmonary resuscitation. *Anesthesiology*, 71(1), 133–149.)

between 1 month and 3 years of age who sustained cardiac arrest while they were invasively monitored in the PICU. Orlowski found that in every patient (when the patient served as the control and with compressions performed in random sequence) compressions performed over the lower third of the sternum resulted in significantly better systolic and mean arterial pressures and stroke volumes than occurred with compressions of the sternum at other locations. These studies are the basis for the recommendation that cardiac compressions be performed in infants by the middle and ring finger, one finger's width below the nipple line and, by the heel of one hand in children, one finger's width above the xiphoid process (AHA, 1986).

Cardiac compression rates are recommended based upon studies that have demonstrated a relationship between the faster rates and higher mean arterial pressures, cardiac index, and cerebral blood flow (Paraskos, 1986). The compression to delivered breath ratio is 5 to 1. It is imperative that the patient receive the delivered breaths by synchronizing ventilation with the upstroke of compressions. Regardless of whether the patient is intubated, a pause at the end of every fifth compression allows the delivery of a breath to facilitate optimal ventilation. Frequent assessment of breath sounds and pulse quality is crucial.

Studies in adults indicate that cardiac compression provides only 25% to 30% of the normal cardiac output, 25% to 33% of the normal mean arterial pressure, and 5% to 10% of the normal cortical blood flow for about the first five minutes of CPR (Koehler & Michael, 1985). Similar data with infants and children do not exist. Considering this, there are many studies investigating the mechanism of blood flow and techniques to improve blood flow during CPR. However, controversy continues regarding the precise mechanism of blood flow during closed chest cardiac compression. It remains unclear whether blood flow occurs as a result of direct compression of

the heart between the sternum and the vertebral column (the cardiac pump theory), or by increased intrathoracic pressure with subsequent extrathoracic arterial to venous pressure gradient caused by chest compressions (the thoracic pump theory), or a combination of both mechanisms (Fig. 33–4).

Studies investigating the duty cycle or the ratio, stated as a percent, of the duration of the compression phase to that of the whole compression-relaxation cycle and the role of sequential opening and closure of cardiac valves during CPR provide support for the cardiac pump theory (Fig. 33–5). The cardiac pump theory may be more important in the pediatric age group. Schleien and coworkers (1986) reported that conventional CPR generated about twice the intrathoracic pressure and volume of cerebral and myocardial blood flow in an infant animal as contrasted to an adult animal model. The researchers attributed their findings to the fact that infants' chests are more pliable, permitting greater cardiac compression.

Data in adults have shown that carotid blood flow can be improved by maneuvers that increase intrathoracic pressures. These maneuvers include high impulse/high rate compressions, simultaneous compression with ventilation, prolonged compressions,

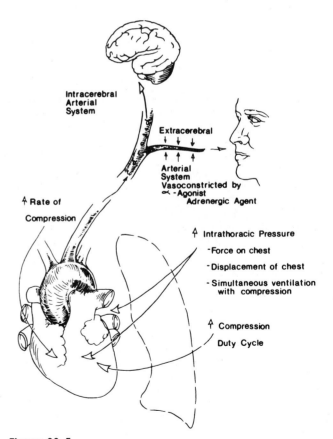

Intracerebral
Arterial
System

Extracerebral

Arterial
System
Vasoconstricted by
∝ - Agonist
Adrenergic Agent

↑ Rate of
Compression

↑ Intrathoracic Pressure

- Force on chest

- Displacement of chest

- Simultaneous ventilation
  with compression

↑ Compression

Duty Cycle

Figure 33–5 ● ● ● ● ● ●

Factors that may increase blood flow from the heart during CPR. (From Schleien, C. L., Berkowitz, I. D., Traysman, R., & Rogers, M. C. (1989). Controversial issues in cardiopulmonary resuscitation. *Anesthesiology*, 71(1), 133–149.)

continuous abdominal binding, and interposed abdominal compressions. Many of these maneuvers improve diastolic pressure and organ perfusion, but none has been linked to improved resuscitation rate or neurologic outcome. Replication of alternative compression methods is required with patients in the pediatric population. The importance of these methods is unclear; in fact, it is conceivable that some of the alternative methods may actually result in injury to children.

Open chest cardiac massage generates better cardiac output and cerebral and myocardial blood flow, but the risk-benefit ratio has not been adequately explored within the pediatric population. In the absence of adequate clinical data this procedure is not recommended except in pediatric patients with penetrating chest trauma, chest deformities (that preclude the performance of effective closed chest compressions), hypothermia (when cardiopulmonary bypass is available), and cardiac tamponade (AHA, 1986).

In the face of high incidence of poor neurologic outcome following cardiopulmonary arrest, it is important to note that closed chest cardiac compressions may result in dramatic increases in intracranial pressure, particularly after volume loading in patients with decreased cerebral compliance. During cardiac compressions some venous reflux into the major veins occurs, producing an increase in the right atrial pressure while cerebral arterial flow continues (Rogers et al., 1979). Goetting and Paradis (1991) reported that a venous valving mechanism exists across the thoracic inlet in the compression phase of CPR. The valving mechanism permits cerebral blood flow to occur during compressions. During the early relaxation phase, the gradient reverses, allowing venous drainage into the chest. The net result is increased cerebral blood volume and intracranial pressure and decreased cerebral perfusion pressure. With this in mind, restoration of spontaneous cardiac activity in children is even more urgent, regardless of the adequacy of pulses generated with cardiac compressions. In addition, this observation may have implications for the continuing development of resuscitation standards for closed chest cardiac compressions in patients with concomitant cerebral hypertension.

Cannulation

Establishing vascular access to administer fluids and drugs is a priority once adequate oxygenation, ventilation, and compressions have been addressed. Obtaining venous access can be difficult and frustrating in the hemodynamically stable pediatric patient and worse in a patient in an arrest situation. During an arrest, the largest and most accessible vein that does not interrupt resuscitation is the preferred site for vascular access.

Attempts at percutaneous peripheral access are limited to several minutes before considering other techniques and routes of administration. Several methods of venous access are commonly used in children. The steel needle (butterfly) is adequate for infants whose condition is stable but is not recommended during resuscitation because of the risk of infiltration, especially when administering caustic medications and fluids at high rates. Over-the-needle catheters are preferred because they can be inserted deep into the vein, thereby decreasing the risk of infiltration. Larger sizes that facilitate more rapid infusion rates are recommended.

Central lines provide access for volume replacement, rapid medication administration close to effector sites, and central venous pressure (CVP) measurement. Complications associated with this access option are more frequently reported in the pediatric age group. Therefore, this procedure should be delegated to the more experienced provider to limit the iatrogenic complications of hemorrhage, pneumothorax, hemothorax, embolism, cardiac injury, or infection (Chameides & Hazinski, 1994).

Supradiaphragmatic central lines, the jugular and subclavian veins, are preferred, based on the theory that higher and more rapid peak serum drug concentrations are produced when medications are administered via this route than via more peripheral sites. However, neckline placement often interferes with the resuscitation attempt, and there is insufficient data to support improved outcomes. Current recommendations still consider long catheters placed above the diaphragm from the femoral vein to be adequate (Chameides & Hazinski, 1994).

The intraosseous route for fluid and drug administration has regained popularity. First described by Drinker in the 1920s, then extensively studied by Trochantis in the 1940s, intraosseous infusion fell into obscurity with the introduction of disposable intravenous cannulas (Spivey, 1987). An intraosseous infusion is recommended as an alternative means to deliver intravenous fluids and medications in children younger than 6 years when vascular access is inadequate or unavailable within three attempts or 90 seconds, whichever comes first (AHA, 1992).

Bone is a noncollapsible structure that allows circulation of blood with little resistance. The medullary cavity of bone is composed of a spongy network of venous sinusoids that drain into a central venous canal. Blood enters the systemic circulation by the nutrient and emissary veins. Intraosseous infusion is accomplished by insertion of a bone marrow needle with stylet into the medullary cavity in a direction away from the epiphyseal plate (Fig. 33–6).

The preferred site is the broad flat portion of the anteriomedial surface of the tibia approximately 1 to 2 cm below the tibial tuberosity or above the femur's external condyles (Fig. 33–7). Loss of resistance from the dense bony cortex usually indicates that the needle is located in the bone marrow. A 15- to 18-gauge short bone marrow needle designed for the purposes of bone marrow aspirations may be used. Various bone marrow needles have been designed with short shafts and protective sheaths that prevent overinsertion and stylets that prevent obstruction of the needle with bone fragments.

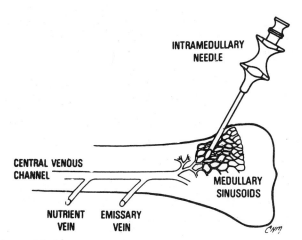

Figure 33–6 ● ● ● ● ● ●

The intramedullary venous system demonstrates position of intraosseous needle in the medullary sinusoids. Blood may be aspirated from the sinusoids to confirm position of the needle. (From Spivey, W. H. (1987). Intraosseous infusions. *Journal of Pediatrics,* 111(5), 639–643.)

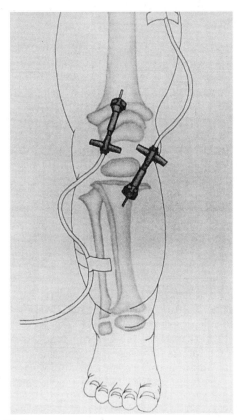

Figure 33–7 ● ● ● ● ● ●

Recommended sites for an intraosseous infusion. (From Manley, L., Haley, K., & Dick, M. (1988). Intraosseous infusion: Rapid vascular access for critically ill or injured infants and children. *Journal of Emergency Nursing*, 14(2), 63–68.)

Successful insertion is demonstrated by (1) the needle standing upright without support, (2) aspiration of bone marrow, and (3) free flow of fluid without extravasation. The interosseous route is acceptable for volume expansion with blood, plasma, colloids, or crystalloid. Average gravity flow rates of 100 mL/hour can be accomplished in the infant, whereas much higher flow rates have been reported when a pressure infuser is used. Drug levels achieved via the intraosseous route are similar to the peripheral venous route (Spivey, et al., 1987) and the central venous route (Orlowski et al., 1990).

Complications associated with intraosseous infusions are few and include leakage from previous sites, extravasation, osteomyelitis, and fat embolus (Rosetti et al., 1985; Spivey, 1987). Compartment syndrome associated with extravasation has been reported (Galpin et al., 1991). The incidence of osteomyelitis is primarily related to the duration of the infusion, presence of concurrent bacteremia, and possibly administration of hypertonic strongly alkaline solutions. Fat embolism is a theoretical complication in older adolescents when yellow marrow has re-

placed red marrow (Rosetti et al., 1985). Complications are limited by brief use of the intraosseous route for emergency measures only, avoiding the use of hypertonic solutions and use in children 6 years of age and older. The only absolute contraindication for the use of intraosseous access is placement within a recently fractured bone. Long-term bone changes or growth disturbances have not been reported.

Arterial lines are useful for direct arterial pressure measurement and evaluation of the ongoing effectiveness of resuscitation through ABG analysis. Various devices are listed in Table 33–4.

Table 33–4. EQUIPMENT USED FOR VENOUS CANNULATION

Age (yr.)	Weight (kg)	Butterfly Needles (gauge)	Over-the-Needle Catheters (gauge)	Intracaths Catheter (gauge)	Intracaths Needle (gauge)	French Size	Length (cm)	Wire Diam. (mm (in.))	Needle (gauge)	French Size	Length (cm)	Wire Diam. (mm (in.))	Needle (gauge)
<1	<10	21, 23, 25	20, 22, 24	22	19	3.0	8	0.46 (.018)	21	4.0	6	0.53 (.021)	20
										4.5	6	0.53 (.021)	20
1–12	10–40	16, 18, 20	16, 18, 20	18	16	4.0	12	0.53 (.021)	20	5.0	13	0.64 (.025)	19
										5.5	13	0.64 (.025)	19
										6.5	13	0.64 (.025)	19
>12	>40	16, 18, 20	14, 16, 18	16	14	5.0	20	0.89 (.035)	18	7.0	13	0.89 (.035)	18
						6.0	20		18	8.0	13	0.89 (.035)	18

Circulatory Support

Most children suffering cardiopulmonary arrest require volume restoration or expansion because of excessive losses, venous pooling, vasodilation, and capillary leak. Frequently, because of hesitancy in administering large volumes of fluid rapidly to small children, too little fluid is administered too late.

Volume restoration precedes the use of vasoactive drugs in resuscitation. The amount of volume administered depends upon the extent of fluid deficit based on an estimate of volume lost and presence of ongoing losses. It is not unusual to note that several 20 mL/kg fluid boluses are required before any improvement in the patient's clinical response is appreciated. In the face of hemorrhage, the volume of red blood cell administration can be approximated by multiplying 4 mL/kg by the difference, in grams, between actual and desired hemoglobin.

It should be noted that while volume *restoration* is essential, volume *loading* is not accompanied by improved vital organ perfusion. Ditchey and Lindenfeld (1984) noted that volume loading produced a disproportionate increase in right atrial pressure relative to aortic pressure, thus reducing the average pressure gradient across the coronary and cerebral circulations.

Controversy surrounds the type of fluid that should be administered during a resuscitation attempt. Colloids and synthetic colloids, such as 5% albumin and hetastarch, are true volume expanders and generally remain within an intact vascular space after administration. Some recommend against colloids in patients with capillary leak syndrome (for example, those patients with trauma, sepsis, and/or burns) because of the high associated risk of adult respiratory distress syndrome (Velanovich, 1988). Approximately 20% to 25% of isotonic crystalloids, such as normal saline and Ringer's lactate, leak from the intravascular space shortly after administration. Therefore, volume replacement with crystalloid may require 20% to 25% more than the estimated loss. The advantage of using crystalloids is that they are relatively inexpensive and readily available.

The routine use of large volumes of high dextrose–containing fluids during fluid resuscitation for hypovolemic shock is avoided. This may result in significant hyperglycemia with resultant osmotic diuresis.

Resuscitation Drugs

Table 33–5 outlines a physiologic approach to resuscitation that helps to organize intervention priorities. Drugs, compared with airway and breathing, are often less essential in resuscitation of infants and children (Melker, 1986). Correction of hypoxemia and acidosis and the restoration of tissue perfusion is primary. However, the child's response to resuscitation efforts is poor in the face of uncorrected imbalances, such as in pH, glucose, potassium, and calcium. Hypothermia further contributes to metabolic acidosis, which renders the myocardium refractory to electrical and pharmacologic intervention. Vagal stimulation may result in refractory bradydysrhythmias. In addition, toxic ingestions may compromise respiratory and cardiac function requiring immediate intervention. Successful resuscitation is dependent on correction of such factors with interventions beyond restoring adequate ventilation.

Variability of Response

It is imperative to note that a great deal of individual physiologic variation, depending upon system maturity, is present in the pediatric population. Children and adolescents are able to maintain cardiac output when heart rate decreases by increasing stroke volume. However, sick infants have relatively fixed stroke volumes so that cardiac output depends primarily on heart rate and rhythm. A relatively fixed stroke volume, characteristic of the infant for the first 6 to 12 months of life, is the result of limited ventricular compliance and contractility. Both are

Table 33–5. PHYSIOLOGIC APPROACH TO RESUSCITATION

A: Airway		
B: Breathing → Oxygenation + Ventilation		
C: Circulation → Perfusion		
Heart Rate & Rhythm	Asystole	Oxygen
	Bradycardia	Epinephrine (bolus → infusion) Atropine
	AV block	Oxygen Atropine or isoproterenol Epinephrine infusion Pacemaker
	PVCs	Oxygen Lidocaine Procainamide
	Ventricular tachycardia	Oxygen Cardioversion @ 0.2-1.0 j/kg Lidocaine
	Ventricular fibrillation	Oxygen Defibrillation @ 2 j/kg May repeat doubling joules Consider: Epinephrine Lidocaine Bretylium
Preload	Volume restoration Decrease excessive intrathoracic pressure Relieve cardiac tamponade Correct asynchronous cardiac rhythms	
Afterload	Correct hypoxemia, acidosis, hypothermia Question congenital outflow obstruction Treat sepsis, drug overdose, anaphylaxis Consider vasodilators if CHF is present	
Contractility	Correct hypoxemia, hypoglycemia, K^+ & Ca^+ Correct acidosis: Ventilation → $NaHCO_3$ Positive inotropic agents: epinephrine, dobutamine, dopamine, amrinone	

Primary management includes correction of hypoxemia, acidosis, hypoglycemia, potassium and calcium imbalance, hypothermia, vagal stimulation, and drug toxicity.

less than in the mature heart because of the greater proportion of noncontractile myocardial tissue relative to contractile myocardial mass (Friedman, 1972). In addition, there is increased interventricular interaction that is especially evident in the small infant. That is, the degree of filling of one chamber affects the degree of filling of another (Friedman, 1972). Therefore, if a large volume of fluid loads the right ventricle or if pulmonary hypertension is present, the interventricular septum will bulge toward the left and compromise left ventricular filling. Knowledge that infants lack myocardial function sufficient to respond to volume loading or overcome excessive afterload is important.

Sympathetic nervous system immaturity is another factor that requires consideration in seriously ill infants. Sympathetic innervation of the myocardium is incomplete at birth; therefore, infants are less responsive to endogenous and exogenous stimulation of the sympathetic nervous system (Zaritisky & Chernow, 1984). As a result, the use of catecholamines in infant resuscitation does not reliably produce the same effect as seen in the older child. Moreover, it is difficult to predict the cardiovascular effect of any dose of any agent. Infants may require higher doses per kilogram of infused catecholamines, but their use requires continuous monitoring and titration of individual hemodynamic affects. Because of sympathetic immaturity, infants are more sensitive to parasympathetic stimulation and experience more vagal-induced bradydysrhythmias than older children.

In summary, determination of how best to individualize the use of catecholamines to improve cardiac output is based on the maturity of the patient. Receptor density and responsiveness, ventricular compliance, and stroke volume all improve with age. Table 33–6 provides a summary of the physiologic responses associated with stimulation of specific adrenergic receptor sites.

Epinephrine. During an asystolic arrest, the *initial* beneficial effect of any catecholamine is mediated through its alpha effect (Zaritisky, 1987). Epinephrine is the catecholamine of choice during resuscitation because it is direct-acting and provides a perfect balance of alpha and beta stimulation. Alpha stimulation causes peripheral vasoconstriction that improves myocardial perfusion pressure generated during closed chest compressions, thus enhancing oxygen delivery to the heart (Micheal et al., 1984). Schleien and coworkers (1986) studied the effects of epinephrine on myocardial and cerebral oxygenation and perfusion in an infant animal model. Epinephrine dramatically increases myocardial blood flow, cerebral blood flow, and subsequent cerebral oxygen uptake. Epinephrine redistributes carotid blood flow to the cerebral circulation and coronary blood flow to the myocardium, which then stimulates spontaneous cardiac contractions. Restoration of coronary artery perfusion pressures is essential for the return of spontaneous circulation (Paradis et al., 1990). This effect is critical in infants and children because most

Table 33–6. ADRENERGIC RECEPTORS: PHYSIOLOGIC RESPONSES AND AGONIST POTENCY

Receptor	Physiologic Response	Agonist
α_1	Vasoconstriction ↑ SVR, PVR Inhibits insulin secretion	E > NE > D
α_2	Vasodilation – Chronotrophy Inhibits NE release	E > NE
β_1	+ Inotrophy + Chronotrophy Enhances renin secretion	I > E ≥ D ≥ NE
β_2	Vasodilation Bronchodilation Enhances glucagon secretion Causes hypokalemia	I ≥ E > D > NE
Dopamine$_1$	Smooth muscle relaxation Renal vasodilation	D
Dopamine$_2$	Inhibits prolactin and β-endorphin	D

E, epinephrine; NE, norepinephrine; D, dopamine; I, isoproterenol
Adapted from Notterman, D.A. (1992). Pharmacology of the cardiovascular system. In B.P. Fuhrman, & J.J. Zimmerman. *Pediatric critical care* (p. 324). St. Louis: Mosby–Year Book.

arrest rhythms are unstable slow rhythms not related to heart block. Pure alpha agonists, like methoxamine and phenylephrine (Neo-Synephrine) may be helpful in restoring a stable rhythm but have failed to show improved outcomes. Pure alpha agonist may also cause adverse effects on organ perfusion once a stable cardiac rhythm is established.

Epinephrine is administered every 5 minutes because of its short duration of action which is depressed by acidosis. The optimal dose of epinephrine is controversial (Paradis & Koscove, 1990). Few human studies adequately describe epinephrine's dose-response effect. Those that suggest higher bolus doses (for example, 10 times the standard dose of 0.01 mg/kg) more often result in the return of spontaneous circulation (Goetting & Paradis, 1991). In addition, higher bolus doses followed by a high-dose continuous infusion may also improve the success of resuscitation in children. However, empirical evidence describing the relationship between the higher epinephrine dose and outcome from cardiac arrest is insufficient at this time (Brown & Kelen, 1991). It is known that the outcome of pediatric arrest is extremely poor if the second standard dose (0.01 mg/kg) of epinephrine fails to revive the asystolic heart (Nichols et al., 1984). Because of this, current standards now recommended that the second dose of epinephrine be increased 10-fold to 0.1 mg/kg in managing asystole in children (e.g., 0.1 mL/kg of the 1:1000 solution [Chameides & Hazinski, 1994]).

Larger epinephrine doses are also recommended when the endotracheal route is used: 0.1 mL/kg of the 1:1000 solution (AHA, 1992). A continuous epinephrine infusion at 20 mcg/kg/minute is used when managing asystole or slow pulseless rhythms that transiently respond to a bolus dose of epinephrine.

This high-dose continuous infusion is titrated down once an effective pulse returns. Low-dose infusions (<0.3 mcg/kg/minute) produce beta effects, whereas higher doses produce alpha stimulation. Side effects of a peripheral epinephrine infusion include compromised skin and extremity blood flow. Previous concerns about the potential for acute renal failure have been unsupported; epinephrine's alpha effect improves vital organ perfusion and, in fact, increases urine output.

Dopamine. This drug is frequently used to improve blood pressure, tissue perfusion, and urine output. If doses higher than 20 mcg/kg/minute are required and the patient is asystolic or bradycardic, a continuous epinephrine infusion is considered. If the patient has a stable rhythm, dobutamine may be considered for its pure beta affect.

Isoproterenol (Isuprel). This drug is used to increase heart rate in patients with second or third degree heart block who are resistant to atropine. The vasodilating effects of isoproterenol decrease tissue perfusion pressures. As a result, myocardial and cerebral perfusion may be compromised. These effects are not desirable during most arrests situations (Chameides, 1990).

Atropine. Atropine, a parasympathetic nervous system blocker, produces both positive chronotropic and dromotropic effects. Slow rhythms during resuscitation most often occur as a result of hypoxemia. As a consequence, it is unlikely that atropine will be efficacious in this situation. Atropine is indicated for slow arrest-related rhythms, that is, bradycardia/arrest and atrioventricular blocks resulting from structural heart disease (Chameides, 1990).

If atropine is used to block vagally mediated bradycardia during an intubation attempt, it is important to understand that atropine also blocks hypoxemia-induced bradycardia. Therefore, careful monitoring of oxygen saturation through pulse oximetry is indicated, and prolonged attempts at intubation are avoided.

Inadequate atropine doses stimulate vagal nuclei and produce paradoxical bradycardia. This affect is avoided by using the full vagolytic dose, which is 0.02 mg/kg, and using a minimum dose of 0.1 mg. Overuse may cause excessive heart rates that shorten ventricular diastolic time and compromise stroke volume. Coronary artery filling may also decrease, compromising myocardial oxygenation as exhibited by ST segment depression. In addition, initial mydriatic effects of atropine may preclude accurate assessment of pupil size and reactivity during postresuscitation neurologic evaluation.

Calcium. The positive inotropic effects of calcium are well known, but it is no longer recommended in the primary management of pediatric arrest. It was thought that calcium, necessary for the excitation-contraction coupling of the heart, was effective in the management of asystole and electromechanical dissociation, but evidence is lacking. Exogenous calcium may cause further problems as calcium enters the cell following ischemia and during reperfusion and produces toxic effects (Katz & Reuter, 1979).

Calcium is still recommended in the management of documented hypocalcemia (commonly seen in stressed infants), and in the management of the adverse cardiac effects associated with hyperkalemia, hypermagnesemia, and calcium channel blocker overdose. Rapid calcium administration is avoided because it may precipitate bradydysrhythmias.

Although further study is required, emphasis is now on the inhibition of calcium accumulation following ischemia through the use of calcium channel blockers. It is thought that the use of calcium channel blockers may prevent the cascade of cytotoxic events leading to reperfusion injuries and thus may preserve myocardial and cerebral function after global ischemic events (Rogers & Kirsch, 1989). However, it appears that the best time to administer the calcium antagonist is before the ischemic episode.

Glucose. This is considered an emergency resuscitation drug in small infants. Infants have limited glycogen reserves and when stressed, particularly in the presence of sepsis, experience acute marked hypoglycemia. Hypoglycemia depresses cardiac contractility and may precipitate seizure activity. Symptoms of hypoglycemia, which include decreased perfusion, diaphoresis, tachycardia, and hypotension, mimic those of hypoxemia.

Conversely, there is some evidence that hyperglycemia, the more common consequence of cardiopulmonary arrest in older children, worsens neurologic outcome (Longstreth et al., 1986). Lactic acidemia produced during anaerobic metabolism is increased when hyperglycemia is present (Pulsinelli et al., 1983). Rapid-response blood glucose screening methods (Chemstrips) should be used to guide intervention strategies. Administration of glucose during resuscitation is avoided unless hypoglycemia is documented.

Management of Acidosis

Management of acidosis during an arrest has been the subject of a great deal of controversy. During an arrest, poor ventilation and low flow states produce mixed respiratory and metabolic acidosis. Inadequate tissue perfusion results in anaerobic metabolism and subsequent lactic acid production. In addition, the circulation of poorly oxygenated blood further contributes to tissue hypoxia and subsequent ischemia. The priority in managing acidosis is restoration of ventilation and tissue perfusion.

Sodium bicarbonate ($NaHCO_3$), described by many as the most overused drug in CPR, is not required in mild to moderate acidosis, which can be managed by volume expansion and proper ventilation. $NaHCO_3$ serves as a buffer by combining with the hydrogen ion (H^+) to form carbonic acid (H_2CO_3), then CO_2 and H_2O:

$$HCO_3 + H \rightarrow H_2CO_3 \rightarrow H_2O + CO_2$$

To correct acidosis by shifting the equation to the *right*, adequate ventilation and pulmonary blood flow must be present. The administration of $NaHCO_3$ in the face of increased tissue CO_2 production and inadequate ventilation and/or pulmonary perfusion may dramatically lower blood pH, worsening metabolic acidosis.

Because CO_2 crosses the blood-brain barrier and cell membranes more rapidly than HCO_3, transient increases in CO_2 produced by $NaHCO_3$ administration can paradoxically worsen cerebral spinal fluid and intracellular acidosis. In hypoxic states, $NaHCO_3$ administration decreases myocardial contractility, cardiac index, and blood pressure, and may worsen electromechanical dissociation. Because respiratory failure is often the precipitating event in cardiopulmonary arrest among infants and children, this population is at greater risk of severe intracellular acidosis because of impaired CO_2 elimination.

Acidic environments promote oxygen release to tissue, as described by the oxyhemoglobin dissociation curve. Excessive $NaHCO_3$ administration shifts the oxyhemoglobin dissociation curve to the left, thereby increasing the affinity between hemoglobin and oxygen and decreasing oxygen release to tissues. Thus, overcorrection of acidosis may eliminate a very effective compensatory mechanism. Although there are no corresponding data among infants and children, survival of adults suffering cardiopulmonary arrest has been related to arterial pH. When pH exceeded 7.55 during the initial 10 minutes an hour after CPR was initiated, there was a sharp decrease in survival (Weil et al., 1985).

A number of other physiologic disturbances occur with excessive $NaHCO_3$ administration. Potassium shifts into the intracellular space; a 0.1 rise in pH typically results in a 0.5 mEq/L decrease in serum potassium. Hypernatremia and hypocalcemia result. Hyperosmolar states may also result from increased serum sodium produced by $NaHCO_3$ administration. The intravascular shift of free water that results from hyperosmolarity may be lethal because it has been implicated in intracranial hemorrhage in infants. To prevent this, $NaHCO_3$ is diluted 1:1 with sterile water in infants younger than 3 months unless 4.2% infant $NaHCO_3$ is available (0.5 mEq/mL). In addition, alkaline solutions inactivate catecholamines and precipitate calcium salts. $NaHCO_3$ *is not recommended* until the patient has been adequately oxygenated and ventilated, CPR has been initiated, epinephrine has been administered without success, and there is documentation of a venous pH 7.0 or less or an arterial pH of 7.2 or less (Chameides & Hazinski, 1994).

Arterial blood gas (ABG) analysis traditionally guides $NaHCO_3$ administration. The formula used to calculate the dose of $NaHCO_3$ to be administered is:

$$\text{dose (mEq)} = 0.3 \times \text{weight (kg)} \times \text{base deficit (mEq/L)}$$

However, there are situations when $NaHCO_3$ administration may precede ABG measurement (for example, when a patient fails to respond to resuscitation efforts despite 10 minutes of adequate ventilation, closed chest compressions, and intravenous epinephrine administration; and when ABG sampling cannot be achieved). The premise is that $NaHCO_3$ administration may improve the patient's response to catecholamines. In this case, $NaHCO_3$ is administered at a dose of 1 mEq/kg. Half of this dose may be repeated every 10 minutes thereafter if the patient continues to be unresponsive to therapy.

In addition, it is unclear whether arterial or venous blood gases are more predictive of patient outcome following cardiopulmonary arrest. During resuscitation from cardiopulmonary arrest, an arterial respiratory alkalosis (high normal pH, low $PaCO_2$) results from a high ventilation/perfusion ratio, whereas a severe venous respiratory acidosis (low pH, high $PvCO_2$ results from poor systemic perfusion. The $PaCO_2$ reflects the adequacy of ventilation and pulmonary perfusion, whereas the $PvCO_2$ reflects tissue CO_2 production and inversely reflects the adequacy of systemic perfusion. Comparison of mixed venous pH and $PvCO_2$ with arterial pH and $PaCO_2$ may more accurately reflect the relationship between tissue oxygenation, ventilation, and perfusion during resuscitation attempts (Weil et al., 1986). Note that the adequacy of ventilation and pulmonary perfusion generated by cardiac compressions can also be assessed by $ETCO_2$ monitoring (Gazmuri et al., 1989; Curley & Thompson, 1990).

The non–CO_2-producing buffer, tromethamine (tris, Tham), holds promise as a replacement for $NaHCO_3$ but has not been sufficiently studied in infants and children (Rosenberg et al., 1989). Its major limitation is that it is excreted by the kidneys. As a consequence, it accumulates when renal blood flow is inadequate. Side effects also include hypoglycemia, hyperkalemia, and respiratory depression.

Routes of Drug Administration

Routes of drug administration for resuscitation include central venous, endotracheal, intraosseous, and intracardiac. Figure 33–8 illustrates a diagram useful in decision-making regarding potential routes for vascular access.

Ideally, resuscitation drugs are administered close to adrenergic receptor sites located on the arterial side of the circulation. To ensure that a bolus medication is delivered into the central circulation rapidly, each medication is followed with a rapid 2- to 5-mL normal saline flush. Continuous infusions of vasoactive medications can be initiated at five to 10 times the usual rate while heart rate and blood pressure are continuously monitored. When the desired effect is evident, the infusion rate is decreased. Another option is to administer the continuous infusion through a Y connector with a faster running intravenous line. Care is taken when titrating either line.

The intraosseous route is acceptable when venous access is delayed. The intraosseous route, considered similar to a peripheral venous route, is acceptable for all resuscitation drugs. Berg (1984) reported a

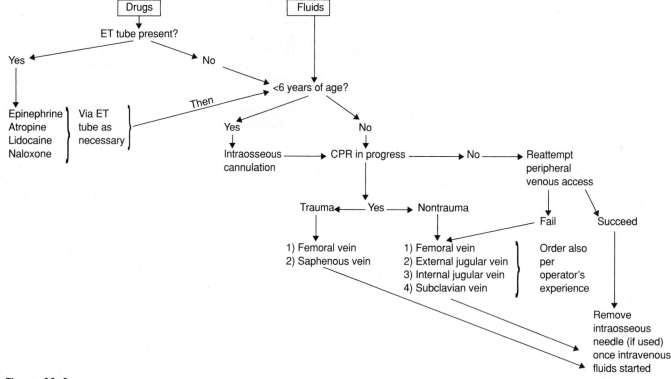

Figure 33–8 ● ● ● ● ● ●

Decision tree for vascular access. (Reproduced with permission.© *Textbook of Pediatric Advanced Life Support,* 1994. Copyright American Heart Association.)

case in which a 6-month-old infant was maintained on both dopamine and dobutamine intraosseous infusions until direct intravenous access could be initiated.

Bone marrow serves as a vascular depot, thus drug flow from the bone is facilitated by following each medication with a 2- to 5-mL normal saline flush. Clotting of the bone marrow can be avoided by adequate flushing or clearing the needle with the stylet. Because the safety of hypertonic and strongly alkaline solutions administered via the intraosseous route requires further study, when used, they should be diluted and flushed well.

Although data in humans are limited, several resuscitation drugs defined by the acronym LEAN (lidocaine, epinephrine, atropine, and Narcan) may be administered by the endotracheal route if intravenous access is unavailable. These drugs are rapidly absorbed when given by the endotracheal route, having a direct cardiac effect. However, optimal dose and mechanism of absorption for medications administered endotracheally are controversial (Chernow et al., 1984). There is data to support larger doses of epinephrine; 10 times the standard intravenous dose is recommended via the endotracheal route (that is, 0.1 mg/kg of the 1:1000 solution) (AHA, 1992). Both epinephrine and atropine have a prolonged effect after endotracheal administration; thus, less frequent administration may be required.

All endotracheal drugs should be diluted with 2 to 3 mL of normal saline and injected deeply into the tracheobronchial tree using a needleless syringe and attached suction catheter or feeding tube. Injection is accomplished after passive exhalation and a resuscitation bag is used to distribute the drug throughout the lung periphery. Sterile normal saline is the only diluent recommended for this procedure in volumes not to exceed 5 mL in infants or 10 mL in adolescents (Greenberg et al., 1981).

The intracardiac route for drug administration is a last resort, primarily because the procedure interrupts cardiopulmonary resuscitation. Other iatrogenic complications include cardiac tamponade, pneumothorax, and coronary artery laceration. If a drug is inadvertently injected into the myocardium it may cause intractable ventricular fibrillation (VF).

Drug Calculations. Various methods have been devised to facilitate rapid calculation and administration of pediatric resuscitation drugs (Table 33–7; Fig. 33–9). The rule of six is often used when weight is known. Precalculated drug dosage reference books with each page representing a different weight are also useful. Optimal systems include a computer program that automatically calculates then prints a resuscitation order sheet when the patient's weight is entered upon admission. When weight is unknown, the Broselow tape may be helpful. Broselow developed a simplified method of estimating weight based upon height and developed a measuring tape with spaces labeled with weight in kilograms instead of units of height (Fig. 33–10). Appropriate doses for many of the resuscitation drugs are printed on one

Table 33–7. PREPARATION OF INFUSIONS

Drug	Calculation
Epinephrine Norepinephrine Isoproterenol Prostaglandin E_1	0.6 × wt (kg) = mgs. to add to diluent to make 100 mL volume

Run at 1 mL/Hr to deliver 0.1 mcg/kg/min

Dopamine Dobutamine Nitroprusside Nitroglycerin	6 × wt (kg) = mgs. to add to diluent to make 100 mL volume

Run at 1 mL/Hr to deliver 1 mcg/kg/min

Lidocaine	120 mg added to diluent to make 100 mL volume

Run at mL/kg/Hr to deliver 20 mcg/kg/min

Alternative Method: Infusion Rate (mL/HR) =

$$\frac{\text{Wt (kg)} \times \text{Dose (mcg/kg/min)} \times 60 \text{ (min/hr)}}{\text{Concentration (mcg/mL)}}$$

May double or triple concentration if excessive volume is an issue. May use 5% dextrose, 5% dextrose normal saline, normal saline, or lactated Ringer's solution as a diluent.

Reprinted with permission from American Heart Association. (1992). Pediatric advanced life support. *JAMA*, 268 (16), 2266 & 2270. Copyright 1992, American Medical Association.

side of the tape; the other side contains equipment sizes for intubation and vascular access. Lubitz and coworkers (1988) found that length was a better predictor of actual weight than estimated weight. They also reported that the Broselow tape is accurate in predicting weight in children from 3.5 to 25 kg, although accuracy considerably decreased in children weighing more than 25 kg. Whatever method is used, it is imperative that it be used consistently so that resuscitation medications can be prepared rapidly.

Electrocardiogram

During a cardiopulmonary arrest in infants and children, hypoxic and acidotic blood circulates through normal coronary arteries under extremely low perfusion pressure. As a consequence, the vast majority of pediatric cardiopulmonary arrest–related dysrhythmias occur as a result of metabolic dysfunction and not from coronary artery disease. The emphasis, therefore, in pediatric resuscitation is on reestablishing adequate oxygenation, ventilation, and tissue perfusion, *not* on complex rhythm analysis and its drug management.

To avoid losing precious time on complex rhythm assessment, the therapeutic approach to pediatric arrest–related dysrhythmias recommended by PALS is to first identify the rhythm's group and then to consider treatment only if the patient's condition is clinically *unstable*. PALS identifies three unstable rhythm groups based upon heart rate and the presence or absence of a pulse. Treatment is basically the

same for dysrhythmias within each group and is based upon whether the patient's cardiac output is, or is likely to become, compromised. In other words, unstable rhythms that require treatment are those that compromise cardiac output and those that have the potential to deteriorate into a lethal rhythm. Rhythms in all three rhythm groups have the potential for inadequate cardiac output. Extremes in heart rate are of no concern unless the effective cardiac output does not match the patient's clinical need. The clinical assessment parameters of blood pressure, heart rate, and end-organ perfusion (specifically to the brain, skin, and kidneys) provide rapid measures of the adequacy of cardiac output and effectiveness of intervention strategies.

Slow Rhythms

Slow rhythms are the most common arrest-related rhythm disturbance in infants and children. Walsh and Krongrad (1983) studied the terminal cardiac rhythms in 100 pediatric patients. Bradycardic arrest occurred in 88% of newborns (birth to 28 days), 67% of infants (28 days to 1 year), and 64% of children (1 to 18 years). In contrast, bradycardia occurs in only 25% to 30% of adult arrests (Iseri et al., 1978).

Because of heart rate dependency, the hemodynamic effect of bradydysrhythmias may be significant in an infant or child. Slow arrest-related dysrhythmias are related to either hypoxic-ischemic insults or structural heart disease (Chameides & Hazinski, 1994). Slow rhythms associated with hypoxic-ischemic insults are often wide QRS complex without p waves. Slow rhythms associated with structural heart disease are often related to heart block or sinus node dysfunction. Priorities for managing bradydysrhythmias start with the resuscitation ABCs then progress if severe cardiopulmonary compromise is present (Table 33–8).

Occasionally, primary bradycardic arrests occur in children with congenital complete heart block or in an infant during procedures that cause vagal stimulation (for example, oral-pharyngeal stimulation or a Valsalva maneuver related to painful procedures).

In an arrest, cardiac pacing may be helpful in managing patients with slow rhythms resulting from structural heart disease. Pacing can be accomplished by external (transcutaneous), transvenous, or epicardial electrodes. Pacing in the hypoxic-ischemic cardiac arrest patient is rarely successful. Even if ventricular capture is accomplished, pacing does not improve myocardial contractility and tissue perfusion.

Fast Rhythms

Fast rhythms are expected in critically ill pediatric patients. Unstable fast rhythms fall into two main categories, those with narrow QRS complexes and those with wide QRS complexes. The differential for narrow fast rhythms include sinus tachycardia (ST), supraventricular tachycardia (SVT), atrial flutter

HARTFORD HOSPITAL
PEDIATRIC RESUSCITATION AND EMERGENCY MEDICATION SHEET

NAME: _____   WEIGHT: _____   BSA: _____   Date: _____

Calculated by: Checked by:

Medication/Dose/kg	Patient Dose	Mode	Interval/Rate	Maximum	Dose Preparation
Resuscitation Meds: Epinephrine 0.1 cc/kg (1:10,000)	____ cc	IV, IO ET	Q5 min	5–10 cc	Prefilled syringe 1:10,000 (0.1 mg/1 cc)
Atropine 0.02 mg/kg minimum dose = 0.1 mg	mg = ____ cc	IV, IO ET	Q5 min	1.0 mg-child 2.0 mg-adol.	Prefilled syringe (0.1 mg/1 cc)
Sodium Bicarbonate 0.5–1 mEq per kg	mEq = ____ cc	IV, IO	By ABG or 0.5 mEq/kg/Q10 min		Prefilled syringe 1 mEq/1 cc 0.5 mEq/1 cc for neonates
Defibrillation 2–4 J/kg	____ Joules	Paddles to chest asynch mode to defib	1 dose @ 2 J/kg double dose, may repeat × 2 if ineffective	4 J/kg × 2	Distinguish between defib. & cardioversion
Other Emergency Meds: Glucose 0.5–1.0 g/kg or 2–4 cc/kg of D25W	g = ____ cc	IV, IO	By chemstrip or failure to respond to resusc. efforts		Dextrose 50% dilute 1:1 with H₂O = D25W
Calcium Chloride 10% 20 mg/kg	mg = ____ cc	IV, IO	1 dose, may repeat in 10 min, further doses based on measured Ca⁺⁺ def.	500 mg = 5 cc	10% solution 100 mg/1 cc
Lidocaine 1 mg/kg	mg = ____ cc	IV, IO ET	Repeat × 1 in 5–10 min, then continuous infusion		2% solution 20 mg/1 cc
Bretylium 5 mg/kg (Bretylol)	mg = ____ cc	IV, IO	1 dose, 5 mg/kg then 1 dose 10 mg/kg with defib. after each dose		5% solution 50 mg/1 cc
Furosemide 1–2 mg/kg (Lasix)	mg = ____ cc	IV, IO			10 mg/1 cc
Naloxone (Narcan) 0.1 mg/kg up to 5 yrs or 20 kg. 2 mg minimum dose for > 5 years	mg = ____ cc	IV, IO ET	Repeat prn to maintain opiate reversal.	0.1 mg/kg	Adult 0.4 mg/1 cc
Propanolol 0.1 mg/kg (Inderal)	mg = ____ cc	Slow IV IO 1 mg/min	Repeat × 1 in 2 min then Q 4–8 hr	3 mg	1 mg/1 cc
Volume Expander 10–20 cc/kg	____ cc	IV, IO	Repeat prn for perfusion		
Succinylcholine 1 mg/kg	mg = ____ cc	IM, IV IO	X 1	2mg/kg/dose	20 mg/1 cc
Vecuronium 0.1 mg/kg	mg = ____ cc	IV, IO	Repeat Q 30 min prn	0.25 mg/kg dose urgent intubation	10 mg/5 cc
Cardioversion 0.5–1 joules/kg	____ Joules	Paddles to chest sync. on			Differentiate between defib. and cardio.

Figure 33–9 ● ● ● ● ● ●

See legend on following page

Medication	Dose Range	Initial Dose	Dose Preparation
Dobutamine	5–20 mcg/kg/min	10 mcg/kg/min = ___ cc/hr	Add 60 mg/100 cc DSW, NS, RL (10 mcg/kg/min = 1 cc/kg/hr)
Dopamine	2–20 mcg/kg/min	10 mcg/kg/min = ___ cc/hr	Add 60 mg/100 cc D5W, NS, RL (10 mcg/kg/min = 1 cc/kg/hr)
Epinephrine	0.1–1.0 mcg/kg/min	0.1 mcg/kg/min = ___ cc/hr	Add 0.6 mg/100 cc D5W, NS, RL (0.1 mcg/kg/min = 1 cc/kg/hr)
Isoproterenol (Isuprel)	0.1–1.0 mcg/kg/min	0.1 mcg/kg/min = ___ cc/hr	Add 0.6 mg/100 cc D5W, NS, RL (0.1 mcg/kg/min = 1 cc/kg/hr)
Lidocaine	20–50 mcg/kg/min	20 mcg/kg/min = ___ cc/hr	Add 120 mg/100 cc D5W, NS, RL (20 mcg/kg/min = 1 cc/kg/hr)
Nitroprusside (Nipride)	0.5–5.0 mcg/kg/min	1 mcg/kg/min = ___ cc/hr	Add 6 mg/100 cc D5W only (1 mcg/kg/min = 1 cc/kg/hr)

Source: American Heart Association. *Textbook of pediatric advanced life support.* L. Chameides (Ed.). Dallas, 1988.

Calculated by _____

Checked by _____

Figure 33–9 ● ● ● ● ● ● *Continued*

Pediatric Resuscitation and Emergency Medication Sheet. (Courtesy of Ann Powers, RN, MSN; The Pediatric Intensive Care Unit, Hartford Hospital, Hartford, Connecticut. Data from American Heart Association. *Textbook of pediatric advanced life support.* L. Chameides (Ed.). Dallas, 1988.)

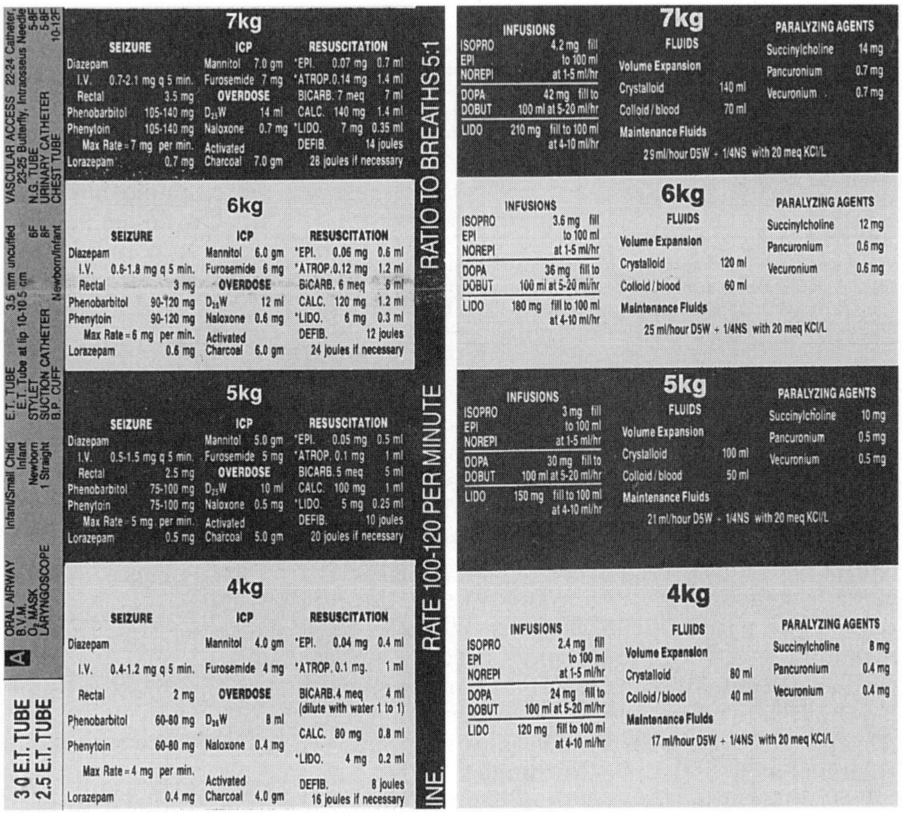

Figure 33–10 ● ● ● ● ● ●

Front and back sides of the Broselow tape. (Courtesy of Vital Signs Inc., Totowa, NJ.)

Table 33–8. BRADYCARDIA DECISION TREE

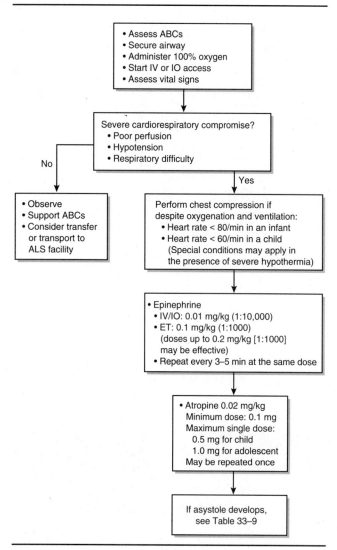

- Assess ABCs
- Secure airway
- Administer 100% oxygen
- Start IV or IO access
- Assess vital signs

↓

Severe cardiorespiratory compromise?
- Poor perfusion
- Hypotension
- Respiratory difficulty

No →

- Observe
- Support ABCs
- Consider transfer or transport to ALS facility

Yes ↓

Perform chest compression if despite oxygenation and ventilation:
- Heart rate < 80/min in an infant
- Heart rate < 60/min in a child
  (Special conditions may apply in the presence of severe hypothermia)

↓

- Epinephrine
- IV/IO: 0.01 mg/kg (1:10,000)
- ET: 0.1 mg/kg (1:1000)
  (doses up to 0.2 mg/kg [1:1000] may be effective)
- Repeat every 3–5 min at the same dose

↓

- Atropine 0.02 mg/kg
  Minimum dose: 0.1 mg
  Maximum single dose:
  0.5 mg for child
  1.0 mg for adolescent
  May be repeated once

↓

If asystole develops, see Table 33–9

ABCs indicates airway, breathing, and circulation; ALS, advanced life support; ET, endotracheal; IO, intraosseous; and IV, intravenous.
From American Heart Association (1992). Pediatric advanced life support. *JAMA* 268(16), 2266. Copyright 1992, American Medical Association.

(AF), or atrial fibrillation (Af). One can easily mistake a rapid sinus tachycardia (ST) for supraventricular tachycardia (SVT). Key diagnostic features of ST include rhythm variability and a heart rate that is congruent with the patient's need for increased cardiac output. Key diagnostic features of SVT include a monotonous rhythm and a heart rate in excess of the patient's clinical need. Whereas ST is a symptom reflecting the patient's need for increased cardiac output, unstable SVT is a primary cardiac rhythm disturbance requiring primary intervention. AF and Af are rare cardiac rhythms in groups other than pediatric patients with complex CHD.

The differential for wide complex fast rhythms is aberrantly conducted SVT or VT. Distinguishing between the two may be impossible in a patient whose condition is unstable. Because wide complex SVT is extremely rare in the pediatric age group, *all wide complex fast rhythms are considered to be VT until proven otherwise.*

Ventricular dysrhythmias occur in approximately 20% of pediatric arrests (Walsh & Krongrad, 1983). Pediatric groups at risk for ventricular tachydysrhythmia as a terminal rhythm include children requiring prolonged resuscitation, infants beyond the neonatal period and/or who weigh more than 2.23 kg, and infants and children with CHD (Walsh & Krongrad, 1983). It is thought that a critical cardiac mass along with sympathetic maturity characteristic of infants beyond 6 to 12 months of age is necessary for ventricular tachydysrhythmias to occur. During prolonged resuscitation attempts many doses of catecholamines, which stimulate the sympathetic nervous system, are often administered. Children with CHD who have arrests more often exhibit bradycardia, but are three times more likely than those without CHD to exhibit ventricular tachydysrhythmias. Supporting the critical mass theory, many children with CHD usually have cardiac enlargement.

Children with CHD are also at risk for sudden primary cardiac death. Krongrad (1984) reported that the incidence of ventricular dysrhythmias increased after cardiac surgery in children who were older at the time of surgery, had a right ventriculostomy, or had residual intracardiac defects. Children with acquired heart disease such as myocarditis may present with fulminating ventricular dysrhythmias. Metabolic causes of ventricular dysrhythmias include hyperkalemia, hypoglycemia, hypothermia, and tricyclic antidepressant overdose.

Treatment of all unstable fast rhythms includes synchronized cardioversion at 0.5 joules/kg (Table 33–9). If unsuccessful, the joules are doubled and cardioversion is repeated. (See Chapter 19 for a thorough discussion of nursing care issues related to cardioversion.)

In VT, lidocaine administration before cardioversion may result in a higher conversion rate. Lidocaine is administered in a dose of 1mg/kg every 10 to 15 minutes. A continuous lidocaine infusion of 20 to 50 mcg/kg/min is useful after conversion to normal sinus rhythm (NSR) if the patient has structural heart disease, has multiple PVCs, or recurrent VT or VF.

Table 33–9. UNSTABLE FAST

MAINTAIN ABCs
↓
Cardioversion 0.5 j/kg*
↓
Cardioversion 1.0 j/kg
↓
Cardioversion 2.0 j/kg
*Lidocaine 1 mg/kg then 20–50 mcg/kg/min infusion

Adapted with permission from AHA. Pediatric advanced life support. (1992). *JAMA*, 268 (16), 2266. Copyright 1992, American Medical Association.

Absent (Collapse) Rhythms

Absent (collapse) rhythms include asystole, VF, and electromechanical dissociation (EMD). These rhythms are considered hemodynamically significant because all three fail to produce cardiac output.

Asystole, like bradycardia, is a common pediatric arrest rhythm. The management goal, to improve oxygenation and perfusion, is similar to that for bradycardia (Table 33–10).

VF and pulseless VT, which are managed in a similar manner, are uncommon pediatric rhythms. *Immediate* defibrillation at 2 joules/Kg is *the* most important determinant of successful conversion to NSR. The pulse and cardiac rhythm are reevaluated after each defibrillation attempt. If unsuccessful, the joules are doubled and the patient is defibrillated twice in rapid succession. Epinephrine may improve coronary artery perfusion pressure, increasing the effectiveness of defibrillation. The epinephrine dose is increased after the first dose as for asystole and repeated every 3 to 5 minutes. Lidocaine may be used to increase the fibrillation threshold but should not delay defibrillation. Metabolic problems such as calcium, potassium, magnesium, or glucose imbalance, and hypothermia or drug intoxication (e.g., with digitalis or tricyclic antidepressants) are continually reassessed and corrected. If VF reoccurs, the previous successful energy level for defibrillation is used.

Bretylium has been found to be very successful in making the fibrillating heart more susceptible to electrical defibrillation in the adult population (Dronen, 1984). Although no pediatric data exist, because of its effectiveness and safety and with establishment of a standard dose in the adult population, bretylium is indicated for the treatment of refractory pediatric VT/VF. In an arrest, 5 mg/kg of bretylium is administered by rapid intravenous bolus followed by defibrillation. If unsuccessful, bretylium is increased to 10 mg/kg followed again by defrillation. Bretylium increases endogenous catecholamine release, thus producing an increase in heart rate and blood pressure within 20 minutes of administration. When endogenous catecholamine stores are depleted, bretylium may then produce hypotension.

EMD or pulseless electral activity is characteristic of organized cardiac electrical activity without effective cardiac output. EMD is usually a slow wide complex rhythm, for example, junctional or idioventricular rhythm. When EMD is caused by hypovolemia, tension pneumothorax, or pericardial tamponade, a narrow-complex, rapid heart rate may be seen. Etiologies also include hypoxia and acidosis.

Table 33–10. ASYSTOLE AND PULSELESS ARREST DECISION TREE

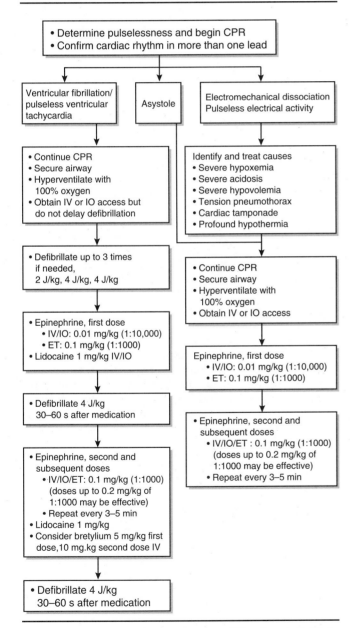

CPR indicates cardiopulmonary resuscitation; ET, endotracheal; IO, intraosseous; and IV, intravenous. From American Heart Association (1992). Pediatric advanced life support. *JAMA,* 268 (16), 2266. Copyright 1992, American Medical Association.

Family Needs

Throughout the crisis of resuscitation, parents require information and support. Information is best provided according to the individual needs of the parents. For example, some parents may want updates every 5 minutes, whereas others may want to know only the outcome when resuscitation attempts are over. Families must be kept accurately informed and assured that everything possible is being done to assist their child.

Providing parents with a private place is essential, both for them and for parents of other critically ill children. A member of the team who has an established relationship with the parents, for example, a nurse, member of the clergy, and/or social worker, ideally stays with the parents, especially if they are alone.

Whether stabilization occurs or attempts to resuscitate are unsuccessful, parents should be given options to see, touch, or hold their child as soon as possible. Some parents may wish to remain at their child's bedside during the resuscitation attempt. Although this may seem difficult for caregivers, each family is assessed individually. Protocols for parents' rights and responsibilities during CPR have been established (Villarreal et al., 1988). Elements include educating staff in resuscitation methods *and* in providing options for parents, especially parents of children whose conditions have been deteriorating over time and in whom CPR can be expected. When death is imminent, the child is allowed to die in the presence or in the arms of parents.

After 2 years of facilitating family visits during resuscitation attempts in the emergency department, Post (1989) reported that 97% of the family members would choose to witness the resuscitation again, 76% felt their grieving was made easier by observing the resuscitation, 67% thought that their presence benefitted the dying person, and all felt confident that everything possible had been done to save their family member. All emergency department staff agreed that having family present during resuscitation made the experience more emotionally stressful for them. Clearly, replication of the study is necessary in the pediatric intensive care population. It seems reasonable to initiate flexible programs to facilitate parental presence during pediatric CPR, especially with parents of chronically critically ill patients. Essential to the success of the program is multidisciplinary staff agreement and support.

Termination of Support

Successful resuscitation results when the patient achieves, or is able to be assisted to achieve, adequate oxygenation, ventilation, cardiac output, and tissue perfusion. Few data exist on when resuscitation maneuvers should be suspended. Until recently, outcome studies were unavailable, especially those that address the quality of neurologic survival. The general consensus is that one should stop when multisystem organ dysfunction is considered irreparable.

Nichols and coworkers (1984) sought to define the variables that predict long-term survival, defined as hospital discharge without neurologic deficit (Table 33–11). There is little optimism when more than two doses of $NaHCO_3$ and epinephrine fail to yield neurologic improvement. This finding was also supported by Zaritsky and coworkers (1987).

Davies and coworkers (1987) described the survival rate and short-term neurologic outcome of 67 children who sustained 81 cardiac arrests in a large pediatric teaching hospital. Cardiac arrest was defined as the need for cardiac compressions. Of those who were resuscitated, none survived to discharge if

Table 33–11. OUTCOME PREDICTORS

Long-term Survival	Parameter
92%	Neurologic improvement after oxygenation and ventilation
78%	Arrest precipitated by airway obstruction
60%	Duration of CPR <15 minutes
50%	Improvement after epinephrine and $NaHCO_3 \times 1$
44%	In-patient arrest
40%	Epinephrine and $NaHCO_3 \times 2$ with neurologic improvement
0%	Epinephrine and $NaHCO_3 \times 2$ without neurologic improvement

Adapted from Nichols, D.G., Kettrick, R.G., Swedlow, D.B., Lee, S., Passman, R., & Ludwig, S. (1984). Factors influencing outcome of cardiopulmonary arrest in children. *Critical Care Medicine, 12*(3), 287. © by Williams & Wilkins, 1984.

CPR lasted longer than 30 minutes. Two patients who required compressions for 24 and 30 minutes survived and were discharged with good neurologic outcome.

Hypothermia, by decreasing metabolic requirements, is commonly thought to protect the patient from hypoxic-ischemic injury. In their study investigating the neurological outcome of near-drowning patients in a region *without* icy water, Quan and coworkers (1990) identified hypothermia to be a risk factor for poor neurologic outcome. In predicting outcome, a critical distinction in the etiology of hypothermia must be made whether hypothermia is due to rapid conductive loss or due to death. Hypothermia resulting from rapid conductive loss may protect the patient against hypoxic injury; hypothermia resulting from death obviously does not.

Documentation

Ongoing documentation of resuscitation events is crucial. Accuracy is enhanced if the person responsible for documentation has no other role in the resuscitation attempt and is positioned in close proximity to the code leader and patient. Figure 33–11 illustrates an example of a resuscitation flow sheet that facilitates documentation. Effective resuscitation flow records provide precise information about code events, include the patient's response to therapy, and minimize the time required for documentation during and after the code (Padilla & Purcell, 1990).

Postresuscitation documentation includes a summary statement including the time and duration of the arrest, ETT size and markings compared with the lip/nare line, catheter sizes and length of insertion, all intravenous fluid administered, blood work and blood loss, drugs and dosages administered, and the patient's and family's response to therapy.

POST-ARREST STABILIZATION

Patient care goals after cardiopulmonary resuscitation include further stabilization of oxygenation, ven-

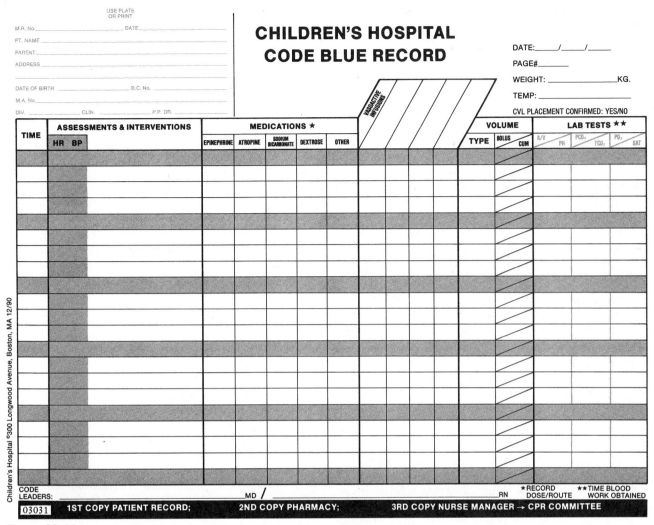

Figure 33-11 ● ● ● ● ● ●

Code Blue record. (Courtesy of Children's Hospital, CPR Committee, Boston, Massachusetts.)

tilation, cardiac output, and tissue perfusion. These goals are vital for neurologic preservation. Two major concerns include the potential of iatrogenic trauma from the resuscitation attempt and multisystem dysfunction resulting from organ hypoperfusion with hypoxic and acidotic blood.

The ABCs are also useful in organizing post-arrest stabilization measures. Assessment starts with an evaluation of the adequacy of the airway. Assessment parameters include the airway size, presence of an ETT leak, and the security of the ETT. If a cuffed ETT was placed, cuff volume and pressures are checked. This is important in pediatrics because cuffed ETTs are infrequently used and can potentially cause a significant amount of airway damage in a short period of time. The placement and patency of the nasogastric tube (NGT) is also assessed. After decompressing the stomach with a large-volume syringe, the NGT is placed to intermittent suction. A chest radiograph is usually indicated to evaluate pulmonary disease, assess for iatrogenic injury, and

check tube placement, that is, ETT, central lines, and/or chest tube positioning.

ABGs are assessed throughout the resuscition attempt. Saturation monitoring resumes when the patient's pulse pressure is adequate. Once the airway is stable, optimal ventilator parameters are identified. Airway pressures sufficient to provide adequate chest excursion and at least 95% saturation are noted during hand ventilation. Keeping the patient on an FiO_2 of 1.0, airway pressures are matched with the ventilator. Once on the ventilator, the patient's ABGs are reanalyzed in 20 minutes and further adjustments in peak inspiratory and positive end-expiratory pressures, tidal volume, and FiO_2 are made.

Vascular access is reassessed for adequacy, patency, and security. Additional vascular access may be indicated and, after fluid resuscitation, can be accomplished in a controlled manner. Intraosseous lines are discontinued as soon as possible after adequate direct vascular access has been obtained. The skin surrounding peripheral intravenous sites requires particular attention. The potential for iatrogenic injury from intravenous infiltration is high. (See Chapter 17 for nursing care issues related to intravenous infiltration.) Immediate consultation to plastic surgery may be indicated.

The initial set of vital signs includes temperature assessment. Patient exposure and administration of large quantities of unwarmed intravenous solutions during the arrest places the patient at risk for post-arrest hypothermia. The hypothermic patient benefits from rewarming measures, for example, warm blankets and overhead radiant warmers or lights.

As soon as possible after resuscitation, a baseline neurologic examination is performed and documented. The neurologic examination is placed in context of the prearrest neurologic status and drugs used during or immediately after resuscitation (for example, atropine, dopamine, and chemical paralyzing agents). Atropine and dopamine act synergistically to cause pupillary dilation, the duration of which cannot be accurately determined because routine half-life calculations are probably invalid following resuscitation (Verna, 1986).

In addition to ABGs, initial post-resuscitation blood work includes studies to evaluate oxygen-carrying capacity, fluid balance, system function (especially renal and liver function), and coagulation profiles. Urine output is evaluated and, if not already present, a Foley catheter is placed.

Patients are usually poorly perfused, acidotic, and hypotensive following a cardiac arrest. The most common reason for poor perfusion in this case is cardiogenic shock, the result of arrest-related myocardial ischemia. Patients may benefit from a 10- to 20-mL/kg fluid bolus administered over several minutes. If ventricular or pulmonary compliance is poor, a fluid bolus is administered with caution. Continuous infusions of inotropic agents (for example, epinephrine, dopamine, dobutamine) can be used to augment contractility and enhance tissue perfusion. Drug therapy is based upon clinical presentation. Inotropes are not indicated for hypovolemic shock.

Dopamine is indicated after volume replacement for the treatment of hypotension and/or poor perfusion in a patient with a stable heart rate and rhythm. Dopamine's effects are dependent on the release of endogenous norepinephrine from sympathetic nerve terminals. Dopamine may not be the agent of choice in infants because of incomplete maturation of the sympathetic nervous system, or in patients with chronic heart failure that depletes norepinephrine stores. Dopamine is started at 5 to 10 mcg/kg/minute, increased if necessary to 20 mcg/kg/minute. If doses higher than 20 mcg/kg/minute are required, dopamine is often associated with tachycardia and excessive vasoconstriction. The addition of an epinephrine infusion may permit administration of both medications at a lower dose. The advantage of low-dose dopamine is selective perfusion of the renal and splanchnic vascular beds. An epinephrine infusion is the drug of choice for patients with persistent bradycardia.

Dobutamine is a positive inotropic agent in patients with poor perfusion and normal blood pressure. Dobutamine is not as effective as dopamine in infants younger than 1 year and those in septic shock states. In cardiogenic shock, dobutamine increases cardiac output, decreases pulmonary capillary wedge pressure, and decreases SVR. Unlike dopamine, dobutamine does not depend upon releasable norepinephrine stores.

The initial priority in septic shock is fluid resuscitation. Ongoing management is then based upon blood pressure. Hypotensive septic patients may require *high* infusion doses of epinephrine or norepinephrine (1.0–1.5 mcg/kg/minute). Renal blood flow improves if pulse pressure increases. Dopamine at 5 to 10 mcg/kg/minute is used when the patient blood pressure is stable. Dobutamine at 5 to 10 mcg/kg/minute is used if the patient is normotensive but in cardiac failure. When poor lung compliance and pulmonary edema are present, dobutamine may worsen hypotension. If more than 20 mcg/kg/minute of dopamine or dobutamine is necessary, a continuous infusion of epinephrine or norepinephrine is helpful.

NEAR DEATH EXPERIENCES (NDE)

Little is known about near death experiences (NDE) among infants and children. In addition to the few retrospective reports that appear sporadically in the lay press, only 13 cases involving children aged 6 months to 16 years have been reported in the professional literature (Morse, 1983; Morse et al., 1986; Herzog & Herrin, 1985).

These reports indicate concerns about the emotional impact of NDEs on younger children. In the adult population, NDEs are generally associated with pleasant feelings of inner peace and love, whereas children report more varied experiences including fears of abandonment and separation. It is conceivable that because separation is difficult for young children, NDEs may be frightening to younger patients. In addition, cognitive immaturity may interfere with a young child's ability to understand, and verbal immaturity inhibits expression of the NDE. Either short- or long-term traumatic stress may result.

What we know about NDEs in the adult population allows us to provide support and comfort to parents of *older* children. The process of dying may not be painful but wondrous and serene despite the critical care environment. Currently, data do not exist to offer the same message for parents of infants and younger children.

Nurses can anticipate that any survivor of resuscitation may have experienced an NDE. Much can be learned by providing an opportunity for patients to talk about the experience. One way is to just ask patients what they can remember when they were very sick. Therapeutic play techniques (for example, drawings used as a communication strategy) have

SIDE 1

Code Blue QI Tool
CONFIDENTIAL MEDICAL PEER REVIEW INFORMATION
Please complete this form <u>immediately</u> after every resuscitation attempt

A. DEMOGRAPHICS

1. Date: _____ Time: _____ Unit: _____

2. Please describe the type of arrest:
   a. respiratory arrest (assisted ventilation required)
   b. cardiac arrest (compressions required)
   c. cardiorespiratory arrest (both a & b required)
   d. other, specify: _____

3. Admission Diagnosis: _____

4. Does the patient have a chronic underlying illness? Yes/No

   If yes, please specify: _____

B. RESPONSE TIME

1. Was the arrest a witnessed event?   Yes/No

2. What time was help called: ___:___ hr

3. What level of response was requested:
   a. "Code Blue"
   b. "Stat Page," specify discipline(s) requested:
   _____

4. How long did it take the team to fully assemble?
   ____minutes

5. Did anyone have difficulty locating the site of the code? Yes/No

   If yes, please identify the service: _____

C. CODE TEAM

Physicians
   ICU: _____

   Anesthesia: _____
Nurses
   ED Nurse: _____

   ICU Nurse: _____

Respiratory Therapist _____

Security Officer _____

Was medical leadership readily identified?   Yes/No

Comments: _____

D. EQUIPMENT

1. Where did you obtain the emergency equipment?
   a. on unit
   b. off unit, specify location: _____
   c. both on and off unit

2. Did you have all the equipment necessary to resuscitate the patient? Yes/No; If no, please specify the deficiencies:
   _____

3. Was all the equipment functioning properly? Yes/No; If no, please specify problem(s):
   _____

SIDE 2

E. PATIENT INFORMATION
1. Was the patient on a cardiac monitor?   Yes/No
2. What was the patient's initial cardiac rhythm?
   a. Asystole
   b. Bradycardia
   c. Fast narrow QRS complex
   d. Fast wide QRS complex
   e. Ventricular fibrillation

F. PATIENT'S OUTCOME
1. What was the patient's immediate outcome?
   a. Survived
   b. Died

2. If the patient *survived* please answer the following questions (if not, continue to E-3):

   a. Was the patient transferred to another unit?

      Yes/No; If yes, specify unit: _____

   b. Were there any delays/problems associated with the transfer? Yes/No; If yes, please describe:
   _____

   c. Please describe the first neuro exam after the arrest:
      1) Exam time _____ (_____ minutes after ending the code)
      2) Pupil response: _____
      3) Does this neuro exam reflect a change from the patient's pre-arrest baseline?   Yes/No

3. Were there any significant family issues?
   Yes/No; If yes, please describe:
   _____

G. OTHER
1. What happened well?

2. Identify one problem, that if addressed, could have significantly impacted the patient's outcome.

3. Were there any critical incidents?
   Yes/No; If yes, please describe:

Recorder's Name: _____

Title: _____ Phone Number: _____

Nurse Manager: _____

THANK YOU!!

Figure 33–12 ● ● ● ● ● ●
Code Blue QI tool. (Courtesy of Children's Hospital, CPR Committee, Boston, Massachusetts.)

been successful in preverbal children. Nursing research is needed to delineate the phenomena of NDE in various age groups so that appropriate interventions can be planned.

QUALITY IMPROVEMENT

Ehrlich and coworkers noted in 1974 that only when a team becomes experienced enough to turn the usual chaos of CPR into an almost routine procedure can patients be saved. Expertise can only be maintained through ongoing practice, yet, fortunately, clinical opportunities for skill development are limited. Adult cardiac arrests occur eight times more frequently than pediatric cardiac arrests (Eisenberg et al., 1983).

Knowledge of emergency procedures and skills is not well retained. Kaye and Mancini (1986) reported a study that evaluated the retention of CPR skills by medical residents, registered nurses, and the public, all of whom were trained 4 to 12 months before testing. No physician or nurse and only one lay person was able to perform basic life support (BLS) correctly and in proper sequence when evaluated. Although medical personnel performed necessary assessments better than lay personnel, all three groups performed ventilation poorly and all had difficulty with rate and depth of compressions.

Coordinated training programs that focus on the code team approach to resuscitation and the special needs of the pediatric patient may be helpful. Yakel (1989) found that detailed and frequent skill instruction coupled with review of past deficiencies helped to improve performance. Monthly interdisciplinary mock codes in which objective criteria are used to evaluate knowledge acquisition and skill performance are excellent ways to do this (Curley & Vaughn, 1987).

As part of a system-wide quality improvement plan, pediatric mock codes help to perfect BLS and PALS skills while also helping to consolidate individual and team roles. In addition, system deficiencies, such as availability of personnel, paging difficulties, impossible drug dilutions, and malfunctioning equipment, can be identified in a benign setting. Mock codes ensure that resuscitation team members are familiar with crash cart contents. Appendix IV (Emergency Cart Contents) contains a list of PICU crash cart contents. It is important that PICU crash cart contents reflect the patient population of the unit. That which may be appropriate for a pediatric cardiovascular surgical unit may be inappropriate for a multidisciplinary PICU. However, standardizing inpatient pediatric unit crash carts is necessary so that code team members can work rapidly from any crash cart in any location. Specialty items, such as cast cutters on an orthopedic unit, can be accommodated in boxes attached to the generic crash cart.

Every resuscitation attempt should be evaluated as a potential opportunity for system-wide improvement. Figure 33–12 illustrates an example of a qual-

ity assessment tool used by a CPR committee to evaluate resuscitation events. A child's potential death represents one of the most stressful experiences any staff member can encounter. Team conferences after successful *and* unsuccessful resuscitation attempts provide the entire healthcare team with an opportunity for mutual support.

SUMMARY

Three major characteristics distinguish cardiopulmonary arrest in infants and children. These are the diverse etiology of the arrest, the fact that most cardiopulmonary arrests can be prevented in infants and children, and certainty that primary cardiac arrest is unusual. Research demonstrates significant differences in overall survival and neurologic outcome in children depending on the type of arrest: survival is better in those who experience only respiratory arrest. Therefore, early recognition and intervention to prevent a pulseless state is critical. Survival rates have been shown to be higher when the interval between cardiac arrest and intervention is shorter. Despite these factors, which would provide the infant and child an apparent advantage, survival among pediatric patients experiencing cardiopulmonary arrest is poor.

Critical care nurses, working collaboratively with other healthcare professionals, are in a unique position to appreciate the anatomic, physiologic, and maturational factors that affect the pediatric patient's response to resuscitation efforts. The essence of caring for the critically ill pediatric patient includes the ability to rapidly identify what compensation looks like, intervene, and prevent cardiopulmonary arrest. Nurses are in a key position to make a critical difference in improving the currently dismal pediatric outcomes.

References

American Heart Association (1986). Standards and guidelines for cardiopulmonary resuscitation and emergency cardiac care; Part IV: Pediatric basic life support; Part V: Pediatric advanced life support. *Journal of the American Medical Association*, 255(21), 2954–2969.

American Heart Association (1992). Standards and guidelines for cardiopulmonary resuscitation and emergency cardiac care; Part V: Pediatric basic life support; Part VI: Pediatric advanced life support. *Journal of the American Medical Association*, 268(16), 2251–2275.

Berg, R.A. (1984). Emergency infusion of catecholamines into bone marrow. *American Journal of Diseases in Children*, 138, 810–811.

Brown, C.G., & Kelen, G.D. (1991). High-dose epinephrine in pediatric cardiac arrest. *Annals of Emergency Medicine*, 20(1), 104.

Chameides, L. (Ed.). (1990). *Textbook of pediatric advanced life support*. Dallas: American Heart Association.

Chameides, L., Hazinski, M.F. (Eds.). (1994). *Textbook of pediatric advanced life support*. Dallas: American Heart Association.

Chernow, B., Holbrook, P., D'Angona, D.S., Zaritsky, A., Casey, L.C., Fletcher, J.R., & Lake, C.R. (1984). Epinephrine absorption after intratracheal administration. *Anesthesia and Analgesia*, 63, 829–832.

Curley, M.A.Q. (1989). *Red flags in the critically unstable pediatric patient*. [Videotape]. NY: American Journal of Nursing.

Curley, M.A.Q., & Thompson, J.E. (1990). End-tidal CO_2 monitoring in critically-ill infants and children. *Pediatric Nursing*, 16(4), 397–403.

Curley, M.A.Q., & Vaughn, S.M. (1987a). Assessment and resuscitation of the pediatric patient. *Critical Care Nurse*, 7(3), 26–45.

Curley, M.A.Q., & Vaughn, S.M. (1987b). Pediatric resuscitation: Mock code. *MCN: The American Journal of Maternal/Child Nursing*, 12(4), 277–280.

Davies, C.R., Carrigan, T., Wright, J.A., Ahmann, P.A., & Watson, C. (1987). Neurologic outcome following pediatric resuscitation. *Journal of Neuroscience Nursing*, 19(4), 205–210.

Ditchey, R.V., & Lindenfeld, J. (1984). Potential adverse effects of volume loading on perfusion of vital organs during closed-chest resuscitation. *Circulation*, 69(1), 181–189.

Dronen, S.C. (1984). Antifibrillatory drugs: The case for bretylium tosylate. *Annals of Emergency Medicine*, 13(9) Part 2, 805–807.

Eisenberg, M., Bergner, L., & Hallstrom, A. (1983). Epidemiology of cardiac arrest and resuscitation in children. *Annals of Emergency Medicine*, 12(11), 672–674.

Ehrlich, R., Emmett, S.M., & Rodriguez-Torres, R. (1974). Pediatric cardiac resuscitation team: A 6 year study. *The Journal of Pediatrics*, 84(1), 152–155.

Fetterolf, G., & Gittings, J.C. (1911). Some anatomic features of a child's thorax and their practical application in physical diagnosis. *American Journal of Diseases in Children*, 1, 6–25.

Finholt, D.A., Ketterick, R.G., Wagner, H.R., & Swedlow, D.B. (1986). The heart is under the lower third of the sternum. *American Journal of Diseases in Children*, 140, 646–649.

Friedman, W.F. (1972). The intrinsic physiologic properties of the developing heart. *Progress in Cardiovascular Disease*, 15, 87.

Friesen, R.M., Duncan, P., Tweed, W.A., & Bristow, G. (1982). Appraisal of pediatric cardiopulmonary resuscitation. *CMA Journal*, 126, 1055–1058.

Galpin, R.D., Kronick, J.B., Willis, R.B., & Frewen, T.C. (1991). Bilateral lower extremity compartment syndromes secondary to intraosseous fluid resuscitation. *Journal of Pediatric Orthopaedics*, 11(6), 773–776.

Gazmuri, R.J., vonPlanta, M., Weil, M.H., & Rackow, E.C. (1989). Arterial pCO_2 as an indicator of systemic perfusion during cardiopulmonary resuscitation. *Critical Care Medicine*, 17(3), 237–240.

Goetting, M.G., & Paradis N.A. (1991a). High-dose epinephrine improves outcome from pediatric cardiac arrest. *Annals of Emergency Medicine*, 20(1), 22–25.

Goetting, M.G., & Paradis, N.A. (1991b). Right atrial-jugular venous pressure gradients during CPR in children. *Annals of Emergency Medicine*, 20(1), 27–30.

Greenberg, M.J., Roberts, J.R., & Baskin, S.I. (1981). Use of endotracheally administered epinephrine in a pediatric patient. *American Journal of Diseases in Children*, 135, 767–768.

Herzog, D.B., & Herrin, J.T. (1985). Near-death experiences in the very young. *Critical Care Medicine*, 13(12), 1074–1075.

Iseri, L.T., Humphrey, S.B., & Siner, E.J. (1978). Prehospital brady-asystolic cardiac arrest. *Annals of Internal Medicine*, 88(6), 741–745.

Katz, A.M., & Reuter, H. (1979). Cellular calcium and cardiac cell death. *American Journal of Cardiology*, 44, 188–190.

Kaye, W., & Mancini, M.E. (1986). Retention of cardiopulmonary resuscitation skills by physicians, registered nurses, and the general public. *Critical Care Medicine*, 14(7), 620–622.

Koehler, R.C., & Michael, J.R. (1985). Cardiopulmonary resuscitation, brain blood flow, and neurologic recovery. *Critical Care Clinics*, 1(2), 205–223.

Krongrad, E. (1984). Postoperative arrhythmias in patients with congenital heart disease. *Chest*, 85(1), 107–113.

Lewis, J.K., Minter, M.G., Eshelman, S.J., & Witte, M.K. (1983). Outcome of pediatric resuscitation. *Annals of Emergency Medicine*, 12(5), 297–299.

Longstreth, W.T., Diehr, P., Cobb, L.A., Hanson, R.W., & Blair, A.D. (1986). Neurologic outcome and blood glucose levels during out-of-hospital cardiopulmonary resuscitation. *Neurology*, 36, 1186–1191.

Lubitz, D.S., Seidel, J.S., Chameides, L., Luten, R.C., Zaritsky, A.L., & Campbell, F.W. (1988). A rapid method of estimating weight and resuscitation drug doses from length in the pediatric age group. *Annals of Emergency Medicine*, 17(6), 576–581.

Melker, R.J. (1986). Alternative methods of ventilation during respiratory and cardiac arrest. *Circulation*, 74[Suppl IV], IV63–IV65.

Micheal, J.R., Guerci, A.D., Koehler, R.C., Shi, A., Tsitlik, J., Chandra, N., Niedermeyer, E., Rogers, M.C., Traystman, R.J., & Weisfeldt, M.L. (1984). Mechanisms by which epinephrine augments cerebral and myocardial perfusion during cardiopulmonary resuscitation in dogs. *Circulation*, 69(4), 822–835.

Morse, M. (1983). A near-death experience in a 7-year-old child. *American Journal of Diseases in Children,* 137, 959–961.

Morse, M., Castillo, P., Venecia, D., Milstein, J., & Tyler, D.C. (1986). Childhood near-death experiences. *American Journal of Diseases in Children*, 140, 1110–1114.

Moynihan, R.J., Brock-Utne, J.G., Archer, J.H., Feld, L.H., & Kreitzman, T.R. (1993). The effect of cricoid pressure on preventing gastric insufflation in infants and children. *Anesthesiology*, 78, 652–656.

Nichols, D.G., Kettrick, R.G., Swedlow, D.B., Lee, S., Passman, R., & Ludwig, S. (1984). Factors influencing outcome of cardiopulmonary arrest in children. *Critical Care Medicine*, 12(3), 287.

Orlowski, J.P. (1984). Optimal position for external cardiac message in infants and children. *Critical Care Medicine*, 12(3), 224A.

Orlowski, J.P., Porembka, D.T., Gallagher, J.M., Lockrem, J.D., & VanLente, F. (1990). Comparison study of intraosseous, central intravenous, and peripheral intravenous infusions of emergency drugs. *American Journal of Diseases in Children*, 144(1), 112–117.

O'Rourke, P.P. (1986). Outcome of children who are apneic and pulseless in the emergency room. *Critical Care Medicine*, 14(5), 466–468.

Padilla, M.C.O., & Purcell, J.A. (1990). Using a structured cardiopulmonary resuscitation flow sheet. *Focus on Critical Care*, 17(6), 490–494.

Paradis, N.A., & Koscove, E.M. (1990). Epinephrine in cardiac arrest: A critical review. *Annals of Emergency Medicine*, 19(11), 1288–1301.

Paradis, N.A., Martin, G.B., Goetting, M.G., Rosenberg, J.M., Rivers, E.P., Appleton, T.J., & Nowak, R.M. (1989). Simultaneous aortic, jugular bulb, and right atrial pressures during cardiopulmonary resuscitation in humans: Insights into mechanism. *Circulation*, 80(2), 361–368.

Paradis, N.A., Martin, G.B., Rivers, E.P., Goetting, M.G., Appleton, T.J., Feingold, M., & Nowak, R.M. (1990). Coronary perfusion pressure and the return of spontaneous circulation in human cardiopulmonary resuscitation. *Journal of the American Medical Association*, 263(8), 1106–1113.

Paraskos, J.A. (1986). External compression without adjuncts. *Circulation*, 74(IV), IV33–IV36.

Phillips, G.W.L., & Zideman, D.A. (1986). Relation of infant heart to sternum: Its significance in cardiopulmonary resuscitation. *Lancet*, 1, 1024–1025.

Post, H. (1989). Letting the family in during a code. *Nursing 89*, March, 43–46.

Pulsinelli, W.A., Levy, D.E., Sigsbee, B., Scherer, P., & Plum, F. (1983). Increased damage after ischemic stroke in patients with hyperglycemia with or without established diabetes mellitus. *American Journal of Medicine*, 74, 540–544.

Quan, L., Wentz, K.R., Gore, E.J., & Copass, M.K. (1990). Outcome and predictors of outcome in pediatric submersion victims receiving prehospital care in King County, Washington. *Pediatrics*, 86(4), 586–593.

Rogers, M.C., & Kirsch, J.R. (1989). Current concepts in brain resuscitation. *Journal of the American Medical Association*, 261(21), 3143–3147.

Rogers, M.C., Nugent, S.K., & Stidham, G.L. (1979). Effects of closed-chest cardiac massage on intracranial pressure. *Critical Care Medicine*, 7(10), 454–456.

Rosenburg, J.M., Martin, G.B., Paradis, N.A., Nowak, R.M., Walton, D., & Welch, K.M.A. (1989). The effect of CO_2 and non-CO_2-generating buffers on cerebral acidosis after cardiac arrest: A ^{31}P NMR study. *Annals of Emergency Medicine*, 18(4), 341–347.

Rosetti, V.A., Thompson, B.M., Miller, J., Mateer, J.R., & Aprahamian, C. (1985). Intraosseous infusions: An alternative route of pediatric intravascular access. *Annals of Emergency Medicine,* 14(9), 885–888.

Schleien, C.L., Berkowitz, I.D., Traysman, R., & Rogers, M.C. (1989). Controversial issues in cardiopulmonary resuscitation. *Anesthesiology,* 71(1), 133–149.

Schleien, C.L., Dean, J.M., Koehler, R.C., Michael, J.R., Chantarojanasiri, T., Traysman, R., & Rogers, M.C. (1986). Effect of epinephrine on cerebral and myocardial perfusion in an infant animal preparation of cardiopulmonary resuscitation. *Circulation,* 73(4), 809–817.

Silka, M. (1991). Sudden death due to cardiovascular disease during childhood. *Pediatric Annals,* 20(7), 360–368.

Spivey, W.H. (1987). Intraosseous infusions. *The Journal of Pediatrics,* 111(5), 639–643.

Spivey, W.H., Lathers, C.M., Malone, D.R., Unger, H.D., Bhat, S., McNamara, R.N., Schoffstall, J., & Tumer, N. (1987). Comparison of intraosseous, central, and peripheral routes of sodium bicarbonate administration during CPR in pigs. *Annals of Emergency Medicine,* 14(12), 1135–1140.

Thaler, M.M., & Stobie, G.H.C. (1963). An improved technic of external cardiac compression in infants and young children. *New England Journal of Medicine,* 269(12), 606–610.

Torphy, D.E., Minter, M.G., & Thompson, B.M. (1984). Cardiorespiratory arrest and resuscitation of children. *American Journal of Diseases in Children,* 138, 1099–1102.

Valdez-Depena, M. (1985). Are some crib deaths sudden cardiac deaths? *Journal of the American College of Cardiology,* 5, 113B–117B.

Velanovich, V. (1989). Crystalloid versus colloid fluid resuscitation: A meta analysis of mortality. *Surgery,* 105(1), 65–71.

Verma, N.P. (1986). Drugs as a cause of fixed, dilated pupils after resuscitation. *Journal of the American Medical Association,* 255(23), 3151.

Villarreal, P., Hansen, M.L., & Middaugh, D. (1988). *Parent's rights and responsibilities during CPR of the hospitalized child.* San Antonio, TX: Children's Hospital Santa Rose Medical Center.

Von Seggern, K., Egar, M., & Fuhrman, B.P. (1986). Cardiopulmonary resuscitation in a pediatric ICU. *Critical Care Medicine,* 14(4), 275–277.

Walsh, C.K., & Krongrad, E. (1983). Terminal cardiac electrical activity in pediatric patients. *American Journal of Cardiology,* 51, 557–561.

Weil, M.H., Rackow, E.C., Trevino, R., Grundler, W., Falk, J.L., & Griffel, M.I. (1986). Difference in acid-base between venous and arterial blood during cardiopulmonary resuscitation. *New England Journal of Medicine,* 315(3), 153–156.

Weil, M.H., Ruiz, C.E., Michaels, S., & Rackow, E.C. (1985). Acid-base determinants of survival after cardiopulmonary resuscitation. *Critical Care Medicine,* 13(11), 888–891.

Yakel, M.E. (1989). Retention of cardiopulmonary resuscitation skills among nursing personnel: What makes the difference? *Heart & Lung,* 18(5), 520–525.

Zaritsky, A. (1993). Pediatric resuscitation pharmacology. *Annals of Emergency Medicine,* 22 (2 part 2), 445–455.

Zaritsky, A. (1988). Selected concepts and controversies in pediatric cardiopulmonary resuscitation. *Critical Care Clinics,* 4(4), 735–754.

Zaritsky, A., & Chernow, B. (1984). Use of catecholamines in pediatrics. *Journal of Pediatrics,* 105, 341–350.

Zaritsky, A., Nadkarni, V., Getson, P., & Kuehl, K. (1987). CPR in children. *Annals of Emergency Medicine,* 16(10), 1107–1111.

Practice Guidelines for Pediatric Critical Care

This three-part section presents practice guidelines for optimal care of critically ill infants, children, and their families. The first part, "Guidelines of Care for the Critically Ill Infant and Child," provides system-based recommendations regarding overall assessment and routine interventions in the care of critically ill infants and children. Nursing research is desperately needed to identify the value-added of traditional care practices. The next part is "Clinical Practice Guidelines," which are derived from the American Association of Critical Care Outcomes Standards. These guidelines were adapted for pediatric use by the Children's Hospital, Boston, Multidisciplinary ICU Council on Nursing Practice. As patients are assessed in the multidisciplinary intensive care unit, the nurse completes a nursing assessment, identifies patient problems, collects copies of the clinical practice guidelines, prioritizes the nursing diagnoses, and then delineates individualized interventions. When complete, the individualized guidelines form the basis of a patient's management plan. These guidelines can also be computerized and then recalled and individualized to again form the basis of an individual's management plan. These guidelines have been helpful in establishing unit-based agreement on common patient problems. The last part replicates the American Academy of Pediatrics and Society of Critical Care Medicine's Guidelines and Levels of Care for Pediatric Intensive Care Units. The guidelines have been helpful in establishing national standards on the overall structure of pediatric intensive care units.

GUIDELINES OF CARE FOR THE CRITICALLY ILL INFANT AND CHILD

Value Statement: Intensive care nurses are responsible for ensuring that all critically ill infants and children and their families receive optimal nursing care. Essential to this process are nursing expertise, nursing autonomy, and multidisciplinary collaboration. This standard is intended to complement all existing institutional standards. Admission assessment and documentation are determined by institutional standards. Ongoing reassessment and documentation will reflect the patient's clinical status and are completed at a frequency determined by the caregiver.

I. NEED: CONTINUOUS RESPIRATORY ASSESSMENT AND MANAGEMENT

Outcome Criteria

The nurse will continually assess all data pertinent to the patient's respiratory system and update/revise the plan of care to promote optimal oxygenation and ventilation.

Process Criteria

1. Nursing assessment of the respiratory system includes the following parameters:
   A. Respiratory rate and depth (degree of chest excursion)
   B. Breath sound characteristics (normal and adventitious)
   C. Color of skin, mucous membranes, and nailbeds
   D. Degree of respiratory distress (e.g., nasal flaring, grunting, retracting, restlessness)
   E. Noninvasive data (SpO_2, $ETcO_2$)
   F. Ventilator parameters
2. Respiratory rate is continuously monitored via bedside monitor or ventilator. High/low limits are set as appropriate for patient's age and acuity. Apnea alarms are set for no more than 20 seconds.
3. Airway patency is protected by positioning, airway adjuncts, and/or suctioning. Frequency of artificial airway and naso/oropharyngeal suctioning is as necessary.
4. If intubated, endotracheal tubes (ETTs) are continuously assessed for adequate stabilization.
5. ETT/tracheostomy size, presence or absence of airleak, and ETT exit markings are documented at the beginning of each shift, and any time the ETT is retaped. If cuffed tubes are used, cuff pressures are monitored/documented with each cuff inflation and maintained <25 mmHg if the minimal leak technique is not used.
6. Ventilatory settings are verified and documented at the beginning of each shift and with each ventilator change.
7. Response to all respiratory treatments/therapy (including IV, enteral, and inhaled medications) is assessed and documented every shift.
8. ABG/VBGs, SpO_2, SvO_2, or $ETcO_2$ baselines are established and trends monitored and documented. SpO_2 and SvO_2 low alarm limits will be set no more than 5% less than expected value. $ETcO_2$ low alarms are set in collaboration with respiratory therapy.
9. Chest tube patency, presence of water seal, level of H_2O suction, and presence or absence of airleak are noted and documented each shift. Unless otherwise stated, suction will be maintained at 20 cmH_2O. Chest tube is banded at all connections. Chest tube dressings are changed every 3 days.
10. If the patient has a tracheostomy, an extra tracheostomy tube is placed within view at the bedside. Daily tracheostomy care is per hospital procedure.
11. The patient is weaned from mechanical ventilation using parameters collaboratively determined by the multidisciplinary team.

II. NEED: CONTINUOUS CARDIOVASCULAR ASSESSMENT AND MANAGEMENT

Outcome Criteria

The nurse will continually assess all data pertinent to the patient's cardiovascular system and update/revise the plan of care to promote optimal tissue perfusion.

Process Criteria

1. Nursing assessment of the cardiovascular system includes the following parameters:
   A. Heart rate and rhythm
   B. Arterial blood pressure and other invasive hemodynamic parameters
   C. Color of skin, mucous membranes, and nailbeds
   D. Capillary refill
   E. Vasopressor parameters
2. The heart rate and rhythm are continuously monitored via bedside monitor. High/low alarm limits are set as appropriate for patient's age and acuity (i.e., 20 above and below current rate). If an arterial line is available, the heart rate is determined by the arterial waveform.
3. Hemodynamic monitoring lines are transduced and the waveform, systolic/diastolic, or mean pressures are continuously monitored. High/low alarm limits for systolic, diastolic, and/or mean are set no more than 20 mmHg above and below current value. Alarms are always on. The trans-

ducer is zeroed and recalibrated at the beginning of the shift and prn. The pressure waveform is continuously monitored.

4. Vital signs are assessed on admission and every 1–4 hours based upon the level of acuity. Baseline cuff blood pressures are obtained and documented at the beginning of the shift. Cuff size is noted upon admission. Heart sounds are auscultated and abnormalities noted with vital signs.

5. Patient temperature is monitored every 1–4 hours.

6. Peripheral perfusion (capillary refill, nailbed color, extremity temperature, pulse quality) is assessed with vital signs.

7. Rhythm strips are obtained whenever there is any question regarding cardiac rhythm. If a dysrhythmia occurs, the effect on the child's perfusion will be assessed and contributing factors considered (e.g., K, Ca, acidosis, hypoxemia).

8. Response to cardiovascular agents is continuously assessed. If a pulmonary artery catheter is in place, cardiac output and hemodynamic measurements are obtained as frequently as warranted by the patient's condition. The pulmonary artery tracing is continuously monitored for fall back to right ventricle or spontaneous wedge.

9. Patients are monitored for evidence of systemic venous engorgement (increased CVP/RAP, periorbital or peripheral edema) and for evidence of pulmonary venous engorgement (tachypnea, decreased lung compliance, alterations in blood gases).

10. Hourly (if acuity necessitates) and running totals will be kept on intake and output.

III. NEED: CONTINUOUS NEUROLOGIC ASSESSMENT AND MANAGEMENT

Outcome Criteria

The nurse will continually assess all data pertinent to the patient's neurologic system and update/revise the plan of care to promote optimal neurologic functioning.

Process Criteria

1. Nursing assessment of the neurologic system includes the following parameters:
   A. Level of consciousness—Glasgow Coma Scale if all parameters can be assessed
   B. Sensory/motor function
   C. Respiratory patterns
   D. Pupil response
   E. Vital signs
   F. Intracranial and cerebral perfusion pressures
   G. Continuous/intermittent electroencephalographs (EEG)
2. Level of consciousness will be assessed with vital signs. A full neurologic assessment is completed when warranted by patient diagnosis/status.

3. To ensure an adequate level of analgesia/sedation, the need for pain/sedation medication will be assessed with vital signs.

4. All infants younger than 1 year of age will have a head circumference done on admission and prn. The anterior fontanelle will be assessed and documented daily (e.g., soft, flat, tense, or bulging). Achievement of developmental milestones is assessed upon admission.

5. Prior to utilizing chemical paralyzing agents, a baseline motor assessment is obtained/documentated. Sedation is always used in conjunction with chemical paralyzing agents.

6. When prescribed, EEG will be documented with suspected seizure activity.

7. Seizure activity (including aura, time of onset, origin and progression of seizure activity, type of activity, level of consciousness, head or eye movement, incontinence of urine or stool, duration of seizure, postictal state) and medications (including doses and their resultant effects) are assessed and documented.

8. Anticonvulsant medications are scheduled to assure therapeutic effectiveness.

9. If ICP monitoring is in place, ICP and CPP are continuously monitored and documented every hour and prn with significant changes. ICP precautions are implemented as indicated (decreased environmental/noxious stimuli, HOB elevated).

IV. NEED: CONTINUOUS GASTROINTESTINAL ASSESSMENT AND MANAGEMENT

Outcome Criteria

The nurse will continually assess all data pertinent to the patient's gastrointestinal system and update/revise the plan of care to promote optimal gastrointestinal functioning.

Process Criteria

1. The abdomen will be inspected and auscultated q4 hours and prn. Baseline abdominal girths are obtained and documented on admission and prn in patients with existing or suspected GI problems.

2. History of usual food intake, food intolerance/allergies is obtained upon admission.

3. Unless specifically noted, all intubated patients will have an NG/OG tube. NG/OG tube placement will be assessed by auscultation and aspiration of gastric contents every shift and before administration of medications or feedings. To prevent skin breakdown, NGTs are isolated and taped down onto the patient's upper lip.

4. All sump tubes are maintained with constant suc-

tion no greater than 60 mmHg. Mucous traps are used in all infants less than 6 months of age.

5. NG/OG tubes are irrigated with NS or sterile water in appropriate volumes prn to maintain tube patency. If the patient is NPO, the gastric pH is measured and documented q4–6 hours. Gastric drainage is tested for blood every shift.

6. Quantity and quality of gastric/bowel outputs will be assessed and documented every shift.

7. Nasojejunal (NJ) tube placement is initially verified by radiographs. Length of NJ tube from nares or mouth to connection is measured and documented at the time of radiograph and every shift.

8. Maintain head of bed (HOB) at 30 degrees while tube feedings are infusing to prevent aspiration. If unable to tolerate HOB elevation, turn right side or prone. Check NG/OG/GT residuals q4 hours. Hold NGT feedings 1/2 hour prior to and during CPT.

9. Assess height, weight, and head circumference on admission; then assess weight at least biweekly or more frequently prn.

V. NEED: CONTINUOUS GENITOURINARY ASSESSMENT AND MANAGEMENT

Outcome Criteria

The nurse will continually assess all data pertinent to the patient's genitourinary system and update/revise the plan of care to promote optimal genitourinary functioning.

Process Criteria

1. All intake and output is recorded with net totals hourly.

2. Unless otherwise noted, trends in urine output less than 0.5 mL/kg/hr are reported to the physician.

3. In all catheterized patients, urine specific gravity and dipstick every shift. Foley bags are emptied every shift and prn. Unless perineal swelling is present, Foley catheters are changed every 2 weeks.

4. Perineal care/Foley care qd and prn. Anchoring tape for Foley catheters is placed on the lower abdomen for boys and inner thigh for girls.

5. Urinary catheters are irrigated to maintain patency.

VI. NEED: CONTINUOUS INTEGUMENTARY ASSESSMENT AND MANAGEMENT

Outcome Criteria

The nurse will continually assess all data pertinent to the patient's integumentary system and update/revise the plan of care to promote/maintain an intact integument.

Process Criteria

1. Unless a newborn, daily baths. Hair is shampooed weekly or prn after EEG leads are removed. ECG leads are changed and dated q3 days with bath.

2. Patient's skin condition will be assessed on admission, every shift, and prn. Skin care every shift and prn turning.

3. Mouth care q4 hours in patients who are NPO, otherwise bid. Vaseline gauze is used to prevent tongue dryness in the comatose intubated patient.

4. Eye care on chemically paralyzed/immobilized patients will include cleansing with sterile NaCl and instillation of a lubricant q4 hours and prn to maintain adequate lubrication. Clear plastic cover may prevent corneal abrasions.

5. Immobilized patients will be turned/tilted every 2–4 hours. If stability prevents total body repositioning, head and extremities are repositioned and measures to protect the torso are implemented. ROM exercise is performed to all extremities every 4 hours on immobilized patients as tolerated. Neutral body position is maintained.

6. Comfort devices are used for immobile patients. Suggestions include eggcrates, air mattresses, and gel pillow/pads.

7. Therapeutic beds may be used on patients with or at high potential for skin breakdown. Reevaluation of the benefits of using the therapeutic bed is documented daily.

8. ICCs are used for thermoregulation in infants developmentally unable to roll over who require invasive monitoring devices. Lotions are used sparingly to avoid altered skin integrity.

9. Heat lamps are maintained at least 18 inches away from the patient.

10. Because of the potential for shivering, cooling blankets are used cautiously on patients not receiving chemical paralyzing agents. When a cooling blanket is used, the condition of dependent skin areas is assessed q2 hours and prn with repositioning.

11. Wound care/surgical dressings are changed as per departmental policy. Nurses are responsible for all dressing changes. Circumferential tape and dressings are avoided.

12. All infusion sites are inspected and documented at the start of the shift for signs of infiltration/infection. Central, arterial, peripheral venous access dressings are changed every 72 hours per departmental policy and procedure. Skin appearance is assessed and documented with all invasive line dressing changes.

VII. NEED: INTENSIVE CARE UNIT ENVIRONMENTAL SAFETY

Outcome Criteria

The incidence of iatrogenic injury will be limited.

Process Criteria

1. Side/cribrails will be kept up at all times except on patients maintained on chemical muscle relaxants. Unless the infant is on ECMO support, siderails on the infant warmer will be kept up at all times to prevent heat loss.
2. Safety restraints will be used on all children when OOB in chairs, infant seats, tumblefoam chairs, highchairs, or go-carts. Physical restraints are used when the patient is assessed to be harmful to himself or others and comfort measures and chemical restraints have been ineffective.
3. Monitor alarms are never deactivated for more than 3 minutes on any bedside monitor.
4. No live plants or flowers will be allowed at the bedside.
5. At beginning of shift, oncoming R.N. will check correctness of all IV solutions and correct rate to deliver desired dosage of drug. Will ensure that all drip cards and medication sheets have been double-checked and co-signed (name, dosage, frequency, route, and hour due [in pen]).
6. Heparin locks are flushed per departmental policy and procedure q6 hours. IV bags/bottles/syringes/intralipid tubings are changed q24 hours; all other tubings are changed every 72 hours and labeled with the patient's name, date, time hung, and initials of the nurse hanging the solution.
7. Unless contraindicated, one distal filter is used on all solutions administered via central line. Albumin and insulin are not filtered.
8. All IV fluids are double-checked for concentration and rate when mixed. Unless contraindicated, unit-standard dilutions will be used. Drip cards are completed on all titratable vasoactive drugs. Two nursing signatures are required to validate that the computation for the infusion is correct. The second nurse will use an alternate method of calculation. All vasoactive drugs are administered on infusion pumps into the most central vascular access site available. Infusion pumps are labeled with the fluid delivered.
9. No more than 2 hours' worth of fluid is placed in a Buretrol. The clamp between the IV bag and Buretrol never remains open except when filling the Buretrol or if the IV rate is greater than 100 mL/hr. A "keep vein open" (KVO) feature should not be disabled.
10. When using a manifold, the order of fluids is determined by infusion rate. The fastest infusion rate is placed distal to the patient.
11. Occlusive caps protect all unused stopcock sidearms. Dead head caps are changed with each line entry.
12. Documentation of continuous narcotic infusions will occur per hospital controlled substance infusion procedure.

VIII. NEED: PSYCHOSOCIAL SUPPORT

Outcome Criteria

The child and family will receive care within the intensive care unit, which is consistent with the philosophy of family-centered care.

Process Criteria

1. Each patient will receive developmentally appropriate stimulation and activities. Consultations with the Child Life therapist are sought as appropriate.
2. Patient and family privacy will be protected at all times. Confidentiality will be ensured. Access to the child's records is limited to the parents/patient and direct care providers.
3. The parents are recognized as vitally important in the care of their child and are invited to participate in all care activities that they find personally rewarding.
4. Information is provided to parents so that they can make informed judgments and actively participate in decision-making regarding their child's plan of care. Nursing staff will advocate for parents' rights to healthcare decision-making.
5. Parents are encouraged to be with their child as soon as possible after admission. Prior to the first visit, anticipatory information regarding their child's appearance and behavior is provided. When the parents are emotionally accessible, they receive an orientation to the unit and a discussion of parental rights.
6. Nursing staff will facilitate visitation and interaction with siblings (without communicable diseases).
7. Multidisciplinary support (including pastoral, social service, and psychiatry) is available to all families as needed.
8. Children and their families will be given time and assistance to come to an appropriate acceptance of the diagnosis, prognosis, treatment, and sequelae with the condition or disease that they face.
9. When necessary, staff will provide an environment that is supportive to the grieving process. Parental wishes and cultural and spiritual beliefs will be supported. Bereavement follow-up will be initiated.

References

American Association of Critical Care Nurses (1989). *Standards for nursing care of the critically ill.* Norwalk, CT: Appleton & Lange.

PICU Clinical Practice Committee and PICU Staff Nurses (1991). *Unit specific standards/guidelines; Pediatric intensive care.* San Diego, CA: San Diego Children's Hospital.

CLINICAL PRACTICE GUIDELINES

Health Perception—Health Management

POTENTIAL FOR INJURY   • • • • • •

Description
The state in which an individual is at risk for bodily injury in the caregiving environment.

Need
To eliminate acquired injury.

Outcome Criteria
Safe passage

Process Criteria
1. Eliminate risk factors where possible (e.g., implement hospital-wide fire safety protocols).
2. Implement individual safety measures (e.g., safety check on flow sheet, cribrails).
3. Adhere to medication precautions (e.g., right patient, right dose).
4. Position to minimize risk of injury (e.g., head turned to side).
5. Implement homeostasis measures (e.g., pressure dressings).
6. Provide adequate lighting with diurnal variation.
7. Provide assistance for sensory impairments (e.g., glasses, hearing aid).
8. Provide assistance to movement as appropriate to condition of patient (e.g., personal assistance by nurse with adequate help, prostheses).
9. Use physical or chemical restraints judiciously.
10. *Teach* developmentally appropriate anticipatory guidance about safety to patient/family.

POTENTIAL FOR INFECTION/ COLONIZATION   • • • • • •

Description
The state in which an individual is at risk for acquiring an infection or becoming colonized with microorganisms.

Need
To limit the patient's risk of infection and colonization.

Outcome Criteria
- Absent signs/symptoms of localized infection (redness, tenderness, swelling).
- Absent signs/symptoms of systemic infection (fever, tachycardia).
- Negative screening cultures for colonization of microorganisms.

Process Criteria
1. Eliminate/modify risk factors where possible (e.g., ineffective airway clearance, impaired skin integrity, altered nutrition).
2. Practice routine infection control measures (e.g., handwashing).
3. Apply infection control measures as appropriate to patient problems and transmission mechanisms of organisms.
4. Adhere to hospital policies/protocols on line/tubing/dressing changes, etc., consistent with Centers for Disease Control and Prevention (CDC) guidelines.
5. Schedule medications to assure therapeutic effectiveness (e.g., maintain blood levels, appropriate relationship to food).
6. Collect specimens for culture where clinical signs and symptoms warrant.
7. Arrange for change of lines/tubes/drains inserted during a crisis when the patient's condition is stable.
8. Ensure care and cleaning of equipment/supplies according to hospital policies/protocols, consistent with CDC guidelines.
9. *Teach* infection control practices to patient/visitors.

Nutritional—Metabolic

ALTERED FLUID VOLUME: DEFICIT   • • • • • •

Description
The state in which an individual experiences vascular, cellular, or intracellular dehydration.

Need
Adequate fluid volume

Outcome Criteria
- Balanced intake and output
- Weight is stable and within normal limits for patient
- Normal serum and urine electrolytes and osmolarity
- Moist mucous membranes
- Normal cardiac filling pressures (CVP, PAWP)
- Absent postural hypotension
- Normal skin turgor

Process Criteria
1. Eliminate/modify etiologies/related factors where possible.
2. Provide adequate fluid intake by
   a. replacing fluid losses.
   b. encouraging oral intake of fluids as appropriate.

c. providing oral fluids appealing to patient.
d. administering free water with tube feedings as appropriate.

3. Maximize physiologic function through titration of IV drug therapy.
4. Avoid postural hypotension by moving patient slowly to a sitting position.
5. Monitor serum electrolytes, serum osmolarity, hemoglobin and hematocrit, and urine specific gravity, and modify fluids as needed.
6. *Teach* the patient and family the need for fluid intake appropriate to physiologic need.

ALTERED FLUID VOLUME: EXCESS • • • • • •

Description
The state in which an individual experiences vascular, interstitial, and/or intracellular fluid retention or overload.

Need
Adequate fluid volume

Outcome Criteria
- Absent acute dyspnea or orthopnea
- Normal serum and urine electrolytes and osmolarity
- Balanced intake and output
- Normal filling pressures (CVP, PAWP)
- Absent or reduced edema
- Absent rales/crackles
- Weight stable within normal limits for patient
- Absent pulmonary congestion

Process Criteria
1. Eliminate/modify etiologies/related factors where possible.
2. Position patient according to physiologic need (e.g., elevate HOB to enhance ventilation).
3. Maximize physiologic function through the scheduling and titration of drug therapy (e.g., inotropes, vasodilators, and diuretics).
4. Limit fluid intake at the prescribed level.
5. Maintain diet appropriate to physiologic need.
6. Monitor electrolytes and osmolarity and modify fluids as needed.
7. *Teach* the patient and family the need for adequate fluid intake and diet appropriate to physiologic need.

ALTERED NUTRITION: LESS THAN BODY REQUIREMENT • • • • • •

Description
The state in which an individual experiences an intake of nutrients insufficient to meet metabolic needs.

Need
To meet metabolic requirements.

Outcome Criteria
- Weight (on the same scale and time of day) stable or increased
- Protein reserves adequate
- Nitrogen balance positive or equal
- Wound healing progressive
- Triceps skin fold measurement within 60% of standard
- Midarm muscle circumference greater than 15th percentile
- Weight:height ratio greater than 5th percentile

Process Criteria
1. Eliminate/modify etiologies/related factors where possible.
2. Provide nutritional requirements that supply adequate concentrations of protein and adequate calories (carbohydrates and fat) to meet energy expenditure.
3. Provide oral hygiene.
4. Provide frequent small meals. Match food texture with the ability to chew.
5. Plan mealtime to avoid interruptions.
6. Consult nutrition support services.
7. Supplement vitamins and trace minerals.
8. Infants:
   - Provide type of nipple normally used for feedings.
   - Encourage breastfeeding or use of breast milk.
   - Offer pacifier during and immediately after tube feeding.
9. Assist with feedings:
   - Encourage family participation.
   - Serve favorite foods.
   - Assist with menu selection.
10. Enteral feed continuously in preference to bolus. Hold tube feedings for signs of intolerance.
11. *Teach* patient/family optimal nutritional practices.

IMPAIRED SKIN INTEGRITY • • • • • •

Description
The state in which an individual's skin is adversely altered.

Need
To improve the skin's integrity.

Outcome Criteria
- Skin color, texture, turgor, moisture, and temperature normal for patient.
- Ulcers, lesions, or erythema improved or absent.
- Tissue epithelialization/granulation at site of impaired skin integrity evident.
- Mucous membranes intact.

Process Criteria

1. Eliminate/modify the etiologies/related factors when possible.
2. Maximize nutritional status.
3. Maintain topical medications for maximal effectiveness.
4. Prevent local skin breakdown by using products that absorb wound drainage.
5. *Teach* the patient and/or the family appropriate ways to prevent pressure, shear, friction, maceration.
6. *Teach* the patient/parents the early signs of skin damage.

POTENTIAL FOR IMPAIRED SKIN INTEGRITY   • • • • • •

Description

The state in which an individual's skin is at risk of being adversely altered.

Need

To maintain the skin's integrity.

Outcome Criteria

• Skin color, texture, turgor, moisture, and temperature remain normal for patient.
• Mucous membranes remain intact.

Process Criteria

1. Eliminate/modify risk factors where possible.
2. Position patient so that all body parts are appropriately supported.
3. Use pressure-dispersing devices as appropriate.
4. Facilitate the highest level of mobility that is possible for the patient (e.g., ROM exercises, frequent turning, assisting patient to get out of bed).
5. Keep skin clean and dry.
6. Select adhesives that are least irritating to patient's skin.
7. Select appropriate measures (alternatives to adhesives) for securing tubes, dressings, other materials.
8. Select soap and lotion according to the patient's skin condition.
9. Provide regular oral hygienic care.
10. *Teach* the patient/family appropriate ways to prevent pressure, shear, friction, maceration, and early signs of skin damage.

ALTERED THERMOREGULATION: HYPERTHERMIA   • • • • • •

Description

The state in which an individual's body temperature is above normal range.

Need

To normalize the patient's temperature.

Outcome Criteria

Body temperature between 36.6 and 37.5°C.

Process Criteria

1. Eliminate/modify etiologies/related factors where possible.
2. Consult with physician regarding collaborative management strategies.
3. Institute measures to increase heat loss (e.g., remove blankets and excess clothing; apply cold cloths, hypothermia blanket, tepid baths, and ice packs; lower environmental temperature).
4. Taper cooling measures at 38°C.
5. *Teach* patient and/or family how to take a temperature and prioritize appropriate interventions.

ALTERED THERMOREGULATION: HYPOTHERMIA   • • • • • •

Description

The state in which an individual's body temperature is below normal range.

Need

To normalize the patient's temperature.

Outcome Criteria

Body temperature between 36.6 and 37.5°C.

Process Criteria

1. Eliminate/modify etiologies/related factors where possible.
2. Reduce or eliminate sources of heat loss:
   • Keep skin dry.
   • Reduce drafts.
   • Increase room temperature.
3. Warm articles used for care (stethoscopes, hands).
4. Add additional blankets or place on warming blanket.
5. Place under warming lights/radiant heater.
6. Neonate:
   • Place cap on head except when under radiant heat source.
   • Use radiant warmer or isolette.
7. Taper warming measures at 36.8°C or adjust to maintain temperature at 36.6–37.5°C.
8. *Teach* patient and/or family how to take a temperature and prioritize appropriate interventions.

Elimination

ALTERED BOWEL ELIMINATION: DIARRHEA   • • • • • •

Description

The state in which an individual experiences a change in normal bowel habits characterized by the frequent passage of loose, fluid, unformed stools.

Need
To eliminate diarrhea.

Outcome Criteria
- Frequency of stools normal for patient
- Consistency of stools normal for patient

Process Criteria
1. Eliminate/modify etiologies/related factors where possible (e.g., remove fecal impactions).
2. Remove food allergens or food to which the patient is intolerant from diet.
3. Schedule medications to control diarrhea/recommend changes or additions in antidiarrheal therapy.
4. Ensure an adequate free water intake.
5. Adjust tube feeding regimen to improve tolerance:
   - Change to continuous drip feedings.
   - Decrease infusion rate.
   - Recommend diluting feedings.
   - Change to a more elemental formula (e.g., Reabilon).
   - Add fiber to formula.
   - Use peptide-based formulas for hypoalbuminemic patients.
6. Infants/toddlers (in addition to the above):
   - Breastfed infants: Discontinue solids; administer clear fluid supplements; continue to breastfeed.
   - Formula- or milk-fed infants: Discontinue formula, milk, and solids; administer clear fluid supplements.
   - Administer small amounts of clear liquids or oral electrolyte solutions every 1/2 to 1 hour for 24 hours.
   - Increase quantity of clear liquids if stools have decreased.
   - Gradually return to regular diet without milk in 2 days.
   - Add one new item at a time and begin with bland foods.
   - Administer bananas, rice, applesauce, and tea (BRAT diet).
7. Consider the effects of medications (e.g., antibiotics, antacids) on stool frequency and consistency.
8. *Teach* the patient/family how to identify the cause of the diarrhea.

ALTERED BOWEL ELIMINATION: CONSTIPATION
• • • • • •

Description
The state in which an individual experiences a change in normal bowel habits characterized by a decrease in frequency and/or passage of hard, dry stools.

Need
To eliminate constipation.

Outcome Criteria
- Frequency of stools normal for the patient
- Consistency of stools normal for the patient

Process Criteria
1. Eliminate/modify etiologies/related factors where possible.
2. Increase activity level.
3. Early ambulation, active and passive range of motion for bedridden patients.
4. Add roughage and bulk to diet.
5. Increase oral fluid intake until urine is clear if not contraindicated by present medical condition.
6. Provide for comfort, privacy, positioning, and sufficient time to enhance defecation attempts (e.g., use bedside commode whenever possible).
7. Consider developmental status.
8. Maintain or establish toileting routine.
9. Select and schedule administration of prn medications: stool softeners, suppositories.
10. Promote stimulation of the defecation reflex (e.g., administer warm oral fluids, direct stimulation of rectal muscle wall).
11. Consider effects of narcotics and other medications on gut motility.
12. *Teach* the patient/family about the role of exercise, diet, fluid intake, and a routine elimination pattern in the prevention of constipation.

ALTERED URINARY ELIMINATION: RETENTION
• • • • • •

Description
The state in which an individual experiences incomplete emptying of the bladder.

Need
To improve or maintain adequate bladder emptying.

Outcome Criteria
- Voids voluntarily every 3–4 hours
- Residual urine amount normal for age and weight
- Sensation of bladder fullness absent
- Bladder distension absent

Process Criteria
1. Eliminate/modify etiologies/related factors where possible.
2. Provide for comfort and privacy during voiding attempts.
3. Provide a timed voiding schedule with voiding attempts every 3–4 hours with intermittent catheterization for postvoid residuals.
4. Maintain adequate fluid intake (appropriate for weight).

5. Perform intermittent catheterization approximately every 4 hours in accordance with the patient's activities.
6. Insert an indwelling Foley catheter (used only when other measures have proved unsuccessful).
7. Provide auditory stimulation (e.g., running water).
8. *Teach* patient methods of initiating voiding (e.g., abdominal strain and Valsalva maneuver, bladder massage), and to void based on a timing schedule or if the symptoms of autonomic dysreflexia are present (headache, flushing, sweating, increased blood pressure).

ALTERED URINARY ELIMINATION: TOTAL INCONTINENCE   • • • • • •

Description
The state in which an individual experiences a continuous or unpredictable loss of urine.

Need
To control urine flow.

Outcome Criteria
- Bladder emptying regular
- Incontinent episodes contained

Process Criteria
1. Eliminate/modify etiologies/related factors where possible.
2. Schedule voiding times at regular intervals (at least once during the night).
3. Provide privacy during voiding attempts.
4. Initiate a bladder-retraining program.
5. Collect urine flow with an external condom catheter, diapers, or incontinent briefs.
6. Maintain fluid intake adequate for weight of patient.
7. *Teach* patient/family maneuvers that facilitate urinary continence.

ALTERED URINARY ELIMINATION: REFLEX INCONTINENCE   • • • • • •

Description
The state in which an individual experiences an involuntary loss of urine, occurring at somewhat predictable intervals, when a specific bladder volume is reached.

Need
To control bladder emptying.

Outcome Criteria
- Urinary continence
- Autonomic dysreflexia absent

- Uses triggering methods to void

Process Criteria
1. Schedule triggered voiding to preempt incontinence or whenever symptoms of autonomic dysreflexia are present.
2. Schedule intermittent catheterization program only as necessary.
3. *Teach* the patient/family methods of triggered voiding (e.g., deep suprapubic tapping, striking the abdomen lightly above inguinal ligaments), use of the Valsalva maneuver during triggered voiding, and to void using Crede's maneuver.

Activity—Exercise

IMPAIRED AIRWAY CLEARANCE   • • • • • •

Description
The state in which an individual is unable to clear the airways of secretions or other obstructing matter.

Need
To clear the patient's airway.

Outcome Criteria
- Rhonchi or localized wheezes are absent after cough
- Peak airway pressure reduced at similar ventilator settings
- Indicates clear airways
- Foreign body absent on subsequent chest film

Process Criteria
1. Eliminate/modify etiologies/related factors where possible.
2. Position and support to enhance cough efficacy.
3. Use alternative cough techniques (e.g., instruct the patient to cough after the 3rd breath).
4. Facilitate deep breathing before coughing (e.g., by request, incentive spirometer, resuscitation bag, or temporary ventilator volume adjustment).
5. Humidify inspired air when upper airway is bypassed.
6. Provide bronchial (postural) drainage treatments (e.g., positioning, vibration, percussion).
7. Schedule analgesia to facilitate airway clearance (cough, bronchial drainage) treatments.
8. Coordinate inhaled bronchodilator administration to facilitate airway (bronchial drainage) treatments.
9. Increase supplemental oxygen during bronchial drainage treatment when indicated.
10. Stabilize artificial airways to limit local irritation or trauma leading to abnormal mucociliary function.
11. Perform tracheobronchial or nasotracheal suctioning.
12. Position to prevent pulmonary aspiration of gastric or pharyngeal contents.

13. Ensure adequate systemic hydration, limit saline instillation during suctioning.
14. *Teach* the patient/family airway clearance therapies and appropriate foods and toys relative to child's age (e.g., no carrots, peanuts, popcorn, balloons for toddlers).

IMPAIRED BREATHING PATTERN • • • • • •

Description
The state in which an individual has an abnormality in the rate, depth, timing, rhythm, or chest wall/abdominal excursion during inspiration, expiration, or both.

Need
To improve/normalize the patient's breathing pattern.

Outcome Criteria
- Normal respiratory rate, depth (volume), timing, and rhythm
- Absent inspiratory retractions/nasal flaring
- Absent accessory muscle use at rest
- Motion of thorax and abdomen synchronous during inspiration
- Absent grunting and/or abdominal end-expiratory contraction
- Excursion of hemithoraces present and symmetric
- Bilateral breath sounds present and normal
- Patient indicates satisfactory breathing

Process Criteria
1. Eliminate etiology/related factors where possible.
2. Maintain upper airway patency (e.g., correct jaw and tongue position, insert nasal or oropharyngeal airway).
3. Administer oxygen.
4. Provide comfort measures to enhance normal respiratory excursion, lung volume, and support of diaphragm in infants (e.g., analgesics, positioning).
5. Provide tactile/auditory stimulation of breathing in apneic/hypopneic infants, and occasionally in children and adults.
6. Provide mechanical support of tidal volume or overall ventilation (e.g., incentive spirometry, manual resuscitation bag, mechanical ventilation).
7. Reduce energy demands.
8. Use airway clearance techniques (e.g., cough, postural drainage, suctioning).
9. Schedule/administer bronchodilators, narcotic antagonists.
10. *Teach* the patient/parents:
    - Deep breathing (e.g., spontaneous, incentive spirometer)
    - Inspiratory muscle training

- Self-administration of medications (e.g., bronchodilators)
- Energy conservation techniques

IMPAIRED GAS EXCHANGE: • • • • • •
HYPOXEMIA

Description
The state in which an individual has a low arterial oxygen pressure (PaO_2) and/or oxygen saturation (SpO_2).

Need
To reduce or eliminate hypoxemia.

Outcome Criteria
- Normal or baseline PaO_2/SpO_2
- Normal respiratory rate and heart rate for patient
- Absent or reduced neurobehavioral abnormalities (e.g., improved response to the environment)
- Resolved cyanosis or pale skin appearance

Process Criteria
1. Assess respiratory status.
2. Eliminate or modify etiologies/related factors where possible.
3. Use tactile or calm vocal stimuli to increase breathing rate/depth.
4. Encourage deep breathing.
5. Position patient so that the unaffected area or side of lung is dependent.
6. Pace activity as tolerated.
7. Administer oxygen.
8. Implement airway clearance techniques; limit suction duration to <15 seconds.
9. Apply or assist with technologic support of arterial oxygenation (e.g., mechanical ventilation, positive end-expiratory pressure, incentive spirometry).
10. *Teach* the patient and family:
    - Signs and symptoms of hypoxemia
    - Interventions for management of hypoxemia
    - Home care for ventilation if required

IMPAIRED GAS EXCHANGE: • • • • • •
HYPERCAPNIA

Description
The state in which an individual has a carbon dioxide pressure ($PaCO_2$) in arterial blood that is greater than normal, with or without acidemia.

Need
To reduce or alleviate hypercapnia.

Outcome Criteria
- $PaCO_2$ <45 mmHg or usual (compensated pH) baseline level

- Headache absent on awakening
- Vision disturbances absent
- Breath sounds present, bilateral, equal
- Breathing rate, depth, negative inspiratory pressures, rhythm normal for age/size
- Arterial oxygenation and bicarbonate level normal or usual (compensated pH) baseline level
- Vasodilation, flushed skin, bounding pulse absent or resolving
- Papilledema, somnolence, stupor, coma absent

Process Criteria

1. Eliminate/modify etiologies/related factors where possible.
2. Maintain upper airway patency by positioning, use of nasal or oral airways.
3. Stimulate (tactile/vocal) breathing/ventilatory effort during postanesthesia period and in neonates with irregular breathing.
4. Assist with measures to promote ventilation and CO_2 elimination (e.g., manual bagging or mechanical ventilation).
5. Provide or assist with secretion clearance therapies, bronchodilator therapy.
6. Schedule medications to avoid ventilatory depression (e.g., narcotics, analgesics, tranquilizers).
7. Notify/consult physician about cause/need for therapy of primary metabolic alkalosis.
8. *Teach* the patient/family:
    - Signs and symptoms of hypercapnia
    - Interventions for airway management
    - Interventions for airway clearance
    - Home care for ventilation, if required

DYSPNEA   • • • • • •

Description

The state in which an individual experiences an unpleasant sensation of increased effort associated with spontaneous or ventilator-assisted breathing.

Need

To reduce or eliminate dyspnea.

Outcome Criteria

- Indicates unpleasant sensation with breathing absent or reduced.
- Completes sentence without stopping for breath.
- Accessory respiratory muscle use appropriate to activity level.
- Respiratory rate normal or reduced.

Process Criteria

1. Assess respiratory status.
2. Remove or limit environmental stimuli.
3. Assist patient to assume a position that may relieve dyspnea.
4. Schedule medications to relieve dyspnea (e.g., bronchodilators, diuretics, narcotics).

5. Administer supplemental oxygen at prescribed levels.
6. Monitor blood gases and oxygen saturations.
7. Use airway clearance techniques.
8. Guide patient through relaxation techniques.
9. Schedule alternating rest and activity periods.
10. *Teach* the patient and family effective use of breathing and relaxation techniques, use of medications, and use of special respiratory equipment.

DECREASED CARDIAC OUTPUT   • • • • • •

Description

A state in which the amount of blood pumped by an individual's heart is sufficiently reduced that it is inadequate to meet the needs of the body's tissues.

Need

To maintain adequate cardiac output to meet the needs of the body's tissues.

Outcome Criteria

- Normal sinus rhythm
- Brisk capillary refill (<2 sec.)
- Normal urine output for age
- Arterial blood pressure within normal limits for age
- Adequate perfusion to major organs
- Warm pink extremities
- Baseline level of consciousness/responsiveness

Process Criteria

1. Eliminate/modify etiologies/related factors where possible.
2. Monitor for dysrhythmias. Titrate antidysrhythmic medications collaboratively with the physician.
3. Monitor heart sounds, assess for the presence of distant heart sounds.
4. Monitor and treat electrolyte abnormalities collaboratively with the physician.
5. Monitor ABGs/VBGs for hypoxemia. Titrate supplemental O_2 therapy collaboratively with the physician.
6. Monitor for hypovolemia (e.g., decreased right atrial pressure, pulmonary artery wedge pressure, left atrial pressure, normal or decreased systolic arterial pressure). Titrate volume expanders collaboratively with the physician.
7. Monitor for inappropriate afterload (e.g., increased systemic vascular resistance index— SVRI). Maintain normothermic environment, titrate afterload reduction therapy collaboratively with the physician.
8. After addressing factors that contribute to a negative inotropic state (e.g., hypoxemia, acidosis, electrolyte abnormalities, hypoglycemia), titrate positive inotropic agent administration collaboratively with the physician.

9. Decrease the workload of the heart (e.g., plan care to allow for rest periods, promote stress reduction, position patient for comfort), titrate analgesics/sedatives within the guidelines established collaboratively with the physician.
10. *Teach* patient adaptive techniques necessary to deal with the effects of decreased cardiac output, stress reduction techniques, and how to cope with and learn about related health problems.

ALTERED TISSUE PERFUSION: CEREBRAL • • • • • •

Description
The state in which an individual experiences a decrease in nutrition or gas exchange at the cerebral cellular level.

Need
To improve or maintain adequate cerebral perfusion.

Outcome Criteria
- Clear or improving level of consciousness
- Cerebral perfusion pressure >50 mmHg in children older than 2 years of age

Process Criteria
1. Eliminate/modify etiologies/related factors where possible.
2. Position head in midline. Position head of bed to optimize cerebral perfusion pressure.
3. Maintain neutral thermal environment.
4. Perform endotracheal suctioning rapidly. Increase oxygen concentration before suctioning. Hyperventilate before activities.
5. Avoid extreme hip flexion.
6. Avoid Valsalva maneuvers.
7. Limit environmental stimuli that increase intracranial pressure.
8. Schedule medications to maintain prescribed levels of cerebral perfusion and intracranial pressure.
9. *Teach* parents how to interact with their critically ill infant/child with increased intracranial pressure (e.g., identify parental activity that decreases the patient's intracranial pressure).

ALTERED TISSUE PERFUSION: MYOCARDIAL • • • • • •

Description
The state in which an individual experiences a decrease in nutrition and gas exchange at the myocardial cellular level.

Need
To optimize myocardial tissue perfusion.

Outcome Criteria
Electrocardiographic manifestations of myocardial ischemia absent or reduced (e.g., ST segment and T wave changes)

Process Criteria
1. Eliminate/modify etiologies/related factors where possible (e.g., medicate before activity or stressful interventions).
2. Minimize or limit activities that increase myocardial oxygen demand:
   - Provide adequate rest
   - Decrease environmental stimuli
   - Decrease anxiety
   - Schedule medications to eliminate or minimize pain
3. Administer supplementary oxygen at prescribed levels.
4. *Teach* the patient and family strategies to decrease personal risk factors for heart disease (e.g., diet, activity level, blood pressure control) and strategies to avoid Valsalva maneuvers during defecation attempts and movement in bed.

ALTERED TISSUE PERFUSION: PERIPHERAL ARTERIAL • • • • • •

Description
The state in which an individual experiences a decrease in nutrition and gas exchange at the peripheral cellular level.

Need
To improve or maintain adequate arterial tissue perfusion.

Outcome Criteria
- Pain absent or reduced
- Capillary refill normal or improved
- Peripheral pulses palpable
- Ulcerations absent or healing

Process Criteria
1. Eliminate/modify etiologies/related factors where possible (e.g., restoration of adequate arterial blood flow to extremity).
2. Release constrictive devices (e.g., dressings, restraints, casts, tourniquets).
3. Maintain extremity in dependent position.
4. Keep pulse points free of pressure.
5. Keep extremity warm without the use of external heating appliances.
6. *Teach* the patient to change position frequently and keep legs uncrossed, strategies to decrease lipid intake, and to increase activity level/exercise.

ALTERED TISSUE PERFUSION: PERIPHERAL VENOUS

Description
The state in which an individual experiences a decrease in peripheral venous flow.

Need
To improve or maintain adequate peripheral venous outflow.

Outcome Criteria
- Circumference of affected extremity is within normal limits or decreased for the patient
- Peripheral edema decreased
- Pain in affected extremity absent or reduced
- Peripheral cyanosis absent or reduced

Process Criteria
1. Eliminate/modify etiologies/related factors where possible.
2. Elevate extremity above the level of the heart or avoid extremity dependence.
3. Limit fluid intake at the prescribed level.
4. Avoid pressure on the popliteal space; apply elastic stockings.
5. *Teach* the patient/family the importance of avoiding crossing legs and the importance of frequent position change.

ACTIVITY INTOLERANCE

Description
A state in which an individual has insufficient physiologic or psychological energy to endure or complete required or desired activities.

Need
To tolerate prescribed level of activity.

Outcome Criteria
During and after activity:
- Heart and respiratory rate normal for patient
- Heart rhythm normal
- Blood pressure normal for patient
- Expresses tolerance to activity
- Diaphoresis absent

Process Criteria
1. Eliminate/modify etiologies/related factors where possible.
2. Schedule activities to decrease energy expenditure.
3. Plan rest periods between activities and after meals.
4. Exhibit confidence in the patient's abilities.
5. Terminate activity sessions at the onset of signs of intolerance.

6. After prolonged bedrest, begin with passive range of motion, then progress to active range of motion and isometric exercises.
7. Maintain supplementary O_2 therapy during activity.
8. Modify or increase assistance with activity in the presence of specific motor deficits.
9. Set realistic activity goals with the patient/family.
10. Provide feedback to the patient regarding his/her progress.
11. *Teach* the patient/family:
    - Self-monitoring techniques (e.g., pulse rate)
    - Rest/activity schedule

IMPAIRED PHYSICAL MOBILITY

Description
The state in which an individual experiences a limitation of ability for independent physical movement.

Need
To maintain or increase mobility.

Outcome Criteria
- Range of motion maintained or increased
- Purposeful movement within the physical environment maintained or increased

Process Criteria
1. Eliminate/modify etiologies/related factors where possible.
2. Provide pain relief measures.
3. Institute progressive mobilization.
4. Change position frequently.
5. Use physical restraint techniques judiciously.
6. Use assistive devices (e.g., trapeze, braces, pillows, splints, ambulation devices).
7. Alternate rest and activity periods.
8. Guide through active ROM exercises, including resistance exercises. Provide passive range of motion.
9. Consult with physical therapist.
10. *Teach* patient how to use adaptive equipment.

SELF-CARE DEFICIT: FEEDING

Description
The state in which an individual indicates an inability or unwillingness to feed self.

Need
To promote the highest level of independence.

Outcome Criteria
- Feeds self appropriately to age/ability
- Cuts food and opens containers
- Brings food from receptacle to mouth

Process Criteria

1. Eliminate or modify etiologies/related factors where possible.
2. Provide opportunities for patient to participate in self-care.
3. Position patient food to minimize energy expenditure.
4. Assist with feeding activities as necessary (e.g., provide straws, weighted cups, special spoons).
5. Develop activity/rest schedule with patient and family.
6. *Teach* parents to identify a patient's readiness to feed self and discuss possible regression of self-feeding ability after hospitalization.

SELF-CARE DEFICIT: TOILETING • • • • • •

Description

The state in which an individual has an impaired ability to perform or complete toileting activities.

Need

Toileting is performed to maximal level of independence.

Outcome Criteria

• Toileting appropriate to age/ability
• Toileting hygiene appropriate to age/ability

Process Criteria

1. Eliminate etiologies/related factors where possible.
2. Ascertain child's word for toileting.
3. Provide opportunities for the patient to participate in self-care.
4. Provide age-appropriate and familiar equipment (e.g., pottychair).
5. Encourage independence; praise successful attempts at toileting.
6. Position patient and equipment to minimize energy expenditure.
7. Assist with toileting and toileting activities as necessary.
8. Provide materials (e.g., tissue, water, soap) for after-toilet hygiene.
9. *Teach* parents to identify a toddler's readiness for toilet training and discuss possible regression of toileting independence after hospitalization.

SELF-CARE DEFICIT: BATHING/HYGIENE • • • • • •

Description

The state in which an individual has an impaired ability to perform or complete bathing/hygiene activities.

Need

To promote the highest level of independence.

Outcome Criteria

• Washes self or body parts appropriate to age/ability.
• Brushes teeth appropriate to age/ability.

Process Criteria

1. Eliminate/modify etiologies/related factors whenever possible.
2. Provide opportunity for patient to participate in self-care.
3. Encourage independence; praise successful attempts.
4. Position patient equipment to minimize energy expenditure.
5. Assist with bathing/hygiene activities as necessary.
6. Develop activity/rest schedule with patient and family.
7. *Teach* the patient and family how to accomplish hygiene measures within the critical care setting.

ALTERED GROWTH AND DEVELOPMENT • • • • • •

Description

The state in which an individual demonstrates deviations in norms from age group.

Need

To demonstrate age- or ability-appropriate activities.

Outcome Criteria

• Age- or ability-appropriate self-care activities performed.
• Cognitive, motor, and social activities normal for age or ability.

Process Criteria

1. Eliminate/modify etiologies/related factors where possible.
2. Support parents/significant others in parental role attainment and maintenance, including participation in care.
3. Maintain age-appropriate developmental activities.
4. Provide continuity in care providers.
5. Use attachment articles (e.g., special blanket, toys).
6. Provide opportunities to meet age-related developmental tasks.
7. Use restraints judiciously; explore alternative methods (e.g., intravenous protectors).
8. Encourage age-appropriate self-care activities.
9. Encourage expression of feelings through play therapy (e.g., fears).
10. *Teach* the patient age-appropriate explanations of procedures and their impact on the body.

Cognitive—Perceptual

ALTERED COMFORT: PAIN   • • • • • •

Description
The state in which an individual has an unpleasant sensory and emotional experience.

Need
To alleviate or control pain.

Outcome Criteria
• Patient states pain is relieved or manageable
• Absent manifestations of pain
• Normal respiratory rate, heart rate, blood pressure
• Body relaxed

Process Criteria
1. Eliminate/modify etiologies/related factors where possible.
2. Tailor pain management program to the patient (e.g., cultural considerations, degree of participation patient desires, history of previous successful pain relief strategies, PCA).
3. Handle gently; position to alleviate pressure, stretch, or strain.
4. Promote rest (e.g., darken room, decrease stimuli).
5. Recommend and/or schedule prescribed pharmacologic agents around the clock to maximize comfort.
6. Schedule pain-associated procedures after administration of pain medication to maximize comfort.
7. Provide sensory and procedural information before any potentially painful techniques.
8. Provide emotional support as well as distraction during painful procedures.
9. *Teach* the patient relaxation methods (e.g., imagery, relaxation, controlled breathing).

ALTERED COMFORT: NAUSEA   • • • • • •

Description
The state in which an individual experiences an unpleasant sensation of sickness or general queasiness in the mouth, throat, epigastrium, or abdomen.

Need
To alleviate or control nausea.

Outcome Criteria
• "Sick to stomach" complaints absent
• Adverse reaction to food absent
• Salivation normal

Process Criteria
1. Eliminate/modify etiologies/related factors where possible.
2. Provide oral care.
3. Apply cool cloths to forehead, neck, and wrist.
4. Decrease odors or unpleasant sights.
5. Restrict liquids with meals.
6. Provide frequent small bland feedings.
7. Schedule antiemetic to promote comfort.
8. Guide through relaxation methods (e.g., controlled breathing, distraction, imagery).
9. *Teach* the patient relaxation methods (e.g., controlled breathing, distraction, imagery).

ALTERED SENSORY PERCEPTION   • • • • • •

Description
The state in which an individual responds adversely to a change in the amount, intensity, and/or pattern of meaningful stimuli (visual, kinesthetic, olfactory, tactile, and/or gustatory).

Need
To promote an appropriate response to sensory-perceptual stimuli.

Outcome Criteria
• Oriented to person, place, and time.
• Accurate description of environment.

Process Criteria
1. Eliminate/modify etiologies/related factors where possible.
2. Provide frequent reorientation to time and place.
3. Provide adequate meaningful stimulation (e.g., clock), avoid overload (e.g., radio).
4. Enhance function of impaired organs (e.g., glasses, hearing aid).
5. Enhance use of other senses to compensate for impaired organs (e.g., provide verbal descriptions to compensate for swollen eyelids).
6. Schedule medications/procedures to minimize sleep interruptions.
7. Provide adequate lighting with diurnal variation.
8. Encourage presence of reassuring family members and/or familiar objects (e.g., toys, pictures).
9. *Teach* the family the source and meaning of unfamiliar stimuli.

Self-perception

ANXIETY   • • • • • •

Description
The state in which an individual experiences feelings of uneasiness (apprehension) and activation of the

autonomic nervous system in response to a vague, nonspecific threat.

Need
To reduce or alleviate anxiety.

Outcome Criteria
- Expresses that anxiety is reduced or absent
- Manifestations of anxiety absent or reduced

Process Criteria
1. Eliminate/modify etiologies/related factors where possible.
2. Support existing coping mechanisms (e.g., allow patient to cry, talk; do not confront rationalizations/defenses).
3. Speak slowly and calmly. Remove excessive stimulation.
4. Convey empathetic understanding.
5. Promote presence of comforting significant others.
6. Anticipate concerns and reinforce standard orientation to environment (e.g., introduce new personnel each shift, describe location of significant others after visiting hours).
7. Guide through relaxation techniques (e.g., breathing techniques, touch, imagery, music).
8. Provide honest information about diagnosis, prognosis, treatment.
9. Schedule pharmacologic agents in anticipation of exacerbations.
10. *Teach* the child relaxation techniques, and teach the family how to help the patient.

FEAR RELATED TO   ● ● ● ● ● ●

Description
The state in which a patient/family experiences a feeling of physiologic or emotional disruption related to an identifiable source that the person perceives as dangerous.

Need
To reduce or alleviate fear.

Outcome Criteria
- Expresses fear as absent or reduced
- Manifestations of fear are absent or reduced

Process Criteria
1. Eliminate/modify etiologies/related factors where possible (e.g., support parental role).
2. Diminish impact of fear (e.g., enforce a consistent routine).
3. Adapt environment to accommodate fear (e.g., provide security objects).
4. Convey empathetic understanding (e.g., quiet understanding, touch).

5. Promote presence of comforting significant others (e.g., parents).
6. *Teach* patient/parent fear management techniques (e.g., identify the source or techniques that the individual used in the past that were effective).

POWERLESSNESS   ● ● ● ● ● ●

Description
The state in which an individual perceives that his/her actions will not significantly alter the outcome; a loss of control over certain events or situations.

Need
To perceive a sense of control.

Outcome Criteria
- Expresses control over present situation and future outcomes, events, and/or situations
- Identifies areas in which individual has control
- Participates in activities of daily living
- Participates in decision-making

Process Criteria
1. Eliminate/modify etiologies/related factors when possible.
2. Provide choices/control whenever possible (e.g., scheduling therapies).
3. Assist in identifying areas in which control remains, despite current losses.
4. Convey understanding (e.g., quiet presence, touch).
5. Arrange for the presence of comforting significant others.
6. Provide frequent updates in progress toward therapeutic goals.
7. *Teach* parents how to function as parents-to-a-critically-ill-child and maintain the basic principles inherent in the Patient's Bill of Rights.

ALTERED SELF-CONCEPT   ● ● ● ● ● ●

Description
The state in which an individual experiences a negative state about the way he/she feels, thinks, or views himself/herself.

Need
To promote a positive self-concept.

Outcome Criteria
- Participates in self-care
- Uses prosthetic/cosmetic devices provided
- Positive expressions about self
- Views and touches affected body part
- Positive reinforcement accepted

Process Criteria

1. Eliminate/modify etiologies/related factors where possible.
2. Spend time with patient to allow expression of feelings and to answer questions.
3. Use therapeutic play to assist with expression of feelings.
4. Assist patient in identifying his/her capabilities. Provide opportunities for early assumption of self-care.
5. Respect privacy and fear of embarrassment.
6. Provide positive feedback. Convey faith in the patient's ability to achieve goals.
7. Involve the patient in the formulation of the plan of care and allow choices between alternatives when possible.
8. Set well-defined limits.
9. Support patient during his/her viewing and touching of disfigured or changed body parts. Discuss the availability of cosmetic and prosthetic devices (e.g., wigs).
10. *Teach* the family their supporting roles.

Role—Relationship

GRIEVING   • • • • • •

Description
The state in which an individual or family is responding to the realization of an actual or anticipated loss/disruption.

Need
To promote/support an adaptive grief response.

Outcome Criteria
- Manifestations of grief appropriate to setting
- Coping mechanisms effective
- Makes decisions
- Effective communication patterns

Process Criteria
1. Acknowledge grief response.
2. Provide emotional support (e.g., touching).
3. Acknowledge individual differences in grief response (e.g., cultural differences).
4. Provide opportunities for the significant others to stay at the bedside and/or participate in the patient's care if desired.
5. Schedule time to spend with significant others to provide information and listen to concerns.
6. Facilitate discussion of mutual feelings and fears between the patient and significant others.
7. Stay connected with the grieving person (avoid withdrawing). Contact clergy if family desires. Refer to community resources or mental health professionals, if needed.
8. Facilitate grief work, depending on response to loss (e.g., denial, depression, anger, guilt).

9. Reinforce adaptive coping mechanisms (e.g., expression of grief).
10. Provide an opportunity for organ and tissue donation, if appropriate.
11. *Teach* the patient/family the grief process.

IMPAIRED COMMUNICATION: VERBAL • • • • • •

Description
The state in which an individual is unable or unwilling to speak at all, or is unable or unwilling to speak so that he/she can be understood by others.

Need
To communicate effectively.

Outcome Criteria
- Acknowledges affirmatively when caregiver correctly repeats content of message sent
- Absent or reduced banging on siderails
- Uses interpreter, communication tool
- Parent indicates pre-verbal child's needs
- Absent or reduced slurred speech
- Decreased level of frustration, anger, anxiety, and fear

Process Criteria
1. Eliminate/modify etiologies/related factors where possible.
2. Plan for/allow increased time to confirm content/meaning, and provide positive feedback for attempts at speech or other forms of communication.
3. Formulate questions, comments so that response requires only yes-no response by head nod or eye-blink code.
4. Provide/use interpreter and/or write selected phrases in patient's language with translation underneath.
5. Include patient in bedside conversations when appropriate.
6. Reduce distraction in environment.
7. Assign caregivers who best understand patient.
8. Initiate referral to speech therapist; ear, nose, and throat specialist for postextubation aphonia.
9. Encourage presence of parent at bedside of pre-verbal child.
10. *Teach* the patient/family use of a communication tool/device appropriate for patient's capability (e.g., picture/word board, specialized "talking" endotracheal or tracheostomy tubes, computer, electrolarynx).

ALTERED ROLE PERFORMANCE   • • • • • •

Description
The state in which there is a disruption in the way an individual perceives one's role performance.

Need

To help alleviate disruption of role performance.

Outcome Criteria

- Expresses acceptance of current/future role performance or role transition
- Uses constructive strategies to cope with situational transition

Process Criteria

1. Eliminate/modify etiologies/related factors where possible.
2. Convey an empathetic understanding about change in role performance.
3. Acknowledge the importance of parents to their critically ill child as soon as possible after admission. Orient parent/family to unit routine and parent/visitor facilities.
4. Encourage information-seeking and provide honest information to parents about their child's current health status at least once a day. Inform promptly about any change in patient status.
5. Assist to identify elements of current role that can persist.
6. *Teach* parent/family how to interact with their critically ill child. Enable parent/family to participate in care activities that they find rewarding.
7. Refer to community resources or mental health professionals as necessary.
8. Suggest participation in an organized support group.
9. *Teach* the parents/family methods of support that are helpful to the patient; about the patient's behavior and trajectory of illness; about the stress of hospitalization/critical illness on family and individuals; and how to use physiologic and spiritual resources.

Coping—Stress Tolerance

IMPAIRED COPING: PATIENT • • • • • •

Description

The state in which a child/adolescent has insufficient adaptive and problem-solving capacities to meet the demands of critical illness.

Need

To support effective coping.

Outcome Criteria

- Participates in decisions regarding health
- Garners support from social network
- Acknowledges physical limitations
- Sleep/wake pattern normal for person and activity in unit
- Decrease in fear, anger, and withdrawal

Process Criteria

1. Eliminate/modify etiologies/related factors where possible.

2. Assist the patient in problem-solving by reducing concerns into small parts.
3. Plan for patient contact with identified significant others (e.g., parents/family/friends).
4. Support adaptive coping responses (e.g., expression of feelings).
5. Provide appropriate levels of environmental stimuli.
6. Encourage expression of feelings through play therapy (e.g., child life specialist).
7. Assist in identification of identified resources (e.g., child-psychology clinical nurse specialist).
8. *Teach* the patient:
   - Current health status, taking cues from patient regarding amount of information desired
   - Relaxation measures (e.g., controlled breathing, guided imagery)

IMPAIRED COPING: PARENT/FAMILY • • • • • •

Description

The state in which a parent or family member has difficulty in providing support, comfort, or assistance that is needed by or for the patient.

Need

To support effective parent/family coping.

Outcome Criteria

- Parents/family members are available to the patient
- Parents/family members express an understanding of patient's health status
- Parents/family members participate in decision-making

Process Criteria

1. Eliminate/modify etiologies/related factors where possible.
2. Orient parent/family to unit routine and parent/visitor facilities.
3. Acknowledge the importance of parents/family members to the critically ill child as soon as possible after admission.
4. Identify contacts (e.g., primary nurse and physician) who will assist parents/family in exploring options for problem-solving.
5. Assist parents/family in garnering social support (e.g., help the parents/family identify personally supportive individuals that are available).
6. Support adaptive coping mechanisms (e.g., expression of feelings, vigilance, use of relaxation techniques).
7. Encourage information-seeking and provide honest information about patient's current health status at least once a day. Hold group education sessions so all family members hear the same information. Inform promptly about any change in patient status.

8. *Teach* parent/family how to interact with the critically ill child. Enable parent/family to participate in care activities that they find rewarding. Provide the parent and child quiet times and privacy when possible.
9. Foster realistic hope (e.g., openly discuss the patient's best outcome).
10. *Teach* the parents/family methods of support that are helpful to the patient; about the patient's behavior and trajectory of illness; about the stress of hospitalization/critical illness on family and individuals; and how to use physiologic and spiritual resources.

Value—Belief

SPIRITUAL DISTRESS   ● ● ● ● ● ●

Description
The state in which an individual experiences conflicts with personal values and/or beliefs.

Need
To reduce or alleviate spiritual distress.

Outcome Criteria
- Comprehends the meaning and purpose of illness/suffering/death
- Conflict between religious beliefs and prescribed health regimen absent or reduced

Process Criteria
1. Listen as patient and/or family shares/talks about feelings related to life and death or religious beliefs.
2. Assist the individual to live fully in the present by focusing on joy, hope, and progress.
3. Respect and acknowledge the individual's religious beliefs.
4. Refer to clergy for prayer, communion, or sacraments (e.g., baptism).
5. Provide support through understanding when a patient/family's recommended care creates a conflict with personal values/beliefs.
6. Provide privacy for reflection or spiritual expression.
7. Assist in identifying previous sources of spiritual strength.
8. Respect presence of religious objects, music, or television programming.
9. Provide substitutes for safety/comfort devices (e.g., hand bell for electric call system for Jewish on Sabbath, kosher food).
10. *Teach* the patient and/or family to identify and utilize sources of spiritual support.

Reference

American Association of Critical Care Nurses (1990). *AACN: Outcome standards for nursing care of the critically ill*. Laguna Niguel, CA: AACN.

GUIDELINES AND LEVELS OF CARE FOR PEDIATRIC INTENSIVE CARE UNITS

The Level I PICU must be capable of providing definitive care for a wide range of complex, progressive, rapidly changing, medical, surgical, and traumatic disorders, often requiring a multidisciplinary approach, occurring in pediatric patients of all ages, excluding premature newborns. Such units are usually found in major medical centers or within children's hospitals. Level II units exist primarily in areas distant from a Level I PICU that do not have the population base to support a Level I unit; these will generally care for fewer severely ill patients. Patients in Level II units will have less complex and more stable disorders whose course is more predictable. As a consequence of the difference in patient population, both the physicians and their specialized services will differ between levels. Level I PICUs will have a complete complement of subspecialists, including pediatric intensivists, whereas Level II PICUs will not require the full spectrum of subspecialists or their services. Each Level II unit must have a well-established communications system with a Level I unit for timely referral of patients who need care unavailable at the Level II PICU.

MINIMUM GUIDELINES AND LEVELS OF CARE

	PICU Facilities and Services*	
	Level I	Level II
General		
Category I facility (AMA guidelines)	R	R
Organization		
PICU committee	R	R
Distinct administrative unit	R	R
Delineation of physician and nonphysician privileges	R	R
Policies		
Admission/discharge	R	R
Patient monitoring	R	R
Safety	R	R
Nosocomial infection	R	R
Patient isolation	R	R
Visitation	R	R
Traffic control	R	R
Equipment maintenance	R	R
Essential equipment breakdown	R	R
System of record-keeping	R	R
Periodic review of		
Morbidity and mortality	R	R
Quality of care	R	R
Safety	R	R
Open admission for all staff MDs	O	O
Medical director		
Appointment by appropriate hospital authority: acknowledgment in writing	R	R
Written documentation of responsibilities	R	R
Qualifications		
Board-certified in CCM (or actively pursuing certification)	R	O
Board-certified in primary specialty (or actively pursuing certification) with residency-level training in pediatric critical care	N/A	R
Participates in development, review, and implementation of PICU policies	R	R
Maintenance of database and/or vital statistics	R	R
Supervises quality control and quality assessment activities (including morbidity and mortality reviews)	R	R
Supervises resuscitation techniques (including educational component)	R	R
Assures policy implementation	R	R
Primary attending MD	O	O
Substitute MD available	R	R
Authority to consult on any PICU patient	R	R
Coordinates staff education	R	R
Participates in budget preparation	R	R
Coordinates research	R	R
Physician staff		
Licensed physician in-house 24 h/d	R	R
PGY 2 or above assigned to the PICU	R	R
PGY 3 or above (in pediatrics or anesthesiology)	R	O
Available in less than 30 min (24 h/d)		
Pediatrician (attending)	R	R
Available in less than 1 h		
Anesthesiologist	R	R
Pediatric anesthesiologist	R	O
Surgeon—general	R	R
Surgical subspecialists		
Pediatric surgeon	R	O
Cardiovascular	R	O
Neurosurgeon	R	R
Pediatric neurosurgeon	O	O
Otolaryngologist	R	R
Orthopedist	R	R
Craniofacial/oral	O/O	O/O
Pediatric subspecialists		
Intensivist	R	O
Cardiologist	R	O
Nephrologist	R	O
Hematologist/oncologist	R	O
Pulmonologist	O	O
Endocrinologist	O	O
Gastroenterologist	O	O
Allergist	O	O
Neonatologist	R	O

Table continued on following page

MINIMUM GUIDELINES AND LEVELS OF CARE *Continued*

	PICU Facilities and Services*	
	Level I	*Level II*
Radiologist	R	R
Pathologist	R	R
Psychiatrist/psychologist	R	O
Nursing staff		
Director—pediatric nursing	R	R
Unit nurse manager	R	O
Training in pediatric critical care	R	O
Nurse to patient ratio (2:1 to 1:3)	R	R
Nursing policies and procedures	R	R
Orientation to intensive care unit	R	R
Nursing skill		
Recognize, interpret, record physiologic parameters	R	R
Administer drugs	R	R
Administer fluids	R	R
Resuscitation, including Pediatric Advanced Life Support certification	R	R
Respiratory care techniques (chest physiotherapy, suctioning, endotracheal tube management, tracheostomy care)	R	R
Preparation/maintenance of patient monitors	R	R
Address psychosocial needs of patient and family	R	R
Nurse educator		
Responsible for pediatric critical care in-service education	R	R
Nurse coordinator for regional continuing education	O	O
Respiratory therapy		
Supervisor responsible for training RRT staff, maintenance of equipment, and quality control/review	R	R
Therapist in-house 24 h/d assigned primarily to unit	R	O
Therapist in-house 24 h/d	R	R
Other team members		
Biomedical technicians (in-house or available within 1 h, 24 h/d)	R	R
Unit clerk 24 h/d—written job description	R	O
Child-life specialist	R	O
Clergy	O	O
Social worker	R	R
Nutritionist/clinical dietician	R	O
Physical therapist	R	O
Occupational therapist	R	O
Pharmacist (24 h/d)	R	R
Radiology technician	R	R
Hospital facilities and services		
Emergency department		
Covered entrance	R	R
Separate entrance	R	R
Adjacent helipad	O	O
Staffed by MD 24 h/d	R	R
Resuscitation area		
Two or more areas with capacity and equipment to resuscitate medical/surgical/trauma pediatric patients	R	O
One or more areas as above	R	R
Intermediate care unit or step-down unit separate from PICU	O	O
Pediatric rehabilitation unit	O	O
Supporting services		
Blood bank		
Comprehensive (for all blood components)	R	R
Type and cross-match within 1 h	R	R
Radiology services/nuclear medicine		
Portable radiograph	R	R
Fluoroscopy	R	O
Computed tomographic scan	R	R
Magnetic resonance imaging	O	O
Ultrasonography	R	O
Angiography	R	O
Nuclear scanning	R	O
Radiation therapy	O	O
Laboratory—microspecimen capability		
Within 15 min		
Blood gases	R	R
Within 1 h		
CBC, platelets, differential count	R	R
Urinalysis	R	R
Chemistry—electrolytes, BUN, glucose, calcium, creatinine	R	R

MINIMUM GUIDELINES AND LEVELS OF CARE *Continued*

	PICU Facilities and Services*	
	Level I	Level II
Clotting studies	R	R
CSF cell count	R	R
Within 3 h		
Ammonia	R	R
Drug screening	R	R
Osmolarity	R	R
Magnesium, phosphorus	R	R
Preparation available—24 h/d		
Bacteriology: culture and Gram stain	R	R
Operating room		
Available within 30 min, 24 h/d	R	O
Available within 60 min, 24 h/d	R	R
Second OR available within 45 min, 24 h/d	R	O
Capabilities		
Cardiopulmonary bypass	R	O
Bronchoscopy, pediatric	R	O
Endoscopy, pediatric	R	O
Radiograph in OR	R	R
Cardiology—pediatric capability		
Electrocardiogram	R	R
Echocardiography		
1. Two-dimensional	R	O
with Doppler	O	O
2. M-mode	R	O
Catheterization laboratory	R	O
Neurodiagnostic laboratory		
EEG	R	O
Evoked potentials	O	O
Transcranial Doppler flow	O	O
Hemodialysis	R	O
Pharmacy—pediatric capability	R	R
24 h/d for all requests	R	R
In close proximity to PICU	O	O
Bedside urgent drug dosage form	R	R
Physical therapy department	R	O
Physical facility: external		
Distinct, separate unit	R	R
Controlled access (no through traffic)	R	R
Proximity to		
Elevators	R	O
Operating room	O	O
Emergency department	O	O
Recovery room	O	O
MD on-call room	R	O
Nurse Manager's office	O	O
Medical Director's office	O	O
Waiting room	R	R
Separate rooms		
Family counseling room	R	R
Conference room	O	O
Staff lounge	O	O
Staff locker room	O	O
Patients' personal effects storage (may be internal)	R	R
Physical facility: internal		
Patient isolation capacity	R	R
Patient privacy provision	R	R
Medication station with drug refrigerator and locked narcotics cabinet	R	R
Emergency equipment storage	R	R
Clean utility (linen) room	R	R
Soiled utility (linen) room	R	R
Nourishment station	R	R
Counter, cabinet space	R	R
Staff toilet	R	R
Patient toilet	R	R
Handwashing facility	R	R
Clocks	R	R
Televisions, radios	R	O
Easy, rapid access to head of bed	R	R
Twelve or more compressed air outlets/bed	R	R
Two oxygen outlets/bed	R	R

Table continued on following page

MINIMUM GUIDELINES AND LEVELS OF CARE *Continued*

	PICU Facilities and Services*	
	Level I	**Level II**
Two or more compressed air outlets/bed	R	R
Two vacuum outlets/bed	R	R
Computerized laboratory reporting or efficient equivalent	R	O
Building code or federal code conforming		
Heating, ventilation, air conditioning	R	R
Fire safety	R	R
Electrical grounding	R	R
Plumbing	R	R
Illumination	R	R
Portable equipment		
Emergency cart	R	R
Procedure lamp	R	R
Doppler ultrasonography	R	R
Infusion pumps (with microinfusion capability)	R	R
Defibrillator/cardioverter	R	R
ECG machine	R	R
Suction machine (in addition to bedside)	R	R
Thermometers	R	R
Expanded scale electronic thermometer	R	R
Automated blood pressure apparatus	R	R
Oto-ophthalmoscope	R	R
Refractometer	R	O
Automatic bed scale	O	O
Patient scales (all weights)	R	R
Cribs (with head access)	R	R
Beds (with head access)	R	R
Infant warmers, incubators	R	R
Heating/cooling blankets	R	R
Bilirubin lights	R	R
Transport monitor	R	O
EEG machine	R	R
Isolation cart	R	R
Blood warmer	R	R
Emergency drugs		
Small equipment		
Tracheal intubation equipment	R	R
Endotracheal tubes (all pediatric sizes)	R	R
Oral/nasal airways	R	R
Vascular access equipment	R	R
Cut-down trays	R	O
Tracheostomy tray	R	O
Respiratory support equipment		
Bag-valve-mask resuscitation devices	R	R
Oxygen tanks	R	R
Respired gas humidifiers	R	R
Air compressor	R	R
Air-oxygen blenders	R	R
Ventilators of all sizes for pediatric patients	R	R
Inhalation therapy equipment	R	R
Chest physiotherapy and suctioning	R	R
Spirometers	R	O
Continuous oxygen analyzers with alarms	R	R
Monitoring equipment		
Capability of continuous monitoring of		
ECG, heart rate	R	R
Respiration	R	R
Temperature	R	R
Systemic arterial pressure	R	R
Central venous pressure	R	O
Pulmonary arterial pressure	R	O
Intracranial pressure	R	O
Esophageal pressure	O	O
Four simultaneous pressure capability	R	O
Five simultaneous pressure capability	O	O
Arrhythmia detection/alarm	O	O
O_2 monitors	R	R
CO_2 monitors	R	R
Monitor characteristics		
Visible and audible high/low alarms for heart rate, respiratory rate, and all pressures	R	R
Hard-copy capability	R	O
Routine testing and maintenance	R	R
Electric patient isolation	R	R

MINIMUM GUIDELINES AND LEVELS OF CARE *Continued*

	PICU Facilities and Services*	
	Level I	Level II
Research and training		
Physician training		
Unit in facility with accredited pediatric residency program	O	O
Unit provides clinical rotation for pediatric residents in pediatric critical care	O	O
Fellowship program in pediatric critical care	O	O
CPR certification	R	R
Ongoing CME for all MDs specific to pediatric critical care	R	R
Staff MDs to attend/participate in regional/national meetings in areas related to pediatric critical care	R	R
Unit personnel training		
CPR certification for nurses and respiratory therapists	R	R
Resuscitation practice sessions	R	R
Ongoing continuing education: on-site and/or off-site workshops/programs for nurses and respiratory therapists	R	R
AACN	O	O
Regional education		
Participation in regional pediatric critical care education	R	R
Service as educational resource center for public education in pediatric critical care	O	O
Prehospital care and interhospital transport		
Integration/communication with EMS	R	R
Transfer arrangements with referral hospital	R	R
Transfer arrangement with Level I PICU	N/A	R
Educational programs in stabilization and transportation for EMS personnel	R	O
Transport system (including transport team)	R	O
24 h/d emergency communication into PICU (ie, phone, radio)	R	R
Communication link to Poison Control	R	R
Quality assessment		
Collaborative quality assessment	R	R
Morbidity/mortality review	R	R
Utilization review	R	R
Medical records review	R	R
Discharge criteria: planning	R	R
Safety review	R	R

*R, required; O, optional but desirable; N/A, not applicable; PICU, pediatric intensive care unit; AMA, American Medical Association; MD, physician; CCM, critical care medicine; PGY, postgraduate year; RRT, Registered Respiratory Therapist; CBC, complete blood cell count; BUN, blood urea nitrogen; CSF, cerebrospinal fluid; OR, operating room; EEG, electroencephalogram; ECG, electrocardiogram; CPR, cardiopulmonary resuscitation; CME, continuing medical education; AACN, American Association of Critical-Care Nurses; EMS, Emergency Medical Services.

Guidelines and Levels of Care for Pediatric Intensive Care Units. Committee on Hospital Care and Pediatric Section of the Society of Critical Care Medicine. Copyright © 1993 by the American Academy of Pediatrics. *Pediatrics* 92 (1):166–175, July 1993.

Policy statements are reviewed and updated as necessary. Please contact the Academy to determine if policy is current.

APPENDIX I
Normal Vital Signs

NORMAL PULSE AND RESPIRATORY RATES FOR SPECIFIC AGES*

Age	Pulse (Beats per Minute)	Average Pulse	Respirations (Breaths per Minute)
Neonate	70–170	120	30–40
2 years	80–130	110	25–32
4 years	80–120	100	23–30
6 years	75–115	100	21–26
8 years	70–110	90	20–26
10 years	70–110	90	20–26
12 years	70–110	85	18–22
14 years	65–105	85	18–22
16 years	60–100	85	16–20
18 years	50–90	80	12–24

*These are averages and vary with the sex of the child.

NORMAL BLOOD PRESSURE GRAPHS

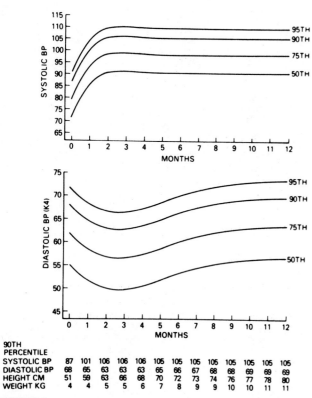

90TH PERCENTILE												
SYSTOLIC BP	87	101	106	106	106	105	105	105	105	105	105	105	105
DIASTOLIC BP	68	65	63	63	63	65	66	67	68	68	69	69	69
HEIGHT CM	51	59	63	66	68	70	72	73	74	76	77	78	80
WEIGHT KG	4	4	5	5	6	7	8	9	9	10	10	11	11

FIGURE 1. ● ● ● ● ●

Age-specific percentiles of blood pressure (BP) measurements in boys—birth to 12 mos of age; Korotkoff phase IV (K4) used for diastolic BP. (From National Heart, Lung, and Blood Institute, Bethesda, MD: Report of the second task force on blood pressure control in children—1987. Reproduced with permission by Pediatrics, vol. 79, p. 1. Copyright © 1987.)

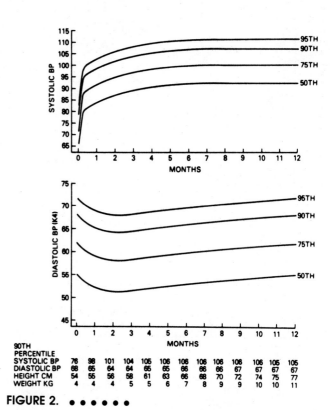

90TH PERCENTILE												
SYSTOLIC BP	76	98	101	104	105	106	106	106	106	106	106	105	105
DIASTOLIC BP	68	65	64	64	65	66	66	66	67	67	67	67	67
HEIGHT CM	54	55	56	58	61	63	66	68	70	72	74	75	77
WEIGHT KG	4	4	4	5	5	6	7	8	9	9	10	10	11

FIGURE 2. ● ● ● ● ●

Age-specific percentiles of BP measurements in girls—birth to 12 mos of age; Korotkoff phase IV (K4) used for diastolic BP. (From National Heart, Lung, and Blood Institute, Bethesda, MD: Report of the second task force on blood pressure control in children—1987. Reproduced with permission by Pediatrics, vol. 79, p. 1. Copyright © 1987.)

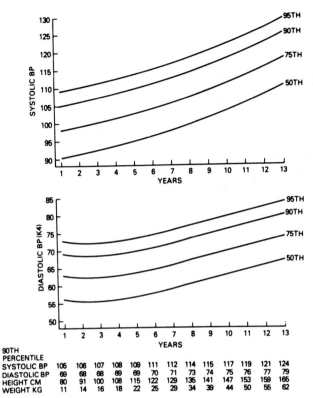

90TH PERCENTILE													
SYSTOLIC BP	105	106	107	108	109	111	112	114	115	117	119	121	124
DIASTOLIC BP	69	68	68	69	69	70	71	73	74	75	76	77	79
HEIGHT CM	80	91	100	108	115	122	129	135	141	147	153	159	165
WEIGHT KG	11	14	16	18	22	25	29	34	39	44	50	55	62

FIGURE 3. ● ● ● ● ● ●

Age-specific percentiles for BP measurements in boys—1 to 13 yrs of age; Korotkoff phase IV (K4) used for diastolic BP. (From National Heart, Lung, and Blood Institute, Bethesda, MD: Report of the second task force on blood pressure control in children—1987. Reproduced with permission of Pediatrics, vol. 79, p. 1. Copyright © 1987.)

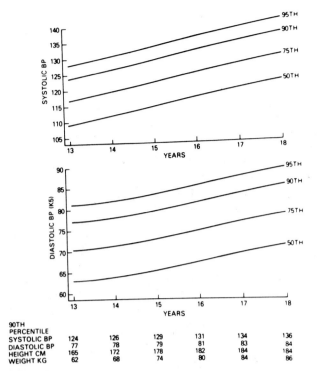

90TH PERCENTILE						
SYSTOLIC BP	124	126	129	131	134	136
DIASTOLIC BP	77	78	79	81	83	84
HEIGHT CM	165	172	178	182	184	184
WEIGHT KG	62	68	74	80	84	86

FIGURE 5. ● ● ● ● ● ●

Age-specific percentiles of BP measurements in boys—13 to 18 yrs of age; Korotkoff phase V (K5) used for diastolic BP. (From National Heart, Lung, and Blood Institute, Bethesda, MD: Report of the second task force on blood pressure control in children—1987. Reproduced by permission of Pediatrics, vol. 79, p. 1, Copyright © 1987.)

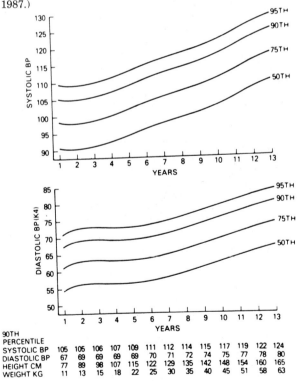

90TH PERCENTILE													
SYSTOLIC BP	105	105	106	107	109	111	112	114	115	117	119	122	124
DIASTOLIC BP	67	69	69	69	69	70	71	72	74	75	77	78	80
HEIGHT CM	77	89	98	107	115	122	129	135	142	148	154	160	165
WEIGHT KG	11	13	15	18	22	25	30	35	40	45	51	58	63

FIGURE 4. ● ● ● ● ● ●

Age-specific percentiles of BP measurements in girls—1 to 13 yrs of age; Korotkoff phase IV (K4) used for diastolic BP. (From National Heart, Lung, and Blood Institute, Bethesda, MD: Report of the second task force on blood pressure control in children—1987. Reproduced by permission of Pediatrics, vol. 79, p. 1. Copyright © 1987.)

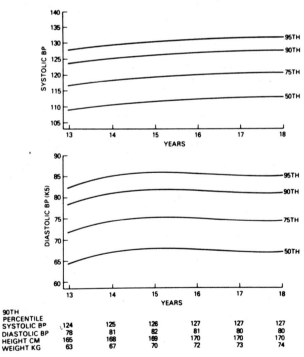

90TH PERCENTILE						
SYSTOLIC BP	124	125	126	127	127	127
DIASTOLIC BP	78	81	82	81	80	80
HEIGHT CM	165	168	169	170	170	170
WEIGHT KG	63	67	70	72	73	74

FIGURE 6. ● ● ● ● ● ●

Age-specific percentiles of BP measurements in girls—13 to 18 yrs of age; Korotkoff phase V (K5) used for diastolic BP. (From National Heart, Lung, and Blood Institute, Bethesda, MD: Report of the second task force on blood pressure control in children—1987. Reproduced with permission of Pediatrics, vol. 79, p. 1. Copyright © 1987.)

APPENDIX II
Growth Charts

GIRLS: BIRTH TO 36 MONTHS
PHYSICAL GROWTH
NCHS PERCENTILES*

NAME_____ RECORD #_____

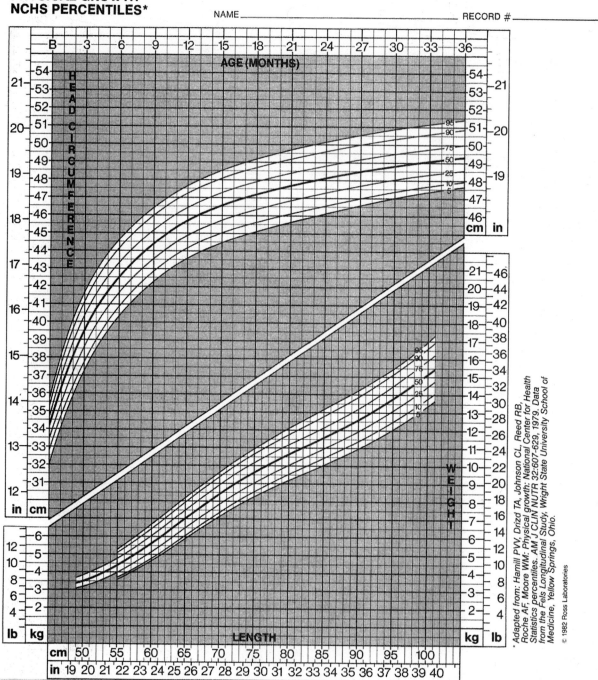

* Adapted from: Hamill PVV, Drizd TA, Johnson CL, Reed RB, Roche AF, Moore WM: Physical growth: National Center for Health Statistics percentiles. AM J CLIN NUTR 32:607-629, 1979. Data from the Fels Longitudinal Study, Wright State University School of Medicine, Yellow Springs, Ohio.

© 1982 Ross Laboratories

Growth charts used with permission of Ross Products Division, Abbott Laboratories, Columbus, OH 43216, from NCHS Growth Charts. © 1982, Ross Products Division, Abbott Laboratories.

GIRLS: BIRTH TO 36 MONTHS
PHYSICAL GROWTH
NCHS PERCENTILES*

NAME_____ RECORD #_____

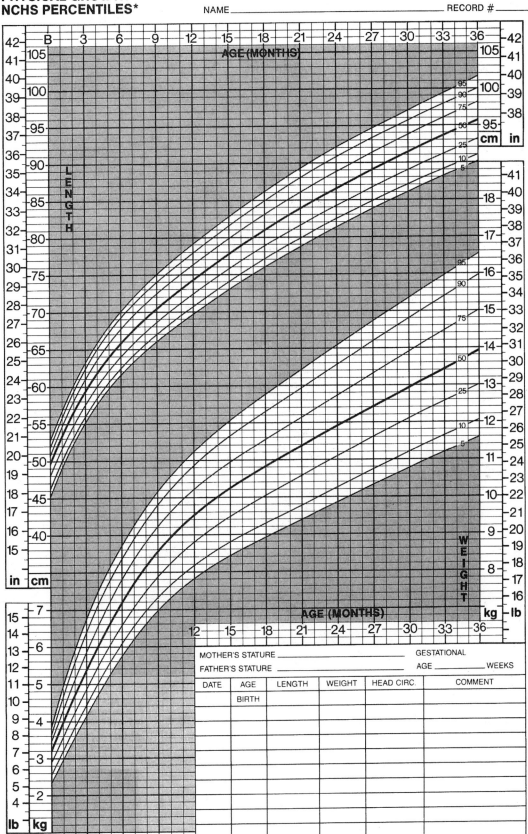

Ross
Growth &
Development
Program

*Adapted from: Hamill PVV, Drizd TA, Johnson CL, Reed RB, Roche AF, Moore WM: Physical growth: National Center for Health Statistics percentiles. AM J CLIN NUTR 32:607-629, 1979. Data from the Fels Longitudinal Study, Wright State University School of Medicine, Yellow Springs, Ohio.

© 1982 Ross Laboratories

MOTHER'S STATURE _____ GESTATIONAL
FATHER'S STATURE _____ AGE _____ WEEKS

DATE	AGE	LENGTH	WEIGHT	HEAD CIRC.	COMMENT
	BIRTH				

BOYS: BIRTH TO 36 MONTHS
PHYSICAL GROWTH
NCHS PERCENTILES* Name_____ Record #_____

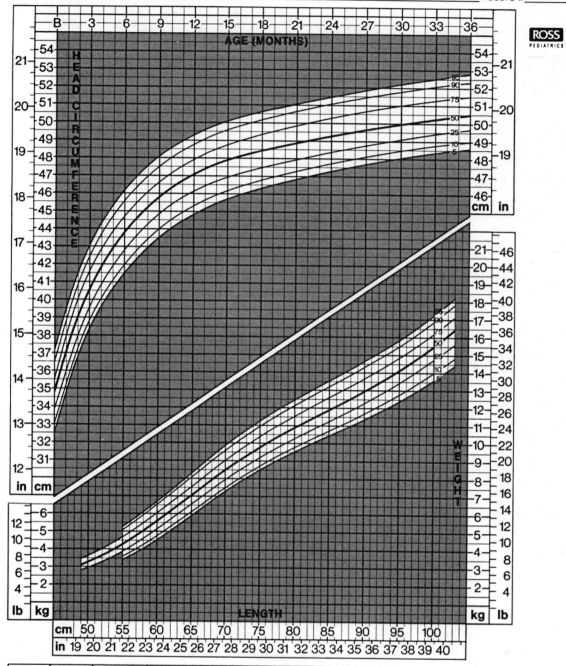

DATE	AGE	LENGTH	WEIGHT	HEAD CIRC.	COMMENT

ROSS **ROSS PRODUCTS DIVISION**
ABBOTT LABORATORIES
COLUMBUS, OHIO 43215-1724

51208 09890WB
(0.05)/SEPTEMBER 1993   LITHO IN USA

**BOYS: BIRTH TO 36 MONTHS
PHYSICAL GROWTH
NCHS PERCENTILES***

Name_____ Record #_____

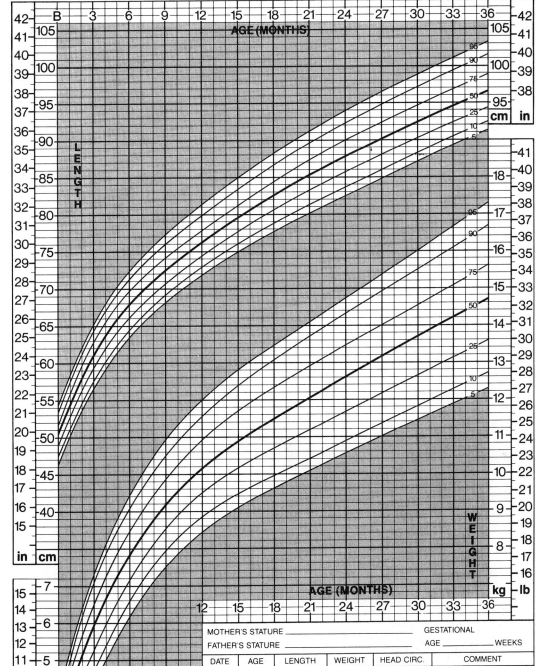

*Adapted from: Hamill PVV, Drizd TA, Johnson CL, Reed RB, Roche AF, Moore WM: Physical growth: National Center for Health Statistics percentiles. AM J CLIN NUTR 32:607-629, 1979. Data from the Fels Longitudinal Study, Wright State University School of Medicine, Yellow Springs, Ohio.

© 1982 Ross Products Division, Abbott Laboratories

MOTHER'S STATURE _____ GESTATIONAL

FATHER'S STATURE _____ AGE _____ WEEKS

DATE	AGE	LENGTH	WEIGHT	HEAD CIRC.	COMMENT
	BIRTH				

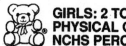

GIRLS: 2 TO 18 YEARS
PHYSICAL GROWTH
NCHS PERCENTILES*

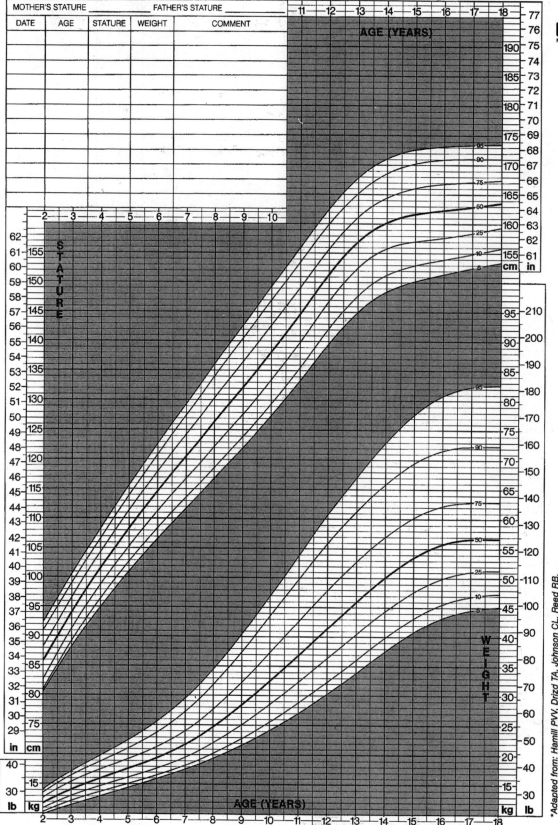

*Adapted from: Hamill PVV, Drizd TA, Johnson CL, Reed RB, Roche AF, Moore WM: Physical growth: National Center for Health Statistics percentiles. AM J CLIN NUTR 32:607-629, 1979. Data from the National Center for Health Statistics (NCHS), Hyattsville, Maryland.

GIRLS: PREPUBESCENT PHYSICAL GROWTH NCHS PERCENTILES*

Name_____ Record #_____

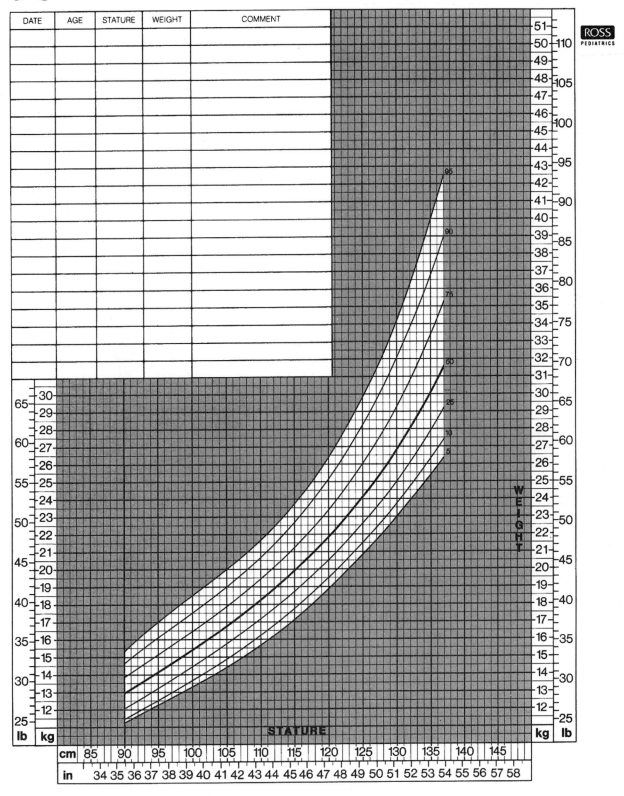

51214 09893WB
(0.05)/SEPTEMBER 1993

ROSS PRODUCTS DIVISION
ABBOTT LABORATORIES
COLUMBUS, OHIO 43215-1724

LITHO IN USA

BOYS: 2 TO 18 YEARS
PHYSICAL GROWTH
NCHS PERCENTILES*

Name_____   Record #_____

ROSS
PEDIATRICS

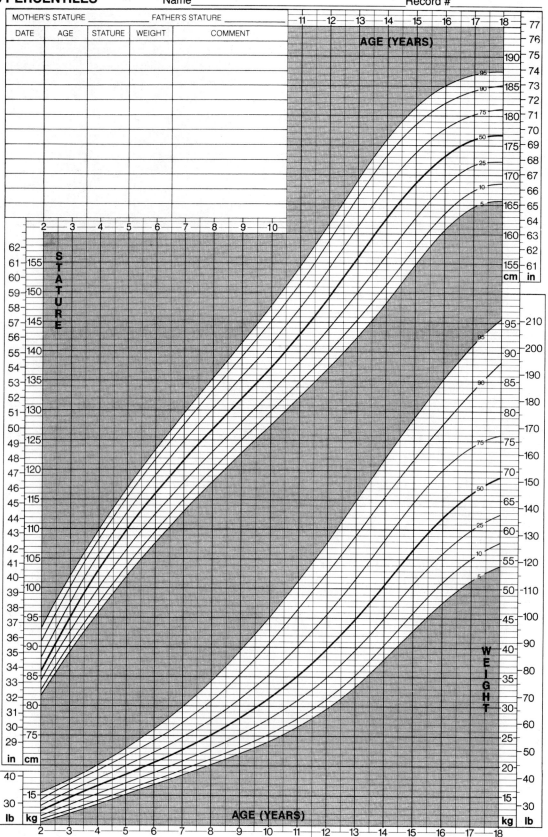

**BOYS: PREPUBESCENT
PHYSICAL GROWTH
NCHS PERCENTILES***

Name_____ Record #_____

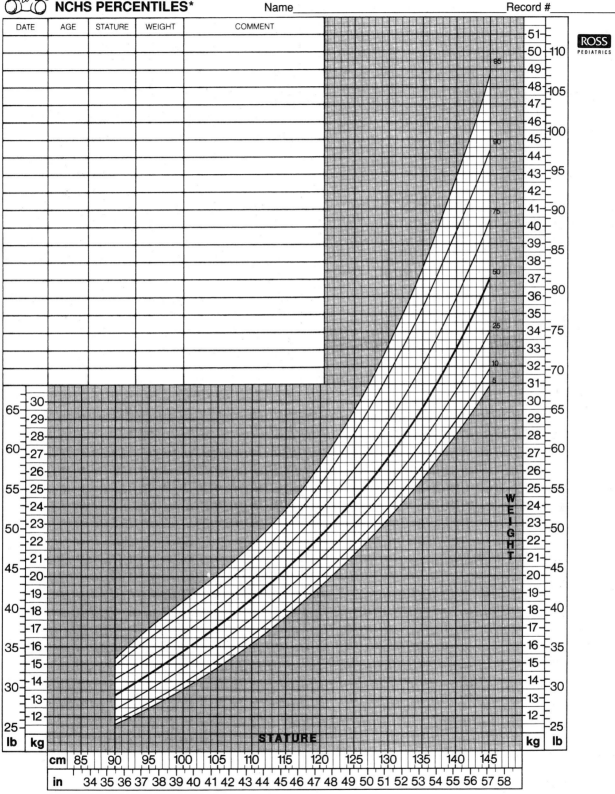

51212 09892WB
(0.05)/JUNE 1994

ROSS PRODUCTS DIVISION
ABBOTT LABORATORIES
COLUMBUS, OHIO 43215-1724

LITHO IN USA

APPENDIX III
Normal Immunization Schedule

Vaccines	Usual Schedule	Comment	True Contraindications	Not True Contraindications
Hepatitis B vaccine (HBV)	Birth, 1–2 months, 6–18 months	Alternate schedule is 1–2 months, 4 months, 6–18 months	None	Pregnancy
Diphtheria-tetanus-pertussis/acellular pertussis with diphtheria and tetanus (DTP/DTaP)	2 months, 4 months, 6 months, 15–18 months, 4–6 years. Tetanus toxoid and reduced dose diphtheria toxoid every 10 years	Can start at 4 weeks in outbreak DTaP licensed for 4th, 5th doses only	Encephalopathy within 7 days of prior dose *Precautions:* case-by-case risk-benefit determinations are made. Give in case of outbreak or foreign travel. Fever > 40.5°C (105°F), collapse or shock-like state, crying more than 3 hours within 48 hours of prior dose Seizures any time within 3 days of prior dose (consider acetaminophen before dose and every 4 hours for 24 hours for children with personal or family history of seizures) Neurologic disorders	Fever < 40.5°C (105°F) after prior dose Family history of SIDS Family history of seizures (consider acetaminophen before dose and every 4 hours for 24 hours for children with personal or family history of seizures) Family history of adverse response

Vaccine	Age to give	Recommendations	Contraindications	Special considerations
H. influenzae type b conjugate vaccine (HIBCV)	2 months, 4 months (6 months), (12 months), (15 months)	Schedule depends on which conjugate is used. Follow manufacturer's insert. Prohibit is given once at 15–59 months	None	Breast feeding; Current antimicrobial therapy; Diarrhea
Oral polio vaccine (OPV)	2 months, 4 months, 12–24 months, 4–6 years	Can start at 4 weeks in outbreak. Minimum of 6-week intervals between doses. A 6-month dose may be added in high-risk areas. Inactivated polio vaccine (IPV) is an alternate to OPV	OPV: HIV, or household contact with HIV-infected person; immunodeficiency, or household contact with immunodeficient person. IPV: anaphylactic reaction to neomycin or streptomycin. Pregnancy	
Measles-mumps-rubella (MMR)	15 months and school entry (or age 11–12)	Can give at 6 months in outbreak, but revaccinate at 15 months if administered at younger than 12 months	Anaphylactic reaction to eggs or neomycin*. Pregnancy. Known immunodeficiency (HIV-infected persons who are asymptomatic may be vaccinated). *Precaution:* if vaccinated within 3 months of receiving blood products, revaccinate 3 months after blood products are given, unless titer is adequate	Tuberculosis (TB) or positive purified protein derivative (PPD) or simultaneous skin test for TB. *Precaution:* MMR may suppress reactivity; either test that day or wait 4–6 weeks. Breast feeding. Pregnancy of household contact. Immunodeficiency of patient or household contact. HIV infection. Nonanaphylactic reaction to eggs or neomycin
General considerations			Anaphylactic reaction to specific vaccine. Anaphylactic reaction to a substance in a specific vaccine. Moderate to severe illness with or without fever contraindicates vaccine during that illness	Mild to moderate local reaction. Mild acute illness with or without low-grade fever. Current antimicrobial therapy. Prematurity: same dose and indications as for normal full-term infant. Recent exposure to infectious disease. Personal or family history of penicillin allergy or nonspecific allergies. Though it is prudent to avoid vaccinations during pregnancy, benefits may outweigh risk.

*Children with history of egg allergy are tested with three intradermal injections: 0.02 mL MMR in a 1:100 dilution; 0.02 mL of physiologic saline as a control, and 0.02 mL of histamine in a 1:100 dilution. A positive reaction is defined as induration and erythema 5 mm or greater than the saline measurements. The MMR test result is read 15–20 minutes after injection. If the child tests positive, the vaccine is administered subcutaneously with increasing increments of 0.05 mL every 15–20 minutes to the full dose of 0.5 mL. Resuscitaton equipment needs to be readily available during testing and vaccine administration.
(See Greenberg, M.A., & Birx, D.L. J. Pediatr. 113:504–506, Sept. 1988; Herman, J.J., et al. J. Pediatr. 102:196–199, Feb. 1983).
Copyright 1994, The American Journal of Nursing Company. Reprinted from *MCN*, 1994;82–84. Used with permission. All rights reserved.

APPENDIX IV
Emergency Cart Contents

STANDARD EMERGENCY CART CHECKLIST

Outside of Cart

Medication labels
Extension cord
Bin with goggles and unsterile gloves
Backboard
IV pole
Checklists, quality assurance and code blue forms on
   clipboard
Needle holder

Top of Cart

Universal precaution kits	3
TB syringes	10
Insulin syringes	10
3-cc syringes	10
10-cc syringes	10
30-cc syringes	6
60-cc syringes	6
Needles: 18-g through 25-g	10 ea
Spinal needles:	
22-g: 3½", 1½"	2 ea
20-g: 3½", 1½"	2 ea
Blood collection tubes:	
Red, purple, blue	2 ea
Green, large red	2 ea
Microtainers	1 box
Chemstrip BG	1 box
Lancets	5
Alcohol wipes	1 box
Sterile normal saline, 10-cc vial	6
ABG kit	5
Calculator	
Albumin 5%, 250-cc, bottle	1

(May be located on bottom shelf if it does not fit here)

Drawer 1

Medications

SMALL BIN

Atropine sulfate	0.4 mg/mL	1-mL vial	5
Sodium bicarbonate	1 mEq/mL	50-mL vial	3

STANDARD EMERGENCY CART CHECKLIST *Continued*

Sodium bicarbonate	1/2 mEq/mL	10-mL vial	3
Calcium chloride	10%	10-mL	3
Dextrose	10%	10-mL vial	3
Dextrose	25%	10-mL syringe	2
Epinephrine (Adrenalin)	50%	50-mL vial	2
Epinephrine (Adrenalin)	1:1000	1-mL vial	5
	1:10,000	10-mL syringe	4

LARGE BIN

Intubation medications			
Ketamine	50 mg/mL	10-mL vial	2
Pancuronium (Pavulon)	1 mg/mL	10-mL vial	1
Succinylcholine	20 mg/mL	10-mL vial	1
Vecuronium	10 mg/10 cc	(Needs to be reconstituted)	2
Midazolam (Versed)	5 mg/mL	1-mL vial	2
Aminophylline	25 mg/mL	10-mL vial	5
Bretylium	50 mg/mL	10-mL amp	2
Dexamethasone	4 mg/mL	5-mL vial	2
Diazepam (Valium)	5 mg/mL	2-mL amp	2
Diphenhydramine (Benadryl)	10 mg/mL	10-mL vial	1
Dobutamine	250 mg/20 mL	20-mL vial	2
Dopamine	40 mg/mL	5-mL vial	3
Esmolol	10 mg/mL	100-mg vial	2
Furosemide (Lasix)	10 mg/mL	2-mL vial	4
Hydralazine (Apresoline)	20 mg/mL	1-mL amp	5
Insulin	100 units/mL—regular	10-mL vial	1
Isoproterenol	1:5000	5-mL amp	4
Lidocaine	20 mg/mL	5-mL syringe	2
Lidocaine	40 mg/mL	25-mL vial	1
Methohexital (Brevital)	500-mg vial		1
Naloxone (Narcan)	0.4 mg/mL	1-mL amp	7
Nitroprusside	50-mg vial		1
Phenobarbital	65 mg/mL	1-mL vial	5
Phenylephrine (Neo-Synephrine)	10-mg/mL	1-mL amp	3
Phenytoin (Dilantin)	50 mg/mL	2-mL amp	5
Procainamide	10 mg/mL	10-mL vial	2
Edrophonium (Tensilon)	10 mg/mL	1-mL amp	2

Division-Specific Drugs:

Drawer 2

Intubation tray	
Benzoin ampules, 1″ tape	2 ea
3 × 3 gauze	2
Stylettes: pediatric and adult	1 ea
Lidocaine jelly	1 tube
Lubrafax	1 tube
Magill forceps: infant and adult	1 ea
Yankauer suction tip	1
Laryngoscope blades:	
Miller: 0, 1, 2, 3	1 ea
Macintosh: 2, 3	1 ea
Wis-Hipple: 1.5	1
Laryngoscope handle	1
Endotracheal tubes: 2.5–8.0	2 ea
Flashlight	1
Batteries: C, D	2 ea
Laryngoscope bulbs	5
Monitor leads: premie, child, adult	2 ea
Ambu masks (clear): Premie, infant, newborn, child (small & medium), adult	1 ea
Oral airways: size 5–11	1 ea
Tongue blades	5

Table continued on following page

STANDARD EMERGENCY CART CHECKLIST *Continued*

Drawer 3

Jelcos: 16-g, 18-g, 20-g, 22-g, 24-g	6 ea
Butterfly needles: 21-g, 23-g, 25-g	4 ea
Intraosseous needles (Cook): small and medium bore	2 ea
T-connectors	4
Extension tubing	4
Stopcocks	4
Solusets: minidrip, macrodrip	1 ea
Sponges 2 × 2	1 box
Adhesive tape: ½″, 1″, 2″	1 ea
Penrose drains (tourniquets) ¼″, ½″, 1″	2 ea
Armboards: small, medium, large	1 ea
IV spike	4
IV tags	4
3.0 silk on curved needle	4
EKG paper and paste	1 ea
Trocar catheters: 10F, 16F	2 ea
20F, 28F, 32F (May be in bottom drawer if doesn't fit here)	1 ea
IVAC syringes (50-cc)	2
IVAC tubing	2
Tubing connectors	2
Kelly clamp	1
Band-Aids, assorted	1 box
Betadine wipes	1 box
Rapid transfusion blood pump set	2

Drawer 4

Self-inflating Ambu bags with oxygen tubing	1 adult, 1 pediatric
Jackson-Reese bags:	
500-mL bag	1
1000-mL bag	1
2000-mL bag (optional)	1
Oxygen flowmeter with nipple adaptor	1
Oxygen tubing and funnel	1 ea
Suction cannister with connecting tubing	1
Nasogastric tubes: Feeding tube: 5F, 8F	1 ea
Salum sump: 10F-18F	1 ea
Suction catheters: 6F–14F	2 ea
Sterile gloves: pairs 6½, 7, 7½, 8	2 ea
Yankauer suction tip catheter	1
Y-connector (for suction)	1
Sodium chloride for instillation 3-mL ampules	5
60-cc catheter tip syringe	2

Bottom Shelf

Cutdown tray	1
Betadine	1 bottle
Central vein cath kit: 16-g, 20-g	1 ea
Cook catheters (with J wire): 2.5F	1
3.0F, 4.0F, 5.0F	2 ea
Various-sized BP cuffs	1 ea
Masks	2
Sterile gloves sizes 7 and 8	2 ea

Bottom Shelf or Inside Doors

Lactated Ringer's, 500 cc	1
Normal saline, 500 cc	1
5% dextrose and water, 500 cc	1
5% dextrose in normal saline, 500 cc	1

Emergency Box Checklist: Ambulatory

Top: Small Compartment

Atropine 0.4 mg/mL, 1-mL vial	3

STANDARD EMERGENCY CART CHECKLIST *Continued*

Bicarbonate 1-mEq/mL, 50-mL syringe	2
Bicarbonate 1-mlEq/mL, 50-mL vial	2
Calcium chloride 10%, 100 mg/mL	3
Dextrose 25%, 10-mL vial or syringe	2
Dextrose 50%, 50-mL vial or syringe	2
Epinephrine 1:1000, 1-mL amp	2
Epinephrine 1:10,000 10-mL syringe	1
Dilantin 50 mg/mL, 1-mL vial	1
Dopamine 40 mg/mL, 5-mL vial	4
Hydralazine 20 mg/mL, 1-mL amp	2
Insulin 100 u/mL, 10-mL vial	2
Lidocaine 20 mg/mL, 5-mL syringe	2
Narcan 0.4 mg/mL, 1-mL amp	2
Normal saline 10-mL vial	1
Phenobarbital 65 mg/mL, 1-mL vial	2
Sterile water 10-mL vial	3
Succinycholine 20 mg/mL, 10-mL vial	1
Valium 5 mg/mL, 2-mL amp	2
Clinic-specific medications:	

Top: Large Compartment

Syringes: 1-cc, 3-cc, 10-cc, insulin	5 ea
Syringes: 30-cc, 50-cc	2 ea
Needles: 18-g, 20-g, 22-g, 25-g	10 ea
Spinal needles: 1½″, 20-g, 22-g	2 ea
Butterflies: 21-g, 23-g, 25-g	4 ea
Jelcos: 16-g through 24-g	4 ea
Armboards	2 (1 small, 1 large)
2 × 2 sponges	10
Alcohol wipes	20
Betadine wipes	20
Extension tubing	2
3-way stopcocks	2
T-connectors	4
Tourniquets	2
Tape, adhesive: ½″, 1″	1 ea
Dextrostix	1 bottle
Lancets	5
ABG kit	2
Blood tubes: red, purple, blue, green, black	3 ea
Microtainers	5
IV tags	5
Intraosseous needles (15- & 18-gauge)	1 ea
Precaution kits (contains mask, disposal gown and gloves)	3

Center Top: Inside

Nasogastric tubes: Feeding 8F	1
Salem 10F–18F	1 ea
Catheter tip syringe, 50-cc	1
Suction catheters: 8F–14F	2 ea
Airways: 00, 0, 1, 2, 3	1 ea
Endotracheal tubes: 2.5–5.0	2 ea: uncuffed
5.5–8.0	1 ea: cuffed
Surgilube	3
Laryngoscope handle	1
Laryngoscope blades:	
Miller 0, 1, 2, 3	1 ea
MacIntosh 2, 3	1 ea
Tongue blades	3
Adhesive tape ½″, pink tape	1 ea
Benzoin bullets	4
Magill forceps, pedi & adult	1 ea
Stylettes, pedi & adult	1 ea
Flashlight	1
Thermometer	1

Table continued on following page

STANDARD EMERGENCY CART CHECKLIST *Continued*

Batteries C & D	2 ea
Laryngoscope bulbs	1
Saline ampules	4
Bottom	
Solusets: Minidrip 150-cc burette	2
Macrodrip 250-cc burette	1
IV solutions: NS	2 500-cc bag
D5NS	1 500-cc bag
Yankauer suction tip	1
Ambu bag with O₂ tubing	1 1000-mL bag, 1 500-cc bag
Anesthesia bag with O₂ tubing	1 1000-mL bag, 1 500-cc bag
Masks: newborn, infant, toddler, child, adult	1 ea
Disposable gloves	10 pairs
Sterile gloves, size 7, 7½	1 pair ea

From Children's Hospital, Boston, CPR Committee, Boston, MA.

APPENDIX V
Resuscitation Drugs

Drugs	Dosage (Pediatric)	Remarks
Adenosine	0.1–0.2 mg/kg Maximum single dose: 12 mg	Rapid IV bolus
Atropine sulfate*	0.02 mg/kg	Minimum dose: 0.1 mg Maximum single dose: 0.5 mg in child, 1.0 mg in adolescent
Bretylium	5 mg/kg; may be increased to 10 mg/kg	Rapid IV
Calcium chloride 10%	20 mg/kg	Give slowly
Dopamine hydrochloride	2–20 µg/kg per min	α-Adrenergic action dominates at ≥15–20 µg/kg per min
Dobutamine hydrochloride	2–20 µg/kg per min	Titrate to desired effect
Epinephrine for bradycardia*	IV/IO: 0.01 mg/kg (1:10 000, 0.1 mL/kg) ET: 0.1 mg/kg (1:1000, 0.1 mL/kg)	Be aware of total dose of preservative administered (if preservatives are present in epinephrine preparation) when high doses are used
Epinephrine for asystolic or pulseless arrest*	**First dose:** IV/IO: 0.01 mg/kg (1:10 000, 0.1 mL/kg) ET: 0.1 mg/kg (1:1000, 0.1 mL/kg) IV/IO doses as high as 0.2 mg/kg of 1:1000 may be effective **Subsequent doses:** IV/IO/ET: 0.1 mg/kg (1:1000, 0.1 mL/kg) • Repeat every 3–5 min IV/IO doses as high as 0.2 mg/kg of 1:1000 may be effective	Be aware of total dose of preservative administered (if preservatives are present in epinephrine preparation) when high doses are used
Epinephrine infusion	Initial at 0.1 µg/kg per min Higher infusion dose used if asystole present	Titrate to desired effect (0.1–1.0 µg/kg per min)
Lidocaine*	1 mg/kg	
Lidocaine infusion	20–50 µg/kg per min	
Naloxone*	If ≤ 5 years old or < 20 kg: 0.1 mg/kg If > 5 years old or > 20 kg: 2.0 mg/kg	Titrate to desired effect
Sodium bicarbonate	1 mEq/kg per dose or 0.3 × kg × base deficit	Infuse slowly and only if ventilation is adequate

*For ET administration, dilute medication with normal saline to a volume of 3 to 5 mL and follow with several positive-pressure ventilations.
Reproduced with permission. © *Textbook of Pediatric Advanced Life Support*, 1994. Copyright American Heart Association.

APPENDIX VI
Drug Compatibility Chart

Key: C = compatible; X = incompatible; Y = compatible in syringe; — = same drug; blank = no data.

Drug	ACETAZOLAMIDE (DIAMOX)	ALBUMIN	AMINOCAPROIC ACID (AMICAR)	AMINOPHYLLINE	AMRINONE (INOCAR)	ATROPINE	BRETYLIUM (BRETYLOL)	BUMETANIDE (BUMEX)	CALCIUM CHLORIDE	CEFAMANDOLE (MANDOL)	CEFTAZIDIME (FORTAZ, TAZIDIME)	CEFAZOLIN (ANCEF, KEFZOL)	CIMETIDINE (TAGAMET)	DEXTRAN	DEXTROSE 5%/WATER	DIAZEPAM (VALIUM)	DIAZOXIDE (HYPERSTAT)	DIGOXIN (LANOXIN)	DOBUTAMINE (DOBUTREX)	DOPAMINE (INTROPIN)	EPINEPHRINE	FUROSEMIDE (LASIX)	GENTAMICIN (GARAMYCIN)	HEPARIN	CALCIPARINE
ACETAZOLAMIDE (DIAMOX)	—												C		C										
ALBUMIN		—											C	C											
AMINOCAPROIC ACID (AMICAR)			—												C										
AMINOPHYLLINE				—	Y		C		X	X		X	X		C	X		C	Y	C	X	C		Y	
AMRINONE (INOCAR)				Y	—	Y	Y		Y				Y		C				C	Y	Y	Y			
ATROPINE					Y	—			X				C						C	C	X	X		X	
BRETYLIUM (BRETYLOL)				C	Y		—		C						C			C	C	C					
BUMETANIDE (BUMEX)								—																	
CALCIUM CHLORIDE				X	Y	X	C		—	X		X			C				C	C					—
CEFAMANDOLE (MANDOL)				X					X	—		X			C								X		
CEFTAZIDIME (FORTAZ, TAZIDIME)											—														X
CEFAZOLIN (ANCEF, KEFZOL)				X					X			—	X		C								X	C	
CIMETIDINE (TAGAMET)	C			X	Y	C			X			X	—		C			C	C		C	C	C	C	
DEXTRAN		C												—					C					C	
DEXTROSE 5%/WATER	C	C	C	C	Y		C		C	C		C	C		—	C<250 mg·l		C	C	C	C		C	C	
DIAZEPAM (VALIUM)				X											C<250 mg·l	—				X	X		X		
DIAZOXIDE (HYPERSTAT)																	—								
DIGOXIN (LANOXIN)				C			C						C		C			—	X					Y	
DOBUTAMINE (DOBUTREX)				Y	Y	C	C		C				C		C			X	—	C	C	X		X	
DOPAMINE (INTROPIN)				C	Y	C	C		C				C		C				C	—			C<"	C	
EPINEPHRINE				X	Y	X							C	C	C	X			C		—			Y	
FUROSEMIDE (LASIX)				C		X							C			X			X			—	X	Y	
GENTAMICIN (GARAMYCIN)									X			X	C		C					C<6°		X	—	X	
HEPARIN				Y		X						C	C	C	C	X		Y	X	C	Y	Y	X	—	
HEPARIN CALCIUM													C		C				C	C					Y
HYDRALAZINE (APRESOLINE)				X				X																	
INSULIN (REGULAR)				X			C						C						X					Y	
ISOPROTERENOL (ISUPREL)				X	Y		C						C		C				C		X		C	C	
LIDOCAINE (XYLOCAINE)				C	Y		C		C	X		X	C		C			C	C	C	X			C	
MEPERIDINE (DEMEROL)				X		C						C<4°			C	X			C			X		X	
METARAMINOL (ARAMINE)				C	Y	X							C	C	C	X			C		C	X		X	
METHYLDOPA (ALDOMET)				C		X									C									C	
METHYLPREDNISOLONE				X	Y								C		C<125 mg·l					C				C in D5W	
MORPHINE				X		X						C<4°	C		C				C					Y	
NAFCILLIN (NAFCIL, UNIPEN)				C									C		C				X	X			X	C	
NALOXONE (NARCAN)																									
NEO-SYNEPHRINE (PHENYLEPHRINE)																									
NITROGLYCERIN				C	Y		C						C						C	C		C			
NITROPRUSSIDE (NIPRIDE)					X		X		C				C		C				C						
NOREPINEPHRINE (LEVOPHED)				X	Y				C				C		C				C					C	
NORMAL SALINE 0.9%	C	C	C	C	C		C		C	C		C	C			C<250 mg·l		C	C	C	C	C	C	C	
PANCURONIUM (PAVULON)																					X				
PENICILLIN G POTASSIUM				X					C	X		X	C		C					X	X		X	C<8°	
PENTAMIDINE																									
PHENOBARBITAL				C					C						C										
PHENYTOIN (DILANTIN)	X	X		X		X	X	X	X	X		X	X	X	X	X		X	X	X	X	X	X	X	X
PIPERACILLIN (PIPRACIL)				X											C						X		X		
POTASSIUM CHLORIDE	C			C	Y		C		C	C		C	C		C	Y		Y	C	C	Y	Y		C	
PROCAINAMIDE (PROCAN)				C	Y		C												C	C				Y	
QUINIDINE							C						C					X					X	X	
RANITIDINE (ZANTAC)									C<6°			C<6°			C			C			C	C	C		
SODIUM BICARBONATE				C	X	X	C		X				C		C	X			X	X				Y	
TOBRAMYCIN (NEBCIN)									X			X	C									Y		X	
TRIMETHOPHAN (ARFONAD)																								Y	
TMP-SMX (BACTRIM)															C<4°										
VERAPAMIL (CALAN, ISOPTIN)		X		C	Y	C	C		C	C		C	C		C				C	C	C	C		C	

Column key (left-to-right across the chart):
1 HYDRALAZINE (APRESOLINE) · 2 INSULIN (REGULAR) · 3 ISOPROTERENOL (ISUPREL) · 4 LIDOCAINE (XYLOCAINE) · 5 MEPERIDINE (DEMEROL) · 6 METARAMINOL (ARAMINE) · 7 METHYLDOPA (ALDOMET) · 8 METHYLPREDNISOLONE · 9 MORPHINE · 10 NAFCILLIN (NAFCIL, UNIPEN) · 11 NALOXONE (NARCAN) · 12 NEOSYNEPHRINE (PHENYLEPHRINE) · 13 NITROGLYCERIN · 14 NITROPRUSSIDE (NIPRIDE) · 15 NOREPINEPHRINE (LEVOPHED) · 16 NORMAL SALINE 0.9% · 17 PANCURONIUM (PAVULON) · 18 PENICILLIN G POTASSIUM · 19 PENTAMIDINE · 20 PHENOBARBITAL · 21 PHENYTOIN (DILANTIN) · 22 PIPERACILLIN (PIPRACIL) · 23 POTASSIUM CHLORIDE · 24 PROCAINAMIDE (PROCAN) · 25 QUINIDINE · 26 RANITIDINE (ZANTAC) · 27 SODIUM BICARBONATE · 28 TOBRAMYCIN (NEBCIN) · 29 TRIMETHOPHAN (ARFONAD) · 30 TMP-SMX (BACTRIM) · 31 VERAPAMIL (CALAN, ISOPTIN)

Drug	1	2	3	4	5	6	7	8	9	10	11	12	13	14	15	16	17	18	19	20	21	22	23	24	25	26	27	28	29	30	31
ACETAZOLAMIDE (DIAMOX)																C				X			C								
ALBUMIN																C				X											X
AMINOCAPROIC ACID (AMICAR)																C															C
AMINOPHYLLINE	X	X	X	C	X	C	C	X	X	C		C		X	C			X		X	X	C	C			C					C
AMRINONE (INOCAR)		Y	Y		Y		Y					Y	X	Y	Y	C		C			Y	Y				X					Y
ATROPINE				C	X	X		X												X						X					C
BRETYLIUM (BRETYLOL)	C		C								C	X			C					X		C	C	C		C					C
BUMETANIDE (BUMEX)																				X											
CALCIUM CHLORIDE		C	C							C	C	C		C		C		C		X		C									C
CEFAMANDOLE (MANDOL)		X												C	X			X		X		C			C<6*		X				C
CEFTAZIDIME (FORTAZ, TAZIDIME)																				X											
CEFAZOLIN (ANCEF, KEFZOL)		X												C	X			X		X		C			C<6*		X				C
CIMETIDINE (TAGAMET)	C	C	C	C<4*	C		C	C<4*	C			C	C	C		C				X		C		C		C			C<4*		C
DEXTRAN					C															X											
DEXTROSE 5%/WATER	C		C	C	C	C	C	C<125mg·l	C	C		C	C	C		C		C		X		C	C	C		C	C	C	C<4*		C
DIAZEPAM (VALIUM)		X	X													C<250mg·l				X	Y		X			X					
DIAZOXIDE (HYPERSTAT)																															
DIGOXIN (LANOXIN)	C		C																	X	Y		C			C					C
DOBUTAMINE (DOBUTREX)	C	X	C	C	C			C		X		C	C	C	C			X		X		C	C			X					C
DOPAMINE (INTROPIN)			C		C	C		X				C			C	X		X		X	X	C	C			X					C
EPINEPHRINE		X	X		C	C						C			C	X		X		X	Y			C							C
FUROSEMIDE (LASIX)			X	X				C				C			C	X		C	X	X	Y		X	C		Y					
GENTAMICIN (GARAMYCIN)		C							X						C	X		X		X	X			C							
HEPARIN	Y	Y	C	C	X	X	C	C in C5W	Y	C			C	C		C<8*		C		X		C	C	Y	X	Y	X	Y			C
HEPARIN CALCIUM											C				C				X	X	X	C									X
HYDRALAZINE (APRESOLINE)																				X											
INSULIN (REGULAR)		—	C					X							Y		X			X	X		Y			C	X				C
ISOPROTERENOL (ISUPREL)			—	X											C					X		C				C					C
LIDOCAINE (XYLOCAINE)	C	X		—		C						C			C		C			X	C	C	C	C		C	X				C
MEPERIDINE (DEMEROL)					—		X	X							C			X	X	X						X					C
METARAMINOL (ARAMINE)		C				—		X							C		X			X		C				C					C
METHYLDOPA (ALDOMET)							—								C					X	C					C					C
METHYLPREDNISOLONE	X			X	X	X	—			X				C	C<250mg·l	C				X	X	X		C							C
MORPHINE		X						—							C				X	X	Y			X							C
NAFCILLIN (NAFCIL, UNIPEN)					X				—		C			C	C				X	C					C	X					
NALOXONE (NARCAN)										—																					C
NEO-SYNEPHRINE (PHENYLEPHRINE)											—									X	X										
NITROGLYCERIN	C		C						C			—			C					X											C
NITROPRUSSIDE (NIPRIDE)													—		C					X						C					C
NOREPINEPHRINE (LEVOPHED)				C					C					—		C				X	X	C				C	X				C
NORMAL SALINE 0.9%	C	Y	C	C	C	C	C	C<250mg·l	C	C		C	C	C		—		C		C	X	C	C	C		C	C		C<4*		C
PANCURONIUM (PAVULON)																—				X											C
PENICILLIN G POTASSIUM		X		C		X		C							C	—				X		C				C	C<8*	X			
PENTAMIDINE																	—														
PHENOBARBITAL	X	X			X				X			X			X	C			—							X					C
PHENYTOIN (DILANTIN)	X	X	X	X	X	X	X	X	X	X	X	X	X	X	X	X	X			—	X	X	X			X	X				X
PIPERACILLIN (PIPRACIL)			C												C		X	—	C			C	X								
POTASSIUM CHLORIDE	C	Y	C	C		C	C	X	Y			C	C	C		—	C		Y	C	Y		C	Y		Y					C
PROCAINAMIDE (PROCAN)		C													C		X	Y	—							C					C
QUINIDINE																	X	—	C												C
RANITIDINE (ZANTAC)	C	C	C		C		C					C	C	C				C	C	—											C
SODIUM BICARBONATE	X		X	X	X	C		X	C				X		C	C<6*	X	X	C	Y		—									X
TOBRAMYCIN (NEBCIN)					X											X	X	X	—					Y							C
TRIMETHOPHAN (ARFONAD)																			Y				—								
TMP-SMX (BACTRIM)							C<4*													—	C										C
VERAPAMIL (CALAN, ISOPTIN)	X	C	C	C	C	C	C	C		C			C	C	C		C	X		C	C	C		X	C		X	C		X	—

Abbreviations: C, compatible for at least 24 hours; X, incompatible; Y, Y-site administration.
Prepared by Susan M. Garabedian-Ruffalo, PharmD. Reprinted with permission of CRITICAL CARE NURSE®, 9 (2), 82–83, 1989.

INDEX

Note: Page numbers in *italics* refer to illustrations; page numbers followed by (t) refer to tables.